Upper Digestive Surgery

Illustrations: Gillian Lee

UPPER DIGESTIVE SURGERY

Edited by

THOMAS V. TAYLOR MDChM MBChB FRCS(ENG) FRCS(ED) FACS FACG
PROFESSOR OF SURGERY, BAYLOR COLLEGE OF MEDICINE;
ASSISTANT CHIEF, SURGICAL SERVICE
AND CHIEF OF GENERAL SURGERY, VETERANS AFFAIRS
MEDICAL CENTER, HOUSTON, TEXAS, USA

ANTHONY WATSON MD FRCS(ENG) FRCS(ED) FRACS
VISITING PROFESSOR OF SURGERY, ROYAL FREE AND UNIVERSITY COLLEGE SCHOOL OF MEDICINE,
ROYAL FREE HOSPITAL, LONDON, UK

and

ROBIN C.N. WILLIAMSON MA MD MChir FRCS(ENG)
PROFESSOR OF SURGERY, DEPARTMENT OF GASTROINTESTINAL SURGERY,
IMPERIAL COLLEGE OF SCIENCE, TECHNOLOGY AND MEDICINE,
THE HAMMERSMITH HOSPITAL, LONDON, UK

W.B. Saunders
London • Edinburgh • New York • Philadelphia • Sydney • Toronto

W.B. SAUNDERS

An imprint of Harcourt Publishers Limited

© Harcourt Publishers 1999

 is a registered trademark of Harcourt Publishers Limited

First published 1999

ISBN 0-7020-1434-6

British Library Cataloguing in Publication Data
A catalogue record for this book is available from the British Library

Library of Congress Cataloguing in Publication Data
A catalog record for this book is available from the Library of Congress

Note
Medical knowledge is constantly changing. As new information becomes available, changes in treatment, procedures, equipment and the use of drugs become necessary. The editors/authors/contributors and the publishers have, as far as it is possible, taken care to ensure that the information given in this text is accurate and up-to-date. However, readers are strongly advised to confirm that the information, especially with regard to drug usage, complies with the latest legislation and standards of practice.

Typeset in England by Phoenix Photosetting, Chatham, Kent
Printed in China

The
Publisher's
policy is to use
**paper manufactured
from sustainable forests**

CONTENTS

PART THREE: SMALL INTESTINE

FOREWORD

The first edition of *Upper Digestive Surgery* is a beautifully edited and magnificently illustrated surgical textbook. Its thoroughness and clarity provides students and surgeons at all levels with an invaluable reference that is highly informative about gastrointestinal physiology and surgery.

The world is changing and so is surgery. The increase in scientific information in the past 30 years has increased the intellectual requirements for surgeons to maintain clinical competence and has increased the technical skills required to integrate expanding science with their practice. This new publication is a means of bringing to the surgical audience, both in practice and in training, the newest aspects of science that bear upon their practice.

Edited by the leaders of this scientific progress, the book will – because of its distinguished list of contributors – become a preeminent reference work. The editors have fulfilled in an exemplary fashion their responsibilities to retain what is important and valuable of the past and to link this with new scientific aspects of surgery destined to carry this specialty into the twenty-first century.

The authors were well chosen for their particular subject. In addition to the academic aspects they bring, it is clear they have had an extensive hands-on experience which they communicate to the reader in a very understandable way. The text is exceptional for its clarity and readability. It contains the information required for understanding a particular problem so that it can be put to clinical use for improved patient care. The various topics are dealt with in sufficient length to provide a thorough understanding without burdening the reader with excessive details. This has allowed the editors to condense an ever expanding body of knowledge into a relatively small and thoroughly practical format.

One of the most appreciated aspects of the text is the extreme clarity and exceptional quality of roentgenographic illustrations and drawings. They could not be improved.

Paul H. Jordan, Jr. MD
Emiritus Professor of Surgery
Baylor College of Medicine
Houston, Texas, USA

PREFACE

There has been an internal revolution in the field of upper digestive surgery over the past decade. Ten years ago laparoscopic therapeutic procedures within the upper abdomen did not exist and acid reducing therapy was the only treatment for peptic ulcer, short of operation. The secretory inhibitors available were not effective of gastro-oesophageal reflux disease and major abdominal surgery was the only feasible approach to the gallbladder or hiatus. Furthermore, the spiral organism, *Helicobacter pylori* had yet to gain the respect it deserves.

Now surgical trainees rarely see vagotomy, only occasionally perform gastrectomy for cancer and treat ninety percent of patients with cholelithiasis and many of those with gastro-oesophageal reflux disease employing a laparoscopic approach. Changes have taken place also in cancer therapy. *Helicobacter pylori* colonization has become, or possibly always was, the most common infectious disease in the world. Its eradication with appropriate therapy can cure some ulcers, treat some lymphomas (maltomas) and may possibly have a major long-term impact on the prevalence of gastric cancer. Hospital practice has changed fundamentally; therapeutic endoscopy has challenged established open surgical therapies in biliary, pancreatic, oesophageal and gastric disorders. Stents, lasers, injection sclerotherapy, snares, balloons and dilators have all impacted on surgical practice. Computerized tomography, magnetic resonance imaging and endoscopic ultrasound have each improved in definition and therefore in accuracy. New avenues such as gene therapy are now on the horizon and surgeons even talk in terms of remote operations performed by telesurgery. The operative surgery of tomorrow might even reach the submicroscopic level of splicing and repairing the DNA molecule.

Also in the last decade, upper gastrointestinal surgery has emerged as a major sub-specialty of general surgery worldwide. Many consultant posts are advertised with a specific interest, and in 1996, the Association of Upper Gastrointestinal Surgeons of Great Britain and Ireland was successfully established to promote high standards of education, training, research and service provision within the specialty.

Against this background of the recognition of and major changes within the specialty, we feel it is timely for a contemporary major volume on *Upper Digestive Surgery* to be launched. In its totality, upper gastrointestinal surgery encompasses surgical disorders of the oesophagus, stomach and duodenum, liver, biliary tract, pancreas, spleen and small intestine. Authoritative texts already exist in the fields of HPB surgery and coloproctology, and we hope that the addition of this volume covering luminal upper gastrointestinal surgery will be seen as fulfilling a need and complementing existing texts to provide authoritative and up-to-date coverage of the entire field of surgical gastroenterology.

In this volume, three sections exist: oesophagus, stomach and duodenum, and small intestine, each edited by one of us. We have chosen a broad range of international specialists in order to give a balanced view of disorders of the upper gastrointestinal tract. In addition to surgery, these specialists include those from the fields of gastroenterology, internal medicine, physiology, pathology, microbiology and radiology. Furthermore, we have incorporated a large section on the paediatric aspects of upper digestive surgery. This diversity has enabled us to discuss the various disease processes from a basic scientific standpoint in terms of aetiology and pathophysiology as well as medical and surgical therapy in children and adults. We have endeavoured to present a holistic approach to the subject matter, in order to give a balanced view of the interaction of the many disciplines within our speciality. We are hopeful that this text will be sufficiently comprehensive to serve as a readable, reliable reference work on upper digestive surgery for a wide range of readers from the medical student to the practising surgeon and particularly for surgical trainees.

We are most grateful to all of our many contributors who have provided us with up-to-date texts of high quality. It is a pleasure to acknowledge the continuous, loyal and hardworking support of Rachel Robson and Sean Duggan, who have provided stability during the many changes in the publishing world, which have impacted on the gestation period of this work. It is our sincere hope that both contributors and readers will agree that the quality of the finished product has justified the wait.

TV Taylor
A Watson
RCN Williamson

CONTRIBUTORS

Derek Alderson MD FRCS, Professor of Gastrointestinal Surgery, Department of Surgery, University of Bristol, Bristol Royal Infirmary, Bristol, UK

Malcolm C Aldridge FRCS FRCS(Ed), Consultant Surgeon, Queen Elizabeth II Hospital, Welwyn Garden City, UK

CP Armstrong MD FRCS(Eng) FRCS(Ed), Consultant Gastrointestinal Surgeon, Department of Surgery, Frenchay Hospital, Bristol, UK

Stephen EA Attwood ChM FRCSI, Department of Surgery, Hope Hospital, Salford, UK

Ralph E Barry BSc MD FRCP, Clinical Dean, Clinical Dean's Office, Bristol Royal Infirmary, Bristol, UK

Scott J Boley MD, Professor of Surgery, Department of Surgery, Montefiore Medical Center, New York, USA

PC Bornman MMED(OFS) FRCS(Ed), Professor of Surgery, Department of Surgery, University of Cape Town, Medical School, South Africa

Cedric G Bremner MD FRCSA, Professor of Surgery, Department of Surgery, Richard K Eamer Medic Plaza, USC Healthcare Consultation Center, Los Angeles, California, USA

Duncan G Colin-Jones MD FRCP, Consultant Physician, Queen Alexandra Hospital, Portsmouth, UK

Kimberly L Collings BS, Clinical Research Co-ordinator, Oklahoma Foundation for Digestive Research, Oklahoma City, USA

Martin J Cooper FRCS, Consultant Surgeon, Department of Surgery, Royal Devon and Exeter Hospital, Exeter, UK

Tom R DeMeester MD, Chairman of Surgery, Department of Surgery, University of Southern California, School of Medicine, Los Angeles, California, USA

Hugh B Devlin CBE FRCS FACS (deceased), formerly Director (Epidemiology and Audit), Royal College of Surgeons, London, UK

Caroline M Doig FRCS, Senior Lecturer in Paediatric Surgery, Booth Hall Children's Hospital, Blackley, Manchester, UK

Philip E Donahue MD FRCS, Professor of Surgery, University of Illinois; Chief, Division of General Surgery, Cook County Hospital, Chicago, USA

John P Dunn FRACS, Consultant Surgeon, Department of Surgery, University of Cape Town, Medical School, Cape Town, South Africa

Peter W Dykes FRCP, Consultant Physician, Chadwick Manor, Bromsgrove, UK

Harold Ellis CBE MD MCh FRCS (retired), formerly Emiritus Professor of Surgery, Charing Cross and Westminster Medical School, London, UK

David F Evans, Senior Lecturer and Research Co-ordinator, The University of London, The London Hospital Medical School, Gastro-Intestinal Science Research, London, UK

John WL Fielding FRCS MD, Consultant Surgeon, Queen Elizabeth Hospital, Queen Elizabeth Medical Centre, Birmingham, UK

WR Fleming FRACS, 8/11 Broomfield Avenue, Fairfield, Victoria, Australia

R Armour Forse MD PhD FRCS(C), Associate Professor of Surgery, Department of Surgery, Harvard Medical School, Beth Israel Deaconess Medical Center, Boston, USA

Gordon M Fraser FRCR, Consultant Radiologist, Department of Radiology, Western General Hospital and Northern General, Edinburgh, UK

Pascal Frileux MD, Chef de Service, Service de Chirurgie Générale et Digestive, Centre Medico-Chirurgical Foch, Paris, France

Robert M Genta MD, Professor of Pathology, Professor of Medicine, Professor of Microbiology and Immunology, Chief of Pathology and Laboratory Medicine, Veterans Affairs Medical Center, Houston, Texas, USA

DY Graham MD, Professor of Medicine and Chief of Gastroenterology, Baylor College of Medicine and Veterans Affairs Medical Center, Houston, Texas, USA

Scott M Graham MD, Lecturer, Department of Surgery, University of Cape Town, Medical School; Consultant Surgeon, Groote Schuur Hospital, Cape Town, South Africa

Teresa Hayes MD PhD, Associate Professor of Medicine, Baylor College of Medicine; Director of Oncology Clinical Services, Veterans Affairs Medical Center, Houston, Texas, USA

Michael J Hobsley TD MChir DSc PhD FRCS, Emiritus Professor, University College London Medical School, London, UK

Stephen Holt MD MRCP(UK) FRCP(C) FACP FACG FACN, Director, Institute of Advanced Medical Sciences, Fairfield, New Jersey, USA

Thomas J Howard MD FACS, Department of Surgery, Indiana University, Indianapolis, USA

J Janssens MD PhD, Department of Medicine, University Hospital, Gasthuisberg, Leuven, Belgium

Hans Eric Jensen MD PhD, formerly Department of Surgery, Bispebjerg Hospital, Copenhagen, Denmark

Alan G Johnson MChir FRCS, Professor of Surgery, University Surgical Unit, Royal Hallamshire Hospital, Sheffield, UK

R Kaleya MD, Department of Surgery, Montefiore Medical Centre, New York, USA

John E Kellow MD FRACP, Department of Medicine, Wallace Freeborn Professional Block, The Royal North Shore Hospital, St Leonards, Australia

T Lerut, Professor, Department of Surgery, Catholic University of Leuven, Leuven, Belgium

Etienne Paul Levy (deceased), formerly Professor and Director of Research, Intensive Care Unit, Department of Digestive Surgery, Hospital Saint-Antoine, Paris, France

Lloyd D MacLean MD, Chairman and Professor of Surgery, McGill University; Consultant Surgeon, Department of Surgery, Royal Victoria Hospital, Montreal, Quebec, Canada

DG Maxton MD, Consultant Physician and Gastroenterologist, Royal Shrewsbury Hospital, Shrewsbury, UK

DB McConnell MD, Department of Surgery, VA Medical Center, Portland, Oregon, USA

John P Miller, Consultant Gastroenterologist, Department of Medicine, Withington Hospital, Manchester, UK

PB Miner Jr, President and Medical Director, Oklahoma Foundation for Digestive Research, Oklahoma City, USA

G Moody, Queen Alexandra Hospital, Portsmouth, UK

James A Morris FRCPath, Consultant Histopathologist, Department of Pathology, Royal Lancaster Infirmary, Lancaster, UK

Daniel J Nolan MD FRCP FRCR, Consultant Radiologist, Department of Radiology, John Radcliffe Hospital, Headington, Oxford, UK

Yann Parc, Intensive Care Unit, Department of Digestive Surgery, Hospital Saint-Antoine, Paris, France

Edward Passaro Jr MD, Professor of Surgery, University College of Los Angeles; Chief of Staff, Surgical Service, West Los Angeles VA Medical Center, Los Angeles, California, USA

Jeffrey H Peters MD FACS, Associate Professor of Surgery, Chief, Section of General Surgery, USC University Hospital, University of Southern California, Los Angeles, California, USA

M Amanda Quine MRCP, Senior Registrar, Queen Alexandra Hospital, Portsmouth, UK

BA Ross MBBS FRCS, Consultant Thoracic Surgeon, East Anglian and Oxford Regional Health Authority, Norfolk, Norwich and Ipswich Hospitals, UK

George Y Saleh MD, Department of Pathology, Veterans Affairs Medical Center, Houston, Texas, USA

Klaus FR Schiller MA DM FRCP, Consultant Gastroenterologist, Woking Nuffield Hospital, Woking, Surrey and Acland Nuffield Hospital, Oxford; Consultant Gastroenterologist (Emiritus), St Peter's Hospital, Chertsey, Surrey, UK

David M Scott-Coombes MS FRCS, Senior Registrar, Hammersmith and St. Mary's Hospitals, London, UK

Thomas Scratcherd MS FRCP (retired), formerly Professor Emeritus of Physiology, Department of Physiological Sciences, Medical School, University of Newcastle-upon-Tyne, Newcastle-upon-Tyne, UK

John Spencer MS FRCS, Reader in Surgery, Department of Surgery, Royal Postgraduate Medical School, Hammersmith Hospital, London, UK

Robert T Spychal MBBS MD FRCS(Ed), Consultant Surgeon, Department of Surgery, City Hospital, Birmingham, UK

Russell JC Steele FRCS, Professor of Surgery, University of Dundee, Ninewells Hospital, Dundee, UK

John GN Studley MS FRCS, Consultant Surgeon, James Paget Hospital, Great Yarmouth, Norfolk, UK

Jan Tack MD PhD, Professor of Medicine, Department of Internal Medicine and Division of Gastroenterology, University Hospital Gasthuisberg, Catholic University of Leuven, Leuven, Belgium

Thomas V Taylor MDChM MBChB FRCS(Eng) FRCS(Ed) FACS FACG, Professor of Surgery, Baylor College of Medicine; Assistant Chief, Surgical Service and Chief of General Surgery, Veterans Affairs Medical Center, Houston, Texas, USA

John G Temple MB FRCS(Ed) FRCS(Eng) ChM FMedSci, Professor of Surgery, Regional Postgraduate Dean, Board of Postgraduate Medical and Dental Education, University of Birmingham, The Medical School, Edgbaston, Birmingham, UK

William EG Thomas MS FRCS, Consultant Surgeon and Clinical Director, Department of Surgery, Royal Hallamshire Hospital, Sheffield, UK

Henry Thompson MD FRCPath, Reader in Pathology, University of Birmingham, Birmingham, UK

B Trunkey MD, Chairman of Department, Department of Surgery, Oregon Health Sciences University, Portland, Oregon, USA

G Vantrappen MD PhD, Professor of Medicine; Head of Department of Medicine, University Hospital Gasthuisberg, Division of Gastroenterology, University of Leuven, Belgium

Robert P Walt MD FRCP, Senior Lecturer in Medicine, University of Birmingham, Birmingham, UK

Anthony Watson MD FRCS(Eng) FRCS(Ed) FRACS, Visiting Professor of Surgery, Royal Free and University College School of Medicine, Royal Free Hospital, London, UK

Elliot Weser MD, Chief, Medical Service, Department of Veterans Affairs, Audi L Murphy Memorial Veterans Hospital, San Antonio, Texas, USA

Robin CN Williamson MA MD MChir FRCS(Eng), Professor of Surgery, Department of Gastrointestinal Surgery, Imperial College of Science, Technology and Medicine, The Hammersmith Hospital, London, UK

Charles P Willoughby MA DM FRCP, Consultant Gastroenterologist, Basildon and Thurrock General Hospital Trust, Essex, London

Bruce G Wolff MD FRCR, Department of Colon, Rectal and General Surgery, Mayo Clinic, Rochester, Minnesota, USA

Andrew R Wright MA MBBS MRCP FRCR, Consultant Radiologist, Department of Radiology, Western General Hospital, Edinburgh, UK

Michael G Wyatt FRCS MD, Consultant and Vascular Surgeon, Freeman Hospital, Newcastle-upon-Tyne, UK

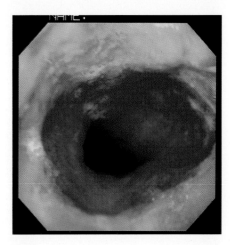

Figure 3.4
Regular dentate line.

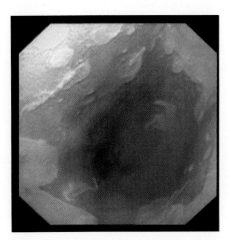

Figure 3.5
Irregular but normal dentate line.

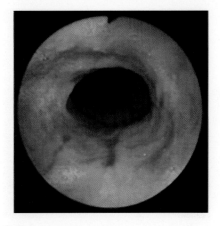

Figure 3.6
Grade I oesophagitis.

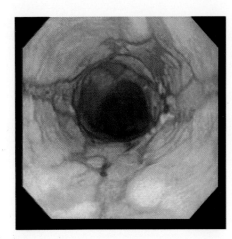

Figure 3.7
Grade II oesophagitis.

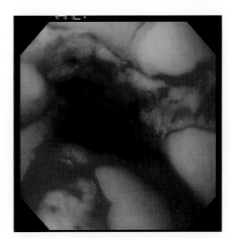

Figure 3.8
Grade III oesophagitis.

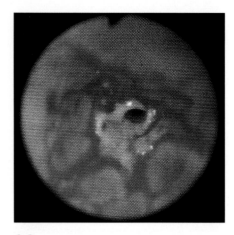

Figure 3.9
Grade IV oesophagitis.

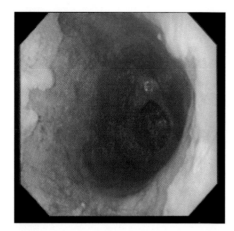

Figure 3.10
Barrett's oesophagus.

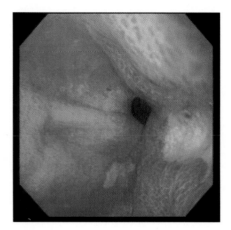

Figure 3.11
Oesophageal ulcer.

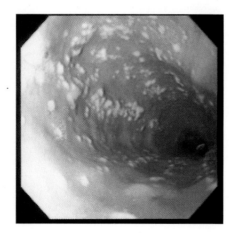

Figure 3.12
Oesophageal candidiasis.

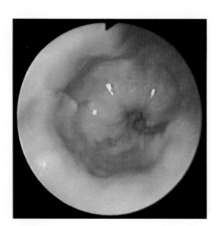

Figure 3.13
Mallory–Weiss tear.

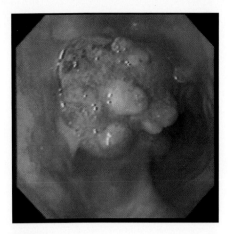

Figure 3.14
Oesophageal cancer.

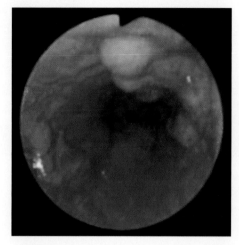

Figure 3.15
Oesophageal varices.

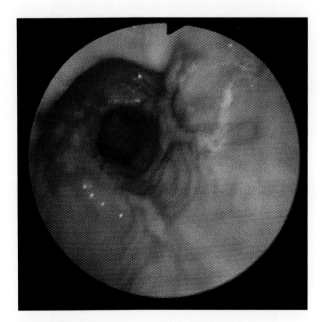

Figure 11.15
Radiographic appearance of a reflux-induced oesophageal
stricture.

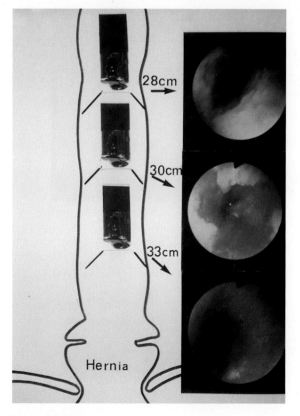

Figure 11.17
Endoscopic appearance of Barrett's metaplastic epithelium at
three levels of the oesophagus. The normal white squamous
epithelium has been replaced by the luxuriant red lining of
Barrett's metaplasia in the lower oesophagus.

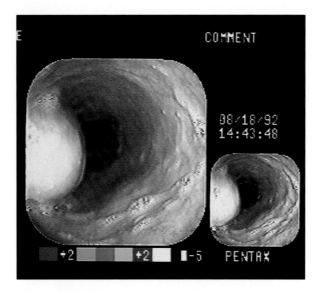

Figure 13.16
Endoscopic view of leiomyoma, diagnosed at endoscopy for reflux sympoms.

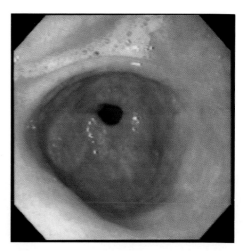

Figure 24.1
Normal gastric antrum and pylorus.

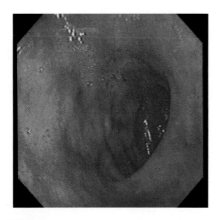

Figure 24.2
Normal proximal duodenum.

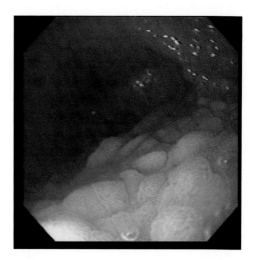

Figure 24.3
Polypoid appearance in the duodenal bulb.

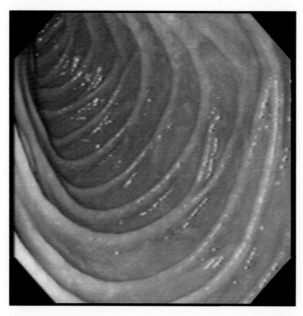

Figure 24.4
Normal second part of duodenum.

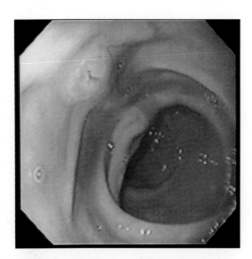

Figure 24.5
Normal duodenal papilla.

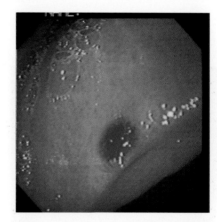

Figure 24.6
Suction artefact.

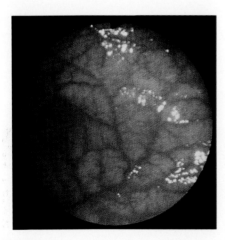

Figure 24.7
Gastric mucosal atrophy. (Reproduced, with permission, from Schiller KFR, Cochel R & Hunt RH. A Colour Atlas of Gastrointestinal Endoscopy. London: Chapman & Hall, 1986.)

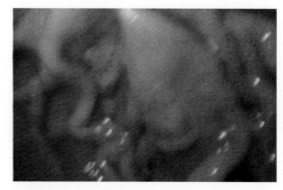

Figure 24.8
Ménètrier's disease. (Reproduced, with permission, from Schiller KFR, Cochel R & Hunt RH. A Colour Atlas of Gastrointestinal Endoscopy. London: Chapman & Hall, 1986.)

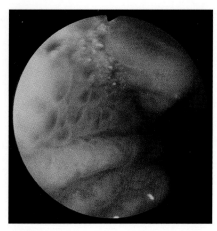

Figure 24.9
Rugal folds in portal gastropathy. (Reproduced, with permission, from Schiller KFR, Cochel R & Hunt RH. A Colour Atlas of Gastrointestinal Endoscopy. London: Chapman & Hall, 1986.)

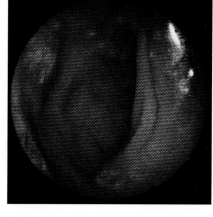

Figure 24.10
Salami-type duodenitis. (Reproduced, with permission, from Schiller KFR, Cochel R & Hunt RH. A Colour Atlas of Gastrointestinal Endoscopy. London: Chapman & Hall, 1986.)

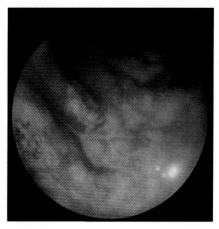

Figure 24.11
Sparsity of small bowel mucosal folds in coeliac disease (illustrated by dye spray).(Reproduced, with permission, from Schiller KFR, Cochel R & Hunt RH. A Colour Atlas of Gastrointestinal Endoscopy. London: Chapman & Hall, 1986.)

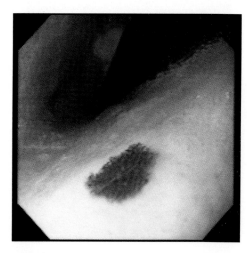

Figure 24.12
Gastric angioma seen on inversion view.

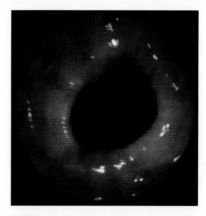

Figure 24.13
Diffuse vascular ectasia – 'watermelon stomach'.

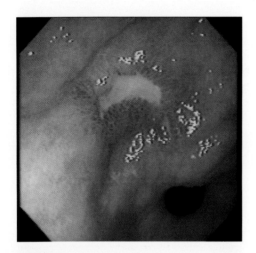

Figure 24.14
Benign gastric ulcer.

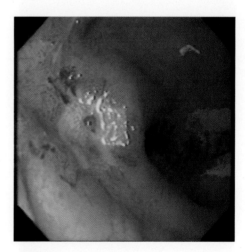

Figure 24.15
Gastric ulcer with visible vessel in its base.

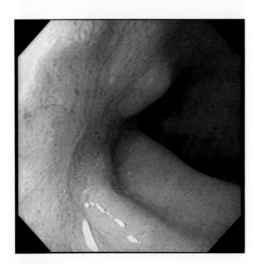

Figure 24.16
Ulcer scar in the duodenum.

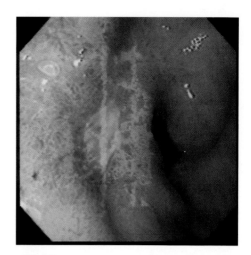

Figure 24.17
Duodenal ulcer.

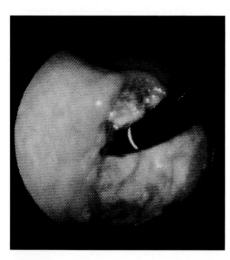

Figure 24.18
Ulcerating gastric carcinoma.

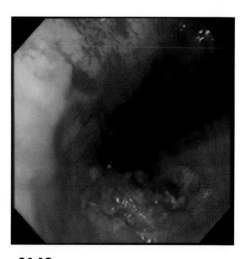

Figure 24.19
Stenosing cancer of the gastric cardia seen on inversion.

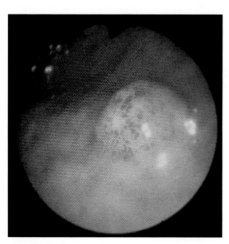

Figure 24.20
Early gastric cancer. (Reproduced, with permission, from Schiller KFR, Cochel R & Hunt RH. A Colour Atlas of Gastrointestinal Endoscopy. London: Chapman & Hall, 1986.)

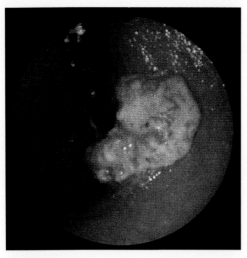

Figure 24.21
Polypoid gastric cancer. (Reproduced, with permission, from Schiller KFR, Cochel R & Hunt RH. A Colour Atlas of Gastrointestinal Endoscopy. London: Chapman & Hall, 1986.)

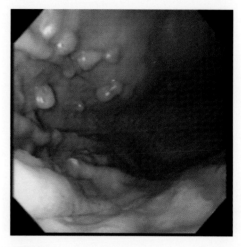

Figure 24.22
Regenerative polyps in the stomach.

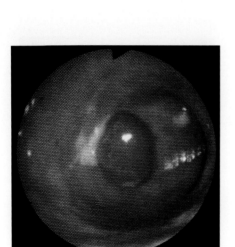

Figure 24.23
Pedunculated benign gastric adenoma. (Reproduced, with permission, from Schiller KFR, Cochel R & Hunt RH. A Colour Atlas of Gastrointestinal Endoscopy. London: Chapman & Hall, 1986.)

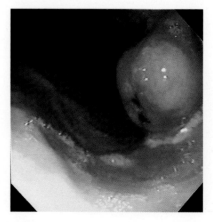

Figure 24.24
Gastric leiomyoma.

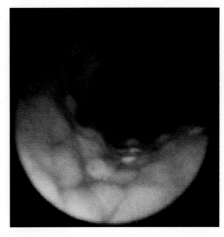

Figure 24.25
Linitis plastica. (Reproduced, with permission, from Schiller KFR, Cochel R & Hunt RH. A Colour Atlas of Gastrointestinal Endoscopy. London: Chapman & Hall, 1986.)

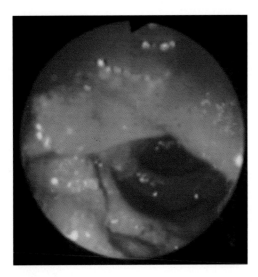

Figure 24.26
Duodenal involvement by pancreatic cancer.

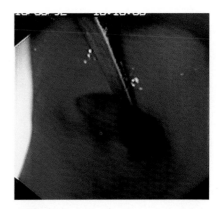

Figure 24.28
Spoon in the stomach – removed with a standard polypectomy snare.

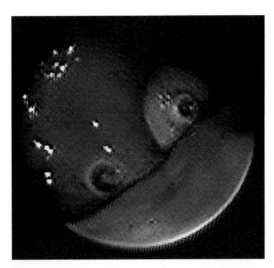

Figure 24.30
Epithelialized gastrostomy, with an adjacent second PEG.

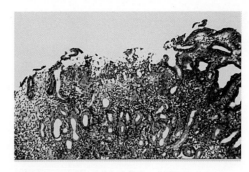

Figure 26.1
Antral erosion. The tissue loss is limited to the epithelium. There is a fibrinopurulent exudate in the area of the eroded surface. A mixed inflammatory infiltrate is visible in the lamina propria immediately subjacent to the erosion (haematoxylin and eosin, ×100).

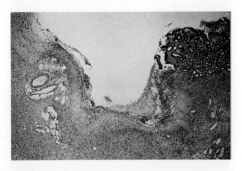

Figure 26.2
Peptic ulcer. The edges of the crater are sharply demarcated and the centre contains a small amount of fibrinopurulent exudate. There is a band of inflammatory infiltrate around the bed of the ulcer; in the lower portions fibrous tissue is beginning to form (haematoxylin and eosin, ×40).

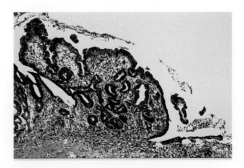

Figure 26.3
High-power photomicrograph of an edge of the ulcer depicted in Figure 26.2. The epithelial cells adjacent to the necrotic border show regenerative activity (large nuclei and increased nucleus : cytoplasm ratio). In contrast to dysplastic or neoplastic cells, however, they remain arranged in an orderly fashion and the nuclear chromatin is fine (haematoxylin and eosin, ×100).

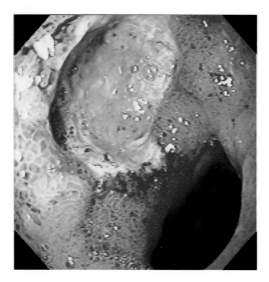

Figure 29.1
Duodenal ulcer. A deep crater can be seen on this endoscopic photograph.

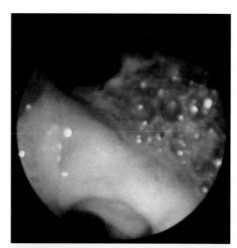
(a)

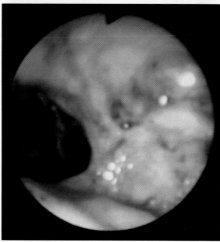
(b)

Figure 29.9
(a) Endoscopic picture of a perforation (dark area, top) above the lumen: the perforation was posterior and had been sealed off. (b) Endoscopic picture of the perforation (same patient as in a) showing a visible vessel (at 2 o'clock). The patient presented with severe pain and a major haemorrhage.

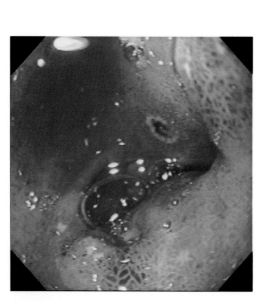

Figure 29.7
Erosive duodenitis as part of duodenal ulcer disease.

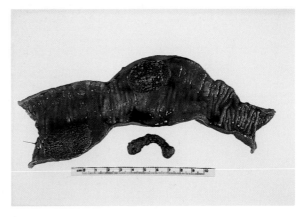

(b)

Figure 52.3
(b) In the opened resection specimen the causative strictures are clearly seen.

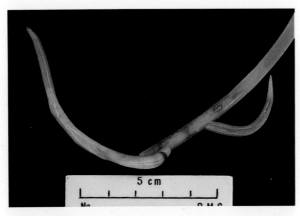

Figure 52.6
Ascaris lumbricodies found on withdrawal of a gastroduodenal tube inserted at vagotomy.

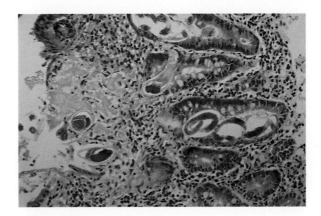

Figure 52.7
Strongyloides stercoralis in duodenal mucosa. The patient presented with an acute abdomen with multiple fluid levels on radiography. Hyperinfestation was treated successfully, but the patient was subsequently found to have a malignant lymphoma.

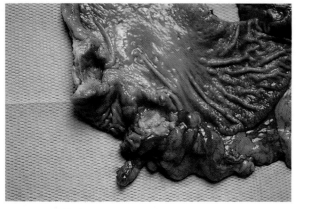
(a)

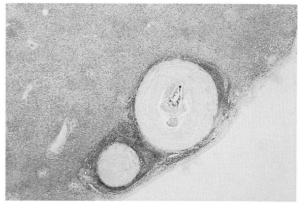
(b)

Figure 52.9
(a) Carcinoma of the antrum; an ulcerated lesion is seen in the prepyloric area. (b) Histological section of a white liver nodule from the same patient. It was not a metastasis, but an encysted larva of *Armillifer armillatus*.

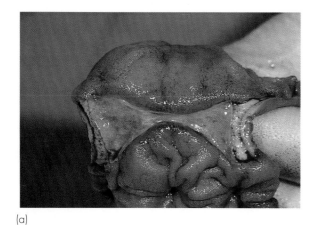
(a)

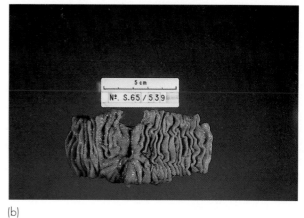
(b)

Figure 52.10
Non-specific ileal ulcers. (a) From a patient who presented with haemorrhage, and (b) From another who presented with ileal obstruction.

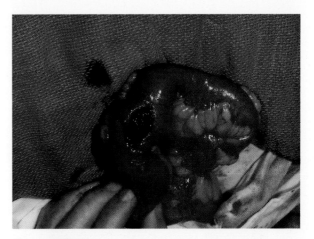

Figure 53.19
Gallstone ileus. A calculus has been exposed through an enterotomy in the ileum.

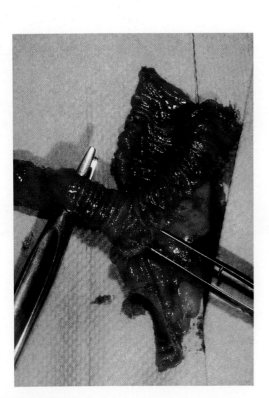

Figure 57.4
A 55-year-old man had recurrent episodes of colicky abdominal pain. He showed evidence of iron-deficiency anaemia with stools that were persistently positive for occult blood. At operation the bleeding lesion proved to be an invaginated Meckel's diverticulum (Figure 57.4), which had led to ulceration of the mucosa and intussusception into the ileum.

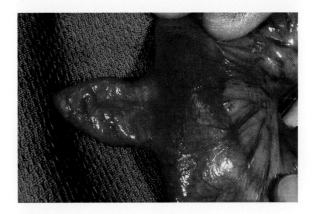

Figure 57.1
Meckel's diverticulum found incidentally at laparotomy in a child of 10 years. The diverticulum was resected uneventfully, although a wide-mouthed diverticulum such as this is unlikely to cause symptoms during life (photograph supplied by Professor RCN Williamson).

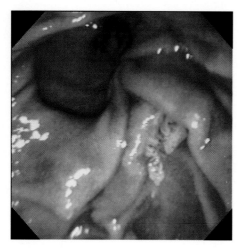

Figure 57.6
Endoscopic photograph showing a large duodenal diverticulum that arises in the typical position in the medial wall just above the papilla.

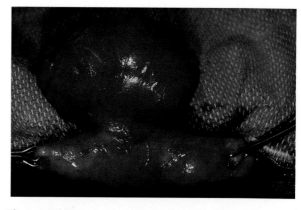

Figure 57.7
A large diverticulum on the antimesenteric border of the descending duodenum was found at laparotomy in a 68-year-old woman with chronic epigastric pain after meals. There was a healed incision in the bowel at this site following an obscure operation forty years earlier (photograph supplied by Professor RCN Williamson).

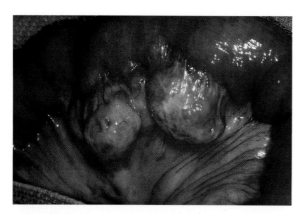

Figure 57.8
Multiple jejunal diverticula found incidentally at laparotomy in an elderly woman. The diverticula arose in the typical site on the antimesenteric border of the bowel.

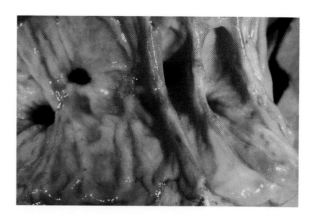

Figure 57.9
Mucosal aspect of a resected segment of jejunum showing multiple jejunal diverticula.

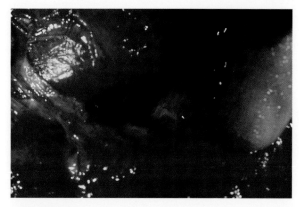

Figure 57.10
Operative findings in a patient with perforated jejunal diverticulitis (photograph supplied by Professor RCN Williamson).

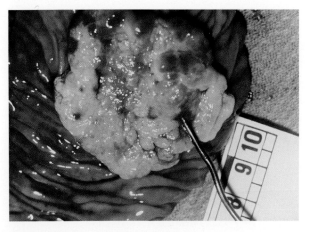

Figure 58.1
Tubulovillous adenoma (5 cm diameter) arising in the second part of the duodenum and surrounding the orifice of the major papilla, which is marked by a probe. There was no evidence of invasive carcinoma. The patient was a woman of 66 years who had presented with acute cholangitis and Gram-negative septicaemia, and the lesion was observed at ERCP. The lesion was excised by means of pylorus-preserving proximal pancreatoduodenectomy.

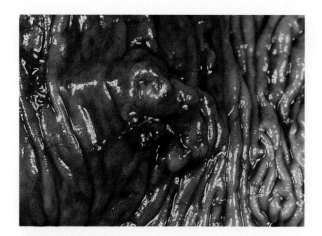

Figure 58.2
Sessile villous adenoma showing histological evidence of moderate-to-severe epithelial dysplasia. The patient was a man of 65 years who had presented with non-specific abdominal pain and heartburn. The lesion was observed during upper gastrointestinal endoscopy and was excised by means of pylorus-preserving proximal pancreatoduodenectomy.

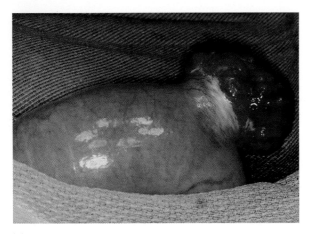

(a)

Figure 58.3
Leiomyoma (stromal tumour) of the jejunum. This lesion was found and resected at emergency laparotomy in a 55-year-old man who presented with shock and the passage of red blood per rectum. (a) Serosal aspect of the bowel with an exophytic tumour; (b) blood clot in a small ulcer on the mucosal surface.

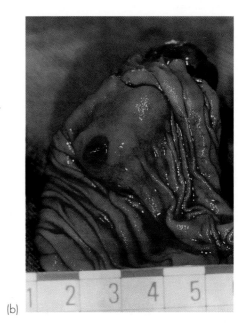

(b)

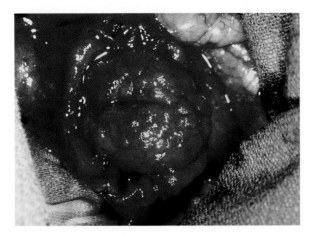

Figure 58.5
Duodenal paraganglioma. The pedunculated lesion which arose in the third part of the duodenum was excised via a duodenotomy.

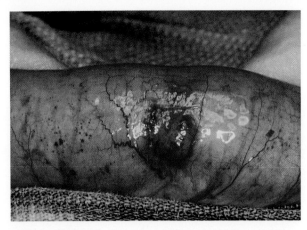

Figure 58.4
Capillary haemangioma of the upper ileum in a 64-year-old woman who presented with persistent iron-deficiency anaemia.

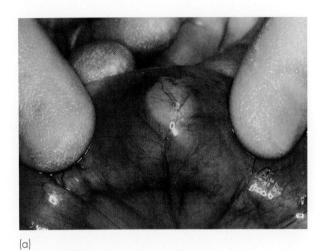

(a)

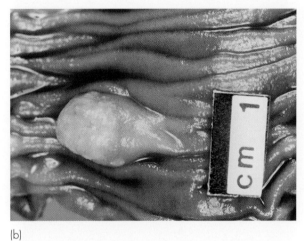

(b)

Figure 58.7
Lymphangioma of the upper ileum. The lesion was found incidentally at laparotomy. The serosal (a) and mucosal (b) aspects are shown.

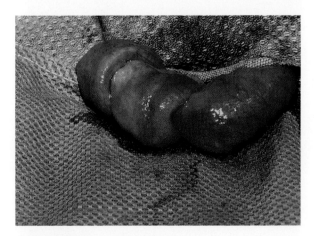

Figure 58.8
Intussusception of the jejunum in a young man with Peutz–Jeghers syndrome who had presented with intermittent attacks of subacute intestinal obstruction.

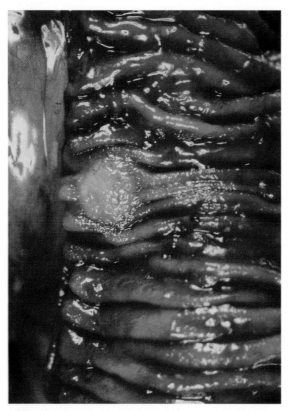

Figure 59.1
A small carcinoid tumour in the ileum. This benign tumour was
an unexpected finding in the ileal wall at laparotomy and was
treated by local resection.

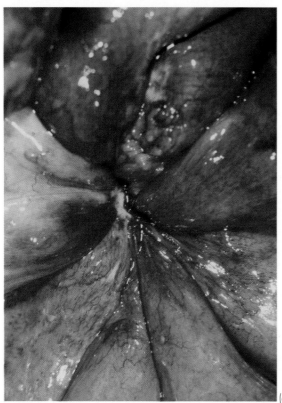

(a)

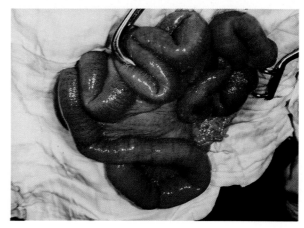

(b)

Figure 59.2
Multiple carcinoid tumours of the ileum with local lymph node
metastases in 69-year-old man who presented with symptoms
of small bowel colic and underwent elective laparotomy.
(a) Desmoplastic reaction involving the ileal mesentery. (b)
Purplish discoloration of the tumour-bearing segment of bowel
following simple handling at laparotomy, presumably due to
the local release of vasoactive substances.

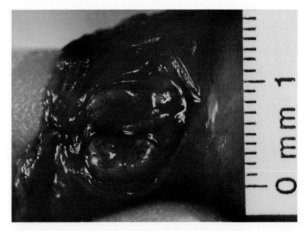

Figure 59.6
Duodenal gastrinoma. This lesion is seen incorporated in the total gastrectomy specimen from a patient who presented with duodenal and oesophageal ulceration and stenosis.

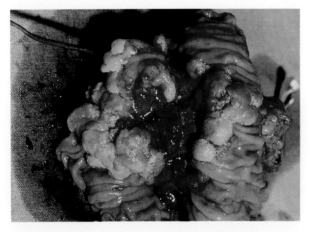

Figure 60.1
Carcinoma of the duodenum in a 71-year-old man treated by pylorus-preserving proximal pancreatoduodenectomy (PPPP). As is frequently the case with primary duodenal cancer, the carcinoma had arisen in an underlying villous adenoma.

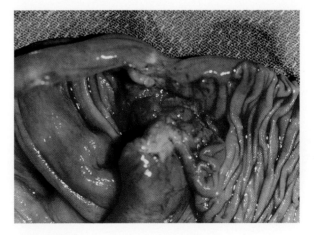

Figure 60.3
Annular carcinoma of the jejunum treated by local excision. The patient had presented with chronic small bowel obstruction, and there is an obvious disparity in size between the obstructed proximal bowel (left) and the collapsed distal bowel (right).

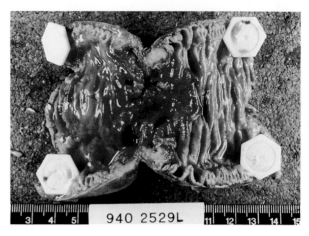

Figure 60.4
Resected carcinoma of the jejunum in an elderly man who had presented with melaena.

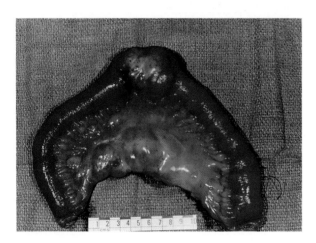

Figure 60.7
Non-Hodgkin's lymphoma involving the ileum in a 37-year-old man who presented with an enormous lower abdominal mass which disappeared after a course of combination chemotherapy. His residual obstructive symptoms were cured by small bowel resection, but he died of cerebral metastases one year later.

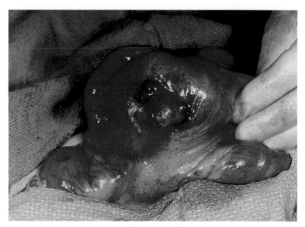

Figure 60.9
Leiomyosarcoma of the jejunum. The patient, a 64-year-old woman, had presented with high small bowel obstruction. Lymph node metastases were present at operation, and she died of disseminated disease two years later.

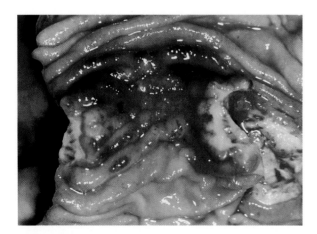

Figure 60.8
Healed stricture resulting from a lymphoma that had been successfully treated with radical chemotherapy four years earlier. There was no evidence of residual tumour in the resection specimen.

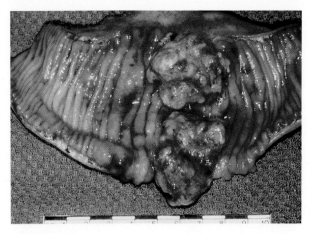

Figure 60.10
Epithelial leiomyosarcoma of the ileum in a 53-year-old man who had symptoms of intermittent small bowel obstruction.

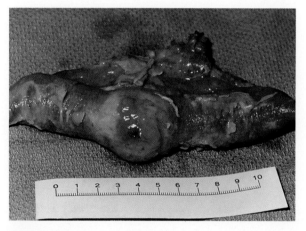

Figure 60.11
Jejunal metastasis from a primary carcinoma of the bronchus. The patient presented with perforation and peritonitis.

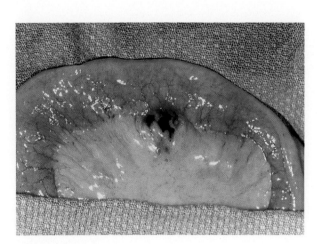

Figure 60.12
Malignant melanoma of the mid small bowel. The patient had iron-deficiency anaemia and stools that were persistently positive for occult blood.

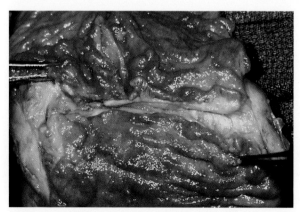

Figure 61.2
Chronic pancreatitis in a 43-year-old man with annular pancreas. The circumferential duct has been opened in the pancreatoduodenectomy specimen. (Professor Williamson's case.)

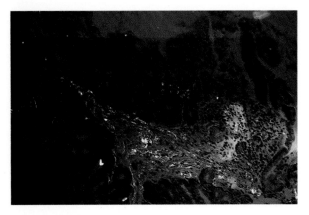

Figure 61.4
A 50-year-old female with chronic intra-abdominal sepsis
developed protein-losing enteropathy. A biopsy of the
duodenum stained with Congo red revealed amyloid deposits
within the duodenal submucosa. Under polarized light these
deposits demonstrate apple-green birefringence (250 ×).
(Courtesy of Dr EM Thompson, Hammersmith Hospital.)

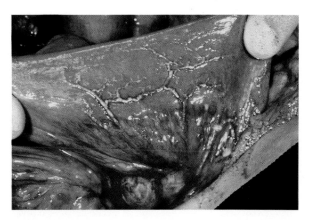

Figure 61.5
Intestinal lymphangiectasia secondary to malignant mesenteric
nodes in a young woman with carcinomatosis. Dilated
lymphatics are seen on the serosal aspect of the bowel.
(Professor Williamson's case.)

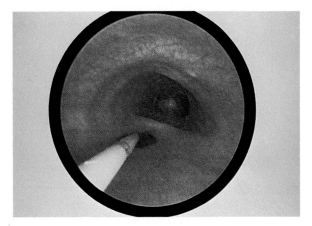

Figure 62.2
Tracheoscopy showing fistula into oesophagus.

PART
ONE

Oesophagus

edited by A. Watson

1

Normal Structure and Function of the Oesophagus

JG Temple

ANATOMY OF THE OESOPHAGUS

The oesophagus is a muscular conduit whose principal function is to convey ingested substances from the mouth to the stomach. It is 23–25 cm long, beginning at the lower border of the cricoid cartilage opposite the sixth cervical vertebra and ending at the cardiac orifice of the stomach opposite the eleventh cervical vertebra (Figure 1.1). It is subdivided into three anatomical segments which are unequal in length:

- cervical
- thoracic
- abdominal

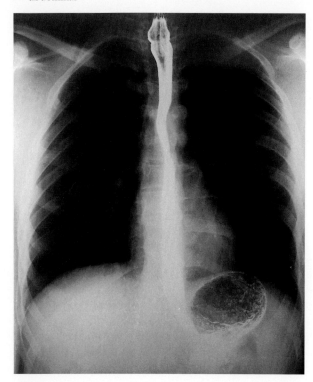

Figure 1.1
P.A. radiograph showing course of the oesophagus.

From its commencement it courses down along the anterior surface of the vertebral column, but high up it deviates slightly from the midline towards the left, as it approaches the root of the neck and, in the lower part of the thorax, as it projects forwards and to the left to pass through the oesophageal opening in the diaphragm. With the exception of the appendix, it is the narrowest part of the alimentary tract and it is constricted slightly at four sites:

- at its commencement
- where it is crossed by the aortic arch
- as it is crossed by the left main bronchus
- where it pierces the diaphragm

These positions are approximately 15 cm, 22.5 cm, 27.5 cm and 37.5 cm from the incisor teeth, respectively (Figure 1.2).

The cervical oesophagus

This is a direct continuation of the pharynx, being bounded above by the cricopharyngeal muscle. It is 5–6 cm in length. It is deeply situated and passes downwards and slightly to the left of the midline. Thus it is not quite totally covered anteriorly by the trachea on the left as it is on the right, and therefore it is slightly easier to approach the oesophagus surgically on the left side (Figure 1.3). The recurrent laryngeal nerves lie on either side in a groove between the trachea and the oesophagus. In the lower part of the neck the thoracic duct ascends for 1–2 cm along the left edge of the oesophagus before it arches anteriorly, forwards and downwards to join the confluence of the internal jugular and subclavian veins.

Posteriorly the oesophagus lies on the prevertebral layer of the deep cervical fascia, to which it is only loosely attached. This enables the oesophagus to move relatively freely upwards and downwards during deglutition.

Laterally the cervical oesophagus is overlapped by the carotid sheath and the posterior part of the lateral lobes of the thyroid.

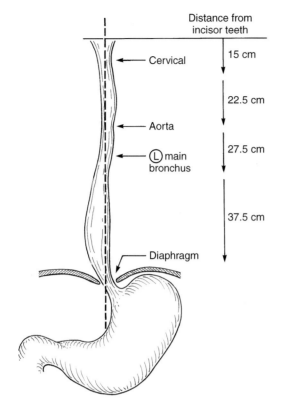

Figure 1.2
Axis deviation of oesophagus and sites of narrowing.

The thoracic oesophagus

This is the longest portion of the oesophagus, commencing at the thoracic inlet opposite the lower border of T1 and ending at the oesophageal hiatus in the diaphragm opposite T10. It is 18 cm in length (Figure 1.1).

It passes medially downwards towards the midline and from the level of T5 and remains in this position behind the heart. It then courses anteriorly and to the left to pass through the oesophageal hiatus of the diaphragm at T10.

It is situated initially in the superior mediastinum between the trachea and vertebral column and then passes behind the aortic arch and descends in the posterior mediastinum along the right side of the descending thoracic aorta (Figure 1.3).

Anteriorly lie trachea, right pulmonary artery, left main bronchus, the left atrium within the pericardium, and finally the diaphragm.

Posteriorly it rests on the vertebral column and is closely related to the thoracic duct, azygos and terminal branches of the hemiazygos vein. Below, close to the diaphragm, it comes to lie on the front of the thoracic aorta.

On the left, in the superior mediastinum lie successively the aortic arch, left subclavian artery, thoracic duct, left pleura and the left recurrent laryngeal nerve, which is situated in a groove between the oesophagus and trachea. In the posterior mediastinum are related the descending thoracic aorta and the left pleura. On the right the pleura is closely applied to the mediastinum and oesophagus all the way down, and the azygos vein arches over it to enter the superior vena cava. The vagus

nerves are closely related to the lower part of the intrathoracic oesophagus, the right coming to lie behind and the left mainly in front as they pass through the oesophageal hiatus in the diaphragm to enter the abdomen (Figure 1.3). The thoracic duct lies behind and to the right in the lower part of the posterior mediastinum. As it ascends it comes to lie immediately posterior to the oesophagus and then, at the level of T5, comes to lie on its left side.

Surgical exposure

Access to the lower end of the intrathoracic oesophagus is possible from either the right or the left side, but for mid- and upper oesophagus, access is easier on the right, as the whole oesophagus can be exposed and the only structure to cross it is the azygos vein.

Abdominal oesophagus

The oesophagus usually passes through the right crus of the diaphragm just to the left of the midline at the level of T10. The abdominal oesophagus is approximately 1.25 cm in length but this can be variable as it frequently prolapses upwards through the diaphragm to form a sliding hiatus hernia. Its direction is downwards to the left and forwards to end at the cardia of the stomach. Its right border is continuous with the

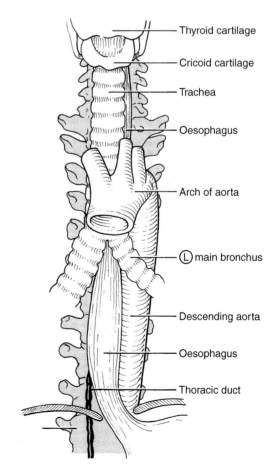

Figure 1.3
Principal relations of the oesophagus.

lesser curvature and its left border is demarcated from the fundus by the oesophagogastric angle of implantation (angle of His). The abdominal oesophagus is covered with peritoneum from the greater sac anteriorly and on the left side. Posteriorly it is not covered by peritoneum, but loose fascia between it and the aorta and crura. The oesophagogastric junction is not demarcated clearly anatomically or macroscopically. Endoscopically, however, the junction between the pale mucosa of the oesophagus and the pink mucosa of the stomach can clearly be seen as the so-called Z line. In 60% of the normal population the Z line is within 1 cm of the position of the gastro-oesophageal sphincter.[1]

Structure of the oesophagus

The oesophageal wall is made up of four coats:

- an outer loose fibrous layer
- a muscular layer – which itself comprises an outer longitudinal layer and an inner circular layer
- a submucosa
- an internal or mucous layer

The oesophagus has no serosa except that covering its abdominal portion, but it is covered throughout its length in loose areolar tissue containing a large network of elastic fibres.

The upper oesophageal sphincter and upper part of the oesophagus comprise striated muscle. The rest of the oesophagus and lower oesophageal sphincter are formed of smooth muscle. The transition from striated smooth muscle occurs usually in the upper 4–5 cm of the oesophagus, but this varies from individual to individual. Furthermore, the position at which this occurs also varies with the striated muscle extending a little further down in the circular than the longitudinal layer.[1] However, the majority of the oesophagus comprises smooth muscle.[2] The submucosa lies between the muscular and mucosal layers. It contains a vascular plexus and mucous glands. The mucous membrane layer is thick and arranged in longitudinal folds – the 'mucosal rosette' – which flattens out on distension of the tube. At the oesophagogastric junction, the striated squamous lining epithelium abruptly changes to columnar epithelium. The mucosa is the strongest layer of the oesophagus anatomically.

Blood supply

The oesophagus does not appear to have an excessively rich blood supply. It has two anastomotic networks, one between muscular and submucosal planes and one on the external surface.

The arterial supply

The cervical part of the oesophagus is supplied by paired branches from the inferior thyroid branch of the thyrocervical trunk. The thoracic oesophagus is vascularized by branches from the descending thoracic aorta and branches from the bronchial arteries. The abdominal part of the oesophagus is supplied by the left gastric artery and left phrenic branches of the abdominal aorta. However, the arterial supply to the oesophagus is not strictly segmental. Thus it is possible to divide all the vessels supplying the intrathoracic oesophagus without infarction resulting.[3]

Venous drainage

This occurs into the inferior thyroid veins in the neck, into the azygos and hemiazygos veins in the thorax, and, most importantly, via the left gastric vein to the portal vein in the abdomen. This provides a communication between the systemic and portal venous systems which can become important clinically in portal hypertension, when it can become manifest as varices in the distal oesophagus and proximal stomach.

Nerve supply

There are two systems which innervate the oesophagus, one extrinsic and the other intrinsic.

The extrinsic network comprises sympathetic and parasympathetic supplies. The sympathetic supply comes from the superior and inferior cervical ganglion in the neck, from the upper thoracic and splanchnic nerves in the thorax, and branches from the coeliac ganglion in the abdomen. The parasympathetic supply comes from the recurrent laryngeal nerves in the neck and from branches of the vagus in the thorax and abdomen.

The intrinsic supply comprises two intramural plexuses, one between the longitudinal and circular muscle layers and one in the submucous layer. The intramural plexus is the larger and contains many ganglion cells, particularly in the smooth muscle part of the oesophagus. The submucous plexus contains no ganglia and fewer nerve fibres.

Lymph drainage

The oesophagus has a very rich lymphatic drainage which originates from two plexuses, one in the submucosal layer and the other within the muscle layer. In general, in the upper two-thirds of the oesophagus the flow of lymph is in a cranial direction, whereas in the lower third of the oesophagus it is in a caudal direction. Once a large lymphatic trunk has penetrated the oesophageal wall, it tends to pass directly into an adjacent lymph node, but there is a very rich anastomotic network of lymphatic trunks up and down the length of the oesophagus. Because of this, submucosal spread of tumours in the oesophagus is common.

PHYSIOLOGY OF THE OESOPHAGUS

The oesophagus has two main functions: active transport of food and fluid boluses from the mouth to the stomach, and the prevention of significant reflux of gastric contents from the stomach back up into the lumen of the oesophagus. It effects these aims principally by emptying and clearing itself rapidly of any contained material, whether by ingestion or reflux.

Swallowing

The initiation of swallowing is voluntary, but subsequent oesophageal clearance of either ingested or refluxed material is entirely involuntary.

Conventionally swallowing is considered in three stages:

- oral
- pharyngeal
- oesophageal

Oral phase

This is the only stage of swallowing which is under voluntary control. Swallowing commences by pressing the tongue and any food or fluid bolus upwards and backwards against the palate. The nasopharynx is closed by the soft palate and the bolus is then projected towards the pharynx. The larynx is closed by the epiglottis to prevent aspiration. Beyond this stage the rest of the swallowing mechanism becomes entirely involuntary. The oral phase of swallowing can be quite vigorous, resulting in liquids arriving into the pharynx and body of the oesophagus before the ensuing peristaltic wave has commenced.[5]

Pharyngeal phase

The pharynx is involved in both deglutition and respiration. When swallowing is commenced, respiration is simultaneously suspended until the bolus has passed from the back of the mouth into the oesophagus. This is a complex involuntary mechanism. Afferent sensory receptors in the pharynx relay impulses to the swallowing centre in the brainstem which initiates this phase of swallowing and which also inhibits the respiratory centre in the medulla to produce the temporary cessation of breathing. The respiratory tract is closed above by the elevation of the soft palate and lower down by protection of the larynx by the epiglottis. This is achieved by contraction of the upper pharyngeal constrictor, elevation of the larynx and inversion of the epiglottis. The cricopharyngeus, together with the lower part of the inferior constrictor of the pharynx and the uppermost part of the circular muscle of the oesophagus, comprise the upper oesophageal sphincter. This is normally tonically contracted, but relaxes at this stage. Contraction of the superior, mid- and upper part of the lower constrictor muscles of the pharynx then initiate the peristaltic wave and the food bolus is projected into the body of the oesophagus.

This whole series of events requires coordination which is mediated by five cranial nerves. Sensory information passes to the mid-brain via the trigeminal, glossopharyngeal and vagus cranial nerves, whereas motor responses are effected by way of the trigeminal, facial, glossopharyngeal, vagus and accessory cranial nerves. This whole process takes 1.5 s and produces coordinated contraction of the pharynx and relaxation of the upper oesophageal sphincter.[6]

Oesophageal stage

This lasts for 7–10 s and involves the generation and propagation of a peristaltic wave which sweeps down the oesophagus

at a rate of 2–3 cm/s, and simultaneous relaxation of the lower oesophageal sphincter to allow the bolus to pass on into the stomach. It is an active process which requires control of both circular and longitudinal muscles of the oesophagus and simultaneous coordination of lower oesophageal sphincter relaxation. The longitudinal muscles contract, thus shortening the oesophagus and the sequential circular muscle contraction produces a peristaltic clearing or wiping wave.

Circular muscle contraction occurs in three typical patterns: namely, primary, secondary and tertiary.

Primary contraction (primary peristalsis) is swallow-initiated. It is centrally mediated and starts in the pharynx. It produces a contractile propulsive wave which lasts for about 9 s and which proceeds aborally down the oesophagus to the oesophagogastric junction. Simultaneously it is associated with relaxation of the lower oesophageal sphincter (Figure 1.4).

Secondary contraction (secondary peristalsis) commences without actual swallowing and thus it is totally involuntary. It is also initiated without any central stimulation. Its origin is in the body of the oesophagus in response to distension.[7] It continues until the oesophagus is emptied and therefore is responsible

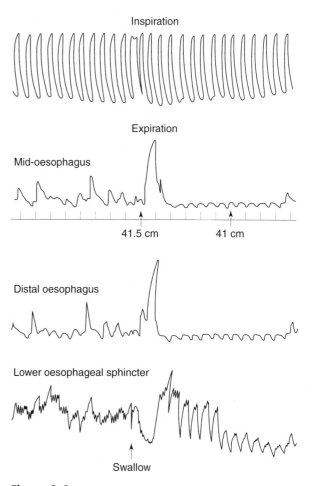

Figure 1.4
Manometry trace showing a peristaltic wave and simultaneous relaxation of the lower oesophageal sphincter. The three recording sites are situated 5 cm apart.

for oesophageal clearance. It represents contraction of the circular muscle. It assumes considerable importance in normal oesophageal function because solid bolus ingestion usually requires more than the single primary peristaltic wave to ensure that the oesophageal lumen is completely emptied in an aboral direction. It is mediated by local neural reflexes. It is manometrically similar to primary peristalsis, except that it starts in the oesophagus itself.

Tertiary contraction (non-peristaltic contraction) is a much less frequent phenomenon in which non-peristaltic contraction of the oesophagus produces segmentation. Such contractions may occur after a swallow or, rarely, spontaneously. They are seen occasionally during normal radiology or manometry examinations, but are much more common in pathological motor dysfunctions of the oesophagus, and in such conditions, they may be the only kind of contractions seen in the body of the oesophagus (Figure 1.5). They may in fact represent only a pathological process in the oesophagus. They certainly play no part in normal peristalsis, either primary or secondary, and when present may actually impede the progress of a food bolus.[8]

Peristalsis and its control

A peristaltic wave has three typical components, initially a small decrease in pressure of a few mm Hg, followed immediately by a similar rise in pressure and then a high-amplitude wave. The initial decrease lasts 0.4 s, the subsequent small rise in pressure 1.5 s and the third wave of high-amplitude, 4–6 s. The wave passes directly from the striated to the smooth muscle of the oesophagus, and its amplitude and duration increases although its speed decreases. It has been suggested that there is a zone of slightly lower peristaltic pressure just below the upper oesophageal sphincter, presumably at the site of the junction of the striated and smooth muscle in the oesophageal wall.[9] In the body of the oesophagus, the amplitude of a wet swallow and the duration of its pressure is

greater than with a dry swallow, and the contraction amplitude also increases distally. Temperature appears to have a considerable effect on contraction, cold substances decreasing peristaltic frequency and amplitude, but prolonging duration and velocity.[10]

Peristalsis appears to be controlled by the swallowing centre in the medulla, and this regulates the events which occur after the initial voluntary act of commencing a swallow.[11] Thus, this centre starts the peristaltic mechanism and momentarily inhibits respiration. The nervous pathways to the pharynx and upper oesophagus appear to be from the nucleus ambiguus in the brainstem to the vagus nerve and then on to the striated muscle. Lower down the body of the oesophagus the pathway is via the dorsal nucleus of the vagus through cholinergic motor nerves in the vagus to the ganglia in the myenteric plexus of the oesophagus.[1] The contractions in this part of the oesophagus, i.e. the smooth muscle of the mid- and lower oesophagus, appear to be largely under the control of the myenteric nervous plexus and as such are a peripheral mechanism. This plexus also receives afferent impulses from the central nervous system and sensory input from the oesophageal wall itself. Following ingestion, this is probably the way in which bolus size has an effect on peristaltic amplitude and duration, and why dry swallows generate lower amplitudes than wet swallows. It would suggest that there is some regulatory mechanism on the involuntary stage of deglutition, presumably related to the impulses carried by the afferent and efferent fibres supplying the myenteric plexus.

Most of the experimental work in understanding peristalsis has been performed on the oesophagus of the opossum.[12] Three typical responses have been identified in the smooth muscle (Figure 1.6). On electrical stimulation of the circular muscle there is a brief small amplitude contraction, the 'on response'. When the stimulus is discontinued, there is a much higher amplitude contraction in the circular muscle, the 'off response'. Both these responses are neural in origin, but whereas the 'on response' is cholinergically based, the 'off response' is not, as it can be inhibited only by nerve toxins such as tetrodotoxin, but not by anticholinergic substances such as atropine or antiadrenergic substances such as hexamethonium. Proceeding aborally, the 'off response' contractions occur at successively longer intervals after the cessation of stimulation – this is the so-called 'latency gradient'. This is the basis of the peristaltic wave. Electrical stimulation of the smooth longitudinal muscles produces a sustained contraction, the 'duration response'. This leads to some shortening of the oesophagus and is probably mediated through a cholinergic pathway. As such it may be controlled by the central nervous system through vagal fibres. Presumably the duration response produces tone in the normally relaxed oesophagus. The 'latency gradient' and 'off response' can thus produce a wiping peristaltic wave and the bolus is propelled down the oesophagus. At the same time an inhibitory neural discharge has allowed the normally tonic lower oesophageal sphincter to relax to receive the bolus.[13] The part played by the initial 'on response' is not physiologically clear. However, if the 'duration

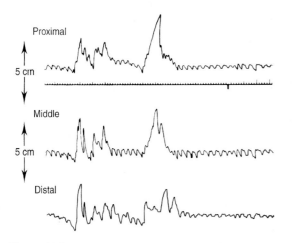

Figure 1.5
Manometry trace showing simultaneous contraction waves in the body of the oesophagus. The three recording sites are situated 5 cm apart.

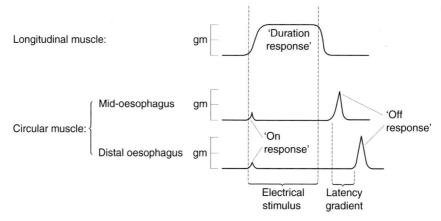

Figure 1.6
Smooth muscle contraction in the opossum. From Castell[6] by kind permission of the author and the publishers: Elsevier, London.

response' of longitudinal muscle did not occur, presumably it would be much more difficult for the circular muscle to propel the bolus down the oesophagus.

Secondary peristalsis produces identical changes in the distal oesophagus. Balloon distension studies in the human oesophagus have confirmed that there is a proximal enhancement of propulsive motor activity mediated by a cholinergic pathway.[8] On balloon inflation a myogenically mediated 'on response' is initiated, and at the same time a cholinergically mediated contraction of the longitudinal muscle, the 'duration response', occurs. On balloon deflation a distally propagated contractile wave starting just above the level of distension, the 'off response', also occurs, this again being mediated by non-adrenergic, non-cholinergic nerves. There also has to be distal inhibition to the contracting wave in the circular muscle and simultaneous relaxation of the lower oesophageal sphincter. This is also mediated by a non-cholinergic, non-adrenergic pathway. This sequence of events is manometrically similar to primary peristalsis. Proximal increase in activity was consistently initiated at a level of distension less than that required for its perception. However, the distal inhibitory response did not occur until greater distension had taken place, and this was sufficient to produce clinical discomfort. The proximal excitation may be the more normal method of initiating secondary peristalsis by stimulation of stress receptors in the oesophagus by retained oesophageal content. This is a phase of normal oesophageal function which is quite subconscious. However, the amplitude of oesophageal contractions and the force stimulating them are not necessarily commensurate. The contractions sufficient to produce peristalsis on manometry are not necessarily sufficient to produce adequate oesophageal clearance. Because of this, manometry may be apparently normal, even in the presence of symptomatic clinical abnormalities of oesophageal function. Equally surprisingly, the progression of the peristaltic wave is not affected by the transition from striated to smooth muscle. Obviously, therefore, the mechanism controlling peristalsis and oesophageal transit is a complex one, for which intact neural pathways and locally mediated reflex mechanisms in the myenteric plexus are all necessary.

The oesophageal sphincters

The upper and lower oesophageal sphincters are situated at the entrance and exit of the thoracic part of the oesophagus, and are therefore subject to pressure gradients between a negative intrathoracic pressure and the positive pressure in the neck, and, to a lesser degree, abdomen. In order to prevent constant ingestion of air from the mouth or reflux of gastric contents from the stomach, these sphincters are normally closed by tonic contraction.

The upper oesophageal sphincter

This is composed of the lower part of the inferior constrictor of the pharynx, cricopharyngeus and the uppermost circular muscle fibres of the oesophagus. It consists of striated muscle and therefore is under voluntary control. The cricopharyngeus is itself attached to the cricoid cartilage and therefore the strongest contractile force in the upper oesophageal sphincter is in the anteroposterior direction. This produces a slit-like opening which has its widest parts facing laterally.

Between the lowermost fibres of the inferior constrictor of the pharynx and the cricopharyngeus muscle itself there exists an area of potential weakness in the posterior wall (Figure 1.7). There is a similar area of weakness between the lower border of cricopharyngeus and the upper circular muscle of the oesophagus posteriorly also. It is at these sites that a pharyngeal diverticulum occasionally develops. Perhaps more importantly, it is here that instrumental damage, and even perforation, can occur during the introduction of an endoscope. This occurs more commonly when a rigid rather than a flexible instrument is used.

The upper oesophageal sphincter is closed at rest as a result of a constant discharge of motor activity mediated through the ninth, tenth and eleventh cranial nerves.[14] The main final pathway is by way of the pharyngeal branch of the vagus, and also the superior and recurrent laryngeal nerves. When a swallow occurs, the action potentials producing this motor activity cease, resulting in relaxation. The upper oesophageal sphincter also relaxes involuntarily in belching and vomiting. The main force in the upper oesophageal sphincter is in the anteropos-

the peak pressure anteriorly occurs approximately 0.5 s before it occurs posteriorly.[9] The high upper oesophageal sphincter pressure protects the oesophagus from filling with air during inspiration. The presence of acid contents just below the sphincter also leads to an increase in pressure, and experimentally, the closer such acid is placed to the sphincter, the greater the rise in pressure.[15] In this way, the upper oesophageal sphincter also acts as a barrier to reflux of oesophageal contents into the pharynx and clearly this prevents aspiration and regurgitation.

Lower oesophageal sphincter

This consists of smooth muscle and is therefore under involuntary control. It is not attached to any bony or cartilaginous structures and therefore it is much rounder when closed than the upper oesophageal sphincter. Dissection does not reveal any anatomical structure at the oesophagogastric junction and therefore the consensus view is that the sphincter is a physiological structure, but an anatomical basis cannot be demonstrated macroscopically or microscopically.

A pressure recording device passed from the lower oesophagus through the oesophagogastric junction into the stomach will identify a definite zone of increased pressure (Figure 1.8). It is 2–4 cm in length and situated in the region of the oesophageal hiatus. It relaxes when a primary or secondary peristaltic wave is initiated, and remains open for several seconds. The main force is not as clearly concentrated in the anteroposterior direction as in the upper oesophageal sphincter, and the actual pressure generated is only in the region of 10–30 mm Hg. This is because the actual pressure gradient between the negative intrathoracic pressure and the positive intra-abdominal pressure is much less than that between the thorax and the neck. There is always a degree of radial asymmetry in the lower oesophageal sphincter, the left and posterior zones recording higher pressures than the right and anterior ones.[16]

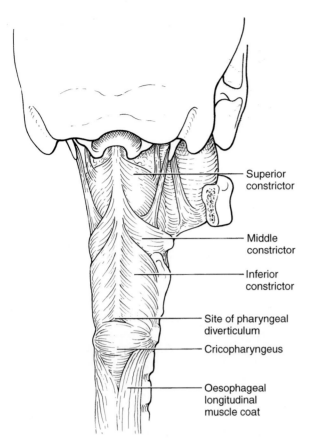

Figure 1.7
The pharynx and upper oesophageal musculature. From Atkinson[5] by kind permission of the author and publishers, Blackwell, Oxford.

terior direction, this being anatomically determined by the configuration of the pharynx.[15] The normal pressure is high, up to 100 mm Hg in this direction, although somewhat less in the lateral direction. There is also a degree of axial asymmetry as

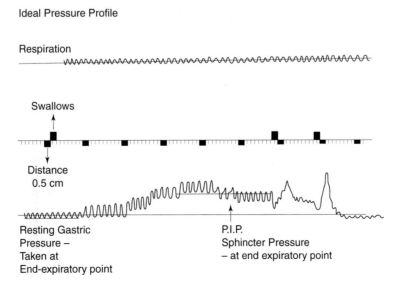

Figure 1.8
Manometry trace showing lower oesophageal sphincter.

The major function of the lower oesophageal sphincter is to prevent gastro-oesophageal reflux and to relax in response to primary or secondary peristalsis, thus aiding oesophageal clearance. The sphincter pressure also increases in response to increased intra-abdominal pressure. Its characteristic response to hormones (peptides), pharmacological agents and distension make it physiologically different from the adjacent muscle in the oesophagus, and thus identify this area as a sphincter. There is no doubt that the lower oesophageal sphincter is under a degree of hormonal control by the gastrointestinal peptides, gastrin and pentagastrin. These produce a rise in sphincter pressure. Fatty meals in the stomach lower pressure, possibly by release of cholecystokinin. All members of the secretin family decrease lower oesophageal sphincter pressure, and vasointestinal peptide (VIP) is thought to be the final chemical mediator for this. Progesterone also decreases sphincter pressure and this is thought to be the mechanism for the development of heartburn in pregnancy. Similarly, women taking oral contraceptives containing progesterone have a reduced lower oesophageal sphincter pressure.[18] Caffeine, nicotine – commonly as a result of smoking – and alcohol all lower sphincter tone. Carminatives also produce a lowering of sphincter tone.[19] They are food substances which, when ingested, produce a sensation of warmth within the abdomen and facilitate eructation. Examples are garlic, onion, herbs and mint extracts, many of which form the aromatic basis of liqueurs (Table 1.1).

Finally, basal smooth muscle tone in the lower oesophageal sphincter is dependent on available calcium ions, and calcium-blocking agents can lower it.[20]

The sphincter is innervated by efferent fibres of the autonomic nervous system, the parasympathetic supply being from the vagus and the sympathetic from the splanchnic nerves. However, the resultant neurogenic control is mediated via the nerve plexuses in the muscle layer itself. Evidence for this can be accrued from the knowledge that the sphincter can function normally above or below the diaphragm, that is, whether there

is or is not a sliding hiatus hernia. Also, sphincter tone appears to be unaffected by truncal or highly selective vagotomy.[21] However, the mechanism by which the lower oesophageal sphincter relaxes is not clear, because in animals it can be reproduced by stimulating the vagus and abolished by a neural toxin such as tetrodotoxin. The tone of the lower oesophageal sphincter is thought to be an intrinsic property of the muscle itself and as such is independent of surrounding structures, but it is influenced by neural and hormonal factors.

Antireflux mechanisms

The lower oesophageal sphincter provides the barrier to gastro-oesophageal reflux. As such it acts as a predominantly one-way valvular system, but this is not to say that reflux of gastric contents up into the body of the oesophagus does not occur. pH monitoring in the distal oesophagus has shown clearly that some reflux is a normal event, but it is usually cleared very quickly by subsequent primary peristalsis, i.e. the arrival of further food and saliva, or secondary peristalsis, which is the normal response to retained substances in the distal oesophagus. Such reflux is termed 'physiological'. 'Pathological reflux' is the condition in which symptoms or pathological changes occur in the lower oesophagus and sphincter area. It occurs when either oesophageal clearance is reduced or impaired, or the volume of the refluxate is increased. The former implies principally a defect in the normal sphincter function and oesophageal clearing mechanisms, the latter usually occurs when the gastric volume increases, most commonly as a result of gastric outlet obstruction associated with chronic peptic ulceration.

Apart from the lower oesophageal sphincter itself, several other factors have been implicated in the antireflux mechanism (Figure 1.9).

1. Intra-abdominal segment of oesophagus;
2. Pinchcock of diaphragmatic crura;
3. The angle of His;
4. Mucosal rosette;
5. Sliding hiatus hernia;
6. Phreno-oesophageal ligament.

All of these other factors can be identified anatomically, whereas the sphincter and its function is a concept which can only be studied physiologically and for which there is no confirmed anatomical basis.[22]

Intra-abdominal segment of oesophagus

The lower oesophageal sphincter normally lies at or very near the oesophageal hiatus in the diaphragm, usually straddling it, with two-thirds lying below and therefore within the abdomen, and one-third above and just within the thorax anatomically. Whenever the sphincter or part of it lies below the diaphragm, it will be subject to positive intra-abdominal pressure, and this will tend to keep it closed. Acting as a flaccid tube, it can therefore be considered as a flutter valve.[23] Thus, the greater the intra-abdominal pressure or its rise, the greater the pressure

Table 1.1 Factors affecting lower oesophageal sphincter pressure (LOSP)

LOSP↑	LOSP↓
Acid in the fundus	Fat in the body and antrum
Gastrin	Secretin
	CCK – pancreozymin
	Glucagon
	VIP
	Progesterone
Cholinergics (bethanechol)	
Metaclopramide	Anticholinergics (atropine)
Domperidone	
Prostigmin	Calcium channel blockers
Cimetidine	
	Caffeine
	Nicotine (smoking)
	Alcohol
	Carminatives

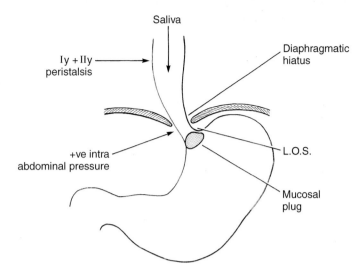

Figure 1.9
Antireflux mechanisms.

on the intra-abdominal oesophagus, and therefore the better its ability to resist reflux.

Diaphragmatic crura

In two-thirds of the population the oesophageal hiatus in the diaphragm is controlled by fibres of the right crus, and these fibres form a kind of sling around the oesophagus and oesophagogastric junction. However, although anatomically they can easily be recognized, it is doubtful whether these sling fibres exert much pressure on the lower oesophagus itself, and therefore have much to do with the prevention of gastro-oesophageal reflux. Further strength to this comes from the knowledge that division of the phrenic nerve, and therefore paralysis of the central part of the diaphragm, has no effect at all on the incidence or severity of gastro-oesophageal reflux.[19] Equally, displacement of the oesophagogastric junction above the diaphragm does not necessarily mean that pathological reflux will occur.

The angle of implantation (angle of His)

It has been postulated that the oblique angle of entry of the oesophagus into the stomach produces a sharp incisura between the oesophagus and the fundus, and that this acts as a flap valve. Increase in intra-abdominal pressure would press this flap against the lesser curvature of the stomach, occluding the oesophageal opening even more. Examinations in cadavers have shown that abolition of the acuteness of the angle of implantation allows reflux to occur more readily.[24] However, this is obviously entirely an anatomical study and does not allow for the physiological function of the sphincter zone at all.

Mucosal rosette

The mucosal rosette has been implicated in the antireflux mechanism. This is a phenomenon seen on endoscopy and results from the excess circumference of mucosa seen when the oesophagus is closed, and which is necessary to allow dilatation of the lower segment to permit passage of a food bolus

and yet maintain an intact mucosa. It is perhaps the final factor in closing and sealing the oesophagogastric junction when the sphincter has contracted.[19,25] Further evidence that it may be important comes from the knowledge that reflux is common in patients with atrophic gastritis, although this is often not symptomatic because these patients are also hypochlorhydric.

Phreno-oesophageal ligament

This represents the confluence of the pleura above and the peritoneum below as each is reflected at the oesophageal hiatus. As such it is not strictly a ligament at all, but merely a condensation of fascia which is quite variable in thickness and tensile strength. It is difficult to identify from below and probably does not play any significant role in the antireflux mechanism.

In conclusion, all the evidence now points to the lower oesophageal sphincter as being the principal factor preventing pathological gastro-oesophageal reflux, coupled with a normal secondary peristaltic mechanism to aid oesophageal clearance. All the other factors may have a summation effect in assisting the competence at the oesophagogastric junction, but without a functioning lower oesophageal sphincter mechanism and adequate peristalsis in the body of the oesophagus, these other factors are collectively ineffective.

REFERENCES

1. Cuschieri A. Anatomy and physiology of the oesophagus. In Hennessy TPJ & Cuschieri A (eds) *Surgery of the Oesophagus.* London; Baillière Tindall, 1986.
2. Meyer GW, Austin RM, Brady CE et al. Muscle anatomy of the human oesophagus. *J Clin Gastroenterol* 1986; **8**: 131.
3. Temple JG. Personal observation, 1989.
4. McKeown KC. Trends in oesophageal resection for carcinoma. *Ann R Coll Surg Engl* 1972; **51**: 213.
5. Atkinson M. Dysphagia. In Misiewicz JJ, Pounder RE & Venables CW (eds) *Diseases of the Gut and Pancreas.* London: Blackwell Scientific Publications, 1987.
6. Castell DO. Anatomy and physiology of the esophagus and its sphincters. In Castell DO, Richter JE & Dalton CB (eds) *Esophageal Motility Testing.* London: Elsevier, 1987.
7. Goyal RK & Cobb BW. Motility of the pharynx, esophagus and

esophageal sphincters. In Johnson LR (ed.) *Physiology of the Gastrointestinal Tract.* New York: Raven Press, 1981.

8. Kendall GPN, Thompson DG, Day SJ & Garvie N. Motor responses of the oesophagus to intraluminal distension in normal subjects and patients with oesophageal clearance disorders. *Gut* 1987; **28:** 272.

9. Katy PO & Castell DO. Function of the normal lumen esophagus. In De Meester TR & Matthews HR (eds) *International Trends in General Thoracic Surgery* Vol. 3. St Louis: CV Mosby, 1987.

10. Windship DH, Viegas de Andrade SR & Zboralske FF. Influence of bolus temperature on human esophagus motor function. *J Clin Invest* 1970; **49:** 243.

11. Weisbrudt NW. Neuromuscular organisation of esophageal and pharyngeal motility. *Arch Intern Med* 1967; **136:** 524.

12. Christensen J & Lund GF. Esophageal responses to distension and electrical stimulation. *J Clin Invest* 1969; **48:** 408.

13. Goyal RK & Ralten S. Nature of the vagal inhibitory innervation to the lower esophageal sphincter. *J Clin Invest* 1975; **55:** 1119.

14. Asoh R & Goyal RK. Manometry and electronmyography of the upper oesophageal sphincter in the opossum. *Gastroenterology* 1978; **74:** 515.

15. Gerhardt DC, Shuck, TJ, Bordeaux RA & Winship DH. Human upper esophageal sphincter: response to volume, osmotic and acid stimuli. *Gastroenterology* 1978; **75:** 268.

16. Winans CS. Manometric asymmetry of the lower esophageal high pressure zone. *Am J Dig Dis* 1977; **22:** 348.

17. Dodals WJ, Dent J & Hogan WJ. Pregnancy and the lower esophageal sphincter. *Gastroenterology* 1978; **74:** 1334.

18. Van Thiel DH, Gavaler JS & Stremple J. Lower esophageal sphincter pressure in women using sequential oral contraceptives. *Gastroenterology* 1976; **71:** 232.

19. Earlam R. Gastro-oesophageal junction. In *Clinical Tests of Oesophageal Function.* London: Crosby Lockwood Hartles, 1976.

20. Goyal RK & Ralton S. Effects of sodium nitroprusside and verapamil on lower esophageal sphincter. *Am J Physiol* 1980; **238:** 40.

21. Temple JG, Goodall RJR & Hay DJ. The effect of highly selective vagotomy upon the lower oesophageal sphincter. *Gut* 1981; **22:** 368.

22. Lendrum FC. Anatomical features of the cardiac orifice of the stomach, with special reference to cardiospasm. *Arch Intern Med* 1937; **59:** 474.

23. Edwards DAW. The anti-reflux mechanism: manometric and radiological studies. *Br J Radiol* 1961; **34:** 474.

24. Marchand P. The gastro-ocsophageal sphincter and the mechanism of regurgitation. *Br J Surg* 1955; **42:** 504.

25. Bocka GSM. *The Gastro-oesophageal Junction: Clinical Applications to Oesophageal and Gastric Surgery.* London, Churchill, 1962.

2

RADIOLOGICAL INVESTIGATIONS OF THE OESOPHAGUS

AR Wright
GM Fraser

There are many radiological techniques available for evaluation of the oesophagus. In this chapter, the roles of plain radiography, barium swallow, radionuclide techniques, computed tomography, magnetic resonance imaging, endoluminal ultrasonography and interventional radiology are discussed, with comments on technique and the strengths and weaknesses of each modality in specific clinical situations.

PLAIN RADIOGRAPHY

Plain films can occasionally be useful in oesophageal disease. A large, fixed hiatal hernia with an air–fluid level is commonly seen behind the heart as an incidental finding on chest radiographs, particularly in the elderly (Figure 2.1). Similarly, marked oesophageal dilatation, due for example to achalasia, scleroderma or obstruction, may be recognized as an increased density (with or without a fluid level) behind the heart or in the superior mediastinum.

Perforation of the oesophagus, which is now seen more frequently due to the increasing use of diagnostic and therapeutic endoscopy, will usually be recognized on plain films.[1] A lateral soft tissue film of the neck will show surgical emphysema with a linear distribution in the vertical plane, and there may also be widening of the retrotracheal soft tissue space. Mediastinal air may be seen on the chest radiograph. In spontaneous rupture of the lower oesophagus (Boerhaave's syndrome), the chest radiograph will also, in the majority of cases, show subcutaneous and mediastinal emphysema. Oesophageal perforation may be complicated by pneumothorax or hydropneumothorax, more commonly on the left side.

Plain radiographs may be useful in detecting foreign bodies in the oesophagus. When opaque, foreign bodies are usually easily recognized on a lateral soft tissue radiograph of the neck (Figure 2.2a). Non-opaque foreign bodies, such as a meat bolus, may separate the walls of the oesophagus, trapping a bubble of air which will persist as a constant feature on a repeat radiograph. Otherwise, non-opaque foreign bodies usually have

to be diagnosed by contrast swallow, where they will appear as a filling defect in the contrast column. The swallow may occasionally be therapeutic by propelling the foreign body into the stomach.

A retropharyngeal abscess will cause widening of the retropharyngeal soft tissue space and mottled air-lucency may also be visible (Figure 2.2b). A pharyngeal pouch (Zenker's diverticulum) may cause widening of the retrotracheal soft tissue space, often with an air-fluid level, and tumours of the cervical oesophagus may also widen the retrotracheal soft tissue space.

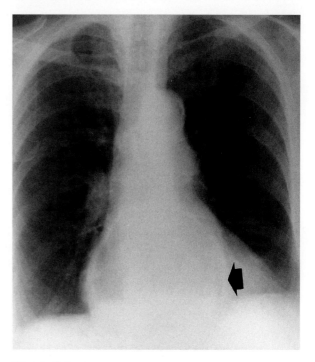

Figure 2.1
Plain chest radiograph showing large, fixed hiatal hernia with air–fluid level (arrowed) behind heart.

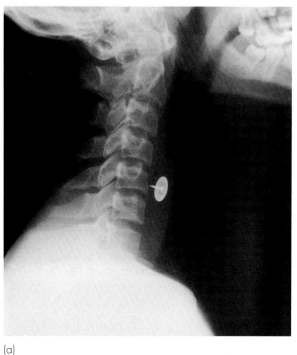

(a)

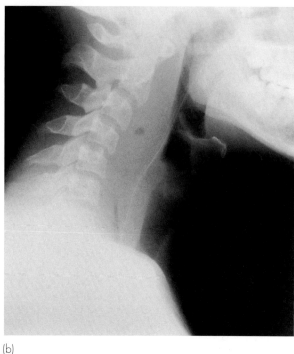

(b)

Figure 2.2

(a) Lateral radiograph of neck showing drawing pin impacted at junction of pharynx and oesophagus. (b) Same patient. Widening of prevertebral space with mottled air-lucency indicating retropharyngeal abscess secondary to perforation by foreign body. (Courtesy of Dr S.A. Moussa.)

Postoperative changes may be recognized on the plain film, including the typical fundal filling defect in the gastric air bubble following Nissen fundoplication, and the saccular opacity (with or without air–fluid level) seen in the mediastinum with gastric or colonic interposition after oesophagectomy.

BARIUM SWALLOW

Technique

This is the most widely used radiological method for examining the oesophagus. The sensitivity for the detection of disease is enhanced by the use of single-contrast, double-contrast and mucosal-relief technique for each examination, along with an assessment of motility. The method for examining the hypopharynx and cervical oesophagus is quite different from that used to examine the lower oesophagus.

The hypopharynx is best demonstrated in the frontal projection with the patient upright and the chin elevated after a bolus of high density (250% w/v) barium has been swallowed and whilst the mucosa of the hypopharynx remains coated with barium (Figure 2.3).[2]

The cervical oesophagus is best demonstrated when the patient swallows a bolus of medium density (100% w/v) barium in the erect position and, with correct timing of the exposure, views of the fully distended cervical oesophagus can be obtained (Figure 2.4). The lateral projection is more informative than the frontal projection, as structural abnormalities such as postcricoid webs (Figure 2.5) and pharyngeal pouches (Figure 2.6) are better demonstrated.

The lateral projection is also best for showing functional abnormalities of the pharynx and cervical oesophagus. Orderly contraction of the superior, middle and inferior constrictor muscles is required to propel the bolus from the pharynx into the oesophagus. At the same time, the larynx is elevated and

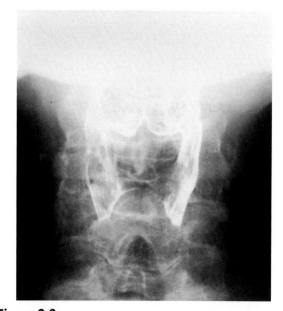

Figure 2.3

Frontal projection of the normal oropharynx showing the paired valleculae and pyriform fossae demonstrated in double contrast.

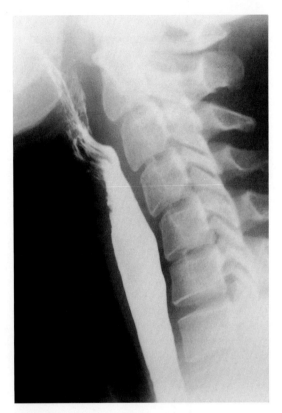

Figure 2.4
Lateral projection of the normal cervical oesophagus demonstrated in single contrast.

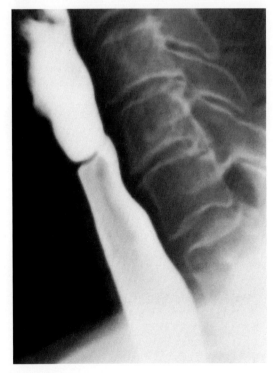

Figure 2.5
A postcricoid web seen as a shelf-like incision on the anterior wall of the cervical oesophagus.

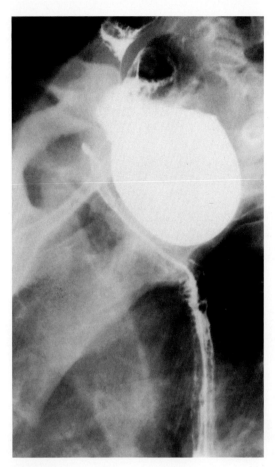

Figure 2.6
A large pharyngeal pouch filled with barium compresses and displaces the cervical oesophagus anteriorly.

the epiglottis tilts down to protect the laryngeal vestibule and deflect the bolus into the lateral food channels. Furthermore, the cricopharyngeus must relax to allow the bolus to pass from the pharynx into the cervical oesophagus. Disruption of these orderly events resulting from pharyngeal constrictor paresis, cricopharyngeal dysfunction or epiglottic dysfunction may lead to aspiration of barium into the laryngeal vestibule and trachea (Figure 2.7). This may be caused by a number of neuromuscular disorders, including cerebrovascular accident, poliomyelitis, multiple sclerosis, Parkinson's disease and muscular dystrophy.

It should be emphasized that the examination in a patient complaining of postcricoid dysphagia is not complete until the whole oesophagus and gastric fundus have been thoroughly examined, as patients presenting with postcricoid dysphagia may in fact have more distal pathology due to inaccurate perception of the level of obstruction.[3]

Much useful information can be obtained about functional abnormalities of the pharynx and cervical oesophagus by careful fluoroscopy and correct film exposure technique as the patient swallows a barium bolus. However, because of the very rapid sequence of events during swallowing, a record of the whole swallow may be required to detect minor functional abnormalities. This may be obtained in one of the following ways:

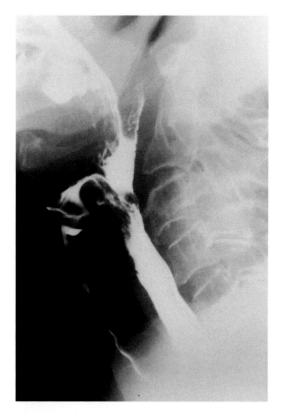

Figure 2.7
Neuromuscular disorder of swallowing with spillage of barium into the laryngeal vestibule and trachea.

- *Video recording.* This is relatively cheap and reliable. The radiation dose to the patient is low and the examination can be played back and studied immediately.

- *Photofluorography.* Serial exposures can be made on 100 mm cut film at up to six exposures per second. The radiographs obtained do not have the same resolution as conventional radiographs but there is less movement blur and less radiation dose per exposure.

- *Digital radiography.* Modern digital radiographic screening units allow rapid exposure at up to six exposures per second. Images can be viewed immediately and selected for transfer to hard copy. Radiation exposure is less than with conventional radiography.

For the examination of the mid- and lower oesophagus, single-contrast views may be obtained initially with the patient in the prone-oblique position. The patient makes several swallows of a large bolus of medium density (100% w/v) barium sucked through a straw. Prior injection of hyoscine-*n*-butylbromide (Buscopan) 20 mg i.v. assists in obtaining maximal distension. Hiatal hernia, lower oesophageal (Schatzki) rings and reflux-induced strictures are well demonstrated with this technique.[3-5] However, the best demonstration of the oesophageal mucosa is obtained with the double-contrast technique. Exposures are made with the patient in the erect position and turned 45° to the left in order to view the oesophagus clear of the dorsal spine and heart. After effervescent tablets or powders have been given, the patient swallows a high-density

(250% w/v) barium suspension as quickly as possible. These repeated rapid swallows interrupt oesophageal peristalsis and this leads to temporary hypotonia.[6] Films should be exposed to demonstrate the oesophageal mucosa coated with high-density barium and distended with swallowed air. The mucosa of the normal oesophagus will be featureless *en face* and will be seen as a thin white line in profile (Figure 2.8). Sometimes double-

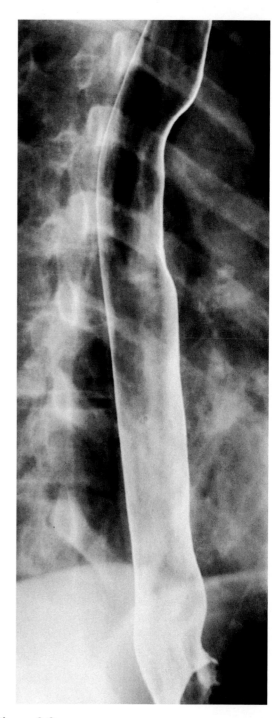

Figure 2.8
Double-contrast view of the normal thoracic oesophagus. The lumen is distended with air and the mucosa coated with barium. The mucosa is featureless *en face* and is seen as a thin white line in profile.

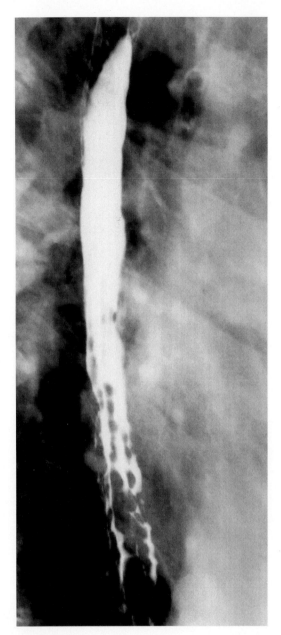

Figure 2.9
Barium swallow showing lobulated filling defects in the distal oesophagus due to varices.

may increase sensitivity. Using this technique, small varices may be detected because of a serpentine or lobulated appearance which they cause in the longitudinal mucosal folds (Figure 2.9). Barium swallow with mucosal-relief films and Buscopan has similar accuracy to endoscopy in the detection of oesophageal varices.[8]

Various additional refinements of the barium swallow technique have been described for different clinical situations and each has its advocate. Acidified barium suspensions, chilled barium and water-siphon provocative tests have been used to demonstrate gastro-oesophageal reflux and oesophagitis with varying degrees of success.[3,9,10] Some radiologists advocate the use of a marshmallow swallow in patents complaining of dysphagia in whom the routine barium swallow shows no abnormality. Half of a 2.5 cm diameter marshmallow is washed down with a bolus of barium. The marshmallow may be held

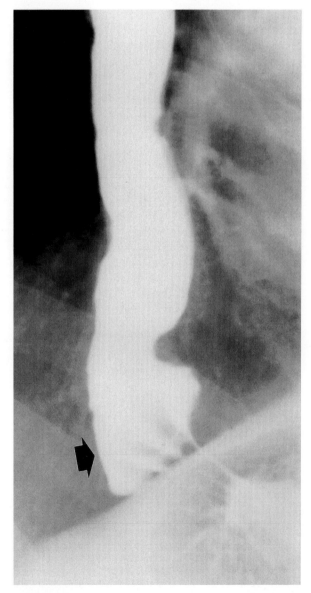

Figure 2.10
Sliding hiatal hernia. Single-contrast barium swallow showing herniation of a portion of the stomach (arrowed) above the diaphragmatic hiatus.

contrast films are not easily obtained with this technique and it may be necessary to repeat the examination after an injection of 20 mg Buscopan has been given intravenously.

Mucosal relief films are obtained after the patient has swallowed a bolus of high density (250% w/v) barium and the oesophageal lumen has collapsed, leaving the longitudinal folds coated with barium. These folds are normally seen as thin parallel lines. Thickened longitudinal mucosal folds with a diameter of greater than 2 mm are considered to be abnormal and are a non-specific sign of oesophagitis from whatever cause.[7] Mucosal relief films are of particular value in the detection of oesophageal varices after the injection of Buscopan 20 mg i.v. to relax the smooth muscle of the oesophagus and allow passive filling of the varices. Prone-oblique positioning

up in the cervical oesophagus by a postcricoid web or in cases of cricopharyngeal dysfunction; and in the lower oesophagus by a reflux-induced stricture or lower oesophageal ring.[11]

Hiatal hernia

Hiatal hernia is a very common finding on the barium swallow in middle-aged patients and its significance is unclear. It is not strongly correlated with the presence of oesophagitis.[12,13] A sliding hiatal hernia is present when the oesophagogastric junction and proximal stomach move into the thorax. This is diagnosed by seeing gastric mucosal folds above the diaphragm. An impression may be present on the herniated stomach from the gastric sling fibres, or from the diaphragmatic hiatus itself. A sliding hiatal hernia may be reducible or fixed (incarcerated) (Figure 2.10). The rarer paraoesophageal or rolling hiatal hernia occurs when the stomach herniates alongside the oesophago-gastric junction, which retains its normal position below the diaphragm. The radiological appearances can be quite dramatic because the herniated stomach often undergoes volvulus within the sac (Figure 2.11).

Oesophagitis

Gastro-oesophageal reflux of barium may frequently be demonstrated during the examination, especially with the patient supine or prone, or when the intra-abdominal pressure is raised. This sign alone is of little clinical significance as a proportion of normal patients have episodes of reflux. However, free and persistent reflux during the examination is more likely to be pathological.[13]

The earliest radiological features of oesophagitis on the barium swallow are abnormal motility, loss of definition and thickening of the mucosal folds and mucosal nodularity or granularity. In more severe cases, ulcers may occur and these are typically linear. Barium may adhere to a linear necrotic

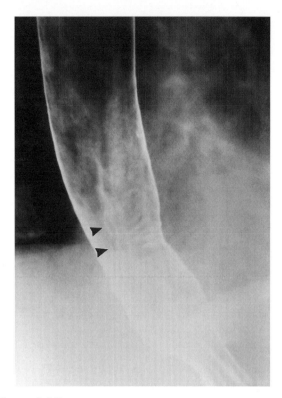

Figure 2.12
Peptic oesophagitis. A linear ulcer (arrowheads) is surrounded by a translucent rim of oedema. Classical radiating mucosal folds are seen at right angles to the ulcer.

slough. With healing, ulcers will demonstrate the characteristic radiating mucosal-fold pattern also seen with gastric and duodenal ulcers (Figure 2.12). Reflux oesophagitis may lead to stricture formation in the distal oesophagus. Classically, these are smooth concentric and tapering, often occurring above a hiatal hernia.[14] Occasionally, reflux-induced strictures are eccentric or irregular, and difficult to distinguish radiologically from carcinoma. In these cases, endoscopic biopsy is essential to exclude neoplasia.[6,15]

In Barrett's oesophagus, a characteristic reticular pattern of the mucosa on double-contrast examinations is seen in a proportion of patients, and may be associated with an adjacent stricture or ulceration (Figure 2.13).[16] Barrett's strictures usually occur at the junction of squamous and columnar epithelium, the position of which can be quite variable. The occurrence of a more proximal benign stricture or ulcer should therefore suggest Barrett's oesophagus, particularly if there is evidence of gastro-oesophageal reflux or hiatal hernia.[17,18] Although the barium swallow is sensitive for the detection of Barrett's oesophagus, the radiological appearance is non-specific, and endoscopic biopsy is necessary to establish the diagnosis. It is important to make the diagnosis as Barrett's oesophagus is regarded as premalignant.[19]

Infective oesophagitis may be suggested by a history of pain on swallowing. In candida oesophagitis, localized areas of plaque formation separated by normal mucosa may be demonstrated on double-contrast views of the oesophagus (Figure 2.14). With more advanced disease, coalescence of plaques

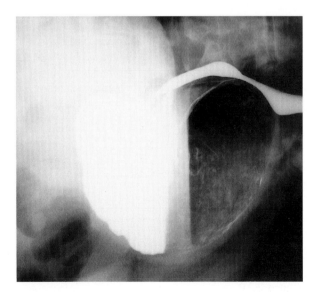

Figure 2.11
Barium swallow showing a large para-oesophageal (rolling) hiatal hernia with gastric volvulus.

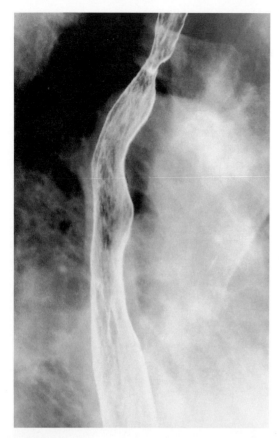

Figure 2.13
Double-contrast swallow showing Barrett's oesophagus. The mucosa has a reticular appearance, and there is a high stricture associated with fine ulceration.

and submucosal oedema leads to a cobblestone appearance, and ulceration may occur. Candida oesophagitis is seen commonly after prolonged antibiotic therapy and in immunosuppressed or otherwise debilitated patients, and may be severe with extensive ulceration in patients with the acquired immune deficiency syndrome (Figure 2.15).[20]

After candidiasis, herpes oesophagitis is the second most common cause of opportunistic infection of the oesophagus and may give similar radiological appearances.[21] However, mild cases may show fine, linear ulcerations against a background of normal mucosa.[22] These cases may thus be distinguished from candidiasis in which ulceration is only seen in advanced disease with a grossly abnormal mucosa.

Cytomegalovirus infection may be similar in appearance to herpes, but occasionally may give rise to large, shallow ulcers which are said to be relatively specific for cytomegalovirus or direct human immunodeficiency virus infection of the oesophagus.[23,24]

Chemical oesophagitis may be caused by deliberate or accidental ingestion of caustic substances or certain drugs, most commonly emepronium bromide, tetracyclines, non-steroidal anti-inflammatory drugs and slow-release potassium. Immediately after ingestion of caustic substances, the contrast swallow should be carried out with caution, using water-soluble agents if perforation is suspected. Radiological findings

are those of non-specific oesophagitis. In the chronic phase, long strictures may develop, even in patients with a previously normal barium swallow. With drug-induced oesophagitis, localized ulceration is usually seen where the oesophagus is indented by the aortic arch, left main bronchus or diaphragmatic hiatus (Figure 2.16). The history of ingestion of the appropriate drug allows the correct diagnosis to be made.

Other types of oesophagitis

In Crohn's oesophagitis, aphthous ulceration may be seen on the double-contrast swallow, usually in conjunction with evidence of Crohn's disease elsewhere. Deeper ulceration may also be present. As with Crohn's disease elsewhere in the gastrointestinal tract, fistulation and stricture formation can occur. Other uncommon types of oesophagitis include: eosinophilic oesophagitis, characterized by mucosal granularity and/or strictures; graft-versus-host disease which may involve the oesophagus with webs and strictures in 15% of patients;[25] Behçet's syndrome where the oesophagus may be ulcerated and strictured; and dermatological conditions such as pemphigoid and epidermolysis bullosa in which the oesophagus is affected by fluid-filled bullae which may rupture, leading to ulceration and stricture formation.

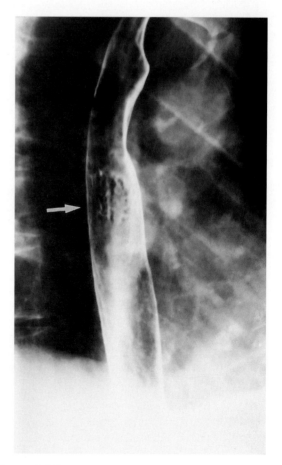

Figure 2.14
Candida oesophagitis. A localized area of elevated plaques (arrowed) seen as translucent defects in the mid-oesophagus.

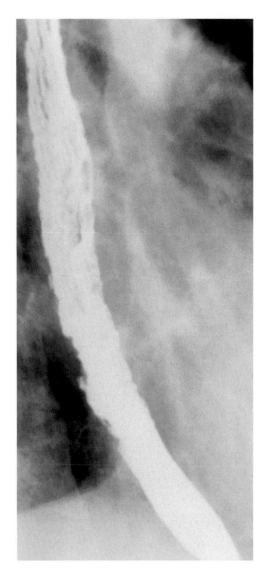

Figure 2.15
Advanced candidiasis in a patient with the acquired immune deficiency syndrome. Barium swallow showing cobblestoning and extensive ulceration. (Courtesy of Dr S.A. Moussa.)

Oesophageal intramural pseudodiverticulosis

This is a rare condition in which small outpouchings appear within the oesophageal wall, best demonstrated on the single-contrast swallow. These are thought to represent dilated mucous gland ducts, and commonly occur in association with evidence of oesophagitis and stricturing. Candidiasis is present in a proportion of patients, but the significance of this is unclear.[26]

Neoplasia

The majority of primary oesophageal neoplasms are squamous cell carcinomas, and these are often advanced by the time of presentation with dysphagia. Early squamous cell carcinoma is usually asymptomatic and detected incidentally as a plaque-like abnormality or sessile polyp (Figure 2.17).[27] More

advanced lesions may produce a typically malignant stricture with irregular mucosa and shouldering; a polypoid, ulcerated appearance; or, due to submucosal infiltration, a smoother stricture with relatively intact mucosa (Figure 2.18). Rigidity of the oesophageal wall on fluoroscopic screening in the region of the tumour may suggest malignancy. Depending on the radiological appearance, squamous cell carcinoma may be confused with benign stricture or ulceration, infective oesophagitis, varices or submucosal haematoma. In advanced cases, contiguous spread into adjacent structures can cause fistulation into the tracheobronchial tree or pleura (Figure 2.19). This can also happen following radiotherapy.

Adenocarcinoma now comprises up to 50% of primary malignant oesophageal neoplasms, and most commonly arises at or near the oesophagogastric junction. The majority arise in Barrett's oesophagus.[19] Early lesions may only show mucosal-fold thickening or small plaques which can be mistaken for oesophagitis. Lesions are usually advanced by the time of diagnosis, and are similar in appearance to squamous

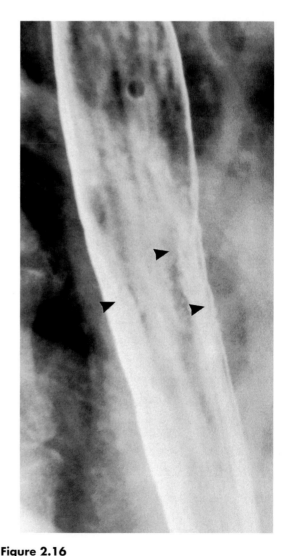

Figure 2.16
Drug-induced oesophagitis caused by tetracycline. Erosions are seen as dots or linear streaks of barium with a surrounding translucent halo of oedema (arrowheads).

polyps (true papillomas and inflammatory polyps), lipomas, haemangiomas and cysts.

Motility disorders

Of the primary oesophageal motor disorders, achalasia is most readily diagnosed radiologically. Achalasia will be best demonstrated during a double-contrast examination as a barium column will build up in the oesophagus during rapid swallowing. Smooth tapering will be seen at the lower end of the oesophagus which never relaxes sufficiently to allow the column of barium to enter the stomach. Instead, barium enters the stomach in short spurts. In the early stage there may be vigorous uncoordinated oesophageal contractions. The term 'vigorous achalasia' is used to describe this appearance. Later the

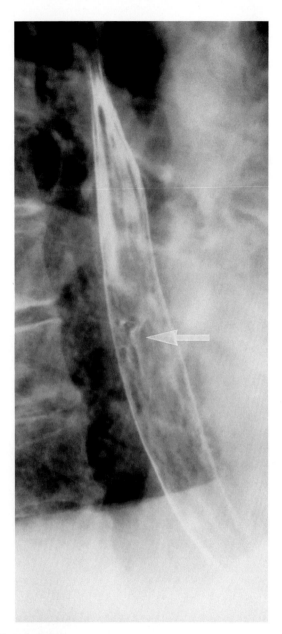

Figure 2.17
Biopsy-proven, early squamous cell carcinoma of oesophagus. Minimal plaque-like abnormality (arrowed) on double-contrast swallow.

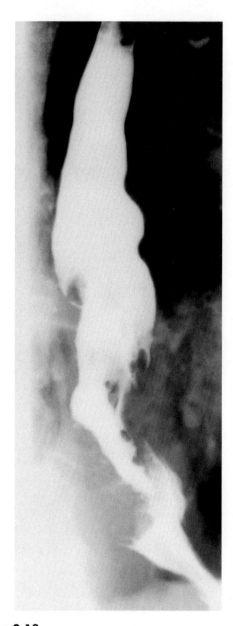

Figure 2.18
Barium swallow showing extensive, stenotic squamous cell carcinoma of distal oesophagus with ulceration.

cell carcinomas. Invasion across the oesophagogastric junction into the gastric fundus is highly suggestive of adenocarcinoma (Figure 2.20).

Other malignant neoplasms include the rare carcinosarcoma, lymphoma (usually of the distal oesophagus), leiomyosarcoma, Kaposi's sarcoma and secondary involvement, either metastatic or due to invasion from carcinoma in adjacent tissues.

Benign tumours are relatively uncommon in the oesophagus. Leiomyomas, being intramural, appear well defined, and smooth or lobulated on the barium swallow (Figure 2.21). The overlying mucosa is usually intact and the lesions may therefore be missed on endoscopy. Other benign lesions include

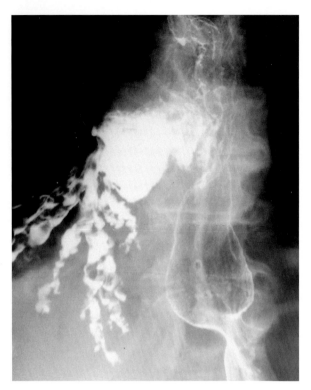

Figure 2.19
Fistulation into tracheobronchial tree from advanced oesophageal cancer. Barium has entered the mediastinum and passed into the right lower lobe bronchus via a fistula from the extensive, ulcerated mid-oesophageal squamous cell carcinoma.

oesophagus will dilate and become aperistaltic and often sigmoid in appearance (Figure 2.22).

Chest pain may be of cardiac or oesophageal origin, and there has been considerable interest in the 'nutcracker' oesophagus as a cause of chest pain. These patients may be referred for radiological evaluation. However, there are no specific radiological findings in this condition and although tertiary contractions may be seen at barium swallow examination, this finding is non-specific. Chobanian et al.[28] have shown that the barium swallow lacks sufficient specificity to screen adequately for the nutcracker oesophagus in patients with atypical angina or dysphagia. Nutcracker oesophagus is a manometric diagnosis characterized by normal primary peristalsis with distal contractions of high amplitude.[29]

Diffuse oesophageal spasm is a primary motility disorder which causes intermittent chest pain and dysphagia. The barium swallow may be normal or may show distal tertiary contractions, giving rise to the so-called 'corkscrew oesophagus'. A similar appearance may be seen in the elderly and may be asymptomatic.[30]

The most common cause of secondary oesophageal motility disorder, after that induced by gastro-oesophageal reflux, is scleroderma. In this condition, atrophy of oesophageal smooth muscle leads to loss of peristalsis, oesophageal atony and gastro-oesophageal reflux, which can be severe.[31] These features are usually easily appreciated on the barium swallow.

Strictures may occur in patients with reflux. Other causes of secondary oesophageal motility problems include other connective tissue diseases and neuromuscular disorders.

Trauma/perforation

As previously stated, plain films may be of help in the diagnosis of perforation but a contrast study is usually required to confirm the diagnosis and show its extent and severity. Barium should not be used in suspected perforation because it may cause mediastinal foreign body granulomas. Instead, a water-soluble contrast medium is preferred. Gastrografin is commonly used but it should be avoided if there is any risk of aspiration as it may cause a severe aspiration pneumonia or pulmonary oedema. Modern non-ionic or low-osmolar contrast

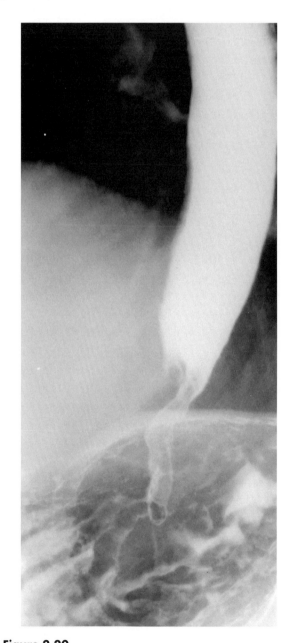

Figure 2.20
Adenocarcinoma of oesophagus. Irregular stenosis of distal oesophagus with invasion of gastric fundus.

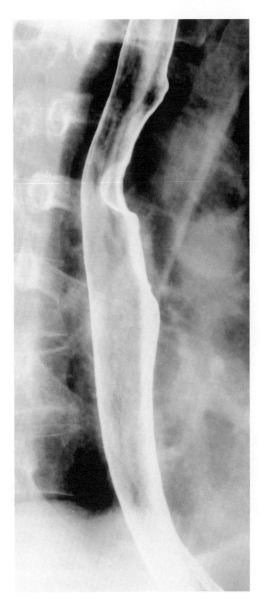

Figure 2.21
Leiomyoma of the oesophagus. Smooth bulge into oesophageal lumen with overlying mucosa intact. Epicentre of lesion lies within the oesophageal wall.

media such as Hexabrix are preferable.[32,33] The technique of the examination is important. Turning the patient from side to side as he or she drinks the contrast will demonstrate most perforations and horizontal-beam radiographs will increase the diagnostic accuracy.[34]

RADIONUCLIDE TECHNIQUES

Radionuclide techniques offer a non-invasive, semiquantitative way of demonstrating oesophageal motility disorders and gastro-oesophageal reflux. Transit studies demonstrate the passage of a bolus of fluid down the oesophagus. For this test, the patient lies under a gamma camera, swallows a 10 ml bolus of technetium-labelled colloid and then 'dry' swallows at regular intervals for 10 minutes. Activity in the oesophagus is documented during the period of the test. Normal transit time is usually less than 15 seconds. Retention of the bolus in the oesophagus indicates defective peristalsis and is seen in achalasia and scleroderma. Abnormally long transit times may be seen in patients with diffuse oesophageal spasm and gastro-oesophageal reflux.

Gastro-oesophageal reflux can be investigated by giving 300 ml of technetium-labelled colloid by mouth and recording episodes of reflux of isotope produced by postural change or abdominal compression. Compared to endoscopy and pH monitoring, the test is non-invasive and the radiation dose is less than with barium swallow. A drawback of these techniques is that neither the transit nor reflux test can demonstrate structural abnormalities and they cannot replace barium radiology or endoscopy.[11]

COMPUTED TOMOGRAPHY

Computed tomography (CT) of the oesophagus is used mainly in the preoperative staging of oesophageal cancer, but is also useful in post-treatment follow-up to assess response to surgery, radiotherapy or chemotherapy, and may be helpful in detecting recurrence. Oesophageal carcinoma accounts for approximately 1% of all malignancies and has the poorest prognosis of all gastrointestinal tumours. As tumour stage has a profound effect on method of treatment and survival, accurate staging is vital prior to treatment.[35] Although definitive staging

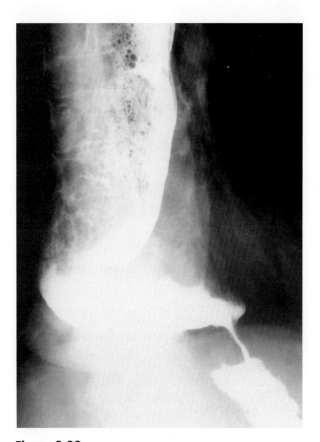

Figure 2.22
Barium swallow showing achalasia. The proximal oesophagus is dilated and tortuous, and contains food debris. Barium spurts through a narrow channel into the stomach.

is based on the TNM system, a modification of this system for CT has been suggested by Moss et al.[36] in an attempt to link CT findings to pathological stage (Table 2.1).

Table 2.1   Staging of oesophageal carcinoma based on CT findings

STAGE	CT FINDINGS
I	Intraluminal mass only without wall thickening
II	Oesophageal wall thickening only (greater than 5 mm)
III	Oesophageal wall thickening with contiguous spread of tumour into adjacent mediastinal structures
IV	Distant metastatic spread (irrespective of local stage)

After Moss et al.[36]

CT is extremely versatile as it allows assessment of the thorax and upper abdomen in a single examination. However, it does have relative strengths and weaknesses. Most of the papers evaluating the efficacy of CT for oesophageal cancer staging were written in the 1980s, and do not take into account major technical advances in CT scanners which have been made since then. In particular, the advent of spiral CT is likely to increase staging accuracy. Spiral CT allows scanning of the chest and upper abdomen in a single breath-hold, and will increase sensitivity by abolishing respiratory misregistration between slices, and allowing optimal timing of scans in relation to delivery of intravenous contrast media.[37] This is known to increase sensitivity for the detection of pulmonary metastases[38,39], and is likely to improve detection of liver metastases as well as subdiaphragmatic nodal metastases.[40]

In oesophageal carcinoma, CT shows thickening of the oesophageal wall and overall tumour size is thus assessed (Figure 2.23). However, it cannot demonstrate individual layers of the oesophageal wall, and so cannot determine the depth of tumour invasion. Tumour stages I and II cannot therefore be

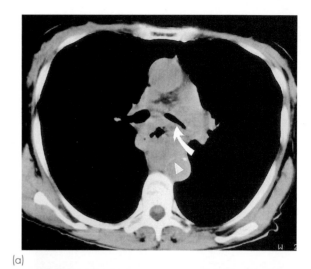

(a)

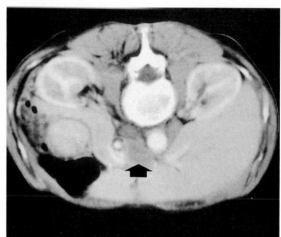

(b)

Figure 2.24

(a) CT scan showing advanced oesophageal carcinoma with mediastinal invasion. The main bronchi are displaced forwards, and there is narrowing of the left main bronchus from behind (arrowed). More than one-quarter of the aortic circumference is contacted by tumour (arrowhead) indicating aortic invasion. (b) Same patient. Contrast-enhanced CT scan showing 3 cm node in coeliac region (arrowed).

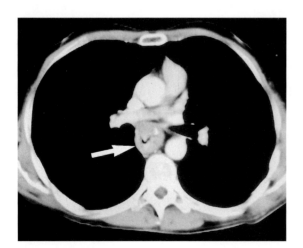

Figure 2.23

CT scan showing concentric wall thickening in oesophageal carcinoma (arrowed). There is no evidence of invasion into the mediastinal fat.

differentiated with CT. This technique is also limited in its ability to detect tumour in mediastinal lymph nodes. It may understage disease by failing to detect small nodes that contain tumour, particularly paraoesophageal nodes.[41] Conversely, it may detect nodes which are not involved with tumour but which are enlarged due to reactive hyperplasia. Sensitivity for involved mediastinal node detection is of the order of 40%, with specificity around 90%. Detection of involved nodes below the diaphragm is more successful, with sensitivity of 61% and specificity 94%.[42]

Mediastinal invasion is diagnosed by seeing extension of soft tissue density from the region of the primary tumour into the mediastinal fat. However, many patients with oesophageal carcinoma are cachectic and have little mediastinal fat, and this may reduce accuracy. In general, local staging of tumours at the oesophagogastric junction is less accurate than with more proximal lesions.[43] Tumour invasion of the tracheobronchial tree is predicted with a high degree of accuracy when tumour masses are seen to abut and compress the trachea or left main bronchus (Figure 2.24). When tumour abuts but does not compress these structures, invasion cannot be diagnosed.[41,44] Tumour invasion of the aorta is predicted when tumour contacts the aorta over a greater than 90° arc (i.e. more than one-quarter of the circumference is contacted). Contact of less than 45° excludes invasion, and contact between 60° and 75° is regarded as indeterminate (Figure 2.24).[41] Using this technique, overall accuracy is 80%, rising to 96% if indeterminate cases are excluded. A more recent study has used tumour invasion of the triangular fat space between the oesophagus, aorta and spine as a criterion of aortic invasion which gives an accuracy of 84%.[45]

Distant metastases are well demonstrated with CT. Lung metastases are best shown with CT, particularly spiral CT.[38,39] Liver metastases and subdiaphragmatic nodes are also well shown by contrast-enhanced CT, and spiral CT is likely to improve sensitivity further.[40,46]

Recurrent local disease is not particularly well assessed with CT due to lack of fat planes, variability in postoperative appearances and artefact due to metallic sutures. It may, however, be useful as a way of demonstrating extensive or metastatic disease, thus influencing therapy, or for treatment planning or monitoring.

MAGNETIC RESONANCE IMAGING

At the present time, magnetic resonance imaging (MRI) does not appear to offer any significant advantages over CT in the staging of oesophageal carcinoma. Sensitivity to motion artefact from vascular pulsation and respiration can reduce spatial resolution, and in some cases can result in non-diagnostic

examinations. The development of faster scanning sequences may improve this. The ability to image in multiple planes may be useful in specific situations, particularly to clarify anatomical relationships (Figure 2.25).

As with CT, MRI is not able to show depth of tumour penetration through the oesophageal wall, and has a similar accuracy in predicting tumour involvement in detected lymph nodes. Although initial reports were disappointing, more recent studies have shown a high accuracy in predicting tracheobronchial, aortic and pericardial invasion.[45,47–49] Liver metastases are well shown by MRI, and sensitivity is similar to CT.[50,51] However, pulmonary metastases are not reliably demonstrated, and small upper abdominal nodes may be missed due to respiration artefact.

Although broadly comparable to CT in terms of accuracy for oesophageal cancer staging, MRI is less versatile, in that several sequences may be required for satisfactory staging of local disease and distant metastases, with a subsequent increase in examination time. A proportion of studies may be non-diagnostic or suboptimal due to motion artefact or claustrophobia experienced by the patient. MRI cannot therefore be currently recommended over the more readily available CT for this indication.

ENDOLUMINAL ULTRASONOGRAPHY

Endoluminal ultrasonography (EUS) is a relatively new technique which shows promise in the staging of oesophageal carcinoma. A high-frequency (7.5 MHz) transducer is attached to a modified endoscope, and comes into direct contact with the oesophageal wall. The images obtained are highly detailed, although the depth of penetration of the ultrasound is limited to a maximum of 10 cm.[52]

Five alternating hyper-/hypoechoic layers can be recognized in the oesophageal wall: (1) hyperechoic – probe–mucosa interface; (2) hypoechoic – deep mucosa–muscularis mucosae;

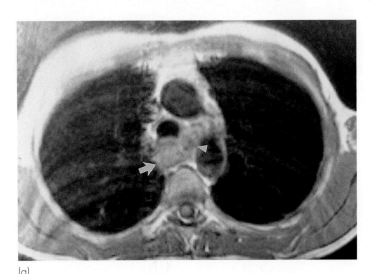

(a)

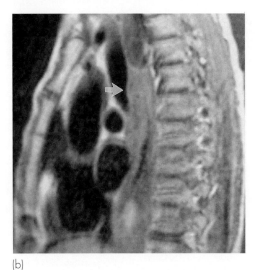

(b)

Figure 2.25

(a) Transverse T1-weighted MRI scan showing recurrent tumour after oesophagectomy (arrowed). Tumour is infiltrating the mediastinal fat in the aortopulmonary window (arrowhead). (b) Sagittal T1-weighted MRI scan in same patient. The longitudinal extent of the tumour is well demonstrated in this plane. Posterior indentation of the trachea (arrowed) is suggestive of invasion.

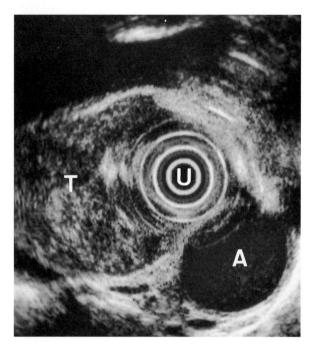

Figure 2.26
Endoluminal ultrasonographic scan showing 3 cm oesophageal tumour invading the adventitia (T3). U, ultrasound probe; T, tumour; A, aorta. (Courtesy of Dr A. McLean, St Bartholomew's Hospital, London.)

(3) hyperechoic – submucosa; (4) hypoechoic – muscularis propria; (5) hyperechoic – adventitia–perioesophageal fat. Tumours are identified as low echogenicity regions which disrupt the characteristic layered pattern. T1–T3 tumours can thus be distinguished by depth of tumour invasion (Figure 2.26).[52-55]

Depth of tumour invasion can be accurately predicted in over 80% when the examination is complete.[53-55] A significant problem is the inability of the probe to pass through malignant strictures of less than 10–13 mm in diameter, which can occur in up to 50% of patients.[53] When this happens, principally in patients with extensive disease, staging is incomplete and therefore less accurate.

Lymph node metastases in the mediastinum can be detected with an accuracy of up to 88% where the examination is technically satisfactory.[53-55] Demonstration of metastatic lymphadenopathy relies on ultrasonographic appearance rather than size criteria, and is more accurate than CT/MRI.[53,55] A hypoechoic, relatively well-defined node is likely to be malignant (Figure 2.27). Direct invasion of mediastinal structures is also well assessed using EUS, with an accuracy of around 90%.[55]

Detection of metastases in the coeliac region and left hepatic lobe is good, although the right hepatic lobe and peritoneum are not well seen due to limitations in sound penetration. The overall accuracy for distant metastases is approximately 70%.[54] Lung metastases cannot be imaged with EUS. CT is more accurate than EUS for demonstration of metastatic disease.

In general, EUS is more suited to the local staging of oesophageal tumours than to the evaluation of extensive or metastatic disease. In this respect, CT and EUS would appear to be complementary, and overall staging accuracy of 86% has been reported from the use of the two techniques together.[54]

EUS is helpful in the demonstration of recurrent, anastamotic tumour (where CT is not very effective).[56] It may also be used in the delineation of submucosal and extraoesophageal lesions as well as oesophageal varices.[57]

INTERVENTIONAL RADIOLOGY

Balloon dilatation of oesophageal strictures is now an accepted and well-documented technique that may be performed under radiological or endoscopic control.[58,59] A barium swallow is performed first to demonstrate the site, length and diameter of the stricture. The oropharynx is anaesthetized with a local anaesthetic spray and a 20 mm diameter, 8 cm length oesophageal catheter passed into the oesophagus. The balloon catheter is introduced over a guide wire and placed across the stricture. The balloon is inflated under fluoroscopic control using a dilute water-soluble contrast medium. Initially, a waist is visible at the site of the stricture and dilatation is continued until the balloon has a smooth contour (Figure 2.28). Dilatation time is initially maintained for 2–5 min.

The total length of dilatation time is dictated by the response of the stricture. Balloon dilatation uses radially applied forces on the stricture and is believed safer than bougienage which exerts longitudinal shearing forces. Complications are unusual. One case of guide-wire perforation of the oesophageal wall has been reported[60] and three cases of oesophageal perforation,[59] but two of these occurred during dilatation of a malignant

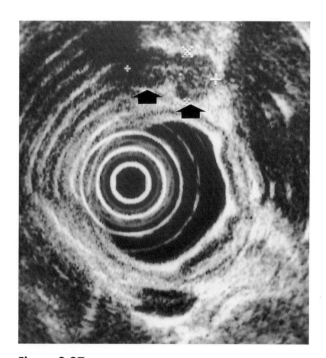

Figure 2.27
Endoluminal ultrasonographic scan in a patient with oesophageal carcinoma. The five layers of the wall are well demonstrated. Small perioesophageal nodes are present anteriorly (arrowed). (Courtesy of Dr A. McLean, St Bartholomew's Hospital, London.)

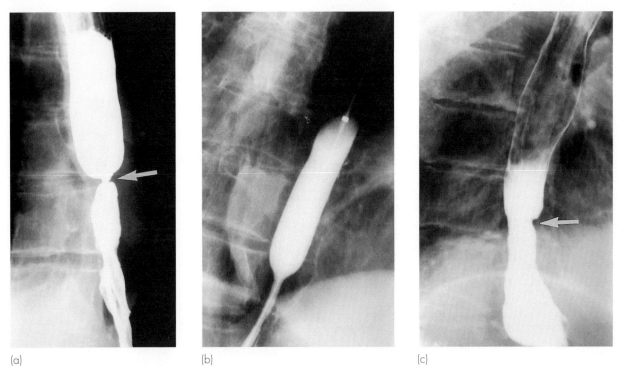

(a) (b) (c)

Figure 2.28
Balloon dilatation of a peptic stricture. (a) A tight stricture demonstrated by barium swallow before dilatation (arrowed). (b) A balloon, inflated with water-soluble contrast medium, is placed across the stricture. (c) Barium swallow after balloon dilatation showing widening of the lumen at the site of the stricture (arrowed).

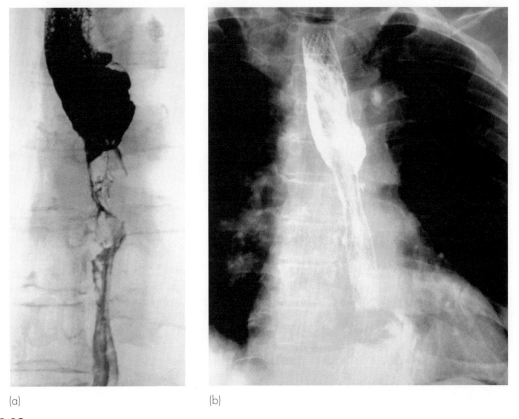

(a) (b)

Figure 2.29
Oesophageal stenting. (a) Before stenting, barium swallow shows extensive, stenotic tumour in mid-oesophagus, with proximal hold-up of barium. (b) After placement of the expanding metallic stent, patency is restored. There is a hiatal hernia below the stent. (Courtesy of Dr D.C. Grieve.)

stricture. However, there is evidence to suggest that bougie dilatation is more effective than balloon dilatation in reducing dysphagia and maintaining stricture patency.[61]

Malignant oesophageal strictures can be treated with radiological placement of expanding metal stents (Figure 2.29). This technique is effective, and is associated with a very low incidence of complications compared with the use of non-expanding oesophageal tubes.[62–64] Malignant fistulas and oesophageal tears have been successfully treated with expanding stents.[63]

REFERENCES

1. Ghahremani GG, Turner MA & Port RB. Iatrogenic intubation injuries of the upper gastrointestinal tract in adults. *Gastrointest Radiol* 1980; **5:** 1–10.
2. Jones B, Kramer SS & Donner MW. Dynamic imaging of the pharynx. *Gastrointest Radiol* 1985; **10:** 213–224.
3. Jones B. & Donner MW. Examination of the patient with dysphagia. *Radiology* 1988; **167:** 319–326.
4. Chen YM, Ott DJ, Gelfand DW & Munitz HA. Multiphasic examination of the oesophagogastric region for strictures, rings and hiatal hernia: evaluation of the individual techniques. *Gastrointest Radiol* 1985; **10:** 311–316.
5. Ott DJ, Gelfand DW, Wu WC & Chen YM. Radiological evaluation of dysphagia. *JAMA* 1986; **256:** 2718–2721.
6. Laufer I. Radiology of oesophagitis. *Radiol Clin North Am* 1982; **20:** 687–699.
7. Kressel HY, Glick SN, Laufer I & Banner M. Radiologic features of esophagitis. *Gastrointest Radiol* 1981; **6:** 103–108.
8. Waldram R, Nunnerly H, Davis M, Laws JW & Williams R. Detection and grading of oesophageal varices by fibreoptic endoscopy and barium swallow with and without Buscopan. *Clin Radiol* 1977; **28:** 137–141.
9. Ott DJ, Gelfand DW, Munitz HA & Chen YM. Cold barium suspension in the clinical evaluation of the oesophagus. *Gastrointest Radiol* 1984; **9:** 193–196.
10. Stevenson GW. Radiology of gastro-oesophageal reflux. *Clin Radiol* 1989; **40:** 119–121.
11. Stevenson GW & Robinson PJ. The normal oesophagus. Methods of examination. Hiatus hernia, gastro-oesophageal reflux and other motility disorders. In Simpkins KC ed. *A Textbook of Radiological Diagnosis* 5th edn. London: HK Lewis, 1988: 52–105.
12. Ott DJ, Gelfand DW, Chen YM, Wu WC & Munitz HA. Predictive relationship of hiatal hernia to reflux esophagitis. *Gastrointest Radiol* 1985; **10:** 317–320.
13. Dodds WJ. The pathogenesis of gastroesophageal reflux disease. *AJR* 1988; **151:** 49–56.
14. McDermott P, Wallers KJ, Holden R & James WB. Double contrast examination of the oesophagus: the radiological changes of peptic oesophagitis. *Clin Radiol* 1982; **33:** 259–264.
15. Fraser GM & Earnshaw PM. The double contrast barium meal: a correlation with endoscopy. *Clin Radiol* 1983; **34:** 121–131.
16. Levine MS, Kressel HY, Caroline DF, Laufer I, Herlinger H & Thompson JJ. Barrett esophagus: reticular pattern of the mucosa. *Radiology* 1983; **147:** 663–667.
17. Shapir J, Dubrow R & Frank P. Barrett's oesophagus: analysis of 19 cases. *Br J Radiol* 1985; **58:** 491–493.
18. Gilchrist AM, Levine MS, Carr RF et al. Barrett esophagus: diagnosis by double contrast esophagography. *AJR* 1988; **150:** 97–102.
19. Levine MS, Caroline D, Thompson JJ, Kressel HY, Laufer I & Herlinger H. Adenocarcinoma of the esophagus: relationship to Barrett mucosa. *Radiology* 1984; **150:** 305–309.
20. Farman J, Tavitian A, Rosenthal LE, Schwarz GE & Raufman JP. Focal oesophageal candidiasis in acquired immune deficiency syndrome (AIDS). *Gastrointest Radiol* 1986; **11:** 213–217.
21. Frager DH, Frager JD, Brandt LT et al. Gastrointestinal complications of AIDS: radiologic features. *Radiology* 1986; **158:** 597–603.
22. Levine MS, Loevner LA, Saul SH, Rubesin SE, Herlinger H & Laufer I. Herpes esophagitis: sensitivity of double contrast esophagography. *AJR* 1988; **151:** 57–62.
23. Balthazar EJ, Megibow AJ, Hulnick D, Cho KC & Beranbaum E. Cytomegalovirus esophagitis in AIDS: radiographic features in 16 patients. *AJR* 1987; **149:** 919–923.
24. Rabeneck L, Popovic M, Gartner S et al. Acute HIV infection presenting with painful swallowing and esophageal ulcers. *JAMA* 1990; **263:** 2318–2322.
25. McDonald GB, Sullivan KM & Plumley TF. Radiographic features of esophageal involvement in chronic graft-vs.-host disease. *AJR* 1984; **142:** 501–506.
26. Levine MS, Moolten DN, Herlinger H & Laufer I. Esophageal intramural pseudodiverticulosis: a reevaluation. *AJR* 1986; **147:** 1165–1170.
27. Levine MS, Dillon EC, Saul SH & Laufer I. Early esophageal cancer. *AJR* 1986; **146:** 507–512.
28. Chobanian SJ, Curtis DJ, Benjamin SB & Cattau EL. Radiology of the nutcracker oesophagus, *J Clin Gastroenterol* 1986; **8:** 230–232.
29. Ott DJ, Richter JE, Wu WC, Chen YM, Gelfand DW & Gastell DO. Radiologic and manometric correlation in 'nutcracker esophagus'. *AJR* 1986; **147:** 692–695.
30. Hollis JB & Castell DO. Esophageal function in elderly man. A new look at 'presbyesophagus'. *Ann Intern Med* 1974; **80:** 371–374.
31. Clouse RE. Motor disorders in gastrointestinal disease. In Sleisenger MH & Fordtran JS (eds) *Gastrointestinal Disease*, 4th edn. Philadelphia: WB Saunders, 1989: 559–593.
32. Parkin GJS. Perforation of the oesophagus. In Simpkins KC (ed.) *A Textbook of Radiological Diagnosis*, 5th edn. London: HK Lewis, 1988: 147–149.
33. Bell KE, McKinstry CS & Mills JOM. Iopamidol in the diagnosis of suspected upper gastrointestinal perforation. *Clin Radiol* 1987; **38:** 165–168.
34. Ginai AZ. Clinical use of Hexabrix for radiological evaluation of leakage from the upper gastrointestinal tract based on experimental study. *Br J Radiol* 1987; **60:** 343–346.
35. Younghusband JD & Aluwihare APR. Carcinoma of the oesophagus: factors influencing survival. *Br J Surg* 1970; **57:** 422–430.
36. Moss AA, Schnyder P, Theoni RF & Margulis AR. Esophageal carcinoma: pretherapy staging by computed tomography. *AJR* 1981; **136:** 1051–1056.
37. Kalender WA, Seissler W, Klotz E & Vock P. Spiral volumetric CT with single-breath-hold technique, continious transport, and continuous scanner rotation. *Radiology* 1990; **176:** 181–183.
38. Remy-Jardin M, Remy J, Giraud F & Marquette C-H. Pulmonary nodules: detection with thick-section spiral CT versus conventional CT. *Radiology* 1993; **187:** 513–520.
39. Collie DA, Wright AR, Williams JR, Hashemi-Malayeri B, Stevenson AJM & Turnbull CM. Comparison of spiral-acquisition CT and conventional CT in the assessment of pulmonary metastatic disease. *Br J Radiol* 1994; **67:** 436–444.
40. Zeman RK, Fox SH, Silverman PM et al. Helical (spiral) CT of the abdomen. *AJR* 1993; **160:** 719–725.
41. Picus D, Balfe DM, Koehler RE, Roper CL & Owen JW. Computed tomography in the staging of esophageal carcinoma. *Radiology* 1983; **146:** 433–438.
42. Trenkner SW, Halvorsen RA & Thompson WM. Neoplasms of the upper gastrointestinal tract. *Radiol Clin North Am* 1994; **32:** 15–24.
43. Thompson WM, Halvorsen RA, Foster WL Jr, Williford ME, Postlethwait RW & Korobkin M. Computed tomography for staging esophageal and gastroesophageal cancer: reevaluation. *AJR* 1983; **141:** 951–958.
44. Inculet RI, Keller SM, Dwyer A & Roth JA. Evaluation of non-invasive imaging tests for the preoperative staging of carcinoma of the esophagus. *Ann Thorac Surg* 1985; **40:** 561–565.
45. Takashima S, Tacheuchi N, Shiozaki H et al. Carcinoma of the esophagus: CT vs MR imaging in determining resectability. *AJR* 1991; **156:** 297–302.
46. Halvorsen RA & Thompson WM. Gastrointestinal cancer: diagnosis, staging and the follow-up role of imaging. *Semin Ultrasound CT MR* 1989; **10:** 467–480.
47. Quint LE, Glazer GM & Orringer MD. Oesophageal imaging by MR and CT: study of normal anatomy and neoplasms. *Radiology* 1985; **156:** 727–731.
48. Heelan RT, Martini N, Westcott JW et al. Carcinomatous involvement of the hilum and mediastinum: computed tomographic and magnetic resonance evaluation. *Radiology* 1985; **156:** 111–115.
49. Petrillo R, Balzarini L, Bidolip J et al. Esophageal squamous cell carcinoma: MRI evaluation of mediastinum. *Gastrointest Radiol* 1990; **15:** 275–278.
50. Heiken JP, Weyman PJ, Lee JK et al. Detection of focal hepatic masses: prospective evaluation with CT, delayed CT, CT during arterial portography, and MR imaging. *Radiology* 1989; **171:** 47–51.

51. Rummeny E, Wernecke K, Saini S et al. Comparison between high field-strength MR imaging and CT for screening of hepatic metastases: a receiver operating characteristic analysis. *Radiology* 1992; **182:** 879–886.

52. Tio TL & Tytgat GN. Endoscopic ultrasonography in the assessment of intra- and transmural infiltration of tumours in the oesophagus, stomach and papilla of Vater and in the detection of extraoesophageal lesions. *Endoscopy* 1984; **16:** 203–210.

53. Vilgrain V, Mompoint D, Palazzo L et al. Staging of esophageal carcinoma: comparison of results with endoscopic sonography and CT. *AJR* 1990; **155:** 277–281.

54. Botet JF, Lightdale CJ, Zauber AG, Gerdes H, Urmacher C & Brennan MF. Preoperative staging of esophageal cancer: comparison of endoscopic US and dynamic CT. *Radiology* 1991; **181:** 419–425.

55. Tio TL, Coene PPLO, Schouwink MH & Tytgat GNJ. Esophagogastric carcinoma: preoperative TNM classification with endosonography. *Radiology* 1989; **173:** 411–417.

56. Lightdale CJ, Botet JK, Kelsen DP, Turnbull AD & Brennan MF. Diagnosis of recurrent upper gastrointestinal cancer at the surgical anastamosis by endoscopic ultrasound. *Gastrointest Endosc* 1989; **35:** 407–412.

57. Tytgat GNJ & Tio TL. Esophageal ultrasonography. *Gastroenterol Clin North Am* 1991; **20:** 659–671.

58. Grundy A & Belli A. Balloon dilation of upper gastrointestinal tract strictures. *Clin Radiol* 1988; **39:** 229–235.

59. Mayner M, Guerra C, Reyes R et al. Esophageal strictures: balloon dilation. *Radiology* 1988; **167:** 703–706.

60. Dawson SL, Mueller PR, Ferrucci JT et al. Severe esophageal strictures: indications for balloon catheter dilatation. *Radiology* 1984; **153:** 631–635.

61. Cox JGC, Winter RK, Maslin SC et al. Balloon or bougie for dilatation of benign oesophageal strictures? An interim report of a randomised control trial. *Gut* 1988; **29:** 1741–1747.

62. Song HY, Choi KC, Kwon HC, Yang DH, Cho BH & Lee ST. Esophageal strictures: treatment with a new design of modified Gianturco stent. *Radiology* 1992; **184:** 729–734.

63. Cwikiel W, Stridbeck H, Tranberg KG et al. Malignant esophageal strictures: treatment with a self-expanding Nitinol stent. *Radiology* 1993; **187:** 661–665.

64. Diamantes T & Mannell A. Oesophageal intubation for advanced oesophageal cancer: the Baragwanath experience 1977–1981. *Br J Surg* 1983; **70:** 555–557.

3

PRINCIPLES OF GASTROINTESTINAL ENDOSCOPY AND ENDOSCOPY OF THE OESOPHAGUS

CP Willoughby
KFR Schiller

HISTORICAL INTRODUCTION

Attempts have been made to visualize the inner recesses of the human body since the time of Hippocrates. The first upper gastrointestinal endoscopy was probably performed in 1868 by Adolf Kussmaul, using a rigid metal tube and a primitive alcohol/turpentine lamp, but early developments in the field were limited both by optical technology and by the lack of a powerful illumination system suitable for medical use. Edison's invention of the incandescent glass bulb in 1879, and its subsequent miniaturization in 1890, was the first major landmark in the evolution of modern endoscopy. In the next 40 years or so, improved varieties of rigid oesophagoscopes and gastroscopes were produced, and in 1932 Wolf and Schindler developed a semiflexible instrument, the first gastroscope suitable for practical clinical use on a large scale.[1] (For discussion of rigid oesophagoscopy see Editor's Note at end of chapter.)

The semiflexible gastroscope was difficult to use, uncomfortable and potentially hazardous for the patient, and only permitted a limited inspection of a part of the stomach and no views of the duodenum. Technical developments in the 1950s led to an interest in photography of the upper gastrointestinal tract using the gastro-camera. However, the information obtained was not immediately available to the operator and this was a considerable disadvantage.

The second major advance in modern endoscopy was the demonstration by Hopkins and Kapany of the practicability of image transmission along coated aligned bundles of flexible glass fibres.[2] This 'fibrescope' was only a few inches long, but further development of the optical system and its incorporation into an instrument

with facilities for directional control, insufflation and suction led to the production of the first usable fibreoptic gastroscope by Hirschowitz and his colleagues in 1958.[3]

During the next 30 years or so, major improvements in instrument design – and particularly the invention of the charge coupled device (CCD) microchip in 1969[4] – have led to the fully immersible and disinfectable video endoscope which is today's workhorse. Although it was once an unusual and complex investigation, endoscopy of the upper gastrointestinal tract – oesophagogastroduodenoscopy (OGD) – has now become widely available in all general hospitals, and increasingly in office practice outside the UK. In England it is estimated that about 1% of the population is currently referred for diagnostic endoscopy each year.[5]

ENDOSCOPIC EQUIPMENT
Outline description

The general appearance of the standard upper gastrointestinal endoscope (Figure 3.1) will be familiar to all practitioners. The great majority of diagnostic and therapeutic endoscopy is performed with a forward-viewing instrument. Side-viewing instruments are occasionally useful in visualizing less accessible areas such as the proximal duodenum just distal to the duodenal bulb, but their major current application is in the performance of endoscopic retrograde cholangiopancreatography (ERCP), although end-viewing instruments are sometimes

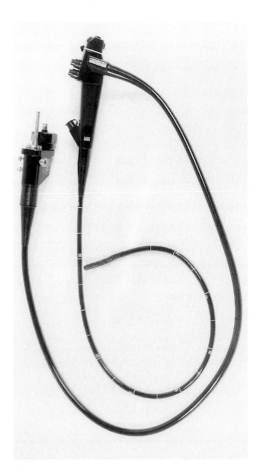

Figure 3.1
Upper gastrointestinal endoscope.

preferable when ERCP is attempted via an afferent duodenal loop after a Polya or Billroth II type gastrectomy.

The typical flexible endoscope consists of three main parts: the insertion tube, the control body and an umbilical universal cord which connects the endoscope to its light source and other ancillary equipment.

The patient insertion tube usually has an overall working length of about 110 cm, the distal 10 cm or so of which is constructed as a specially manoeuvrable bending section. Full-length control wires within the sheath of the endoscope produce vertical and lateral movements of the distal tip, which can usually be angulated 100° each way in the horizontal plane, 200° upwards and about 90° downwards. By using this range of angulation, together with torqued rotational movements of the more proximal shaft, it is possible to inspect any desired area in the upper gastrointestinal tract, including the oesophagus, stomach and upper duodenum, comprehensively and with relative ease.

The tip of the endoscope (Figure 3.2) bears an image gathering system, either optical or electronic. In addition, one or more efferent light guides end at the tip and carry illumination from a cold light source outside the patient via a non-coherent glass fibre bundle or bundles (see below). Finally, there are the openings of channels for suction and air insufflation or water instillation, the latter as a cleaning spray across the distal lens or microchip cover.

The endoscope body contains several distinct groups of instrument controls. Two wheels mounted on the right side of the body produce distal tip movements by tensioning the shaft control wires as mentioned above. These wheels can be locked in any chosen position by lever ratchet mechanisms. Two or more valves or microswitches on the upper surface of the body control suction, insufflation and water blowing. Additional microswitches are often present at the proximal end of the instrument head, particularly in electronic endoscopes, and are used to operate image storing systems such as video printers and recorders. In the optical fibrescope, a lens array and eyepiece at the end of the instrument body allow direct examination by the operator of the transmitted image.

The umbilical tube of the endoscope contains suction and insufflation channels and also the efferent light guide bundles carrying illumination from an external light source. In video endoscopes it also transmits information by a wire from the distally sited CCD microchip to a computer system, which uses this information to build up a high quality televised image.

The valved entry port of the biopsy channel is usually situated on the control body. The biopsy channel, which joins the suction channel, runs the length of the insertion tube so that there is a common opening at the endoscope tip. Diagnostic and therapeutic appliances, e.g. biopsy forceps, cytology brushes and balloon dilators, may be passed through this channel.

All modern gastrointestinal endoscopes are constructed so

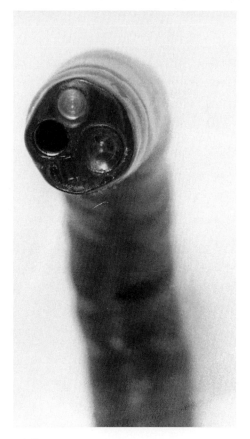

Figure 3.2
Endoscope tip.

that their components are completely sealed and impervious to fluid. This fully immersible property of the instruments is essential to allow for adequate cleaning and disinfection as described later. With proper care and maintenance, the working life of an endoscope is about seven years although, depending on intensity of use, many instruments remain in service for significantly longer.

Ancillary equipment

A wide range of accessory equipment is necessary for the provision of an adequate diagnostic and therapeutic upper gastrointestinal service. First, a suitable light source is required, whether a fibreoptic or electronic endoscope is used. Most current models employ a xenon arc lamp powerful enough for endoscopy with or without an add-on video camera. With electronic endoscope systems, the light source may be combined with a video processor and may also allow the use of fibreoptic instruments transformed to video by a suitable CCD converter.

With fibreoptic endoscopy, the image may be displayed on a television monitor when the appropriate television camera is attached to the eyepiece. If video endoscopy is carried out, such a monitor is an essential part of the system. It can conveniently be mounted at eye level on a purpose-designed trolley which will also hold image storing systems such as video recorders or printers as desired. A typical system is illustrated in Figure 3.3 where other accessories such as portable suction and endoscopic diathermy equipment are also evident. The entire kit is ideally sited in a purpose-designed suite so that facilities such as wall-mounted suction, piped oxygen and ample power points are readily available.

A large variety of through-endoscope flexible accessories is now routinely used in diagnostic and therapeutic practice. For example, a multitude of different biopsy forceps is available and other devices such as injection needles, dilators, balloons, snares and retrieval instruments will be needed to provide an adequate service. In addition, there are numerous more specialized accessories ranging from heater probes to lasers, and kits to enable the introduction of gastric or jejunal feeding tubes.

An endoscopy service will also require adequate cleaning and disinfection equipment. A dedicated computer system is highly desirable for generating legible and rapid reports of investigations, for booking lists, organizing recall appointments for check examinations and building up a database for audit and research purposes.

Fibreoptic versus video endoscopy

The relative advantages of the two types of endoscope are summarized in Table 3.1.

Table 3.1 Relative advantages of fibrescopes and electronic endoscopes

FIBRESCOPES	VIDEO ENDOSCOPES
Wide availability	Better image
Familiarity to many users	More robust
Less expensive	Easier to manoeuvre
Cheaper accessories	Less strain on user
More portable	Image storage
Better still photographs	Teaching
	Possibly safer

Fibreoptic endoscopes are available in most general hospitals. These instruments are usually cheaper than their electronic counterparts, as are some of their accessories such as light sources. A fibreoptic system is relatively more mobile and hence advantageous for bedside examination outside the main endoscopy suite.

In contrast, video endoscopes provide a better image to the observer. As they do not have to be held up to the eye, they

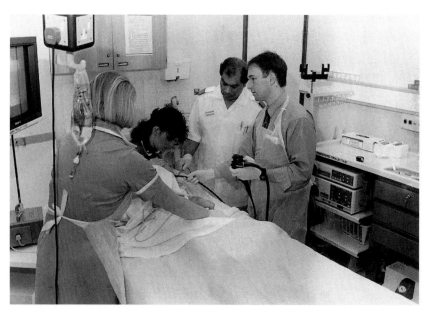

Figure 3.3
Typical endoscopy system.

are more manoeuvrable, easier to learn to use, and tend to cause less muscular strain to the examiner. The increased distance of the endoscope from the user's face and eyes reduces the risk of infection from contaminated body fluids. Electronic instruments have substantial advantages in terms of ease of image storage onto tape or disk and are particularly appropriate for demonstration and teaching.

Where to perform endoscopic examinations

At present, in the UK, the great majority of gastrointestinal endoscopies are performed on a day case basis in the hospital setting. Units serving a population of 300,000 will deal with up to 3000 day patients per year. This figure excludes emergency OGDs, ERCPs and colonoscopies. This implies a minimum of ten routine half-day sessions per week, and use of at least two procedure rooms so that parallel lists can be run as necessary.[5] The endoscopy unit should be sited either close to the hospital's general day care facilities, or have its own day stay beds; easy access to the wards is desirable to facilitate the investigation of in-patients. Proximity to the X-ray department or provision of a dedicated screening unit in the endoscopy suite is important for some interventional procedures.

Full access to resuscitation facilities is mandatory as emergency situations such as cardiorespiratory arrest, haemorrhage or anaphylaxis may occasionally arise.

In addition to the examination rooms and day beds, the endoscopy unit will require a suitable waiting area for patients and relatives, changing and toilet facilities, secretarial offices and instrument cleaning and storage space.

Exceptionally, endoscopies may need to be performed in other areas, for example in the operating theatres, in the intensive care unit or at the patient's bedside. However, routine work should be concentrated in the endoscopy unit both to maximize safety by the use of optimal facilities, and to reduce unnecessary and costly duplication of endoscopic equipment.

Outside the United Kingdom, and especially in the United States, many upper intestinal endoscopies are carried out in office practice.[6] It has been suggested that a similar change might occur in the UK, with at least diagnostic OGDs being carried out in general practice if suitably qualified practitioners were to be provided with appropriate equipment and premises.[7] The potential problems in ensuring satisfactory levels of expertise, staffing and safety have been investigated by the British Society of Gastroenterology.[8] Quite apart from these considerations, the financial burden of setting up and running a basic diagnostic service to proper standards is appreciable, the start-up costs alone amounting to about £80,000 at 1994 UK prices.[8]

STAFFING CONSIDERATIONS

The endoscopist: training and experience

Currently in Britain about two thirds of upper gastrointestinal diagnostic endoscopy is performed by physicians and one third by surgeons.[9] Detailed recommendations for adequate training in endoscopy have been formulated[10] but there is at present in the UK no mandatory accreditation scheme ensuring that practitioners have fulfilled the suggested requirements.

In essence, the suggestion is that formal training should be undertaken in a busy unit where endoscopy forms part of a broadly based gastroenterology service, and should be supplemented by attendance at approved external courses. A training unit should carry out at least 1000 OGDs per year so that a full range of conditions and procedures may be encountered by the trainee. Suitable teaching equipment, particularly video endoscopes, should be available. Training is expected to take at least six months, the trainee endoscopist participating in at least one weekly list and undertaking 150–200 supervised diagnostic examinations before being judged competent to work alone. Therapeutic procedures should only be started after diagnostic expertise is properly established.

Similar standards have been proposed in the US as part of the formalized and already established fellowship training programmes in gastroenterology.[11,12]

Once basic training is complete, continued experience in a busy unit is essential if skill levels are to be maintained. Adequate access to specialized units and courses is necessary if the endoscopist is to develop expertise in more complex diagnostic and therapeutic procedures, and is to remain abreast of new developments.

Support staff

In addition to medical staff, the endoscopy unit needs secretarial and nursing support. Depending on the work throughput, at least one experienced secretary will be required to manage the clerical side of the service. Specially trained endoscopy nurses are essential, the overall number again being dependent on case load. Trained nurses are necessary to assess patients on arrival, to care for and monitor them during the endoscopic procedure, and to supervise their recovery and discharge from the unit. Specialist courses are run by bodies such as the English National Board and cover both the nursing and technical aspects of endoscopy.

A minimum of two endoscopy assistants is required in each procedure room, one to care for the patient and one to help with the instruments. Further staff are needed to supervise recovering patients and to organize instrument cleaning and disinfection. A senior nurse (in the UK of Sister grade) should be in administrative charge of the endoscopy unit and be responsible for its day to day activities, for the training of nursing and technical staff, and for care of the equipment.

STERILIZATION AND SAFETY CONSIDERATIONS

Instrument disinfection

Gastrointestinal endoscopy carries an obvious risk of transmission of infection from one patient to another. In addition to the common gut bacteria which may contaminate the endoscope, there are also the less common organisms such as mycobacteria and viruses including hepatitis B (HBV) and human immunodeficiency virus (HIV). Although the likelihood of encountering these will vary from practice to practice, scrupulous attention to instrument cleaning and disinfection is mandatory to reduce the chance of disease transmission via the endoscope from undiagnosed asymptomatic carriers. Even organisms of low pathogenicity may give rise to serious disease if inoculated into an immunocompromised patient by a contaminated instrument.[13,14] To minimize infection risks, units should have a defined cleaning and disinfection policy and regular audit of the results.

Prior to disinfection, mechanical cleaning of the endoscope is obligatory and removes the majority of organisms present. All accessible channels should be flushed through and brushed vigorously. The outside of the instrument should be washed thoroughly with detergent. Adequate cleansing implies that endoscopes which are not completely fluid immersible should no longer be used. Detailed instructions for cleaning procedures are provided by the various instrument manufacturers.

After mechanical cleaning, the endoscope should be disinfected according to the manufacturer's specifications. A number of automated endoscope washing machines are now available which can handle one or more immersible instruments simultaneously, provide a uniform and controlled disinfection cycle and reduce staff exposure to toxic disinfectant chemicals. Some machines have considerable design flaws, and careful microbiological monitoring and cleaning of the units is important if the washing machines themselves are not to constitute an extra infection hazard.[15] Furthermore, the autodisinfectors are usually not sealed and may still allow undue staff exposure to chemical fumes; this danger can be obviated if the machines are housed in a fume cupboard system and if automated transfer pumps are used to fill and empty the disinfectant reservoirs.

Currently it is accepted that the only generally satisfactory endoscope disinfectants are 2% glutaraldehyde or equivalent aldehyde chemicals. These will inactivate vegetative bacteria and viruses during a 10 minute instrument exposure period, which is adequate between patients during a list. Including automated washing before disinfection and a rinsing period after, the minimum total cleaning cycle between patients is 25 min or so, which implies that at least three endoscopes are necessary for one endoscopist to run a satisfactory list. At the beginning and end of such a list, a longer 40 min disinfection period is conventionally used, either to remove contaminants which may have multiplied during endoscope storage, or to reduce the chance of this occurring prior to the next list. In special circumstances, for example investigation of immunosuppressed and HIV-positive patients, more prolonged instrument disinfection times have been advised.[16]

Instrument accessories

There is an increasing tendency to use disposable through-endoscope accessories where possible. Non-disposable accessories can be washed in detergent and brushed or flushed through as appropriate, further cleaned in an ultrasonic bath and finally either cold disinfected or preferably, and where possible, autoclaved.

Protection of staff

Protection from infection

The endoscopy unit is a hazardous environment where staff may regularly encounter infectious patients. In the UK it is recommended that all medical, nursing and technical staff should be immunized against HBV and receive booster injections as necessary. The unit must have strictly observed precautions to minimize the risk of needle stick or similar injuries. There should be written protocols for handling and disposal of blood, body fluids and suction bottle wastes. Where appropriate, and particularly when dealing with HIV-positive patients, protective clothing, including masks and visors to protect eye splashes, should be worn; the take-up rate of such advice is, however, poor.[17]

Protection from disinfectant

Although glutaraldehyde and similar substances are the only microbiologically satisfactory agents for endoscope disinfection, they are toxic chemicals and constitute appreciable hazards to the staff handling them. Direct contact may produce dermatitis or respiratory irritation, sensitization may induce allergic asthma, and other adverse effects include headaches, dizziness and nausea. When precautions to minimize exposure are not rigorously followed, between one-third and three-quarters of endoscopy units experience staff problems related to aldehyde-related damage.[18,19] In the UK, the Control of Substances Hazardous to Health (COSHH) Regulations require employers to ensure that safe working systems are in place to minimize staff exposure to hazardous chemicals such as glutaraldehyde, and furthermore to ensure that appropriate health surveillance is undertaken.[20] Detailed recommendations as to how endoscopy units can comply with these regulations have been produced by the British Society of Gastroenterology.[21]

INDICATIONS AND CONTRAINDICATIONS

It is often difficult in the first instance to be certain of the site of origin of a presenting gastroenterological symptom. Dyspepsia-like symptoms and acute upper gastrointestinal bleeding are good examples. It seems appropriate, therefore, to consider the oesophagus, stomach and duodenum together.

Indications

The main indications for the endoscopy of the upper gastrointestinal tract are shown in Table 3.2. With regard to suspected oesophageal disease, the principal symptoms for which endoscopy is indicated are dysphagia, odynophagia and symptoms suggestive of gastro-oesophageal reflux. Dysphagia is a potentially serious symptom and warrants early investigation. Whereas this symptom may reflect an underlying motility disorder, benign stricture, neurological problem or even a functional disorder (Chapter 14), it is a cardinal symptom of a malignant obstructing lesion of the oesophagus, which must be regarded as a likely diagnosis until excluded by endoscopy. Endoscopy has advantages over radiology in that it provides direct vision, the facility to obtain a histological diagnosis and frequently gives better assessment of the length of an obstructing lesion, often underestimated by radiology. However, some workers prefer to perform a barium swallow prior to endoscopy in patients with dysphagia to exclude pharyngeal pouch (Zenker's diverticulum) as a cause, to obtain a working 'road map' prior to endoscopy and to allow visualization downstream of an obstructive lesion in case it should prove impassable at endoscopy. However, an apparently normal contrast swallow should not influence the decision to perform endoscopy.

Table 3.2   Indication for endoscopy of the upper gastrointestinal tract

DIAGNOSTIC ENDOSCOPY	THERAPEUTIC ENDOSCOPY
Dyspepsia and upper abdominal pain	Gastrointestinal bleeding
Heartburn and reflux symptoms	Treatment of tumours
Dysphagia	Removal of foreign bodies
Gastrointestinal bleeding	Dilatation of strictures and in
Anaemia or positive faecal occult blood tests	achalasia
Malabsorption states – for duodenal biopsy	Insertion of feeding tubes
Anorexia and weight loss	
Nausea and vomiting	
Gastric ulcer – follow-up	
Equivocal barium meal findings	
Screening and monitoring	

Much progress has been made in recent years in the management of gastro-oesophageal reflux disease. It has therefore become increasingly important to to be able to diagnose this disorder accurately, to be aware of its complications and to be able to monitor progress. The grading of the severity of oesophagitis is based on endoscopic appearances (Table 3.3): radiology is less relevant in this respect. It is becoming increasingly recommended that endoscopy need not be performed in all patients with reflux symptoms, but should be reserved for those whose symptoms begin over the age of 40, those who have potentially alarming symptoms such as dysphagia, odynophagia or bleeding, or those whose symptoms do not resolve on a short course of an appropriate acid-suppressing agent.

Endoscopic appearances do not help greatly in the diagnosis and assessment of motility disorders. In the oesophagus, for

Table 3.3   Savary–Miller endoscopic grading of reflux oesophagitis[52]

Grade I	Single or non-confluent multiple erythematous streaks with or without minor degrees of erosion extending proximally from the dentate line.
Grade II	Discrete linear erosions not involving the whole circumference of the oesophagus.
Grade III	Confluent erosions involving the whole oesophageal circumference but without stenosis.
Grade IV	Severe inflammation with chronic ulceration and stricture formation.

example, achalasia is better diagnosed by radiology and manometry, though there is a place for long-term monitoring for the development of a complicating carcinoma. In the stomach, endoscopy cannot be used to make a diagnosis of non-ulcer dyspepsia, though many endoscopists regard it as useful in such patients to be able to reassure them that no organic cause for their symptoms is present.

Recent onset of dyspepsia in patients over the age of about 40 years is an important indication for endoscopy; the prevalence of significant organic gastroenterological disease is well known to increase steadily with age. In younger patients, endoscopic examination may be unnecessary, as typical symptom patterns often exclude serious disease reasonably accurately, and malignant tumours are uncommon.[22] However, it is arguable that even in younger subjects endoscopy may give helpful negative information, or may allow biopsy screening for *Helicobacter pylori* in patients with gastritis or duodenal ulceration.[23] It should, however, be stressed that 'gastritis' is not easily recognized visually at OGD. In duodenal ulceration, biopsy material for the identification of *H. pylori*, be it for a urease test, histopathology or bacteriological culture, should be taken from the antrum. The endoscopic workload in younger dyspeptic subjects may be reduced if adequate management protocols can be devised based on symptom patterns and less invasive tests for *H. pylori* such as the ^{13}C-urease breath test[24] or benchtop antibody assays.[25]

Upper gastrointestinal endoscopy is the investigation of choice in cases of frank haematemesis or melaena. In addition to its purely diagnostic role, various endoscopic intervention manoeuvres are possible which can both stop the haemorrhage and reduce the rebleeding rate (see Chapter 38).

Radiology is unreliable in the differentiation between benign and malignant gastric ulcers.[26] Endoscopy with target biopsy achieves an accurate diagnosis in about 98% of cases provided that multiple tissue specimens are taken from both the edge and the base of the lesion.[27] Even in apparently benign gastric ulcers (GUs) the conventional advice is to repeat endoscopy and biopsy after a course of medical treatment in order to check for healing and to take further biopsies if healing is incomplete. The previously recommended interval between endoscopies of six weeks is too short to achieve complete healing in a significant proportion of benign ulcers, and a treatment course of 8–12 weeks is preferable. A check endoscopy may be inappropriate in frail, elderly patients in whom the initial biopsies are benign and where the symptomatic response to treatment is satisfactory.

Upper gastrointestinal endoscopy is often requested to check equivocal barium meal findings. In many instances, endoscopy would have been preferable as an initial investigation but the choice may be influenced by local availability of tests. Endoscopy is certainly more appropriate in patients who have had previous benign ulceration or gastroduodenal surgery, as radiological appearances may be difficult to interpret in the presence of postinflammatory or postoperative scarring.

Endoscopy has a useful role to play in monitoring or surveillance of disorders of the upper gastrointestinal tract.

Examples would include Barrett's oesophagus and in the stomach, perhaps in patients with Addisonian pernicious anaemia, both conditions being premalignant. It is also advisable, as is already common practice in the colon, to place patients who have undergone removal of an adenomatous polyp of the upper gastrointestinal tract under long-term endoscopic surveillance.

Contraindications

Contraindications to upper gastrointestinal endoscopy tend to be relative rather than absolute. Even diagnostic endoscopy carries an appreciable morbidity and the 30-day mortality in elderly, unfit subjects is not negligible (0.04%).[28] The main hazards are cardiorespiratory depression or hypotension secondary to over-sedation, cardiac arrhythmia and pulmonary aspiration.

The patients most at risk are elderly subjects with severe cardiorespiratory disease. Endoscopy may be impossible in a patient with heart failure or orthopnoea who cannot lie reasonably flat. The risk of respiratory depression can be reduced if sedation is minimized or avoided completely, and the procedure performed under topical analgesia only. Indeed, endoscopy without sedation is entirely feasible, and in some countries is employed routinely in patients of all ages. Because of the risks of cardiac dysrhythmias,[29] non-urgent endoscopy is inadvisable within three months of an acute myocardial infarction.

Patients who have recently had orthopaedic surgical procedures, particularly hip replacement, may be difficult to endoscope because of positioning problems. Care must be taken to maintain artificial hips in abduction because of the risks of dislocation.

The particular problems relating to patients with HBV or HIV have already been mentioned. Investigation of these patients does not present insuperable difficulties in investigation, and dedicated endoscopes are not necessary, provided the proper disinfection procedures are carried out.

PROCEDURE OF ENDOSCOPY

Patient preparation

Before diagnostic or therapeutic endoscopy, a patient needs to have adequate information about the reasons for and the actual performance of the procedure. This may be provided in the form of a booking letter from the endoscopy unit, discussion with a doctor or nurse, a suitably designed information leaflet, or even as video tapes.[30] The use of a 'named nurse' system within the unit – where a particular nurse talks to the patient before endoscopy, accompanies the patient during the test and supervises recovery afterwards – facilitates the provision of information about the investigation, its results and any planned treatment, though most clinicians prefer to discuss the procedure, the results and further management themselves. Any system must ensure that a pre-endoscopy check list can easily be completed, relating to important factors such as relevant previous illnesses, drug treatments and allergies, and that written and verbal informed consent for the planned procedure(s) is obtained.

To minimize the chance of aspiration, and to achieve satisfactory visualization of the upper gastrointestinal tract, the patient's stomach must be empty; a pre-endoscopy starvation period of four to six hours is usually adequate. In patients with suspected outlet obstruction, gastric lavage can be performed before the test. If an urgent endoscopy is necessary in a patient who has eaten recently or who has bled, a prokinetic agent such as intravenous metoclopramide may accelerate gastric emptying.

In any patient, but especially patients who have had a previous partial gastrectomy, foaming and bubbles within the gastric remnant and the duodenum may impair the view. The use of oral liquid dimethicone before or during endoscopy in such cases can be helpful.[31]

Intravenous or transdermal anticholinergics are sometimes given routinely, both to reduce salivation and gastroduodenal motor activity and to prevent vagally mediated bradiarrhythmias. However, there are doubts as to whether such drugs are either useful or necessary.[32] Indeed, it is often helpful to see the pattern of gastroduodenal contractions as they may be abnormal, e.g. in antral carcinoma. It is therefore recommended that an anticholinergic to reduce these movements should only be given, if at all, after the movements have been studied endoscopically.

Endoscopy-related bacteraemia with both aerobic and anaerobic organisms from the upper gastrointestinal tract is well recognized, particularly after therapeutic procedures.[33] In patients at risk, and particularly those with artificial heart valves, antibiotic prophylaxis is advisable.[34, 35]

Analgesia, sedation and monitoring

At present, the majority of upper gastrointestinal endoscopies in the UK are carried out using 'conscious sedation' induced by an intravenous benzodiazepine such as diazepam or midazolam.[36] Both drugs carry a risk of cardiorespiratory depression, which is substantially increased if an opiate such as pethidine is used in combination.[37]

Although sedation is necessary for prolonged procedures, especially therapeutic endoscopies, there is an increasing tendency for simple diagnostic gastroscopies to be performed under local analgesia only, or without even employing this. In expert hands and using small diameter endoscopes, this approach is acceptable to the majority of patients. It carries the additional advantages that the results can be discussed with the patient immediately, and that he/she is fit to leave the unit on completion of the examination and resume normal activities.

If sedation is employed, the smallest necessary drug dose should be administered by a practitioner experienced in sedation techniques.[38] Excessive drug doses increase the risk of hypoxia, as do pre-existing cardiorespiratory disease, prolonged endoscopic procedures, the use of large-bore therapeutic instruments, and the performance of tests by inexperienced operators.[39] Hypoxia in turn is probably the commonest cause of cardiac dysrhythmias during endoscopy.[40]

Pre-oxygenation of patients, and continued supplementation at 2–4 l/min via mask or nasal cannula, reduces the chance of oxygen desaturation.[41] Clinical observation is unreliable in the early detection of respiratory depression, and pulse oximetry monitoring is now mandatory for all endoscopic procedures where sedation is used.[38,42,43] If oversedation does result in hypoxia, the effects of opiates and benzodiazepines can be reversed with competitive antagonists such as naloxone and flumezanil, respectively. Flumezanil should be used with caution as it can, very rarely, provoke epileptic seizures.[44] Full resuscitation facilities should be immediately available in endoscopy rooms and endoscopy unit recovery areas.

Performing a diagnostic endoscopy

The patient lies on the left side, supervised by a trained nurse, and is sedated and monitored as appropriate. A mouthguard is placed between the teeth if present, both to protect them and to prevent damage to the endoscope; in edentulous patients the mouthguard is usually difficult to retain and unnecessary.

With the subject's neck in slight flexion, the endoscope is inserted gently over the back of the tongue and into the pharynx, while monitoring the tip position visually. Some operators intubate 'blind' and guide the endoscope digitally into the upper oesophagus. This is not universally recommended for two reasons: first, unexpected problems are occasionally present in the throat and will be missed if the 'blind' method is used;[45] and secondly a precipitate 'blind' intubation in a patient with a pharyngeal pouch or a high oesophageal obstruction may result in avoidable perforation.

As the endoscope tip passes over the posterior tongue, the larynx is usually clearly visible. By gentle caudad pressure in the mid-line behind the larynx, the upper oesophagus can be entered against minimal resistance. The endoscope is then passed slowly down the oesophagus and the level of the oesophagogastric junction noted. If a fixed hiatal hernia is suspected, the patient can be instructed to sniff; this opposes the crura of the diaphragm, causing a constriction at the lower limit of the hernia.

At the oesophagogastric junction, the endoscope tip should be deflected slightly to the left and advanced into the stomach. Air insufflation separates the gastric rugae and allows inspection of the body mucosa at this stage, although the area may be better seen during withdrawal. If the stomach is of the 'cup and spill' variety and the instrument tip is allowed to deviate to the right, the inexperienced endoscopist can find himself trapped in an apparent blind sac formed by the gastric fundus.

Once the body of the stomach has been examined, the endoscope is advanced following the line of the rugae and swinging round to the right along the lesser curve; this movement is most easily achieved if the operator simply turns to the right and thus rotates the instrument shaft by torque into the correct direction, rather than making excessive use of the control wheels. The antrum is relatively free from rugal folds. Next, the pylorus will come into view, sometimes fairly high up under the angulus.

At this stage of the examination, an inversion or J-manoeuvre can be used to examine the gastric angle, cardia and the fundus of the stomach. Once the antrum has been inspected,

the upward control of the endoscope is turned to full deflection, thus retroverting the instrument tip. This brings the gastric angle into clear view, and withdrawal of the endoscope in the retroflexed attitude, together with rotation if necessary, allows visualization of the high lesser curve, the cardia and the fundus, and the gastro-oesophageal junction, and of a hiatal hernia if present.

Once this phase of the examination is complete, the tip deflection is returned to neutral, the pylorus located again and the endoscope advanced into the proximal duodenum. Circumferential movements permit full examination of the duodenal bulb, although inspection of the area just distal to the pyloric ring may be difficult, in which case retroflexion of the tip may be tried with care. At the far end of the first part of the duodenum, the endoscope tip is turned to the right, the shaft rotated clockwise and the instrument gently advanced while simultaneously angling upwards and later, sometimes, a little downwards and allowing the clockwise rotation to come back to the vertical. This simple manoeuvre slides the tip around into the second part of the duodenum where the peri-ampullary area and often the duodenal papilla can be inspected.

After the furthest practicable insertion of the endoscope has been achieved (which is usually the second or at best the third part of the duodenum), a slow withdrawal with continued examination of the various duodenal, gastric, oesophageal and pharyngeal areas is undertaken. Careful inspection of the upper oesophagus and pharynx is particularly important if the 'blind' method of intubation has been used. Air insufflation during the test should not be excessive, and subsequent patient comfort is increased if the duodenum and stomach are deflated by continuous suction as the endoscope is withdrawn.

The above scheme is clearly subject to modification according to the practices of individual endoscopists, but provides a reasonable framework for a comprehensive diagnostic inspection. A full negative examination, not including the time required for preparation of the patient, should take little more than five minutes or so in the hands of an experienced operator.

ENDOSCOPIC DIAGNOSIS IN THE OESOPHAGUS

There is a wide range of normal and abnormal appearances in the oesophagus which the trainee endoscopist must learn to recognize. Standard endoscopic atlases[47-48] and latterly an atlas available on CD-ROM[49] can be useful sources of information and reference. Here it is only possible to mention a few of these appearances.

Normal variant appearances

The typical normal oesophagus appears as a pale pink tube with variable prominence of longitudinal ridges particularly towards its lower extremity. These ridges may be confused with small oesophageal varices by the inexperienced endoscopist, but are whitish-pink rather than bluish in colour and become less obvious as the organ is insufflated with air.

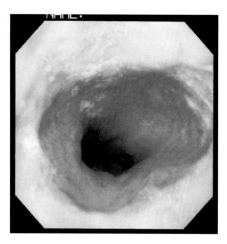

Figure 3.4
Regular dentate line.

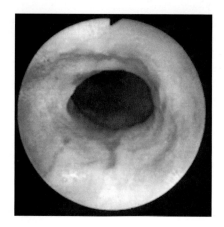

Figure 3.6
Grade I oesophagitis.

Peristaltic activity is most easily seen in the lower third of the gullet and no food or other debris should normally be present, unless the patient has been inadequately starved prior to the examination. The pulsatile aortic indentation is usually clearly visible in the middle third, and transmitted cardiac pulsation is commonly seen below this level. If the patient retches during the endoscopy, reddened gastric mucosal folds may momentarily prolapse into the lower oesophagus. Various trivial lumps and bumps can occur in the oesophageal wall, the most frequent being small pale nodules due to subepithelial glycogen, so-called glycogenic acanthosis.

The dentate or Z-line at the oesophagogastric junction is very variable in appearance. It commonly presents as a sharply defined, regular, circular demarcation between the pale squamous oesophageal epithelium and the thicker redder gastric mucosa (Figure 3.4, see colour plate also), but may be irregular with wavy figure-like processes extending in a cephalad direction (Figure 3.5, see colour plate also), or sometimes incorporate paler mucosal islands mimicking oesophagitis with ulceration.

An inordinate amount of symptomatology is attributed by patients to the presence of a hiatal hernia, but many, if not most such radiologically diagnosed 'abnormalities' are probably of little symptomatic or clinical importance. Many sliding hiatal hernias confidently reported following X-ray examination are inapparent on endoscopic inspection. A true fixed hiatal hernia appears as a chamber lined with gastric mucosa, lying above the impression of the diaphragmatic crura, with the dentate line displaced well proximal from its usual distance of about 40 cm from the incisors. The position of the hiatus proper can be demonstrated if the patient is asked to sniff; opposition of the crura during this manoeuvre is clearly visible to the endoscopist. It is arguable that in most symptomatic patients, the clinical problem is really attributable to acid reflux damage rather than to the presence of a hiatal hernia as such, and in elderly subjects hernias are so frequent as to be virtually a normal variant. Their only major practical importance to the endoscopist arises if they are very large, and especially if they are in part paraoesophageal in configuration. In these circumstances, it is quite easy for the novice to become lost in the hernial sac and to find visualization of the subdiaphragmatic portion of the stomach difficult or even impossible.

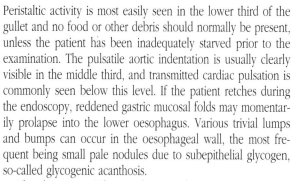

Figure 3.5
Irregular but normal dentate line.

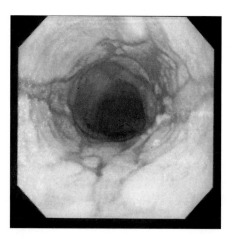

Figure 3.7
Grade II oesophagitis.

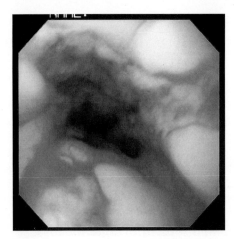

Figure 3.8
Grade III oesophagitis.

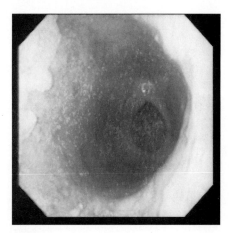

Figure 3.10
Barrett's oesophagus.

Superficial lesions

Oesophagitis

Oesophagitis is the most commonly identified abnormality at diagnostic upper gastrointestinal endoscopy. Several attempts at classification of oesophagitis have been made on anatomical, functional or pathological grounds[50,51] and none has proved entirely satisfactory. It has become conventional to score oesophagitis endoscopically using some modification of the Savary–Miller grading system[52] (Table 3.3). Examples of the various grades are shown in Figures 3.6–3.9 (see colour plates also). In general, symptoms of oesophagitis correlate poorly with the visual appearances. Up to 50% of patients with true reflux problems have no demonstrable endoscopic abnormality, and patients with relatively mild symptoms may have grade 3 or 4 oesophagitis.

Barrett's oesophagus

This is a relatively common abnormality, where the lower oesophagus becomes lined by columnar rather than squamous epithelium.[53] Conventionally, Barrett's change is considered to be present when columnar mucosa extends more than 3 cm proximal to the cardia although the importance of 'short segment' Barrett's is now being realized. Such patients may or may not have a history of chronic reflux, and the mucosal change is suggested to develop as healing of acute or long-term ulceration proceeds, with progressive upwards replacement of the oesophageal lining by gastric-type mucosa; this theory, though attractive, remains unproven.

The typical endoscopic appearance is of a tubular lower oesophagus lined with dull red gastric mucosa extending well above the hiatus (Figure 3.10, see colour plate also). The change can easily be confirmed by biopsy, which is additionally important as the condition carries a small risk of malignant change.[54] In many units, younger patients with Barrett's mucosa are followed-up with an annual endoscopy and biopsy to detect premalignant dysplasia. For those preoccupied by such matters, it may be of interest that the cost/benefit ratio of this approach has not been conclusively established.

Oesophageal ulcer

Discrete oesophageal ulcers (Figure 3.11, see colour plate also) may occur in areas of squamous epithelium, in Barrett's mucosa or within a hiatal hernia. They are usually a consequence of

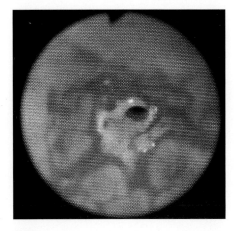

Figure 3.9
Grade IV oesophagitis.

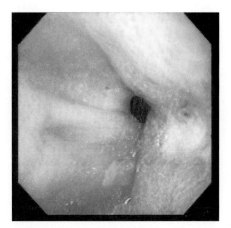

Figure 3.11
Oesophageal ulcer.

acid reflux, but may result from local epithelial trauma and particularly from direct contact with ulcerogenic tablets, such as slow-release potassium supplements and some urinary antispasmodics. As in the stomach, apparently benign ulcers may be carcinomatous and it is advisable therefore that multiple biopsies and possibly a cytological smear are taken at diagnostic endoscopy.

Benign stricture

Again, this commonly develops as a late effect of long-term reflux, when ulceration and consequent fibrosis lead to progressive constriction and luminal narrowing. A degree of oesophagitis is usually present in relation to the stricture, but may be minimal or even absent in chronic cases or where the patient has recently received powerful acid-suppressant therapy. As the appearances of a carcinoma may mimic those of benign stricture, biopsy examination is important even where a stricture appears radiologically or endoscopically benign. Benign strictures may also develop as a result of the accidental or deliberate ingestion of caustic materials; management of such cases is discussed elsewhere.

Oesophageal candidiasis

Yeast infections of the oesophagus are relatively common in the elderly, in immunocompromised patients such as those with AIDS, and in asthmatic patients using corticosteroid inhalers. *Candida* forms discrete white spots or confluent white or dirty-looking patches on the oesophageal lining, with friable inflamed tissue beneath the plaques. The endoscopic appearance is typical (Figure 3.12, see colour plate also) but can be confirmed histologically or microbiologically if desired.

Viral oesophagitis

The oesophageal epithelium is occasionally infected by viruses such as *Herpes simplex*, papillomaviruses or cytomegalovirus, particularly in patients who are therapeutically or naturally immunosuppressed. Such infections result in oesophageal erosions, ulcers or vesicles, and accurate diagnosis depends on the microscopic examination of biopsy specimens.

Mucosal tears

So-called Mallory–Weiss tears may develop at the oesophago-gastric junction, particularly after multiple retching episodes. They are a relatively common cause of haematemesis, particularly in young male patients after overindulgence in alcohol, and account for 1–2% of admissions for upper gastrointestinal bleeding in most series. The typical endoscopic appearance is of a longitudinal split in the mucosa at the cardia, surrounded by an erythematous flare and often with signs of recent or active bleeding (Figure 3.13, see colour plate also). The bleed is usually self-limiting, but may rarely be severe and require endoscopic or even surgical intervention to obtain control.

Uncommon superficial abnormalities

Crohn's disease can occasionally affect the oesophagus, usually when the disorder is already known to be present elsewhere in the gastrointestinal tract; the appearances are similar to Crohn's disease elsewhere, with areas of ulceration or cobblestoning.

Spontaneous haematomas sometimes occur and appear as rounded bluish swellings below the epithelium.

Oesophagitis dissecans is a rare abnormality where apparently normal non-inflamed epithelium sloughs away from the underlying oesophageal wall and is shed as a membranous cast visible at endoscopy.

Mass lesions

Oesophageal carcinoma

Cancer of the oesophagus usually appears as either a typical malignant ulcer, or as an exophytic circumferential mass causing luminal obstruction (Figure 3.14, see colour plate also). In the lower third of the oesophagus, the tumour is likely to be an adenocarcinoma arising from gastric-type mucosa (from the cardia or a short-segment Barrett's), while in the upper two-thirds squamous carcinomas are more common. The histology of the growth may have an important bearing on treatment, but cannot be determined with any accuracy purely from the endoscopic appearances; assessment of biopsy and cytological specimens is therefore an essential component of the examination.

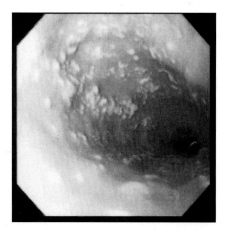

Figure 3.12
Oesophageal candidiasis.

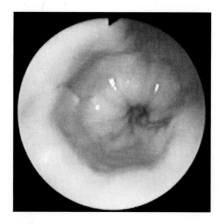

Figure 3.13
Mallory–Weiss tear.

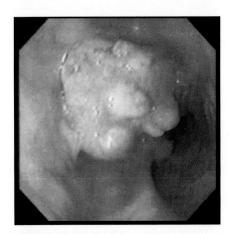

Figure 3.14
Oesophageal cancer.

Other tumours

Many other tumour types can be found in the oesophagus, but diagnosis usually depends on biopsy examination or examination of the whole specimen rather than on specific visual appearances. Extrinsic oesophageal involvement from an infiltrating bronchial carcinoma is relatively common, and dysphagia may be the presenting complaint in such patients. In patients with AIDS, lesions of Kaposi's sarcoma are a fairly frequent finding in the oesophagus.

Other abnormalities

Oesophageal varices

In patients with portal hypertension, oesophageal varices are usually easily recognized by the endoscopist as bluish, sometimes tortuous or beaded, venous columns running upwards from the oesophagogastric junction (Figure 3.15, see colour plate also). Very large varices may virtually fill the oesophageal lumen. Where bleeding has occurred, one or more columns may show superficial ulceration, adherent blood clot, or active

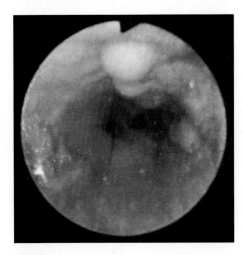

Figure 3.15
Oesophageal varices.

haemorrhage. As the pressure in the varices is high, bleeding may be torrential and may cause problems in both diagnosis and therapy because of poor visualization of the underlying oesophageal wall. Small varices may occasionally be confused with the normal longitudinal folds seen in the undistended oesophagus, and even large varices may collapse and be difficult to identify with certainty after a large bleed which has resulted in hypovolaemia and shock.

Achalasia

Abnormalities of motility may be difficult to judge by endoscopy, when barium, and especially manometric studies may be more helpful. However, in advanced cases of achalasia the oesophagus is typically dilated, tortuous, aperistaltic and contains a large volume of old food and fluid despite the usual preparation for endoscopy. The oesophagogastric junction, when it can be seen in these circumstances, appears normal and does not resist passage of the endoscope despite the radiological appearance and the obvious retention of debris. Achalasia-like appearances can occur in infiltrating tumours of the cardia; biopsy specimens should therefore be obtained from this area during the examination. Furthermore, long-standing achalasia is a premalignant condition; histological assessment by multiple biopsy is therefore important when a very long-standing case of the disorder is encountered and especially if appearances raise the question of malignant change. Accurate further assessment of achalasia by both radiology and manometry is mandatory if endoscopic or surgical therapy is to be undertaken.

Webs and rings

Pharyngeal and oesophageal webs, particularly in the post-cricoid area, are not infrequently reported on barium swallow examinations and may be associated with chronic iron-deficiency states. The lesions are often flimsy, and the higher webs in particular are often broken during endoscopic intubation or not seen at all by the endoscopist.

A musculofibrous contraction ring (Schatzki ring) can develop in the lower oesophagus, particularly at the upper extremity of a fixed hiatal hernia. To the endoscopist this appears as a smooth circumferential ridge covered by normal epithelium. The condition can be associated with dysphagia and sometimes responds to standard dilatation procedures. In contradistinction to benign oesophageal stricture, there is no firm association with gastro-oesophageal reflux disease or oesophagitis.

Pouches and diverticula

As already mentioned, unsuspected pharyngeal pouches can be a hazard in upper gastrointestinal endoscopy because the instrument tends to enter the pouch preferentially during intubation and perforation into the mediastinum is an appreciable risk. A known pharyngeal pouch is therefore a relative contraindication to endoscopy, and the examination should certainly only be performed by an experienced operator if the test is mandatory.

Shallow mid-oesophageal diverticula are common and of little significance. They are usually sited at the level of the pulmonary hilum and may possibly arise in consequence of external traction forces from adjacent fibrotic lung tissue. So-called pulsion diverticula, which may be single or multiple, are most frequently seen just proximal to peptic strictures. They can be a problem when oesophageal dilatation is necessary, and it is obviously important to select the true lumen of the oesophagus when positioning the guide wire or balloon, and not to attempt to enter or dilate a diverticulum.

THERAPEUTIC ENDOSCOPIC PROCEDURES IN THE OESOPHAGUS

This section is concerned in the main with the principles underlying the techniques of various therapeutic endoscopic procedures in oesophageal disease. These techniques are more fully described elsewhere in this volume. Indications, contraindications, complications and results are only touched on. In particular, no attempt is made rigorously to compare the results of one treatment with another.

Dilatation of benign oesophageal strictures

The advent of the fully flexible endoscope improved the management of this condition especially with regard to the incidence of perforation. Prior to dilatation, it is advisable to take biopsies of any lesion which at endoscopy does not look entirely typical of a benign stricture, though some endoscopists advise that such biopsies should always be obtained. Dilating a malignant stricture has no lasting effect, but dilatation often precedes other therapeutic procedures such as the placing of an endoprosthesis. The tip of the endoscope is placed a little above the stricture, and a wire with a flexible tip is passed through the biopsy channel of the endoscope under direct vision through the stricture so that the wire lies well in the stomach. Some operators prefer to use radiological screening to check the position of the guide wire. The next step will vary according to which method of dilatation is to be used. For rigid dilators, the endoscope is withdrawn, leaving the wire *in situ*. A variety of graded dilators is available. Olive-shaped dilators of increasing size, mounted on a stave, can be passed in ascending order of size until, by feel, the stricture is deemed to have been sufficiently dilated. Alternatively, stepped dilators can be passed along the wire. With both these methods, the actual procedure of dilatation is 'blind' to the endoscopist. Some endoscopists prefer the use of balloons which are threaded down the biopsy channel of the endoscope, introduced into the stricture under direct endoscopic vision, and are filled with water or air after being sited in the stricture. Theoretically, this may be a safer procedure but no conclusive results of clinical trials are available. Whatever method of dilatation is used, the site should be inspected after dilatation is completed. Some local bleeding and mucosal damage are commonplace. The endoscope can usually be passed through a dilated benign stricture at completion. It is advisable to check for free mediastinal or pleural air an hour or so after completion of dilatation, in case of perforation. Under normal circumstances, dilatation is an outpatient or day patient procedure.

Forced pneumatic dilatation in achalasia

The endoscopist has a choice of specially constructed balloons for this procedure. Balloons are usually a few centimetres in length and sometimes waisted, to minimize the risk of slipping out of position when inflated. Many contain radio-opaque rings, a useful adjunct for correct positioning. A balloon should be of a plastic material making it impossible to expand beyond the desired width. Under X-ray control, it is correctly placed, collapsed, over a previously introduced guide wire (see above), and inflated. Inflation pressure and length of time *in situ* will vary with the manufacturer's specifications and the endoscopist's wishes. Postdilatation endoscopic and radiological checks are mandatory.

Placing of endoprostheses (stents)

Endoprostheses are commonly used in the management of oesophageal carcinoma, particularly if there is an oesophago-pleural or an oesophagobronchial fistula. The endoscopist can choose from a large variety of uncuffed and cuffed semirigid endoprostheses, made from various latex-based or plastic materials, and often containing a strengthening coiled wire core. Semi-rigid endoprostheses are usually removable. Recently there has been growing interest in expandable metal-mesh endoprostheses.[55] These are easier to introduce but are irremovable. They are prone to carcinomatous ingrowth, and like all endoprostheses, liable to overgrowth. Tumour ingrowth may be reduced if a new type of sheathed metal-mesh stent is used. Prior to introducing any type of endoprosthesis, the affected portion of the oesophagus may be dilated using the methods described above. Metal-mesh expandable stents must be placed using the introducer supplied by the manufacturer. There are a variety of ways of placing a semi-rigid endoprosthesis, e.g. using a special introducer, or sliding it with a 'pusher' over an endoscope *in situ*, enabling the procedure to be conducted under visual control. The operation site must be carefully inspected on completion, more especially to check on the correct positioning of the prosthesis and an X-ray check for perforation – a common complication – is essential.

Laser therapy

Malignant oesophageal tumours can be treated by laser in two ways.

First, a powerful neodymium yttrium–aluminium–garnet (Nd-YAG) laser source may be used to destroy tumour tissue by direct application of thermal energy using a contact or non-contact technique. The laser light is transmitted to the tumour along a quartz fibre introduced through the biopsy channel of the endoscope. This technique is particularly useful in debulking exophytic growths, as oesophageal patency can be restored by vaporization and coagulation of tumour tissue.[56] Careful control of the amount of energy applied is important to minimize the risk of perforation. In experienced hands, the procedure improves dysphagia scores at least as well as if not better than intubation, but relief of symptoms tends to be rather short-lived and repeated treatments are usually needed, often every few weeks.[57] The necessary equipment is expensive and in general only available in tertiary referral centres.

Non-thermal tumour destruction is achievable by laser activation of a previously injected photosensitizing agent. Photodynamic therapy (PDT) relies on the relatively selective accumulation within tumour tissue of agents such as haematoporphyrins, which release cytotoxic singlet-oxygen when exposed to laser light of an appropriate wavelength.[58-60] The technique is at present experimental, but has been shown to reduce tumour size and improve swallowing, particularly with superficial growths.[59,61] Haematoporphyrin administration results in prolonged skin sensitization, and patients receiving PDT must avoid sunlight for several months after treatment. Newer agents, associated with only transitory skin sensitization, are currently under evaluation.

Endoscopic therapy for oesophageal varices

There continues to be a dispute as to whether oesophageal varices should be treated merely because they have been found to be present, and may over a period of time become more marked and eventually bleed, i.e. whether such varices should be treated prophylactically, or whether treatment should be reserved for varices which are bleeding or have recently bled.[62] The principles of endoscopic therapy are, however, similar. If much blood is present, visualization will be poor and diagnosis uncertain, and will make sclerotherapy or banding impossible. General supportive methods should therefore be employed until the endoscopist can work in a more or less clean field. The relative advantages of sclerotherapy and banding are discussed in detail elsewhere (see Chapter 17).

Sclerotherapy

Some years ago it was fashionable to use a Williams overtube, a device with a terminal longitudinal slot through which a varix would bulge into the lumen of the tube. Injections were then performed via an oblique-viewing endoscope. This method has been largely superseded in favour of the 'free-hand' method. The endoscope is placed with its tip low in the oesophagus so as to enable injections to be placed as close as possible to the origin of the varices, which is usually at the oesophagogastric junction. Injections are made through a retractable needle passed through the biopsy channel of the endoscope. There is some dispute as to whether intravasal or paravasal injections should be used. It is probable that most endoscopists will find it difficult to deliver the whole injection according to one or the other method, though an attempt at intravasal injection is advisable. Again, there are differences of opinion as to the best sites and most desirable number of injections. It may be best to inject each major vein at two or three points at perhaps 2 cm intervals progressing in a cephalad direction. However, some bleeding may ensue from one or more sites making exact visualization difficult, and limiting the number of sites attempted.

Bleeding is usually self-limited. Various preparations, including sodium morrhuate, ethanolamine oleate, sodium tetradecyl sulphate (STD) and absolute alcohol are in common use. Complications of sclerotherapy include bleeding, transient chest pain, perforation and mediastinitis, and the later occurrence of oesophageal strictures. The development of superficial ulcers at the injection sites is common and should not be regarded as a significant complication; such ulcers heal in a matter of days.

Banding of varices

Endoscopic ligation of oesophageal varices was first described in 1988. The technique uses a special applicator preloaded with an elastic O-ring and fitted to the distal end of a standard endoscope. Under direct vision, the band can be applied to an epithelial fold over an oesophageal varix, occluding the underlying vein when it is released and halting haemorrhage or preventing re-bleeding.[63,64] Endoscopic banding is claimed to have less late complications than sclerotherapy, and to be a more effective treatment for varices in that fewer treatment sessions are usually needed to produce complete obliteration of the abnormal vessels.[65] The speed of the process is increased if one of the newer applicators preloaded with five or six bands is employed. The late results of sclerotherapy and band ligation are similar.[66]

Foreign bodies in the oesophagus

Impaction of foreign material in a normal oesophagus is very rare. Sudden complete dysphagia due to food bolus obstruction, often a piece of unchewed meat, may be the presenting symptom of a serious disorder such as an oesophageal tumour. After removal of any foreign body from the oesophagus, a full diagnostic endoscopy is mandatory to exclude benign or malignant lesions contributing to the blockage.

Food impaction

Complete oesophageal obstruction by a food bolus requires urgent treatment. Undue delay may result in pressure necrosis of the oesophageal wall. Recently swallowed lumps of meat can be retrieved using tripod forceps, a snare or a stone retrieval basket. Partly digested food that has been impacted for some hours can often be broken up by biopsy forceps and the fragments then pushed distally to the stomach. After clearing the obstruction, the oesophagus must be carefully inspected, and any suspicious area biopsied. Any stricture present may then be dilated using one of the standard methods (q.v.), though some endoscopists advise that further therapy, following the removal of the impacted material, should await the results of the biopsies and additional investigations as appropriate. In cases of known or suspected achalasia, removal of old food debris from the oesophagus by naso-oesophageal suction may be necessary prior to diagnostic or therapeutic endoscopy, in order to allow visualization of the oesophago-gastric junction. Any residual debris will usually clear spontaneously after balloon dilatation of the cardia, and further specific removal measures are seldom required.

Where an inoperable oesophageal cancer has been treated by palliative intubation, the patient may later present with stent obstruction. Sometimes this is by tumour overgrowth of the prosthesis, but more commonly the lumen is occluded by impacted food. Strict adherence to a dietary regimen of liquidized or soft foods, together with fizzy drinks after each meal, can help to avoid the problem and patients should be provided with a detailed advice sheet after the prosthesis has been inserted. A blocked tube can usually be disimpacted endoscopically using biopsy forceps or a dilator, but occasionally the stent has to be removed and replaced. With the increasing use of expanding metallic mesh endoprostheses, which cannot be removed, preventive measures will assume particular importance.

Other foreign bodies

Very occasionally, swallowed objects such as tablets, coins or safety pins lodge in the oesophagus and require removal. In general, foreign bodies should only be extracted endoscopically when they are unlikely to pass spontaneously through the gastrointestinal tract, and to prevent probable damage to the oesophagus.

Particularly in children, the procedure may be more safely performed under general anaesthesia and with the airway protected by an endotracheal tube. In both children and adults an endoscope overtube technique can be helpful, both for protecting the airway and for avoiding damage to the oesophageal wall during removal of sharp or pointed objects such as razor blades or open safety pins. However, the use of an overtube can produce its own problems, particularly by making adequate insufflation of the upper gastrointestinal tract more difficult. Foreign objects in the oesophagus can be grasped and recovered either by using general purpose devices, including snares and baskets, or specially designed accessories such as coin retrieval forceps; these are available from endoscopic instrument suppliers.

For a more detailed discussion on this topic, and for useful practical hints, the reader is referred to standard texts.[67-69]

Miscellaneous procedures

Obstructing oesophageal cancers which are irresectable or recurrent after earlier treatment can be palliated by injection of a few millilitres of absolute alcohol into the tumour tissue. Such injections are carried out under direct vision using a standard varices needle, and result in immediate blanching of the treated area, with later necrosis. Dysphagia can be improved for several weeks and the procedure then repeated as necessary to maintain luminal patency.[70] This technique can be particularly useful as a rescue measure when tumour tissue is growing over and blocking the proximal end of an oesophageal endoprosthesis.

A cheaper and potentially more widely available alternative to laser therapy for oesophageal tumours is electrocoagulation using a thermal probe. Dilators incorporating a bipolar electrode array can produce much the same improvement in dysphagia as laser treatment but at a much lower cost, although damage to the oesophageal wall occurs if used in non-circumferential tumours.[71] As with laser therapy, repeated applications are necessary in order to maintain symptom relief.

EDITORS NOTE: RIGID OESOPHAGOSCOPY

Kussmaul was the first surgeon to look inside the oesophagus in 1868. He passed a lighted tube through the entire length of the oesophagus, with the patient in a 'sword swallowing' position. In 1881, Von Mickulicz refined the design of the oesophagoscope, when, for the first time, lesions could be biopsied and strictures dilated without the need for surgical exploration. With further refinements in instrumentation by Chevalier Jackson and Negus in the first half of the 20th century, rigid oesophagoscopy was the mainstay of enabling visualization, biopsy, dilatation of strictures, insertion of prosthesis and removal of foreign bodies until the advent of fibreoptic endoscopy, and indeed variceal sclerotherapy was developed using rigid endoscopes.

At the present time, some thoracic surgeons still prefer to use rigid oesophagoscopy, but most surgeons, and particularly gastrointestinal surgeons prefer the superior visualization of fibreoptic endoscopy, the difference being magnified even more with the advent of video endoscopy. Protagonists of rigid endoscopy claim that it has advantages over fibreoptic endoscopy in providing better visualization of lesions proximal to and involving the cricopharyngeal sphincter, by allowing the passage of larger instruments for suction, biopsy and removal of foreign bodies and by enabling dilatation of strictures under direct vision. Disadvantages include the significantly inferior optical system and visualization, the necessity for general anaesthesia, the higher rate of perforation and inability to perform the procedure in patients with rigid cervical spines or with mandibular or dental abnormalities.

If rigid oesophagoscopy is undertaken, careful attention to technique is vital in order to reduce the risk of perforation. Full general anaesthesia with endotracheal intubation is necessary. The patient is positioned supine, with the shoulders slightly raised and facilities to change the position of the head, preferably by an assistant. With the neck flexed, the instrument is introduced over the dorsum of the tongue and is gradually advanced under direct vision as the neck is slightly extended. The instrument passes behind the endotracheal tube, and its tip is brought gently forward. The anterior lip of the instrument is advanced until it lies just behind the interarytenoid fold and then into the cervical oesophagus. Once in the oesophagus, the lumen must be kept in view at all times, which is aided by elevation of the dorsal spine.

REFERENCES

1. Gibbs DD. The history of gastrointestinal endoscopy. In Schiller KFR & Salmon PR (eds). *Modern Topics in Gastrointestinal Endoscopy*. London: Heineman Medical, 1976: 1.
2. Hopkins HH & Kapany NG. A flexible fibrescope using static scanning. *Nature* 1954; **173:** 39.
3. Hirschowitz BJ, Curtis LE, Peters CW & Pollard HM. Demonstrations of a new gastroscope, the fiberscope. *Gastroenterology* 1958; **35:** 50.
4. Sivak MV Jr. Videoendoscopy, the electronic endoscopy unit and

integrated imaging. In Carr-Locke DL (ed.) *Baillières Clinical Gastroenterology*, Vol. 5, no. 1, *Endoscopy Update*. London: Baillière Tindall, 1991: 1.

5. Special Report: Provision of gastrointestinal endoscopy and related services for a district general hospital. *Gut* 1991; **32:** 95.
6. Report: Guidelines for office endoscopic services. *Surg Endos* 1993; **7:** 371.
7. *GP Fundholding Practices: The Provision of Secondary Care.* (HSG 93 14) NHS Management Executive 1993.
8. Report: Gastro-intestinal endoscopy in general practice. *Gut* 1994; **35:** 1342.
9. Hobsley M. Training for digestive surgery. *Gut* 1994; **35:** 1007.
10. Report of a working party on the staffing of endoscopy units. *Gut* 1987; **28:** 1682.
11. Vennes JA, Ament M & Boyce HW Jr. et al. Principles of training in gastrointestinal endoscopy. American Society for Gastrointestinal Endoscopy. Standards of Training Committees. 1989–1990. *Gastrointestinal Endoscopy* 1992; **38(6):** 743–6.
12. Cass OW, Freeman ML, Peine CJ et al. Objective evaluation of endoscopy skills during training. *Ann Intern Med* 1993; **118:** 40.
13. O'Connor HJ & Axon ATR. Gastrointestinal endoscopy: infection and disinfection. *Gut* 1983; **24:** 1067.
14. Axon ATR. Disinfection of endoscopy equipment. In Carr-Locke DL (ed.) *Baillières Clinical Gastroenterology*, Vol. 5, no. 1, *Endoscopy Update*. London: Baillière Tindall, 1991: 61.
15. Lynch DAF, Porter C, Murphy L & Axon ATR. Evaluation of four commercial automated endoscopy washing machines. *Endoscopy* 1992; **24:** 766.
16. Report: Cleaning and disinfection of equipment for gastrointestinal flexible endoscopy. *Gut* 1988; **29:** 1134.
17. Kim-Deobald J, Kozarek R, Ball T et al. Compliance and costs associated with OSHA mandated changes in colonoscopy practice. *Gastroenterology* 1993; **99:** A257.
18. Axon ATR, Banks J, Cockel R, Deverill CFA & Neumann C. Disinfection in upper digestive tract endoscopy in Britain. *Lancet* 1981; **1:** 1093.
19. McAdam JG & Leicester RJ. Incidence of aldehyde sensitivity in endoscopy units. *Gut* 1992; **33:** 852.
20. Control of Substances Hazardous to Health Regulations 1988. Approved code of practice control of substances hazardous to health and approved code of practice control of carcinogenic substances. London: HMSO, 1988.
21. Special report: Aldehyde disinfectants and health in endoscopy units. *Gut* 1993; **34:** 1641.
22. Mansi C, Savarino V, Mela GS, Picciotto A, Mele MR & Celle G. Are clinical patterns of dyspepsia a valid guideline for appropriate use of endoscopy? A report on 2253 dyspeptic patients. *Am J Gastroenterol* 1993; **88:** 1011.
23. McNulty CAM, Dent JC, Uff JS, Gear MWL & Wilkinson SP. Detection of *Campylobacter pylori* by the biopsy urease test: an assessment in 1445 patients. *Gut* 1989; **30:** 1058.
24. Graham DY, Evans DJ, Alpert LC et al. *Campylobacter pylori* detected noninvasively by the 13-C urea breath test. *Lancet* 1987; **i:** 1174.
25. Sobala GM, Crabtree JE, Pentith JA et al. Screening dyspepsia by serology to *Helicobacter pylori*. *Lancet* 1991; **338:** 94.
26. Mountford RA, Brown P, Salmon PR, Alvarenga C, Newman CS & Read AE. Gastric cancer detection in gastric ulcer disease. *Gut* 1980; **21:** 9.
27. Classen M & Roesch W. Gastroscopy, biopsy and cytology in early detection of stomach cancer. In: Grundmann E, Grunze H & Witte S (eds). *Early Gastric Cancer: Current States of Diagnosis*. Berlin. Springer-Verlag. 1974: 113.
28. Quine MA, Bell GD, McCloy RF, Charlton JE, Devlin HB & Hopkins A. Prospective audit of upper gastrointestinal endoscopy in two regions of England: safety, staffing and sedation methods. *Gut* 1995; **36:** 462.
29. Hart R & Classen M. Complications of diagnostic gastrointestinal endoscopy. *Endoscopy* 1990; **22:** 229.
30. Probert CSJ, Jayanthi V, Quinn J & Mayberry JF. Information requirements and sedation preferences of patients undergoing endoscopy of the upper gastrointestinal tract. *Endoscopy* 1991; **23:** 218.
31. Bertoni G, Gumina C & Conigliaro R et al. Randomized placebo-controlled trial of oral liquid simethicone prior to upper gastrointestinal endoscopy. *Endoscopy* 1992; **24:** 268.
32. Hedenbro JL, Frederiksen SG & Lindblom A. Anticholinergic medication in diagnostic endoscopy of the upper gastrointestinal tract. *Endoscopy* 1991; **23:** 199.
33. Sontheimer J, Salm R, Friedrich G, von Wahlert J & Pelz K. Bacteraemia

following operative endoscopy of the upper gastrointestinal tract. *Endoscopy* 1991; **23:** 67.
34. Safrany L. Antibiotic prophylaxis in endoscopy: a new round in old discussion. *Endoscopy* 1991; **23:** 91.
35. Antibiotic prophylaxis in gastrointestinal endoscopy. In: *Guidelines in Gastroenterology*. British Society of Gastroenterology, 1996.
36. Daneshmend TK, Bell GD & Logan RFA. Sedation for upper gastro-intestinal endoscopy: results of a nationwide survey. *Gut* 1991; **32:** 12.
37. Bell GD. Premedication and intravenous sedation for upper gastrointestinal endoscopy. *Aliment Pharmacol Ther* 1990; **4:** 103.
38. Bell GD, McCloy RF, Charlton JE et al. Recommendations for standards of sedation and patient monitoring during gastrointestinal endoscopy. *Gut* 1991; **32:** 823.
39. Lavies NG, Creasy MB, Harris K & Hanning CD. Arterial oxygen saturation during upper gastrointestinal endoscopy: influence of sedation and operator experience. *Am J Gastroenterol* 1988; **83:** 618.
40. Fleischer D. Monitoring the patient receiving conscious sedation for gastrointestinal endoscopy: issue and guidelines. *Gastrointest Endosc* 1989; **35:** 262.
41. Bell GD, Morden A, Bown S, Coady T & Logan RFA. Prevention of hypoxaemia during upper gastrointestinal endoscopy by means of oxygen via nasal cannulae. *Lancet* 1987; **i:** 1022.
42. Murray AW, Morran CG, Kenny GNC & Anderson JR. Arterial oxygen saturation during upper gastrointestinal endoscopy: the effects of a midazolam/pethidine combination. *Gut* 1990; **31:** 270.
43. Thompson AM, Park KGM, Kerr F & Munro A. Safety of fibreoptic endoscopy: analysis of cardiorespiratory events. *Br J Surg* 1992; **79:** 1046.
44. O'Connor HJ. Status epilepticus following administration of flumazenil after endoscopy. *Endoscopy* 1990; **23:** 53.
45. Rai AS & Steer H. The first 15 cm are important in upper gastrointestinal endoscopy. *BMJ* 1993; **306:** 1742.
46. Blackstone MO. *Endoscopic Interpretation: Normal and Pathologic Appearances of the Gastrointestinal Tract*. New York: Raven Press, 1984.
47. Schiller KFR, Cockel R & Hunt RH. *A Colour Atlas of Gastrointestinal Endoscopy*. London: Chapman and Hall, 1986.
48. Silverstein FE & Tytgat GNJ. *Gastrointestinal Endoscopy* (3rd ed.). London: Mosby-Wolfe, 1997.
49. Misiewicz JJ, Forbes A, Price A, Shorvon P, Triger D & Tytgat GNJ. *CD-Atlas of Clinical Gastroenterology*. Aylesford, UK: Times–Mirror International Publishers Ltd, 1994.
50. Bancewicz JH, Matthews HR, O'Hanrahan T & Adams A. A comparison of surgically treated reflux patients in two surgical centres. In Little AG, Ferguson DB & Skinner DB (eds) *Diseases of the Oesophagus*, vol. II. Mount Kiscoe, NY: Futura, 1990: 177.
51. Armstrong D, Monnier PH, Nicolet M, Blum AC & Savary M. Endoscopic assessment of oesophagitis. *Gullet* 1991; **1:** 63.
52. Savary M & Miller G. *The Oesophagus*. Solothurn, Switzerland: Gassmann, 1978.
53. Barrett NR. The lower oesophagus lined by columnar epithelium. *Surgery* 1957; **41:** 881.
54. Atkinson M. Barrett's oesophagus – to screen or not to screen. *Gut* 1989; **30:** 2.
55. Cotton PB. Metallic mesh stents – is the expanse worth the expense? *Endoscopy* 1992; **24:** 421.
56. Lambert R. Endoscopic therapy of esophago-gastric tumours. *Endoscopy* 1992; **24:** 24.
57. Hagenmuller F, Sander C, Sander R, Ries G & Classen M. Laser and endoluminal 192-Iridium radiation. *Endoscopy* 1987; **19** Suppl. 1: 16.
58. Dougherty TJ & Marcus SL. Photodynamic therapy. *Eur J Cancer* 1992; **28A:** 1734.
59. McCaughan JS. Photodynamic therapy of skin and esophageal tumours. *Cancer Invest* 1990; **8:** 407.
60. McCaughan JS, Nims TA, Guy GT et al. Photodynamic therapy for esophageal tumours. *Gastrointest Endosc* 1990; **36:** 85.
61. Sander RR & Poesl H. Cancer of the oesophagus – palliation, laser treatment and combined procedures. *Endoscopy* 1993; **25:** 679.
62. Greig JD, Garden OJ & Carter DC. Prophylactic treatment of patients with oesophageal varices: is it ever justified. *World J Surg* 1994; **18:** 176.
63. Stiegmann GV, Goff JS, Sun JH, Hruza D & Reveille RM. Endoscopic ligation of esophageal varices. *Am J Surg* 1990; **159:** 21.
64. Williams SG & Westaby D. Management of variceal haemorrhage. *BMJ* 1994; **308:** 1213.
65. Gimson AE, Ramaje JK, Panos MZ, Hayllar K, Harrison PM & Williams R. Randomised trial of variceal banding ligation versus injection sclerotherapy for bleeding oesophageal varices. *Lancet* 1993; **342:** 391.

66. Burroughs AK & McCormick PA. Prevention of variceal rebleeding. *Gastroenterol Clin North Am* 1992; **21:** 119.

67. Chung RS. *Therapeutic Endoscopy in Gastrointestinal Surgery.* New York: Churchill Livingstone, 1987.

68. Sanowski RA. Foreign body extraction in the gastrointestinal tract. In Sivak MV Jr (ed.) *Gastroenterologic Endoscopy.* Philadelphia: WB Saunders, 1987: 321.

69. Schiller KFR & Forgacs IC. Foreign bodies in the upper gastrointestinal tract. In Bennett JR & Hunt RH (eds) *Therapeutic Endoscopy and Radiology of the Gut* (2nd edn). London: Chapman & Hall, 1990: 91.

70. Payne-James JJ, Spiller RC, Misiewicz JJ & Silk DBA. Use of ethanol-induced tumour necrosis to palliate dysphagia in patients with esophagogastric cancer. *Gastrointest Endosc* 1990; **36:** 43.

71. Nava HR, Schuh ME, Nambisan R, Clark JL & Douglass HO. Endoscopic ablation of esophageal malignancies with the neodymium-YAG laser and electrofulguration. *Arch Surg* 1989; **124:** 225.

INVESTIGATION OF OESOPHAGEAL FUNCTION

DF Evans

INTRODUCTION

Recent advances in medical technology have had a major impact on diagnostic investigations in the upper gastrointestinal (GI) tract. The scope of this chapter is to outline the wide spectrum of techniques now available to the clinician to aid the diagnosis of diseases of the oesophagus. It is impossible to discuss each method in depth and there are consequently, key references made to the techniques in the various sections which the reader may consult in order to obtain more detail regarding equipment, protocols and interpretation of data from the various investigations available.

General background

Investigation of the oesophagus has progressed somewhat further than that of the remainder of the GI tract. Being the most accessible part of the gut, the oesophagus was soon found to be suitable for examination under direct vision. Crude, rigid telescopes, illuminated by oil lamps were used to examine the oesophageal lumen almost 100 years ago. The discovery of X-rays at the turn of the century also made limited examination of the oesophagus possible but this was greatly enhanced by the development of liquid contrast materials to outline the soft tissues of the GI tract.

Manometric techniques using balloons were utilized when Bayliss and Starling[1] discovered that peristalsis was the force required to drive food into the stomach. Manometry became more accurate and popular with the introduction of water-perfused catheters in the 1950s.

The next major advance in oesophageal investigations did not come until the 1960s with the development of flexible fibreoptic endoscopes, allowing direct vision of the upper GI tract and the additional benefit of tissue sampling and more recently therapeutic procedures; pH measurement for gastro-oesophageal reflux disease was another major step. Described initially in Great Britain,[2,3] developed in the USA[4] and refined to the ambulatory techniques available today,[5] this was another major milestone in oesophageal investigation. Ultrasonography,

magnetic resonance, impedance tomography and radioisotopic methods are other newer techniques developed in the last 20 years which are now in current use by gastroenterologists.

OESOPHAGEAL SYMPTOMS

Oesophageal symptoms can be divided into three major categories. These relate to impairment of the normal passage of food into the stomach, reflux of gastric juice and a variety of symptoms which can be described collectively as motility disorders or perceived sensory abnormalities in the pharynx or oesophagus (functional).

Dysphagia

Dysphagia is a common symptom and may be related to obstructive or functional lesions in the oesophagus. Swallowing difficulties may arise suddenly as the condition progresses to a point where the oesophageal lumen becomes smaller than will allow the unimpeded passage of food by normal peristalsis. Symptoms may worsen progressively, the rate of change often being determined by the type of obstruction. In benign conditions such as reflux stricture or achalasia, symptom progression may be slow, over one or more years. With malignant lesions, symptom progression is often more rapid as the tumour mass encloses the oesophageal lumen. Dysphagia is associated in many patients with accompanying weight loss, sometimes severe and up to 10–15% of body weight before presentation.

Dysphagia can be associated with gastro-oesophageal reflux disease (GORD), in which case it is often secondary to other more typical symptoms such as heartburn and weight loss is rarely present.

Regurgitation

Regurgitation of non-acid material (swallowed food) is often associated with dysphagia and is a result of retained food contained within the oesophageal body above an obstruction or lower oesophageal sphincter incompetence. Some patients complain of regurgitation of white, frothy mucous. This is probably a mixture of swallowed saliva and oesophageal mucous possibly lying on the surface of other retained food. A perception of heartburn with dysphagia may be attributed to retained food fermenting in the oesophageal lumen producing lactic acid (pH4–5).[6,7]

Pain

In some obstructive oesophageal diseases, chest pain, sometimes radiating to the back, is reported. This is thought to be caused by oesophageal wall spasm induced by the presence of retained food and saliva entrapped above the obstruction. The pain can be severe and debilitating and often mimics angina-like cardiac pain and may be mistaken for ischaemic heart disease (IHD). The term 'irritable oesophagus' has been used to describe patients who, as a result of luminal oesophageal stimulation, experience chest pain.[8]

Heartburn

Heartburn is the classical oesophageal symptom related to gastro-oesophageal reflux of gastric juice (GOR). Burning retrosternal pain is synonymous with the term heartburn and is also described in relation to GOR. Occasionally, chest pains may be described as 'crushing' and dull and misdiagnosed as angina. A significant proportion of patients with angina-like chest pain may have been initially investigated by cardiologists suspicious of IHD.[9]

Epigastric pain

Epigastric pain is another common symptom experienced in patients with GORD. The pain probably originates from the sensory nerves in the mucosa or deeper tissues at the gastro-oesophageal junction and is directly related to local pain transmission caused by direct contact with acidic gastric juice.

Pain and heartburn may also result from luminal exposure to other corrosive substances. Pepsin and refluxed duodenal juices, containing proteolytic enzymes and bile, have been found in oesophageal refluxate in some patients. The severity and progression of acid-related diseases may well be related to the nature of the refluxate,[10,11] but as yet acid remains the major culprit.

Symptom progression

In the early, acute phase of the acid-related oesophageal diseases, heartburn and burning epigastric pain are common but these are often replaced by regurgitation, chest pain and dysphagia as the disease progresses. This change may come about by some reduction in the sensitivity of the oesophageal mucosa as tissue is constantly exposed to gastric juice and undergoing the process of inflammation and healing. Replacement of mucosa with fibrous tissue may give rise to stricture formation in advanced disease or in the elderly and in some cases the damaged oesophageal mucosa may be replaced by columnar type gastric epithelium, 'Barrett's oesophagus', first described by Norman Barrett in 1950.[12]

Pharyngeal symptoms

High oesophageal, pharyngeal and laryngeal symptoms may be caused by disorders of the respiratory system, neurological problems or diseases of the oropharynx or larynx. However, some oesophageal disorders are experienced as upper oropharyngolaryngeal symptoms due to referred sensation from below, or as a secondary manifestation of the oesophageal disorder. For example, dysphagia is often perceived as a sensation of globus (a lump in the throat) even though the obstruction may be lower in the oesophagus.[13] Acid regurgitation into the mouth can damage the oropharynx and vocal cords and has also recently been associated with tooth wear.[14] GORD has also been associated with hoarseness, chronic wheeze and nocturnal asthma, these symptoms being associated with aspiration of gastric refluxate into the respiratory tree.[15]

In children in particular, some respiratory problems in infancy have been shown to have a definite association with regurgitation and aspiration of gastric contents and investigation for GOR is often undertaken when children present with apnoea, cyanosis, respiratory arrest or even near-miss sudden infant death.[16] Intraoesophageal pH measurement for GOR is often the first non-respiratory investigation undertaken when a cause for these symptoms is in doubt. A 24 h pH study is less hazardous, technically less demanding and can, in some cases, lead to a positive diagnosis, whether the investigation is positive or negative, than other more hazardous tests in young children. Barium radiology and endoscopy are more difficult to perform in the very young and a diagnosis by exclusion is therefore more likely to be sought if the investigation is safe and easy to perform.[17]

OESOPHAGEAL MANOMETRY

The measurement of motility for functional studies of the oesophagus has become an increasingly useful investigation in recent years. Motility of oesophageal smooth muscle is controlled by the myenteric plexus and is responsible for efficient transport of a food bolus from the pharnyx into the stomach. Abnormal oesophageal motility may result in dysphagia chest pain, often mistaken for cardiac pain and regurgitation of swallowed food with the complication of aspiration into the airways in some cases.

Oesophageal manometry was first developed in its present form in the 1950s[18] and at one stage was heralded as a means of diagnosis of GORD by measurement of lower oesophageal sphincter (LOS) pressure. However, with the advent of endoscopy and pH monitoring, manometry is now considered to be more useful in identifying LOS position and function for pH electrode positioning and to investigate patients in whom a motility disorder is suspected. The major role for oesophageal manometry in clinical use is the investigation of dysphagia and chest pain and other symptoms undiagnosed by radiology, endoscopy or pH monitoring. Recently, the development of ambulatory manometry is proving useful in patients with intermittent or infrequent symptoms suggestive of oesophageal spasm.

Techniques

Perfused tube

The mainstay technique for measurement of motility of the upper GI tract in humans involves the water perfused tube. This method is suitable for measurements not only in the oesophagus but also in the antrum, small intestine, biliary tract and colon.[19]

A soft, usually plastic, multilumen tube with side holes placed along its length is positioned at the desired site by intubation per oram or transnasally. Each port is simultaneously perfused with water or saline by a pneumohydraulic pump[20] at a flow rate determined by the desired frequency response of the system (faster flow rates for higher frequency detection, as in the oesophagus). Occlusion of the side hole in any pressure channel by contraction of the oesophageal wall causes a rise in pressure in that channel. The diameter of the catheter is usually determined by the number of recording ports (typically 2–3 mm for up to four channels and 3–5 mm up to eight channels). However, the diameter of the catheter is also important in the resultant pressure measured and larger diameter catheters will overestimate pressure when compared with smaller diameter types.[21] The pressure rise is detected by an in-line pressure transducer connected to a recording device (analogue pen recorder or computer-driven system supported by an analogue to digital conversion unit).

Figure 4.1 illustrates the essential parts of the water perfused system. These systems are almost exclusively used as static measuring systems due to the bulky nature of the pressure detection apparatus. Modified perfused tube systems can be used in a portable recording apparatus in which case the perfusion pump is replaced by a battery-operated microsyringe infusion pump. This technique is not widely used as telemetry capsules and microtransducers offer a more convenient and easy to use alternative.

Radiotelemetry capsules

Radiotelemetry capsules (RTC) have been available since the 1960s and offer the potential for less-invasive monitoring of motility in the GI tract in comparison with intubation methods. They also offer the potential for ambulatory recordings, a trend that has become increasingly attractive in recent years.[22] RTCs are small pressure-sensitive radio transmitters that are swallowed. If untethered, they move through the GI tract unhindered, transmitting information relating to intraluminal pressure. If tethered, they behave in a similar way to a perfused tube. Two or more RTCs can be tethered together to detect propulsion and peristalsis. Untethered RTCs are more useful in the colon where movement of luminal content is slow and infrequent. New methods are being developed to implant RTCs in the gut lumen using an endoscopically guided sewing machine.[23]

Signals from RTCs are detected by a body-borne aerial belt,

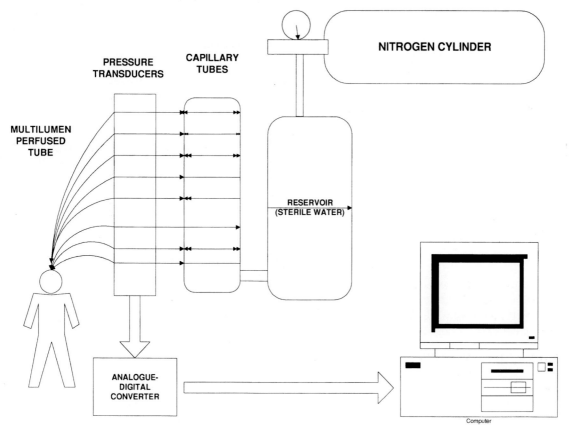

Figure 4.1
Schematic diagram illustrating the essential parts of a water-perfused oesophageal manometry system.

decoded by a dedicated radioreceiver and recorded on to pen recorders or ambulatory data loggers (see below). In the oesophagus, the use of RTCs is either tethered to prevent caudad movement of the device or by implantation. Neither of these methods is particularly suitable for human studies but implanted capsules are at present being used in animal research where they can be used at any site within the GI tract as semipermanent pressure sensors, transmitting pressure information for several months.[24]

Strain gauge microtransducers

Miniature strain gauges mounted on small, flexible catheters are becoming increasingly popular in the measurement of oesophageal motility. Although expensive (£500–1000 per channel), they obviate the need for water perfusion and can be used more easily in ambulatory measurements.[25] Even in static systems, they have some advantages over perused tubes. The requirement for supine measurements in pull-through studies is overcome as the zero pressure reference is not dependent on the catheter position and transducer height remaining constant

Electrical strain gauges deform when a positive or negative pressure is applied to the surface. This deformation is generally produced by contracting smooth muscle (and corresponding gut wall movement), but a pressure rise in the lumen is required to alter the electrical output. In organs with a large viscus (i.e. gastric fundus) other techniques may be more representative of motor function such as the barostat.[26] In the oesophagus, barostat studies are possible but are not currently being widely used outside research applications.

Sleeve sensors

Dent sleeve During certain manoeuvres such as deep breathing, after food and during oesophageal peristalsis, there is a tendency for the position of the LOS to alter in relation to a fixed point and this makes accurate siting of a pressure sensor in the LOS difficult, especially for prolonged measurements. To overcome this problem, Dent devised a thin, 6 cm, open-ended, silastic sleeve which surrounds the most distal perfused port of a multilumen catheter, specifically to facilitate LOS measurements.[27] The function of the sleeve is to straddle the high pressure zone of the LOS to record the average circumferential and axial pressure as a resultant of all forces acting on the sleeve. The LOS may move by up to ± 2 cm in relation to the sleeve without compromising the pressure detection (Figure 4.2). The Dent sleeve is recommended for all prolonged measurements of LOS pressure where the catheter is fixed, i.e. no pull-through measurements. Clearly, the sleeve is perfused and is therefore used mainly in non-ambulant studies.

Sphinctometer For prolonged ambulatory studies of LOS pressure, a device called a 'sphinctometer' has been developed[28] and subsequently commercially manufactured (Gaeltec Ltd, Isle of Skye, Scotland). This device is sited at the most distal port of a multichannel microtransducer catheter and consists of a side-mounted strain gauge surrounded by a silicone oil-filled silastic tube of 6 cm in length of the same diameter as the catheter.

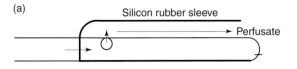

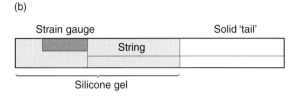

Figure 4.2
Schematic diagram illustrating the principles of the Dent sleeve (a) and sphinctometer (b).

The oil-filled segment detects both circumferential and radial forces, in a similar way to the Dent sleeve, and the length of the detecting segment helps to overcome the possibility of positional changes in LOS position (Figure 4.2). The device has been fully evaluated both technically[28] and clinically[29] and is currently in use by many gastroenterologists in the UK in pathophysiological studies of oesophageal dysfunction.[30]

Motility measurement techniques

Three main techniques are employed using the above types of transducers.

Static sensor

Transducers are sited in the desired part of the oesophagus and tethered from without. Recordings of function are made for the required period on suitable recording devices. Figure 4.3 is an example from a 24 h combined pH and pressure recording derived from a three-channel strain gauge catheter and two channel pH catheter sited in the oesophagus. The sensors are sited in the (LOS), and at 7.5 & 15 cm proximal in the oesophageal body. pH channels are at 5 and 20 cm proximal to the LOS. The figure depicts a series of water swallows demonstrating normal peristalsis and LOS relaxation, which is detected by the sphinctometer as described above.

Pull-through

These techniques are most useful for LOS measurements. Technically, the most important property of the measuring catheter is the ability to detect pressure at different points around its circumference. This is achieved with either radially mounted sensors at the same level (minimum 3 (120°), maximum 8 (45°)), or staggered along the length of the catheter where the radial LOS measurement is achieved during station pull-through. These catheters are essential to accurately map LOS pressure as it is well known that the LOS is radially asymmetrical.[31] Single measurements at only one point on the circumference of the LOS will almost certainly over-or underestimate the true sphincter pressure.

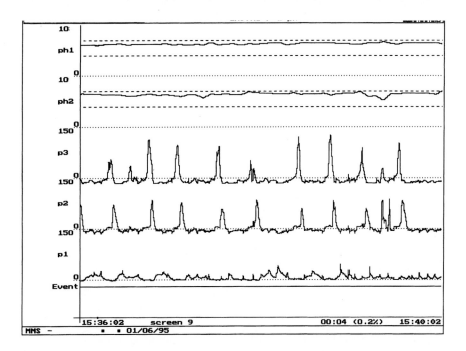

Figure 4.3
Section of a 24 h recording of oesophageal motility using a three channel strain gauge transducer incorporating a sphinctometer (P1) and two oesophageal body channels (P3 proximal and P2 distal). Two pH channels at 5 (pH2) and 20 cm (pH1) detect GOR. Swallowing is associated with LOS relaxation and peristalsis. No GOR is evident in this trace.

Station pull-through

The recording ports are passed beyond the LOS and withdrawn in small increments (usually 0.5–1 cm), recordings being made at each station for a sufficient period to give a stable reading. Figure 4.4 is an example of a station pull-through the lower oesophageal sphincter and oesophageal body using a three-channel water-perfused catheter with 5 cm separation between sensors. The figure illustrates the response of the LOS and oesophageal body to 5 ml water swallows.

Rapid pull-through

This technique, using similar equipment to that above, requires a steady, continuous withdrawal of the recording ports through the sphincter. This is best achieved by a mechanical puller. The technique is to pull the catheter through the LOS at a continuous steady rate (0.5–1 cm/s) while the patient holds their breath. This allows LOS pressure to be measured without the interference of respiration. Technically, the measurement is more demanding as it requires a higher frequency responsive system to accurately detect the rapid rise and fall in pressure.

Sphincter measurements

LOS

LOS pressure measurements are used to document pressure, length and relaxation and as such give the majority of information required to characterize the sphincter functionally. The recording of radial pressures from many ports at the same level has facilitated the production of three-dimensional images of

LOS morphology in addition to the other data referred to as 'vector volume'.[32,33] The technique, first developed in the anorectum can be used to produce three-dimensional visual images of LOS pressure profiles which may be useful where sphincter defects are to be corrected.

Upper oesophageal sphincter

The upper oesophageal sphincter (UOS) is morphologically derived from the striated crycopharyngeus muscle located behind the hyoid bone. This sphincter has a tonic pressure substantially higher than the LOS and a dynamic response in keeping with striated muscle in the high velocity of opening and closure in response to swallowing. In consequence, measurement of UOS function requires higher fidelity measuring equipment in comparison to the other parts of the oesophagus.

Manometric assessment of the UOS comprises measurements of position, intrinsic tone with due attention paid to radial asymmetry, relaxation and the relationship of relaxation to pharyngeal and oesophageal contractions. The perfused tube catheter does not have a frequency response fast enough to follow UOS dynamics so micro strain-gauge transducers are recommended for the accurate assessment of this sphincter. Static and station pull-through protocols are the most widely used methods to examine the function of the UOS and detailed information regarding the equipment and methodology have been well described.[34]

In relation to the investigation of the UOS in patients with dysphagia, UOS abnormalities are rarely found in the majority of swallowing problems and most are limited to patients with neurological problems in spite of the frequency of globus type

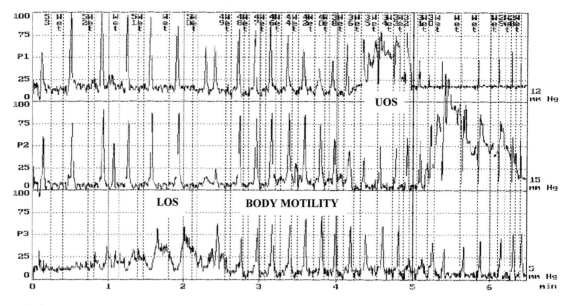

Figure 4.4

Computer generated oesophageal station pull-through manometry. A three lumen perfused catheter, 5 cm spacing (ch 1- proximal (15 cm from tip), ch2- middle, ch3-distal (5 cm from tip)) is progressively pulled through the LOS and oesophageal body (stations in cm at top of trace – all measurements from tip of catheter). Wet swallows (marked 'wet') 5 ml water are associated with peristalsis (channels 1 and 2) and LOS relaxation (first 3 min of channel 3). The upper sphincter (UOS) pull through (sustained high pressure in ch1 and 2) appears towards the end of the trace.

symptoms and high dysphagia reported by patients at consultation.

Prolonged ambulatory recordings

In recent years, gastroenterologists have recognized that the symptoms of disordered GI function are often intermittent and that representative measurements may be better obtained by prolonged recordings. Furthermore, circadian changes in gut biorhythms require that measurements are made to span a normal daily cycle. This requirement, together with the rapid

development in computer technology has seen the introduction of digital recording systems. These have sufficient memory capacity and on-board computer processing power to allow high fidelity recordings from multichannel sensors for long periods, in some cases over many days. Equipment is battery powered, lightweight and portable and allows for almost total ambulation during measurement.[35] This means that not only are recordings made in near-physiological conditions, but also that patients can undergo studies in their homes and workplace. Event markers also allow for correlation between symptoms and abnormalities in the measured parameter.

(a)

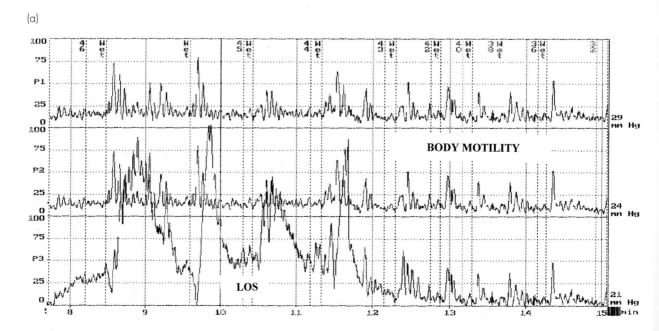

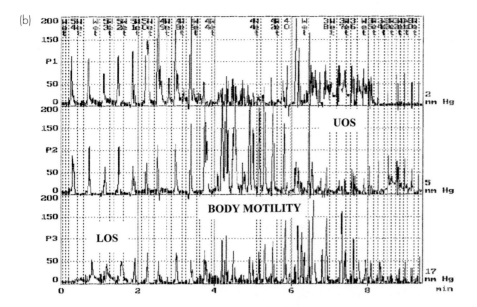

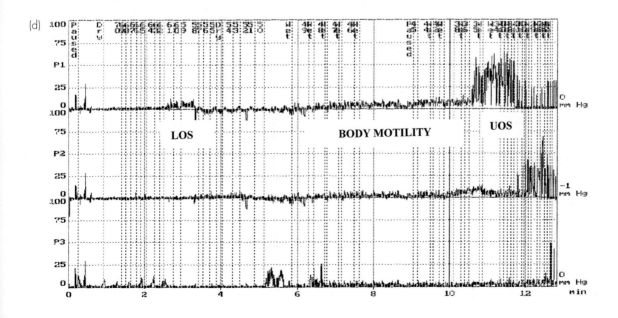

Figure 4.5
Computer generated oesophageal station pull-through manometry of four specific oesophageal motor disorders. (a) Achalasia; high pressure, non-relaxation in LOS. Simultaneous, repetitive oesophageal body motility. (b) Diffuse oesophageal spasm: Normal LOS. Mixed simultaneous and peristaltic body motility with repetive waves. Very high amplitude (max. 240 mmHg). (c) 'Nutcracker' oesophagus: normal LOS. High pressure (max. 210 mmHg) body motility but normal peristaltic sequences in response to liquid and solid swallows. (d) Scleroderma: total absence of all LOS and body motility. Some residual contractility in striated oesophagus (20–22 cm from nose). Normal UOS function.

The development of such technology has also added the ability to analyse recordings with sophisticated computer software programs providing further benefits of both time-savings and the rapid acquisition of accurate, repeatable, unbiased information derived from large quantities of data.[36,37]

Diagnostic yield

Oesophageal manometry is most useful in the diagnosis or confirmation of motility disorders. It is not a substitute for radiology, endoscopy or pH monitoring, but, when used in conjunction with these investigations can yield important information which is relevant in diagnosis and management. In general, static studies are most useful in detection of motility abnormalities that are continuously present and not readily diagnosed by radiology or endoscopy, such is achalasia. Prolonged ambulatory studies are best used for diagnosis of diffuse oesophageal spasm where abnormal motor patterns may be only present for brief periods and may be missed by the 'snapshot' view seen during static studies.[38,39]

Table 4.1 lists the disorders best diagnosed with oesophageal manometry and Figure 4.5(a–d) illustrates examples of manometric patterns of the four commonest abnormalities, achalasia, diffuse oesophageal spasm (DOS), nutcracker oesophagus and scleroderma.

OESOPHAGEAL pH MEASUREMENTS

Gastro-oesophageal reflux disease (GORD) is the commonest acid-related disorder of the oesophagus affecting 35–60% of the adult population of the Western world at some time in their lives.[40] The accurate diagnosis of GORD can be complicated by the absence of endoscopic oesophagitis in up to 40% of patients[41] and in some cases, a poor correlation with symptoms. Many investigations have been developed to aid diagnosis, including manometry and endoscopy but neither of these detect the presence of gastric juice in the oesophagus. Intraoesophageal pH recording was first described in the late 1960s, refined by DeMeester and colleagues and subsequently developed as an ambulatory technique. Ambulatory pH measurement, is now thought to be the best discriminator between physiological and pathological reflux[42] and is regarded as the gold standard in the diagnosis of reflux disease. pH monitoring is simple and inexpensive to perform, with little discomfort to the patient and requires a minimum of specialized skills.[43]

In acid disorders such as GORD or in gastric or duodenal acid-related conditions, it is sometimes useful to measure gastric pH. Some years ago, when peptic ulcer disease posed a serious problem, it was common to measure acid secretion by aspiration of gastric content. In recent years it is now accepted that prolonged intraluminal pH measurements give a more representative picture of acid status and the methodology developed for the oesophagus has been adapted for gastric measurement.[44,45] In association with simultaneous oesophageal pH monitoring, gastric acid measurements can yield additional information regarding alkaline reflux[46] and the efficacy of acid suppression therapy.[47,48]

Methodology

Sensors

Miniature (< 2 mm), glass or antimony electrodes are available with either combined or external reference electrodes. Combined electrodes are usually larger in diameter (> 3 mm diameter) and more expensive. Antimony electrodes are constructed from monocrystalline or polycrystalline antimony, but both types appear to function effectively in clinical practice. Most antimony electrodes have a working life of around 5 days of continuous measurement due to oxidation of the surface of the sensor. Glass electrodes have a longer life but are more fragile. Some electrodes are semidisposable and are inexpensive, but reusable glass electrodes with a combined reference are probable more accurate, especially in a highly acidic environment such as the stomach and sometimes, the oesophagus. A glass, cable-free radiotelemetry capsule is also available but is mainly used for research purposes. This device is, however, essential if pH profiles of the small intestine beyond the duodenum are made. In this case, a free-fall RTC recording on to a dedicated receiver–recorder system is used.[49]

Recorders

Recorders, like those for pressure, have seen much development. Most are digital, portable and solid-state.[50] Ambulatory, out-patient recordings are desirable in order to express acid states physiologically. Most recorders incorporate event markers to document symptoms, meals and upright and supine periods, all important for the accurate diagnosis and categorization of pathological GOR.

Procedure

The pH sensor is introduced transnasally or orally and the distal oesophageal sensor (or tip sensor if only one sensor is used) is positioned 5 cm proximal to the lower oesophageal sphincter, this being determined by manometry. Some workers position the sensor by measurements taken at endoscopy, radiology or by a pH withdrawal technique, but manometry is the

Table 4.1 Common disorders of motility best diagnosed by manometry

Achalasia of the cardia
Diffuse oesophageal spasm
Scleroderma
'Nutcracker' oesophagus
Hypertensive/hypotensive lower oesophageal sphincter
Non-specific motility disorder (NSMD)

Figure 4.6
Prolonged pH traces from distal oesophagus. Traces (a)–(c) illustrate increasing severity of GOR. Symptoms are indicated by the vertical dotted lines and sometimes correlate with reflux episodes. Meals ■ and sleep ▨ are indicated on the upper border.

(a)
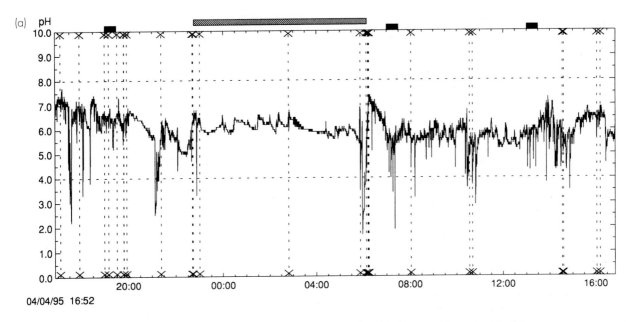
04/04/95 16:52

(b)
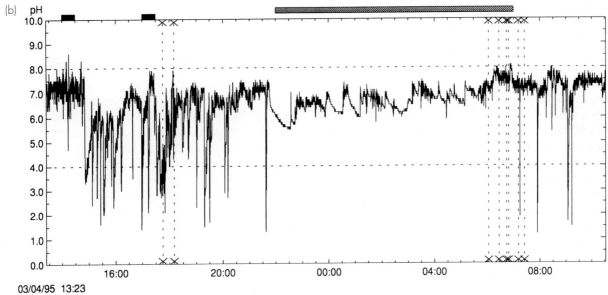
03/04/95 13:23

(c)
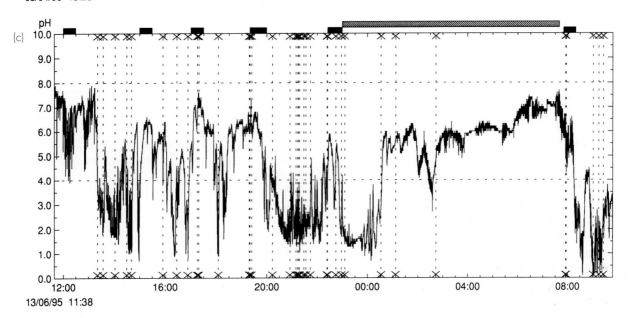
13/06/95 11:38

most accurate positioning method and is the only recommended technique. For investigators without manometry facilities, there are commercially available LOS finders which consist of portable pressure indicators which detect the LOS high pressure zone. An alternative, inexpensive method to determine LOS position comprises a small, graduated catheter with an inflatable balloon at the tip to locate the gastro-oesophageal junction.[51] This technique is perfectly satisfactory but does require an additional intubation.

pH sensors may have an internal reference, but when an external reference is used, this is sited high on the chest over a bony area and secured with adhesive tape. The pH sensor lead is usually brought out nasally, fixed to the cheek with waterproof adhesive tape and connected to the recorder by routing the cable underneath the clothing. This enables the patient to undress without disconnection and is also more cosmetically acceptable.

pH measurements should be performed for 24 h ideally but shorter periods are permitted. It is essential to include at least one or two meals and the nocturnal period, so the minimum period is probably around 18 h. This is to ensure that postprandial and nocturnal GOR is assessed. Studies should be performed under near physiological conditions and patients should be encouraged to perform normal daily activities where possible. During diagnostic tests, free access to normal meals, smoking and alcohol should be allowed, but these events should be documented. Antireflux medication is usually withdrawn for up to 5 days prior to study (5 days proton pump inhibitors, 2 days H_2 receptor antagonists and prokinetics, 24 h antacids and alginates), but in some circumstances may be continued, in which case the investigation may be useful in assessing the efficacy of treatment. This is particularly helpful when medication appears ineffective in controlling symptoms. Dual oesophageal and gastric pH recordings are particularly useful to detect failure of acid inhibitors and to document alkaline reflux, although the latter is not common (see below).

Figure 4.6 illustrates three 24 h recordings taken from patients with symptoms of GOR. Figure 4.6a–c illustrate increasing severity of GOR. In Figure 4.6(a) a reflux episodes are infrequent and of short duration. They are also limited to the daytime period. Figure 4.6(b) shows a greater frequency and duration of daytime GOR but again, nothing of note at night. Figure 4.6(b) is taken from a patient with severe GORD. GOR is seen during both day and night and acid clearance is also poor. This patient is more likely to become a candidate for surgery.

Multichannel pH measurement

Many recorders now have the capability of recording two or more channels of pH. With two or more sensors, the reference sensor is always the distal oesophageal site (5 cm above LOS) and the other sensors may then be positioned above or below at intervals set by the interelectrode distance (usually 5, 10, 15 or 20 cm). These studies are particularly useful in more detailed examinations of acid and alkaline levels around the

Table 4.2   Indications for multichannel pH recording

ADULT	PAEDIATRICS
Oesophageal – Distal and proximal measurements	
Regurgitation	Vomiting
Hoarseness	Cyanosis/apnoea
Wheeze/asthma	Near miss cot death
Palatal tooth wear	Chest infection
Duodenogastric or gastro-oesophageal	
Acid suppression treatment failures (on therapy)	
Suspected duodenogastric alkaline reflux	

gastro-oesophageal junction. Table 4.2 outlines a number of combinations of multisite electrode positions that may prove useful in investigation of pH around the gastro-oesophageal junction. The choice of electrode position is dictated by the specific requirement of the measurement, but up to four sites can be chosen with currently available technology. A number of important areas of measurement are worthy of more detailed description.

Combined pH and pressure measurements

With recent advances in computer technology, the last few years have seen the introduction of data loggers with high capacity solid-state memory and multichannel recording facilities. This type of equipment is useful in the investigation of unexplained, non-cardiac chest pain (NCCP). Prior to this, combined, ambulatory, oesophageal pressure and pH recordings could only be achieved using a tape-based system.[35]

The objective of such recordings is the simultaneous monitoring of oesophageal motility, LOS function and pH. This enables a comparison of abnormalities of motility and GOR and any correlation with symptoms. Technically, the recordings can be achieved easily, using solid-state multichannel microtransducers, either combined with one or two pH channels, or as is more common, separate from the pH electrode. The investigation is more demanding for the patient due to the presence of a larger single catheter, or two catheters and for the investigator because of the more complex analysis and interpretation of the recording.

Some publications[36,37] have suggested that the major use of combined recordings is the investigation of NCCP caused by diffuse oesophageal spasm. The test is also useful for exclusion of oesophageal pain as a cause of NCCP as, sometimes, patients with microvascular angina can be missed on initial cardiological investigations. At present, in our practice, combined recordings are limited to patients who have no oesophagitis, normal pH and stationary manometry, but who remain symptomatic.

Figure 4.7 illustrates a patient with high pressure contractions in the oesophageal body with simultaneous GOR and associated symptoms. The abnormal motility is consistent with diffuse oesophageal spasm. The infrequency of the abnormal motility with GOR is not likely to be detected by conventional stationary manometry.

(a)

(b)

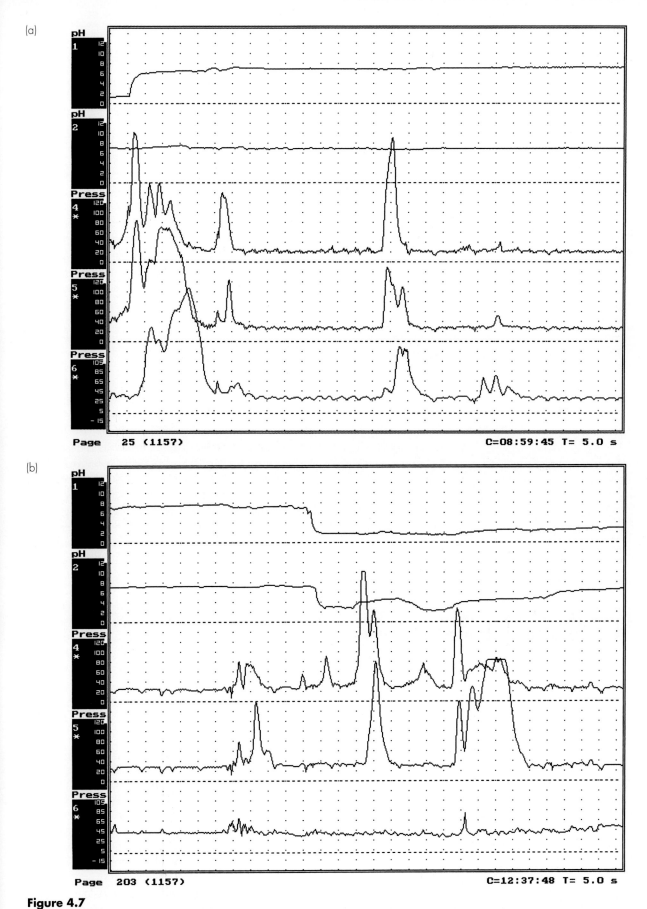

Figure 4.7
Combined pressure (ch4–6 prox to distal oesophageal body) and pH recordings (pH1 – 5 cm prox to LOS and pH 2 at 10 cm) showing oesophageal spasm with (a) and without (b) associated GOR. (Courtesy of Dr A Raimundo, Central Middlesex Hospital, London.)

Acid suppression efficacy

A significant cohort of patients respond poorly to acid suppression medication, even at high doses. It has been suggested that about one in six patients with long-standing, chronic, relapsing GORD may require continuous long-term treatment with acid suppression drugs (H₂ receptor antagonists or proton pump inhibitors) in order to obtain acceptable symptom relief.[47] Before embarking on such a strategy, pH studies of gastric and oesophageal pH can be helpful in establishing the degree of acid suppression achieved with a particular treatment regime and may also be useful in titration of the optimal dose of therapy in individual patients.

Prolonged dual-channel pH studies are performed with the distal sensor sited 10 cm below the gastro-oesophageal junction and the proximal sensor in the standard position (5 cm above LOS) while the patient continues to take acid suppression therapy. The degree of acid suppression as measured by gastric pH (% time <pH4), the amount of GOR (% time <pH4) and the symptom profile and correlation will determine how efficient the acid suppression is in a particular individual. Figure 4.8 shows a 24 h dual gastric and oesophageal pH trace in a patient taking 40 mg omeprazole nocte, but with continuing symptoms. In this case, the patient is seen to continue to experience symptomatic GOR because the degree of acid inhibition is insufficient to maintain gastric pH>4 for a significant time period during the study.

A systematic study from our own group showed a variable response to high dose acid-suppressing drugs in 15% of patients undergoing investigation for GORD (n=20). In this group, acid suppression was suboptimal with a median percentage (%) time gastric pH<4 of 37.5%. GOR was reduced in some, the median % time pH<4 being 1.5% (0–58), although symptoms continued to be experienced in spite of therapy.[48] Alkaline reflux or duodenogastric alkaline reflux may be another reason, which is detectable by dual oesophageal and gastric pH monitoring and Bilitec™ monitoring.

Oropharyngo-oesophageal pH measurement

Multisite pH measurements in the oesophageal body have been advocated as a more sensitive measurement than single site alone, especially where reflux is thought to cause atypical symptoms. A good example of this is where patients complain of regurgitation with associated sore throat, dysphonia, wheeze and hoarseness of voice. A small group of patients suffering from nocturnal asthma have been shown to have coincidental GORD and in these, GOR may be contributory to the asthma.[52]

A dual channel pH study, with the proximal site positioned high in the oesophagus or above the upper sphincter in the pharynx will determine whether reflux into the distal oesophagus migrates proximally and also whether this proximal spread is associated with the symptoms outlined above. Figure 4.9 illustrates such a recording in a patient with symptoms of regurgitation of gastric juice into the mouth with associated chronic hoarseness of voice and laryngitis. The distal probe is sited 5 cm above the LOS and the proximal site of 15 cm above, high in the oesophagus or pharynx. A proportion of

GOR episodes are seen to migrate to the proximal site in spite of the patient being asymptomatic for most of the time.

In dentistry, tooth erosion, particularly at the palatal surface of the incisor teeth, is regarded as being associated with regurgitation of gastric juice into the mouth[53] and recent research has shown a clear correlation with GOR and toothwear in patients with symptoms of regurgitation.[14] Bartlett et al. have shown that measurements of oral, pharyngeal and distal oesophageal pH are useful in the detection of GOR in dental patients with tooth erosion but who are not necessarily undergoing consultations for GORD. Oral acidification with associated distal reflux showed good evidence for an association between the two events. They also demonstrated good correlation between oral and pharyngeal acidification suggesting that a high level of GOR in the pharynx is strongly suggestive of oral regurgitation and toothwear. If this is the case, then dual site oesophageal pH studies can be a useful tool to detect GOR as a possible cause for tooth wear.

Alkaline reflux

A small proportion of patients with GOR symptoms may be refluxing either alkaline or mixed alkaline and acid secretions. Alkaline reflux emanates from the duodenum and may contain bile and has been shown to reflux into the stomach with the potential for further reflux into the oesophagus. The combination of acid and pepsin together with bile and pancreatic enzymes may be a more corrosive mixture than acid alone and may therefore be more injurious than acid alone, producing the most severe form of mucosal injury.[54] In terms of therapy, acid inhibitors may actually worsen symptoms as any neutralization of alkaline secretions will be lost by the acid suppression of alkaline reflux. Single site, distal oesophageal pH measurement was initially advocated as a method of detecting alkaline reflux[42] but multisite (gastric and pH) methods are preferable.

In the early days of pH measurement, alkaline reflux was said to exist if oesophageal pH rose above pH 8 for any time period. Two difficulties exist here. First, some ingested food may be >pH8 (for example tea and milky drinks) and without a careful diary may lead to inaccuracies. Secondly, it is conceivable that a mixture of alkaline secretions from the duodenum and acid juice may result in a slightly acidic (pH4–6) or even neutral pH and this mixture refluxing into the oesophagus will be ignored by standard analytical criteria as being within normal limits (>pH4 and <pH8). The refluxate may, however, be highly corrosive to the oesophageal mucosa and give rise to symptoms thus confusing diagnosis and symptom correlation. Iftikhar et al.[55] measured oesophageal bile acids, pH and symptoms in Barrett's oesophagus, a condition known to be more prone to alkaline reflux. They measured the pH of various mixtures of bile and gastric juice and determined that large quantities of alkaline juice are required to raise the pH to >8.

Oesophageal pH measurement alone is, therefore, of limited use in the detection of alkaline reflux and alternative methods have been tested. The simultaneous measurement of gastric

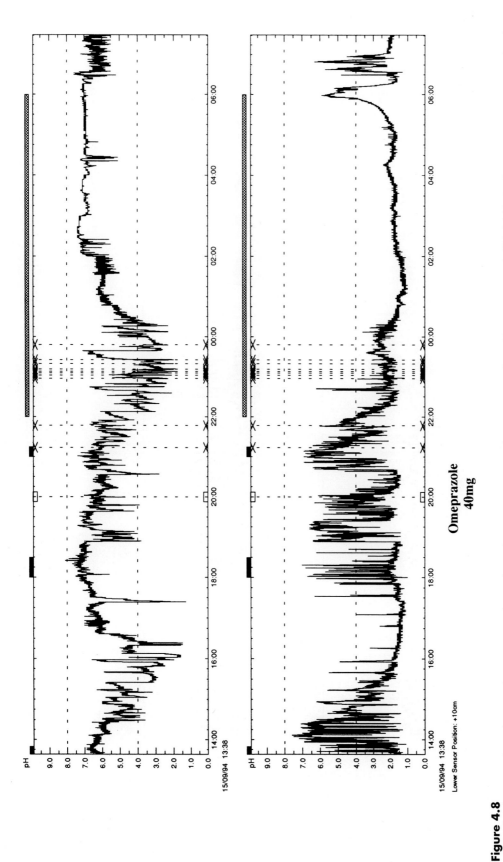

Figure 4.8

Twenty four hour two-channel gastric (lower trace) and oesophageal (upper trace) pH study in a patient taking 40 mg omeprazole (20.00 h). Acid suppression is not optimal and symptomatic reflux continues to be symptomatic, especially at night.

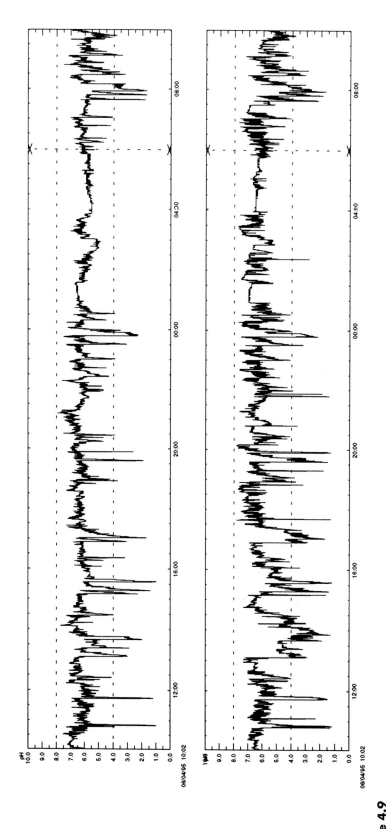

Figure 4.9

Two-channel distal oesophageal (5 cm from LOS) and proximal oesophageal (20 cm from LOS) pH recording the migration of asymptomatic GOR into the pharynx in a patient with dysphonia, globus and wheeze.

and oesophageal pH has been put forward as a viable alternative, whereby the simultaneous detection of either acid–alkaline mixture in the stomach (pH>4 and <7) or true alkaline juice (>pH7) in the stomach, together with alkacid (pH>4 and <7) or alkaline (pH>8) in the oesophagus, reflects true alkaline reflux as measured by pH alone. Mattioli et al.[46,56] have produced convincing evidence of this phenomenon and have advocated a minimum of three pH measurement sites as being necessary (gastric body and fundus and distal oesophagus). Figure 4.10 illustrates a three channel pH measurement (after Mattioli) showing periods of alkaline reflux that affect both gastric and oesophageal pH.

Other methods of oesophageal bile measurement Because the detection of oesophageal alkaline reflux by pH alone is difficult, a number of alternative methods have been developed. Gotley et al.[51,58] described an aspiration method whereby oesophageal aspirates were examined by higher performance liquid chromatography (HPLC) for the presence of bile salts. The methodology is difficult because of the simultaneous presence of gastric acid, which contaminates the refluxate and makes chemical analysis difficult and also the requirement of an additional aspiration catheter and continuous suction to collect samples.

However, this group and others[55] have shown high concentrations of oesophageal bile acid in specific patient groups and it is likely in clinical practice that a small but significant group of patients with reflux symptoms may need some form of alkaline reflux assessment in order to determine the correct diagnosis.

Sodium ion sensor A novel method has been developed which consists of an oesophageal catheter incorporating a sodium ion selective electrode sensitive to the high sodium content in bile salts.[59] The results of validation studies were encouraging but there is a problem with sensitivity and specificity as the acidic contents of the stomach can influence the recordings and sodium also rises in the stomach in response to meals.

Ambulatory spectrophotometric bile sensor Recently, a new apparatus has been developed which has been specifically designed to detect oesophageal bilirubin which would be expected to be present in alkaline reflux. The 'Bilitec' (Synectics Medical, Stockholm) consists of a bile-sensitive probe incorporated into an oesophageal catheter, which utilizes a spectrophotometric sensor which is set to the optimum absorbance for bilirubin. Signals from the sensor are recorded on to a dedicated data logger and replayed after the recordings through specialized software.

The equipment has been evaluated in patients with known bile reflux and shows great promise.[60] Figure 11.4 illustrates the ability of the device to detect oesophageal bilirubin in an ambulatory measurement and its relation to symptoms.

This new system may be particularly useful in the investigation of patients with oesophageal reflux symptoms who have normal pH studies but who are resistant to high dose acid suppression. In these, it is possible that alkaline reflux may be the cause of their symptoms and a reliable, continuous method of detection of reflux with bile as one of its components will be helpful in establishing a diagnosis.

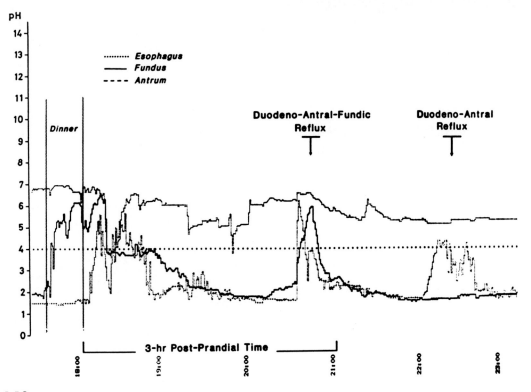

Figure 4.10
Three-channel pH recording to investigate duodenogastro-oesophageal reflux. Gastric (fundic and antral) pH and distal oesophageal pH show simultaneous alkaline changes in a patient with dyspepsia. (Reproduced, with permission, from ref. 56.)

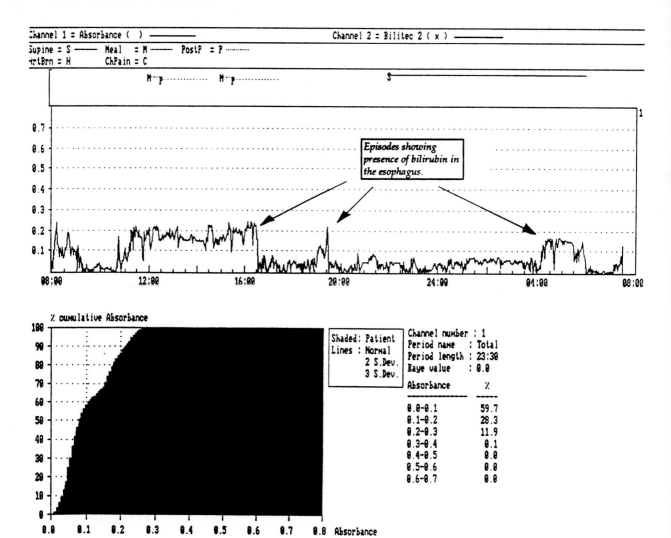

Figure 4.11

Twenty four hour recording of the output from the Bilitec device showing bilirubin reflux into the oesophagus. (Courtesy of Synectics Medical.)

Clinical indications for pH investigation

Oesophageal pH monitoring is most useful in patients with atypical symptoms or who have had a poor response to treatment. Thus patients with a good history and typical symptoms of GOR, with visible oesophagitis on upper GI endoscopy, will not require pH studies unless treatment fails. Table 4.3 outlines the common indications for pH investigations for both adults and children. This is not a hard and fast dictum but avoids the temptation to 'overinvestigate' that is often the case when new technology becomes available in a particular centre.

pH monitoring does not have a 100% sensitivity and specificity. Some patients with oesophagitis may have a normal pH study, possibly due to the cyclical nature of the disease and the strong influence of dietary and other factors. Some asymptomatic controls will have pathological levels of reflux on occasions, again, probably induced by dietary excesses or other reflux-provoking factors. Most estimates report an 85–90% sensitivity and specificity.[61] It is probable that some patients may require repeat pH studies when in a symptomatic period to demonstrate pathological reflux and define a cause for their symptoms. A high degree of symptom correlation, even in the presence of only minor pathological reflux, is still useful information in the diagnosis of GORD.

Table 4.3   Indications for intraoesophageal pH monitoring

ADULT	PAEDIATRIC
Angina-like (non-cardiac) chest pain	Vomiting
Dysphagia with normal motility	Failure to thrive
Nocturnal asthma or wheeze	Haematemesis
Reflux symptoms without endoscopic oesophagitis	Near – miss sudden infant death
Globus hystericus	Anaemia
Other symptoms suspicious of GOR	Apnoea/cyanosis
	Chest infection/wheeze

Symptoms unresponsive to therapy or frequent relapse
Patients being considered for surgery

Paediatric pH measurements

Oesophageal pH measurements are now widely used in paediatrics to investigate a variety of symptoms related to GORD. Table 4.3 illustrates some of the gastrointestinal and non-gastrointestinal symptoms which may be associated with GOR in children. In fact, the use of intraoesophageal pH monitoring has been found to be so useful in this group that it is probably now more widely used in paediatrics than in adult gastroenterology.

In general, the pH catheters and recording equipment are similar to those used in adults but there are some differences in procedures and analysis due to the nature of the patient group.

Electrodes and positioning

In all but the smallest infants, pH electrodes are the same as used for adults, excluding the larger (>3 mm) combined glass and antimony types. In neonates, it may be preferable to use a smaller than standard electrode (<2 mm).

pH electrode positioning is rarely gauged by prior manometry as this is often not available and is also more difficult and distressing to perform in children. Nomograms have been devised[62] to calculate oesophageal length in children but the two widest used methods are radiological positioning[63] and the pH withdrawal technique.[64] Radiological positioning of the electrode tip with a plain thoracic X-ray film obviously involves radiation and relies on the anatomical identification of the diaphragm to identify the gastro-oesophageal junction. Unless barium is also used during X-rays, the presence of a hiatus hernia may give rise to errors in accurate placement of the pH electrode.

The pH withdrawal technique involves passing the pH electrode into the stomach while monitoring pH and then withdrawing the electrode slowly until the pH changes abruptly from acid to neutral. The electrode is then further withdrawn 2–5 cm, depending on the size of the child, to site it in the optimum position for detecting GOR. The presence of GOR at the time of positioning, or a hiatus hernia, may lead to errors in accurate siting of the electrode using this method and a two-electrode system can be helpful to reduce this problem.

Recording protocols

In infants and small children, feeds are frequent and sleep is not only restricted to the night time period. In addition, the LOS and oesophageal motility may not be fully developed until some months after birth.[65] Consequently, the recording protocol will vary according to the age of the child and the analysis of the recordings will need to be adjusted accordingly.

Analysis and interpretation of pH recordings

Since 1974, when Johnson and DeMeester published their analysis of 24h pH recordings and introduced the DeMeester scoring system,[4] debate has continued as to the most sensitive analytical methods used in the interpretation of GOR and the separation of physiological from pathological reflux. Initially, all analyses of GOR were performed manually[5], but currently, with computer regeneration of data, calculations of GOR data are totally automated. In the last year few years, pH programs are being presented in Microsoft Windows format which brings the whole technique of pH investigations into the hands of those with few computing skills.

Recordings are replayed using laser or other digital printer facilities, either compressed, or as detailed hour by hour plots of oesophageal pH. Figure 4.6 shows Three prolonged oesophageal pH traces taken from acutal recordings. The 24 h plots are from a Windows-based program (Flexsoft, Oakfield Instruments, Oxon). The pH traces are from patients with mild (a), moderate (b) and severe (c) GOR.

Analysis of numerous previously published parameters of GOR is totally automated as part of all of the commercially available systems and Table 4.4 highlights the major parameters that have been suggested as being useful in the discrimination of pathological from physiological reflux. Various scoring systems have also been devised in an attempt to simplify the discriminative process and these may also be used in the interpretation of results (Table 4.4). Although %time <pH4 has been widely accepted as the single most important criterion used to determine pathological reflux, other parameters also give useful information regarding individual cases and should not be completely disregarded.

GOR analysis: adult

Records are normally analysed for total time and also divided into epochs of upright, supine, and also postprandial periods. This enables separation between nocturnal (supine) and daytime (erect) GOR. A further subdivision of inter- and postprandial periods allows inclusion or exclusion of meal-related reflux and a correlation analysis between meals and GOR.

Summary analyses can calculate numerous variables which have been suggested as useful discriminants between physiological and pathological GOR. The percentage time below pH4 was initially advocated by DeMeester and Johnson as the best discriminant between physiological and pathological GOR and this single figure remains the most widely recommended parameter in reflux assessment.[66] All commercially available equipment has facilities to calculate all GOR parameters, direct and derived and reflux totals can also be compared with previously published upper physiological limits taken from asymptomatic controls. Most systems will produce a full analytical summary in a few minutes.

Table 4.4 Analytical parameters and scoring systems used in analysis of GOR

BASIC DATA	DERIVED SCORES
Frequency (episodes/hr)	DeMeester Scores
Duration (mins/hr)	Frequency Duration Index
Longest episode (mins)	Kaye Score (Post-prandial)
No episodes > 5 min	Cumulative pH plots
% time <pH4	
Total symptom score	Reflux Index
Post-prandial GOR time	Meal Reflux Index

pH analysis: paediatrics

In paediatrics, basic analysis is performed as in adult studies, although some differences exist. Normal ranges for physiological GOR vary according to development. The LOS and oesophageal motility are not fully developed until at least 100 days after birth and in premature babies may be even later.[65] Upper physiological limits have been calculated in children and stratified by age[67] to achieve a better discriminant analysis taking development into account.

The influence of postprandial and nocturnal GOR is also more difficult in paediatrics due to the nature and timing of feeds and the frequent interfood sleep cycles. In addition, the greater supine periodicity may also affect the normal calculation based on adult values.

PROVOCATION TESTS

When oesophageal symptoms are intermittent, especially where pain is a factor, there may be doubt about the diagnostic accuracy of the oesophageal tests described so far in relation to detection of the cause of the symptoms. As most tests at best only examine the possible abnormality for up to 24 h, and where even prolonged studies fail to detect a causal relationship between the measurement and the patient's symptoms, provocation manoeuvres have been devised to stimulate symptoms during a controlled, supervised period of investigation.

Bernstein test

In 1958, Bernstein and Baker[68] described a procedure whereby symptoms of possible oesophageal origin related to GOR were investigated by infusing the oesophagus with hydrochloric acid. The onset of pain provoked by the presence of HCl was tested as follows.

The patient was intubated with a small nasogastric catheter such that the tip was sited in the middle third of the oesophageal body, 30 cm from the nose. The catheter was connected to three infusion bags containing 0.1 M HCl, sodium bicarbonate and normal saline. Without the patient knowing, the physician instilled first saline, then acid into the oesophagus at a controlled rate. The stimulation of pain by acid and subsequent relief by instillation of alkali and saline signified a positive association between oesophageal pain and the presence of acid. Any pain experienced during saline infusion or when bicarbonate was present was regarded as a false positive. The overall sensitivity and specificity of the test has been variably cited over the years, but on average sensitivity is 78% and specificity 84%.[69]

The Bernstein test was popular among gastroenterologists during the 10–15 years following its introduction but is now not widely used due to the introduction of prolonged intraoesophageal pH measurement.

Acid clearance test

The acid clearance test, first described in 1968,[70] examines oesophageal acid clearance by measuring pH changes after the instillation of 15 ml of 0.1M HCl into the mid-oesophagus. Acid clearance is detected by a pH electrode sited 5 cm above the LOS. A positive result is achieved if the subject fails to raise oesophageal pH > 5 in 1–10 swallows made at 30 s intervals. Patients with GORD and poor acid clearance require greater numbers of swallows than controls. The test has a low sensitivity and specificity[71] and is now rarely used, having been replaced by prolonged, ambulatory pH measurement.

Standard acid reflux test (SART) and Acid reflux provocation test (ARPT)

Tuttle and Grossman[72] tested the competence of the LOS antireflux mechanism by introducing a bolus of HCl into the stomach after which patients with GOR symptoms performed various physical manoeuvres (Valsalva, Muller, coughing and deep breathing) in four different postures. The test (SART) was advocated as a means of demonstrating GOR under standard laboratory conditions. Pathological reflux, assessed by intraoesophageal pH, was positive if the pH fell below 4 for two or more of the 20 manoeuvres. A high reported false positivity and negativity[73] stimulated others to develop more sensitive provocation tests.

Branicki et al.[74] modified the SART in an attempt to increase the diagnostic yield. The ARPT increased the range of reflux provocative manoeuvres by raising intra-abdominal pressure with weight lifting, floor scrubbing in a crouched position and head-down posture and leg raising exercises. Acid secretion and GOR were stimulated with a small meal prior to provocation. The test has a higher sensitivity and specificity than the SART but as with all the provocative tests has been largely superseded by 24th ambulatory pH monitoring.

Acid reflux provocation tests are time-consuming, labour intensive and rather unphysiological and although still possibly useful in a research setting, have now become part of history in the development of investigations for GORD.

Investigation of chest pain

Intermittent chest pain of non-cardiac origin continues to be the most difficult symptom to diagnose in relation to acid-related disorders of the upper GI tract. Development of provocative tests of chest pain of oesophageal origin have been advocated as an aid to diagnosis of a somewhat difficult symptom pattern associated with both GORD and oesophageal motility disorders. Two tests are occasionally used to investigate patients with intermittent chest pain of non-cardiac origin, although again, prolonged, combined, manometry and pH are tending to replace these investigations as technology advances and equipment and methodology become more widely available.

Edrophonium provocation or 'Tensilon' test

Edrophonium bromide (Tensilon) is a cholinometic agent that increases the contractility of oesophageal smooth muscle. The compound can be used to provoke oesophageal pain in some patients after intravenous administration of the drug. The technique was first described by London et al.[75] and has been used sporadically by a number of gastroenterologists with some success.[76,77]

The procedure is usually combined with oesophageal

manometry in order to investigate the relationship between symptoms and manometric abnormalities provoked after edrophonium stimulation. The patient is intubated with a standard oesophageal manometry catheter with pressure ports placed at the LOS and at intervals along the oesophageal body.

Edrophonium is administered intravenously after baseline measurements and the resultant effects monitored. The patient is asked to press an event marker and document the frequency and type of symptoms experienced during the examination. The test has a high false negative rate and in some patients may cause cardiac arrhythmias. It is not now widely used having been replaced by other tests but is occasionally useful when all other investigations have been negative.

Balloon distension

Oesophageal pain can be provoked in some patients by distension of the oesophageal lumen. This attempts to stimulate the passage of a large food bolus and may cause oesophageal wall spasm with associated pressure changes and symptoms. The balloon distension test,[78] involves naso-oesophageal intubation with a balloon catheter into the mid-oesophagus, The balloon is inflated in steps until symptoms are perceived or until maximum balloon volume is achieved. Simultaneous manometry detects oesophageal motility changes associated with the distension and correlates these changes with symptoms. A positive test is reported if pain is experienced during the test. The sensitivity and specificity of this test has been variably reported in the literature[79,80] and is clearly useful in the few patients where diagnosis has proven difficult. The test is useful if combined pH and pressure studies fail to show any abnormalities or if patients persistently fail to exhibit symptoms during non-provocative ambulatory studies.

RELATED OESOPHAGEAL INVESTIGATIONS

Gamma scintigraphy

Radionuclide scanning is now widely used by gastroenterologists for imaging and functional studies in the GI tract. The development of radiolabelled scintigraphic compounds has increased the versatility of the technique in gastroenterology. For imaging, the differential uptake of certain radiolabelled compounds by malignant tumours allows identification of primary, secondary and metastatic spread of cancers in the GI tract. Of equal usefulness is the ability to use scintigraphy to examine GI function.

Functional studies of transit in the upper GI tract rely on the principle that the passage of radiolabelled substances can be followed by the detection of gamma emissions from a test meal labelled with a suitable isotope as it transits the gut. Site-specific uptake or the use of colloidal isotopes also enables studies in selected organs within the gut, such as the liver and biliary system.

Oesophageal transit

Gamma scintigraphy has been used to qualify transit of both liquid and solid meals in oesophageal investigations.[81,82] It offers some advantages over radiographic techniques as it allows the quantification of flow and velocity with the use of computer-aided analysis. The technique is similar in principle to a barium swallow. The patient swallows solid or liquid boluses of radiolabelled materials in front of a gamma camera. Continuous acquisition and storage of images facilitates subsequent replay and analysis of oesophageal transit of the bolus. Computer analysis facilitates the production of temporal transit plots to produce profiles of liquids and solids during swallows.[83] The advantage of scintigraphy over the barium swallow is the ability easily and objectively to evaluate the velocity of movement of the bolus and relate this to other factors in the clinical history of the patient.

Gastric emptying

Gastric emptying disorders may predispose to symptoms of GOR and other oesophageal symptoms (globus, regurgitation, vomiting) and gastric emptying abnormalities in GORD have been reported in varying numbers of patients.[84,85] Gamma scintigraphy is now widely recognized as the 'gold' standard technique in the evaluation of gastric emptying.

Numerous reports in the medical literature describe the various techniques whereby liquid and solid components of normal foods are radiolabelled with short half-life gamma isotopes.[86] These isotopes are incorporated into meals and then located in the stomach by the gamma camera. By selecting isotopes with different emission characteristics, it is possible to label the solid and liquid components of a meal separately such that both can be simultaneously monitored. Intermittent, sequential images of the isotopes are acquired and stored as the meal gradually empties from the stomach. Graphical plots of emptying curves of liquids and solids can be obtained by processing the images. In patients with suspected small intestinal involvement, it may be useful to continue imaging to display transit through the small bowel, although this is relatively rare, and can mostly be detected by other tests.

Tests of gastric emptying may be useful in patients with oesophageal symptoms if there is a suspicion of gastric pathology to suggest that GOR is secondary to retained food. For example, patients who experience postprandial GOR and who also complain of early satiety, bloating and nausea may be suitable for gastric emptying studies in addition to the other investigations described in this chapter.

HIDA Scan

Scintigraphy is also useful in measurement of bile flow. Derivatives of iminodiacetic acid (HIDA) labelled with[99m] technetium allow high quality images of the biliary system to be obtained.[87] This technique has been used in sphincter of Oddi dysfunction,[88] suspected bile duct obstruction[89] and in oesophageal reflux diseases where duodenogastric reflux (DGR) is suspected.[90]

The HIDA scan for duodenogastric reflux investigates the appearance of isotope in the oesophagus after intravenous injection. The stimulation of DGR may be further provoked by the administration of a fatty meal to increase bile flow from the gal bladder. Recently, a technique has been described whereby the investigation can be performed by prolonged, ambulatory recording. Washington et al.[91] described a technique using a cadmium telluride gamma isotope detector placed over the distal oesophagus, with simultaneous oesophageal pH measurement. Continuous radioactive counts from the detector and pH were recorded on a portable data logger after administration of i.v. HIDA and a test meal. The presence of DGR and GOR was monitored by a rise in radioactive counts and GOR in healthy volunteers.

Gamma scintigraphy for GI tract investigations is safe, non-invasive and the radiation exposure is minimal. The type of investigation, the selection of a specific isotope and the method of radiolabelling are all determined by the specific requirements of the test.

Impedance methods

Two specific methods of detection of transit using impedance have been developed and show promise. Both rely on the principle that the GI tract acts as an electrically non-conducting hollow lumen lying within a conductive cavity. The impedance within the gut lumen can be detected by passing a small a.c. current across the abdomen and measuring the resultant voltage on the opposite surface. By filling the lumen with a substance of either greater or lower conductance than the viscera, a change in impedance can be detected. If the change in impedance over time is plotted, movement of luminal content can be detected from one area to another, i.e. gastric emptying and oesophageal transit.

Although the technique is in its infancy, potentially, it offers a safe, non-invasive method of measurement. It is ideal for patients who are not suitable for imaging with X-rays or isotopes, i.e. children and pregnant women. The equipment is inexpensive and portable and does not require undue skills to operate or expensive consumables. At present, research has concentrated mainly on techniques of gastric emptying, although some research in oesophageal function has been described.

Epigastrography

This system utilizes two electrodes per channel (usually two channels). A current is passed anterior to posterior across the gastric region and a voltage plot drawn of the underlying resistance across the gastric lumen. Gastric filling and emptying of selected test-meals (mainly liquids and semisolids) is plotted as a change in impedance with a gradual return to baseline.[92] The technique is highly sensitive to movement artefacts and gastric acid secretion.

Electrical impedance tomography (EIT)

This technique produces a two-dimensional tomogram of a 4–6 cm transverse section across the abdomen underlying 16 surface electrodes positioned in a horizontal ring. Each electrode pair sequentially acts as a current generator and receiver and the resultant impedance tomogram is plotted as a full colour impedance 'contour' picture. Movement of luminal content can

be plotted as impedance changes in the contour map. Quantification of data can be achieved by drawing regions of interest over specific areas and luminal movement against time plotted.[93] The technique is also sensitive to gastric acid and has been advocated as a non-invasive measure of acid secretion.[94] Because of the acid sensitivity, it has been suggested that EIT may be a more physiological measurement of gastric function than other methods because it detects luminal volume, i.e. ingested food content plus secretions.[95]

Recent advances in EIT have demonstrated its potential in the investigation of the oesophagus. Ravelli and Milla[96] have suggested that EIT can detect GOR and DGR in children. Recent work in our own laboratories has confirmed this in adults. Some attempts have been made with EIT to study oesophageal transit[97] although this work is again still in its infancy.

The major drawback with EIT for oesophageal studies has been the orientation of imaging. The nature of the technique has dictated that only transverse images can be obtained. Recently, a modification of EIT has been described whereby coronal images have been achieved using a rosette of electrodes placed over the surface of the abdomen.[98] This technique holds much promise in the investigation of oesophageal function.

REFERENCES

1. Bayliss WM & Starling EH. The movement and the innervations of the small intestine. *J Physiol* 1899; **24:** 229–240.
2. Pattrick FG. Investigation of gastro-oesophageal reflux in various positions with a two-line pH electrode. *Gut* 1970; **11:** 659–667.
3. Spencer J. Prolonged pH recording in the study of gastro-oesophageal reflux. *Br J Surg* 1969; **56:** 912–915.
4. Johnson LF & DeMeester TR. Twenty four hour pH monitoring of the distal oesophagus. a quantitative measure of gastro-esophageal reflux. *Am J Gastroenterol* 1974; **62:** 325–331.
5. Branicki FJ, Evans DF, Hardcastle JD, Ogilvie AL & Atkinson M. Ambulatory monitoring of oesophageal pH in reflux oesophagitis using a portable radiotelemetry system. *Gut* 1982; **23:** 992–998.
6. Smart HL, Foster PN, Evans DF, Slevin B & Atkinson MA. Twenty four hour oesophageal acidity in achalasia before and after pneumatic dilatation. *Gut* 1987; **28:** 883–887.
7. Shoenut JP, Micflikier AB, Yaffe CS, Den Boer B & Teskey JM. Reflux in untreated achalasia patients. *J Clin Gastroenterol* 1995; **20:** 6–11.
8. Vantrappen G, Janssens J & Ghilbert G. The irritable oesophagus. *Lancet* 1987; **i:** 1232.
9. De Caestecker J, Blackwell J, Brown J & Heading RC. The oesophagus as a cause of recurrent chest pain. *Lancet* 1985; **ii:** 1143–1146.
10. Gillen P, Keeling P, Byrne PJ, Healy M, O'Moore RR & Hennessy TPJ. Implications of duodenogastric refluxate in the pathogenesis of Barrett's oesophagus. *Br J Surg* 1988; **75:** 540–543.
11. Gotley DC, Morgan AP, Ball D, Owen WR & Cooper MJ. Composition of gastro-oesophageal refluxate. *Gut* 1991; **32:** 1093–1097.
12. Barrett NR. Chronic peptic ulcer of the oesophagus and oesophagitis. *Br J Surg* 1950; **38:** 175–182.
13. Hennessy TPJ. Clinical features of reflux. In Hennessy TPJ, Cuschieri A & Bennett JR (eds) *Reflux Oeosphagitis.* London: Butterworths, 1989: 37–53.
14. Bartlett D, Angiansah A, Owen W, Evans DF & Smith BGN. Dental erosion – a presenting feature of gastro-oesophageal reflux disease. *Eur J Gastroenterol Hepatol* 1994; **6:** 895–900.
15. Iverson LIG, May IA & Salmon PC. Pulmonary complications in benign oesophageal disease. *Am J Surg* 1973; **126:** 223–228.
16. Jolly SG, Halpern LM, Sterling CE & Feldman BE. The relationship of respiratory complications from gastro-oesophageal reflux to prematurity in infants. *J Paedia Surg* 1990; **25:** 755–757.
17. Kapila L & Evans DF. Gastro-oesophageal reflux. In Freeman NV, Burge DM, Griffiths DM & Malone PSJ (eds) *Surgery of the Newborn.* Churchill New York: Livingstone, 1994: 375–393.

18. Fyke FE, Code CF & Schlegel JF. The gastro-oesophageal sphincter in healthy humans. *Gastroenterologia* 1956; **86:** 135–150.

19. Malagelada JR, Camilleri M & Staghellini V. *Manometric Diagnosis of Gastrointestinal Motility.* New York: Thieme, 1986.

20. Arndorfer RC, Stef JJ, Dodds WJ et al. Improved infusion system for intraluminal oesophageal manometry. *Gastroenterology* 1977; **73:** 23.

21. Biancani P, Zabinski MP & Behar J. Pressure, tension and force of closure of the human lower oesophageal sphincter and oesophagus. *J Clin Invest* 1975; **56:** 476–483.

22. Evans DF. Radiotelemetry. In Kumar D & Wingate DL (eds) *An Illustrated Guide to Gastrointestinal Motility;* 2nd edn, London: Churchill Livingstone, 1993: 211.

23. Swain CP, Evans DF, Glynn M, Brown G & Mills T. Endoscopic sewing machine used to achieve continuous non-invasive monitoring of gastric pH for 3 months in man. *Gastrointest Endosc* 1992; **38:** 278.

24. Dahlgren S & Thoren L. Intestinal motility in low small bowel obstruction. *Acta Chir Scand* 1967; **33:** 417–422.

25. Gill RC, Kellow JE, Browning C & Wingate DL. The use of intraluminal strain gauges for recording ambulant small bowel motility. *Am J Physiol* 1990; **258:** G610.

26. Azpiroz F & Malagelada JR. Physiological variations in canine gastric tone measured by an electronic barostat. *Am J Physiol* 1985; **248:** G229.

27. Dent J. A new technique for continuous sphincter pressure measurement. *Gastroenterology* 1976; **71:** 263–267.

28. Gotley DC, Barham CP, Miller RJ, Arnold R & Alderson D. The sphinctometer: a new device for measurement of lower oesophageal function. *Br J Surg 1991;* **78:** 933–935.

29. Barham CP, Gotley DC, Miller R, Mills A & Alderson D. Ambulatory measurement of oesophageal function: clinical use of a new pH and motility recording system *Br J Surg* 1992; **79:** 1056.

30. Anggiansah A, Taylor G, Bright N et al. Primary peristalsis is the major acid clearance mechanism in reflux patients. *Gut* 1994; **35:** 1536–1542.

31. Welch RW & Gray GE. The influence of respiration on recordings of lower oesophageal sphincter pressure in humans.*Gastroenterology* 1982; **83:** 590–594.

32. Welch RW, Luckmann K, Ricks PM, Drake ST & Gates GA. Manometry of the normal oesophageal sphincter and its alteration in laryngectomy. J Clin Invest 1979; **63:** 1036–1041.

33. Stein HJ, DeMeester TR Naspetti R, Jamieson J & Perry RE. Three-dimensional imaging of the lower oesophageal sphincter in gastro-oesophageal reflux disease. *Ann Surg* 1991; **214:** 374–383.

34. Wilson J & Heading RC. The proximal sphincters. In Kumar D & Wingate DL (eds) *An Illustrated Guide to Gastrointestinal Motility,* (2nd edn), London: Churchill Livingstone, 1993; 211.

35. Janssens J, Vantrappen G & Ghillebert G. 24-hr recording of esophageal pressure and pH in patients with non cardiac chest pain. *Gastroenterology* 1986; **90:** 1978–1984.

36. Castillo FD, Benson MJ, Wingate Dl, Samaras T & Spyrou NM. Evaluation of computerised analysis of propagation of human duodenjejunal contractions. *J Neurogastroenterol Mot* 1994; **6:** 11.

37. Emde C, Armstrong D, Bumm R, Kaufhold HJ, Riecken EO & Blum AL. Twenty four hour continuous ambulatory measurement of oesophageal pH and pressure; a digital recording system and computer aide manometric analysis. *J Amb Mon* 1990; **3:** 47–62.

38. Barham CP, Gotley DC, Miller RE, Mills A & Alderson D. Ambulatory measurement of oesophageal function: clinical use of a new pH and pressure recording system. *Br J Surg* 1992; **79:** 1056–1060.

39. Bortolotti M, Annese V, Coccia G et al. Twenty four hour ambulatory oesophageal manometry in normal subjects (co-operative study). *J Neurogastroenterol Motil* 1994; **6:** 311–320.

40. Jones R & Lydeard S. Prevalence of dyspepsia in the community. *BMJ* 1989; **298:** 30.

41. Richter JE & Castell DO. Gastroesophageal reflux. Pathogenesis, diagnosis and therapy. *Ann Intern Med* 1982; **97:** 93–103.

42. DeMeester TR, Johnson LR, Joseph GJ, Toscano MS, Hall AW & Skinner DB. Patterns of gastroesophageal reflux in health and disease. *Ann Surg* 1976; **184:** 459–469.

43. Evans DF. Twenty-four hour ambulatory oesophageal pH monitoring: an update. *Br J Surg* 1987; **74:** 157–161.

44. Rohmel O, Merki HS, Wilder-Smith CH & Walt RP. Analytical and statistical evaluation of intragastric pH recordings. *Dig Dis Sci* 1990; **8** (supp): 87.

45. Walt RP, Reynolds JR, Langman MJ et al. Intravenous omeprazole rapidly raises intragastric pH. *Gut* 1985; **26:** 902.

46. Mattioli S, Pilotti V, Felice V et al. Ambulatory 24 hour pH monitoring of

47. Klinkenberg – Knol EC & Meuwissen SG. Combined gatric and oesophageal 24 hour pH monitoring and oesophageal manometry in patients with reflux disease resistant to treatment with omeprazole. *Aliment Pharmacol Ther* 1990; **4;** 485–490.

48. Evans DF, Kadirkamanathan SS & Wingate DL. The effectiveness of acid suppression in patients with refractory GORD. *Gastroenterology* 1994; **106:** A75.

49. Evans DF, Pye G, Bramley R, Clark AG, Dyson TJ & Hardcastle JD. Measurement of gastrointestinal pH in normal ambulant human subjects. *Gut* 1988; **29:** 1035.

50. Evans DF. Ambulatory pH systems – Product review. J Amb Monit 1988; **1:** 127.

51. Angiannsah A, Bright N, McCullagh M, Sumboonanonda K & Owen WJ. Alternative method of positioning the pH probe for oesophageal pH monitoring *Gut* 1992; **33:** 111–114.

52. Mansfield LE & Stein MR. Gastroesophageal reflux and asthma: a possible reflex mechanism. *Ann Allergy* 1981; **47:** 431–434.

53. Smith BGN & Knight JK. A comparison of patterns of toothwear with aetiological factors. *Br Dent J* 1984; **157:** 16–19

54. Attwood SEA, Ball CS, Barlow AP, Jenkrison LR, Norris TL & Watson D. Role of intra-gastric and intra-oesophageal olkalinisation in the genesis of complications in Barrett's columnorised oesophagus. *Gut* 1993; **34:** 11–15.

55. Iftikhar YF, Ledingham SJ, Evans DF et al. Bile reflux in columnar lined Barrett's oesophagus. *Ann R Coll Surg Eng* 1993; **75:** 411–416.

56. Mattioli S, Felice V, Pilotti V, Bacchi ML, Pastina M & Gozzetti G. Indications for 24 hr gastric pH monitoring with single and multiple pH probein clinical research and practice. *Dig Dis Sci* 1992; **37:** 1793–1801.

57. Gotley DC, Morgan AP & Cooper MJ. Bile acid concentrations in the refluxate of patients with reflux oesophagitis. *Br J Surg* 1988; **75:** 587–590.

58. Gotley DC, Appleton GV & Cooper MJ. Bile acids and trypsin are unimportant in gastro-oesophageal reflux. *J Clin Gastroenterol* 1992; **14:** 2–7.

59. Smythe A, O'Leary D Johnson AG. Duodenogastric reflux after gastric surgery and in gastric ulcer disease: continuous measurement with a sodium ion electrode. *Gut* 1993; **34:** 1047–1050.

60. Vaezi MF, Lacamera RG & Richter J. Validation studies of Bilitec 2000: an ambulatory duodenogastric reflux monitoring system. *Am J Physiol* 1994; **267:** G1050–1057.

61. Johnson F & Joelsson B. The reproducibility of ambulatory pH monitoring. *Gut* 1988; **29:** 886–889.

62. Strobel CT. Correlation of oesophageal lengths in children with height: application of the Tuttle test without prior esophageal manometry. *J Pediatr* 1979; **94:** 81–84.

63. DeMeester TR, Wang CI, Wernly JA et al. Technique, indications and clinical use of 24 hour esophageal pH monitoring. *J Thorac Cardiovasc Surg* 1980; **79:** 656–670.

64. Dehn TCB & Kettlewell M. 24 hour monitoring of oesophageal pH in outpatients. *Lancet* 1987; **1:** 625–626.

65. Boix-Ochoa J & Canals J. Maturation of the lower oesophagus. J Pediatr Surg 1976; **11:** 749–756.

66. Emde C, Garner A & Blum AL. Technical aspects of intraluminal pH metry in man: current status and recommendations. *Gut* 1987; **28:** 1187–1188.

67. VandenPlas Y & Sacre L. Continuous 24 hour pH monitoring in 285 asymptomatic infants 0–15 months old. *J Paediatr Gastroenterol Nutr* 1987; **6:** 220–224.

68. Bernstein LM & Baker L. A clinical test for oesophagitis. *Gastroenterology,* 1958; **34:** 760–781.

69. Jamieson GG & Duranceau A. The investigation and classification of reflux disease. In Jamieson GG (ed) *Surgery of the Oesophagus;* Edinburgh; Churchill Livingstone, 1988: 201–210.

70. Booth DJ, Kemmerer WT & Skinner DB. Acid clearing from the distal esophagus. *Arch Surg* 1968; **96:** 731–734.

71. Little AG, DeMeester TR, Kirchner PT, O'Sullivan GC & Skinner DB. Pathogenesis of esophagitis in patients with gastroesophageal reflux. *Surgery* 1980; **88:** 101–107.

72. Tuttle SG & Grossman MI. Detection of gastroesophageal reflux by simultaneous measurement of pressure and pH. *Proc Soc Exp Biol Med* 1958; **98:** 225–227.

73. Grande L, Pujol A, Garcia-Valdecasas JC, Fuster J, Visa J & Pera C. Intraesophageal pH monitoring after breakfast and lunch in gastroesophageal reflux. *J Clin Gastroenterol* 1988; **10:** 373–376.

74. Branicki FJ, Evans DF, Jones JA & Hardcastle JD. The evaluation of oesophageal reflux using a frequency duration index (FDI). *Br J Surg* 1984; **71:** 425–430.

75. London RL, Ouyang A, Snape Jr W, Goldberg S, Hirshfield Jr JW & Cohen S. Provocation of esophageal pain by ergonovine or edrophonium. Gastroenterology 1981; **81:** 10–14.

76. Richter JE, Hackshaw BT, Wu W & Castell DO. Edrophonium: a useful provocation test for esophageal chest pain. *Ann Intern Med* 1985; **103:** 14–21.

77. Linsell J, Owen WJ, Mason RC & Anggiansah A. Edrophonium provocation test in he diagnosis of diffuse oesophageal spasm. *Br J Surg* 1987; **74:** 688–689.

78. Baylis JH, Kauntze R & Trounce JR. Observations on distension of the lower end of the oesophagus. *Q J Med* 1955; **14:** 143–154.

79. Barish CF, Castell DO & Richter JE. Graded oesophageal balloon distension: a new provocative test for non-cardiac chest pain. *Dig Dis Sci* 1986; **31:** 1292–1298.

80. DeCaestecker JS, Pryde A & Heading RC. Site and mechanism of pain perception with oesophageal balloon distension and intravenous edrophonium in patients with oesophageal chest pain. *Gut* 1992; **33:** 580–586.

81. Fisher RS, Malmud LS, Roberts GS & Lobis IF. Gastro-esophageal (GE) scintiscanning to detect and quantitate GE reflux. Gastroenterology 1976; **70:** 301.

82. Cranford CA, Sutton D, Sadek SA, Kennedy N & Cuschieri A. A new physiological method of evaluating oesophageal transit. *Br J Surg* 1987; **74:** 411–415.

83. Harding LK & Robinson PJA. *The Clinicians Guide to Nuclear Medicine – Gastroenterology.* Edinburgh: Churchill Livingstone, 1991.

84. McCallum RW, Berkowitz DM & Lerner E. Gastric emptying in patients with gastroesophageal reflux. *Gastroenterology* 1981; **80:** 285–291.

85. Shay SS, Eggli D, McDonald C & Johnson LF. Gastric emptying of solid in patients with gastroesophageal reflux. *Gastroenterology* 1987; **92:** 459–465.

86. Harding K & Notghi A. Radioscintigraphy. In Kumar D & Wingate DL (eds) *An Illustrated Guide to Gastrointestinal Motility*, 2nd edn, London; Churchill Livingstone, 1993: 228–242.

87. Krishnamurthy GT, Bobbs VR & Kingston E. Radionuclide ejection fraction: a technique for the quantitative analysis of motor function of the human gall bladder. *Gastroenterology* 1981; **80:** 482.

88. Shaffer EA, Hershfield NB, Logan K et al. Cholescintigraphic detection of functional obstruction of the sphincter of Oddi. *Gastroenterology* 1986; **90:** 728.

89. Darweesh RMA, Dodds WJ, Hogan WJ et al. Efficacy of quantitative hepatobiliary scintigraphy and fatty meal sonography for evaluating patients with suspected partial common bile duct obstruction. *Gastroenterology* 1988; **94:** 779.

90. Shaffer EA, McOrmond P & Duggan H. Quantitative choliscintigraphy: assessment of gallbladder filling and emptying in duodenogastric reflux. *Gastroenterology* 1980; **79:** 899.

91. Washington N, Moss HA, Greaves JL, Steele RJ & Wilson CG. Non-invasive detection of GOR using an ambulatory system. *Gut* 1993; **34:** 1482–1486.

92. Sutton JA, Thompson S & Sobnack R. Measurement of gastric emptying by radioactive isotope scintigraphy and epigastric impedance. *Lancet* 1985; **2:** 898.

93. Avill R, Mangnall YF, Bird NC et al. Applied potential tomography: a new non-invasive technique for measuring gastric emptying. *Gastroenterology* 1987; **92:** 1019.

94. Baxter AJ, Mangnall YF, Loj EJ et al. Evaluation of applied potential tomography as a new non-invasive test of gastric secretion. *Gut* 1988; **29:** 1730.

95. Wright JW, Evans DF, Bush D & Ledingham SJ. The effect of nutrient and non-nutrient test meals on gastric emptying using EIT. In Holder D (ed.) *Clinical and Physiological Applications of Electric Impedance Tomography,* London; UCL Press, 1993: 100.

96. Ravelli AM & Milla PJ. Detection of gastro-oesophageal reflux by EIT. In Holder D (ed.) *Clinical and Physiological Applications of Electric Impedance Tomography.* London: UCL press, 1993: 159–165.

97. Hughes TAT, Liu P, Griffiths CM, Lawrie BW & Wiles CM. An analysis of studies comparing EIT and x-ray videofluoroscopy in the assessment of swallowing. Physiol Meas 1994; **15(2a):** 199–209.

98. Smallwood RH, Mangnall YF & Leathard AD. Transport of gastric contents. *Physiol Meas* 1994; **15:** A175–188.

5

OESOPHAGEAL MOTILITY DISORDERS

J Tack
J Janssens
G Vantrappen

Primary oesophageal motility disorders constitute a spectrum including achalasia, diffuse oesophageal spasm and intermediate conditions.[1] In addition, non-specific oesophageal motility disorders have been described, which include conditions such as hypertensive lower oesophageal sphincter and the nutcracker oesophagus.[2,3] The latter two conditions have been identified on the basis of high resting or contractile pressures not accompanied by abnormalities of peristalsis or sphincteric relaxation. The relationship between these manometric findings and clinical symptoms remains controversial. The irritable oesophagus denotes a condition in which the gullet appears hypersensitive to various stimuli, such as acid or motility disorders.[4]

Secondary oesophageal motility disorders include secondary forms of achalasia (due to malignancy, Chagas' disease or pseudo-obstruction), postsurgical conditions, amyloidosis, sarcoidosis, etc. Severe gastro-oesophageal reflux may induce oesophageal motility disturbances mimicking the manometric picture of diffuse oesophageal spasm. Diabetic and alcoholic neuropathy, and striated and smooth muscle diseases, may also produce secondary motility disturbances.

PRIMARY OESOPHAGEAL MOTILITY DISORDERS

Achalasia

Typical achalasia is a disease of unknown aetiology characterized by aperistalsis in the body of the oesophagus and defective relaxation of the lower oesophageal sphincter, which is often hypertonic. Loss of propulsive peristaltic contractions, together with defective sphincter relaxations, cause stasis of food in a progressively dilating gullet. The oesophageal stasis is the common factor in most of the symptoms and complications of achalasia.

Incidence

The incidence of achalasia is in the range of 1 per 100 000 population per year. The disease can occur at any age, but only 5% of the patients have onset of symptoms before the age of 14 years.

Pathology and pathophysiology

The pathology of achalasia is still incompletely understood. Lesions have been demonstrated in the dorsal vagal nucleus, in the vagal nerve fibres, in Auerbach's plexus and in the oesophageal muscle.[5-7] Histological studies revealed inflammation of the myenteric plexus and a marked decrease in the number of myenteric ganglion cells in the oesophagus.[8] There is compelling evidence that the non-adrenergic, non-cholinergic inhibitory intrinsic innervation is impaired in achalasia patients. This system mediates sphinter relaxation in the opossum and may also have a role in the peristaltic progression of oesophageal contractions.[9,10] Inhibitory neurones containing nitric oxide and vasoactive intestinal polypeptide are lost from the myenteric plexus of the oesophagus.[11] Cholinergic neurones seem to be (relatively) preserved, and they may be responsible for the high resting lower oesophageal sphincter tone in achalasia. Administration of a cholinesterase inhibitor (edrophonium) will increase the pressure in the lower oesophageal sphincter,[12] whereas atropine or local injection of botulinum toxin will decrease the lower oesophageal sphincter pressure in patients with achalasia.[13,14] There is, however, pharmacological evidence of some cholinergic denervation too, as direct cholinergic stimulation by methacholine (Mecholyl) results in a strong contractile reaction in both the oesophageal body and the lower oesophageal sphincter.[15]

The aetiology of achalasia is unknown. Infection with a neuropathic virus has been proposed as a possible candidate, but the available data are conflicting. In a subset of achalasia patients, antimyenteric neuronal antibodies can be found, staining both nitrergic and non-nitrergic neurones.[16] Their role in the pathophysiology of achalasia is presently unclear.

Clinical features

Dysphagia, regurgitation, weight loss and pain are the most important symptoms of achalasia.[17] Characteristically, the patients has dysphagia for liquids as well as solids from the onset of the disease. This 'funtional dysphagia' differs from organic dysphagia, which is initially for solids, and only later for both solids and liquids. The degree of swallowing difficulty varies considerably from day to day, but tends to get worse with time. Prandial or postprandial regurgitation is often mistaken for vomiting. Retention of large quantities of food in a dilated gullet may lead to regurgitation when the patient is in the recumbent position, or to aspiration in the airways and bronchopulmonary complications. The degree of weight loss is related to the severity of the dysphagia. Retrosternal pain occurs more often in the younger age groups and in the initial stages of the disease. The frequency of these various symptoms is summarized in Figure 5.1.

Investigations

The diagnosis can be made in most instances by radiological examination. However, manometry allows a better appreciation and a quantitative evaluation of the diagnostically important motor disorders.

Radiology and scintigraphy Cineradiography may visualize the absence of peristaltic contraction waves and the disorganized and non-propulsive nature of the contractions. Because the lower oesophageal sphincter fails to open normally following deglutition, the head of the barium column takes a smoothly tapered 'bird's beak' appearance (Figure 5.2). The oesophageal body gradually becomes dilated, and eventually elongated and tortuous; the gastric air bubble disappears. Radionucleotide transit studies may demonstrate impaired passage of the bolus in the distal oesophagus and at the level of the lower oesophageal sphincter. However, in a prospective study,

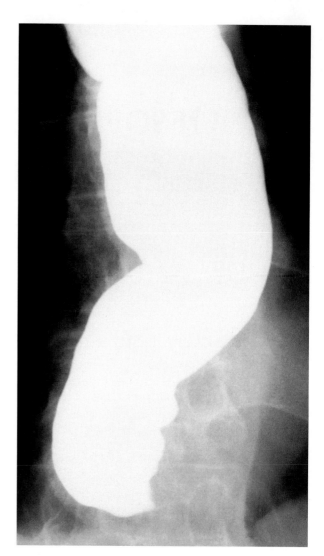

Figure 5.2
Barium swallow showing classical achalasia.

radionucleotide and fluoroscopic studies were found to lack sensitivity in detecting achalasia.[18]

Manometry The diagnosis of achalasia has traditionally been a manometric diagnosis. On manometric examination the deglutitive pressure peaks develop shortly after swallowing and occur simultaneously throughout the oesophageal body (Figure 5.3). In some patients progressive contractions still occur in the upper few centimetres of the gullet, corresponding to the striated muscle portion. After treatment the oesophageal diameter decreases in nearly one-third of the patients and peristaltic contractions may reappear.[1]

The amplitude of the pressure waves decreases when the oesophagus becomes dilated and they assume a typical broad-based shape. When the amplitude of the contraction waves is high, the pressure waves are repetitive and spontaneous contractions occur, the condition is called 'vigorous achalasia'.[19] The hyperactive deglutitive motility response of the oesophageal body and some clinical features of vigorous achalasia resemble the pattern of symptomatic diffuse oesophageal

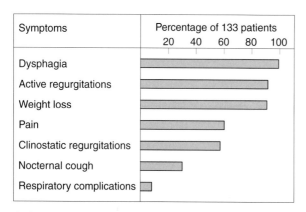

Symptoms	Percentage of 133 patients				
	20	40	60	80	100
Dysphagia					
Active regurgitations					
Weight loss					
Pain					
Clinostatic regurgitations					
Nocternal cough					
Respiratory complications					

Figure 5.1
Frequency of symptoms of achalasia.

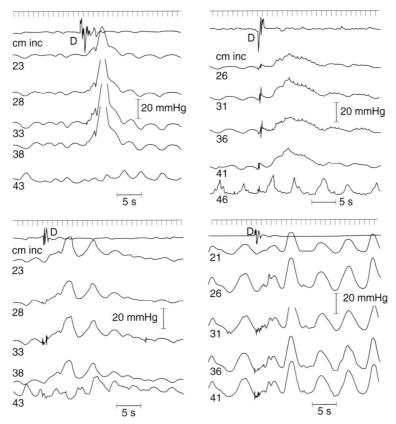

Figure 5.3

Manometric patterns in achalasia (D = deglutition): simultaneous waves of normal amplitude (upper left); simultaneous waves in dilated oesophagus (upper right); simultaneous repetitive waves (lower left); vigorous achalasia (lower right).

spasm. As in achalasia, however, peristaltic waves are not seen, and the sphincteric relaxations are defective.

The resting pressure of the lower oesophageal sphincter is increased in achalasia.[20] Pressures above 30 mmHg have been measured in 40–90% of the patients.[20,21] Furthermore, sphincter relaxation upon swallowing is incomplete (about 30% relaxation), in contrast to the normal sphincter, which relaxes completely. The residual sphincter pressure seems responsible for the obstruction to the passage from the oesophagus into the stomach.

Differential diagnosis

A mega-oesophagus with a smooth distal narrowing has been found in children with familial dysautonomia (Riley–Day syndrome), but in these patients oesophageal peristalsis is preserved.[22] Amyloidosis may cause a mega-oesophagus which resembles achalasia on both radiological and manometric examination. Bulbar paralysis and intestinal pseudo-obstruction can also cause an atonic oesophagus. In these instances extraoesophageal manifestations will point to the diagnosis. In scleroderma, the skeletal muscle portion of the oesophagus is usually not involved, some degree of peristalsis may be preserved in the smooth muscle portion, the oesophageal contractions are weak and the tone of the lower oesophageal sphincter is decreased. Barium is readily evacuated in the upright position, but not in the recumbent position.

Carcinoma of the cardia may pose a difficult diagnostic problem (pseudo-achalasia). Oesophagoscopy, with biopsy if necessary, is performed to rule out carcinomatous involvement of the distal oesophagus. Endoscopy is also the best way to recognize carcinomatous change (usually in the body of the oesophagus), which may complicate long-standing achalasia.

Pancreatic, bronchial and gastric cancer, and lymphoma of the distal oesophagus, may produce an achalasia-like picture.[23,24] The manometric features are identical to those in idiopathic achalasia, but the clinical history is slightly different. Patients are usually more than 50 years old, have a short duration of dysphagia (less than one year) and weight loss is prominent. The mechanism of this type of secondary achalasia is unknown.

Diffuse oesophageal spasm

Symptomatic diffuse oesophageal spasm is characterized by clinical symptoms of intermittent chest pain, dysphagia or both in the absence of a demonstrable organic lesion, and by abnormal, non-peristaltic contractions on manometry or radiological examination.[25–27]

Incidence

Typical diffuse spasm is a rare disorder, being less than one-fifth as frequent as achalasia. It can occur in either sex and at any age, but is more common in individuals over 50 years of age.

Pathology

The pathology of diffuse oesophageal spasm is not well known. Oesophageal wall thickening has been ascribed to both hyperplasia and hypertrophy of smooth muscle cells.[6,28] The nervous tissue changes are less pronounced than in achalasia, but show the same pattern, i.e. decreased number of ganglion cells, degenerative nerve endings and inflammation.[6,29,30]

Pathophysiology

The oesophageal motility disorders of patients with diffuse oesophageal spasm are less severe than those of achalasia. The oesophagus has not completely lost the capacity to produce normal peristaltic contractions and normal lower oesophageal sphincter relaxation. In the typical patient peristalsis progresses in a normal way from the pharynx along the oesophagus over a length of several centimetres. In the middle third of the gullet, the peristaltic contraction is replaced by 'tertiary contractions' which develop simultaneously over the entire length of the remaining distal oesophagus. The tertiary contractions of diffuse oesophageal spasm often produce pressure waves of high amplitude and longer duration. Not infrequently, deglutition results in repetitive contractions (several waves in response to a single swallow).[31] Sometimes, the peristaltic progression seems to be interrupted in a segment of several centimetres and reappears in the more distal part of the oesophagus. The propulsion of the swallowed bolus may be hindered by 'spastic' tertiary contractions which obliterate the lumen prior to the passage of the bolus. This is one mechanism for dysphagia, another being defective relaxation of the lower oesophageal sphincter. Pain is probably produced by strong contractions following deglutition or occurring 'spontaneously'.

The creation of an artificial high pressure zone in the body of the oesophagus, by inflating an intraoesophageal balloon to a critical level, allows the study of deglutitive inhibition in the oesophageal body in humans.[32] This deglutitive inhibition is likely to express the activation of inhibitory neurones in response to swallowing. In patients with primary motor disorders of the oesophagus, the degree of inhibition after swallowing is inversely related to the progression velocity of the contraction. Absence of inhibition results in simultaneous contractions. This observation, together with the favourable response to nitrergic agents, suggests that patients with primary oesophageal motor disorders may have a deficient inhibitory innervation of the oesophagus. However, so far, loss of inhibitory neurones has only been documented in achalasia. Described in 1960,[33] when oesophageal manometry was still performed with an unperfused catheter system, the 'hypertensive lower oesophageal sphincter' syndrome remains a controversial issue. The mean resting pressure in these syndromes was 49.8 mmHg, as compared with 18 mmHg in a control series. A hypertensive sphincter may occur as an isolated finding, or it may be accompanied by distal oesophageal body contraction abnormalities, which may range from the nutcracker oesophagus (abnormally increased distal oesophageal body contraction amplitude)[20,34] to diffuse oesophageal spasm.[20,35–37] Most,[3,38,39] but not all[40] manometric studies in patients with the hypertensive lower oesophageal sphincter syndrome have shown that the percentage relaxation of the sphincter after swallowing does not differ significantly from that of controls. Consequently, the residual pressure after swallowing is higher than in controls, which may contribute to the development of dysphagia.

The symptoms that have been ascribed to a hypertensive lower oesophageal sphincter include chest pain and dysphagia. As for the nutcracker oesophagus, it is unclear whether the hypertensive lower oesophageal sphincter is merely an abnormal manometric finding, or whether it constitutes a clinically important abnormality. It is possible that a hypertensive lower oesophageal sphincter is an epiphenomenon from an exaggerated response to various stimuli such as chest pain or environmental stress.[41]

Clinical features

Most patients have both pain and dysphagia; these occur intermittently and vary from mild and occasional to severe and daily. The pain is precipitated by a meal in approximately 50% of patients, is often associated with dysphagia, and may worsen during periods of emotional stress. However, the pain may also be unrelated to meals, occur at night and mimic pain of myocardial origin. Both types of pain are relieved by glyceryl trinitrate. The dysphagia is of variable severity and lacks the persistence seen in achalasia or organic stenosis.

Investigations

The diagnosis of diffuse oesophageal spasm is based on a combination of clinical symptoms and a poorly defined complex of manometric abnormalities (Figure 5.4) in an oesophagus which has not completely lost its ability to produce peristaltic contractions and lower oesophageal sphincter relaxations.

One of the main problems is the relationship between symptomatic diffuse oesophageal spasm and acid sensitivity. Both conditions may coexist. Pressure monitoring and 24-hour pH may prove to be useful for the recognition of pain of oesophageal origin and for the identification of gastro-oesophageal reflux or spasm as the cause of pain.

Manometry There are no uniform, generally accepted criteria for the manometric diagnosis of diffuse oesophageal spasm. According to Richter and Castell,[42] more than 10% of wet swallows should produce simultaneous pressure peaks. For others, 30% of the deglutitive responses should consist of simultaneous waves of high amplitude and long duration.[25,43] A duration of more than 6 s has been proposed as the definition of prolonged contractions, because this value is greater than the mean + two standard deviations in normal subjects.[2,43,44] However, with intraluminal transducers or a low compliance perfusion system and wet swallows, pressure peaks in the distal oesophagus of 190 mmHg or more are generally considered to be of high amplitude. Repetitive waves (several pressure peaks in response to a single swallow) are seen in the majority (56–95%) of patients and spontaneous contractions (not

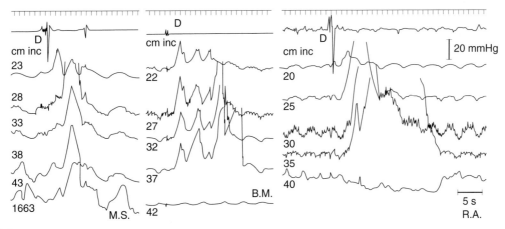

Figure 5.4

Manometric patterns in diffuse oesophageal spasm (D = deglutition): peristaltic waves becoming simultaneous in the distal oesophagus (left); repetitive waves (centre); peristaltic 'giant' waves (right).

induced by swallows) occur in more than half of these patients.[27,45] Incomplete (< 75%) lower oesophageal sphincter relaxations and high (> 50 mmHg) sphincter pressures may also be seen.

Radiology The radiological appearance of symptomatic diffuse oesophageal spasm (Figure 5.5) is described as curling, segmental spasm, ladder spasm, rosary bead oesophagus, spastic pseudodiverticulosis, corkscrew oesophagus, etc. These terms refer to segmental, non-peristaltic contractions, which may trap the barium and push it back and forth. This is best demonstrated when the patient is in the recumbent position. A second, but less common picture, is a tight contraction of the oesophagus over a length of several centimetres or a slight diffuse narrowing of the lower half of the oesophagus with a slightly dilated upper segment.[37] Marked dilatation of the oesophagus and prolonged stasis of food and fluids are rare in diffuse spasm.

The extent and severity of the radiological abnormalities may vary widely from patient to patient, and from one time to another in the same patient.[46] The severity of the radiological changes correlates poorly with the clinical, manometric or pathological findings. Patients with diffuse oesophageal spasm may appear normal on routine radiological examination and typical radiological pictures may occur in asymptomatic patients (mainly in the elderly) or in a patient with diffuse spasm at a symptom-free moment.

Diagnostic tests The lack of strict diagnostic criteria, and the need to distinguish diffuse spasm from achalasia on the one hand and from non-specific or asymptomatic motor disorders on the other hand, make provocation tests highly desirable. The oesophagus of many patients with symptomatic diffuse oesophageal spasm is hypersensitive to cholinergics such as methacholine and bethanechol,[43,47] and is also hypersensitive to the cholinesterase inhibitor edrophonium chloride.[43] However, the methacholine test is also positive in patients with primary achalasia, those with Chagas' disease and in some patients with carcinomatous infiltration of Auerbach's plexus.[48] The test can be useful in distinguishing diffuse spasm from asymptomatic

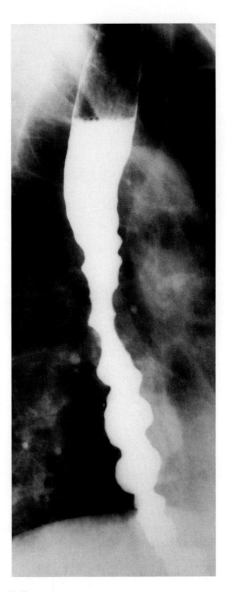

Figure 5.5

Radiograph of diffuse oesophageal spasm.

motor disorders and from reflux-related spasm.[43,47] The oesophagus of patients with diffuse spasm has been reported to be supersensitive to pentagastrin or gastrin administration.[49,50] The pentagastrin test has proved to be disappointing because it is often negative in patients with symptomatic diffuse oesophageal spasm and positive in patient with achalasia and in some elderly patients.[51,52]

Ergometrine maleate (Ergonovine), an alpha-adrenergic agonist, has been used as a provocative test for coronary artery spasm and for oesophageal spasm.[53,54] However, serious side-effects may occur and the test should not be used routinely.

Almost 5% of patients taking the serotonin-1D receptor agonist sumatriptan for migraine have chest discomfort. These symptoms are most frequently not associated with changes in cardiac function or enzymes. In healthy subjects, administration of sumatriptan in supratherapeutic doses causes small but significant increases in the amplitude and duration of deglutitive contractions, and an increased frequency of repetitive contractions can be observed.[55] These data suggest that sumatriptan might provoke diffuse oesophageal spasm in susceptible patients. However, until now, no temporal association has been observed between chest symptoms and abnormal oesophageal motility after sumatriptan.

Primary oesophageal motility disorders of the intermediate type

Although achalasia and symptomatic diffuse oesophageal spasm have distinctive properties, a number of patients do not fit into this simple classification. Some patients who would otherwise fit the criteria have occasional peristaltic waves or sphincter relaxations. Up to 24% of those with motility disorders severe enough to justify treatment with dilatation did not fit well into the two classic categories.[1] Furthermore, after dilatation as many as 45% of the patients fell into the intermediate category. These patients presented with either complete absence of peristalsis and the presence of (at least some) normal lower oesophageal sphincter relaxations, or with some degree of peristalsis and complete absence of normal lower oesophageal sphincter relaxation. These observations suggest that the primary oesophageal motility disorders constitute a spectrum of motor disorders composed of achalasia, diffuse spasms and intermediate types (Figure 5.6).[1] Moreover, transition from symptomatic diffuse oesophageal spasm to achalasia has been documented,[1,56] although most patients with diffuse spasm remain unchanged over long periods of time. Radiological examination shows an oesophagus that resembles achalasia rather than diffuse spasm. Treatment with pneumatic dilatation results in a success rate comparable to that of achalasia.

Nutcracker oesophagus (symptomatic oesophageal peristalsis)

The development of measurement systems able to pick up rapid pressure rises has led to the description of a syndrome characterized clinically by angina-like chest pain and/or dysphagia and manometrically by oesophageal peristaltic

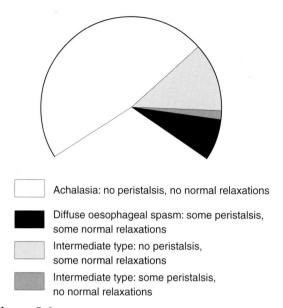

☐ Achalasia: no peristalsis, no normal relaxations

■ Diffuse oesophageal spasm: some peristalsis, some normal relaxations

▨ Intermediate type: no peristalsis, some normal relaxations

▨ Intermediate type: some peristalsis, no normal relaxations

Figure 5.6
Spectrum of primary oesophageal motility disorders.

contractions of markedly increased amplitude and/or duration.

Originally identified by Brand et al.,[57] this condition has been the subject of intensive investigation and is usually termed 'nutcracker oesophagus'.[2,39,58,59] The manometric criteria proposed for the diagnosis of nutcracker oesophagus are a mean amplitude of deglutitive pressure peaks above 180 mmHg in the lower one-third of the oesophagus after swallowing 5 ml liquid boluses.[58,60] The most common symptom is angina-like chest pain. High-amplitude, distal oesophageal body contractions have been reported in 27–48% of patients with non-cardiac chest pain. Others have doubted the relationship between the amplitude of the contraction peaks and symptoms in patients with nutcracker oesophagus, because calcium channel blockers may decrease the amplitude without improving the symptoms.[60,61] Because the amplitude of oesophageal contractions increases during psychological stress, particularly in patients with the nutcracker oesophagus, high amplitude contractions may simply be an epiphenomenon from an exaggerated response to various stimuli such as chest pain or environmental stress. Oesophageal ischaemia could be another contributing factor: after oesophageal cooling, the rewarming time was found to be longer in patients with nutcracker oesophagus, suggesting oesophageal ischaemia as a possible cause of chest pain.[62]

Irritable oesophagus

The irritable oesophagus concept was derived from the observation that some patients with non-cardiac chest pain, when studied by 24-hour pH and pressure measurements, sometimes developed pain associated with reflux alone (without motor disorders), and on other occasions during the same study experienced the same pain together with motility disorders alone (without acid reflux).[4] The oesophagus of these patients appears to be hypersensitive to a variety of stimuli. The diagnosis of irritable oesophagus is therefore based on the demonstration that the patient's familiar chest pain can be elicited by both mechanical and chemical stimuli.

To demonstrate the association of pain with endogenous stimuli (acid reflux, motor disorders), 24-hour pH and pressure measurements are used. The optimal time window in symptom analysis of 24-hour oesophageal pressure and pH data begins at 2 minutes before the onset of the pain and ends at the onset of the pain.[63]

Provocation tests can also be used as exogenous stimuli. These include the acid perfusion test of Bernstein, the edrophonium test, the balloon distension test and the vasopressin test.[64-67] A positive acid perfusion test indicates that the oesophagus is acid sensitive, but does not prove that the spontaneous pain attacks are induced by acid reflux.[68] Likewise, a positive edrophonium test or a positive balloon distension test indicates that the oesophagus is mechanosensitive, but does not prove that motor disorders are the cause of the spontaneous chest pain episodes. Moreover, provocation tests may be influenced by the style of test administration and the interaction between the tester and the patient.[69] At present, the best way to determine the cause of spontaneous pain attacks of non-cardiac chest pain is by 24-hour intraoesophageal pH and pressure recordings.[64] Finally, a belching disorder may be the mechanism responsible for chest pain in patients with abnormal sensitivity to intraoesophageal balloon distention, as shown by the intraoesophageal injection of air.[70]

The use of extensive oesophageal testing in patients with non-cardiac chest pain has been controversial. In a prospective study, patients who underwent oesophageal testing showed a decline in utilization of health care resources.[71] It is obviously important to identify the specific abnormality that causes the chest pain because this will determine the type of treatment. Patients with chest pain due to acid reflux will be treated primarily by measures that reduce or eliminate acid exposure of the oesophageal mucosa. Hyperactive motility disturbances will be treated by muscle relaxants such as nitrates or calcium channel blockers. Patients with an irritable oesophagus constitute a difficult management problem. These patients may need drugs that reduce pain perception rather than drugs that combat gastro-oesophageal reflux or motor disturbances. Clouse et al.[72] have successfully used the non-tricyclic antidepressant trazodone in patients with chest pain.

SECONDARY OESOPHAGEAL MOTOR DISORDERS

Various generalized diseases may cause motor disorders of the oesophagus (Table 5.1), but only some of these are discussed here.

Systemic sclerosis and other collagen diseases

The oesophagus is abnormal in 50–80% of patients with scleroderma.[73] The degree of oesophageal involvement bears no rela-

Table 5.1 Diseases causing oesophageal motility disorders

Collagen diseases
  Systemic sclerosis
  Systemic lupus erythematosus
  Polymyositis–dermatomyositis

Muscle diseases
  Myotonic dystrophy
  Ocular and oculopharyngeal myopathy
  Myasthenia gravis

Central nervous system diseases
  Brainstem lesions
  Poliomyelitis
  Motor neurone disease
  Extrapyramidal disturbances
  Stiff-man (Moersch–Woltmann) syndrome
  Dysautonomia
  Intestinal pseudo-obstruction

Peripheral neuropathies
  Diabetic neuropathy
  Alcoholic neuropathy

tion to the degree of involvement of other organs. Sometimes the skin lesions improve while the oesophageal involvement progresses. Histological studies of the oesophagus show that the smooth muscle layers are atrophied with some fibrous replacement, whereas striated muscle fibres are remarkably well preserved.[74-77] Inflammatory and fibrous changes also occur in the mucosa and submucosa. At least some of the mucosal lesions are due to gastro-oesophageal reflux. Intraluminal pressure measurements indicate that peristalsis usually remains normal in the upper, striated portion of the gullet, whereas in the smooth muscle portion the contractions are often non-peristaltic, weak and may eventually disappear completely (Figure 5.7).[78,79] The lower oesophageal sphincter pressure is frequently lower than normal, which may lead to gastro-oesophageal reflux and oesophagitis. The loss of coordinated peristalsis in the distal oesophagus is fairly well correlated with the development of Raynaud's phenomenon.[80]

Oesophageal motility disorders may be present in early scleroderma, in the presence of normal oesophageal smooth muscle at autopsy.[77] Moreover, some patients with scleroderma have a preserved response to muscle stimulants but not to agents requiring intact cholinergic innervation.[81] Although these observations suggest that smooth muscle atrophy is a secondary phenomenon, ultrastructural and light microscopic studies have failed to provide morphological supporting evidence.[82]

The oesophagus is involved in 10–25% of patients with systemic lupus erythematosus. The motility disorders resemble those of systemic sclerosis, but are less pronounced.[8] In Sjögren's syndrome, oesophageal motor abnormalities are found in one-third of the patients.[83]

More than 60% of patients with dermatomyositis or polymyositis complain of high dysphagia.[84,85] The degree of dysphagia parallels the course and severity of the muscle involvement. Initially, the motility disorders are most prominent

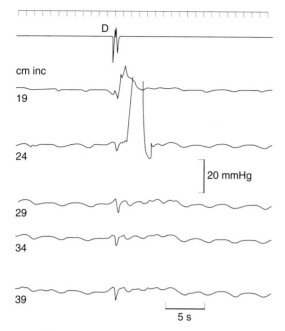

Figure 5.7
Manometric pattern of oesophageal motility in scleroderma.
Normal peristaltic contractions in the upper part; absence of
deglutitive response in the lower part.

in the pharynx and upper oesophagus; later, smooth muscles
are also involved. Weakness of oesophageal contractions often
leads to tracheal aspiration and nasal reflux. Radiological examination reveals an atonic upper oesophageal sphincter and
pooling of barium in the valleculae and pyriform sinuses. When
the lower oesophagus is involved, the contractions become
weak and non-peristaltic and the lower oesophageal sphincter
pressure decreases, predisposing the patient to reflux
oesophagitis.

REFERENCES

1. Vantrappen G, Janssens J, Hellemans J & Coremans G. Achalasia, diffuse esophageal spasm, and related motility disorders. *Gastroenterology* 1979; **76**: 450.
2. Benjamin SB, Gerhardt DC & Castell DO. High amplitude peristaltic esophageal contractions associated with chest pain and/or dysphagia. *Gastroenterology* 1979; **77**: 478–483.
3. Freidin N, Traube M, Mittal RK & McCallum RW. The hypertensive lower esophageal sphincter. Manometric and clinical aspects. *Dig Dis Sci* 1989; **34**: 1063–1067.
4. Vantrappen G, Janssens J & Ghillebert G. The irritable esophagus – a frequent cause of angina-like pain. *Lancet* 1987; **i**: 1232–1234.
5. Cassella RR, Brown AL Jr, Sayre GP & Ellis FH Jr. Achalasia of the esophagus: pathologic and etiologic considerations. *Ann Surg* 1964; **160**: 474–486.
6. Cassella RR, Ellis FH Jr & Brown AL. Fine-structure changes in achalasia of the esophagus. I. Vagus nerves. *Am J Pathol* 1965; **46**: 279–288.
7. Trounce JR, Deucher DC, Kauntze R & Thomas GA. Studies in achalasia of the cardia. *Q J Med* 1957; **28**: 433–443.
8. Goldblum JR, Whyte RI, Orringer MB & Appelman HD. Achalasia: a morphologic study of 42 resected specimens. *Am J Surg Pathol* 1994; **18**: 327–337.
9. Diamant NE & El-Sharkawy TY. Neural control of esophageal peristalsis. A conceptual analysis. *Gastroenterology* 1977; **72**: 546–556.
10. Goyal RK & Rattan S. Neurohumoral, hormonal and drug receptors for the lower esophageal sphincter. *Gastroenterology* 1978; **84**: 589–619.
11. Mearin F, Mourelle M, Guarner F et al. Patients with achalasia lack nitric oxide synthase in the gastro-oesophageal junction. *Eur J Clin Invest* 1993; **23**: 724–728.
12. Cohen S, Fisher R & Tuch A. The site of denervation in achalasia. *Gut* 1972; **13**: 556–558.
13. Holloway RH, Dodds WJ, Helm JF, Hogan WJ, Dent J & Arndorfer RC. Integrity of cholinergic innervation to the lower esophageal sphincter in achalasia. *Gastroenterology* 1986; **90**: 924.
14. Pasricha PJ, Ravich WJ, Hendrix TR, Sostre S & Kalloo AN. Intrasphincteric botulinum toxin for the treatment of achalasia. *N Engl J Med* 1995; **332**: 774–778.
15. Kramer P & Ingelfinger FJ. Esophageal sensitivity to mecholyl in cardiospasm. *Gastroenterology* 1951; **19**: 242–253.
16. Verne GN, Sallustio JE & Eaker EY. Anti-myenteric neuronal antibodies in patients with achalasia. A prospective study. *Dig Dis Sci* 1997; **42**: 307–313.
17. Vantrappen G & Hellemans J. Achalasia. In Vantrappen G & Hellemans J (eds) *Diseases of the Oesophagus.* Berlin, Heidelberg, New York: Springer-Verlag, 1975: 287–354.
18. Stacher G, Schima W, Bergmann H et al. Sensitivity of radio nuclide bolus transport and video fluoroscopic studies compared with manome-try in the diagnosis of achalasia. *Am J Gastroenterol* 1994; **89**: 1484–1486.
19. Sanderson DR, Ellis FH Jr, Schlegel JF & Olsen AM. Syndrome of vigorous achalasia: clinical and physiologic observations. *Dis Chest* 1967; **52**: 508–517.
20. Cohen S & Lipschutz W. Lower esophageal sphincter dysfunction in achalasia. *Gastroenterology* 1971; **61**: 814–820.
21. Berger K & McCallum RW. The hypertensive lower esophageal sphincter: a clinical and manometric study. *Gastroenterology* 1980; **80**: 1109.
22. Joseph R & Job JC. Dysautonomie familiale et mégaoesophage. *Arch Fr Pédiatr* 1963; **20**: 25–33.
23. Kolodny M, Schrader ZR, Rubin W, Hochman R & Sleisenger MH. Esophageal achalasia probably due to gastric carcinoma. *Ann Intern Med* 1968; **69**: 569–573.
24. Tucker HJ, Snape WJ Jr & Cohen S. Achalasia secondary to carcinoma: manometric and clinical features. *Ann Intern Med* 1978; **89**: 315–318.
25. DiMarino AJ Jr & Cohen S. Characteristics of lower esophageal sphincter function in symptomatic diffuse esophageal spasm. *Gastroenterology* 1974; **66**: 1–6.
26. Fleshler B. Diffuse esophageal spasm. *Gastroenterology* 1967; **52**: 559–564.
27. Gillies M, Nicks R & Skyring A. Clinical, manometric and pathological studies in diffuse oesophageal spasm. *BMJ* 1967; **2**: 527–530.
28. Friesen DL, Henderson RD & Hanna W. Ultrastructure of the esophageal muscle in achalasia and diffuse esophageal spasm. *Am J Clin Pathol* 1983; **79**: 319–325.
29. Adams CWM, Brain RHF & Trounce JR. Ganglion cells in achalasia of the cardia. *Virchows Arch* 1976; **327**: 75–79.
30. Sloper JC. Idiopathic diffuse muscular hypertrophy of the lower oesophagus. *Thorax* 1954; **9**: 136–146.
31. Creamer B, Donoghue FE & Code CF. Pattern of esophageal motility in diffuse spasm. *Gastroenterology* 1958; **34**: 782–796.
32. Sifrim D, Janssens J & Vantrappen G. Failing deglutitive inhibition in primary esophageal motility disorders. *Gastroenterology* 1994; **106**: 875–882.
33. Code CF, Schlegel JF, Kelly ML, Olsen AM & Ellis JH. Hypertensive gastroesophageal sphincter. *Mayo Clin Proc* 1960; **35**: 391–399.
34. Traube M & McCallum RW. Comparison of esophageal manometric characteristics in asymptomatic subjects and symptomatic patients with high-amplitude esophageal peristaltic contractions. *Am J Gastroenterol* 1987; **82**: 831–835.
35. Garrett JM & Goodwin DH. Gastroesophageal hypercontracting sphincter. *JAMA* 1969; **208**: 992–998.
36. Pederson SA & Alstrup P. The hypertensive gastroesophageal sphincter. A manometric and clinical study. *Scand J Gastroenterol* 1972; **7**: 531–534.
37. Vantrappen G & Hellemans J. Diffuse muscle spasm of the oesophagus and hypertensive oesophageal sphincter. *Clin Gastroenterol* 1976; **5**: 59–72.
38. Orr WC & Robinson MG. Hypertensive peristalsis in the pathogenesis of chest pain: further exploration of the 'nutcracker' esophagus. *Am J Gastroenterol* 1982; **77**: 604–607.
39. Traube M, Aaronson RM & McCallum RW. Transition from nutcracker esophagus to diffuse esophagus spasm. *Arch Intern Med* 1987; **146**: 1844–1847.
40. Waterman DC, Dalton CB, Ott DJ et al. Hypertensive lower esophageal sphincter: What does it mean? *J Clin Gastroenterol* 1989; **11**: 139–146.

41. Anderson KO, Dalton CB, Bradley LA & Richter JE. Stress induces alteration of esophageal pressures in healthy volunteers and non-cardiac chest pain patients. *Dig Dis Sci* 1989; **34**: 83–91.

42. Richter JE & Castell DO. Diffuse esophageal spasm: a reappraisal. *Ann Intern Med* 1984; **100**: 242–245.

43. Mellow M. Symptomatic diffuse esophageal spasm. Manometric follow-up and response to cholinergic stimulation and cholinesterase inhibition. *Gastroenterology* 1977; **73**: 237–240.

44. Richter JE, Wu WC, Johns DN et al. Esophageal manometry in 95 healthy adult volunteers. Variability of pressures with age and frequency of abnormal contractions. *Dig Dis Sci* 1987; **32**: 583–592.

45. Roth HP & Fleshler B. Diffuse esophageal spasm. *Ann Intern Med* 1964; **61**: 914–923.

46. Bennett JR & Hendrix TR. Diffuse esophageal spasm: a disorder with more than one cause. *Gastroenterology* 1970; **59**: 273–279.

47. Kramer P, Fleshler B, McNally E & Harris LD. Oesophageal sensitivity to mecholyl in symptomatic diffuse spasm. *Gut* 1967; **8**: 120–127.

48. Herrera AF, Colon J, Valdes-Dapena A & Roth JLA. Achalasia or carcinoma? The significance of the mecholyl test. *Am J Dig Dis* 1970; **15**: 1073–1081.

49. Eckhardt VF, Kruger J, Holtermuller KH & Ewe K. Alteration of esophageal paeristalsis by pentagastrin in patients with diffuse eosophageal spasm. *Scand J Gastroenterol* 1975; **10**: 475–479.

50. Lane WH, Ippoliti AF & McCallum RW. Effect of gastrin heptadecapeptide (G17) on oesophageal contractions in patients with diffuse oesophageal spasm. *Gut* 1979; **20**: 756–759.

51. Guelrud M, Simon C, Gomez G & Villalta B. Pentagastrin supersensitivity of the lower esophageal sphincter (LES) in the elderly. *Gastroenterology* 1981; **80**: 1165.

52. Orlando RC & Bozymski E. The effects of pentagastrin in achalasia and diffuse esophageal spasm. *Gastroenterology* 1979; **77**: 472–477.

53. Dart AM, Alban Davies H, Lowndes RH, Dalal J, Ruttley M & Henderson AH. Oesophageal spasm and 'angina': diagnostic value of ergonovine provocation. *Eur Heart J* 1980; **1**: 91–95.

54. Heupler FA Jr, Proudfit WL, Razavi M, Shierley EK, Greenstreet R & Sheldon WC. Ergonovine maleate provocative test for coronary arterial spasm. *Am J Cardiol* 1978; **41**: 631–640.

55. Houghton L, Foster JM, Whorwell PJ, Morris J & Fowler P. Is chest pain after sumatriptan esophageal in origin? *Lancet* 1994; **344**: 985–986.

56. Kramer P, Harris LD & Donaldson RM Jr. Transition from symptomatic diffuse spasm to cardiospasm. *Gut* 1967; **8**: 115–118.

57. Brand DL, Martin D & Pope CE. Esophageal manometries in patients with angina-like chest pain. *Am J Dig Dis* 1977; **22**: 300–304.

58. Dalton CB, Castell DO & Richter JE. The changing faces of the nutcracker esophagus. *Am J Gastroenterol* 1988; **83**: 623–628.

59. Traube M, Abibi R & McCallum RW. High amplitude peristaltic contractions associated with chest pain. *JAMA* 1983; **250**: 2655–2659.

60. Richter JE, Dalton CB, Bradley LA & Castell DO. Oral nifedipine in the treatment of non-cardiac chest pain in patients with the nutcracker esophagus. *Gastroenterology* 1987; **93**: 21–28.

61. Cohen S. Esophageal motility disorders: the sphinx revisited. *Gastroenterology* 1987; **93**: 201–203.

62. MacKenzie J, Belch J, Land D, Park R & McKillop J. Oesophageal ischaemia in motility disorders associated with chest pain. *Lancet* 1988; **ii**: 592–595.

63. Lam HGT, Breumelhof R, Roelofs JMM, Van Berge Henegouwen GP & Smout AJPM. What is the optimal time window in symptom analysis of 24-hour esophageal pressure and pH data? *Dig Dis Sci* 1994; **39**: 402–409.

64. Bernstein LM & Baker LA. A clinical test for esophagitis. *Gastroenterology* 1958; **34**: 760–781.

65. Ghillebert G, Janssens J, Vantrappen G, Nevens F & Piessens J. Ambulatory 24 hour intraoesophageal pH and pressure recordings vs provocation tests in the diagnosis of chest pain of oesophageal origin. *Gut* 1990; **31**: 738–744.

66. Richter JE, Barish CF & Castell DO. Abnormal sensory perception in patients with esophageal chest pain. *Gastroenterology* 1986; **91**: 845–852.

67. Richter JE, Hackshaw BT, Wu WC & Castell DO. Edrophonium: a useful provocative test for esophageal chest pain. *Ann Intern Med* 1985; **103**: 14–21.

68. Janssens J, Vantrappen G & Ghillebert G. 24-hour recording of esophageal pressure and pH in patients with noncardiac chest pain. *Gastroenterology* 1984; **90**: 1978–1984.

69. Rose S, Achkar E, Falk GW, Flesher B & Revta R. Interaction between patient and test administrator may influence the results of edrophonium provocative testing in patients with non-cardiac chest pain. *J Gastroenterol* 1994; **88**: 20–24.

70. Gignoux C, Bost R, Hostein J et al. Role of upper esophageal reflex and belch reflex dysfunctions in non-cardiac chest pain. *Dig Dis Sci* 1993; **38**: 1909–1914.

71. Rose S, Achkar E & Easly KA. Follow-up of patients with noncardiac chest pain: value of esophageal testing. *Dig Dis Sci* 1994; **39**: 2069–2073.

72. Clouse RE, Lustman PJ, Eckert TC, Ferney DM & Griffith LS. Low dose trazodone for symptomatic patients with esophageal contraction abnormalities. *Gastroenterology* 1987; **92**: 1027–1036.

73. Hellemans J & Vantrappen G. Motor disorders due to collagen diseases. In Vantrappen G & Hellemans J (eds) *Diseases of the Esophagus*. Berlin: Springer, 1974; 383–393.

74. Atkinson M & Summerling MD. Oesopahgal changes in systemic sclerosis. *Gut* 1966; **7**: 402–408.

75. d'Angelo WZ, Fries JF, Masi AT & Schulman LE. Pathologic observations in systemic sclerosis (scleroderma). *Am J Med* 1969; **46**: 428–440.

76. Dornhorst AC, Pierce JW & Whimsler IW. The esophageal lesion in scleroderma. *Lancet* 1954; **i**: 698–699.

77. Treacy WL, Baggenstoss AH, Slocumb CH & Code CF. Scleroderma of the esophagus. A correlation of histologic and physiologic findings. *Ann Intern Med* 1963; **59**: 351–356.

78. Garrett JM, Winkelmann RK, Schlegel JF & Code CF. Esophageal deterioration in scleroderma. *Mayo Clin Proc* 1971; **46**: 92–96.

79. Turner R, Lipshutz W, Miller W, Rittenberg G, Schumacher HR & Cohen S. Esophageal dysfunction in collagen disease. *Am J Med Sci* 1973; **265**: 191–199.

80. Stevens MB, Hookman P, Siegel CI, Esterly JR, Shleman LE & Hendrix TR. Aperistalsis of the esophagus in patients with connective-tissue disorders and Raynaud's phenomenon. *N Engl J Med* 1964; **270**: 1218–1222.

81. Cohen S, Fisher R, Lipshutz W, Turner R, Myers A & Schumacher R. The pathogenesis of esophageal dysfunction in scleroderma and Raynaud's disease. *J Clin Invest* 1972; **51**: 2663–2668.

82. Russel ML, Friezen D, Henderson RD & Hanna WM. Ultrastructure of the esophagus in scleroderma. *Arthritis Rheum* 1982; **25**: 1117–1123.

83. Palma R, Freire A, Freitas J et al. Esophageal motility disorders in patients with Sjogren's syndrome. *Dig Dis Sci* 1994; **39**: 758–761.

84. Christianson HB, Brunsting LA & Perry HL. Dermatomyositis: unusual features, complications, and treatment. *Arch Dermatol* 1956; **74**: 581–589.

85. Donoghue F, Winkelmann R & Moersch H. Esophageal defects in dermatomyositis. *Ann Otol* 1960; **69**: 1139–1145.

6

MEDICAL TREATMENT OF OESOPHAGEAL MOTILITY DISORDERS

J Tack
J Janssens
G Vantrappen

Primary oesophageal motility disorders constitute a spectrum including achalasia, diffuse oesophageal spasm and intermediate conditions.[1] Equally vague is the border between these primary motility disorders and so-called non-specific oesophageal motility disorders (NEMD), which include conditions such as the nutcracker oesophagus and the hypertensive lower oesophageal sphincter.[2,3] The latter two conditions have been identified on the basis of high contractile pressures not accompanied by abnormalities of peristalsis or sphincteric relaxation. The relationship between this manometric finding and clinical symptoms remains controversial.

Dysphagia and chest pain are the main symptoms of primary motility disorders of the oesophagus. Dysphagia is the prime symptom in achalasia although chest pain may be present as well, especially in the early stage of the disease. Patients with symptomatic diffuse oesophageal spasm mainly complain of chest pain together with some degree of dysphagia; it rarely, if ever, leads to significant oesophageal stasis. Chest pain may also occur in patients with NEMD, as a consequence of gastro-oesophageal reflux, as a result of oesophageal wall ischaemia or as part of the irritable oesophagus syndrome.[4]

Secondary oesophageal motility disorders include secondary forms of achalasia (due to malignancy, Chagas' disease or pseudo-obstruction), postsurgical conditions, amyloidosis, sarcoidosis, etc. Severe gastro-oesophageal reflux disease may induce oesophageal motility disturbances mimicking the manometric picture of diffuse oesophageal spasm. Diabetic and alcoholic neuropathy, and striated and smooth muscle diseases may also produce secondary motility disturbances. Medical treatment of secondary oesophageal motility disorders should aim at correcting the underlying condition; if not possible, symptoms should be treated in the same way as in primary oesophageal motility disorders.

ACHALASIA

Most symptoms and complications of achalasia are due to retention of food and fluid in the oesophagus, as a result of defective relaxation of an often hypertensive lower oesophageal sphincter, together with loss of propulsive peristalsis in the oesophageal body.[1-3] This is caused by the loss of intrinsic inhibitory neurones in the lower oesophageal sphincter, while intrinsic excitatory (cholinergic) neurones are preserved.[4,5] The current treatment of achalasia and related motor disorders is at best palliative. It is still impossible to restore the disordered motility of the achalatic oesophagus to normal. Therefore, treatment should aim to improve oesophageal emptying by decreasing the resistance at the cardia sufficiently to allow easy aboral flow, thereby taking care that the sphincter continues to present a pressure barrier to prevent free gastro-oesophageal reflux. Non-surgical means of diminishing resistance at the cardia consist of drugs, forceful dilatation of the cardia, and endoscopic injection of botulinum toxin.

Drug treatment

Several pharmacological agents have been used in an attempt to decrease lower oesophageal sphincter pressure in patients with achalasia. Most studies, however, have evaluated only relatively short-term effects, often in patients with only mild or moderate degrees of achalasia. There are very few studies devoted to the long-term evaluation of medical therapy for achalasia, or to the comparison of drug therapy with other means of treatment.

Earlier therapeutic trials with anticholinergic agents and adrenergic blockers failed to show a substantial benefit.[6-8] More recently, cimetropium bromide, an anticholinergic, was shown to reduce lower oesophageal sphincter pressure significantly and accelerate oesophageal transit in patients with achalasia.[9] One study reported a decrease in lower oesophageal sphincter pressure in patients with achalasia following administration of high doses of loperamide.[10] No data on clinical use of these drugs have been published so far.

In the 1980s, nitrates and calcium antagonists were found to decrease lower oesophageal sphincter pressure and they have been used in an attempt to relieve achalasia symptoms.

Calcium channel blockers

Calcium entry blockers have a relaxant effect on vascular and gastrointestinal smooth muscle. Nifedipine (10–20 mg) has been shown to reduce significantly resting lower oesophageal sphincter pressure (maximum reduction 56%) and, at higher doses, the amplitude of oesophageal body contractions (maximum reduction 35%) in healthy volunteers.[11–13]

Administration of 10–20 mg nifedipine in achalasia patients significantly reduces lower oesophageal sphincter pressure (maximum reduction 47%).[14,15] In a dose of 10–20 mg given sublingually before each meal, nifedipine improved the symptoms of dysphagia in 14 of 20 patients with mild to moderate achalasia (stage I and II according to Adam's criteria) during a follow-up period of 6–18 months.[14] In a non-randomized follow-up study, treatment with nifedipine 10–20 mg sublingually 30 minutes before each meal, was compared with pneumatic dilatation in a randomized trial in 30 patients. Both treatments proved equally effective: excellent or good clinical results were observed in 75% of dilated patients and 77% of nifedipine treated patients.[16] Again, this trial was carried out in patients with mild to moderate achalasia. In another study (a crossover trial with nitrates), 15 patients with achalasia were treated with nifedipine 20 mg sublingually before meals.[15] This study also included nine patients with a dilated oesophagus (stage III). Only eight patients (53%) noted relief of dysphagia by nifedipine.

In a double-blind placebo-controlled study, nifedipine 10–30 mg sublingually in 10 achalasia patients was found to significantly reduce the frequency of dysphagia, but substantial symptoms remained during drug therapy.[17] Chronic nifedipine treatment decreased lower oesophageal sphincter pressure only moderately (by 28%, still leaving lower oesophageal sphincter pressures of 30–35 mmHg) whereas the radionuclide measurement of oesophageal emptying remained unchanged.[17] Side-effects, such as peripheral oedema, headache, flushing and hypotension, were relatively common, but did not usually require discontinuation of the drug.

Finally, a double-blind crossover study with oral nifedipine (20 mg orally 1 h before each meal), verapamil (160 mg orally 1 h before each meal) and placebo in eight patients with stage II achalasia failed to demonstrate statistically significant differences in the overall clinical symptomatology with any of the drugs.[18] This study used oral instead of sublingual nifedipine, but adequate nifedipine plasma levels were documented. The effect of diltiazem (120 mg orally) on lower oesophageal sphincter pressure and on symptoms in patients with achalasia (60–90 mg orally QID) was only marginal.[19]

Nitrates

Nitrates have a relaxant effect on smooth muscle of a variety of species and tissues, including the gastrointestinal tract in man. Early radiographic studies demonstrated relaxation of the cardia of achalasia patients in response to nitrite inhalation or sublingual nitroglycerin.[20–22] However, this effect was short-lived (4–30 minutes) and associated with several side-effects. The long-acting form of nitroglycerin, isosorbide dinitrate, was found to reduce mean lower oesophageal sphincter pressure by 66% in patients with achalasia, for at least 60 minutes.[15,23] In a dose of 5 mg given sublingually before each meal, isosorbide dinitrate improved symptoms of dysphagia in 19 of 23 patients during a follow-up period of 2–19 months, but side-effects (mainly headaches) were very common (8/24 patients).[15]

A randomized cross-over study compared the effect of two weeks of treatment with isosorbide dinitrate 5 mg sublingually before meals with that of nifedipine 20 mg in 15 patients with achalasia.[15] Isosorbide dinitrate induced a more pronounced acute reduction in lower oesophageal sphincter pressure when compared with nifedipine (63% versus 47%), resulted in a larger degree of subjective improvement (13 versus eight patients), but also had a higher rate of side-effects (six versus two patients). However, radionuclide measurement of oesophageal emptying still demonstrated considerable oesophageal retention in four patients with subjective benefit. Therapeutic failure necessitated pneumatic dilatation in six of the 15 patients.

Studies investigating pharmacological treatment of achalasia have yielded conflicting results. The apparent differences may reflect differences in patient selection and outcome measures. Studies in patients without a dilated oesophagus seem to yield better results, and patients with marked oesophageal dilatation may respond less well to pharmacological treatment. It seems that pharmacological treatment has at least some clinical efficacy in diminishing symptoms of dysphagia: even negative studies report improved symptoms in a subset of patients. However, the response is considerably less when symptom criteria other than dysphagia are taken into account.

In view of the limitations of the currently available drug therapy (limited reduction in lower oesophageal sphincter pressure, frequent failure to improve oesophageal emptying rate, high failure rate due to insufficient potency, side-effects or progression of the disease), it seems hard to justify their life-long use when other treatment modalities, i.e. pneumatic dilatation or surgery, result in excellent or good long-term results in over 80% of patients. It seems reasonable, therefore, to restrict drug therapy to the following indications: (a) as a temporary measure until more definitive treatment is performed; (b) as an adjuvant therapy for patients in whom dilatation or surgery was only partially successful; and (c) as a palliative therapy in patients with an unacceptably high risk for more invasive therapy and with no response to botulinum toxin. In these instances, nifedipine (10–20 mg) or isosorbide dinitrate (5 mg) sublingually before each meal seems appropriate. Transcutaneous nerve stimulation has been reported to relieve dysphagia in a small number of patients with achalasia,[24,25] but further studies are required.

Forceful dilatation

Forceful (pneumatic or hydrostatic) dilatation is still the most effective non-surgical treatment modality in achalasia. Although details of the dilatation procedure vary from institution to institution, they all aim at mechanical disruption of the muscle fibres at the oesophagogastric junction. There is some controversy about the frequency at which dilatation should be repeated, about the parameters of dilatation that should be used, and whether or not the procedure should be carried out under general anaesthesia. Several types of dilators have been proposed. They consist of a balloon of a fixed diameter (usually 3 cm) which is filled under high pressure (up to 500 mm Hg) with water or air.[26–29] However, some of these dilators are difficult to pass through the cardia if the oesophagus is tortuous and dilated, which is not the case with the Sippy pneumatic dilator used by our group. This system consists of several bags of increasing diameter (3–4.5 cm) which are used in consecutive dilatations[30] (Figure 6.1). More recently, the Rigiflex achalasia dilator (a design similar to that of a Grunzig angioplasty catheter), and the Witzel endoscopic piggyback pneumatic dilators have become available, which allow placement across the gastro-oesophageal junction under direct vision. Endoscopically guided pneumatic dilation, in the absence of fluoroscopic control, seems to be both safe and efficient.[31–35] According to one randomized study, the use of pneumatic or

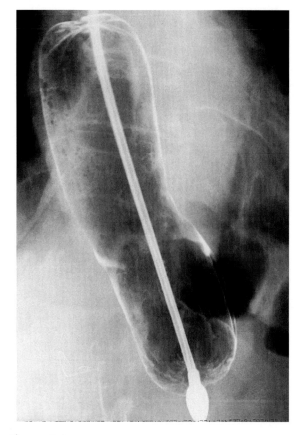

Figure 6.1
Pneumatic dilatation of the cardia. The indentation of the left lateral border of the inflated balloon at the level of the cardia is almost flattened.

metallic dilators does not seem to have an impact on the results and complication rate.[36]

Technique of pneumatic dilatation

Since 1958, over 1200 patients have been treated in our unit by the same technique of pneumatic dilatation.[30,37,38] The basic principles of this method are (1) the guided introduction of the dilator and its positioning under fluoroscopic control, (2) progressive dilatation in consecutive sessions with balloons of increasing diameter and (3) determination of the number of dilatation sessions by the results of lower oesophageal sphincter manometry. Before dilatation, the patient swallows a mercury-filled latex bag to which a nylon string is attached. As soon as the mercury-filled bag has passed into the small intestine, the nylon wire can be used as a guide-wire. At the start of each dilatation session, a metal wire with an eye at the end is threaded over the nylon string into the stomach to provide a rigid guide for the introduction of the dilator. The dilatation procedure is performed with the patient in the upright position. Fluoroscopic control of the position of the dilator is required before inflation. The balloon is then inflated to a pressure of 200 mmHg for 1 minute and to 300 mm Hg for an additional minute. Usually pain disappears or diminishes considerably within two minutes after completion of the dilatation. In most patients, three or four dilatations are performed until the manometric criteria for adequate dilatation are met, i.e. until the lower oesophageal sphincter pressure is reduced to 6–7 mm Hg. Contraindications to pneumatic dilatation are:

- inability of the patient to cooperate because of age, such as in small children, or the presence of psychosis;
- inability to rule out an organic stenosis;
- the presence of lesions at the cardia or stomach, which makes surgery mandatory;
- the presence of an epiphrenic diverticulum, which increases the risk of perforation.

Old age, poor cardiopulmonary condition, a grossly dilated and sigmoid-shaped oesophagus or previous cardiomyotomy do not constitute contraindications for pneumatic dilatation.

Results of forceful dilatation

Published results have shown that after a single dilatation with a hydrostatic or pneumatic bag, excellent or good results are obtained in 67% of patients, whereas some 18% are not improved. Treatment by repeated dilatation with progressively larger diameter yields excellent or good results in about 77%, whereas only 7% are not improved. Thus, progressive dilatation may increase the success rate by 10%, without increased risk of complications[30,37–39] (Figure 6.2).

Only few studies have assessed the effect of clinical and dilatation parameters on outcome in patients undergoing pneumatic dilation for achalasia. In one prospective study, oesophageal transit, symptoms, and diameter did not predict the symptomatic response to pneumatic dilatation.[40] Furthermore, the size of the dilator, the frequency of dilation

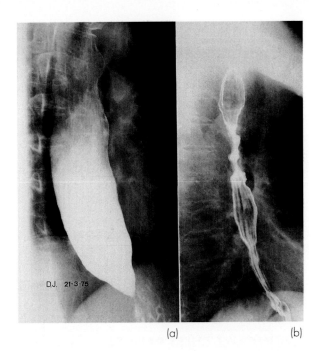

Figure 6.2
Radiological picture of achalasia (a) before and (b) after pneumatic dilatation.

and the duration of inflation of the balloon had no effect on the success of pneumatic dilatation. In another study, the only treatment characteristic predicting long-term clinical response was postdilation lower oesophageal sphincter pressure.[41] Young age adversely influenced outcome.

Complications of forceful dilatation

The major immediate complication of dilatation is perforation at the lower end of the oesophagus, which occurs in 1–5% of patients according to the literature. In our experience, perforation occurred in 2.6%. The risk of perforation is higher if patients had undergone previous dilatations or when inflation pressures of above 11 psi are used.[42] Despite widely held opinion to the contrary, perforation after pneumatic dilatation can usually be treated safely and effectively by parenteral nutrition, broad-spectrum antibiotics and continuous oesophageal aspiration, provided that perforation is recognized early and that the patient remained fasted.[30] The most troublesome late complication after forceful dilatation is reflux oesophagitis and reflux-induced stricture formation. In our experience, stricture formation was seen in only 0.7% of patients.

Injection of botulinum toxin

Botulinum toxin blocks the presynaptic release of acetylcholine at the neuromuscular junction. Animal data have indicated that intrasphincteric injection of botulinum toxin is able to lower oesophageal sphincter pressure.[43] In subsequent studies, it was established that intrasphincteric administration of botulinum toxin is able to decrease lower oesophageal sphincter pressure in patients with achalasia.[44,45] In a double-blind, placebo-controlled trial, it was shown that intrasphincteric injection of botulinum toxin in patients with achalasia is able to decrease manometric abnormalities and to provide significant improvement in symptoms in about two-thirds of patients.[44,45] The duration of response is on average more than one year. Higher success rates are seen in patients over 50 years of age and in patients with vigorous achalasia. Because of its simplicity, injection of botulinum toxin has the potential to become the non-surgical treatment of choice for achalasia, although the necessity for repeated treatments is a disadvantage.

Choice of therapy

Cardiomyotomy yields good results in 63–95% of patients.[46-54] A full discussion of surgical treatment can be found in Chapter 7. As good prospective trials are lacking, a reasonable choice between forceful dilatation and surgery must be based on retrospective studies.[55] In a retrospective analysis, comparing the effect of surgery with pneumatic dilation, the overall success rate of pneumatic dilation was comparable to that of surgery (88% versus 89%). Symptomatic relief was comparable in both groups, but heartburn occurred more frequently after myotomy.[1] The total cost for initial oesophagomyotomy was calculated to be 2.4 times higher than for initial pneumatic dilatation.[56,57] The only prospective study published so far yielded excellent or good long-term results in 95% of patients after myotomy, compared with 65% after dilatation, which is, however, an abnormally low success rate for pneumatic dilatation in comparison to results reported by other groups.[58] The two retrospective studies which are reasonably comparable in several aspects are the Mayo Clinic myotomy study and the Leuven dilatation study[30,37,55,59] (Table 6.1). The number of excellent or good results is higher in the Mayo clinic study (85% versus 77%), whereas early morbidity and mortality are similar. Late strictures occurred in only 0.7% of the Leuven patients, compared with 3% in the Mayo Clinic series.

Therefore, it seems reasonable to perform forceful dilatation as the initial treatment and to reserve cardiomyotomy for those patients who fail to benefit from dilatation. Due to its less invasive nature and low risk compared to other therapies, treatment of achalasia using botulinum toxin appears to be an interesting alternative in patients who are not suitable for or

Table 6.1 Comparison of myotomy and forcible dilatation

	MYOTOMY (MAYO CLINIC)	PROGRESSIVE DILATATION (LEUVEN)
Number of patients	427	403
Duration of follow-up (years)	6.5	7.8
Results		
Excellent or good (%)	58	77
Fair (%)	9	8.7
Poor (%)	6	14.4
Improved (%)	94	93
Early morbidity (%) (surgical oesophageal leak; perforation)	1	2.6
Mortality (%)	0.21	0.17
Late stricture (%)	3	0.7

who refuse conventional therapy. However, definition of its final role in the treatment of achalasia will depend on long-term results, especially as pneumatic dilatation or surgery may result in excellent or good long-term results in over 80% of patients.

SYMPTOMATIC DIFFUSE OESOPHAGEAL SPASM

Medical treatment of symptomatic diffuse oesophageal spasm is often disappointing, both for the patient and for the physician, but so is surgical treatment. Reassurance about the non-serious nature of the disease is especially important in patients in whom angina-like chest pain is the predominant symptom.

A variety of medical treatments have been offered to these patients, but few have proved to be very efficient. Anticholinergics are not indicated because they worsen the peristaltic performance of the oesophagus and predispose to gastro-oesophageal reflux, which in itself may trigger motor abnormalities. Long-term symptomatic and manometric improvement has been reported with the use of long-acting nitrates, but the tolerated dose is usually low because of side-effects, especially headache.[60,61] The favourable long-term effects reported in a small group of patients with symptomatic diffuse spasm need confirmation.[62] Calcium channel blockers have been suggested as potentially beneficial, mainly because they reduce lower oesophageal sphincter pressure and the amplitude of oesophageal body contractions in healthy subjects. Nifedipine is able to reduce the amplitude and the frequency of non-peristaltic contractions in patients with diffuse oesophageal spasm, but the results of long-term trials have been controversial. No significant effect on symptoms has been obtained in double-blind studies prolonged for more than one month.[63,64]

It has been suggested that interaction between oesophageal and psychological symptoms may induce an alteration of sensory perception in some patients. Anecdotal reports have shown sedatives, tranquillizers and antidepressants to be effective in patients whose symptoms were precipitated by stress. In a placebo-controlled study, low doses of the antidepressant trazodone improved symptomatic perception (but not the oesophageal motor abnormalities) in a group of patients with non-cardiac chest pain, including some patients with diffuse oesophageal spasm, but the authors did not specify individual responses to therapy.[65] The beneficial effect of biofeedback reported in a case study awaits confirmation.[66]

Symptomatic diffuse oesophageal spasm should only be treated by pneumatic dilatation if the lower oesophageal sphincter is functioning poorly and if dysphagia is the main symptom. The same technique as used in achalasia is used, but the results are less favourable. In our own limited experience, only 45% of patients treated in this manner reported excellent or good long-term results.[30] Relief of dysphagia was clearly better than relief of pain. The same holds true for cardiomyotomy. In a non-controlled study, the efficacy of minimally invasive surgical therapy for primary oesophageal motility disorders was superior to that of medical therapy.[67] However, this study only shows that surgery may be beneficial in a highly selected population of patients. In our view, long oesophageal myotomy is indicated only exceptionally.

There is evidence that primary oesophageal motility disorders constitute a spectrum of conditions comprising achalasia, diffuse oesophageal spasm and intermediate types. The last are characterized by complete absence of peristalsis with preservation of normal lower oesophageal relaxation, or by complete absence of normal relaxation but with preservation of some degree of peristalsis.[2] In a series of 156 consecutive patients with dysphagia of such degree that dilatation seemed necessary, the nature of the motility disorder was typical achalasia in 70%, typical diffuse spasm in 11% and an intermediate type in 19%. On radiological examination, a typical picture of early achalasia is seen. Progressive pneumatic dilatation in these intermediate types yielded similar results as in typical achalasia: excellent or good in 78.5% and fair or poor in 21.5% of patients.[30]

ANGINA-LIKE CHEST PAIN OF OESOPHAGEAL ORIGIN

Chest pain of non-cardiac origin is now the most frequent indication for oesophageal manometry.[68,69] About 20–30% of patients with suspected angina pectoris do not seem to have significant coronary artery stenosis or spasm on cardiac catheterization and coronary arteriography. In 20–60% of these patients, the oesophagus has been considered to be the cause of the chest pain. A crucial problem remains the careful exclusion of a cardiac origin of the pain, which may be difficult in patients with abnormalities of the heart microcirculation (microvascular angina or syndrome X) but normal coronary arteries on coronary angiography. The picture has become even more complex since a high incidence of oesophageal motor abnormalities was reported in patients with proven microvascular angina, and a common smooth muscle abnormality has been suggested as underlying both conditions.[70,71]

Angina-like chest pain may be present in patients which achalasia, diffuse spasm and intermediate-type motility disorders. Some patients with gastro-oesophageal reflux may interpret the sensation produced by reflux as angina-like chest pain rather than heartburn. Chest pain is also reported in patients with non-specific oesophageal motility disorders and especially in those with nutcracker oesophagus. Some studies have reported the presence of nutcracker oesophagus in 27–58% of patients with non-cardiac chest pain.[72,73] More recent studies have thrown some doubt on the clinical value of the finding of nutcracker oesophagus because a clear relationship between the amplitude of the oesophageal contraction and the presence of symptoms could not be established in such patients.[74] One study assessed the association of gastro-oesophageal reflux with nutcracker oesophagus in patients with non-cardiac chest pain.[75] In a subset of patients with nutcracker oesophagus, evidence of gastro-oesophageal reflux disease was found, and 83% of these responded well to antireflux treatment, with symptomatic improvement, but generally not with normalization of the manometric findings.

The best and probably the only way to establish the oesophageal origin of the chest pain is to prove a correlation in time between the occurrence of chest pain and the abnormal oesophageal event, i.e. oesophageal motor abnormalities or reflux. This may be achieved by oesophageal provocation tests such as the acid perfusion and the edrophonium tests.[72,76–81] In order to determine the nature of the underlying disorders (reflux or motility disturbance), combined intra-oesophageal pH and pressure measurements over 24 hours or more should be performed, enabling the patient to indicate the occurrence of chest pain episodes and allowing the investigator to correlate symptoms with oesophageal events.[82–84] In up to 40% of patients with angina-like chest pain of oesophageal origin, the oesophagus is sensitive to a variety of stimuli. This condition has been called the irritable oesophagus (Figure 6.3).[85] More recent studies have also implicated oesophageal ischaemia and inability to belch in the production of chest pain in some patients with oesophageal motility disorders.[86,87]

The medical therapy of angina-like chest pain of oesophageal origin remains controversial. Many patients may improve with confident reassurance alone, although it seems important for many patients not only to prove the absence of cardiac disease or malignancy but also to establish a definite cause for the symptoms to avoid ongoing concern.[88,89]

Anticholinergics have been suggested for the treatment of chest pain ascribed to underlying motility abnormalities, but at the present time there are no controlled studies to justify this therapy. In a single-blind acute study, cimetropium bromide produced a dramatic decrease in oesophageal contraction amplitude in patients with nutcracker oesophagus, but data about pain relief were lacking.[90] Nitroglycerin and long-acting nitrates have been shown to be beneficial in patients with symptomatic diffuse oesophageal spasm, but to date no data have been published on the effect of these agents in patients with non-cardiac chest pain without a manometric picture of diffuse spasm.

Several studies have examined the effect of the calcium channel blocker diltiazem on non-cardiac chest pain, but the results are conflicting with regard to symptom relief as well as the effect on oesophageal contraction amplitude.[19,91–93] Nifedipine was shown to decrease the amplitude of oesophageal contractions in patients with nutcracker oesophagus, but it was no better than placebo in symptom relief after 6 weeks of treatment.[91,94] In patients with non-cardiac chest pain and proven gastro-oesophageal reflux, intensive antireflux therapy with high doses of H_2-blockers or with proton pump inhibitors, is able to improve symptoms.[95,96]

The treatment of patients with an irritable oesophagus is even more difficult. Acid-blocking agents will at best only partially relieve symptoms, whereas motor inhibitory drugs may aggravate reflux. Drugs which interfere with pain perception may well be indicated in these patients. Such a mechanism

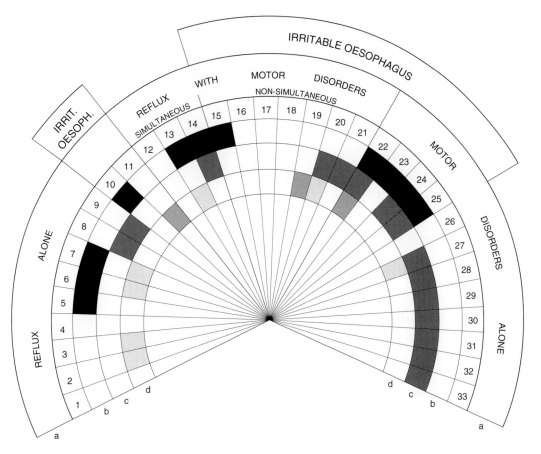

Figure 6.3
Patients with an irritable oesophagus are sensitive to both acid and mechanical stimuli.

could explain the beneficial effect on symptom relief obtained with a low dose of the antidepressant trazodone in symptomatic patients with oesophageal contraction abnormalities.[65] Imipramine, a tricyclic antidepressant helpful in the management of patients with chronic pain syndromes, was evaluated in the treatment of patients with chest pain and normal coronary angiograms.[97] Imipramine reduced by approximately 50% the number of chest pain episodes, and it also reduced the sensitivity to cardiac pain during electrical stimulation. Oesophageal motility testing did not identify patients who were likely to respond to imipramine.

More work needs to be done before an efficient treatment strategy for chest pain of oesophageal origin can be established. The long-term follow-up of patients with non-cardiac chest pain has been inadequate. The use of oesophageal testing and diagnosis has been controversial. Rose et al.[98] studied prospectively the effect of oesophageal testing on patient well-being in subjects with non-cardiac chest pain. There was a decline in hospital utilization in all patients, suggesting that oesophageal testing by itself is useful in reassuring patients of a non-cardiac aetiology of their symptoms.

REFERENCES

1. Vantrappen G, Van Goidsenhoven GE, Verbeke S, Van Den Berghe G & Vandenbroucke J. Manometric studies in achalasia of the cardia, before and after pneumatic dilations. *Gastroenterology* 1963; **45**: 317–325.
2. Vantrappen G, Janssens J, Hellemans J & Coremans G. Achalasia, diffuse esophageal spasm, and related motility disorders. *Gastroenterology* 1979; **76**: 450.
3. Vantrappen G & Hellemans J. Achalasia. In Vantrappen G, Hellemans J (eds) *Diseases of the Oesophagus*. Berlin, Heidelberg, New York: Springer-Verlag, 1975: 287–354.
4. Mearin F, Mourelle M, Guarner F et al. Patients with achalasia lack nitric oxide synthase in the gastro-oesophageal junction. *Eur J Clin Invest* 1993; **23**: 724–728.
5. Holloway RH, Dodds WJ, Helm JF, Hogan WJ, Dent J & Arndorfer RC. Integrity of cholinergic innervation to the lower esophageal sphincter in achalasia. *Gastroenterology* 1986; **90**: 924.
6. Christensen J. Effects of drugs on esophageal motility. *Arch Intern Med* 1976; **136**: 532–537.
7. Lobis JB & Fischer RS. Anticholinergic therapy for achalasia. A controlled study. *Gastroenterology* 1976; **70**: 976.
8. Nickerson M & Call LS. Treatment of cardiospasm with adrenergic blockade. *Am J Med* 1957; **11**: 123–127.
9. Marzio L, Grossi L, DeLaurentis MF, Cennamo L, Lapenna D & Cucurullo F. Effect of cimetropium bromide on esophageal motility and transit in patients affected by primary achalasia. *Dig Dis Sci* 1994; **39**: 1389–1394.
10. Penagini, Bartesaghi B, Negri G & Bianchi PA. Effect of loperamide on lower oesophageal sphincter pressure in idiopathic achalasia. *Scand J Gastroenterol* 1994; **29**: 1057–1060.
11. Blackwell JN, Holt S & Heading RC. Effect of nifedipine on oesophageal motility and gastric emptying. *Digestion* 1981; **21**: 50–56.
12. Hongo M, Traube M, McAllister RG & McCallum RW. Effects of nifedipine on esophageal motor funciton in humans: correlation with plasma nifedipine concentration. *Gastroenterology* 1984; **84**: 8–12.
13. Weiser HF, Lepsien G, Golenhofen K & Siewert R. Clinical and experimental studies on the effect of nifedipine on smooth muscle of the oesophagus and LES. In Duthie (ed.) *Gastrointestinal Motility in Health and Disease*. Lancaster: MTP Press, 1978; 565–574.
14. Bortolotti M & Labo G. Clinical and manometric effects of nifedipine in patients with esophageal achalasia. *Gastroenterology* 1981; **80**: 39–44.
15. Gelfond M, Rozen P & Gilat T. Isosorbide dinitrate and nifedipine treatment of achalasia: a clinical, manometric and radionuclide evaluation. *Gastroenterology* 1982; **83**: 963–969.
16. Coccia G, Bortolotti M, Micheti P & Dodero M. Prospective clinical and manometric study comparing pneumatic dilatation and sublingual nifedipine in the treatment of oesophageal achalasia. *Gut* 1991; **32**: 604–606.
17. Traube M, Dubovik R, Lange RC & McCallum RW. The role of nifedipine therapy in achalasia: results of a randomized, double-blind placebo-controlled study. *Am J Gastroenterol* 1989; **84**: 1259–1262.
18. Triadafilopoulos G, Aaronson M, Sackel S & Burakoff R. Medical treatment of esophageal achalasia. Double-blind crossover study with oral nifedipine, verapamil, and placebo. *Dig Dis Sci* 1991; **36**: 260–267.
19. Silverstein BD, Kramer CM & Pope CE. Treatment of esophageal motor disorders with a calcium blocker, diltiazem. *Gastroenterology* 1982; **81**: 1181 (abstract).
20. Lorber SM & Shay H. Roentgen studies of esophageal transport in patients with dysphagia due to abnormal motor function. *Gastroenterology* 1955; **28**: 697–714.
21. Field CE. Octyl nitrite in achalasia of the cardia. *Lancet* 1944; **ii**: 848–851.
22. Douthwaite AJ. Achalasia of cardia. Treatment with nitrites. *Lancet* 1943; **ii**: 353–354.
23. Gelfond M, Rozen P, Keren S & Gilat T. Effect of nitrates on LOS pressure in achalasia: a potential therapeutic aid. *Gut* 1981; **22**: 312–318.
24. Guelrud M & Ramirez M. The effect of transcutaneous nerve stimulation on lower esophageal sphincter pressure in patients with achalasia. *Gastroenterology* 1989; **96**: 188.
25. Kaada B. Successful treatment of esophageal dysmotility and Raynaud's phenomenon in systemic sclerosis and achalasia by transcutaneous nerve stimulation. *Scand J Gastroenterol* 1987; **22**: 1137.
26. Bennett JR & Hendrix TR. Treatment of achalasia with pneumatic dilatation. *Mod Treat* 1970; **7**: 1217.
27. Browne DC & McHardy G. A new instrument for use in esophagospasm. *JAMA* 1929; **113**: 1963–1964.
28. Csendes A & Strauszer T. Long term clinical, radiological and manometric follow up period of patients with achalasia treated with pneumatic dilatation. *Digestion* 1974; **11**: 128–134.
29. Rider JA, Moeller HC, Puletti EJ & Desai DC. Diagnosis and treatment of diffuse esophageal spasm. *Arch Surg* 1969; **99**: 435.
30. Vantrappen G & Hellemans J. Treatment of achalasia and related motor disorders. *Gastroenterology* 1980; **79**: 144–154.
31. Cox J, Buckton GK & Bennet JR. Balloon dilatation in achalasia: a new dilator. *Gut* 1986; **57**: 986.
32. Kadakia SC & Wong RK. Graded pneumatic dilation using Rigiflex achalasia dilators in patients with primary esophageal achalasia. *Am J Gastroenterol* 1993; **88**: 34–38.
33. Lambroza A & Schuman RW. Pneumatic dilation for achalasia without fluoroscopic guidance: safety and efficacy. *Am J Gastroenterol* 1995; **90**: 1226–1229.
34. McLean TR, Bombeck CT & Nyhus LM. Endoscopic piggyback pneumatic dilation in the initial management of patients with achalasia. *Gastrointest Endosc* 1986; **32**: 290.
35. Witzel L. Treatment of achalasia with a pneumatic dilator attached to a gastroscope. *Endoscopy* 1981; **13**: 176–177.
36. Mearin G, Armengol JR, Chicharro L, Papo M, Balboa A & Malagelada JR. (1994) Forceful dilatation under endoscopic control in the treatment of achalasia: a randomized trial of pneumatic versus metallic dilator. *Gut* 1994; **35**: 1360–1362.
37. Tack J, Janssens J & Vantrappen G. Non-surgical treatment of achalasia. *Hepatogastroenterology* 1991; **38**: 493–497.
38. Vantrappen G, Hellemans J, Deloof W, Valembois P & Vandenbroucke J. Treatment of achalasia with pneumatic dilatations. *Gut* 1971; **12**: 268–275.
39. Reynolds JC & Parkman HP. Achalasia. *Gastroenterol Clin North Am* 1989; **18**: 223.
40. Kim CH, Cameron AJ, Hsu JJ et al. Achalasia: prospective evaluation of relationship between lower esophageal sphincter pressure, esophageal transit, and esophageal diameter and symptoms in response to pneumatic dilation. *Mayo Clinic Proc* 1993; **68**: 1067–1073.
41. Eckardt VF, Aignherr C & Bernhard G. Predictors of outcome in patients with achalasia treated by pneumatic dilation. *Gastroenterology* 1992; **103**: 1732–1738.
42. Nair LA, Reynolds JC, Parkman HP et al. Complications during pneumatic dilation for achalasia or diffuse esophageal spasm. Analysis of risk factors, early clinical characteristics, and outcome. *Dig Dis Sci* 1993; **38**: 1893–1904.
43. Pasricha PJ, Ravich WJ & Kalloo AN. Effects of intrasphincteric botulinum toxin on the lower esophageal sphincter in piglets. *Gastroenterology* 1993; **105**: 1045–1049.
44. Pasricha PJ, Ravich WJ, Hendrix TR, Sostre S & Kalloo AN. Intrasphincteric botulinum toxin for the treatment of achalasia. *N Engl J Med* 1995; **332**: 774–778.

45. Pasricha PJ, Rai R, Ravich WJ, Hendrix TR & Kalloo AN. Botulinum toxin for achalasia: long-term outcome and predictors of response. *Gastroenterology* 1996; **110**: 1410–1415.
46. Black J, Vorbach AN & Collis JL. Results of Heller's operation for achalasia of the esophagus. The importance of hiatal repair. *Br J Surg* 1976; **63**: 949–953.
47. Csendes A, Larrain A, Strauszer T & Ayala M. Long term clinical, radiological and manometric follow up period of patients with achalasia of the esophagus treated with esophagomyotomy. *Digestion* 1975; **13**: 141–145.
48. Effler DB, Loop FL, Groves LK & Favaloro AG. Primary surgical treatment for esophageal achalasia. *Surg Gynecol Obstet* 1971; **132**: 1057–1063.
49. Ellis FH, Gibb SP & Grozier RE. Esophagomyotomy for achalasia of the esophagus. *Ann Surg* 1980; **192**: 157–161.
50. Jara FM, Toledo-Pereyra LH, Lewis JW & Magilligan DJ. Long-term results of esophagomyotomy for achalasia of esophagus. *Arch Surg* 1979; **114**: 935–936.
51. Menguy R. Management of achalasia by transabdominal cardiomyotomy and funduplication. *Surg Gynecol Obstet* 1971; **133**: 482–484.
52. Menzies-Gow N, Gummer JWP & Edwards DAW. Results of Heller's operation for achalasia of the cardia. *Br J Surg* 1978; **65**: 483–485.
53. Rees JR, Thorbjarnarson B & Barnes WH. Achalasia: results of operations in 84 patients. *Ann Surg* 1970; **171**: 195–201.
54. Wingfield MV & Karwowski A. The treatment of achalasia by cardiomyotomy. *Br J Surg* 1972; **59**: 281–284.
55. Vantrappen G & Janssens J. To dilate or to operate? That is the question. *Gut* 1983; **24**: 1013.
56. Parkman HP, Reynolds JC Ouyang A, Rosato EF, Eisenberg JM & Cohen S. Pneumatic dilatation or esophagomyotomy treatment for idiopathic achalasia: clinical outcomes and cost analysis. *Dig Dis Sci* 1993; **38**: 75–85.
57. Csendes A, Velasco N, Braghetto I & Henriquez A. A prospective randomized study comparing forceful dilatation and oesophagomyotomy in patients with achalasia of the oesophagus. *Gastroenterology* 1981; **80**: 789–795.
58. Csendes A, Braghetto I, Henriquez A & Cortes A. Late results of a prospective randomised study comparing forceful dilatation and oesophagomyotomy in patients with achalasia. *Gut* 1989; **30**: 299–304.
59. Okike N, Spencer Payne W, Neufeld DM, Bernatz PE, Pairolero PC & Sanderson DR. Oesophagomyotomy versus forceful dilatation for achalasia of the oesophagus: results in 899 patients. *Ann Thorac Surg* 1979; **28**: 119–125.
60. Orlando RC & Bozymski EM. Clinical and manometric effects of nitroglycerin in diffuse esophageal spasm. *N Engl J Med* 1973; **289**: 23.
61. Swamy N. Esophageal spasm: clinical and manometric responses to nitroglycerine and long acting nitrites. *Gastroenterology* 1977; **72**: 23.
62. Mellow MH. Effect of isosorbide and hydralazine in painful primary esophageal motility disorders. *Gastroenterology* 1982; **83**: 364.
63. Nasrallah SM, Tommaso CT, Singleton RT and Backhaus EA. Primary esophageal motor disorders: clinical response to nifedipine. *South Med J* 1985; **78**: 312.
64. Davies HA, Lewis M, Rhodes J & Henderson A. Nifedipine for relief of esophageal chest pain? *N Engl J Med* 1982; **307**: 1274.
65. Clouse RY, Lustman PJ, Eckert TC, Ferney DM & Griffith LS. Low dose trazodone for symptomatic patients with esophageal contraction abnormalities. A double-blind, placebo-controlled trial. *Gastroenterology* 1987; **92**: 1027.
66. Latimer PR. Biofeedback and self regulation in the treatment of diffuse esophageal spasm: a single case study. *Biofeedback Self Regul* 1981; **6**: 181.
67. Patti MG, Pellegrini CA, Arcerito M, Tong J, Mulwihill SJ & Way LW. comparison of medical and minimally invasive surgical therapy in primary esophageal motility disorders. *Arch Surg* 1995; **130**: 609–615.
68. Richter JE, Bradley LA & Castell DO. Esophageal chest pain: current controversies in pathogenesis, diagnosis and therapy. *Ann Intern Med* 1989; **110**: 66.
69. Janssens J & Vantrappen G. Angina like chest pain of oesophageal origin. *Balliere's Clin Gastroenterol* 1988; **1**: 843.
70. Ducrotte PH, Berland MJ, Denis PH et al. Coronary sinus lactate estimation and esophageal motor abnormalities in angina with normal coronary angiograms. *Dig Dis Sci* 1985; **29**: 305.
71. Catteau EL, Hirzel R, Benjamin SB & Cannon RO. Esophageal motility disorders in patients with abnormalities of coronary flow reserve and atypical chest pain. *Gastroenterology* 1987; **92**: 1339.
72. Katz PO, Dalton CB, Richter JE, Wu WC & Castell DO. Esophageal testing of patients with noncardiac chest pain or dysphagia. *Ann Intern Med* 1987; **106**: 593.
73. Herrington JP, Burns TW & Balart LA. Chest pain and dysphagia in patients with prolonged peristaltic contractile durations of the esophagus. *Dig Dis Sci* 1984; **29**: 134.
74. Cohen S. Esophageal motility disorders and their response to calcium channel antagonists. The sphinx revisited. *Gastroenterology* 1987; **93**: 201.
75. Achem SR, Kolts BE, Wears R, Burton L & Richter JE. Chest pain associated with nutcracker esophagus: a preliminary study of the role of gastro-esophageal reflux. *Am J Gastroenterol* 1993; **88**: 187–192.
76. Demeester TR, O'Sullivan GC, Bermudez G, Midell AI, Cimochowski GE & O'Drobinak J. Esophageal function in patients with angina-type chest pain and normal coronary angiograms. *Ann Surg* 1982; **196**: 488.
77. Bernstein LM & Baker LA. A clinical test for esophagitis. *Gastroenterology* 1958; **34**: 760.
78. Ghillebert G, Janssens J, Vantrappen G, Nevens F & Piessens J. Ambulatory 24 hour intra-esophageal pH and pressure recordings versus provocation tests in the diagnosis of chest pain of oesophageal origin. *Gut* 1990; **31**: 738.
79. London RL, Ouyang H, Snape WJ, Goldberg S, Hirstfeld JW & Cohen S. Provocation of esophageal pain by ergonovine or edrophonium. *Gastroenterology* 1981; **81**: 10.
80. De Caestecker JS, Pryde A & Heading RC. Comparison of intravenous edrophonium and oesophageal acid perfusion during oesophageal manometry in patients with noncardiac chest pain. *Gut* 1988; **29**: 1029.
81. Hewson EG, Dalton CB & Richter JE. Comparison of esophageal manometry, provocative testing, and ambulatory monitoring in patients with unexplained chest pain. *Dig Dis Sci* 1990; **35**: 302.
82. Vantrappen G, Servaes J, Janssens J & Peeters T. 24 hour esophageal pH and pressure recording in out patients. In Wienbeck M (ed.) *Motility of the Digestive Tract.* New York: Raven Press, 1982: 293.
83. Janssens J, Vantrappen G & Ghillebert G. 24 h recording of esophageal pressure and pH in patients with non-cardiac chest pain. *Gastroenterology* 1986; **90**: 1978.
84. Peters L, Maas L, Patty D et al. Spontaneous non-cardiac chest pain: evaluation by 24 h ambulatory esophageal motility and pH monitoring. *Gastroenterology* 1988; **94**: 878.
85. Vantrappen G, Janssens J & Ghillebert G. The irritable esophagus – a frequent cause of angina-like pain. *Lancet* 1987; **i**: 1232–1234.
86. MacKenzie J, Belch J, Park R & McKillip J. Oesophageal ischemia in motility disorders associated with chest pain. *Lancet* 1988; **ii**: 592.
87. Gignoux C, Rost B, Hostein J et al. Role of upper esophageal reflex and belch reflex dysfunction in noncardiac chest pain. *Dig Dis Sci* 1993; **38**: 1909–1914.
88. Ockene IS, Shay MJ, Alpart JA, Weiner BH & Dalen JE. Unexplained chest pain in patients with normal coronary arteriograms. A follow-up study of functional status. *N Engl J Med* 1980; **303**: 1249.
89. Van Dorpe A, Piessens J, Willems JL & De Geest H. Unexplained chest pain with normal coronary arteriograms. A follow-up study. *Cardiology* 1987; **74**: 436.
90. Bassotti G, Gaburri M, Imbimbo BP et al. Manometric evaluation of cimetropium bromide activity in patients with nutcracker esophagus. *Scand J Gastroenterol* 1988; **23**: 1079.
91. Richter JE, Spurling TJ, Cordova CM & Castell DO. Effects of oral calcium blocker, diltiazem, on esophageal contractions. Studies in volunteers and patients with nutcracker esophagus. *Dig Dis Sci* 1984; **29**: 649.
92. Spuring TJ, Cattau EL, Hirszel R, Richter JE, Chobanian SJ & Castell DL. A double blind crossover study of the efficacy of diltiazem in patients with esophageal motility dysfunction. *Gastroenterology* 1985; **88**: 1596.
93. Frachtman RL, Botoman VA & Pope CE. A double blind crossover trial of diltiazem shows no benefit in patients with dysphagia and/or chest pain of esophageal origin. *Gastroenterology* 1986; **90**: 1420.
94. Richter JE, Dalton CB & Castell DO. Nifedipine: a potent inhibitor of esophageal contractions. Is it effective in the treatment of non cardiac chest pain? *Dig Dis Sci* 1985; **30**: 790.
95. Singh S, Richter JE, Hewson EG, Sinclair JW & Hackshaw BT. The contribution of gastro-esophageal reflux to chest pain in patients with coronary artery disease. *Ann Intern Med* 1992; **117**: 824–830.
96. Stahl WG, Beton R, Johnson CS, Brown CO & Waring JP. Diagnosis and treatment of patients with gastro-esophageal reflux and non-cardiac chest pain. *South Med J* 1994, **87**: 739–742.
97. Cannon RO, Quyyumi AA, Mincemoyer R et al. Imipramine in patients with chest pain despite normal coronary angiograms. *N Eng J Med* 1994; **19**: 1411–1417.
98. Rose S, Achkar E & Easly KA. Follow-up of patients with noncardiac chest pain: value of esophageal testing. *Dig Dis Sci* 1994; **39**: 2063–2068.

7

SURGICAL MANAGEMENT OF MOTILITY DISORDERS

T Lerut

Although oesophageal function has been discussed in Chapter 1, it is important in considering surgical treatment of disorders of motility to recapitulate some important principles. The first is that to transport a food bolus from the oesophageal cavity to the stomach requires perfect co-ordination of the often delicate and complex mechanisms responsible for this transport. The swallowing mechanism can basically be divided into the following parts:

- Pharyngeal impeller
- Upper oesophageal sphincter mechanism
- Oesophageal pump
- Lower oesophageal sphincter mechanism.

Primary and secondary peristalsis are the most important components of the transport function. The upper oesophageal sphincter prevents constant air entry into the upper gastrointestinal tract and also prevents constant regurgitation and aspiration. The lower oesophageal sphincter has to protect the oesophageal mucosa from damage by reflux of gastric acid into the oesophagus. Any abnormality of peristalsis or sphincter function that is not secondary to another systemic or local organic pathological condition has to be considered as an oesophageal motility dysfunction.[1] Motility disorders secondary to such causes as tumours, neurological disorders and systemic diseases will not therefore be discussed here.

Although the classical subdivision between motility disorders of the upper oesophageal sphincter, the oesophageal body and the lower oesophageal sphincter will be followed in this chapter, it cannot be overemphasized that the swallowing act involves all the above-mentioned mechanisms and has therefore to be considered as one entity in which the different parts may interact in normal and abnormal conditions. All too often an artificial distinction is made between the different parts of the swallowing mechanism as if the components were to be considered almost as separate and specific entities. This distinction is often reflected in the different specialists to which patients with swallowing disorders are referred, such as gastroenterologists, gastrointestinal surgeons, thoracic surgeons and ENT surgeons.

In any functional abnormality of a particular segment of the oesophagus it is essential to investigate the entire swallowing tract from mouth to stomach. In so doing, all structures participating in deglutition will be evaluated and the contribution of each component related to the patient's swallowing problems assessed. This is of paramount importance before any therapeutic attempt is undertaken,[2] and especially before surgical intervention is contemplated.

CRICOPHARYNGEAL DISORDERS

The upper oesophageal sphincter zone is a distinct entity. It performs the useful function of protecting the upper end of the oesophagus from exposure to inappropriate ingested substances, and inappropriate volumes of normal ingested substances. It is also an important barrier to reflux of oesophageal or gastric contents into the hypopharynx.

Hypertonicity of the upper sphincter has been described as cricospasm or upper oesophageal sphincter achalasia. It is thought to be caused by incoordination of the cricopharyngeal muscle, either as incomplete relaxation, premature contraction or delayed relaxation. These abnormalities can result in dysphagia, regurgitation or pulmonary aspiration, and will be considered in more detail when the problem of Zenker's diverticulum is discussed.[3,4]

Cricopharyngeal function may be impaired in a variety of circumstances, such as bulbar poliomyelitis, cerebrovascular accidents, muscular dystrophy and idiopathic dysfunction.[5] If cricopharyngeal dysfunction is well documented by X-ray investigation or manometry, cricopharyngeal myotomy is likely to result in a reasonable chance of improvement provided the patient has maintained the ability to move the bolus through the oral and pharyngeal phase of deglutition, and has enough sensation necessary to initiate the swallowing reflex.[6]

In our institution we have performed cricopharyngeal myotomy in six patients with cricopharyngeal dysfunction.

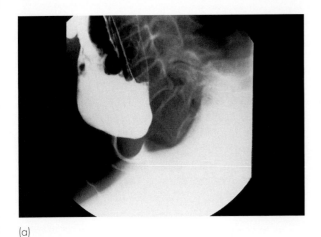
(a)

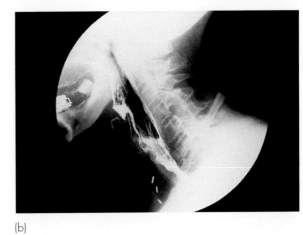
(b)

Figure 7.1
Cricopharyngeal dysfunction. (a) Preoperative radiograph: 'thumb-like' impression of the cricopharyngeal muscle and atonic 'decompensated' hypopharynx leading to total dysphagia in an 80-year-old woman. (b) Postoperative radiograph 3 months after unilateral left 5 cm long myotomy of the cricopharyngeal muscle and cervical muscle wall. Disappearance of cricopharyngeal bar and hypopharyngeal atonia. Free passage of contrast bolus into the cervical oesophagus. The patient is swallowing without difficulty.

Amytrophic lateral sclerosis, cerebrovascular accident and bulbar palsy were the underlying causes in three patients. The three other cases were considered as idiopathic. Myotomy was performed in all six patients through a left cervical approach resulting in improvement in all of them, three having an excellent result (Figure 7.1). Cricopharyngeal dysfunction is frequently reported to be associated with gastro-oesophageal reflux, which is thought to increase the tone of the sphincter. This increased pressure seems to decrease after surgical correction of the reflux. In these cases, correction of gastro-oesophageal reflux, and not cricopharyngeal myotomy, is suggested as the treatment of choice, resulting in restoration of normal cricopharyngeal function.[7] However, further investigation is needed to substantiate this hypothesis.

ACHALASIA

In this condition peristalsis of the oesophageal body is characteristically absent, at least in the distal two-thirds. The other pathognomonic feature is an absent or incomplete relaxation of the lower oesophageal sphincter, with an abnormal high resting pressure in a substantial proportion of patients.[8] An accurate diagnosis can be made in the majority of patients by a combination of clinical history, barium swallow and manometry.[9] Endoscopy is mandatory to rule out other diseases, such as carcinoma causing pseudoachalasia.[10] The aim of treatment of achalasia is not to cure patients of their condition but to relieve dysphagia and, more importantly, to prevent regurgitation and aspiration, which are still the major causes of morbidity and mortality in these patients.

It is accepted that achalasia has to be considered as a premalignant condition in the long term, with an average prevalence of subsequent carcinoma of 5%.[11] It remains unclear whether any form of treatment, with the exception of oesophagectomy, can reduce the incidence of malignancy. At the present time there are two principal therapeutic options in the management of achalasia: endoscopic treatment by pneumatic dilatation or injection of Botulinum toxin and cardiomyotomy, with or without an antireflux procedure, both options aiming at an improvement of oesophageal emptying by reducing the resistance of the lower oesophageal sphincter.[12] Endoscopic methods have been described in Chapter 6 and the surgical approach will be discussed in more detail here.

There is a general agreement that good long-term results can be obtained with both pneumatic dilatation and cardiomyotomy. Improvement following pneumatic dilatation has been reported in between 46 and 90% of cases, with an average of 76%.[13-17] The corresponding figures for myotomy are 65 and 96%, with an average of 87%[18-28] (Table 7.1). The indications for, and effectiveness of, the two methods therefore remain, even today, highly controversial, and thus far there is only one really randomized trial. In this study the surgical group fared better, but at a price of a higher incidence of gastro-oesophageal reflux. Moreover, the results of pneumatic dilatation were not as good as in other reports in the literature, which casts some doubt on the efficacy of the technique used by that group.[29]

Pneumatic dilatation has traditionally been a less attractive option to surgeons as they feel that disruption of the circular muscle fibres of the lower oesophageal sphincter eventually results in scar tissue formation that might render myotomy more difficult, should it be required in the event of failure or recurrence. However, in our own experience in patients previously treated by pneumatic dilatation we have never experienced such a problem. We therefore believe that this consideration should not be used as an argument against pneumatic dilatation. The development of laparoscopic and thoracoscopic surgery has led to a new approach to surgical treatment of achalasia.[30] The single definitive treatment by this minimally invasive means appears to provide a viable option

Table 7.1 Results of treatment of achalasia

STUDY	YEAR	NO. OF PATIENTS	IMPROVED (%)
Pneumatic dilatation			
Kurlander et al.[13]	1963	62	84
Von and Christensen[14]	1975	48	46
Van Trappen and Hellemans[15]	1980	403	85.7
Fellows et al.[16]	1983	63	90
Csendes et al.[17]	1989	37	70
Oesophagomyotomy			
Payne and Donoghue[18]	1970	268	91
Effler et al.[19]	1971	95	87
Belsey[20]	1972	149	90
Gavriliu[21]	1975	256	96
Black et al.[22]	1976	108	65.5
Okike et al.[23]	1978	468	94
Jara et al.[24]	1979	145	89
Pal et al.[25]	1984	16	94
Ellis et al.[26]	1984	113	91
Little et al.[27]	1988	57	84
Author's series	1991	18	82
Bonavina et al.[28]	1992	206	94

to pneumatic dilatation, which frequently necessitates often multiple sessions to obtain prolonged control of symptoms.

Surgical technique of cardiomyotomy

Heller[31] performed the first myotomy for achalasia in 1913, with both an anterior and posterior incision confined to the lower oesophageal sphincter. Later, Zaaijer[32] simplified the technique by omitting the posterior myotomy, claiming equally good results, but the technique is still referred to as Heller's myotomy. Despite further refinements in the subsequent seven decades there are still different areas of controversy.

Transabdominal versus transthoracic approach

Some surgeons, especially those who are less familiar with thoracic surgical techniques, prefer an abdominal approach and claim less postoperative morbidity compared with the transthoracic approach. However, the transthoracic approach is currently favoured by many oesophageal surgeons. It permits a long myotomy, offers better possibilities for correcting recurrent symptoms following failed previous surgery, enables a wider range of antireflux procedures to be performed concomitantly (see below) and, finally, in the case of concomitant reflux stricture or suspicion of malignancy, enables a synchronous oesophageal resection and reconstruction to be performed.[33] It is claimed that the necessity for a concomitant antireflux procedure is likely to be less if the myotomy is performed transthoracically, because of less disruption to the normal attachments at the cardia.[26]

Extent of myotomy

It is clear that an incomplete myotomy of the muscle of the lower sphincter is doomed to failure. On the other hand, continuing the myotomy well into the stomach may lead to the destruction of the lower sphincter mechanism, especially in those cases (approximately 10%) in which a concomitant type 1 hiatal hernia is present. This leads to the complication of gastro-oesophageal reflux.

Proximally, the myotomy is performed until total division of the hypertrophied muscle is ensured. However, some authors advocate routine extension of the myotomy up to the aortic arch, especially in patients in whom pain is a predominant symptom. Up to 50% of patients with classic achalasia are reported to suffer from chest and epigastric pain. The pain is bursting in quality, often occurring at night, and may or may not be related to eating. When prolonged manometric studies are performed, these pain episodes seem to correlate with spastic contractions of the body of the oesophagus. These factors are associated with the fact that achalasia is not always a clear-cut entity and transitional forms ranging across a spectrum from achalasia to diffuse spasm have been well documented.[34,35] Postoperatively, it can be anticipated that with progressive decrease in the diameter of the oesophagus, if dilatation was not excessive, hyperkinetic spastic contractions may return, causing pain and relative obstruction in the infra-aortic smooth muscle part of the oesophageal body. For these reasons we believe that a long myotomy up to the aortic arch is preferable.[36] Preoperative manometric recordings may be useful in determining the length of the myotomy, which may, if necessary, have to be extended above the level of the aortic arch.

Concomitant antireflux procedures

Reports from the literature indicate an incidence of postoperative gastro-oesophageal reflux caused by iatrogenic destruction of the lower oesophageal sphincter ranging from 3 to 48%, leading in some patients to reflux-induced stricture and recurrence of dysphagia.[22-26,37] There is evidence that the incidence of reflux after myotomy is related to the experience of the surgeon. Very experienced surgeons in this field seem to obtain excellent results with a myotomy alone,[26] but for the less experienced it is more difficult to judge the precise extent of the myotomy into the stomach. If the myotomy is too long, the antireflux barrier is jeopardized, with an increased risk of gastro-oesophageal reflux. If insufficiently long, lower sphincter relaxation may still be incomplete, resulting in persistent dysphagia. For the surgeon dealing only occasionally with the surgical treatment of achalasia it is preferable to advise a sufficiently long extension of the myotomy on the gastric side and to perform a concomitant antireflux procedure.

With regard to the type of antireflux procedure, because of the major peristaltic defect in patients with achalasia, one of the partial fundoplication procedures, such as the Belsey Mark IV, is preferable. In these circumstances, a complete 360° wrap, such as the Nissen, has a greater risk of producing obstruction and dysphagia, and it would appear logical to use one of the partial fundoplication procedures which has been shown to be as effective in reflux control as the Nissen procedure.[33,36,38] There are therefore many points of debate related to the technical aspects of the surgical treatment of achalasia. It is thus impossible to designate a universally agreed optimal form

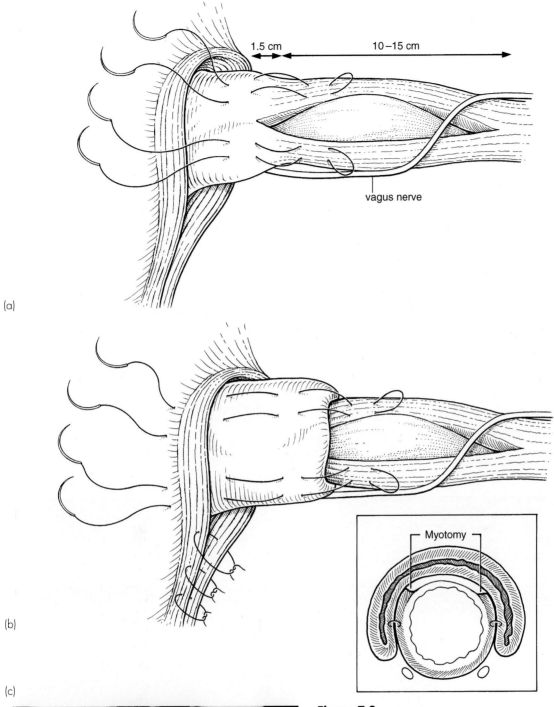

(a)

1.5 cm

10–15 cm

vagus nerve

(b)

(c)

Myotomy

Figure 7.2

Surgical technique of extended myotomy and Belsey Mark IV antireflux procedure in achalasia. (a) First row of two mattress sutures passing through stomach and oesophagus. (b) Second row of two mattress sutures passing through diaphragm, fundic wrap and oesophagus. (c) Peroperative view of extended myotomy (arrow) and first row of Belsey Mark IV antireflux procedure. The chest is entered through the left sixth intercostal space.

of surgical management. The description of surgical technique which follows is that preferred in our institution and subsequently a brief description of transabdominal cardiomyotomy with a Dor antireflux procedure is presented.

Technique of transthoracic extended myotomy and antireflux procedure (Figures 7.2 and 7.3)

The chest is entered through a sixth left interspace thoracotomy. After mobilization of the oesophagus up to the aortic arch, the cardia is mobilized as for the classical Belsey Mark IV antireflux procedure. The phreno-oesophageal membrane is opened, giving access to the greater sac of the peritoneal cavity. The upper limit of the gastrohepatic ligament is divided between clamps. After full mobilization of the cardia, two traction sutures are placed on the muscle layer of the distal oesophagus, elevating the muscle layer from the underlying mucosa. The myotomy starts on the anterolateral aspect of the oesophagus: the muscle layers down to the submucosa are incised, with the division of all muscle fibres over the lower oesophageal sphincter zone. The myotomy is extended into the stomach in order to make sure that the lower oesophageal sphincter is completely divided after division of the fat-pad. When the stomach is reached, an abrupt increase in the vascularity of the submucosa is noted and the structure of the muscle layer changes. It is very important to divide all circular muscle fibres because leaving only a few circular muscle fibres intact can prevent satisfactory relief of dysphagia. Proximally, the myotomy is extended up to the aortic arch, with careful preservation of the vagus nerves and their branches. There is usually an oblique vagal branch connecting the right and the left vagus nerves. This branch is elevated from the muscle to facilitate the myotomy. A biopsy specimen of the muscle layer is usually removed as a vertical strip of muscle from one margin of the myotomy. The muscle layer is dissected off the underlying mucosa in the submucosal plane, for about half the surface of the organ, in order to prevent reconstitution of the muscle layer by healing of the myotomy incision.

The antireflux repair is a modification of the Mark IV procedure. Instead of two rows of three mattress sutures, only two mattress sutures are placed in each of the two rows on each side of the myotomy. This produces as firm a repair as is achieved by the two rows of three mattress sutures in the classical Mark IV procedure, because of the marked muscular hypertrophy in the lower oesophagus. In this way a 240° fundoplication is obtained around the distal 4–5 cm of the oesophagus. After reduction underneath the diaphragm of the distal 4–5 cm of the oesophagus, embraced over two-thirds of its circumference by the fundoplication, a posterior buttress is created by approximating the two limbs of the right crus by knotting previously placed sutures. It is very important to avoid excessive narrowing of the hiatus in view of the absence of the oesophageal body peristalsis.

Technique of transabdominal cardiomyotomy and Dor antireflux procedure

Access is via an upper midline incision, employing both a self-retaining abdominal retractor and a sternal-elevatory retractor of the Goligher type to facilitate access to the hiatal area. The left

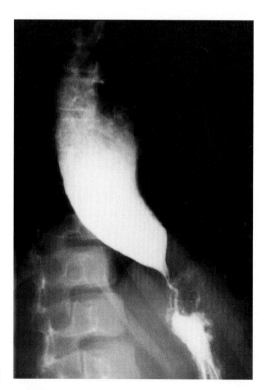

(a)

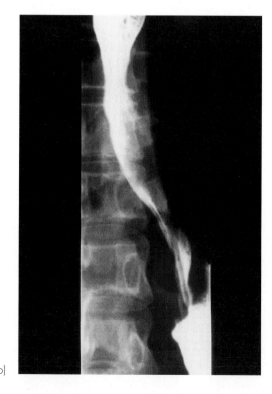

(b)

Figure 7.3
Surgical treatment of achalasia: extended myotomy and Belsey Mark IV antireflux procedure. (a) Preoperative and (b) postoperative barium swallow.

lobe of the liver is retracted which may be facilitated if the lobe is large, by division of the left triangular ligament. The phreno-oesophageal ligament is divided and the plane around the oesophagus achieved by gentle blunt dissection, taking care to identify and preserve the vagal trunks and branches. Division of the oesophageal attachments and oesophageal mobilization is more restricted than during antireflux surgery in order to minimize disruption of the antireflux mechanism, although most surgeons perform a prophylactic antireflux procedure in association with transabdominal cardiomyotomy. It is considered by many surgeons that a myotomy length of 7–8 cm on the oesophagus is sufficient, with extension for 1–2 cm across the gastric sling fibres. As with transthoracic myotomy, an incision is made through both longitudinal and circular muscle layers, the correct plane being readily identified by spreading the incised muscle layers laterally with Denis Browne or blunt-jawed forceps. This enables the myotomy to be extended proximally by first elevating the muscle layers from the submucosa and then dividing them with McIndoe's scissors, although the distal part of the myotomy, where the muscle layers thin out, is best done by scalpel dissection. The Dor anterior fundoplication is performed by covering the anterior aspect of the intra-abdominal oesophagus with the anterolateral aspect of the gastric fundus. This is sutured by a longitudinal row of sutures, between each muscular edge of the myotomized segment and the stomach wall. Alternatively, one of the other partial fundoplication procedures, such as the Hill, Toupet or Watson procedures, may be used (see Chapter 10).

We would not necessarily advocate a standardized technique as long as certain basic principles are adhered to; indeed, different procedures may be justified according to circumstances. For instance, in the small proportion of cases of achalasia where coexisting reflux may be present as an intermittent phenomenon, a concomitant antireflux procedure should be performed routinely, providing that both conditions have been documented by objective studies. If a surgeon's preference is to dissect the hiatus extensively, as may be the case in a transabdominal myotomy, or if the myotomy is carried for more than 1 cm over the stomach, then it is preferable to perform an antireflux procedure. Conversely, if the myotomy is performed with minimal hiatal dissection, and extends for 1 cm or less across the stomach, an antireflux procedure is not usually necessary.

Videoscopic treatment of ochalesia

Recent developments in video-assisted and minimally invasive technology have opened a new dimension to surgeons. Stimulated by the excellent results of laparoscopic cholecystectomy minimally invasive techniques have been rapidly applied to the treatment of different oesophageal conditions including motor disorders of the oesophagus.

Minimal invasive treatment of achalasia can be performed either via a thoracoscopic (VATS) or laparoscopic approach.

Thoracoscopic myotomy (Figure 7.4).

For this procedure the patient is positioned in right lateral decubitus position. Single lung ventilation is essential and made possible by the placement of a double lumen endotracheal tube. Usually, five thoracoports are used: one for the camera and four working channels. Two of these channels are used by the surgeon and two by the assistant who is responsible for retracting the lung. An initial port is inserted just below and anterior to the tip of the scapula in the midaxillary line to introduce the thoracoscope. A 10-mm 0° thoracoscope is most frequently used.

After introducing the scope, the surgeon can inspect the pleural cavity for adhesions. Dense adhesions may preclude thoracoscopy and necessitate conversion to open thoracotomy. If no dense adhesions are present, three of four additional 10-mm ports are made under direct vision, one port in the anterior axillary line and two in the posterior axillary line.

Once the lung has been deflated, the mediastinal pleura over the oesophagus is opened to allow mobilization of the oesophagus.

Exposure of the lateral aspect of the oesophagus is achieved with anterior and mediastinal distraction of the oesophagus, which allows exposure and clipping of the branches from the aorta. When the oesophagus is deflected posterolaterally, a dissection plane can be developed between the oesophagus and the pericardium.

After this manoeuvre, attachments to the posterior mediastinum are divided so that a sling or Penrose drain may be passed around the oesophagus, usually from medial to lateral. The sling is brought out of the chest alongside one of the thoracoports and is used to exert traction on the oesophagus when necessary.

After exposure of the muscular wall of the oesophagus, the myotomy is begun midway between the oesophageal hiatus and the inferior pulmonary vein. With a 90° hook electrocautery or spatula the longitudinal and circular layers of the oesophagus are progressively elevated and divided while the underlying mucosa is protected. Transillumination with a fibreoptic endoscope may be helpful in identifying the layers of the oesophagus. The myotomy is extended distally under endoscopic guidance until the endoscopically visible constriction at the lower oesophageal sphincter is completely divided. This part of the dissection is facilitated with cephalad retraction on the oesophagus and depression of the diaphragm. After complete division of the lower oesophageal sphincter, gastric muscle fibres with a different orientation and increased vascularity are encountered. In most patients the myotomy is extended only a short distance (0.5 cm) onto the gastric cardia to reduce the risk of bleeding and postoperative reflux.

After longitudinal completion of the myotomy, the submucosal plane is dissected along each muscle edge. A third or more of the mucosa may be mobilized circumferentially by this technique, which allows the mucosa to pouch out through the myotomy and prevents reapproximation of the muscle margins. Thoracoscopic and endoscopic inspection ensures that there is no bleeding and that the mucosa has not been injured. A chest drain is passed through the lowest trocar site and positioned posteriorly. The lung is re-expanded and all ports are removed and closed under direct vision.

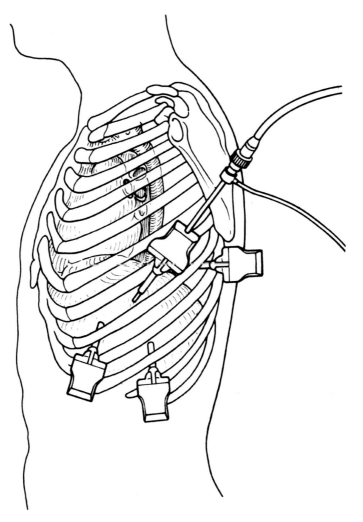

Figure 7.4
Placement of thoracoports for VATS treatment of achalasia.

Laparoscopic myotomy

The patient is positioned in low lithotomy with steep anti-Trendelenberg. The pattern of port placement is the same as for most procedures performed at or around the gastro-oesophageal junction (see Chapter 10). During the procedure, the 30° telescope is placed through the supraumbilical port. After exploration of the abdomen, the left lobe of the liver is elevated superiorly and the stomach retracted inferiorly with instruments inserted through the right and left subcostal ports. After passage of the endoscope to verify the location of the oesophagus, the anterior portion of phreno-oeosophageal ligament is divided. This exposes the oesophagus anteriorly, after which its anterior wall is cleared for a distance of 5 cm from hiatus to cardia, serving the anterior vagus nerve. Division of the phreno-oesophageal ligament during laparoscopic myotomy does increase the risk of postoperative reflux compared with that of thoracoscopic myotomy. For this reason, the procedure should be completed with the addition of one of the partial fundoplication procedures. Therefore, the posterior attachments of the oesophagus are divided and the fundus is freed in preparation for the antireflux procedure that will be done later. The endoluminal endoscope is then used to locate the narrowed section of the lumen and to elevate the oesophagus for initiation of the myotomy. Using the hook cautery or spatula technique, longitudinal and circular muscle layers are divided beginning in the middle third of the exposed oesophagus to the left of the vagus. It is usually necessary to carry the myotomy onto the stomach for a distance of up to 1 cm to relieve all endoscopically visible narrowing.

The operation is then completed by a partial fundoplication procedure.

As thoracoscopic and laparoscopic management is a relatively new procedure only early results are available from literature.

Pellegrini et al.[39] in a series of 24 patients with achalasia treated through VATS, found good relief in 21 patients (88%) with a median follow-up of 12 months. However, in 16 of their patients 24 h pH monitoring showed mild abnormal reflux thus questioning the necessity of adding an antireflux procedure in the treatment of achalasia.

Rosati et al.[40] using a laparoscopic approach and adding a Dor anterior fundoplication obtained complete symptom relief in 87% in a series of 43 patients with a median follow-up of 17 months. Asymptomatic gastro-oesophageal reflux was detected at postoperative 24 h pH monitoring in only 8% of the series.

These results are comparable with those obtained of open surgery, but with the usual advantages of shorter hospital stay and earlier return to normal activity. If these early results are maintained into the long term, cardiomyotomy will become a strongly competing option to pneumatic dilatation for treatment of a mucosine proportion of patients with achalasia.

When to resect?

In the case of a totally decompensated oesophagus and end-stage achalasia, an entity termed dolichomegaoesophagus, the chances of sufficient recovery of the function after myotomy preventing oesophageal stasis and concomitant symptoms are small.[42] In these cases resection of the thoracic oesophagus is the treatment of choice. Continuity can be restored either by a long segment isoperistaltic colon interposition (Figure 7.5) or by a gastroplasty, provided the anastomosis is performed at the level of the neck, in order to obviate postoperative reflux.

Results of surgical treatment

Analysis of the results of most surgical series shows an overall improvement ranging from 65% to almost 100%. In our own experience of 18 patients we observed improvement in 82% of the patients, 66% having excellent or good results. One patient is suffering from severe reflux. Because of the many differences in technique it is almost impossible to compare results from different series, particularly as many authors do not give precise technical details of their procedure.

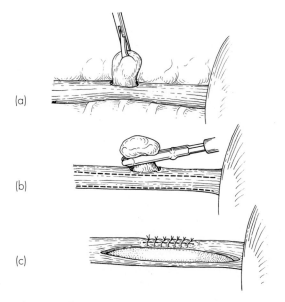

(a)

(b)

(c)

Figure 7.5
Principles of VATS treatment of oesophageal diverticula. (a) Diverticulum is identified and grasped. (b) A Maloney bougie or endoscope is passed endoluminally; Resection of the diverticulum with the endostapler. (c) Closure of the myotomy above the resected diverticulum and contralateral myotomy of the oesophageal body.

Complications of surgical treatment and their management

Inadequate myotomy

The myotomy may be too short proximally or distally or it may not be deep enough, leaving circular muscle fibres undivided. Persistence of dysphagia and failure to gain weight are the main symptoms. Endoscopic pneumatic dilatation may be successful but in a small proportion of cases a second myotomy will be required. This can be done either through an abdominal or a thoracic approach. It is preferable to dismantle completely the previous operation, identify the myotomy and perform the necessary corrections. The main danger is, of course, mucosal perforation. For these reasons, some authors prefer to perform a myotomy on the opposite side.[42] Because of the necessity for greater dissection, an antireflux procedure is considered necessary in these reinterventions. It should be noted that there are other causes of persistence of original symptoms besides an inadequate myotomy. Abnormal scar tissue formation within the fundoplication may occasionally lead to stenosis, as we observed in one patient. This also requires reintervention involving dismantling the antireflux procedure and division of the fibrous band, followed by a revisional fundoplication. Some patients will develop a 'diverticulization' of the mucosa through the myotomy. This may lead to stasis and fermentation, producing regurgitation and an acid taste in addition to dysphagia. If symptoms are disabling, oesophagectomy is recommended. In order to prevent the occurrence of this unpleasant complication we cover the myotomy site by stitching the mediastinal edges of the pleura to the medial edge of the myotomy.

Gastro-oesophageal reflux

The second most common cause of failure is the development of severe oesophagitis, which may eventually lead to stenosis. The treatment of this complication is difficult. Optimal medical treatment should always be instituted as the initial treatment of choice but this is not always successful, especially in cases of stenosis or ulcer. If antireflux surgery has not been performed it is worth considering it in the event of failed medical treatment. However, if there is considerable scarring, or an antireflux procedure has already been performed, oesophagectomy followed by colon interposition is recommended. Fekete[42] obtains excellent results with total duodenal diversion consisting of antrectomy, Roux-en-Y jejunal anastomosis and truncal vagotomy.

Complications of concomitant antireflux procedure

Some patients may develop dysphagia related to the antireflux procedure. The reason for this, especially in megaoesophagus, is the reduction of too long a segment of distal oesophagus below the diaphragm, creating a long high-pressure zone that may lead to dysphagia, irrespective of the type of antireflux procedure. However, the most common reason for this type of complication is the use of the 360° Nissen fundoplication which, in the absence of the oesophageal peristaltic pump mechanism, may obstruct the cardia.[43] Pneumatic dilatation is usually unhelpful in this situation and reintervention converting the 360° fundoplication into a partial antireflux procedure is usually successful.

Malignant change

Cancer may occur as a complication, even after a successful myotomy, causing dysphagia and giving the impression of a failed operation. The treatment of choice is oesophagectomy if the disease has not spread beyond the limits of surgical treatment.[44]

DIFFUSE OESOPHAGEAL SPASM AND OTHER MOTILITY DISORDERS

Diffuse oesophageal spasm is characterized typically by sudden and often intense episodes of chest pain.[45] The cause is unknown. Some authors believe that diffuse oesophageal spasm is a part of the spectrum of achalasia. Although the classic manometric features of this condition are well described, the diagnosis is not always easy. With modern refinements of manometric techniques many variations are described, including nutcracker oesophagus (supersqueezer oesophagus). It is also generally accepted that there is some overlap between the different disorders, according to their manometric features, as in hypertensive lower oesophageal sphincter and vigorous achalasia and non-specific oesophageal motility disorders.[46–50] The common denominator of these conditions is the characteristic symptom complex of chest pain and dysphagia. Medical and supportive therapy is the first choice of treatment for most symptomatic patients. Bougienage may be of value, as reported by some authors.[15] Surgery may be the treatment of choice, especially when chest pain is the dominant symptom, and consists of a long myotomy from the aortic arch to the lower oesophageal sphincter. Controversy exists as to whether the myotomy should be done through the lower sphincter when manometry shows normal sphincter function, and whether a concomitant antireflux procedure should be performed.[51] The technique of myotomy and antireflux procedures is similar to that described for achalasia and a thoracoscopic approach has also been described.[52] Improvement after surgery is observed in around 75% of patients.

DIVERTICULA OF THE OESOPHAGEAL BODY

Diverticula of the oesophageal body can be found at any level of the oesophagus. Generally they are classified as traction and pulsion diverticula. Traction diverticula are true diverticula caused by a mediastinal inflammatory process, e.g. tuberculosis. They are often asymptomatic and not associated with any motility disorder. Specific treatment is not therefore usually necessary. Pulsion diverticula are false diverticula, as only mucosa and submucosa protrude. It is now accepted that they are an expression of an underlying motor disorder. Pulsion diverticula are seen at three levels: at the pharyngo-oesophageal junction (Zenker's diverticulum) and in the mid-thoracic and the distal (epiphrenic) oesophagus.[53] Dysphagia,

regurgitation and aspiration are the most common symptoms; associated chest pain is mainly caused by the underlying disorder. Zenker's diverticulum will be discussed separately. Mid-oesophageal diverticula comprise 10–15% of all oesophageal diverticula. Manometric studies in patients with mid-oesophageal diverticula frequently show the classic features of diffuse oesophageal spasm or nonspecific motor disorders.[54] Lower oesophageal sphincter pressure in these cases is usually normal although sphincter relaxation abnormalities are frequently seen.[55,56] From these data it is clear that a correct diagnosis of a possible underlying motor disorder should be made before any surgical treatment is attempted. The natural history of mid-oesophageal diverticula may lead to severe complications, such as erosions of the oesophageal wall, causing haemorrhage or perforation. Fistulation into the pericardium has been described[57] and occasional neoplastic transformation has been reported.

Treatment

The necessity for, and method of, treatment of oesophageal diverticula depends on the presence of symptoms and the size of the diverticula. Asymptomatic diverticula, which are usually small, normally require no treatment. In general terms, treatment should be orientated towards the cause of the symptoms, i.e. the underlying motor disorder. Conservative treatment will usually be unsuccessful. The objective of the operative technique is the elimination of the underlying functional disorder by a long myotomy. The myotomy must be extended proximally above the level of the diverticulum, or the highest diverticulum when multiple diverticula are present. Distally, the myotomy may or may not be extended on to the stomach, according to the manometric features of lower oesophageal sphincter function.[58] If the myotomy is extended on to the stomach, consideration needs to be given to the previously discussed issues relating to the risk of gastro-oesophageal reflux and the necessity of performing a concomitant antireflux procedure. Small diverticula that are unlikely to cause food retention do not usually require any further specific treatment as they tend to regress in size following the myotomy.

For larger diverticula which are likely to result in food retention treatment has also to be directed to the diverticulum itself. The choice of treatment lies between diverticulopexy or diverticulectomy. The introduction of stapling devices has greatly facilitated diverticulectomy, substantially decreasing the risk of suture line leaks. As a result of this, very large diverticula or diverticula with a very narrow communication between sac and oesophageal lumen are indications for resection of the diverticulum.[59] In the latter circumstances, diverticulopexy would result in inadequate drainage of the diverticulum. An additional argument in favour of diverticulectomy is the possible risk, albeit small, of malignant change within the diverticulum due to chronic stasis.

Epiphrenic diverticula comprise approximately 20% of all oesophageal diverticula.[55] They are frequently alluded to as separate pathological entities from pulsion diverticula. There is, however, sufficient evidence to show that the same underlying mechanisms as in mid-thoracic pulsion diverticula are present. Hypertensive lower oesophageal sphincter and increased tone within the oesophagus create a high-pressure area above the sphincter, resulting in outpouching of the mucosa through what is thought to be a weak area of muscle.[60] Epiphrenic diverticula may also be seen in association with achalasia as well as with diffuse oesophageal spasm. The natural history, complications and principles of treatment are, therefore, the same as for mid-oesophageal diverticula. However, in epiphrenic diverticula it is mandatory for the myotomy to include the whole of the lower oesophageal sphincter, and a concomitant non-obstructing partial fundoplication is therefore advised.

The importance of performing myotomy is well-illustrated by a study, performed at the Mayo Clinic by Allen and Clagget[61] in which two series of patients were compared. In a first series of 21 patients, only a diverticulectomy was performed. Five patients suffered from suture line leakage and four had a documented recurrence of the diverticulum. In a subsequent series, myotomy was added to the diverticulectomy in ten patients. No leakage was observed.

Our own experience is of 12 patients (Table 7.2). Diffuse

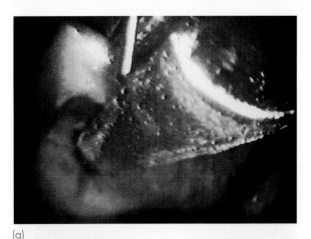
(a)

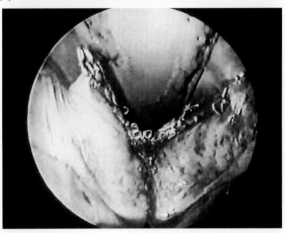
(b)

Figure 7.6
Principles of videoscopic treatment of Zenker's diverticulum.
(a) Application of endostapler; (b) oesophagodiverticulostomy after firing of the endostapler. U shape aspect caused by the retraction of the cricopharyngeal muscle.

Table 7.2 Oesophageal thoracic diverticula: morphological characteristics

CHARACTERISTIC	NUMBER
Localization	
Distal third epiphrenic	8
Middle third (all multiple)	4
Multiple diverticula	4
Associated hiatal hernia	4
Gastric prolapse in diverticulum with strangulation	1

oesophageal spasm was documented in six, achalasia in two and nutcracker oesophagus in one patient. Eight patients had an epiphrenic diverticulum. Four patients had multiple diverticula extending up to the level of the aortic arch. In one patient the stomach was prolapsing in a giant diverticulum, with symptoms of strangulation being the indication for surgery (Figure 7.6). In four patients a hiatal hernia was documented. Surgical treatment consisted of a simple diverticulectomy in one patient. In all other patients a myotomy was performed. Diverticulopexy was performed in four patients and diverticulectomy in six (Table 7.3). One patient with a giant diverticulosis showed an intense peridiverticulitis in the entire mediastinium at the time of surgery. The operation comprised a myotomy only, resulting in complete symptomatic relief until the patient died from lung carcinoma 12 years later (Figure 7.7). In five patients including the four with hiatal hernia, myotomy was accompanied by a Belsey Mark IV antireflux procedure.

There was no postoperative mortality, no incidence of leakage and no major complications (Table 7.4). In 11 patients follow-up was longer than 1 year, with a maximum of 16 years. Early and transient postoperative dysphagia was seen in three patients. One patient required several dilatations for a stenosis

at the oesophagogastric junction, probably reflux induced. Another patient was treated for an episode of food impaction requiring endoscopic extraction. The final result was judged excellent in six patients, very good in four and good in one patient. No patient had a bad result.

Table 7.3 Oesophageal thoracic diverticula: type of operation

OPERATION	NUMBER
Left side	11
Right side	1
Without resection ($n = 5$)	
Myotomy	1
Myotomy + pexy	2
Myotomy + pexy + Belsey Mark IV	2
With resection ($n = 7$)	
Diverticulectomy	1
Diverticulectomy + myotomy	3
Diverticulectomy + myotomy + Belsey Mark IV	3

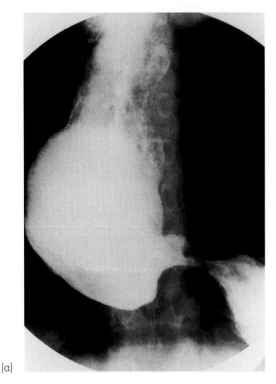
(a)

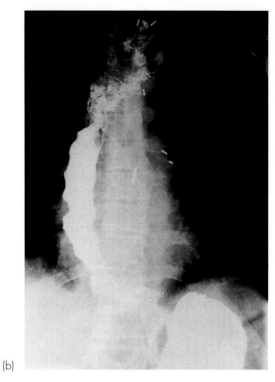
(b)

Figure 7.7
Achalasia. (a) Barium swallow showing development of a megaoesophagus after two failed surgical procedures: abdominal Heller myotomy (1965); thoracic myotomy and Belsey Mark IV (1974). (b) Barium swallow after resection and coloplasty (1982).

Minimally invasive management of diverticula (Figure 7.8)

The access for VATS treatment depends on the localization of the diverticula. The approach is left-sided for distal diverticula and right-sided for more proximal diverticula. In these cases division of the azygos vein may be necessary using an endostapler.

A diverticulum is usually easy to identify and is grasped by an endoscopic Babcock retractor or an Endograsp. With upward traction the sac can be freed from surrounding structures circumferentially. At the level of the neck, the surrounding muscle fibres are gently pushed away to free the entire base of the neck. The diverticulum can be removed with either a standard linear stapler introduced through a widened intercostal port or with a linear endostapler. Use of a linear endostapler requires the introduction of the instrument through the lowest posterior thoracoport in such a way that the stapler is parallel to the neck of the diverticulum. This manoeuvre can be cumbersome and difficult to perform.

When the neck of the diverticulum is small, the application on one 35-mm stapler suffices. If the diverticulum has a broad base, two or more applications or the use of a 60-mm endostapler are needed. To avoid narrowing of the oesophageal lumen, it is advisable to introduce either an oesophagoscope or a 50 F Maloney bougie into the oesophagus before the diverticulum is stapled.

After the diverticulum is resected, the surgeon begins the myotomy by marking the area of the muscle to be divided with an electrocautery. The longitudinal fibres are incised in an area at least 90° away from the diverticular staple line. The underly-ing circular muscle layer is incised with the electrocautery hook. Great care is taken to lift the fibres during coagulation to avoid injury to the mucosa.

The myotomy is continued caudad to or across the gastro-oesophageal junction according to the manometric findings. The myotomy is taken cephalad to a level proximal to the neck of the diverticulum. After an adequate myotomy, the mucosa should bulge fully between the cut edges of the muscular wall. Insufflation of air through a nasogastric tube rules out mucosal perforation. The procedure ends with approximation of the two edges of the muscular wall to cover the diverticular staple line. In the event of mucosal perforation, the defect can usually be closed with a simple fine-needle suture.

Table 7.4 Oesophageal thoracic diverticula: results

RESULT	NUMBER
Postoperative mortality	0
Fistulas	0
Major complications	0
Long-term follow-up ($n = 11$)	
Early postoperative dysphagia	3
Dilatations for stenosis of gastro-oesophageal junction (reflux?)	1
Episode of food impaction	1
Final score	
Excellent	6
Very good	4
Good	1

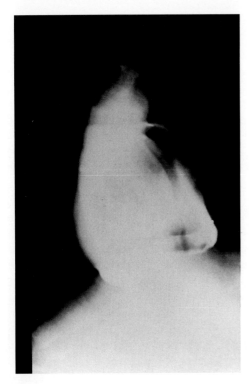
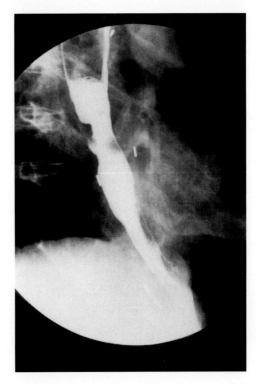

(a)

(b)

Figure 7.8
Diverticulum of the oesophageal body. (a) Epiphrenic diverticulum and prolapse of gastric fundus with strangulation in a patient with achalasia. (b) Postoperative barium swallow after extended myotomy, diverticulectomy and Belsey Mark IV antireflux procedure.

ZENKER'S DIVERTICULUM

A pharyngeal diverticulum (Zenker's diverticulum) is a protrusion of the hypopharyngeal mucosa posteriorly between the oblique fibres of the inferior pharyngeal constrictor and the transverse fibres of the cricopharyngeus muscles. Its origin still remains unclear. For a long time this condition was considered as a strictly mechanical entity, with the diverticulum obstructing the oesophagus by virtue of its volume and dependent position. Manometric studies have, however, revealed the delicate and coordinated sequence of the swallowing act in which relaxation of the upper oesophageal sphincter seems to play a major role. In this respect several theories have been proposed to explain the genesis of a Zenker's diverticulum. Premature contraction of the upper sphincter is one of the mechanisms that might account for upper oesophageal dysphagia and pharyngo-oesophageal diverticula. According to Knuff et al.,[62] however, there is no incoordination at all, the sphincter pressure being normal in patients with pharyngo-oesophageal diverticula. More recent studies[63] have demonstrated that in Zenker's diverticulum there seems to be an apparent loss of elasticity of the UES that results in a restricted opening of the sphincteric segment during the passage of a barium bolus despite normal muscle relaxation. As a result, increased intrabolus pressure is generated during swallowing suggesting that in patients with Zenker's diverticulum, diverticulum formation is the eventual consequence of increased stress on the hypopharynx resulting from this increased intrabolus pressure. The mechanism

of Zenker's diverticulum could then be seen as being a 'blow out' of the pharyngeal mucosa at a weakened point above the relative obstruction.

Several different studies also mention the association between pharyngo-oesophageal diverticula and gastro-oesophageal reflux.[64,65] Hunt et al.[7] demonstrated a higher basal upper sphincter pressure in patients with gastro-osophageal reflux, returning to normal values after antireflux surgery, suggesting that pharyngo-oesophageal pouches are a consequence of cricopharyngeal dysfunction caused by reflux. Henderson and Marryatt[66] showed an incoordination at the upper sphincter in the form of a premature contraction in patients with gastro-oesophageal reflux complaining of upper dysphagia. In a study of 200 patients with reflux they noticed the presence of pharyngo-oesophageal dysphagia in 100 patients, which disappeared in 90% of them after antireflux surgery.

Belsey[67] made a clear distinction between diverticula resulting from primary dysfunction of the upper sphincter and diverticula resulting from spasm secondary to gastro-oesophageal reflux. In this second group, when a small diverticulum occurs, the correction of the reflux can be sufficient to enable the diverticulum to resolve.

Symptomatology and associated pathology

Since 1976 we have treated 225 patients with Zenker's diverticulum; 100 consecutive cases, operated before June 1988, were analysed. This series comprised 57 men and 43 women with a mean age of 68 years (range 38–92 years). Fifty per cent of patients were more than 70 years old and 22% were more than 80 years old. All patients were symptomatic, with a mean duration of symptoms of 37.4 months. The cardinal symptom was dysphagia (85%), followed by regurgitation (76%) and hoarseness (8%). In addition to the symptoms directly related to the diverticulum, other clinical features were present in the majority of patients (Table 7.5): the most important were cachexia (19%), chronic pulmonary infection (37%), hiatal hernia (36%) and/or gastro-oesophageal reflux in 30%.

In 27 patients, 24 h pH monitoring was performed and found to be pathological in 13 (48%). Manometry of the oesophageal body and lower oesophageal sphincter was performed in 31 patients. Only eight (26%) patients had a normal recording. If gastro-oesophageal reflux as a possible cause was excluded, seven patients showed clear evidence of a motility disorder, there was diffuse spasm in four, a nutcracker oesophagus in two and achalasia in one patient who had experienced long-standing symptoms suggestive of this condition. Thus, overall, 60% of patients showed some form of synchronous or metachronous upper gastrointestinal tract pathology.

As regards the upper oesophageal sphincter itself, manometry was possible in 13 patients. In eight (61.5%) a probable incoordination in the function of the cricopharyngeal muscle was suggested. The recorded pressures were normal in six, elevated in two and abnormally low in five patients. These findings could not be related to age, motility disorder of the oesophageal body or to gastro-oesophageal reflux.

Table 7.5 Zenker's diverticulum: associated pathology

PATHOLOGY	NUMBER
Cachexia	19
Pulmonary infection	37
Porforated diverticulum	1
Gastrointestinal	
Hiatus hernia	36
Reflux	30
Diverticulum of oesophageal body	1
Diffuse spasm*	4
Nutcracker oesophagus*	2
Achalasia	1
Gastroduodenal ulcer	27
Gastric polyp	1
Duodenal diverticulum	2
Internal herniation	1
Cholelithiasis	11
Hepatitis	1
Colon carcinoma	1
Volvulus	5
Ulcer	1
Endocrine	9
Cardiac	10
Urological	5
Neurological	8

*Manometric diagnosis.

Treatment: surgical technique
(Figures 7.9 and 7.10)

In symptomatic patients treatment is surgical. Controversy exists between several therapeutic options. Firstly, there is debate as to whether cricopharyngeal myotomy should be performed and, if so, to what extent this should be continued into the cervical oesophagus. Most authorities currently favour myotomy, which will usually suffice if the diverticulum is small but, if large, then attention to the diverticulum itself is also necessary. There are three possible options in dealing with the diverticulum. These comprise either suspension or resection of the sac, and endoscopic myotomy with electrocoagulation, which was first described by Dohlman[69] in 1949, and has more recently been refined by the use of laser and microsurgical technology.[70]

The surgical treatment of choice in our institution is an extramucosal myotomy of the cricopharyngeal muscle with extension into the cervical oesophageal wall, combined with diverticulopexy. This has been performed in 94 patients. In five patients the diverticulum was judged too small for diverticulopexy to be performed and in one patient a resection was undertaken because of a suspicion of malignancy. Surgery was performed under general anaesthesia in all patients, the operation being carried out through a left cervical incision. The pouch is completely freed up to its neck and an extramucosal myotomy incision is made over the anterolateral aspect of the upper oesophagus, starting at the cricopharyngeal muscle and extending upwards for 0.5–1 cm through the inferior constrictor of the pharynx, above the neck of the pouch and downward for 4–5 cm into the upper oesophagus. Small diverticula of 2 cm or less are left untouched. All other diverticula are suspended behind the pharynx, with sufficient tension to eliminate any prolapse of the pouch below the neck of the sac, and firmly sutured to the anterior vertebral ligament with a series of interrupted mattress 4/0 monofilament sutures. These sutures are passed through the flattened diverticulum, right through its lumen near its periphery, in the form of an inverted horseshoe, and serve to obliterate the pouch as well as to maintain its inversion and dependent drainage.

Results (Table 7.6)

There was no postoperative mortality and only minimal morbidity. One patient had a transient fistula which resolved spontaneously after a short period of parenteral feeding. The most frequently encountered problem (six patients) was a temporary change in phonation, which was probably a consequence of post-manipulation oedema. In three patients there was a temporary recurrent nerve paralysis. Four patients had wound infections and in two patients surgical drainage of a haematoma was required. There was no incidence of mediastinitis. Oral feeding was usually commenced on the first day after operation. Early in our experience we left a nasogastric tube in situ for 48 hours but our current practice is to remove it immediately after the operation (64 patients). The mean duration of hospitalization was 7 days, but later in our experience patients have been discharged earlier, 39 patients being able to leave hospital within 5 days.

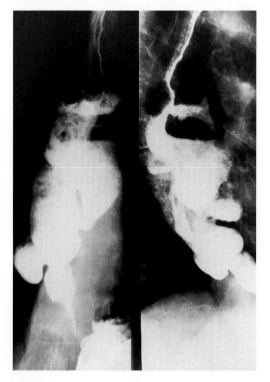
(a)

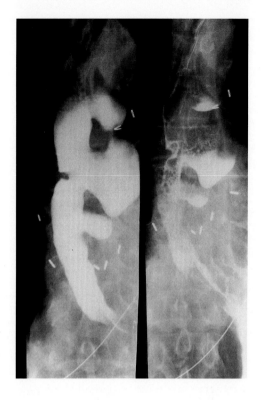
(b)

Figure 7.9
Diverticula of the oesophageal body. (a) Barium swallow showing giant diverticulosis in a patient with diffuse oesophageal spasm. At operation an intense peridiverticulitis of the entire mediastinum was found. A long myotomy was performed. (b) Postoperative barium swallow showing free passage of the contrast bolus. The patient remained asymptomatic until death 12 years after operation.

Long-term follow-up (Table 7.7)

All patients have been followed-up until the present time or until death, either in the clinic or by a detailed questionnaire. The mean follow-up is 4 years (range 1–12 years). Ninety patients (90%) have remained completely asymptomatic. Four patients have residual oesophageal symptoms: occasional choking while drinking in three and in one patient we had to perform a second myotomy on the contralateral side. This patient showed strong evidence of a primary muscular disease on pathological examination. Five patients had respiratory symptoms: three patients developed a single episode of bronchitis and two others developed pneumonia (one obstructive pneumonia due to a lung carcinoma and one pneumonia as a sequel to a cerebrovascular accident). There was no incidence of aspiration pneumonia due to gastro-oesophageal reflux. Of all the patients who had associated gastro-oesophageal reflux, two were treated surgically simultaneously (one Belsey Mark IV, one Toupet + highly selective vagotomy and two underwent a Belsey Mark IV at a subsequent procedure). The remaining patients are all controlled by medical treatment.

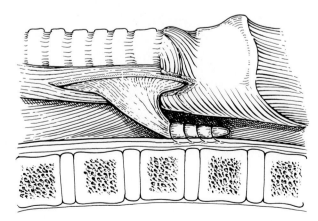

Figure 7.10
Zenker's diverticulum. Extramucosal myotomy of the upper oesophageal sphincter zone and diverticulopexy.

Table 7.6   Zenker's diverticulum: postoperative complications

COMPLICATION	NUMBER
Temporary phonetic symptoms	6
Infection/abscess	4
Pneumonia	3
Recurrent nerve paralysis	3
Haematoma	2
Fistula	1
Respiratory insufficiency	1
Thoracic duct leak	1
Other	3
Postoperative mortality	0

Table 7.7   Zenker's diverticulum: follow-up[a]

FINDING	NUMBER
Clinical	
Oesophageal symptoms	4
Insufficient myotomy (1° muscular disease?)	
treated by contralateral myotomy	1
Intermittent choking on liquids	3
Tracheopulmonary symptoms	6
Impression of foreign body in throat	1
Bronchitis	3
Pneumonia (cerebrovascular accident, Ca bronchus)	2
X-ray: cine-fluoroscopy	
Insufficient diverticulopexy → (asymptomatic)	1
Aspiration of contrast material (meningioma →	
N. glossopharyngeus paralysis)	1
Patient's judgement	
Very good – excellent: 92%	

[a]Mean (range) duration 4 (1–12) years.

Many of the patients have had follow-up cine-fluoroscopic barium swallows. In most patients, an additional trickle of contrast can be seen behind the oesophagus at the level of the diverticulopexy, and in only one patient who had a very large diverticulum was there an insufficient diverticulopexy. However, this patient was asymptomatic 12 years postoperatively, perhaps illustrating in an indirect way the value of the extramucosal myotomy.

Endoscopic management of Zenker's diverticulum (Figure 7.11)

The development of endostaplers has provided an opportunity for treating Zenker's diverticulum with endoscopic assistance. The introduction into the pharynx of a Weerda diverticuloscope (Storz; Karl Storz, Tuttlingen, Germany) offers good visualization of the mouth of the diverticulum, the oesophageal orifice, and the cricopharyngeal bar, which separates them. The endostapler is applied by insertion of one limb, or jaw, of the stapler into the diverticulum whereas the second limb is passed into the oesophageal lumen. When closed, the jaws of the stapler compress the wall of the oesophagus and the wall of the diverticular sac for a distance of 3 cm. When the stapler is fired, this wall, which includes the cricopharyngeus muscle, is divided between two rows of staples. This division results in a myotomy and forms a common space between the sac and the oesophageal lumen, which allows easy passage of swallowed food. With endoscopy, one can visualize the retracted, stapled edges of the cricopharyngeus muscle and the common opening of diverticulum and oesophagus. This procedure is quick and simple and allows the patient to eat and drink on the first postoperative day.[68]

In a prospective study, undertaken to evaluate endoscopic diverticulo-oesophagostomy, 20 patients (mean age 64 years) with symptomatic Zenker's diverticulum underwent either endoscopic treatment ($n=11$) or a standard cervical approach with a diverticulopexy and extramucosal myotomy ($n=9$). There were two perioperative complications in the endoscopic treatment group, including one case of subcutaneous emphysema (but no leak on contrast study) and one case of temporary vocal cord paralysis. In the open myotomy group, one patient with a history of having undergone an operation on the carotid artery had an incisional haematoma that required drainage. The long-term follow-up period ranged from 1 to 16 months. No patient in the open myotomy group had new symptoms, and all had excellent functional results (Table 7.8).

In the endoscopy group, one patient had an episode of unexplained haematemesis. Another patient experienced slight dysphagia after eating dry meat and reported vocal weakness. Two patients experienced return of moderate dysphagia after

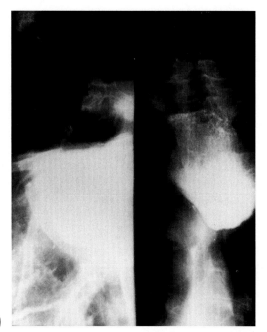

(a)

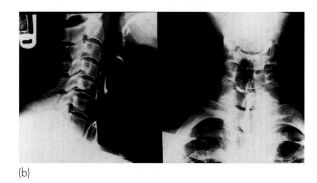

(b)

Figure 7.11
Zenker's diverticulum. (a) preoperative barium swallow. (b) Postoperative barium swallow showing free passage of contrast bolus. The lateral view shows a trickle of contrast outlining the remainder of the suspended diverticulum.

Table 7.8 Results of a prospective study to evaluate diverticulo-oesophagostomy

TYPE OF PROCEDURE	NO. OF PEROPERATIVE COMPLICATIONS	NO. OF POSTOPERATIVE COMPLICATIONS	LATE COMPLICATIONS	FINAL OUTCOME
Open (n = 9)	–	Haematoma: 1	–	Excellent 9
Endoscope (n = 11)	Subcutaneous emphysema: 1	Left vocal cord paresis : 1	Haematemesis 1 Dysphagia Slight 1 Moderate 2	Excellent 4 Good 5 Fair 2

an initial period of excellent functional recovery. At endoscopy, it seemed that the U-shaped suture line had been transformed into a web-like ridge of scar tissue that impaired passage of a solid bolus of contrast material. In both patients, endostapler application was repeated, and the patients had an excellent early outcome.

Peracchia (personal communication) reported a series of 90 patients with Zenker's diverticulum treated with the endostapler technique. In his experience five patients required a reintervention by the same technique. All patients were asymptomatic after a median follow-up of 23 months. The endosurgical approach is, however, not recommended in small diverticula of less than 2 cm, as insufficient length of myotomy will be obtained resulting in persisting dysphagia. In large diverticula, there is a risk of creating a residual common cavity which interferes with emptying of the bolus.

Conclusions

Our results demonstrate that Zenker's diverticulum is essentially a condition of old age. Symptoms are usually long standing; it should be emphasized that symptoms are not only confined to the oesophagus, but that many patients, 37% in our series, suffer from chronic pulmonary infection due to chronic aspiration. This, combined with old age and suboptimal nutritional status may result in a life-threatening condition which is, unfortunately, all too often underestimated.

The most important form of associated pathology is the presence of a coexisting hiatal hernia or gastro-oesophageal reflux. This has been emphasized previously by several authors.[65,68,71] In our series, 40% of patients had a hiatal hernia and evidence of gastro-oesophageal reflux, which was diagnosed in 48% of

those patients who underwent 24 h pH monitoring. It is interesting that our study revealed that 60% of our patients were found to have associated upper gastrointestinal tract disease. Moreover, manometric studies were normal in only eight of 31 patients investigated, and seven patients (with no evidence of reflux) showed clear evidence of diffuse spasm or nutcracker oesophagus. None of these patients had gastro-oesophageal reflux confirming that the motility disorder was a primary phenomenon. These findings raise the possibility of Zenker's diverticulum being one expression of a more complex pathology in which disturbed vagal function could be the common denominator. In this larger context, cricopharyngeal incoordination could be considered as just one expression of a more complex functional disease rather than a single disease entity.

This concept is endorsed by the clear pathological changes found in the muscle biopsies of 62 patients compared with biopsies from 19 controls (Table 7.9). Although some suggested myogenic degeneration, many were suggestive of neurogenic disease, not only confined to cricopharyngeal muscle but also affecting the striated muscles of the cervical oesophagus, resulting in a weaker and slower contractility, as we have demonstrated previously.[72]

From this changed morphology and contractility compared with controls, it can be assumed that the so-called upper sphincter is more than just the cricopharyngeal muscle, and that perhaps the whole of the striated oesophageal wall acts as a sphincter of which the cricopharyngeal muscle is only a locally thickened and more pronounced part. This concept is supported by the fact that manometry of the upper oesophageal sphincter reveals not a well-defined sphincter but, as in the lower oesophageal sphincter, a high-pressure zone extending over the proximal oesophagus.

Table 7.9 Zenker's diverticulum: Enzyme histochemical and immunological findings in specimens from 62 patients and 19 controls

DOMINANT FIBRE TYPE	HYPERTROPHY	ATROPHY	NECROSIS	SIZE VARIATION	FIBROSIS	CENTRAL NUCLEUS	INFLAMMATION	NEMALINE RODS	RAGGED RED FIBRES	ACETYLCHOLIN ESTERASE	NEURO FILAMENTS
Controls I 9 II 3	1/15	1/15	0/15	2/15	2/15	1/15	0/15	0/15	2/15	0/9	0/9
Zenker I 40	32/41	37/41	33/41	40/41	31/41	30/41	21/41	4/41	23/41	33/44	33/44

The denominator gives the number of patients in which a given parameter was examined.

As a result of our morphological studies we feel that it is necessary to extend the myotomy distally well into the high-pressure zone over a distance of at least 4–5 cm. It is perhaps surprising in these circumstances that there is not a much higher incidence of recurrence after simple diverticulectomy. A possible explanation may be that recurrence, like the primary process, takes a long time to develop and, as 50% of patients with Zenker's diverticulum are over 70 years old at the time of their surgical correction, there is insufficient time for a recurrence to become symptomatic.

The involvement of the entire upper oesophageal sphincter zone, as suggested by our morphological studies, may also explain why, after a Dohlman endoscopic short (0.5 cm) myotomy, up to 25% of patients require more than one session before symptoms disappear,[70] whereas with a single-step diverticulopexy and myotomy, no symptomatic recurrences have been observed in our experience.

As far as the treatment of the diverticulum itself is concerned, we prefer a diverticulopexy because it avoids opening the oesophageal lumen and the consequent risk of leakage, which is greater following excision[73,74] and is frequently described with the Dohlman procedure.[70] Furthermore, diverticulopexy allows immediate oral feeding from the first postoperative day resulting in earlier hospital discharge, now usually within 5 days, and therefore decreased morbidity within the elderly group of patients. This is perhaps the reason why there was no mortality in our series. The only criticism of diverticulopexy is the risk of malignant degeneration[75] but this is extremely rare, the incidence being estimated at around 0.4%. We routinely perform a careful preoperative endoscopic examination after lavage of the sac, together with careful palpation. We have not observed any concomitant or subsequent malignant degeneration in our series.

Postoperative manometric studies confirm the persistence of a residual pressure at the level of the upper oesophageal sphincter which probably suffices to prevent aspiration of gastric juice in the case of coexisting reflux. Some authors have advocated a concomitant antireflux procedure in such cases.[1] There has been no evidence, in our series, of aspiration pneumonitis after myotomy and diverticulopexy when coexisting gastro-oesophageal reflux is present, and we would advocate concomitant antireflux surgery according to the usual indications in refractory gastro-oesophageal reflux. In the long-term evaluation of results of treatment of Zenker's diverticulum it is important not to confine the assessment to oesophageal symptoms, as is often implied in the literature, but to include the pulmonary aspects, which are perhaps of greater importance because of their life-threatening potential.

REFERENCES

1. Belsey RH. Functional disease of the oesophagus. *J Thorac Cardiovasc Surg* 1966; **52**: 164–188.
2. Jones G, Ravics WJ, Donner MW, Kramer SW & Hendrix TR. Pharyngoesophageal interrelationships: observations and working concepts. *Gastrointest Radiol* 1985; **10**: 222–223.
3. Palmer ED. Disorders of the cricopharyngeus muscle: a review. *Gastroenterology* 1976; **71**: 510–519.
4. Kilman WJ & Goyal RK. Disorders of pharyngeal and upper oesophageal sphincter motor function. *Arch Intern Med* 1976; **136**: 592–601.
5. Hellemans J, Agg HO, Pelemans W & Vantrappen G. Pharyngoesophageal swallowing disorders and the pharyngo-oesophageal sphincter. *Med Clin North Am* 1981; **65**: 1149–1170.
6. Hurwitz AL & Duranceau A. Upper-esophageal sphincter dysfunction: pathogenesis and treatment. *Dig Dis Sci* 1978; **23**: 275–281.
7. Hunt PS, Connell AM & Smiley TB. The cricopharyngeal sphincter in gastric reflux. Gut 1970; **11**: 303–306.
8. Wooler GH. Cardiospasm. In Jones FA (ed.) *Modern Trends in Gastroenterology.* London: Butterworth, 1952: 179–198.
9. Little AG & Skinner DB. Treatment of motility abnormalities of the esophagus. *Adv Surg* 1987; **20**: 265–278.
10. Swamy N & Rayl JE. Functional disease of the esophagus: role of endoscopy. *Ann Otol* 1987; **87**: 523–527.
11. Hankin JR & McLaughlin JS. The association of carcinoma of the esophagus with achalasia. *J Thorac Cardiovasc Surg* 1974; **69**: 355–360.
12. Vantrappen G & Janssens J. To dilate or to operate? That is the question. Gut 1983; **24**: 1013–1019.
13. Kurlander D, Raskin HF, Kirsner JB & Palmer WL. Therapeutic value of the pneumatic dilator in achalasia of the esophagus; long term results in sixty-two living patients. *Gastroenterology* 1963; **45**: 604–613.
14. Von J & Christensen J. An uncontrolled comparison of treatments for achalasia. *Ann Surg* 1975; **182**: 672–676.
15. Vantrappen G & Hellemans J. Treatment of achalasia and related motor disorders. *Gastroenterology* 1980; **79**: 144–154.
16. Fellows IW, Ogilvie AL & Atkinson M. Pneumatic dilatation in achalasia. Gut 1983; **24**: 1020–1023.
17. Csendes A, Braghetto I, Henriquez A et al. Late results of a prospective randomized study comparing forceful dilatation or oesophagectomy in patients with achalasia of the oesophagus. Gut 1989; **30**: 299–302.
18. Payne WS & Donoghue FE. Surgical treatment of achalasia. *Mod Treat* 1970; **7**: 1229–1240.
19. Effler DB, Loop FD, Groves LK & Favaloro RG. Primary treatment for esophageal surgery. *Surg Gynecol Obstet* 1971; **132**: 1057–1063.
20. Belsey R. Recent progress in oesophageal surgery. *Acta Chir Belg* 1972; **71**: 230–238.
21. Gavriliu D. Operation for functional obstruction of the cardia (cardiospasm achalasia). *Curr Probl Surg* 1975; **12**: 29–36.
22. Black J, Vorbach AN & Collis JL. Results of Heller's operation for achalasia of the esophagus. The importance of hiatal repair. *Br J Surg* 1976; **63**: 949–953.
23. Okike N, Payne WS, Neufeld DM et al. Esophagomyotomy versus forceful dilatation for achalasia of the esophagus; results in 899 patients. *Ann Thorac Surg* 1978; **28**: 119–125.
24. Jara FM, Toledo-Pereyra LH, Lewis JW & Magilligan DJ Jr. Long-term results of esophagotomy for achalasia of the esophagus. *Arch Surg* 1979; **114**: 935–936.
25. Pai GP, Ellison RG, Rubin JW et al. Two decades of experience with modified Heller's myotomy for achalasia. *Ann Thorac Surg* 1984; **38**: 201–210.
26. Ellis FH Jr, Crozier RE & Watkins E Jr. Operation for esophageal achalasia: results for esophagomyotomy without an anti-reflux operation. *J Thorac Cardiovasc Surg* 1984; **88**: 344–351.
27. Little AG, Soriano A, Ferguson MK et al. Surgical treatment of achalasia: results with esophagomyotomy and Belsey repair. *Ann Thorac Surg* 1988; **45**: 489–494.
28. Bonavina L, Nosadini A, Bardini R et al. Primary treatment of esophageal achalasia: long term results of myotomy and Dor fundoplication. *Arch Surg* 1992; **127**: 222–226.
29. Csendes A, Velasco N, Braghetto I & Hewiques A. A prospective randomized study comparing forceful dilatation and oesophagomyotomy in patients with achalasia of the oesophagus. *Gastroenterology* 1981; **80**: 789–795.
30. Shimi S, Nathanson LK & Cuschieri A. Laparoscopic cardiomyotomy for achalasia. *J R Coll Surg Edinb* 1991; **36**: 152–154.
31. Heller E. Extramuose Kardiaplastik mit chronischen Cardiospasmus mit Dilatation des Oesophagus. *Grenzgeb Med Chir* 1913; **27**: 141–149.
32. Zaaijer JH. Cardiospasm in the aged. *Ann Surg* 1923; **77**: 615–617.
33. Belsey RH. Operative treatment of achalasia. In Wu YK & Peters RM (eds) *International Practice in Cardiothoracic Surgery.* Beijing: Science Press, 1985: 530–539.
34. Kramer P, Lauran DH, Donaldson RM Jr. Transition from symptomatic diffuse spasm to cardiospasm. Gut 1967; **8**: 115–116.
35. Vantrappen G, Janssens J, Hellemans J et al. Achalasia, diffuse

esophageal spasm and related motility disorders. *Gastroenterology* 1979; **76**: 450–457.

36. Little AG. Esophageal motility disorders. In Cameron JL (ed.) *Current Surgical Therapy*. Toronto: Decker, 1986: 3–6.

37. Ellis FH Jr. Surgery for achalasia – how do I do it. In Wu YK & Peters RM (eds) *International Practice in Cardiothoracic Surgery*. Beijing: Science Press, 1985: 524–529.

38. Thomson D, Shoenut JP, Trenholm BG & Teskey JM. Reflux patterns following limited myotomy without fundoplication for achalasia. *Ann Thorac Surg* 1987; **43**: 550–553.

39. Pellegrini CA, Leichter R, Patti M et al. Thoracoscopic esophageal myotomy in the treatment of achalasia. *Ann Thorac Surg* 1993; **56**: 680–682.

40. Rosati R, Fumagalli U, Bonavina L et al. Laparoscopic paroscopic approach to esophageal achalasia. *Am J Surg* 1995; **169**: 424–427.

41. Skinner DB & Belsey RHR. Achalasia of the cardia. In Skinner DB & Belsey RHR (eds) *Management of Esophageal Disease*. Philadelphia: WB Saunders, 1988: 453–484.

42. Fekete F. Management of failed Heller's operation. In DeMeester TR & Matthews HR (eds) *International Trends in General Thoracic Surgery*, vol. 3, Benign Oesophageal Disease. St Louis: C V Mosby, 1987: 293–303.

43. Duranceau A, Cardin JL & Taillefer R. Long-term effects of total fundoplication on the myotomized esophagus. In Siewert JR & Holscher RM (eds) *Diseases of the Esophagus*. New York: Springer, 1988: 1206–1209.

44. Wychulis AR, Woolam GL, Howard AA & Ellis FH. Achalasia and carcinoma of the esophagus. *JAMA* 1971; **215**: 1638–1641.

45. Osgood H. A peculiar form of oesophagismus. *Boston Med Surg J* 1889; **120**: 401–405.

46. Sanderson DR, Ellis FH Jr, Schelger JF et al. Syndrome of vigorous achalasia: clinical and physiological observations. *Chest* 1967; **52**: 508–517.

47. Benjamin JB, Gerhardt DC & Castell DO. High amplitude peristaltic contraction associated with chest pain and/or dysphagia. *Gastroenterology* 1979; **77**: 478–483.

48. Berger K & McCallum RW. The hypertensive lower esophageal sphincter: a clinical and manometric entity. *Gastroenterology* 1980; **80**: 119 (abstract).

49. Douglas WS, Wu WC & Ott DJ. Transition from non-specific motility disorder to achalasia. *Am J Gastroenterol* 1980; **73**: 325–328.

50. Henderson RD. Extended oesophageal myotomy in the management of diffuse oesophageal spasm. DeMeester TR & Matthews HR (eds) In *International Trends in General Thoracic Surgery*, vol. 3, Benign Oesophageal Disease. St Louis: CV Mosby, 1987; 305–315.

51. DeMeester RR. Surgery for esophageal motor disorders. *Ann Thorac Surg* 1982; **34**: 225–229.

52. Shimi SM, Nathanson LK, Cuschieri A. Thoracoscopic sling myotomy for nutcracker oesophagus: initial experience of a new surgical approach. *Br J Surg* 1992; **29**: 533–536.

53. Giuli R, Estienne B, Richard CA & Lortat-Jacob JL. Les diverticules de l'oesophage. A propos de 221 cas. *Ann Chir* 1974; **28**: 435–443.

54. Cross FS, Johnson GF & Gerein AN. Oesophageal diverticula. *Arch Surg* 1961; **83**: 525–533.

55. Kaye MD. Oesophageal motor dysfunction in patients with diverticula of the mid-thoracic oesophagus. *Thorax* 1974; **29**: 666–672.

56. Di Marino AJ & Cohen S. Characteristics of lower esophageal sphincter function in symptomatic diffuse esophageal spasm. *Gastroenterology* 1974; **66**: 1–6.

57. Balthazar EM. Esophagobronchial fistula secondary to ruptured traction diverticulum. *Gastrointest Radiol* 1977; **2**: 119–121.

58. Fegiz G, Paolini A, Di Marchi C & Torato F. Surgical management of oesophageal diverticula. World J Surg 1984; **8**: 757–765.

59. Skinner DB & Belsey RHR. Esophageal spasm and diverticulum. In *Management of Esophageal Disease*. Philadelphia: WB Saunders, 1988: 431–452.

60. Hurwitz AL, Way LW & Haddad JK. Epiphrenic diverticulum in association with an unusual motility disturbance: report of surgical correction. *Gastroenterology* 1975; **68**: 795–798.

61. Allen TH & Clagget OT. Changing concepts in the surgical treatment of pulsion diverticula of the lower oesophagus. *J Thorac Cardiovase Surg* 1965; **50**: 455–462.

62. Knuff TE, Benjamin SB & Castell DO. Pharyngo-esophageal (Zenker's) diverticulum: a reappraisal. *Gastroenterology*.

63. Cook JP & Blumbergs P. Zenker's diverticulum: evidence for a restrictive cricopharyngeal myopathy. *Hepatol* 1992; **7**: 556–562.

64. Smiley TB. Pressure studies in the upper oesophagus in relation to hiatus hernia. In Smith RA & Smith RE (eds) *Surgery of the Esophagus*. London: Butterworth, 1972: 152–158.

65. Delahunty JE, Margulis SI, Alonso WA & Knudson DH. The relationship of reflux esophagitis to pharyngeal pouch (Zenker's diverticulum) formation. *Laryngoscope* 1971; **81**: 570–577.

66. Henderson RD & Marryatt G. Cricopharyngeal myotomy as a method of treating cricopharyngeal dysphagia secondary to gastro-oesophageal reflux. *J Thorac Cardiovasc Surg* 1977; **74**: 721–725.

67. Belsey RHR. Disorders of function of the oesophagus. In Smith RA & Smith RE (eds) *Surgery of the Esophagus*. London: Butterworth, 1972: 193–207.

68. Collard JP, Otte J, Kestens PJ. Endoscopic stapling technique of esophagodiverticulostomy for Zenker's diverticulum. *Ann Thorac Surg* 1993; **56**: 573–576.

69. Dohlman GL. & Mattson O. The endoscopic operation for hypopharyngeal diverticula: a roentgencinematographic study. *Arch Otolaryngol* 1949; **71**: 744–752.

70. Knegt PP, de Jong PC & van der Schans EJ. Endoscopic treatment of hypopharyngeal diverticulum with CO_2 laser. *Endoscopy* 1985; **17**: 205–206.

71. Duranceau A & Jamieson G. Cricopharyngeal myotomy for pharyngo-oesophageal diverticula. In DeMeester TR & Matthews HR (eds) In *International Trends in General Thoracic Surgery*, vol. 3, Benign Esophageal Disease. St Louis: CV Mosby, 1987: 358–363.

72. Lerut T, Guelinckx P, Dom R, Geboes K & Gruwez J. Does the musculus cricopharyngeus play a role in the genesis of Zenker's diverticulum? Enzyme histochemical and contractility properties. In Siewert JR & Holscher AM (eds) *Diseases of the Esophagus*. New York: Springer, 1988: 1018–1023.

73. Lerut T, Vandekerkhof J, Leman G, Guelinckx P, Dom R & Gruwez JA. Cricopharyngeal myotomy for pharyngo-oesophageal diverticula. In DeMeester TR & Matthews HR (eds) *International Trends in General Thoracic Surgery*, vol. 3, Benign Esophageal Disease. St Louis: CV Mosby, 1987: 351–357.

74. Payne WS & King RM. Pharyngo-esophageal (Zenker's) diverticulum. *Surg Clin North Am* 1983; **63**: 815–824.

75. Huang B, Unni KK & Payne WS. Long-term survival following diverticulectomy for cancer in pharyngo-oesophageal (Zenker's) diverticulum. *Ann Thorac Surg* 1984; **38**: 207–210.

8

GASTRO-OESOPHAGEAL REFLUX

SEA Attwood
TR DeMeester

DEFINITION OF GASTRO-OESOPHAGEAL REFLUX DISEASE

Gastro-oesophageal reflux disease is a condition in which gastric juices reflux into the oesophagus and result in symptoms or tissue damage. The primary pathophysiological abnormality is the presence of excessive gastric juice in the oesophageal lumen. This may occur secondary to increased quantity of refluxed material, changes in the quality of the refluxed juice, decreased ability to clear refluxed material or, as is usually the case, a combination of these factors.[1]

The effects of gastric juice in the oesophagus are quite variable depending on the individual and include the induction of symptoms and the development of complications of the disease. Defining the disease either by symptoms or the development of complications is unreliable because of the variability of these effects and the most objective definition is to describe the abnormal exposure of the oesophagus to gastric juice.[2]

Symptoms thought to be indicative of gastro-oesophageal reflux disease, such as heartburn or acid regurgitation, are very common in the general population and many individuals consider them to be normal and do not seek medical attention. An epidemiological study has shown that approximately 7% of the population in the USA have heartburn on a daily basis, whereas 33% have this symptom at least once a month.[3] Even when excessive, these symptoms are not specific for gastro-oesophageal reflux and can be caused by other diseases such as achalasia, diffuse spasm, oesophageal carcinoma, pyloric stenosis, cholelithiasis, gastritis, gastric or duodenal ulcer and coronary artery disease. Furthermore, gastro-oesophageal reflux may also present with atypical symptoms, especially when there is associated duodenogastric reflux[4] or oesophagopharyngeal reflux.[5] The symptoms of the former are more suggestive of gastric disease, such as epigastric pain, nausea, vomiting, postprandial fullness and belching, the latter are more respiratory in character, such as choking, chronic cough, wheezing and hoarseness. The severity of these symptoms can override or modify the typical symptoms of heartburn and regurgitation that are necessary to diagnose gastro-oesophageal reflux disease on a symptomatic basis. This is clearly illustrated in the work of Klauser et al.[6] who examined 304 patients referred for pH monitoring and identified a specificity of 89% and 95% for heartburn and acid regurgitation but these symptoms showed remarkably low sensitivity at 38% and 6% for gastro-oesophageal reflux disease. In their study, one-third of the patients reported such inconclusive symptomatology that no preliminary diagnosis could be made about the presence or absence of gastro-oesophageal reflux.

The presence of symptoms does not correlate well with the presence of tissue damage in the oesophagus. For example, significant complications, such as Barrett's oesophagus, even with a developing adenocarcinoma, can occur in the absence of symptoms. Conversely, the observation of a complication such as endoscopic oesophagitis is not necessarily related to the presence of excessive gastric juice in the oesophagus. Although this is the case in 90% of patients, in at least 10% the oesophagitis is caused by other factors, the most common being unrecognized chemical injury from drug ingestion.[7] Also, many patients have symptoms of gastro-oesophageal reflux but do not have endoscopic oesophagitis. This occurs in 40% of patients with typical symptoms of gastro-oesophageal reflux.[8] Obtaining a biopsy is of little help since the sensitivity and specificity of epithelial biopsy is 0.75 and 0.9, respectively and depends on an interested pathologist for proper interpretation. Consequently, a large number of patients with complaints of sufficient severity to seek medical advice do not have endoscopic oesophagitis and are treated expectantly. Oesophagitis is a tissue injury that occurs as a complication of gastro-oesophageal reflux but is not necessarily synonymous with the presence of disease.

By measuring the basic pathophysiological abnormality of the disease, that is, increased exposure of the oesophagus to gastric juice, it is possible objectively to define gastro-oesophageal reflux disease. In the past, reflux of gastric juice was inferred by the presence of a hiatal hernia, later by endoscopic oesophagitis, and more recently by a hypotensive lower oesophageal sphincter pressure. Now, with the use of modern pH electrodes it is a relatively simple matter to quantitate the pH in the oesophagus over prolonged periods.[9] The pH profile in symptomatic patients can be compared to normal individuals and increased exposure of the oesophagus to gastric juice can be documented most commonly by the presence of excessive acid pH and, in some situations, an excessive alkaline pH. Thus, today, the definition of gastro-oesophageal reflux disease rests on the demonstration of potentially harmful exposure of the oesophagus to gastric juice.

EPIDEMIOLOGY

Foregut symptoms are among the most common encountered by physicians in Western society. This is substantiated by the amount of profit recorded by the major pharmaceutical companies who supply this market. The degree to which gastro-oesophageal reflux contributes to these symptoms is difficult to evaluate because there is no one symptom complex that can be used to indicate its presence. The prevalence of endoscopic oesophagitis is high in symptomatic patients as shown recently in Norway where 12% of patients with dyspepsia had endo-

scopic oesophagitis compared to only 6% who had peptic ulcer disease.[10] Furthermore, many individuals consider the sensation of typical heartburn to be normal and do not seek medical attention. The prevalence of gastro-oesophageal reflux disease is estimated to be as high as 0.36% of the general population and it accounts for approximately 75% of oesophageal pathology.

PHYSIOLOGICAL REFLUX IN NORMAL SUBJECTS

Healthy individuals have occasional episodes of gastro-oesophageal reflux. When reflux of gastric juice occurs, normal subjects rapidly clear the refluxate from their oesophagus. This physiological reflux is more common when awake and in the upright position than during sleep in the supine position.[11] A typical example is shown in Figure 8.1. There are several explanations for this observation. Firstly, reflux episodes occur in healthy volunteers during transient losses of the gastro-oesophageal barrier. These may be due to a relaxation of the

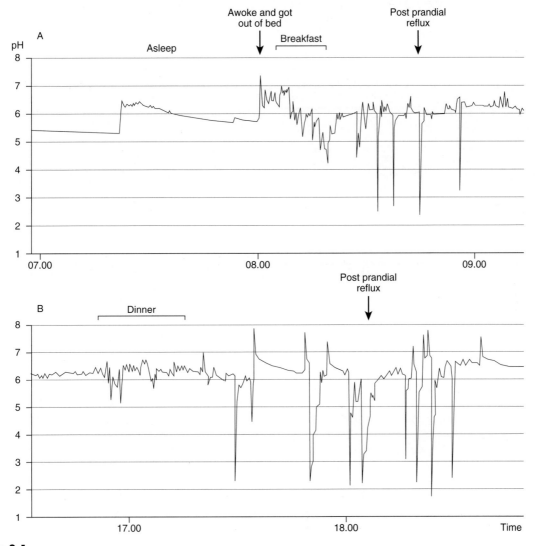

Figure 8.1
Excerpts from a 24-h pH tracing of a subject with episodes of reflux to a pH below 4 occurring predominantly in the postprandial period.

lower oesophageal sphincter or a rise in intragastric pressure overcoming the resistance of the sphincter.[12,13] Gastric juice may also reflux when a swallow-induced relaxation of the lower oesophageal sphincter is not protected by an oncoming peristaltic wave. The average frequency of these unguarded moments is far less while asleep and in the supine position than while awake and in the upright position.[14] Secondly, in the upright position there is a 12 mmHg pressure gradient between the resting, positive intra-abdominal pressure measured at mid-thoracic level.[15] This gradient favours the flow of gastric juice up into the thoracic oesophagus when upright. The gradient diminishes in the supine position.[16] Thirdly, the lower oesophageal sphincter pressure in normal subjects is significantly higher in the supine position than in the upright position. This is due to the hydrostatic pressure of the upper abdomen on the abdominal portion of the lower oesophageal sphincter when supine. In the upright position, the abdominal pressure surrounding the sphincter is negative compared to atmospheric pressure, and the abdominal pressure gradually increases the more caudally it is measured (Table 8.1).[17] This pressure gradient tends to move the gastric contents toward the cardia and encourages the occurence of reflux into the oesophagus when the individual is upright. In contrast, in the supine position this gradient diminishes, and the hydrostatic pressure under the diaphragm increases causing a rise in sphincter pressure and increasing competence of the cardia.

Table 8.1 Intra-abdominal pressure (cm H_2O)

| POSITION | UNDER DIAPHRAGM | | IN LOWER |
	INSPIRATION	EXPIRATION	PART OF ABDOMEN
Supine	3.0	3.5	5.5
Erect	−3.5	−3.0	10.0
Head down	11.0	16.0	0.5
Head up 45°C	−2.5	−2.0	8.0
Head down 45°C	6.0	5.5	2.0
Supine (second reading)	3.0	3.5	5.5

Reproduced from Lam[17] Copyright 1939, American Medical Association.

DETECTION OF INCREASED OESOPHAGEAL EXPOSURE TO GASTRIC JUICE

Prolonged oesophageal pH monitoring

The most direct method of measuring increased oesophageal exposure to gastric juice is by an indwelling pH electrode. Prolonged monitoring of oesophageal pH is performed by placing a pH probe 5 cm above the upper border of the lower oesophageal sphincter for 24 hours. It enables quantitation of the actual time the oesophageal mucosa is exposed to gastric juice, measurement of the ability of the oesophagus to clear refluxed acid and correlation of oesophageal acid exposure with the patient's symptoms. A 24-hour period is necessary so that measurements are made over one complete circadian cycle. This allows for measuring the effect of physiological activity, such as eating or sleeping, on the pattern of reflux of gastric juice into the oesophagus.[9]

It is important to emphasize that 24-hour oesophageal pH monitoring should not be considered a test for reflux, but rather a measurement of the oesophageal exposure to gastric juice. The measurement is expressed as the time the oesophageal pH is below a given threshold during the 24-hour period. This single assessment, although concise, does not reflect how the exposure has occurred; that is, did it occur in a few long episodes or several short episodes? This aspect is important as the effect of a single long episode can be more significant than several short episodes, analogous to rapidly passing one's hand in and out of a candle flame which causes no pain, in contrast to leaving the hand in the flame for an equivalent continuous period which will produce a serious burn. To describe this aspect, two other assessments are necessary: the frequency of the reflux episodes and their duration.

The units used to express oesophageal exposure to gastric juice are:

1. The cumulative time the oesophageal pH is below a chosen threshold expressed as a percentage of the total, upright and supine time;

2. The frequency of the reflux episodes expressed as the number of episodes per 24 hours; and

3. The duration of the episodes expressed as the number of episodes greater than 5 minutes per 24 hours and the time in minutes of the longest episode recorded.

Normal values for these six components of the 24-hour cycle at each whole number pH threshold were derived from 50 asymptomatic control subjects. The upper limits of normal were established at the 95th percentile. Figure 8.2 shows the median and the 95th percentile of the normal values for each component. Patient values are shown in black. If the values of a symptomatic patient are outside the 95th percentile of normal subjects he or she is considered abnormal for the component measured. Most centres use pH 4 as the threshold. Using this threshold there is a remarkable uniformity in the normal values of the six components from centres around the world, indicating that oesophageal acid exposure can be quantitated and compared to normal subjects despite variations in nationality or dietary habits.

During initial analysis of 24-hour oesophageal pH records obtained from patients with typical symptoms of gastro-oesophageal reflux it was noted that not all of the six parameters measured were uniformly abnormal. For instance, the component most commonly abnormal was acid exposure during the recumbent period whereas the total number of reflux episodes per 24 hours had the lowest incidence of abnormality. This observation indicated a need to define when the 24-hour pH record was abnormal. In other words, even though the six components that were measured provided a means for quantitating gastric juice exposure, some were abnormal and others normal at the same time, and it was unclear as to when an individual should be considered to have increased exposure to gastric juice. To solve this problem, the standard deviation of the mean of each of the six components in the 50 normal subjects was used as a weighing factor (Table 8.2). In order to

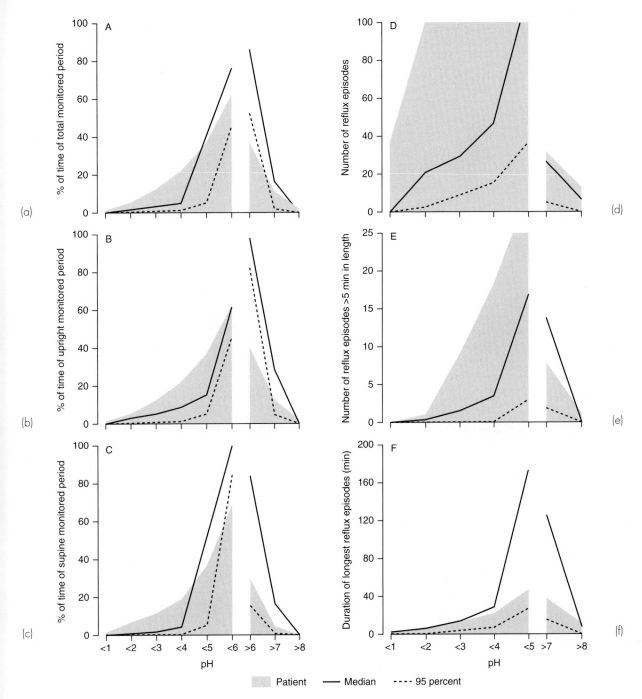

Figure 8.2

Graphic display of ESOpHOGRAM showing the median and 95th percentile levels in 50 normal individuals using whole pH values above and below 6 as thresholds. The shaded area represents measurements made in the patient. The lower line shows the median and the upper line the 95th percentile value for the 50 normal subjects. When the shaded area exceeds the 95th percentile line for a given pH threshold the patient has an abnormal value for the component being measured. (a) % cumulative exposure for total time; (b) % cumulative exposure for upright time; (c) % cumulative exposure for supine time; (d) number of episodes; (e) number of episodes greater than 5 min; (f) length of longest episode.

use standard deviation in this manner it is necessary to deal with the data as though they were parametric. To do so, a zero point was established two standard deviations below the mean value measured for each particular component. This technique allowed a scoring system to be built around the standard deviation as a weighting unit, while treating the data as if they had a normal distribution. Thus, any measured value could be

referenced to this zero point and, in turn, be awarded points based on whether it was below or above the normal mean value for that component (Figure 8.3). The formula used in this calculation is:

$$\text{Patient's value} \times \frac{1}{\text{SD}} + 1 - \left(\frac{\text{mean} - \text{SD}}{\text{SD}}\right)$$

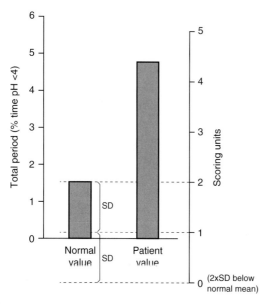

Figure 8.3
Concept of using the standard deviation as the scoring unit.
Note the establishment of an abstract zero point 2 standard
deviations below the mean for the parameter being measured.
Theoretically that allows scoring the measurement as though the
normal values were parametric.

Mathematical reorganization of this formula gives a simpler
version by the following steps:

$$Component\ score = \frac{Pt\ value}{SD} + \frac{SD}{SD} - \frac{(mean - SD)}{SD}$$

$$= \frac{Pt\ value - mean + 2SD}{SD}$$

$$= \frac{Pt\ value - mean}{SD} + 2$$

The use of the constant 2 is not essential as it alters the magnitude of the score by the same value in every case. However, in
our practice we have used a constant for the convenience of
maintaining a positive value when scoring each component.
The minimum value of that constant was one scoring unit. So

Table 8.2   Normal values for oesophageal exposure to
pH < 4 (n = 50)

COMPONENT	MEAN	SD	95%
Total time	1.51	1.36	4.45
Upright time	2.34	2.34	8.42
Supine time	0.63	1.0	3.45
No. of episodes	19.00	12.76	46.9
No. > 5 min	0.84	1.18	3.45
Longest episode	6.74	7.85	19.8

Source: DeMeester TR & Stein HJ. Gastroesophageal reflux
disease. In Moody FG (ed.) *Surgical Treatment of Digestive
Disease*, 2nd edn. Chicago: Year Book Medical, 1989,
with permission.

the simplified formula for scoring each component in practice
is:

$$Component\ score = \frac{Patient\ value - mean}{SD} + 1$$

This formula is used to weight each component of the 24-hour
pH record according to the dependability and reliability of the
measurement. For example, in normal subjects the number of
reflux episodes per 24 hours had a very wide standard deviation, resulting in a large number being used to weigh the measured value in patients. This rewarded few points for that
particular component. In contrast, normal individuals rarely
reflux at night: therefore, the standard deviation for supine
reflux is small. Consequently, an increase in nocturnal acid
exposure is given greater weight and therefore more points. In
summary, the standard deviation of the measurements in normal individuals was used as a weighting unit to score the pH
record of symptomatic patients in a manner that appropriately
weights each component of their exposure in regard to the
accuracy of measuring that component in normal subjects.

A 24-hour pH composite score was obtained by adding the
scores calculated for each of the six components.[18] The composite score was considered abnormal when it exceeded the
95th percentile of the composite scores calculated from the 50
normal subjects. The upper limit of normal (95th percentile) for
the composite score for each pH threshold is shown in Table
8.3.

Recently the process of reading the pH record has been
computerised and the amount of oesophageal acid exposure
at each whole number pH threshold has been measured. The
data are expressed as the percentage time the oesophageal
pH is below 1, 2, 3 or 4 or above 7 or 8. The number of
reflux episodes, the number of episodes lasting longer than 5
minutes and the longest reflux episode are also measured for

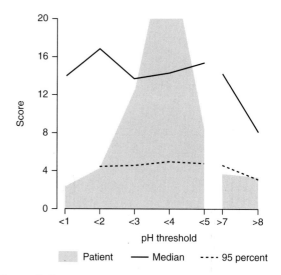

Figure 8.4
The composite score used to express the overall pH result. The
lower line represents the median score and the upper line the
95th percentile of 50 normal subjects. The shaded area
represents the composite score of the patient, with an increased
oesophageal acid exposure measured at pH <4.

Table 8.3 Normal composite score

pH THRESHOLD	UPPER LEVEL OF NORMAL VALUE (95TH PERCENTILE)
< 1	14.2
< 2	17.37
< 3	14.10
< 4	14.72
< 5	15.76
< 6	12.76
< 7	14.90
< 8	8.50

Source: DeMeester TR & Stein HJ. Gastro-oesophageal reflux disease. In: Moody FG (ed.) *Surgical Treatment of Digestive Disease*, 2nd edn. Chicago: Year Book Medical, 1989, with permission.

each pH threshold. The data for each component are shown graphically as shown in Figure 8.2. A composite score calculated from all the components for each pH threshold can also be expressed graphically (Figure 8.4). An IBM-compatible program to perform this function is available from Gastrosoft Inc, Texas, USA.

24-hour pH monitoring is a highly reproducible and reliable investigation for objective assessment of the presence or absence of abnormal reflux in symptomatic adults.[27] The objectivity of this investigation is even more important in children in whom symptoms are difficult to evaluate. A number of studies have clearly shown the value of 24-hour pH monitoring in infants and children[19–21] with excellent reproducibility. Although short studies are considered convenient in children most studies emphasize the need for prolonged monitoring in order to achieve accurate results.

The detection of increased oesophageal exposure to acid gastric juice is more dependable than alkaline gastric juice.[22] The latter is suggested by an alkaline exposure above pH 7 or 8. Increased exposure in this range can be caused by abnormal calibration of the pH recorder, the presence of dental infection which increases salivary pH, the presence of oesophageal obstruction which results in static pools of saliva with an increase in pH secondary to bacterial overgrowth, or the presence of regurgitation of alkaline gastric juice into the oesophagus.

Contrast radiology

The definition of radiographic gastro-oesophageal reflux varies depending on whether reflux is spontaneous or induced by various manoeuvres. In only about 40% of patients with classic symptoms of gastro-oesophageal reflux is spontaneous reflux observed by the radiologist, i.e. reflux of barium from the stomach into the oesophagus with a patient in the upright position.[23] In most patients who show spontaneous reflux on radiograph, the diagnosis of increased oesophageal acid exposure is confirmed by 24-hour pH monitoring. Therefore, the demonstration of spontaneous regurgitation of barium into the oesophagus in the upright position is a reliable indicator that reflux is present. Failure to see this

does not indicate the absence of disease. Some have advocated observing for reflux while the patient is sipping water and pressure is applied to the abdomen.[24] This so-called 'water-sipping' test is not an accurate test of pathological reflux. Normal people will frequently demonstrate reflux of barium under these conditions since swallowing during sipping causes relaxation of the lower oesophageal sphincter, permitting reflux of barium to occur.

Scintigraphy

A scintigraphic test for the detection of gastro-oesophageal reflux disease was introduced in 1976.[25] In this test 100 µCi of ^{99m}Tc-sulphur colloid is mixed with 300 ml of physiological saline and drunk by the patient or instilled into the stomach by nasogastric tube. The patient is placed supine and an abdominal binder may be placed to raise the abdominal pressure. Gastro-oesophageal reflux can be quantitated with a gamma camera. A major disadvantage of the test is the short duration of the monitoring period and the unphysiological means by which reflux is induced. The sensitivity and specificity of this test for the diagnosis of gastro-oesophageal reflux disease have been questioned.[26] One helpful feature is the ability to detect radioactive material in the lungs that may have been aspirated after an episode of gastro-oesophageal reflux. This may be helpful in establishing reflux as the cause of recurrent pneumonitis in atypical cases.

Bile reflux monitoring

The presence of duodenal juice in the stomach or oesophagus can be detected by direct measurement using a continuous monitoring system, similar in application to the ambulatory pH monitoring system described above. The use of an alkaline pH to infer the presence of duodenal juice is neither sensitive nor specific. A highly specific spectrophotometric device can be used to detect bilirubin in the stomach or duodenum[28] (Bilitec Synectics, Stockholm). A small probe with a reflective tip is passed transnasally to lie in the oesophagus or stomach. Light from a small portable source is passed down the probe and across a gap near its tip. The reflected light is detected by a sensor and the absorption of light of the wavelength of bilirubin is determined and recorded continuously over a 24-hour period. A record can then be obtained describing the pattern of bilirubin exposure during the monitoring period. The presence of bilirubin is an accurate marker of the presence of bile. The degree of absorbance bears some correlation with the concentration of bilirubin but there are a number of factors which confound the relationship, including pH, particulate matter, and the poor correlation at very high concentrations.[29] Also there may well be times when refluxed duodenal juice does not contain bile. In addition, the normal values for bile exposure in the stomach and oesophagus are not known for individuals in the relevant age ranges to allow accurate discrimination between normality and abnormality. The detection of bilirubin exposure by the spectrophotometric method is therefore possible but caution should be exercised in the interpretation of results.

Summary of methods for detecting gastro-oesophageal reflux

When analysed according to the above principles 24 h oesophageal pH monitoring is the most accurate means of detecting increased oesophageal exposure to gastric juice. The use of the scoring system allows reproducible assessments to be made on patients which are more accurate than using single parameter analysis alone.[18] It is essential to allow analysis of supine and upright positions separately as there is a significant bimodal distribution of reflux events in normal subjects[30] and the differentiation of these patterns is important in clinical practice.[1] Several studies in institutions around the world have shown the clinical value of pH monitoring.[29–34] We have used it in more than 2000 patients with foregut symptoms and have substantiated it as a safe, useful and accurate investigation. It does not, however, determine the reason for the abnormal exposure. In each patient this requires further investigation.

AETIOLOGY AND PATHOPHYSIOLOGY

There are three main causes of increased oesophageal exposure to gastric juice in patients with gastro-oesophageal reflux disease. The first is a mechanically defective lower oesophageal sphincter.[35] The other two are inefficient oesophageal clearance of refluxed gastric juice and abnormalities of the gastric reservoir that augment the effects of physiological reflux (Figure 8.5).[36,37] In addition to these defects Dent et al.[38] have proposed that transient lower oesophageal sphincter relaxations may occur and contribute to gastro-oesophageal reflux disease. Using manometry and pH measurements Dent et al. have correlated these relaxations to symptomatic episodes of gastro-oesophageal reflux. The mechanism is very similar to a belch and the relaxations are related to a vagal reflex which has an identical pattern to that seen during relaxations of the lower oesophageal sphincter during belching.[39]

The antireflux mechanism of the cardia consists of both the sphincter and the clearance function of the body of the oesophagus. Failure of either component can be compensated for by the other. Failure of both inevitably leads to abnormal exposure of the oesophagus to gastric juice. The identification of a defective sphincter is important since it is the one aetiology that antireflux surgery is designed to correct. This accounts for about 60% of the causes of gastro-oesophageal reflux disease. In about 40% the cardia is manometrically normal. In these patients there may be either an abnormal clearance of refluxed material or an abnormality of gastric function. The presence of an isolated abnormality of oesophageal clearance is rare and it is more usual to find it in association with a mechanically defective cardia where it augments the oesophageal exposure to gastric juice by prolonging the duration of each reflux episode. The effect of abnormalities in gastric function may alter the quality as well as the quantity of the refluxed juice. In any patient with gastro-oesophageal reflux disease abnormalities in the quantity, quality and clearance of refluxed gastric juice combine to produce the damage to the oesophagus and the subsequent complications, and any assessment should include all of these considerations.

A mechanically defective cardia

Failure of the lower oesophageal sphincter is caused by inadequate pressure, overall length or abdominal length, that is the portion exposed to the positive pressure environment of the abdomen (Figure 8.6). The probability of increased exposure to gastric juice is 69–76% if one component of the sphincter is abnormal, 65–88% if two components are abnormal, and 92% if all three are abnormal. This indicates that the failure of one or two of the components may be compensated for by other

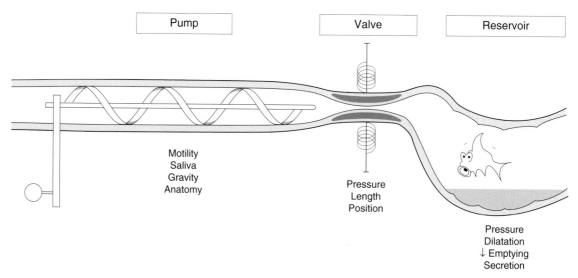

Pump | Valve | Reservoir

Motility
Saliva
Gravity
Anatomy

Pressure
Length
Position

Pressure
Dilatation
↓ Emptying
Secretion

Figure 8.5
Mechanical model of the oesophagus as a propulsive pump, the lower oesophageal sphincter as a valve and the stomach as a reservoir. (From DeMeester TR, Attwood SE: Gastroesophageal reflux disease, hiatus hernia, achalasia of the oesophagus and spontaneous rupture. In Schwarz SI and Ellis H (eds) *Maingot's Abdominal Operations*, 9th edn, 1989, New York: Appleton & Lange with permission.)

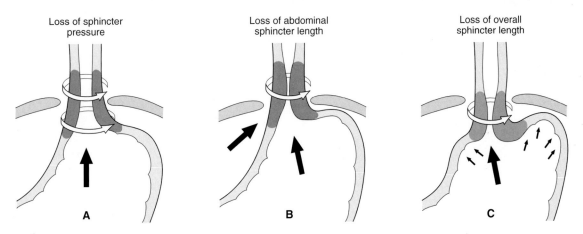

Figure 8.6

Causes of a mechanically defective cardia. Deficiency in any one of these sphincter characteristics – pressure, abdominal length or overall length – may result in an incompetent cardia.

mechanisms, such as clearance function of the oesophageal body, but failure of all three sphincter components inevitably leads to increased oesophageal exposure to gastric juice.[40–42]

The most common cause of a mechanically defective lower oesophageal sphincter is an inadequate sphincter pressure. The explanation for the reduced pressure is most likely due to an abnormality of myogenic function. This is supported by two observations. First, the location of the lower oesophageal sphincter, either in the abdomen or the chest is not a major factor in the genesis of the sphincter pressure since it can be measured when the chest and abdomen have been opened surgically, and the distal oesophagus is held freely in the surgeon's hand.[43] Secondly, it has been shown that the response of the muscle of the distal oesophageal sphincter to stretch is reduced in patients with an incompetent cardia. This suggests that sphincter pressure depends on the length/tension characteristics of the sphincter's smooth muscle.[44] Surgical fundoplication has been shown to restore the mechanical efficiency of the sphincter to normal. In addition to an intrinsic muscular sphincter, a certain amount of pressure is developed by the effect of the diaphragm on the oesophagus. The studies by Mittal et al.,[45] which showed that diaphragmatic contraction enhances the lower oesophageal sphincter pressure in humans, is supported by experiments in the dog which demonstrate that there is both an intrinsic muscular component to the lower oesophageal sphincter and a contribution from the muscular fibres of the diaphragm.[46]

Various factors have been suggested to explain the decrease in sphincter pressure in gastro-oesophageal reflux disease. These include neural, humoral and myogenic influences and sphincter location. A neural excitatory mechanism for the maintenance of basal sphincter pressure was questioned, since truncal vagotomy has no effect on sphincter pressure.[47] Cholinergic agents have the ability to increase sphincter pressure and anticholinergics to decrease it, but the relevance of these observations to the physiological tone of the sphincter has not been explained.[48] The influence of many hormones on the distal oesophageal sphincter has been investigated, but the effects noted are associated with pharmacological doses, and

probably do not represent the true physiological situation. Secretin, cholecystokinin, glucagon and prostaglandins reduce the pressure of the lower sphincter, whereas exogenous gastrin, bombezin and motilin augment the pressure, but the role of these agents in the pathogenesis of gastro-oesophageal reflux has not been defined. Progesterones and oestrogen decrease the sphincter pressure and these are thought to be of relevance to the hypotensive lower oesophageal sphincter seen in pregnancy.

Dietary agents that lower the sphincter pressure to a degree that their effect is clinically significant include chocolate,[49] fatty foods, alcohol and nicotine. The mechanisms of acid reflux associated with cigarette smoking have been investigated by Kahrilas and Gupta[50] who showed that although there were major changes in relative pressures in the abdominal and thoracic compartments during the act of smoking a cigarette, the primary mechanism of reflux was a general lowering of the tone of the lower oesophageal sphincter in smokers. Reflux was increased throughout the day and not specifically related to the act of smoking an individual cigarette. In addition, the chronic coughing that occurred in smokers exacerbated episodes of acid gastro-oesophageal reflux. For these reason it is usual to advise patients with reflux to avoid these substances. Unfortunately such advice is often unheeded.

Although an inadequate sphincter pressure is the most common cause of a mechanically defective cardia, the efficiency of a normal pressure can be nullified by an inadequate abdominal length or an abnormally short overall resting length of the sphincter.[34,35,51] The importance of an abdominal length to the lower oesophageal sphincter was first explained by the anatomical measurements by Bombeck and co-workers,[52] who showed a correlation between the level of insertion of the phreno-oesophageal membrane on the oesophagus and the presence of oesophagitis. Patients with oesophagitis had a statistically shorter portion of the sphincter exposed to the abdominal environment than those who did not. Even when a hiatal hernia was present, this held true. Subsequent studies have shown that in this situation a portion of the distal sphincter is still exposed to the abdominal pressure because of the presence of the hernia sac, which acts as a conduit to transmit changes in intra-abdominal pressure around the abdominal portion of the sphincter.[53] This structural arrangement allows for extrinsic compression of that portion of the sphincter and provides protection against reflux secondary to changes in intra-abdominal pressure.

It remained to be discerned whether the extrinsic pressure acted directly on the intra-abdominal segment of the sphincter or through an adaptive neural reflex response intrinsic to the stomach and distal oesophagus. In the former, the behaviour of the lower oesophageal sphincter could be explained simply on extrinsic mechanical factors, whereas the latter implies the presence of complex neural reflexes with less emphasis on the mechanical function of the cardia. To differentiate between these two possibilities we challenged the lower oesophageal sphincter with variations in intra-abdominal and intrathoracic pressure to determine their effect on the thoracic and abdominal segments of the sphincter in patients whose reflux status was defined by the standard acid reflux test and 24-hour pH monitoring.[54] The results showed that each portion of the distal oesophagus, whether abdominal or thoracic, was markedly affected by changes in environmental pressure and each was affected independently. An increase in abdominal pressure caused an increase in the luminal pressure of the abdominal portion of the sphincter and stomach, whereas the thoracic portion of the sphincter and oesophagus remained unaffected and vice versa.

This behaviour suggests that changes in sphincter pressure occurring with changes in environmental pressure are due simply to extrinsic mechanical factors rather than to complex

neural reflexes. The oesophagus is a soft muscular tube and, as such, the intraluminal pressure of the sphincter results both from applied extrinsic environmental pressure and from intrinsic myogenic tone. Consequently, only that portion of the intragastric pressure due to gastric muscle tone must be exceeded by the muscle of the distal oesophageal sphincter to prevent reflux from occurring. This study further showed that at least 1 cm of the lower oesophageal sphincter must be exposed to the positive pressure of the abdomen in order for this aspect of the antireflux mechanism to function adequately. Lesser amounts place the cardia at a mechanical disadvantage, and reflux is likely to occur when there is an increase in intra-abdominal pressure secondary to straining or changing body position.

To understand the relationship between the amplitude of the lower oesophageal sphincter pressure and the length of sphincter exposed to abdominal pressure, an *in vitro* model was developed which enabled study of the function of these two components individually and together[55] (Figure 8.7). This study showed that the competence of the cardia to challenges of intra-abdominal pressure was solely the function of the length of the lower oesophageal sphincter exposed to the positive pressure environment of the abdomen. If the intrinsic sphincter pressure was negligible, i.e. less than 6 mmHg, greater than 4 cm of abdominal sphincter was necessary to achieve competence. The shorter the length of the sphincter exposed to the abdominal pressure environment, the greater the intrinsic pressure of the sphincter had to be in order to maintain competence. The model further demonstrated, as the earlier clinical study suggested, that under ideal conditions a

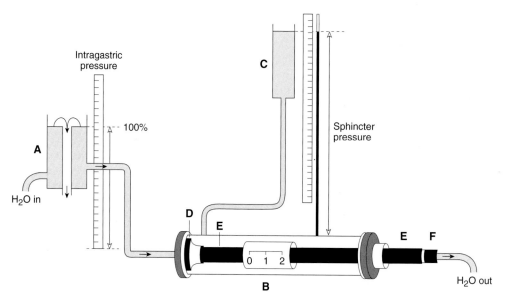

Figure 8.7

In vitro model designed to simulate the forces acting on the distal oesophageal sphincter. A gastric reservoir (A) is connected to a chamber (B) where the specimen is located. A second reservoir (C) is attached to this chamber. The gastric end of the specimen is connected to an adjustable ring (D) representing the circumference of the cardia, and the oesophageal end is attached to a metal tube (E). The length of the oesophagus exposed to the pressure within chamber B is adjusted by sliding a watertight stent (F) through the specimen. Competence is determined by a comparison of fluid levels in reservoir A and the manometer. (From Bonavina L, DeMeester TR and Evander A. Role of the overall length of the distal esophageal sphincter in the antireflux mechanism. In JR Siewert and AH Holscher (eds) *Diseases of the Esophagus* Springer-Verlag 1987; 1031–1036, with permission.)

minimum length of 1 cm was required to protect against challenges of increases in intra-abdominal pressure. The reason for this was that the mechanical advantage was lost with less than 1 cm of abdominal sphincter and, as a consequence, the amplitude of intrinsic sphincter pressure necessary to achieve competence became infinite. The predictions of the *in vitro* model were evaluated in patients with abnormal oesophageal exposure to gastric juice using oesophageal manometry and simultaneous 24-hour monitoring of their oesophageal pH and intra-abdominal pressure.[35] This study showed that when normal mechanical components of the lower oesophageal sphincter are present, the cardia is more resistant to intra-abdominal pressure challenges than when they are absent.

Table 8.4 shows the results of a clinical study confirming these observations.[40] A total of 391 consecutive patients with symptoms suggestive of gastro-oesophageal reflux had both oesophageal manometry and 24-hour oesophageal monitoring. Table 8.4 was constructed by stratifying the patients as to the length of sphincter exposed to the positive pressure environment of the abdomen, and the amplitude of its intrinsic pressure. The competence of the cardia was evaluated using 24-hour oesophageal pH monitoring and revealed that competence is related to the level of pressure in the lower oesophageal sphincter, the length of sphincter exposed to the positive pressure environment in the abdomen and an interaction between both. A high incidence of incompetence occurred when either the intrinsic sphincter pressure was below 6 mmHg, or a length of sphincter exposed to abdominal pressure was less than 1 cm. A secondary observation from these data is that a sphincter pressure below 6 mmHg can occur when an adequate length of sphincter is exposed to abdominal pressure, and a normal amplitude of pressure (15–20 mmHg) can occur when a sphincter length of less than 1 cm is exposed to abdominal pressure. This indicates that the intrinsic sphinc-ter pressure is not caused by the positive pressure of the abdomen acting extrinsically on the intra-abdominal segment, but rather is due to an intrinsic myogenic property as previously discussed.

It was noteworthy that several patients refluxed who had adequate sphincter pressure and abdominal length, although the incidence of such reflux was low. These patients had a short overall length. We hypothesized that under these conditions reflux could occur because the length over which the pressure was exerted was insufficient to provide enough resistance to the flow of gastric contents into the oesophagus.

We made use of an *in vitro* model, similar to the one described earlier, to study the relationship between intragastric pressure and distal oesophageal sphincter pressure.[56,57] The results of the study showed that the ratio of lower oesophageal sphincter pressure to intragastric pressure necessary to maintain competence is inversely related to the overall length of the sphincter. When the sphincter length is 2 cm or less, a pressure in excess of two to three times the resting intragastric pressure, or 16–14 mmHg above an intragastric pressure of 8 mmHg, is necessary to prevent reflux. Since this represents high normal sphincter pressure, most patients with lower oesophageal sphincters of only 2 cm in length would be expected to have an incompetent cardia when studied by 24-hour oesophageal pH monitoring.

This hypothesis was again tested in the clinical situation. A total of 448 consecutive patients with symptoms suggestive of gastro-oesophageal reflux were classified according to lower oesophageal sphincter pressure and overall length. The incidence of an abnormal pH test was calculated for each of the groups (Table 8.5). The importance of the lower oesophageal pressure in maintaining competence was again shown, and occurred even when the overall length of the sphincter was normal. Patients with an overall sphincter length of less than 2 cm had a high incidence of abnormal 24-hour pH monitoring, regardless of the resting lower oesophageal sphincter pressure. Progressive increases in lower oesophageal sphincter pressure or in the overall length of the sphincter resulted in decreases in the prevalence of gastro-oesophageal reflux. This is similar to the relationship of the abdominal sphincter length to sphincter pressure shown in Table 8.4, in that the relationship between overall length and sphincter pressure in reflux control was not strictly additive but included an interactive effect, i.e. changes in either influenced the contribution of each to the competence of the sphincter.

In summary, the resistance to gastro-oesophageal reflux provided by the cardia depends on the lower oesophageal sphincter pressure, the length of the sphincter exposed to the positive pressure environment of the abdomen and the overall length of the sphincter. The most common cause of a mechanically defective lower oesophageal sphincter is an inadequate lower oesophageal sphincter pressure, but the efficiency of a sphincter with normal pressure can be nullified by an inadequate abdominal length or an abnormally short overall length. An adequate abdominal length is important in preventing reflux caused by increases in intra-abdominal pressure.

Patients with a low sphincter pressure, or those with a

Table 8.4 Incidence of increased oesophageal acid exposure in patients classified according to abdominal length and pressure measurements of lower oesophageal sphincter (n = 391)

| PRESSURE (MMHG) | ABDOMINAL LENGTH (CM) | | |
	0–2	> 2–4	>4
0–5			
%	92%	88%	87.5%
n	34/37	22/35	7/8
>5–10			
%	90%	58%	68%
n	19/21	29/50	17/25
>10–15			
%	86%	77%	76%
n	14/16	34/44	26/34
>15–20			
%	67%	60%	71%
n	4/6	15/25	20/28
>20			
%	90%	40%	19%
n	9/10	10/25	7/37

Reproduced from O'Sullivan GC et al.,[40] with permission.

Table 8.5 Incidence of abnormal pH test in patients classified according to overall length and pressure measurements of lower oesophageal sphincter (n=448)

PRESSURE (mmHg)	OVERALL LENGTH (cm)		
	0–2	> 2–4	>4
0–6			
%	74%	79%	81%
n	14/19	46/58	25/31
>6–12			
%	82%	51%	69%
n	18/22	59/116	20/29
>12–18			
%	65%	63%	40%
n	11/17	42/67	4/10
>18–24			
%	80%	46%	30%
n	4/5	12/26	3/10
>24			
%	67%	36%	29%
n	2/3	10/28	2/7

Reproduced from DeMeester TR and Stein HJ. Gastro-oesophageal reflux disease. In: Moody FG (ed.) *Surgical Treatment of Digestive Disease*, 2nd edn. Chicago: Year Book Medical 1989, with permission.

normal pressure but a short abdominal length, are unable to protect against reflux caused by fluctuations of intra-abdominal pressure that occur with daily activities or changes in body position. An adequate overall length is important in increasing the resistance to reflux caused by rises in intragastric pressure independent of intra-abdominal pressure. Patients with a low sphincter pressure, or a normal sphincter pressure but a short overall length, are unable to protect against increases in gastric pressure caused by outlet obstruction, aerophagia or gluttony. Individuals who have a short overall length are at a disadvantage in protecting against normal fluctuations in gastric pressure secondary to eating, and suffer postprandial reflux.

Detection of a mechanically defective cardia

Oesophageal manometry is the most accurate method of assessing the function of the lower oesophageal sphincter.[58] It is performed by using a catheter containing a series of five transducers or ports located at regular intervals along its length, and orientated radially around the circumference. The catheter is passed through the nose and oesophagus and into the stomach and then pulled back stepwise across the gastro-oesophageal junction to obtain a pressure profile of the lower oesophageal sphincter.[59]

The characteristics of the lower oesophageal sphincter which are measured include its upper and lower borders, the respiratory inversion point – that is, the point at which positive excursions that occur with breathing change to negative – and its height above gastric baseline pressures. From these measurements, the sphincter's pressure, overall length and abdominal length, that is, the length below the respiratory inversion point, can be determined. Table 8.6 shows the normal values for these parameters obtained from 50 healthy subjects.[35] The

level at which incompetence occurs has been defined by comparing the frequency distribution of the values of these sphincter characteristics to a population of patients with symptoms of gastro-oesophageal reflux disease, a portion of whom had reflux documented by increased oesophageal exposure to acid gastric juice on 24-hour pH monitoring. Based on these studies, a mechanically defective sphincter has one or more of the following characteristics: an average resting pressure of less than 6 mmHg, an average length of less than 2 cm, or an average length exposed to the positive pressure environment of the abdomen of less than 1 cm. Compared to normal subjects, these values are below the 2.5th percentile for sphincter pressure and overall length, and below the 5th percentile for abdominal length. As expected, these values are also two standard deviations below the mean measurements in normal subjects. A patient who has any one or a combination of these characteristics, has a mechanically defective cardia which an antireflux procedure is designed to correct.

Inadequate oesophageal clearance

The four factors important in oesophageal clearance are gravity, oesophageal motor activity, salivation, and anchoring of the distal oesophagus in the abdomen. The loss of any one of these factors can augment the effects of a refluxed bolus of gastric juice by delaying the return of oesophageal pH to normal. In the upright position, gravity enhances oesophageal emptying and this explains why prolonged reflux episodes in the supine position occur in patients who are nocturnal refluxers. Refluxed gastric juice is cleared from the oesophagus by a primary peristaltic wave initiated by a pharyngeal swallow, or by a secondary peristaltic wave initiated by either distension of the lower oesophagus, or a fall in the luminal pH.[60] The oesophageal contractions initiated may have a normal peristaltic pattern or an abnormal pattern consisting of broad-based powerful and synchronous contractions. The latter reduce the efficiency of oesophageal clearance and encourage the regurgitation of refluxed material into the pharynx, predisposing to aspiration. Such disorders include diffuse oesophageal spasm and the abnormal motility may, in some circumstances, be induced by the reflux of gastric juice into the oesophagus. A much more common motility disturbance is an inadequate amplitude of peristaltic contraction which fails to propel the refluxed bolus back into the stomach. Clinically, it is difficult to determine whether this weakness is a cause of gastro-oesophageal reflux disease, or is a result of the tissue damage from excessive reflux of gastric juice.[61,62]

Table 8.6 Normal values of the distal oesophageal sphincter (n = 50)

		PERCENTILES	
	MEDIAN	2.5TH	97.5TH
Pressure (mmHg)	13.8	5.8	27.7
Overall length (cm)	3.6	2.1	5.6
Abdominal length (cm)	2.2	0.9	4.7

Salivation contributes to oesophageal clearance by neutralizing the minute amount of acid that is left after a peristaltic wave.[63,64] Return of oesophageal pH to normal is significantly longer if salivary flow is reduced, such as after radiotherapy, and is shorter if saliva is stimulated by sucking lozenges. Saliva production may also be increased by the presence of acid in the lower oesophagus and, when present clinically, the patient experiences excessive mucus in the throat, referred to as waterbrash.

The presence of a hiatal hernia can also contribute to an oesophageal propulsion defect due to the loss of anchorage of the oesophagus within the abdomen. This results in reduction in the efficiency of muscle contraction.[53,65] This hypothesis has been confirmed by Kahrilas and colleagues[66] who used simultaneous manometry and videofluoroscopy to analyse oesophageal emptying during barium swallows in 22 patients with axial hiatal hernias and in 14 volunteers. They showed that the presence of the hiatal hernia severely reduced the efficiency of oesophageal emptying and indicated a mechanism whereby hiatal hernia is involved in the pathogenesis of reflux disease.

Detection of poor oesophageal clearance

Delay in oesophageal clearance of refluxed acid can be assessed from the 24-hour pH measurements using the number of reflux episodes greater than 5 min and the length in minutes of the longest reflux episode. Manometry of the oesophageal body can also detect failure of oesophageal clearance by analysis of the pressure, amplitude and speed of progression of the peristaltic wave through the oesophagus. The work of Kahrilas et al.[66] has shown that the amplitude of an oesophageal contraction required to clear the oesophagus of a bolus of barium varies according to the level, lower segments requiring a greater amplitude than upper. Inadequate amplitude results in ineffective clearance (Figure 8.8). Oesophageal clearance can also be measured with a radiolabelled liquid by calculating the time to clear a swallowed bolus from the area of the oesophagus.

Abnormalities of gastric function

Gastric abnormalities that increase oesophageal exposure to gastric juice include gastric dilatation, increased intragastric pressure, impaired gastric emptying and increased gastric acid secretion.[56,67–71] The effect of gastric dilatation is to shorten the overall length of the lower oesophageal sphincter resulting in a decrease in the sphincter resistance to reflux. As the stomach dilates, the sphincter gets shorter in a manner similar to the neck of a balloon on inflation. Excessive gastric dilatation most commonly results from aerophagia due to increased pharyngeal swallowing. Each swallow results in the propulsion of 1–2 ml of air into the stomach. This occurs in chronic gum chewers, patients with decreased saliva from Sjögren's syndrome, or previous head and neck radiation, patients who are unable to initiate secondary peristalsis and require multiple pharyngeal swallows to propel food into the stomach, and patients who reflux and swallow to clear the oesophagus.

Increased intragastric pressure occurs as a result of outlet obstruction by a scarred pylorus or as a consequence of previous vagotomy, which interferes with the normal active relaxation of the stomach. The increase in intragastric pressure can overcome the sphincter resistance and result in reflux. The causes of increased gastric pressure may relate to a loss of gastric adaptive relaxation which allows expansion of the stomach after a meal without increasing the intragastric pressure. This has been shown to be abnormal in patients with gastro-oesophageal reflux compared to normal volunteers although the underlying cause of this motility disturbance is poorly understood.[69]

Delayed gastric emptying results is persistence of the gastric reservoir, which increases oesophageal exposure to gastric juice by accentuating physiological reflux.[70] Delayed gastric emptying may be secondary to myogenic abnormalities, such as gastric atony in advanced diabetes, diffuse neuromuscular disorders and postviral infections. Non-myogenic causes are vagotomy, pyloric dysfunction and duodenal dysmotility. The latter may result in duodenogastric reflux of bile and pancreatic juice, with consequent gastritis and gastroparesis secondary to inflammation.[4] Reflux of this mixture of pancreatic and duodenal enzymes together with bile into the oesophagus may result in severe tissue damage which may result in Barrett's oesophagus and its complications.[72] However, because the pH of this refluxate may lie within the normal range after it has been buffered by gastric acid, it is difficult to detect unless there are prolonged periods of pH>7 in the oesophageal lumen. Such duodenogastro-oesophageal reflux is of primary importance in influencing the quality of the refluxed material and its potential to produce tissue destruction in the oesophagus.

Gastric hypersecretion can increase oesophageal exposure to acid gastric juice by physiological reflux of concentrated gastric acid.[71] Barlow et al.[73] has recently shown that in patients with increased oesophageal exposure to gastric juice measured by 24-hour pH monitoring, 28% had gastric hyper secretion. They noted that a mechanically defective sphincter was more important than gastric hypersecretion in the development of complications of the disease. In this respect, gastro-oesophageal reflux disease differs from duodenal ulcer disease as the latter is specifically related to gastric hypersecretion. However, the presence of gross hypersecretion of acid as seen in Zollinger–Ellison syndrome is associated with a very high incidence of oesophageal symptoms (61%) and endoscopic oesophagitis (43%).[74]

Detection of abnormal gastric function

Delayed gastric emptying as a cause of increased oesophageal exposure to gastric juice can be assessed by endoscopy and radioactive studies. The observation of retained food after a 12-hour fast indicates delayed gastric emptying.[75] The presence of gastritis or excessive bile on endoscopy suggests delayed emptying on the basis of an inflammatory gastroparesis or gastro-duodenal dysmotility. Radionuclide studies quantitate the rate of gastric emptying by measuring the time it takes to evacuate ^{99m}Tc- or ^{111}In-labelled solid and liquid test meals.[76]

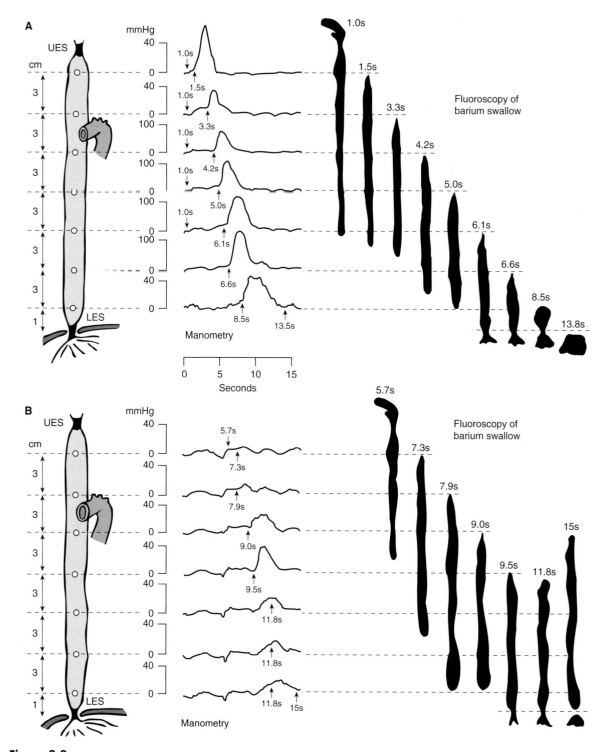

Figure 8.8
Correlation of manometry and the passage of a barium bolus. The tracings from the video images on the right depict the distribution of the barium bolus at the times indicated by arrows on the manometric record. (a) Normal; (b) abnormal. In this example minimal volume clearance occurs due to a failed peristaltic wave. In the distal oesophagus the simultaneous waves, recorded in the three distal recording sites were of low amplitude and nearly identical waveform. (From Kahrilas PJ et al.,[66] with permission.)

As discussed, the measurement of duodenogastric reflux is less precise. If the time the oesophageal pH is above pH 7 or 8 exceeds normal values, then duodenogastric reflux may be inferred. However, significant duodenogastric reflux can occur without this pH change due to buffering by gastric contents and the pH is indistinguishable from normal. In such situations, duodenogastric reflux may be assessed by using continuous ambulatory 24-hour gastric pH monitoring which may identify abnormal gastric alkalinization,[77] or by using a TcHIDA scan and cholecystokinin infusion and scanning the stomach for any radiolabelled isotope refluxed from the biliary tract through the duodenum into the stomach.[78] More recently, the availability of a portable spectrophotometric system has enabled the ambulatory detection and quantitation of bilirubin.[28] This has been clinically tested in patients with gastro-oesophageal reflux disease.[79-81] These studies conclude that bile is present in juices refluxing into the oesophagus. Interpretation of the exposure of the oesophagus or stomach to bile is hampered by a lack of normal values and a lack of correlation with disease processes.[82] Whether the bile which has been detected in patients with gastro-oesophageal reflux disease can be reduced by medical therapy is debated and Vaezi et al.[82] argue that reduction of the volume of refluxed juice by proton pump inhibition may bring about a reduction in refluxed bile. The role of bile diversion surgery is still uncertain. Further understanding of the role of bile in the aetiology of reflux or cancer in the lower oesophagus and cardia depends on adequate studies of the range of bile reflux in health and in disease.

Gastric hypersecretion is confirmed by the presence of increased basal and maximal acid output on gastric aspiration studies following pentagastrin stimulation. The presence of a duodenal ulcer on endoscopy raise the clinical suspicion of increased acid secretion. The presence of increased gastric pressure or gastric dilatation as a cause for increased oesophageal exposure to gastric juice is suggested by the complaint of belching, but is difficult to quantitate.

RELATIONSHIP TO HIATAL HERNIA

The frequency with which a sliding (Type 1) hernia is demonstrated on an upper gastrointestinal barium study in patients with gastrointestinal symptoms varies with the examiner and his technique. The finding of a hiatus hernia does not indicate that the patient's symptoms are necessarily caused by reflux.

Incompetence of the cardia in patients with a hiatus hernia is still dependent on the presence of mechanical defects.[54] Although the presence of a hiatus hernia would seem to indicate that the lower oesophageal sphincter is not under the influence of positive intra-abdominal pressure, this is not so. Studies have shown that in such patients, a portion of the distal oesophageal sphincter is still exposed to positive intra-abdominal pressure because of the presence of the hernial sac which acts as a conduit to transmit intra-abdominal pressure around the sphincter (Figure 8.9). Shortening of the abdominal portion of the lower oesophageal sphincter, whether in a hernial sac or not, results in an incompetent sphincter, because the sphincter cannot be affected extrinsically by changes in the intra-abdominal pressure. The presence of a hiatal hernia also affects the function of the oesophageal body, as has been mentioned previously. Figure 8.10 gives a dramatic example of the result of an oesophagus losing its anchorage at the lower end, because of the presence of a hiatus hernia. The peristaltic wave deforms the shape of the oesophageal body without effectively clearing its contents.

The rare paraoesophageal (Type 2) and mixed (Type 3) herniae deserve special mention. The majority of patients with paraoesophageal herniae complain of epigastric fullness and dysphagia, due to entrapment of air and distension of the intrathoracic portion of the stomach with compression of the oesophagus. In 60% of patients there is associated increase in oesophageal exposure to gastric juice, indicating that in this condition reflux can also be a problem[83] but, as with the sliding type, competence depends on the status and position of the sphincter. Of patients with paraoesophageal herniae, 20% whether symptomatic or not, are prone to the complications of gastric ischaemia resulting in bleeding, infarction and perforation.[84] When a paraoesophageal hernia is discovered, early surgical repair should be encouraged to prevent these complications.

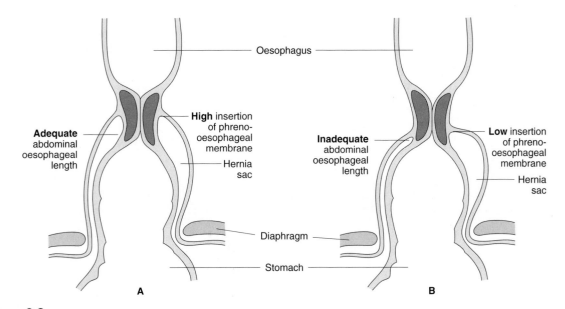

Figure 8.9

High (a) and low (b) insertion of the phreno-oesophageal ligament in sliding hiatus hernia, resulting in sphincter competence in the former, and failure of the sphincter in the latter.

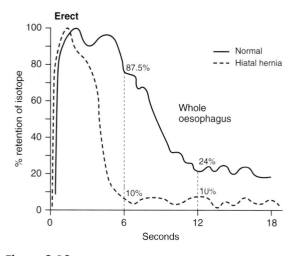

Figure 8.10
Clearance of a radioisotope swallow showing a marked delay of isotope transit in a patient with hiatal hernia compared to a normal subject.

PATTERNS OF OESOPHAGEAL GASTRIC JUICE EXPOSURE

Patients with gastro-oesophageal reflux disease do not appear to be an homogenous population with regard to their reflux patterns. When compared to asymptomatic normal subjects, some patients have excessive upright exposure while awake, but a normal supine acid exposure while asleep. These are 'upright refluxers' and contrast with the 'supine refluxers' who have excessive oesophageal acid exposure only in the supine position while asleep. A third group have excessive acid exposure in both postures and are 'combined' or 'bipositional' refluxers.[1]

A retrospective comparison of the results of surgical antireflux procedures on patients with upright reflux compared to those with supine reflux suggested that each had a different mechanism of reflux. It is our view that upright refluxers are habitual air swallowers and repetitive belchers, each belch causing a reflux episode. The pH tracing from such a patient is illustrated in Figure 8.11. Bipositional refluxers have a mechanically defective cardia and the resulting reflux stimulates multiple dry pharyngeal swallows to clear the refluxed acid from the oesophagus, leading to a secondary form of aerophagia. This leads to a cyclic process of gastric dilatation, belching and recurrent reflux. In our experience an antireflux procedure does not correct the abnormality in pure upright refluxers and may result in severe postoperative gas bloat syndrome. Bipositional refluxers, on the other hand, eventually lose the swallowing habit and become free of the gas bloat problem.

Supine refluxers have excessive supine acid exposure due to a different aetiology. In normal subjects, swallowing during sleep occurs with arousal and occasionally induces reflux episodes. However, reflux episodes occur due to a mechanically defective lower oesophageal sphincter, or if the sphincter is competent, during cyclic periods of loss of the gastro-oesophageal barrier lasting for 5–30 seconds. Studies have shown that these patients do rouse more quickly than normal subjects when acid is infused into their oesophagus, but have difficulty in initiating oesophageal contractions to clear the refluxed material. Normal subjects, although less likely to be aroused, do respond with more oesophageal contractions and, as the waves are secondary, i.e. without a pharyngeal component, gastric dilatation is not a problem.[85]

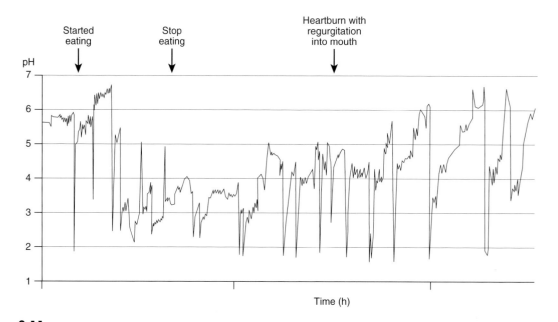

Figure 8.11
pH tracing from a patient with severe reflux associated with air swallowing. Reflux is most frequently seen in the postprandial period associated with belching. These patients are usually upright refluxers and rarely suffer night time or supine reflux. Antireflux surgery in this group may be associated with a higher incidence of gas bloat.

INCREASED OESOPHAGEAL SENSITIVITY TO GASTRIC JUICE

There are two primary symptoms resulting from oesophageal dysfunction: dysphagia and chest pain. Heartburn is considered part of the latter and is a form of chest pain that is typically oesophageal in origin. Because patients are evaluated more frequently than normal subjects, physicians become programmed into thinking that the experience of heartburn indicates that acid has contacted the oesophageal mucosa. This may not be true. Rather the studies by Jones[86] showed that the symptoms of heartburn can arise from a variety of oesophageal stimuli that are unrelated to the presence of regurgitated gastric acid in the oesophagus. Jones recorded the sensation experienced by subjects during the distension of a balloon at different levels of the oesophagus (Table 8.7). The majority of subjects felt a sensation of choking or fullness in the upper portion of the oesophagus and a small percentage reported a burning sensation. As the point of stimulation descended, there was an increasing frequency in the burning sensation, but a decrease in the feelings of choking. Over half the subjects examined felt definite burning the moment the balloon was distended in the region of the cardia. Also, in a few instances, in addition to the sensation of burning, subjects felt as if something hot or sour was being carried up toward the mouth. Such findings explain why heartburn can be experienced by patients with achlorhydria and that heartburn can occur from causes other than irritation of the lower oesophagus by reflux of gastric acid.

Table 8.7 Predominant symptom experienced with balloon distension of the oesophagus

SIGN	UPPER OESOPHAGUS	MID OESOPHAGUS	LOWER OESOPHAGUS
Choking or fullness	62% (18/29)	20% (5/25)	10% (3/29)
Heartburn	14% (4/29)	44% (11/25)	59% (17/29)[a]
Chest pain	10% (3/29)	8% (2/25)	10% (3/29)
Uncomfortable	14% (4/29)	20% (7/25)	21% (6/29)

Adapted from Jones.[86]
[a]Seven patients also complained of chest pain.

In additional studies, Jones placed a nasogastric tube just above the cardia in eight normal subjects and made repeated observations on the effects of introducing various amounts of warm water, cold water, 0.1 M sodium hydroxide, 0.1 M hydrochloric acid and gastric juice into the oesophagus. There was a wide variation in the amount of fluid that could be introduced into the oesophagus before heartburn or any other sensation was experienced. The speed with which the fluid was introduced was also an in important factor, with rapid introduction producing an in almost instantaneous sense of discomfort or pain. Table 8.8 shows the findings in these normal subjects related to the infusion of different fluids. With warm water, five out of eight subjects noted a cool sensation and

Table 8.8 Sensation noted in eight normal subjects following infusion of the lower oesophagus with various fluids (n = 8)

FLUID EMPLOYED	SUBJECTS EXPERIENCING COLD	SUBJECTS EXPERIENCING 'HEARTBURN'
Cold water	0/8	8/8
Warm water	5/8	3/8
0.1 M HCl	1/6	5/6
0.1 M NaOH	1/7	6/7
Gastric juice	1/3	2/3

Adapted from Jones.[86]

three had a feeling of heartburn, whereas with iced water all eight subjects had a distinct sensation of heartburn. Introduction of HCl produced a sensation of coolness in one subject, and in five subjects caused a definite feeling of heartburn. In six out of seven subjects, NaOH had the same effects but to a greater degree. From a clinical standpoint these studies indicate that the experience of heartburn by a normal subject is more dependent on the speed of oesophageal distension, and the repetition of the event, than on the chemical composition of the fluid in the lower oesophagus. Consequently, in patients who complain of heartburn, chemical neutralization cannot be expected to bring about a universal relief of the discomfort. Although the presence of acid within the oesophagus is central to the pathophysiology of gastro-oesophageal reflux, the symptoms that it elicits can be variable. The development of an acid-sensitive mucosa appears to be largely dependent on the volume of each reflux episode and the rapidity with which the episodes occur.

For these reasons the acid-perfusion test, introduced by Bernstein and Baker in 1952, is unreliable.[87] The purpose of the test is to determine whether a patient's symptoms can be reproduced by the infusion of acid into the oesophagus. If positive, the test indicates that the oesophagus is sensitive to acid. Increased oesophageal acid exposure is assumed. In the original technique, the distal oesophagus was perfused with 0.1 M HCl at 6–8 ml/min with the patient sitting upright. Ideally, a placebo is also infused alternately with the acid and the patient is asked to report any symptoms that develop during the infusion. Consistent reproduction of the patient's usual symptoms only during acid infusion and rapid abatement during saline perfusion, or after antacid administration, indicates a positive test. Development of symptoms during both the saline and acid perfusion, or development of symptoms different from the patient's usual experience represents an equivocal test. Failure to develop any symptoms during a 30-minute acid perfusion indicates a normal test.

Various investigators have reported that 34–100% of patients with typical symptoms of gastro-oesophageal reflux disease have a positive acid perfusion test. Failure to include certain components of gastric juice that may be responsible for the symptoms (such as pepsin, bile, pancreatic enzymes) in the perfusate may account for some of the negative results. A false negative result can also occur in patients who have an insensitive oesophagus, which has been exemplified in those patients who have severe haemorrhagic oesophagitis in the absence of pain. False positive results are seen in 15% of asymptomatic subjects.[88–92] It is of concern that symptomatic subjects whose pain is not due to reflux may have a similar incidence of false positive tests resulting in an erroneous diagnosis. Patients with duodenal ulcer may have heartburn and indeed gastro-oesophageal reflux as well and often develop symptoms during oesophageal acid perfusion. This can cause diagnostic confusion if the ulcer is overlooked.

The mechanism by which refluxed acid provokes pain has been a matter of controversy. Some investigators suggest that the pain associated with reflux is due to acid-induced muscle spasms.[92,93] Others believe that induced motility changes are not an integral part of the pain mechanism.[94] The work of Atkinson and Bennett[95] suggests that the presence of acid in the oesophagus has two independent effects: (1) to produce pain, and (2) to increase non-propulsive muscular activity, and the motor changes are not an in essential part of the pain mechanism. The latter is based on the observation that pain and non-peristaltic contractions may each occur in the absence of the other, and when both pain and a change in motility occur together, sodium bicarbonate infusion will relieve the pain without affecting the motility, and propantheline will abolish the motility without relieving the pain.

PATHOGENESIS OF OESOPHAGEAL TISSUE DAMAGE

Tissue damage in the oesophagus may be objectively documented only by endoscopy. In the most commonly used modification of the Savary and Miller grading system reddening of the mucosa without ulceration is scored as grade 1. Endoscopically the sensitivity of detecting grade 1 oesophagitis varies, depending on the observer. Grade 2 oesophagitis is recorded when linear ulcerations are noted. These are usually lined with granulation tissue and bleed easily on touch. Grade 3 oesophagitis represents a more advanced stage where the ulcerations coalesce leaving islands of epithelium, which on endoscopy appear as a cobblestone oesophagus. Grade 4 oesophagitis is the presence of a stricture, ulcer or Barrett's columnar-lined oesophagus (CLO). When a stricture or CLO is observed, the severity of the oesophagitis above it should be recorded. The absence of inflammation above a stricture suggests a chemical-induced injury, or a neoplasm, as the cause for the stricture. The latter should always be considered and is ruled out only by tissue biopsies.

Oesophageal biopsy is a useful method of confirming the presence or absence of oesophageal tissue injury. Chronic exposure of the oesophageal mucosa to gastric juice has been implicated as the cause of the loss of surface epithelial cells, and changes in the architecture of the epithelium seen in biopsy specimens from patients with gastro-oesophageal reflux disease.[96,97] This is reflected by a closer approximation of the apex of the papillae to the luminal surface and hyperplasia of the basal zone layer. In some, but not all patients, an inflammatory infiltrate can be seen with intraepithelial polymorphs and low concentrations of eosinophils. The presence of high concentrations of eosinophils has not, in our experience, been associated with marked acid gastro-oesophageal reflux and may represent an allergic reaction to some other form of irritant. This form of marked hyperplastic eosinophilic oesophagitis seems to represent a distinct clinical syndrome in which there is a severe dysphagia in the absence of mechanical obstruction and no detectable acid reflux[98].

Recently, the effect of early epithelial cell damage has been indicated by the presence of large vacuolated cells in which structural protein degradation has been demonstrated. These pale cells have been termed 'balloon cells' on account of their histological appearance.[99]

Oesophageal mucosal exposure to acid gastric juice has been correlated with the above histological parameters of oesophageal tissue damage using 24-hour pH monitoring.[100] For each of the parameters, the degree of histological change correlates directly with increasing exposure to gastric juice. However, the specificity is poor when the changes are small. Receiver operator curve analysis has shown that with increasing severity of histological change there is a marked reduction in sensitivity for the diagnosis of gastro-oesophageal reflux. Indeed, these changes will occur after chemical or drug injury, and a variety of infectious disorders, such as moniliasis and the infective oesophagitis seen in patients with AIDS. Thus, these criteria cannot be used to make the diagnosis of gastro-oesophageal reflux disease but, in the presence of documented increased oesophageal exposure to gastric acid, the histological changes can be used to assess the effect of this exposure on the epithelium.

A noteworthy effect is observed when the patterns of reflux are related to the severity of histological oesophagitis. Papillary height was found to exceed 60% of the width of the epithelium in supine and bipositional refluxers, that is, those patients whose acid exposure resulted from few reflux episodes, but ones of long duration. Of importance is the finding that although the total duration of the upright reflux episodes significantly exceeded the total duration of the recumbent episodes, the upright acid exposure was less damaging because of rapid clearance. The concept appears to be that low frequency, long duration exposure to gastric juice is more damaging than high frequency, short duration exposure.[101]

A similar effect is observed when the patterns of reflux are related to the incidence and severity of endoscopic oesophagitis. Figure 8.12 shows that isolated supine gastric juice exposure is associated with a higher incidence of oesophagitis and more severe oesophagitis than is isolated upright exposure. Thus, supine reflux appears to be the most critical factor in the development of oesophagitis. Bipositional refluxers have the highest incidence of endoscopic oesophagitis, as well as the more severe grades, which probably reflects a severe form of gastro-oesophageal reflux disease that started as isolated supine reflux.

Considerable differences of opinion exist in regard to what ingredient in the refluxed gastric juice produces oesophagitis. Ingredients in both gastric and duodenal secretions have been

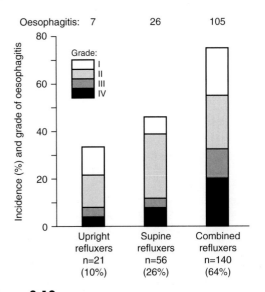

Figure 8.12

Percentage incidence and grade of oesophagitis related to the pattern of reflux as detected by 24-h pH monitoring in patients with increased oesophageal exposure to gastric juice.

implicated. Twenty-four hour oesophageal pH monitoring has shown that when pH profiles from patients with symptoms of gastro-oesophageal reflux disease are compared with those from asymptomatic controls, patients have excessive exposure to acid (pH less than 4), alkali (pH greater than 7) or both. Interestingly, the three types of pH exposure patterns are associated with a comparable incidence and severity of oesophagitis. These findings suggest that gastric contents as a whole, rather than hydrochloric acid in particular, are injurious to squamous oesophageal mucosa.

Quincke, in 1879, was the first to record the correlation between oesophagitis and the digestive action of acid gastric juice.[102] Subsequently, several studies were designed to identify the offensive agent in the gastric juice. These consisted of infusion experiments in which the substance under question was dripped continuously into the oesophagus of an anaesthetized animal,[103] or experiments in which surgical manipulations resulted in chronic reflux of a variety of digestive juice components.[104,105] The results of these studies showed that a combination of acid and pepsin had a damaging effect on the oesophageal mucosa of the species tested. However, in all the experiments prolonged continuous exposure of the oesophageal mucosa to the substance tested was necessary to produce a damaging effect. The time required was in excess of that measured in patients with severe reflux oesophagitis. In these patients, oesophageal pH was below 4 for only 20–30% of the 24-hour period, and the exposure was not continuous but broken up into several episodes. These findings suggested that factors in addition to hydrochloric acid and pepsin were involved in the development of oesophagitis in humans.

The occurrence of oesophagitis in patients with achlorhydria[106] or after total gastrectomy[107] is a well-established clinical observation and indicates that an injurious agent must also be present in duodenal juice. In support of this concept, several authors have demonstrated a concomitant increase in duodenogastric reflux in patients with symptomatic gastro-oesophageal reflux disease.[106-111] Bile, pancreatic secretions, and duodenal secretions are all potentially injurious ingredients in duodenal juice. Bile salts are considered to be the corrosive component of bile, and their presence in the oesophagus has been correlated with symptomatic heartburn.[112] The corrosive components of pancreatic juice are activated enzymes, such as trypsin, lipase and carbopeptidase, all of which have been shown to produce epithelial changes when incubated with strips of oesophageal mucosa.[113] These proteolytic enzymes are generally thought to be rapidly inactivated in the stomach. Experiments have demonstrated that the inactivation of trypsin by pepsin takes place at a pH below 3.5.[114] In the absence of pepsin, trypsin is stable in acid solution and present in active form.[115] Active trypsin has been demonstrated in the human stomach at pH values between 3, 5 and 7 for as long as 90 minutes after a test meal.[116]

The elegant experiments of Johnson and Harmon involving *in vivo* perfusion of rabbit oesophagi have shed considerable light on the pathogenesis of mucosal injury and have explained the seemingly conflicting clinical observations regarding reflux of gastric and duodenal juice.[117] These studies have shown that oesophageal squamous mucosa is resistant to hydrogen ion injury at pH 2 or above, and damaged when the pH drops below this level (Figure 8.13). Bile salts at concentrations found in gastric juice are potentially damaging to the oesophageal mucosa, depending on the pH of the solution. When the pH of gastric juice is less than the pK_a of bile acid, the batter is no longer damaging to the mucosa. For example, at a pH of 2 taurine-conjugated bile salts with pK_a values slightly less than 2 remain in solution and are damaging to the mucosa, whereas unconjugated bile salts with pK_a values much

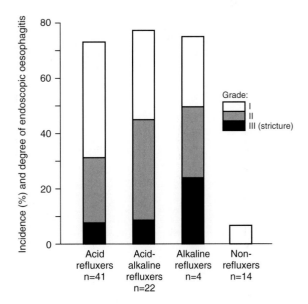

Figure 8.13

Incidence and degree of endoscopic oesophagitis in patients with either excessive acid and/or alkaline oesophageal exposure.

greater than 2 are precipitated and non-injurious. When the pH of the gastric juice rises to 7, the unconjugated bile salts go into solution and injure the mucosa whereas taurine-conjugated bile salts precipitate out and are non-injurious.

An important observation from the experiments of Johnson and Harmon was that acid or bile could produce oesophageal mucosal barrier abnormalities, including changes in potential difference, hydrogen ion flux and permeability defects, yet neither alone nor in combination could they produce morphological lesions consistent with clinical reflux oesophagitis. When the enzyme pepsin or trypsin was present in physiological concentrations, significant gross and microscopic oesophagitis resulted, depending on the pH of the perfusate. These observations appear relevant to humans in that increased concentrations of pepsin have been found in oesophageal aspirates of patients with severe ulcerative oesophagitis, compared to those without oesophagitis,[118] and erosive oesophagitis comparable to that observed with excessive acid reflux has been observed following total gastrectomy.[107]

The studies by Johnson and Harmon suggested that trypsin may be a major injurious agent in an alkaline refluxate, and pepsin in an acid refluxate.[117] It appears that the pH of refluxed juice dictates which enzyme, if present, would be the injurious agent by providing the optimal pH range for its activity. Johnson and Harmon also pointed out an interaction between bile salts and pepsin or trypsin activity. They observed that bile salt taurodeoxycholate significantly diminished the degree of oesophagitis caused by pepsin in an acid environment in a dose-dependent manner. In contrast, soluble unconjugated bile salts significantly potentiated the degree of oesophagitis caused by trypsin in an alkaline environment. Figure 8.14 illustrates these interactions graphically.

The variation in oesophageal mucosal injury across this spectrum of refluxed material provides an explanation for the poor correlation between the symptoms of heartburn and endoscopic oesophagitis. The reflux of acid gastric juice

contaminated with duodenal contents could break the oesophageal mucosal barrier, irritate nerve endings in the papillae close to the luminal surface, and cause severe heartburn. Despite the presence of intense heartburn, the bile salts would destroy pepsin, the acid pH would inactivate trypsin and the patient would have little or no evidence of oesophagitis. In contrast, the patient who refluxes alkaline gastric juice may have minimal heartburn because of the absence of hydrogen ions in the refluxate, but severe endoscopic oesophagitis because of bile salt potentiation of trypsin activity on the oesophageal mucosa. Consequently, changing the pH of the refluxed gastric juice from acid to less acid juice by the administration of H_2 blockers, may intensify the mucosal injury, and at the same time giving the patient a sense of security by alleviating the symptom of heartburn. The results of clinical studies with H_2 blockers suggest that this may occur in that their administration markedly reduces symptoms, but has a lesser effect in improving the endoscopic grade of oesophagitis.[119] However, near-complete acid suppression with the new powerful proton pump inhibitors does allow increased levels of healing of endoscopic oesophagitis. This may be a consequence of reduction in the total volume of refluxed gastric juice regardless of its chemical composition (Figure 8.15).

When the composition of the refluxed gastric juice is such that sustained or repetitive oesophageal injury occurs, two sequences can result. First, a luminal stricture can develop from submucosal and eventually intramural fibrosis. Secondly, Barrett's columnar-lined oesophagus (CLO) can develop by replacement of repetitively damaged squamous mucosa by columnar epithelium. The columnar epithelium, although acid-resistant and therefore associated with alleviation of the complaint of heartburn, is subject to the complications of stricture in 50%, deep ulceration in 15%[72] and dysplasia with possible adenocarcinomatous change. The incidence of adenocarcinoma has yet to be determined, but studies to date show a range from 1 in 441 to 1 in 56 patient years.[120–123] Although this appears to be a small risk it can be placed in better perspective when compared to the risk of lung cancer in a population of men between the ages of 55 and 64 who have smoked one pack of cigarettes per day for 20 years. The incidence of lung cancer in such a population is 227 per 100 000 individuals. In patients with Barrett's CLO the incidence is between 500 and 1000 per 100 000. This is over 30 times more frequent than the risk of developing oesophageal carcinoma in the general population in the USA. When placed in this perspective, the risk of adenocarcinoma resulting from reflux emerges as a serious problem but one that has the potential for earlier recognition and appropriate therapy.

The development of extensive oesophageal damage, such as a stricture or Barrett's CLO, is usually associated with a profound mechanical defect of the cardia and decreased acid clearance by the body of the oesophagus.[127] Studies have shown that patients with reflux-induced stricture or Barrett's CLO have a more profound defect in sphincter pressure than patients with simple oesophagitis and, as expected, this results in a greater exposure of the distal oesophagus to gastric juice.[124]

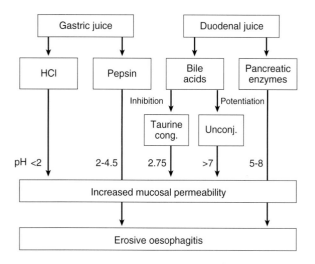

Figure 8.14
Schematic diagram of the interaction of injurious agents refluxed into the oesophagi of patients with gastro-oesophageal reflux disease.

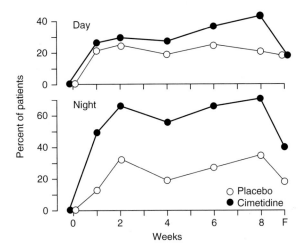

Figure 8.15
Percentage of patients with gastro-oesophageal reflux disease
who became pain free during the study period while receiving
the H, blocker cimetidine or a placebo. Altering the pH of the
refluxed gastric juice with H, blockers resulted in a significant
decrease in symptoms (*P*<0.05).

Those patients with Barrett's CLO who develop the complications of stricture, ulcer or dysplasia do not have a greater
exposure to gastric acid than those who have a relatively quiescent columnarized segment (Figure 8.16).[72] Although this
may seem surprising, it may be a feature of the protective
value of the columnar epithelium to injury by gastric acid. In
contrast, those patients who develop complications of their
Barrett's CLO have a markedly elevated oesophageal exposure
to alkaline gastric juice. These studies were supported by the

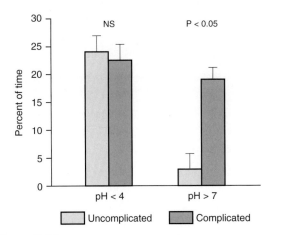

Figure 8.16
The exposure of the oesophagus in Barrett's oesophagus to
acid and alkaline pH: patients with Barrett's oesophagus
complicated by ulcer, stricture or dysplasia showed no
difference in acid exposure to those without complications in
their Barrett's oesophagus, but the exposure to a pH > 7 was
significantly greater in those Barrett's patients with
complications. (From Attwood SEA et al. Alkaline
gastroesophageal reflux – implications in the development of
complications in Barrett's columnar lined lower esophagus.
Surgery **106**: 1989; 764–770, with permission.)

observations of duodenogastric reflux on TcHIDA scans during
continuous gastric pH monitoring and during ambulatory
Bilitec monitoring. Thus, duodenal juices are implicated in the
development of complications in Barrett's CLO. It is not known
whether this exposure to duodenal juices is responsible for the
development of adenocarcinoma but the role of bile in the
development of adenocarcinoma elsewhere in the gastrointestinal tract is well established. In patients with genetic predisposi-
tions to carcinoma of the colon, bile has been implicated as a
cofactor in the carcinogenesis and these patients after total
colectomy are still at an increased risk of developing adenocarcinoma of the duodenum, ampulla and stomach in comparison
to normal subjects.[10,126]

Bile as a cofactor in the carcinogenesis of adenocarcinoma
of the oesophagus has recently been clearly shown in a rat
model with gastro-oesophageal reflux and duodeno-
oesophageal reflux but its effect in humans with Barrett's
columnar-lined oesophagus awaits further study.[127]

REFERENCES

1. DeMeester TR, Johnson LF, Joseph GJ, Toscano MS, Hall AW & Skinner DB. Patterns of gastro-oesophageal reflux in health and disease. *Ann Surg* 1976; **184**: 459.
2. DeMeester TR & Johnson LF. The evaluation of objective measurements of gastro-oesophageal reflux and their contribution to patient management. *Surg Clin North Am* 1976; **56**: 39.
3. Nebel OR, Fornes MF & Castell DO. Symptomatic gastro-oesophageal reflux: incidence and precipitating factors. *Am J Dig Dis* 1976; **21**: 953.
4. Kaye MD & Showalter JP. Pyloric incompetence in patients with symptomatic gastro-oesophageal reflux. *J Lab Clin Med* 1974; **83**: 198.
5. Pellegrini CA, DeMeester TR & Johnson LF. Gastro-oesophageal reflux and pulmonary aspiration: incidence, functional abnormality and results of surgical therapy. *Surgery* 1979; **86**: 110.
6. Klauser AG, Schindlbeck NE & Muller-Lissner SA. Symptoms in gastro-oesophageal reflux disease. *Lancet* 1990; **335**: 205.
7. Bonavina L, DeMeester TR, Chesney L, Schwizer W, Albertucci M & Bailey RT. Drug-induced oesophageal strictures. *Ann Surg* 1987; **206**: 173.
8. Fuchs KH, DeMeester TR & Albertucci M. Specificity and sensitivity of diagnosis of gastro-oesophageal reflux disease. *Surgery* 1987; **102**: 575.
9. Johnson LF & DeMeester TR. 24-hour pH monitoring of the distal oesophagus: a quantitative measure of gastro-oesophageal reflux. *Am J Gastroenterol* 1974; **62**: 325.
10. Johnsen R, Bernersen B, Straume B, Forde O, Bostrad L & Burhol P. Prevalence of endoscopic and histological findings in subjects with and without dyspepsia. *BMJ* 1991; **302**: 749.
11. Mittal RA & McCallum RW. Characteristics and frequency of transient relaxations of the lower oesophageal sphincter in patients with reflux oesophagitis. *Gastroenterology* 1988; **95**: 593.
12. Leon CSC, Flanagan JBL & Moorrees CFA. The frequency of deglutition in man. *Arch Oral Biol* 1965; **10**: 83.
13. Orr WC, Robinson MG & Johnson LF. Acid clearing during sleep in patients with oesophagitis and controls. *Dig Dis Sci* 1981; **26**: 423.
14. Johnson LF, Lin TC, Hong SK. Gastro-oesophageal dynamics during immersion in water to the neck. *J Appl Physiol* 1975; **38**: 449.
15. Banchero N, Schwartz PE & Wood EH. Intra-oesophageal pressure gradient in man. *J Appl Physiol* 1967; **22**: 1066.
16. Babka JC, Hagar GW & Castell DO. The effect of body position on lower oesophageal sphincter pressure. *Am J Dig Dis* 1973; **18**: 441.
17. Lam CR. Intra-abdominal pressure: a critical review and an experimental study. *Arch Surg* 1939; **39**: 1006.
18. DeMeester TR. Prolonged oesophageal pH monitoring. In Read NW (ed.) *Gastrointestinal Motility: Which Test?* Petersfield, UK: Wrightson Biomedical, 1989.
19. Vandenplas Y, Helven R, Goyvaerts H & Sacre L. Reproducibility of continuous 24 hour oesophageal pH monitoring in infants and children. *Gut* 1990; **31**: 374.
20. Colson DJ, Campbell CAG, Wright VA & Watson BW. Predictive value

of oesophageal pH variables in children with gastro-oesophageal reflux. *Gut* 1990; **31**: 370–373.

21. Cucchiara S, Staiano A, Gobio-Casali L, Boccieri A & Paone FM. Value of 24 hour intraoesophageal pH monitoring in children. *Gut* 1990; **30**: 129.

22. Pellegrini CA, DeMeester TR, Wernley JA et al. Alkaline gastro-oesophageal reflux. *Am J Surg* 1978; **135**: 177.

23. Battle WS, Nyhus LM & Bombeck CT. Gastro-oesophageal reflux: diagnosis and treatment. *Ann Surg* 1973; **177**: 560.

24. Linsman JF. Gastro-oesophageal reflux elicited while drinking water (water siphonage test). Its clinical correlation with pyrosis. *AJR* 1965; **94**: 325.

25. Fisher RS, Malmud LS, Roberts GS et al. Gastro-oesophageal (GE) scintiscanning to detect and quantitate GE reflux. *Gastroenterology* 1976; **70**: 301.

26. Hoffman GC & Vamsant HH. The gastro-oesophageal scintiscan: comparison of methods to demonstrate gastro-oesophageal reflux. *Arch Surg* 1979; **114**: 727.

27. Wiener GJ, Morgan TM, Copper JB et al. Ambulatory 24-hour oesophageal pH monitoring. Reproducibility and variability of pH parameters. *Dig Dis Sci* 1988; **33**: 1127.

28. Bechi P, Pucciani F, Daldini F et al. Long term ambulatory enterogastric reflux monitoring. Validation of a new fibreoptic technique. *Dig Dis Sci* 1993; **38**: 1297.

29. Caldwell MTP, Byrne P, Brazil N et al. An ambulatory bile reflux measuring system – an in vitro appraisal. *Physiol Meas* 1994; **15**: 57.

30. Cheadle WG, Vitale GC, Sadek SA & Cushieri A. Computerised ambulatory oesophageal pH monitoring in 50 asymptomatic volunteer subjects; results and clinical implications. *Am J Surg* 1988; **155**: 503.

31. Klauser AG, Heinrich C, Schindlback NE & Muller-Lissner SA. Is long-term oesophageal pH monitoring of clinical value? *Am J Gastroenterol* 1989; **84**: 362.

32. Pujol A, Grande L, Ros E & Pera C. Utility of inpatient 24-hour intra-oesophageal pH monitoring in the diagnosis of gastro-oesophageal reflux. *Dig Dis Sci* 1988; **33**: 1134.

33. Rokkas T & Sladen GE. Ambulatory oesophageal pH recording in gastro-oesophageal reflux: relevance to the development of oesophagitis. *Am J Gastroenterol* 1988; **83**: 629.

34. Weiser HF, Lange R & Bollschweiler, E. Intra-oesophageal 24-hour pH-metry: an in indispensable tool for the diagnosis of reflux disorders. In: Siewert JR & Holscher AH (eds) *Diseases of the Oesophagus*. Berlin: Springer Verlag, 1987: 800.

35. Zaninotto G, DeMeester TR, Schwizer W, Johansson KE & Cheng SC. The lower oesophageal sphincter in health and disease. *Am J Surg* 1988; **155**: 104.

36. Joelsson BE, DeMeester TR, Skinner DB, LaFontaine E, Waters PF & O'Sullivan GC. The role of the oesophageal body in the antireflux mechanism. *Surgery* 1982; **92**: 417.

37. Ahtaridis G, Snape WJ & Cohen S. Lower oesophageal sphincter pressure as an index of gastro-oesophageal reflux. *Dig Dis Sci* 1981; **26**: 993.

38. Dent J, Holloway RH, Toouli J & Dodds WJ. Mechanisms of lower oesophageal sphincter incompetence in patients with symptomatic gastro-oesophageal reflux. *Gut* 1988; **29**: 1020–1028.

39. Holloway RH & Orenstein SR. Gastro-oesophageal reflux disease in adults and children. *Ballieres Clin Gastroenterol* 1991; **5**: 337–370.

40. O'Sullivan GC, DeMeester TR, Joelsson et al. Interaction of lower oesophageal sphincter pressure and length of sphincter in the abdomen as determinants of gastro-oesophageal competence. *Am J Surg* 1982; **143**: 40.

41. Wernley JA, DeMeester TR, Bryant GH, Wang CI, Smith RB & Skinner DB. Intra-abdominal pressure and manometric data of the distal oesophageal sphincter. *Arch Surg* 1980; **115**: 534.

42. Bonavina L, DeMeester TR & Evader A. Role of the overall length of the distal oesophageal sphincter in the antireflux mechanism. In: Siewert JR & Holscher AH (eds) *Diseases of the Oesophagus*. Berlin: Springer-Verlag, 1987; 1031.

43. DeMeester TR. What is the role of intra-operative manometry? *Ann Thorac Surg* 1980; **30**: 1.

44. Biancini P, Zabinsky MP & Behar J. Pressure, tension and force of closure of the human lower oesophageal sphincter and oesophagus. *J Clin Invest* 1975; **56**: 476.

45. Mittal RK, Rochester DF & McCallum RW. Effect of the diaphragmatic contraction on lower oesophageal sphincter pressure in man. *Gut* 1987; **28**: 1564.

46. Radmark T & Pettersson GB. The contribution of the diaphragm and an intrinsic sphincter to the gastro-oesophageal antireflux barrier. An experimental study in the dog. *Scand J Gastroenterol* 1989; **24**: 85.

47. Mann CV & Hardcastle JD. The effect of vagotomy on the human gastro-oesophageal sphincter. *Gut* 1968; **9**: 688.

48. Castell DO. The lower oesophageal sphincter: physiological and clinical aspects. *Ann Intern Med* 1975; **83**: 390.

49. Murphy DW & Castell DO. Chocolate and heartburn: evidence of increased acid exposure after chocolate ingestion. *Am J Gastroenterol* 1988; **83**: 633.

50. Kahilras PJ & Gupta RR. Mechanisms of acid reflux associated with cigarette smoking. *Gut* 1990; **31**: 4.

51. Johnsson F, Joelsson B & Gudmundsson K. Determinants of gastro-oesophageal reflux and their inter-relationships. *Br J Surg* 1989; **76**: 241.

52. Bombeck CT, Dillard DH & Nyhus LM. Muscular anatomy of the gastro-oesophageal junction and role of phreno-oesophageal ligament: autopsy study of sphincter mechanism. *Ann Surg* 1966; **164**: 643.

53. DeMeester TR, LaFontaine E, Joelsson BE et al. Relationship of a hiatal hernia to the function of the body of the oesophagus and the gastro-oesophageal junction. *J Thorac Cardiovasc Surg* 1981; **82**: 547.

54. Pellegrini CA, DeMeester TR & Skinner DB. Response of the distal oesophageal sphincter to respiratory and positional manoeuvres in humans. *Surg Forum* 1976; **27**: 380.

55. Sloan S & Kahilras PJ. Impairment of oesophageal emptying with hiatal hernia. *Gastroenterology* 1990; **100**: 596.

56. DeMeester TR, Wernley JA, Bryant et al. Clinical and *in vitro* analysis of gastro-oesophageal competence. A study of the principles of antireflux surgery. *Am J Surg* 1979; **137**: 39.

57. DeMeester TR. Experimental and clinical evidence for mechanical factors in the competency of the cardia. In Van Heukelem HA, Gooszen HG, Perpestra JB et al. (eds) *Pathological Gastro-oesophageal Reflux*. Amsterdam; Zuid Nederlandse Uitgevers Maatschappij BV, 1982; 17.

58. Castell DO, Richter RE & Dalton CB (eds) *Oesophageal motility testing*. New York: Elsevier, 1987.

59. Winans CS & Harris LD. Quantitation of the lower oesophageal sphincter competence. *Gastroenterology* 1967; **52**: 773.

60. Helm JF, Dodds WJ & Hogan WJ. Salivary responses to oesophageal acid in normal subjects and patients with reflux oesophagitis. *Gastroenterology* 1987; **93**: 1393.

61. Eriksen CA, Sadek EK, Cranford C, Sutton D, Kennedy N & Cushieri A. Reflux oesophagitis and oesophageal transit: evidence for a primary oesophageal motor disorder. *Gut* 1988; **29**: 448.

62. Stanciu C & Bennett JR. Oesophageal acid clearing: one factor in the production of reflux oesophagitis. *Gut* 1974; **15**: 852.

63. Johnson LF. Saliva in health and disease. *J Clin Gastroenterol* 1986; **8** (Suppl. 1): 26.

64. Helm JF, Dodds WJ, Pelc LR, Palmer DW, Hogan DW & Teeter BC. Effect of oesophageal emptying and saliva on clearance of acid from the oesophagus. *N Engl J Med* 1984; **310**: 284.

65. Mittal RK, Lange RC & McCallum, RW. Identification and mechanism of delayed oesophageal acid clearance in subjects with hiatus hernia. *Gastroenterology* 1987; **92**: 130.

66. Kahrilas PJ, Dodds WJ & Hogan WJ. Effect of peristaltic dysfunction on oesophageal volume clearance. *Gastroenterology* 1988; **94**: 73.

67. Bonavina L, Evader A, DeMeester TR et al. Length of the distal oesophageal sphincter and competence of the cardia. *Am J Surg* 1986; **151**: 25.

68. Malagelada JR. Physiological basis and clinical significance of gastric emptying disorders. *Dig Dis Sci* 1979; **24**: 657.

69. Hartley MN, Walker SJ & Mackie CR. Abnormal gastric adaptive relaxation in patients with gastro-oesophageal reflux. *Gut* 1990; **31**: 500.

70. McCallum RW, Berkowitz DM & Levin E. Gastric emptying in patients with gastro-oesophageal reflux. *Gastroenterology* 1980; **80**: 285.

71. Boesby S. Relationship between gastro-oesophageal acid reflux, basal gastro-oesophageal sphincter pressure and gastric acid secretion. *Scand J Gastroenterol* 1977; **12**: 547.

72. Attwood SEA, DeMeester TR, Bremner CG, Barlow AP & Hinder RA. Alkaline gastro-oesophageal reflux: implications in the development of complications in Barrett's columnar lined lower oesophagus. *Surgery* 1989; **106**: 764.

73. Barlow AP, DeMeester TR, Ball CS & Eypasch EP. The significance of the gastric secretory state in gastro-oesophageal reflux disease. *Arch Surg* 1989; **124**: 937.

74. Miller LS, Vinayek R, Frucht H, Gardner JD, Jensen RT & Maton PN.

Reflux esophagitis in patients with Zollinger–Ellison syndrome. *Gastroenterology* 1990; **98**: 341.

75. Schwizer W, Hinder RA & DeMeester TR. Does delayed gastric emptying contribute to gastro-oesophageal reflux disease? *Am J Surg* 1989; **157**: 74.

76. Maddern GJ, Chatterton BE, Collins PJ, Horowitz M, Shearman DJC & Jamieson GG. Solid and liquid gastric emptying in patients with gastro-oesophageal reflux. *Br J Surg* 1985; **72**: 344.

77. Fuchs KH, DeMeester TR, Schwizer W & Albertucci M. Concomitant duodenogastric and gastro-oesophageal reflux: the role of 24-hour gastric pH monitoring. In Siewert JR & Holscher AH (Eds) *Diseases of the Oesophagus*. Berlin: Springer Verlag, 1988: 1073.

78. Wickremesinghe PC, Dayrit PQ, Manfredi OL, Faio RA & Fagel VL. Quantitative evaluation of bile diversion surgery utilising [99m] TcHIDA scintigraphy. *Gastroenterology* 1983; **84**: 354.

79. Vaezi MF & Richter JE. Synergism of acid and duodenogastric reflux in complicated Barrett's oesophagus. *Surgery* 1995; **177**: 699–704.

80. Caldwell MTP, Lawler P, Byrne PJ, Walsh TN & Hennessy TPJ. Ambulatory oesophageal bile reflux monitoring in Barrett's oesophagus. *Br J Surg* 1995; **82**: 657–660.

81. Kauer WKH, Burdiles P, Ireland AP et al. Does duodenal juice reflux into the esophagus of patients with complicated GERD. Evaluation of a fiberoptic sensor for bilirubin. *Am J Surg* 1995; **169**: 98–104.

82. Vaezi MF, Lacamera RG & Richter JE. Validation studies of Bilitec 2000 – an ambulatory duodenogastric reflux monitoring system. *Am J Physiol* 1994; **30**: 1050–1057.

83. Walther B, DeMeester TR, LaFontaine E, Courtney JF, Little AG & Skinner DB. Effect of paraoesophageal hernia on sphincter function and its implication on surgical therapy. *Am J Surg* 1984; **147**: 111.

84. Mercer DC, Velasco N, Hill, LD. Paraoesophageal hernia. In: Hill LD, Kozarek R, McCallum RW & Mercer DC (eds) *The Oesophagus: Medical and Surgical Management*. 1988; 148. Philadelphia: WB Saunders.

85. Helm JF, Dodds WJ, Riedel DR et al. Determinants of oesophageal acid clearance in normal subjects. *Gastroenterology* 1983; **85**: 607.

86. Jones CM. *Digestive Tract Pain*. New York: Macmillan, 1938.

87. Bernstein LM & Baker CA. A clinical test for oesophagitis. *Gastroenterology* 1957; **34**: 760.

88. Behar J, Biancini P & Sheahan DG. Evaluation of oesophageal tests in the diagnosis of reflux oesophagitis. *Gastroenterology* 1976; **71**: 9.

89. Bennett JR & Atkinson M. Oesophageal acid-perfusion in the diagnosis of praecordial pain. *Lancet* 1966; **ii**: 1150.

90. Ben LJ, Hootkin LA, Margulies S et al. A comparison of clinical measurements of gastro-oesophageal reflux. *Gastroenterology* 1972; **62**: 1.

91. Breen KJ & Whelan G. The diagnosis of reflux oesophagitis: an evaluation of five investigative procedures. *Aust NZ J Surg* 1978; **46**: 156.

92. deMoraes-Filho JPP & Bettarello A. Lack of specificity of the acid perfusion test in duodenal ulcer patients. *Am J Dig Dis* 1974; **19**: 785.

93. Edwards DAW. Oesophageal pain and motility. *Am J Dig Dis* 1968; **13**: 340.

94. Siegel CI & Hendrix TR. Oesophageal motor abnormalities induced by acid perfusion in patients with heartburn. *J Clin Invest* 1963; **42**: 686.

95. Atkinson M & Bennett JR. Relationship between motor changes and pain during oesophageal acid perfusion. *Am J Dig Dis* 1968; **13**: 346.

96. Ismael Beigi F & Pope CE. Distribution of histological changes of gastro-oesophageal reflux in the distal oesophagus of man. *Gastroenterology* 1975; **66**: 1109.

97. Johnson LF, DeMeester TR & Haggitt RC. Oesophageal epithelial response to gastro-oesophageal reflux; a quantitative study. *Am J Dig Dis* 1978; **23**: 498.

98. Attwood SEA, Smyrk TC, DeMeester TR & Jones JB. Esophageal eosinophilia: a distinct clinical syndrome. *Dig Dis Sci* 1993; **38**: 109.

99. Jerssurun J, Yardley JH, Giardiello FM & Hamilton SR. Intracytoplasmic plasma proteins and distended oesophageal squamous cells (balloon cells). *Modern Pathol* 1988; **1**: 175.

100. Smyrk T, Barlow AP, Attwood TR & DeMeester TR. Reflux oesophagitis: the sensitivity and specificity of histological parameters. *Modern Pathol* 1989; **2**: 89a.

101. DeMeester TR, Wang CI, Wernley JA et al. Technique, indications and use of 24-hour oesophageal pH monitoring. *J Thorac Cardiovasc Surg* 1980; **79**: 656.

102. Quincke H. Ulcus oesophagi ex digestione. *Deutsch Arch Klin Med* 1879; **24**: 72.

103. Henderson RD, Mugashe F, Jeejeebhoy KN et al. The role of bile and acid in the production of oesophagitis. *Ann Thorac Surg* 1972; **14**: 465.

104. Gillison EW, deCastro VAM, Nyhus LM et al. The significance of bile in reflux oesophagitis. *Surg Gynecol Obstet* 1972; **134**: 419.

105. Kranendonk SE. Reflux oesophagitis: an experimental study in rats. Thesis. Rotterdam 1980, Erasmus University.

106. Palmer ED. Subacute erosive ('peptic') oesophagitis associated with achlorhydria. *N Engl J Med* 1960; **262**: 927.

107. Helsingen N. Oesophagitis following total gastrectomy. *Acta Chir Scand Suppl* 1961; **273**: 5.

108. Donovan IA, Harding LK, Keighley MRB et al. Abnormalities of gastric emptying and pyloric reflux in uncomplicated hiatus hernia. *Br J Surg* 1977; **64**: 847.

109. Stol DW, Murphy GM & Collis JL. Duodenogastric reflux and acid secretion in patients with symptomatic hiatal hernia. *Scand J Gastroenterol* 1974; **9**: 97.

110. Crumplin MKH, Stol DW, Murphy GM et al. The pattern of bile salt reflux and acid secretion in sliding hiatal hernia. *Br J Surg* 1974; **61**: 611.

111. Clemencon G. Nocturnal intragastric pH measurements. *Scand J Gastroenterol* 1972; **7**: 293.

112. Gillison EW & Nyhus LM. Bile reflux, gastric secretion and heartburn. *Br J Surg* 1971; **58**: 864.

113. Bateson MC, Hopwood D, Milne G et al. Oesophageal ultrastructure after incubation with gastrointestinal fluids and their components. *J Pathol* 1981; **133**: 33.

114. Heier WD, Cleveland CR & Iber FL. Gastric inactivation of pancreatic supplements. *Johns Hopkins Med J* 1965; **116**: 261.

115. Northop JH, Nunitz M & Herriot RM. *Crystalline Enzymes*, 2nd edn. New York: Columbia University Press, 1948.

116. Wenger J & Towbridge CG. Bile and trypsin in the stomach following a test meal. *South Med J* 1971; **64**: 1063.

117. Johnson LF & Harmon JW. Experimental oesophagitis in a rabbit model. *J Clin Gastroenterol* 1986; **8** (Suppl): 26.

118. Alwin JA. The physiological basis of reflux oesophagitis in sliding hiatal diaphragmatic hernia. *Thorax* 1952; **8**: 38.

119. Behar J, Brand DL, Brown FC et al. Cimetidine in the treatment of symptomatic gastro-oesophageal reflux. *Gastroenterology* 1978; **74**: 441.

120. Cameron AJ, Ott BJ & Spencer Payne W. The incidence of adenocarcinoma in columnar-lined (Barrett's) oesophagus. *New Engl J Med* 1985; **313**: 857.

121. Spechler SJ, Robbins AH, Rubins HB et al. Adenocarcinoma and Barrett's oesophagus. An over-rated risk? *Gastroenterology* 1984; **87**: 927.

122. Hammeetman W, Tytgat GNJ, Houthoff HJ & van den Tweel. Barrett's oesophagus: development of dysplasia and adenocarcinoma. *Gastroenterology* 1989; **96**: 1249.

123. Robertson CS, Mayberry JF, Nicholson DA, James PD & Atkinson M. Value of surveillance in the detection of neoplastic change in Barrett's oesophagus. *Br J Surg* 1988; **75**: 760.

124. DeMeester TR, Attwood SEA, Smyrk TC, Therkildsen DH & Hinder RA. Surgical therapy in Barrett's esophagus. *Ann Surg* 1990; **212**: 528.

125. Iascone C, DeMeester TR, Little AG et al. Barrett's oesophagus: functional assessment, proposed pathogenesis and surgical therapy. *Arch Surg* 1983; **118**: 543.

126. Jagelman JG, Decosse JJ & Bussey HJ. Upper gastrointestinal cancer in familial polyposis. *Lancet* 1988; **i**: 1149.

127. Attwood SEA, Smyrk TC, DeMeester TR, Mirvish SS, Stein HJ & Hinder RA. The effects of duodeno-oesophageal reflux on the development of esophageal adenocarcinoma in nitrosamine treated rats. *Surgery* 1992; **111**: 503.

9

MEDICAL MANAGEMENT OF UNCOMPLICATED GASTRO-OESOPHAGEAL REFLUX

JE Kellow

The term gastro-oesophageal reflux disease (GORD) encompasses pathological gastro-oesophageal reflux occurring in the absence of endoscopic oesophagitis, as well as reflux oesophagitis demonstrated at endoscopy.[1] In patients who have sought medical attention because of troublesome symptoms, however, there do not appear to be major differences in symptom severity between those with and without oesophageal inflammation. The aims of medical therapy of uncomplicated GORD are therefore: (1) to control reflux symptoms; (2) to prevent reflux-induced mucosal damage; and (3) to heal, and to maintain healing of, any mucosal damage, thereby preventing progression to *complicated* GORD.

Based on considerations of the several proposed pathophysiological factors,[2] the theoretical principles of medical therapy of GORD can be summarized as follows: (1) to reduce the incidence of transient lower oesophageal sphincter relaxations – which are considered to be the major pathophysiological abnormality in mild disease; (2) to improve lower oesophageal sphincter competence and diminished lower oesophageal sphincter pressure (LOSP), which are more relevant in severe disease; (3) to enhance oesophageal clearance and oesophageal acid neutralization by swallowed saliva; (4) to decrease the volume and potency of refluxed material (acid, pepsin and duodenal contents); (5) to protect the oesophageal mucosa from refluxed material; and (6) to improve any delay in gastric emptying or other gastroduodenal dysmotility.

Although renewed attention has been given to agents which modify oesophageal motor activity, there is, as yet, no drug which appears able to affect or reduce the incidence of inappropriate lower oesophageal sphincter relaxation. Therefore, therapy aimed at neutralizing or inhibiting gastric acid secretion remains the most well-established and effective line of treatment when drug therapy is indicated. It is important to appreciate that the vast majority of drug studies in GORD have been confined to the group with reflux oesophagitis. It is

appropriate to consider both healing and maintenance therapy in these patients. Unfortunately, conflicting results may well have resulted from differences in study design, patient selection and duration of treatment.

When a patient presents to a physician with reflux symptoms, these are usually interfering significantly with his or her life-style and have often not responded to over-the-counter preparations. Once an accurate diagnosis of GORD has been made, therapy should be initiated in a step-wise fashion, according to the severity of symptoms, the stage or progression of the disease, and in some cases the patient's age and preference for treatment. This type of approach is particularly relevant to the primary case setting. In one such scheme, 'phase 1' therapy involves a variety of general measures with or without the use of antacids or antacid–alginate combinations, 'phase 2' includes the use of systemic drugs, such as H_2-receptor antagonists or prokinetic agents, 'phase 3' involves the use of proton pump inhibitors or combinations of such drugs, including mucosal protective agents, and 'phase 4' therapy implies surgical intervention. In gastroenterological practice, where more advanced cases of GORD are seen, another effective approach is where treatment is initiated with a proton pump inhibitor, and then stepped down to continuing or maintenance therapy with an H_2-receptor antagonist or prokinetic agent, if symptoms remain uncontrolled. Each of these classes of therapy or drugs will be considered in detail; other agents[3–5] which have received occasional or limited attention, and which are not routinely prescribed, will not be considered.

GENERAL MEASURES

Surprisingly, environmental or life-style factors may not have been considered or identified by the patient as conditions which provoke symptoms, and an explanation of the mechanisms of reflux and suggestions for modifying these factors are often helpful. Gastro-oesophageal reflux may occur mainly at night (supine reflux), mainly during the day (postprandial or upright reflux), or during both day and night (combined reflux);[6] an attempt to determine, at least historically, which pattern is present may enable more appropriate advice to be given. The rationale and efficacy of conservative therapy for GORD has been reviewed in detail.[7] Weight loss in obese individuals, avoidance of bending, stooping and straining to lift heavy objects, limiting strenuous exercise, removal of tight clothing and avoidance of excessive straining at stool are simple time-honoured recommendations which do have a pathophysiological basis and may improve symptoms; scientific studies on their efficacy, however, are scarce. Dietary alterations include the avoidance of substances which appear to decrease LOSP or act as oesophageal irritants, such as fatty foods, alcohol, chocolate, peppermint, spicy foods and caffeinated beverages. Alcohol ingestion may also impair normal acid clearance.[8] Beverages such as orange and tomato juice may provoke symptoms, presumably on the basis of their hyperosmolarity.[9] Several of these foodstuffs have received renewed investigation recently. For example it has been confirmed that ingestion of chocolate results in a significant increase in oesophageal acid exposure in the first postprandial hour in patients with reflux oesophagitis,[10] whereas ingestion of raw onions can provoke heartburn and episodes of reflux in patients with chronic reflux symptoms.[11] Also, fat ingestion prolongs oesophageal acid exposure for up to 3 hours postprandially.[12] Eating smaller, more frequent meals, avoiding liquids with solid food, and eating at least 3 hours before exercising or retiring, all tend to decrease the volume of gastric contents available for reflux, to reduce gastric overdistension, and to limit the rate of nocturnal acid production. Promotion of postprandial salivary flow by using chewing gum or lozenges should, on a theoretical basis, improve oesophageal clearance of refluxate.

Cigarette smoking should be avoided or reduced as it produces a marked decrease in LOSP, reduces oesophageal clearance and salivary function, and acutely reduces the rate of gastric emptying of both liquids and solids.[13,14] The frequency of reflux episodes is clearly increased after smoking.[15] Various medications should be avoided in GORD as they may affect, at least theoretically, LOSP, and potentiate gastro-oesophageal reflux (Table 9.1). Such medications should only be used in patients with GORD if effective alternative therapies are not available.[2] The advent of 24 h pH monitoring has led to more detailed study of some of these agents; for example an increase in reflux duration and symptoms in chronic asthmatics was demonstrated with theophylline.[16] Elevation of the head of the bed by 15 cm (6 inches) has been shown to decrease total overnight acid exposure time significantly.[17] This manoeuvre is more effective than propping up the head and shoulders on pillows, and may potentiate the efficacy of H_2-receptor antagonists;[18] it appears to be of particular value in smokers. On the basis of oesophageal pH monitoring, a foam wedge 25 cm (10 inches) high has been shown to be as effective as elevation of the bed head and may be preferred by some patients.[19] Unfortunately, little information is available regarding the efficacy of each of these conservative measures on a long-term or

Table 9.1 Drugs which may aggravate GORD

Anticholinergics
Calcium-channel blockers
Theophylline
Progesterone
β-Adrenergic agonists
Dopamine
Opioids
Nitrates
α-Adrenergic agonists
Diazepam
Prostaglandins

maintenance basis; although there is no reason to suggest any diminishing benefit in terms of symptomatic control, the major problem encountered is that of continued patient compliance. Given the expense and potential side-effects of long-term drug therapy, however, every effort should be made to continue these measures irrespective of the requirement for more potent therapy.

ANTACIDS

Antacids remain the most widely used agents for symptomatic therapy of GORD.[20] Their principal action is to neutralize gastric contents and thereby diminish the availability of acid for reflux; inactivation of pepsin may also occur.[21] Symptoms can be relieved by taking antacids (as required) but their overall duration of action is relatively short lived and they have little effect on intragastric acidity during the night.[22] Their duration of action varies according to when they are taken; thus postprandial administration prolongs their activity by up to 2 hours. Other possible mechanisms of action in GORD include a binding effect on bile acids[23] and an elevation of resting LOSP.[24]

Several placebo-controlled studies have been performed with antacids as short-term therapy in reflux oesophagitis.[25–29] In none of these studies has there been a significant improvement in endoscopic oesophagitis or histological grade, or oesophageal sensitivity to acid, after 4–6 weeks of therapy with liquid antacid, in doses ranging from 560 to 850 mmol/day neutralizing capacity, when compared with placebo. Only in the two most recent studies[28,29] was an improvement in heartburn demonstrated; for example in 47 patients with grade I or II oesophagitis, treatment with one chewable antacid tablet four times daily for 2 weeks did produce symptomatic improvement. There were significantly lower global symptom scores, less acid regurgitation, and fewer days and nights with heartburn than during placebo therapy.[29] For more long-term use, only one study is available: antacids were able to relieve symptoms in less than 20% of patients with severe reflux oesophagitis.[30]

There are no established guidelines regarding the dosage or timing of administration of antacids (preprandial, postprandial such as one and then again 3 hours after meals, or at bedtime), or regarding the most effective formulation. Although antacid tablets are more convenient, they may be less effective than liquid formulations. Commonly used antacid preparations are magnesium hydroxide, aluminium hydroxide and sodium bicarbonate; calcium carbonate is seldom used these days. Side-effects are few but in high doses diarrhoea may occur with magnesium hydroxide, and constipation with aluminium hydroxide. When given in combination, such as single preparations of magnesium and aluminium hydroxide, however, altered bowel habit is not usually a clinical problem. Interference with the absorption of other drugs may occur, while aluminium-containing antacids have been shown to bind phosphate in the gut and result in damage to bone.[31] Aluminium compounds may also result in some aluminium absorption[32] and therefore their long-term use should be prudent, because of the possible, although unsubstantiated, effect of aluminium on the central nervous system.[33] At the present time, cost and poor patient compliance, together with the availability of more potent drugs, limit the use of antacids to little more than symptomatic relief. Thus in mild cases, or in patients whose symptoms are reasonably well controlled by conservative measures or by other medications, the use of antacids before events known to precipitate symptoms may be of value in the continuing control of GORD. It is clear that antacids should not be used as the sole therapy when there are persistent or nocturnal symptoms, or in the presence of erosive oesophagitis and/or sphincter incompetence.

ALGINIC ACID

Alginic acid, a gelatinous polysaccharide derived from marine algae, may provide symptomatic relief in GORD by the creation of a mechanical barrier to reflux. It is available in combination with antacids (for example Gaviscon, a combination of sodium bicarbonate, aluminium hydroxide, magnesium trisilicate and alginic acid), in tablet or liquid form, and is usually administered after meals and at bedtime. Alginates react with sodium bicarbonate in the presence of saliva to form a highly viscous solution or foam which appears to float like a raft on the surface of the gastric pool. When reflux occurs, this protective layer is the first to contact the oesophageal mucosa, theoretically limiting acid-peptic damage. The buffering capacity of these substances is minimal, however, and whether alginates reduce total acid exposure in the distal oesophagus is not established. As with antacids, their value in improving symptoms in GORD is controversial, and no effect on endoscopic oesophagitis has been demonstrated. Thus in four of five placebo-controlled studies symptoms were alleviated to a significantly greater extent than placebo, in 55–95% of cases, when a dose of 4–8 tablets daily was employed for 2–6 weeks.[34-38] When compared with standard antacids only one study, using a liquid formulation of alginate, has demonstrated superiority with respect to symptom relief;[39] the largest of several such comparative studies (133 patients treated for 4 weeks) showed no benefit with respect to alginates.[40]

H₂-RECEPTOR ANTAGONISTS

Since the mid-1980s, H$_2$-receptor antagonists have been regarded widely as the treatment of choice when drug therapy is deemed necessary in GORD. There are four generally available drugs in this class: cimetidine, ranitidine, famotidine and nizatidine. They differ chiefly in regard to their relative potencies. Each of these agents inhibits gastric acid secretion for prolonged periods by competitive blockade of the H$_2$-receptors located on the parietal cells; they may also reduce oesophageal sensitivity to acid.[41] They do not affect LOSP[42] or modify the incidence of transient lower oesophageal sphincter relaxations.[43] Recently, however, an increase in postprandial LOSP was reported after prolonged therapy with ranitidine, in the absence of other demonstrable effects on oesophageal motility.[44] With respect to gastric motor function, until recently H$_2$-receptor antagonists were not thought to affect gastric emptying. Oral ranitidine (300 mg), however, but not cimetidine, may increase liquid emptying rate, at least in healthy volunteers,[45] whereas each of the H$_2$-receptor antagonists, when administered intravenously, appears to prolong gastric emptying of a solid meal.[46] The side-effects of these agents are not usually a clinical problem, with an incidence of about 4%.[47] Cimetidine, more than the other agents, may theoretically interact with the metabolism of several drugs (e.g. theophylline, warfarin) by inhibition of the cytochrome P$_{450}$ enzymes.[48]

Several detailed reviews regarding the effectiveness of H$_2$-receptor antagonists in GORD have been published;[49-51] it is now clear that an insufficiently high dosage of these agents was used in the initial clinical trials where dosages were based on those effective in peptic ulcer disease. The multitude of clinical trials involving these agents are especially difficult to compare because of variations in factors such as the criteria for symptomatic and endoscopic assessment of severity or healing.[51] Moreover, the lack of information provided in these reports on what instructions patients were given regarding concomitant changes in life style during the treatment period is also a problem. A further deficiency in such studies is that little or no information is available regarding cost-effectiveness, for example comparing drug costs against days lost from work, etc.

It is pertinent to consider data relating to these various agents both as short-term or healing courses and as maintenance therapy.

Short-term therapy

Cimetidine

Cimetidine was the first widely available H$_2$-receptor antagonist. Some controlled trials of cimetidine versus placebo in uncomplicated GORD, many well over 10 years old, are detailed in Table 9.2. The majority of these studies report significant improvement in the frequency and severity of symptoms, especially for heartburn; this was often despite a reduced intake of antacids. In contrast, only a few studies demonstrate either endoscopic healing or a significant improvement in endoscopic severity, and histological improvement was even less frequent.[53,60] In the most recent assessment,[65] relatively low healing rates of 30 and 38% were observed after 8 weeks therapy with low-dose antacids and cimetidine 400 mg twice daily, respectively, in patients with reflux oesophagitis. The dosage regimen does not appear to be of great importance. Thus no

Table 9.2 Short-term cimetidine versus placebo in uncomplicated GORD

REFERENCE	NO. OF PATIENTS	DOSE (MG/DAY)	MAXIMUM DURATION (WEEKS)	SIGNIFICANT EFFECT IN FAVOUR OF CIMETIDINE	
				SYMPTOMATIC IMPROVEMENT	ENDOSCOPIC HEALING
Behar et al. (1975)[30]	84	1200	8	+	−
Ferguson et al. (1979)[52]	26	1600	6	−	+
Wesdorp et al. (1978)[53]	24	1600	8	−	+
Powell-Jackson et al. (1978)[54]	27	1600	6	+	−
Lepsien et al. (1979)[55]	36	1600	6	+	+
Brown (1979)[56]	22	1200	8	+	−
Thanik et al. (1982)[57]	43	1200	4	+	+
Bright-Asare and El-Bassoussi (1980)[58]	30	1200	8	+	−
Festen et al. (1980)[59]	20	1600	8	−	−
Fiasse et al. (1980)[60]	34	1600	8	+	−
Druguet and Lambert (1980)[61]	82	1600	4	+	+
Greaney and Irvin (1981)[62]	20	1600	4	−	−
Breen et al. (1983)[63]	27	1000	8	−	−
Frank et al. (1989)[64]	250	1600	8	+	+

Modified from Meuwissen and Klinkenberg-Knol.[50]

major therapeutic differences have been observed between doses of 800 and 1600 mg cimetidine per day in divided doses, between cimetidine 600 mg twice daily and 300 mg four times daily, or between 800 mg as a single dose (either after the evening meal or before bed) and 400 mg four times daily,[66–68] although symptomatic relief was better using the last regimen in one study. Duration of therapy is important as treatment for 12 weeks clearly appears to be better than 6 weeks.[67,68] In summary, 65–70% of unselected patients with mild reflux oesophagitis will heal after 6 weeks of therapy, and 80–90% will heal after 12 weeks therapy.[50] These figures decline as the severity of oesophagitis increases: thus for severe reflux oesophagitis, the figures will be 20–30% (6 weeks) and 40–50% (12 weeks). Symptomatic improvement can be expected to be considerably higher than these percentages.

Ranitidine

It has been shown, using pH monitoring, that both the number and duration of discrete reflux episodes can be reduced by ranitidine in patients with GORD, seemingly in a dose-dependent manner; intragastric acidity may also be reduced more than by cimetidine. Controlled trials have indicated symptom relief to be significantly greater with ranitidine, in 'standard' doses of 150 mg twice daily for 6–12 weeks, than with placebo (Table 9.3). Improved rates of endoscopic healing have also been observed in virtually all studies; as with cimetidine, however, patients with more severe disease tend to respond less well. Once daily dosage of ranitidine (300 mg) appears to be as effective as twice daily dosage (150 mg).[77–79] In a recent large multicentre study, however, ranitidine 300 mg twice daily offered a significant advantage over 300 mg nocte, or 300 mg after the evening meal, with respect to symptom relief, although there were no differences in endoscopic healing rates at 4, 8 or 12 weeks.[80] Even higher doses have been employed in an attempt to obtain further inhibition of gastric acid secretion and improved efficacy. Thus greater healing and symptomatic improvement occurred in patients given ranitidine 300 mg four times daily compared with 150 mg twice daily;[81] after 8 weeks, 54% of those on the twice-daily regimen had complete endoscopic healing of lesions, compared with 75% of

Table 9.3 Short-term ranitidine versus placebo in uncomplicated GORD

REFERENCE	NO. OF PATIENTS	DOSE (MG/DAY)	MAXIMUM DURATION (WEEKS)	SIGNIFICANT EFFECT IN FAVOUR OF RANITIDINE	
				SYMPTOMATIC IMPROVEMENT	ENDOSCOPIC HEALING
Berstad (1982)[69]	39	300	6	+	+
Goy et al. (1983)[70]	37	300	6	+	+
Wesdorp et al. (1983)[71]	36	300	6	+	+
Sherbaniuk et al. (1984)[72]	73	300	6	+	+
Hine et al. (1984)[73]	46	300	6	+	+
Lehtola et al. (1986)[74]	41	450	12	+	+
Johansson et al. (1986)[75]	38	300	8	+	+
Sontag et al. (1987)[76]	237	300	6	+	+

Modified from Meuwissen and Klinkenberg-Knol.[50]

those taking the four times daily regimen, and 64 and 84% respectively had symptomatic relief. In another study, however, healing rates at 8 weeks were not different between ranitidine 300 mg four times daily (62%) and 150 mg four times daily (69%).[82] Side-effects do not appear to be increased with such regimens, and thus higher dose treatment with ranitidine may be of value in patients with severe oesophagitis or for those with milder disease who do not respond rapidly to lower doses. Ranitidine has also been compared directly with cimetidine[83] on several occasions. In these studies, when cimetidine was given in a dose of 800 mg once or twice daily, as well as in a dose of 1000 mg daily, and when ranitidine was given in a dose of 150 mg twice daily or 300 mg once daily, for treatment periods of 6–12 weeks, no major differences in therapeutic efficacy emerged between the two drugs.

Famotidine and nizatidine

Fewer clinical data in GORD are available at present for the newer agents famotidine and nizatidine than for cimetidine and ranitidine. When given in doses of 40 mg nocte, or 20 mg twice daily or 40 mg twice daily, famotidine was shown to decrease oesophageal acid contact time, but only the twice daily regimens decreased the proportion of upright acid exposure.[84] This suggests that twice daily dosage may be necessary for symptom control during the daytime, a situation confirmed in a large multicentre placebo-controlled study which compared famotidine 20 mg twice daily with 40 mg nocte.[85] Both doses were superior to placebo for global symptomatic response and for complete healing; famotidine 20 mg twice daily, however, had a significantly greater effect than the single nocte dose on the relief of daytime heartburn. Higher doses of famotidine, e.g. 40 mg twice daily, do not appear to produce significantly greater healing rates compared with 20 mg twice daily.[86,87] Famotidine 40 mg nocte has been compared with ranitidine 150 mg twice daily;[88] both produced similar symptom relief (approximately 75% good or excellent global improvement) but only 50–60% of patients were healed endoscopically at 12 weeks with no differences observed between the two drugs. In an elderly population with oesophagitis, one other comparative study of famotidine and ranitidine found that after 8 weeks of therapy 12 of 27 (45%) patients were healed with famotidine compared with 7 of 27 (26%) with ranitidine.[89]

With respect to nizatidine, two dose levels (150 mg twice daily and 300 mg twice daily) were compared with placebo during 6 weeks in 515 patients.[90] Six-week healing rates were 39% for nizatidine dose level 300 mg, 41% for dose level 150 mg and 26% for placebo. These rates were higher for nizatidine 150 mg three times daily (81%) and 300 mg twice daily (68%) in another study,[91] indicating that nizatidine is an effective alternative to the other H_2-receptor antagonists for short-term use.

Maintenance therapy

Far less data are available regarding maintenance therapy with H_2-receptor antagonists in GORD than for short-term therapy. After healing therapy has been discontinued, the rate of relapse appears to be related to the initial grade of oesophagitis as well as to the initial rate of healing. Cimetidine in a dose of 400 mg nocte has been shown to be ineffective in preventing symptomatic relapse after completion of 12 weeks initial therapy with higher doses,[92] although another much smaller study did report an effect at this dose.[66] A group of patients with oesophagitis followed for more than 2 years continued to require cimetidine regularly, at least at bedtime, to maintain a satisfactory level of symptomatic improvement,[93] and it is clear that many patients will require continuing therapy with full dose H_2-receptor antagonists.[94] Higher than usual daily (especially evening) doses of ranitidine appear to be effective in preventing relapse,[72,95] whereas a dose of 150 mg nocte does not.[96] In the case of famotidine, nocturnal doses of either 40 mg or 20 mg were no more effective than placebo in preventing relapse of oesophagitis.[97]

PROTON PUMP INHIBITORS

The substituted benzimidazoles omeprazole, pantoprazole and lansoprazole are members of a new class of gastric antisecretory agents which specifically inhibit the enzyme hydrogen potassium adenosine triphosphatase, the final step in the formation of hydrochloric acid in the parietal cell. They result in more complete and long-lasting supression of both basal and stimulated gastric acid secretion than H_2-receptor antagonists.[98–101] In patients with duodenal ulcer, either 40 or 60 mg of omeprazole daily produces a 96–98% reduction in intragastric acidity, whereas 20 mg produces a 90% reduction.[102,103] Because a 10 mg daily dose shows wide interindividual variation in acid inhibition,[103,104] 20 mg appears to be the lowest dose for routine clinical use. Omperazole does not appear to affect oesophageal motility or to improve disordered oesophageal motility, such as the reduced LOSP, reduced peristaltic amplitude, or reduced peristaltic duration which may be present in patients with reflux oesophagitis.[105]

Elevation of gastric pH with omeprazole was demonstrated to heal reflux oesophagitis initially in a small group of patients.[106] Episodes of gastro-oesophageal reflux were assessed[107] in seven patients with reflux oesophagitis before and during crossover treatment with omeprazole 60 mg daily or ranitidine 150 mg twice daily, and the pH profile of five patients on omeprazole, and one on ranitidine, returned to normal. Importantly, omeprazole produced significant improvement in the range of pH parameters measured, whereas during ranitidine treatment these values were not significantly different from baseline measurements. Ruth et al.[108] assessed 22 patients with erosive oesophagitis in a similar fashion. Omeprazole significantly reduced the number of reflux episodes, the number of episodes of more than 5 minutes duration, and the total reflux time; in contrast, ranitidine significantly reduced the total reflux time only. When the two treatment groups were compared, a significant difference in favour of omeprazole was found for daytime and total reflux values, except for those reflux episodes of more than 5 minutes duration.

The safety aspects of the proton pump inhibitors have

attracted a great deal of attention. The incidence of serious adverse events reported in comparative short-term studies with H_2-receptor antagonists and with placebo have been similar; and no specific pattern can be ascribed to omeprazole. In longer-term studies no serious specific drug-related effects have been reported, the spectrum of mild subjective side-effects does not appear to differ between the proton pump inhibitors and the H_2-receptor antagonists and no clinically significant changes in laboratory variables have been observed. The effects of long-term omeprazole treatment on the gastric endocrine cell population were assessed in 36 patients with refractory peptic ulcer or reflux disease.[109] A small number of patients demonstrated a significant increase in the argyrophilic cell volume density during the first year of treatment, probably mediated by hypergastrinaemia; no further increase was observed after this time. In other studies, no pathological changes in the argyrophilic cell population of the gastric mucosa have been observed in hundreds of patients treated with omeprazole for several years. Concerns about the possible consequences of prolonged elevation of serum gastrin and the other long-term effects of profound acid inhibition, as well as the risk–benefit profile, will need to be re-evaluated after further long-term usage studies of omeprazole. In the interim, it can be concluded that, in man, omeprazole is as safe as H_2-receptor antagonists if administered in recommended doses.[110]

Short-term therapy

Sixty-four patients were assessed in the first major placebo-controlled study of omeprazole;[111] after 4 weeks 81% of the omeprazole-treated group (40 mg daily) were endoscopically healed compared with only 6% of the placebo-treated patients. A further 132 patients were then randomized to receive either 20 or 40 mg omeprazole; in those with grade II oesophagitis, after 4 weeks of therapy, endoscopic healing (confirmed by histology) occurred in 80% of those receiving 20 mg omeprazole, and in 97% of those receiving 40 mg omeprazole. Healing rates for grades III and IV oesophagitis were 67% and 88% respectively, but it should be noted that the more widely used Savary–Miller grading system was not employed, grades III and IV corresponding to grades II and III in the latter system. In the omeprazole-treated group, healing was influenced only by the initial severity of the oesophagitis and by the dose of omeprazole. Omeprazole has also been shown to be superior to H_2-receptor antagonists for the short-term treatment of reflux oesophagitis (Table 9.4). For example when compared to ranitidine 150 mg twice daily, omeprazole in the relatively high dose of 60 mg daily produced greater symptom relief and endoscopic healing rates in over 50 patients with erosive oesophagitis,[113] and the majority of patients who were resistant to ranitidine healed after switching to omeprazole. Omeprazole was especially superior to ranitidine in patients with severe ulcerative lesions (grade III oesophagitis). A daily dose of 20–40 mg of omeprazole thus appears to be substantially superior in terms of endoscopic healing and symptomatic relief to ranitidine in doses of both 300 and 600 mg per day, and to cimetidine in a dose of 1600 mg per day, when therapy is continued for at least 4 weeks. In summary, these comparative studies have demonstrated relief of heartburn after 4 weeks in 66–90% of patients given omeprazole and in 24–46% given ranitidine or cimetidine. For endoscopic healing, the figures are 63–81% for omeprazole versus 17–53% for ranitidine or cimetidine after 4 weeks, and 74–95% omeprazole versus 28–65% ranitidine at 8 weeks. Omeprazole also has been shown to produce better healing, better symptom relief and lower treatment-related withdrawals than the combination of ranitidine and metoclopramide, although the newer prokinetic agents have not been studied in this fashion.[122]

Lansoprazole has been shown to produce healing of reflux oesophagitis in 63–68% of patients after 4 weeks at a dose of 30 mg, compared with 39–53% with ranitidine; after 8 weeks, healing rates were 85–92% with lansoprazole and 53–70% with ranitidine.[123] There were no differences in healing rates with 20 mg omeprazole and 30 mg lansoprazole, although lansoprazole produced greater relief from heartburn at 4 weeks.[124] In 103 patients with reflux oesophagitis resistant to H_2-receptor antagonist therapy, lansoprazole was significantly more effective then ranitidine with respect to healing and symptom relief at 2, 4, 6 and 8 weeks.[125]

Table 9.4   Short-term omeprazole versus H_2-receptor antagonists in uncomplicated GORD

REFERENCE	NO. OF PATIENTS	DOSE (MG/DAY)		MAXIMUM DURATION (WEEKS)	SIGNIFICANT EFFECT IN FAVOUR OF OMEPRAZOLE	
		Om	H_2RA		SYMPTOMATIC IMPROVEMENT	ENDOSCOPIC HEALING
Blum et al. (1986)[112]	164	40	R300	3	+	−
Klinkenberg-Knol et al. (1987)[113]	51	60	R300	8	+	+
Havelund et al. (1988)[114]	162	40	R300	12	+	+
Vantrappen et al. (1988)[115]	61	40	R300	8	+	+
Sandmark et al. (1988)[116]	152	20	R300	8	+	+
Dehn et al. (1990)[117]	67	40	C1600	8	+	+
Zeitoun et al. (1989)[118]	156	20	R300	8	+	+
Lundell et al. (1990)[119]	98	40	R600	12	+	+
Blum (1990)[120]	177	20	R300	4	+	+
Bate et al. (1990)[121]	272	20	C1600	8	+	+

Om, omeprazole; H_2 RA, H_2-receptor antagonist;   R, ranitidine;   C, cimetidine.

The place of proton pump inhibitors in relation to H_2-receptor antagonists for short-term therapy of GORD can be summarized as follows: for grade I and grade II reflux oesophagitis, the H_2-receptor antagonists are a safe and effective treatment resulting in good levels of symptomatic relief and acceptable levels of healing. For patients not responding to H_2-receptor antagonists, however, and in severe GORD, the proton pump inhibitors have superseded even high-dose H_2-receptor antagonist therapy.

Maintenance therapy

The rate of endoscopic relapse after initial healing with, and subsequent cessation of, omeprazole was determined in the study of Hetzel et al.[111] Erosive or ulcerative oesophagitis recurred in 88 of 107 (82%) patients by 6 months. The initial dose of omeprazole (20 or 40 mg), the initial grade of oesophagitis or the presence of smoking were not shown to influence relapse rates. The physiological effects of cessation of omeprazole maintenance treatment (20–60 mg daily for 18–42 months) have been studied in patients with resistant reflux oesophagitis.[126] After cessation of omeprazole, basal acid output increased significantly within 10 days and the serum gastrin levels returned to normal. All patients had symptomatic recurrence within 2 days and endoscopic recurrence was observed in more than half the patients at day 10. Koop and Arnold[127] have recently demonstrated that two-thirds of 31 patients with GORD remained in remission with maintenance therapy of 20 mg omeprazole; those who relapsed did so within 6 months and were rapidly healed when the dose was increased to 40 mg daily. When compared with ranitidine, omeprazole therefore appears to be superior for the prevention of recurrence of reflux oesophagitis, at least over a 12-month period.[128]

Different maintenance treatment regimens have also been examined, for example low-dose omeprazole therapy (10 mg) daily was compared with omeprazole 20 mg daily given for only 3 consecutive days per week ('weekend' therapy) in 87 patients over a 6-month period.[129] Of those receiving daily omeprazole, 75% remained in remission after 6 months, compared with 44% of those on 'weekend' therapy. Also, in a larger multicentre study,[130] more than 200 patients with erosive or ulcerative reflux oesophagitis were treated for 8 weeks with omeprazole 20 mg daily. After 8 weeks endoscopic healing occurred in 81% and these patients were then randomized to one of three maintenance treatment regimens: omeprazole 20 mg daily, omeprazole 20 mg daily on 'weekends' or ranitidine 150 mg twice daily. After 12 months the cumulative proportion of patients in remission was 89% for omeprazole 20 mg daily, in contrast to 32% for 'weekend' omeprazole therapy, and 25% for ranitidine. These findings have been confirmed in patients with severe refractory oesophagitis[131] even against high dose H_2-receptor antagonist therapy, indicating that remission in this group of patients is best maintained by sustained acid inhibition with omeprazole. The interaction of long-term acid suppression with *Helicobacter pylori* is an area of current interest. Although more data are required, it may be appropriate to eradicate the organism in patients with GORD who will require such treatment.

PROKINETIC AGENTS

Bethanechol

Although not a true prokinetic agent, the cholinergic agonist bethanechol does increase LOSP[132] and improves oesophageal clearance of acid by increasing oesophageal peristalsis and by increasing the rate of salivary flow.[133–135] Oesophageal acid exposure, assessed using 24 h pH monitoring, has also been shown to be reduced with bethanechol. Although gastric emptying is not affected,[136] gastric acid secretion is stimulated and other cholinergic side-effects such as abdominal cramping, urinary frequency, blurred vision and diarrhoea often occur. Two studies, using bethanechol 25 mg four times daily, have demonstrated it to be effective in improving symptoms and producing endoscopic healing when compared with either placebo or antacid therapy only.[137,138] Two other studies, however, have failed to show benefit with bethanechol plus antacid when compared with antacid alone.[139,140] Bethanechol has also been compared with cimetidine and no differences in rates of endoscopic or symptomatic improvement were observed.[57] Despite this, with the development of agents with fewer side-effects there is now no role for bethanechol in the routine management of GORD.

Metoclopramide

The dopamine antagonist metoclopramide increases the amplitude of oesophageal contractions and raises LOSP,[141,142] and also accelerates delayed gastric emptying in GORD patients, without affecting gastric secretion.[143] Two studies, using metoclopramide 10 mg four times daily, have observed a decrease in symptoms in patients with GORD but not healing of oesophagitis.[58,144] Other investigators, however, have reported no significant benefit with treatment by metoclopramide when compared with placebo.[145,146] When compared with ranitidine, metoclopramide has not proved as effective; in one study,[147] symptomatic improvement was equal but objective improvement was less, while in another[148] ranitidine (150 mg twice daily) was greatly superior to metoclopramide (10 mg four times daily) in reducing oesophageal acid contact time and both the frequency and severity of heartburn, especially during the daytime. On the other hand, adding metoclopramide (40 mg daily) to treatment with cimetidine has been associated with greater rates of symptomatic and endoscopic improvement.[149] Thus, no clinical trials have demonstrated significant endoscopic improvement with metoclopramide therapy alone, and side-effects limit the use of the medication: fatigue, anxiety, agitation and restlessness may occur in up to 30% of patients.

Domperidone

The newer dopamine antagonist domperidone also has properties which theoretically may be useful in the therapy of GORD, such as an increase in oesophageal peristalsis, LOSP and gastric emptying.[150] The effect on LOSP is, however, controversial, with some investigators concluding that oral domperidone does not influence oesophageal function.[151,152] Some studies have demonstrated domperidone to be more effective than placebo in relieving dyspeptic symptoms consistent with GORD.[152-154] In a double-blind crossover study in 22 patients with reflux oesophagitis, Blackwell et al.[151] reported that, after 2 weeks of therapy, domperidone in a dose of 80 mg daily in divided doses (with concomitant alginate) was superior to placebo in relieving symptoms. Masci et al.[155] compared domperidone therapy (60 mg daily) with ranitidine (300 mg daily) in GORD and found no significant difference between the two drugs after 6 weeks of therapy, for either symptom improvement (83%) or endoscopic healing (domperidone 66%, ranitidine 73%). The same overall conclusion was reached when domperidone was compared with famotidine.[156] Domperidone does not cross the blood–brain barrier to an appreciable degree[157] and thus the risk of extrapyramidal side-effects is very low. It may, however, produce symptoms related to the development of a hyperprolactinaemic state such as galactorrhoea and amenorrhoea.

Cisapride

The prokinetic agent cisapride is a substituted benzamide which acts to enhance directly the release of acetylcholine at the myenteric plexus. It also appears to act through serotonergic pathways and is devoid of antidopaminergic and direct cholinergic effects. Cisapride has been shown to consistently raise LOSP in healthy volunteers in a dose-dependent fashion after 5–20 mg orally;[158] it also appears to increase the amplitude and duration of contractions in the oesophageal body.[159,160] In patients with GORD, cisapride also raised LOSP when given in doses of 5–10 mg orally[161] and improved clearance of oesophageal contents.[162] Studies examining the effect of cisapride on intraoesophageal pH in patients with GORD have demonstrated that the total time of acid exposure in the oesophagus is reduced; cisapride also enhances gastric emptying in those GORD patients with delayed emptying. Side-effects are extremely uncommon, primarily consisting of occasional mild diarrhoea.

Short-term therapy

In the short-term treatment of GORD, several studies have demonstrated cisapride in a dose of 5–10 mg three times daily to be superior to placebo in terms of symptomatic improvement, and in a dose of 10 mg four times daily to heal oesophagitis effectively over 6–12 weeks (Table 9.5). Cisapride also appears to be as effective as the H_2-receptor antagonists in healing grades I–III oesophagitis (Table 9.5). In terms of adjunctive therapy, in one study[175] 47 patients with grade II–III oesophagitis were randomized to therapy with placebo or cisapride 10 mg three times daily, added to cimetidine 200 mg three times daily and 400 mg nocte. After 6–12 weeks healing occurred in 46% of patients on cimetidine alone and 70% of patients on combined therapy. There was a significantly greater decrease in severity of daily and nocturnal heartburn with combination therapy. Wienbeck et al.,[176] however, did not demonstrate significant differences in symptomatic or endoscopic improvement between ranitidine 150 mg twice daily together with cisapride 10 mg twice daily versus ranitidine alone in 93 patients.

Thus cisapride appears to be a valid alternative to the H_2-receptor antagonists of mild to moderate disease. Whether it is most useful in those GORD patients with a delay in gastric emptying is not established. Further studies are also necessary to determine the role of combination therapy using cisapride and H_2-receptor antagonists in GORD; in those patients not responding to H_2-receptor antagonist therapy after 6 weeks the addition of cisapride is a reasonable course of action. Certainly, with the introduction of cisapride there is little role for domperidone or metoclopramide in the therapy of GORD.

Table 9.5 Short-term cisapride versus placebo and other agents in uncomplicated GORD

REFERENCE	NO. OF PATIENTS	DOSE (MG/DAY)	MAXIMUM DURATION (WEEKS)	SIGNIFICANT EFFECT IN FAVOUR OF CISAPRIDE	
				SYMPTOMATIC IMPROVEMENT	ENDOSCOPIC HEALING
Hutteman et al. (1988)[163]	39	15 or 30	6	+	N/A
Nicolaidis et al. (1987)[164]	40	15 or 30	4	+	N/A
Van Outryve et al. (1987)[165]	55	15 or 30	4	+	N/A
Baldi et al. (1988)[166]	63	40	12	+	+
Lepoutre et al. (1990)[167]	19	40	16	+	+
Robertson et al. (1993)[168]	48	40	12	+	N/A
Manousos et al. (1987)[169]	30	Cis30,M30	4	+	N/A
Janisch et al. (1988)[170]	56	Cis40,R300	12	Cis=R	Cis=R*
Galmiche et al. (1990)[171]	73	Cis40,C1600	12	Cis=C	Cis=C*
Maleev et al. (1990)[172]	63	Cis20,C800	12	Cis=C	Cis=C*
	62	Cis40, C1600	12	Cis=C	Cis=C*
Arvanitakis et al. (1993)[173]	37	Cis40,R300	8	Cis=R	Cis=R*
Geldof et al. (1993)[174]	155	Cis40(b.d. or q.i.d.), R300	12	Cis=R	Cis=R*

Cis, cisapride; M, metoclopramide; R, ranitidine; C, cimetidine; N/A, not available:
* Similar complete healing rates (55–89%) for Cis and R or C.

Maintenance therapy

Cisapride is theoretically a particularly attractive agent for the maintenance therapy of GORD and reports suggest that it may have an important role in such therapy. Verlinden and Devis[177] studied 138 patients with oesophagitis (62% grade II or III) who were given an open dose of cisapride 10 mg four times daily for 8–16 weeks and in whom healing was obtained in 69%. Eighty of the healed patients were included in the second phase of the study of 6 months duration, and were randomly assigned to double-blind treatment with either cisapride 10 mg twice daily or placebo. The cumulative percentage of patients in remission was higher in the cisapride group than the placebo group, the relapse rates being 20 and 30% respectively. Reflux symptoms, especially nocturnal heartburn and regurgitation, continued to improve in the cisapride group and deteriorated in the placebo group. In the other European study,[178] 304 patients with healed reflux oesophagitis endoscopically were evaluated after double-blind maintenance treatment with one of two regimens of cisapride (10 mg twice daily or 20 mg nocte) or placebo. The cumulative percentage of patients in remission at 12 months was significantly higher in the cisapride group (relapse rates 33% for the cisapride twice daily and nocte regimens) than in the placebo group (51%). In two other studies, similar results were obtained at 6 months follow-up.[179,180]

SUCRALFATE

Sucralfate, the basic aluminium salt of sucrose octahydrogen sulphate, appears to afford mucosal protection by forming a viscous material which in vivo binds protein exudate in areas of ulceration and inflammation. It also absorbs bile salts in vitro and has been shown to stimulate synthesis and release of prostaglandin E_2 from gastric mucosa.[181] Even though it has only minimal acid neutralizing capacity,[182] it thus provides protection from aggressive substances such as pepsin and hydrochloric acid, and possibly bile acids. In a rabbit model, sucralfate prevented experimentally induced oesophagitis, as well as preventing pepsin induced changes in mucosal permeability.[183] The compound adheres to inflamed mucosa such that it cannot be removed by scraping with biopsy forceps, and when administered in the form of a slurry remains in the oesophagus for longer than normal in the presence of oesophagitis.[184] It is very well tolerated, with only occasional mild side-effects such as nausea, abdominal distension and constipation. Although sucralfate has been shown to produce greater symptomatic and endoscopic improvement than placebo or antacids for GORD (Table 9.6), these differences have not usually been statistically significant. Sucralfate has been shown, however, to be similar in efficacy to H_2-receptor antagonists (Table 9.6), for example Elsborg and Jorgenson[192] compared sucralfate granulate with cimetidine over a 12-week treatment period. The healing rate at 12 weeks was 62% for sucralfate and 59% for cimetidine, and half of the patients in each group were relieved of symptoms.

Sucralfate as adjunctive therapy to H_2-receptor antagonists has also been examined recently. Herrera et al.[193] treated 18 patients, with oesophagitis of grade II or higher and an abnormal oesophageal acid exposure on 24 h pH monitoring, with cimetidine 300 mg four times daily and sucralfate suspension 1 g four times daily for a 12-week period; another 18 similar patients were treated with cimetidine alone. Endoscopic healing occurred in seven patients on the combination regimen but in only two treated with monotherapy. On the other hand, the combination of full-dose sucralfate and low-dose cimetidine (400 mg nocte) was not superior to sucralfate alone in acute healing of oesophagitis.[194] Moreover, low-dose sucralfate (2 g daily) was not superior to placebo in preventing relapse over a 6-months period; further maintenance studies with full-dose sucralfate are required. Data on the use of sucralfate in

---

Table 9.6   Short-term sucralfate versus placebo and other agents in uncomplicated GORD

REFERENCE	NO. OF PATIENTS	DOSE (G/DAY)	MAXIMUM DURATION (WEEKS)	SIGNIFICANT EFFECT IN FAVOUR OF SUCCRALFATE	
				SYMPTOMATIC IMPROVEMENT	ENDOSCOPIC HEALING
Weiss et al. (1983)[185]	47	S4	12	–	+
Williams et al. (1987)[186]	68	S5	8	–	–*
Carling et al. (1988)[187]	138	S4	12	+	–*
Evreux (1987)[188]	45	S4 AA20	6	–	–
Laitinen et al. (1985)[189]	68	S4 AA8	6	–	–*
Simon and Mueller (1987)[190]	41	S4 R0.3	8	S = R	S = R†
Hameeteman et al. (1987)[191]	40	S4 C1.6	8	S = C	S =C†
Elsborg and Jorgensen (1991)[192]	60	S4 C0.8	12	S = C	S = C†

S, sucralfate;   AA, alginate–antacid;   R, ranitidine;   C, cimetidine.
* Greater complete healing rates for S (36–72%) but not significant over placebo or AA.
† Similar complete healing rates (14–68%) for S and R or C.

oesophagitis refractory to therapy with H_2-receptor antagonists are also conflicting. Ros et al.[195] demonstrated that complete healing occurred after 4–6 months of uninterrupted sucralfate therapy in a group of such patients, whereas Pace et al.[196] found that famotidine, but not sucralfate, was useful in this situation. The precise place of sucralfate thus requires further study but, in view of the other available drugs, it appears at present to have only a relatively small role in the practical management of patients with GORD.

REFERENCES

1. Castell DO, Wu WC & Ott DJ (eds). *Gastroesophageal Reflux Disease*. Mount Kisco, NY: Futura, 1985: 5.
2. Castell DO & Richter J. Gastroesophageal reflux. Pathogenesis, diagnosis and therapy. *Ann Intern Med* 1982; **97**: 93–103.
3. Smart HL, James PD, Alkinson M & Hawkey CJ. Treatment of reflux oesophagitis with trimoprostil. *Digestion* 1989; **44**: 52–56.
4. Maxton DG, Heald J. Whorwell PJ & Haboubi NY. Controlled trial of pyrogastrone and cimetidine in the treatment of reflux oesophagitis. *Gut* 1990; **31**: 351–354.
5. Sato JL, Wu WC & Castell DO. Randomized, double-blind, placebo controlled crossover trial of pirenzepine in gastro-oesophageal reflux patients. *Gastroenterology* 1990; **98**: A119.
6. DeMeester TR, Johnson LF, Joseph GJ et al. Patterns of gastroesophageal reflux in health and disease. *Ann Surg* 1976; **184**: 459–470.
7. Kitchin LI & Castell DO. Rationale and efficacy of conservative therapy for gastro-oesophageal reflux disease. *Arch Intern Med* 1991; **151**: 448–454.
8. Vitale G, Cheadle WG, Patel B et al. The effect of alcohol on nocturnal gastroesophageal reflux. *JAMA* 1987; **258**: 2077–2079.
9. Lloyd DA & Borda IT. Food-induced heartburn: effect of osmolality. *Gastroenterology* 1981; **80**: 740–741.
10. Murphy DW & Castell DO. Chocolate and heartburn: evidence of increased esophageal acid exposure after chocolate ingestion. *Am J Gastroenterol* 1988; **83**: 633–636.
11. Allen ML, Mellow MH, Robinson MG & Orr WC. The effect of raw onions on acid reflux and reflux symptoms. *Am J Gastroenterol* 1990; **85**: 377–380.
12. Becker DJ, Sinclair J, Castell DO & Wu WC. A comparision of high and low fat meals on postprandial esophageal acid exposure. *Am J Gastroenterol* 1989; **84**: 782–786.
13. Dennish GW & Castell DO. Inhibitory effect of smoking on the lower esophageal sphincter. *N Engl J Med* 1971; **284**: 1136–1137.
14. Scott AM, Kellow JE, Shuter B et al. Acute effects of cigarette smoking an intragastric distribution and gastric emptying of solids and liquids. *Gastroenterology* 1993; **104**: 410–416.
15. Kahrilas PJ & Gupta RR. Mechanisms of acid reflux associated with cigarette smoking. *Gut* 1990; 31: 4–10.
16. Ekstrom T & Tibbling L. Influence of theophylline on gastro-oesophageal reflux and asthma. *Eur J Clin Pharmacol* 1988; **35**: 353–356.
17. Johnson LF & DeMeester TR. Evaluation of elevation of the head of the bed, bethanechol, and antacid foam tablets on gastroesophageal reflux. *Dig Dis Sci* 1981; **26**: 673.
18. Harvey RF, Hadley N, Gill TR et al. Effects of sleeping with the bed-head raised and of ranitidine in patients with severe peptic oesophagitis. *Lancet* 1987; **ii**: 1200–1203.
19. Hamilton JW, Boisen RJ, Yamamoto DT et al. Sleeping on a wedge diminishes exposure of the esophagus to refluxed acid. *Dig Dis Sci* 1988; **33**: 518–522.
20. Graham DY, Smith JL & Patterson DJ. Why do apparently healthy people use antacid tablets? *Am J Gastroenterol* 1983; **78**: 257–260.
21. Scarpignato C. Pharmacological bases of the medical treatment of gastroesophageal reflux disease. *Dig Dis* 1988; **6**: 117–148.
22. Keenan RA, Hunt RH, Vincent D, Wright B & Milton-Thompson GJ. The case for high dose antacid therapy in duodenal ulcer. *Gut* 1978; **19**: A974.
23. Clain JE, Malagelada JR, Chadwick VS & Hoffman AF. Binding properties in vitro of antacids for conjugated bile acids. *Gastroenterology* 1977; **73**: 556–559.
24. Higgs RH, Smyth RD & Castell DO. Gastric alkalinisation: effect of lower-esophageal sphincter pressure and serum gastrin. *N Engl J Med* 1974; **291**: 486–490.
25. Meyer C, Berenzweig H, Kuljian B et al. Controlled trail of antacid versus placebo on relief of heartburn. *Gastroenterology* 1979; **76**: 1201.
26. Graham DY & Patterson DJ. Double-blind comparison of liquid antacid and placebo in the treatment of symptomatic reflux esophagitis. *Dig Dis Sci* 1983; **28**: 559–563.
27. Furman D, Mensh R, Winan G et al. A double-blind trial comparing high dose liquid antacid to placebo and cimetidine in improving symptoms and objective parameters in gastroesophageal reflux. *Gastroenterology* 1982; **82**: 1062.
28. Grove O, Bekker C, Jeppe-Hansen MG et al. Ranitidine and high dose antacid in reflux oesophagitis: a randomized, placebo-controlled trail. *Scand J Gastroenterol* 1985; **20**: 457–461.
29. Weberg R & Berstad A. Symptomatic effect of a low-dose antacid regimen in reflux oesophagitis. *Scand J Gastroenterol* 1989; **24**: 401–406.
30. Behar J, Brand DL, Brown FC et al. Cimetidine in the treatment of symptomatic gastroesophageal reflux. *Gastroenterology* 1975; **74**: 441–448.
31. Spencer H & Lender M. Adverse effects of aluminium-containing antacids on mineral metabolism. *Gastroenterology* 1979; **76**: 603–606.
32. Kaehny WD, Hegg AP & Alfrey AC. Gastrointestinal absorption of aluminium from aluminium-containing antacids. *N Engl J Med* 1977; **296**: 1389–1393.
33. Perl DP & Brody AR. Alzheimer's disease: X-ray spectrometric evidence of aluminium accumulation in neurofibrillary tangle-bearing neurons. *Science* 1980; **208**: 297–299.
34. Beeley M & Warner JO. Medical treatment of symptomatic hiatus hernia with low-density compounds. *Curr Med Res Opin* 1972; **1**: 63–69.
35. Stanciu C & Bennett JR. Alginate/antacid in the reduction of gastro-oesophageal reflux. *Lancet* 1974; **i**: 109–111.
36. Grossman AE, Klotz AP, Rhodes JB & Korb T. Reflux esophagitis: a comparison of old and new medical treatment. *J Kansas Med Soc* 1973; **74**: 423–424.
37. Barnardo DE, Lancaster-Smith M, Strickland ID & Wright JT. A double-blind controlled trial of Gaviscon in patients with symptomatic gastro-oesophageal reflux. *Curr Med Res Opin* 1975; **3**: 388–391.
38. Lanza FL, Smith V, Page-Castell JA & Castell DO. Effectiveness of foaming antacid in relieving induced heartburn. *South Med J* 1986; **79**: 327–330.
39. Chevrel B. A comparative crossover study on the treatment of heartburn and epigastric pain: liquid Gaviscon and a magnesium–aluminium antacid gel. *J Int Med Res* 1980; **8**: 300–302.
40. McHardy G. A multicentre randomized clinical trial of Gaviscon in reflux esophagitis. *South Med J* 1978; **71**(Suppl. 1): 16–21.
41. Behar J & Sheanan DC. Histologic abnormalities in reflux esophagitis. *Arch Pathol* 1975; **99**: 387–391.
42. Freeland GR, Hlggs RH & Castell DO. Lower esophageal sphincter response to oral administration of cimetidine in normal subjects. *Gastroenterology* 1977; **72**: 28–30.
43. Smout AJ, Bogaard JW, van Hattum J et al. Effects of cimetidine and ranitidine on interdigestive and postprandial lower esophageal sphincter pressures and plasma gastrin levels in normal subjects. *Gastroenterology* 1985; **88**: 557.
44. Baldi F, Ferrarini F, Longanesi A, Angeloni M, Ragazzini M & Barbara L. Oesophageal function before, during and after healing of erosive oesophagitis. *Gut* 1988; **29**: 157–160.
45. Houghton LA & Read NW. A comparative study of the effect of cimetidine and ranitidine on the rate of gastric emptying of liquid and solid test meals in man. *Aliment Pharmacol Ther* 1987; **1**: 401–408.
46. Stamm CP, Maydonovitch CL & Peura DA. Comparison of intravenous H_2 antagonists influence on gastric emptying in humans. *Gastroenterology* 1990; **98**: A130.
47. Freston JW. Safety perspectives on parenteral H_2-receptor antagonists. *Am J Med* 1987; **83**(Suppl. 6A): 58–67.
48. Rendic S, Kajfez F & Ruf HH. Characterization of cimetidine, ranitidine, and related structures' interaction with cytochrome P-450. *Drug Metab Dispos* 1983; **11**: 137–142.
49. Boyd EJS & Wood JR. H_2-receptor antagonists in the treatment of reflux oesophagitis. *Scand J Gastroenterol* 1989; **24**(Suppl. 171): 136–143.
50. Meuwissen SGM & Klinkenberg-Knol EC. Treatment of reflux oesophagitis with H_2-receptor antagonists. *Scand J Gastroenterol* 1988; **23**(Suppl. 146): 201–213.

51. Stalnikowicz-Darvasi R. H$_2$-antagonists in the treatment of reflux oesophagitis: a critical analysis. *Am J Gastroenterol* 1989; **83**: 245–248.

52. Ferguson R, Dronfield MW & Atkinson M. Cimetidine in treatment of reflux oesophagitis with peptic stricture. *BMJ* 1979; **2**: 472–474.

53. Wesdorp E, Bartelsman J, Pape K et al. Oral cimetidine in reflux esophagitis: a double-blind controlled trial. *Gastroenterology* 1978; **74**: 821–824.

54. Powell-Jackson P, Barkley H & Northfield TC. Effect of cimetidine on symptomatic gastro-oesophageal reflux. *Lancet* 1978; **ii**: 1068–1069.

55. Lepsien G, Sonnenberg A, Berges W et al. Die Behandlung der Refluxosophagitis mit Cimetidin. *Dtsch Med Wochenschr* 1979; **104**: 21–26.

56. Brown P. Cimetidine in the treatment of reflux oesophagitis. *Med J Aust* 1979; **2**: 96–97.

57. Thanik K, Chey WY, Shak A, Hamilton D & Nadelson N. Bethanechol or cimetidine in the treatment of symptomatic reflux esophagitis. *Arch Intern Med* 1982; **142**: 1479–1481.

58. Bright-Asare P & El-Bassoussi M. Cimetidine, metolopramide or placebo in the treatment of symptomatic gastro-oesophageal reflux. *J Clin Gastroenterol* 1980; **2**: 149–156.

59. Festen HPM, Driessen WMM, Lamers CHB & van Tongeren JHM. Cimetidine in the treatment of severe ulcerative reflux oesophagitis: results of an 8-week double-blind study and of subsequent long-term maintenance treatment. *Neth J Med* 1980; **23**: 237–240.

60. Fiasse R, Hanin C, Lepot A et al. Controlled trial of cimetidine in reflux esophagitis. *Dig Dis Sci* 1980; **25**: 750–755.

61. Druguet M & Lambert R. Oral cimetidine in reflux oesophagitis: a double-blind controlled trial. In Dress A, Barbier F, Harvengt C & Tytgat GN (eds) *Cimetidine Tagamet*. Proceedings of the Second National Symposium, October 1979, Brussels. Amsterdam: Excerpta Medica, 1980: 30–36.

62. Greaney MG & Irvin TT. Cimetidine for the treatment of symptomatic gastro-oesophageal reflux. *Br J Clin Pract* 1981; **35**: 21–24.

63. Breen KJ, Desmond PV & Whelan G. Treatment of reflux oesophagitis. A randomized, controlled evaluation of cimetidine. *Med J Aust* 1983; **2**: 555–556.

64. Frank WO, Wetherington J, Palmer RH & Young MD. Cimetidine – effective therapy for reflux esophagitis (RE). *Gastroenterology* 1989; **96**: A156.

65. Farup PG, Weberg R, Berstad A et al. Low-dose antacids versus 40 mg cimetidine twice daily for reflux oesophagitis. *Scand J Gastroenterol* 1990; **25**: 315–320.

66. Kaul B, Petersen H, Ericksen H et al. Gastroesophageal reflux disease. Acute and maintenance treatments with cimetidine. *Scand J Gastroenterol* 1986; **21**: 139–145.

67. Dawson J, Barnard J & Delattre G. Cimetidine 800 mg at bedtime in reflux oesophagitis: a multicentre trial. In Siewert JR & Hölscher AH (eds) *Proceedings of the International Esophageal Week*, September 1986, Munich. Gräfelfing: Demeter, 1986: 189.

68. Tytgat GNJ, Nicolai JJ & Reman FC. Efficacy of different doses of cimetidine in the treatment of reflux esophagitis. *Gastroenterology* 1990; **99**: 629–634.

69. Berstad A. Overview of ranitidine in reflux oesophagitis: its effect on symptoms, endoscopic appearance and histology. In Misiewicz J & Wormsley K (eds) *The Clinical Use of Ranitidine*. Second Ranitidine Symposium, October 1981, London. London: Medical Publications Foundation, 1982: 297–304.

70. Goy SG, Maynard JH, McNaughton WM et al. Ranitidine and placebo in the treatment of reflux oesophagitis. A double-blind randomized trial. *Med J Aust* 1983; **2**: 558–561.

71. Wesdorp ICE, Dekker W & Klinkenberg-Knol EC. Treatment of reflux oesophagitis with ranitidine. *Gut* 1983; **24**: 921–924.

72. Sherbaniuk R, Wensel R, Bailey R et al. Ranitidine in the treatment of symptomatic gastroesophageal reflux disease. *J Clin Gastroenterol* 1984; **6**: 9–15.

73. Hine KR, Holmes G, Melikian V et al. Ranitidine in reflux oesophagitis. *Digestion* 1984; **29**: 119–123.

74. Lehtola J, Niemela S, Martikainen J et al. Ranitidine, 150 mg three times a day, in the treatment of reflux oesophagitis. A placebo-controlled, double-blind study. *Scand J Gastroenterol* 1986; **21**: 175–180.

75. Johansson KE, Boeryd B, Johansson K & Tibbling L. Double-blind crossover study of ranitidine and placebo in gastro-oesophageal reflux disease. *Scand J Gastroenterol* 1986; **21**: 769–778.

76. Sontag S, Robinson M, McCallum RW et al. Ranitidine therapy for gastroesophageal reflux disease. Results of a large double-blind trial. *Arch Intern Med* 1987; **147**: 1485–1491.

77. Bovero E, Cheli R, Barbara L et al. Short-term treatment of reflux oesophagitis with ranitidine 300 mg nocte. Italian multicentre study. *Hepatogastroenterology* 1987; **34**: 155–159.

78. Rohner HG & Wienbeck M. Zwei oder eine Tagesdosis Ranitidine zur Behandlung der Refluxöesophagitis. *Z Gastroenterol* 1986; **24**(8): 396–402.

79. Halvorsen L, Lee FI, Wesdorp ICE, Johnson NJ, Mills JG & Wood JR. Acute treatment of reflux oesophagitis: a multicentre study to compare 150 mg ranitidine twice daily with ranitidine 300 mg at bedtime. *Aliment Pharmacol Ther* 1989; **3**: 171–182.

80. Johnson NJ, Laws S, Mills JG, McMahon A & Wood JR. Effect of ranitidine dose and administration time on reflux oesophagitis: results of a multi-centre study. *Gastroenterology* 1990; **98**: A66.

81. Johnson NJ, Boyd EJS, Mills JG & Wood JR. Acute treatment of reflux oesophagitis: a multicentre trial to compare 150 mg ranitidine b.d. with 300 mg ranitidne q.d.s. *Aliment Pharmacol Ther* 1989; **3**: 259–266.

82. Euler AR, Murdock RH, Wilson TH, Silver MT, Parker SE & Powers L. Ranitidine is effective therapy for erosive esophagitis. *Am J Gastroenterol* 1993; **88**: 520–524.

83. Fielding JF & Doyle GB. Comparison between ranitidine and cimetidine in the treatment of reflux oesophagitis. *Ir Med J* 1984; **77**: 356–357.

84. Orr WC, Robinson MG, Humphries TJ, Antonello J & Cagliola A. Dose response effects of famotidine on patterns of gastroesophageal reflux. *Aliment Pharmacol Ther* 1988; **2**: 229–235.

85. Sabesin SM, Schaffer JA, Bradstreet K, Walton-Bowen K & Humphries TJ. Famotidine – symptomatic relief and healing in patients with reflux esophagitis: results of a US multicenter trial. *Gastroenterology* 1990; **98**: A128.

86. Simon TJ, Berlin RG, Tipping R & Gilde L for the Famotidine Erosive Esophagitis Study Group. Efficacy of twice daily doses of 40 or 20 milligrams famotidine or 150 milligrams ranitidine for treatment of patients with moderate to severe erosive esophagitis. *Scand J Gastroenterol* 1993; **28**: 375–380.

87. Wesdorp ICE, Dekker W & Festen HPM. Efficacy of famotidine 20 mg twice a day versus 40 mg twice a day in the treatment of erosive or ulcerative reflux oesophagitis. *Dig Dis Sci* 1993; **38**: 2287–2293.

88. Berlin R, Ebel D & Cook T. Famotidine (F) 40 HS vs ranitidine (R) in the treatment of reflux oesophagitis: the results of a multicentre trial. *Gastroenterology* 1989; **96**: A39.

89. Dickinson RJ, Royston CMS & Sutton DR. A comparison of famotidine and ranitidine in an elderly population: a multicentre study. *Postgrad Med J* 1986; **62**(Suppl. 2): 63–65.

90. Cloud ML & Offen WW. Nizatidine versus placebo in gastroesophageal reflux disease: a six-week multicenter, randomized double-blind comparison. *Dig Dis Sci* 1992; **37**: 865–874.

91. Baldi F, Longamesi A, Ferrarini F, et al. Italian Gord study Group. Nizatidine in the treatment of reflux oesophagitis: Italian Multicentre Study. *Eur J Gastroenterol Hepatol* 1993; **5**: 475–478.

92. Ottenjann R, Siewert JR, Heilmann K, Neiss A & Dopfer H. Treatment of reflux oesophagitis: results of a multicentre study. In Siewert JR & Hölscher AH (eds) *Diseases of the Oesophagus*. Berlin: Springer, 1988: 1123–1129.

93. Lieberman DA. Medical therapy for chronic reflux oesophagitis. Long-term follow-up. *Arch Intern Med* 1987; **147**: 1717–1780.

94. Bright-Asare P, Behar J & Brand DL. Effect of long-term maintenance cimetidine (CIM) therapy on gastroesophageal reflux disease (GERD). *Gastroenterology* 1982; **82**: 1025.

95. McCallum RW, Sontag SJ, Vlahcevic ZR et al. Ranitidine versus placebo in long-term treatment of gastroesophageal reflux. *Am J Gastroenterol* 1985, **80**: 864.

96. Koelz HR, Birchler R, Bretholz A et al. Healing and relapse of reflux oesophagitis during treatment with ranitidine. *Gastroenterology* 1986; **91**: 1198–1205.

97. Berlin R, Ebel D & Cook T. Famotidine (F) 20 HS & 40 HS vs placebo in the maintenance therapy (MT) of reflux oesophagitis (RE): results of a double-blind multi-centre trial. *Gastroenterology* 1989; **96**: A39.

98. Lind T, Cederberg C, Ekenved G, Haglund U & Olbe L. Effect of omeprazole – a gastric proton pump inhibitor – on pentagastrin stimulated acid secretion in man. *Gut* 1983; **24**: 270–276.

99. Walt RP, Gomes MdeFA, Wood EC, Logan LH & Pounder RE. Effect of daily oral omeprazole on 24 hour intragastric acidity. *BMJ* 1983; **287**: 12–14.

100. Hongo M, Ohara S, Hirasawa Y et al. Effect of lansoprazole on intragastric pH: comparison between morning and evening dose. *Dig Dis Sci* 1990; **37**: 882–890.

101. Sanders SW, Tolman KG, Greski PA et al. The effects of lansoprazole, a new H⁺, K⁺–ATPase inhibitor, on gastric pH and serum gastrin. *Aliment Pharmacol Ther* 1990; **6**: 359–372.

102. Naesdal J, Bodemar G & Walan A. Effect of omeprazole, a substituted benzimidazole, on 24-h intragastric acidity in patients with peptic ulcer disease. *Scand J Gastroenterol* 1984; **19**: 916–922.

103. Sharma BK, Walt RP, Pounder RE, Gomes M deFA, Wood EC & Logan LH. Optimal dose of oral omeprazole for maximal 24 hour decrease of intragastric acidity. *Gut* 1984; **25**: 957–964.

104. Prichard PJ, Yeomans ND, Shulkes A et al. The effect of omeprazole on 24 h intragastric pH and fasting plasma gastrin during low dosage (10 mg) in the morning or the evening. *J Gastroenterol Hepatol* 1986; **1**: 289–295.

105. Howard JM, Frei JV, Flowers M, Bondy DC, Tilbe K & Reynolds RPE. Omeprazole heals esophagitis but does not improve abnormal esophageal motility in reflux esophagitis. *Gastroenterology* 1990; **98**: A61.

106. Downton J, Dent J, Heddle R et al. Elevation of gastric pH heals peptic oesophagitis. *J Gastroenterol Hepatol* 1987; **2**: 317–324.

107. Klinkenberg-Knol EC, Festen HPM & Meuwissen SGM. The effects of omeprazole and ranitidine on 24-hour pH in the distal oesophagus of patients with reflux oesophagitis. *Aliment Pharmacol Ther* 1988; **2**: 221–227.

108. Ruth M, Enbom H, Lundell L, Lönroth H, Sandberg N & Sandmark S. The effect of omeprazole or ranitidine treatment on 24-hour esophageal acidity in patients with reflux esophagitis. *Scand J Gastroenterol* 1988; **23**: 1141–1146.

109. Lamberts R, Creutzfeldt W, Stöckmann F, Jacubaschke U, Maas S & Brunner G. Long-term omeprazole treatment in man: effects on gastric endocrine cell populations. *Digestion* 1988; **39**: 126–135.

110. Arnold R & Koop H. Omeprazole long-term safety. *Digestion* 1989; **44**: 77–86.

111. Hetzel DJ, Dent J, Reed WD et al. Healing and relapse of severe peptic esophagitis after treatment with omeprazole. *Gastroenterology* 1988; **95**: 903–912.

112. Blum AL, Riecken EO, Dammann HG et al. Comparison of omeprazole and ranitidine in the treatment of reflux oesophagitis. *N Engl J Med* 1986; **314**: 716.

113. Klinkenberg-Knol EC, Jansen JMBJ, Festen HPM, Meuwissen SGM & Lamers CBHW. Double blind multicentre comparison of omeprazole and ranitidine in the treatment of reflux oesophagitis. *Lancet* 1987; **i**: 349–351.

114. Havelund T, Laursen LS, Skoubo-Kristensen E et al. Omeprazole and ranitidine in treatment of reflux oesophagitis: double blind comparative trial. *BMJ* 1988; **296**: 89–92.

115. Vantrappen G, Rutgeerts L, Schurmans P & Coenegrachts J-L. Omeprazole (40 mg) is superior to ranitidine in short-term treatment of ulcerative reflux esophagitis. *Dig Dis Sci* 1988; **33**: 523–529.

116. Sandmark S, Carlsson R, Fausa O & Lundell L. Omeprazole or ranitidine in the treatment of reflux esophagitis. *Scand J Gastroenterol* 1988; **23**: 625–632.

117. Dehn TCB, Shepherd HA, Colin-Jones D, Kettlewell MGW & Carrol NJH. Double blind comparison of omeprazole (40 mg od) versus cimetidine (400 mg qd) in the treatment of symptomatic erosive reflux oesophagitis, assessed endoscopically, histologically and by 24 h pH monitoring. *Gut* 1990; **31**: 509–513.

118. Zeitoun P, Rampal P, Barbier P, Isal J-P, Eriksson S & Carlsson R. Omeprazole (20 mg o.m.) versus ranitidine (150 mg b.i.d.) in reflux esophagitis. Results of a double-blind randomised trial. *Gastroenterol Clin Biol* 1989; **13**: 457–462.

119. Lundell L, Westin IH, Sandmark S et al. Omeprazole or high dose ranitidine in the treatment of patients with reflux oesophagitis not responding to standard doses of H₂-receptor antagonists. *Aliment Pharmacol Ther* 1990; **4**: 145–153.

120. Blum AL. Treatment of acid related disorders with gastric acid inhibitors: the state of the art. *Digestion* 1990; **47**(Suppl. 1): 3–10.

121. Bate CM, Keeling PWN, O'Morrain C, Wilkinson SP, Foster DN & Mountford RA. Comparison of omeprazole and cimetidine in reflux oesophagitis: symptomatic, endoscopic and histological evaluations. *Gut* 1990; **31**: 968–972.

122. Robinson M, Decktor DL, Maton PN et al. Omeprazole is superior to ranitidine plus metoclopramide in the short-term treatment of erosive oesophagitis. *Aliment Pharmacol Ther* 1993; **7**: 67–73.

123. Barradell LB, Faulds D & McTavish D. Lansoprazole. A review of its pharmacodynamic and pharmacokinetic properties and its therapeutic efficacy in acid-related disorders. *Drugs* 1992; **44**: 225–250.

124. Hatlebakk JG, Berstad A, Carling L et al. Lansoprazole versus omeprazole in short-term treatment of reflux oesophagitis: results of a Scandinavian multicentre trial. *Scand J Gastroenterol* 1993; **28**: 224–228.

125. Feldman M, Harford WV, Fisher RS et al. Lansoprazole Study Group: treatment of reflux esophagitis resistant to H₂-receptor antagonists with lansoprazole, a new H⁺/K⁺ATPase inhibitor: a controlled, double-blind study. *Am J Gastroenterol* 1993; **88**: 1212–1217.

126. Klinkenberg-Knol EC, Jansen JMBJ, Lamers CBHW, Nelis F & Meuwissen SGM. Temporary cessation of long-term maintenance treatment with omeprazole in patients with H₂-receptor antagonist resistant reflux oesophagitis: effects on symptoms, endoscopy, serum gastrin levels and gastric acid output. *Scand J Gastroenterol* 1990; **25**: 1144–1150.

127. Koop H & Arnold R. Long-term maintenance treatment of reflux esophagitis with omeprazole: prospective study in patients with H₂-blocker-resistant esophagitis. *Dig Dis Sci* 1991; **36**: 552–557.

128. Lundell L, Backman L, Ekstrom P et al. Prevention of relapse of reflux oesophagitis after endoscopic healing: the efficacy and safety of omeprazole compared with ranitidine. *Scand J Gastroenterol* 1991; **26**: 248–256.

129. Zeitoun P, Barbier P, Cayphas J-P et al. Comparison of two dosage regimens of omeprazole 10 mg once-daily and 200 mg weekends as prophylaxis against recurrence of reflux oesophagitis. *Hepatogastroenterology* 1989; **36**: 279–280.

130. Dent J. Australian clinical trials of omeprazole in the management of reflux oesophagitis. *Digestion* 1990; **47** (Suppl. 1): 69–71.

131. Bardhan KD, Morris P, Thompson M et al. Omeprazole in the treatment of erosive oesophagitis refractory to high dose cimetidine and ranitidine. *Gut* 1990; **31**: 745–749.

132. Humphries TJ & Castell DO. Effect of oral bethanechol on parameters of esophageal peristalsis. *Dig Dis Sci* 1981; **26**(2): 129–132.

133. Helm JF, Dodds WJ, Pelc LR et al. Effects of esophageal emptying and saliva on clearance of acid from the esophagus. *N Engl J Med* 1984; **310**: 284.

134. Boesby S, Brandsberg M, Larsen NK & Pedersen SA. The effect of carbachol on resting gastroesophageal sphincter pressure and serum gastrin in normal human subjects. *Scand J Gastroenterol* 1976; **11**: 171–175.

135. Dhaosowasdi K, Malmud LS & Tolin RD. Cholinergic effects on esophageal transit and clearance. *Gastroenterology* 1981; **81**: 915–920.

136. McCallum RW, Fink SM, Lerner E et al. Effects of metoclopramide and bethanechol on delayed gastric emptying present in gastroesophageal reflux patients. *Gastroenterology* 1983; **84**: 1573.

137. Farrell RL, Roling GT & Castell DO. Cholinergic therapy of chronic heartburn. *Ann Intern Med* 1974; **8**: 573–576.

138. Thanik K, Chey WY, Shah AS & Guiterrez JG. Reflux esophagitis: effect of oral bethanechol on symptoms and endoscopic findings. *Ann Intern Med* 1980; **93**: 805–808.

139. Saco LS, Orlando RC, Levinson SL et al. Double-blind controlled trial of bethanechol and antacid versus placebo and antacid in the treatment of erosive esophagitis. *Gastroenterology* 1982; **82**: 1369.

140. Miller WN, Komoranahalli PG, Dodds WJ, Hogan WJ, Barreras RF & Arndorfer RC. Effect of bethanechol on gastroesophageal reflux. *Am J Dig Dis* 1977; **22**: 230–234.

141. Dilawari JB & Misiewicz JJ. Does oral metoclopramide increase cardiac sphincter pressure? *Gut* 1972; **13**: 856.

142. Baumann HW, Sturdevant RAL & McCallum RW. L-Dopa inhibits metoclopramide stimulation of the lower oesophageal sphincter in man. *Dig Dis Sci* 1979; **24**: 289–295.

143. Behar J & Ramsby G. Gastric emptying and antral motility in reflux esophagitis: effect of oral metoclopramide. *Gastroenterology* 1978; **74**: 253–256.

144. McCallum RW, Ippoliti AF, Cooney C & Sturdevant RAL. A controlled trial of metoclopramide in symptomatic gastro-esophageal reflux. *N Engl J Med* 1977; **296**: 354–357.

145. Venables CW, Bell D & Eccleston D. A double-blind study of metoclopramide in symptomatic peptic oesophagitis. *Postgrad Med J* (Suppl. 4) 1973; **49**: 73–76.

146. Paull A & Kerr Grant A. A controlled trial of metoclopramide in reflux oesophagitis. *Med J Aust* 1974; **2**: 627–629.

147. Guslandi M, Testoni PA, Passaretti S et al. Ranitidine vs metoclopramide in the medical treatment of reflux oesophagitis. *Hepatogastroenterology* 1983; **30**(3): 96.

148. Orr WC, Finn AL, Twaddel T & Russell J. Comparative effects of ranitidine and metoclopramide on gastro-esophageal reflux and heartburn. *Am J Gastroenterol* 1990; **85**: 697–700.

149. Lieberman DA & Keeffe EB. Treatment of severe reflux esophagitis with cimetidine and metoclopramide. *Ann Intern Med* 1986; **104**: 21.

150. Jacobs F, Akkermans LMA, Yol OH & Wittebol P. Effect of domperidone on gastric emptying of semi-solid and solid food. Progress with domperidone. *R Soc Med (Int Cong Symp Ser)* 1981; **36**: 21–29.

151. Blackwell JN, Heading RC & Fetter MR. Effect of domperidone on lower esophageal sphincter pressure and gastroesophageal reflux in patients with peptic oesophagitis. Progress with domperidone. *R Soc Med (Int Cong Symp Ser)* 1981; **36**: 57–61.

152. Valenzuela JE. Effects of domperidone on the symptoms of reflux oesophagitis. Progress with domperidone. *R Soc Med (Int Cong Symp Ser)* 1981; **36**: 51–57.

153. Englert W & Schlich D. A double blind crossover trial of domperidone in chronic postprandial dyspepsia. *Postgrad Med J* 1979; **55**: 28–29.

154. Nagler J & Miskovitz P. Clinical evaluation of domperidone in the treatment of chronic postprandial upper gastrointestinal distress. *Am J Gastroenterol* 1981; **76**: 495–499.

155. Masci E, Testoni PA, Passaretti S, Guslandi M & Tittobello A. Comparison of ranitidine, domperidone maleate and ranitidine plus domperidone maleate in the short-term treatment of reflux oesophagitis. *Drugs* 1985; **11**: 687–692.

156. Guslandi M, Dell'Oca M, Molteni V, Romano R, Passaretti S & Ballarin E. Famotidine versus domperidone, versus a combination of both in the treatment of reflux esophagitis: interim report. *Gastroenterology* 1989; **96**: A191.

157. Broekaert A. Effect of domperidone on gastric emptying and secretion. *Postgrad Med J* 1979; **55**: 11–14.

158. Janssens J. Effect of cisapride on oesophageal motility. In Johnson AG & Lux G (eds) *Progress in the Treatment of Gastrointestinal Motility Disorders: the Role of Cisapride*. Amsterdam: Excerpta Medica, 1988: 48–55.

159. Janssens J, Ceccatelli P & Vantrappen G. Cisapride restores the decreased lower oesophageal sphincter pressure in reflux patients. *Digestion* 1986; **34**: 139–140.

160. Smout AJPM, Bogaard JW, Grade AC, Ten Thije OJ, Akkermans LMA & Wittebol P. Effects of cisapride, a new gastrointestinal prokinetic substance, on interdigestive and postprandial motor activity of the distal oesophagus in man. *Gut* 1985; **26**: 246–251.

161. Corazziari E, Bontempo I & Anzini F. Effect of cisapride on primary peristalsis and lower oesophageal sphincter pressure. *Gut* 1984; **25**: A1318.

162. Horowitz M, Maddox A, Harding PE et al. Effect of cisapride on gastric and esophageal emptying in insulin-dependent diabetes mellitus. *Gastroenterology* 1987; **92**: 1899–1907.

163. Hutteman W. Cisapride in gastro-oesophageal reflux disease. In Johnson AG & Lux G (eds) *Progress in the Treatment of Gastrointestinal Motility Disorders: the Role of Cisapride*. Amsterdam: Excerpta Medica, 1988: 56–62.

164. Nicolaidis CL, Kehegioglou K, Mantzaris G et al. Cisapride relieves reflux symptoms in oesophagitis patients. Double-blind placebo-controlled comparison of two dosages. *Prog Med* 1987; **43** (Suppl. 1): 43–48.

165. Van Outryve M, Vanderlinden I, Dedullen G & Rutgeerts L. Dose response study with cisapride in gastro-oesophageal reflux disease *Curr Ther Res* 1988; **43**: 1059–1061.

166. Baldi F, Bianchi Porro G, Dobrilla G et al. Cisapride versus placebo in reflux esophagitis. *J Clin Gastroenterol* 1988; **10**: 614–618.

167. Lepoutre L, Van Der Spek P, Vanderlinden I, Bollen J & Laukens P. Healing of grade II and III oesophagitis through motility stimulation with cisapride. *Digestion* 1990; **45**: 109–114.

168. Robertson CS, Evans DF, Ledingham SJ & Atkinson M. Cisapride in the treatment of gastro-oesophageal reflux disease. *Aliment Pharmacol Ther* 1993; **7**: 181–190.

169. Manousos ON, Mandidis A & Michailidis D. Treatment of reflux symptoms in esophagitis patients: a comparative trial of cisapride and metoclopramide. *Curr Ther Res* 1987; **42**: 807–813.

170. Janisch HD, Huttemann W & Bouzo MH. Cisapride versus ranitidine in the treatment of reflux esophagitis. *Hepatogastroenterology* 1988; **35**: 125–127.

171. Galmiche JP, Fraitag B, Filoche B et al. Double-blind comparison of cisapride and cimetidine in treatment of reflux esophagitis. *Dig Dis Sci* 1990; **35**: 649–655.

172. Maleev A, Mendizova A, Popov P et al. Cisapride and cimetidine in the treatment of erosive esophagitis. *Hepatogastroenterology* 1990; **37**: 403–407.

173. Arvanitakis C, Nikopoulos A, Theoharidis A et al. Cisapride and ranitidine in the treatment of gastro-oesophageal reflux disease: a comparative randomized double-blind trial. *Aliment Pharmacol Ther* 1993; **7**: 635–641.

174. Geldof H, Hazelhoff B & Otten MH. Two different dose regimens of cisapride in the treatment of reflux oesophagitis: a double-blind comparison with ranitidine. *Aliment Pharmacol Ther* 1993; **7**: 409–415.

175. Galmiche J-P, Brandstatter G, Evreux M et al. Combined treatment with cisapride and cimetidine in severe reflux oesophagitis. A double-blind controlled trial. *Gut* 1988; **29**: 675–681.

176. Wienbeck M. and the Ranprid Study Group. Therapeutic effect of cisapride added to ranitidine in patients with reflux esophagitis. *Dig Dis Sci* 1986; **31**: 97.

177. Verlinden M & Devis G. Healing and prevention of relapse of reflux oesophagitis by cisapride. *Gastroenterology* 1990; **98**: A144.

178. Blum AL, Adami B, Bouzo MH et al and the Italian Eurocis Trialists. Effect of cisapride on relapse of esophagitis. A multinational, placebo-controlled trial in patients healed with an antisecretory drug. *Dig Dis Sci* 1993; **38**: 551–560.

179. Tytgat GNJ, Anker Hansen OJ, Carling L et al. Effect of cisapride on relapse of reflux oesophagitis, healed with an antisecretory drug. *Scand J Gastroenterol* 1992; **27**: 175–183.

180. Toussaint J, Gossuin A, Deruyttere M, Huble F & Devis G. Healing and prevention of relapse reflux oesophagitis by cisapride. *Gut* 1991; **32**: 1280–1285.

181. Konturek SJ, Kwiecien N, Obtulowicz W, Kopp B & Olesky J. Double-blind controlled study on the effect of sucralfate on gastric prostaglandin formation and microbleeding in normal and aspirin-treated man. *Gut* 1986; **27**: 1450–1456.

182. Nagashima R. Mechanisms of action of sucralfate. *J Clin Gastroenterol* 1981; **3**(Suppl. 2): 117–127.

183. Schweitzer EJ, Bass BL, Johnson LF & Harmon TW. Sucralfate prevents experimental peptic oesophagitis in rabbits. *Gastroenterology* 1985; **88**: 611–619.

184. Pleet D, Malmud LS, Maurer A et al. Sucralfate binding to inflamed esophageal mucosa. *Gastroenterology* 1985; 88: 1540.

185. Weiss W, Brunner H & Buttner GR. Therapie der Refluxoesophagitis mit Sucralfat. *Dtsch Med Wochenschr* 1983; **108**: 1706–1716.

186. Williams RM, Orlando RC, Bozymski EM et al. Multicenter trial of sucralfate for the treatment of reflux esophagitis. *Am J Med* 1987; **83** (Suppl. 3B): 61–66.

187. Carling L, Cronstedt J, Engqvist A, Kagari I, Nystrom B & Svedberg L-E. Sucralfate versus placebo in reflux esophagitis. *Scand J Gastroenterol* 1988; **23**: 1117–1124.

188. Evreux M. Sucralfate versus alginate-antacid in the treatment of peptic oesophagitis. *Am J Med* 1987; **83**: 48–50.

189. Laitinen S, Stahlberg M & Kajralnoma MI. Sucralfate and alginate/antacid in reflux oesophagitis. *Scand J Gastroenterol* 1985; **20**: 229–234.

190. Simon D & Mueller P. Comparison of the effect of sucralfate and ranitidine in reflux oesophagitis. *Am J Med* 1987; **83** (Suppl. 3B): 43–47.

191. Hameeteman W, Boomgaard DM, Dekker W, Schrijver M, Wesdorp ICE & Tytgat GNJ. Sucralfate versus cimetidine in reflux esophagitis, a single blind multicentre study. *J Clin Gastroenterol* 1987; **9**: 390–394.

192. Elsborg L & Jorgensen F. Sucralfate versus cimetidine in reflux oesophagitis. A double-blind clinical study. *Scand J Gastroenterol* 1991; **26**: 146–150.

193. Herrera JL, Shay SS, McCabe M, Peura DA & Johnson LF. Sucralfate used as adjunctive therapy in patients with severe erosive peptic esophagitis resulting from gastroesophageal reflux. *Am J Gastroenterol* 1990; **85**: 1335–1338.

194. Schotborgh RH, Hameeteman W, Dekker W, Boomgard DM, Van Olffen GH & Schriver M. Combination therapy of sucralfate and cimetidine in patients with peptic reflux oesophagitis. *Am J Med* 1989; **86** (Suppl. 6A): 77–78.

195. Ros E, Pujol A, Bardas JM & Grande L. Efficacy of sucralfate in refractory reflux oesophagitis. *Scand J Gastroenterol* 1989; **24**: 49–55.

196. Pace F, Lazzaroni M & Bianchi-Porro G. Failure of sucralfate in the treatment of refractory oesophagitis versus high-dose famotidine. *Scand J Gastroenterol* 1991; **26**: 491–494.

10

SURGICAL MANAGEMENT OF UNCOMPLICATED GASTRO-OESOPHAGEAL REFLUX DISEASE

A Watson

HISTORICAL ASPECTS OF ANTIREFLUX SURGERY

The early history of antireflux surgery was clouded by some confusion between the entities of gastro-oesophageal reflux and hiatal hernia. It would appear that the first published report of repair of a hiatal or diaphragmatic hernia for reflux-like symptoms was by Soresi in 1919.[1] Subsequently, the entity of 'symptomatic hiatal hernia' appeared to be recognized more frequently, and more operations of an anatomical nature were undertaken. In 1938, Harrington reported surgical treatment of 131 cases at the Mayo clinic.[2] The operation comprised narrowing the oesophageal hiatus, crushing the phrenic nerve to produce eventration and ensuring the gastro-oesophageal junction lay within the abdomen, together with excision of the hernial sac, if present. This description suggested that some of these patients had para-oesophageal herniae. Somewhat surprisingly, 84% of patients had complete relief of their symptoms. The next major milestone was the realization by Allison, from Oxford, in 1951 that reflux of gastric contents rather than the presence of a hiatal hernia was the major problem, and he introduced the term 'reflux oesophagitis'.[3] Nonetheless, the operative procedure he described to alleviate this problem was very much an anatomical repair, although abandoning the phrenic nerve crush. Through a left thoracotomy and an incision into the diaphragm, he fixed the oesophagogastric junction within the abdomen using plicating sutures through the phreno-oesophageal ligament. This resulted in short-term symptomatic relief in 91% of patients and became the operation of choice over the next 15–20 years, with minor modifications such as avoidance of an incision in the diaphragm and performance by a transabdominal technique. However, subsequent clinical and radiological follow-up in patients who had been operated on more than 10 years previously showed an anatomical recurrence of the hiatal hernia in approximately 50% of patients and the symptomatic satisfaction rate had fallen to 66%.[4] This was believed to relate to the fact that the Allison repair did not address any other factors to control reflux, other than placing the oesophagogastric junction within the abdomen. Because of the unsatisfactory long-term results and the contemporaneous development of antireflux procedures which addressed other factors known to be relevant to the antireflux mechanism, the Allison repair fell into disrepute.

Belsey in Bristol had, during this period, been developing a transthoracic antireflux procedure which aimed not only to restore the oesophagogastric junction to within the abdomen, but to create a long intra-abdominal segment to be exposed to positive intra-abdominal pressure, and a partial fundoplication to further augment external pressure on the long intra-abdominal segment, particularly during raised intragastric pressure, such as occurs in the postprandial period. Between 1949 and 1967, the procedure underwent several modifications, the final version being referred to as the Belsey Mark IV procedure which is still performed today by many thoracic surgeons with excellent results. In 1956, Rudolf Nissen in Basel reported a transabdominal antiflux procedure involving a total fundoplication of 3–6 cm in length.[5] This procedure proved to be effective in the correction of gastro-oesophageal reflux and gained popularity because of this and the fact that it was a relatively straightforward transabdominal procedure. However, it became apparent that there was a significant incidence of mechanical complications, including slippage, disruption, troublesome dysphagia, gas-bloat syndrome and inability to belch or vomit. The belief that many of these complications were associated with over-tightness of the wrap led to various technical modifications. The first was by Donahue and Bombeck in 1976,[6] who advocated a loose, floppy wrap around a 50 FG bougie. This resulted in some improvement, but incomplete abolition of mechanical complications. In 1967, Hill described a transabdominal partial fundoplication procedure in an attempt to overcome these problems.[7] In 1979, Angelchik and Cohen described the use of a prosthetic silcone collar placed around the gastro-eosophageal junction at laparotomy[8] with the aim of correcting gastro-oesophageal reflux relatively simply and without mechanical complications. Although it proved to be very effective in reflux control, the prosthesis was itself subject to a variety of complications, necessitating its removal in 10–17% of patients, which prejudiced its popularity. In 1986, DeMeester and colleagues recommended further modifications to the Nissen fundoplication, including the use of a larger (60 FG) bougie, a shorter (1–2 cm) wrap and division of the short gastric vessels, which resulted in a further diminution in incidence of some of the mechanical complications, and this is the type of Nissen fundoplication most frequently performed at present.[9]

An alternative approach to reducing the mechanical complications associated with total fundoplication was advocated by several workers, with the common principle of combining a partial fundoplication with a valvuloplasty procedure, based on the success of the Belsey Mark IV procedure with its 270° wrap, but with the disadvantage of necessistating thoracotomy. In addition to the Hill procedure, transabdominal partial fundoplication procedures have been described by Lind et al.,[10] Toupet[11] and Watson.[12] All have been shown to produce similar results to total fundoplication in terms of reflux control, but with a lower incidence of mechanical complications demonstrated in several prospective randomized studies. Although the Nissen fundoplication remains the most popular procedure at the present time, there is increasing interest in the partial fundoplication procedures and the concept of 'tailored' antreflux surgery is gaining support,[13,14] with increasing use of these procedures in patients with significant oesophageal dysmotility, in whom it is believed that mechanical complications following total fundoplication are more prevalent.

Finally, in 1991, the first laparoscopic antireflux procedure was reported by Dallemagne,[15] which was a Nissen fundoplication. Since then, each of the principal antireflux procedures has been the subject of published series of its laparoscopic use, many having shown both subjective and objective success in reflux control similar to that at open surgery, but with some shortening of the recovery period. In many early reports, the incidence of troublesome mechanical complications after laparoscopic Nissen fundoplication appears to be more marked than after open surgery,[16,17] which has resulted in a further increase in interest in partial fundoplication procedures.

INDICATIONS FOR ANTIREFLUX SURGERY

The majority of patients with gastro-oesophageal reflux have mild disease and many are not even referred to hospital. Such patients with mild disease often have normal lower oesophageal sphincter characteristics, but exhibit transient relaxations and at least half will not have endoscopic oesophagitis. These patients can usually be managed quite satisfactorily by a combination of life-style changes and pharmacological agents as described in Chapter 9. As the disease severity increases, the proportion of patients with abnormal lower oesophageal sphincter characteristics, including low resting pressure and a short intra-abdominal length, together with disordered oesophageal body 'pump' function increases, as does the incidence of oesophagitis, although, as discussed in Chapter 8, the nature of the refluxate as well as the severity of the pathophysiological defect is an important determinant of the development of oesophagitis. Those patients who have both a severe pathophysiological defect of the antireflux mechanism and those with a significant alkaline component to the refluxate are most likely to progress to the complications of gastro oesophageal reflux disease, including stricture, ulcer and Barrett's columnar-lined oesophagus (CLO). Antireflux surgery is, at present, the only effective way of totally correcting the major pathophysiological defects of lower oesophageal sphincter failure and alkaline reflux.

The principal groups of patients in whom antireflux surgery should be considered are those who are considered to have failed on medical treatment, younger patients who require long-term maintenance treatment with proton pump inhibitors and those developing complications of the disease.

Failed medical treatment

Failure of medical treatment may relate to persistent symptoms, persistent oesophagitis and intolerance of medication.

Persistent symptoms

It is well recognized that there is an imperfect relationship between symptoms and grade of endoscopic oesophagitis[18,19] and in some patients who have mild or even no oesophagitis, the symptoms may be sufficiently severe and uncontrolled by pharmacological means to warrant antireflux surgery. There are three principal groups of patients in whom this situation may arise. The first is those in whom regurgitation is a predominant symptom. These patients often have a mechanically defective cardia, often in association with a hiatal hernia, who may be refluxing a bland refluxate, which may not result in oesophagitis, or even heartburn, but who regurgitate frequently large amounts of fluid, which may be aggravated by bending and stooping and by the supine posture. The second group of patients is those who have been labelled as having a 'sensitive' oesophagus. These patients have very severe heartburn, often in the absence of oesophagitis, and sometimes in the absence of pathological acid exposure on 24 h pH monitoring. In these patients, short-lived reflux episodes within the physiological range may produce dramatic symptoms, and although the majority of these patients will respond to acid suppression, a minority will not. The third group of patients in whom symptoms may be disproportionate to the presence or degree of oesophagitis comprises those with atypical symptoms of gastro-oesophageal reflux such as non-cardiac chest pain, atypical respiratory symptoms and laryngeal symptoms. Again the symptoms may be dramatic and inadequately controlled by pharmacological means.

Persistant oesophagitis

Although omeprazole has been shown to result in healing of endoscopic oesophagitis in 90% of cases,[20] most series have not stratified between the various grades of oesophagitis, and as the minor grades are the most common, it is most likely that these grades comprise the majority of patients in published series. One series which has stratified between various grades of oesophagitis has shown that the healing rate on omeprazole 40 mg daily for 2 months is less than 67% with the more severe grades of oesophagitis.[21] About 82% of all cases relapse within 6 months of treatment, but this proportion can be reduced to 33% at the end of one year if 20 mg of omeprazole is maintained.[22] There are no data about recurrence rates within the different grades of oesophagitis, but it is likely that the more severe grades have a higher recurrence rate and it can be calculated on the basis of available data that approximately 50% of patients with Savary and Miller grade 3 oesophagitis will be unhealed at the end of one year of treatment with omeprazole, using 40 mg daily for 2 months in order to achieve healing and 20 mg daily as maintenance treatment.

Intolerance of medication

Intolerance due to major side-effects of H_2 receptor antagonists and protom pump inhibitors are relatively rare, but do occur. Reported side-effects of H_2 receptor antagonists include diarrhoea, dizziness, rashes and gynaecomastia and rarely blood dyscrasias, hepatocellular damage and confusional states. Similar side-effects have been reported with proton pump inhibitors, although these occur less frequently.

In patients who are intolerant of proton pump inhibitors, it is likely that a proportion of patients with moderate to severe disease may be controlled on H_2 receptor antagonists, but this is in a minority of all cases because of the lesser degree of efficacy. A small proportion of patients referred for surgery exhibit side-effects to both H_2 receptor antagonists and proton pump inhibitors, and in these circumstances, in the presence of severe disease, antireflux surgery can offer complete control.

Failure of medical treatment, therefore, still remains a significant indication for surgery. By looking at various characteristics of reflux patients who have been followed longitudinally, being treated initially by conservative means and with surgery reserved for failure, predicative factors can be identified in those patients not responding to medical treatment, which include manometric evidence of oesophageal sphincter failure, severe 'pump' function impairment, grade 3–4 oesophagitis, very high levels of acid exposure and pathological alkaline exposure[23] (Table 10.1). In addition to these factors, another study has shown that a small subset of patients demonstrate resistance to omeprazole, possibly related to increased enzymic in vivo destruction of the compound and decreased bioavailability.[24] In a study which compared the characteristics of patients referred for antireflux surgery before and after the availability of proton pump inhibitors, 40% had failed to

Table 10.1 Pathophysiological factors influencing response to acid suppression

- LOS failure
- Peristaltic failure
- Grade III–IV oesophagitis
- High acid exposure
- Alkaline exposure

respond to omeprazole.[25] The mean grade of oesophagitis was higher than in the preomeprazole era, as was the incidence of dysphagia associated with concomitant motility disturbances, of lower oesophageal sphincter failure and of alkaline reflux (Table 10.2). These factors demonstrate that those patients not responding to omeprazole comprise the most extreme end of the pathopysiological spectrum of reflux disease. There is some evidence that these resistant patients may achieve symptomatic control by doses of omeprazole up to 120 mg daily for healing and 60 mg daily for maintenance therapy,[26] which may be of practical value in older patients or those with contraindications to surgery. However, such doses result in significant elevation in serum gastrin levels, increased micronodular hyperplasia in the argentaffin cells and increased prevalence of atrophic gastritis, which should signal a cautious approach to long-term treatment at these levels in young patients.

Antireflux surgery as an alternative to long-term maintenance therapy

In patients who can only be maintained in remission by the administration of continuous and life-long proton pump inhibition, antireflux surgery should be considered as an alternative form of maintenance therapy, particularly in younger patients. Arguments in support of this view include concern about the long-term effects of profound acid suppression, the fact that acid suppression does not address the root cause of the problem, the disadvantages and cost consequences of life-long proton pump inhibitor administration and concern that if compliance or bioavailability of acid suppression therapy is less than optimal, the effects of damaging bile salts in the refluxate may be potentiated (see below).

Although serious consequences of hypergastrinaemia, particularly neoplasia, and altered bacterial colonization are largely theoretical or confined to animal studies, nonetheless

Table 10.2 Characteristics of patients referred for antireflux surgery before and after the availability of omeprazole

	PREOMEPRAZOLE	POSTOMEPRAZOLE
Failure of medical treatment (%)	84	39
Concern about long-term medication (%)	8	32
Associated dysphagia (%)	22	53
LOS failure (%)	18	47
Mean % supine time pH<4	3.6	11.6
Alkaline DGR and GOR (%)	14	37

the desirability of life-long virtual anacidity, particularly in young patients, is questionable. As a consequence, many patients and gastroenterologists express some concern at this prospect in young patients, and in the study which compared the characteristics of patients referred for antireflux surgery since the advent of omeprazole, 32% of patients were referred because of concern regarding long-term medication, compared to 8% prior to the availability of omeprazole.[25] Conceptually, antireflux surgery has the advantage of addressing the root cause of the problem, which is not usually gastric hypersecretion, and is the only modality which can completely correct lower oesophageal sphincter failure and alkalkine reflux. These factors may explain the superiority of antireflux surgery over acid suppression in the only published prospective randomized study,[27] although this was using H₂ receptor antagonists, and clearly a similar study has to be repeated using proton pump inhibition. To some patients, the administration of long-term medication is unacceptable, and there are also cost implications. One study has calculated the cost of omeprazole 20 mg daily over a 10-year period at approximately £4250, when the concurrent NHS costing of a laparoscopic antireflux procedure corrected to include treatment costs of the 7% requiring further treatment was £1746.[28] Of particular concern is a study by Kauer et al. using simultaneous ambulatory pH and bilirubin (Bilitec) monitoring which showed that 58% of patients with gastro-oesophageal reflux disease had a mixed acid and alkaline refluxate and 87% of the alkaline exposure occurred in the range pH 4–7.[29] It is within this pH range that some bile salts are in non-ionized form and therefore capable of crossing the cell membrane and causing cellular damage. Therefore, if during acid suppression therapy, the pH lapses into the 4–7 range because of poor compliance or diminished bioavailability, severe mucosal damage may ensue.

There are, therefore, several reasons to consider antireflux surgery as an alternative form of maintenance therapy, particularly in younger patients. The availability of laparoscopic antireflux surgery in centres where good results are being obtained makes antireflux surgery an even more attractive alternative than when performed openly, and, increasingly, patient preference is becoming an indication for surgery in this group of patients. The outcome of prospective randomized studies of proton pump inhibition and antireflux surgery, incorporating economic and quality of life measures are awaited with interest.

Antireflux surgery in complications of gastro-oesophageal reflux disease

Complications of gastro-oesophageal reflux disease, such as Barrett's ulcer, reflux-induced stricture or Barrett's columnar-lined oesphagus are relative indications for antireflux surgery, particularly in young patients. Because these patients represent the most severe end of the pathophysiological spectrum in gastro-oesophageal reflux disease, with a high proportion of the predictive factors mentioned above, pharmacological treatment is less likely to be successful. Athough many patients with reflux stricture are elderly and surgical treatment will be

inappropriate, in younger patients, antireflux surgery has proved superior to high dose H₂ receptor antagonists from the standpoint of reducing dilatation requirement and in resolution of strictures.[30] Similar controlled studies using omeprazole have not, as yet, been reported.

The optimal management of uncomplicated Barrett's CLO is controversial. Many workers advocate no specific treatment in the absence of symptoms and acid suppression therapy in the presence of symptoms or in patients with endoscopic oesophagitis above the columnarized segment. However, many patients with Barrett's CLO are asymptomatic because of impaired or absent sensation of acid exposure[31] and in many Barrett's patients, particularly those with complications, there is frequently a significant degree of alkaline exposure,[29,32] which will not be abolished by acid suppression. Although many patients with Barrett's CLO are elderly and surgical treatment would be inappropriate, in younger patients, this has been shown to be more effective in controlling symptoms and reducing the incidence of complications.[33,34] Antireflux surgery has also been shown to arrest progression of the columnarized segment[35] and is the only form of treatment which has repeatedly shown regression of the columnarized segment, albeit often only partially, and in a minority of patients.[33,34,36,37] However, no study has yet shown that antiflux surgery reduces the incidence of adenocarcinoma. An international prospective randomized study of the effect of optimal conservative therapy, including endoscopic mucosal ablation, and antireflux surgery on the natural history of the columnarized segment, with particular reference to the incidence of adenocarcinoma, is currently being established jointly between the Oesophageal Section of the British Society of Gastroenterology and OESO (Organisation Internationale d'Etudes Statistiques pour les maladies d'Oesophage).

A summary of the indications for antireflux surgery is shown in Table 10.3.

OBJECTIVES OF ANTIREFLUX SURGERY

These can be subdivided into clinical and pathophysiological objectives.

Table 10.3   Indications for antireflux surgery

- Poor response to proton pump inhibitors
  - persistent symptoms
  - persistent oesophagitis
  - regurgitation
  - micro-aspiration

- Young patients with severe disease requiring continuous maintenance therapy

- Intolerance to medication
  - side-effects
  - patient preference

- Complications of GORD
  - unhealed ulcers
  - bleeding
  - stricture in young patients
  - Barrett's columnar lined oesophagus (controversial)

Clinical objectives

The primary aim of treatment of symptomatic gastro-oesophageal reflux disease is clearly to relieve symptoms. However, as with peptic ulcer disease, there is an imperfect correlation between symptoms and endoscopic findings.[18,19] Indeed, patients with the more severe degrees of gastro-oesophageal reflux resulting in complications such as reflux-induced stricture and Barrett's columnar-lined oesophagus often have fewer symptoms than those with erosive oesophagitis,[38,39] which is likely to be due to diminished sensitivity to oesophageal acid perfusion in these patients.[31] As the presence of significant erosive oesophagitis may lead to such complications as ulceration and stricture formation, it is clearly of paramount importance that successful antireflux surgery enables oesophagitis to heal as well as relieving symptoms, in those patients who have endoscopic oesophagitis. Once healed, it is also important that both healing of oesophagitis and symptomatic relief is maintained over the long term, and therefore durability of results is an important objective of antireflux surgery. Finally, it is important that the surgical procedure is not complicated by unwanted side-effects.

Pathophysiological objectives

The principal pathophysiological objective of antireflux surgery is the correction of pathological acid or alkaline exposure to the oesophageal mucosa and in addition to the clinical criteria of success in relief of symptoms and in healing of oesophagitis, restoration of a physiological pH profile is an essential prerequisite for success. In order to achieve this, it is necessary to correct the pathophysiological defect(s) around the cardia, which are responsible for the pathological acid/alkaline exposure, such as excessive transient lower oesophageal sphincter relaxations, a mechanically incompetent cardia or a hiatal hernia. In achieving these objectives, it is essential to ensure that the cardia is not rendered supracompetent, which may result in inability to vent gas and consequent abolition of physiological reflux, impairment of physiological relaxation of the lower oesophageal sphincter on swallowing and the creation of a high pressure zone, the resistance of which may exceed the propulsive force of the oesophageal body, which may already exhibit peristaltic impairment. Such situations are responsible for the principal mechanical complications of antireflux surgery, namely dysphagia, gas-bloat and inability to belch or vomit.

Another pathophysiological objective which receives little attention in the literature, but which is considered to be of importance, is restoration of the distal fixation of the oesophagus. In the normal situation, the oesophagus, and indeed the whole of the gastrointestinal tract, is fixed posteriorly by the dorsal mesentery, and the intra-abdominal oesophagus is fixed anterolaterally by the phreno-oesophageal membrane. Studies have shown that attenuation or loss of these factors is associated with more severe degrees of gastro-oesophageal reflux and associated with peristaltic dysfunction.[40-43] Although loss of the intra-abdominal segment of oesophagus is an important consequence of loss or attenuation of the distal fixation of the

oesophagus, it seems likely that ineffective peristaltic ability of the oesophageal body is an equally important consequence. Therefore, the restoration of distal oesophageal fixation may well be an important objective, which is an integral component of two of the commonly practised antireflux procedures.

MECHANISM OF ACTION OF ANTIREFLUX PROCEDURES

The range of available antireflux procedures is as varied as the complex of factors responsible for competence at the cardia. The various antireflux procedures which have shown to be effective rely to differing degrees on the principal factors in the antireflux mechanism, either augmenting lower oesophageal sphincter pressure or enhancing one or more of the various valvuloplasty components of competence. In this context, it is apposite to review the relative roles of these factors (Table 10.4) (see also Chapter 1).

Lower oesophageal sphincter

Addressing lower oesophageal sphincter (LOS) tone is clearly an important component of the antireflux mechanism. Since its discovery by Fyke et al. in 1956,[44] it has received considerable attention in terms of the various factors modulating its tone and how these may be responsible for impairment of function and predispose towards gastro-oesophageal reflux disease. However, several factors suggest that the lower oesophageal sphincter is but one component of a complex and multifunctional antireflux mechanism. First, it is well recognized that resting lower oesophageal sphincter pressure, in individual cases, correlates poorly with the presence or absence of pathological acid exposure[45] and postoperative measurements of lower oesophageal sphincter pressure also bear an imperfect relationship to correction of reflux.[46] Furthermore, with a normal range of resting lower oesophageal sphincter pressure (LOSP) of 10–25 mmHg, it clearly cannot operate alone in preventing reflux during sudden increases in intra-abdominal pressure such as during coughing or sneezing, when intra-gastric pressure may be as high as 100 mmHg.[47] Studies have shown that whereas 73% of subjects with a resting LOSP less than 6 mmHg have pathological acid exposure, 27% do not[48] and conversely 40–55% of patients with pathological acid exposure have normal LOS characteristics.[42,48] These observations, together with those indicating that a competent antireflux mechanism can be created in the absence of the myogenic influence of the LOS in animals,[49] in humans[50] and even in the autopsy room,[51] indicate clearly that other factors are involved.

Table 10.4 Relevant factors in the antireflux mechanism

FUNCTIONAL	STRUCTURAL
Lower oesophageal sphincter tone 'Peristaltic pump'	Intra-abdominal length Crural diaphragm Angle of His Mucosal rosette Phreno-oesophageal ligament

These include the intra-abdominal segment of oesophagus, the crural sling, the acute angle of implantation (His), the mucosal rosette and the gastric sling fibres, which together comprise the valvuloplasty component of competence. Although for many years, hypotheses supporting the role of these mechanical factors were largely based on theorectical considerations, there is now increasing objective evidence to support the role of these factors.

Intra-abdominal segment of oesophagus

In reflux patients, it has been shown that the level of acid exposure is inversely proportional to the length of the intra-abdominal segment of oesophagus. The probability of reflux is 19% when the length is greater than 2 cm, but rises to 90% when the length is 1 cm or less in the presence of normal lower oesophageal sphincter pressure.[52,53] In an experimental model, DeMeester et al.[54] demonstrated a progressive increase in competence with increasing length of the intra-abdominal segment, reaching 100% competence when the intra-abdominal length was 5 cm, irrespective of other factors, including lower oesophageal sphincter pressure. In the normal situation, the effect of positive intra-abdominal pressure on the intra-abdominal segment maintains apposition of its walls, as shown by the flattened cross-sectional appearance of the oesophagus on CT-scanning.[55] It would appear logical that the greater the length of intra-abdominal segment subject to this phenomenon and accentuated by negative intrathoracic pressure above the diaphragm, the greater the intragastric pressure needed to overcome this mechanism and result in reflux.

Diaphragmatic crural sling

The crural sling has long been felt to be a relevant component of the antireflux mechanism, but it is only relatively recently that objective data have supported this hypothesis. The crural diaphragm has a different embryological derivation from its costal counterpart. Animal studies have shown that the crural diaphragm contracts momentarily before the costal component and causes an increase in resting LOS pressure during inspiration, whereas contraction of the costal component causes a decrease.[56] Simultaneous oesophageal manometry using a perfused sleeve catheter and crural EMG recording in humans has shown that the augmentation of resting LOS pressure which occurs during deep inspiration and increased intra-abdominal pressure is associated with and proportional to the magnitude of crural diaphragmatic contractions.[57] Furthermore, this effect persisted even when the LOS was relaxed by balloon distension, and relaxation of the crural diaphragm was observed during transient lower oesophageal sphincter relaxations. Studies in patients with gastro-oesophageal reflux disease have shown that the augmentation of LOS pressure by the crural diaphragm during deep inspiration is deficient in such patients, particularly in the presence of a hiatal hernia, but is restored by an antireflux procedure which incorporates a crural repair.[58] These studies have shown that during deep inspiration or sudden increases in intra-abdominal pressure such as during coughing or sneezing, pressures of 50–100 mmHg challenge the anti-

reflux mechanism, which would clearly overwhelm a lower oesophageal sphincter with a maximum tone of 25 mmHg if this were the only factor, but in such circumstances a similar level of augmentation of resting LOSP occurs by virtue of crural contraction.

Angle of His and mucosal rosette

The acute angle of implantation is believed to be important in providing the abrupt insertion into the stomach and constant small diameter necessary to enable Laplace's law governing the behaviour of soft tubes to operate.[59] This states that for a given wall tension, the pressure generated within a tube is inversely proportional to its radius. Thus, during raised intragastric pressure, which predisposes to reflux, it would require a massive increase in pressure in the large diameter stomach to overcome distal intra-oesophageal pressure, even in the absence of LOS tone, assuming that the intrinsic pressure on the the two structures was equal (i.e. there was an intra-abdominal oesophageal segment) and that there was an abrupt insertion of oesophagus into the stomach, as in the presence of an acute angle of His. An acute angle of implantation also maximizes the effect of the mucosal rosette or choke, the loose mucosal folds at this site providing a 'mucosal sealing' component to the valvuloplasty when increased intra-abdominal or intragastric pressure results in apposition of the walls of the intra-abdominal oesophageal segment.[55]

Although most research has been concentrated on the sphincteric component of competence, the relatively low values of resting LOS pressure compared to the magnitude of distracting forces applied to the cardia, suggest that the mechanical factors comprising the valvuloplasty component are probably at least as important and can effectively compensate for absence of sphincteric function.[59] This is exemplified by the ability previously referred to, to create a competent antireflux mechanism in the absence of the myogenic influence of the lower oesophageal sphincter. This explains the finding that different antireflux procedures which rely on different degrees of augmentation of the high pressure zone and correction of mechanical factors can be equally successful in control of gastro-oesophageal reflux.

Mode of action of Nissen fundoplication

The most important principle of the Nissen fundoplication is the complete encirclement of the region of the lower oesophageal sphincter by the gastric fundus over a length which has progressively reduced since first described by Nissen, from 4–5 cm to 1–2 cm currently. This results in circumferential compression of the distal oesophagus during raised intragastric pressure when reflux is most likely to occur, and produces a buttressing effect on distensibility of the cardia, which both increases opening pressure[60] and reduces the incidence of transient lower oesophageal sphincter relaxations.[61] There is no doubt that Nissen fundoplication restores resting high pressure zone (HPZ) pressure, which is more accurate than referring to LOS pressure in this context, since a functioning LOS is not necessary to generate this effect. Many studies have shown that the resulting HPZ pressure is considerably higher than preoperatively[61-63] and often higher than in control subjects.[64] Lower oesophageal sphincter vector volume, which is believed to be a more accurate measure of LOS function and correlates better with reflux status, is significantly greater following Nissen fundopliction than in control subjects.[65] Several other studies have alluded to another unphysiological consequence of Nissen fundoplication, namely impairment of relaxation of the LOS on swallowing,[61,62,66,67] the lowest pressure at full relaxation ranging from 2 to 12 mmHg, which is associated with virtual abolition of gas reflux[66] and associated physiological reflux.[65,68]

Thus, there is considerable evidence that Nissen fundoplication produces a supracompetent antireflux mechanism, interfering with normal LOS relaxation on swallowing and with physiological reflux, which is apparent in many published pH studies.

Mode of action of partial fundoplication procedures

The philosophy underlying partial fundoplication procedures is the attempt to achieve reflux control by placing more emphasis on mechanical factors in the antireflux mechanism and less on achieving an extreme degree of competence by augmentation of lower oesophageal sphincter pressure, by reducing the degree of fundoplication. Each of the commonly used partial fundoplication procedures was designed with the aim of minimizing the mechanical complications associated with total fundoplication, without compromising the degree of reflux control by increased emphasis on mechanical factors, and this has turned out to be the case, although simple anatomical repairs without accentuation of the mechanical factors proved unsuccessful.[4]

The Belsey procedure involves a 240° fundoplication, with creation of a long intra-abdominal segment of oesophagus and a posterior buttress created by approximation of the two limbs of the crural sling. The principle of providing a buttress for the portion of the intra-abdominal oesophagus uncovered by the partial fundoplication is an important one. In total fundoplication, the intra-abdominal segment is completely buttressed by the surrounding gastric fundus. In partial fundoplication procedures, the creation of a buttress against which the uncovered portion of intra-abdominal oesophagus can be compressed during increased intragastric pressure has been shown to prevent bulging of the uncovered portion and consequent loss of valvular function and competence which would otherwise occur.[69] However, the fact that the intra-abdominal segment is not circumferentially squeezed during raised intragastric pressure means that normal eructation and indeed normal physiological reflux can occur.

The Hill repair relies principally on intra-abdominal fixation of the cardia to the median arcuate ligament of the diaphragm and augmentation of the effect of the lower oesophageal sphincter by plication of the cardia to a varying degree, calibration being controlled by intraoperative manometry. Although the procedure does not specifically describe the creation of a long intra-abdominal segment of oesophagus, fixation of the cardia to the median arcuate ligament is believed to be important not only in ensuring its exposure to positive intra-abdominal pressure and creation of a valvuloplasty effect, but also to enable more effective oesophageal body peristalsis by restoring the normal distal fixation of the cardia. There is no fundoplication component described to the repair, although fixation of the anterior and posterior phreno-oesophageal bundles to the median arcuate ligament does result in a short segment of oesophagus being partially covered by gastric fundus.

The Toupet fundoplication comprises a 180° posterior partial fundoplication, with fixation of the wrap to each limb of the crural sling over a length of 2–3 cm. This results in maintenance of the cardia within the abdomen, restoration of distal fixation of the cardia and ensures an acute angle of implantation. The partial fundoplication ensures some augmentation of LOS function during raised intragastric pressure, although the anterior aspect of the intra-abdominal oesophagus is unbuttressed, despite which the repair produces equivalent reflux control to Nissen fundoplication,[70,71] emphasizing the importance of mechanical factors in competence.

The 'physiological' antireflux procedure described by Watson[72] was designed with the specific aim of correcting and accentuating each of the known physical factors relevant to the antireflux mechanism and minimizing the fundoplication to 120° in an attempt to provide effective reflux control whilst preserving physiological LOS function, in order to obviate mechanical complications. The procedure involves creation of a 5 cm segment of intra-abdominal oesophagus by blunt transhiatal dissection. The limbs of crural sling are then opposed routinely, for three reasons. The first is because of the known influence of the crural sling on competence, its diminished influence in reflux patients and its restorability by crural repair.[57,58] The second is to provide an easily accessible structure to which the long intra-abdominal segment can be fixed and maintained, and thirdly to provide a posterior buttress for the intra-abdominal segment during raised intragastric pressure. The angle of implantation is rendered extremely acute to enhance the valvuloplasty effect, and finally the 120° anterolateral fundoplication produces augmentation of LOS function during gastric distension. This procedure has been studied in considerable detail, and at operation, when the stomach is distended by insufflating air down a nasogastric tube, the fundus is seen to distend so that the whole anterior aspect of the intra-abdominal oesophageal segment is covered by gastric fundus and buttressed against the crural repair, but normal gas venting can occur. When studied manometrically, LOS characteristics including resting pressure, intra-abdominal length and particularly relaxation on swallowing are comparable to physiological levels, unlike after Nissen fundoplication, which is believed to account for the extremely low incidence of mechanical complications associated with the 'physiological' repair.

PREOPERATIVE ASSESSMENT FOR ANTIREFLUX SURGERY

Most patients will, by the time of referral for surgery, have had an accurate diagnosis made, although this may, in some circumstances, need to be verified. It is particularly important in patients who fail to respond to proton pump inhibitors that the diagnosis of gastro-oesophageal reflux disease is unequivocally made. If the history is typical and there is clear endoscopic evidence of oesophagitis, in the absence of any other cause such as drug ingestion, then further confirmatory tests are not mandatory, although most specialist units would, in practice, perform pH monitoring as a baseline for subsequent postoperative pH studies to confirm effective reflux control. However, up to 30% of patients requiring antireflux surgery will have no endoscopic oesophagitis and in these circumstances, pH monitoring is mandatory, as it is unwise to operate without some objective confirmation of the diagnosis. Patients with atypical symptoms of gastro-oesophageal reflux disease, such as non-cardiac chest pain and respiratory or laryngeal symptoms frequently fall into this category and it is vital where there is neither a typical history nor endoscopic oesophagitis that the diagnosis is substantiated. It needs to be remembered, however, that pH monitoring is a marker of acid reflux only, and in around 20% of patients with demonstrable endoscopic eosophagitis, the level of intraoesophageal acid exposure will be within the normal range.[73] This does not mean necessarily that no pathological reflux is occurring, but rather that the pH of the reflux may be greater than 4, which can occur if there is an alkaline component to the refluxate, which is now known to be present in 58% of reflux patients.[29] Therefore, if gastro-oesophageal reflux disease is strongly suggested in the presence of a normal endoscopy and normal pH monitoring, an alkaline refluxate should be sought either by simultaneous oesophageal and gastric pH monitoring or preferably by ambulatory bilirubin (Bilitec) monitoring.

The role of oesophageal manometry in the preoperative assessment of patients undergoing antireflux surgery is, to some extent, controversial, but nonetheless it is conducted in most specialist units. The most important role of oesophageal manometry in this context is to ensure that there is not a primary motility disorder of the oesophagus, particularly achalasia, in which circumstances, antiflux surgery would inevitably result in severe dysphagia. Patients with achalasia frequently complain of reflux-type symptoms and indeed pH monitoring has shown that around 40% of patients with achalasia have pathological acid exposure.[74] Manometry is the only reliable means of diagnosing achalasia and although the incidence of this in patients referred for antireflux surgery is relatively low, an inappropriate operation in such circumstances is a disaster, which will inevitably lead to the need for revisional surgery and a dissatisfied patient.

A more frequent association between gastro-oesophageal reflux disease and oesophageal motility disorders is that of the so-called secondary motility disorders, occurring in approximately 40% of reflux patients. These comprise a mixture of peristaltic abnormalities, including low amplitude peristalsis, particularly in the lower third of the oesophagus, occasionally high amplitude peristalsis, simultaneous, non-propagated peristalsis and the complex known as non-specific motility disorder. Controversy exists as to whether these disorders are truly secondary to gastro-oesophageal reflux or a predisposing

condition because of impaired peristaltic efficacy, resulting in diminution or loss of the secondary peristalsis mechanism. Some series report reversal of motility abnormalities after fundoplication, suggesting that they may be secondary to reflux[67,75] but others report no change, suggesting that they are a primary phenomenon.[76] This controversy has extended into debate about whether patients with significantly disordered oesophageal body peristalsis should undergo total fundoplication on the basis that they are at greater risk of developing mechanical complications, thus making preoperative manometry mandatory in the decision-making process, as to whether a total or partial fundoplication procedure should be performed. This concept has both protagonists[77–80] and antagonists,[81,82] but in the practical setting, there is increasing support for the concept of 'tailored' antireflux surgery, whereby the 60% or so of patients with normal oesophageal body motility are offered total fundoplication and those with impaired motility undergo a partial fundoplication procedure, in the belief that these patients are at greater risk of development of mechanical complications, which is significantly reduced by this approach.[13,14,83] Such an approach is predicted on the hypothesis that total fundoplication is the better approach for reflux control and should be offered to those at least risk of mechanical complications, but it should be noted that firstly three prospective randomized studies have shown equivalent reflux control with partial fundoplication procedures (see below) and secondly, it is well recognized that those patients with gastro-oesophageal reflux disease and motility disturbances comprise the most severe group of refluxers, whether measured by the level of acid exposure[42] or grade of oesophagitis.[41,52] The fact that the 'tailored' approach to antireflux surgery has not led to any diminution in efficacy of reflux control in those series which have employed this, reversing partial fundoplication for the most severe group of refluxers, militates against the perceived superiority of total fundoplication in reflux control. Preoperative assessment for antireflux surgery is summarized in Table 10.5.

OPERATIVE TECHNIQUE OF ANTIREFLUX PROCEDURES

Antireflux procedures are divisible into total fundoplication procedures, partial fundoplication procedures and prosthetic

---

Table 10.5 Preoperative assessment for antireflux surgery

- Accurate history
- Endoscopy
- pH monitoring
  - no oesophagitis
  - atypical symptoms
- Manometry
  - pH probe placement
  - exclusion of primary motility disorder
  - ? influence decision re-Antireflux Surgery

Table 10.6 Antireflux procedures

TOTAL FUNDOPLICATION	PARTIAL FUNDOPLICATION	PROSTHETIC INSERTION
Nissen	Hill	Angelchik
Rosetti–Hell	Toupet	
	Watson	
	Lind	
	Belsey	

insertion (Table 10.6). Each of the commonly performed antireflux procedures may be conducted using a minimally invasive approach, and this is described separately.

Approach to and exposure of the oesophagus

Before each of the trans-abdominal antireflux procedures, the principles of access and exposure of the distal oesophagus and hiatal region are similar. It is of vital importance in the safe conduct of effective antireflux surgery that the hiatal region and its component structures are carefully and clearly exposed. Access is usually by an upper midline incision between the sternum and the umbilicus, which may be extended superiorly along the left border of the sternum or inferiorly around and below the umbilicus, if necessary. Effective liver retraction is necessary, particularly of the left lobe. Some workers advocate division of the left triangular ligament and retraction of the folded left lobe towards the right lateral side of the upper abdomen. Alternatively, the left lobe can be retracted superiorly. Access to the hiatal region may be enhanced considerably by the use of a Goligher sternal-elevating retractor and by using some 20° of anti-Trendelenberg tilt. Exposure of the anterior aspect of the intra-abdominal oesophagus is achieved by dividing the phreno-oesophageal ligament, together with the contiguous structures which are the anterior layer of the gastrohepatic omentum on the right and the phrenogastric ligament on the left (Figure 10.1). It is the author's preference to commence dissection at the phreno-oesophageal ligament, although some prefer to commence to the right of the oesophagus through the anterior layer of the gastrohepatic omentum. There are several important technical points in this stage of exposure. Firstly, there may be vessels running just beneath the phreno-oesophageal ligament, which are best divided, ensuring that the anterior wall of the oesophagus is not damaged by diathermy. Secondly, the hepatic branch of the anterior vagus nerve traverses the anterior layer of the gastrohepatic omentum and this should be preserved. Thirdly, there is occasionally an aberrant hepatic artery crossing the anterior aspect of the gastrohepatic omentum, having arisen directly from the coeliac axis, and this vessel, when present, should be preserved to obviate the risk of segmental hepatic infarction. Once the anterior aspect of the oesophagus has been exposed, blunt dissection of the loose areolar tissue on either side of the oesophagus, extending posterolaterally, exposes the plane between the oesophagus and the two limbs

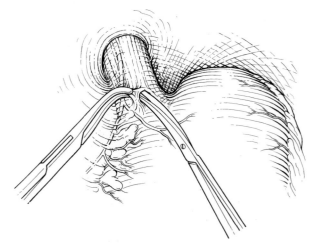

Figure 10.1
Exposure of the anterior aspect of the oesophagus is commenced by incision of the phreno-oesophageal ligament.

of the crural sling. The plane posterior to the oesophagus is then developed by blunt dissection, which is extended proximally through the oesophageal hiatus to the posterior mediastinum and distally to be decussation of the limbs of the crural sling in front of the abdominal aorta. Loose areolar tissue may also need to be divided by blunt dissection on the anterolateral aspect of the oesophagus superiorly, between the oesophagus and the reflected phreno-oesophageal ligament. During exposure and mobilization of the oesophagus, it is important to preserve the vagus nerves. The anterior vagus nerve and some of its terminal branches lie closely applied to the musculature of the anterior aspect of the oesophagus, whereas the posterior vagal trunk lies in areolar tissue 2–3 mm away from the posterior oesophageal musculature. Once the oesophagus has been exposed and mobilized, a sling of latex or silastic is passed around the posterior aspect of the oesophagus (Figure 10.2), preferably with the posterior vagal trunk

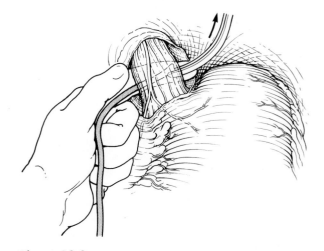

Figure 10.2
Once the plane behind the oesophagus has been achieved, a silastic sling is passed around the oesophagus to aid subsequent retraction.

between the sling and the oeosophagus, and the two ends of the sling are held between a clamp anteriorly in order to provide anterior and downward retraction on the oesophagus.

In situations where an anatomical hiatal hernia is present, the phreno-oesophageal ligament is often attenuated and the trans-hiatal dissection is performed around the margins of the hernia. Reduction is usually very straightforward and once this has been done and the plane behind the oesophagus achieved by blunt dissection, exposure of the intra-abdominal oesophagus and crural sling continues as described above.

Once the oesophagus has been exposed and mobilized and the crural sling exposed and held via a sling, any of the trans-abdominal antireflux procedures can now be performed, and the length of intra-abdominal oesophagus can be increased to the desired length by continuing the trans-hiatal dissection, by a combination of sharp and blunt dissection, as necessary. This process is facilitated by gentle retraction of the oesophagus using either a Kocher's retractor, or a specially designed retractor for this purpose. If necessary, some of the small vessels supplying the oesophagus within the posterior mediastinum may be coagulated or clipped.

Total fundoplication procedures

Nissen fundoplication

The majority of workers advocate thorough mobilization of the gastric fundus by division of the short gastric vessels, in order to achieve a loose, floppy wrap, with the aim of reducing the incidence of mechanical complications. Division of the short gastric vessels is usually started superiorly at the gastrosplenic ligament where the most proximal vessels pass between the fundus and the splenic hilum. Moving distally, the gastroepiploic mesentery is arranged in anterior and posterior leaves, each containing vessels, and it is preferable to divide and ligate each individually, in order to avoid bunching and compromising the length and mobility of the fundus.

Approximation of the limbs of the crural sling is somewhat controversial in Nissen fundoplication. It did not form part of the original description of the procedure by Nissen[5] nor of the 'floppy' modification by Donahue and Bombeck.[6] However, many prefer to incorporate this manoeuvre in order to reduce the incidence of proximal migration of the fundoplication into the mediastinum (see below). If performed, crural approximation is achieved by retracting the oesophagus anteriorly, and by commencing just above the inferior decussation of the limbs of the crural sling, a series of three or four interrupted sutures of 0 or 2/0 silk sutures are tied loosely so as to avoid either cutting out or strangulation of the muscle. It is important that the closure does not extend too far proximally as to unduly narrow the oesophageal hiatus, and it should be possible to insert the tip of an index finger between the oesophagus and hiatus, otherwise dysphagia will result.

Prior to constructing the fundoplication, a bougie (size 50–60 FG depending on operator preference) is passed by the anaesthetist and its distal position guided by the operating surgeon. Some workers meticulously dissect off the fat-pad from the anterior aspect of the gastro-oesophageal junction,

although there is no evidence to support the necessity for this, and it frequently results in troublesome oozing from small vessels or damage to branches of the anterior vagal fibres. The freed posterior wall of the gastric fundus is passed posteriorly in the plane between the posterior aspect of the oesophagus and the crural sling (Figure 10.3), and the anterior wall of the mobilized fundus is pulled across the anterior wall of the oesophagus, so that the two walls can be opposed close to the midline of the anterior aspect of the oesophagus (Figure 10.4). The length of the opposed anterior and posterior walls has become progressively reduced, from some 4 cm in length when the procedure was first described, most workers currently advocating a short wrap of 1–2 cm in an attempt to reduce the incidence of mechanical complications. Approximation is achieved either by two or three interrupted non-absorbable sutures, such as silk or prolene, or using a single horizontal mattress suture placed over teflon pledgets as described by DeMeester.[9] The tension should be sufficiently lax as to enable passage of the index finger between the wrap and the oesophagus containing a bougie. Some workers advocate the placement of a suture between the wrap and the anterior aspect of the oesophagus in order to maintain its position.

Rosetti–Hell fundoplication

This modification of Nissen fundoplication was described by Rosetti and Hell.[85] It involves the use of the anterior aspect of the gastric fundus only, bringing the superomedial part of this around the back of the oesophagus, over the anterior aspect of the oesophagus and placing sutures between it and the anterior aspect of the gastric fundus adjacent to the left side of the oesophagus. The degree of fundal mobility necessary to achieve this type of fundoplication is much less than that described above, and advocates of this procedure do not

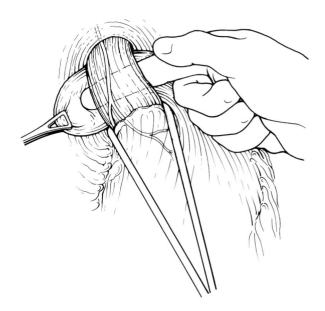

Figure 10.3

Nissen fundoplication. The mobilized posterior wall of the gastric fundus is passed posteriorly in the plane between the posterior aspect of the oesophagus and the crural sling.

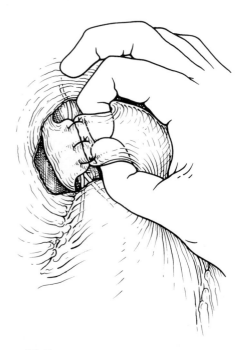

Figure 10.4
Nissen fundoplication. The anterior wall of the mobilized gastric fundus has been pulled across the anterior wall of the oesophagus and the two walls loosely apposed such that an index finger will easily pass between the wrap and the oesophagus.

At this stage, the limbs of the crural sling are loosely approximated, as described previously (Figure 10.6). Babcock clamps are then placed on the anterior and posterior phreno-oesophageal bundles to permit the posterior wall of the stomach, including the seromuscular layer, to be visualized. A fixation suture is placed through the posterior phreno-oesophageal bundle and passed through the preaortic fascia. Care must be taken to avoid damage to the posterior vagus nerve. A suture is then placed deep in the anterior phreno-oesophageal bundle, taking care to avoid the anterior vagus nerve. This suture is carried deeper through the posterior phreno-oesophageal bundle and beneath the median arcuate ligament (Figure 10.7). Two or more additional imbricating sutures are placed deeper through the anterior and posterior phreno-oesophageal bundles, including the seromuscular layer of the stomach, and are carried beneath the median arcuate ligament. The first imbricating suture is tied, and at this stage, intraoperative measurement of lower oesophageal sphincter pressure is made. If the suture has been correctly placed, the tension it creates tightens the oesophageal hiatus such that resting lower oesophageal sphincter pressure is at least 40 mmHg. If this pressure is not reached, an additional imbricating suture is placed, and if the pressure is too high, the initial suture is loosened. The remaining sutures are tied, which securely anchor the oesophagogastric junction to the preaortic

routinely divide the short gastric vessels, unless this appears necessary in individual cases. The wrap is secured with three or four interrupted sutures over a length of 2.5–4 cm.

Partial fundoplication procedures

Hill median arcuate ligament repair

After exposure of the oesophagus and hiatal region as previously described, the proximal few short gastric vessels are divided in order to provide some mobility to the gastric fundus. The proximal part of the stomach is then rotated anticlockwise in order to visualize the posterior phreno-oesophageal bundle, which includes the posterior seromuscular layer of the stomach. The stomach is then retracted to the patient's left, exposing the pre-aortic fascia. The coeliac axis and aorta are identified by palpation, and the coeliac nerve plexus, lying superficial to the coeliac axis is exposed. The median arcuate ligament is palpated by depressing the aorta posteriorly along with the coeliac axis. After dissecting the fibro-areolar tissue off the coeliac axis, the coeliac plexus is retraced caudally. Dissection should be confined to the midline, as a branch goes from each side of the coeliac axis to the diaphragmatic crura. Once the nerve and fibro-areolar tissue have been dissected from the coeliac axis, the median arcuate ligament can be readily visualized. It is elevated from the coeliac axis and a Goodall cervical dilator placed beneath the median arcuate ligament (Figure 10.5). The dilator should pass proximally with ease if the correct plane is entered. Any attempt to exert pressure may cause damage to the aorta, coeliac axis or plexus.

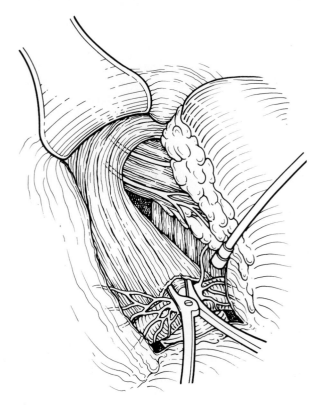

Figure 10.5
Hill repair. The proximal part of the stomach has been rotated anticlockwise and the stomach retracted to the left, exposing the preaortic fissure. The coeliac nerve plexus lying superficial to the coeliac access and the median arcuate ligament have been displayed.

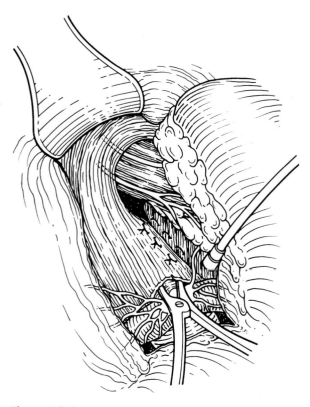

Figure 10.6
Hill repair. Crural repair has been performed whilst elevating the median arcuate ligament by a Goodall cervical dilator.

fascia and the median arcuate ligament, and the 3 cm segment of intra-abdominal oesophagus is visualized. Further measurements of lower oesophageal sphincter pressure are made to ensure that the final pressure is 40–50 mmHg, which equates to 15–25 mmHg at standard laboratory manometry. The tension of the sutures is adjusted appropriately if the level is outside this range, and this process has been described as 'calibration of the cardia', which is an integral part of the Hill repair, as is distal fixation of the cardia.

Although the whole repair is an effective antireflux procedure, its disadvantages are that it is technically difficult to perform, with risk of damage to the coeliac axis and coeliac plexus, and intraoperative manometry is necessary.

Toupet posterior partial fundoplication

This procedure involves a posterior hemifundoplication, leaving the anterior aspect of the oesophagus uncovered and unbuttressed. Mobilization of the gastric fundus is not as extensive as during total fundoplication, and is usually confined to division of the gastrosplenic ligament and the vessels contained therein. The fundus is passed behind the mobilized oesophagus, but only enough fundus is used to reach the right lateral aspect of the oesophagus. Four rows of sutures are used. These comprise two interrupted sutures on each side between the posterolateral aspect of the mobilized fundus and the right and left limbs of the crural sling, (Figure 10.8). Two further layers of three interrupted sutures are used to oppose

the anterolateral aspect of the mobilized fundus to the antero-lateral aspect of the oesophagus on each side (Figure 10.9). The length of the partial fundoplication is usually 2–3 cm.

'Physiological' anterolateral (Watson) fundoplication

This is the most recently described antireflux procedure, being first described in 1984[12] and designed with the specific aim of achieving as effective reflux control as total fundoplication but minimizing mechanical complications, utilizing available knowledge which has accumulated in respect of relevant components of the antireflux mechanism, the pathophysiology of fundoplication and of mechanical complications. The philosophy underpinning the procedure, which was subsequently confirmed in clinical studies,[72] was that by restoring and accentuating the various factors which have been shown to be relevant to the antireflux mechanism, total fundoplication could be avoided without detriment to the efficacy of reflux control, and the incidence of mechanical complications reduced by creating a more physiological high pressure zone. The principles utilized are the achievement of a long intra-abdominal segment of oesophagus, accentuating the angle of His and opposing the limbs of the crural sling in all cases. This latter manoeuvre is believed to be important firstly in utilizing the role of a 'snug' crural sling in competence, secondly to provide a strong and easily identifiable structure to which the intra-abdominal oesophagus may be fixed and thirdly to provide a structure

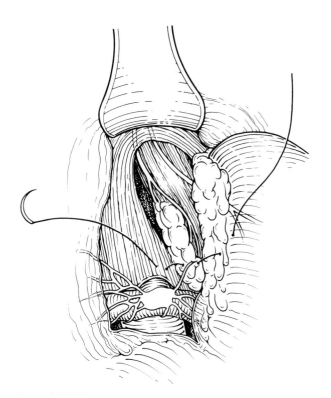

Figure 10.7
The Hill posterior gastropexy. The median arcuate ligament is elevated by the forceps, beneath which lies the coeliac plexus. The anterior and posterior phreno-oesophageal bundles are being sutures to the median arcuate ligament.

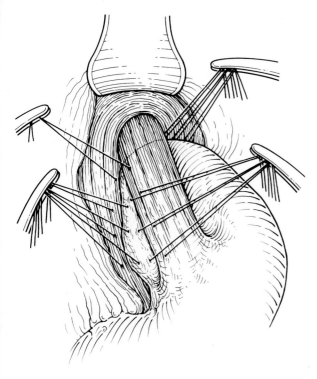

Figure 10.8
Toupet procedure. The gastric fundus has been passed behind the posterior aspect of the oesophagus and the first two layers of sutures inserted between the fundus and the right limb of the crural sling and the fundus and right margin of the oesophagus.

Exposure of the oesophagus and cardia is as described previously, although particular attention is paid to achieving at least 5 cm of intra-abdominal oesophagus (Figure 10.10). This is readily achievable, except when fibrotic shortening is present, by extending the trans-hiatal dissection more proximally in the mediastinum, which at open operation is performed by blunt dissection as in trans-hiatal oesophagectomy, but at laparoscopy can be performed under direct vision. Once achieved, the intra-abdominal segment, together with the posterior vagal nerve, is retracted anteriorly, using a Kocher's or specially designed retractor to expose the crural sling, which is very often attenuated to some degree even in the absence of an anatomical hiatal hernia (Figure 10.11). The limbs of the crural sling are then opposed with interrupted 2–0 silk sutures, tied relatively loosely; three or four sutures are usually adequate. A bougie is not required. Care should be taken to ensure that the tip of an index finger can pass comfortably alongside the oesophagus through the oesophageal hiatus. After tying these sutures, the needles are retained, and used to suture the posterolateral aspect of the oesophagus to the crural repair (Figure 10.12). These sutures should incorporate the muscular layers of the oesophagus only, and again should be tied relatively loosely in order to avoid cutting or necrosis of the muscle. These sutures are placed from above downwards and retraction of the oesophagus gradually relaxed as each suture is placed (Figure 10.13).

In performing the anterolateral fundoplication, because of

against which the portion of intra-abdominal oesophagus uncovered by fundus can be buttressed during raised intragastric pressure.

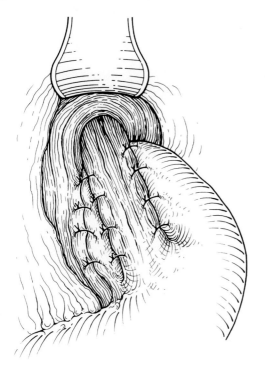

Figure 10.9
Toupet fundoplication. The completed procedure.

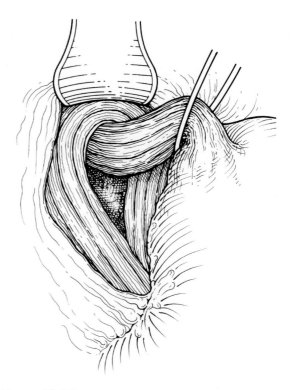

Figure 10.10
'Physiological' anterolateral (Watson) fundoplication. The crural sling has been exposed and a 5 cm segment of intra-abdominal oesophagus achieved by blunt trans-hiatal dissection.

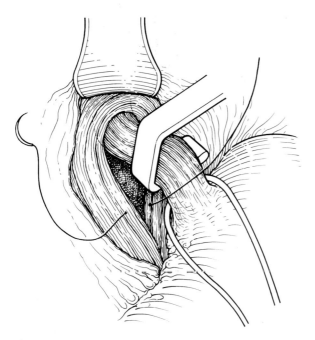

Figure 10.11
'Physiological' anterolateral (Watson) fundoplication. The oesophagus is retracted anteriorly and a posterior crural repair commenced.

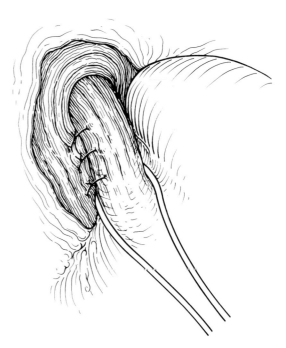

Figure 10.13
'Physiological' anterolateral (Watson) fundoplication. The intra-abdominal oesophagus has been fixed to the posterior crural repair.

the limited nature of the wrap, no mobilization of the fundus is necessary. The most superomedial point of the gastric fundus is initially sutured to the crural diaphragm by two interrupted silk sutures, the first being at the mid-point of the arch of the

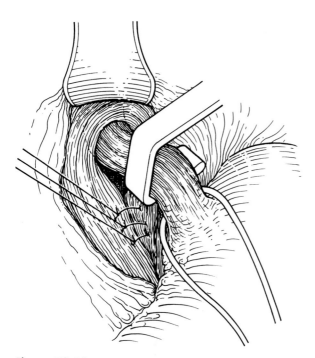

Figure 10.12
'Physiological' anterolateral (Watson) fundoplication. The posterior crural repair has been commenced, the needles having been retained on the three interrupted sutures in order to fix the long intra-abdominal segment to the crural repair.

crural sling over the oesophagus, and the second just lateral to that. These two sutures result in a very acute angle of His and bring the medial aspect of the fundus into line with the anterior aspect of the oesophagus, in preparation for the fundoplication sutures. A point on the anterior aspect of the oesophagus is selected for the row of usually four interrupted sutures to suture the medial aspect of the gastric fundus to the anterolateral aspect of the oesophagus, usually to the right of the midline, such that the anterior vagus nerve is not damaged and a small segment of the right anterolateral aspect of the oesophagus is left uncovered. The interrupted sutures are placed between the suture in the crural arch and the region of the fat-pad, such that the length of the partial fundoplication equates to the length of the intra-abdominal oesophagus (Figure 10.14). It has been observed that when the nasogastric tube is insufflated with air intraoperatively, resulting in increased intragastric pressure, the fundus distends to cover the entire anterior aspect of the intra-abdominal oesophagus and buttress it against the crural sling repair, returning to its former position on deflation. Technical advantages of this procedure are that division of the short gastric vessels and passage of a bougie are not required. It is relatively easy and expeditious to perform, and fixation of the cardia can be achieved to a structure which is easily identified and does not incur a risk of damage to other structures. Possible disadvantages are the number of sutures necessary, which is less than required in the Toupet procedure and more than compensated for by the time saved in not having to fully mobilize the fundus in total fundoplication. There is a theoretical risk of mucosal damage by the intraoesophageal sutures, but this does not appear to be a problem in practice.

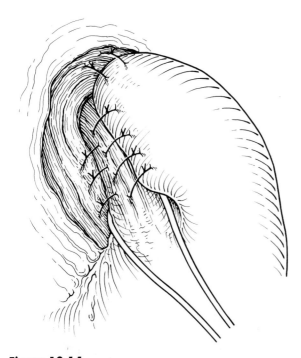

Figure 10.14

'Physiological' anterolateral (Watson) fundoplication. The completed procedure.

Lind partial fundoplication procedure

This is not a commonly practised procedure, but was a procedure used in one of the important prospective randomized studies of partial versus total fundoplication.[84] It consists of both anterior and posterior partial fundoplication, of 300° in all, leaving a 60° bare area on the anterior aspect of the oesophagus. A bougie is not used routinely and proponents of this procedure usually divide the short gastric vessels selectively, when it is felt that a 300° wrap cannot be achieved without tension. Three rows of interrupted sutures are used, one on each side between the fundus and each lateral aspect of the oesophagus, with a third layer between the most anterior part of the fundus and the anterior aspect of the oesophagus.

Belsey Mark IV fundoplication

This procedure is performed transthoracically, and consequently is used predominantly by thoracic surgeons. It is claimed by its originator that thoracotomy is necessary to achieve adequate mobilization of the oesophagus to the level of the aortic arch, which may have been true at the time of its description in 1967, when antisecretory drugs were not available and a high proportion of cases requiring surgery had complications, particularly significant oesophageal shortening. Access is through a left posterolateral thoracotomy incision through the sixth intercostal space. Once into the mediastinum, the oesophagus is mobilized from the level of the diaphragm to the aortic arch, care being taken to preserve the vagal nerves. It is necessary to divide and ligate the left superior and inferior bronchial arteries and the oesophageal vessels coming directly from the distal thoracic aorta. The cardia and hiatal

hernia (if present) are then freed from the diaphragm. With experience, this can be performed without making an incision in the central tendon or enlarging the oesophageal hiatus. Entry into the peritoneal cavity is achieved by division of the phreno-oesophageal ligament. This is the key to achieving the correct plane from which to be able fully to mobilize the cardia by a combination of blunt and sharp dissection. When all the attachments between the cardia and hiatus have been divided, the fundus and body of the stomach are then drawn up through the hiatus into the mediastinum. In order to achieve this, it is necessary to divide most, if not all of the short gastric vessels. The fat-pad is usually dissected free, as described under Nissen fundoplication. The objective is to produce a 270° partial fundoplication around the anterior two thirds of the lower 3–4 cm of the oesophagus. The partial wrap is held in place by two rows of three mattress sutures placed equidistantly between the seromuscular layers of the stomach and the muscular layers of the oesophagus. A posterior buttress is constructed by a series of interrupted sutures through the limbs of the crural sling (Figure 10.15). The first row of mattress sutures is placed 1.5 cm above the cardia and tied loosely just to obtain tissue apposition. It is necessary to rotate the oesophagus to the left in order to place the right anterolateral suture sufficiently to the right. A second row of sutures is placed 1.5–2 cm above the first row, using the previously placed sutures in the first row as a guide to position (Figure 10.16). Once again, the sutures are tied so as just to achieve tissue apposition without strangulation. Needles are retained on these sutures and passed 0.5 cm distant from each other through the diaphragm from abdominal to mediastinal surface, 1–1.5 cm from the edge of the hiatus. The diaphragmatic sutures are placed at the 4, 8 and 12 o'clock positions, orientated with the 6 o'clock position placed posteriorly between the right and left limbs of the crural sling, just anterior to the aorta. Care must be taken when placing these sutures in order to avoid injury to

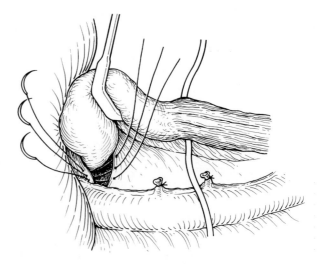

Figure 10.15

Belsey-Mark IV repair. The posterior buttress is created by placing interrupted sutures between the limbs of the crural sling, which are not tied at this stage.

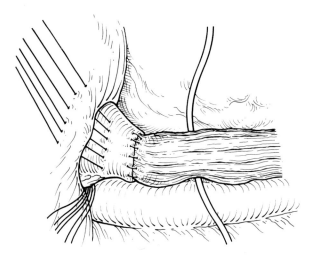

Figure 10.16
Belsey–Mark IV repair. The three mattress sutures of the second row have been placed but not tied.

the abdominal structures; this may be achieved by using a spoon retractor.

The reconstructed cardia is gently pushed through the hiatus and placed in the abdomen, manually manoeuvring the fundal wrap through the hiatus. Once in the abdomen, the cardia remains there without tension on the holding sutures. Once the repair sits comfortably within the abdomen, the previously placed crural sutures are tied. The holding sutures are then tied, approximating the knot against the previously tied knot now located under the diaphragm, so as to avoid redundancy in the suture between the repair and the diaphragm. The final remaining stitch to the diaphragm is sufficient to hold the cardia in position.

The principal disadvantages of the Belsey repair are that it requires a thoracotomy to achieve, and it is technically a difficult procedure, having gone through three technical modifications since it was first described. Other than surgeon preference among thoracic surgeons, there can be no particular advantage of performing an antireflux procedure via a thoracotomy in the majority of cases, because of the greater metabolic insult, increased incidence of respiratory complications, prolonged hospital stay and convalescence and the risk of post-thoracotomy pain. The vast majority of antireflux surgery can be performed very adequately by a transabdominal or minimally invasive route, although some workers prefer the transthoracic approach in certain complex situations. These include the presence of gross oesophageal shortening, a fixed hiatal hernia, the presence of gross obesity and for revisional antireflux surgery.

Prosthetic insertion

Despite the general principle in surgery that artificial materials should only be implanted where there is no satisfactory alternative approach, prosthetic insertion, and particularly the use of the Angelchik prosthesis achieved a period of popularity because of its relative ease of performance, and a belief among many of its advocates that despite the availability of several

traditional antireflux procedures, there was still room for improvement.

Insertion of Angelchik prosthesis

The Angelchik prosthesis is a C-shaped silicone elastomer shell filled with silicone gel. It is held in place by a polyster-reinforced Dacron tape, which contains a radio-opaque marker. After mobilizing the hiatal area and oesophagus as described previously, the prosthesis is passed behind the oesophagus so that the open part of the 'C' lies anteriorly (Figure 10.17a). The tapes are tied and the knot may be retained in place with a ligaclip. The procedure is performed over a bougie, and the prosthesis should be loosely tied such that a finger can easily be passed between the oesophagus and the prosthesis (Figure 10.17b). Crural repair does not form an integral part of the procedure, although some surgeons perform this either selectively or routinely.

The principal advantage of the Angelchik prosthesis is that it is relatively easy to perform and is an effective antireflux procedure. However, there have been many complications associated with the procedure, including severe dysphagia due principally to angulation and migration of the prosthesis, either within the peritoneal cavity, or, less commonly, into the gastrointestinal tract. As a consequence of these problems, the early re-operation rate was 10–17%[86,87] and a recently published long-term study showed that eventually, 25% had to be

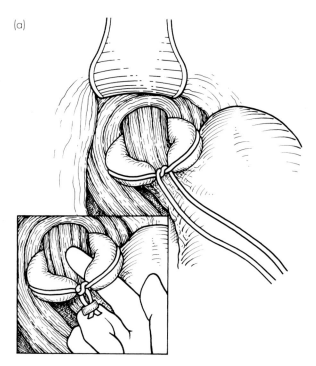

(a)

Figure 10.17
(a) Angelchik prosthesis. After achievement of the plane behind the oesophagus, the prosthesis is placed behind, so that the open 'C' and the tapes lie anteriorly. (b) The tapes have been tied and the knot secured with a Liga-clip. It should be possible to pass an index finger between the prosthesis and the oesophagus.

removed.[88] For these reasons, the procedure has largely fallen into disrepute.

POSTOPERATIVE MANAGEMENT FOLLOWING ANTIREFLUX SURGERY

It is the author's practice not to use a nasogastric tube postoperatively and to commence small amounts of clear fluids as soon as the patient is awake. Oral fluid intake is gradually increased over 48 h, and when adequate amounts of fluid are taken by mouth, intravenous fluids are discontinued and a soft diet is commenced, usually on the third day. Patients are counselled about the likelihood of some transient dysphagia for extremes of solids during the first 2 or 3 weeks until perioperative oedema has resolved, and are advised to adhere to a soft diet within that period. Patients are discharged home on the fourth or fifth day, with dissolvable subcuticular skin sutures. Most advocates of total fundoplication employ a nasogastric tube, as there is a greater risk of gastric dilatation with such procedures. DeMeester advocates retaining a nasogastric tube for 5 days following which a barium swallow is performed to ensure free transit across the cardia prior to commencing diet.[9]

RESULTS OF ANTIREFLUX SURGERY

In assessing the results of antireflux surgery, it is pertinent to consider its level of success in fulfilling the clinical and pathophysiological objectives referred to previously, how these results compare with medical treatment when surgery is offered as an alternative for maintainence therapy, comparison of results between the various antireflux procedures and the complications associated with antireflux surgery.

In terms of fulfilment of clinical and pathophysiological objectives, much more information is now available with an increasing number of good prospective studies and increased emphasis on objective as well as symptomatic criteria for success. In general terms, results from specialist units relating to reflux control currently report symptomatic improvement (Visick grades 1 and 2) around 90%, correction of pathological acid exposure on pH monitoring in around 85% and healing of endoscopic oesophagitis in 85–90% of patients for most of the commonly performed procedures.

With regard to Nissen fundoplication, DeMeester et al.[9] reported 91% success in control of reflux symptoms in 100 patients with no evidence of stricture or significant motility disturbance, representing 49% of patients undergoing Nissen fundoplication over a 12-year period. Median follow-up was 3 years, three patients being followed to 10 years. pH monitoring was performed in just over one third of patients, of whom 83% had a normal pH profile. In a group of 40 patients undergoing Nissen fundoplication who were all followed for 5 years, with independent symptomatic assessment and endoscopy as well as pH monitoring, 80% of patients were Visick grades 1–2, the patients being equally divided between the two grades.[66] Of the patients with endoscopic oesophagitis, healing occurred in 82%. pH monitoring was normal in 92% of 36 patients studied, the results being similar at 6 months and 5 years.

Similar results in terms of reflux control have been reported

after partial fundoplication procedures. Belsey[89] reported a symptomatic success rate of 90%, although this was reduced to 75% at 10 years. Hill et al.[40] have reported 88% symptomatic satisfaction up to 20 years after the Hill repair. Lundell et al.[70] studied the Toupet procedure up to 5 years in 72 patients and found this to be effective in reflux control as defined by clinical and endoscopic parameters in 94% of patients. pH monitoring was performed and acid exposure for all patients was within the physiological range and comparable to a similar group of patients studied following Nissen fundoplication, although the actual percentage of patients with abnormal acid exposure was not stated. The Watson 'physiological' procedure has been studied by symptomatic scoring by a non-surgical observer, endoscopy, manometry and 24 h pH monitoring in 100 patients.[72] Symptomatic satisfaction occurred in 96%, 85% being Visick 1. Healing of endoscopic oesophagitis occurred in 86% and restoration to physiological acid exposure in 84% (Table 10.7). These were short-term studies, although long-term clinical studies in 452 patients operated on over a 15-year period revealed a re-operation rate of only 3.8% for recurrent, troublesome reflux. A recent study in another institution confirmed objective durability, with pH profile at 5 years comparable with that after Nissen fundoplication.[89a]

Complications of antireflux surgery

Antireflux procedures are currently associated with low mortality of 1% or less and a relatively low, but variable incidence of complications. There is a small incidence (less than 5%) of chest and wound complications, although this is higher if a transthoracic procedure is performed. Complications directly related to the antireflux procedure vary depending on the procedure performed. Nissen fundoplication is most frequently associated with mechanical complications because of the completely circumferential wrap, the degree of tension which may be associated with this and the effect on lower oesophageal sphincter characteristics, particularly the ability to relax on swallowing. Complications which require re-operation include slippage, where the wrap migrates distally to encircle the stomach, resulting in an 'hourglass' obstruction of the stomach proximal to the wrap,[90,91] disruption, where the wrap becomes undone, resulting in recurrent reflux[90,92] and proximal migration of the wrap or the development of a paraoesophageal hernia, associated with tension and absence of distal fixation and crural repair.[93] Intrathoracic fundoplication appears to be a particularly dangerous situation, with the risk of gastric ulceration

---

Table 10.7 'Physiological' antireflux procedure: clinical results

	SYMPTOMATIC IMPROVEMENT (%)	SYMPTOMATIC CURE (%)	HEALING OF OESOPHAGITIS (%)	NORMAL pH PROFILE (%)
'Physiological'	94	82	86	84
Range of results: reported for Nissen fundoplication	65–96	32–80	63–91	67–85

and potentially fatal intrathoracic rupture of the wrap.[94] Technical modifications, including crural repair where the hiatus is unduly large and the production of a loose, floppy wrap with increased mobilization of the greater curve of the stomach has reduced the incidence of some of these complications, although some series still report disruption rates of 7%[92] and greater curve mobilization brings its own attendant risk of splenic trauma, the incidence of incidental splenectomy during Nissen fundoplication being reported at 7–10%.[95]

In addition to these rather dramatic, but relatively uncommon complications which usually require corrective surgery, there is a series of more subtle mechanical complications of a functional nature, associated with the production of a supracompetent cardia with impaired relaxation, and therefore most frequently associated with Nissen fundoplication. These include the gas-bloat syndrome, which should be defined as troublesome bloating which was not present preoperatively, and which occurs in up to 25% of patients postoperatively.[96] Troublesome persistent dysphagia, requiring either dilatation, significant dietary modification and occasionally re-operation occurs in up to 10% of patients after Nissen fundoplication. It should be noted that a degree of transient dysphagia lasting 2–4 weeks after surgery and believed to be due to oedema is relatively common after all antireflux procedures but this resolves spontaneously and adherence to a soft diet during this time should obviate problems. Dysphagia which persists beyond 6 weeks postoperatively is unlikely to resolve spontaneously and usually requires attention. Where re-operative surgery is required, usually after Nissen fundoplication, most authors recommend taking down the fundoplication and converting to one of the partial fundoplication procedures.[90,91,97] Other mechanical complications include inability to belch or to vomit which are more frequent sequelae of Nissen fundoplication than gas-bloat or dysphagia (Table 10.8).[9] Severe gas-bloat occasionally necessitates revisional surgery[70] although for the most part, these particular complications are usually managed conservatively.

The occurrence of these mechanical complications, which are predominantly associated with Nissen fundoplication, has resulted in a series of modifications to the technique as described previously. In the series of DeMeester et al.,[9] the incorporation of a very loose, short wrap with adequate mobilization of the short gastric vessels resulted in reduction of the incidence of gas-bloat from 15% to 11% and of troublesome dysphagia from 14% to 3%, but inability to belch or vomit

Table 10.9 Complications of Nissen fundoplication

MECHANICAL	FUNCTIONAL
Slippage	Dysphagia
Disruption	Gas-bloat
Proximal migration	Inability to belch
Splenic damage	Inability to vomit

remained unchanged at 36% and 63%, respectively. These complications are extremely uncommon with partial fundoplication procedures[40,70–72] (Table 10.9). It should be borne in mind that the quality of life following antireflux surgery can only be improved when the symptoms of reflux are eliminated without the production of postoperative symptoms created by the procedure itself.[98]

Controlled trials in antireflux surgery

A large number of longitudinal studies has suggested firstly that a well-conducted partial fundoplication procedure is as effective as Nissen fundoplication in control of reflux and secondly that mechanical postoperative complications are greater after Nissen fundoplication. However, there is undoubtedly a prejudice among enthusiasts of Nissen fundoplication that partial fundoplication procedures are less effective and less durable than the Nissen procedure, largely because of the reported long-term failure following the anatomical repair of Allison[4] which, unlike many current antireflux procedures, did not address the valvuloplasty factors in the antireflux mechanism. Prospective randomized control trials are the only way to replace prejudice by objectivity, and four have been reported. The first was conducted by DeMeester et al.[99] colleagues over 20 years ago, which studied only short-term reflux control and found the Nissen to be superior to the Hill and Belsey procedures. It is noteworthy that only 15 patients were randomized to each arm and all the operative procedures were performed by residents, which is in conflict with the more modern belief that antireflux surgery is a specialist activity and should be performed by experts in order to obtain the best results. Two prospective randomized studies have compared Nissen fundoplication with the Toupet procedure. Thor and colleagues performed a small study, randomizing 31 patients but following for 5 years and documenting the incidence of mechanical complications as well as reflux control.[71] Reflux control was similar in both groups, although because of a higher incidence of mechanical complications in the Nissen group, some requiring re-operation, overall good or excellent results occurred in 67% compared to 95% following the Toupet procedure. In a much larger study comparing the Rossetti–Hell modification of Nissen fundoplication with the Toupet procedure, Lundell et al.[70] randomized 137 patients and documented reflux control and mechanical complications to five years.[70] Both procedures controlled reflux equally well with 94% objective durability, but both early and late mechanical complications were significantly greater in the Nissen group. About 9% required re-operation, mostly because of intrathoracic migration of the wrap, despite crural repair being selectively performed. Walker et al.[84]

Table 10.8 'Physiological' antireflux procedure: mechanical complications

	GAS-BLOAT (%)	INABILITY TO BELCH/VOMIT (%)	TRANSIENT DYSPHAGIA (%)	TROUBLESOME DYSPHAGIA (%)
'Physiological'	0	0	11	2
Range of results: reported for Nissen fundoplication	11–54	5–63	19–86	4–24

randomized 52 patients between Nissen fundoplication and a Lind partial fundoplication procedure. Once more, symptomatic and objective reflux control was equivalent with both procedures. Although they reported no statistically significant advantage from either procedure, the authors found that dysphagia and gas-bloat occurred more frequently and persisted longer after Nissen fundoplication. In a subsequent follow-up at 10 years, there was a mild deterioration in satisfactory control of reflux symptoms in both groups, but in the Nissen group alone there was a significant deterioration in reflux control measured by pH monitoring.[100]

On the balance of evidence from prospective randomized studies, therefore, it is apparent firstly that partial fundoplication procedures are at least as effective and durable as Nissen fundoplication and secondly they are associated with a lower incidence of mechanical complications and consequently a lower incidence of re-operation. In spite of these factors, Nissen fundoplication is the most commonly performed antireflux procedure, which is perhaps surprising in this era of evidence-based medicine.

Comparison of medical and surgical treatment of gastro-oesophageal reflux disease

It may seem inappropriate to compare the results of medical and surgical treatment of gastro-oesophageal reflux disease, since the majority of patients can be effectively controlled by conservative means, at least on symptomatic evaluation. However, the question becomes relevant first, if other endpoints than symptomatic satisfaction are considered as criteria of success and second, in considering how the best interests may be served in patients who require continuous life-long medical treatment in order to maintain symptomatic remission.

The imperfect correlation between symptoms and endoscopic oesophagitis has been referred to, and data are beginning to emerge on the natural history of oesophagitis treated conservatively. In one study in which 25 patients with grade 2–3 reflux oesophagitis were followed-up after a mean of 38 months on medical treatment, three patients (12%) developed Barrett's oesophagus and five patients (10%) had grade 2 oesophagitis. pH monitoring in 19 patients showed that two had changed from a normal to an abnormal pH profile, three had changed from abnormal to normal and 14 were abnormal on both occasions.[101]

In a non-randomized study of 105 patients with endoscopic oesophagitis, 37 who failed to respond adequately to acid suppression with H$_2$ receptor antagonists or omeprazole underwent antireflux surgery.[102] At long-term follow-up with a mean of 11 years, 84% of those undergoing antireflux surgery had either no heartburn or experienced it only very occasionally and 11% had oesophagitis, the corresponding figures being 53% and 55%, respectively, in the medically treated group. However, Barrett's oesophagus was subsequently diagnosed in 15% of patients, being equally distributed between both treatment groups. In a prospective randomized study of 247 predominantly male veterans with erosive oesophagitis, including

ulcer, stricture and Barrett's CLO, antireflux surgery was compared with conservative treatment, which including H$_2$ receptor antagonists and prokinetic drugs (but not proton pump inhibitors), antireflux surgery was significantly more effective in controlling symptoms and healing of oesophagitis.[27] Similar studies involving proton pump inhibitors are currently in progress.

Therefore, there is a suggestion that antireflux surgery may offer more effective reflux control than conservative treatment, particularly in the presence of severe disease, which probably reflects the permanent and constant nature of reflux control which is independent of compliance, together with the fact that in patients with lower oesophageal sphincter failure and a significant alkaline refluxate, only antireflux surgery can totally correct these problems. However, randomized studies comparing the best conservative treatment with the best in antireflux surgery, with quality of life analysis are necessary to provide a definitive answer and these studies are currently in progress.

LAPAROSCOPIC ANTIREFLUX SURGERY

It was inevitable that the advantages accruing from laparoscopic cholecystectomy in terms of reduced metabolic upset, diminished wound and respiratory complications, short hospital stay and early return to normal activity would be applied to antireflux surgery, and in 1991, Dallemagne reported the first laparoscopic Nissen fundoplication.[15] Since then, many series have been published describing most of the commonly performed procedures adapted to a laparoscopic approach. These series, which cumulatively have totalled many thousands of patients, show that the benefits of shorter hospital stay and early return to normal activity remain valid, although a little less marked than after laparoscopic cholecystectomy, since the ratio of trauma of access compared to trauma of the surgical procedure, is less. Furthermore, the potential for major complications is higher and the 'learning curve' steeper, emphasizing the necessity for expertise both in oesophageal surgery and laparoscopic surgery, together with formal training in laparscopic antireflux surgery.

Operative technique

The principles of access and exposure of the hiatal region are similar, whichever antireflux procedure is performed. The patient is positioned with the hips gently flexed using Lloyd Davis stirrups, and with about 30° of anti-Trendelenberg tilt (Figure 10.18). Most surgeons position themselves between the patient's legs; a typical operating theatre layout is shown in Figure 10.19. Five ports are utilized, a supraumbilical one for the telescope, a left subcostal port in the anterior axillary line for retraction of the stomach and subsequent sling retraction of the oesophagus, right and left subcostal ports in the midclavicular line for dissection and suturing and a subxyphoid port for the liver retractor (Figure 10.20). Once pneumoperitoneum has been established to a pressure of 10–12 mmHg, the left lobe of the liver is retracted using an inflatable fan retractor or a Nathenson retractor, and the proximal stomach is retracted distally using an atraumatic forceps inserted through the left

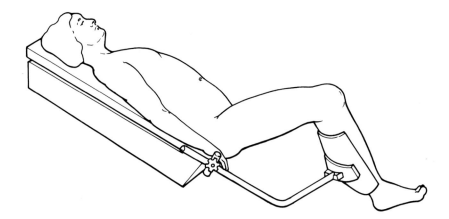

Figure 10.18

Laparoscopic antireflux surgery. The patient is positioned with the hips gently flexed using Lloyd–Davis stirrups, with about 30° of anti-Trendelenberg tilt, the operating surgeon is standing between the legs of the patient.

lateral subcostal port. Although dissection may commence as in the open procedure by division of the phreno-oesophageal ligament and exposure of the plane between the oesophagus and the right and left limbs of the crural sling, many workers believe that the risk of oesophageal trauma is minimized by commencing dissection in the gastrohepatic omentum above

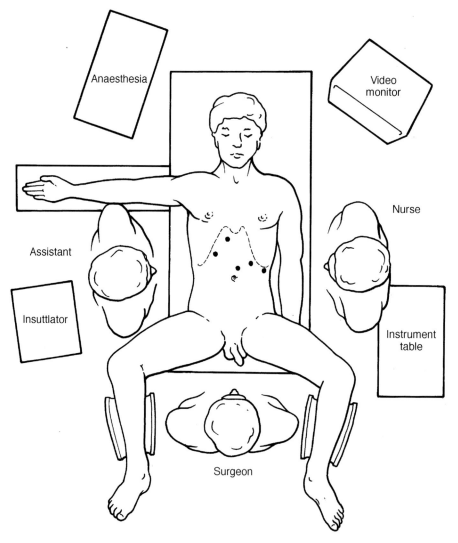

Figure 10.19

A typical layout of equipment and personnel for laparoscopic antireflux surgery.

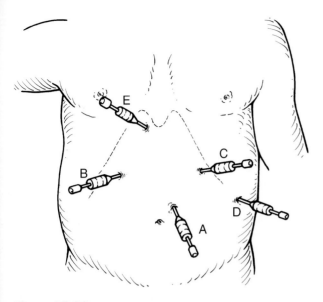

Figure 10.20
Port placement for laparoscopic antireflux surgery. A, camera;
B and C, operating ports; D, port for initial retraction of cardia
and subsequent sling retraction of the oesophagus; E, port for
liver retractor

the hepatic branch of the vagus nerve, exposing the right limb
of the crural sling and dividing the peritoneum along the
length of the limb until the decussation of the right and left
limbs is seen inferiorly, at which level a posterior window is
created behind the cardia and a sling passed around the
oesophagus, which is now retracted by the forceps previously
retracting the proximal stomach. The peritoneum is then
incised along the length of the left limb of the crural sling and
planes are developed between the oesophagus and each limb
of the crural sling, and posteriorly the oesophageal window is
enlarged by a combination of blunt and sharp dissection,
under direct vision. The phreno-oesophageal ligament is then
divided if not done so initially, so that the oesophagus is fully
mobilized. The steps of the various antireflux procedures are
then performed as in the open approach. In those procedures
where a long intra-abdominal segment is a major feature, such
as the Watson fundoplication, the trans-hiatal dissection and
mobilization performed bluntly at open operation can be performed under direct vision well into the mediastinum to ensure
that an intra-abdominal segment can be achieved, which is at
least as long as obtained by the open approach. Crural repair
may be performed exactly as in the open approach, and in
Nissen fundoplication, division of the short gastric vessels can
be achieved either by division between clips using an automatic clip applier, or simply divided using a harmonic scalpel.

Complications of laparoscopic antireflux surgery

The complications of laparoscopic antireflux surgery include
those complications previously described following open
antireflux surgery, complications of laparoscopy, including
haemorrhage, visceral perforation and cardiovascular complications, and those specific to laparoscopic fundoplication. The

latter include pneumothorax, especially on the left side during
completion of the posterior oesophageal window, the risk of
which is minimized by commencing dissection at the level of
the decussation of the right and left limbs of the crural sling.
Perforation of both the oesophagus and proximal stomach
have been reported, sometimes with a fatal outcome, the risk
being increased when there is dense perioesophagitis. In those
procedures, particularly Nissen fundoplication, where insertion
of a bougie is necessary, bougie perforation has been reported,
due to diminished ability of the operating surgeon to guide the
distal tip of the bougie as it is passed from above. As a result
of these complications, most of the published series have
reported perioperative morbidity of 8–15%, compared to 4–5%
after open surgery, although with increasing experience, this
figure appears to be diminishing.

It is noteworthy that when performed laparoscopically,
Nissen fundoplication appears to be associated with a higher
incidence both of proximal wrap migration and of troublesome
dysphagia than is the case at open operation. The incidence of
proximal wrap migration requiring re-operation has been
reported at between 1 and 7%,[17,103] which has been attributed
possibly to the larger posterior oesophageal window necessary
to bring the fundus posterior to the oesophagus laparoscopically, and to earlier mobilization after surgery. Troublesome
dysphagia requiring re-operation has been reported to be
1–3%.[16,103] Peters et al.[17] compared the results of laparoscopic
with open Nissen fundoplication in a non-randomized study.
They found comparable results in terms of reflux control, but a
threefold incidence of troublesome dysphagia in the laparoscopic group (9% versus 3%), with only one third of patients in
the laparoscopic group exhibiting normal high pressure zone
relaxation. Possible reasons for this increased incidence of
troublesome dysphagia include inadequate fundal mobilization,
use of the anterior gastric wall and altered geometry in terms
of performing the fundoplication with laparoscopic instruments
some distance from the fundus, resulting in some obliquity in
the fundoplication, placing traction forces on the wrap.[104]
Where dysphagia is sufficiently severe to require re-operation,
conversion into one of the partial fundoplication procedures is
generally recommended.[97,103] Interestingly, in the laparoscopic
context, division of the short gastric vessels has been shown
not to influence the incidence of troublesome dysphagia and
other mechanical complications in a prospective randomized
study performed by Jamieson et al.[105]

Results of laparoscopic fundoplication

Although the results of randomized and long-term studies are
awaited, most short-term non-randomized studies report symptomatic and objective reflux control in over 90% of cases and a
shorter hospital stay and earlier return to normal activity than is
traditionally reported in open series. However, perioperative
morbidity and re-operation rate is higher for the reasons
described previously (Table 10.10).

In one of the larger series of laparoscopic Nissen fundoplication, Hinder et al.[106] reported 198 cases with one death (0.5%),
morbidity 5%, and re-operation rate 1.5%. Syptomatic relief was

Table 10.10 Large published series of laparoscopic fundoplication

	CUSCHIERI (1993)[107]	JAMIESON (1994)[16]	HINDER (1994)[106]	ANVARI (1995)[114]	GOTLEY (1996)[103]
Number	116	155	198	168	200
Mortality (%)	0	0.7	0.5	0	0
Morbidity (%)	13	15	7.5	9	8
Re-operation (%)	0	7	3.5	2.5	3
Median hospital stay (days)	2	4	3	3	3
Return to work (weeks)	–	2	3	–	–
Symptomatic success (%)	91	97	97	92	93
Physiological pH profile (%)	–	100	87	98	–

obtained in 92% and restoration to a physiological pH profile occurred in 87%. Median hospital stay was 3 days and median return to work 3 weeks. However, 31% experienced mild or moderate dysphagia at late assessment at 6–32 months. The incidence of gas-bloat was 36%. Cuschieri et al.[107] reported 116 patients in a multicentre study in which 80 underwent Nissen fundoplication and 36 a Toupet partial fundoplication. There was no mortality and morbidity was 13%. Clinical and objective success in reflux control was over 90%. Of the 14 patients (13%) who developed mechanical complications of troublesome dysphagia or gas-bloat, 13 patients were in the Nissen group. In a non-randomized study, McKernan[108] compared the Nissen and Toupet procedures, and found equivalent reflux control, but a 14% incidence of troublesome dysphagia in the Nissen group; no patients in the Toupet group experienced mechanical complications. In a similar study, Bell et al.[109] compared the Nissen–Rosetti with the Toupet procedure, finding significantly higher incidence of troublesome mechanical complications, predominantly dysphagia, in the Nissen–Rosetti group. Re-operation was necessary in half the patients with troublesome mechanical complications, conversion from Nissen–Rosetti to Toupet resulting in complete resolution of symptoms. In a preliminary study of the first 26 patients undergoing the laparoscopic Watson procedure, 91% had documented symptomatic and objective success by pH monitoring.[110] There was no gas-bloat or inability to belch or vomit and no dysphagia lasting beyond two weeks. Lower oesophageal sphincter characteristics, including resting pressure, ability to relax and intra-abdominal length were compar-able both with controls and with values obtained in patients undergoing the open procedure. These results have been maintained in 84 patients treated subsequently. Similar results have been reported by Krukowski and Munro (personal communication).

The apparent increase in mechanical complications following laparoscopic Nissen fundoplication over and above the incidence at open operation has led both to advocation of the 'tailored' approach to laparoscopic antireflux surgery as previously described and an increased deployment of partial fundoplication procedures. In Liege, Belgium, where laparoscopic antireflux surgery started, the incidence of partial fundoplication procedures has increased from 1% in 1992 to 13% in 1993 and 33% in 1994.[97] Prospective randomized trials of laparoscopic total and partial fundoplication procedures are currently

in progress and the results are awaited with interest. Preliminary results are available from a randomized study between laparoscopic Nissen fundoplication and on anterior partial fundoplication similar to the Watson procedure. Reflux control was similar, but the incidence of troublesome dysphagia was higher in the Nissen group and overall patient satisfaction was lower. The Nissen group had greater impairment of LOS relaxation, higher levels of resting OSP and prolonged oesophageal emptying time.[97a]

Laparoscopic antireflux surgery, particularly when performed by experts in specialist centres, offers an attractive approach to long-term management of severe gastro-oesophageal reflux disease, particularly in patients refractory to medical treatment. However, it also offers a more attractive option to open antireflux surgery in young patients who need continuous medical therapy, particularly at high dosage, and increasingly since the advent of laparoscopic reflux surgery, patient preference is becoming an indication for surgery in this group. Prospective randomized studies are in progress in such patients, in which quality of life and health economic outcomes are being studied. It seems likely that laparoscopic antireflux surgery will have an advantage in the latter parameter, as 10 years of maintainance therapy on 20 mg omeprazole daily currently costs over £4000 and at current NHS costs of laparoscopic antireflux surgery, the break-even point is at approximately 3 years of treatment (including treatment of recurrences).[28] However, in countries where hospitalization is more expensive, the cost advantage may be less apparent.[28]

In terms of suitability for a laparoscopic approach in those patients in whom antireflux surgery is indicated, the vast majority of patients are suitable. Contraindications include those of laparoscopy in general, such as pregnancy, bleeding diatheses and extensive previous upper abdominal surgery. Conversion rates in the literature from laparoscopic to open approach range from 0 to 15% and in general terms, the lower the conversion rate the higher the rate of complications, although this is not necessarily the case in experienced hands as the conversion rate is decreasing with increasing experience. Reasons for conversion include extensive perioesophagitis, oesophageal shortening such as associated with reflux stricture, large fixed hiatal herniae, previous hiatal surgery and gross obesity. Many would advocate an open approach in these circumstances, or at least advise patients of the significant likelihood of conversion if an attempt at a laparoscopic approach is preferred.

A mature approach to laparoscopic antireflux surgery offers a real alternative to life-long medication, which addresses the root cause of the problem and preserves normal gastric acid secretion. Before this stage is reached, it is essential that we establish firstly which antireflux procedure offers the best results in terms of efficacy of reflux control, durability, freedom from mechanical complications and overall improvement in quality of life. This will set the scene for a prospective randomized study in eligible patients requiring long-term maintenance therapy, between the best of laparoscopic antireflux surgery and the best of conservative treatment, encompassing independent assessment, quality of life and health economic outcomes.

These studies should be of sufficient duration in order to establish which approach has the greatest influence on the natural history of the disease in the long term.

TREATMENT OF FAILURES FOLLOWING ANTIREFLUX SURGERY

Revisional surgery for failed antireflux procedures is required in the event of recurrent reflux uncontrolled by medical means or complications of the initial antireflux procedure which are sufficiently severe as to require remedial surgery. The former indication is common to a small proportion of patients irrespective of the primary antireflux procedure, but the latter relate predominantly to Nissen fundoplication or prosthetic insertion, the latter being rarely performed nowadays.

Skinner[80] reviewed 117 patients undergoing revisional antireflux surgery over a 16-year period and evolved a classification of the reasons for revisional surgery. These comprised sphincter mechanism failure leading to recurrent reflux, oesophageal clearance failure, a combination of both of these, alkaline reflux and non-reflux causes arising out of an incorrect diagnosis or other complications of the fundoplication. Recurrent gastro-oesophageal reflux disease was present in 55% of their patients and clearance failure in 52%, 37% having both disorders. About 18% of patients had no reflux present, but complications of the initial antireflux procedure.

Low et al.[95] reviewed 305 patients undergoing revisional antireflux surgery a mean of 51.4 months after the primary procedure, although the mean interval before onset of symptoms was only 12.8 months. Recurrent reflux was again the most common indication for revisional surgery in 65% of patients, most of the remainder having severe dysphagia and 6% having intrathoracic migration of Nissen fundoplication, half of whom had developed a gastric ulcer in the wrap, which occasionally perforated and penetrated into contiguous structures.

In terms of the primary operation, Nissen fundoplication was commonest in both series, accounting for 57% in Skinner's series, no other procedure accounting for more than 13%. There are relatively few series which specifically address the frequency of necessity for revisional surgery to correct recurrent gastro-oesophageal reflux disease in a large cohort of patients with long follow-up. In Skinner's series of 298 patients undergoing primary antireflux surgery, 6% of patients undergoing Nissen fundoplication and 2% of those undergoing Belsey partial fundoplication required surgical correction of recurrent reflux.[80] If the indication for primary surgery was stricture, the overall incidence rose to 9.6%. O'Hanrahan et al.[92] also reported a 6% incidence of revisional surgery for recurrent reflux in 125 patients undergoing Nissen fundoplication. In 452 patients reported by Watson et al. having undergone a 'physiological' partial fundoplication procedure, median follow-up was 6 years with a maximum of 15 years and the incidence of revisional surgery for recurrent reflux was 4%.[46] Where the indication for revisional surgery is dysphagia or other mechanical problems, the vast majority of patients in both Skinner's and Low's series had undergone Nissen fundoplication as the primary procedure. In Skinner's series, clearance failure with dysphagia was present in 86% of patients with a failed Nissen, compared to 32% after other procedures, including partial fundoplication and insertion of Angelchik prosthesis. In Low's series, 60% of patients having previously undergone Nissen fundoplication had dysphagia and 40% had manometrically diagnosed dysmotility which had not been present preoperatively. The complications of slippage, intrathoracic migration and gastric ulceration were specific to Nissen fundoplication.

In the era of laparoscopic antireflux surgery, mechanical complications have overtaken recurrent reflux as the major indication for revisional surgery, reflecting principally the higher incidence of mechanical complications following laparoscopic Nissen fundoplication referred to previously. In a series of 26 cases of laparscopic fundoplication requiring revisional surgery reported by Dallemagne et al.[97] 35% required revisional surgery for recurrent reflux, compared to 54% for severe dysphagia. In 65% of cases, the first operation was Nissen fundoplication, and indeed the complication of wrap migration and severe dysphagia have been referred to as 'Nissen-specific' complications, as they are relatively uncommon after other procedures. The incidence of re-operation following laparoscopic Nissen fundoplication in large series varies between 1.5 and 7%,[93,103,106] which is considerably higher than after open operation. Where severe dysphagia is the indication for revisional surgery, most workers recommend conversion to a partial fundoplication procedure, particularly where impaired oesophageal body motility is present.[97,103] Of four series reporting laparoscopic partial fundoplication procedures, there has been no incidence of revisional surgery for correction of mechanical complications, and reflux control has been equivalent to that reported following laparoscopic Nissen fundoplication.[107-110] Prospective randomized studies between laparoscopic partial and total fundoplication procedures are currently in progress.

Surgical approach to revisional antireflux surgery

The majority of published data relate to open antireflux surgery, and indeed most, but not all workers would recommend that revisional surgery after failed laparoscopic antireflux surgery should be approached by open operation. Both Skinner[80] and Little et al.[112] recommend a transthoracic approach, in order to achieve greater mobility of the oesophagus, particularly if more than one procedure has been performed previously. If there is difficulty in achieving a sufficient length of mobilized oesophagus to give a tension-free repair, then a Collis gastroplasty should be performed (see Chapter 11). However, if the primary repair has been performed laparoscopically, which results in minimal adhesion formation, it is reasonable to approach at least the first revisional procedure transabdominally.

Factors influencing the choice of revisional procedure include the reason for failure according to Skinner's[80] classification, the number of previous surgical procedures and the extent of functional oesophageal damage. It is therefore of paramount importance to perform a full functional evaluation of such patients, including endoscopy, manometry, pH monitoring and preferably acid secretory status, Bilitec monitoring and gastric emptying studies. Any associated gastric hypersecretion and impairment of gastric emptying need to be addressed as part of the revisional procedure.

If the reason for failure is recurrent reflux in the presence of good oesophageal body function, it is reasonable to perform the repair of choice based on individual preference, particularly if there is evidence of disruption or inadequacy of the primary repair. However, if there is significant functional impairment of the oesophageal body, as is frequently the case after Nissen fundoplication, then most authorities recommend that the revisional procedure should be a partial fundoplication procedure, obviously checking for over-tightness of the hiatus and correcting this, if present. Purely mechanical complications resulting in obstructive symptoms should be managed similarly, and other mechanical complications of slippage or transthoracic migration of a Nissen fundoplication require attention to the specific abnormality, with no absolute necessity to modify the initial antireflux procedure, although if these complications occurred once, it may be more logical to perform an antireflux procedure which carries only a minimal risk of these complications. In particularly resistant patients, who have had several operative procedures, and particularly where there is evidence of gross peristaltic failure, transhiatal oesophagectomy or resection with colonic replacement may provide the only chance of a successful outcome.

When alkaline reflux is an indication for revisional surgery, careful assessment is necessary in relation to the type of symptoms experienced and the presence of significant antral alkaline gastritis. If duodenogastric and gastro-oesophageal alkaline reflux are detected by Bilitec monitoring, and there is no significant antral gastritis and associated symptoms of nausea, epigastric discomfort and occasional bile vomiting, then attention should be directed towards performing an effective antireflux procedure. If the latter complex is present, then a bile-diversion procedure in the form of a Roux-en-Y duodenal diversion should be performed with an efferent loop 60 cm in length. Such a procedure has been advocated as a routine in the management of failure following antireflux surgery on the basis that both acid and alkaline reflux are obviated when performed with a vagotomy or antrectomy, without involvement in the dense adhesions in the hiatal region,[113] but it has largely fallen into disrupte as an option in this context, as it fails to prevent regurgitation of gastric contents. However, good results follow its use in conjunction with revisional antireflux surgery in the circumstances described above.

Results of revisional antireflux surgery

The results of revisional antireflux surgery depend on the number of previous antireflux procedures, the degree of loss of oesophageal functional reserve and the complexity of the revisional procedure required. Little et al.[112] classified results according to whether patients had undergone one, two or more than three previous repairs. Good and excellent results were achieved in 85%, 66% and 42%, respectively, and corresponding morbidity was 27%, 26% and 75%, respectively. Mortality increased with the number of previous operations also reflecting both increased complexity and greater incidence of resection and interposition from 3% in patients with one previous operation, to 5% with two previous operations and 30% with three or more previous operations.

These results emphasize the importance of obtaining as high a success rate as possible with the primary antireflux procedure. The hallmarks of success include careful patient selection and preoperative assessment so as to detect significant oesophageal body motility disorders, alkaline reflux and concomitant gastric pathology, such as impaired emptying and biliary gastritis. The choice of primary procedure is critical and there is increasing evidence that Nissen fundoplication is associated with a significantly higher incidence of mechanical complications than many partial fundoplication procedures, particularly in the presence of oesophageal body dysmotility and when the procedure is performed laparoscopically.

Finally, meticulous attention to technique is mandatory in order to reduce the incidence of preventable complications. Particular attention should be directed towards avoiding an overtight wrap or hiatal closure, avoiding an oblique wrap or one which incorporates the body of the stomach rather than the fundus if Nissen fundoplication is used, and closure of the hiatus to an appropriate degree in order to prevent proximal migration of Nissen fundoplication, while avoiding overtightness which may result in obstructive symptoms. Finally, if oesophageal shortening is present, the judicious use of a Collis gastroplasty will reduce the risk of failure. It will follow, therefore, that the safe and effective conduct of antireflux surgery requires considerable judgement, expertise and back up with appropriate investigational facilities and best results will be obtained from specialist centres possessing all these attributes. Fortunately, in this era of evidence-based medicine, good prospective randomized studies comparing the various antireflux procedures performed by both open and laparoscopic approaches are in progress, with independent symptomatic assessment together with studies of both objective and quality of life parameters, looking not only at efficacy of reflux control, but also functional assessment of oesophagogastric function and the incidence of mechanical complications. Hopefully, when these are completed, it should be possible to place the rational choice of antireflux procedure on a scientific footing, based on accumulated knowledge of the pathophysiology of reflux control and the genesis of mechanical complications, rather than one based on dogma and prejudice.

REFERENCES

1. Soresi AL. Diaphragmatic hernia: its unsuspected frequency, diagnosis; technique for radical care. *Ann Surg* 1919; **69:** 254–270.
2. Harrington SW. Esophageal hiatus diaphragmatic hernia; etiology, diagnosis and treatment in 123 cases. *J Thorac Surg* 1938; **8:** 127–135.
3. Allison PR. Reflux oesophagitis, sliding hiatal hernia and anatomy of repair. *Surg Gynecol Obstet* 1951; **92:** 419–431.
4. Allison PR. Hiatus hernia; a 20 year retrospective survey. *Ann Surg* 1973; **178:** 273–276.
5. Nissen R. Gastropexy and fundoplication in surgical treatment of hiatal hernia. *Am J Dig Dis* 1961; **10:** 954–961.

6. Donahue PF, Bombeck PT. The modified Nissen fundoplication – reflux prevention without gas bloat. *Chir Gastroenterol* 1977; **11:** 15–27.

7. Hill LD. An effective operation for hiatal hernia: an 8-year appraisal. *Ann Surg* 1967; **166:** 681–692.

8. Angelchik JP, Cohen R. A new surgical procedure for the treatment of gastro-esophageal reflux and hiatal hernia. *Surg Gynecol Obstet* 1979; **148:** 246–248.

9. DeMeester TR, Bonavina L, Albertucci M. Nissen fundoplication for gastroesophageal reflux disease. *Ann Surg* 1986; **204:** 9–20.

10. Lind JF, Burns CM, MacDougall JT. 'Physiological' repair for hiatal hernia – manometric study. *Arch Surg* 1965; **91:** 233–237.

11. Toupet A. Technique d'oesophago-gastroplastie avec phreno-gastropexic appliquée dans la cure radicalc des hernies hiatales et comme complément de l'operation d'Heller dans les cardiospasmes. *Mém Acad Chir Paris* 1963; **89:** 384–389.

12. Watson A. A clinical and pathophysiological study of a simple effective operation for the correction of gastro-oesophageal reflux. *Br J Surg* 1984; **71:** 991.

13. Fuchs K-H, Heimbucher J, Freys SM, & Thiede A. Management of gastro-esophageal reflux disease: tailored concept of anti-reflux operations. *Dis Esophagus* 1994; **7:** 250–254.

14. Kauer WKH, Peters JH, DeMeester TR, Heimbucher J, Ireland AP and Bremner CG. A tailored approach to antireflux surgery. *J Thorac Cardiovasc Surg* 1995; **110:** 141–147.

15. Dallemagne B, Weerts JM, Jehaes C, Markiewicz S & Lombard R. Laparoscopic Nissen fundoplication: preliminary report. *Surg Laparosc Endosc* 1991; **1:** 138–143.

16. Jamieson GG, Watson DI, Britten-Jones R, Mitchell PC & Anvari M. Laparoscopic Nissen fundoplication. *Ann Surg* 1994; **220:** 137–145.

17. Peters JH, Heimbucher J, Kauer WKH, Incarbonc R, Bremner CG & DeMeester TR. Clinical and physiologic comparison of laparoscopic and open Nissen fundoplication. *J Am Coll Surg* 1995; **180:** 385–393.

18. Green JRB. Is there such an entity as mild oesophagitis? *Eur J Clin Res* 1993; **4:** 29–35.

19. Bate CM, Keeling PWN, O'Morain C et al. Comparison of omeprazdeacinetidine in reflux oesophagitis: symptomatic, endoscopic histological evaluations. *Gut* 1990; **31:** 968–972.

20. Klinkenberg-Knol EC, Jansen JMBJ, Festen HPM et al. Double-blind multicentre comparison of omeprazole and ranitidine in the treatment of reflux oesophagitis. *Lancet* 1987; **i:** 349–351.

21. Hetzel DJ, Dent J, Reed WD et al. Healing and relapse of severe peptic oesophagitis after treatment with omeprazole. *Gastroenterology* 1988; **95:** 903–912.

22. Lundell L, Beckman L, Ekström P et al. Prevention of relapse of reflux esophagitis after endoscopic healing: the efficacy and safety of omeprazole compared with ranitidine. *Scand J Gastroenterol* 1991; **26:** 248–256.

23. Barlow AP, Norris TL, Watson A. Can failure of medical treatment be predicted in gastro-oesophageal reflux? *Gut* 1989; **30:** 730.

24. Cederberg C, Andersson T & Skanberg I. Omeprazole: pharmacokinetics and metabolism in man. *Scand J Gastroenterol* 1989; **24** (suppl 166): 33–40.

25. Watson A, Peck N, Callander N. The role of anti-reflux surgery in the post-omeprazole era. *Proceedings 5th World Congress, International Society for Diseases of the Esophagus.* 1992; 242.

26. Klinkenberg-Knol EC. The management of severe, therapy-resistant, reflux oesophagitis. *Gullet* 1993; **3:** Suppl 70–75.

27. Spechler SJ & the Department of Veterans Affairs Gastroesophageal Reflux Disease Study Group. Comparison of medical and surgical therapy for complicated gastroesophageal reflux disease in veterans. *N Engl J Med* 1992; **326:** 786–792.

28. Watson A. Is laparoscopic fundoplication a more attractive option than long-term omeprazole in gastro-oesophageal reflux disease? *Gut* 1995; **36:** A14.

29. Kauer WKH, Peteres JH, DcMeester TR, Ireland AP, Bremner CG and Hagen JA. Mixed reflux of gastric and duodenal juices is more harmful to the esophagus than gastric juice alone: the need for surgical therapy re-emphasized. *Ann Surg* 1995; **222:** 525–533.

30. Watson A. Controlled trial of medical versus surgical reflux control in the management of peptic oesophageal stricture treated by intermittent dilatation. *Gut* 1985; **26:** 553–554.

31. Ball CS & Watson A. Acid sensitivity in reflux oesophagitis with and without complications. *Gut* 1988; **29:** 729.

32. Attwood SEA, Ball CS, Barlow AP, Jenkinson L, Norris TL & Watson A. Role of intragastric and intraoesophageal alkalinisation in the genesis of complication in Barrett's columnar lined oesophagus. *Gut* 1993; **34:** 11–15.

33. Attwood SEA, Barlow AP, Norris TL & Watson A. Barrett's oesophagus: effect of antireflux surgery on symptom control and development of complications. *Br J Surg* 1992; **79:** 1050–1053.

34. Ortiz A, Martinez De Haro LF, Parilla P et al. Conservative treatment versus anti-reflux surgery in Barrett's oesophagus: long-term results of a prospective study. *Br J Surg* 1991; **78:** 274–278.

35. Bremner CG. Barrett's oesphagus. *Br J Surg* 1989; **76:** 995–996.

36. Sagar PM, Ackroyd R, Hosïe KB, Patterson JE, Stoddard CJ and Kingsnorth AN. Regression and progression of Barrett's oesophagus after the antireflux surgery. *Br J Surg* 1995; **82:** 806–810.

37. Williamson WA, Ellis FH, Gibb SP et al. Effect of anti-reflux operations on Barrett's mucosa. *Ann Thorac Surg* 1990; **49:** 537–542.

38. Jenkinson LR, Norris TL, Watson A. Symptoms and endoscopic findings – can they predict abnormal nocturnal gastro-oesophageal reflux? *Ann R Coll Surg Eng* 1989; **71:** 117–119.

39. Watson A. A clinical study of the role of anti-reflux surgery combined with endoscopic dilatation in peptic esophageal stricture. *Am J Surg* 1984; **148:** 346–349.

40. Hill LD, Aye RW & Ramel S. Antireflux surgery: a surgeon's look. *Gastroenterol Clin North Am* 1990; **19:** 745–775.

41. Kahrilas PJ, Dodds WJ, Hogan WJ et al. Esophageal peristaltic dysfunction in peptic esophagitis. *Gastroenterology* 1986; **91:** 897–904.

42. Jenkinson IR, Ball CS, Barlow AP, Norris TL & Watson A. A re-evaluation of the manometric assessment of oesophageal function in reflux oesophagitis. *Gullet* 1991; **1:** 135–142.

43. Bombeek CT, Dillard DH & Nyhus LM. Muscular anatomy of the gastroesophageal junction and the role of the phrenoesophageal ligament: autopsy study of sphincter mcchanism. *Ann Surg* 1966; **164:** 643–654.

44. Fyke FE Jr, Code CF & Schlegel JF. The gastroesophageal sphincter in healthy human beings. *Gastroenterologia* 1956; **86:** 135–150.

45. Pope CE, Micyer GW & Castell DO. Is measurement of lower esophageal sphincter pressure clinically useful? *Dig Dis Sci* 1981; **26:** 1025–1030.

46. Bancewicz J, Mughal M & Marples M. The lower oesophageal sphincter after floppy Nissen fundoplication. *Br J Surg* 1987; **974:** 162–164.

47. Mittal RK, Fisher MJ, McCallum RW, Dent J, Rochester DF & Sluss J. Human lower esophageal sphincter pressure response to increased intra-abdominal pressure. *Am J Physiol* 1990; **258:** G624–G630.

48. Zaninotto G, DeMeester TR, Schwizer W, Johansson K-E & Cheng S-C. The lower oesophageal sphincter in health and disease. *Am J Surg* 1988; **155:** 104–111.

49. Higgs RH, Castell DO & Farrell RL. Evaluation of the effect of fundoplication on the incompetent lower esophageal sphincter. *Surg Gynecol Obstet* 1975; **141:** 571–575.

50. Bombeck CT, Coeltro RGP & Nyhus LM. Prevention of gastro-esophageal reflux after resection of the lower esophagus. *Surg Gynecol Obstet* 1970; **136:** 1035–1043.

51. Butterfield WC. Current hiatal hernia repairs. Similarities, mechanisms and extended indications – an autopsy study. *Surgery* 1971; **69:** 910–916.

52. Johnsson F, Joelsson B & Gudmundsson K. Determinants of gastro-oesophageal reflux and their intra-relationships. *Br J Surg* 1989; **76:** 241–244.

53. O'Sullivan GC, DeMeester TR, Joelsson BE et al. Interaction of lower esophageal sphincter pressure and length of sphincter in the abdomen as determinants of gastroesophageal competence. *Am J Surg* 1982; **143:** 40–47.

54. DeMeester TR, Wernly JA, Bryant GH, Little AG & Skinner DB. Clinical and in vitro determinants of gastroesophageal competence: a study of the principles of antireflux surgery. *Am J Surg* 1979; **137:** 39–46.

55. Clark J. Hiatal hernia and reflux oesophagitis. In Hennessy TPJ & Cuschieri A (eds) *Surgery of the Oesophagus.* London: Ballière Tindall 1986; 173–240.

56. DeTroyer A, Sampson M, Sigrist S & Macklem P. Action of costal and crural parts of the diaphragm on the rib cage in dog. *J Appl Physiol* 1982; **53:** 30–39.

57. Mittal RK, Rochester DF & McCallum RW. Electrical and mechanical activity in the human lower esophageal sphincter during diaphragmatic contraction. *J Clin Invest* 1988; **81:** 1182–1189.

58. Peck N, Callander N & Watson A. Manometric assessment of the effect of the diaphragmatic crural sling in gastro-oesophageal reflux: implications for surgical management. *Br J Surg* 1995; **82:** 798–801.

59. Skinner DB. Pathophysiology of gastroesophageal reflux. *Ann Surg* 1985; **202:** 546–556.

60. Little AG. Mechanisms of action of antireflux surgery: theory and fact. *World J Surg* 1992; **16:** 320–325.

61. Ireland AC, Holloway RH, Toouli J & Dent J. Mechanisms underlying the anti-reflux action of fundoplication. *Gut* 1993; **33:** 303–308.

62. Lundell L, Abrahamsson H, Ruth M, Sandberg N & Olbe LC. Lower esophageal sphincter characteristics and esophageal acid exposure following partial or 360 degrees fundoplication: results of a prospective, randomized, clinical study. *World J Surg* 1991; **15:** 115–120.

63. Jamieson GG. Anti-reflux operations: how do they work? *Br J Surg* 1987; **74:** 155–156.

64. DeMeester TR, Johnson LF. Evaluation of the Nissen anti-reflux procedure by esophageal manometry and 24 hour pH monitoring. *Am J Surg* 1975; **129:** 94–100.

65. Zaninotto G, Costantini M, Anselmino M, et al. Excessive competence of the lower oesophageal sphincter after Nissen fundoplication: evaluation by three-dimensional computerised imaging. *Eur J Surg* 1995; **161:** 241–246.

66. Johnsson F, Holloway RH, Ireland AC, Jamieson GG & Dent J. Effect of fundoplication on transient lower oesophageal sphincter relaxation and gas reflux. *Br J Surg* 1997; **84:** 686–689.

67. Gill RC, Bowes KL, Murphy PD & Kingma YJ. Esophageal motor abnormalities in gastroesophageal reflux and the effects of fundoplication. *Gastroenterology* 1986; **91:** 364–369.

68. Weiser HF, Wu YO & Siewert JR. Supercontinence following antireflux surgery – evaluation by pH-metry. *Dig Surg* 1984; **1:** 185–189.

69. Alday ES & Goldsmith HS. Efficacy of fundoplication in preventing gastric reflux. *Am J Surg* 1973; **126:** 322–324.

70. Lundell L, Abrahamsson H, Ruth M, Rydberg L, Lönroth H & Olbe L. Long-term results of a prospective randomized comparison of total fundic wrap (Nissen–Rossetti) or semifundoplication (Toupet) for gastro-oesophageal reflux. *Br J Surg* 1996; **83:** 830–835.

71. Kjell BA, Thor MD & Silander T. A long-term randomized prospective trial of the Nissen procedure *versus* a modified Toupet technique. *Ann Surg* 1989; **210:** 719–724.

72. Watson A, Jenkinson LR, Ball CS et al. A more physiological alternative to total fundoplication for the surgical correction of resistant gastro-oesophageal reflux. *Br J Surg* 1991; **78:** 1088–1094.

73. Ball CS, Norris JL & Watson A. Dual gastric pH monitoring for the detection of duodenogastric reflux. *Gut* 1990; **31:** 598.

74. Ferraro P, Perrault LP, Emond & Filion R & Beauchamp G. Preoperative 24-hour pH monitoring in achalasia patients. *Dis Esophagus* 1985; **8:** 200–204.

75. Escandell AO, de Haro LFM, Paricio PP, Albasini JLA, Marcilla JAG & Cuenca GM. Surgery improves defective oesophageal peristalsis in patients with gastro-oesophageal reflux. *Br J Surg* 1991; **78:** 1095–1097.

76. Russell COH, Pope CE, Gannan RM, Allen FD, Velasco N & Hill LD. Does surgery correct esophageal motor dysfunction and gastroesophageal reflux? *Ann Surg* 1981; **194:** 290–296.

77. Pope CE. Esophageal motility – who needs it? *Am Gastroenterol Assoc* 1978; **74:** 1337–1338.

78. Richter JE. Surgery for reflux disease – reflections of a gastro-enterologist. *N Eng J Med* 1992; **326:** 825–827.

79. Lundell LR, Myers JJ & Jamieson GG. The influence of preoperative oesophageal motor function in the long-term outcome of anti-reflux surgery. *Gullet* 1993; **3:** 50–53.

80. Skinner DB. Surgical management after failed antireflux operations. *World J Surg* 1992; **16:** 359–363.

81. Bancewicz J, Mughal M & Marples M. The lower oesophageal sphincter after floppy Nissen fundoplication. *Br J Surg* 1987; **74:** 162–164.

82. Baigrie RJ, Watson DI, Myers JC & Jamieson GG. Outcome of laparoscopic Nissen fundoplication in patients with disordered preoperative peristalsis. *Gut* 1997; **40:** 381–385.

83. Hunter JG, Trus TL, Branum GD, Waring JP & Wood WC. A physiologic approach to laparoscopic fundoplication for gastroesophageal reflux disease. *Ann Surg* 1996; **223:** 673–687.

84. Walker SJ, Holt S, Sanderson CJ & Stoddard CJ. Comparison of Nissen total and Lind partial trans-abdominal fundoplication in the treatment of gastro-oesophageal reflux. *Br J Surg* 1992; **79:** 410–414.

85. Rosetti N, Hell K. Fundoplication for treatment of gastro-esophageal reflux in hiatal hernia. *World J Surg* 1977; **1:** 439–443.

86. Durrans D, Armstrong CP & Taylor RV. The Angelchik anti-reflux prosthesis – some reservations. *Br J Surg* 1985; **72:** 525–527.

87. Wale RJ, Royston CMS, Bennett JR et al. Prospective study of the Angelchik anti-reflux prosthesis. *Br J Surg* 1985; **72:** 520–525.

88. Maxwell-Armstrong CA, Steele RJC, Amar SS et al. Long-term results of the Angelchik prosthesis for gastro-oesophageal reflux. *Br J Surg* 1997; **84:** 862–864.

89. Belsey R. Mark IV repair of hiatal hernia by the transthoracic approach. *World J Surg* 1977; **1:** 475–483.

89a. Campbell KL & Munro A. Efficacy and incidence of postfundoplication symptoms at a median of 5 years following open Watson fundoplication. *Br J Surg* 1998; **85**(Suppl 1): 8.

90. Low DE, Mercer CD, James EC & Hill LD. Post Nissen syndrome. *Surg Gynecol Obstet* 1988; **167:** 1–5.

91. Leonardi HK, Corzier RE & Ellis FH. Re-operation for complications of the Nissen fundoplication. *J Thorac Cardiovasc Surg* 1981; **81:** 50–56.

92. O'Hanrahan T, Marples M & Bancewicz J. Recurrent reflux and wrap disruption after Nissen fundoplication: detection, incidence and timing. *Br J Surg* 1990; **77:** 545–547.

93. Watson DI, Jamieson GG, Devitt PG, Mitchell PC & Game PA. Paraoesophageal hiatus hernia: an important complication of laparoscopic Nissen fundoplication. *Br J Surg* 1995; **82:** 521–523.

94. Mansour KA, Burton HG, Miller JI & Hatcher CR Jr. Complications of intrathoracic Nissen fundoplication. *Ann Thorac Surg* 1981; **32:** 173–178.

95. Rogers DM, Herrington JL Jr & Morton C. Incidental splenectomy associated with Nissen fundoplication. *Ann Surg* 1980; **191:** 153–166.

96. Negre JR. Postfundoplication syndromes. Do they restrict the success of Nissen fundoplication? *Ann Surg* 1983; **198:** 698–700.

97. Dallemagne B, Weerts JM, Jehaes C & Markiewicz S. Causes of failures of laparoscopic antireflux operations. *Surg Endosc* 1996; **10:** 305–310.

97a. Davies N, Watson DI, Pike GK, Devitt R, Britten-Jones R & Jamieson GG. Laparoscopic Nissen vs anterior fundoplication: a randomized trial. *Br J Surg*; **85**(Suppl 1): 7.

98. Pope CE. The quality of life following antireflux surgery. *World J Surg* 1992; **16:** 355–358.

99. DeMeester TR, Johnson LF & Kent AH. Evaluation of current operations for the prevention of gastroesophageal reflux. *Ann Surg* 1974; **180:** 511–523.

100. Baxter ST, Walker SJ & Sutton R. Randomised controlled trial of Nissen versus Lind fundoplication: results at ten year follow-up. *Gut* 1995; **36:** A14.

101. McDougall NJ, Johnston BT, Collins JSA, McFarland RJ and Love AHG. Three year follow-up of oesophagitis with endoscopy and oesophageal pH monitoring. *Gut* 1995; **36:** A15.

102. Isolauri J, Luostarinen M, Viljakka M, Isolauri E, Keyrilä O & Karvonen A-L. Long-term comparison of antireflux surgery *versus* conservative therapy for reflux esophagitis. *Ann Surg* 1997; **225:** 295–299.

103. Gotley DC, Smithers BM, Rhodes M, Menzies B, Branicki FJ & Nathanson L. Laparoscopic Nissen fundoplication – 200 consecutive cases. *Gut* 1996; **38:** 487–491.

104. Hunter JG, Swanstrom L & Waring JP. Dysphagia after laparoscopic antireflux surgery: the impact of operative technique. *Ann Surg* 1996; **224:** 51–57.

105. Watson DI, Pike JK, Bangrie RJ, et al. Prospective double-blind randomized trial of Laparoscopic Nissen fundoplication with division and without division of short gastric vessels. *Ann Surg* 1997; **226:** 642–652.

106. Hinder RA, Filipi CJ, Wetscher G, Neary P, DeMeester TR & Perdikis G. Laparoscopic Nissen fundoplication is an effective treatment for gastroesophageal reflux disease. *Ann Surg* 1994; **220:** 472–483.

107. Cuschieri A, Hunter J, Wolfe B, Swanstrom LL & Hutson W. Multicenter prospective evaluation of laparoscopic antireflux surgery. *Surg Endosc* 1993; **7:** 505–510.

108. McKernan JB. Laparoscopic repair of gastroesophageal reflux disease: Toupet partial fundoplication versus Nissen fundoplication. *Surg Endosc* 1994; **8:** 851–856.

109. Bell RCW, Hanna P, Powers B, Sabel J & Hruza D. Clinical and manometric results of laparoscopic partial (Toupet) and complete (Rosetti–Nissen) fundoplication. *Surg Endosc* 1996; **10:** 724–728.

110. Watson A, Spychal RT, Brown MG, Peck N & Callander N. Laparoscopic 'physiological' antireflux procedure: preliminary results of a prospective symptomatic and objective study. *Br J Surg* 1995; **82:** 651–656.

111. Heudebert GR, Marks R, Wilcox CM & Centor RM. Choice of long-term

strategy for the management of patients with severe esophagitis: A cost-utility analysis. *Gastroenterology* 1997; **112:** 1078–1086.

112. Little AG, Ferguson MK & Skinner DB. Reoperation for failed antireflux operations. *J Thorac Cardiovasc Surg* 1986; **91:** 511–517.

113. Herrington JL & Mody B. Total duodenal diversion for treatment of reflux esophagitis uncontrolled by repeated antireflux procedures. *Ann Surg* 1976; **183:** 636–644.

114. Anvari M, Allen C & Borm A. Laparoscopic Nissen fundoplication is a satisfactory alternative to long-term omeprazole therapy. *Br J Surg* 1995; **82:** 938–942.

11

COMPLICATIONS OF GASTRO-OESOPHAGEAL REFLUX

JH Peters
CG Bremner

NATURAL HISTORY OF GASTRO-OESOPHAGEAL REFLUX DISEASE

Studies on the natural history of gastro-oesophageal reflux disease (GORD) are difficult to perform because of the mobility of modern society. Those that have been done indicate that most patients have relatively mild disease responsive to simple lifestyle, dietary and medical therapy and do not go on to develop complications. Investigations of the natural history of GORD in the absence of oesophagitis have demonstrated return of symptoms in the majority of patients following cessation of medical therapy.[1] Furthermore, progression to a more severe form of the disease occurs in 10–20% of patients.[2] Increasingly, GORD is recognized as a chronic disease requiring lifelong medical treatment to prevent symptomatic recurrence, with the potential for progressive oesophageal injury and dysfunction. The response of severe oesophagitis (grade iv) to acid inhibition by omeprazole therapy (40 mg daily) has been disappointing and in one study fewer than half of the patients healed on this dosage.[2] Moreover, erosive or ulcerative oesophagitis recurred in 82% of patients within 6 months of cessation of therapy. The response to medical therapy gives some guidance as to the indications for anti-reflux surgery. Surgery provides the only known means of altering the natural history of the disease and is more likely to be required in those patients with more severe disease who have greater potential to develop complications. The principal complications of GORD are listed in Table 11.1.

The Swiss population tends to be less mobile and their lifestyle is highly organized. This has allowed the opportunity for physicians at the University of Lausanne, Switzerland to follow longitudinally a large number of patients with reflux oesophagitis. In the Lausanne region the prevalence of oesophagitis at endoscopy rose from 190 per 100 000 population in 1970 to 1058 per 100 000 in 1980. Although the major reason for this is likely to be the wider availability and use of upper gastrointestinal endoscopy, increased consumption of

Table 11.1 Complications of gastro-oesophageal reflux

Oesophageal
Oesophagitis
Stricture
Columnar lining (Barrett's)

Oral/pharyngeal
Glossitis
Loss of dental enamel
Pharyngitis

Laryngeal
Laryngitis
Vocal cord granuloma
Subglottic and tracheal stenosis

Pulmonary
Chronic cough
Aspiration pneumonia
Non-allergic asthma
Apnoeic episodes (child)

alcohol, tobacco, large fatty meals and perhaps even antisecretory agents may have played a role. Ollyo and colleagues[3] have investigated the natural history of grade I–III oesophagitis in 701 patients receiving medical therapy including omeprazole (Figure 11.1). About 46% of patients had an isolated episode of oesophagitis, 31% had recurrent episodes of oesophagitis but no increase in their severity and 23% developed recurrent and progressive mucosal damage.

At present, there is no reliable method for identifying which patients will develop progressive disease. Although the concept of endoscopic surveillance has largely centred on those patients with Barrett's oesophagus, it seems prudent to suggest intermittent upper gastro-intestinal endoscopy as a means of detecting patients with progressive or recurrent disease. Patients who fall into these categories should be offered early antireflux surgery as a means of preventing the development of

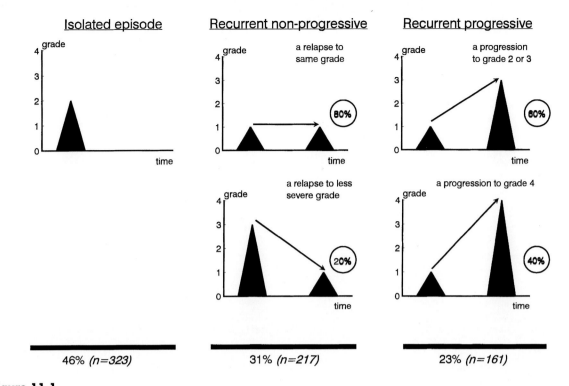

Figure 11.1

Natural history of erosive oesophagitis in patients with gastro-oesophageal reflux disease. This study was carried out in Lausanne, Switzerland, with a relatively fixed population of patients who underwent serial endoscopy over the course of several years. (Reproduced from Ollyo et al.[3].)

the irreversible complication of Barrett's oesophagus or the progressive deterioration of oesophageal function.

INCREASED OESOPHAGEAL EXPOSURE TO ACID

In normal individuals, the intraoesophageal pH, measured by ambulatory oesophageal pH monitoring (Figure 11.2) is above 4 for 98.5% of the time.[4] A pH threshold of 4, therefore, has a

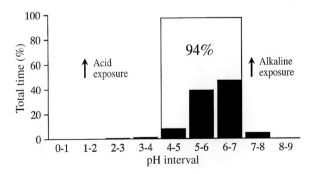

Figure 11.2

Normal range of oesophageal pH expressed as the median percentage of the total time spent at each pH interval in 50 normal volunteers. Note that 94% of the time is spent within pH 4.0–7.0. (Reproduced from DeMeester TR & Stein HJ. In Richter JE (ed.) *Ambulatory Esophageal pH Monitoring: Practical Approach and Clinical Applications.* New York: Igaku-Shoin, 1991; 81–92.)

high sensitivity and specificity in detecting increased acid exposure to the oesophagus. This threshold, however, is not useful in predicting which patients are more likely to develop complications of GORD. The 24-hour oesophageal pH data for 50 normal subjects and 154 patients with proven GORD were analysed for time spent at different pH intervals. The greatest prevalence of mucosal damage (oesophagitis, stricture, Barrett's) was found in those patients with increased oesophageal exposure time of pH 0–2, corresponding to the known pK_a of pepsin (Figure 11.3).[5] According to this study, an oesophageal exposure time to pH 0–2 for more than 1.32% of the time is likely to result in mucosal injury.[6] This exposure was not, however, related to a hypersecretory state. An increased prevalence of oesophagitis has also been reported in patients with acid hypersecretion, and oesophagitis occurs in about 50% of patients with the Zollinger–Ellison syndrome.[7] Basal acid secretion[8] and gastrin-stimulated acid secretion are also raised in Barrett's oesophagus.[9] The mechanism of mucosal breakdown of the squamous epithelium has also received much attention. The major resistance to H^+ diffusion into the squamous epithelial layer is provided by intracellular lamellar lipids and glycoconjugates in the intercellular spaces of the stratum corneum and spinosum layers.[10] H^+ ions do not diffuse into the mucosa unless the luminal pH falls below a pH of 2.0 for prolonged periods of time (>30–60 min).[11] Other luminal factors such as pepsin, bile salts and alcohol can potentiate H^+ ion injury by decreasing paracellular resistance.[11] Patients with mucosal injury have a higher prevalence of a defective sphincter than patients with a normal mucosa.

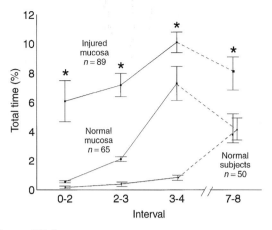

Figure 11.3

Mean percent time of oesophageal exposure to different pH intervals for normal subjects and patients with normal or injured mucosa. Normal values are included for reference.
(* = P <0.01 versus no injury). Data expressed as mean ± s.e.m. (Reproduced from Bremner et al.[5].)

IMPORTANCE OF ALKALINE REFLUX

Reflux of alkaline duodenal contents into the stomach and oesophagus is increasingly recognized as an important pathophysiological factor in GORD.[12] Pure alkaline reflux, that is increased oesophageal exposure to gastric juice with a pH >7, is an uncommon though well documented event occurring almost exclusively after cholecystectomy or surgical disruption of the pyloric mechanism. The vast majority of patients reflux either pure acid gastric juice or a mixture of gastric and duodenal juice. Pellegrini et al.[13] investigated reflux patterns by simultaneously monitoring antral, fundic and oesophageal pH in 67 patients with symptoms suggestive of GORD and no previous history of gastric surgery. Patients were classified as acid, acid/alkaline or alkaline refluxers, based on the characterization of their reflux patterns over 24 h; 42% of the patients were found to have acid reflux, 40% acid/alkaline reflux and 18% alkaline reflux. Fiorucci et al.[14] performed a similar study using both a fundic and oesophageal probe and related the type of reflux episode to the severity of oesophagitis (Figure 11.4). They found that severe oesophagitis was related to a high prevalence of mixed reflux episodes (Figure 11.5). They further showed that patients who had mixed reflux episodes had a higher average gastric pH, suggesting that the mixed reflux episodes were due to duodenogastric reflux (Figure 11.6).

Recognition of alkaline gastro-oesophageal reflux

The term alkaline gastro-oeosophageal reflux is somewhat of a misnomer as the pH in the lower eosophagus rarely exceeds 8. By convention, alkaline reflux is said to be present when there is excessive oesophageal exposure to a pH >7, due to repetitive rises in oesophageal pH to above 7 during a time when the gastric pH is above 4. The quantification of this exposure is based on six measurements: the percentage of total, upright and supine time the oesophagus has a pH greater than 7; the

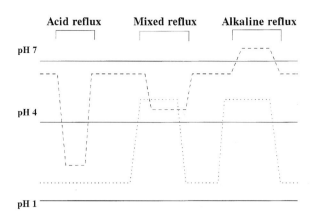

Figure 11.4

Criteria used for the simultaneous analysis of gastric (broken line) and oesophageal (dotted line) pH. Oesophageal reflux is a decrease in the oesophagus pH to <4 associated with an acid gastric pH. Mixed refluxes are characterized by a decrease in oesophageal pH from the baseline to a value >4 associated with increases in the gastric pH to >4. Alkaline refluxes are those with increases of oesophageal pH to >7 associated with an increase in the gastric pH to >4. (Reproduced from Fiorucci et al.[14].)

number of episodes that pH of the oesophagus exceeds 7; the number of episodes lasting longer than 5 minutes; and the longest episode during which the pH remained above 7.[15] Normal values for these six components have been derived from study of 50 asymptomatic control subjects. The upper limits of normality were established at the 95th percentile. If patients' values are above this level, they are considered abnormal for the component measured. The six components are combined into one expression of the overall oesophageal alkaline exposure by calculating a composite alkaline pH score.[16]

The presence of increased oesophageal exposure to pH >7 must be interpreted carefully. Increased exposure in this pH range can be caused by abnormal calibration of the pH

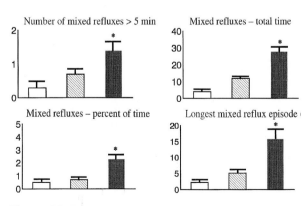

Figure 11.5

Pattern of mixed reflux in healthy subjects (☐), patients with mild oesophagitis (▨) and patients with severe-complicated oesophagitis (■). *P <0.01 versus both healthy subjects and patients with mild esophagitis. (Reproduced from Fiorucci et al.[14].)

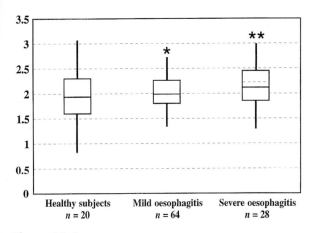

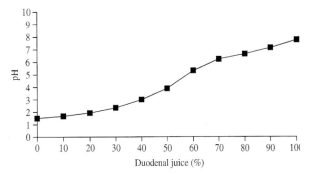

Figure 11.7

Titration curve of 0.1 mmol/l hydrochloric acid with duodenal juice obtained by aspiration from a patient. Over 50% duodenal content is required to raise the pH above 4 and over 90% to elevate the pH to above 7. (Reproduced from Kauer WKH, Burdiles P, Ireland AP et al. Does duodenal juice reflux into the oesophagus of patients with complicated GERD? Evaluation of a fibreoptic sensor for bilirubin. *Am J Surg* 1995; **169:** 98–104.)

Figure 11.6

Box – Whisker plots of gastric pH and gastric acidity in healthy subjects and patients with mild oesophagitis or severe-complicated oesophagitis. Gastric pH was determined from 540 individual pH values obtained by determining the mean of 2-minute intervals. Postprandial pH values (2 h) were not considered. Mean 18-hour gastric pH was significantly higher in patients with severe oesophagitis than in healthy subjects ($P < 0.001$) or patients with mild oesophagitis ($P < 0.01$). **$P < 0.001$ vs. healthy subjects; *$P < 0.01$ vs. severe oesophagitis. (Reproduced from Fiorucci et al.[14].)

recorder, the presence of dental infection, which increases salivary pH,[17] the presence of oesophageal obstruction resulting in static pools of saliva with an increase in pH secondary to bacterial overgrowth,[18] or the regurgitation of a mixture of gastic and duodenal juice that results in a rise in pH of the oesophagus to above 7. When using a properly calibrated probe, in the absence of dental infection or oesophageal obstruction, the percentage of time the pH is measured above 7 has been shown to correlate with the concentration of bile acids continuously aspirated from the oesophagus over a 24-hour period.[19]

Recently it has been shown that gastric juice, with a pH of 1.5, must contain at least 70% of duodenal juice in order to raise the pH to >7 (unpublished data) (Figure 11.7), although somewhat less if some saliva is present. It is important to understand that increased oesophageal exposure to pH >7 only infers increased oesophageal exposure to duodenal juice, that is bile and/or pancreatic juice. When present, it represents only the tip of the iceberg of the total time the oesophagus is actually exposed to duodenal contents.

Newer tests which can directly measure the components of duodenal juice in the oesophagus have shown that reflux episodes containing components of duodenal juice can occur when the oesophageal pH remains in its normal range of 4–7 or even when the oesophageal pH drops below 4, as during acid reflux episodes. Data from 24-hour oesophageal aspiration studies indicate that, compared with normal subjects, abnormal amounts of bile are detected in patients with proven acid reflux during the postprandial and supine periods (Figure 11.8).[20] Studies using a fibreoptic probe which recognizes intraluminal bilirubin as a marker of duodenal juice have shown that bile, and hence duodenal juice, is commonly present in the refluxate, independent of its pH. This is well demonstrated

in patients with Barrett's oesophagus who have an increased oesophageal exposure to acid (Figure 11.9). Thus, the measurement of increased oesophageal acid exposure does not exclude the presence of components of duodenal juice in the refluxate. In general, there appears to be a direct relationship between the degree of duodenal juice present in the refluxate and the severity of mucosal injury; that is, a mixture of duodenal and gastric juice is more injurious than gastric juice alone. Patients with Barrett's oesophagus, for example, had a significantly higher amount of bilirubin in their refluxate than patients with uncomplicated reflux disease (Figure 11.10). The latter group showed higher amounts of bilirubin than normal subjects, but the increase is not statistically significant. The reflux of a high percentage of duodenal and gastric juice in Barrett's oesophagus is presumably due to excessive duodenogastric reflux present in these patients. When the mixed gastric and duodenal juice refluxes into the oesophagus, there

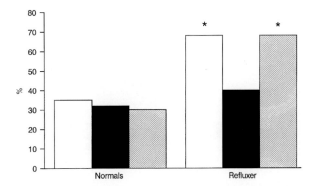

Figure 11.8

Percentage of subjects with bile on oesophageal aspiration during postprandial (☐), upright (■) and supine (▨) period in normals and patients with reflux disease (*$P<0.01$ versus normals). (Reproduced from Peters JH, Kauer WKH & DeMeester TR. *Dis Esoph* 1994; **7:** 94.)

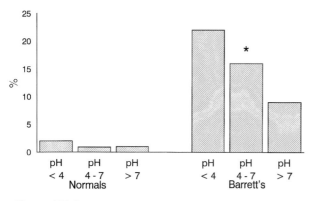

Figure 11.9
Median percentage time of pH <4, 4–7, >7 spent at bilirubin absorbance >0.14 in normals and patients with Barrett's oesophagus (*P < 0.01 versus normals). (Reproduced from Peters JH, Kauer WKH & DeMeester TR. *Dis Esoph* 1994; 7: 95.)

is little change in the oesophageal pH, and consequently minimal heartburn. Despite the lack of symptoms, mucosal damage still appears, probably from activated pancreatic enzymes.

Duodenogastric reflux as the cause of increased oesophageal alkaline exposure

Several authors have demonstrated concomitant increases in duodenogastric reflux in patients with symptomatic GORD.[21–24] Combined oesophageal and gastric pH monitoring has shown that the alkaline component is probably due to excessive reflux of duodenal contents through the stomach and into the distal oesophagus (Figure 11.11). In normal subjects, 24- h gastric pH monitoring with multiple gastric probes has shown that elevation in antral pH typically occurs in the early hours of the morning and progresses from the pylorus into the proximal stomach.[15] Aspiration studies have confirmed the presence of

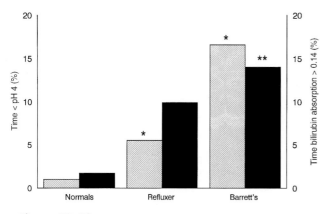

Figure 11.10
Oesophageal acid (▨) and duodenal juice (■) exposure expressed as percentage total time pH < 4 and percentage total time bilirubin absorption > 0.14 in normals, patients with reflux disease and patients with Barrett's oesophagus (*P <0.03 and **P <0.01 versus normals). (Reproduced from Peters JH, Kauer WKH & DeMeester TR. *Dis Esoph* 1994; 7: 94.)

bile during the same periods, when elevation in gastric pH was noted.[25,26] Consequently, the reflux of a limited amount of duodenal content into the stomach, particularly in the early morning hours, is a normal physiological event.[16,27]

Excessive reflux of duodenal contents into the stomach occurs after cholecystectomy, pyloroplasty/pyloromyotomy, pylorectomy, antrectomy or gastroenterostomy. The typical symptom complex includes epigastric pain, nausea and bilious vomiting. Peristomal gastritis is often seen and may progress to intestinalization of the gastric mucosa and possibly even malignant change.[28,29] Abnormal duodenogastric reflux is also known to occur as a primary disease process due to disordered motility of the antropyloroduodenal complex. When excessive duodenogastric reflux occurs in a patient with a mechanically defective lower oesophageal sphincter, increased oesophageal exposure to components of duodenal juice can be expected to occur. Furthermore, this exposure may occur at the normal pH interval of the oesophagus, resulting in very few symptoms.

Consequences of increased oesophageal acid and alkaline exposure

The complications of gastro-oesophageal reflux result from the damage inflicted by gastric juice on the oesophageal mucosa or respiratory epithelium and changes caused by subsequent repair and fibrosis (Table 11.1). Complications of reflux are oesophagitis, stricture and Barrett's oesophagus and from repetitive aspiration and progressive pulmonary fibrosis. The observation that complications of gastro-oesophageal reflux can occur in patients with a mechanically normal sphincter and that some patients who have a mechanically defective sphincter can be free of complications indicates that factors other than sphincter competence, such as the composition of the refluxed gastric juice, are important in the development of complications.

The prevalence of reflux complications, i.e. oesophagitis, stricture and Barrett's oesophagus, are related to the presence of a mechanically defective sphincter together with an increased oesophageal exposure to both acid and alkali (Figure 11.12).[30] Furthermore, the prevalence of complications is significantly higher in patients with acid/alkali reflux as compared with those with acid reflux alone (Figure 11.13). These estimations come from measuring an increase in oesophageal exposure to pH >7 and pH <4 and represent the most severe forms of mixed reflux. Obviously, in other patients, the oesophagus is exposed to mixed reflux but the degree of the duodenal component is not sufficient to push the oesophageal exposure to pH >7 to abnormal levels.

Differences of opinion exist as to what ingredient in the refluxed gastric or duodenal juice produces the mucosal injury. Components from both have been implicated. Our current knowledge regarding the noxious component in the refluxed juice is based on the elegant studies of Harmon and colleagues[31] (Figure 11.14). Hydrogen ion injury to the oesophageal squamous mucosa occurs mainly at a pH below 2. It results in injury to the mucosal barrier but rarely produces mucosal lesions or inflammatory changes. In an acid refluxate,

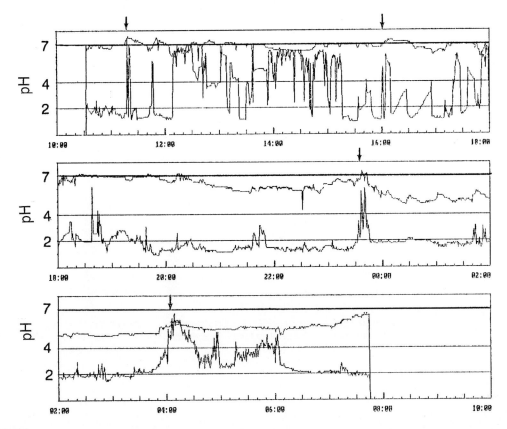

Figure 11.11
Combined ambulatory oesophageal (upper tracing) and gastric (lower tracing) pH monitoring showing duodenogastric reflux (arrows) with propagation of the alkaline juice into the oesophagus of a patient with complicated Barrett's oesophagus. The gastric tracing is taken from a probe lying 5 cm below the lower oesophageal sphincter. The oesophageal tracing is taken from a probe lying 5 cm above the lower oesophageal sphincter. Note that in only a small proportion of time does duodenogastric reflux move the pH of the oesophagus above the threshold of 7, causing the iceberg effect. (Reproduced from DeMeester TR, Stein HJ & Fuchs KH. In Zuidema GD & Orringer MB (eds) *Shackelford's Surgery of the Alimentary Tract*, 3rd edn, vol. I. Philadelphia: WB Saunders, 1991: 123.)

the enzyme pepsin appears to be the major injurious agent. Reflux of bile and pancreatic enzymes into the stomach can either protect or augment oesophageal mucosal injury. For instance, in a patient whose gastric acid secretion maintained an acid environment, the presence of bile salts would attenuate the injurious effect of pepsin and the acid gastric environment would inactivate the trypsin. Such a patient would have bile-containing acid gastric juice that, when refluxed into the oesophagus, would injure the mucosal barrier and the epithelial cells, but would be less noxious than the reflux of acid gastric juice containing pepsin. In contrast, a patient with significant duodenogastric reflux may create an alkaline intragastric environment that supports optimal trypsin activity and encourages the dissolution of bile salts with a high pK_a that potentiate the enzyme's effect. Reflux of this juice into the oesophagus causes severe oesophagitis. Hence, duodenogastric reflux and the acid secretory capacity of the stomach interrelate by altering the pH and enzymatic activity of the refluxed juice to modulate the injurious effects of the enzymes on the oesophageal mucosa.[32]

Similarly, the disparity in injury, or mucosal barrier abnor-malities caused by acid and bile alone, as opposed to oesophagitis caused by pepsin and trypsin, explains the poor correlation between severity of heartburn and mucosal pathology. The reflux of acid gastric juice contaminated with duodenal juice can readily break the oesophageal mucosal barrier, irritate nerve endings in the papillae close to the luminal surface, and cause severe heartburn. The bile salts in the duodenal juice would inhibit pepsin, the acid pH environment of the stomach would inactivate trypsin, and the patient would have severe heartburn with little or no gross evidence of oesophagitis. In contrast, the patient who refluxed alkaline gastric juice may have minimal heartburn because of the reduction of hydrogen ions in the refluxed juice, but have endoscopic oesophagitis due to bile salt potentiation of trypsin activity on the oesophageal mucosa. This suggests that the combination of duodenogastric reflux and gastro-oesophageal reflux may be more detrimental than gastro-oesophageal reflux alone and may explain the impaired sensation of acid infusion into the squamous-lined oesophagus in patients with Barrett's oesophagus (who have pathological alkaline exposure) compared with patients with grade I–III erosive oesophagitis.[33]

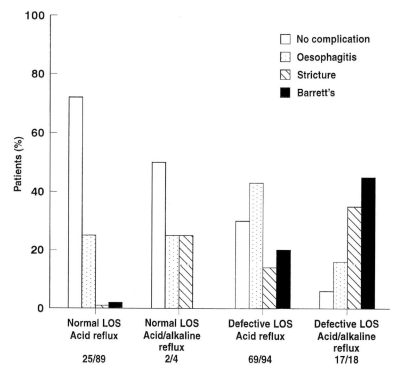

Figure 11.12
Severity of complications in patients with GORD and acid reflux or acid/alkaline reflux with and without a mechanically defective lower oesophageal sphincter (LOS). (Reproduced from Stein et al.[30].)

Sequelae of mucosal injury

When the composition of the refluxed gastric juice is such that sustained or repetitive oesophageal injury occurs, four sequelae can result: oesophagitis, stricture, ulcer or Barrett's meta-plasia (Figure 11.15, see colour plate also). Oesophagitis of varying degrees of severity precedes stricture formation or Barrett's oesophagus. A luminal stricture can develop from submucosal and eventually intramural fibrosis (Figure 11.16), whereas Barrett's oesophagus can develop by replacement of destroyed squamous mucosa by a peculiar form of healing with columnar

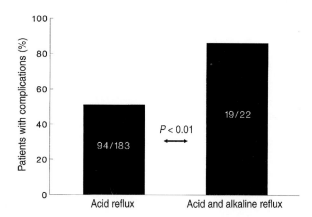

Figure 11.13
Prevalence and severity of oesophageal mucosal injury in patients with acid reflux alone and acid/alkaline reflux. (Reproduced from DeMeester TR & Stein HJ. In Castell DO (ed.) *The Esophagus.* Boston: Little Brown, 1992: 592.)

epithelium (Figure 11.17, see colour plate also).[34,35] The columnar epithelium is resistant to acid and is associated with alleviation of the symptom of heartburn. Endoscopically, the Barrett's changes can be quiescent or associated with complications of oesophagitis, stricture, Barrett's ulceration and dysplasia. Clinical evidence suggests that the complication associated with Barrett's may be due to the continuous injury and repair from refluxed alkalinized duodenogastric juice.[12] Recently Fein et al. demonstrated that bile reflux added a noxious component to the oesophageal refluxate and potentiated the injurious effects of acid gastro-oesophageal reflux. Of 120 patients studied by 24 h pH studies, 82 had increased acid exposure, which was high in 36 patients. The prevalence of injury in this group was related more to oesophageal bile exposure than acid exposure. The most important complication is the development of dysplastic changes in the Barrett's epithelium which initiates the progression to adenocarcinoma. The incidence of this occurring in patients with Barrett's oesophagus is yet to be determined, but is predicted to be between 0.5 and 10%.[36]

It appears that the healing of mucosal lesions by Barrett's metaplasia can occur at any time during the course of the disease and is not an event that occurs only in patients with severe long-standing disease. As columnar epithelial healing occurs, it gives the impression that the metaplasia is advancing into the area of inflammation, as a slow progressive process. This may not be so; rather, the whole process may occur suddenly. An oesophageal stricture can be associated with severe oesophagitis or Barrett's oesophagus.[37] In the latter situation, it occurs at the site of maximal inflammatory injury, i.e. the squamocolumnar epithelial interface. Patients who have

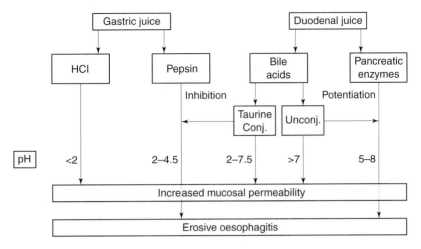

Figure 11.14
Interaction of injurious agents refluxed into the oesophagi of patients with GORD. Conj., conjugated; Unconj., unconjugated. (Reproduced from DeMeester TR & Stein HJ. In Moody FG, Carey LC, Jones RC et al. (eds) *Surgical Treatment of Digestive Diseases*, 2nd edn. Chicago: Year Book, 1989: 82.)

a stricture in the absence of Barrett's oesophagus should have the presence of gastro-oesophageal reflux documented before the aetiology of the stricture is ascribed to reflux oesophagitis. In patients with normal acid exposure, the stricture may be due to a drug-induced chemical injury resulting in the lodgement of a capsule or tablet in the distal oesophagus.[38] In such patients, dilatation usually corrects the problem of dysphagia. Heartburn, which may have occurred only because of the chemical injury, need not be treated. It is also possible for drug-induced injuries to occur in patients who have underlying oesophagitis and a distal oesophageal stricture secondary to gastro-oesophageal reflux.

When the refluxed gastric juice is of sufficient quantity it can reach the pharynx, with the potential for pharyngeal tracheal aspiration, causing symptoms of repetitive cough, choking, hoarseness and recurrent pneumonia.[39] This is often an unrecognized complication of GORD because either the pulmonary or the gastrointestinal symptoms may predominate in the clinical situation and focus the physician's attention on one to the exclusion of the other. Studies have identified three factors that are important in the pulmonary complication of reflux. Firstly, the loss of respiratory epithelium secondary to the aspiration of gastric contents can take up to 7 days to heal and may give rise to a chronic cough between episodes of aspiration.[40] When studied during this time, the cough may not be related to a reflux episode. Secondly, the presence of an oesophageal motility disorder is observed in 75% of patients with reflux-induced aspiration and is believed to promote the aboral movement of the refluxate toward the pharynx. Finally, if the pH in the cervical oesophagus is below 4 for 3% of the time, the respiratory symptoms have a high probability of being caused by aspiration.[40] Caution must be exercised in treating the patient with an abnormal motility disorder by surgery because a component of their aspiration may be retained oesophageal secretions and their cough will persist.

TREATMENT OF COMPLICATED REFLUX DISEASE

Reflux oesophagitis

Pathological acid reflux will cause macroscopic oesophagitis in about 50% of patients. Macroscopic grading of oesophagitis into grades I–IV[41] is useful as a predictor for response to medical therapy. Grades I and II oesophagitis will respond well to continued proton pump inhibition of acid output, but reports of the response rate in grades III and IV have been less satisfactory. Hetzell et al.[2] reported on a 97% healing rate of grades I and II oesophagitis after 4 weeks of treatment with 40 mg omeprazole daily, but healing occurred in only 88 and 44% of grades III and IV, respectively.

According to Ollyo et al.[3] approximately 23% of patients with grades I–III oesophagitis will have progressive disease on

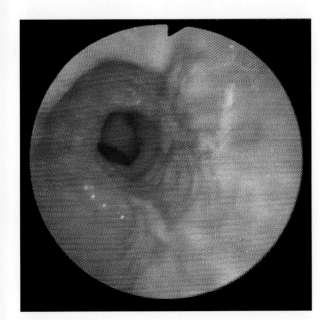

Figure 11.15
Radiographic appearance of a reflux-induced oesophageal stricture.

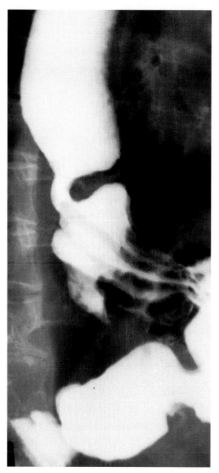

Figure 11.16
Endoscopic appearance of grade III oesophagitis. Note the linear streaks of inflamed mucosa. The patient probably also has a stricture which is visible in the distance. This would be grade IV.

medication. Lieberman[42] has identified a group of patients with a manometrically incompetent lower oesophageal sphincter (mean pressure 4.9 mmHg) who did not respond well to medical therapy (Figure 11.18). Kuster et al.[43] had a similar experience with a group of patients who had GORD related to a poor lower oesophageal sphincter pressure, and in whom surgical treatment was recommended. Sixteen patients accepted the surgical option and at follow-up 3 years later 91% were symptom free and were not using medication. On the other hand, the group which chose medical therapy were still symptomatic and required continuous therapy. Patients who did not respond to medical therapy or who relapse on medical therapy should be considered for an antireflux operation. The exact cause of the reflux should be carefully elucidated by manometry and pH testing, and in patients with a normal sphincter mechanism an alternative cause for the reflux should be investigated by gastric function and duodenogastric reflux studies.

Indications for surgical treatment

The need for continuous medical therapy in patients who have a mechanically incompetent lower oesophageal sphincter is the prime indication for surgery, providing they have oesophageal

body motility adequate for the surgical procedure of choice. Young patients are best treated by operation to avoid a lifetime of medication. Young female patients with significant reflux require surgery prior to pregnancy to avoid disastrous antenatal reflux complications. Patients who have respiratory symptoms related to gastro-oesophageal reflux are best treated surgically before respiratory function deteriorates.

In the presence of adequate oesophageal body motility and an incompetent lower oesophageal sphincter, a modified Nissen fundoplication procedure is our procedure of choice. If body motility is inadequate (pressure response to swallowing <20 mmHg), as occurs in a high proportion of patients with stricture or Barrett's oesophagus, the Belsey Mark IV procedure will have less tendency to cause obstruction and dysphagia. The Toupet[44] or Watson[45] procedures are alternatives which can be performed by the abdominal route, but we have not evaluated these options. Watson et al.[45] reported relief symptoms (Visick 1 and 2) in 96% at 3.5 years, including patients with peristaltic impairment. The modified Nissen fundoplication can be expected to give a 90% 10-year good result[46,47]

Technique of the modified Nissen fundoplication[46]

The procedure is usually performed by the abdominal route. Indications for the transthoracic route are: (1) suspected short

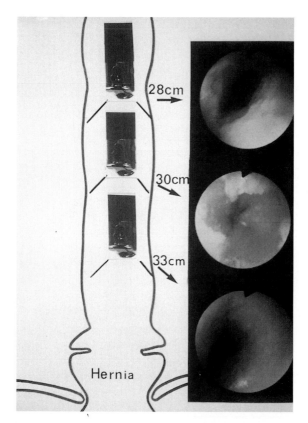

Figure 11.17
Endoscopic appearance of Barrett's metaplastic epithelium at three levels of the oesophagus. The normal white squamous epithelium has been replaced by the luxuriant red lining of Barrett's metaplasia in the lower oesophagus.

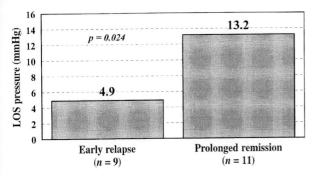

Figure 11.18

Comparison of mean lower oesophageal sphincter (LOS) pressures in patients with severe reflux oesophagitis on prolonged medical therapy. Patients experiencing early relapse of reflux symptoms had significantly lower mean LOS pressures than those on long-term medical therapy without symptomatic relapse ($P = 0.024$). (Modified from Lieberman[42].)

oesophagus which may require a Collis lengthening procedure; (2) obesity; and (3) previous unsuccessful operation. The laparoscopic technique is performed in the same way as that used at open operation.

Stricture

Although some patients with stricture will have a good response to endoscopic dilatation and acid suppression, a randomized controlled study has shown that surgical control of reflux results in a significant reduction in dilatation requirements.[48] However, as the mean age of patients with stricture is 70 years,[49] a conservative approach is appropriate for many patients.

The surgical approach to a reflux stricture will depend on the length of the stricture, the length of the oesophagus, the response to prior stricture dilatation and the motility of the oesophageal body. The majority of reflux strictures which are short and 'soft' are easy to dilate and respond well to dilatation and antireflux surgery[50-52]. Approximately 11% of reflux strictures are long.[53] Long strictures (>2 cm) may be related to a columnar-lined oesophagus,[54] prolonged nasogastric intubation or caustic pill damage. Such strictures may be as long as 10 cm and have a narrow lumen. The exact cause of a stricture which uncommonly follows nasogastric intubation is unclear but it is possibly a reflux stricture exacerbated by an intense period of gastro-oesophageal reflux. About 20% of patients who first present with a stricture give no history of heartburn,[3] and it is important in this group of patients to exclude a caustic-induced stricture from medication. In one series,[38] approximately 20% of strictures were caustic pill induced. The importance of a complete evaluation by reflux testing and motility in these patients cannot be overstressed.

The development of a stricture in a patient with a mechanically defective sphincter who is on acid suppression therapy represents a failure of medical therapy, and is an indication for a surgical antireflux procedure. Before surgery, a malignant aetiology of the stricture should be excluded by biopsy and cytology, and the stricture progressively dilated up to a 60 Fr

bougie. If dysphagia is relieved and the amplitude of oesophageal contractions and length of the oesophagus are adequate, a total fundoplication can be performed. In a patient with adequate oesophageal length in whom dysphagia persists or oesophageal contractility is compromised, a partial fundoplication procedure should be performed. If in either of these situations the oesophagus is shortened by the disease process, a Collis gastroplasty and partial fundoplication (Belsey Mark IV) should be performed (Figure 11.19). When oesophageal acid exposure is normal in a patient with a stricture, the aetiology is most likely to be a drug-induced injury and dilatation is usually all that is necessary.

Long strictures, usually those >2 cm in length which are difficult to dilate preoperatively, can be dilated intraoperatively after mobilization of the oesophagus. This technique should be tried first if it is felt that there is a reasonable chance of dilating the stricture. The dilatation can be performed by an assistant using guided bougies (Eder–Puestow, Savary or Celestin). Oesophageal lengthening will usually be necessary in this situation. Undilatable strictures are usually associated with poor oesophageal motility and our preference is resection with gastric or colon interposition. Short segment colon or jejunal interposition is a further option if the proximal oesophageal motility is adequate (swallow response pressures >30 mmHg).[55]

Barrett's oesophagus

The condition whereby the tubular oesophagus is lined with columnar epithelium rather than squamous epithelium was first described by Norman Barrett in 1950.[56] He incorrectly believed it to be congenital in origin. It is now realized that it is an acquired abnormality, occurring in 7–20% of patients with GORD, and representing a peculiar form of healing of the mucosal ulceration produced in this disease. It is also understood to be distinctly different from the congenital condition, in which islands of mature gastric columnar epithelium are found in the upper half of the oesophagus. In the spectrum of GORD, Barrett's oesophagus stands out as being associated with profound mechanical deficiency of the lower oesophageal sphincter, severe impairment of oesophageal body function, increased oesophageal exposure to both acid and alkaline juice, and excessive duodenogastric reflux.[22]

Patients with longer segments of columnar lining (>5 cm) have significantly lower pressure responses to swallowing than patients with shorter segments, suggesting a progressive deterioration of function with advancing disease.[57] Gastric hypersecretion occurs in 44% of patients.

The typical complications in Barrett's oesophagus include ulceration in the columnar lined segment (20%), stricture formation (62%) and a dysplasia–cancer sequence.[58] Ulceration is unlike the erosive ulceration of reflux oesophagitis, in that it more closely resembles peptic ulceration in the stomach or duodenum and has the same propensity to bleed, erode or perforate. The strictures found in Barrett's oesophagus occur at the squamocolumnar junction, typically at a higher level than 'peptic' strictures in the absence of Barrett's. The risk of adenocarcinoma developing in Barrett's mucosa is variously estimated

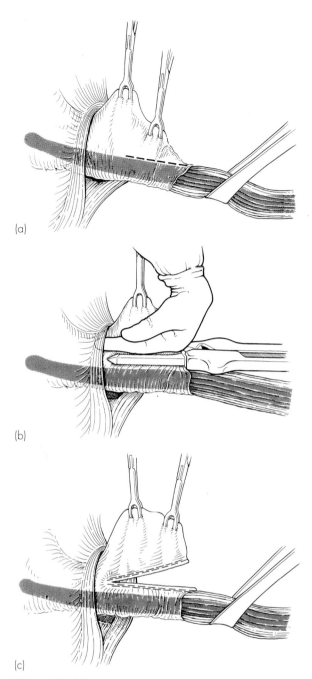

Figure 11.19

(a) Construction of a Collis gastroplasty. A 48 Fr bougie is passed into the stomach. The dotted line indicates the site of division of the gastric wall for construction of the gastric tube in continuity with the oesophagus. (b) Continued construction of the Collis gastroplasty. The stomach is divided with a GIA stapler. Traction is exerted on the greater curvature side of the fundus before the jaws of the stapler are closed. This ensures that the gastric tube closely approximates the diameter of the indwelling 48 Fr bougie throughout its length. (c) After stapling and division of the stomach, a 5 cm gastric tube is formed along the proximal portion of the lesser curvature. This effectively lengthens the oesophagus and allows the construction of a Belsey partial fundoplication which can be placed below the diaphragm without tension. (Reproduced from Pearson FG, Cooper JD, Patterson GA, Ramirex J & Todd TR. *Ann Surg* 1987; 206: 473–481.)

at 1 in 50 to 1 in 400 patient-years of follow-up. By conservative estimates, this represents a risk 40 times that of the general population. Most adenocarcinomas of the oesophagus arise in Barrett's oesophagus. Conversely, about 10–30% of all patients with Barrett's present with malignancy.

The development of complications is believed to be related to the reflux of gastric juice mixed with duodenal juice secondary to the concomitant excessive duodenogastric reflux. Nearly 60% of patients with complications of Barrett's oesophagus had abnormal oesophageal alkaline exposure, compared with 6% of patients without complications (Figure 11.20). The columnar mucosal insensitivity, the diminished sensation in the squamous mucosa of patients with Barrett's oesophagus and the higher pH of the mixed reflux may be the reasons why tissue damage may continue without worsening of the patient's symptoms.

The approach to the patient with suspected Barrett's oesophagus begins with an upper gastrointestinal barium contrast examination and endoscopy. The contrast study may show a hiatus hernia which, if it fails to reduce in the upright position, may indicate a shortened oesophagus. It may also show a high oesophageal stricture or a penetrating ulcer. Endoscopically, Barrett's oesophagus is recognized by the appearance of gastric-type mucosa extending into the tubular oesophagus. Shorter segments of Barrett's mucosa have been discovered by biopsy and are prone to the same risks of cancer. The columnar mucosa may be in the form of one or more tongues, and need not be circumferential. The endoscopic diagnosis must be confirmed histologically. To avoid sampling errors, we recommend performing at least four biopsies for every 1 cm interval along the length of the Barrett's segment. The most important feature is to identify the presence of intestinalization of the mucosa and whether dysplasia has occurred, and if so, whether of high or low grade.

Elderly patients, those with a low risk of developing complications and those whose symptoms are readily controlled by medication may be considered for medical therapy. H_2 blockers and omeprazole often bring symptomatic improvement, especially if hypersecretion of acid is an aetiological factor. Objective healing of ulcers and stabilization of strictures is not as reliably achieved. The value of prokinetic agents, such as bethanechol or cisapride, is usually minimal because of the loss of oesophageal body function. The principal problem with medical treatment is that acid reduction therapy does nothing to correct the underlying mechanically defective sphincter, and therefore does nothing to reduce the reflux of neutralized gastric juice or the prevention of aspiration. Indeed the symptomatic relief may allow tissue damage to progress unnoticed, so that advancement of the disease continues to occur. For this reason, surgery is appropriate earlier in the course of the disease when it is first evident that the oesophagitis is resistant to healing by usual measures.

In uncomplicated Barrett's oesophagus, the loss of oesophageal body function can still occur but the patients are less frequently referred for surgery. However, one comparative study showed better symptom control and a lower incidence of complications of Barrett's oesophagus in patients treated by

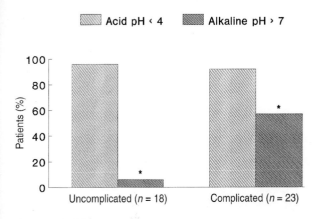

Figure 11.20

Prevalence of abnormal oesophageal acid and alkaline exposure in patients with or without complications of Barrett's oesophagus (*P<0.01 Fisher's exact test). (Reproduced from DeMeester TR, Attwood SEA, Smyrk TC et al. *Ann Surg* 1990; 212: 528–542.)

antireflux surgery compared with high-dose ranitidine.[59] More often, patients with complicated Barrett's oesophagus are referred for surgery and the status of oesophageal function renders it necessary to modify the operative strategy. This includes oesophageal body shortening, loss of peristaltic propulsive force, stricture formation and a large penetrating ulcer.

In these circumstances, it is wiser to use a transthoracic approach as it allows thorough mobilization of the infra-aortic oesophagus and provides the option of performing a Collis gastroplasty if shortening of the oesophagus persists despite full mobilization. It also puts the surgeon in the best position to deal with mediastinal inflammation secondary to a penetrating ulcer, where there is a risk of creating a full-thickness defect in the oesophageal wall after mobilization. If this occurs, oesophageal replacement is usually necessary.

Since Barrett's oesophagus is a premalignant condition and Barrett's patients represent the extreme end of the pathophysiological spectrum in GORD, there are strong theoretical grounds for considering early antireflux surgery in all but the elderly and unfit patient. The goal of antireflux surgery is to prevent progression of the disease rather than produce regression of the Barrett's epithelium. Regression of Barrett's epithelium after surgery has been reported,[59-61] in some patients, but it is possible that some of the more enthusiastic reports may have included artefacts related to surgical relocation of the oesophagogastric junction. Despite the small incidence of regression, there is a growing body of evidence to attest to the ability of fundoplication to protect against dysplasia and invasive malignancy. Although some cancers have developed after antireflux surgery, the absence of pre-existent dysplasia or the efficacy of the operative procedure in reducing 24-hour oesophageal acid exposure to normal has not been documented. A long-term registry maintained on patients with Barrett's free of dysplasia on entry recently reported that the development of dysplasia and cancer in patients healed medically was 19.7 and 1.3%, respectively, whereas in those treated by fundoplication, dysplasia emerged in only 3.4% and no

cancers developed.[62] This information has been used to recommend surgery as a prophylactic measure in patients with a segment of Barrett's mucosa free of dysplasia. It is not known what effect antireflux surgery has when dysplasia is already present. The situation is more clear when high-grade dysplasia is discovered at biopsy. If this is confirmed by two knowledgeable pathologists, oesophagectomy is recommended because 50% of the operative specimens from these patients will show early invasive carcinoma.

Surveillance requirements

Regular yearly endoscopic surveillance with biopsies has been incorporated into the practice of most gastroenterologists. Biopsies should be reviewed by a pathologist with expertise in this field.

If low-grade dysplasia is confirmed, biopsies should be repeated after 12 weeks of antisecretory therapy. If high-grade dysplasia is evident on more than one biopsy, resectional surgery is advisable because of the high risk that invasive cancer is already present.[63] Early detection and resection will decrease the mortality rate from oesophageal cancer in these patients. Among 16 patients who had undergone oesophageal resection for Barrett's adenocarcinoma, there were no deaths in five patients in whom the malignancy was detected by endoscopic surveillance, whereas 11 patients who had cancer not detected during a surveillance programme died of the tumour.[64] Williamson et al.[65] and Lerut et al.[66] have reported on similar good results after resection of early cancer diagnosed during surveillance procedures. The 5-year survival in nine patients without lymph node metastases in Lerut's series was 91.7%.

The short oesophagus

Failure to recognize and plan appropriate surgical therapy for the short oesophagus will inevitably result in failure. The so-called 'slipped' Nissen fundoplication probably represents a surgical error from the outset when the fundoplication is mistakenly placed around a stomach which is tubularized by excessive traction.

Recognition of the short oesophagus which requires a Collis lengthening procedure may be difficult, and the need for oesophageal lengthening may only be evident during surgery. An irreducible hernia assessed radiologically is an inaccurate predictor of reducibility. It is sometimes possible to assess reducibility of the hernia at the endoscopy evaluation. During surgery, the oesophagus must be mobilized completely to the aortic arch, and if the hernia cannot be reduced well into the abdominal cavity without tension, a Collis gastroplasty must be added to the antireflux procedure. Oesophageal motility in patients with reflux stricture is usually poor, and this precludes a 360° fundoplication (Figure 11.21). In such cases, our preference has been to use the Belsey Mark IV procedure.

Atypical reflux symptoms

Chronic respiratory symptoms, such as chronic cough, recurrent pneumonias, episodes of nocturnal choking, waking up with gastric contents in the mouth, or soilage of the pillow,

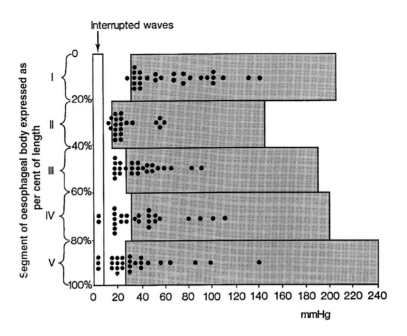

Figure 11.21
Individual distribution of amplitude of oesophageal contractions in 28 consecutive patients with reflux-induced oesophageal stricture. The shaded area represents the normal range (2.5–97.5 percentile) of amplitude for each segment of the oesophageal body. In patients with short oesophagi, only three or four segments could be measured. (From: Zaninotto G, DeMeester TR, Bremner CG et al. *Ann Thorac Surg* 1989; 47: 367.)

may also indicate the need for surgical therapy. The chest radiograph in patients suffering from repetitive pulmonary aspiration secondary to gastro-oesophageal reflux often shows signs of pleural thickening, bronchiectasis and chronic interstitial pulmonary fibrosis. If 24-hour pH monitoring confirms the presence of increased oesophageal acid exposure and manometry shows a mechanical defect of the lower oesophageal sphincter and normal oesophageal body motility, an antireflux procedure can be performed, with an expected good result. Usually these patients have, however, a non-specific motor abnormality of the oesophageal body which tends to propel the refluxed material towards the pharynx. In some of these patients the motor abnormality will disappear after a surgical antireflux procedure. In others, the motor disorder will persist and contribute to postoperative aspiration of swallowed saliva and food. Consequently, the results of an antireflux procedure in patients with a motor disorder of the oesophageal body are variable.

Chest pain may be an atypical symptom of gastro-oesophageal reflux and is often confused with coronary artery disease. Fifty per cent of patients in whom a cardiac aetiology of the chest pain has been excluded will have increased oesophageal acid exposure as a cause of the episode of pain. An antireflux procedure provides relief of the chest pain with greater constancy than will occur with medical therapy.

Dysphagia, regurgitation and/or chest pain on eating in a patient with normal endoscopy and oesophageal function studies can be an indication for an antireflux procedure. These symptoms are usually related to the presence of a large para-oesophageal hernia, an intrathoracic stomach or a small hiatal hernia with a narrow diaphragmatic hiatus. A Schatzki ring

may be present with the last. All these conditions are easily identified with an upper gastrointestinal barium examination performed by a knowledgeable radiologist. These patients may have no heartburn because the lower oesophageal sphincter is usually normal and reflux of gastric acid into the oesophagus does not occur. The surgical repair of the hernia usually includes an antireflux procedure because the competence of the cardia has a high probability of being destroyed by the surgical dissection. If a Schatzki ring is identified in a patient with dysphagia, a hiatus hernia, a normal size of hiatus and normal oesophageal acid exposure, dilatation with a 60 Fr often gives relief of dysphagia. The symptoms, however, may reoccur and repeat pH testing is necessary to exclude gastro-oesophageal reflux and the possible need for antireflux surgery.

Scleroderma

Gastro-oesophageal reflux in association with scleroderma is a particularly difficult situation due to the complete absence of the lower oesophageal sphincter and contractility in the distal oesophagus. Intensive medical therapy should be used initially until symptoms or severe oesophagitis can no longer be controlled. When this occurs a Belsey Mark IV partial fundoplication in association with a gastroplasty can be done, with the expectation that this will reduce oesophageal acid exposure but not return it to normal. The gastroplasty is added because of the shortening of the oesophagus that occurs as a consequence of the disease. About 50% of patients receive excellent to good results with this approach. If the oesophagitis is severe or there has been a previous failed antireflux procedure and the disease is associated with delayed gastric emptying, a gastric resection with Roux-en-Y oesophagojejunostomy and a Hunt–Lawrence pouch has provided the best option.

Previous gastric surgery

The presence of a mechanically defective sphincter after vagotomy and gastric resection or pyloroplasty can allow reflux of gastric and pancreaticobiliary secretions into the oesophagus. This problem is usually manifest by symptoms of regurgitation and pulmonary aspiration. Heartburn may be present. Endoscopic oesophagitis can occur and is usually mild. Medical therapy designed to control both acid and alkaline reflux usually fails, and a bile-diverting procedure, without reconstruction of the cardia, is of little benefit in preventing the symptoms of aspiration and may contribute to delayed gastric emptying. A simple antireflux procedure may be difficult when a gastric resection has been done. In this situation, the proper surgical therapy usually requires a complete gastric resection with a Roux-en-Y oesophagojejunostomy and a Hunt–Lawrence pouch. Bile diversion procedures such as antrectomy, vagotomy and Roux-en-Y will give a failure rate of 15–20%.[67] Exceptionally, a primary bile diverting procedure (suprapapillary duodenojejunostomy)[68] should be considered.

Reflux in association with oesophageal motor disorders

The presence of reflux oesophagitis after balloon dilatation for achalasia that persists despite medical therapy is an indication for early surgical intervention because oesophagitis in the presence of a severe motility disorder progresses rapidly to stricture formation. A Belsey Mark IV partial fundoplication or a transabdominal partial fundoplication procedure, such as the Toupet or Watson, should be performed in this situation because their low outflow resistance makes them particularly suitable to an oesophageal body that has no propulsive activity. Once a stricture has developed under these conditions, oesophageal resection and a colon interposition is usually necessary to re-establish alimentation. In this situation, a vagal sparing oesophagectomy should be done because postoperative function of the reconstructed foregut is much improved if the vagal function is preserved.

REFERENCES

1. Pace F, Santalucia F & Porro GB. Natural history of gastro-oesophageal reflux disease without esophagitis. *Gut* 1991; **32:** 845–848.
2. Hetzel DJ, Dent J, Reed WD et al. Healing and relapse of severe peptic esophagitis after treatment with omeprazole. *Gastroenterology* 1988; **95:** 903–912.
3. Ollyo JB, Monnier P, Fontolliet C & Savary M: The natural history, prevalence and incidence of reflux esophagitis. *Gullet* 1993; **3**(Suppl.): 3–10.
4. Jamieson JR, Stein HJ, DeMeester TR et al. Ambulatory 24-hour esophageal pH monitoring: normal values, optimal thresholds, specificity, sensitivity and reproducibility. *Am J Gastroenterol* 1992; **87:** 1102–1111.
5. Bremner RM, Crookes PF, DeMeester TR, Peters JH & Stein HJ. Concentration of refluxed acid and esophageal mucosal injury. *Am J Surg* 1992; **164:** 522–526.
6. Zaninotto G, DiMario F, Costantini M et al. Oesophagitis and pH of refluxante: an experimental and clinical study. *Br J Surg* 1992; **79:** 161–164.
7. Richter JE, Pandol SJ, Castell DO & McCarthy DM. Gastroesophageal reflux disease in the Zollinger–Ellison syndrome. *Ann Intern Med* 1981; **95:** 37–43.
8. Collen MJ, Lewis JH & Benjamin SB. Gastric acid hyposecretion in refractory gastroesophageal reflux disease. *Gastroenterology* 1990; **98:** 654–661.
9. Mulholland MW, Reid BJ, Levine DS & Rubin CE. Elevated gastric acid secretion in patients with Barrett's metaplastic epithelium. *Dig Dis Sci* 1989; **34:** 1329–1334.
10. Goldstern JL, Watkins JL, Greager JA & Layden TJ. The esophageal mucosal resistance: structure and function of a unique gastroesophageal epithelial barrier. *J Lab Clin Med* 1994; **123:** 653–559.
11. Salo J & Kivilaakso E. Role of luminal H⁺ in the pathogenesis of experimental esophagitis. *Surgery* 1982; **92:** 61–68.
12. Bremner CG & Mason RJ. Bile in the esophagus. *Br J Surg* 1993; **19:** 1374–1376.
13. Pellegrini CA, DeMeester TR, Wernly JA et al. Alkaline gastroesophageal reflux. *Am J Surg* 1978; **135:** 177–184.
14. Fiorucci S, Santucci L, Chiucchiu S & Morelli A. Gastric acidity and gastroesophageal reflux patterns in patients with esophagitis. *Gastroenterology* 1992; **103:** 855–861.
15. Fuchs KH & DeMeester TR. Intragastric pH pattern analysis in patients with duodenogastric reflux. *Dig Dis* 1990; **9**(Suppl. 1): 54–59.
16. Fuchs KH, DeMeester TR, Hinder RA et al. Computerized identification of pathologic duodenogastric reflux using 24-hour gastric pH monitoring. *Ann Surg* 1991; **213:** 13–20.
17. Jaervinen V, Meurman JH, Hyvaerinen H et al. Dental erosion and upper gastrointestinal disorders. *Oral Surg Med Pathol* 1988; **65:** 298–303.
18. DeVault KR, Georgeson S & Castell DO. Salivary stimulation mimics esophageal exposure to refluxed duodenal contents. *Am J Gastroenterol* 1993; **88:** 1040–1043.
19. Stein HJ, Feussner H, Kauer W et al. 'Alkaline' gastroesophageal reflux assessment by ambulatory esophageal aspiration and pH monitoring. *Am J Surg* 1994; **167:** 163–168.
20. Kauer WKH. *Langzeitrefluxzspirationstest – eine neue Methode zur qualitativen und quantitativen Refluatanalyse bei 'nicht saurem' Reflux.* Doctoral thesis, Technical University of Munich, 1994.
21. Singh S, Bradley LA & Richter JE. Determinants of oesophageal alkaline: pH environment in controls and patients with gastro-oesophageal reflux disease. *Gut* 1993; **34:** 309–316.
22. Stein JH, Hoeft S & DeMeester TR. Functional foregut abnormalities in Barrett's esophagus. *J Thorac Cardiovasc Surg* 1993; **105:** 107–111.
23. Attwood SE, DeMeester TR, Bremner CG et al. Alkaline gastroesophageal reflux: implications in the development of complications in Barrett's columnar-lined lower esophagus. *Surgery* 1989; **106:** 764–770.
24. Attwood SEA, Ball CS, Barlow AP, Jenkinson LR, Norris TL & Watson A. Role of intragastric and intra-oesophageal alkalinisation in the genesis of complications in Barrett's columnar-lined oesophagus. *Gut* 1993; **34:** 11–15.
25. Gotley DC, Ball DE, Ownen RW et al. Evaluation and surgical correction of esophagitis after partial gastrectomy. *Surgery* 1992; **111:** 29–36.
26. Gotley DC, Morgan AP, Ball DE et al. Composition of gastro-oesophageal refluxate. *Gut* 1991; **32:** 1093–1099.
27. Stein JH, Hinder RA & DeMeester TR. Clinical use of 24-hour gastric pH monitoring vs. o-diisopropyl iminiodiacetic acid (DISIDA) scanning in the diagnosis of pathologic duodenogastric reflux. *Arch Surg* 1990; **125:** 966–970.
28. Ritchie WP. Alkaline reflux gastritis: an objective assessment of its diagnosis and treatment. *Ann Surg* 1980; **92:** 288–298.
29. Offerhaus GJ, Tersmette AC, Tersmette KW et al. Gastric, pancreatic and colorectal carcinogenesis following remote peptic ulcer surgery. *Mod Pathol* 1989; **1:** 352–356.
30. Stein JH, Barlow AP & DeMeester TR. Complications of gastroesophageal reflux disease. Role of the lower esophageal sphincter, esophageal acid and acid/alkaline exposure, and duodenogastric reflux. *Ann Surg* 1992; **216:** 35–43.
31. Harmon JW, Johnson LF & Maydonovitch CL. Effect of acid and bile salts in the rabbit esophageal mucosa. *Dig Dis Sci* 1981; **26:** 65–72.
32. Harmon JW, Doang T & Gadacz TR. Bile acids are not equally damaging in the gastric mucosa. *Surgery* 1978; **84:** 79–86.
33. Ball CS, Jenkinson LR, Watson A & Norris TL. Acid sensitivity in reflux oesophagitis with and without complications. *Gut* 1988; **29:** 729.
34. DeMeester TR. Barrett's esophagus. *Surgery* 1993; **113:** 239–240.
35. Richardson JD, Williams RA, Ackerman DM, Wheller M, Cornett D &

Benjamin S. Mechanisms involved in the development of Barrett's esophagus: an experimental rat model. *Dis Esoph* 1994; **7:** 53–59.

36. Sarr MG, Hamilton SR, Marone GC et al. Barrett's esophagus: its prevalence and association with adenocarcinoma in patients with symptoms of gastroesophageal reflux. *Am J Surg* 1985; **149:** 187–193.

37. Zaninotto G, DeMeester TR, Bremner CG, Smyrk TC & Cheng SC. Esophageal function in patients with reflux induced strictures and its relevance to surgical treatment. *Ann Thorac Surg* 1989; **47:** 352–370.

38. Bonavina L, DeMeester TR, McChesney L et al. Drug-induced esophageal strictures. *Ann Surg* 1987; **206:** 173–183.

39. Pellegrini CA, DeMeester TR, Johnson LF et al. Gastroesophageal reflux and pulmonary aspiration: incidence, functional abnormality, and results of surgical therapy. *Surgery* 1979; **86:** 110–119.

40. Patti MG, Debas HT & Pellegrini CA. Clinical and functional characterization of high gastroesophageal reflux. *Am J Surg* 1993; **165:** 163–168.

41. Savary M & Miller G. The esophagus. *Handbook and Atlas of Endoscopy.* Solothurn, Switzerland: Gassman, 1979; 135–139.

42. Lieberman DA. Medical therapy for chronic reflux esophagitis. *Arch Intern Med* 1987; **147:** 1717–1720.

43. Kuster E, Ros E, Toledo-Pimentel Y et al. Predictive factors of the long-term outcome in gastroesophageal reflux disease: six year follow-up of 107 patients. *Gut* 1994; **35:** 8–14.

44. Toupet A. Technique d'oesophago-gastroplastie aver phrénogastropexie appliquée dans la cure radicale des hernies histales et comme complément de l'opération d'Heller dans les cardiospismes. *Mem Acad Chir* 1963; **89:** 394.

45. Watson A, Jenkinson LR, Ball CS, Barlow AP & Norris TL. A more physiological alternative to tal fundoplication for the surgical correction of resistant gastro-oesophageal reflux. *Br J Surg* 1991; **78:** 1088–1094.

46. DeMeester TR, Bonavina L & Albertucci M. Nissen fundoplication for gastroesophageal reflux disease – evaluation of primary repair in 100 consecutive patients. *Ann Surg* 1986; **204:** 9–20.

47. Stein HJ, Bremner RM, Jamieson J & DeMeester TR. Effect of Nissen fundoplication on esophageal motor function. *Arch Surg* 1992; **127:** 288–291.

48. Watson A. Controlled trial of medical versus surgical reflux control in the management of peptic oesophageal stricture treated by intermittent dilatation. *Gut* 1985; **26:** 553–554.

49. Watson A. Reflux stricture of the oesophagus. *Br J Surg* 1987; **74:** 443–448.

50. Watson A. A clinical study of the role of anti-reflux surgery combined with endoscopic dilatation in peptic oesophageal stricture. *Am J Surg* 1984; **148:** 346–349.

51. Bremner CG. Benign strictures of the esophagus. *Curr Prob Surg* 1982; **19:** 401–489.

52. Bremner CG. Current management of benign esophageal strictures. *J Coll Surg Edinb* 1989; **34:** 297–301.

53. Ott DJ, Gelfand DW, Lane TG & Wu WC. Radiologic detection and spectrum of appearance of peptic esophageal strictures. *J Clin Gastroenterol* 1982; **4:** 11–15.

54. Bremner RM & Bremner CG. Barrett's oesophagus – radiological features in 100 cases. *S Afr Med J* 1990; **78:** 660–664.

55. Kahrilas PJ, Dodds WJ & Hogan WJ. Effect of peristaltic dysfunction on esophageal volume clearance. *Gastroenterology* 1988; **94:** 73–80.

56. Barrett NR. Chronic peptic ulcer of the oesophagus and oesophagitis. *Br J Surg* 1950; **38:** 175–182.

57. Mason RJ & Bremner CG. Motility differences between long-segment and short-segment Barrett's esophagus. *Am J Surg* 1993; **165:** 686–689.

58. Bremner CG. The management of the columnar-lined esophagus. In Jamieson GG (ed.) *Surgery of the Oesophagus.* Edinburgh: Churchill Livingstone, 1988: 223–232.

59. Attwood SEA, Barlow AP, Norris TL & Watson A. Barrett's oesophagus: effect of antireflux surgery on symptom control and development of complications. *Br J Surg* 1992; **79:** 1050–1053.

60. Skinner DB, Walther BC, Riddell RH, Schmidt H, Iascone C & DeMeester TR. Barrett's esophagus: comparison of benign and malignant cases. *Ann Surg* 1983; **198:** 554–565.

61. Brand DL, Ylvisaker JT, Gelfand M & Pope CE. Regression of columnar esophageal (Barrett's) epithelium after antireflux surgery. *N Engl J Med* 1980; **302:** 844–848.

62. McCallum RW, Palepalle S, Davenport K, Frierson H & Boyd S. Role of antireflux surgery against dysplasia in Barrett's esophagus. *Gastroenterology* 1991; **100:** A121.

63. Dent J, Bremner CG, Collen MJ, Haggitt RC & Spechler SJ. Working party report to the World Congress of Gastroenterology, Sydney 1990. Barrett's esophagus. *J Gastroenterol Hepatol* 1991; **6:** 1–22.

64. Duhaylongsod FG & Wolfe WG. Barrett's esophagus and adenocarcinoma of the esophagus and gastroesophageal junction. *J Thorac Cardiovasc Surg* 1991; **102:** 36–42.

65. Williamson WA, Ellis FH, Gibb SP et al. Barrett's esophagus: prevalence and incidence of adenocarcinoma. *Arch Intern Med* 1991; **151:** 2212–2216.

66. Lerut T, DeLeyn P, Coosemans W et al. Surgical strategies in esophageal carcinoma with emphasis on radical lymphadenectomy. *Ann Surg* 1992; **216:** 583–590.

67. Hinder RA & Bremner CG. The uses and consequences of the Roux-en-Y operation. *Surg Annu* 1987: 151–174.

68. DeMeester TR, Fuchs KH, Ball CS, Albertucci M, Smyrk TC & Marcus JN Experimental and clinical results with proximal end-to-end duodenojejunostomy for pathologic duodenogastric reflux. *Ann Surg* 1987; **206:** 414–426.

12

DIAPHRAGMATIC HERNIA

RT Spychal

ANATOMY

The diaphragm

The diaphragm is a domed, musculotendinous septum that separates the thorax from the abdomen and is pierced by the structures that pass between them. It consists of a skeletal muscular part arising from the margins of the body wall and a centrally placed tendon. The muscular fibres take origin peripherally and insert into the margin of the trefoil shaped central tendon. The origin of the diaphragm may be divided into three parts; a sternal part consisting of small slips arising from the posterior surface of the xiphisternum, a costal part arising from the lower six costal cartilages and a vertebral part arising by means of crura and from the arcuate ligaments (Figure 12.1).

The right crus arises from the bodies of the upper four lumbar vertebrae and their intervening discs, whereas the left crus arises from the first two or three lumbar vertebrae. Lateral to the crura, the diaphragm arises from the medial and lateral arcuate ligaments, which are the thickened upper margins of the fascia overlying the psoas and quadratus lumborum muscles. The fibrous medial borders of the two crura are connected by the median arcuate ligament which crosses over the front of the aorta. The crura pass upwards and forwards to form a sling that forms the margin of the oesophageal opening with the median arcuate ligament behind. The fibres of the right crus usually form the boundaries of the oesophageal opening although there is considerable variation in the relative contribution of the left crus[1] (Figure 12.2). The crura are musculotendinous, being more tendinous posteriorly, from their vertebral origin, and medially.[2]

The oesophageal opening is 2–3 cm to the left of the midline at the level of the tenth thoracic vertebra. It transmits the oesophagus, the right and left vagus nerves, the oesophageal branches of the left gastric vessels and the lymphatics of the lower oesophagus. The aortic opening is in the midline at the

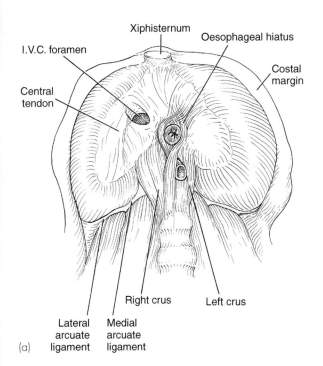

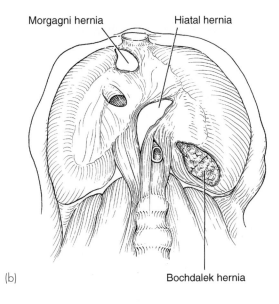

Figure 12.1

The diaphragm seen from below. (a) Origins from the body wall. (b) Sites of congenital and hiatal herniation.

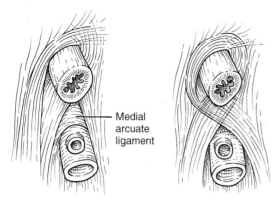

Figure 12.2
The variation of the crural sling. (a) Most common arrangement, in 50% of cases, with the right crus providing the sling. (b) Left crus contributes to the right limb of the sling.

level of the twelfth thoracic vertebra behind the crura. It transmits the aorta, the thoracic duct and azygos vein. The foramen for the vena cava is in the central tendon 3 cm to the right of the midline opposite the eighth thoracic vertebra and transmits the inferior vena cava with terminal branches of the right phrenic nerve.

The left phrenic nerve travels on the lateral border of the heart to pierce the muscular part of the diaphragm in front of the central tendon. The phrenic nerves provide the motor supply on the abdominal surface of the diaphragm. They split into branches that fan out to supply the sternal, costal, lateral and crural parts of the diaphragm.

Other structures which pierce the crura include the splanchnic nerves, the sympathetic trunk which passes posterior to the medial arcuate ligament, the subcostal nerves and vessels which run behind the lateral arcuate ligament, and the superficial epigastric vessels which pass between the sternal and costal origins of the diaphragm on either side.

Phreno-oesophageal membrane

The phreno-oesophageal membrane is an arrangement of elastic and collagenous fibres that derive from peridiaphragmatic tissue and fan out to penetrate the distal 2–3 cm of the oesophageal muscle.[3] Most of the membrane is derived from the transversalis fascia on the undersurface of the diaphragm with a smaller contribution from the endothoracic fascia above (Figure 12.3). This structure is thought to tether the distal oesophagus within the hiatal tunnel and maintains the oesophagogastric junction in its correct intra-abdominal position. As it has an elastic component, it allows the normal physiological movement of the lower oesophagus.

During fetal development the diaphragm and oesophagus are bound at the hiatus by connective tissue[4] but in postnatal life the oesophagus needs to be more mobile and the space between the two becomes filled with looser connective tissue. With increasing age this membrane becomes less pronounced, and in patients with hiatal hernia the structure is particularly attenuated or may be absent.[3,4]

The importance, or even the presence of this structure

appears to polarize opinion much as does the question of whether the diaphragm and its afflictions should be approached from above or below. Harrington[5] and Allison[6] were believers in its importance whereas Barrett dismissed it as '... strands of tissue, which can be dissected out with the eye of faith ... they can be ignored'.[7]

Oesophagogastric junction and hiatal hernia

Hiatal hernia describes an anatomical abnormality whereby part of the stomach protrudes above the oesophageal hiatus. In a sliding hiatus hernia, the lower oesophagus and upper stomach form a tubular structure at the cardia which slides above the hiatus. In paraoesophageal hiatal hernia, the fundus and greater curvature of the stomach bulge above the hiatus into the posterior mediastinum but with the cardia normally situated. When the cardia is also displaced upwards the hernia is termed a mixed sliding and paraoesophageal hernia (Figure 12.4).

The definition of the site of the oesophagogastric junction and hence hiatal hernia depend upon the anatomical, histological, radiological, surgical and endoscopic perspective.

Anatomically, the junction lies at the end of the tubular oesophagus as it joins the saccular stomach. The histological junction is the irregular boundary between the stratified squamous and the simple columnar junctional epithelium, with the true gastric epithelium commencing more distally. The oesophageal mucosa moves easily over the underlying muscle layer and hence makes the precise relationship between these junctions somewhat variable. The histological mucosal junction is usually 1–3 cm above the anatomical junction.

Radiologically, the junction is assessed by various landmarks including the upper level of the transverse rugal gastric folds, the notch from the gastric sling fibres and an imaginary transverse line drawn from the angle of implantation of the oesophagus to the lesser curve of stomach. The lower end of the oesophagus may balloon slightly to form the vestibule or phrenic ampulla before joining the stomach. If the radiological oesophagogastric junction is seen to lie above the level of the

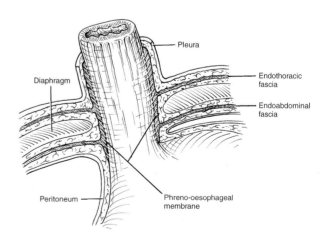

Figure 12.3
The phreno-oesophageal membrane. Origins and attachments.

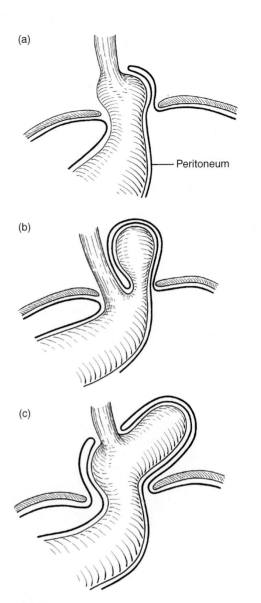

Figure 12.4

Types of hiatal hernia. Relationship to peritoneal sac and site of oesophago-gastric junction. (a) Siding hiatal hernia. (b) Para-oesophageal hiatal hernia. (c) Mixed hiatal hernia.

diaphragm, then a sliding hiatal hernia is diagnosed. As the oesophageal hiatal sling is more vertical than horizontal, this makes the radiological assessment somewhat inprecise, particularly if not based on lateral views. The distinction between a reducible and fixed hiatal hernia is made if the gastric folds are not visible above the diaphragm at the start of a swallow. The mobility of the oesophagogastric junction is readily seen during fluoroscopic screening and provocative testing, such as sucking through a straw. From a surgical perspective, the oesophago-gastric junction is the upper border of the peritoneal reflection from the stomach onto the oesophagus. At laparoscopy the increased intra-abdominal pressure of a pneumoperitoneum may accentuate the appearance of a hiatus hernia.

Endoscopically, the mucosal junction, ora serrata or Z-line, is seen where the pale pink oesophageal mucosa abuts darker red gastric mucosa. The depth of colour is variable between

subjects. The mucosal junction is seen to be mobile during respiration and on movement of the endoscope and distension of the stomach. The diaphragm normally clasps the oesophagogastric junction and can be seen to contract during respiration. Sniffing and deep breaths will accentuate this diaphragmatic hiatal closure. The site of the hiatus and degree to which it contracts to obliterate the lumen can be visualized endoscopically. The site of the Z-line and the diaphragmatic closure are recorded from the markings on the endoscope and the difference is the length of the sliding hiatus hernia, although differences less than 2 cm may not be significant. Retrograde views of the oesophagogastric junction with the endoscope retroflexed in the stomach (J manoeuvre) will visualize a patulous hiatus and a gastric pouch. This view can also identify a paraoesophageal component to the hiatal hernia.

The classification of hiatal hernia and gastro-oesophageal reflux proposed by the International Society for Diseases of the Esophagus[8] takes into account some of the variables discussed above and recognizes that there is usually no difficulty in the diagnosis of a sliding hiatal hernia greater than 3 cm for either radiologist or endoscopist. This simple grading is as follows.

0. No hiatal herniation identified

1. Small and/or reducing sliding hiatal hernia

2. Constant sliding hiatal hernia, not reducing on barium studies or with the oesophagogastric junction fixed more than 3 cm above the diaphragm on endoscopy

3. Mixed or para-oesophageal hiatal hernia.

SLIDING HIATAL HERNIA

A sliding hiatal hernia occurs when the gastro-oesophageal junction is displaced upwards through the oesophageal hiatus into the posterior mediastinum (Figures 12.4 and 12.5). This carries with it a peritoneal sac from the front and left side of the stomach. The right and posterior aspect of the sliding hiatal hernia is not covered with peritoneum as it is derived from the bare area of the stomach. The sac is always empty with its apex lying close to the level of the oesophago-gastric junction.[4] The anatomical analogy with a sliding inguinal hernia is a good one in that in both an organ herniates out of the abdomen and itself forms part of the hernial sac.

Varying amounts of the stomach may be above the diaphragm depending on the size of the crural defect, posture and the intra-abdominal pressure. Mobility of the oesophagogastric junction is needed to facilitate normal swallowing, vomiting and belching. As the oesophagus shortens during swallowing, the gastric cardia tents upwards through the hiatus. The ease with which herniation can be visualized during provocative radiological contrast studies is a testament to this. This phenomenon provided convincing evidence against hiatal hernia alone being important in gastro-oesophageal reflux disease.

Quite how a sliding hiatal hernia develops is unclear. As it can occur in infancy and childhood a congenital cause is feasible. In the rare cases of congenital oesophageal shortening there is no sac present and the oesophagogastric junction lies

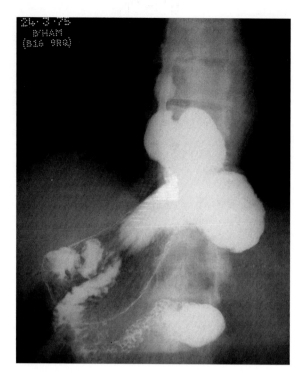

Figure 12.5
Barium study demonstrating a sliding hiatal hernia.

fixed in the chest, presumably due to failure of elongation of the embryological oesophagus. Hiatal hernias diagnosed in early childhood persist into adulthood in about 50% of cases.[9] There is a 10% incidence of hiatal hernia after repair of congenital diaphragmatic hernia in neonates which may represent relative shortening of the oesophagus when the hypoplastic lungs expand.[10]

Overt hiatal hernia formation may result from progressive degeneration of the phreno-oesophageal membrane.[11] The membrane becomes less definite with age, contains fewer elastic fibres and subperitoneal fat accumulates in its vicinity thus making the oesophagogastric junction less firmly fixed.[3,6] When the normal fan-like distribution of its fibres is lost it forms a single layer attached proximally that may allow the formation of a sliding hernia.[4] The phrenic ampulla, or vestibule, is thought to represent that part of the oesophagus encompassed by the phreno-oesophageal membrane. It is analogous to a small reducing hiatal hernia; at times the distinction between the two is arbitrary.[11] There is no relationship between the type of configuration of the crural sling and frequency of hiatal hernia.[1]

It is possible that hiatal hernia may occur as a consequence of reflux. The longitudinal muscle of the oesophagus, which connects the base of skull to the oesophagogastric junction via the median raphe of the pharynx, may contract as a result of reflux events which provoke mucosal irritation. As the intra-abdominal oesophageal length progressively shortens the cardia elevates above the diaphragm. Animal work on oesophageal shortening by acute mucosal acid exposure lends support to the concept that oesophagitis could contribute to shortening of the long axis of the oesophagus.[12] In the later

stages of severe reflux damage, oesophageal shortening may have the effect of pulling more stomach into the chest.

The natural history of sliding hiatal hernias is variable. In an asymptomatic population, 30% may have a hiatal hernia although this does depend on how the diagnosis is made.[13,14] The oesophageal hiatus increases in size with age[15] as does the incidence of hiatal hernia.[16] Some hernias could remain stable and undiagnosed over years, however once diagnosed hiatal hernias have a tendency to become larger with time.[17]

Relationship to gastro-oesophageal reflux

The symptoms associated with sliding hiatal hernia, when present, are essentially those of gastro-oesophageal reflux, mechanical symptoms being uncommon, in contradistinction to paraoesophageal hernias. About 50% of patients with upper gastrointestinal symptoms and a hiatal hernia will have evidence of gastro-oesophageal reflux, whereas 60–90% of all those with reflux will have a coexisting hiatal hernia.[18-22]

Sliding hiatal hernia is one of the many contributing factors in the development and pathogenesis of gastro-oesophageal reflux and as such should not be considered in isolation. Much of the confusion about the relationship between hiatal hernia and reflux may be due to considerable variation in the prevalence of oesophagitis and in the radiological criteria used for the diagnosis of hiatal hernia.[14] The case against hiatal hernia being solely responsible for gastro-oesophageal reflux was polarized by Cohen and Harris[23] who demonstrated, in a large group of selected subjects with reflux, that symptoms only occurred in the presence of a hypotensive lower oesophageal sphincter, irrespective of whether a hernia was present or not. Other studies have shown that resting lower oesophageal sphincter pressure alone correlates poorly with the presence or absence of reflux.[24] and that the presence of a hiatal hernia, but not a hypotensive sphincter, is the prime predictor of frequency of reflux, acid contact time and hence oesophagitis.[21] The importance of transient lower oesophageal sphincter relaxation in reflux episodes[25] and the action of the crural diaphragm in protecting against stress reflux[26] only serve to illustrate the multifactorial nature of gastro-oesophageal reflux disease.

Although the presence of a hiatal hernia in reflux may make little difference to the manometric evaluation of the lower oesophageal sphincter, exposure to refluxate is increased by poor clearance.[27] Hiatal hernias may act as a reservoir for refluxate thereby facilitating reflux.[28,29] During acid clearance a small amount is trapped in the hernial sac and refluxes into the oesophagus when the lower oesophageal sphincter relaxes on swallowing. These repeated episodes account for the delayed clearance in hiatus hernia with reflux.[29] The retrograde flow of reflux during the swallowing cycle can occur early during relaxation of the lower oesophageal sphincter and late when the sac empties. The increased acid clearance found in larger hiatal hernias is due to early retrograde flow.[28] The severity of reflux oesophagitis is strongly related to the presence and size of a sliding hiatal hernia.[18,20,30] Increasing size of hiatal hernia has also been correlated with poorer lower oesophageal sphincter function, poorer acid clearance, greater reflux and more severe oesophagitis.[30,31]

In conclusion gastro-oesophageal reflux can occur without the presence of a hiatal hernia and hiatal hernia can exist without reflux. Large sliding hiatal hernias, however, are more likely to be found in the more severe forms of gastro-oesophageal reflux.

Non-reflux features of sliding hiatal hernia

Symptomatic hiatal hernia usually relates to the symptoms of gastro-oesophageal reflux which are not different from those without hiatal hernia.[22] Benign ulceration and bleeding can occur with or without associated symptoms of reflux. Such ulcers occur in 1% of sliding hiatal hernias and account for 10% of benign gastric ulcers overall.[32] One series of large incarcerated hernias with complications requiring surgery found 10 of 17 to be sliding hiatal hernias alone.[33] The ulceration may be at the diaphragmatic constriction, the riding ulcer,[34] or within the herniated stomach. Haemorrhage presents either acutely or with chronic anaemia in half of the cases. Ulceration seems to be more common in larger hernias[17] and is associated with elderly females and non-steroidal anti-inflammatory drug use.[32]

As they have a high complication rate surgery may be most appropriate to relieve the mechanical cause of the ulceration.[17,32,33] The mechanical factors include trauma to the gastric mucosa at the site of constriction during respiration and relative ischaemia due to diaphragmatic pressure. An acid-reducing procedure is probably not necessary with repair of the hernia although an antireflux procedure is advisable[33,35] particularly if gastro-oesophageal reflux has been objectively demonstrated.

Management

The management of sliding hiatal hernia is really that of gastro-oesophageal reflux disease and is covered in depth in earlier chapters.

PARAOESOPHAGEAL HIATAL HERNIA AND MIXED HIATAL HERNIA

Paraoesophageal hiatal hernia is a true hernia with a peritoneal sac lying in the posterior mediastinum anterior to the oesophagus (Figure 12.4). The sac has the potential to contain any mobile intra-abdominal organ but initially contains the gastric fundus. The most mobile parts of the stomach will herniate anteriorly, but ultimately the whole stomach may herniate when the attachments of the gastrohepatic, gastrophrenic and gastrosplenic ligaments are stretched. Omentum, spleen and bowel can also enter the sac (Figures 12.6 and 12.7). Alternative terminology for para-oesophageal hiatal hernia includes rolling hiatal hernia, parahiatal hernia, intrathoracic stomach and upside-down stomach. The term parahiatal hernia should be restricted to the rare situation of a defect separate to the hiatus with a small part of the diaphragm intervening.[36] The distinction between a pure paraoesophageal hernia and a mixed paraoesophageal and sliding hernia is made based on whether the oesophagogastric junction is below or above the diaphragm (Figures 12.7 and 12.8). In the latter situation, gastro-oesophageal reflux is more likely.

Paraoesophageal hernia rarely occurs in childhood although the basic defect of a widened hiatus may be congenital rather like the Bochdalek or Morgagni foramina.[6,36,37] Barrett[7] believed that paraoesophageal herniation was into a

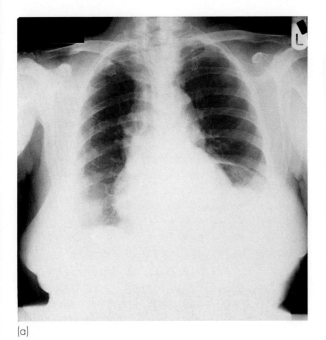

(a)

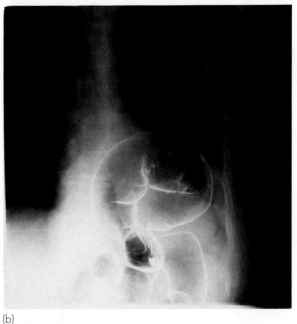

(b)

Figure 12.6
Paraoesophageal hernia. (a) Chest X-ray demonstrating a retrocardiac shadow. (b) Barium study of same patient showing colon within the hernia.

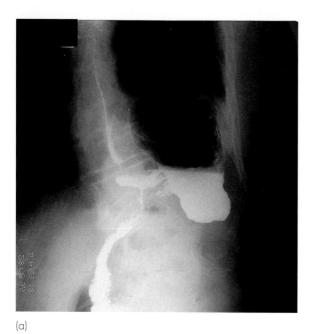

(a)

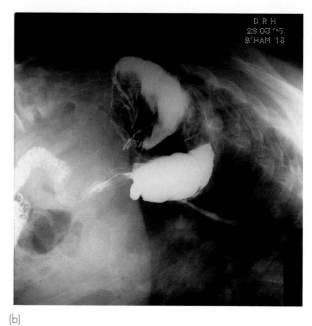

(b)

Figure 12.7
Barium meal showing intra-thoracic stomach with intermittent volvulus. (a) AP view. (b) Lateral view.

preformed congenital mediastinal sac which was an embry-ological remnant of the pneumoenteric recess. The presentation of paraoesophageal hernias in adult life and often in the elderly suggests that acquired factors are relevant also. Theories include an increase in intra-abdominal pressure from

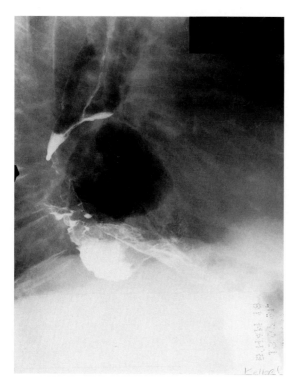

Figure 12.8
Barium study showing a mixed paraoesophageal and sliding hiatal hernia.

distension, coughing, straining and trauma, or possibly degeneration of the musculotendinous fibres of the crura. The phreno-oesophageal membrane remains intact and functional posteriorly, whilst being attenuated anteriorly thus allowing the paraoesophageal sac to develop, the posterior fibres being considered the strongest and hence tether the oesophagogastric junction.[36] Some authors believe that all paraoesophageal hernias represent an advanced stage of a sliding hiatal hernia.[35]

Iatrogenic paraoesophageal herniation is an important subgroup and occurs after both open and laparoscopic gastro-oesophageal surgery. Aetiological factors include disruption of the phreno-oesophageal membrane, lack of crural closure, unrecognized oesophageal shortening, postoperative gastric distension and too rapid a return to normal activity.[38–41]

The incidence of para-oesophageal hernia varies between series and accounts for 0.5–19% of all hiatal hernias seen in various units.[6,36,42–46] The incidence depends on whether the denominator is for surgically treated patients or allcomers, whether pure paraoesophageal hernias only are included, or whether the series only includes large hernias with a massive intrathoracic component. The relative incidence of pure and mixed hiatal hernia depends on different authors and their definitions.

Gastro-oesophageal reflux is classically said not to occur with pure paraoesophageal hernia, this being attributed to the oesophagogastric junction retaining its normal position.[6,36,47] In mixed sliding and paraoesophageal hernia reflux may be more common due to the displacement of the oesophagogastric junction. As competence of the oesophagogastric junction is not dependent on its position alone, this must represent a simplistic view. The reported rates of reflux symptoms in para-oesophageal hernia vary as does the incidence of the hernia, being anywhere between 7 and 72% with an average of 30% between series.[35,36,42,46,48-51]

Clinical features

The clinical presentation of paraoesophageal hernia may range from the asymptomatic to the catastrophic. Although it is usually seen late in life it can present at any age. An incidental finding on chest radiology is not an uncommon presentation. The most commonly reported clinical features include postprandial discomfort in 70%, nausea and vomiting in 40%, dysphagia in 40%, symptoms of reflux in 30% and gastrointestinal haemorrhage either acute or chronic in 30%.[35,42,44,46,48-51] The symptoms often appear intermittently and may seem vague. Early symptoms of epigastric discomfort and fullness may be ignored whereas hiccough, belching and chest gurgling may be embarrassing symptoms reported by partners rather than the patient. Respiratory difficulties and cardiac type pain may occur, symptoms that are probably more likely as the hernia enlarges particularly if there is a sudden increase.

Acute presentation of a paraoesophageal hernia may signify a potentially serious complication, including bleeding, perforation, gastric and oesophageal obstruction, gastric torsion or volvulus, strangulation and infarction. Ulceration from repeated trauma and torsion of the congested mucosa of an incarcerated stomach could bleed or perforate. Perforation from ulceration or infarction may result in contamination of the mediastinum, pleura or peritoneum and present with severe sepsis.

The presentation of gastric volvulus is characterized by Borchardt's triad of severe epigastric pain with vomiting, followed by retching with inability to vomit and difficulty in passing a nasogastric tube. Examination may reveal minimal abdominal signs apart from retraction, respiratory signs, a succussion splash in the chest and cardiorespiratory collapse.[52] Cardiorespiratory and haemodynamic embarrassment will accompany many of these acute presentations. Some may masquerade as pneumonia or cardiac pain.

Radiological examination is the main aid to diagnosis. Plain chest films may demonstrate a retrocardiac mass with air–fluid levels (Figure 12.6). Contrast studies can distinguish between the types of hiatal herniation and the amount of stomach involved in the hernia (Figures 12.7 and 12.8). Incarceration is diagnosed by an irreducible hernia on standing and volvulus may be demonstrated during the examination.

In acute cases, obstruction at the oesophageal or a gastric level may be evident (Figure 12.9). Occasionally a barium enema may reveal the presence of colon in the defect (Figure 12.6) although this is usually an incidental finding during investigation of colonic symptoms.[53]

Endoscopy is useful in the assessment of oesophageal symptoms and anaemia, in determining the level of the diaphragm and the mucosal junction and assessing the presence of oesophagitis or peptic ulceration. An unsuspected paraoesophageal hernia with an intrathoracic twist of stomach may cause orientation difficulties with inability to either enter or leave the stomach. With smaller hernias, the relative contribution of a sliding or paraoesophageal component will be visualized on retroversion of the endoscope within the abdominal stomach. Oesophageal manometry and 24 h pH monitoring may be useful in the elective management of patients about to undergo surgery particularly if they have reflux symptoms. The knowledge gained about the motility of the oesophagus and the degree of acid exposure should be used to influence the type of surgical repair. The obstructive features of paraoesophageal hernia can make manometry difficult to perform and may also accentuate the degree of measured acid exposure.[54]

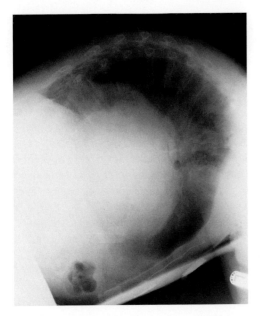
(a)

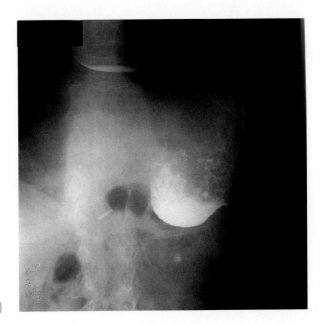
(b)

Figure 12.9
Massive intrathoracic gastric distension from a strangulated paraoesophageal hiatal hernia. (a) Lateral chest X-ray. (b) Oral contrast study showing gastric dilatation.

Indications for surgery

The mortality of paraoesophageal hernia is largely dependent on its mode of presentation. In aggregated emergency surgical series the mortality rate of 12% compares very badly to the rate of less than 1% when surgery is performed electively.[42,44,46,48,51,52,55] Acute presentation should certainly warrant surgical treatment. Prior to surgical intervention, the successful passage of a nasogastric tube and subsequent decompression may allow time to deliver adequate resuscitation and to plan elective repair providing perforation and infarction can be confidently excluded.

In general, symptomatic patients should undergo elective repair although a conservative approach may be adopted in the presence of mild symptoms in a high-risk patient. Repair of asymptomatic hernias is controversial. Hayward stated that 'most patients with a para-oesophageal hernia have no symptoms and need no treatment'[56] and Shackleford[57] felt that an elderly patient with a short life expectancy without troublesome symptoms could be left alone as the risks of the procedure may be greater than the development of complications. The risk of elective surgery even in the very elderly, however, is low. Skinner,[45] Hill[55] and others feel that a paraoesophageal hernia should be repaired on diagnosis to avoid life-threatening complications. Belsey's experience of six deaths from 21 complications among patients with minimal symptoms managed conservatively[45] has questioned the advisability of withholding repair if the patient is fit for surgery. In a series adopting an approach of performing elective surgery only when symptoms worsen, 13 of 24 eventually required operation without mortality.[46] A series from the Mayo clinic found that four of 23 developed worsening symptoms, one dying of aspiration, but the likelihood of gastric strangulation developing with time was low. They felt that high-risk patients should be managed conservatively.[42]

Once the decision to operate has been made the question of whether to perform an antireflux procedure needs to be addressed, a choice which will often be dictated by the surgical approach. The centres that rely on the thoracic route will invariably perform an antireflux procedure.[35,42,44] Those that favour an abdominal approach provide more flexibility regarding the inclusion of an antireflux procedure.[48,49,51]

The best evidence in favour of including an antireflux procedure is found in a study of 15 patients with pure paraoesophageal hernia.[50] Nine had pathological reflux on 24 h pH monitoring and the lower oesophageal sphincter, although of normal pressure, was very short. Two thirds experienced some degree of reflux symptoms although symptoms were not helpful in determining competence of the cardia. It would appear reasonable, if time permits, to investigate for the presence of reflux, and to add an antireflux procedure in those in whom this is demonstrated. Another series with a very high proportion of patients with reflux symptoms,[46] argues for a concomitant antireflux procedure as a routine, as most treated by anatomical repair alone had recurrent reflux symptoms compared to 20% of those who had a fundoplication. Such an approach obviates the frequent difficulty in intubating such patients in order to perform manometry and pH monitoring.

Ellis[47] states that a concomitant antireflux procedure is seldom required. His group favour objective testing of symptomatic patients before adopting an antireflux procedure.[51] Myers et al.[40] found that those with pure paraoesophageal hernias had a 20% chance of reflux, based on symptoms, endoscopy and objective testing whereas those with mixed hernias had a 50% chance. Menguy[48] reported that when paraoesophageal hernia is accompanied by a complete intrathoracic stomach, pre-existing symptoms of reflux are uncommon.

In the emergency situation, the type of surgical procedure undertaken is based on the management of the complication of the paraoesophageal hernia, and the question of whether an antireflux procedure is performed is of secondary importance.

Principles of surgical repair

Many techniques have been described in the management of paraoesophageal hiatal hernia. The majority involve the basic steps of reduction of the hernial contents, excision of the hernial sac and a crural closure. A gastropexy or a gastrostomy is often added in an attempt to maintain fixation and prevent further rotation. An antireflux procedure may be added both as a means of fixation and to prevent gastro-oesophageal reflux. Whether a thoracic or abdominal approach is used is dictated by surgical preference and the individual patient's pathology. The thoracic route may facilitate the management of cases with oesophageal shortening, iatrogenic hernias and in the very obese. The abdominal route may be most appropriate in the emergency situation and will allow other abdominal pathologies to be dealt with. Although large hernias, particularly with an intrathoracic gastric volvulus, appear very dramatic radiologically, the vast majority reduce easily and can be adequately repaired by a transabdominal route.

Abdominal approach

Through an upper midline incision a sternal retractor is inserted and the left lobe of liver is retracted upward away from the hiatus. The paraoesophageal defect will be seen to contain its herniated viscus, usually the stomach, most of which may not actually be visible within the abdomen. The stomach or other organs are gently reduced by downward traction using fingers or tissue forceps. A small degree of head-up tilt may help in this process and in keeping the contents reduced. The peritoneal hernia sac is dissected from its margins anteriorly and freed from the posterior mediastinum by a mixture of sharp and blunt dissection and traction and subsequently excised. The sac is usually more vascular on its posterior margin arising from the stomach. In pure paraoesophageal hernia without evidence of reflux, the oesophagus is not dissected from its posterior attachments. The hernial defect is closed anteriorly with heavy interrupted non-absorbable sutures buttressed with felt pledgets. The completed repair should allow the insertion of the operator's index finger alongside the oesophagus. In a hernia with a sliding component, the oesophagogastric junction will need to be mobilized, a step facilitated by the presence of a nasogastric tube, and fixed posteriorly, combining this with a posterior crural repair prior to anterior crural closure. A standard partial or full fundoplication can be combined with this step. A gastropexy is then performed by suturing the fundus to the diaphragm with four or five interrupted sutures in front of the oesophagus and close to the crural repair. Further fixation of the anterior wall of the stomach to the left anterior abdominal wall with a continuous suture completes the procedure prior to abdominal wall closure.

Thoracic approach

Through a left posterolateral thoracotomy in the seventh intercostal space, the pleura is opened and the left lung selectively deflated by the use of a double lumen endobronchial tube. The inferior pulmonary ligament is divided and the lung retracted upwards. The hernial sac is then exposed fully and opened to display its contents which are reduced into the abdominal cavity avoiding rotation. The peritoneal sac is then excised fully. The oesophagus need not be dissected if the oesophagogastric junction lies in its correct place. The hernial defect can then be closed both anteriorly and posteriorly using interrupted non-absorbable sutures. The inclusion of a antireflux procedure whether of the Nissen or Belsey variety follows standard techniques (as described in earlier chapters). If there is oesophageal shortening a Collis–Belsey or an uncut Collis–Nissen technique may be advisable.

Laparoscopic approach

Treatment of paraoesophageal hiatal hernia can be accomplished using laparoscopic techniques.[41,58-61] The same principles that have been developed in open repair are used although the excision of the peritoneal sac is more troublesome than in open surgery and there is a greater tendency to use a prosthetic mesh to facilitate hiatal closure. The patient is placed supine with the legs spread on leg boards or on stirrups and the surgeon stands between the legs with the first assistant on the left and cameraman to the right of the patient. Five trocars are used. A supraumbilical port is inserted after open dissection and capnoperitoneum at a pressure of 10 mmHg is initiated. The remaining ports are inserted under direct vision, right and left subcostal operating ports and lateral ports for liver retraction and stomach, and oesophageal sling retraction. Their respective sizes will depend upon the types of instruments used. Either a forward-viewing or oblique-viewing telescope can be used; the latter may be more helpful when dissecting the hernial sac. Head-up tilt of the patient will facilitate hernia reduction and improve comfort for the operator.

The left lobe of the liver is elevated with an expandable retractor passed via the right subcostal port. The herniated stomach is reduced by sequential traction with atraumatic grasping forceps although with mixed paraoesophageal hernias, complete reduction may not be possible until the hernial sac is excised from the mediastinum. The whole peritoneal sac is removed if possible by a mixture of scissor, blunt and diathermy dissection. By attempting to keep a relatively bloodless field during this dissection, vagal fibres and the pleural reflections are identified and preserved. Diathermy should be

minimized in the vicinity of the vagi. An alternative strategy with the hernial sac may be to leave it *in situ* or merely incise it at the diaphragmatic edge to expose the crura. If the sac is left, this may provide a potential space for a serous fluid collection.

The hernial defect is closed in front of the oesophagus with interrupted sutures of 00 non-absorbable material. The passage of an endoscope or a flexible lighted bougie can ensure that the crural closure is not too tight. Alternatively, a prosthetic mesh can be stapled around the defect with a 3 cm clearance. The fundus can then be sutured or stapled to the diaphragm to act as a gastropexy and to cover the mesh if used. A gastrostomy is an alternative option, the tube being inserted percutaneously via the gastroscope.

If the gastro-oesophageal junction has been fully mobilized during the dissection or an antireflux procedure is required, the distal oesophagus can be retracted by a sling and a short, loose 360° fundoplication or a partial fundoplication procedure fashioned over the bougie after a posterior crural repair has been performed. The need for mobilization of the short gastric vessels will be dictated by the ease with which the wrap can be formed, although the fundus will usually be mobile because of a long gastrosplenic ligament. The wrap is then sutured to the diaphragm by three or four sutures. An endoscope can be used to visualize the oesophageal and gastric mucosa to assess any damage prior to closure of the trocar sites.

Emergency management

In the emergency management of the complications of paraoesophageal hernia, each case will need to be approached individually. The overall condition of the patient together with the pathological state of the stomach will dictate the necessary procedure. The range of options will include minimal intervention, such as reduction and fixation of the herniated stomach alone, or major resection. Resuscitation of the patient may be facilitated by decompression of the stomach via a nasogastric tube, hence buying valuable time. If the stomach is thought to be compromised, or if the patient's condition dictates, emergency surgery is indicated. An abdominal approach is probably the best option. If reduction of the hernial contents is difficult, either manipulation of the nasogastric tube or a gastrotomy in a visible, viable part of the stomach may allow decompression and subsequent reduction. The stomach may be full of food matter which can make decompression difficult. Reduction is usually accomplished by gentle downward traction on that part of the stomach or other viscus that is seen entering the defect. Reduction difficulties may be due to adhesions within the sac or constriction at the neck of the sac, which is dealt with by enlarging the muscular defect. The viability of the hernial contents is then assessed after decompression and reduction of the torsion. Infarction or necrosis may be dealt with by segmental resection if localized, or a major oesophagogastric resection may be needed particularly if there is gross mediastinal contamination.

If the indication for surgery is bleeding, a gastrotomy may be required to identify the source which is then under-run. If no focal source is found, relief of the strangulation may be all that is required. A perforated ulcer will need to be over-sewn after its excision and lavage performed to the contaminated area.

If the situation permits, excision of the sac and repair of the defect should be added in most cases. In the particularly high-risk patient, simple reduction of the hernia combined with an anterior gastropexy or a high gastrostomy may be the most sensible option.

An antireflux procedure should be considered if there has been extensive dissection around the lower oesophagus and cardia, if the hernia is of the mixed variety or if there were pre-operative reflux symptoms. A posterior crural repair with posterior fixation of the oesophagus and cardia combined with a partial anterior fundoplication that fixes the stomach to the diaphragm is a simple reliable technique.

Postoperative Management

A nasogastric tube, if a gastrostomy was not fashioned, is kept in place for at least 24 hours until a contrast study is performed to ensure that there is no leakage and that there is adequate gastric drainage. Oral fluids can then be introduced followed by a light diet over the following few days. The recovery period may be shorter with a laparoscopic approach and more prolonged in the emergency setting.

Complications will largely relate to whether emergency or elective surgery was undertaken and to whether the repair was for an iatrogenic or primary hernia. Mortality greater in emergency surgery and for re-operations, as are septic complications and distal oesophageal injury. Recurrent herniation may occur in up to 10%, the rate being similar for an abdominal or thoracic route.[44,51]

CONGENITAL DIAPHRAGMATIC HERNIA

This is considered in Chapter 62.

Eventration of the diaphragm

Eventration of the diaphragm is an abnormally high intact hemidiaphragm which can be congenital or acquired. Congenital eventration is a developmental abnormality resulting in muscular aplasia, whereas in acquired eventration a normally formed diaphragm becomes atrophic.[62] Congenital eventration is found more commonly on the right side and bilateral involvement is rare. The incidence is about one quarter that of congenital diaphragmatic hernia. In acquired eventration, phrenic nerve injury may be due to a difficult delivery or to a thoracic or cervical surgical procedure. If the nerve has not been severed, paralysis may be temporary. Other causes of acquired eventration include neuropathies and myopathies.

Pulmonary function testing will show decreased functional residual capacity and forced vital capacity and an increased respiratory rate. The improvement in respiratory mechanics following plication of the eventrated diaphragm is largely due to the contralateral normal diaphragm.[63]

Diagnosis and treatment

The two main indications for surgical intervention are respiratory distress and the abdominal complication of gastric volvulus.

Presentation in neonates may be similar to congenital diaphragmatic hernia with respiratory distress. The outlook after surgery is good in the absence of lung hypoplasia. Difficulty in weaning from ventilation can be a problem in infancy, childhood and in adult life which may be alleviated by diaphragmatic plication. In childhood, respiratory symptoms with repeated bronchitis or pneumonia may occur as may occasional upper gastrointestinal symptoms.

Acute gastric volvulus in childhood is associated with diaphragmatic eventration which commonly leads to a mesenteroaxial twist.[64] Symptoms are mainly vomiting, abdominal pain and distension although respiratory distress can occur. Eventration is also a cause of gastric volvulus in adults.[65]

Eventration is readily diagnosed on chest radiography, although ultrasound is useful in assessing mobility of the diaphragm.

Surgical management

Repair via a transthoracic route is preferable for eventration which is not complicated by gastric volvulus or other abdominal pathology. The access afforded for right-sided defects is particularly superior to the abdominal approach. There are a number of techniques available to deal with the diaphragm (Figure 12.10).

A lateral thoracotomy is made on the affected side through the seventh intercostal space with 45° table tilt. The lung is collapsed or retracted superiorly and the diaphragm is elevated between tissue forceps. A series of interrupted non-absorbable plication sutures are placed from front to back each taking three or four bites of diaphragm. The sutures are clipped and then tied when all have been placed. Alternatively, an ellipse of central redundant diaphragmatic tissue may be excised, taking care not to injure the underlying liver and abdominal organs, and an overlapping two-layered repair performed, giving the final result of a flat sheet. Another option is to use a linear stapling device to form the pleat of an overlapping repair which is then sutured to the underlying diaphragm.[66] Any repair may be augmented by a prosthetic patch which is sutured to the periphery of the diaphragm. A chest drain is inserted before layered closure of the thoracic incision to remain *in situ* for 2 or 3 days.

In cases of gastric volvulus associated with left-sided eventration, nasogastric decompression should be attempted prior to surgery. An upper abdominal incision will facilitate reduction of the torsion of the stomach. The diaphragmatic eventration is plicated prior to fixation of the stomach to the anterior abdominal wall, with or without a gastrostomy.

Potential alternative strategies for gastric fixation in a non-rotated position involve gastropexy or gastrostomy by open, endoscopic or laparoscopic means, without plication of the diaphragm.

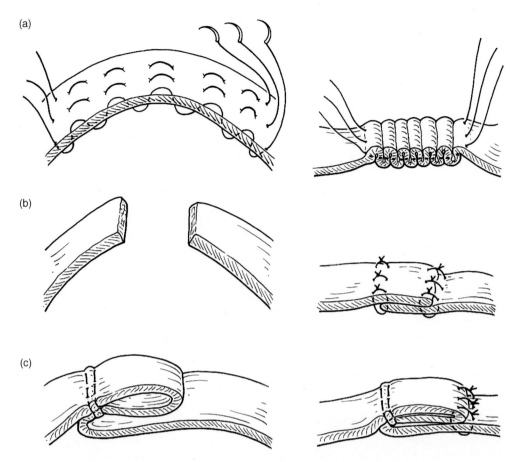

Figure 12.10
Three methods of diaphragmatic plication for eventration.

TRAUMATIC DIAPHRAGMATIC HERNIA

Rupture of the diaphragm can occur as a result of both blunt and penetrating abdominal and chest trauma and may lead to acute or chronic herniation of abdominal contents into the chest. Acute traumatic diaphragmatic hernia may be diagnosed early or late. Chronic herniation may represent either a missed acute hernia or develop at a time remote from the initial diaphragmatic injury. Traumatic diaphragmatic hernias occur most commonly on the left side. Blunt trauma is mostly associated with acute visceral herniation whereas penetrating trauma is more likely to lead to a delayed presentation of a hernia.

Direct injury may be a result of wounds from stabbings, firearms and fragments of fractured ribs as well as surgical incisions. Herniation is uncommon in the early aftermath of penetrating wounds but an initially small defect by creating a pressure differential may allow the sucking in of abdominal viscera into the chest.[67]

Small defects which develop into chronic hernias may be more dangerous than large ones as they are associated with increased mortality and morbidity from obstruction and strangulation.[68] Iatrogenic trauma is a result of surgical incisions in the diaphragm or inadvertent damage during surgery. Such hernias may occur through the hiatus or through a sutured or unrecognized surgical injury to the diaphragm. Indirect injury to the diaphragm via blunt trauma results from a sudden increase in abdominal pressure which is dissipated through the diaphragm, the most common example being motor vehicle accidents. Although any portion of the diaphragm may be injured, tears are usually radial and preferentially affect the left posterolateral diaphragm, which is its weakest point.[69,70] The reason for the higher incidence of left-sided defects in penetrating trauma may be that most assailants are right handed.

Diagnosis and management

The diagnosis of a traumatic diaphragmatic hernia relies on a high index of suspicion. Features to heighten awareness include the mode of injury, a history of chest or abdominal trauma, fractures of the pelvis or lumbar spine, compression injury to the torso, clinical features such as dyspnoea and hypoxia, pain in the lower chest or upper abdomen with referral to the shoulder, physical signs in the lower chest, mediastinal shift and bowel sounds in the chest.[68,71] Clinical assessment may be less sensitive when diaphragmatic rupture occurs without visceral herniation.[72]

The presentation of chronic traumatic diaphragmatic hernia may be many years after the original injury with epigastric pain and fullness, nausea and vomiting, chest pain and exertional dyspnoea. Bowel obstruction or gastric volvulus are particularly dangerous presentations.

Chest radiology alone may reveal the diagnosis in a majority

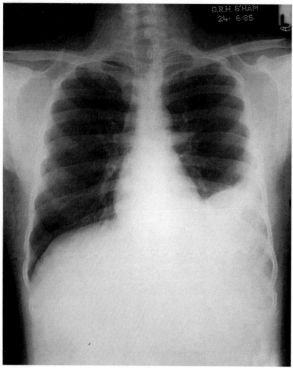

(a)

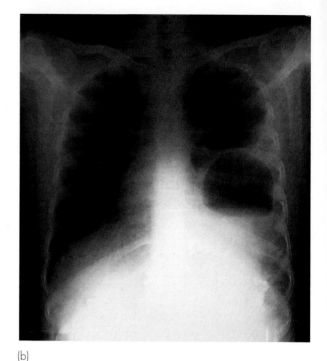

(b)

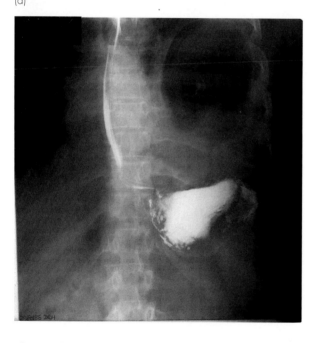

(c)

Figure 12.11

Development of a traumatic diaphragmatic hernia. (a) Chest X-ray on admission after a stab wound to the left chest. Note raised, blurred left hemidiaphragm. (b) Chest X-ray after 2 days with gas filled viscus in left chest producing mediastinal shift. (c) Oral contrast study showing herniation of stomach into chest.

of cases[73] (Figure 12.11). Radiological signs include an elevated or indistinct diaphragm, an effusion or presence of bowel in the chest, compressed lung and mediastinal shift together with rib, spine or pelvic fractures. Computed tomography is valuable in the management of the acute trauma patient and contrast studies are particularly helpful in chronic cases.

Nasogastric tube insertion, will decompress gastric distension and may be visible in the thorax on plain radiology. Peritoneal lavage can be a sensitive indicator of abdominal injuries associated with the diaphragmatic injury, although a negative result does not exclude the diagnosis.[72]

In the surgical treatment of any intra-abdominal injury, a thorough laparotomy should include inspection and palpation for a potential diaphragmatic injury. Thoracic injury may lead to pneumo- or haemothorax which is managed by chest drainage alone, but if thoracotomy is required for control of blood loss or management of bronchial or cardiac wounds the diaphragm must be inspected.

Surgical management

The choice of surgical approach in traumatic diaphragmatic hernia depends on whether the presentation is acute or chronic and on the presence or suspicion of coexisting pathology above or below the diaphragm. In acute diaphragmatic hernia, a midline abdominal incision allows a thorough laparotomy to diagnose and repair any associated abdominal injuries, reduction of the hernia and repair of the diaphragmatic defect. If thoracic injury is suspected or if the diaphragmatic trauma affects the right side, the patients position may be adjusted to allow a thoracotomy and laparotomy.[69] Diaphragmatic incision either through the chest or abdomen should be avoided, as it will weaken the repair without significantly enhancing the exposure.

In the elective management of chronic traumatic diaphragmatic hernia, a transthoracic approach may be simpler because of the difficulty often encountered while freeing the adhesions between the herniated viscera and the lung and pleura. However, when a preoperative diagnosis of incarcerated bowel or a gastric volvulus is made, an abdominal approach is preferable. A thoracoscopic or laparoscopic repair is feasible as an adjunct to a diagnostic procedure particularly in stable patients. Repair can be by suturing, stapling or mesh placement.[74,75]

A peritoneal sac is not present in traumatic hernias. In acute cases, the herniated viscera are easily reduced and repair of the diaphragmatic defect is usually effected by suture closure with synthetic non-absorbable material using an interrupted technique either in one or two layers. There is seldom need to use a prosthetic mesh to close the defect in open surgery although this may change as thoracoscopic or laparoscopic repair become more common.

In transthoracic repair, a double-lumen endobronchial tube will facilitate collapse of the lung on the operative side thereby allowing maximal exposure of the hernia and the diaphragmatic defect. A posterolateral thoracotomy through the seventh intercostal space is made, the pleura opened and the lung allowed to collapse and a rib spreader is inserted. The herniated viscera may be densely attached to the pleura and lung. These adhesions are divided with as little damage to the coapted abdominal and thoracic organs as possible by sharp dissection. The hernial contents are freed from the diaphragmatic edges and reduced. The defect in the diaphragm is then repaired with interrupted non-absorbable sutures using a two-layered technique of an initial horizontal mattress and a second simple over and over suture. A patch of prosthetic mesh is sutured to the diaphragm if there is difficulty in closing the defect primarily.

Recurrence of herniation is generally low, although in one series six out of 21 repairs for chronic hernia had had a previous repair.[68] The morbidity and mortality is related to the presence and severity of associated major injuries and to strangulation of the gut.

REFERENCES

1. Listerud MB & Harkins HN. Anatomy of the esophageal hiatus. Anatomical studies on two hundred and four fresh cadavers. *Arch Surg* 1958; **76:** 835–842.
2. Skandalakis JE, Gray SW, Rowe JS Jr & Skandalakis LJ. Surgical anatomy of the diaphragm. In Nyhus LM, Baker RJ (eds) *Mastery of Surgery*, 2nd edn. Boston: Little Brown and Company, 1992: 377–396.
3. Peters PM. Closure mechanisms at the cardia with special reference to the diaphragmatico-oesophageal elastic ligament. *Thorax* 1955; **10:** 27–36.
4. Eliska O. Phreno-oesophageal membrane and its role in the development of hiatal hernia. *Acta Anat* 1973; **86:** 137–150.
5. Harrington SW. Diagnosis and treatment of various types of diaphragmatic hernia. *Am J Surg* 1940; **50:** 381–446.
6. Allison PR. Reflux esophagitis, sliding hiatal hernia and the anatomy of repair. *Surg Gynecol Obstet* 1951; **92:** 419–431.
7. Barrett NR. Hiatus hernia: a review of some controversial points. *Br J Surg* 1954; **42:** 231–243.
8. Matthews HR. A proposed classification for hiatus hernia and gastroesophageal reflux. *Dis Esoph* 1996; **9:** 1–3.
9. Johnston BT, Carre IJ, Thomas PS & Collins BJ. Twenty to 40 year follow up of infantile hiatal hernia. *Gut* 1995; **36:** 809–812.
10. Nagaya M, Akatsuka H & Kato J. Gastroesophageal reflux occuring after repair of congenital diaphragmatic hernia. *J Pediatr Surg* 1994; **29:** 1447–1451.
11. Lin S, Brasseur JG, Ponderoux P & Kahrilas PJ. The phrenic ampulla: distal oesophagus or potential hiatal hernia? *Am J Physiol* 1995; **268:** G320–327.
12. Paterson WG & Kolyn DM. Esophageal shortening induced by short-term intraluminal acid perfusion in opposum: a cause for hiatus hernia? *Gastroenterology* 1994; **107:** 1736–1740.
13. Pridie RB. Incidence and coincidence of hiatus hernia. *Gut* 1966; **7:** 188–189.
14. Ott DJ, Gelfand DW, Chen YM et al. Predictive relationship of hiatal hernia to reflux esophagitis. *Gastrointest Radiol* 1985; **10:** 317–320.
15. Caskey CI, Zerhouni EA, Fishman EK & Rahmouni AD. Aging of the diaphragm: a CT study. *Radiology* 1989; **171:** 385–389.
16. Wolf BS. Sliding hiatal hernia: the need for redefinition. *A J R* 1973; **117:** 231–247.
17. Sprafka JL, Azad M & Baronofsky ID. Fate of esophageal hiatus hernia: a clinical and experimental study. *Surgery* 1954; **36:** 519–524.
18. Berstad A, Weberg R, Froyshov Larsen I et al. Relationship of the hiatus hernia to reflux oesophagitis. A prospective study of coincidence, using endoscopy. *Scand J Gastroenterol* 1986; **21:** 55–58.
19. Gregorie HB, Cathcart RS & Gregorie RJ. Surgical treatment of intractable esophagitis. *Ann Surg* 1984; **199:** 580–589.
20. Petersen H, Johannessen T & Sandvik AK. Relationship between endoscopic hiatus hernia and gatroesophageal reflux symptoms. *Scand J Gastroenterol* 1991; **26:** 921–926.
21. Sontag SJ, Schnell TG, Miller TQ et al. The importance of hiatal hernia in reflux esophagitis compared with lower esophageal sphincter pressure or smoking. *J Clin Gastroenterol* 1991; **13:** 628–643.
22. Stilson WL, Sanders I, Gardiner GA et al. Hiatal hernia and gastroesophageal reflux: a clinico-radiological analysis of more than 1000 cases. *Radiology* 1969; **93:** 1323–1327.
23. Cohen S & Harris LD. Does hiatus hernia affect the competence of the gastroesophageal sphincter? *N Engl J Med* 1971; **284:** 1053–1056.
24. Pope CE II, Meyer GW & Castell DO. Is measurement of lower oesophageal sphincter pressure clinically useful? *Dig Dis Sci* 1981; **26:** 1025–1031.
25. Dodds WJ, Dent J, Hogan WJ et al. Mechanisms of gastroesophageal reflux in patients with reflux esophagitis. *N Engl J Med* 1982; **307:** 1547–1552.
26. Mittal RK, Rochester DF & McCallum RW. Sphincteric action of the diaphragm during a relaxed lower esophageal sphincter in humans. *Am J Physiol* 1989; **256:** G139–G144.
27. DeMeester TR, Lafontaine E, Joelsson BE et al. Relationship of a hiatal hernia to the function of the body of the esophagus and the gastroesophageal junction. *J Thorac Cardiovasc Surg* 1981; **82:** 547–558.
28. Sloan S & Kahrilas PJ. Impairment of esophageal emptying with hiatal hernia. *Gastroenterology* 1991; **100:** 596–605.
29. Mittal RK, Lange RC & McCallum RW. Identification and mechanism of delayed esophageal acid clearance in subjects with hiatus hernia. *Gastroenterology* 1987; **92:** 130–135.
30. Patti MG, Goldberg HI, Arcerito M et al. Hiatal hernia size affects lower esophageal sphincter function, esophageal acid exposure and the degree of mucosal injury. *Am J Surg* 1996; **171:** 182–186.
31. Jenkinson LR, Ball CS, Barlow AP et al. An evaluation of the manometric assessment of oesophageal function in reflux oesophagitis. *Gullet* 1991; **1:** 135–142.
32. Boyd EJ, Penston JG, Russell RI & Wormsley KG. Hiatal hernial ulcers: clinical features and follow-up. *Postgrad Med J* 1991; **67:** 900–903.
33. Cathcart RS, Gregorie HB & Holmes SL. Nonreflux complications of hiatal hernia. *Am Surg* 1987; **53:** 320–324.
34. Windsor CWO & Collis JL. Anaemia and hiatus hernia: experience in 450 patients. *Thorax* 1967; **22:** 73–78.

35. Pearson FG, Cooper JD, IIves R et al. Massive hiatal hernia with incarceration: a report of 53 cases. *Ann Thorac Surg* 1983; **35:** 45–51.
36. Hill LD & Tobias JA. Para-esophageal hernia. *Arch Surg* 1968; **96:** 735–744.
37. Bremer JL. Diaphragm and diaphragmatic hernia. *Arch Pathol* 1943; **36:** 539–549.
38. Mira-Navarro J, Bayle-Bastos F, Frieyro-Segui M et al. Long-term follow up of Nissen fundoplication. *Eur J Pediatr Surg* 1994; **4:** 7–10.
39. Parikh D & Tam PKH. Results of fundoplication in a UK paediatric centre. *Br J Surg* 1991; **78:** 346–348.
40. Streitz JM Jr & Ellis FH Jr. Iatrogenic paraesophageal hiatus hernia. *Ann Thorac Surg* 1990; **50:** 446–449.
41. Watson DI, Jamieson GG, Devitt PG et al. Para-oesophageal hiatus hernia: an important complication of laparoscopic Nissen fundoplication. *Br J Surg* 1995; **82:** 521–523.
42. Allen MS, Trastek VF, Deschamps C & Pairolero PC. Intrathoracic stomach: presentation and results of operation. *J Thorac Cardiovasc Surg* 1993; **105:** 253–259.
43. Gahahan T Hiatus hernia without esophageal reflux. *Arch Surg* 1967; **95:** 595–605.
44. Ozdemir IA, Burke WA & Ikins PM. Paraesophageal hernia: a life threatening disease. *Ann Thorac Surg* 1973; **16:** 547–554.
45. Skinner DB & Belsey RHR. Surgical management of esophageal reflux and hiatus hernia. Long term results in 1,030 patients. *J Thorac Cardiovasc Surg* 1967; **53:** 33–54.
46. Treacy PJ & Jamieson GG. An approach to the management of para-oesophageal hiatus hernias. *Aust N Z J Surg* 1987; **57:** 813–817.
47. Ellis FH Jr. Controversies regarding the management of hiatus hernia. *Am J Surg* 1980; **139:** 782–788.
48. Menguy R. Surgical management of large paraesophageal hernia with complete intrathoracic stomach. *World J Surg* 1988; **12:** 415–422.
49. Myers GA, Harms BA & Starling JR. Management of paraesophageal hernia with a selective approach to antireflux surgery. *Am J Surg* 1995; **170:** 375–380.
50. Walther B, DeMeester TR, Lafontaine E et al. Effect of para-esophageal hernia on sphincter function and its implication on surgical therapy. *Am J Surg* 1984; **147:** 111–116.
51. Williamson WA, Ellis FH Jr, Streitz JM & Shahian DM. Paraesophageal hiatal hernia: is an antireflux repair necessary? *Ann Thorac Surg* 1993; **56:** 447–452.
52. Carter R, Brewer LA & Hinshaw DB. Acute gastric volvulus. A study of 25 cases. *Am J Surg* 1980; **140:** 99–106.
53. Jewel FM, Tesar PA & Virjee J. Diaphragmatic herniation of the large bowel. *Clin Radiol* 1994; **49:** 469–472.
54. Landreneau RJ, Johnson JA, Marshall JB et al. Clinical spectrum of paraesophageal herniation. *Dig Dis Sci* 1992; **37:** 537–544.
55. Hill LD. Incarcerated para-esophageal hernia. A surgical emergency. *Am J Surg* 1973; **126:** 286–291.
56. Hayward J. Paraesophageal hernia. In Nyhus LM & Harkins HN (eds) *Hernia.* Philadelphia: Lippincott, 1964: 522–526.
57. Shackleford RT. Paraesophageal (type II) hiatal hernia and parahiatal hernia. In Shackelford RT (ed.) *Surgery of the Alimentary Tract,* 2nd edn. Philadelphia: WB Saunders, 1978: 489–499.
58. Kuster GGR & Gilroy S. Laparoscopic technique for repair of paraesophageal hiatal hernias. *J Laparoendosc Surg* 1993; **3:** 331–338.
59. Mosnier H, Leport J, Aubert A et al. A 270 degree laparoscopic posterior fundoplasty in the treatment of gastroesophageal reflux. *J Am Coll Surg* 1995; **181:** 220–224.
60. Pitcher DE, Curet MJ, Martin DT et al. Successful laparoscopic repair of paraesophageal hernia. *Arch Surg* 1995; **130:** 590–596.
61. Oddsdottir M, Franco AL, Laycock WS et al. Laparoscopic repair of paraesophageal hernia. New access, old technique. *Surg Endosc* 1995; **9:** 164–168.
62. Puri P. Congenital diaphragmatic hernia. In Freeman NV, Burge DM, Griffiths DM & Malone PSJ (eds) *Surgery of the Newborn.* Edinburgh: Churchill Livingstone, 1994: 331–352.
63. Takeda S, Nakahara K, Fujii Y et al. Effects of diaphragmatic plication on respiratory mechanics in dogs with unilateral and bilateral phrenic nerve paralysis. *Chest* 1995; **107:** 798–804.
64. McIntyre RC, Bensard DD, Karrer FM et al. The pediatric diaphragm in acute gastric volvulus. *J Am Coll Surg* 1994; **178:** 234–238.
65. Askew AR. Treatment of acute and chronic gastric volvulus. *Ann R Coll Surg Engl* 1978; **60:** 326–328.
66. Maxson T, Robertson R & Wagner CW. An improved method of diaphragmatic plication. *Surg Gynecol Obstet* 1993; **177:** 620–621.
67. Gourin A & Garzon A. Diagnostic problems in traumatic diaphragmatic hernia. *J Trauma* 1974; **14:** 20–31.
68. Payne JH & Lellin AE. Traumatic diaphragmatic hernia. *Arch Surg* 1982; **117:** 18–24.
69. Lucido JL & Wall CA. Rupture of the diaphragm due to blunt trauma. *Arch Surg* 1963; **86:** 989–999.
70. Bekassy SM, Dave KS, Wooler GH & Ionescu MI. 'Spontaneous' and traumatic rupture of the diaphragm. *Ann Surg* 1973; **177:** 320–324.
71. Lee WC, Chen RJ, Fang JF et al. Rupture of the diaphragm after blunt trauma. *Eur J Surg* 1994; **160:** 479–483.
72. Aronoff RJ, Reynolds J & Thal ER. Evaluation of diaphragmatic injuries. *Am J Surg* 1982; **144:** 671–675.
73. de la Rocha AG, Creel RJ, Mulligan GWN & Burns CM. Diaphragmatic rupture due to blunt abdominal trauma. *Surg Gynecol Obstet* 1982; **154:** 175–180.
74. Koehler RH & Smith RS. Thoracoscopic repair of missed diaphragmatic injury in penetrating trauma. *J Trauma* 1994; **36:** 424–427.
75. Thomas P, Moutardier V, Ragni J et al. Video-assisted repair of a ruptured right hemidiaphragm. *Eur J Cardiovasc Thorac Surg* 1994; **8:** 157–159.

13

TUMOURS OF THE OESOPHAGUS

JA Morris
A Watson

Although carcinoma of the oesophagus is the most common and most important tumour to affect the oesophagus, there is a whole range of tumours, divisible into epithelial and non-epithelial, benign and malignant, which may arise in the oesophagus, albeit rarely in many cases. The first part of this chapter deals with the classification and pathological features of the whole spectrum of tumours arising in the oesophagus, but concentrates on carcinoma, dealing with epidemiology, aetiological factors and premalignant lesions. The second part deals with clinical features and diagnosis, whereas Chapters 14 and 15 deal with management of oesophageal carcinoma.

BENIGN EPITHELIAL TUMOURS

Glycogenic acanthosis

Glycogenic acanthosis is a common benign lesion of the oesophagus. The reported prevalence varies from 6 to 15% in endoscopy series[1,2] but the condition is found in the majority of adults at necropsy.[3] It was first described in 1908 by Lindemann[4] as pachyderma nodosa. Macroscopically there are discrete, oval, slightly elevated grey–white plaques of 0.2–1.5 cm diameter (Figure 13.1). The long axis of the plaques usually follows the longitudinal axis of the oesophagus and they are superimposed on the summits of mucosal folds.[3] Occasionally the lesions form diffuse confluent islands of raised white areas which give the mucosa a cobblestoned appearance. They are most common and most extensive in the lower third of the oesophagus.

Microscopically there is both hyperplasia and hypertrophy of squamous cells forming a raised squamous plaque. The cells of the prickle cell layer are distended due to their cytoplasmic content of glycogen. This causes the cell cytoplasm to appear clear on ordinary histological sections but it stains intensely with glycogen stains such as periodic acid–Schiff (PAS). There is no epithelial dysplasia and these lesions are completely benign with no malignant potential.

Glycogenic acanthosis must be clearly distinguished from leukoplakia. In fact the latter condition is extremely rare in the oesophagus but, if there is any doubt, the lesion should be biopsied so that the distinction can be made. Monilia is another possible source of confusion but it is usually associated with inflammation which does not occur in glycogenic acanthosis.

Squamous papilloma

Squamous cell papillomas of the oesophagus are rare.[5-7] In one series only six cases were found in 14,900 gastrointestinal endoscopies.[7] Macroscopically the tumours are pale, warty,

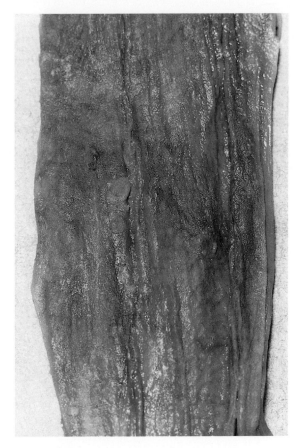

Figure 13.1
Oval plaque of glycogenic acanthosis.

sessile lesions. They can be single or multiple. The majority have been found in men, and the lower oesophagus is the site of predilection. A number of authors have pointed to an apparent association with gastro-oesophageal reflux. Microscopically, there is papillary growth of squamous epithelium. The cores of the papillae are formed by connective tissue. The epithelium is thickened due to an increase in the number of squamous cells, but these show regular differentiation and there is no epithelial dysplasia.

A possible aetiological role for viruses in squamous cell papilloma is of considerable theoretical interest. Viral-induced papillomas occur in the oesophagi of cattle.[8] Human papilloma viruses (HPV), of which there are a large number of subtypes, are implicated in viral warts of the skin, cervix, larynx and oesophagus.[9,10] These viruses are responsible for widespread papillomatosis of the larynx and trachea in children, and this can occasionally extend to involve the oesophagus. In one study using the polymerase chain reaction 13 of 26 oesophageal squamous papillomas were positive for human papilloma virus, most commonly type 16 and less often type 18 and type 6b/11.[11]

Squamous cell papillomas of the oesophagus have been induced in experimental animals with benzopyrene[12] and nitrosamines.[13]

The patients present with epigastric pain, dysphagia and symptoms of reflux oesophagitis. The lesions are benign and resection is curative.

Adenoma

The oesophageal submucosal glands are a possible site for the origin of adenomas. Their occurrence, however, is exceptionally rare. There is a range of possible histological types as seen in salivary glands and bronchi.

A second site for adenomas is Barrett's mucosa. Indeed, some early reports of oesophageal adenomas probably represent hyperplastic Barrett's mucosa rather than true neoplasms. Neoplasms can arise, however, in Barrett's glandular epithelium and they resemble adenomas seen in the stomach, and small and large intestine. They have a villous or tubular pattern and show varying degrees of dysplasia. They are premalignant lesions.[14]

MALIGNANT EPITHELIAL TUMOURS

Carcinoma of the oesophagus is more common in men than in women. The incidence rises with age and the disease shows marked geographical variation. In 1985 it was the ninth most common cancer in the world with 90% of new cases arising in developing countries in Asia, Africa and Latin America.[15,16]

The USA, Canada, and most of Europe, apart from France, are relatively low-risk areas, the mean incidence being 26 per 100,000. In the UK, cancer of the oesophagus forms 1.9% of all cancers and 3.1% of all cancer deaths.[17] Within Europe, France has the highest mortality rate for males and the highest male preponderance at 12:1.[18] There are also marked geographical variations within France. The male mortality rate is twice as high in Normandy and Brittany than in the rest of France.

Within parts of Brittany and Normandy, the incidence is as high as 50 per 100,000. Since the early 1970s there has been an increase in oesophageal cancer in the former communist countries of central Europe.[16] This could be related to increased tobacco and alcohol consumption and seasonal unavailability of fresh fruit and vegetables. In the USA the rate of oesophageal cancer is higher in Blacks.[16]

There are several regions of the world in which the incidence is very high. In China, deaths from cancer of the oesophagus form 26% of all cancer deaths in men and 20% in women. These figures exceed those in all other countries.[19] The incidence of oesophageal cancer, however, varies greatly within China. In some provinces, up to 70% of all cancer deaths are due to carcinoma of the oesophagus. The highest rate is in Linxian County in Henan Province of Northern China. The age-adjusted mortality fluctuated between 100 and 150 per 100,000 over a 30-year period to 1970. The maximum mortality for men is 645 times the minimum and for women 790 times the minimum. In general, in China, the male to female ratio is 2:1. In high-risk areas, men and women tend to have a similar incidence, but in low-risk areas the male to female ratio is increased. There is, however, some evidence that these very high rates are starting to fall as the general nutritional status of the population improves.[20]

There are similar epidemiological patterns in the littoral zone around the Caspian sea.[21] The crude prevalence rate in these areas of Russia and Iran is as high as 195 per 100,000. In the population aged 35–64 years in the Guriev District of Kazakhstan Province in Russia, the disease prevalence is 547 per 100,000 and is the major cause of death in this population. In general, the disease is more common in men than women, although one district in Northern Iran has a reversal of this ratio.

There are also areas of high incidence in South Africa. These occur in the black population around the City of Durban and from Transkei.[22] The disease is more common in men than women. The age-specific incidence rates for the whole of Transkei rise to 270 per 100,000 in men aged 60–69 years. In certain areas within Transkei, however, the incidence in men over 35 years is as high as 357 per 100,000.

Age incidence

The incidence of carcinoma of the oesophagus rises steeply with age in both high-risk and low-risk areas (Figures 13.2 and 13.3). This is usually explained in terms of multihit models of carcinogenesis.[23] The concept is that a single cell only undergoes malignant change after suffering a series of rare events. In which case, if n events are required for neoplasia, then it can be shown that:

$$I = ct^{n-1}$$

where I = incidence at time t, t = age in years, c = a constant and n = number of events for malignancy. Thus the incidence rises exponentially with age. Taking logarithms in the above equation gives:

$$\log I = \log c + (n - 1) \log t$$

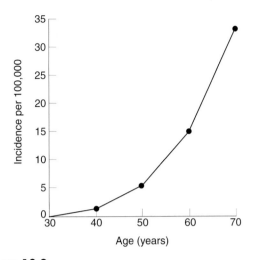

Figure 13.2
Age incidence of carcinoma of the oesophagus.

In other words a plot of log incidence against log age gives a straight line with a slope of $n - 1$.[24]

This is the simplest multistage model. There are more complex models in which the first event gives a cell a proliferative advantage so that it produces a clone of altered cells and further events affecting single cells in the clone lead to malignant change. With these models, two or three hits can be sufficient to produce a steeply rising exponential curve.

These ideas were formulated on the basis of epidemiological data but they have received considerable support in recent years from advances in molecular biology.[25–27] All cells contain a number of growth control genes, called proto-oncogenes, which when activated lead to cell division. The transcription products of these genes are directly involved in the pathways which trigger mitosis. In addition, cells contain antioncogenes

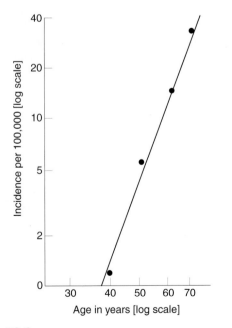

Figure 13.3
A plot of log incidence against log age gives a straight line with a slope of 5.

whose products suppress growth. It appears that the antioncogenes are recessive and it is thought that in certain cases their transcription products suppress the activity of growth-promoting genes. Proto-oncogene expression is normally suppressed in differentiated cells. These genes could be activated, however, by mutations which inactivate antioncogenes or damage control sequences of the proto-oncogene. It requires the loss of at least two antioncogenes before a growth control system is activated, and it is possible that for many cancers more than one growth-control system needs to be active. Thus, a malignant clone will only arise after several rare mutations have occurred in a single cell.

The environmental factors that increase the chance of mutation include viruses, radiation and chemical carcinogens. Even in the absence of these mutagens, however, there is a finite chance of mutation with every cell division which is of the order of 1×10^{-7} per gene per cell division.[28] In particular cellular metabolism generates free radicals which can directly damage DNA. This will be more marked if there is a relative dietary deficiency of certain natural antioxidants.

Aetiological factors in oesophageal cancer

From the above discussion it is clear that aetiological agents in carcinogenesis can act in a number of ways. Radiation and chemical carcinogens can directly damage DNA. Conditions which increase cell turnover, such as chronic inflammation, will increase the frequency of spontaneous mutation. In addition dietary deficiency of antioxidants will increase spontaneous mutation through damage by free radicals. Viruses can damage DNA both directly and indirectly. Integration of viral DNA adjacent to a suppressed oncogene could cause its activation, whereas cellular hyperplasia caused by viruses will increase spontaneous mutation. It is an interesting exercise to try to relate the known aetiological agents in oesophageal cancer to these primary factors.

Alcohol

In the Western world, alcohol is a major risk factor for oesophageal cancer.[16,29–32] In one study, drinkers of alcoholic beverages had 6.4 times the risk of non-drinkers. The risk increased steadily with the amount of alcohol consumed and was highest in those who drank spirits.[31] Epidemiological studies in France also support the importance of alcohol consumption as an important aetiological factor.[18,29] France has a high per capitum alcohol consumption, and the highest rates of oesophageal cancer and cirrhosis of the liver in Europe. The incidence of oesophageal cancer and cirrhosis of the liver fell as a result of decreased alcohol consumption during World War II. Since 1966, the rate of oesophageal cancer, cirrhosis of the liver and alcohol consumption have stopped rising. In Normandy and Brittany, the incidence of oesophageal cancer is higher than the national average. This distribution correlates with mortality from other diseases related to alcohol consumption.

The mechanism by which alcohol increases the risk of cancer is not known but a number of hypotheses have been advanced.[32] There is no evidence that alcohol is a direct carcinogen or mutagen in experimental animals. Increased alcohol consumption, however, is associated with a decreased intake of essential nutrients and vitamins and these dietary factors could be important in causing cancer. In other high-risk areas of the world, such as China and Iran, poor diet is thought to contribute to the cancer incidence.[33] Other suggested possibilities for the mode of action of alcohol include irritation of the mucosal lining leading to increased cell division and increased spontaneous mutation, facilitation of the transport of tobacco-associated carcinogens into cells, damage to the liver's ability to detoxify carcinogens, and suppression of the immune response.

Alcohol is certainly not an essential factor for oesophageal carcinogenesis because the high incidence in Northern China and Iran is not associated with alcohol consumption. There is, however, a noteworthy association of alcohol consumption and oesophageal cancer in South Africa. In this case, the association is with home-brewed maize beer. Maize is not an indigenous African crop and its introduction and gradual replacement of the traditional kaffir beer, which is made from sorghum, has been associated with a marked increase in the incidence of oesophageal carcinoma over the last 60 years. It is probably not the ethanol content but the contamination of maize kernels by *Fusarium* mycotoxins that is the important aetiological factor.

Tobacco

The second major risk factor in developed countries is tobacco.[16] There is an increased risk in those who smoke cigarettes, cigars or pipe tobacco.[30] This has been confirmed in Europe and South Africa.[34] Alcohol and tobacco appear to act in synergy to increase the rate of carcinogenesis.

Auerbach and colleagues[35] performed detailed studies on oesophagi from 1203 American men whose smoking history was known. In non-smokers, only 6.6% showed atypical nuclei in the basal layer and none had carcinoma in situ. In smokers, atypical nuclei were found in 79.8% and carcinoma in situ in 1.9%.

Cigarette smoke is a direct carcinogen with a systemic effect. It has recently been shown, for instance, that the frequency of mutations in lymphocytes is increased in people who smoke.[36] This is presumably due to systemic absorption of mutagens. In addition, it is possible that tobacco smoke could act directly on oesophageal mucosal cells due to absorption from the oesophageal lumen.

The habit of chewing tobacco and betel nuts is common in some parts of the world, such as Ceylon, India and Burma. This could contribute to oesophageal cancer in these areas.[37]

Dietary factors

The high-risk areas of Northern China, Russia, Iran and South Africa are characterized by poor socioeconomic conditions and a poor diet. The latter is probably the major factor in oesophageal carcinogenesis in these areas, and although the relationship between diet and cancer is complex, there are two main aspects.[38] These are: dietary deficiency of trace elements and vitamins, and dietary excess of nitrosamines and other carcinogens.

In Northern China, the diet is deficient in vitamins A and C and riboflavine.[39] In South Africa, changes in the diet of the Zulu people over 60 years have led to deficiencies of riboflavine and niacin.[40,41] Vitamin A has a role in the control of epithelial differentiation and deficiencies led to epithelial metaplasia. This vitamin will protect against experimentally induced epithelial neoplasms in animals.[38] Vitamin C has a complex role in connective tissue metabolism and there is some experimental evidence that it can block nitrosamine synthesis and thereby protect against carcinogenesis. Riboflavine is essential for maintaining the integrity of epithelial surfaces. Deficiency of this vitamin in experimental animals leads to increased oesophageal tumour yield induced by methylbenzyl nitrosamine.[38]

There is a negative correlation between the incidence of oesophageal cancer and the soil content of certain minerals in China, the former Soviet Union and South Africa. The deficient minerals are manganese, zinc, molybdenum and magnesium.[42,43] Zinc deficiency in rats leads to increased production of oesophageal neoplasms induced by methylbenzyl nitrosamine.[44] Evidence from epidemiological and experimental studies also indicates that magnesium has an anticarcinogenic effect.[45]

A number of dietary factors in high-risk areas lead to increased exposure to nitrosamines. This group of chemicals had a major carcinogenic potential.[46] Nitrosamines will induce oesophageal tumours in experimental animals. The precursors of nitrosamines (nitrates, nitrites and secondary amines) are widespread in nature. Contamination of food by bacteria and fungi and molybdenum deficiency in soil are important factors in increasing nitrosamine concentration.

Molybdenum is a cofactor of the enzyme nitrate reductase, and deficiency leads to a modified balance between nitrates and nitrites in plants. Bacterial contamination of food leads to reduction of nitrates to nitrites and increases the generation of nitrosamines. Contamination of food by fungi such as *Fusarium* and *Aspergillus* has a similar effect, reducing nitrates and promoting the formation of nitrosamines.

Traces of nitrosamines have been found in several Chinese dishes, and practices such as curing fish with raw salt greatly increase the nitrosamine content.[47,48] In high risk areas in Northern China, the practice of pickling cabbage and other foods is common. The pickled foods become contaminated with *Geotrichum candidum* and *Fusarium* species as well as other bacteria and fungi. Extracts of this material fed to rats induce oesophageal epithelial dysplasia.[39] In the Caspian littoral, cereal grains and alcoholic beverages have been shown to be contaminated with *Fusarium* species.[34]

A number of other aspects of nutrition might be important in oesophageal carcinogenesis. Irritation of oesophageal mucosa by diets containing abrasive pariculate minerals has been suggested as a factor in the Transkei, South Africa. High-incidence regions have soil with a high quantity of silica and quartz. The silica is absorbed by plants and enters the diet. The cutting edge of the silica particles could then damage the oesophageal epithelium and lead to chronic inflammation. In Iran, bread is contaminated by silica due to a weed which contaminates wheat flour.[49]

Another possible factor is thermal damage due to the practice of drinking hot tea. This is common among the inhabitants of Iran, Puerto Rico and China.[50] Hirayana[33] has reported that those who feed on chagayu, a mixture of hot tea and boiled rice, have an increased risk of oesophageal cancer, especially if they also have nutritional deficiencies.

There are a large number of opium consumers in areas at high risk for oesophageal cancer.[51] The resinous residue in the pipes of addicts is mutagenic.[52]

A noteworthy aspect of the epidemiology of oesophageal carcinoma in high-risk areas is that there is also a high incidence of tumours of the upper alimentary tract in animals in the same areas. For instance, tumours of the pharynx and upper part of the oesophagus are found in chickens. They are mostly squamous cell carcinomas with rare adenocanthomas and adenocarcinomas. Carcinoma of the oesophagus in goats is also common in Linxian County.[19]

Trials of the effects of vitamin and mineral supplementation on histological dysplasia and early cancer of the oesophagus are underway in high risk areas in China, but to date the results are inconclusive.

Viruses

There is considerable interest in the role of viruses in squamous cell carcinoma. It has long been known that papilloma viruses are the cause of warts in man and a wide range of animals. Their possible relationship to human cancer is under investigation in the cervix. The epidemiology of cervical cancer points to an infective agent and there is evidence that infection of cervical squamous cells by human papilloma viruses is common. The use of in situ hybridization techniques in which specific genetic probes are used to visualize viral DNA in cells has shown that types 6 and 11 are associated with low-grade intraepithelial cervical lesions, whereas types 16, 18 and 31 are more often associated with high-grade lesions.[53] There is much less information on the relationship of human papilloma virus infection to squamous cell carcinoma of the oesophagus, but this is a subject of current research activity in a number of centres. Loke et al.[54] failed to demonstrate human papilloma virus 6, 11, 16 and 18 in cases of oesophageal carcinoma using in situ hybridization. Kiyabu et al.[55] were unable to detect human papilloma virus 16 or 18 in invasive squamous cell carcinoma of the oesophagus in North American patients using the polymerase chain reaction. But Chen et al.[56] studied squamous cell carcinomas in a high risk population with PCR and found evidence of HPV types 6 and 16, but not 11 and 18, in 60% (24 of 40) of cases.

Premalignant lesions

Plummer–Vinson syndrome

The Plummer–Vinson syndrome, or Paterson–Kelly syndrome,[57-61] probably results from a complex deficiency of vitamins and iron.[57] Therapy with iron usually alleviates the symptoms, although it can develop without iron deficiency and anaemia.

The condition is characterized by atrophy of the oral, pharyngeal and oesophageal mucosae. There is functional spasm of the oesophagus and cardia leading to dysphagia. Hypochromic anaemia is common.

There is a greatly increased risk of carcinoma of the upper alimentary tract, especially the upper part of the oesophagus and hypopharynx.[62] In Sweden, a significant percentage of females with carcinoma of the oesophagus have had Plummer–Vinson syndrome. In fact, it has been calculated that carcinoma of the oesophagus will develop in one of every ten females with the syndrome. In 1940, iron was introduced into bread by statute in Sweden. Since then there has been a marked fall in the incidence of Plummer–Vinson syndrome and a marked reduction in chronic iron deficiency. In addition, in more recent years, the incidence of carcinoma of the oesophagus and hypopharynx in females has also decreased.[62]

Cicatricial stricture

Cicatricial strictures are a late complication of acid or lye burns in the oesophagus. This condition predisposes to oesophageal carcinoma.[63,64] In a study of 63 patients with oesophageal carcinoma after lye burns, the mean latent interval to occurrence of carcinoma was 41 years.[64] This type of carcinoma is localized mainly to the middle third of the oesophagus, the position in which most cicatricial strictures occur.

It has been shown that if rats are subjected to a surgically induced oesophageal stenosis, they develop more tumours in response to nitrosamines than controls without stenosis. The tumours were induced earlier in the rats with stenosis and they developed within the area of stenosis.[65]

Achalasia

Achalasia of the oesophagus is due to neuromuscular dysfunction in which there is a failure of relaxation of the cardia. This leads to functional stenosis with progressive dilatation of the middle and upper oesophagus. It occurs as a consequence of an acquired impairment of ganglion cells of unknown cause.[66] Squamous cell carcinoma of the oesophagus is an important late complication of achalasia. It can develop with a latent interval of 20–35 years, although these patients usually develop carcinoma 10–15 years earlier than patients without achalasia.[57]

Diverticula

The most common oesophageal diverticulum is a pulsion diverticulum of the posterior wall of the hypopharynx directly above the oesophageal orifice. This is designated Zenker's diverticulum. Traction diverticular are found at the level of the bifurcation of the trachea and develop due to fibrous contraction following chronic inflammation of the mediastinal lymph nodes. The most common cause of this in the recent past was tuberculosis. Epiphrenic diverticula in the terminal oesophagus arise as pulsion diverticula secondary to distal oesophageal obstruction.[67]

Carcinoma in Zenker's diverticulum was first reported in 1933.[68] Over 20 cases have now been described. Most authors have suggested that chronic irritation due to retained food is a pathogenic factor.[69]

Genetic factors

Tylosis palmaris et plantaris is an autosomal dyskeratosis with dominant inheritance. It is characterized by severe epithelial thickening and hyperkeratosis of the palms of the hands and soles of the feet. There is an increased incidence of carcinoma of the oesophagus in this condition.[70,71] In two families with dominant inheritance and high penetrance, there were 18 carcinomas of the oesophagus in 48 family members with tylosis, but only one carcinoma of the oesophagus in 37 family members without tylosis.[72]

There are reports of familial clustering of oesophageal cancer in the high-risk areas of Northern China and the Caspian littoral.[57] It is not possible, however, to tell to what extent this is due to genetic factors or a shared environment in areas of high incidence.

There have been a number of reports linking oesophageal cancer with certain HLA haplotypes. In these investigations, however, a large number of different antigens are tested and it is possible for a statistically significant association to arise by chance. If the convention is adopted of using a significance level of 0.05 divided by n where n is the number of independent tests performed, then most series give non-significant results.[73]

Neoplastic development of squamous cell carcinoma

Work in Northern China, and other areas of high incidence, has shown the importance of preneoplastic changes in oesophageal cancer.[39,74–76] Two separate mass-screening studies of over 30,000 people were conducted between 1961–1969 and 1971–1972. Regions with a high incidence of carcinoma were found to have a high incidence of dysplasia. The patients with dysplasia were on average 7–8 years younger than patients with carcinoma. All of the 67 early carcinomas had associated areas of dysplasia.

In a study done in Linxian County 21,581 patients were studied over a 9-year period. Of these cases, 12.7% had mild dysplasia, and 12.1% had severe dysplasia.[39] It should be noted that the prevalence of dysplasia greatly exceeded the expected incidence of oesophageal carcinoma. A total of 184 patients with dysplasia were followed for an average of 4 years. Of 79 patients with severe dysplasia, 26.5% proceeded to invasive carcinoma, 32.9% varied from mild to severe and 40.5% reverted to normal or mild dysplasia. The subsequent incidence of invasive carcinoma in the severely dysplastic group was 140 times that in the normal population of the same region. Of the 105 patients with mild dysplasia, 15.2% progressed to severe dysplasia, 40% remained unchanged and 44.8% reverted to normal. Thus, at any stage, dysplastic lesions can revert to normal, remain the same or progress. The more severe the lesion, the more likely it is to progress.

The other consistent finding in high-risk areas is a high prevalence of chronic oesophagitis.[76] This is found in up to 70% of inhabitants of Northern China. The relationship of chronic inflammation to the dysplasia–carcinoma sequence is not clear but chronic inflammation will increase cell turnover and thereby increase the frequency of mutation. It should be noted that this oesophagitis is in the middle third of the oesophagus, unlike reflux oesophagitis which usually involves the lower third, and indeed reflux oesophagitis is uncommon in China.

Microscopic changes

The histological spectrum of preinvasive neoplastic change of squamous epithelium is continuous from normal through mild, moderate and severe dysplasia, to carcinoma in situ. The use of this terminology, however, can cause confusion as it implies a qualitative distinction between dysplasia and carcinoma in situ, whereas they form part of a spectrum. In the cervix, these terms have been replaced by intraepithelial neoplasia grades I–III. Grade I corresponds to mild dysplasia and grade III to carcinoma in situ.[77] This terminology has not yet been used for the oesophagus. Consequently, in the following discussion the term dysplasia will be retained but only three grades will be recognized, and severe dysplasia will be synonymous with carcinoma in situ.

In mild squamous cell dysplasia, the nuclear and cellular changes are confined to the lower third of the epithelium. There is a slight increase in nuclear size and an increased nuclear:cytoplasmic ratio. There is also an alteration in the nuclear chromatin pattern with increased density of chromatin staining (hyperchromatism). The nuclei may show more prominent nucleoli and some irregularity of nuclear contour. Mitotic activity within the zone is increased and mitotic figures can be abnormal.

In moderate dysplasia, these changes are found in the lower third and middle third of the epithelium. The cytological abnormalities are more marked and mitotic figures are found at a higher level than the proliferative zone.

In severe dysplasia, these changes involve the whole thickness of the epithelium and there is a failure of cell maturation at the surface. The cytological features can be bizarre and abnormal mitotic figures are seen at all levels of the epithelium (Figure 13.4).

In summary, progression along the dysplastic spectrum is associated with (1) increasing cytological abnormality, and (2) increased loss of cell maturation, as shown by the proportion of the epithelium occupied by abnormal cells.

Progression from severe dysplasia to invasive carcinoma occurs when groups of squamous epithelial cells appear to breach the basement membrane and are found as irregular clumps extending into the underlying connective tissue (Figure 13.5).

Squamous carcinoma

Gross appearance

Squamous cell carcinoma of the oesophagus can be polypoid or fungating (60%), ulcerative (25%), or infiltrative (15%) on

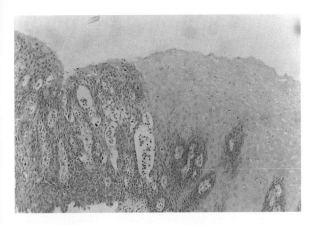

Figure 13.4
The junction between normal squamous epithelium and epithelium showing the changes of carcinoma in situ.

gross appearance.[78] Fungating carcinomas have a large polypoid intraluminal growth with a varying degree of central ulceration. Ulcerating tumours have a large central ulcer with little intraluminal tumour. The borders of the ulcer are irregular, raised and rolled. These tumours often invade deeply and involve adjacent viscera. Purely infiltrative tumours are uncommon. They can be difficult to diagnose by gross inspection. There is usually a small central ulcer, but the bulk of the disease is in the submucosa and muscularis propria. This causes abnormal distensibility and proximal dilatation of the oesophagus.

Early carcinoma Early carcinomas are more difficult to recognize on gross inspection and at endoscopy. In China, where a relatively large number have been seen, the following gross types have been described.[79]

Plaque-like The oesophageal mucosa is slightly elevated and swollen and has a coarse granular surface which may show small areas of erosion. The longitudinal and transverse ridges are interrupted. Most early oesophageal carcinomas removed by surgery are of this type.

Erosive The oesophageal mucosa is slightly depressed. The lesion is map-like with irregular margins but it is sharply demarcated from the surrounding mucosa. The depressed area is finely granular. The transverse and longitudinal folds are interrupted.

Occult The mucosa is neither protruded nor depressed. It is pink in fresh specimens with dilated and congested capillaries. In fixed specimens it is barely perceptible to the naked eye. This type of early carcinoma is rarely seen in surgical specimens.

Papillary There is a papillary protrusion 1–3 cm in diameter. There is clear demarcation between the edge of the cancer and the surrounding normal mucosa. Small areas of erosion occur on the surface with associated inflammatory debris. This type is the least common.

Microscopic features

The following are described:

- Intraepithelial carcinoma (synonyms – carcinoma in situ, severe dysplasia): cancer cells occupy the entire thickness of the oesophageal epithelium but the basement membrane is intact.
- Intramucosal carcinoma: small groups of cancer cells escape from the intraepithelial location. They penetrate the basement membrane and infiltrate the lamina propria.
- Submucosal carcinoma: cancer cells have penetrated the muscularis mucosa but have not reached the muscularis propria.

The invading islands of squamous cell carcinoma retain features of squamous cell differentiation to a variable degree. This forms the basis of classification into well, moderately well and poorly differentiated types. Differentiation is most easily assessed by the degree of keratin production and whether or not intercellular bridges can be seen.

Site

The American Joint Committee for Cancer Staging and End Results Reporting has recommended the following three anatomical divisions of the oesophagus:[80]

1. The cervical oesophagus starts at the inception of the oesophagus in the pharynx and extends to the thoracic inlet, approximately 18 cm from the incisor teeth.
2. The upper and mid-thoracic oesophagus extends from the thoracic inlet to a point 10 cm above the gastro-oesophageal junction. This is opposite the lower edge of the eighth thoracic vertebra, approximately 31 cm from the incisor teeth.
3. The lower thoracic oesophagus extends from the lower edge of the eighth thoracic vertebra to the gastro-oesophageal junction. It is 10 cm long and the junction is approximately 40 cm from the incisor teeth.

Using these definitions and extrapolating from the literature, 55% of squamous cell carcinomas occur in the upper and mid-thoracic oesophagus, 34% in the lower thoracic oesophagus,

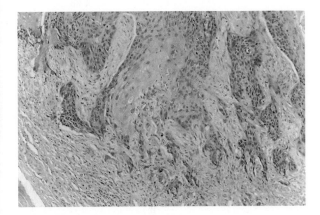

Figure 13.5
Islands of invasive squamous cell carcinoma arising from overlying epithelium showing carcinoma in situ.

8% in the cervical oesophagus, with 3% unspecified.[21] In parts of the world where Plummer–Vinson syndrome is more common, more cases occur in the cervical oesophagus and more cases are found in women.

Spread

In Ming's[78] series, 38% of cases were found to extend to paraoesophageal soft tissue, 41% to lymph nodes and 16% to both at the time of initial diagnosis. The bronchial tree and aorta are involved in 13 and 6% of cases, respectively. This can lead to catastrophic events. Indeed, the close proximity of the oesophagus to mediastinal structures contributes to its poor prognosis.

The patterns of nodal spread vary with the site of the tumour.[81] Tumours of the cervical oesophagus spread to deep cervical, paraoesophageal and posterior mediastinal lymph nodes. Tumours in the middle third drain to paraoesophageal, posterior mediastinal and tracheobronchial nodes. Those in the lower third spread to paraoesophageal, coeliac and splenic nodes. However, spread can occur to groups of nodes distant from the primary tumour (see Chapter 14). Metastatic spread occurs to liver, lungs, adrenals and kidneys.

Adenocarcinoma

Adenocarcinoma of the oesophagus could, in theory, arise from areas of glandular heterotopia,[82] from oesophageal submucosal glands or in areas of glandular metaplasia. In fact, the most common origin is glandular metaplasia in Barrett's oesophagus (Figure 13.6).

Barrett, and other early workers, noted that the lower oesophagus could be lined by columnar epithelium. Barrett[83] thought that this was due to a congenital short oesophagus with part of the gastric cardia pulled into the thorax. It is now realized, however, that this is a metaplastic process in which part of the squamous epithelial lining of the lower oesophagus, above the physiological sphincter, is replaced by glandular epithelium which can differentiate to gastric or intestinal cell types.[84–86] The pathogenic sequence is reflux of gastric acid[87] or duodenal contents[88,89] leading to oesophageal ulceration and subsequent regeneration with glandular epithelium.

An experimental model of Barrett's metaplasia has been produced in dogs.[87] Three groups of animals were studied. In one group the squamous mucosa of the distal oesophagus was excised. The injured segment healed with squamous epithelium. In the second group, the squamous mucosa was excised and a hiatus hernia was formed. In this case, healing resulted in either squamous epithelium or glandular epithelium. In the third group, mucosal excision was performed, a hiatus hernia was produced and the animals were given histamine to increase gastric acid production. In this group, healing was predominantly with glandular epithelium. Thus ulceration, reflux and gastric acidity are all important in the pathogenesis of Barrett's metaplasia. Barrett's oesophagus, however, can also arise in patients who have undergone a total gastrectomy.[88,89] In this situation, it is thought that bile reflux is an important factor.

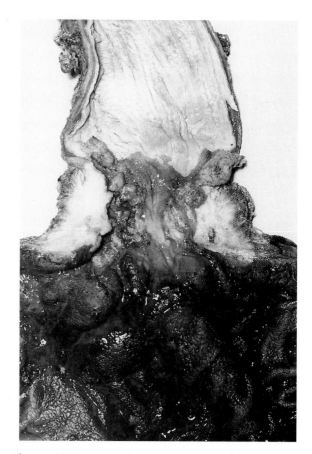

Figure 13.6
Adenocarcinoma arising at the oesophagogastric junction in an area of Barrett's metaplasia.

A number of clinical observations also support the thesis that Barrett's metaplasia is an acquired lesion consequent on gastro-oesophageal reflux. The prevalence of glandular metaplasia in patients with chronic gastro-oesophageal reflux is 10–12%.[86,90,91] Furthermore, transformation to Barrett's metaplasia and proximal progression has been demonstrated in a number of series.[84,92,93] Most patients with columnar metaplasia complain of long-standing symptoms of reflux oesophagitis.

Barrett's columnar-lined oesophagus: macroscopic appearance

In the region of the lower oesophageal sphincter, there is a transition from white squamous epithelium of the oesophagus to the pink columnar epithelium of the stomach. The line of transition is termed the ora serrata or Z line, because of its undulating course. In Barrett's columnar-lined oesophagus, the ora serrata is relocated proximally so that there is a metaplastic zone between it and the lower oesophageal sphincter. The metaplastic zone is pink–red in colour and is quite distinct from the adjacent squamous epithelium. Ulceration is commonly seen at the junction and in the metaplastic zone. It is also not uncommon to find irregular squamous islands within the area of metaplasia.[85,86,91,94]

Barrett's columnar-lined oesophagus: microscopic appearances

The glandular epithelium of Barrett's oesophagus is a variable admixture of gastric and intestinal cell types (Figure 13.7). The surface cells can be mucus-secreting columnar cells, as seen in the stomach, mucus-secreting goblet cells, as seen in the small intestine, or, less commonly, intestinal absorptive cells with a microvillous brush border. The gastric-type surface cells contain neutral mucins, whereas the intestinal cells contain acidic, non-sulphated mucins. The latter are stained by alcian blue at pH 2.5. The underlying glands most commonly resemble the simple gastric glands seen in the cardiac and pyloric regions of the stomach. In addition, however, there is commonly a variable admixture of other cell types. These include Paneth cells, neuroendocrine cells and parietal cells. Immunoperoxidase techniques have shown that the endocrine cells may contain gastrin, somatostatin, serotonin, secretin and pancreatic polypeptide.[94-96]

Neoplastic potential (see also Chapter 11)

The majority of cases of adenocarcinoma of the lower oesophagus are associated with Barrett's metaplasia.[85,91,97-99] In the metaplastic zone adjacent to the invasive carcinoma, it is often possible to demonstrate high-grade dysplasia. In the case of adenocarcinoma of the gastro-oesophageal junction, foci of Barrett's metaplasia are found in up to 50% of cases.[85,91,100,101] It is obviously likely that in many other cases the tumour has overgrown and destroyed a pre-existing metaplastic area. These observations have led to the concept that adenocarcinomas of the lower oesophagus and of the oesophagogastric junction have a common aetiology related to Barrett's metaplasia.

More recently it has been realized that adenocarcinoma of the lower oesophagus, oesophagogastric junction and gastric cardia have features in common which differentiate them from other gastric adenocarcinomas and that they might have a common pathogenesis.[101-103] If adenocarcinoma of the oesophagus and gastric cardia are compared with those of the rest of the stomach, there is a higher male to female ratio, the patients are more likely to have experienced symptoms of acid reflux, to have a hiatus hernia and to have demonstrable Barrett's metaplasia. A family history of gastric cancer is less common. Furthermore, although the overall incidence of gastric carcinoma has fallen in recent years in the USA and in the UK, the relative proportion of adenocarcinomas of the gastric cardia has risen. The overall incidence of gastric carcinoma is higher in Blacks than in Whites in the USA, but carcinoma of the gastric cardia, like oesophageal adenocarcinoma, is more common in Whites.[104]

Adenocarcinoma of the lower oesophagus, which does not involve the gastric cardia, is relatively uncommon accounting for only 2.4–4% of cases of carcinoma of the oesophagus in low incidence areas.[85] If all cases of adenocarcinoma of the lower oesophagus and oesophagogastric junction are considered, however, then the total equals that of squamous carcinoma. If carcinoma of the gastric cardia is also included, then adenocarcinoma in association with Barrett's oesophagus is more common than squamous cell carcinoma of the oesophagus in low incidence countries. Several reports have alluded to the increasing incidence of oesophageal adenocarcinoma since the early 1960s, which is increasing by 5% per annum.[16]

There is no doubt that patients with Barrett's metaplasia have an increased risk of adenocarcinoma, but the magnitude of the risk has not been precisely determined. The prevalence of adenocarcinoma in patients with Barrett's metaplasia detected at endoscopy is 8–15%.[105] Patients with adenocarcinoma, however, are more likely to be symptomatic and undergo endoscopy. Consequently, the true prevalence is likely to be less than this figure. The incidence of adenocarcinoma in patients under surveillance with Barrett's metaplasia has varied between one adenocarcinoma per 46 to one per 441 patient years of follow-up.[105] If the six series from which these figures are taken are combined,[105] the incidence is one adenocarcinoma per 166 patient years based on 478 patients followed for a mean of 4.6 years, which considerably exceeds the risk in the general population by a factor of at least 150.

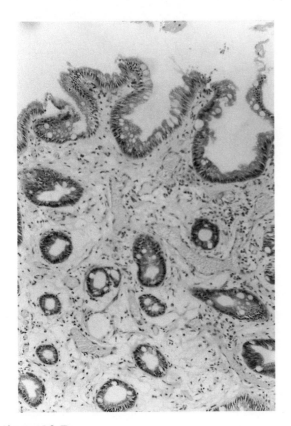

Figure 13.7

Barrett's mucosa showing goblet cells as seen in intestinal mucosa.

Dysplasia

One possible marker of malignant potential is the presence of dysplasia. This is a neoplastic alteration of the glandular epithelium assessed by changes in cytology and architecture (Figures 13.8 and 13.9). There is good evidence that high-grade dysplasia is a premalignant lesion because retrospective

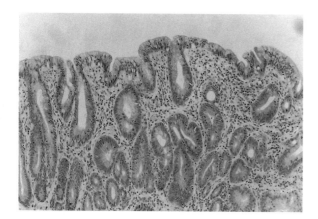

Figure 13.8
Barrett's mucosa with low-grade dysplasia.

studies demonstrate dysplasia in the mucosa adjacent to adenocarcinoma.[106]

Secondly, some patients who have undergone oesophagectomy because of high-grade dysplasia are found to have previously unrecognized adenocarcinoma. The significance of low-grade dysplasia is less clear. In other neoplastic systems, such as the cervix, dysplastic lesions can regress, remain the same or progress. High-grade dysplasia has a high chance of progression, whereas low-grade dysplasia is less likely to progress. These rules also apply to squamous cell carcinoma of the oesophagus and they probably operate in oesophageal adenocarcinoma (Figure 13.10).

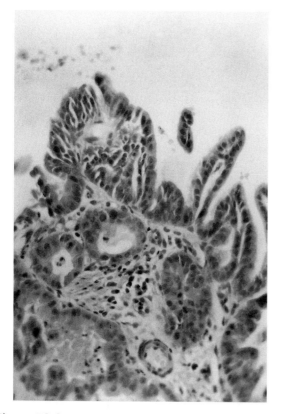

Figure 13.9
Barrett's mucosa with high-grade dysplasia.

The assessment of glandular dysplasia, however, is subjective and there is both interobserver and intraobserver variation. In one study, glandular epithelium was classified as (1) negative for dysplasia, (2) indefinite for dysplasia, (3) low-grade dysplasia, (4) high-grade dysplasia and (5) intramucosal carcinoma.[107] There was good interobserver agreement (85–87%) for the diagnosis of intramucosal carcinoma and high-grade dysplasia, but much less agreement in the diagnosis of low-grade dysplasia, and the groups indefinite for dysplasia.

Criteria for the diagnosis of dysplasia depend on assessment of glandular architecture and epithelial cytology. Architectural abnormalities include budded, branched crowded or irregularly shaped glands, papillary extensions into glandular lumina and villiform configurations of the mucosal surface. Cytological features include variation in nuclear size and shape, increased nuclear cytoplasmic ratio, hyperchromatism, increased mitotic rate and abnormal mitoses.

There is a consensus of opinion that the diagnosis of high-grade dysplasia is an indication for oesophagectomy in suitable surgical candidates, whereas a diagnosis of low-grade dysplasia is an indication for careful follow-up with regular endoscopic surveillance.

Flow cytometry

The technique of flow cytometry enables measurement of the DNA content of a large number of individual cells. A single cell suspension is prepared from tissue fragments stained by a fluorescent dye and then the cells are passed in single file where they interact with a beam of light, and the amount of DNA per cell is assayed.[108] In general, the development of cancer is associated with genomic instability and a variable proportion of cancer cells show DNA aneuploidy. This technique has been used to investigate Barrett's glandular mucosa.[109–112] Patients with high-grade dysplasia and carcinoma have abnormal flow cytometry patterns with aneuploid cell populations. Most patients without dysplasia have normal flow cytometry. However, a few patients with aneuploidy but no histological evidence of dysplasia do progress during follow-up to high-grade dysplasia or carcinoma.

Immunohistochemistry

Immunohistochemical investigation of Barrett's mucosa is an active area of current research. There is particular interest in the p53 gene which normally functions as a tumour suppressor gene.[113] Mutations in this gene are the most commonly identified genetic abnormalities associated with many human cancers. Certain of the mutations lead to an abnormal protein product with an extended half life which can be recognized with immunohistological staining techniques. Younes et al.[114] investigated 114 specimens of Barrett's epithelium and found positive staining for p53 in none of those negative for dysplasia, 9% of those with low-grade dysplasia, 55% of those with high-grade dysplasia and 87% of those with adenocarcinoma.

Other studies have concentrated on protein markers of cell proliferation. The proliferating cell nuclear antigen is an auxiliary protein to DNA polymerase, which is expressed in dividing

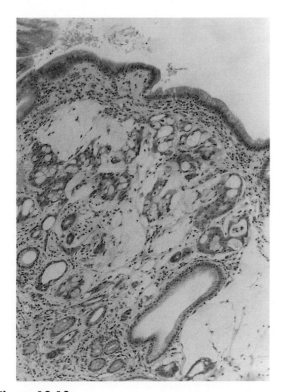

Figure 13.10
Mucus-secreting adenocarcinoma infiltrating Barrett's mucosa.

cells. The Ki67 protein is expressed in cells in the G_1 phase of the cell cycle. Both of these antigens show increased expression in Barrett's specialized epithelium which is negative for dysplasia.[112,115]

Another area of current investigation is that of cell adhesion molecules and their relationship to metastasis. The process of metastatic spread, which is the main determinant of poor prognosis in cancer, involves complex biochemical changes. There is decreased expression of adhesion molecules linking epithelial cells but increased expression of molecules involved in adherence to endothelial cells and migration into tissues. For instance, the E-cadherin-catenin complex expressed by epithelial cells is important for cell-to-cell adhesion. Decreased expression of these proteins, demonstrated by immunohistochemistry, is found in oesophageal adenocarcinoma and correlates with poor prognosis.[116] Conversely, the CD44 cell surface glycoprotein, which is implicated in lymphocyte homing and cell-extracellular matrix interactions, shows increased expression in dysplastic Barrett's glandular mucosa and oesophageal carcinoma.[117]

Endoscopic surveillance

Although endoscopically detected high-grade dysplasia appears to be a precursor to the development of adenocarcinoma, there is no direct evidence that endoscopic surveillance of patients with Barrett's mucosa reduces the mortality or morbidity associated with adenocarcinoma. It has been calculated that 2000 patients would have to be followed for 10 years to demonstrate a 50% reduction in mortality at a significance level of 0.05.[118] If the reduction in mortality was less than 50%, the number of patient years of follow-up would need to be greater, and it is unlikely that studies of this size will be feasible.

It is clear, therefore, that the search for reliable markers of increased malignant potential should continue, so that high-risk cases can be targeted. In the meantime, the consensus view is that endoscopic surveillance should be used for patients with Barrett's mucosa of 8 cm or more,[105] as the risk of neoplastic potential is considerably higher in such patients.[119]

Polypoid tumour of the oesophagus

This tumour has been described by a variety of terms, including carcinosarcoma, pseudosarcoma and pseudosarcomatous carcinoma. The differing terms reflect differing views on its histogenesis. These tumours are polypoid, they contain spindle cell areas which are morphologically indistinguishable from sarcoma and a variable admixture of carcinoma. They occur in the mouth, pharynx, larynx, oesophagus, renal pelvis and bladder.[120-126] They are, however, rare in the oesophagus. There were only 51 reported cases up to 1979,[127] and since then only a few reports of small groups of cases have been added.[128-130]

Within the oesophagus, the site and age of presentation is similar to that of squamous cell carcinoma. They are also more common in males than females.[124,127] The presenting symptoms are usually those of progressive dysphagia and weight loss.

The tumours are usually large pedunculated masses growing into and distending the oesophageal lumen from a narrow base (Figure 13.11). They rarely present as ulcerating or constricting lesions. Radiological examination reveals a characteristic cupola sign in which barium forms a dome over the smooth-surfaced tumour.[131]

Histologically, the carcinomatous component is usually squamous. It can be purely in situ or form part of the invasive mass. The sarcomatous component consists of spindle cells showing varying degrees of nuclear pleomorphism and mitotic activity (Figure 13.12). The spindle cell areas may show bizarre giant cells, strap-like cells resembling rhabdomyoblasts and

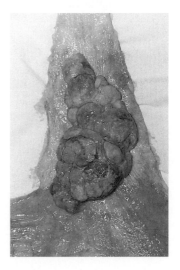

Figure 13.11
A large polypoid tumour of the oesophagus.

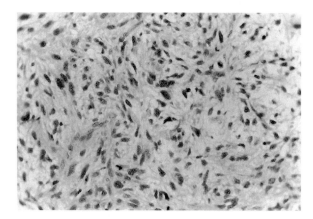

Figure 13.12
Sarcomatous component of a polypoid tumour of the oesophagus.

areas of osteoid or cartilaginous differentiation. The polypoid tumours seen in the renal pelvis and bladder have shown areas resembling malignant osteoclastoma.[124,125]

The tumours can invade deeply through the wall of the oesophagus, but in general the depth of invasion is less than for squamous cell carcinomas of equivalent size. In the series of 36 cases reported by Osamura and colleagues,[124] invasion was confined to the mucosa in 12 (33.3%) and submucosa in 10 (28%). The polypoid appearance is presumably a consequence of tumour growth with relatively limited invasion. Metastases of these tumours may be carcinomatous or sarcomatous.

The histogenesis of these tumours was in doubt for a number of years and this is reflected in the varied terms that have been used to describe the entity. It is now accepted, however, that the tumours are epithelial in origin and that the sarcomatous area is derived by a process of dedifferentiation or mesenchymal metaplasia. Detailed ultrastructural studies have shown that there is a gradual transition from cells showing epithelial features, through intermediate cells showing both epithelial and mesenchymal features to cells which are indistinguishable from mesenchymal cells.[123,125,132] The ultrastructural markers of squamous cells are tonofilaments and specialized desmosomes, whereas mesenchymal cells have less specialized desmosomes, intermediate filaments and variable dilated rough endoplasmic reticulum.

In recent years, a number of epithelial and mesenchymal markers have been recognized using specific antibodies and immunohistological techniques. For instance, epithelial cells express epithelial membrane antigen and have cytokeratin filaments in the cytoplasm, whereas mesenchymal cells have intermediate filaments which are recognized by antibodies to vimentin. Only a few studies of spindle cell carcinomas have been performed with these techniques.[127,129,130] It appears that cells which resemble squamous cells or epithelial cells by light and electron microscopy show epithelial markers, whereas cells that resemble mesenchymal cells by light and electron microscopy express mesenchymal markers.

The prognosis of polypoid carcinomas of the oesophagus is probably better than that of more typical squamous cell carci-

nomas, which is a consequence of a lesser degree of invasion. In the cases reviewed by Hinderlieder and colleagues,[127] of 18 cases available for follow-up after resection, only four patients died with recurrence within 3 years and three survived for over 5 years.

Verrucous carcinoma

Verrucous carcinoma is a variant of squamous cell carcinoma which was first described by Ackerman.[133] These tumours have a verrucous, cauliflower-like appearance. They are slow growing and locally invasive, but rarely metastasize. Histologically, they are extremely well differentiated papillary lesions with only minimal cytological atypia towards the base. The surface squamous cells can be indistinguishable from those of squamous cell papillomas. These tumours occur on squamous-lined mucosal surfaces, such as the oral cavity, larynx, vagina and anus. They have been described in the oesophagus, but are very rare.[134-136] Radical surgical excision is regarded as the treatment of choice. Radiation therapy does not control the growth and there is some evidence that it may increase the malignancy of the lesion.[137,138]

Oat cell carcinoma

Oat cell carcinoma of the oesophagus was first described by McKeown in 1952.[139] In 1983, Briggs and Ibrahim reported 23 cases and reviewed another 34.[140-147] The age range was 29–88 years. Oat cell carcinoma comprised 2.4% of the 955 unselected consecutive oesophageal carcinomas examined by Briggs and Ibrahim.[140] In their series of 23 cases, 15 of the patients were female and only eight were male. This compares with a male to female ratio in the 955 cases of 1.5:1. The majority of reported cases had arisen in the lower third of the oesophagus (57%), with 39% in the middle third and 4% in the upper third. In the majority of cases the tumours have been large, ulcerating and fungating.

The histological appearance of these tumours is identical to that of oat cell carcinoma of the bronchus. The constituent cells have round or ovoid hyperchromatic nuclei with inconspicuous nucleoli. The cells occur in sheets, cords or trabeculi and can show streaming and rosette formation (Figure 13.13). Areas of squamous, nodular and carcinoid differentiation may occur.

Ultrastructural examination reveals membrane-bound dense core granules, termed neurosecretory granules in some but not all cases. The granules are characteristic of neuroendocrine cells.[148] Even after a thorough search of many blocks, however, these granules can be absent from cases which are otherwise typical of oat cell carcinoma. A similar argument applies to the demonstration of argyrophil granules using silver stains on formalin-fixed paraffin-embedded sections. A positive argyrophil reaction is found in some but not all cases. Positive staining for neurone-specific enolase, using an immunoperoxidase technique, is seen in some cases and can be helpful in diagnosis.[149] More recently chromogranin has proved to be a useful marker of neuroendocrine cells and this can be demonstrated by immunoperoxidase staining techniques in formalin-fixed tissue.

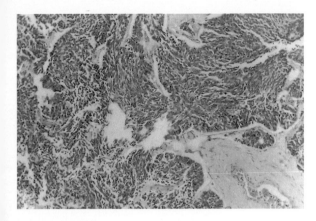

Figure 13.13
Oat cell carcinoma of the oesophagus.

The diagnosis of primary oat cell carcinoma of the oesophagus depends on the typical histological appearance and the demonstration that the tumour has not spread from the bronchus. Electron microscopy, argyrophil stains and immuno-histological techniques can provide supportive evidence, but negative results do not exclude the diagnosis.

The histogenesis of oat cell tumours is controversial. Neuroendocrine cells are found in the oesophageal mucosa[94,150] and these could be the cell of origin for oat cell carcinoma. This is analogous to the situation in the bronchus.[151] Alternatively, it is possible that basal stem cells of squamous epithelium could differentiate into cells of the neuroendocrine system.

It is important to recognize this entity because it tends to behave differently from squamous carcinoma. These tumours are aggressive and have a poor prognosis. They metastasize widely and have a rapid clinical course. Paraendocrine syndromes are associated with this cell type, and at least in the lung these tumours can respond to cytotoxic therapy.

Metastatic malignant melanoma

The gastrointestinal tract is a common site for metastases from cutaneous malignant melanoma, but metastasis to the oesophagus is rare.[152,153] When it occurs, the typical finding is a nodule on the crest of a rugal fold or a submucosal nodule with a deep ulcerated crater. These ulcers produce a so-called 'bull's eye' effect radiologically due to trapping of barium.

Primary malignant melanoma

Primary malignant melanoma of the oesophagus is uncommon. A convincing diagnosis can only be made when the tumour arises from an area of mucosa showing junctional activity. However, some tumours will overgrow their site of origin prior to diagnosis so that cases are accepted if there is no other possible primary site.[154–156]

Benign melanocytes have been identified in 48% of oesophagi using silver staining techniques,[150,157,158] and are thought to be the precursor cells of malignant melanoma. They have been shown to increase in number as a result of chronic inflammation. Occasionally, gross patches of pigmentation due to junctional proliferation of benign melanocytes are seen. These are usually found in association with malignant melanoma.[153,159]

Primary malignant melanomas are usually polypoid growths which show central ulceration.[160] They may or may not be grossly pigmented. In a review of 65 cases[154] the age range was 7–82 years, but the vast majority of cases occurred in the later decades. The male to female ratio was 2:1. The site of origin was upper third 16%, middle third 40% and lower third 44%. The prognosis is poor due to early lymphatic and systemic metastasis.

Adenoid cystic carcinoma

Adenoid cystic carcinoma occurs in salivary gland, breast, bronchus and skin, and extremely rarely in the oesophagus. Akamatsu and colleagues[161] found only 23 cases in a review of the world literature between 1950 and 1983.

These tumours have a characteristic histological appearance in which glandular cells form a cribriform pattern (Figure 13.14). The cribriform spaces between the cells may be true acini but are more commonly pseudoacini composed of reduplicated basement membrane and stroma.[162,163] The stroma stains positively with PAS and alcian blue.

Most authors believe that these tumours arise from intercalated ducts of submucosal oesophageal glands. Indeed, some of the reported cases have been intimately associated with submucosal glands and have shown minimal involvement of the mucosa.[163] Furthermore, ultrastructural examination reveals epithelial and myoepithelial cells with a relationship similar to that seen in normal salivary gland and salivary gland tumours.[163]

In one series,[163] the age range of cases was 51–72 years and the male to female ratio was 19:1. The tumours occurred most commonly in the middle third. The patients presented with progressive dysphagia and the tumours were usually advanced with invasion through the wall, spread to mediastinal lymph nodes and widespread metastases. These tumours seem to have a poor prognosis and seem to be more aggressive than adenoid cystic carcinoma in other sites. This might be partly because they present late and also because of their anatomical

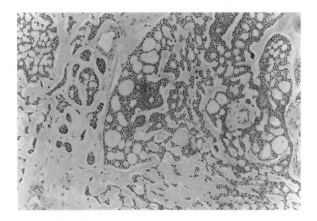

Figure 13.14
Adenoid cystic carcinoma.

location close to major mediastinal structures. However, it should be realized that poorly differentiated adenocarcinomas can occasionally produce a cribiform pattern resembling adenoid cystic carcinoma. Inclusion of these cases would bias data.

Mucoepidermoid carcinomas

Mucoepidermoid carcinomas are rare salivary gland tumours which arise from oesophageal submucosal glands. The histological diagnosis depends on the recognition of mucin-secreting cells, squamous cells and intermediate cells.[164,165] They must, however, be differentiated from (1) adenocanthomas – which are adenocarcinomas with foci of bland squamous metaplasia, and (2) adenosquamous carcinomas in which there are malignant glandular and squamous elements.

Mucoepidermoid carcinomas of the oesophagus have a worse prognosis than similar tumours at other sites. This is probably because they present late and are situated close to the mediastinal structures. This is analogous to the findings in adenoid cystic carcinoma.

Secondary malignant epithelial tumours

Secondary invasion of the oesophagus by carcinoma can be direct, by lymphatic spread or by the haematogenous route. In a series of disseminated carcinoma, the oesophagus is involved in 1–3%.[166–168] In a review of 82 cases of metastasis to the oesophagus, 28 cases were from the breast, 26 from the pharynx, ten from the stomach and three from the lung.[169] If direct extension is excluded, the breast and the lung are the major sites. It is possible that as many as 99% of fatal breast cancer cases and 4% of lung cancer cases invade the oesophagus.[170] However, because spread to the oesophagus is late in the disease, symptoms of dysphagia are rare, occurring in only 10 of 2500 cases of advanced breast cancer in one series.[171]

The most common gross change is a short segment, smooth-contoured, circumferential stenosis of the mid-oesophagus. The mucosa is usually intact and endoscopic biopsy fails to reveal the tumour.

NON-EPITHELIAL TUMOURS

Leiomyoma

Leiomyomas are the most common non-epithelial tumours of the oesophagus. Takubo and colleagues[172] examined 342 oesophagi by a serial block technique and found 38 minute smooth muscle tumours in 27 of the cases. None of the tumours was more than 7 mm in diameter and most arose in the inner circular muscle. Of the 38 tumours, 25 were located at the oesophagogastric junction.

The tumours that present clinically are usually 2–5 cm diameter[173] but can be over 1000 g in weight.[174,175] The most common location is the lower oesophagus, and the male to female ratio is 2.5:1. The majority of the tumours are firm, encapsulated, round to oval masses which are usually submucosal but can form pedunculated polyps. Microscopically, they are composed of interlacing bundles of smooth muscle cells. The cells lack

nuclear pleomorphism and there are few mitotic figures.

Many cases are asymptomatic and may be demonstrated radiologically or endoscopically during investigation of upper digestive symptoms. When they do present clinically, the symptoms are usually dysphagia, substernal pain or heartburn. Bleeding is a rare complication, unlike the situation with leiomyomas of the stomach or intestine. The typical radiological appearance of an intramural leiomyoma is a crescent-shaped filling defect with a smooth mucosal border.

There are a number of reports of leiomyomas occurring in association with epiphrenic diverticula,[176–178] and osteoarthropathy and clubbing of digits.[179]

Leiomyomatosis

In this condition the oesophagus, and often the gastric cardia, is distorted by confluent myomatous nodules which merge with hypertrophied smooth muscle. The condition must be distinguished from multiple oesophageal leiomyomas and idiopathic muscular hypertrophy. The latter is the morphological expression of diffuse oesophageal spasm in which the muscular hypertrophy is diffuse, as opposed to nodular.

Leiomyomatosis may affect either one or both muscle layers of the oesophagus and/or the muscularis mucosa.[180] The condition is rare. Fernandes and colleagues[181] reviewed 15 cases in 1975. The age range was 17–74 years but one-third of the cases presented before 25 years of age, and these were mainly women. The patients suffered from progressive dysphagia which sometimes started in childhood. The condition has been described in association with leiomyomas of the vulva,[182,183] and with Alport's syndrome.[184]

Leiomyosarcoma

Leiomyosarcoma is rare, comprising less than 0.5% of oesophageal tumours.[185] It is more common in males and most patients are elderly. The presenting symptoms are dysphagia, weight loss and substernal pain. The tumours are slightly more frequent in the distal oesophagus. Macroscopically they form polypoid intraluminal masses or infiltrating intramural masses. The histological features are similar to those of malignant smooth muscle tumours elsewhere in the body. The distinction from leiomyoma, however, can be difficult. The features of nuclear pleomorphism and mitotic activity are not completely reliable, casting doubt on reports of transformation from a benign leiomyoma to a leiomyosarcoma. In view of these difficulties, some authors recommend that the term 'leiomyomatous tumour', or more recently stromal tumour of uncertain malignant potential (STUMP), should be used for all smooth muscle tumours of the gastrointestinal tract. Prognosis can then be based on the size, character of the margins, degree of excision, presence of nuclear pleomorphism and mitotic frequency.

Fibrovascular polyps

Fibrovascular polyps are smooth-surfaced, pedunculated intraluminal masses. Microscopically, there is a connective tissue core which is commonly myxoid and vascular with a variable admixture of fibroadipose tissue. The mucosa is usually intact but can be ulcerated. The majority arise in the upper oesophagus, usually the postcricoid region.[186] They are usually large, most cases being over 1 cm in diameter and they can be up to 20 cm diameter. The tumours usually occur in middle-aged to elderly males who present with dysphagia or a globus sensation. The tumours can regurgitate into the mouth, or even out of the mouth.[187] The mass can be aspirated into the larynx causing asphyxiation. A further possible complication is torsion, with subsequent rapid growth due to congestion and oedema.

Lipoma

On occasions the connective tissue core of a lesion which otherwise resembles a fibrovascular polyp is formed entirely or predominantly of mature adipose tissue. These lesions are then designated as lipomas.[188]

Inflammatory fibroid polyp

These lesions are more common in the stomach but can occur in the oesophagus. They form intraluminal pedunculated masses covered by mucosa which may be ulcerated. The core is composed of connective tissue in which there is a characteristic arrangement of fibroblasts around small blood vessels. There may be a pronounced infiltrate of eosinophils.[189]

Inflammatory reflux polyps

These are small polyps occurring in the lower oesophagus close to the gastro-oesophageal junction. They develop in the presence of reflux oesophagitis and consist of granulation tissue. Severe bleeding can occur.[190,191]

Granular cell tumours

Granular cell tumours are relatively uncommon lesions found in the skin, tongue, breast, upper respiratory tract and gastrointestinal tract. Approximately one-third of the gastrointestinal lesions occur in the oesophagus.[192] The majority of these occur in the distal third.[192,193] They present as small, firm, solid, submucosal nodules which are white or yellow on section. Microscopically they are composed of diffuse sheets of cells with abundant granular cytoplasm which stains positively with PAS (Figure 13.15). There is often pseudoepitheliomatous hyperplasia of the overlying squamous epithelium. Ultrastructural examination shows that the characteristic cystoplasmic granularity is due to the presence of numerous large secondary lysosomes.

The histogenesis of this tumour has been a matter of dispute.[194,195] At one time these lesions were called granular cell myoblastomas because of a presumed origin from muscle cells. Recent immunohistological studies, however, have shown that these tumours express the antigen S100 which is a marker of neural cells.[195]

Granular cell tumours can be asymptomatic or can present with dysphagia or substernal pain. They are more common in men than women. The tumours are occasionally multiple within the oesophagus, and they occasionally occur in association with granular cell tumours elsewhere in the body. Very rarely they behave in a malignant fashion.[196]

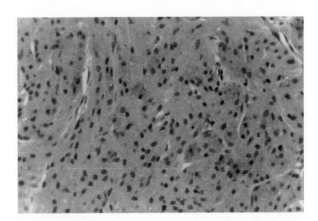

Figure 13.15
A granular cell tumour.

Other neoplasms

The many different types of soft tissue neoplasm which are found elsewhere in the body can occur in the oesophagus. Reported examples include rhabdomyosarcoma,[197] chondroma,[198] osteogenic sarcoma,[199] cavernous haemangioma,[200,201] lymphangioma[202,203] and Kaposi's sarcoma.[204,205] Osteosarcomas are of note in that although they are extremely rare in man, they do occur in dogs in South Eastern USA where the oesophageal nematode, *Spirocerca lupi* is endemic.[206]

Lymphoma

Primary lymphoma of the oesophagus is extremely rare. There are only a few well-documented cases including nodular sclerosing Hodgkin's disease[207] and non-Hodgkin's lymphoma.[208,209]

The gastrointestinal tract is commonly secondarily involved in malignant lymphoma, but the oesophagus is the least common organ in which secondary lymphoma is found. In one series, only 7.4% of gastrointestinal malignant lymphomas involved the oesophagus. When the oesophagus is involved, it is usually secondary to spread from mediastinal lymph nodes. Interestingly, in patients with malignant lymphoma who develop oesophageal bleeding, the cause is most commonly non-tumorous ulceration.[210]

CLINICAL FEATURES OF TUMOURS OF THE OESOPHAGUS

The mode of presentation of oesophageal tumours depends on the size and consequently the type of tumour. Benign tumours rarely achieve a significant size, with the exception of leiomyomas, and consequently are often chance findings at endoscopy. Very rarely, benign tumours may produce minor degrees of dysphagia and are detected during investigation of this, but more usually, they are detected during endoscopy to investigate upper gastrointestinal symptoms. Leiomyomas, which occur most commonly in the region of the cardia, may result in reflux symptoms because of interference with the antireflux mechanism, but more usually are asymptomatic. The fact that reflux symptoms are so common in the general population has led some authors to suggest an association between benign oesophageal tumours, particularly squamous papilloma,

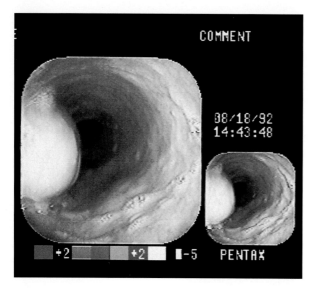

Figure 13.16
Endoscopic view of leiomyoma, diagnosed at endoscopy for reflux sympoms.

and gastro-oesophageal reflux. Once leiomyomas achieve a large size (Figure 13.16, see colour plate also, and Figure 13.17) they may produce a sensation of certain foods sticking on the way down, although they rarely present with frank dysphagia, as they are not usually circumferential. It is in malignant tumours, and particularly in carcinoma, that dysphagia becomes a predominant symptom.

Indeed the classical presenting symptom of oesophageal carcinoma is dysphagia. This usually begins as an awareness of the passage of particularly solid foods such as bread and meat, progressively followed by an inability to swallow these foods. As the growth of the tumour progressively encroaches on the oesophageal lumen, the degree of dysphagia increases, such that there may be hold up of all solids, at which time many

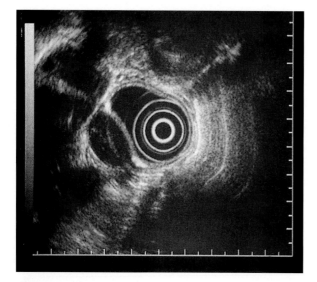

Figure 13.17
Endoluminal ultrasound in the same patient as in Figure 13.16 showing gross distortion of the muscle layers but with intact mucosa over the lesion.

patients modify the consistency of their diet in order to maintain nutrition, and it is for this reason that, somewhat surprisingly, the delay between first onset of symptoms and clinical presentation varies from 4 to 7.5 months.[211,212] A small proportion of patients do not present until they have dysphagia for liquids and even in swallowing their own saliva, in which circumstances there is usually considerable weight loss and dehydration.

There is frequently an imperfect correlation both between the site of the obstruction and the sensation of dysphagia, and between the degree of dysphagia and the degree of luminal obstruction. Edwards and Lobello[213] showed that up to 30% of patients described their dysphagia at a considerable distance from the site of the obstruction. With regard to the degree of dysphagia and its relationship to the degree of luminal obstruction, any impaction of a lump of meat, a fruit stone or vegetable matter may produce virtually complete dysphagia. However, in most circumstances, the degree of dysphagia is relentlessly progressive with time, in distinction to that associated with motility disorders, which is often very variable and paradoxical, i.e. worse for liquids than for solids. It is also invariably associated with significant weight loss, in distinction to patients with reflux-induced stricture. Whenever there is a severe degree of luminal narrowing, food or fluid are retained above it. This may lead to regurgitation, particularly when the patient is supine. The oesophageal contents may spill over into the larynx and trachea, giving rise to coughing bouts or, at night when the cough reflex is inhibited, to aspiration pneumonia. The cough may be productive, with particles of food within the sputum. Similar symptoms, with severe cough and even dyspnoea may result from a fistula between the oesophagus and the trachea or a main bronchus.

Although dysphagia is the classical symptom of oesophageal cancer, and every patient with dysphagia should be considered as possibly suffering from this disease until proved otherwise, there are many other causes of dysphagia, which may be structural, associated with inflammatory conditions or may be functional, due either to neurological disorders, disorders of innervation or muscle and connective tissue disorders. The differential diagnosis of dysphagia is shown in Table 13.1.

An inevitable consequence of reduced dietary intake, consequent on progressive and oesophageal narrowing, is impaired nutrition and weight loss, most patients having lost some 10% of their body weight at the time of presentation.[214] This may be exacerbated by the metabolic effects of the tumour itself, and hypoalbumenaemia is common at presentation, which is an unwelcome prelude to the prospect of major surgical intervention.

Pain is an uncommon, but often distressing symptom of oesophageal cancer. Acute obstruction by an impacted food bolus may produce excruciating oesophageal pain or odynophagia, felt retrosternally and radiating into the back and occasionally the jaws and arms. More seriously, pain may reflect very advanced disease, with local infiltration into the aorta, spine or intercostal nerves, producing a severe, boring type of pain.

Table 13.1 Differential diagnosis of dysphagia

Mechanical obstruction
Fibrous stricture
   Reflux-induced
   Schatzki ring
   Corrosive ingestion
   Drugs e.g. doxycycline, ascorbic acid
   Postradiotherapy
   Behcet's disease
Webs
Diverticulum
Food bolus obstruction
Foreign bodies
Inflammatory conditions
   Refluxoesophagitis
   Candidiasis
   Herpes
   Crohn's disease
Neoplasms
   Carcinoma – oesophagus, pharynx, cardia
   Leiomyoma
   Sarcoma
Extrinsic compression
   Bronchogenic carcinoma
   Hilar lymphadenopathy
   Retrosternal goitre
   Aortic aneurysm
   Aberrant right subclavicular artery
   Postoperative – Nissen, Angelchik
   Pharyngeal pouch (Zenker's diverticulum)
   Rolling paraoesophageal hiatal hernia

Motility disorders
Achalasia
Chagas' disease
Diffuse oesophageal spasm
Hypertensive LOS
Non-specific motility disorder

Muscle and collagen disorders
Scleroderma
Systemic lupus erythematosus
Dystrophia myotonica

Neurological disorders
Multiple sclerosis
Cerebrovascular accident
Autonomic neuropathy, e.g. diabetes

Rarely, oesophageal tumours may present with bleeding. This may be in the form of occult bleeding producing anaemia, but exceptionally, oeosophageal carcinoma may present with an acute gastrointestinal bleed due to ulceration of the neoplasm, in the absence of dysphagia. In some circumstances, oesophageal tumours may be detected relatively early in these circumstances. Massive bleeding due to erosion of a major vessel is an unusual circumstance, except as a terminal event.

Very occasionally, oesophageal tumours may present by virtue of extension into contiguous organs or by the development of metastases. Hoarseness or respiratory problems may indicate recurrent laryngeal nerve paresis or tracheo-oesophageal fistula. More rarely, metastatic nodes in the neck or hepatic metastases may have their primary origin in an oesophageal tumour, but the vast majority of patients have local manifestations before this stage is reached.

Physical signs are usually few in oesophageal carcinoma, and by the time they develop, the tumour is usually already very advanced. Supraclavicular gland enlargement can occur on either side, and extension of a primary cervical cancer or secondary lymph nodes may result in a palpable mass in the neck. Narrowing or displacement in the trachea may occur, leading to stridor. Tumours or glands in the thoracic inlet or in the mediastinum can cause venous congestion, or even superior vena caval obstruction. Extensive liver metastases may result in hepatomegaly, and advanced distal oesophageal lesions may result in an epigastric mass. Transperitoneal spread may result in ascites, or palpable nodules in the rectovesical or rectovaginal pouch on pelvic examination. Occasionally, blood borne spread may result in skin lesions and metastases in bone, lung and brain.

REFERENCES

1. Clemencon G & Gloor F. Benign epithelial hyperplasia of the esophagus: glycogenic acanthosis. *Endoscopy* 1974; **6:** 214–217.
2. Stern Z, Sharon P, Ligumsky M, Levij IS & Rachmilewitz D. Glycogenic acanthosis of the esophagus. *Am J Gastroenterol* 1980; **74:** 261–263.
3. Rywlin AM & Ortega R. Glycogenic acanthosis of the esophagus. *Arch Pathol* 1970; **90:** 439–443.
4. Lindemann A. Zur pathologie der Menschlichen Osophaguschleimhaut. *Virchow Arch Pathol Anat* 1908; **193:** 258–269.
5. Adler RH, Carberry DM & Ross CA. Papilloma of the oesophagus. *J Thorac Surg* 1959; **37:** 625–635.
6. Colina F, Salis JA & Munoz MT. Squamous papilloma of the esophagus.
7. Fernandez-Rodriguez CM, Badia-Figuerola N, Ruiz del Arbol L, Fernandez-Seara J, Dominguez F & Aviles-Ruiz JF. Squamous papilloma of the oesophagus: report of six cases with long term follow up in four patients. *Am J Gastroenterol* 1986; **81:** 1059–1062.
8. Jarrett WFH, Murphy J, O'Neil BW et al. Virus induced papillomas of the alimentary tract of cattle. *Int J Cancer* 1978; **22:** 323–328.
9. Mounts P & Shah KV. Respiratory papillomatosis: etiological relation to genital tract papilloma viruses. *Prog Med Virol* 1984; **29:** 90–114.
10. Anon. Papillomavirus invades oesophagus: incidence seems to be increasing. *JAMA* 1984; **25:** 2185–2187.
11. Odze R, Antonioli D, Shocket D et al. Esophageal squamous papillomas: a clinicopathologic study of 38 lesions and analysis for human papillomavirus by the polymerase chain reaction. *Am J Surg Pathol* 1993; **17:** 803–812.
12. Dunham L & Sheets R. Effects of oesophageal constriction on benzopyrene carcinogenesis in hamster oesophagus and forestomach. *J Natl Cancer Inst* 1974; **53:** 875–881.
13. Nakamura T, Matsuyama M & Kismimoto M. Tumors of oesophagus and duodenum. Methyl-*N*-nitro-*N*-nitrosoguanidine. *J Natl Cancer Inst* 1974; **52:** 519–522.
14. Paraf F, Flejou JF, Potet F, Molas G & Fekete F. Adenomas arising in Barrett's oesophagus with adenocarcinoma: report of three cases. *Pathol Res Pract* 1992; **188:** 1028–1032.
15. Parkin DM, Pisani P & Ferley J. Estimation of the worldwide incidence of eighteen major cancers in 1985. *Int J Cancer* 1993; **54:** 594–606.
16. Day NE & Varghese C. Oesophageal cancer. *Cancer Surv* 1994; **19/20:** 43–53.
17. Doll R & Peto R. Epidemiology of cancer. In Weatherall DJ, Ledingham JGG & Warrell DA (eds) *Oxford Textbook of Medicine.* Oxford: Oxford Medical Publications, 1987: 4.100.
18. Tuyns AJ. Epidemiology of oesophageal cancer in France. In Pfeiffer CJ (ed.) *Cancer of the Esophagus*, Boca Raton, Florida: CRC Press, 1982: 3–18.
19. Liu BQ & Li B. Epidemiology of carcinoma of the esophagus in China. In Huang GJ & Kai WY (eds) *Carcinoma of the Esophagus, and Gastric Cardia*. New York: Springer, 1984: 1–24.
20. Lu XB, Yang WX, Liu JM, Li YS & Qin YM. Trends in morbidity and mortality for oesophageal cancer in Linxian county. *Int J Cancer* 1985; **36:** 643–645.

21. Enterline H & Thompson J. *Pathology of the Esophagus.* New York; Springer, 1984.

22. Rose EF. Esophageal cancer in Transkei – the pattern and associated risk factors. In Pfeiffer CJ (ed.) *Cancer of the Esophagus,* vol 1, Boca Raton, Florida: CRC Press, 1982: 19–28.

23. Peto R. Epidemiology, multistage models and short term mutangenicity tests. In Hiatt HH, Watson JD & Winsten JA (eds) *Origins of Human Cancer.* Cold Spring Harbor, NY: Cold Spring Harbor Laboratory, 1977: 1403–1428.

24. Burch PRJ. *The Biology of Cancer: a New Approach.* Lancaster; MTP Press, 1976.

25. Paul J. Oncogenes. *J Pathol* 1984; 143: 1–10.

26. Weiss RA & Marshall CJ. Oncogenes. *Lancet* 1984; ii: 1138–1142.

27. Spandidos DA & Anderson MLM. Oncogenes and onco-suppressor genes: their involvement in cancer. *J Pathol* 1989; 157: 1–10.

28. Morris JA. A mutational theory of leukaemogenesis. *J Clin Pathol* 1989; 42: 337–340.

29. Tuyns AJ. Alcohol. In (Schottenfield D & Fraumeni JF (eds) *Cancer Epidemiology and Prevention.* Philadelphia: Saunders, 1982: 293–303.

30. Wynder EL & Bross IJ. A study of etiological factors in cancer of the oesophagus. *Cancer* 1961; 14: 389–413.

31. Pattern LM, Morris LE, Blot WJ, Ziegler RG & Fraumeni JK. Esophageal cancer among black men in Washington DC. 1. Alcohol, tobacco and other risk factors. *J Natl Cancer Inst* 1981; 67: 777–783.

32. Ziegler RG Alcohol nutrient interactions in cancer etiology. *Cancer* 1986; 58: 1942–1948.

33. Hirayana T. Diet and cancer. *Nutr Cancer* 1979; 1: 67–81.

34. Warwick GP & Harrington JS. Some aspects of epidemiology and aetiology of oesophageal cancer with particular emphasis on the Transkei, South Africa. *Adv Cancer Res* 1973; 17: 218–229.

35. Auerbach O, Stout AP, Hammond EC & Garfinkle L. Histologic changes in oesophagus in relation to smoking habits. *Arch Environ Health* 1965; 11: 4–15.

36. Cole J, Green MHL, James SE, Henderson L & Cole H. A further assessment of factors influencing measurements of thioguanine resistant mutant frequency in circulating T lymphocytes. *Mutat Res* 1988; 204: 493–507.

37. Stephens SJ & Uragoda CG. Some observations on oesophageal carcinoma in Ceylon including its relation to betel chewing. *Br J Cancer* 1970; 24: 11–15.

38. Pera M, Cardesa A, Pera C & Mohr U. Nutritional aspects in oesophageal carcinogenesis (review). *Anticancer Res* 1987; 7: 301–308.

39. Yang CHS. Research on oesophageal cancer in China: a review. *Cancer Res* 1980; 40: 2633–2644.

40. Van Rensburg SJ, Bradshaw ES, Bradshaw D & Rose EF. Oesophageal cancer in Zulu men, South Africa. A case control study. *Br J Cancer* 1985; 51: 399–405.

41. Ming Xin Li & Shu Jun Cheng. Etiology of carcinoma of the esophagus. In Huang GJ & K'ai WY (eds) *Carcinoma of the Esophagus and Gastric Cardia.* Berlin: Springer, 1984: 26–47.

42. Burrel RJW, Roach WA & Schadwell A. Esophageal cancer in the Bantu of the Transkei associated with mineral deficiency in garden plants. *J Natl Cancer Inst* 1966; 36: 204–214.

43. Lin HJ, Chan WC & Fong YY. Zinc levels in serum, hair and tumours from patients with oesophageal cancer. *Nutr Rep Int* 1977; 15: 635–643.

44. Fong LYY, Sivak A & Newberne PM. Zinc deficiency and methylbenzylinitrosamine induced esophageal cancer in rats. *J Natl Cancer Inst* 1978; 61: 145–150.

45. Blondell J M. The anticarcinogenic effect of magnesium. *Med Hypotheses* 1980; 6: 863–871.

46. Lijinsky N. Nitrosamines and nitrosamides in the etiology of gastrointestinal cancer. *Cancer* 1977; 40: 2446–2449.

47. Fong YY & Chan WC. Nitrate, nitrite, dimethyl nitrosamine and N-nitrosopyrrolidine in some Chinese food products. *Food Cosmet Toxicol* 1977; 15: 143–145.

48. Fong YY & Chan WC. Dimethylnitrosamine in Chinese marine salt fish. *Food Cosmet Toxicol* 1973; 11: 841–845.

49. Rose EF. The effects of soil and diet on disease. *Cancer Res* 1968; 28: 2390–2392.

50. Mahboubi E & Aramesh B. Epidemiology of esophageal cancer in Iran, with special reference to nutritional and cultural aspects. *Prev Med* 1980; 9: 613–621.

51. Tuyns AJ, Pequinot G & Jensen DM. Role of diet, alcohol and tobacco in esophageal cancer as illustrated by two contrasting high incidence

52. areas in the North of Iran and Western France. *Front Gastrointest Res* 1979; 4: 101–110.

52. Hewer T, Rose E, Chadirian P et al. Ingested mutagens from opium and tobacco pyrolysis products and cancer of the oesophagus. *Lancet* 1978; ii: 494–496.

53. Bonfiglio TA & Stoler MH. Human papillomavirus and cancer of the uterine cervix. *Hum Pathol* 1988; 19: 621–622.

54. Loke SL, Ma L, Womg M, Srivastawa G, Lo I & Bird CC. Human papillomavirus in oesophageal squamous cell carcinoma. *J Clin Pathol* 1990; 43: 909–912.

55. Kiyabu MT, Shibata D, Arnheim N, Martin WJ & Fitzgibbons PL. Detection of human papillomavirus in formalin fixed invasive squamous carcinoma using the polymerase chain reaction. *Am J Surg Pathol* 1989; 13: 221–224.

56. Chen B, Yin H & Dhurandhar N. Detection of human papillomavirus DNA in oesophageal squamous cell carcinomas by the polymerase chain reaction using general consensus primers. *Hum Pathol* 1994; 25: 920–923.

57. Sons HU. Etiologic and epidemiologic factors of carcinoma of the esophagus. *Surg Gynecol Obstet* 1987; 165: 183–189.

58. Plummer HS. Diffuse dilatation of the oesophagus without anatomic stenosis (cardiospasm). A report of ninety one cases. *JAMA* 1912; 58: 2013–2015.

59. Vinson PP. A case of cardiospasm with dilatation and angulation of the esophagus. *Med Clin North Am* 1919; 3: 623–627.

60. Paterson DR. A clinical type of dysphagia. *Br J Laryngol Rhinol Otol* 1919; 24: 289–291.

61. Kelly AB. Spasm of the entrance of the oesophagus. *Br J Laryngol Rhinol Otol* 1919; 34: 285–289.

62. Larson LG, Sandstrom A & Westling P. Relationship of Plummer–Vinson disease to cancer of the upper alimentary tract in Sweden. *Cancer Res* 1975; 35: 3308–3316.

63. Hopkins RA & Roslethwaite RW. Caustic burns and carcinoma of the oesophagus. *Ann Surg* 1981; 194: 146–148.

64. Appelquist P & Salmo M. Lye corrosion carcinoma of the oesophagus. *Cancer* 1980; 45: 2655–2658.

65. Sons HU, Burchard F, Muller-Jah K & Sandmann H. Accelerated tumour induction by distal oesophageal constriction in the rat under the influence of N-ethyl-N-butyl-nitrosamine. *Cancer* 1985; 56: 2617–2621.

66. Adams CWM, Brian RHF & Trounce JR. Ganglion cells in achalasia of the cardia. *Virchows Arch* 1976; 371: 75–79.

67. Tucker JA. Oesophageal diverticula. In Bockus HL (ed.) *Gastroenterology,* 3rd edn. Philadelphia: WB Saunders, 1974: 319–328.

68. Sarks JW. Report of a case of pharyngeal diverticulum containing a neoplasm in its wall. *Br J Radiol* 1933; 6: 233–236.

69. Nanson EM. Carcinoma in a long standing pharyngeal diverticulum. *Br J Surg* 1976; 63: 417–419.

70. Harper PS, Harper RMJ & Howel-Evans AW. Carcinoma of the oesophagus with tylosis. *Q J Med* 1970; 39: 317–333.

71. Ashworth MT, Nash JRG, Ellis A & Day DW. Abnormalities of differentiation and maturation in the oesophageal squamous epithelium of patients with tylosis: morphological features. *Histopathology* 1991; 19: 303–310.

72. Howel-Evans W, McConnel RB, Clarke CA & Sheppard PM. Carcinoma of the oesophagus with keratosis palmaris et plantaris (tylosis). *Q J Med* 1958; 27: 413–417.

73. Hammond MG. HLA and cancer of the oesophagus. In Pfeiffer CJ (ed.) *Cancer of the Esophagus,* vol. 1, Boca Raton, Florida: CRC Press, 1982: 139–148.

74. Miller RW. Cancer epidemics in the People's Republic of China. *J Natl Cancer Inst* 1978; 60: 1195–1203.

75. Li FP & Shiang EL. Screening for oesophageal cancer in 62,000 Chinese. *Lancet* 1979; ii: 804.

76. Guanrei Y & Songliang Q. Endoscopic surveys in high risk and low risk populations for esophagel cancer in China with special reference to precursors of esophageal cancer. *Endoscopy* 1987; 19: 91–95.

77. Buckley CH, Butler EB & Fox H. Cervical intraepithelial neoplasia. *J Clin Pathol* 1982; 35: 1–13.

78. Ming SC. Tumours of the oesophagus and stomach. In *Atlas of Tumor Pathology,* Series 2, Fascide 7 Washington DC: Armed Forces Institute of Pathology, 1973: 30–36.

79. Liu FS & Zhou CN. Pathology of carcinoma of the oesophagus. In Huang GJ & K'ai WY (eds) *Carcinoma of the Oesophagus and Gastric Cardia.* New York: Springer, 1984: 77–116.

80. The American Joint Committee for Cancer Staging and End Results

Reporting: clinical staging system for carcinoma of the esophagus. *Cancer* 1975; **25**: 50.

81. Nishimaki T, Tanaka O, Suzuki T, Aizawa K, Hatakeyama K & Muto T. Patterns of lymphatic spread in thoracic oesophageal cancer. *Cancer* 1994; **74**: 4–11.

82. Christensen WN & Sternberg SS. Adenocarcinoma of the upper oesophagus arising in ectopic gastric mucosa. *Am J Surg Pathol* 1987; **11**: 397–402.

83. Barrett NR. The lower oesophagus lined by columnar epithelium. *Surgery* 1957; **41**: 881–894.

84. Ozello L, Savang M & Roethlisberger B. Columnar mucosa of the distal oesophagus in patients with gastro-oesophageal reflux. *Pathol Annu* 1977; **12**: 11–86.

85. Thompson JJ, Zinsser KR & Enterline HT. Barrett's metaplasia and adenocarcinoma of the oesophagus and gastro-oesophageal junction. *Hum Pathol* 1983; **14**: 42–61.

86. Reid BJ. Barrett's oesophagus and adenocarcinoma. *Annu Rev Med* 1987; **38**: 477–492.

87. Bremner CG, Lynch VP & Ellis FH. Barrett's oesophagus: congenital or acquired? An experimental study of oesophageal mucosal regeneration in the dog. *Surgery* 1970; **68**: 209–216.

88. Hamilton SR & Yardley JH. Regeneration of cardiac type mucosa and acquisition of Barrett mucosa after oesophagogastrectomy. *Gastroenterology* 1977; **72**: 669–675.

89. Meyer W, Vollmar F & Bar W. Barrett oesophagus following total gastrectomy. *Endoscopy* 1979; **2**: 121–126.

90. Sjogren RW & Johnson LF. Barrett's oesophagus: a review. *Am J Med* 1983; **74**: 313–321.

91. Thomspon JJ. Oesophageal cancer and the premalignant changes of oesophageal disease. In Cohen S & Soloway RD (eds) *Disease of the Oesophagus*. New York, London: Churchill Livingstone, 1982: 239–276.

92. Barrie J & Goldwater L. Columnar cell lined oesophagus: assessment of etiology and treatment. *J Thorac Cardiovasc Surg* 1976; **71**: 825–834.

93. Naef AP & Ozello L. Columnar lined lower oesophagus: an acquired lesion with malignant predisposition. *J Thorac Cardiovasc Surg* 1975; **70**: 826–835.

94. de Nard FG & Riddell RH. The normal oesophagus. *Am J Surg Pathol* 1991; **15**: 296–309.

95. Bucahn AMJ, Granst S & Freeman HJ. Regulatory peptides in Barrett's oesophagus. *J Pathol* 1985; **146**: 227–234.

96. Griffin M & Sweeney EC. The relationship of endocrine cells, dysplasia and carcinoembryonic antigen in Barrett's mucosa to adenocarcinoma of the oesophagus. *Histopathology* 1987; **11**: 53–62.

97. Belladonna JA, Hajdu SI, Bains MS & Winawer SJ. Adenocarcinoma in situ of Barrett's oesophagus diagnosed by exfoliative cytology. *N Engl J Med* 1974; **291**: 895–896.

98. Haggitt RC, Tryzelaar J, Ellis FH & Cocker H. Adenocarcinoma complicating columnar epithelium lined (Barrett's) oesophagus. *Am J Clin Pathol* 1978; **70**: 1–5.

99. Berenson MM, Ridell RH, Skinner DB & Freston JW. Malignant transformation of oesophageal columnar epithelium. *Cancer* 1978; **41**: 554–561.

100. Webb JN & Busuttil A. Adenocarcinoma of the oesophagus and of the oesophagogastric junction. *Br J Surg* 1978; **65**: 475–479.

101. Hamilton SR, Smith RL & Cameron JL. Prevalence and characteristics of Barrett's oesophagus in patients with adenocarcinoma of the oesophagus or oesophagogastric junction. *Hum Pathol* 1988; **19**: 942–948.

102. Roger EL, Goldkind SF, Iseri OA et al. Adenocarcinoma of the lower oesophagus. *J Clin Gastroenterol* 1986; **8**: 613–618.

103. Macdonald WC & MacDonald JB. Adenocarcinoma of the oesophagus and or gastric cardia. *Cancer* 1987; **60**: 1094–1098.

104. Hesketh PJ, Clapp RW, Doos WG & Spechler SJ. The increasing frequency of adenocarcinoma of the esophagus. *Cancer* 1989; **64**: 526–530.

105. Atkinson M. Barrett's oesophagus – to screen or not to screen. *Gut* 1989; **30**: 2–5.

106. Hamilton SR & Smith RRL. The relationship between columnar epithelial dysplasia and invasive adenocarcinoma arising in Barrett's oesophagus. *Am J Clin Pathol* 1987; **87**: 301–312.

107. Reid BJ, Haggitt RC, Rubin CE et al. Observer variation in the diagnosis of dysplasia in Barrett's oesophagus. *Hum Pathol* 1988; **19**: 166–178.

108. Quirke P & Dyson JED. Flow cytometry: methodology and applications in pathology. *J Pathol* 1986; **149**: 79–87.

109. Reid BJ, Haggitt RC, Rubin CE & Rabinovitch PS. Barrett's oesophagus: correlation between flow cytometry and histology in detection of patients at risk for adenocarcinoma. *Gastroenterology* 1987; **93**: 1–11.

110. Haggitt RC, Reid BJ, Rabinovitch PS & Rubin CE. Barrett's oesophagus: correlation between mucin histochemistry, flow cytometry and histologic diagnosis for predicting increased cancer risk. *Am J Pathol* 1988; **131**: 53–61.

111. Reid BJ, Blount PL, Rubin CE, Levine DS, Haggitt RC & Rabinovitch PS. Flow cytometric and histological progession to malignancy in Barrett's esophagus: prospective endoscopic surveillance of a cohort. *Gastroenterology* 1992; **102**: 1212–1219.

112. Reid BJ, Sanchez CA, Blount PL & Levine DS. Barrett's oesophagus: cell cycle abnormalities in advancing stages of neoplastic progression. *Gastroenterology* 1993; **105**: 119–129.

113. Levone DS. Barrett's oesophagus and p53. *Lancet* 1994; **344**: 212–213.

114. Younes M, Leboutz RM, Lechago LV & Lechago J. p53 protein accumulation in Barrett's metaplasia, dysplasia and carcinoma: a follow up study. *Gastroenterology* 1993; **105**: 1637–1642.

115. Gray MR, Hall PA, Nash J, Ansari B, Lane DP & Kingsworth AW. Epithelial cell proliferation in Barrett's oesophagus by proliferating cell nuclear antigen immunolocalisation. *Gastroenterology* 1992; **103**: 1769–1776.

116. Krishnadath KK, Tilanus HW, Blankenstein MV et al. Reduced expression of the Cadherin-catenin complex in oesophageal adenocarcinoma correlates with poor prognosis. *J Pathol* 1997; **182**: 331–338.

117. Castella E, Ariza A, Fernandez-Vasalo A, Roca X, Ojanguren I. Expression of CD44H and CD44v3 in normal oesophagus, Barrett mucosa and oesophageal carcinoma. *J Clin Pathol* 1996; **49**: 489–492.

118. Editorial. Endoscopic surveillance for patients with Barrett's oesophagus: does the cancer risk justify the practice? *Ann Intern Med* 1987; **106**: 902–904.

119. Iftikhar SY, James PD, Steele RJ, Hardcastle JD & Atkinson M. Length of Barrett's oesophagus: an important factor in the development of dysplasia and adenocarcinoma. *Gut* 1992; **33**: 1155–1158.

120. Lane N. Pseudosarcoma (polypoid like masses) associated with squamous cell carcinoma of the mouth, fauces and larynx. *Cancer* 1957; **10**: 19–41.

121. Leifer C, Miller AS, Putong PB & Min BH. Spindle cell carcinoma of the oral mucosa. A light and electron microscopic study of apparent sarcomatous metastasis to cervical lymph nodes. *Cancer* 1974; **34**: 597–605.

122. Lichtinger BG, Mackay B & Tessmer CF. Spindle cell variant of squamous carcinoma. A light and electron microscopic study of 13 cases. *Cancer* 1970; **26**: 1311–1320.

123. Battifora H. Spindle cell carcinoma: ultrastructural evidence of squamous origin and collagen production by tumour cells. *Cancer* 1976; **37**: 2275–2282.

124. Osamura RY, Watanabe K, Shimamura K et al. Polypoid carcinoma of the oesophagus: a unifying term for carcinomsarcoma and pseudosarcoma. *Am J Surg Pathol* 1978; **2**: 201–208.

125. Borg-Grech A, Morris JA & Eyden BP. Malignant osteoclastoma-like giant cell tumour of the renal pelvis. *Histopathology* 1987; **11**: 415–425.

126. Holtz F, Fox JE & Abell MR. Carcinosarcoma of the urinary bladder. *Cancer* 1972; **29**: 294–304.

127. Hinderlieder CO, Aguam AS & Wilder JR. Carcinosarcoma of the oesophagus: a case report and review of the literature. *Int Surg* 1979; **64**: 13–19.

128. Du Boulay CEH & Isaacson P. Carcinoma of the oesophagus with spindle cell features. *Histopathology* 1981; **5**: 403–414.

129. Linder J, Stein RB, Roggli VL et al. Polypoid tumour of the oesophagus. *Hum Pathol* 1987; **18**: 692–700.

130. Guarino M, Reale D, Micoli G & Forlini B. Carcinosarcoma of the oesophagus with rhabdomyoblastic differentiation. *Histopathology* 1993; **22**: 493–498.

131. McCort JJ. Oesophageal carcinosarcomas and pseudosarcomas. *Radiology* 1972; **102**: 519–524.

132. Harris M. Spindle cell squamous carcinoma: ultrastructural observations. *Histopathology* 1982; **6**: 197–210.

133. Ackerman LV. Verrucous carcinoma of the oral cavity. *Surgery* 1948; **23**: 670–678.

134. Agha FP, Watherbee L & Sams JS, Verrucous carcinoma of the oesophagus. *Am J Gastroenterol* 1984; **79**: 844–849.

135. Barbier PA, Luder PJ, Wagner HE et al. Verrucous acanthosis – so called verrucous carcinoma of the oesophagus. *Z Gastroenterol* 1987; **25**: 93–97.

136. Jasin KA & Bateson MC. Verrucous carcinoma of the oesophagus – a diagnostic problem. *Histopathology* 1990; **16**: 473–475.
137. Kraus FT & Perez-Mesa C. Verrucous carcinoma. Clinical and pathological study of 105 cases involving oral cavity, larynx and genitalia. *Cancer* 1966; **19**: 26–38.
138. Perez CA, Kraus FT, Evans JC et al. Anaplastic transformation in verrucous carcinoma of the oral cavity after radiation therapy. *Radiology* 1966; **86**: 108–115.
139. McKeown F. Oat cell carcinoma of the oesophagus. *J Pathol Bacteriol* 1952; **64**: 889–891.
140. Briggs JC & Ibrahim NBN. Oat cell carcinoma of the oesophagus: a clinico-pathological study of 23 cases. *Histopathology* 1983; **7**: 261–277.
141. Turnbull AD, Rosen P, Goodner JT & Beattie EJ. Primary malignant tumours of the oesophagus other than typical epidermoid carcinoma. *Ann Thorac Surg* 1973; **15**: 463–473.
142. Matsusaka T, Watanabe H & Enjoji M. Anaplastic carcinoma of the oesophagus. Report of three cases and their histogenetic consideration. *Cancer* 1976; **37**: 1352–1358.
143. Tateishi R, Taniguchi K, Horai T et al. Argyrophil cell carcinoma (apudoma) of the oesophagus. A histopathologic entity. *Virchows Arch [A]* 1976; **371**: 183–294.
144. Cook MG, Eusebi V & Betts CM. Oat cell carcinoma of the oesophagus: a recently recognised entity. *J Clin Pathol* 1976; **29**: 1068–1073.
145. Imai T, Sannohe Y & Okano H. Oat cell carcinoma (apudoma) of the oesophagus. *Cancer* 1978; **41**: 358–364.
146. Reid HAS, Richardson WW & Corrin B. Oat cell carcinoma of the oesophagus. *Cancer* 1980; **45**: 2342–2347.
147. Reyes CV, Wellington J & Gould VE. Neuroendocrine carcinoma of the oesophagus. *Ultrastruct Pathol* 1980; **1**: 367–376.
148. Gould VE. Neuroendocrinomas and neuroendocrine carcinomas. APUD cell system neoplasms and their aberrant secretory activities. *Pathol Annu* 1977; **12**: 33.
149. Heimann R, Dehou MF, Lentrebecq B et al. Anaplastic small cell (oat cell) carcinoma of the tonsils. Report of two cases. *Histopathology* 1989; **14**: 67–74.
150. Tateishi R, Taniguchi H, Wada A et al. Argyrophil cells and melanocytes in oesophageal mucosa. *Arch Pathol* 1974; **98**: 87–89.
151. Bensch KG, Corrin B, Pariente R & Spencer H. Oat cell carcinoma of the lung – its origin and relationship to bronchial carcinoid. *Cancer* 1968; **22**: 1163–1172.
152. Beardsmore GL, Davies MC, McLeod R et al. Malignant melanoma in Queensland: a study of 219 deaths. *Aust J Dermatol* 1969; **10**: 158–168.
153. Das Gupta TK & Brusfield RD. Metastatic melanoma of the gastrointestinal tract. *Arch Surg* 1964; **88**: 969–973.
154. Kreuser ED. Primary malignant melanoma of the oesophagus. *Virchows Arch [A]* 1979; **385**: 49–59.
155. Takubo K, Kanda Y, Ishii M et al. Primary malignant melanoma of the oesophagus. *Hum Pathol* 1983; **14**: 727–730.
156. de Mik JI, Kooijman CD, Hoekstra JBL & Tytgat GNJ. Primary malignant melanoma of the oesophagus. *Histopathology* 1992; **20**: 77–79.
157. De La Pava S, Nigogosyan G, Pickren JW et al. Melanosis of the oesophagus. *Cancer* 1963; **16**: 48–50.
158. Ohashi K, Kato Y, Kanno J & Kasuga T. Melanocytes and melanosis of the oesophagus in Japanese subjects – analysis of factors affecting their increase. *Virchows Arch [A]* 1990; **417**: 137–143.
159. Piccone VA, Klopstock R, Le Veen HH et al. Primary malignant melanoma of the oesophagus associated with melanosis of the entire oesophagus. *J Thorac Cardiovasc Surg* 1970; **59**: 864–870.
160. Di Costanzo DP & Urmacher C. Primary malignant melanoma of the oesophagus. *Am J Surg Pathol* 1987; **11**: 46–52.
161. Akamatsu T, Honda T, Nakayana J et al. Primary adenoid cystic carcinoma of the oesophagus. *Acta Pathol Jpn* 1986; **36**: 1707–1717.
162. Azzopardi JG & Smith OD. Salivary gland tumour and their mucins. *J Pathol Bacteriol* 1959; **77**: 131–140.
163. Sweeney EC & Cooney T. Adenoid cystic carcinoma of the oesophagus. A light and electron microscopic study. *Cancer* 1980; **45**: 1516–1522.
164. Osamura RY, Sato S, Miwa M et al. Mucoepidermoid carcinoma of the oesophagus. Report of an unoperated autopsy case and review of the literature. *Am J Gastroenterol* 1978; **69**: 467–470.
165. Woodward BH, Shelburn JD, Vollmer RT et al. Mucoepidermoid carcinoma of the oesophagus: a case report. *Hum Pathol* 1978; **9**: 352–354.
166. Toreso WE. Secondary carcinoma as a cause of dysphagia. *Arch Pathol* 1944; **38**: 82–84.
167. Abrams HL, Spiro R & Goldstein N. Metastases in carcinoma. Analysis of 1000 autopsy cases. *Cancer* 1950; **3**: 74–85.
168. Fisher MS. Metastases to the oesophagus. *Gastrointest Radiol* 1976; **1**: 249–251.
169. Garusi G & Conati E. Carcinoma metastatico cell esofago. *Fracastero* 1969; **52**: 117–138.
170. Anderson MF & Harell GS. Secondary oesophageal tumors. *AJR* 1980; **135**: 1243–1246.
171. Holyoke ED, Nemota T & Dao TL. Oesophageal metastases and dysphagia in patients with carcinoma of the breast. *J Surg Oncol* 1979; **1**: 97–107.
172. Takubo K, Nakagawa H, Tsuchiya S et al. Seedling leiomyoma of the oesophagus and oesophagogastric junction zone. *Hum Pathol* 1981; **12**: 1006–1010.
173. Serenetis MG, Lyond WS, DeGuzman VC et al. Leiomyomata of the oesophagus. *Cancer* 1976; **38**: 2166–2177.
174. Kramer MD, Gibb P & Ellis FH. Giant leiomyoma of the oesophagus. *J Surg Oncol* 1986; **33**: 166–169.
175. Tsuzuki T, Kakegawa T, Arimori M et al. Giant leiomyoma of the oesophagus and cardia weighing more than 1,000 gms. *Chest* 1971; **60**: 396–399.
176. Bozorgi S, Migliorelli F & Cook WA. Leiomyomas of the oesophagus presenting as a bleeding epiphrenic diverticulum. *Chest* 1973; **63**: 281–284.
177. Gothlin J, Block R & Sundgren R. Intraphrenic oesophageal leiomyoma associated with diverticula. Pre-operative diagnosis by angiography. *Acta Radiol Scand* 1975; **16**: 673–678.
178. Hodge GB. Oesophageal leiomyoma associated with epiphrenic diverticulum and hiatus hernia. *Am J Surg* 1970; **36**: 538–543.
179. Ullal SR. Hypertrophic osteoarthropathy and leiomyoma of the oesophagus. *Am J Surg* 1972; **123**: 356–358.
180. Heald J, Moussalli H & Hasleton PS. Diffuse leiomyomatosis of the oesophagus. *Histopathology* 1986; **10**: 755–759.
181. Fernandes JP, Mascarenhas MJ, da Costa JD et al. Diffuse leiomyomatosis of the oesophagus – a case report and review of the literature. *Am J Dig Dis* 1975; **20**: 684–690.
182. Wahlen J, Astedt B. Familial occurrence of co-existing leiomyomas of vulva and oesophagus. *Acta Obstet Gynecol Scand* 1965; **44**: 197–203.
183. Schapiro RL & Sandrock AR. Oesophagogastric and vulvar leiomyomatosis. A new radiologic syndrome. *J Can Assoc Radiol* 1973; **24**: 184–187.
184. Lonsdale RN, Roberts PF, Vaughan RV & Thiru S. Familial oesophageal leiomyomatosis and nephropathy. *Histopathology* 1992; **20**: 127–133.
185. Rainer WG & Brus R. Leiomyosarcoma of the oesophagus. Review of the literature and report of 3 cases. *Surgery* 1965; **58**: 343–350.
186. Tolten RS, Stout AP, Humphries GH et al. Benign tumours and cysts of the oesophagus. *J Thorac Surg* 1953; **25**: 606–622.
187. Jang GC, Clouse ME & Fleischer FG. Fibrovascular polyp – a benign intraluminal tumour of the oesophagus. *Radiology* 1969; **92**: 1196–2000.
188. Nora AF. Lipoma of the oesophagus. *Am J Surg* 1964; **108**: 353–356.
189. LiVolsi VA & Perzi KH. Inflammatory pseudotumours (inflammatory fibrous polyps) of the oesophagus. A clinicopathologic study. *Am J Dig Dis* 1975; **20**: 475–481.
190. Rabin MS, Bremner CG & Botha JR. The reflux gastro-oesophageal polyp. *Am J Gastroenterol* 1980; **73**: 451–453.
191. Branski D, Gardner RV, Risher JE et al. Gastro-oesophageal polyp as a cause of haematemesis in adolescence. *Am J Gastroenterol* 1980; **73**: 448–450.
192. Johnston J & Helwig FB. Granular cell tumours of the gastrointestinal tract and perianal region. *Dig Dis Sci* 1981; **26**: 807–816.
193. Coutinho DS, de Soga J, Yoshikaura T et al. Granular cell tumours of the oesophagus: a report of two cases and review of the literature. *Am J Gastroenterol* 1985; **80**: 758–762.
194. Aparicio SR & Lumsden CE. Ligh and electron-microscopic studies on the granular cell myoblastoma of the tongue. *J Pathol* 1969; **97**: 339–355.
195. Stefansson K & Wollmann RL. S-100 protein in granular cell tumours (granular cell myoblastoma). *Cancer* 1982; **49**: 1934–1938.
196. Ohmori T, Anta N, Urago N et al. Malignant granular cell tumour of the oesophagus. *Acta Pathol Jpn* 1987; **37**: 775–783.
197. Vartio T, Nickels J, Hockerstedt K. Rhabdomyosarcoma of the oesophagus. *Virchows Arch [A]* 1980; **386**: 357–361.
198. Mahow GA & Hamsum EG. Osteochondroma (tracheobronchial choristoma) of the oesophagus. *Cancer* 1967; **20**: 1489–1493.
199. McIntyre M, Webb JN & Browning GCP. Osteosarcoma of the oesophagus. *Hum Pathol* 1982; **13**: 680–682.

200. Gentry RW, Dockerty MB & Clagett OT. Vascular malformations and vascular tumours of the gastrointestinal tract. *Int Abs Surg* 1949; **88:** 281–323.

201. Hariel K, Tally NA & Hunt DR. Haemangioma of the oesophagus: an unusual cause of upper gastrointestinal bleeding. *Dig Dis Sci* 1981; **26:** 257–263.

202. Armengal-Miro JR, Ramental F, Salford J et al. Lymphangioma of the oesophagus. *Endoscopy* 1979; **3:** 185–189.

203. Brady PG & Milligan FD. Lymphangioma of the oesophagus. Diagnosis by endoscopic biopsy. *Dig Dis Sci* 1973; **18:** 423–425.

204. Siegal JH, Janis R, Alper JC et al. Disseminated visceral Kaposi's sarcoma – appearance after human renal allograft operation. *JAMA* 1969; **207:** 1493–1496.

205. Umerh BC. Kaposis sarcoma of the oesophagus. *Br J Radiol* 1980; **53:** 807–808.

206. Ribelin WE & Bailey WS. Oesophageal sarcoma associated with *Spirocerca lupi* infection in the dog. *Cancer* 1958; **11:** 1242.

207. Stein H, Murray D & Warner HA. Primary Hodgkins of the oesophagus. *Dig Dis Sci* 1981; **26:** 457–461.

208. Bemar MD, Falchuk KR, Trey C et al. Primary histiocytic lymphoma of the oesophagus. *Dig Dis Sci* 1979; **24:** 883–886.

209. Ahmed N, Ramos S, Sika J et al. Primary extramedullary oesophageal plasmacytoma: first case report. *Cancer* 1976; **38:** 943–947.

210. Ehrlich AN, Stalder G, Geller W et al. Gastrointestinal manifestations of malignant lymphoma. *Gastroenterology* 1968; **54:** 1115–1121.

211. Watson A. A study of the quality and duration of survival following resection, endoscopic intubation and surgical intubation in oesophageal carcinoma. *Br J Surg* 1982; **69:** 585–588.

212. Earlam R & Cunha-Melo JR. Oesophageal squamous cell carcinoma. 1. A critical review of surgery. *Br J Surg* 1980; **67:** 381–390.

213. Edwards DAW & Lobello R. Site of referral of the sense of obstruction to swallowing. *Gut* 1982; **23:** 435.

214. Watson A. Carcinoma of the oesophagus. In McArdle CS (ed.) *Surgical Oncology.* London: Butterworths, 1990; 1–27.

14

SURGICAL MANAGEMENT OF CARCINOMA OF THE OESOPHAGUS

A Watson

HISTORICAL ASPECTS OF RESECTION FOR CARCINOMA OF THE OESOPHAGUS

In 1871, Theodore Billroth discussed the possibility of resection of a carcinoma of the oesophagus, and performed a successful cervical resection and anastomosis in dogs. It was not until six years later, in 1877, that Czerny performed the first successful resection of a carcinoma of the cervical oesophagus in a patient. Anastomosis was not performed, however, the proximal and distal ends being brought out as cervical oesophagostomies, the excision therefore being very localized, although the patient lived for 15 months. In 1886, Mikulicz made the first attempt to resect an intrathoracic oesophageal carcinoma by the extrapleural route. This, and many other attempts over the next 25 years, were unsuccessful in that there were no survivors, although Mikulicz did sucessfully resect a cervical oesophageal carcinoma with reconstruction using skin flaps. It was not until 1913 that Torek in New York performed the first successful open resection of an intrathoracic oesophageal carcinoma through a left thoracotomy. The proximal and distal ends were brought out as a cervical oesophagostomy and gastrostomy, with a view to subsequent reconstructive surgery. However, the patient declined this procedure, and the two stomas were connected by a rubber tube, with which the patient survived for the next 13 years. The same year, Denk performed the first blunt transhiatal oesophagectomy through abdominal and cervical incisions, once more bringing the cervical oesophagus and stomach to the surface. In 1933, Grey-Turner revived interest in blunt transhiatal oesophagectomy, but it was not until 1938 that Adams and Phemister performed the first successful transthoracic resection with anastomosis in America.

Once it had been shown that transthoracic resection with anastomosis was feasible, attention was turned to achieving as much longitudinal clearance as possible, and landmark descriptions of the two-phase procedure of laparotomy and right thoracotomy were made by Ivor Lewis in 1946 and Tanner in 1947. A third cervical phase was added by Ong in 1969 and McKeown in 1972. This latter approach resulted in a resurgence of interest in blunt transhiatal resection with a cervical oesophagogastric anastomosis, by Kirk in 1974 and Orringer in 1978. An attempt to achieve even greater radicality in resection was the 'radical en-bloc' procedure described by Skinner in 1983, involving excision of the whole intrathoracic oesophagus, both pleural surfaces, the pericardium and azygos vein, with re-establishment of continuity by a colon interposition. The early 1990s have seen the advocation of extensive mediastinal and bilateral cervical nodal dissections by Japanese workers and thoracoscopic mobilization of the intrathoracic oesophagus. Hopefully the place of these techniques will be defined as a result of prospective randomized studies.

INDICATIONS FOR RESECTIONAL SURGERY

Radical resection is the only treatment modality which has been repeatedly associated with long survival in the literature, and, with or without adjuvant therapy, must be considered the treatment of choice in a relatively fit patient with a relatively localized tumour. As oesophageal tumours tend to present relatively late in the Western world, and the majority occur in patients over the age of 60, against a long background of tobacco and alcohol abuse, careful tumour staging and patient assessment is necessary before a rational decision on the most optimal therapy can be taken. Obvious contraindications to radical resection are advanced age, serious intercurrent disease, a tumour which has metastasized to viscera or distant lymph nodes such as the axillary group, or advanced local infiltration such as involvement of contiguous structures including the bronchi, great vessels or recurrent laryngeal nerve.

In a series of 396 patients with oesophageal carcinoma

referred from a well-defined catchment population of high incidence to a single unit for assessment, 82 patients were felt to be inappropriate for resectional surgery on account of advanced age, infirmity or severe intercurrent disease. A further 153 patients (38%) were considered to be unsuitable for resection on the basis of disseminated metastases or locally advanced disease. This left only 164 patients (41%) who satisfied the criteria for an attempt at curative resection.[1] This emphasizes the importance of tumour staging and pretreatment patient assessment.

Tumour staging

The principal aims of tumour staging are to identify the presence of metastatic disease and the extent of local tumour invasion. The desirability of staging oesophageal tumours as accurately as possible before embarking on a decision to identify the optimal therapeutic approach was illustrated by the large, historical review by Earlam and Cunha-Melo, which showed that one third of patients in accrued published series between 1953 and 1979, underwent needless surgical exploration, only to find the tumour was too advanced or too widespread to warrant any therapeutic procedure.[2] With the current availability of several endoscopic modalities for palliation of such patients, it is of paramount importance that surgical exploration is reserved for those patients with a high likelihood of undergoing resection. Furthermore, some workers believe that there is a place for treating patients with locally advanced disease with chemotherapy and/or radiotherapy in order to render them operable,[3] although results of prospective randomized studies to support such an approach are not, as yet, available.

Of the several staging systems available, the two most frequently used in oesophageal cancer are the TNM classification as used for tumours in other sites and the simpler clinical-diagnostic system (Table 14.1). The latter system is commonly used in clinical decision making, as a general rule Stages I and II representing relatively localized disease in which surgical resection should be undertaken with a possibility of cure, and Stages III and IV generally representing incurable disease in which surgery is best avoided. The TNM system is, however, much more precise and enables communication at an international level between research groups wishing to correlate tumour stage with patient outcome for various therapeutic strategies.

There are several investigations which have been used to help stage oesophageal cancers, ranging from the simple to the highly sophisticated.

Chest radiography

Although most clinicians would perform a chest radiograph relatively early in the investigation of patients with oesophageal carcinoma, it can only reveal gross abnormalities and those which can be detected by other means. Pulmonary metastases may be visible on chest radiograph, and pleural ones inferred by the presence of pleural effusion. Severe inflammatory changes or consolidation may suggest the possibility of a

Table 14.1 TNM and clinical-diagnostic staging classification for oesophageal tumours

Primary tumour (T)

T0	No evidence of primary tumour
T1S	Carcinoma in situ
T1	Tumour invades lamina propria or submucosa
T2	Tumour invades muscularis propria
T3	Tumour invades adventitia
T4	Tumour invades adjacent structures

Regional lymph nodes (N)

N0	No regional lymph node metastasis
N1	Local (paraoesophageal) node metastasis
N2	More extensive node metastasis, e.g. subcarinal, tracheobronchial
N3	Distant node metastasis (e.g. coeliac for proximal lesions; cervical for distal lesions)

Distant metastases (M)

M0	No distant metastases
M1	Distant metastases present

clinical, diagnostic-classification

Stage I	T1, N0, M0
Stage II	T1, N1–2, M0 or T2, N0–2, M0
Stage III	T2, any N, M0 or any T, N3, M0
Stage IV	Any T, any N, M1

respiratory fistula and a large hilar shadow may suggest extensive nodal metastases.

Barium swallow

It is generally considered wise practice to perform a barium swallow prior to endoscopy in patients with dysphagia to obtain a working 'road map', which may be helpful in identifying a pharyngeal pouch, if present, and in the case of strictures which may prove impassable at endoscopy, in giving information about the length of the lesion and the presence or absence of pathology downstream from the obstructing lesion. From the standpoint of staging, a barium swallow may identify a respiratory fistula. Otherwise, the staging information obtained by barium swallow is relatively crude and indirect, being related to tumour length and axis deviation.

Barium swallow gives a fairly accurate indication of macroscopic tumour length, which has an indirect, although imperfect correlation with tumour staging. Rosenberg et al.[4] showed that 40% of tumours 5 cm or less in length were localized to the oesophagus, although 25% extended beyond the oesophagus and 35% were unresectable or had distant metastases. For tumours longer than 5 cm, 37% were localized to the oesophageal wall, 15% extended beyond the oesophagus and 75% were unresectable or had distant metastases. In a series of 241 resected patients reported by Postlethwait[5] a curative resection was feasible in almost 50% of patients with tumours 4 cm or less in length, whereas this rate fell to around 8% for tumours longer than 8 cm, largely because of lateral extension into contiguous structures. With regard to survival, Huang[6] found in a series of 976 patients with an overall five-year survival rate of 30.3%, that the 8% of patients with tumours less than 3 cm in length had a five-year survival rate of 43.3%

compared to the 92% of patients with tumours longer than 3 cm, in whom the corresponding figure was 28.9%. In our own series,[7] five-year survival only occurred in tumours less than 6 cm in length, although survival between one and two years occurred in some patients with tumours of 8–10 cm in length. In two multivariate analyses, tumour length itself did not correlate with survival, although greater tumour length was more frequently associated with greater depth of invasion and nodal involvement.[3,8]

Deviation of the long axis of the oesophagus either in the anteroposterior or lateral plane as shown on barium swallow is frequently associated with advanced disease. In a series reported by Akiyama et al.[9] 74% of patients who could not be completely resected had evidence of axis deviation. However, 26% had a normal axis, and 10% of patients who were totally resected had axis deviation. Similar results were reported from a series by Mori et al.[10] who reported that 19% of patients with lesions limited to the wall had positive axis deviation. Thus, like tumour length, axis deviation has some relationship to tumour staging, but this is insufficiently accurate in itself to use as a basis for determining operability.

Endoscopy

Upper gastrointestinal endoscopy should be performed in all patients in whom a diagnosis of oesophageal cancer is suspected, and indeed in all patients with dysphagia. The principal advantage is to enable a positive tissue diagnosis to be made, and indeed the cell type to be identified, which may influence the therapeutic strategy employed. It is important to take multiple biopsies from the lumen of the tumour as well as the proximal margin, but 5–10% of tumours will be impassable by the endoscope, although this proportion may be reduced by dilatation. Particularly in such cases, brush cytology should be employed, passing a retractable brush in a polythene sheath through the biopsy channel of the endoscope. The combination of brush cytology with punch biopsy leads to an accurate diagnosis in over 90% of cases.[11] With regard to assessment of operability, endoscopy has similar limitations to barium swallow, in that tumour length, axis deviation and obstructing lesions do not correlate totally with operability. As with barium swallow, the site of a respiratory fistula may be visible, although endoscopy may be more reliable than barium swallow in detecting distant satellite deposits or unsuspected metachronous primary tumours, which occur in 6% of cases.[12]

Computed tomographic scanning

Computed tomographic (CT) scanning is able to provide information relating to the primary tumour, the regional lymph nodes and the presence of distant metastases, predominantly in the lungs and liver.

With regard to the primary tumour, it can be seen on the CT scan as a thickening of the oesophageal wall, which is initially eccentric and becoming circumferential with advanced lesions. Although this information is obviously not very different from that obtained by barium studies or endoscopy, it is the detection of extraoesophageal extension of the tumour which gives CT scanning a definite advantage. The early stages of extraoesophageal spread are seen as blurring of the normally well-defined outer oesophageal wall, progressing to obvious extension of the tumour mass beyond the confines of the oesophagus and ultimately to encroachment of the tumour mass onto contiguous structures, particularly the tracheobronchial tree and the thoracic aorta.

The demonstration of extraoesophageal spread of tumours depends on blurring or obliteration of the fat planes between the oesophagus and contiguous structures, but as these fat planes are often lost in cachectic patients, reliability becomes diminished as the disease becomes advanced. Consequently, the mere appearance of proximity between the tumour and surrounding structures does not necessarily imply invasion, and by the same token, lesser degrees of invasion may be undetected on CT scanning. For this reason, the overall accuracy of staging of the primary tumour by CT is approximately 60%.[13]

Once invasion of contiguous structures is sufficiently advanced to produce certain characteristic features, accuracy increases considerably. Significant tracheobronchial invasion results in indentation or bowing inwards of the posterior wall of the trachea or a main bronchus, and in these circumstances, the sensitivity of CT scanning in the detection of tracheobronchial invasion is 98% and specificity 95%.[14] With regard to aortic invasion, contact between the tumour and the aortic wall over an arc greater than 90° predicts invasion with an accuracy of around 80%.[14] However, an arc of contact of 45° or less is considered normal, and between 45° and 90°, indeterminate. Because of this, and the fact that CT scanning is unable to distinguish between neoplastic and inflammatory adherence, the latter being important in determining resectability, the overall accuracy of CT scanning in determining aortic invasion falls to about 55%.[15] Although relatively uncommon, extensive transmediastinal spread denotes absolute unresectability, and in this situation, the accuracy of CT scanning is much greater, exceeding 90%.[16]

Although CT scanning is frequently used in an attempt to determine lymph node involvement, its accuracy is somewhat limited in this regard. First, the resolution is such that nodes less than 1 cm in diameter cannot be reliably detected, and metastatic nodes may certainly be smaller than this. Secondly, CT scanning is unable to distinguish reliably between enlarged metastatic nodes and those which are the seat of reactive hyperplasia.[17] As a consequence, the accuracy of CT scanning in the detection of nodal metastases is low at around 50%.[13,18]

With regard to detection of metastatic disease, oesophageal tumours metastasize most frequently to liver (32%) and lungs (21%), and a search for metastases may generally be restricted to these organs. CT scanning is currently the most accurate modality in detecting metastatic disease in both these organs, accuracy being of the order of 95%.[14]

Magnetic resonance imaging

The need for greater accuracy than can be provided by CT scanning has led to the evaluation of magnetic resonance imaging (MRI) as a staging modality. However, it is generally believed that the additional expense does not produce any improvement in accuracy over that of CT scanning[19,20] which has restricted its value in clinical decision making.

Ultrasonography

Both transcutaneous and endoluminal ultrasonography have been used to help stage oesophageal tumours. Transcutaneous ultrasonography is almost as accurate as CT scanning in the detection of liver metastases but as most units now perform routine CT scans, its use in this context has diminished. Transcutaneous ultrasonography has also been used in the evaluation of cervical node metastases, in which its accuracy is at least as good as CT scanning, and considerably greater when combined with ultrasound-guided fine needle aspiration biopsy.[21] Such information is currently sought only in selected centres where it is felt that nodal status may influence a decision to perform a three-field lymphadenectomy or to precede surgery with chemoradiation (see later).

Endoluminal ultrasonography has attracted considerable attention in recent years as a much more accurate staging modality than CT scanning or MRI. The most widely used systems comprise a rotating ultrasonic transducer built into the tip of a dedicated endoscope, the transducer scanning a field of 360° at at a frequency of 7.5–12 mHz. The ability to scan in close proximity to the oesophageal wall, gland fields and contiguous structures confers considerable advantages over alternative staging modalities, in that the individual layers of the oesophageal wall are clearly discernible, and the detailed resolution of lymph nodes frequently enables a distinction to be made between normal and metastatic nodes on the basis of the echogenic pattern of the node. Disadvantages include the capital costs of the equipment and the size and rigidity of the probe preventing passage in a proportion of stenotic lesions.

There are now many comparative studies which report significantly greater accuracy of endoluminal ultrasonography (EUS) over CT scanning[24] (Table 14.2) in staging of the primary tumour. The overall accuracy of EUS is around 90%, compared to 60% for CT scanning. Corresponding figures for nodal involvement are approximately 75% for EUS and 50% for CT scanning. As would be expected, however, EUS is less accurate than CT scanning in the detection of distant metastases, accuracy being in the order of 70 and 95%, respectively.

These excellent figures for the reliability of EUS in staging local disease are somewhat offset by the inability to pass the echoendoscope in 26–40% of patients.[22,25] However, in our experience, this figure can be brought down to 12% by performing endoscopic dilatation of stenotic lesions prior to EUS.[26] Furthermore, microtransducers are being evaluated which can pass down the biopsy channel of a conventional endoscope, which should virtually eliminate this problem as well as reducing capital costs.

Bronchoscopy

The use of bronchoscopy in staging oesophageal cancer varies considerably from unit to unit. In those units where

Table 14.2 Reported accuracy of endoluminal ultrasonography compared to CT scanning for T and N staging of oesophageal cancer

| | | ACCURACY (%) | |
REFERENCE	NO.	EUS	CT
T stage			
Tio, 1990[13]	74	89	59
Botet, 1991[22]	50	92	60
Grimm, 1991	49	89	62
Ziegler, 1991[23]	37	89	51
Heintz, 1991	22	77	64
Schuder, 1990	22	86	57
Watson, 1995[24]	33	91	64
Total	287	86	59
N stage			
Tio, 1990[13]	74	80	51
Vilgrain, 1990	51	50	48
Botet, 1991[22]	50	88	74
Ziegler, 1991[23]	37	69	51
Heintz, 1991	22	86	50
Schuder, 1990	22	81	48
Watson, 1995[24]	33	86	45
Total	289	77	52

oesophageal cancer is managed predominantly by thoracic surgeons, bronchoscopy tends to be used more frequently than in gastrointestinal surgical units. Invasion of the respiratory tree is, in fact, a relatively unusual occurrence, the incidence being less than 10% in those patients in whom surgery is initially considered appropriate. In these circumstances, it is difficult to justify performing routine bronchoscopy on all such patients, and many workers believe it is best reserved for those patients in whom involvement of the respiratory tree is suspected on clinical grounds, chest radiography or CT scanning.

Laparoscopy

The recent increase in the use of laparoscopy has led to its deployment in the staging of gastric and pancreatic cancer, but to a much lesser extent in oesophageal cancer. However, one study has compared the accuracy of laparoscopy with that of ultrasonography and CT scanning in the detection of intra-abdominal spread of oesophageal cancer.[27] The accuracy of laparoscopy in the detection of liver metastases was 96%, compared to 83% by ultrasonography and 85% by CT scanning. The corresponding figures for nodal metastases were 72% for laparoscopy, 52% for ultrasound and 57% for CT scanning. Laparoscopy diagnosed peritoneal metastases (which occurred in 10% of patients) with an accuracy of 98%, peritoneal deposits not being identified by either ultrasound or CT. It does appear, therefore, that laparoscopy has a place in the preoperative staging of oesophageal cancer, certainly in the diagnosis of peritoneal deposits, and possibly in identifying liver and nodal metastases, although the accuracy of laparoscopy in these latter two situations was equivalent to that generally reported in the literature for CT scanning. However, the advantage of laparoscopy is that a tissue diagnosis can be obtained and its use is increasing.

Thoracoscopy

As with laparoscopy, the use of thoracoscopy is increasing, and it has potential attractions in staging of oesophageal tumours, from the standpoint of assessing fixity and nodal status, with the potential of nodal biopsy. However, at the time of writing, there are no published series of the accuracy compared to other modalities.

Patient selection

Resection of the oesophagus by a thoracoabdominal route is the most common 'curative' approach to oesophageal cancer. It is one of the most complex elective surgical procedures which can be undertaken, and one that is associated with significant morbidity and mortality. This, coupled with the fact that the majority of patients with oesophageal cancer are over the age of 60 and are chronic smokers with a high incidence of cardiorespiratory pathology, makes careful selection of patients of paramount importance. The two principal considerations in selection of patients with a view to undergoing a 'curative' resection are age and intercurrent disease.

Age

It is well recognized that for all surgical procedures, and particularly major ones, such as oesophageal resection, morbidity and mortality increase with increasing age. Elderly people have decreased cardiopulmonary reserve, and one large study of a wide range of over 15,000 surgical cases showed progressive increase in morbidity and mortality with advancing age, particularly over the age of 75 years.[28] Wong[29] showed that for oesophageal resection, the mortality in patients over the age of 70 years was double that of the 40–60 age group. In a more recent multivariate analysis, the same group found increasing age to be a risk factor for increased morbidity and mortality, being associated with relatively poor pulmonary reserve, and an increased incidence of respiratory complications.[30] Another mechanism which may be relevant is a reduction in the maximum response of the stress hormones to oesophageal resection, with an increased incidence of multiorgan dysfunction in patients over 70.[31]

For these reasons, many centres would not advocate radical resectional surgery in patients over the age of 75, unless they were exceptionally fit for their age or had a relatively favourable tumour, although this is by no means universal. A series from Dublin[32] reported similar results in a group of patients aged 70–84 years as in those below 70 years, although hospital mortality was 21% in the elderly group and the incidence of cardiorespiratory complications was higher than in those under 70. Peracchia and colleagues[33] showed that patients over 70 had a higher risk of complications due to concomitant disease and poor physiological reserve, but with stringent patient selection, complications and mortality were similar to those of younger patients. This shows clearly that biological age is more important than chronological age, and that age alone should not preclude an attempt at curative resection, but it must be borne in mind that over the age of 75, particularly in the type of patients suffering from oesophageal cancer, life expectancy is limited, and reducing the risk of such a patient dying from oesophageal cancer will only increase the chance of death from heart disease or stroke.[34]

Intercurrent disease

The fact that the majority of patients with oesophageal cancer are aged over 60 years and have a high tobacco and alcohol intake results in a significant incidence of intercurrent disease in these patients, reaching 20–40% for pulmonary disease.[35] It has been shown that the incidence of postoperative pulmonary complications increases significantly when the FEV$_1$ is reduced by 20% or more,[30] and as pulmonary complications represent the most common cause of death in most series, adequate pulmonary function is clearly necessary. An operation of the magnitude of thoracoabdominal oesophageal resection also requires adequate cardiac function, which may also be impaired in a significant proportion of patients with oesophageal cancer. Some workers believe that the ejection fraction should be measured routinely, and if this falls below 40%, then 'curative' resection is contraindicated.[36] It has also been shown that the mortality of thoracoabdominal resection is increased in the presence of increasing degrees of liver disease (principally cirrhosis), renal impairment and diabetes.[29]

Clearly, therefore, careful patient selection is of the utmost importance if morbidity and mortality are to be reduced. We would recommend that pulmonary function tests are performed on all potential candidates for resectional surgery, and a full cardiological work-up performed on all patients with a history of cardiac disease or who present with suggestive symptoms, or in whom abnormalities are detected on physical examination. Where any intercurrent disease is detected, providing its severity does not obviously contraindicate surgery, it is essential that the patient is assessed by a specialist in the appropriate discipline to fully investigate the problem in question from the standpoint of optimizing the condition of the patient and assisting in the risk-analysis process.

THE ROLE OF TUMOUR STAGING AND PATIENT SELECTION IN CLINICAL DECISION MAKING

In the clinical context, some patients will present with clinically obvious advanced disease in whom it is readily apparent that an attempt at 'curative' resection is inappropriate, and detailed assessment unnecessary. These include patients with obvious metastatic disease, or those with such locally advanced disease as is clearly incurable, such as vocal cord paresis or an easily detected tracho-oesophageal fistula. Similarly, a proportion of patients will be very elderly or have a severe degree of intercurrent disease as to make an attempt at resectional surgery an unacceptable risk. However, in the majority of patients it is necessary to go through a selection process, firstly to stage the tumour to assess whether an attempt at 'curative' resection is appropriate, and in some circumstances, whether this should be preceded by chemoradiation, followed by a detailed assessment of fitness for surgery.

Once endoscopy has been performed and a tissue diagnosis

made, the next investigation will normally be a CT scan of the thorax and abdomen. Although, as discussed above, CT scanning has some shortcomings in accurately staging the tumour and detecting nodal involvement, it is a useful initial screening investigation to exclude hepatic or pulmonary metastases or the presence of extensive transmediastinal spread or gross involvement of contiguous structures, such as the bronchial tree, aorta or pericardium. If there is unequivocal evidence of incurable disease by any of these parameters, then further staging investigations are inappropriate and palliation should be the principal aim. If invasion of the bronchial tree is suspected, then bronchoscopy should be performed in order to confirm or exclude this, and if confirmed, once more palliation should be the principal objective. In all other circumstances, the next logical step is to perform endoluminal ultrasound which provides a more accurate indication of the T stage of the tumour, involvement of contiguous structures and nodal involvement. Only if the tumour is unequivocally invading aorta or pericardium should the patient be denied a chance of resectional surgery, as in doubtful cases, particularly in relation to the aorta, adherence may be inflammatory rather than neoplastic, and in such circumstances adequate resection is almost always feasible. With regard to nodal status, positive nodes in relation to a squamous carcinoma, unless extensive and involving all groups from cervical to coeliac, should not be a contra-indication to resectional surgery, as 10% of patients with node-positive squamous lesions survive five years with resectional surgery accompanied by an adequate lymphadenectomy.[37] However, there is increasing evidence to suggest that such patients should undergo preoperative chemoradiation,[38] although results of prospective randomized studies are awaited before benefit can be confirmed. The situation is rather different in relation to adenocarcinomas, particularly with extensively involved coeliac nodes, in which circumstance cure is unlikely.

If the tumour appears resectable based on these criteria, the next step should be a detailed assessment of fitness for surgery, particularly in relation to cardiovascular and respiratory systems as previously described. If the patient is deemed fit to withstand a thoracoabdominal resection, then it would be wise to plan for preresection laparoscopy and possibly thoracoscopy in order to convincingly exclude peritoneal metastases, small hepatic metastases, dense coeliac nodal involvement and extreme tumour fixity which conventional staging modalities may not have detected, and by so doing some patients will be spared unnecessary surgical intervention. If the tumour is deemed resectable but the patient found unfit to undergo major surgery, then consideration should be given to a local debulking procedure such as laser photocoagulation, followed by an aggressive course of chemoradiation. In those patients who are deemed fit to undergo resectional surgery, their subsequent management can be categorized into preoperative, operative and postoperative.

PREOPERATIVE MANAGEMENT

Thoracoabdominal resection for oesophageal cancer is one of the most major elective surgical procedures and the fact that it is often performed on patients who are heavy smokers and tend to be malnourished as a result of their disease, provides the potential for considerable morbidity and mortality. Preoperative care is an unimportant aspect of management in which the potential for morbidity can be reduced. The majority of patients with oesophageal cancer have lost some weight at the time of presentation, both because of restriction of the ability to eat and the metabolic effects of the tumour. It is our policy to perform endoscopic dilation of the tumour at the time of the initial endoscopy to obtain a tissue diagnosis, which improves the patient's eating capacity while the staging investigations and assessment of fitness for surgery are being conducted, as well as increasing the likelihood of the endoluminal ultrasound probe to traverse the tumour. Once the tumour has been dilated, the patient is advised to take a high protein, high calorie diet, which, with the help of the hospital dietician, can be provided in semisolid or liquid form, depending on the patient's swallowing capacity. This approach is satisfactory for the majority of patients, although there are two clinical situations where this may be inadequate. The first is if the tumour is causing virtually complete obstruction and is not readily dilatable, and the other is when the patient has lost in excess of 20% of body weight. In both these circumstances, active nutritional support is necessary either by enteral nutrition following passage of a fine bore feeding tube, or parenteral nutrition. Whichever is used, it should be continued for at least 10–14 days in order to confer measurable benefit.

Other aspects of preoperative care include correction of specific deficiencies, such as transfusion if the patient is anaemic and correction of any electrolyte or trace metal deficiencies. Chest physiotherapy is best commenced preoperatively after insisting that those patients who smoke have discontinued this. Immediately preoperatively, prophylactic antibiotics and low-dose heparin should be administered and continued over the perioperative period in order to reduce the risk of infection and thromboembolic disease.

OPERATIVE MANAGEMENT

There are several surgical techniques used in the management of patients with oesophageal cancer. Which one is deployed depends on several factors, including whether the procedure is performed with curative or palliative intent, whether a total or subtotal oesophagectomy is performed, whether stomach, colon or jejunum is used as the replacement organ, and the route chosen for access. The range of procedures is shown in Table 14.3, and each will be discussed in turn.

'CURATIVE' PROCEDURES

There are two important factors in the biological behaviour of oesophageal tumours which govern the principles underlying 'curative' resection. The first is the propensity for both squamous and adenocarcinomas to extend microscopically both by direct extension and lymphatic embolization, to a considerable distance from the apparent macroscopic tumour limits. This process can extend as much as 6 cm, particularly proximally, and may manifest as microscopic tumour deposits

Table 14.3   Surgical procedures for oesophageal cancer

'CURATIVE'	PALLIATIVE
Lewis–Tanner oesophagogastrectomy	Palliative resection
Three-phase total oesophagectomy	(using any technique listed under 'curative')
Synchronous combined three-phase technique	Oesophagogastrostomy
Left thoracic approach	Reversed gastric tube (Heimlich)
Left thoracoabdominal approach	Kirschner procedure
Blunt transhiatal (abdominal-cervical) oesophagectomy	Surgical intubation
Endoscopic transmediastinal oesophagectomy	
Thoracoscopically assisted oesophagogastrectomy	

submucosally, or occasionally satellite nodules which may reach the mucosa some distance from the primary tumour. There may be areas of normality between the upper margin of the macroscopically apparent tumour and the upper limit of this process, leading to the possibility that frozen section may not necessarily be a reliable guide to adequacy of longitudinal excision. The safest policy is to plan to resect at least 8 and preferably 10 cm of 'normal' oesophagus proximal to the upper margin of the macroscopically apparent tumour. It has been shown that when longitudinal clearance is less than 5 cm, the incidence of anastomotic recurrence is 20%. This is reduced to 7% when the resection margin is 8–10 cm and 0 when the resection margin is over 10 cm.[39]

The other important consideration is the pattern of lymphatic spread of oesophageal tumours, as demonstrated by Akiyama and colleagues.[40] They showed that oesophageal tumours, irrespective of their location, are capable of metastasizing to lymph nodes over a wide region from the superior mediastinal to the coeliac nodes, with significant involvement, particularly with distal tumours, of nodes along the lesser curvature of the stomach. They therefore advocated a wide lymphadenectomy and excision of the lesser curvature of the stomach in all resected cases, and demonstrated overall 5-year survival of 35%, and 15% of patients with positive nodes so treated. It follows, therefore, that in order to obtain the best results, resection should include longitudinal clearance of 10 cm or more, resection of the lesser curvature of the stomach and an adequate lymphadenectomy including not only the paraoesophageal nodes, but also superior mediastinal, tracheobronchial and subcarinal nodes and left gastric and coeliac nodes. There have been recent suggestions, again emanating from Japan, that even more extensive lymphadenectomy including bilateral cervical nodal dissections should be performed (see below). However, this is associated with a significant increase in morbidity, and as yet there is no firm evidence of increased survival, and this practice has not been adopted routinely in the West.

Most of the established dissection techniques embody the principles of adequacy of both longitudinal clearance and lymphadenectomy. However, there are those that fall short of these principles, including transhiatal oesophagectomy and transmediastinal endoscopic oesophagectomy, and those that go further, particularly the radical en-bloc resection, which in addition to these essential prerequisites also involves resection of the azygos vein, the pericardium and both pleural surfaces, and replaces the oesophagus with a colonic conduit. There is evidence to suggest that the former procedures may well be inadequate in many patients, but little evidence to suggest that increasing radicality, as with the en-bloc procedure confers additional survival benefit. However, this debate is being re-opened with the advent of three-field dissection (see below).

Lewis–Tanner oesophagogastrectomy

This is currently the most widely practised surgical procedure for oesophageal cancer, having been developed almost simultaneously by Lewis in 1946[41] and Tanner in 1947.[42] This is essentially a two-phase procedure, the first comprising laparotomy in which, assuming there are no contraindications found to resection, the entire stomach and distal oesophagus are mobilized and a gastric tube prepared. The patient is then turned and a full right thoracotomy is performed, at which the intrathoracic oesophagus is mobilized, the gastric tube brought up into the mediastinum, and oesophagogastrectomy performed together with the oesophagogastric anastomosis.

Operative technique

There are several important anaesthetic considerations in patients undergoing thoracoabdominal resectional procedures, and it is essential if good results are maintained that the skills of an anaesthetist who is regularly involved in such procedures are deployed. Endotracheal intubation should be performed using a double-lumen tube in order to allow for subsequent selective collapse of the right lung during the right thoracotomy. A thoracic epidural catheter should be inserted, usually at T5 level, as per- and postoperative epidural analgesia has been shown to have a dramatic influence on the incidence and severity of postoperative respiratory complications.[43] Careful monitoring of haemodynamic parameters, including central venous pressure, together with oxygen saturation and urinary output are essential.

The abdominal phase is performed first, with the patient supine, through an upper midline or left upper paramedian incision (Figure 14.1). The abdomen is first examined for evidence of intra-abdominal disease, particularly hepatic metastases or lymph node metastases, especially around the left gastric artery and coeliac axis. In distally placed lesions, the lower margin of the tumour may be palpable, and the degree of adherence to the diaphragm and posterior abdominal wall can be assessed. Assuming there is no contraindication to resection, the stomach is mobilized by entering the lesser sac and dividing all vessels between the pylorus and the cardia, but preserving the right gastroepiploic artery on the greater curve side and the right gastric artery on the lesser curve aspect. All other vessels including the left gastroepiploic, left gastric and short gastric vessels are divided, and dissection performed of the left gastric, coeliac axis and lesser curvature perigastric nodes, together

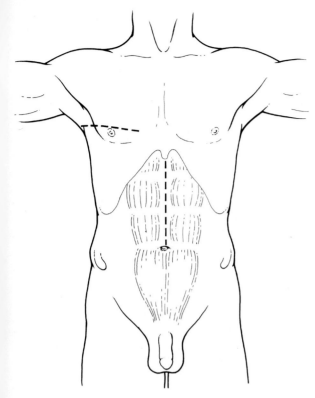

Figure 14.1
Incisions for Lewis–Tanner oesophagogastrectomy, i.e. upper midline and right thoracotomy through 5th or 6th interspace.

factors as to whether the resection is potentially curative or palliative. As with gastric cancer, there has been considerable debate as to the value of performing splenectomy, and it is generally believed that in the absence of direct or nodal involvement of the spleen or hilum, the immunological advantages of retaining the spleen probably outweigh those of removing it for the perceived benefit of greater clearance.

Having mobilized the stomach along both of its curvatures on right gastric and right gastroepiploic pedicles, the duodenum is then mobilized by dividing the peritoneum along its lateral border (Kocher's manoeuvre) so that the inferior vena cava is exposed, and the hand can then be placed under the duodenum and head of the pancreas to lift the structures forward, which aids mobility of the distal stomach towards the oesophageal hiatus. Proximally, the distal oesophagus is mobilized by blunt trans-hiatal dissection, although this may need to be supplemented by sharp dissection should the distal portion of the tumour be adherent within the hiatus. Ideally, 5–7 cm of distal oesophagus should be mobilized during the abdominal phase. Attention is now turned to the pylorus, which should be assessed for the presence of pyloric or duodenal ulceration, in which case pyloroplasty is necessary because of the inevitable truncal vagotomy which will be performed subsequently during transection of the intrathoracic oesophagus. In the absence of pyloroduodenal pathology, opinion is divided as to the necessity for pyloroplasty. A prospective randomized study by Fok and colleagues[44] showed that from the standpoint of gastric emptying, patients with pyloroplasty fared better than those with no drainage procedure. However, pyloroplasty is known to facilitate duodenogastric alkaline reflux, and this predisposes to the risk of alkaline oesophageal exposure following oesophagogastrectomy. Those who argue against pyloroplasty[45,46] maintain that the situation following oesophagogastrectomy is

with those along the splenic artery (Figure 14.2). Such a dissection will obviously not be feasible in all cases depending on the degree and extent of nodal involvement, although the ability to perform such a lymph-adenectomy will be one of the deciding

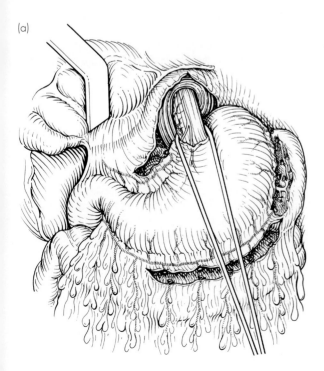
(a)

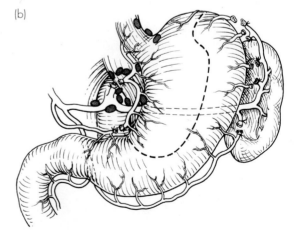
(b)

Figure 14.2
(a) Mobilization of the stomach, showing division of the greater omentum, with preservation of the right gastroepiploic and the right gastric artery. (b) Showing the area of the stomach to be resected along with the oesophagus, together with dissection of the left gastric, coeliac and paraoesophageal nodes. The right gastric vessels have been divided at the level of the incisura in preparation for formation of the greater curve gastric tube.

not analogous to that of truncal vagotomy when it was used for the treatment of duodenal ulcer disease, in that the pyloroduodenal region is normal in the majority of patients undergoing oesophagogastrectomy, and because of the subsequent anatomy, with the pylorus coming to lie vertically in the region of the oesophageal hiatus, gravity aids emptying of the gastric remnant.[47] A compromise position is the performance of a pyloric procedure falling short of pyloroplasty and thus hopefully obviating duodenogastric alkaline reflux, while facilitating gastric emptying. Some have used a standard pyloromyotomy.[48,49] Our practice in over 200 resections over the past 20 years has been to perform a blunt pyloromyotomy by finger and thumb invagination of the pylorus; this has been associated with a 5% incidence of symptomatic impairment of gastric emptying, which in the majority of cases can now be treated adequately by endoscopic balloon dilatation.[50]

Preparation of the gastric tube is performed during the abdominal phase, and the author's preferred technique is by using linear staplers. The first is applied at right angles to the lesser curvature at the level of the incisura, having divided the ascending branch of the right gastric artery. Subsequent staple lines are then applied parallel to the greater curvature of the stomach and approximately 4 cm from it (Figure 14.3). The staple line can be taken as far up the greater curvature towards the fundus as is necessary to produce a greater curve gastric tube, vascularized by the right gastric and right gastric-epiploic arteries, the upper margin of which will reach the neck if necessary. Most of the cardia and the lesser curvature of the stomach, including most of the intra-abdominal lymphatic pathways will subsequently be resected along with the oesophagus. The abdomen is closed at this stage, nothing irrevocable having been done if the oesophageal tumour is subsequently found to be unresectable within the chest. The patient is then turned into a full right thoractomy position, entry being achieved through

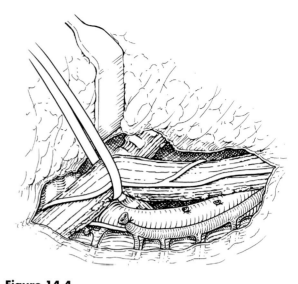

Figure 14.4
At right thoracotomy, the oesophagus has been mobilized from its bed and the arterial branches from the aorta and the arch of the azygos vein have been divided.

the fifth or sixth interspace depending on the level of the lesion. The right lung is collapsed by the anaesthetist by clamping off the right limb of the double lumen endobronchial tube, which allows excellent access to the whole intrathoracic oesophagus. The proximal margin of the trans-hiatal dissection should be clearly visible at this stage. The inferior pulmonary ligament is divided such that the collapsed right lung can be adequately retracted. The pleura overlying the intrathoracic oesophagus is incised posteriorily and anteriorly from the diaphragmatic hiatus to the apex of the mediastinum. The arch of the azygos vein is divided between ligatures. The plane behind the normal oesophagus above and below the tumour is achieved by blunt dissection, and silastic slings may be passed to enable retraction of the oesophagus (Figure 14.4). This facilitates identification of the segmental blood vessels from the aorta and intercostal vessels, which should be ligated or clipped close to their origins to facilitate an adequate lymphadenectomy of the paraoesophageal nodes. Anteromedially, the tracheobronchial, subcarinal and hilar nodes should also be dissected, and if necessary, the tumour should be dissected free from adherence to contiguous structures. Once the oesophagus has been fully mobilized, the stomach can be brought into the mediastinum, and the final attachment between the fundus of the stomach and the prepared gastric tube is divided. A Satinsky clamp is lightly applied across the oesophagus at the apex of the mediastinum, assuming there is at least 8 cm clearance from the upper limit of the tumour, and the oesophagus is divided and resected along with the cardia and lesser curvature of the stomach. If there is less than 8 cm of clearance from the proximal margin of the tumour, then a three-phase resection with a cervical oesophagogastric anastomosis will need to be performed, and the oesophageal dissection is continued in the superior mediastinum along the posterior wall of the oesophagus until the retropharyngeal space is found (see below). Attention is now turned to the oesophagogastric anastomosis.

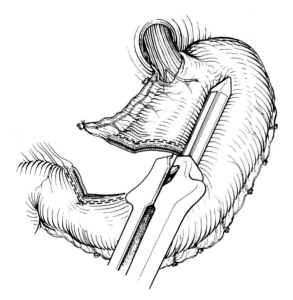

Figure 14.3
The linear stapler has firstly been applied at right angles to the lesser curvature at the level of the incisura, and subsequently parallel to the greater curvature.

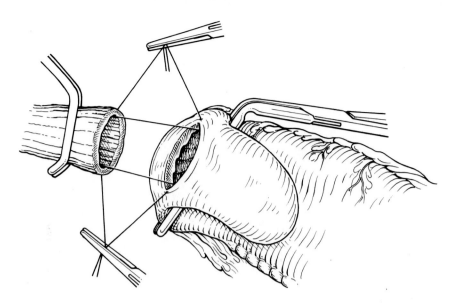

Figure 14.5
Satinsky clamps have been applied to the divided oesophagus and mobilized gastric tube, and an incision made in the posterior aspect of the latter, 4 cm from its upper margin.

Oesophageal anastomoses have a greater propensity for leakage than most other gastrointestinal anastomoses, because of the relatively poor vascularity of the oesophagus, the absence of a serous layer and the high intraluminal pressures generated on swallowing. Consequently, great care must be exercised in ensuring that vascularity is preserved and that the anastomosis is performed with adequate access and without tension. It is the author's preference to perform a hand-sewn anastomosis with a single layer of interrupted 3/0 silk sutures. A second Satinsky clamp is placed 4 cm distal to the upper margin of the gastric tube, and a horizontal incision is made in the posterior aspect of the stomach just above the clamp, the length of the incision being equivalent to the diameter of the divided oesophagus (Figure 14.5). The anastomosis is performed using the 'parachute' technique, placing the stay sutures and posterior layer of sutures with the two clamps held some distance apart to facilitate access (Figure 14.6). When all sutures in the posterior layer have been placed, the clamp on the gastric tube is approximated to the oesophageal clamp and the posterior layer of sutures are tied (Figure 14.7). Because of the particular features of oesophageal anastomoses already discussed, it is important that the sutures include a good bite of

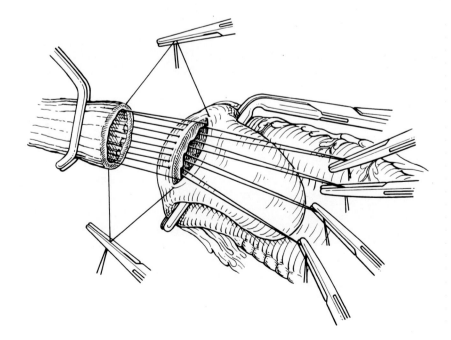

Figure 14.6
Stay sutures have been applied to the divided oesophagus and mobilized gastric tube, and the posterior layer of sutures has been placed using the 'parachute' technique.

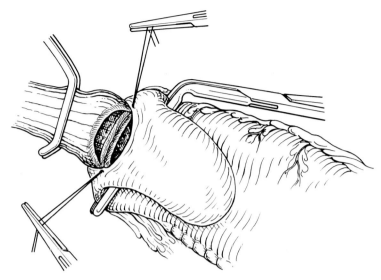

Figure 14.7
The clamps have been approximated and the posterior layer of sutures tied and cut.

the oesophageal mucosa and submucosa (being the strongest layers of the oesophageal wall), which have a tendency to retract if there is undue tension. Also, because of the delicate vascularity, the sutures should be placed about 3 mm apart, and not tied unduly tightly. A nasogastric tube is then passed into the proximal oesophagus and then into the gastric tube, and the anterior layer of interrupted sutures placed and tied (Figure 14.8). The 4 cm segment of the gastric tube which lies proximal to the oesophagogastric anastomosis is sutured to the apical medastinal pleura, which serves both to relieve tension from the anastomosis and to seal it anteriorly (Figure 14.9). Some surgeons prefer to perform the anastomosis using a circular stapler passed via the gastric tube. However, comparative studies have shown no significant difference in the rate of anastomotic dehisence,[52,53] although stapled anastomoses are associated with a higher rate of anastomotic stricture, particularly when the smaller staple heads are used.[54]

Once the anastomosis has been satisfactorily completed, the chest is closed with underwater seal drainage, using one apical and one basal drain.

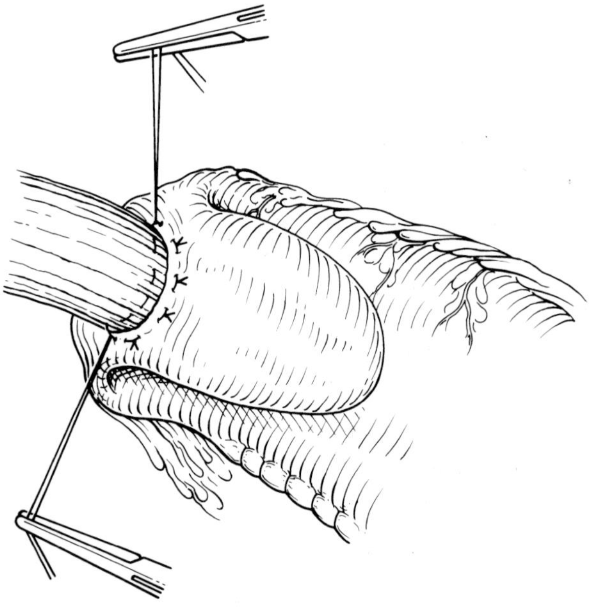

Three-phase oesophagogastrectomy

The addition of a third, cervical phase to the Lewis–Tanner procedure was described by Ong and Kwong in 1969[55] and by McKeown in 1972.[56] This involved closure of the chest at the stage when the oesophagus had been fully mobilized, including at the apex of the mediastinum and into the retropharyngeal space, and then, through a right cervical incision, the oesophagus was mobilized, the thoracic oesophagus and gastric fundus brought into the neck, and resection performed as in the Lewis–Tanner procedure, but including most of the cervical oesophagus in addition, and the oesophagogastric anastomosis was performed in the neck. The rationale of this approach was first to achieve greater longitudinal clearance and secondly to site the anastomosis in the neck, where the blood supply is somewhat better and, in theory, the consequences of leakage would be less serious. In practice, there is no difference in anastomotic leakage rate between cervical and intrathoracic anastomoses, and most leaks from anastomoses constructed in the neck actually occur into the mediastinum.[57] Although some centres favour this approach, our policy is in agreement with that of Wong,[39] to perform a Lewis–Tanner procedure, providing 8–10 cm proximal clearance can be achieved, and the anastomosis is performed at the apex of the mediastinum, thus avoiding adding a third phase to what is already a major procedure. However, if the tumour is proximally sited, such that the requisite clearance cannot be achieved by these means, then a three-phase procedure is performed.

Figure 14.8
The anterior layer of sutures has been placed.

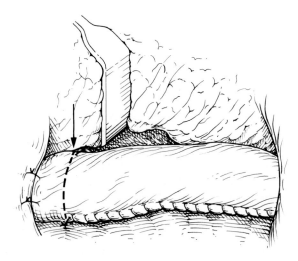

Figure 14.9

The apex of the gastric tube is sutured to the mediastinal pleura so as to lie over the anastomosis anteriorly and to relieve tension from it.

Operative technique

The abdominal and thoracic phases are performed as in the Lewis–Tanner procedure. A skin-crease incision or one along the anterior border of sternomastoid is made in the right side of the neck (Figure 14.10). The anterior border of sternomastoid is freed and retracted laterally and the right lobe of the thyroid is retracted medially after division of the middle thyroid vein. The cervical oesophagus is identified by dissection in the plane between the carotid sheath and the thyroid gland (Figure 14.11). The plane of dissection is kept close to the oesophagus so as to avoid damage to the recurrent laryngeal nerve which lies between it and the trachea. Once the plane behind the cervical oesophagus has been achieved and the distal segment mobilized, the distal cervical oesophagus, together with the thoracic oesophagus and the mobilized stomach can be delivered into the neck (Figure 14.12). The remaining attachment between the mobilized stomach and prepared gastric tube is

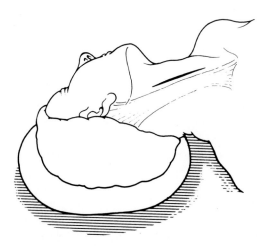

Figure 14.10

Right cervical incision, either parallel to the anterior border of sternum mastoid or a right transverse skin crease incision.

divided, and the specimen removed. The oesophagogastric anastomosis is then constructed as described previously, except that it is often easier to perform a straightforward end to end anastomosis in the neck. The cervical wound is then closed, with a small drain placed alongside the anastomosis.

Synchronous combined three phase technique

This modification of the three phase procedure was described by Nanson in 1975[58] with the aim of overcoming the criticism of significant prolongation of operating time by the addition of a cervical phase. Nanson's technique involves slight elevation of the right chest on a sandbag, so that the abdominal approach and a thoracic approach through an anterior right thoracotomy can be performed simultaneously by two teams of operators. This technique has been adopted by some centres, the advantages being reduction in operating time and the ability to confirm resectability within the mediastinum at an early stage. Disadvantages include a slight compromise of access for both thoracic and abdominal teams because of the patient position and the fact that the operating surgeons occasionally get in each other's way. A recent randomized study showed that the period of single lung anaesthesia was longer using this technique and the incidence of significant complications higher than with the Lewis–Tanner technique.[59]

Left thoracic approach

This is the preferred approach of many thoracic surgeons. Entry is made usually via the sixth intercostal space, and access to the abdomen either through the oesophageal hiatus or by a tangential incision through the central tendon of the diaphragm, posterior to the phrenic nerve. This approach has the advantages of a single incision and avoidance of repositioning the patient during operation. The disadvantages are that access to abdominal structures is less than with formal laparotomy, and dissection of the upper intrathoracic oesophagus as well as an adequate lymphadenectomy may be less easy than through a right thoracotomy because of the heart and great vessels. This approach can also be used for total oesophagectomy by adding a cervical phase.

Left thoracoabdominal approach

This approach is attractive to some workers in dealing with distal oesophageal lesions, in that it affords good access to both abdominal and thoracic cavities, but by employing a single incision and avoiding the need to reposition the patient.

Operative technique

The patient is placed in a semilateral position, with the left side of the chest elevated with sandbags. An oblique left upper abdominal incision is made, commencing approximately midway between the xiphisternum and the umbilicus, and continued obliquely towards the left costal margin. Laparotomy is then performed to assess operability, and to perform the gastric mobilization and preparation of the gastric tube as previously described. The incision is then carried across the costal margin,

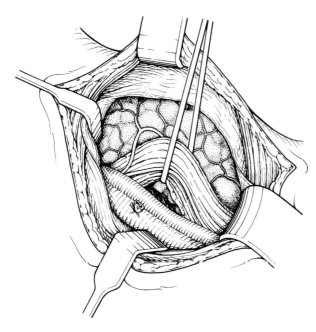

Figure 14.11

The right lobe of the thyroid is retracted medially, and the cervical oesophagus mobilized from its bed between the thyroid and the carotid sheath.

and into the seventh or eighth interspace, extending as far posteriorly as required. The costal margin itself is divided and the diaphragm is separated from its costal attachment and incised into the oesophageal hiatus. The thoracic phase is performed as described previously, and the diaphragm repaired with dissolvable sutures. The chest and abdomen are closed in routine fashion and the skin closed as a single continuous incision.

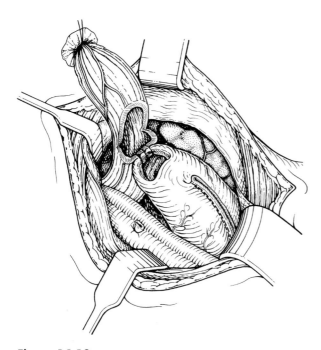

Figure 14.12

The gastric tube is brought into the neck for an end-to-end oesophagogastric anastomosis.

Although operating time is considerably shorter than the Lewis–Tanner approach, the principal disadvantage of the left thoracoabdominal approach is that access within the left chest is considerably more restricted because of the presence of the heart and great vessels. It is relatively easy to perform an oesophagogastric anastomosis low in the left chest, but if 8–10 cm of longitudinal clearance are to be achieved, the anastomosis for the most distally situated oesophageal tumours will be at least at the level of the aortic arch. In the author's experience, it is more difficult to achieve a high anastomosis without tension and without adequate exposure than in the right chest, and this approach is more frequently associated with cardiac dysrhythmias.[60]

Radical en-bloc oesophagectomy

This procedure was described by Skinner[61] as a more radical, ablative approach to oesophageal resection than other procedures. Fundamental to this approach is the belief that in tumours which appear localized to the oesophageal wall, there will be many in which the tumour is beginning to penetrate outside the oesophageal wall, or has undergone microscopic spread to regional lymph nodes, and that it is only by removing an envelope of tissue, including the embryological dorsal meso-oesophagus, which will be curative in these circumstances. Such resection entails an en-bloc removal of the entire mesentery, including the oesophagus, and consisting also of a block of tissue limited by the membraneous trachea and pericardium anteriorly, the right and left mediastinal pleura laterally, and intercostal arteries, aorta and anterior vertebral ligaments posteriorly. Thus, the thoracic oesophagus is removed together with its surrounding areolar tissue containing the paratracheal, subcarinal, paraoesophageal and cardiac lymph nodes, the thoracic duct and the azygos vein down to the level of the oesophageal hiatus, and a collar of muscle surrounding the latter. Although Skinner's original description allowed for a choice of replacement organ, including a gastric tube, others believe that the en-bloc dissection should be continued into the abdomen, removing all the posterior peritoneal and periaortic areolar tissue down to the coeliac axis and superior to the common hepatic artery.[62] This necessitates removal of the distal three-quarters of the stomach and greater omentum, continuity being re-established by colon interposition.

Operative technique

The radical en-bloc procedure is based on a three-phase technique, the thoracic and abdominal phases often being performed simultaneously by two teams of surgeons. A right thoracotomy is performed through the fifth or sixth interspace. The azygos vein is divided close to its junction with the superior vena cava and distally at the oesophageal hiatus, together with each of the intercostal branches between these points. The mediastinum is entered through a longitudinal pleural incision made anterior to the oesophagus and parallel to the posterior margin of the trachea, hilum and pericardium down to the diaphragm. A posterior pleural incision is made parallel to the spine along the line of the previously ligated intercostal branches of the azygos vein. The anterior incision is deepened by extending it across to the left mediastinal pleura, following the posterior surface of the trachea, left bronchus and pericardium. The posterior incision is extended across to the left mediastinal pleura following the intercostal arteries over the spine to the aorta and over its anterior surface. The hemiazygos vein is identified and ligated, as is the thoracic duct. The pericardium is entered on the back of the pulmonary veins and left atrium and the pleuropericardial reflection on the left side is incised from the pulmonary hilum down to the diaphragm. The reflection of the pericardium from the right pulmonary vein is identified by traction on the incised pericardium, and incision through this leads to entry into the right pleural cavity. The right pleuropericardial reflection is incised from within the pericardium. The right pulmonary ligament is then divided and the oesophagus is now completely mobilized and transected at the apex of the mediastinum, the proximal stomach being temporarily oversewn for subsequent anastomosis in the neck. Where a gastric tube is used as the replacement organ, the abdominal dissection is performed as described previously, and the proximal end of the gastric tube attached to the transected proximal oesophageal stump. The abdomen and chest are closed and a cervical oesophagogastric anastomosis fashioned as described previously. However, in the majority of instances a colon inter position is used.

Technique of colonic interposition

The most widely used colonic interposition is an isoperistaltic segment of left colon on a left colic artery pedicle, although it is possible to use either a right or transverse colon segment based on the middle colic artery. It is important preoperatively to exclude colonic disease by colonoscopy, and many workers advocate arteriography in order to confirm integrity of the vascular supply. The left colon, splenic flexure and transverse colon are initially mobilized from their attachments by dividing the peritoneal reflection and detaching the greater omentum. It is important to mark an appropriate length of colon to be isolated and subsequently anastomosed to the gastric remnant distally and the upper oesophagus proximally. This is best achieved by gentle upward traction on the mobilized colon, such that the upper left colic artery points in a cephalad direction, and the part of the colon adjacent to the most cephalad point of the left colic artery will become the distal level of the conduit and can be marked by a Babcock's forceps or a suture. A tape can then be used to measure from this point to a few centimetres beyond the anticipated site of the proximal anastomosis, and a second Babcock's forceps or suture placed on the proximal colon, this distance away from the previous marker (Figure 14.13). In preparation for transection of the colon at this point, the main trunks of the middle colic vessels are divided, as are the marginal vessels at the site of transection. The route to be taken by the colonic conduit and the proximal anastomotic site are then prepared. If the posterior mediastinal route is chosen, the conduit will need to pass through the oesophageal hiatus and into the posterior mediastinum, and subsequently into the neck for a cervical anastomosis. If the

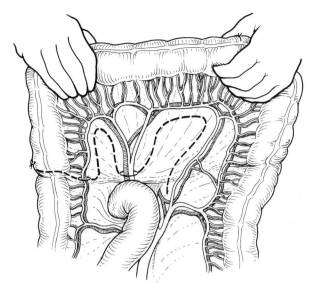

Figure 14.13
The colon is retracted to identify the site of the marking sutures to form the colonic conduit. The sites of mesocolic and vascular division are shown, the conduit being vascularized by the left colic artery and marginal arcade.

substernal route is chosen, the conduit will need to pass through the gastrohepatic ligament, into a substernal tunnel prepared by blunt dissection, and for cervical anastomoses, the medial end of the first rib, the sternal end of the clavicle and half of the manubrium sterni will need to be excised. The proximal colon is then transected and guided to the site of the proposed oesophagocolic anastomosis, taking care to ensure the mesocolon does not become twisted (Figure 14.14). The proximal anastomosis is then fashioned. Attention is now directed towards the distal end of the conduit, which is initially anchored by a few sutures to one margin of the oesophageal hiatus, ensuring that the mediastinal portion of the conduit is neither under too much tension, nor too lax. The distal colonic transection can then be made at an appropriate distance to comfortably perform the cologastric anastomosis. In performing the transection, care must be taken to preserve the marginal artery, on which the conduit depends for its blood supply. After performing the cologastric anastomosis (Figure 14.15), a pyloroplasty, pyloromyotomy or blunt myotomy may be performed according to preference and finally, colonic continuity is restored by performing a colocolic anastomosis.

Additional indications for colonic interposition, other than as part of a radical en-bloc oesophagectomy, are during oesophagectomy for carcinoma when the stomach is not available as a replacement organ by virtue of disease or previous surgery, in which case the distal end of the conduit may be anastomosed to a Roux-en-Y jejunal loop, and following oesophagectomy for severe benign disease of the oesophagus, e.g. following caustic ingestion, in which the distal anastomosis is performed end to side into the posterior aspect of the upper third of the stomach, the main vagal trunks being preserved, if possible.

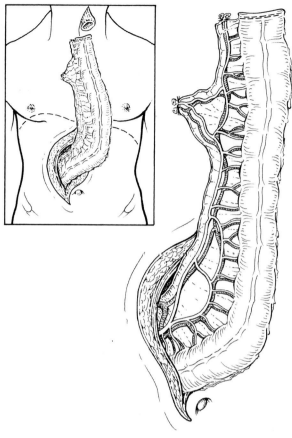

Figure 14.14

The prepared colonic conduit, adequacy of length being confirmed. The middle colic vessels have been divided and ligated, vascularity being through the upper left colic artery and marginal arcade.

Transhiatal (abdominocervical) oesophagectomy

This technique was first described by Grey Turner in 1933 as a means of performing oesophageal resection without the dangers of thoracotomy. It has undergone a revival in the last two decades following further reports of its use by Kirk in 1974[63] and Orringer and Sloane in 1978.[64] The perceived advantage of this approach when first performed was that it enabled oesophageal resection to be undertaken without the hazards of thoracotomy. More recently, it was believed that the morbidity and mortality of oesophageal resection could be reduced by the avoidance of thoracotomy.

Operative technique

A preliminary laparotomy is performed and the stomach mobilized as in the Lewis–Tanner procedure. At the time of mobilizing the distal oesophagus within the oesophageal hiatus, an attempt should be made to determine any fixity of the oesophageal tumour, assuming that it can be palpated. If there is no undue fixity, or the tumour cannot be palpated, the cervical phase of the procedure is commenced. The cervical oesophagus is exposed as described previously (Figures 14.10 and 14.11). Mobilization of the oesophagus is continued

directly posterior to the prevertebral fascia, which is followed bluntly with the index finger into the superior mediastinum. The plane between the trachea and oesophagus is developed by sharp dissection, keeping posterior to the tracheo-oesophageal groove in order to avoid injury to the recurrent laryngeal nerve. The cervical oesophagus is then bluntly mobilized circumferentially, and a sling or rubber drain is passed around the oesophagus. Gentle proximal traction on this enables continuation of blunt dissection well into the superior mediastinum, and mobilization from the carina. For proximal lesions, it may be necessary to assess the degree of fixity from this aspect. In certain middle third tumours, it may not be possible to assess the degree of fixity either from the abdominal or cervical aspect, and in these circumstances many would feel this approach to be contraindicated, as there is a risk of significant haemorrhage if unsuspected fixity to contiguous structures is present.

Once a decision has been taken to proceed, the mediastinal dissection is performed, initially from the abdominal aspect. While applying downward traction to the sling around the gastro-oesophageal junction, blunt finger dissection is continued with the palmar surface of the fingers towards the oesophagus, initially posteriorly, then laterally on each side, and finally anteriorly until the hand can be inserted through the oesophageal hiatus (Figure 14.16). Care must be taken to maintain the dissection close to the oesophagus so as not to injure the pleura or trachea, and the final stage of the mediastinal dissection is assisted by passing a swab on a stick posterior to the oesophagus through the cervical incision (Figure 14.17). Once the fingers from below meet the swab on a stick, the oesophagus can be gently avulsed from its bed, and the

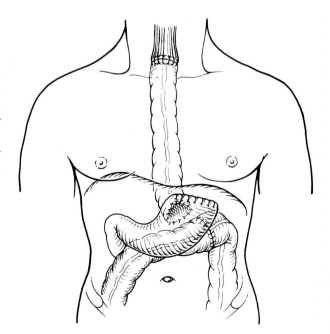

Figure 14.15

The conduit has been anastomosed to the oesophagus proximally and the stomach distally, and the colocolic anastomosis has been performed.

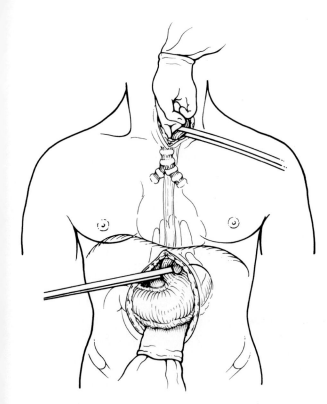

Figure 14.16
Abdominocervical (transhiatal) oesophagogastrectomy showing initial proximal and distal dissection.

posterior dissection is complete. The anterior dissection is then commenced, again with the palmar aspect of the hand towards the oesophagus, gently breaking down the adhesions between the oesophagus and the posterior aspect of the pericardium and the carina. Once more, dissection must be kept very close to the oesophagus in order to avoid damage to these structures. The lateral dissection is then completed, being facilitated by initially retracting the upper thoracic oesophagus into the cervical wound and subsequently gently stripping the lateral attachments from either side of the oesophagus from below, while traction is applied to the distal sling. Once the oesophagus has been completely mobilized, the upper thoracic oesophagus is drawn into the cervical wound and transected, and a rubber drain is sutured to the distal part of the divided oesophagus. The thoracic oesophagus and attached drain are then withdrawn into the abdominal cavity, the gastric tube completed and the oesophagus, lesser curvature and cardia resected, cutting the rubber drain just above its insertion into the thoracic oesophagus, the drain then being sutured to the apex of the gastric tube (Figure 14.18). After ensuring there is no significant bleeding, gentle traction on the proximal end of the rubber drain from outside the cervical incision with simultaneous gentle feeding of the stomach through the oesophageal hiatus enables the gastric tube to be placed into the mediastinum and its apex to be delivered into the cervical wound. The oesophagogastric anastomosis is then performed as described previously.

The principal advantage of the transhiatal approach is that it avoids thoracotomy and therefore reduces operating time. However, it does have certain disadvantages. First, by necessity, dissection must be kept close to the oesophagus, which precludes what many would consider to be an adequate lymphadenectomy and risks leaving tumour behind in T3 lesions. Secondly, it is associated with a higher incidence of some complications than the Lewis–Tanner procedure, because of technical factors. Blunt dissection with the hand and lower forearm in the mediastinum can result in haemodynamic instability. Although the terminal branches of vessels supplying the oesophagus are relatively small and likely to thrombose readily,[65] avulsion as opposed to division of these vessels between ligatures or clips is usually associated with increased blood loss, and certainly the incidence of major bleeding is higher than after a thoracoabdominal approach.[66] There is also a higher incidence of complications not normally associated with the Lewis–Tanner approach, namely recurrent laryngeal nerve paresis, tracheobronchial injuries and damage to the thoracic duct.[67,68] The results of several series show that the incidence of pulmonary complications, is, in fact, no less than after thoracotomy, because of the risk of pleural and tracheobronchial injury.[66–69] The reported perioperative mortality is also similar to that following thoracoabdominal resection, although one series reported a hospital mortality of 2.4% when the procedure was applied to adenocarcinomas of the oesophagogastric junction only.[69] Although survival equivalent to that following thoracoabdominal resection is claimed by advocates of the transhiatal technique, in the belief that it is the biology of the tumour rather than radicality of the procedure which determines

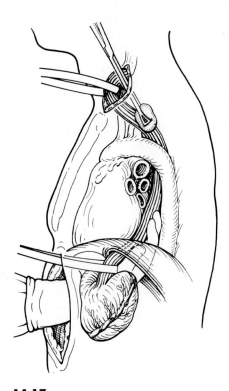

Figure 14.17
Proximal dissection extended using a swab on a stick. Distal dissection continued until the hand and the swab on a stick meet.

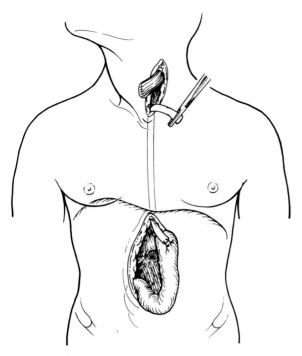

Figure 14.18
Drain attached to proximal end of the mobilized stomach, which is then drawn into the neck for the oesophagogastric anastomosis.

survival, there are few good long-term studies comparing each approach with tumours of equivalent staging. Some preliminary results are emerging to suggest that in T3 and node-positive tumours, survival is less favourable following transhiatal resection, but these need to be confirmed. It is generally believed that transhiatal resection may have a place in early oesophageal cancer and in proximal and distal lesions where there is a contraindication to thoracotomy and the tumour itself can be dissected under direct vision. There is a general consensus that transhiatal resection is inappropriate for middle third tumours which may be locally advanced, because of the

risks of bleeding and damage to contiguous structures by blind, blunt dissection.

Endoscopic trans-mediastinal oesophagectomy

This is a variant of blunt abdominocervical oesophagectomy in which the mediastinal dissection is performed through a specially designed endoscope which is inserted into the mediastinum through a left cervical incision[70] (Figure 14.19). It has the advantage that the entire dissection is performed under direct vision, and bleeding of significant sized vessels can be coagulated and suction applied. Early reports suggest that this technique is associated with less morbidity than open transhiatal oesophagectomy. It suffers the same theoretical disadvantage of being limited to a localized and less radical dissection and lymphadenectomy than the Lewis–Tanner technique, but long-term studies are awaited.

Operative technique

The abdominal phase of the procedure is performed as previously described. A left cervical incision is made, and the mediastinoscope is inserted into the retropharyngeal space. The dissection is kept close to the oesophagus, and areolar tissue surrounding it can be separated by blunt dissection. Blood vessels can be grasped by appropriately insulated forceps and coagulated using monopolar diathermy, and denser adhesions can be divided with scissors. As with transhiatal dissection, the dissection is initiated posterior to the oesophagus, then moving to the lateral and anterior aspects. A plastic tube is fed by the abdominal operator between the jaws of a grasping forceps passed down the mediastinoscope, which is then withdrawn into the neck. After transection of the oesophagus, the plastic tube is sutured to the thoracic oesophagus immediately distal to the transection, and delivered into the abdomen by traction on the distal end of the tube. After completion of the gastric tube and resection of the specimen, the mediastinoscope is then passed from above, checking that haemostasis is

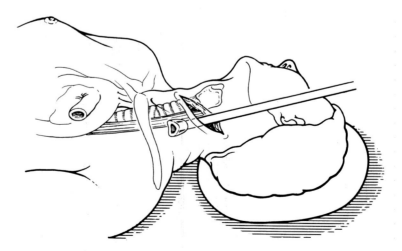

Figure 14.19
The mediastinoscope being inserted through a cervical incision, and blunt dissection posterior to the oesophagus being commenced.

complete, and by suturing the plastic tube to the apex of the gastric tube, a similar manoeuvre delivers the proximal stomach into the neck for the oesophagogastric anastomosis.

Thoracoscopically assisted oesophagogastrectomy

The recent advent of video-assisted laparoscopic and thorascopic surgery has been applied to mobilization of the intrathoracic oesophagus as part of a three-phase oesophagogastrectomy (Figure 14.20). The perceived advantages are the avoidance of morbidity associated with thoracotomy and the ability to perform a similar oesophageal and nodal dissection to that performed at thoracotomy.

Operative technique

The thoracoscopic phase is performed first, through the right chest with the patient in a prone or semiprone position, and with a double-lumen endobronchial tube to facilitate collapse of the right lung. Although some workers advocate insufflation of CO_2 at low pressure, this is not strictly necessary. Several port positions have been described, but usually four ports are used, a posterior and posterolateral port in the upper thorax and similarly placed ports in the lower thorax. The dissection is performed on similar principles to that at thoracotomy, with division of the mediastinal pleura on either side of the oesophagus, and division of the arch of the azygos vein using a miniature linear stapler. Dissection is performed in the standard way, with a mixture of sharp and blunt dissection under direct vision, and individual vessels are divided between clips. It is claimed that equivalent nodal dissection can be performed to that at thoracotomy. Once thoracoscopic mobilization has been completed, the abdominal and cervical phases are performed simultaneously as described previously and apical and basal chest drains are inserted through two of the port sites.

Early experience with thoracoscopic oesophageal mobilization suggests that it is feasible in the majority of cases,

although time consuming, taking 2–3 h. Early reports have suggested hospital mortality up to 25%, with bleeding and thoracic duct injuries being the major complications. Although these figures may relate to the 'learning curve', progress must be made with extreme caution, as thoracotomy, particularly in the era of thoracic epidural analgesia, is no longer associated with significant morbidity and mortality, hospital mortality for thoracoabdominal resection being around 5% in most specialist units. Furthermore, it remains to be proven whether long term survival is equivalent to that achieved by conventional surgery.

POSTOPERATIVE MANAGEMENT

It is advisable to manage patients in the early stages after oesophageal resection in the intensive therapy unit (ITU) where careful monitoring of cardiorespiratory parameters can be undertaken. The duration of stay in ITU depends on many factors, including the type of procedure undertaken, the policy regarding elective ventilation, the incidence of postoperative complications and staffing issues. Prior to 1985, it was our practice to electively ventilate all patients following thoracoabdominal oesophagogastrectomy for 24 h, which was inevitably associated with several days stay in the ITU. Since 1985, we have routinely used thoracic epidural analgesia, both peroperatively and postoperatively, and have extubated the vast majority of patients soon after the end of the operative procedure.[43] This has resulted in a considerable reduction in the time spent in the ITU, the majority of patients currently staying only overnight. Other recent reports of early extubation have resulted in similar trends.[71] Advocates of the radical en-bloc oesophagectomy recommend elective ventilation for 3–4 days postoperatively, necessitating a much longer stay in ITU. Somewhat paradoxically, one of the recent communications regarding thoracoscopic oesophageal mobilization reported a mean ITU stay of 7 days.

The mainstays of postoperative management comprise fluid replacement, prevention and management of pulmonary complications and care of the anastomosis. Adequate fluid replacement is monitored by recording central venous pressure, urinary output and haematocrit values. With regard to respiratory complications, intensive physiotherapy is necessary, and we have found this to be much more effective with a fully conscious and cooperative patient with adequate pain relief by epidural analgesia without the depressant effect of systemic opiates on respiration and conscious level. Since adopting this practice, we have noticed a dramatic reduction in the incidence of respiratory complications (see below). In patients who are ventilated, regular endobronchial suction is necessary. The apical chest drain can usually be removed 48 h postoperatively, although it is a wise precaution to precede this by clamping the tube and ensuring that radiological expansion is maintained thereafter. It is our practice to retain the basal drain until anastomotic integrity has been demonstrated.

In view of the rather delicate nature of oesophageal anastomosis, most workers advocate avoidance of oral fluids until anastomotic integrity has been demonstrated. The stomach is kept decompressed by nasogastric aspiration, and it is our

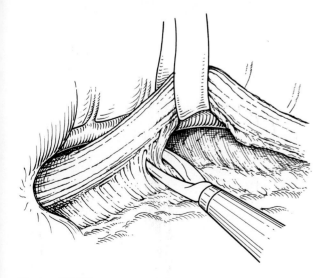

Figure 14.20
Thoracoscopic mobilization. The oesophagus is being mobilized from its bed, aided by sling retraction.

practice to withhold oral fluids until a water-soluble contrast swallow on the fifth postoperative day has confirmed anastomotic integrity. At this stage, oral fluids are commenced and the basal chest drain is removed. The nasogastric tube is removed once it is evident that gastric emptying is occurring satisfactorily. A soft diet is commenced the following day and the patient gradually progressed onto a normal diet, although being advised to take small meals frequently on account of reduced gastric capacity and the possibility of temporary impairment of gastric emptying. Many patients are able to go home by the tenth postoperative day, and the majority within 14 days.

Opinion is divided on the question of nutritional support in the postoperative period. Preoperative correction of nutritional deficiencies has already been discussed, but most patients with oesophageal cancer have suffered some nutritional impairment, and given the fact that it may be a week before a significant oral intake is re-established, it would seem logical on general nutritional and immunological grounds to provide nutritional support during this period. Several studies have addressed this issue,[72-74] and the conclusions of these and a meta-analysis[75] have shown that although there may be some benefit in nutritional status, there is no measurable benefit in clinical parameters, such as incidence of complications and mortality, except in a subset of the most severely malnourished patients. This may relate to the fact that most of these studies have involved nutritional support for 7-10 days, which may be insufficient time for adequate assimilation and translation into measurable clinical benefit. Over the past 20 years, we have variously used total parenteral nutrition, enteral nutrition by percutaneous jejunostomy feeding and by a transoral jejunostomy tube, as well as no nutritional support in all but the most severely malnourished patients. We too have observed no difference in clinical outcome, apart from both mechanical and metabolic complications associated with nutritional support, and our policy over the last 5 years has been not to administer nutritional support routinely, but to administer it preoperatively in the most severely malnourished patients, and postoperatively only if there is any anxiety about anastomotic integrity on the contrast swallow, in which case oral alimentation may be delayed.

COMPLICATIONS OF OESOPHAGEAL RESECTION

Oesophageal resection is one of the most major elective procedures and consequently the potential for complications is high, particularly in centres where these procedures are not performed regularly.[76] Complications of oesophageal resection are divisible into general complications associated with any major surgical procedure, such as haemorrhage, infection, thromboembolic disease and cardiovascular problems, and those specific to the procedure itself. Only this latter group of complications will be discussed here.

Pulmonary complications

Although pulmonary complications may follow any major operative procedure, there is a particular predilection for these following oesophageal resection. These may range from a simple chest infection or basal collapse, through to florid pneumonia, segmental or total pulmonary collapse, persistent pneumothorax, haemothorax or damage to the trachea or bronchus. The pain associated with thoracotomy generally militates against achieving and maintaining full expansion and clearance of secretions, and the administration of systemic opiates only diminishes conscious and respiratory effort. Experience has shown that elective ventilation carries its own problems, associated with the mechanical effects of prolonged intubation, the respiratory depressant effect of drugs administered to enable tolerance of an endotracheal tube, and the haemodynamic effects of prolonged ventilation. In our experience, the greatest advance in this area has been the advent of thoracic epidural analgesia, and since its routine use in our unit since 1985, patients are usually alert and pain-free the morning following surgery, and able to cooperate fully with physiotherapy. This has been associated with a reduction in respiratory complications from 36 to 13%, and in fatal respiratory complications from 5% to 0.[43]

Anastomotic leakage

This has traditionally been one of the most serious risks associated with oesophageal resection. In the 1970s, clinically significant anastomotic dehiscence rates of around 20% were reported, but this had fallen to around 10% in a meta-analysis of over 120 series published during the 1980s.[77] This is undoubtedly associated with improved surgical technique and greater understanding of the factors influencing anastomotic healing, namely preservation of the vascularity and avoidance of tension, together with extremely careful tissue handling. This trend has continued, with specialized centres reporting clinically relevant anastomotic leakage rates of less than 5%.[37,39] The incidence of anastomotic dehiscence does not seem to relate to whether a single-layer or two-layer anastomosis is performed, although anastomoses with absorbable sutures have a higher incidence of leakage than those performed with nonabsorbable material.[78] There is also no evidence that performing a stapled anastomosis reduces the incidence of anastomotic leakage in experienced hands.[54,78] There is no evidence that cervical anastomoses have a lower leakage rate than intrathoracic anastomoses,[58,79] indeed it may be higher.[80] When leakage does occur, the meta-analysis of Muller et al.[78] suggested that it was more likely to be fatal if the anastomosis was intrathoracic, although this was not borne out by a prospective study from a specialist unit.[79]

The clinical presentation of anastomotic leakage is variable, and probably relates to the size of the defect and whether the leakage occurs early or late in the postoperative course. Clinically relevant leaks most commonly occur between the second and seventh postoperative day. If the defect is relatively large, the presentation is usually quite dramatic, with collapse, often severe pain and overwhelming sepsis consequent on mediastinitis, which has a high mortality rate. Smaller defects may present less dramatically with fever and tachycardia. Some very small leaks may only become apparent when the contrast swallow is performed, but these small, subclinical leaks almost invariably heal spontaneously if fasting is continued and nutritional support given. A multicentre study of 339 anastomotic leaks developing in 2400 patients undergoing resection, revealed an inverse relationship between time of development of the leak after surgery and mortality.[81] Mortality for leaks developing within the first week to 10 days postoperatively was 93%, with no survivors when the leak developed before the fourth day. Those presenting later ran a somewhat more benign course, usually presenting as a localized perianastomotic abscess as late as 4 months after surgery, although the mortality associated with 'late' leaks was still 40%. This phenomenon is probably closely related to the size of the original defect, as a study from the same centre reported that as the size of the defect increased from a small punctate one to a large defect and to an almost complete separation, the respective mortality was 19%, 55%, and 71%.[57]

Diagnosis and management of an anastomotic leak relies on awareness of this possibility in a patient with local or systemic signs of sepsis or who becomes haemodynamically unstable. If there is a connection with the pleural cavity, gastric content may be seen emanating from the chest drain and if doubt exists, the pH of the drainage fluid can be tested or the patient given a small amount of methylene blue by mouth. Radiologically, evidence of mediastinal air or fluid may be seen, and, if a pleural fistula occurs, this will be evident also. If the patient's condition is sufficiently stable, confirmation of the existence and size of the leak should be obtained by a limited contrast study using a small dose of a water-soluble contrast medium.

Management of an anastomotic leak depends on the size of the defect, its clinical relevance and the general condition of the patient, against the background of the likely prognosis from the standpoint of tumour staging. Very small defects, and particularly those only detected at routine contrast swallow should be managed conservatively, with continuance of nil by mouth, nasogastric aspiration and nutritional support. Further contrast swallows should be obtained at intervals of 5–7 days, and once healing is complete, oral fluids and subsequent feeding can be administered. Larger defects, but without significant systemic upset or local abscess formation, can be treated by gentle endoscopic intubation, using either a standard oesophageal prosthesis, one fitted with a balloon to isolate the defect, or one of the more recently devised covered Wallstents. Where the defect is large and there is significant systemic upset, mortality is likely to be high and only major reoperative surgery has a chance of salvaging the situation. In this context, the age and likely prognosis must be considered and weighed against the prospect of further surgery, which may involve multiple procedures. If a decision to reoperate is taken, this should be performed as soon as the patient has been resuscitated. The aim of revisional surgery, whatever the level of the anastomosis, must be to remove non-viable tissue, to drain exuded fluid and associated abscesses, to divert proximal and distal to the anastomosis and to provide effective drainage. As with anastomotic leakage elsewhere, it is unlikely in the presence of inflamed and possibly devascularized tissue and sepsis

that primary repair will be successful. Some success has been claimed for covering the defect with an adjacent muscle flap, particularly in patients with incomplete disruption who are operated on within 6 h of dehiscence.[82] However, for major disruptions, most workers agree that the only option is to perform a cervical oesophagostomy, a draining gastrostomy and a feeding jejunostomy, together with drainage of any abscess cavities and excision of any devitalized tissue as indicated previously. Mortality is high, but if the patient survives, subsequent reconstruction will be necessary, with the possibility of having to bridge the defect with a colonic or jejunal interposition.

Chylothorax

Injury to the thoracic duct can occur during any type of oesophageal resection, particularly with the recent emphasis on performing an adequate lymphadenectomy. It is more likely to occur during transhiatal oesophagectomy, particularly in the case of adherent tumours, and of course excision of the thoracic duct is an integral part of radical en-bloc oesophagectomy, and care must be taken to ensure that each end is firmly ligated. During oesophagectomy under direct vision, it is important to identify the thoracic duct, which lies on the vertebral bodies and is related to the azygos vein and the aorta until it reaches the left side of the oesophagus in the upper thorax. It is covered by mediastinal pleura, and becomes smaller as it ascends through the thorax, and therefore may be difficult to see. The difficulty is compounded by the numerous anatomical variations in up to 50% of cases, particularly with several accessory channels and lymphaticovenous anastomoses. Damage to the thoracic duct or a lymphatic channel may be apparent at the time of operation, in which case ligation is necessary. However, many such injuries go unrecognized, which results in the clinical development of chylothorax. In one series of 537 oesophageal resections, the incidence of chylothorax was 0.2% following transthoracic procedures and 10.5% following transhiatal oesophagectomy.[83]

The onset of chylothorax is often insidious, as leakage of chyle initially occurs into the posterior mediastinum and may form a localized collection. It may only be after many days that the collection becomes large enough to leak into the pleural cavity, although if a chest drain is still in situ, an increase in drainage may be noted, together with the characteristic milky appearance, although under fasting conditions, the chest drainage fluid may assume a pale yellow appearance. If the leak is a major one, drainage of up to 2–3 l/day is possible, which soon results in fluid and electrolyte depletion, and particularly a marked fall in serum proteins.

The management of chylothorax depends on the size of the injury, the volume of drainage and whether or not an intrapleural chest drain is already present. If a pleural effusion occurs, this clearly requires drainage. Supportive treatment should be commenced with cessation of feeding, if this has been commenced, and total parenteral nutrition. If a chest drain is present, the volume of chylous drainage can be monitored, and if this is relatively small (less than 400 ml/day), such leaks will often heal spontaneously. However, for large volume leaks, or others which do not resolve, then thoracotomy should be performed together with double ligation of the duct above and below the severed portion, before the patient becomes too fluid and protein depleted. If operation is undertaken, identification of the site of the leakage may be facilitated by administering intralipid via the nasogastric tube preoperatively. The mortality of chylothorax is high, being reported as 46% whether managed conservatively or by surgical intervention.[83]

Injuries to other intrathoracic structures are less common, although injury to the recurrent laryngeal nerve, and tracheobronchial injuries have been described, particularly following transhiatal oesophagectomy.

Impaired gastric emptying

Clinically relevant impairment of gastric emptying is a relatively uncommon complication of oesophagogastrectomy, particularly if attention is directed towards the pylorus. In the study by Fok and Wong,[79] 13% of patients without a pyloroplasty developed frank gastric outlet obstruction whereas no patients who had pyloroplasty developed this complication. In this study, symptomatic reflux of either acid or bile was not a problem, although duodenogastric alkaline reflux is a frequent complication of pyloroplasty used in other situations.[84,85] In our experience using blunt myotomy of the pylorus, the incidence of clinically relevant impairment of gastric emptying has been 5%. Since the availability of endoscopic balloon dilatation of the pylorus, all such patients have been satisfactorily treated by this means, and we have taken the view that we would prefer to treat the 5% who have problems by this relatively non-invasive means rather that run the risk of alkaline reflux, which is now known to be relevant to the development of Barrett's columnar-lined oesophagus and particularly the complications of Barrett's columnar-lined oesophagus including stricture and adenocarcinoma.[86]

Recent studies have demonstrated the benefit of erythromycin and other macrolide analogues in improving gastric motility and gastric emptying following oesophagogastrectomy,[87,88] and this may prove to be another therapeutic option in patients who develop transient impairment of gastric emptying.

Anastomotic stricture

The incidence of benign anastomotic stricture varies depending on the technique used to perform the anastomosis. In sutured anastomosis, the stricture rate is fairly constant in reported series at 7–8%.[1,39] In Wong's[39] study, the incidence of anastomotic stricture following stapled anastomosis was 25%. However, further analysis of the data depending on the size of staple head used showed that when the 25 mm head was used, the incidence of stricture was 43%. It fell to 12.5% when the 25 mm head was used and there were no cases of stricture when the 33 mm head was used. Clearly, therefore, there are advantages to using the largest staple head possible if a stapled anastomosis is used, although it is only usually when the

oesophagus is dilated that the 33 mm head is feasible. This phenomenon is clearly related to the small defect in mucosa to mucosa apposition that occurs with stapled anastomoses, healing taking place by fibrous tissue.

The benign anastomotic strictures that occur following either sutured or stapled anastomosis are usually easily treated by endoscopic dilatation, which should always be accompanied by biopsy to exclude anastomotic recurrence. Rarely, repeated dilatations are necessary, and in such cases, gastro-oesophageal reflux may play a part. Benign anastomotic strictures tend to present within the first three months of surgery, unless they are induced by reflux. Strictures presenting later than this should be regarded as highly suspicious of local anastomotic recurrence. As discussed previously, this should be relatively uncommon if there is adequate longitudinal clearance at the time of surgery, but nonetheless the incidence is about 5%. Management of anastomotic recurrence should be by either intubation, self-expanding metallic stents or laser therapy, which may be supplemented by radiotherapy or chemotherapy depending on the histology of the lesion, the presence of metastatic disease, and the general condition of the patient.

Gastro-oesophageal reflux

The fact that the lower oesophageal sphincter is excised during oesophagogastrectomy, and the stomach brought into the chest, produces a theoretical situation in which gastro-oesophageal reflux might be expected to be a troublesome complication. In reality, the incidence of troublesome reflux symptoms is relatively uncommon, although the actual incidence varies according to the degree of enthusiasm with which the presence of reflux is sought. It also seems to vary with the level of the oesophagogastric anastomosis. In one study which followed-up two groups of patients following oesophagogastrectomy, one of which had a supra-aortic anastomosis and the other having an infra-aortic anastomosis, the incidence of reflux symptoms was 12 and 19%, respectively, half of the patients in each group having an associated stricture.[89] The incidence of gastro-oesophageal reflux was higher in this study when evidence was sought by endoscopy. Endoscopic oesophagitis was present in 29% of patients with a high anastomosis, compared to 95% of those with a low anastomosis. It follows, therefore, that as in gastro-oesophageal reflux disease in the unoperated patient, symptoms are not necessarily a guide to the presence of reflux or oesophagitis, which once more may have bearing on the question of performing pyloroplasty, with its risk of duodenogastric alkaline reflux. All patients in this study had, in fact, undergone pyloroplasty. The lower incidence of reflux with high anastomoses may seem, at first sight, paradoxical, but has been reported by others.[90] The mechanism appears to relate to the translocated stomach acting as a pressure equalizing reservoir between the higher intra-abdominal and lower intrathoracic pressure. When studied in a mechanical model simulating positive intra-abdominal and negative intrathoracic pressure with the anastomosis at various levels, it was found that when the anastomosis was low in the chest, the intragastric pressure was positive, and little different from intra-abdominal pressure. However, as the anastomosis was placed more proximally, the intragastric pressure became negative, to a degree proportional to the height of the anastomosis.[89]

As most workers now perform a high anastomosis, either at the apex of the mediastinum, or in the neck for reasons of clearance, the incidence of reflux symptoms is relatively low. In our experience, the overall incidence was 8%, and only half of these patients had troublesome symptoms, but all were satisfactorily managed by conservative means.

Nutritional problems

Nutritional problems following oesophageal resection have not been studied in great detail. Certainly, the majority of patients with oesophageal cancer have lost weight preoperatively, and more is likely to be lost perioperatively, irrespective of whether nutritional support is given. In our experience, following oesophagogastrectomy 91% of patients are able to swallow entirely normally[12] and the vast majority gain weight postoperatively, although by no means all are restored to their previously normal weight.[1] This is likely to relate to the consequences of vagotomy, gastric resection and transposition of the stomach on its motility and reservoir function. Although it was believed for a long time that a transposed gastric tube behaved as an inert conduit, more recent studies have shown that it is capable of function, albeit diminished, and that this can be enhanced by erythromycin and other macrolide analogues[88,91] There is obviously considerable scope for further studies of nutritional status following oesophagogastrectomy and the possibility of influencing this.

RESULTS OF RESECTION OF OESOPHAGEAL CANCER

The principal criteria used to assess the results of resection include perioperative mortality and morbidity, duration of survival and quality of life. Each of these is discussed in turn.

Mortality and morbidity

With improvements in preoperative preparation, operative and anaesthetic technique and postoperative management, there has been a significant decline in postoperative mortality and morbidity. At the time of the first meta-analysis in 1980,[2] the mean hospital mortality following oesophageal resection was reported as 29%, although this review included cases performed up to 40 years previously. By the time of the next meta-analysis published in 1990,[78] mean hospital mortality was reported as 16%, this review being restricted to series reported in the 1980s. This included many series from specialized centres with hospital mortality less than 10%. In our series of 156 resections performed over a 15-year period, hospital mortality was 8.3% overall, and 6.6% in the period 1985–1990 since the routine use of thoracic epidural analgesia.[1,43] Review of the various series shows that there is little difference in hospital mortality between the various operative procedures performed, be it a Lewis–Tanner procedure, a three-phase oesophagectomy, a radical en-bloc resection or transhiatal resection. Currently, the

Table 14.4 Causes of hospital 30 day mortality in 156 resected patients 1975–1990

CAUSE OF DEATH	NUMBER
Respiratory failure	4
Anastomotic leakage	2
Cardiac failure	2
Septicaemia	2
Pulmonary embolus	1
Peritonitis (dislodgment of feeding jejunostomy)	1
Massive haemorrhage (from pulmonary vessel after Swan–Ganz insertion)	1
Total	13 (8.6%)

early reports of thoracoscopic mobilization have increased, rather than decreased this mortality. In the meta-analysis of Muller and colleagues,[78] hospital mortality did not appear to relate to cell type or the level of the tumour. However, tumour stage *per se* did not seem to have an influence on hospital mortality, although this was significantly higher for palliative resections compared to those performed with curative intent. Two other factors which have been shown to have a bearing on hospital mortality are the experience of the operating surgeon[76] and geography – Japanese and Chinese centres consistently reporting very low hospital mortality.[78] The most frequent causes of death are cardiorespiratory problems, anastomotic dehiscence and sepsis, the causes of death in 13 patients in our series being shown in Table 14.4.

Perioperative morbidity associated with oesophagectomy is, as discussed previously, related both to the general morbidity associated with major surgery, as well as specific problems relating to oesophageal resection, particularly respiratory complications and anastomotic dehiscence, the incidence of which have been discussed. The incidence of perioperative morbidity is variously reported at 30–50%, depending on the criteria used to define morbidity, such as whether simple chest infections or wound infections are included. However, in general terms, the incidence of perioperative morbidity, as with mortality, appears to be falling with improvement in pre- and postoperative care and surgical and anaesthetic technique. The influence of the use of thoracic epidural analgesia and early extubation following resection on respiratory complications are shown in Table 14.5.

Risk factors for the development of fatal and non-fatal

Table 14.5 Influence of thoracic epidural analgesia

PARAMETER	1975–1985 (NO THORACIC EPIDURAL)	1985–1990 (THORACIC EPIDURAL USED ROUTINELY)
Number of patients	81	75
Postoperative ventilation	81	5 (6.7%)
Respiratory complications	29 (36%)	10 (13.3%)
Fatal respiratory complications	4 (4.9%)	0
Fatal anastomotic leakage	1 (1.2%)	1 (1.3%)
30 day/hospital mortality	8 (9.9%)	5 (6.7%)

complications can be divisible into preoperative, operative and postoperative. Preoperative factors have been discussed in detail under **Patient Selection**, and comprise principally age, nutritional status and the presence of intercurrent disease, principally of the cardiovascular and respiratory systems. Operative factors obviously include operative technique, particularly in fashioning the anastomosis. The type of operation performed for tumours of equivalent stage has only a limited influence. Clearly, radical en-bloc oesophagectomy is a more major undertaking than a Lewis–Tanner procedure, requiring multiple anastomoses and care in preserving the vascularity of the colonic conduit, but in skilled hands, the morbidity and mortality is only marginally higher than that following the Lewis–Tanner procedure. Procedures which have been designed to be less invasive, such as transhiatal oesophagectomy and thoracoscopic mobilization as part of a three-phase procedure have not been shown to reduce morbidity or mortality. The stage of the disease, however, is an important factor in determining morbidity and mortality. The risk of major haemorrhage or damage to contiguous structures is considerably greater if the tumour or its metastatic lymph nodes are densely adherent to those structures, especially if a blunt transhiatal dissection is performed. In a multivariate analysis by Law and colleagues,[30] stage of the disease was the major variable which predicted morbidity and mortality, and in particular whether the surgical procedure was regarded as potentially curative or palliative. Presumably this relates not only to technical factors of adherence to contiguous structures, but also to nutritional and immunological consequences of advanced disease, as those patients undergoing a palliative bypass procedure have the highest morbidity and mortality.[30,78] In the postoperative phase, the combination of thoracic epidural analgesia and early extubation has been associated with a significant decrease in morbidity and mortality,[43,71] which relates to the increasing evidence that mechanical ventilation is associated with alveolar trauma and pulmonary oedema.[92,93] The other major factor in the postoperative course is the necessity to reoperate following thoracoabdominal resection, which is associated with a high mortality whether for bleeding, chylothorax or anastomotic leakage.

Survival

In general terms, there appears to have been little improvement in overall survival following resection for oesophageal carcinoma over the last four decades. Although the various improvements in pre- and postoperative care, operative technique and staging have reduced morbidity and mortality and increased resectability rate, there does not appear to have been any concomitant improvement in overall five-year survival, which was 18% in the first meta-analysis[2] and 20% in the most recent.[78] Strict comparison is difficult because of the wide variation in tumour staging and relative proportions of adenocarcinoma and squamous lesions in reported series.

With regard to determinants of survival, the stage of the disease is the overriding factor. T1 lesions are universally reported with excellent five-year survival rates ranging from 68 to 83%

for both Eastern and Western series.[1,94,95] Such lesions, however, are relatively uncommon in the West, comprising only 10% of our series compared to around 30% in collective series from Japan[95] and 70% in areas of high incidence, such as the Linxian province in Northern China where screening programmes exist.[96] As the degree of wall penetration increases, so does the likelihood of nodal metastases, resulting in an inverse relationship to survival.

In a multicentre prospective study conducted by OESO (Organisation Internationale d'Etudes Statistiques pour les Maladies de l'Oesophage) involving over 700 reported cases, the incidence of nodal metastases rose progressively from 14% in T1 lesions to 72% in T3 lesions.[57] This is reflected in survival; 5-year survival for T3 lesions rarely exceeding 10%.[97,98] Although the more advanced the T stage of the tumour, the greater the likelihood of nodal involvement, the fact that each of these parameters has been identified as independent prognostic variables in several multivariant analyses[3,95] is illustrated by the finding that the relatively few patients with T3 tumours but no nodal metastases have a 5-year survival of 34% compared to 8% for the majority with nodal metastases.[97] In addition to the presence or absence of nodal metastases, both the number of involved nodes and their distribution appear relevant. Roder and colleagues[99] showed a gradual reduction in survival with increasing numbers of nodal metastases, 5-year survival in node negative cases exceeding 40%, falling to around 10% with up to seven involved nodes and with no 5-year survival if the number of positive nodes exceeded seven.

As an extension to the influence of the number of involved nodes, Roder and colleagues[99] found the ratio of involved to excised nodes to be a highly significant predictor of survival, the higher the ratio the poorer the survival, which provides theoretical support for the concept of performing an adequate lymphadenopathy. Other factors relating to the influence of nodal involvement on prognosis include the size and distribution of the nodal metastases. Patients with positive nodes greater than 1 cm in diameter and those with nodes in two or three fields had a poorer prognosis than those with smaller nodes, or nodes confined to a single field.[95] The distance of the nodal involvement from the site of the primary tumour seems to play a part, no 5-year survival being reported by Ide and colleagues[95] for lower third tumours with cervical nodal metastases, and extensive coeliac lymphadenopathy being rarely associated with 5-year survival, particularly with more proximally situated tumours.[98]

The influence of cell type on survival is somewhat controversial. In the meta-analysis by Muller and colleagues[78] it was noted that the series reporting only results of squamous cell carcinoma had a mean 5-year survival rate of 24% compared to 18% for those series comprising both squamous and adenocarcinomas. Other studies have reported no difference in survival between adenocarcinoma and squamous lesions.[3] In our series, although there was no difference in survival according to cell type for tumours of equivalent staging, adenocarcinomas tended to be more advanced at the time of presentation, 85% having nodal involvement compared to 60% with squamous lesions. Of 81 resected patients followed-up for more than 5 years, overall 5-year survival was 17.3%, the figure for squamous lesions and adenocarcinoma being 23% and 9.1%, respectively. The mean 5-year survival for T1 lesions was 75% and for node-negative lesions 47%, there being little difference between squamous and adenocarcinomas. However, for node-positive lesions, 10% of patients with squamous lesions survived 5 years, whereas none of our node-positive adenocarcinomas, all of whom had extensive coeliac nodal involvement, survived 5 years (Tables 14.6 and 14.7).

Other factors which may influence survival are the type of resection performed and the use of adjuvant therapy, either chemotherapy, radiotherapy or both. With regard to the surgical resection, debate has centred around whether a transhiatal resection is oncologically sound and associated with survival as good as with a two- or three-phase oesophagectomy, whether survival is increased with a radical en-bloc resection, and whether extensive lymphadenectomy confers additional benefit. It is consistently agreed that resections considered to be curative after completion of the procedure are associated with a better prognosis than those considered to be palliative, with residual tumour or involved nodes left behind. In the meta-analysis by Muller et al.[78] the 5-year survival rate of patients undergoing what was felt to be 'curative' surgery was 23%, compared to 2% when the procedure was considered to be palliative. In specialized centres, the trend is the same although the actual results are better; Roder and colleagues[3] reported 5-year survival of 31% for patients with complete macroscopic and microscopic (R0) resection compared with 7% for patients with residual microscopic disease (R1 resection) and 0 in those with residual macroscopic tumour following resection (R2 resection). On this basis, doubt has been cast on the ability of a transhiatal resection to be adequate in all but the earliest tumours. Although there have been no strictly randomized prospective studies. looking at 5-year survival, Peracchia et al.[100] observed equivalent survival following transhiatal and thoracoabdominal oesophagectomy with lymphadenectomy following a curative (R0) resection, but in the absence of nodal metastases, 5-year survival after thoraco-abdominal resection was 41% compared to 29% after transhiatal resection. Furthermore, the incidence of locoregional occurrence was greater after transhiatal oesophagectomy suggesting that an inadequate lymphadenopathy was performed during transhiatal oesophagectomy, leading to tumour understaging. There is also evidence that patients with intermediate stage disease (clinical stage II) had a lower 5-year survival after transhiatal oesophagectomy than after thoracoabdominal resection, particularly for tumours of the upper thoracic oesophagus.[100]

Table 14.6 Five-year survival according to tumour characteristics (%)

	ALL TUMOURS	SQUAMOUS	ADENO
All stages	17.3	23	9.1
Node positive	6.1	10.3	0
Node negative	46.8	47.4	40
Superficial	75	71	100

Table 14.7 Distribution according to tumour characteristics (%)

	ALL TUMOURS	SQUAMOUS	ADENO
All stages	100	59	41
Node Positive	70.4	60.4	84.4
Node Negative	27.2	39.6	15.1
Superficial	9.9	14.6	3

The radical en-bloc resection was proposed as a means of obtaining greater clearance and hence improving survival.[61] This procedure would appear to be more likely to achieve the objectives of increasing the likelihood of an R0 resection and increasing the ratio of non-involved to involved nodes, and therefore improve survival. Skinner et al.[101] compared survival following radical en-bloc resection between two time periods: one when all resectable patients were treated with a radical en-bloc oesophagectomy, and one where only lesions staged pre-operatively as T1, N0–1 were so treated, patients with more advanced disease being treated with a standard oesophagectomy. There was little difference in 5-year survival of around 20% between the time periods when radical en-bloc oesophagectomy was used for all resectable cases, and that when it was reserved for the most favourable. In the latter period, when standard oesophagectomy was reserved for relatively unfavourable cases, this was associated with a very low 5-year survival rate, which probably reflects the advanced stage of the disease as well as the different surgical procedures. Indeed, when the more favourable cases treated by radical en-bloc resection were analysed stage for stage, 5-year survival for T1, N0 tumours was 60%, for all node-negative patients 40% and all node-positive patients 6%. These figures are little different from our results for two- or three-phase oesophagogastrectomy shown in Table 14.6, and it has been suggested that whereas radical en-bloc oesophaectomy may result in less mediastinal recurrences, the evidence in favour of improved 5-year survival over two- or three-phase oesophagogastrectomy with lymphadenectomy for tumours of equivalent staging, is inconclusive.[3,102] It appears, therefore, that for all but the very earliest of tumours, there is a minimal acceptable standard of resection which comprises subtotal or total oesophagectomy and lymphadenectomy, and that currently proposed more radical alternatives do not significantly improve 5-year survival. This difficulty in improving overall survival despite genuine attempts based on sound oncological principles has led to evaluation of ultraradical or three-field lymphadenectomy and multimodal therapy.

Three-field dissection

The fact that nodal metastases from oesophageal cancer can occur in nodal groups at some considerable distance from the primary lesion has been known for some time, since the classic studies of Akiyama et al.[40] They showed that involvement of the superior mediastinal nodes was present in almost 30% of patients with upper thoracic tumours, 11% with mid-thoracic tumours and even in 10% of patients with tumours of the distal oesophagus. More recently, studies from the same centre with more extensive nodal dissection and staging showed that in 182 patients, 34.1% had cervical nodal metastases, 60% had positive mediastinal nodes and 50% had positive abdominal nodes.[103] The incidence of positive cervical nodes was even higher with proximally situated tumours, being 43%, and even 29% with tumours of the lower third. Furthermore, nodal metastases may 'skip' groups of nodes in almost 50% of cases; for example there may be metastases in the N2 and N3 nodes, with no involvment of the N1 group.[104] These data have clearly shown that many tumours are, firstly, understaged, and, secondly, may be undertreated unless attention is directed towards the superior mediastinal and cervical nodes.

Most centres from the West have restricted lymphadenectomy to the abdominal and lower and mid-mediastinal nodes in the belief that gross and distant nodal involvement signify systemic disease, but several recent studies, emanating mostly from Japan, have suggested that more extensive lymphadenectomy involving the superior mediastinal and cervical nodes may be associated with improved survival. Ide and colleagues[95] reported a 60% actuarial 5-year survival when a two-field dissection was performed and extended to involve the superior mediastinal nodes. In addition to the abdominal dissection which included the lesser curvature, left gastric and coeliac nodes and those around the origin of its branches, together with the mid- and lower mediastinal group, including the paraoesophageal, subcarinal, hilar and tracheobronchial nodes, the dissection extended to the superior mediastinal nodes, including the paratracheal groups and those related to the brachiocephalic artery, which are in close proximity to the right and left recurrent laryngeal nerves. The 5-year survival among 223 such cases was 38.3%, compared to 23.5% among historical controls who did not undergo superior mediastinal dissection. Subsequently, three-field dissection was advocated, including bilateral cervical dissection of the deep lateral nodes, situated along the accessory nerve of the lower part of the neck, the deep external nodes around the internal jugular vein and including the supraclavicular nodes and the deep internal nodes including the paraoesophageal and paratracheal nodes of the neck closely related to the recurrent laryngeal nerve. Kato and colleagues[105] reported a 5 year survival of 49% after three-field dissection, compared to 34% for patients undergoing two-field dissection, although the two groups were not strictly comparable. A Japanese nationwide study compared approximately 1800 patients undergoing three-field lymphadenectomy with approximately 800 undergoing a two-field dissection.[106] Overall 5-year survival for the three-field group was 34% compared with 27% for the two-field group, the figures in node-positive patients being 33% and 29%, respectively and for node-negative patients 57% and 45%. This study was not randomized, but the apparent improvement in survival in both groups is noteworthy. This is despite an incidence of 73% of node-positive patients in the three-field group and 59% in the two-field group, the difference possibly reflecting more accurate staging with extensive lymphadenectomy.

As may be expected, extended two- and three-field lymphadenectomy is a somewhat time-consuming procedure, all studies having reported, particularly with three-field dissection, increased operating time of the order of 8 h. Such patients usually require postoperative ventilation, which carries its own morbidity, and in general the incidence of recurrent laryngeal nerve injury appears to be increased. The Japanese nationwide study reported a 14% incidence of nerve injury for extended two-field dissection and 20% for three-field, compared to an incidence of less than 5% for standard two-field dissection. However, very low perioperative mortality is reported, that of Kato and colleagues[105] being 2.6%, and the Japanese nationwide study reporting a figure of 2.8%.[106] Peracchia and colleagues[100] have reported the use of a three-field dissection in a Western series of 40 patients, with a perioperative mortality of only 5% and recurrent laryngeal nerve injury in 7.5%. The long-term survival data are awaited with interest, although this procedure has been performed in selected patients only. Although the preliminary results of three-field dissection give grounds for optimism, a true survival advantage has yet to be confirmed by prospective randomized studies, as has the exact place of this extensive procedure. Currently, there are conflicting reports as to whether the survival advantage is confined to those patients with negative cervical nodes, those with positive cervical nodes or for all patients with oesophageal cancer.[102] What does seem clear is that three-field dissection results in improved staging, the incidence of locoregional recurrence is reduced, and it does appear to improve overall survival in lesions of the upper thoracic oesophagus.

Multimodal therapy

An alternative means of addressing the concept of oesophageal cancer as a systemic disease and the importance of eradication of distant nodal metastases is by adjuvant therapy. There is no evidence that adjuvant chemotherapy or radiotherapy alone, given pre- or postoperatively improves survival. However, there has been interest in various multimodality regimens which combine both chemotherapy and radiotherapy, usually administratered preoperatively, with resectional surgery, on the basis that some chemotherapeutic agents act as sensitizers and potentiate the effects of radiotherapy. Several phase II studies have been performed, combining preoperative radiotherapy with a dose of around 30 Gy with chemotherapy with 5-fluorouracil and cisplatin in combination, although adriamycin, mitomycin and bleomycin have been used. Complete pathological and histopathological response often occurs, the reported frequency of this being 18–40%.[107,109] Wolfe and colleagues[109] reported 5-year survival in excess of 40% in patients receiving multimodal therapy, compared to 25% in historical controls. Other studies have suggested no survival benefit,[107] and several studies have alluded to significant morbidity or even mortality from the chemotherapeutic regimens.[108] Another problem is that in patients who do not respond to chemoradiation, their tumour may progress and they may become unresectable in the interval between initial staging and eventual resection.[109]

As a result of the doubt as to whether a complete

histopathological response equates with prolonged survival, and whether this is influenced by the toxicity of the regimes, a series of prospective randomized trials has begun in many centres. In one such study using preoperative chemotherapy only, there was no survival advantage, but a higher incidence of post operative septic and pulmonary complications in those receiving chemotherapy.[110] In another multicentre study involving 186 patients with squamous cell carcinoma of the oesophagus, there was no survival advantage in patients receiving preoperative chemotherapy or chemoradiation.[111] One recently reported study has suggested a survival advantage for adenocarcinomas,[112] 5-year survival in those receiving multinodal therapy being 32% compared to 6% for those undergoing resection alone, although the latter figure is lower than in many reported series.

Quality of life

With a disease as disabling as oesophageal cancer, and operations of the magnitude of oesophagogastrectomy, which frequently may only be palliative, it is clearly important to measure success of treatment by quality of life as well as duration of survival, particularly with an increasing array of available palliative modalities. Until relatively recently, only restoration of the ability to swallow has been measured and documented. Most oesophageal surgeons agree that resection is the modality which best restores the ability to swallow normally, and as such, offers the best palliation, even if the disease cannot be cured.[12,32,39] In one series which directly compared restoration of normal swallowing between resection, endoscopic intubation and surgical intubation, 91% of patients undergoing resection were able to swallow normally, compared to 33% undergoing endoscopic intubation and 15% undergoing surgical intubation.[12] The procedures were obviously not performed in comparable groups of patients, but the results illustrate that resection can restore the ability to swallow in the vast majority of patients.

The ability to continue in gainful employment following resection has also being documented.[1] As might be expected, this is dependent on age and prognosis. Among patients surviving less than 1 year, only 34% previously in employment returned to work, all of these patients being under the age of 60 years. None of those over the age of 60 who survived less than 1 year returned to work. However, of patients surviving longer than 1 year, 88% of those previously in employment who were below the age of 60 returned to work, this proportion falling to 28% for those over 60 years.

Roder and colleagues[113] reported a more structured quality of life assessment in an attempt to evaluate a variety of physical complaints, psychological complaints and general satisfaction with life. Patients who had undergone oesophagogastrectomy were compared with a group of patients suffering from various types of malignancy and with healthy controls. As might be expected, specific physical complaints in the patients undergoing oesophagectomy were higher than in controls, but no different from patients with other tumours or indeed patients with other illnesses such as coronary artery disease.

These complaints were generally related to postoperative organ dysfunction, such as bloating, nausea and occasionally weakness. Psychological complaints were generally less than those in patients with other tumours, and somewhat surprisingly, overall satisfaction with life was significantly higher than in controls. This was felt to reflect the changed perception of values among patients with potentially fatal illnesses which has been observed in other such situations. The authors concluded that although the quality of life measurements were as good in patients who had undergone oesophagogastrectomy compared to patients with other malignancies or other significant illnesses, this only obtained when the procedure was performed with curative intent. In patients undergoing palliative resection, the scores in all categories were considerably lower.

Fortunately, there are several ongoing studies of quality of life assessment following various forms of treatment for oesophageal cancer. It is clearly important to be aware of these, and with improvements in palliation, such as covered Wallstents and combination of laser with radiotherapy, it will be important to consider such data in planning treatment for those patients in whom a cure is thought to be unlikely.

PALLIATIVE SURGICAL PROCEDURES

With improvements in non-operative palliative modalities (Chapter 15), the use of surgery as a planned means of palliation is decreasing. However, as discussed previously, many resections which begin with curative intent have to be regarded as palliative because of the tumour being more extensive than expected on the basis of staging investigations, particularly where residual tumour is left behind. Furthermore, 5–10% of patients deemed operable at the time of staging investigations will be found to be unresectable at operation. In these circumstances, the surgeon may choose to employ one of the surgical palliative options.

Palliative resection

As overall 5-year survival following resection for oesophageal cancer, certainly in the Western world, rarely exceeds 25%, the view can be taken that some three-quarters of resections undertaken are palliative. Even in node-negative disease, unless with a T1 tumour, 5-year survival of around 50% means that approximately half of such resections are palliative. The difficulty is that in both node-negative disease and even node-positive disease, except where nodal involvement is gross and extensive, it is impossible to predict in an individual case which patients will be cured and which will not. Several factors have been studied with a view to predicting prognosis, including aneuploidy on DNA flow cytometry, expression of the tumour suppressor gene *P53*, amplification of proto-oncogenes and overexpression of epidermal growth factor, but to date only in relatively limited groups of patients and unfortunately with conflicting results.[3] Furthermore, it is believed that patients with resectable disease fare better from the standpoints of both quality of swallowing and mean survival following resection than after any of the currently available palliative modalities. In our series, 1-year survival following resection was 57%, mean survival 24.2 months overall and 36.3 months for squamous lesions, in which the majority of tumours were T3, N1. In published series of laser photocoagulation or intubation, many of which considered T3–4 and node-positive tumours to negate a surgical approach, 1-year survival is usually below 10% and mean survival 5–8 months.[114–116]

At operation, it is usually possible to make a reasonable judgement as to whether the operation will be purely palliative or may be performed with curative attempt. In extreme cases, where tumours are locally advanced and cannot be completely removed, and where lymph nodes are obviously grossly involved and at several sites, most surgeons will consider these as incurable and would only modify the extent of their resection. In less extreme cases, some surgeons would adopt the approach as enunciated by Skinner[61] in performing an ultraradical procedure in those with very early disease who may be considered to be curable, and a less extensive resection in others. Our practice is in accord with that of Wong[29] in performing subtotal oesophagectomy and lymphadenectomy in all cases, and the operation is deemed to be palliative or 'curative' depending on whether an R₀ resection has been achieved.

Surgical bypass procedures

The principal objective of surgical bypass procedures is to achieve a similar degree of palliation to that obtained by resection, in circumstances where the tumour is unresectable. Where it is possible to determine by preoperative staging that the tumour is unlikely to be resectable, or has metastasized, most workers would favour a non-operative approach to palliation, although surgical bypass has retained greater popularity in the Far East and the US. However, despite increased emphasis on preoperative staging, there are still 5–10% of patients initially felt to be operable whose tumours prove to be unresectable at operation. In these circumstances, a palliative bypass procedure may be considered a reasonable alternative, in that the surgery is not of a greater magnitude once the chest is open, and the quality of palliation is comparable to that following resection. Bypass procedures may also provide useful palliation in tracheo-oesophageal fistula, although there is no evidence that this is superior to that provided by endoscopic intubation. A variety of surgical bypass procedures has been employed.

Oesophagogastrostomy

The simplest form of bypass procedure is to anastomose the mobilized gastric fundus end-to-side to the oesophagus proximal to the tumour, although superior results are claimed by dividing the oesophagus proximally, closing the distal end and performing an end-to-end anastomosis between the proximal oesophagus and the gastric fundus.[117] Lam and colleagues[118] described a side-to-side bypass procedure, access being achieved by an incision in the left hemidiaphragm. Good palliation was achieved, but the problems of performing major surgery on those with advanced malignancy were reflected in the 30-day mortality which was close to 40%.

Reversed gastric tube

Heimlich and Winfield[119] described the construction of a tube from the greater curvature of the stomach, based on the left gastroepiploic vessels, of sufficient length to bypass the entire oesophagus and perform an oesophagogastric anastomosis in the neck. Postlethwait[5] reported the use of this technique in 20 patients in whom the gastric tube was placed substernally, with good functional results. The commonest complication was anastomotic leakage.

Kirschner operation

This procedure was initially described in 1920 for the surgical management of benign oesophageal stricture. The stomach is initially mobilized on right gastric and right gastro-epiploic pedicles, following which the oesophagogastric junction is divided and the cardia closed. The stomach is brought up retrosternally or subcutaneously and anastomosed to the cervical oesophagus. The oesophagus is then anastomosed to a Roux-en-Y jejunal loop.

Results of surgical bypass

The main disadvantage of surgical bypass procedures is the application of major surgery to patients who, by definition, have advanced tumours and are usually debilitated and have a limited lifespan. This is reflected in reported results of these procedures with operative mortality in the range 21–41% and a mean survival of approximately 5 months.[5] It is debatable whether such high mortality is justified when the subsequent survival is poor, particularly when other less-invasive means of palliation are now available.

Surgical intubation

This technique is rarely used nowadays, since the advent of fibreoptic endoscopic intubation and self-expanding metallic stents. However, it may be used when tumours are found to be unresectable at operation, and in the small proportion of patients with such locally advanced obstructing and tortuous tumours in whom it is impossible to pass a guide-wire endoscopically or radiologically. In these circumstances, it is usually possible to pass a fine gum-elastic bougie from below at gastrotomy; the bougie is then passed proximally through the mouth, the tail of a Mousseau–Barbin or Celestin tube sutured to the end of the bougie and gradually drawn back into the stomach.

The surgical intubation technique was popularized by Mousseau and colleagues[120] and Celestin,[121] the principle of intubation being the passage of a narrow pilot guide through the tumour. This is passed peroram into the stomach, and at gastrotomy gentle traction is applied until the tube is felt to pass through the tumour and the proximal funnel to rest at the upper margin of the tumour. The tube is then cut to the appropriate length in the stomach and usually sutured at two points to the gastric wall.

The mortality of surgical intubation is little different from palliative surgical bypass, even though the procedure is more minor. This probably reflects the immunodepressive effects of surgery and anaesthesia on already debilitated patients, but it is likely also that perforation, due to splitting of the tumour, occurs more frequently than is realized. The quality of palliation following surgical intubation is inferior to that following resection or surgical bypass; only 15% of patients are restored to normal swallowing, although over 60% are able to take a soft or pureed diet.[12] As might be expected, the mean survival is similar at 5–8 months.

REFERENCES

1. Watson A. Operable esophageal cancer: current results from the West. *World J Surg* 1994; **18:** 361–366.
2. Earlam R & Cunha-Melo JR. Oesophageal squamous cell carcinoma: I. Critical review of surgery. *Br J Surg* 1980; **67:** 381–390.
3. Roder JD, Stein HJ & Siewert JR. Prognostic markers in patients with carcinoma of the oesophagus. *Eur J Gastroenterol Hepatol* 1994; **6:** 663–669.
4. Rosenberg JC, Franklin R & Steiger Z. Squamous cell carcinoma of the thoracic esophagus: an interdisiciplinary approach. *Curr Probl Cancer* 1981; **5:** 1.
5. Postlethwait RW. *Surgery of the Esophagus*, New York: Appleton-Century-Crofts, 1979: 341–414.
6. Huang KC. Surgical treatment of carcinoma of the esophagus: results in 1647 patients. In Stipa S, Belsey RHR & Moraldi A (eds) *Medical and Surgical Problems of the Esophagus.* New York; Academic Press, 1981: 353–359.
7. Watson A. Pathologic changes affecting survival in esophageal cancer. In Delarue NC, Wilkins EW & Wong J (eds) *International Trends in General Thoracic Surgery: Esophageal Cancer.* St Louis: Mosby, 1990: 90–96.
8. Galandiuk S, Hermann RE, Gassman JJ et al. Cancer of the oesophagus. *Ann Surg* 1986; **203:** 101.
9. Akiyama H, Kogure T & Itayi Y. The esophageal axis and its relationship to the resectibility of carcinoma of the esophagus. *Ann Surg* 1972; **176:** 30–36.
10. Mori S, Kasai M, Watanabe T et al. Preoperative assessment for resectability for carcinoma of the thoracic esophagus. I. Esophagram and azygogram. *Ann Surg* 1979; **190:** 100–105.
11. Tytgat GNJ. Non-radiological investigation of the oesophagus. In Watson A & Celestin LR (eds) *Disorders of the Oesophagus.* London: Pitman, 1984: 24–36.
12. Watson A. A study of the quality and duration of survival following resection, endoscopic intubation and surgical intubation in oesophageal carcinoma. *Br J Surg* 1982; **69:** 585–588.
13. Tio TL, Coene PPLO, den Hartog Jager FCA & Tytgat GNJ. Preoperative TNM-classification of oesophageal carcinoma by endosonography. *Hepatogastroenterology* 1990; **37:** 376.
14. Halvorsen RA & Thompson WM. Critical review: oesophageal carcinoma CT findings. *Invest Radiol* 1987; **22:** 84–87.
15. Quint LE, Glazer GM & Orringer MB. Esophageal imaging by MR and CT: study of normal anatomy and neoplasms. *Radiology* 1985; **156:** 727–731.
16. Moss AA, Schnyder P, Thoeni RF & Marguilis AR. Esophageal carcinoma: pre-therapy staging by computed tomography. *A J R* 1981; **136:** 1051–1056.
17. Watson A. Is CT demonstration of enlarged nodes a contra-indication to resection in oesophageal cancer? *Gut* 1989; **30:** 750.
18. Laas J, Scheller E, Haverich A et al. How accurate is the pre-operative staging with computed tomography in esophageal cancer? In *Proceedings of the Third World Congress of the International Society of Diseases of the Esophagus*, 1986: 40.
19. Petrillo R, Balzarini L, Bidoli P et al. Esophageal squamous cell carcinoma: MRI evaluation of mediastinum. *Gastrointest Radiol* 1990; **15:** 275.
20. Takashima S, Takeuchi N, Shiozaki H et al. Carcinoma of the esophagus: CT vs. MR imaging in determining resectability. *A J R* 1991; **156:** 297.
21. Van Overhagen H, Lameris JS, Berger MY et al. Supraclavicular lymph node metastases in carcinoma of the esophagus and gastroesophageal junction: assessment with CT, US and US-guided fine-needle aspiration biopsy. *Radiology* 1991; **179:** 155.
22. Botet JF, Lightdale CJA, Zauber G et al. Preoperative staging of esophageal cancer: comparison of endoscopic US and dynamic CT *Radiology* 1991; **181:** 419.
23. Ziegler K, Sanft C, Zeitz M et al. Evaluation of endosonography in TN staging of oesophageal cancer. *Gut* 1991; **32:** 16.
24. Watson A & Cope C. Endoluminal ultrasonography in staging of oesophageal cancer – the influence of endoscopic dilatation. *Gut* 1995; **36:** 55.
25. Fok M & Wong J. Treatment of oesophageal cancer: curative modalities. *Eur J Gastroenterol Hepatol* 1994; **6:** 676–683.
26. Watson A. Oesophageal cancer – overview. *Eur J Gastroenterol Hepatol* 1994; **6:** 645–648.
27. Watt I, Stewart I, Anderson E et al. Laparoscopy, ultrasound and computed tomography in cancer of the oesophagus and gastric cardia: a prospective comparison for detecting intraabdominal metastases. *Br J Surg* 1989; **76:** 1036.
28. Sikes ED, Jr & Detmer DE. Aging and surgical risk in older citizens of Wisconsin. *Wis Med J* 1979; **78:** 27–30.
29. Wong J. Management of carcinoma of the oesophagus: Art or Science? *J R Coll Surg Edinb* 1981; **26:** 138–148.
30. Law SYK, Fok M & Wong J. Risk analysis in resection of squamous cell carcinoma of the esophagus. *World J Surg* 1994; **18:** 339–346.
31. Nishi M, Hiramastu Y et al. Pulmonary complications after subtotal oesophagectomy. *Br J Surg* 1988; **75:** 527.
32. Keeling P, Gillen P & Hennessy TPJ. Oesophageal resection in the elderly. *Ann R Coll Surg Engl* 1988; **70:** 34–37.
33. Peracchia A, Bandini R, Ruol A et al. Carcinoma of the esophagus in the elderly (70 years of age or over): indications and results of surgery. *Dis Esophagus* 1988; **1:** 147.
34. Maloney JV. The limits of medicine. *Ann Surg* 1981; **194:** 247–255.
35. Little AG. Oesophageal cancer: staging and selection of treatment. *Eur J Gastroenterol Hepatol* 1994; **6:** 670–675.
36. DeMeester TR & Barlow AP. Surgery and current management of cancer of the esophagus and cardia. *Curr Probl Surg* 1988; **25:** 541.
37. Watson A. Surgery for carcinoma of the oesophagus. *Postgrad Med J* 1988; **64:** 860.
38. Holscher AH, Dittler HJ & Siewert JR. Staging of sqamous esophageal cancer: accuracy and value. *World J Surg* 1994; **18:** 312–320.
39. Wong J. Esophageal resection for cancer: the rationale of current practice. *Am J Surg* 1981; **153:** 18–24.
40. Akiyama H, Tsurumaru M, Kawamura T & Ono Y. Principles of surgical treatment for carcinoma of the esophagus. Analysis of lymph node involvment. *Ann Surg* 1981; **194:** 438–446.
41. Lewis I. The surgical treatment of carcinoma of the oesophagus with special reference to a new operation for growths of the middle third. *Br J Surg* 1946; **34:** 18–20.
42. Tanner NC. The present position of carcinoma of the oesophagus. *Postgrad Med J* 1947; **23:** 109–139.
43. Watson A. Influence of thoracic epidural analgesia on outcome after resection for esophageal cancer. *Surgery* 1994; **115:** 429.
44. Fok M, Cheng SWK & Wong J. Pyloroplasty versus no drainage in gastric replacement of the esophagus. *Am J Surg* 1991; **162:** 447–452.
45. Holscher AH, Voit H, Buttermann G & Siewert JR. Function of the intrathoracic stomach as esophageal replacement. *World J Surg* 1988; **12:** 835–844.
46. Mannell A, McKnight A & Esser JD. Role of pyloroplasty in the retrosternal stomach: results of a prospective, randomised, controlled trial. *Br J Surg* 1990; **77:** 57–59.
47. Hinder RA. The effects of posture on the emptying of the intrathoracic vagotomized stomach. *Br J Surg* 1976; **63:** 581–584.
48. McKeown KC. Total oesophagectomy – three staged resection. In Jamieson GG (ed.) *Surgery of the Oesophagus.* Edinburgh: Churchill Livingstone, 1988: 677–686.
49. Orringer MB. Esophageal replacement after transhiatal esophagectomy without thoracotomy. In Nyhus LM & Baker RJ (eds) *Mastery of Surgery.* Boston: Little, Brown, 1992: 569–584.
50. Watson A. Esophogastrectomy for carcinoma. In Nyhus LM & Baker RJ (eds) *Mastery of Surgery.* Boston: Little, Brown 1992: 541–550.
51. Watson A. Sutured oesophageal anastomosis. In Jamieson GG & Debas HT (eds) *Rob & Smith's Operative Surgery: Surgery of the Upper Gastrointestinal Tract.* London: Chapman & Hall, 1994: 79–83.
52. Hopkins RA, Alexander JC & Postlethwait RW. Stapled esophago-gastric anastomosis. *Am J Surg* 1984; **147:** 283–287.
53. Wong J, Cheung H, Lui R et al. Oesophagogastric anastomosis performed with a stapler: the occurrence of leakage and stricture. *Surgery* 1987; **101:** 408.

54. Paterson IM & Wong J. Anastomotic leakage: all avoidable complication of Lewis–Tanner oesophagectomy. *Br J Surg* 1989; **76:** 127–129.

55. Ong GB & Kwong KH. The Lewis–Tanner operation for cancer of the oesophagus. *J R Coll Surg Edinb* 1969; **14:** 3–19.

56. McKeown KC. Trends in oesophageal resection for carcinoma. *Ann R Coll Surg Engl* 1972; **51:** 213–238.

57. Giuli R (ed.) *Cancer of the esophagus (Proceedings of First Polydisciplinary International Congress of OESO),* Paris: Maloine SF Editeur, 1984.

58. Nanson EM. Synchronous combined abdomino-thoraco-cervical oesophagectomy. *Aust NZ J Surg* 1975; **45:** 340–348.

59. Hayes N, Shaw IH, Raimes SA & Griffin SM. Comparison of conventional Lewis–Tanner two-stage oesophagectomy with the synchronous two-team approach. *Br J Surg* 1995; **82:** 95–97.

60. Watson A. Therapeutic options and patient selection in the management of oesophageal carcinoma. In Watson A & Celestin LR (eds) *Disorders of the Oesophagus.* London: Pitman, 1984; 167–186.

61. Skinner DB. En bloc resection for neoplasms of the oesophagus and cardia. *J Thorac Cardiovasc Surg* 1983; **85:** 59–69.

62. DeMeester TR & Lafontaine ER. Surgical therapy. In DeMeester TR & Levin D (eds) *Cancer of the Esophagus.* Orlando: Grune & Stratton, 1985: 141.

63. Kirk RM. Palliative resection of oesophageal carcinoma without formal thoracotomy. *Br J Surg* 1974; **61:** 689–690.

64. Orringer MB & Sloane HE. Esophagectomy without thoracotomy. *J Thorac Cardiovasc Surg* 1978; **76:** 643–654.

65. Leibermann-Meffert D, Luscter U, Neff U et al. Esophagectomy without thoractomy: is there a risk of intramediastinal bleeding? A study on blood supply of the esophagus. *Ann Surg* 1987; **206:** 184–188.

66. Hankins JR, Attor J, Coughlin TR et al. Carcinoma of the esophagus: a comparison of the results of transhiatal versus transthoracic resection. *Ann Thorac Surg* 1989; **47:** 700–705.

67. Giuli R & Sancho-Garnier H. Diagnostic, therapeutic and prognostic features of cancers of the esophagus: results of the international prospective study conducted by the OESO group (790 patients). *Surgery* 1986; **99:** 614–622.

68. Shahian EM, Neptune WB, Ellis FH & Watkins E. Transthoracic versus extra-thoracic esophagectomy: mortality, morbidity and long-term survival. *Ann Thorac Surg* 1986; **40:** 321–322.

69. Finley RJ & Inculet RI. The results of esophagogastrectomy without thoracotomy for adenocarcinoma of the esophagogastric junction. *Ann Surg* 1989; **210:** 535–543.

70. Buess G & Maddern GJ. Endoscopic oesophagectomy. In Jamieson G & Debas HT (eds) *Rob & Smith's Operative Surgery: Surgery of the Upper Gastrointestinal Tract.* London: Chapman & Hall, 1994: 601–606.

71. Caldwell MTP, Murphy PG, Page R et al. Timing of extubation after oesophagectomy. *Br J Surg* 1993; **80:** 1537–1539.

72. Fan ST, Lau WY, Wong KK & Chan YPM. Pre-operative parenteral nutrition in patients with oesophageal cancer: a prospective randomised clinical trial. *Clin Nutr* 1989; **8:** 23–27.

73. Woolfson AMJ & Smith JAR. Elective nutritional support after major surgery: a prospective randomised trial. *Clin Nutr* 1989; **8:** 15–21.

74. Buzby GP, Blovin G, Colling CL et al. Perioperative total parenteral nutrition in surgical patients. *N Engl J Med* 1991; **325:** 525–532.

75. Detzky AS, Baker JP, O'Rourke K & Goel V. Perioperative parenteral nutrition: a meta-analysis. *Ann Intern Med* 1987; **107:** 195–203.

76. Matthews HR, Powell DJ & McConkey CC. Effect of surgical experience on the results of resection for oesophageal carcinoma. *Br J Surg* 1986; **73:** 621–623.

77. Chassin JL. Oesophago-gastrectomy: data favouring end-to-end side anastomosis. *Ann Surg* 1987; **188:** 22–26.

78. Muller JM, Erasmi H, Stelzner M et al. Surgical therapy of oesophageal carcinoma. *Br J Surg* 1990; **78:** 845–857.

79. Fok M, Ah-Chong AK & Wong J. Comparison of a single layer continious hand-sewn method and circular stapling in 580 oesophageal anastomoses. *Br J Surg* 1991; **78:** 342–345.

80. Lerut T, De Leyn P, Goosemans W et al. Surgical strategies in esophageal carcinoma with emphasis on radical lymphadenectomy. *Ann Surg* 1992; **216:** 583–590.

81. Giuli R & Gignoux M. Treatment of carcinoma of the esophagus. *Ann Surg* 1980; **192:** 44–52.

82. Richardson JD, Martin LF, Borzotta AP & Polk HC, Jr. Unifying concepts in treatment of oesophageal leaks. *Am J Surg* 1985; **149:** 157–162.

83. Bolger C, Walsh TN, Tanner WA et al. Chylothorax after oesophagectomy. *Br J Surg* 1991; **78:** 587–588.

84. Meshkinpour H, Marks JW, Schoenfield LJ et al. Reflux gastritis syndrome: mechanism of symptoms. *Gastroenterology* 1980; **79:** 1283–1287.

85. Tytgat GNJ, Offerhaus GJA, Mulder CJJ & van den Berg BTJ. Consequences of gastric surgery for benign conditions: an overview. *Hepatogastroenterology* 1988; **35:** 271–278.

86. Attwood SEA, Barlow AP, Norris TL & Watson A. Barrett's oesophagus: effect of anti-reflux surgery on symptom control and development of complications. *Br J Surg* 1992; **79:** 1050–1053.

87. Hill ADK, Walsh TN, Hamilton D et al. Erythromycin improves emptying of the denervated stomach after oesophagectomy. *Br J Surg* 1993; **80:** 879–881.

88. Walsh TN, Caldwell MTP, Fallon C et al. Gastric motility following oesophagectomy. *Br J Surg* 1995; **82:** 91–94.

89. Hetzer R, Ennker J, Dragojevic D & Borst HG. Management and complications of surgery of the oesophagus – reflux. In Jamieson GG (ed.) *Surgery of the Oesophagus.* Edinburgh: Churchill Livingstone, 1988: 877–892.

90. McKeown KC. Surgical treatment of carcinoma of the oesophagus. *J R Coll Surg Edinb* 1979; **24:** 253–274.

91. Casson AG, Powe J, Inculet R & Finley R. Functional results of gastric interposition following total oesophagectomy. *Clin Nucl Med* 1991; **16:** 918–922.

92. Haake R, Schlichtig R, Ulstad DR & Herischen RR. Barotrauma: pathophysiology, risk factors and prevention. *Chest* 1987; **91:** 608–613.

93. Tsund K, Prato P & Kolobow T. Acute lung injury from mechanical ventilation at moderately high airway pressures. *J Appl Physiol* 1990; **69:** 956–961.

94. Huang GJ. Recognition and treatment of the early lesion. In Delarue NC, Wilkins EW & Wong J (eds) *International Trends in General Thoracic Surgery: Esophageal Cancer.* St Louis: CV Mosby, 1988: 149–154.

95. Ide H, Nakamura T, Hayashi K et al. Esophageal squamous cell carcinoma: pathology and prognosis. *World J Surg* 1994; **18:** 321–330.

96. Wong P & Chein K. Surgical treatment of carcinoma of the esophagus and cardia among the Chinese. *Ann Thorac Surg* 1983; **35:** 143–147.

97. Mannell A. Carcinoma of the esophagus. *Curr Probl Surg* 1982; **557:** 1.

98. Siewert JR, Holscher AH & Dittle HJ. Preoperative staging and risk analysis in esophageal carcinoma. *Hepatogastroenterology* 1990; **37:** 382–387.

99. Roder JD, Busch R, & Stein HJ et al. Ratio of invaded to removed lymph nodes as a predictor of survival in squamous carcinoma of the oesophagus. *Br J Surg* 1994; **81:** 410–413.

100. Peracchia A, Ruol A, & Bordini R et al. Lymph node dissection for cancer of the thoracic esophagus: how extended should it be? Analysis of personal data and review of the literature. *Dis Esophagus* 1992; **5(i)** 69.

101. Skinner DB, Little AG, Ferguson MK et al. Selection of operation for esophageal carcinoma based on staging. *Ann Surg* 1986; **204:** 391–401.

102. Hennessy TPJ. Expectations of oesophageal resection. In Paterson-Brown S & Garden OJ (eds) *Surgical Laparoscopy.* London; WB Saunders, 1994; 351–373.

103. Tsurumaru M, Akiyama H, & Udagawa H et al. Cervical–thoracic–abdominal lymph node dissection for intrathoracic esophageal carcinoma. In Ferguson MK, Little AG & Skinner DB (eds) *Diseases of the Esophagus: Malignant Diseases.* New York: Futura; 1990: 187–196.

104. Fekete F, Gayet B & Molas GJM. Prophylactic operative techniques: thoracic esophageal squamous cell cancer surgery, with special reference to lymph node removal. Delarue NC, Wilkins EW & Wong J (eds) *Esophageal Cancer: International Trends in General Thoracic Surgery.* Louis: Mosby, 1988: 133.

105. Kato H, Tachimori Y, Watanabe H et al. Lymph node metastasis in thoracic esophageal carcinoma. *J Surg Oncol* 1991; **48:** 106–111.

106. Isono K, Sato H & Nakayama K. Result of a nationwide study on the three-field lymph node dissection of esophageal cancer. *Oncology* 1991; **48:** 411.

107. Poplin E, Fleming T, & Leichman L et al. Combined therapies for carcinoma of the esophagus; a Southwest Oncology Group Study (SWOG 8037). *J Clin Oncol* 1987; **5:** 622–628.

108. Forastiere AA, Orringer MB, Perez-Tamayo C et al. Preoperative chemoradiation followed by transhiatal esophagectomy for carcinoma of the esophagus: final report. *J Clin Oncol* 1993; **11:** 1118–1123.

109. Wolfe WG, Vaughn AL & Seigler HF et al. Survival of patients with carcinoma of the esophagus treated with combined-modality therapy. *J Thorac Cardiovasc Surg* 1993; **105:** 749–756.

110. Schlag PM. Randomized trial of preoperative chemotherapy for squamous cell cancer of the esophagus. *Arch Surg* 1992; **127:** 1446–1450.
111. Nygaard K, Hagen S, & Hansen HS et al. Pre-operative radiotherapy prolongs survival in operable esophageal carcinoma: a randomized multicenter study of pre-operative radiotherapy and chemotherapy. The second Scandinavian trial in esophageal cancer. *World J Surg* 1992; **16:** 1104–1110.
112. Walsh TN, Noonan N, Hollywood D et al. A comparison of multinodal therapy and surgery for esophageal adenocarcinoma. *N Engl J Med* 1996; **335:** 462–467.
113. Roder JD Herschach P, Sellschopp A & Siewert JR. Quality of life following oesophagectomy. *Theor Surg* 1991; **6:** 206.
114. Ogilvie AL, Dronfield MW, Ferguson R et al. Palliative intubation of oesophagogastric neoplasms at fibreoptic endoscopy. *Gut* 1982; **23:** 1060–1067.
115. Krasner N & Beard J. Laser irradiation of tumours of the oesophagus and cardia. *Br Med J* 1984; **288:** 829.
116. Loizou LA, Grigg D, Atkinson M et al. A prospective comparison of laser therapy and intubation in endoscopic palliation for malignant dysphagia. *Gastroenterology* 1991; **100:** 1303–1310.
117. Johnson CL & Clagett OT. Palliative esophagogastrectomy for inoperable carcinoma of the esophagogastric junction. *J Thorac Cardiovasc Surg* 1970; **60:** 269–274.
118. Lam KH, Wong J, Lim STK & Ong GB. Intrathoracic gastric bypass of the esophagus found unresectable at exploration. *Br J Surg* 1982; **69:** 71–73.
119. Heimlich HJ & Winfield JN. The use of a gastric tube to replace or bypass the esophagus. *Surgery* 1955; **37:** 540–559.
120. Mousseau M, LeForestier J, Barbin J et al. Place de l'intubation a demeure dans le traitement palliative du cancer de l'oesophage. *Arch Mal Appar Digest* 1956; **45:** 208–216. (In French)
121. Celestin LR. Permanent intubation in inoperable cancer of the oesophagus and cardia. A new tube. *Ann R Coll Surg Engl* 1959; **25:** 165–170.

15

NON-SURGICAL MANAGEMENT OF CARCINOMA OF THE OESOPHAGUS

TG Hayes

INTRODUCTION

Oesophageal carcinoma is a rapidly growing cancer, with a tumour doubling time as short as 5 days.[1] As a consequence most patients in Western countries present with advanced inoperable tumours. Of the remaining patients with potentially operable tumours, a significant proportion have serious medical conditions that make them poor surgical risks. Often there are concurrent cardiac and pulmonary problems caused by the very habits (tobacco and alcohol use) that predisposed them to oesophageal cancer.[2] Thus, non-surgical techniques are very important in the management of oesophageal cancer.

When deciding on the optimal therapy for cancer of the oesophagus, it is important to determine the goals for the patient as an individual. In good performance patients with early stage lesions, therapy with curative intent is possible. In patients with advanced disease and a short life expectancy, the goal should be palliation of dysphagia with the least possible morbidity.

Non-surgical techniques are appropriate in patients with advanced disease. Surgically incurable malignancy is suggested by the presence of distant metastases, tracheo-oesophageal fistula, paralysis of the recurrent laryngeal nerve, or invasion of the aorta or bronchial tree. Non-surgical techniques can also be very effective in management of early oesophageal lesions, with much less morbidity than oesophagectomy, and may be suitable for patients with contraindications to surgery. The many treatment options available for non-surgical management of oesophageal cancer include radiation therapy, chemotherapy and a variety of endoscopic methods for palliating dysphagia that can be used alone or in combination.

RADIOTHERAPY

Patients with unresectable disease or serious comorbid medical conditions have been traditionally referred for external beam radiation therapy as the primary treatment modality. Radiation is administered through a multiple field technique. There are several possible ways in which the fields can be set up. In one

commonly used plan, the beam is initially directed antero-posteriorly and postero-anteriorly (AP–PA fields). Later, oblique fields are used to minimize exposure of the spinal cord and mediastinum.[3] Treatment of the cervical oesophagus requires more complicated techniques because of the changing contour from the neck to the thoracic inlet. Three-dimensional treatment planning using a CT scanner is useful in selecting the optimal beam angles and ports that will give maximal treatment to cancerous tissues while avoiding sensitive normal structures.[4]

There is no relationship between radiation field size and 5-year survival.[5] However, because of the known propensity of oesophageal cancer to have 'skip' lesions, radiation fields are designed to cover the known tumour length plus a margin of 4–6 cm above and below the tumour, with 2–3 cm lateral margins.[3,6] For upper oesophageal cancers, the supraclavicular nodes are typically included in the radiation field. The coeliac axis is included for middle and lower oesophageal tumours, although the incidence of nausea and vomiting increases when irradiating abdominal nodes.[3] The cone down target volume ('boost') should be at least 2.5 cm beyond the tumour in all dimensions. During the boost, positioning the patient in the prone position increases the distance between the oesophagus and spinal cord, allowing the spinal cord to be spared from excessive radiation.

Treatment is delivered using high energy (6–24 mV) photon beams.[3] Older studies in the literature generally used total doses of 50–60 Gy given in approximately 2 Gy fractions.[5,7,8] Doses as high as 70 Gy have been used, but higher doses induce increased toxicity without significant survival benefit.[9] Current recommendations for definitive treatment of oesophageal cancer ('radical radiotherapy') are radiation therapy 5 days a week using 1.8–2 Gy per fraction to a total dose of 60–66 Gy, without scheduled breaks. A dose of 45–50 Gy is used for palliation of dysphagia.[3]

There is radiographic evidence of improvement in 50–60% of patients after radiation therapy. Up to 85% of patients will achieve good palliation of their dysphagia lasting from 5 to 10 months.[4,7] There is no difference in the response of squamous cell carcinomas and adenocarcinomas to radiotherapy. Early stage lesions (less than 5 cm long or not penetrating through the oesophageal wall) have a better prognosis than cancers that are more advanced.[5,8] Lesions in the cervical oesophagus respond better to radical radiotherapy than do lesions in the middle or lower oesophagus. For reasons that are not well understood, the prognosis in females is better than that in males.[7,8]

Despite initial symptomatic improvement, most oesophageal cancer patients treated with radiation eventually develop progressive local disease and distant metastases, leading to death.[10] Five-year survival is below 10% in many series, with a median survival of about 12 months.[5,7,8] No prospective randomized studies have yet been done that directly compare surgery and radiotherapy. Such a trial was attempted by the British Medical Research Council, but closed due to lack of patient accrual.[11]

Side-effects of radiation therapy include oesophagitis, stomatitis, neutropenia, anorexia, nausea and generalized malaise.[5,8] Dysphagia often worsens during the first week of therapy because of inflammation and oedema around the tumour. Patients may need nutritional support during treatment if they lose more than 10% of their body weight. Long-term complications include symptomatic oesophageal strictures in 30–44% of patients and pulmonary fibrosis in 9%.[5,8,12] Radiation myelitis should rarely occur if careful attention is paid to total spinal cord dose. The mean time to development of benign (fibrotic) oesophageal stricture is 14 weeks to 6 months after radiotherapy.[13] It is important to remember, however, that more than half the oesophageal strictures that develop after radiation will be due to recurrent malignancy.

Hyperfractionated radiotherapy has been used in an attempt to shorten the duration of treatment time, lessen costs and improve outcome. By giving more than one radiation treatment each day, there is theoretically less time for the malignant cells to repair sublethal DNA damage. Accelerated fractionation schemes increase local control, especially in early lesions.[14] However, in most studies there is no statistically significant difference in long-term survival between conventional dosing and hyperfractioned radiotherapy. There are more acute complications with hyperfractionated radiation, especially mucositis and oesophagitis. Delayed stricture formation also occurs.[13]

Brachytherapy, or intraluminal application of a radioactive source, has been studied extensively in oesophageal cancer. To perform this technique, a hollow 'afterloading' catheter containing radio-opaque markings is inserted into the oesophagus. After ensuring proper positioning by radiography, a radioactive source is placed into the catheter for a variable amount of time and then removed. The use of the afterloading catheter reduces exposure of medical personnel to radioactivity and allows for fine adjustments in dosimetry. Various radioisotopes can be used for brachytherapy. Cesium-137 provides a moderate dose rate of approximately 160–170 cGy/h.[15] For higher dose rate radiation, iridium-92 wire or cobalt-60 pellets can be used.[16,17] The use of ^{92}Ir has the advantage of a much shorter time of application (15–30 min vs 2–12 h), which lessens the period that the patient must have the intraluminal catheter in place.[15,16] However, the low dose rate application has a greater margin of safety and fewer side-effects.[18]

Intraluminal application of radioactivity ensures that a very high radiation dose is delivered directly to the tumour, as much as 15 Gy in one sitting.[16] Brachytherapy is best suited for circumferential tumours, as radiation is distributed in a cylindrical fashion around the radiation source and might otherwise damage healthy tissue. The American Brachytherapy Society considers patients to be good candidates for definitive treatment with brachytherapy if they have unifocal thoracic adenocarcinoma or squamous cell carcinoma under 10 cm in length, with no evidence of intra-abdominal or metastatic disease. Contraindications include cancer of the cervical oesophagus, tracheal or bronchial involvement, or stenosis that cannot be bypassed. They recommend high dose radiotherapy, 10 Gy in 2 weekly fractions of 5 Gy each, or low dose radiation 20 Gy in a single course at 0.4–1 Gy/h.[19]

Brachytherapy gives faster results than external beam radiation therapy. Dysphagia and odynophagia improve in more than two-thirds of patients, and the mean duration of response is about 5 months.[16] Acute reactions occur in approximately half the patients, consisting of mild to moderate oesophagitis one week after therapy. However, there is a significant risk of complications including ulceration, haemorrhage, stricture and fistula formation.[15,16]

Brachytherapy can be used by itself either for definitive treatment or for tumour palliation.[16,19] It is frequently used in combination with external beam radiotherapy to improve local control and a modest survival advantage is reported compared to external beam treatment alone.[20,21] Such therapy can result in complete pathological remissions as determined by subsequent surgery in up to 43% of patients.[22] Brachytherapy should not be given concurrently with chemotherapy, as there is increased toxicity from the combined treatments.

CHEMOTHERAPY

Several chemotherapy drugs are active against oesophageal cancer, including bleomycin, cisplatin, etoposide, 5-fluorouracil, mitoguazone, mitomycin C, methotrexate, paclitaxel, vindesine, peplomycin and vinorelbine. Most of these drugs have been studied in squamous cell carcinoma of the oesophagus, with relatively little information available about adenocarcinoma. Single drug response rates are generally 15–35% in untreated patients and lower in patients with advanced disease.[23,24] Slightly better response rates are produced using continuous infusion therapy with 5-fluorouracil, methotrexate or cisplatin in patients with no previous treatment.[25,26]

Responses to single chemotherapy drugs are usually of brief duration, and the medications themselves often have undesirable side-effects. This may improve with the development of newer drugs. Recent trials with paclitaxel[27] and vinorelbine[28] demonstrate that these well-tolerated chemotherapy agents induce median response durations of 17 and 21 weeks, respectively. Lobaplatin, a less toxic analogue of cisplatin, is under investigation in Europe, where it has shown activity in treatment of squamous cell carcinoma of the oesophagus.[29]

Numerous types of combination chemotherapy regimens have been tried. Most of them use 5-fluorouracil combined with either cisplatin or mitomycin C. Historically, trials often incorporated bleomycin, but pulmonary toxicity proved too high, especially when chemotherapy was coupled with surgery or radiation therapy. In general, response rates of 35–58% have been observed with combination chemotherapy in metastatic oesophageal cancer, with response durations of under 6 months.[23,24] Recent trials incorporating paclitaxel in combination with 5-fluorouracil and cisplatin look promising,[30] and further studies are in progress.

In general, single agent or combination chemotherapy by itself has not been very successful in the treatment of oesophageal cancer. Debilitated patients with significant dysphagia may not be able to tolerate side-effects from chemotherapy or maintain oral intake long enough for chemotherapy to have an effect. There are no randomized trials demonstrating whether combination chemotherapy is better than best supportive care in advanced oesophageal cancer. Local palliative treatment options such as endoscopic therapy or radiation are usually preferred for patients with poor performance status.

COMBINED CHEMOTHERAPY AND RADIOTHERAPY

Combined chemotherapy and radiation is the current standard for primary therapy of unresectable cancer of the oesophagus in patients with good performance status, and is being increasingly studied in the neoadjuvant setting prior to resectional surgery. There are theoretical advantages to using chemotherapy and radiation therapy at the same time. The use of both modalities allows the treatment of local and distant disease simultaneously. Certain chemotherapy agents act as radiation sensitizers, potentiating the effect of radiation therapy. Chemotherapy can prevent cells from repairing sublethal radiation damage and might kill cells that are resistant to the effects of radiotherapy, and vice versa.[9,30] Some investigators feel that for cervical oesophageal carcinoma, definitive chemoradiotherapy is preferable to surgery even in early stage patients, as there is more chance of being able to preserve the larynx.[31]

The ability to eradicate oesophageal carcinoma cells by combined chemotherapy and radiation therapy has been amply demonstrated in studies where the chemoradiotherapy treatment was designed to be followed by surgical resection. At least 35 small trials have used combined chemotherapy and radiation with various stages of oesophageal cancer.[32–35] Most showed complete clinical or pathological responses in 30–55% of patients. Complete responses are sometimes seen even in patients with bulky abdominal lymphadenopathy.[36] Median survival after preoperative chemoradiotherapy ranges from 6 to 22 months.[23]

Patients who achieve complete pathological responses prior to surgery have a clear survival benefit. For example, in the study by Bates et al.,[6] 51% of the patients had complete pathological responses. The median survival was 36.8 months for patients with complete responses, 12.9 months for patients

with residual tumour and 22 months overall. However, the fact that most patients with complete pathological response in their resected specimen ultimately die with recurrent oesophageal cancer demonstrates that current regimens do not completely eliminate residual cancer cells from the body.[37] In the only prospective randomized study to compare neoadjuvant chemoradiation prior to surgical resection with resection alone in oesophageal adenocarcinoma, the administration of 5-fluorouracil and cisplatin with 40 Gy of external beam radiotherapy resulted in 3-year survival of 32% compared to 6% for surgery alone.[38]

Chemoradiotherapy for primary treatment of unresectable oesophageal cancer has been tested in multiple trials. Similar to the preoperative studies, they are mostly non-randomized phase I or II protocols involving small numbers of patients at various stages of cancer.[12,21,31] In general, palliation of dysphagia is excellent using combined chemotherapy and radiation therapy,[39] and there is a moderate improvement in survival with the combined modalities.

The following are some representative examples of combined chemoradiotherapy protocols. Coia et al. used external beam radiation therapy 60 Gy plus bolus mitomycin C and infusional 5-fluorouracil. The overall median survival of Stage I and II patients was 18 months. Patients with Stage III and IV disease survived 9 and 7 months, respectively, with relief of dysphagia in 77%. There were severe acute toxicities in 12%, mostly due to moderate oesophagitis.[40] Kagami et al. treated patients with Stage II and III oesophageal cancer with alternating chemotherapy (cisplatin, methotrexate and peplomycin) and radiation. Radiation was either external beam alone (50–55 Gy) or external beam plus brachytherapy (14–20 Gy). There were 60% complete responses with an overall response rate of 95%, and a 5-year survival of 25%. Toxicity was modest, and there were no treatment-related deaths.[41] Using a regimen of cisplatin, 5-fluorouracil, and paclitaxel with hyperfractionated radiotherapy followed by surgery, the 2-year survival was 61%, although toxicity was substantial.[42] The above studies illustrate that symptoms and overall survival are improved with the use of combined chemotherapy and radiotherapy, at the cost of increased toxicity.

Four prospective randomized studies compared combined chemotherapy and radiation therapy to definitive radiation therapy in oesophageal cancer. The Eastern Cooperative Oncology Group randomized Stage I and II oesophageal cancer patients between radiation alone or radiation with concurrent 5-fluorouracil and mitomycin C chemotherapy. The median survival increased from 9.1 to 14.8 months with the combined regimen. The results in this study are somewhat difficult to interpret, however, because some patients in the study had the choice of surgical resection.[43] Another study randomized 59 patients to radiotherapy 50 Gy or radiotherapy 50 Gy plus chemotherapy with 5-fluorouracil, bleomycin and mitomycin C. Although not statistically significant because of the small number of patients, the 5-year survival in the combined therapy group was 16% compared to 6% with radiotherapy alone. Oesophagitis and myelosuppression were worse in the chemoradiation group.[44] The Radiation Therapy Oncology

Group (RTOG) with the Southwestern Oncology Group (SWOG) and North Central Cancer Treatment Group compared treatment with radiotherapy 64 Gy to treatment with radiotherapy 50 Gy plus cisplatin and 5-fluorouracil chemotherapy. Median survival was 9.3 months in the radiation alone group and 14.1 months in the combined treatment group (P<0.0001).[45] Five-year survival was 30% in the combined modality group compared to 0 in the radiation alone arm, and the local failure rate was 44% vs 65%. Of the patients receiving chemoradiotherapy, 64% had life-threatening side-effects from the treatment, mostly myelosuppression and mucositis.[46] Finally, the European Organization for the Research and Treatment of Cancer (EORTC) randomized 221 patients with inoperable squamous cell carcinoma of the oesophagus to split course radiation therapy of 40 Gy versus the same radiation plus concomitant and subsequent cisplatin chemotherapy. Preliminary analysis shows a trend towards greater overall survival in the combined modality group, which has not yet reached statistical significance.[47] The randomized studies confirm that there can be modest improvement in survival in unresectable oesophageal cancer treated with combined chemoradiotherapy. However, toxicity is significant, even in the good performance status patients accepted into such trials.

Sequential chemotherapy followed by radiotherapy does not seem to be as effective as concurrent chemotherapy and radiation. In a phase II trial, Sharma et al.[48] gave four cycles of chemotherapy with 5-fluorouracil and cisplatin followed by external beam radiation of 60 Gy. There were 11 partial responses (85%) and one complete response (8%), with a median survival of only 9.8 months. Three cycles of cisplatin and bleomycin followed by radiotherapy 50 Gy resulted in a median survival of 8 months.[49] Induction chemotherapy with cisplatin, folinic acid, bleomycin and mitomycin C for 2 weeks followed by chemoradiotherapy (radiation therapy of 60 Gy plus cisplatin, 5-fluorouracil and folinic acid) produced a median survival of 32 months in 60 patients.[50] Other approaches include alternating chemotherapy and radiation,[41] long-term infusional low-dose 5-fluorouracil administered before and concomitantly with radiotherapy,[25] and radiation along with daily low-dose cisplatin, carboplatin or carboplatin/5-fluorouracil plus monthly vindesine.[51] The daily low-dose chemotherapy/radiotherapy approach appears to be highly effective and relatively non-toxic, but awaits confirmation in larger prospective trials.

Attempts at increasing response rates by using more intensive chemotherapy or radiotherapy have produced added toxicity without a clear survival advantage. In a phase II Intergroup Trial, Minsky et al. gave three cycles of chemotherapy with cisplatin and 5-fluorouracil followed by two more cycles of chemotherapy combined with radiotherapy 64.8 Gy. The incidence of grade 3 or greater toxicity was 72%, and there were 13% treatment-related deaths, most because of sepsis or dehydration. Overall median survival was 20 months.[52]

It is clear that much work remains to be done towards the development of effective, non-toxic combined modality regimens. The answer may be in some of the newer chemotherapeutic agents under study. In a small study of 13 patients given paclitaxel, carboplatin and concurrent radiotherapy using 45 Gy as a preoperative treatment, the complete pathological response rate was 69%, with only mild to moderate toxicity.[53]

Brachytherapy has been added to combined chemotherapy/radiotherapy protocols in an attempt to improve local control. The addition of a 10 Gy high dose-rate brachytherapy boost to conventional radiation of 60 Gy plus cisplatin, 5-fluorouracil and mitomycin C chemotherapy gave a one-year local control rate of 74% and overall median survival of 17 months, but with moderately severe toxicity.[54] Gaspar et al. used cisplatin/5-fluorouracil chemotherapy, external beam radiotherapy 50 Gy, and high-dose rate brachytherapy 15 Gy. Of the patients receiving brachytherapy 17% developed tracheo-oesophageal fistulas, and the median survival was only 11 months.[55] Because of the increased toxicity, it is not recommended to give brachytherapy concurrently with chemotherapy.

Overall, the addition of chemotherapy to definitive radiotherapy results in better local control and overall survival than radiotherapy alone,[32] although the results are far from optimal in terms of acute toxicity and survival. Whether chemoradiation followed by surgery is any better than chemoradiation alone remains to be tested in clinical trials.

ENDOSCOPIC THERAPY

Recent improvements in endoscopic techniques have produced a wide range of methods useful in treatment of oesophageal cancer. The endoscope can be used for definitive therapy of oesophageal cancer in early lesions, but is mostly used for palliation of advanced tumours.

Very early lesions may be resected endoscopically for cure with a 95% 5-year survival after endoscopic resection of superficial lesions.[56,57] Patients should be carefully staged with endoscopic ultrasonography before attempting endoscopic mucosal resection. To be successfully resected, lesions should be confined to the mucosa or submucosa and be no more than 2–3 cm in diameter. Once tumour has penetrated through the submucosa, there is a 35–39% chance of lymph node involvement, and curative endoscopic resection is unlikely.[56,57] Superficial lesions can also be treated endoscopically using Nd:YAG laser or photodynamic therapy (see below).[58,59]

Palliation of symptoms is a major application of endoscopic treatment. Malignant strictures, or benign strictures that form after surgical anastomosis or radiation therapy, can be dilated using bougies or balloons.[60] Dilation is done slowly in a stepwise fashion, using bougies with progressively larger diameter, until an adequate oesophageal lumen is established. No more than three successively larger dilators (in 1 mm or 3 Fr increments) should be used at one sitting, to avoid perforation of the oesophagus.[61]

In patients who have had previous radiation therapy, oesophageal strictures can be very firm and fibrotic, and may split or fissure into the mediastinum during the dilation procedure. The rate of perforation in this circumstance is 3–5% per procedure.[61,62] Other risks of dilation include haemorrhage and pulmonary aspiration. Transient chest pain and bacteraemia are common, and patients with prosthetic heart valves or artificial joints should receive antibiotic prophylaxis.[61]

Dilation may result in rapid relief of obstruction, which can be very effective for benign strictures caused by radiation therapy. Unfortunately, in malignant strictures the alleviation of obstruction by dilation alone is short-lived. In most cases dilation of malignant obstruction must be followed by another treatment modality such as radiation, laser therapy, or stenting (see below).

Laser therapy

Endoscopic laser therapy was first used for cancer of the oesophagus in 1982.[63] Lasers are high-energy beams of monochromatic light. When the light energy interacts with biological tissue, it is converted into heat energy, which kills cells. Using flexible endoscopes, a quartz waveguide carries the laser light beam from the laser source to the treatment site. The depth of penetration and the heat produced depend on the individual laser wavelengths. Commonly used types of lasers in endoscopy include the neodymium:yttrium-aluminum-garnet (Nd:YAG) laser, which has the deepest penetration, and the argon laser, which penetrates more superficially.[64]

An exophytic tumour mass of the middle or distal oesophagus is the type of lesion most appropriate for laser therapy. Cervical oesophageal malignancy, flat or submucosal tumour, lesions more than 6 cm long, or complex strictures of the gastro-oesophageal junction are difficult to treat with the laser.[61,65] Laser therapy should not be attempted in patients with extrinsic compression of the oesophagus or tracheo-oesophageal fistula.[61,66]

Laser therapy can be done in either a prograde or a retrograde fashion. In the prograde technique, the laser is used to burn a channel through the obstructed tissue, starting in the centre of the lumen. If tumour stenosis is too small to allow passage of an endoscope, a laser-resistant guide probe can be used. The probe is required to prevent accidental misdirection of the beam, which might cause oesophageal perforation. Treatment continues until an adequate lumen has been re-established. With particularly long tumours, it may not be possible to treat the whole obstruction at one session. In such circumstances, treatments may be spaced every 2–3 days to allow for maximal tissue necrosis. At subsequent treatments, necrotic tissue is removed before proceeding with further laser therapy.[64] An average of three to five sessions may be required before full patency of the oesophagus is established.[1,65]

In the retrograde technique, the oesophagus is first dilated using Savary–Gilliard or balloon dilators until a small calibre endoscope can be passed to the distal margin of the tumour. The laser is then slowly advanced proximally until the entire tumour is treated. The advantage of the retrograde technique is that tissue oedema during treatment occurs distal to the laser tip and does not prevent visualization of the lumen or advancement of the laser. Treatment often can be accomplished in one sitting, and there is less risk of perforation since the location of the oesophageal lumen has been established. It is helpful to remove soft, exophytic portions of the tumour with a polypectomy snare and electrosurgical cutting current before laser therapy.

Laser photocoagulation is very effective in achieving palliation; 70–85% of treated patients have relief of dysphagia and improvement in quality of life.[67,68]

Laser therapy is relatively safe. Complications are generally minor and include mild fever, chest pain and abdominal distention during the procedure. There may be a transient worsening of dysphagia due to oedema of the treated tissues. Major complications of laser therapy include oesophageal perforation in 2–6% of patients, tracheo-oesophageal fistula in 1.3–7%, bleeding and late stricture formation in up to 21%.[61,65,67,69,70] There are potential hazards to the endoscopist, including heated gases and smoke generated during the procedure, and the possible vaporization and inhalation of infectious biological substances including papillomavirus. Risks can be minimized by using commercially available smoke evacuators.

Recurrence of dysphagia after laser therapy typically occurs after 4–8 weeks, necessitating repeat procedures, which is the principal disadvantage of the technique.[66,71] After multiple laser treatments the oesophagus often becomes fibrotic, and stenting may be required.[72] Laser therapy has been combined with external beam radiotherapy or brachytherapy in an attempt to extend the duration of palliation, with encouraging results.[69,73,74] Insertion of a plastic oesophageal stent after laser therapy is not helpful, as it increases the complication rate and the rate of recurrent dysphagia.[69,75] Whether the newer expandable metal stents will prove to be more useful remains to be determined.

Heater probe

The BICAP heater probe is an endoscopic device that destroys tissue through the use of electrocoagulation. A guidewire is placed endoscopically, and the tumour is dilated to a diameter sufficient to pass the tumour probe. The probe is then passed over the guidewire. Bipolar electrode tips are used to apply an electric current in an antegrade or retrograde fashion, causing a circumferential treatment burn. After 48 h, necrotic tissue is removed by repeat endoscopy.

The heater probe is used on circumferential tumours, both exophytic and submucosal. It is very helpful for long stenotic tumours, and is technically easier to use than laser therapy in lesions of the cervical oesophagus.[64,76] It is not recommended in non-circumferential tumours, as there will be too much thermal damage to normal tissue. Treatment is generally effective and well tolerated, with mild side-effects such as transient fevers and chest pain.[76] Major complications are uncommon and include delayed haemorrhage, tracheo-oesophageal fistula, and delayed stricture formation.[64] Symptomatic relief usually lasts from 4 to 10 weeks.[64,76] The equipment required for BICAP heater probe therapy is much less expensive than laser equipment.

Photodynamic therapy

Photodynamic therapy is a means of destroying malignant tissue by a photochemical reaction induced by a photosensitizer exposed to specific wavelengths of low intensity light. The most commonly used photosensitizers are haematoporphyrin derivatives, especially porfimer sodium (Photofrin II). The photosensitizer is administered systemically to the patient and is taken up preferentially by malignant tissue. Two days after administration, when the difference in uptake between normal and malignant cells is maximal, the patient's tumour is irradiated through an endoscope with light at a wavelength of 630 nm, supplied by an argon-pumped dye laser.

The laser light causes the formation of toxic oxygen free radicals in the sensitized cells, leading to cell death. The depth of tissue necrosis depends on the dose of light delivered per square centimetre of tissue.[77] There is less danger of oesophageal perforation with photodynamic therapy than with other techniques, because photodynamic therapy has no effect on tissue collagen. If necrosis occurs in normal tissue, it heals and regenerates new epithelium, often without scarring.

This technique is very effective in the therapy of small, superficial or multifocal tumours.[59] Areas of Barrett's mucosa treated with photodynamic therapy sometimes revert to squamous epithelium.[78,79] Lesions difficult to treat with Nd:YAG laser, including long tumours and previously treated areas, can be effectively palliated with photodynamic therapy.[71] After one or two treatments, most patients achieve a complete or partial improvement in dysphagia lasting a median of 4–11 weeks.[71,77]

Because the drug accumulates in the skin, there is an increase in skin sensitivity for several weeks after therapy. Patients must avoid sunlight and other strong light for 4–6 weeks after therapy, or significant sunburn may result. Other complications include nausea, fever, fistula formation, oesophageal strictures, and post-treatment bleeding.[59,71]

A significant problem with photodynamic therapy is less than perfect tumour selectivity of the photosensitizing agent. Newer agents are being developed that have a shorter half-life, cause less skin sensitization, and/or are more selective for cancer cells. These include *m*-tetra (hydroxyphenyl) chlorin and 5-aminolaevulinic acid.[80,81] Photodynamic therapy is not yet widely available due to the expense of the photosensitizing agent and the special laser required. Where it is available, its principal use lies in the treatment of high-grade dysplasia and early adenocarcinomas arising in Barrett's metaplasia. Studies are in progress to assess its effect in ablating segments or Barrett's metaplasia.

Other endoscopic techniques

Local injection of toxic substances through the endoscope can be used to induce necrosis of obstructing oesophageal tumours. Dehydrated ethanol injections are inexpensive, well tolerated and require no specialized equipment. They produce effective palliation lasting a few weeks, although it is sometimes difficult to control the treatment field because of diffusion of ethanol through tissues.[82] In a prospective randomized trial between laser photocoagulation and injection of the sclerosant polidocanol, both methods were effective, with 80% of patients being relieved of dysphagia after the first treatment course.[82] Multiple treatments were required with both, but the cost of sclerosant injection is much less than laser therapy.

Combined chemotherapy and sclerotherapy with 5-fluorouracil and sodium morrhuate injected directly into the tumour using a sclerotherapy catheter has been used, but has not yet shown durable responses.[83] Other substances such as OK-432, a potent biological response modifier, are under investigation.[84]

Stents

Oesophageal stents are tubes that are inserted through an obstructed oesophageal lumen to provide immediate relief of dysphagia. Their rigid walls keep the oesophageal lumen open so that food and secretions can pass through. They are the treatment of choice for tracheo-oesophageal fistula, as they occlude the perforation and prevent aspiration.[1]

The first oesophageal stents were rigid plastic tubes with an external diameter of up to 14 mm and an internal diameter of 10–11 mm. Only 10–15% of patients with plastic stents were able to eat a normal diet, and patients often had the persistent sensation of a foreign body in the oesophagus. Plastic stents have a significant complication rate, with a procedure-related mortality of 4–16%.[61,85,86] One of the major problems with the plastic stents is that because of their large outside diameter and the bulky semirigid introducing systems, dilation of the oesophagus to a diameter of over 15 mm (45 Fr) is required for stent placement. This form of intubation results in oesophageal perforation in up to 10% of patients, approximately half of which prove fatal.[86] Other early complications include haemorrhage, aspiration pneumonia, pressure necrosis and airway obstruction. Late complications are common and consist of tube migration, gastro-oesophageal reflux, food impaction and tumour overgrowth.[69,85,86]

Recently, flexible, self-expanding metal stents (SEMS) have been developed that overcome some of the disadvantages of the plastic tubes. Metal stents are inserted in a semicollapsed state with small introducing systems of 8–12 mm and then slowly expand to 20–25 mm after having been placed in the oesophageal lumen.[87] Due to their small diameter at the time of insertion, they require less oesophageal dilation compared to plastic stents. The metal used is either stainless steel or nitinol, a flexible titanium-nickel 'memory' alloy that is considered to be particularly useful for long and tortuous malignant strictures.[88] Stents are available in knitted wire (nitinol: Ultraflex, Microinvasive, Watertown, MA), wire mesh (Wallstent: Schneider, Minneapolis, MN), coil (EsophaCoil: Instent, Eden Prairie, MN), or expandable Z-stent (Gianturco: Wilson-Cook, North Salem, NC) design.[61] The different stent types vary in their radial force, with the Esophacoil > Wallstent > Gianturco Z-stent > nitinol Ultraflex.[61] Large tumours and tumours with significant extrinsic compression of the oesophagus require a stent with more radial force to keep the lumen open. In the upper oesophagus, it is important to ensure that the trachea is not compressed as the stent expands, and a less forceful stent such as the nitinol Ultraflex may be more appropriate. Except for the Gianturco Z-stent, all types of metal stent shorten as they expand, up to a 20% decrease in length.[61,88] This characteristic must be remembered when choosing the stent size.

The open structure of the metal stents allows for good

adherence to the oesophageal wall, as granulation tissue grows between the wires and holds them in place. However, it is also easy for tumour ingrowth to occur through the metal wires, and the rate of reocclusion by tumour is high. More recently, metal stents coated with polyethylene, polyurethane, or silicone have been developed.[87,89] The coating prevents tumour ingrowth and also allows the metal stents to be used for occlusion of tracheo-oesophageal fistulas. The disadvantage of the coated stents is that they anchor less well to the oesophageal wall than do the uncoated ones. Consequently, stent migration occurs more frequently.[90] Attempts at overcoming this difficulty include placing barbs at the centre of the stent to anchor it to oesophageal tissue, or using a longer stent length.

All the expandable metal stents have very high rates of successful placement and relief of dysphagia.[61,88,89] The acute perforation rate is low, both because dilation is less frequently required prior to insertion and because of the small diameter, flexible introducing system. Problems which may occur during or soon after insertion include incomplete stent expansion, retrosternal pain and heartburn. Late complications include bleeding, stent migration, perforation or fistula formation due to pressure necrosis, and occlusion by food impaction or tumour overgrowth.[61,88,89,91] A stent which traverses the cardia predisposes to reflux, so patients must remain in an upright position for at least 2 h after eating. Stent wires or mesh may also fracture, erode into the aorta, or be destroyed during subsequent laser treatment for tumour ingrowth.[88,89] Since many self-expanding metal stents are not easily removable, a second stent must sometimes be placed to overcome problems that develop.[85,88]

In a prospective randomized trial involving 60 patients, placement of metal stents provided better palliation of dysphagia for oesophageal cancer patients than endoscopic laser therapy.[90]

In a randomized study which compared conventional plastic prostheses with uncovered Wallstents, relief of dysphagia and 30-day mortality were similar.[91] Despite a 10-fold increase in cost of the Wallstents over plastic prostheses, the overall cost of palliation was less because of a mean hospital stay of 12.5 days for plastic prostheses. This is higher than in many reported series and may relate to their insertion under general anaesthesia in this study.

CONCLUSIONS

The choice of therapy in oesophageal cancer must be individualized for each patient. For early stage oesophageal cancer, several potentially curative non-surgical procedures are available, including endoscopic mucosal resection, Nd:YAG laser therapy, and photodynamic therapy. Multimodality treatment with chemoradiation is being used as adjunctive treatment to resection in patients with operable disease and indeed locally advanced tumours may be down-staged prior to resection. In more advanced disease, combined chemoradiation offers the best chance for long-term survival and palliation of dysphagia, although at the cost of significant toxicity. For frail patients with limited life expectancy, procedures such as stent place-

ment, endoscopic laser therapy or brachytherapy offer rapid relief of symptoms without excessive morbidity. The choice of modalities will depend on the patient's health status and preferences, and what resources are locally available.

REFERENCES

1. Ponec RJ & Kimmey MB. Endoscopic therapy of esophageal cancer. *Surg Clin North Am* 1997; **77**: 1197–1217.
2. Launoy G, Milan CH, Faivre J et al. Alcohol, tobacco and oesophageal cancer: effects of the duration of consumption, mean intake and current and former consumption. *Br J Cancer* 1997; **75**: 1389–1396.
3. Drinkard L, Ferguson MK, Mundt AJ et al. Therapy of esophageal cancer. In Aisner J, Arriagada R, Green MR et al. (eds) *Comprehensive Textbook of Thoracic Oncology.* Philadelphia: Williams and Wilkins, 1996; 606–629.
4. Roth, JA, Putnam, JB Jr, Rich, TA et al. Cancer of the esophagus. In DeVita VT Jr, Hellman S & Rosenberg SA (eds) *Cancer: Principles and Practice of Oncology,* 5th edn. Philadelphia: Lippincott-Raven, 1997: 980–1021.
5. Beatty JD, DeBoer G & Rider WD. Carcinoma of the esophagus: pretreatment assessment, correlation of radiation treatment parameters with survival, and identification and management of radiation treatment failure. *Cancer* 1979; **43**: 2254–2267.
6. Bates BA, Detterbeck FC, Bernard SA et al. Concurrent radiation therapy and chemotherapy followed by esophagectomy for localized esophageal carcinoma. *J Clin Oncol* 1996; **14**: 156–163.
7. Pearson JG. The value of radiotherapy in the management of esophageal cancer. *Am J Roentgenol* 1969; **105**: 500–513.
8. Newaishy GA, Read GA, Duncan W et al. Results of radical radiotherapy of squamous cell carcinoma of the esophagus. *Clin Radiol* 1982; **33**: 347–352.
9. Herskovic A, Al-Sarraf M. Combination of 5-fluorouracil and radiation in esophageal cancer. *Semin Rad Oncol* 1997; **7**: 283–290.
10. Sun D-R. Ten year follow-up of esophageal cancer treated by radical radiation therapy: analysis of 869 patients. *Int J Radiat Oncol Biol Phys* 1989; **16**: 329–334.
11. Earlam R. An MRC prospective randomized trial of radiotherapy versus surgery for operable squamous cell carcinoma of the oesophagus. *Ann R Coll Surg Engl* 1991; **73**: 8–12.
12. John MJ, Flam MS, Mowry PA et al. Radiotherapy alone and chemoradiation for nonmetastatic esophageal carcinoma: a critical review of chemoradiation. *Cancer* 1989; **63**: 2397–2403.
13. Ng TM, Spencer GM, Sargeant IR et al. Management of strictures after radiotherapy for esophageal cancer. *Gastrointest Endosc* 1996; **43**: 584–590.
14. Powell ME, Hoskin PJ, Saunders MI et al. Continuous hyperfractionated accelerated radiotherapy (CHART) in localized cancer of the esophagus. *Int J Radiat Oncol Biol Phys* 1997; **38**: 133–136.
15. Fleischman EH, Kagan AR, Bellotti JE et al. Effective palliation for inoperable esophageal cancer using intensive intracavity radiation. *J Surg Oncol* 1990; **44**: 234–237.
16. Jager J, Langendijk H, Pannebakker M et al. A single session of intraluminal brachytherapy in palliation of oesophageal cancer. *Radiother Oncol* 1995; **37**: 237–240.
17. Sur RK, Singh DP, Sharma SC et al. Radiation therapy of esophageal cancer: role of high dose rate brachytherapy. *Int J Radiat Oncol Biol Phys* 1992; **22**: 1043–1046.
18. Micaily B, Miyamoto CT, Freire JE et al. Intracavitary brachytherapy for carcinoma of the esophagus. *Semin Surg Oncol* 1997; **13**: 185–189.
19. Gaspar LE, Nag S, Herskovic A et al. American Brachytherapy Society (ABS) consensus guidelines for brachytherapy of esophageal cancer. Clinical Research Committee, American Brachytherapy Society, Philadelphia, PA. *Int J Radiat Oncol Biol Phys* 1997; **38**: 127–132.
20. Caspers, RJ, Zwinderman AH, Griffioen G et al. Combined external beam and low dose rate intraluminal radiotherapy in oesophageal cancer. *Radiother Oncol* 1993; **27**: 7–12.
21. Hyden EC, Langholz B, Tilden T et al. External beam and intraluminal radiotherapy in the treatment of carcinoma of the esophagus. *J Thorac Cardiovasc Surg* 1988; **96**: 237–241.
22. Keyes M, Haylock B & Hay JH. An evaluation of pathological effect of pre or post external beam brachytherapy in radical radiotherapy of carcinoma of the esophagus. *Clin Invest Med* 1994; **17**: 681, B115.
23. Vogl SE, Greenwald E & Kaplan BH. Effective chemotherapy for esophageal cancer with methotrexate, bleomycin and *cis*-diammine dichloroplatinum. *Cancer* 1981; **48**: 2555–2558.

24. Ilson, DH & Kelson, DP. Management of esophageal cancer. *Oncology* 1996; **10**: 1385–1402.

25. Lokich JJ, Shea M & Chaffey J. Sequential infusional 5-fluorouracil followed by concomitant radiation for tumors of the esophagus and gastroesophageal junction. *Cancer* 1987; **60**: 275–279.

26. Miller JI, McIntyre MD & Hatcher CR. Combined treatment approach in surgical management of carcinoma of the esophagus: a preliminary report. *Ann Thorac Surg* 1985; **40**: 289–293.

27. Ajani JA, Ilson DH, Daugherty K et al. Activity of Taxol in patients with squamous cell carcinoma and adenocarcinoma of the esophagus. *J Natl Cancer Inst* 1994; **86**: 1086–1091.

28. Conroy T, Etienne P-L, Adenis A et al. Phase II trial of vinorelbine in metastatic squamous cell esophageal carcinoma. *J Clin Oncol* 1996; **14**: 164–170.

29. Schmoll HJ, Köhne CH, Papageorgiou E et al. Single agent lobaplatin is active in patients with esophageal carcinoma: a phase II evaluation. *Proc Am Soc Clin Oncol* 1995; **14**(483): 201.

30. Kelsen D, Ginsberg R, Bains M et al. A Phase II trial of paclitaxel and cisplatin in patients with locally advanced metastatic esophageal cancer: a preliminary report. *Semin Oncol* 1997; **24**(Supp 19): S19-77–S19-81.

31. Soto PH, Valente M, Bidoli P et al. Definitive chemoradiotherapy in cervical esophageal carcinoma. *Proc Am Soc Clin Oncol* 1997; **16**(929): 262a.

32. Thomas CR Jr. Biology of esophageal cancer and the role of combined modality therapy. *Surg Clin North Am* 1997; **77**: 1139–1167.

33. Ganem G, Dubray B, Raoul Y et al. Concomitant chemoradiotherapy followed, where feasible, by surgery for cancer of the esophagus. *J Clin Oncol* 1997; **15**: 701–711.

34. Forastiere AA, Heitmiller RF & Kleinberg L. Multimodality therapy for esophageal cancer. *Chest* 1997; **112**(4 Suppl): 195S–200S.

35. Forastiere AA, Heitmiller RF, Lee DJ et al. Intensive chemoradiation followed by esophagectomy for squamous cell and adenocarcinoma of the esophagus. *Cancer J Sci Am* 1997; **3**: 144–152.

36. Sueyama H, Sakai K, Sugita T et al. Neoadjuvant chemotherapy followed by concurrent chemotherapy and radiotherapy for locally advanced esophageal carcinoma with bulky upper abdominal lymphadenopathy. *Am J Clin Oncol* 1997; **20**: 580–584.

37. Kavanagh B, Anscher M, Leopold K et al. Patterns of failure following combined modality therapy for esophageal cancer, 1984–1990. *Int J Radiat Oncol Biol Phys* 1992; **24**: 633–642.

38. Walsh TN, Noonan N, Hollywood D et al. A comparison of multimodal therapy and surgery for esophageal adenocarcinoma. *N Engl J Med* 1996; **335**: 462–467.

39. Wolfe WG, Burton GV, Seigler HF et al. Early results with combined modality therapy for carcinoma of the esophagus. *Ann Surg* 1987; **205**: 563–571.

40. Coia LR, Engstrom PF, Paul AR et al. Long-term results of infusional 5-FU, mitomycin-C, and radiation as primary management of esophageal carcinoma. *Int J Radiat Oncol Biol Phys* 1991; **20**: 29–36.

41. Kagami Y, Nishio M, Narimatsu N et al. Treatment of squamous cell carcinoma of the esophagus with alternating radiotherapy and chemotherapy (cisplatin, methotrexate, and peplomycin). *Am J Clin Oncol* 1997; **20**: 16–18.

42. Wright CD, Wain JC, Lynch TJ et al. Induction therapy for esophageal cancer with paclitaxel and hyperfractionated radiotherapy: a phase I and II study. *J Thorac Cardiovasc Surg* 1997; **114**: 811–815.

43. Sischy B, Ryan L, Haller D et al. Interim report of EST 1282 Phase III protocol for the evaluation of combined modalities in the treatment of patients with carcinoma of the esophagus, stage I and II. *Proc Am Soc Clin Oncol* 1990; **9**: 105.

44. Araujo C, Souhami L, Gil R et al. A randomized trial comparing radiation therapy versus concomitant radiation therapy and chemotherapy in carcinoma of the thoracic esophagus. *Cancer* 1991; **67**: 2258–2261.

45. Herskovic A, Martz K, Al-Sarraf M et al. Combined chemotherapy and radiotherapy compared with radiotherapy alone in patients with cancer of the esophagus. *N Engl J Med* 1992; **326**: 1593–1598.

46. Al-Sarraf M, Martz K, Herskovic A et al. Superiority of chemo-radiotherapy (CT-RT) vs radiotherapy (RT) in patients with esophageal cancer. Final report of an intergroup randomized and confirmed study. *Proc Am Soc Clin Oncol* 1996; **15**(464): 206.

47. Roussel A, Haegele P, Paillot B et al. Results of the EORTC-GTCCG phase III trial of irradiation vs irradiation and CDDP in inoperable esophageal cancer. *Proc Am Soc Clin Oncol* 1994; **13**: 199.

48. Sharma D, Krasnow SH, Davis EB et al. Sequential chemotherapy and radiotherapy for squamous cell esophageal carcinoma. *Am J Clin Oncol* 1997; **20**: 151–153.

49. Izquierdo MA, Marcuello E, Gomez de Segura G et al. Unresectable nonmetastatic squamous cell carcinoma of the esophagus managed by sequential chemotherapy (cisplatin and bleomycin) and radiation therapy. *Cancer* 1993; **71**: 287–292.

50. Roca E, Pennella E, Sardi M et al. Combined intensive chemoradiotherapy for organ preservation in patients with resectable and non-resectable oesophageal cancer. *Eur J Cancer* 1996; **32A**: 429–432.

51. Ohno S, Kuwano H, Morita M et al. Simultaneous combination therapy of carboplatin and radiation for patients with carcinoma of the esophagus. *Hepatogastroenterology* 1997; **44**: 181–186.

52. Minsky B, Neuberg D, Kelsen D et al. Neoadjuvant chemotherapy plus concurrent chemotherapy and high dose radiation for squamous cell cancer of the esophagus – a preliminary analysis of the phase II intergroup trial 0122. *J Clin Oncol* 1996; **14**: 149–155.

53. Meluch AA, Hainsworth JD, Thomas M et al. Preoperative therapy with paclitaxel, carboplatin, 5-FU and radiation yields 69% pathologic complete response (CR) rate in the treatment of local esophageal carcinoma. *Proc Am Soc Clin Oncol* 1997; **16**: 927, p. 261a.

54. Calais G, Dorval E, Louisot P et al. Radiotherapy with high dose rate brachytherapy boost and concomitant chemotherapy for Stages IIB and III esophageal carcinoma: results of a pilot study. *Int J Radiat Oncol Biol Phys* 1997; **38**: 769–775.

55. Gaspar LE, Qian C, Kocha WI et al. A phase I/II study of external beam radiation, brachytherapy and concurrent chemotherapy in localized cancer of the esophagus (RTOG 92-07): preliminary toxicity report. *Int J Radiat Oncol Biol Phys* 1997; **37**: 593–599.

56. Endo M. Endoscopic resection as local treatment of mucosal cancer of the esophagus. *Endoscopy* 1993; **25**: 672–674.

57. Takeshita K, Tani M, Inoue I et al. Endoscopic treatment of early oesophageal or gastric cancer. *Gut* 1997; **40**: 123–127.

58. Yang GR, Zhao LQ, Li SS et al. Endoscopic Nd-YAG laser therapy in patients with early superficial carcinoma of the esophagus and the gastric cardia. *Endoscopy* 1994; **26**: 681–685.

59. Sibille A, Lambert R, Souquet JC et al. Long-term survival after photodynamic therapy for esophageal cancer. *Gastroenterology* 1995; **108**: 337–344.

60. Cox J & Bennett JR. Light at the end of the tunnel? Palliation for oesophageal carcinoma. *Gut* 1987; **28**: 781–785.

61. Reed CE. Pitfalls and complications of esophageal prosthesis, laser therapy, and dilation. *Chest Surg Clin North Am* 1997; **7**: 623–636.

62. O'Rourke IC, Tiver K, Bull C et al. Swallowing performance after radiation therapy for carcinoma of the esophagus. *Cancer* 1988; **61**: 2022–2026.

63. Fleischer D & Kessler F. Endoscopic Nd-YAG laser therapy for carcinoma of the esophagus: a new palliative approach. *Am J Surg* 1982; **143**: 280–283.

64. Reilly HF, Fleischer DE. Palliative treatment of esophageal carcinoma using laser and tumor probe therapy. *Gastroenterol Clin North Am* 1991; **20**: 731–742.

65. Naveau S, Chiesa A, Poynard T et al. Endoscopic Nd-YAG laser therapy as palliative treatment for esophageal and cardial cancer: parameters affecting long-term outcome. *Dig Dis Sci* 1990; **35**: 294–301.

66. Bown SG, Hawes R, Matthewson K et al. Endoscopic laser palliation for advanced malignant dysphagia. *Gut* 1987; **28**: 799–807.

67. Krasner N, Barr H, Skidmore C et al. Palliative laser therapy for malignant dysphagia. *Gut* 1987; **28**: 792–798.

68. Loizou LA, Rampton D, Atkinson M et al. A prospective assessment of quality of life after endoscopic intubation and laser therapy for malignant dysphagia. *Cancer* 1992; **70**: 386–391.

69. Bown S. Palliation of malignant dysphagia: surgery, radiotherapy, laser, intubation alone or in combination? *Gut* 1991; **32**: 841–844.

70. Mathus-Vliegen EMH & Tytgat GNJ. Analysis of failures and complications of neodymium: YAG laser photocoagulation in gastrointestinal tract tumors. *Endoscopy* 1990; **22**: 17–23.

71. Lightdale CJ, Heier SK, Marcon NE et al. Photodynamic therapy with porfimer sodium versus thermal ablation therapy with Nd:YAG laser for palliation of esophageal cancer: a multicenter randomized trial. *Gastrointest Endosc* 1995; **42**: 507–512.

72. Shmueli E, Myszor MF, Burke D et al. Limitations of laser treatment for malignant dysphagia. *Br J Surg* 1992; **79**: 778–780.

73. Renwick R, Whitton V & Moghissi K. Combined endoscopic laser therapy and brachytherapy for palliation of oesophageal carcinoma: a pilot study. *Gut* 1992; **33**: 435–438.

74. Sargeant IR, Loizou LA, Tobias JS et al. Radiation enhancement of laser palliation for malignant dysphagia: a pilot study. *Gut* 1992; **33**: 1597–1601.

75. Barr H, Krasner N, Raouf A et al. Prospective randomised trial of laser therapy only and laser therapy followed by endoscopic intubation for the palliation of malignant dysphagia. *Gut* 1990; **31**: 252–258.

76. Jensen DM, Machicado G, Randall G et al. Comparison of low-power YAG laser and BICAP tumor probe for palliation of esophageal cancer strictures. *Gastroenterology* 1988; **94**: 1263–1270.

77. Heier SK, Rothman KA, Heier LM et al. Photodynamic therapy for obstructing esophageal cancer: light dosimetry and randomized comparison with Nd:YAG laser therapy. *Gastroenterology* 1995; **109**: 63–72.

78. Overholt BF & Panjehpour M. Barrett's esophagus: photodynamic therapy for ablation of dysplasia, reduction of specialized mucosa, and treatment of superficial esophageal cancer. *Gastrointest Endosc* 1995; **42**: 64–70.

79. Holscher AH, Bollschweiler E, Schneider PM et al. Early adenocarcinoma in Barrett's oesophagus. *Br J Surg* 1997; **84**: 1470–1473.

80. Regula J, MacRobert AJ, Gorchein et al. Photosensitisation and photodynamic therapy of oesophageal, duodenal, and colorectal tumours using 5 aminolaevulinic acid induced protoporphyrin IX – a pilot study. *Gut* 1995; **36**: 67–75.

81. Gossner L, Sroka R, Hahn E et al. Photodynamic therapy: successful destruction of gastrointestinal cancer after oral administration of aminolevulinic acid. *Gastrointest Endosc* 1995; **41**: 55–58.

82. Payne-James JJ, Spiller RC, Misiewicz JJ et al. Use of ethanol-induced tumor necrosis to palliate dysphagia in patients with esophagogastric cancer. *Gastrointest Endosc* 1990; **36**: 43–46.

83. Wright RA & O'Connor KW. A pilot study of endoscopic injection chemo/sclerotherapy of esophageal carcinoma. *Gastrointest Endosc* 1990; **36**: 47–48.

84. Mukai M, Kubota S, Morita S et al. A pilot study of combination therapy of radiation and local administration of OK-432 for esophageal cancer. *Cancer* 1995; **75**: 2276–2280.

85. Angueira CE & Kadakia SC. Esophageal stents for inoperable esophageal cancer: which to use? *Am J Gastroenterol* 1997; **92**: 373–376.

86. Cusumano A, Ruol A, Segalin A et al. Push-through intubation: effective palliation in 409 patients with cancer of the esophagus and cardia. *Ann Thorac Surg* 1992; **53**: 1010–1014.

87. Watkinson AF, Ellul J, Entwisle K et al. Esophageal carcinoma: initial results of palliative treatment with covered self-expanding endoprostheses. *Radiology* 1995; **195**: 821–827.

88. Grund KE, Storek D, Becker HD. Highly flexible self-expanding meshed metal stents for palliation of malignant esophagogastric obstruction. *Endoscopy* 1995; **27**: 486–494.

89. Ell C, May A, Hahn EG. Gianturco-Z stents in the palliative treatment of malignant esophageal obstruction and esophagotracheal fistulas. *Endoscopy* 1995; **27**: 495–500.

90. Adam A, Ellul J, Watkinson AF et al. Palliation of inoperable esophageal carcinoma: a prospective randomized trial of laser therapy and stent placement. *Radiology* 1997; **202**: 344–348.

91. Knyrim K, Wagner H-J, Bethge N et al. A controlled trial of an expansile metal stent for palliation of esophageal obstruction due to inoperable cancer. *N Engl J Med* 1993; **329**: 1302–1307.

16

OESOPHAGEAL PERFORATION

BA Ross

Perforation of any alimentary viscus is potentially a life-threatening disaster. Perforation of the intrathoracic oesophagus is a particularly lethal condition, especially if diagnosis and treatment are delayed. The condition is not common, and it is unlikely that any one surgeon or surgical unit will accumulate a vast experience of the various types and complications of oesophageal perforation. For this reason, treatment should be tailored to the individual patient rather than to expound a common policy for all patients. For example, small perforations can be managed conservatively and large perforations, presenting late for various reasons, may also not be suitable for major surgical intervention. However, excision of necrotic tissue, local and regional toilet together with primary closure should be the gold standard to which surgeons should strive. One facet on which all clinicians involved with the disrupted oesophagus would agree is that the earlier the diagnosis is made and treatment is instituted, the more favourable the outcome.

Table 16.1 summarizes the types and sites of oesophageal perforation.

Table 16.1 Types and sites of oesophageal perforation

Spontaneous
  Complete rupture
  Intramural rupture of haematoma
Instrumental
  Cervical
  Intrathoracic
    Above aortic arch
    Below aortic arch
  Intra-abdominal
  Foreign bodies
Postoperative
  Resection and anastomosis
  Other oesophageal operations
Miscellaneous

SPONTANEOUS PERFORATION

Complete disruption (Boerhaave's syndrome)

In 1946, Barrett[1] reviewed Boerhaave's classical description of the death of Grand Admiral Wassanaer following spontaneous rupture of the oesophagus in 1723. As no patient had survived to this date, Barrett prophesied that 'there was no fundamental reason why this unsatisfactory position should not be improved upon in the future'. A year later, the same author described the first successful repair of this condition[2] and Olson and Clagett[3] similarly reported a successful repair.

Clinical features

Unfortunately, the diagnosis of spontaneous oesophageal rupture is often delayed, many patients with this serious condition being admitted to the coronary care unit or to a general surgical ward, and recognition of the true diagnosis dawning only with the relentless deterioration of the patient's condition, or the observation of cervical or mediastinal emphysema.

The condition invariably follows ingestion of a large meal, as in Baron Wassanaer's case, or a considerable amount of alcohol. The patient then vomits and may violently attempt to restrain this action for social reasons. A crushing central chest pain ensues which may mimic that of myocardial infarction. On examination, some of the features of myocardial infarction may indeed be present, such as tachycardia, sweating, hypotension and oliguria. There may be no other physical signs at an early stage, but after 4–6 hours surgical emphysema may be detected in the neck. The diagnosis hinges on the severe chest pain being accompanied by or preceded by vomiting. If this combination is correctly elicited and recorded, the diagnosis of spontaneous perforation must be accepted until proved incorrect.

Investigations

Chest radiography With these presenting symptoms, chest radiography is mandatory and should include sufficient of the soft tissues above the clavicles to identify early surgical emphysema in the neck. Mediastinal emphysema may be seen, but in the early stages it may be absent or difficult to recognize. Mediastinal pleural elevation from the lateral pericardial border is a classical radiological sign.

Cervical spine radiography The presence of surgical emphysema in the neck is most easily recognized, even at an early stage, by a lateral X-ray view of the cervical spine (Figure 16.1). The

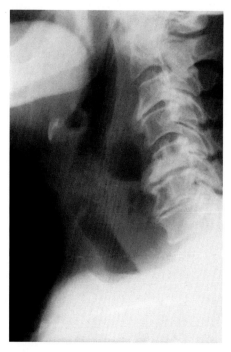

Figure 16.1
Lateral view of cervical spine – showing retropharyngeal air.

stippled appearance of the post-tracheal space is diagnostic of extraoesophageal air and will be detected long before air is seen on the AP view of the spine or PA/AP views of the chest.

Contrast swallow This investigation is mandatory if the diagnosis is even considered. A negative contrast swallow could provide considerable reassurance, as distinct from the problems that arise if the condition is not recognized at an early stage. There is, however, a small risk of a negative contrast study even in the presence of a small perforation. Non-ionic contrast media are preferred by many radiologists who consider this type of contrast to be less harmful to the mediastinum. However, definition is not as good as with barium, and anxiety regarding mediastinal granuloma formation may be more apparent than real, as a positive diagnosis will result in early thoracotomy and mediastinal drainage.[4] It is important not only to establish the presence of a leak but also to localize its site as accurately as possible.

If, as frequently happens, the diagnosis is delayed beyond 12 hours, surgical emphysema will be obvious – certainly radiologically and invariably on clinical examination as well. Pyrexia will be present and cardiac dysrhythmia may be noted. In addition, a pneumothorax or hydropneumothorax may be seen on chest radiograph. If the perforation has extended below the peritoneal reflection of the oesophagus, subphrenic air may also be seen, although perforation at this site is uncommon.

Aetiology

Vomiting is a common phenomenon, which fortunately is only rarely accompanied by rupture of the oesophagus. To achieve rupture, the high retrograde pressure wave, which can exceed

200 mmHg, is potentiated by failure of the upper oesophageal sphincter to relax. This severe force meeting the proverbial immovable object results in such increase in wall tension that a longitudinal tear develops in the oesophagus. This tear varies in length between 1–2 cm and 10–15 cm in a variety of positions around the circumference of the organ. The position of the tear will determine whether the air and fluid collection will remain central within the mediastinum, or rupture through the mediastinal pleura to contaminate one or other or both pleural cavities. The mediastinal collection may remain outside the pleural space for some time but will eventually break through the pleura to produce pneumothorax or hydropneumothorax.

Management

Having completely documented the position of the perforation, there are four alternatives for treatment, all of which involve a surgical procedure of varying magnitude. These are summarized in Table 16.2 Preliminary resuscitation with intravenous fluids and antibiotics is mandatory.

Table 16.2   Surgical treatment modes

Primary closure + Pleural and mediastinal drainage
Oesophageal intubation (Pulsion) + Pleural drainage
Immediate oesophageal resection
T – Tube drainage
Draining gastrostomy and feeding jejunostomy

Before any of the various procedures, all patients should undergo aspiration oesophagoscopy, preferably using a fibre-optic instrument, at which time the defect may be visualized. It is also recommended that before attempting to close the defect by suture, a Maloney oesophageal bougie (size 36–40) is left within the oesophageal lumen together with a nasogastric tube.

Operative procedures

Primary closure The most satisfactory treatment is to close the defect by primary suture. However, the patient must be fit enough to withstand a thoracotomy and laparotomy and the tissues must be reasonably healthy to achieve satisfactory healing. Both these factors are prejudiced by delayed diagnosis and late presentation, and the method is the preferred option when the perforation is less than 6 hours old but should always be attempted unless there is a significant contraindication to a major operation.

It is preferable, but not essential, to obtain unilateral lung ventilation by insertion of one of the many available double-lumen endobronchial tubes, thus facilitating the approach to the posterior mediastinum. Through the appropriate posterolateral thoracotomy the pleural space is entered and all free fluid removed by suction. The lung should be mobilized to give sufficient access to the posterior mediastinum, revealing the oedematous and blood-stained mediastinal pleura, which is opened widely to evacuate all extraneous debris, including food, saliva, barium and any other collected material. Even after 4 hours, the perforated oesophagus is oedematous and the tear may not be immediately obvious. The presence of the Maloney bougie aids the identification of the defect and allows the easy passage of a tape around the oesophagus. It is vital to demarcate accurately the upper and lower margins of the tear before closure is started. The mucosal tear often extends above or below the defect in the muscle coat. The mucosa is approximated with interrupted sutures, the material being a matter of personal preference of the surgeon. The author advocates 3/0 PDS (Ethicon Ltd). Ideally, the muscle layers should be closed over the mucosa. If the oesophageal wall is particularly friable and oedematous, it is preferable to close with a single layer of interrupted sutures, taking great care to close the extremities of the tear. It is often helpful to lay all sutures in a perfect position before tying any of them. The completed closure should be reinforced using vascularized adjacent tissue, such as pleura as advocated by Grillo and Wilkins,[5] or a strip of diaphragm or pericardium, whichever is the most conveniently situated to the suture line. Having cleared the perioesophageal space, a careful inspection of the other side of the oesophagus should be made to exclude a second tear. This eventuality will require full mobilization of the oesophagus from the aorta to the diaphragm to enable satisfactory rotation to be performed for further sutures to be inserted. Large-bore (36Fr) drains are laid in the mediastinum and the supradiaphragmatic pleural space and brought out through stab incisions below the skin wound, before closure of the chest.

The next stage is debatable but strongly recommended. Many workers would advocate that at the completion of the thoracotomy, the patient is turned into the supine position for a laparotomy. Through a small incision in the upper abdomen, a draining gastrostomy is performed using the traditional Stamm technique and a large bore (26Fr) Foley catheter which is brought out through a stab incision in the left upper abdomen. A feeding jejunostomy is inserted using a smaller (16Fr) silastic Foley catheter, or a fine-bore feeding tube. This is inserted into the proximal jejunum and a seromuscular tunnel is constructed, the jejunum being sutured to the anterior abdominal wall at the site of exit from the peritoneum, again through a stab incision below the gastrostomy tube. A feeding gastrostomy does not keep the lower oesophagus empty, particularly if a nasogastric tube has rendered the oesophagogastric junction incompetent. Insertion of the feeding line into the proximal jejunum avoids this, but the draining gastrostomy allows more satisfactory dependent emptying of the stomach and thus lessens gastro-oesophageal reflux and thus further autodigestion. The nasal tube should be withdrawn until the tip lies just above the upper extremity of the perforation. Some surgeons favour an exclusion cervical oesophagostomy but the author does not believe this to be necessary, except in advanced cases. Intubated cervical oesophagostomies are not to be recommended as there is a high incidence of erosion of a major vessel if this tube remains in place for weeks, as is so often required for complete healing to occur (see below).

Postoperative care includes antibiotic cover, metronidazole by suppository and a broad-spectrum third generation cephalosporin, such as cefotaxime or cefuroxime intravenously. H2 receptor antagonists or proton pump inhibitors are recommended to reduce gastric acid production and thus lessen the autodigestion which manifests so rapidly before surgical closure can be effected. The patient is denied oral fluids and food, nutrition being maintained enterally through the jejunostomy using one of the proprietary feeds introduced through a mechanical roller pump. The chest drains are retained until satisfactory closure has been confirmed by a contrast study around 10 days after operation. Immediately before this, 100 ml of a concentrated solution of Ribena® blackcurrant juice (R) may be administered orally. Persistence of the leak may result in the appearance of the dye in the chest drain, thus obviating the necessity for a contrast swallow. A negative 'Ribenagram' (R) should be followed by contrast radiography which should confirm successful healing, enabling full oral feeding to be recommenced. The chest drains and gastrostomy tube can be removed and lastly, when the patient is managing a satisfactory calorie intake, the jejunostomy tube may be removed.

In the unhappy event of the leak persisting, it is recommended that the supportive measures outlined above are continued and a further 'Ribenagram' performed at a suitable interval depending on the size of the residual defect. If the leak is persistent, the chest drains can be cut flush with the skin and allowed to drain into dressings or a bag, thus enabling the patient to be completely ambulant. Depending on the size of the residual leak, solid food can be taken by mouth and fluids inserted into the jejunostomy as before. A leak continuing beyond three weeks is a good indication for endoscopy and sodium hydroxide cautery to the fistula as advocated by McCluskie (personal communication, 1975) and later by Gunning and Kingsnorth.[6] Parry et al.[7] have reported successful use of this controversial treatment in a patient with an acquired broncho-oesophageal fistula who was unfit for any surgical exploration. The caustic agent in their patient, being applied to both the oesophageal and bronchial aspects of the fistula resulted in closure of the communication and good palliation. It is always difficult to determine whether this intervention has accelerated the healing of a fistula, but it is the author's opinion based on many uncontrolled procedures that it is highly beneficial, and should not be dismissed as anecdotal.

Usually, spontaneous perforation of the oesophagus occurs only once in a lifetime, but Reeder et al.[8] record an example of a second episode 30 years after the first in an alcoholic!

Intubation Having identified the site and extent of the leak, the patient's age or general condition may preclude the formidable undertaking described above. In these patients, a pulsion tube can be inserted into the oesophagus to lie across the area of the perforation thus diverting saliva and even ingested fluids into the stomach, allowing the perforation to heal spontaneously. The Wilson–Cooke tube (Cooke UK) associated with an inflatable sponge tampon has been found to be very useful in this situation.

In the presence of significant pleural or mediastinal contamination, large-bore tube drainage of these areas – usually associated with a small segment rib resection – will be mandatory to lessen the risk of septicaemia, which is frequently a fatal complication in this situation.

The endo-oesophageal tube will need to be in place for at least eight weeks before removal is attempted. This in itself is dangerous, as withdrawing the bulbous proximal end of the tube may result in further damage to the oesphagus. Occasionally, the leak may not have closed but it would be difficult to detect this even by contrast radiography until the tube has been removed. A small residual leak at this stage could be treated with sodium hydroxide cautery.

Oesophagectomy Kerr[9] and Matthews et al.[10] have described removal of the damaged oesophagus by subtotal oesophagectomy. The radical subtotal oesophagectomy, advocated by Matthews,[11] is an attractive procedure performed through a left thoracotomy, mobilizing the stomach to pass either orthotopically or through the anterior mediastinum to the neck and constructing an oesophagogastrostomy in the neck, the pleura and mediastinum being drained as described previously. Orringer and Stirling[12] advocate transhiatal resection in this situation, describing 24 patients so treated with three deaths. It is of note that they advocate feeding jejunostomy in all patients. However postoperative feeding can be achieved through a nasogastric tube, the distal end being placed well below the diaphragm. Alternatively, intravenous feeding may be used although this is more expensive and prone to complications.

T-tube drainage Exposure of the perforation, attempted primary closure and insertion of a T-tube oesophagostomy has been described.[13] This has the advantage of allowing a granulation-lined track to develop between the oesophagus and chest wall. Repeated contrast studies are necessary to determine the progress of closure, the T-tube being clamped before removal when it is obvious radiologically that contrast, and therefore food, is passing into the stomach without extravasation.

Exclusion and oesophageal diversion Urschel et al.[14] have advocated since 1974 an 'improved management of oesophageal perforation'. They recommend a policy of exclusion and diversion of the oesophagus which accelerates healing of the oesophagus and resolution of mediastinitis. To support this contention, they described six selected patients, in whom this technique was used. To bring this technique up to date Urschel, discussing a presentation on pleural wrap for the support of oesophageal perforations by Gouge et al.[15] reported 58 patients undergoing this procedure with only five deaths.

The operative procedure advocated entails a cervical oesophagostomy in continuity, i.e. a side hole in the oesophagus, the mucosa being sutured to the subcutaneous tissues and skin. Some surgeons might be tempted to intubate the cervical oesophagus for long-term drainage. This is likely to be disastrous as secondary haemorrhage from a major cervical blood vessel, either carotid artery or jugular vein will provide a fatal outcome of this misguided procedure. The patient is fed through a gastrostomy and the lower oesophagus is partially obstructed by the placement of one or two umbilical tapes around the oesophagus, deep to the vagus nerves, just above the oesophagogastric junction. The object of this manoeuvre is to lessen or abolish reflux from the stomach to the sutured perforation. Survivors of this procedure need to undergo further

operations, certainly to close the cervical fistula. In the early patients, the oesophageal tape was removed at a subsequent laparotomy, which itself could result in further damage to the oesophagus, even perforation! The current technique advocated by its authors entails a prolene suture encircling the oesophagus which itself is protected by a silastic sleeve to prevent the suture eroding into the wall. This is simply removed by external traction after 3–4 weeks.

Abolition of gastro-oesophageal reflux can be simply achieved by the placement of a large bore (24 Fr) Foley catheter into the stomach as a draining gastrostomy as described above. Continuous suction applied through a low pressure pump will keep the stomach empty. The gastrostomy is inserted at the same time as the feeding jejunostomy, both procedures in the author's opinion being mandatory in the management of significant oesophageal leaks, irrespective of cause. The stomach should not be used for feeding purposes in this situation as the feed and gastric secretions will undoubtedly reflux into the damaged oesophagus.

In conclusion, spontaneous complete rupture of the oesophagus is a life-threatening disaster but accurate and early diagnosis can be attended by a high survival rate. The ideal method of surgical treatment is immediate closure with suture line support from local tissues, associated with pleural and mediastinal drainage and enteral feeding. If the diagnosis is delayed beyond 12 hours, this is unlikely to be successful and one of the alternative methods should be considered. The mortality will be much higher in these circumstances, Nesbitt and Sawyers[16] reporting an increase in mortality from 13% to 56% when treatment is delayed.

Intramural rupture of the oesophagus

The presentation of this fascinating condition is similar to that of complete rupture. It is usually associated with vomiting, when severe pain in the chest is followed by difficulty and pain on swallowing.[17] The difference between this condition and spontaneous rupture is that complete perforation does not occur, but rather a dissection between the muscular layers, which results in the development of a large haematoma. Early endoscopy may be confusing as the mucosa is oedematous and distorted, a carcinoma being likely to be suspected. Biopsy at this stage will not contribute to the diagnosis and might be positively harmful. Contrast studies are usually diagnostic; the typical appearance of this condition at barium swallow is shown in Figure 16.2. The use of barium gives far superior results to imaging with water soluble contrast media. CT screening is also helpful in making the diagnosis.

Treatment

Having confidently established the diagnosis and, in particular, having excluded complete rupture, treatment is totally conservative and supportive. If the patient is unable to swallow, either on account of obstruction or severe pain, intravenous fluids will be required for a few days until the acute episode has subsided. A further barium swallow performed ten days later will probably be perfectly normal. The patient will be able to take

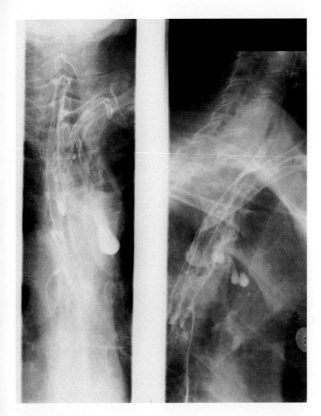

Figure 16.2
Barium swallow showing typical appearance of intramural haematoma.

a soft diet without difficulty from this stage, even if the contrast study is not completely normal.

INSTRUMENTAL PERFORATION

It is unfortunate that the passage of any endoscope is attended by a recognized incidence of varying severity of trauma. Perforation applies particularly to the oesophagus, the reported incidence being generally less than 1% of all endoscopic procedures. As with spontaneous perforation, iatrogenic damage is associated with mortality which has been reported as high as 13%,[18,19] particularly if treatment is delayed. The American Society of Gastrointestinal Endoscopy[20] in a very large survey of over 200,000 endoscopies reported perforation in 0.03% of simple endoscopic examinations. The risk is increased by performing therapeutic procedures endoscopically, the American Society reporting a 0.25% incidence of perforation. The British Society of Gastroenterology Endoscopy Committee following a questionnaire survey of over 800 procedures, reported a 9% incidence of perforation after pulsion intubation. The greatest risk of oesophageal trauma is associated with the passage of a rigid oesophagoscope, the cervical portion being particularly vulnerable. However, it is regrettable that even fibreoptic endoscopes can perforate the cervical region at the initiation of the procedure. The passage of an endotracheal tube can also traumatize the wall of the pharynx or proximal oesophagus. In order to discuss the implications and management of instrumental perforation, it is convenient to divide the organ into cervical, thoracic and abdominal segments. Michel et al.[21] reporting their experience with oesophageal perforations indicate that 68% of perforations were iatrogenic. Sandrasagra and colleagues[22] reviewed 28 patients with perforations of which 21 were instrumental in origin. These occurred in 1052 endoscopies and despite aggressive surgical treatment the overall mortality was 32%. A review of other series with a total of over 14,000 endoscopies showed an incidence of perforation of 0.6%. Bladergroen et al.[23] in a retrospective survey over 47 years report 114 perforations diagnosed before death, of which 55% were iatrogenic.

Cervical oesophagus

As suggested above, the cervical oesophagus is prone to damage at the time of insertion of the rigid oesophagoscope, particularly in inexperienced hands. To gain the cricopharyngeus, excessive leverage applied to the instrument may result in either laceration of the posterior pharyngeal wall itself, or tearing of the oesophagus anterior to the cervical spine, particularly in the elderly in whom osteophytes may be present. It cannot be emphasized too strongly that in rigid oesophagoscopy the single-handed endoscopist must obey the rules of intubation – the neck should be flexed on the trunk and the head extended at the atlanto-occipital joint. This is a perfectly safe technique, often made easier by the passage of a 30 Fr Maloney bougie through the endoscope and into the proximal oesophagus, allowing the rigid endoscope to then pass over the bougie. Having obtained entry into the lumen of the thoracic oesophagus, the bougie is withdrawn and the patient's head extended to allow the further passage of the instrument which must be under direct vision from this point. Some endoscopists still prefer the Chevalier Jackson technique, requiring an assistant to hold the head and shoulders in the correct position. Modern operating tables should have made the use of this technique quite unnecessary. Although the risk of perforation and the necessity of indulging in these complex measures is much less with fibreoptic endoscopy, the cervical oesophagus is still at risk of perforation if excessive pressure is applied, particularly in the presence of a pharyngeal pouch.

Patients frequently complain of a sore throat after endoscopy, the majority responding to reassurance and simple analgesics. However, persistence of the soreness, particularly if associated with fever and tachycardia, should alert the clinician to the possibility of minor damage to the pharyngeal mucosa. In these circumstances, a lateral radiograph of the cervical spine may show the characteristic stippling of extraoesophageal air (Figure 16.1). Untreated, this may develop into a retropharyngeal abscess; this is characterized by a change in voice, stridor, and very severe dysphagia, the neck exhibiting marked tenderness on palpation. Contrast radiography is quite unnecessary to confirm this diagnosis and spontaneous healing can be confidently anticipated following drainage of the abscess.

Treatment

The diagnosis of a cervical oesophageal tear having been established at an early stage, the majority will respond to conservative treatment with oral food and fluids being denied, hydration being by intravenous fluids. Antibiotics should be given, in a regime similar to that described for spontaneous rupture. The regression of pain and the ability to take oral fluids with decreasing discomfort will be accompanied by a reduction of local neck tenderness. Persistence of the pain and tenderness and the features listed above suggest the development of a collection of infected saliva in the postoesophageal space, the precursor of an abscess. Failure to resolve within four or five days, with persisting symptoms and signs, is an indication for drainage of the retro-oesophageal space.

Operative technique As the laryngopharynx may be oedematous, particularly if the perforation is some days old, endotracheal intubation during anaesthetic induction should be performed with great care. The approach should be on the side of the neck with maximum tenderness or swelling. If doubt exists, the left side gives the easiest access to the retro-oesophageal space. A short transverse incision is made from the mid-line extending to the external jugular vein, which is preserved. The investing layer of cervical fascia is opened along the line of the sternomastoid muscle. The traditional approach is to make this incision anterior to this muscle, but the author prefers to split the muscle between its heads. This leaves the surgeon in a more posterior position and ideally placed to expose the abscess. The middle thyroid vein is divided and blunt dissection lateral to the thyroid gland will reveal the abscess which is readily opened, as it has no wall at this stage. Air, purulent fluid and saliva will be immediately apparent and a soft drain should be left in the retro-oesophageal space and brought out through the wound. No attempt need be made to find the perforation unless it is suspected that the hole in the oesophagus is large. However, repair of the laceration is advocated by some,[21] but by the time the exploration is performed, usually later than 48 h after the endoscopy, the oesophageal tissues are unlikely to retain sutures and more damage may be caused in mobilizing the organ to find the defect. The wound is closed with loose approximation of the heads of sternomastoid, platysma being closed before skin closure with either interrupted sutures or clips. Moghissi and Pender[24] reports no mortality in patients with cervical perforation treated by drainage.

The effect on the patient's condition is dramatic with immediate relief of pain and respiratory obstruction, and the salivary fistula closes spontaneously within a few days. Meanwhile, the patient is supported with antibiotics and intravenous fluids. Should the fistula persist for more than 14 days, it is reasonable to use sodium hydroxide[6] on the defect to cauterize the area and encourage the proliferation of granulation tissue. The drain can be removed when the salivary leak has stopped and a 'Ribenagram' is negative. Occasionally an iatrogenic intramural dissection of the oesophageal wall can be seen. This can be caused by a fibreoptic instrument perforating the oesophageal or pharyngeal wall in the neck, the endoscope being driven all the way down the oesophagus without further perforation (Figure 16.3). In this instance, it is usually easy to find the true lumen at careful endoscopy. In these circumstances, a nasogastric tube can be passed into the stomach for feeding, and the

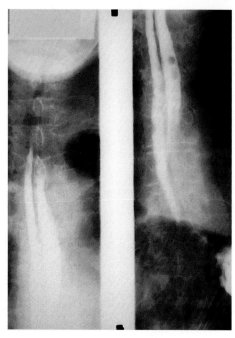

Figure 16.3
Barium swallow showing a 'double barrel' oesophagus. The false lumen starts in the neck and ends blindly in the lower mediastinum. No extravasation is seen.

cervical laceration will usually heal spontaneously. If there is no extravasation, no other operative drainage is required.

Although perforation may follow fibreoptic endoscopy, the risk is considerably less than that following rigid oesophagoscopy. Once the gastroscope or duodenoscope has left the lumen of the oesophagus, it is often driven a long way into or down the mediastinum before the error is suspected. This may result in an abscess at any level in the mediastinum, drainage of which through the neck may be far from ideal. It may be preferable to use a latex rubber tube drain to which suction can be applied, thereby aiding the evacuation of the abscess. In the presence of a significant mediastinal collection below the neck, resumption of oral feeding must be delayed until contrast radiography has confirmed that the leak is completely healed. If this is prolonged, a feeding gastrostomy will allow the patient to return home before the fistula has fully healed, even with the cervical drain still in place.

Thoracic oesophagus

Aetiology

The commonest cause of intrathoracic oesophageal perforation is endoscopy associated with either dilatation of strictures, or attempted pulsion intubation of a carcinoma. This complication was more commonly seen before the advent of malleable dilators and fibreoptic endoscopes. Using a rigid endoscope, the stricture could readily be reached and visualized. Passage of rigid gum elastic and Chevalier–Jackson bougies enabled the proximal aspect of the stricture to be entered. The rigidity of the endoscope, the relative rigidity of the bougie and the natural curve of the oesophagus associated with kyphosis, so often encountered in middle-aged and elderly patients, determined the onward passage of the bougie. This did not necessarily follow the lumen either of the stricture or, more importantly, of the oesophagus immediately distal to the stricture, potential existing for the bougie to be driven out into the mediastinum through the posterior or lateral walls. The use of Maloney bougies has largely eliminated this problem and must be recommended as the bougie of choice for use with a rigid endoscope. However Orringer[12] cites six of nine bougie injuries to the oesophagus being caused by Maloney bougies.

When a fibreoptic instrument is used to view and dilate strictures, it is recommended that a guide wire be passed through the stricture into the stomach, its passage and final position ideally being confirmed under fluoroscopic control. Dilatation of the stricture can be easily effected using warmed Celestin bougies (Duromed Ltd) passed over the guide wire, under the control of C-arm image intensification. These simple precautions have reduced the risk of perforation to a minimum but, unfortunately, perforation may still occur because of incorrect passage of the guide wire. Even these precautions have not eliminated the risk of perforation of a stricture which could occur in the case of very rigid or fibrous benign strictures, or carcinomatous strictures, which may give way on dilatation, like an unripe pear. This is particularly a hazard of pulsion tube insertion for palliation of inoperable oesophageal tumours as identified by The British Society of Gastroenterology.

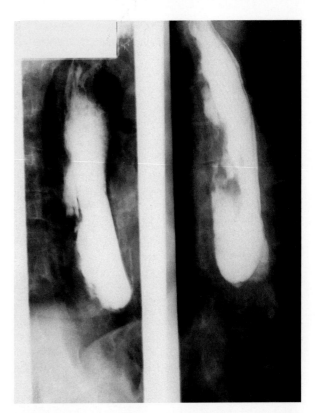

Figure 16.4
Barium swallow showing a mediastinal abscess below the level of the clavicle.

Clinical features and investigation

Following dilatation or intubation, the patient awakes with severe unremitting back pain. This symptom alone should arouse suspicion of the likelihood of perforation. Mediastinal pain following stretching of the stricture does occur, but this symptom should be viewed with great suspicion and the minimum investigation is chest radiography. The pain is usually accompanied by fever and tachycardia. Surgical emphysema may be detected clinically in the neck, but this is sometimes a late sign. The absence of mediastinal emphysema is reassuring, but persistent pain must be investigated by a contrast study using either dilute barium or a water-soluble opaque medium in the first instance. In this situation, it might be necessary to treat the patient conservatively, even though a perforation is confirmed; nevertheless, barium need not be avoided as the definition of the anatomy is far superior to that obtained with water-soluble media.[4] In addition, retained barium in the lung or mediastinum is less harmful.

The finding of mediastinal emphysema must be considered as the cardinal feature of a post-dilatation perforation. Once again, the soft tissues of the neck may provide this evidence, the air being invisible on chest radiograph. Confirmation and localization of the leak must be provided by contrast studies as discussed above. If the perforation is not recognized at this early stage, the patient's condition will quickly deteriorate and a purulent mediastinitis will supervene. Pneumothorax or pyopneumothorax will inevitably follow if the diagnosis is delayed.

Treatment

The age and general fitness of the patient together with the underlying pathology and the size of the perforation have to be considered in formulating the definitive treatment. Small perforations frequently heal on conservative treatment with antibiotics, nil by mouth and intravenous fluids if instituted early, healing being confirmed by contrast swallow on the seventh to tenth day. In the unlikely event of a large perforation of a normal oesophagus, there can only be one approach – immediate thoracotomy and suture of the perforation. This procedure performed at an early stage, ideally at the time of perforation, will be rewarded by complete success. Perforation at or above a stricture, whether benign or malignant, will be unlikely to heal even if closed surgically, due to the unrelieved obstruction distal to the perforation or the pathology of the tissue perforated. Management alternatives are as follows.

Conservative treatment Antibiotics, intravenous feeding and pleural drainage may be applicable to frail elderly patients with only minor degrees of extravasation. The mortality in this group must be expected to be high.

Further endoscopy and intubation This might also be contemplated in the unfit patient, but it is axiomatic that the true lumen of the oesophagus must be intubated, which will be more difficult because of the perforation. It is, however, often surprisingly easy to find the normal lumen on the second occasion, a guide wire left in the stomach facilitating the insertion of an endo-oesophageal tube using a standard pulsion technique. The Wilson–Cooke (R) tube has been a useful stent for this purpose, as described above, the latex sponge providing excellent tamponade for the area of trauma. Pleural drainage will undoubtedly be required. After a suitable interval, usually not before two months, the tube can be removed if the underlying stricture was benign. If malignant, it would be reasonable to leave the tube and offer the patient radiotherapy to the tumour.

Immediate resection Resection would be the treatment of choice in the fit patient with either a benign or malignant stricture, as described by Kerr,[9] Matthews[10] and Orringer and Stirling[12]. The choice of approach would depend entirely on the level of the stricture; the indications and the operative technique used are described elsewhere in this volume. Such a procedure carries a significant mortality and considerable morbidity, depending on the interval between perforation and diagnosis. Immediate resection has the advantage of ablation of the underlying pathology and at the same time allowing drainage of the mediastinum and pleura. Damage to the oesophagus at or above the arch of the aorta will entail resection of the whole oesophagus with either a very high intrathoracic anastomosis or, preferably, a cervical anastomosis.

Abdominal oesophagus

Since the advent of fibreoptic endoscopic dilatation of oesophageal strictures, not only is the risk of perforation much less, but many of the perforations which do occur are guide wire perforations, and hence small. A large proportion of these perforations will heal on conservative treatment, including withholding oral food and fluids, intravenous fluids and antibiotics, providing there is no systemic upset to the patient. Contrast radiography should always attempt to confirm the presence and site of perforation.

Perforation below the diaphragm is the least common site, the finding of subphrenic air after endoscopy often being attended by no constitutional disturbance whatever. Recognition and treatment at this level is very similar to the methods described above for intrathoracic perforations. Once again, it is vital to assess the condition of the patient as a number will respond to gastric drainage through a nasal tube and intravenous fluids, particularly if the stomach has been perforated with a guide wire. If the intra-abdominal oesophagus is damaged, this can only be delineated by contrast studies, as described above. Treatment for perforations at this level will depend on the underlying pathology, carcinoma being resected, if feasible.

FOREIGN BODY PERFORATION

Ingestion of hard or sharp foreign bodies is likely to damage the oesophagus to a varying degree. Extraction of these may also further damage the wall of the oesophagus. Patients in long-stay psychiatric hospitals commonly swallow knives, forks, leather shoe soles or other movable objects. Bones, both meat and fish, are common culprits, becoming lodged in the oesophageal wall, the meat associated with the bone causing intraluminal obstruction. Meat bones are often difficult to remove on account of their multifaceted surface. Fish bones are often difficult to see and can easily be overlooked at a first inspection, particularly if this is performed by an inexperienced endoscopist. Another unusual impacting agent is a half set of dentures which, when incomplete, may present so many facets that any one of them may become impacted. Many are not radio-opaque, thus making endoscopy mandatory. If acrylic, it may be possible to divide the plate with specialized instruments before it can be safely removed. It is often necessary to resort to oesophagotomy to remove a foreign body of this size. Occasionally, such large foreign bodies might impact in a pharyngeal pouch and remain undetected for a long time. The clinical features and management of perforation following ingestion or removal of foreign bodies is similar to that described above for instrumental perforation.

POSTOPERATIVE PERFORATION (ANASTOMOTIC LEAKAGE)

No commentary on oesophageal perforation would be complete without brief reference to leaks which might occur as a result of a definitive surgical operation.

Following oesophageal resection

The complications of oesophageal resection have been fully discussed elsewhere (Chapter 14). Leaks may occur at any suture line following oesophagotomy, oesophageal resection and excision of a pharyngeal pouch. Leakage following reconstruction of the foregut may occur at the anastomosis, the reconstructed lesser curve of stomach, or the gastrotomy used for insertion of a circumferential stapling cartridge. Those leaks manifesting on the second or third day after operation should be regarded as technical inadequacies of the original operation, and re-operation and closure is clearly indicated if the patient's condition will tolerate the procedure. Those leaks occurring at or after the tenth day after operation should generally be treated conservatively initially, aided by adequate pleural drainage and nutritional support, either enteral or parenteral. Revisional surgery may be considered if healing does not occur or if the defect is large, although the mortality of such intervention is high.

Following other oesophageal operations

Operative procedures on the oesophagus are not without risk of perforation, irrespective of whether the mucosa has been surgically breached. These procedures include oesophagotomy, for enucleation of leiomyomata and myotomy, for achalasia or cricopharyngeal or diffuse oesophageal spasm (see below).

Cardiomyotomy or cervical myotomy may damage the fragile mucosa, commonly as a result of injudicial use of surgical diathermy, causing necrosis which results in a leak. Such a problem in the neck results in an abscess which drains or can readily be drained through the original incision without significant disturbance to the patient. Leakage after cardiomyotomy is far more serious, resulting in the problems of diagnosis and treatment discussed above in relation to other oesophageal perforations at this level.

Fundoplication whether complete (Nissen) or partial (Belsey) may be complicated by suture penetration of the oesophageal lumen giving rise to leakage, occult or overt (usually the former), presenting as dysphagia due to abscess formation within the wrap. Antibiotics may resolve this problem, a few patients requiring further exploration and drainage of the collection.

The technique favoured by some in which the Angelchik prosthesis is used for prevention of gastro-oesophageal reflux may occasionally be complicated by erosion and perforation of the oesophagus.[25]

Injection of ethanolamine oleate to control variceal haemorrhage may be followed by quite severe mediastinal pain. This is due to a degree of oesophageal extravasation into and sometimes through the wall of the oesophagus. Fortunately, necrosis and free perforation is very rare.

MISCELLANEOUS CAUSES OF PERFORATION

Mallory–Weiss tears

This is not a true oesophageal perforation but is, however, a cause of approximately 10% of haematemeses. This may follow an episode of vomiting, resulting in a tear in the gastric mucosa just distal to the oesophagogastric junction which may extend cephalad to cause disruption of the lower oesophageal mucosa. Although the presentation is dramatic, the prognosis with conservative treatment is excellent once the diagnosis is confirmed by endoscopy, and other causes of haematemeses are excluded.

Post-traumatic perforation

Closed chest injuries

Rupture of the oesophagus is perhaps not such an uncommon complication of blunt chest trauma as any one surgeon may think.[26] A review of many series of oesophageal injury quotes an incidence as high as 19%.[27]

Penetrating injury

Any penetrating wound to the neck or posterior mediastinum may injure the oesophagus. Damage to this organ following gunshot wounds or knife injuries is uncommon, but must always be borne in mind when such an injury presents and an active process of exclusion must be performed.

The clinical features and management of post-traumatic perforation are similar to those described above for large instrumental perforations.

SUMMARY

Oesophageal perforation, whether spontaneous or instrumental is potentially a highly dangerous condition requiring rapid and accurate diagnosis. Treatment is attended by a varying degree of success, inversely related to the time elapsing before treatment is instituted. Surgical treatment is mandatory in most cases, taxing the ingenuity of general and thoracic surgeons alike. If appropriate expertise is not available locally, referral to a specialized centre experienced in the management of this complex situation is strongly recommended.

REFERENCES

1. Barrett NR Spontaneous perforation of the oesophagus. *Thorax* 1946; **1**: 48–70.
2. Barrett NR Report of a case of spontaneous perforation of the oesophagus successfully treated by operation. *Br J Surg* 1947; **35**: 216–218.
3. Olsen AM & Clagett OT. Spontaneous rupture of the oesophagus. Report of a case with immediate diagnosis and successful surgical repair. *Postgrad Med J* 1947; **2**: 417–419.
4. Appleton DS, Sandrasagra FA & Flower CDR. Perforated oesophagus: review of 28 consecutive cases. *Clin Radiol* 1979; **30**: 493–497.
5. Grillo HC & Wilkins EW. Oesophageal repair following late diagnosis of intrathoracic perforation. *Ann Thorac Surg* 1975; **20**: 387–399.
6. Gunning AJ & Kingsnorth A. Treatment of chronic oesophageal perforations with special reference to an endoscopic method. *Br J Surg* 1979; **66**: 226–229.
7. Parry GW, Juma A & Dussek JE. Broncho-oesophageal fistula treated effectively without surgical resection. *Thorax* 1993; **48**: 189–190.
8. Reeder LB, Warren SE & Ferguson MK Recurrent spontaneous perforation of the oesophagus. *Ann Thorac Surg* 1995; **59**: 221–222.
9. Kerr WF. Emergency oesophagectomy. *Thorax* 1968; **23**: 204–209.
10. Matthews HR, Mitchell IM & McGuigan JA Emergency subtotal oesophagectomy. *Br J Surg* 1989; **76**: 918–920.
11. Matthews HR & Steel A Left sided subtotal oesophagecomy for carcinoma. *Br J Surg* 1987; **74**: 1115–1117.
12. Orringer MB & Stirling MC: Oesophagectomy for oesophageal disruption. *Ann Thorac Surg* 1990; **49**: 35–43.
13. Abbott OA, Manson KA, Logan WD, Hatcher CR & Symbas PN. Atraumatic so-called 'spontaneous' rupture of the oesophagus. A review of 47 personal cases with comments on a new method of surgical therapy. *J Thorac Cardiovasc Surg* 1970; **59**: 67–82.
14. Urschel HC, Razzuk MA & Wood RE. Improved management of oesophageal perforation: exclusion and diversion in continuity. *Ann Surg* 1974; **179**: 587–592.
15. Gouge TH, Depan HJ & Spencer FC. Experience with the Grillo pleural wrap procedure in 18 patients with perforation of the thoracic oesophagus. *Ann Surg* 1989; **209**: 612–617.
16. Nesbitt JC & Sawyers JL. Surgical management of esophageal perforation. *Am Surg* 1987; **53**: 183–187.
17. Kerr WF. Spontaneous intramural rupture and intramural haematoma of the oesophagus. *Thorax* 1980; **35**: 890–897.
18. Berry BE & Ochsner JL. Perforation of the oesophagus. *J Thorac Cardiovasc Surg* 1973; **65**: 1–7.
19. Triggiani E & Belsey R. Oesophageal trauma: incidence, diagnosis and management. *Thorax* 1977; **32**: 241–249.
20. Silvis SE, Nebel O, Rogers C, Sugava C & Mandelstam P. Endoscopic complications: result of the 1974 American Society of Gastrointestinal Endoscopy survey. *JAMA* 1976; **235**: 928–930.
21. Michel L, Grillo HC & Malt RA. Operative and non operative management of oesophageal perforations. *Ann Surg* 1981; **194**: 57–63.
22. Sandrasagra FA, English TAH & Milstein BB. (1978) The management and prognosis of oesophageal perforations. *Br J Surg* 1978; **65**: 629–632.
23. Bladergroen MR, Lowe JE & Postlethwait RW. Diagnosis and recommended management of oesophageal perforation and rupture. *Ann Thorac Surg* 1986; **42**: 235–239.
24. Moghissi K & Pender D. Instrumental perforations of the oesophagus and their management. *Thorax* 1988; **43**: 642–646.
25. Lilly MP, Slafsky SF & Thompson WR. Intraluminal erosion and migration of the Angelchik anti-reflux prosthesis. *Arch Surg* 1984; **119**: 849–851.
26. Young CP, Large SR & Edmonson SJ. Blunt traumatic rupture of the thoracic oesophagus. *Thorax* 1988; **43**: 794–795.
27. Jones WG & Ginsberg RJ. Oesophageal perforation: a continuing challenge. *Ann Thorac Surg* 1992; **53**: 534–543.

17

OESOPHAGEAL VARICES

AG Johnson

Oesophageal varices are one manifestation of portal hypertension. They are the result, not the cause, of a disease process and, although they frequently develop at a late stage of the disease, haemorrhage may be the first sign the patient has of an underlying problem. Throughout the world, bleeding oesophageal varices are an important cause of mortality because portal hypertension caused by liver damage due to schistosomiasis or hepatitis B is common in the large populations of Africa and Asia. However, the prevalence of oesophageal varices is uncertain because large numbers of asymptomatic patients have not been endoscoped. The incidence is easier to determine as patients present either with a bleed or with the complications of their liver disease.

CLINICAL PRESENTATION

In Britain, bleeding oesophageal varices account for less than 5% of upper gastrointestinal haemorrhage in an unselected population, but this is far higher in units which act as referral centres and figures from such units can be misleading. If all patients with established cirrhosis without ascites are endoscoped, 25–30% are found to have oesophageal varices. If there is ascites the figure rises to 35–40%, and with alcoholic cirrhosis it is as high as 80%. Untreated oesophageal varices do not give dysphagia or pain and are only rarely accompanied by reflux oesophagitis. Dysphagia may result from repeated injection of varices, particularly if sclerosant is injected into the muscle layer, producing fibrosis. However, varices can coexist with other conditions which cause bleeding, such as peptic ulcer, and it is not safe to assume that a patient with known varices who bleeds is always bleeding from that site. Table 17.1 gives the sites of first bleed in patients with portal hypertension and the sites of recurrent bleeding once treatment of oesophageal varices has been started.

UNDERLYING CAUSES OF PORTAL HYPERTENSION

Oesophageal varices, whether or not they bleed, are the result of an underlying disease. Portal hypertension can be caused by liver disease or venous occlusion, or both; the causes are classified in Table 17.2.

Table 17.1 Source of gastrointestinal bleeding in patients with portal hypertension on first presentation and subsequent episodes (over 4 years)

SITE	PRESENTING BLEEDS		SUBSEQUENT BLEEDS	
	NO.	%	NO.	%
Oesophageal varices	88	77	64	31.7
Gastric varices	6	5.3	11	5.5
Gastropathy	9	8	71	35.2
Peptic ulcer	4	3.6	3	1.5
Postinjection slough	—	—	16	7.9
Rectal varices	3	2.5	2	0.9
Others	4	3.6	36	17.3

Unpublished data from the Sheffield Portal Hypertension Unit, The Royal Hallamshire Hospital, where emergency and long-term injection sclerotherapy was the mainstay of treatment.

The *cause* of portal hypertension is relevant to gastrointestinal surgeons for the following reasons:

Table 17.2 Classification of the causes of portal hypertension

A. Presinusoidal
  1. Extrahepatic obstruction
    (a) Intrinsic thrombosis — neonatal sepsis
                    – pyelophlebitis
                    – increased coagulability
    (b) Extrinsic compression — pancreatic tumour
                    – pancreatitis
                    – enlarged lymph nodes
  2. Intrahepatic — schistosomiasis
                    – congenital hepatic fibrosis
                    – sarcoidosis
                    – reticuloendothelial disease
                    – early stages of primary biliary cirrhosis
B. Intrahepatic – mainly cirrhosis, e.g. alcohol, viral, haemochromatosis, chemical poisons, idiopathic
C. Postsinusoidal – obstruction of hepatic veins or inferior vena cava (Budd–Chiari syndrome)
D. Increased portal flow — AV fistula
                       – increased hepatic flow

1. The prognosis largely depends on the underlying disease, in that most patients with cirrhosis eventually die of liver failure, especially as methods of controlling acute bleeding have improved.

2. Some causes can be treated, or at least contained, e.g. by a patient with alcoholic cirrhosis abstaining. All long-term studies of different treatments of bleeding varices show better results in those who stop drinking than in those who do not.

3. The long-term treatment e.g. portosystemic shunting, may be indicated in some, but not in others.

4. Prevention must be directed to the underlying cause.

The causes of liver damage vary greatly in their relative incidence in different parts of the world and also in different parts of the same country. In the USA and France, over 90% of cases of cirrhosis are alcoholic in origin, whereas in Sheffield fewer than 50% are alcoholic and the rest have several different causes. In South-East Asia, hepatitis B is the most common cause, whereas in Egypt over 90% of cases are due to schistosomiasis with or without hepatitis B. Vaccination against hepatitis B and not standing in static water, thereby preventing infection with schistosomiasis, may have a profound influence on reducing the prevalence of the problem in the future.

WHY DO OESOPHAGEAL VARICES BLEED?

This is one of the important unsolved questions. Some patients present with bleeding apparently early in the natural history of their portal hypertension, whereas others have cirrhosis and varices for many years and die of liver failure, their varices never having bled. As a broad generalization, the larger the varices and higher the portal pressure, the more likely they are to bleed, but there is not a direct linear relationship between pressure and risk of bleeding. However, it is unlikely that varices will bleed when the portal (wedge hepatic venous) pressure is below 13 mmHg.[1]

The other fascinating clinical observation is that oesophageal varices nearly always bleed in the lower 4–5 cm of the oesophagus, even though they may extend much further up than that. Over the years, there has been debate about whether 'erosive' or 'eruptive' forces are mainly responsible for initiating a bleed. The evidence for foreign bodies, such as fish bones or overcooked toast damaging the varix is rather sparse and it is rare to find associated reflux oesophagitis accompanying varices. The weight of evidence[2] favours *eruptive* forces, perhaps sudden changes within the varix itself and the overlying mucosa. Sudden changes in intravariceal pressure may occur with coughing or straining or with a sudden rise in portal venous pressure, as with acute alcoholic hepatitis. There are important anatomical and physiological features of the lower oesophagus which are relevant to variceal rupture. They are:

1. The mucosal junction zone between squamous and gastric mucosa.

2. The unique venous arrangement in the lower oesophagus.

3. The diaphragm crossing the region, with the difference in pressure above and below.

4. The physiological lower oesophageal sphincter, which occupies the lower 4 cm of the oesophagus.

VENOUS ANATOMY OF THE LOWER OESOPHAGUS

The main venous drainage from the upper stomach and lower oesophagus into the portal system comprises the short gastric vein, the left gastric (coronary) vein and a constant 'polar' vein, not usually described, which drains into the middle of the splenic vein and forms an arcade with the left gastric vein (Figure 17.1). There have been several descriptions[3–5] of the venous anatomy, all of which use slightly different names. In summary, there are, in longitudinal section (Figure 17.2), three layers of vessels, each of which connect with a similar plexus in or around the stomach. The *subepithelial* layer drains the small vessels in the epithelium, which do not have valves, and these are connected by perforating veins through the muscularis mucosa to the *submucosal* veins, which have valves at their lower end directing flow down to the stomach. These in turn are connected by perforating veins through the main oesophageal muscle to the *perioesophageal* vessels, which join the azygos (or hemiazygos) vein above or the gastric vessels below. The perforating veins have valves just outside the oesophageal wall which direct blood *outwards*. The other important discovery by image analysis studies[6] is that, in both normal subjects and in patients with portal hypertension, the

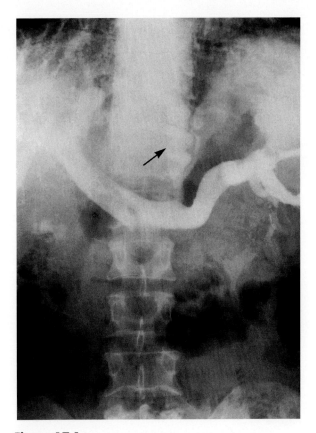

Figure 17.1
Portal venogram of patient with portal hypertension showing varicosity of posterior gastric ('polar' vein (arrow).

Oesophageal veins

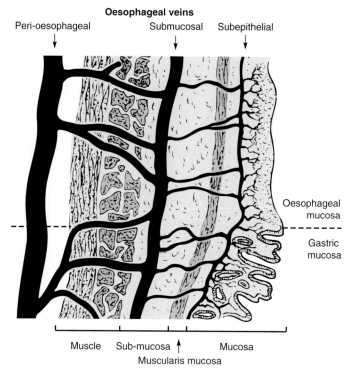

Figure 17.2

Longitudinal section through gastro-oesophageal junction showing three layers of vessels connected by perforating veins. POS, paraoesophageal; SMV, submucosal; SEV, subepithelial; MM, muscularis mucosae. (Reproduced with permission from McCormack T. ChM thesis, University of Dublin.)

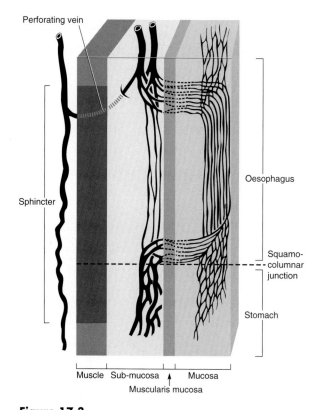

Figure 17.3

Venous channels lying superficially in the lower few centimetres of the oesophagus. (From De Carvalho CAF. *Acta Anat* 1966; **64:** 125–162.)

subepithelial channels are larger and more numerous in the lower 4–5 cm than are the submucosal channels – whereas these form the largest channels more proximally (Figure 17.3). Therefore, in the area where varices nearly always bleed, the main venous channels are lying just beneath the epithelium, unprotected by the muscularis mucosa.

The gastric and lower oesophageal veins can be classified into four zones (Figure 17.4): the gastric, pallisade, perforating and truncal zones. The pallisade zone consists of many small venous channels lying superficially; these join above to form four or five major channels with the main perforating zones at the junction. Both Doppler and anatomical studies have confirmed that there is nearly always one or more perforating vessel 2–3 cm above the gastro-oesophageal mucosal junction. The normal direction of flow is outwards. In portal hypertension, the veins dilate, the valves become incompetent and flow partially reverses. Consequently, blood is directed from outside towards the lumen, leading to a greater risk of bleeding – a situation very analogous to the constant perforating vein above the medial malleolus, which becomes incompetent and important in varicose veins of the leg (the common site of ulceration and bleeding). In portal hypertension, one or more main vessels sometimes dilate across the pallisade zone (Figure 17.5a), and sometimes only the oesophageal vessels in the truncal zone dilate (Figure 17.5b), hence filled through the perforators. When the small vessels in the epithelium also dilate they give rise to the endoscopic appearance of 'cherry-red' spots (see below).

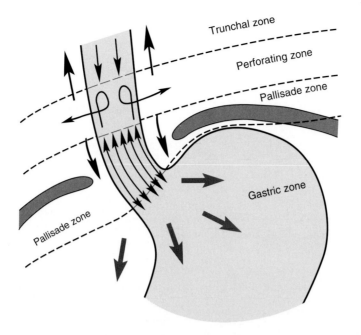

Figure 17.4
Normal venous pattern of lower oesophagus and upper stomach with direction of blood flow. gz, gastric zone; plz, pallisade zone; pfz, perforating zone; tz, truncal zone. (From Carter, Russell et al. *Operative Surgery* (5th edn) London: Chapman and Hall.)

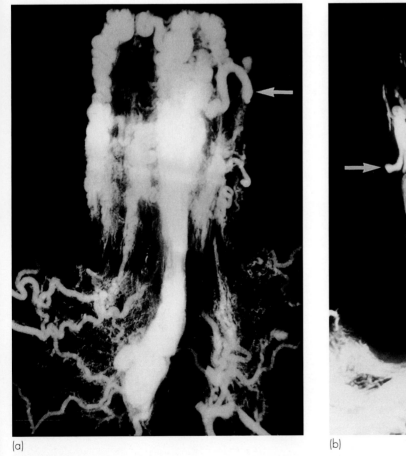

(a)

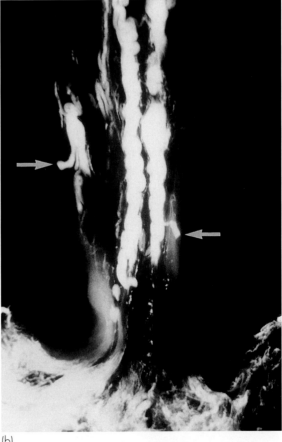

(b)

Figure 17.5
Radiograph of corrosion cast in portal hypertension showing dilatation of (a) pallisade zone vessels and perforator (arrow), and (b) truncal zone vessels filled through perforators (arrows) without dilatation of pallisade zone. (Reproduced with permission from Vianna A. PhD thesis, University of London.) (Figure 5(a) from Carter, Russell et al. *Operative Surgery* (5th edn) London: Chapman and Hall.)

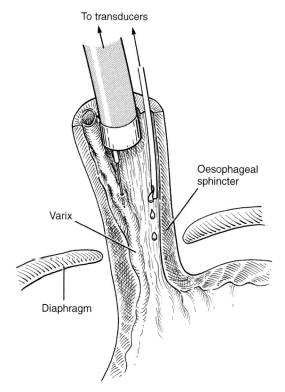

Figure 17.6
Apparatus used with endoscope to measure transvariceal wall pressure by comparing intravariceal pressure and oesophageal lumen pressure. (Adapted from Hosking SW, Robinson P & Johnson AG. The effect of Valsalva's manoeuvre and hyoscintylbromide on the pressure gradient across the wall of the oesophageal varices. *Gut* 1987; **28:** 1151.)

PHYSIOLOGICAL CHANGES

If 'eruptive' forces are important in the initiation of bleeding, this must relate to a local or general rise in pressure in the portal system. The important measurement is the *differential* pressure across the variceal wall, i.e. the difference between the intravariceal pressure and the pressure in the oesophageal lumen. This has been measured in patients using a perfused catheter in the lumen and a perfused needle in the varix (Figure 17.6)[7] and by high resolution endoluminal sonography.[8]

General increase in portal pressure

A general rise in portal pressure is produced by the following changes:

- Increased splanchnic arterial inflow. Initially, drug therapy of variceal bleeding was aimed at reducing splanchnic flow, e.g. vasopressin (see below).
- Increasing 'hepatic' resistance. This may be produced by acute swelling of the liver, such as after an acute alcoholic 'binge' or portal vein thrombosis or obstruction or even obstruction of the hepatic veins (Budd–Chiari syndrome). Recent research on drug therapy for bleeding has concentrated on dilatation of these vessels, thereby reducing resistance.

Local changes in pressure

Alterations of pressure in the oesophageal varices are produced by respiratory changes and the effect of the lower oesophageal sphincter.

Respiratory changes and manoeuvres

The Valsalva manoeuvre (attempted expiration against a closed glottis) might be expected to increase intrathoracic pressure and so 'burst' the varices, but clinical evidence does not support this concept because bleeding in patients with portal hypertension is very uncommon during the second stage of labour. Studies in patients undergoing sclerotherapy using the apparatus illustrated in Figure 17.6 show that, although the intravariceal pressure does indeed rise during a Valsalva manoeuvre, so does the intraoesophageal pressure, and in only a minority of patients is there a rise in *trans-variceal* pressure. The Müller manoeuvre on the other hand – the opposite of the Valsalva (i.e. attempted inspiration against a closed glottis) – leads to large negative pressure within the chest and could tend to encourage blood flow into the varices. So far we have been unable to train patients to do this with an endoscope in place, but during a barium swallow it has been shown that the varices distend markedly (Figure 17.7). This suggests that a sudden forced *in*spiration, as at the end of a cough, could cause changes which would tend to rupture the varices.

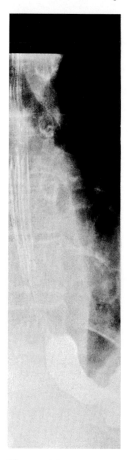
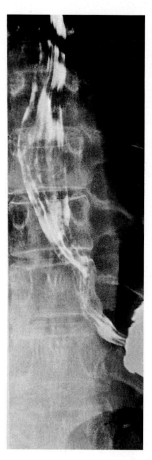

Figure 17.7
Barium swallow before (left) and after (right) Müller manoeuvre showing distension of varices. (Courtesy of the Radiology Department, Erasmus University, Rotterdam.)

Effect of the lower oesophageal sphincter

As discussed in Chapter 1, the physiological lower oesophageal sphincter surrounds the lower 4 cm of the oesophagus. Its contractions will therefore affect blood flow through the wall and also the lowermost perforating veins. Studies have shown that drugs which produce contraction of the sphincter for a shorter (pentagastrin) or longer (metoclopramide) time greatly reduce the net variceal pressure just above the sphincter (Figure 17.8). A controlled trial in patients with active bleeding has found that contraction of the sphincter with metoclopramide (20 mg) is effective in stopping active bleeding.[9]

In conclusion, the following factors are important in the site, initiation and control of a bleed.

- The overall level of the portal pressure, and especially sudden increases.
- Sudden increases in negative intrathoracic pressure.
- The superficial position of the varices in the lower oesophagus.
- The presence of perforating veins in the lower oesophagus.
- The effect of the lower oesophageal sphincter.

It is, however, still not clear what the initiating event really is for any one patient.

ENDOSCOPIC CLASSIFICATION OF VARICES

Nowadays, the diagnosis of oesophageal varices is made endoscopically rather than by barium swallow, which can be misleading. They may be classified by the height to which they extend up the oesophagus, their diameter and protrusion into the lumen (grades I–III) and their colour and appearance of the surface. It must be admitted that size is rather subjective and may be affected by the patient straining. The Japanese group[10,11] first proposed a classification of endoscopic appearances as a way of predicting

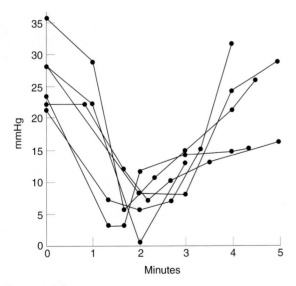

Figure 17.8
Effect of a bolus pentagastrin injection on transvariceal wall pressure. (Adapted from Hosking SW, Doss W, El-Zeiny H, Robinson P, Barsoum M & Johnson AG. Pharmacological constriction of the lower oesophageal sphincter – a simple method of controlling variceal haemorrhage. *Gut* 1988; **19:** 1098.)

Table 17.3 Classification of the appearance of oesophageal varices

COLOUR	RED SIGNS
Blue	Cherry-red spot
White	Red wale (weal) marking
	Haemocystic spot
	Diffuse redness

the risk of bleeding and hence selecting patients for prophylactic treatment (Table 17.3). Calès and colleagues[12] from Paris looked at observer variability and the relationship of the signs to the degree of hepatic dysfunction. There was good agreement amongst observers for all features in the oesophagus except extent, and these related well to the degree of hepatic dysfunction.

Large varices with cherry-red signs appear to predict a high risk of bleeding. Indeed, the North Italian Endoscopic Club criteria[13] include Pugh's grading of liver function, variceal size and red weal markings and can reliably identify the probability of a patient bleeding within 1 year.

INVESTIGATIONS OF PORTAL HYPERTENSION

Measurement of portal pressure

Portal pressure can be measured by direct puncture of the spleen, by cannulation of a tributary of the portal vein at operation, or indirectly by inserting a cannula into a hepatic vein via the vena cava ('wedged hepatic venous pressure'). This last method is only valid in cirrhotic patients and even then may be inaccurate in some types of cirrhosis. However, we must first ask whether measuring portal pressure has any clinical significance – and whether it alters decisions about treatment. The answer is generally 'no', but we do know that if the wedged pressure hepatic venous pressure is below 12 mmHg above the inferior vena caval pressure (or can be reduced to this level pharmacologically), varices are very unlikely to bleed. This may be important in choosing patients for clinical trials or measuring the effect of drugs, but not in the ordinary management of patients.

Ultrasonography

This is an important non-invasive investigation which can show focal lesions in the liver, such as tumours and dilated bile ducts.

Portal vein patency

In the overall prognosis and management of patients with portal hypertension it is very important to distinguish hepatic causes from portal vein thrombosis or the rare Budd–Chiari (posthepatic) syndrome. This can now usually be done by duplex ultrasonographic scanning which not only demonstrates patency of the portal vein but also whether the flow is towards the liver (hepatopedal) or away from the liver (hepatofugal). If a portosystemic shunt is being considered, then the venous phase of an arteriogram should be used to show the anatomy of the veins clearly, and this can also be used to assess the patency of a shunt.

The prognosis of portal vein thrombosis is usually better than that of cirrhosis and the mortality of a bleed far lower because liver function and the clotting system are normal; if, however, a shunt is being considered, a portacaval shunt is obviously not possible, and alternative methods have to be used (e.g. splenorenal or mesocaval).

Liver biopsy and liver function tests

As has been stressed above, bleeding oesophageal varices are the result of a disease process rather than a disease in themselves. Once acute bleeding has been controlled and portal vein thrombosis excluded, a liver biopsy should be performed to establish the nature of the liver disease, which will determine prognosis, possible treatment and advice to the patient – to stop drinking alcohol, for example. The prothrombin time must be corrected and severe ascites treated before liver biopsy. Liver 'function' tests indicate the degree of liver damage and activity of inflammation, and are used, together with the presence or absence of encephalopathy and ascites, to grade the liver disease A, B or C (Pugh's modification of Child's grading).[14] This grading has prognostic value and is also a guide to the risks of operation. If a hepatoma is suspected, a greatly raised alpha α-fetoprotein level confirms the diagnosis, but it is not always raised. Hepatomas are common in areas such as Africa and South-East Asia where hepatitis B is endemic, but are being found increasingly in patients in the West with long-standing cirrhosis from other causes.

PROPHYLACTIC TREATMENT OF VARICES

At first sight it would seem sensible to try to prevent variceal bleeding because, when it does occur, it is life threatening. However, further investigation shows that in the Western world only about one-third of patients with cirrhosis and varices will eventually bleed, and in one-third of these the bleed will be a terminal event. Prophylactic treatment was abandoned 20 years ago after several controlled trials of portacaval shunts[15] found that operated patients fared worse than controls. However, this involved a major operation; the concept of prophylaxis has been revived, now that endoscopic sclerotherapy is a standard treatment and so much less invasive. A number of controlled trials of prophylactic sclerotherapy have been published (Table 17.4). Three in Europe showed an improved mortality in patients with alcoholic cirrhosis but not in others,[21,23,24] and this may be due to patients reducing their alcohol intake as well as to the sclerotherapy. The Veterans study in the USA[19] found that the sclerotherapy group fared worse, but this was due to complications of sclerotherapy which were unacceptably high. The consensus view from all the trials does not support the concept of *widespread* prophylactic sclerotherapy,[25] although there may be some indications in the future for selected, high-risk patients, especially those with alcohol-related cirrhosis.

Prophylactic drug therapy is an even more attractive option and five trials have shown that beta blockers are safe for patients with large varices who have not bled and who do not have ascites. However, many patients cannot tolerate the doses required to reduce portal pressure significantly because of

Table 17.4 Prospective randomized trials of prophylactic sclerotherapy for oesophageal varices

AUTHOR(S)	DATE	COUNTRY	RESULT
Paquet[14]	1982	W. Germany	Benefit in selected patients
Witzel et al.[15]	1985	W. Germany	Benefit
Koch et al.[16]	1986	W. Germany	No benefit
Gregory et al.[17]	1987	USA	Harm
Santangelo et al.[18]	1988	USA	No benefit
Sauerbruch et al.[19]	1988	W. Germany	Benefit in alcoholics
Piai et al.[20]	1988	Italy	Benefit in high-risk patients
Triger et al.[21]	1991	England	Benefit in alcoholics
Potzi et al.[22]	1989	Austria	Benefit in alcoholics

systemic hypotension; therefore beta blockers are not recommended for general prophylaxis. There may be particular high-risk patients in whom they are justified.

Prophylactic devascularization procedures, as practised in Japan, are not supported by controlled evidence,[26] despite a very low operative mortality.

MANAGEMENT OF BLEEDING VARICES

All bleeding from oesophageal varices is life threatening and there is no place for waiting and hoping that the bleeding will stop or not recur. Management can be divided into five phases, and clear decisions must be made at each stage. If the medical attendants are not experienced in methods of definitive treatment, patients must be transferred to a suitable unit as soon as their condition is stable, rather than waiting for a further bleed. Drug treatment using intravenous infusion of a somatostatin analogue or metoclopramide should be used to control bleeding during transfer.

Resuscitation

The sooner the patient can reach hospital and be transfused, the better, and we now give patients with known varices a letter to carry with them which requests the emergency services to bring them to the specialist unit immediately. Resuscitation consists of intravenous fluids (colloids) and blood as soon as possible. If liver disease is suspected, high sodium containing fluids (eg. 'normal' saline) and opiate drugs should be avoided or increased ascites and lengthy sedation may result. A prolonged prothrombin time is likely and can be helped by vitamin K (10 mg) intravenously. Approximately one-third of patients will have stopped bleeding on admission, one-third will be bleeding slowly and one-third will be bleeding rapidly. It is this last group which needs effective and rapid diagnosis and control. In order to control the bleeding from the lower oesophagus and clear the stomach of blood to make diagnosis easier, metoclopramide (20 mg i.v.) is recommended.[9]

Endoscopy

It is frequently assumed that a patient with known cirrhosis must be bleeding from oesophageal varices. This is not necessarily so, especially if treatment to the varices has already been started, when a minority of bleeds are from the oesophagus. Patients with portal hypertension may bleed from gastric varices, gastric and duodenal ulcers, gastropathy or gastric erosions. Correct identification of the bleeding site is essential because a Sengstaken–Blakemore tube, however well positioned, does nothing for a bleeding duodenal ulcer! Endoscopy, under as little sedation as possible, may have to be repeated after 1–2 hours once the stomach has cleared of blood; occasionally bleeding from oesophageal varices may have to be inferred from absence of bleeding in other sites. The endoscopist does not always see a spurting varix, a clot or a mucosal defect overlying the varix (Figure 17.9). Fundal varices are particularly difficult to see if there is blood in the stomach, and the gastroscope must be retroflexed in order to inspect the area just around the cardia. Sometimes fresh blood can be seen dripping down from the oesophagus alongside the gastroscope. Barium meal examination has no place in the acute assessment of varices.

Arresting bleeding

Sometimes a varix can be injected (just below the bleeding point) whilst it is actively bleeding, and the other varices can be injected 24–48 h later. Although metoclopramide usually produces brief control, it is short acting and bleeding may recur on endoscopy. Occasionally, if there is torrential bleeding which has not stopped and nothing can be identified on endoscopy because of the bleeding, tamponade may have to be used on the assumption that the bleeding is variceal. The technique of tamponade is described below and, if correctly applied, is the most certain way of controlling oesophageal and upper gastric varices. However, it is *not* a treatment and the balloons should not be inflated for more than 24 hours – ideally not more than 12 hours. If they are deflated at the end of this time, rebleeding is very likely, so the time must be used to bring up the patient's blood pressure, clear out the old blood in the bowel and plan definitive treatment.

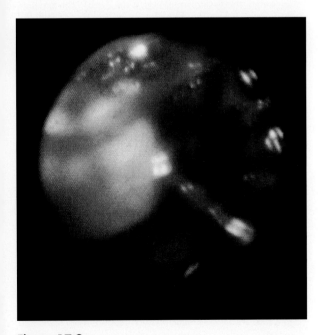

Figure 17.9
Endoscopic view of a spurting oesophageal varix.

Other drugs have been used to arrest bleeding. Vasopressin alone is probably of no overall benefit because of its cardiac side-effects in older patients. Vasopressin plus glyceryl trinitrate is a possibility,[27] and glypressin is safer and better than vasopressin, but beta blockers have no place in the immediate control of variceal bleeding. There has recently been interest in somatostatin and its analogues (octreotride) which can be continued for several days.

Recent randomized controlled trials[28] have found it as effective as injection (although only a proportion of patients were actively bleeding). For the minority who fail to respond to immediate injection, temporary tamponade followed by injection is the most certain method of arresting bleeding (effective in 90–95% of cases).

Temporary control of bleeding

At the present time, injection sclerotherapy by various techniques or banding are the best methods of controlling bleeding from oesophageal varices. Sclerotherapy is easier when there is active bleeding but banding may be more definitive. The newer banding devices allow several bands to be placed without having to withdraw the gastroscope. Possibly injection of the bleeding point followed by banding 24 h later may be the best combination. If tamponade has been used the balloon(s) should be kept inflated until just before the endoscope is inserted. There is no value in deflating the balloon and risking a further bleed obscuring the view for injection. The injection may be repeated 24 hours later if complete control has not been achieved, and tamponade used for a few hours afterwards. If bleeding still persists and is still coming from the oesophagus, an open operation must be considered. Only about 5% of patients come into this category but repeatedly failed injection leads to disaster. The best operation in this situation is an oesophageal transection with or without a devascularization, but it becomes hazardous if the lower oesophagus is oedematous from repeated injections, and is contraindicated if there is an oesophageal ulcer. In this case a portacaval shunt may be preferred (p 277).

Unfortunately, there are no criteria so far to select this small group of patients when they first present; otherwise surgery could be considered as the first option. However, the general opinion of experienced surgeons and gastroenterologists is that if two adequate injection sessions have failed to stop the bleeding, that is the time for surgery. Figure 17.10 shows an algorithm for the management of actively bleeding oesophageal varices.[29] A recent prospective, randomized trial found that an H graft shunt was better than TIPSS (p 278) unless the patients were especially poor risks for operation.[30]

Long-term prevention of rebleeding

Whereas there is general agreement about the acute treatment of bleeding varices, there is more uncertainty about long-term management. The options are: repeated sclerotherapy, banding devascularization and/or transection, some form of shunt surgery and, possibly, drugs such as beta blockers.

Repeated sclerotherapy depends on patient compliance and

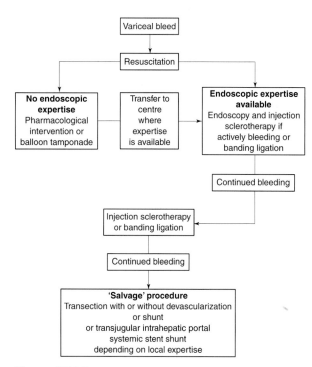

Figure 17.10
Algorithm for management of actively bleeding oesophageal
varices. (Reproduced with permission from Williams SGJ &
Westaby D. *BMJ*; 308: 1213.)

needs an average of 3–4 sessions to achieve complete thrombosis, followed by yearly or half-yearly checks, and further injections if varices reappear. This regimen certainly reduces bleeding episodes but may not improve mortality when compared with initial injection and further injections if and when bleeding occurs.[31,32]

There have been controlled trials between sclerotherapy and a distal splenorenal (Warren) shunt, and one trial found that sclerotherapy was the best initial option, with recourse to a shunt if this regimen 'failed',[33] whereas another[34] showed no advantage for sclerotherapy alone. The addition of propanolol to sclerotherapy appears to reduce rebleeding.[35]

We have completed a controlled trial between long-term sclerotherapy and devascularization/transection in Child's A and B patients, once the initial bleeding has been controlled and the patient's condition has been stabilized. Results[36] showed a higher early mortality but better 5-year survival after surgery, with identical survival at 2.5 years. A trial of endoscopic sclerotherapy versus TIPPS[37] found no difference in rebleeding but a superior survival after sclerotherapy.

A trial in patients with bilharzia between devascularization, standard splenorenal and distal splenorenal shunt showed devascularization with splenectomy to be the best.[38]

In summary, the long-term management will depend on whether patients can be reviewed easily and regularly, the progression and nature of the underlying liver disease and the local surgical expertise. Unless the surgeon is performing shunts frequently, it is wiser to do a portacaval shunt rather than the more complicated distal splenorenal in a patient with good liver function. Shunt surgery still has a role in the treatment of carefully selected patients, but surgery of any type should be avoided in grade C patients if at all possible.

TECHNIQUES AND COMPLICATIONS

Tamponade

Tamponade is safe and effective provided that the balloons are in the right place at the right pressure. Placing these balloons is a life-saving or life-threatening procedure and, as such, must be studied carefully and learnt. There are two types of tube: the Linton, with just a gastric balloon, which relies on traction to compress the lower oesophageal veins; and the Sengstaken–Blakemore, with gastric and oesophageal balloons, and its Minnesota modification (which has an oesophageal suction channel to stop saliva accumulating above the oesophageal balloon, thereby avoiding inhalation). Controlled trials have shown the Sengstaken type to be superior to the Linton for oesophageal, but not for gastric, varices.

The steps in passing the tube are as follows:

1. Check that the balloon functions satisfactorily by inflation and deflation. The gastric balloon is inflated with 300–400 ml of air and the balloon pressure is measured and recorded by attaching the inflation channel to a standard manometer. Similarly, the oesophageal balloon is inflated until it is evenly and firmly distended (but not distorted) and the volume and pressure are recorded (usually 110–120 ml of air and 50–60 mmHg).

2. With the balloon completely deflated, the well-lubricated tube is passed through the mouth and well down into the stomach, to the 50 cm mark on the tube. A lubricated guide wire or a period in the refrigerator sometimes helps to stiffen the tube, enabling it to pass more easily.

3. The gastric balloon is then inflated and the tube drawn back until the gastric balloon is at the cardia. The pressure is measured (and should be very little higher than it was before insertion). The distance from the teeth should now read 35–40 cm on the tube, depending on the position of the cardia.

4. With gentle traction on the tube, the oesophageal balloon is slowly inflated to the previously measured volume, unless there is pain, when inflation is stopped. The pressure is measured and should be 20–25 mmHg higher than the pressure before insertion (due to counterpressure exerted by the oesophageal wall). This difference equates to the pressure transmitted to the varices.

5. Once the position and pressures are satisfactory, the tube is either taped to the cheek or kept in position using a split tennis ball against the side of the mouth. The balloon pressure and the tube position are checked every 0.5–1 hour and adjusted if necessary.

6. The oesophageal aspiration channel is attached to continuous low pressure suction and the gastric aspiration channel to a bag, with manual aspiration being performed from time to time. Fresh bleeding from the stomach suggests that either the balloon pressure or the position is inappropriate,

or bleeding is occurring from the stomach or duodenum below the gastric balloon. If there is doubt, it is safer to deflate the oesophageal balloon and reinflate from the beginning – or even regastroscope the patient, rather than progressively inflating it without a definite diagnosis.

Once the tube is in position, the balloon pressures and positions must be checked half-hourly, the oesophageal aspiration channel must be on continuous low-pressure suction and the gastric aspiration channel attached to a bag and aspirated half-hourly. This will detect any new bleeding into the stomach. The balloon positions can be checked radiographically (Figure 17.11).

As stressed above, once the tube has controlled the bleeding, plans must be made for injection at the next convenient time with the patient resuscitated, or for transfer to an appropriate specialist unit.

Complications of tamponade

The gastric balloon may be inflated in the wrong position, which may be in the duodenum, the oesophagus or even the right lower lobe bronchus if consciousness is impaired. This can obviously result in serious damage. If the oesophageal

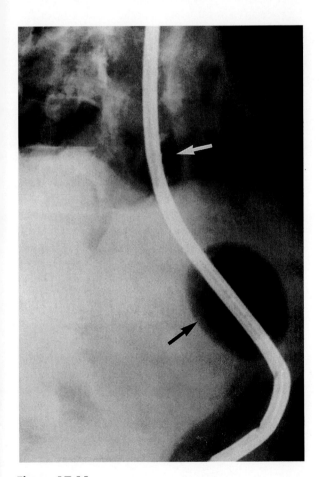

Figure 17.11
Plain abdominal radiograph showing gastric (black arrow) and oesophageal (white arrow) balloons in correct positions. From Carter, Russell et al. *Operative Surgery* (5th edn) London: Chapman and Hall.

balloon is inflated too much it can rupture the oesophagus, and if left inflated for more than 24 hours it can cause pressure ulceration or necrosis. If there is concern about rebleeding at night, the oesophageal balloon, but not the gastric balloon, may be deflated after 12 h and the tube left in position; the oesophageal balloon can then be reinflated easily should bleeding recur. It is important to empty the balloons completely by suction before attempting to remove the tube.

Occasionally a very restless or violent patient may try to pull the tube out with the balloons inflated, which can be disastrous. Probably the safest treatment is a general anaesthetic with positive pressure ventilation for 24–48 h until the acute confusion (or delirium tremens) has passed. Inhalation of saliva is a danger, especially if the patient is unconscious, and continuous aspiration is essential.

Sclerotherapy

Instruments

A flexible fibreoptic instrument is used and various balloons or oversheaths may be employed to control any bleeding immediately after injection. A 'freehand' technique with the flexible instrument is usually satisfactory.

Intravariceal or paravariceal?

There is sometimes confusion about these two techniques. The majority of clinicians use the intravariceal method, in which 3–6 ml of sclerosant is injected into each of 3–4 variceal columns, and this has been shown in one trial to be the better method.[39] Siting of the needle is helped by a simple pressure measuring device which significantly reduces complications.[40] Paravariceal injections are of small volume (0.5 mg) and are placed into the grooves on either side of the variceal column, producing fibrosis around the varices rather than thrombosis inside. The injecting of several millilitres of sclerosant into the submucosa on the *surface* of the varices has not been advocated; this can only lead to slough and ulceration, which can be dangerous, *especially if the underlying varix is not thrombosed.*

Sclerosants

Several different sclerosants are used according to their availability in different countries. Some are more potent than others and cause more damage if they leak outside the varix.

The following sclerosants are in common use:

- 5% Ethanolamine oleate
- Sodium morrhuate
- Polidocanol
- Sodium tetradecyl sulphate
- Absolute alcohol.

Phenol in almond oil is *not* safe for intravenous injection. Tissue adhesives and thrombins have also been used (especially for gastric varices) but adhesives may damage the endoscope and there are reports of serious neurological complications. They should be used as a last resort if surgery is strongly contraindicated.

The end-point of sclerotherapy is not well defined in the literature. Some papers refer to 'obliteration', some to 'disappearance' and some to 'thrombosis'. Sometimes the varices do disappear altogether, leaving no trace and an apparently normal oesophagus on endoscopy. At other times the variceal column becomes firm, thrombosed and triangular shaped rather than semicircular. With the paravasal technique the submucosa becomes thickened and whiter and the vessels become obscured even if not thrombosed. It is important, when reporting results, to describe the appearance of the lower oesophagus, and the word 'obliteration' may mean either disappearance or thrombosis.

Complications of sclerotherapy

Inhalation A confused or heavily sedated patient may inhale saliva or blood during the procedure. Sedation should be as little as possible and carefully controlled; oral and pharyngeal suction must be available continuously.

Injection ulcer These can be large and very slow to heal and may give rise to slow bleeding, and occasionally even massive haemorrhage, if the neighbouring varix is not thrombosed. It can be avoided by stopping an intravariceal injection as soon as the mucosa blanches, or by using a pressure device (see above). Treatment is by omeprazole 20 mg o.d.

Systemic reactions There have been very few reports of any systemic reactions to intravariceal injections, but it is wise not to give more than 25 ml of ethanolamine at one session.

Late oesophageal stricture If injections are performed carefully and precisely, stricturing of the lower oesophagus should be rare, but some series report an incidence of 10–20%. Once the varices are obliterated, the oesophagus can be dilated in the standard way, as for benign fibrotic strictures. Mild alterations in lower oesophageal motility are common but do not seem to be of clinical importance.

Mediastinitis Although some temporary chest pain is quite common, if it persists and is accompanied by a prolonged fever, a chemical, and sometimes infected, mediastinitis must be suspected. This is a rare complication but may be due to an injection being given too deep or the sclerosant passing into the perioesophageal tissues via the perforating veins. A tear is very rare with the fibreoptic gastroscope, but a chest x-ray to show any air in the mediastinum is required if there is any doubt. If a fever persists for more than 12 hours after sclerotherapy it is wise to give antibiotics as a precaution.

Endoscopic banding ligation

In this technique a cylinder is attached to the distal end of a forward viewing endoscope, which enables the varix to be sucked into it using the normal endoscopic channel. A second cylinder containing the elastic band on its distal circumference is held in place by a trip wire running up the biopsy channel of the endoscope. Pulling on this wire 'fires' the band around the base of the varix which has been sucked into the cylinder. In earlier models, for each individual banding, the endoscope

had to be brought out and 'reloaded', and this process is aided by a sheath across the mouth, pharynx and upper oesophagus. Now there are multiple banding apparatus. As could be inferred from a comparison of banding and injection of haemorrhoids, there is little to choose between the two techniques in the effective control of bleeding and long-term outcome. However, one trial has shown that banding requires fewer sessions to produce obliteration.[41] There is a danger, if suction is inadequate and only a superficial part of the large varix is banded, that when the area sloughs a massive haemorrhage could result.

SURGICAL TREATMENT OF VARICES

Surgical operations for oesophageal varices can be divided into two main groups: direct ligation, devascularization or transection on the one hand, and some form of portosystemic shunt on the other. It must be remembered that the risks of any surgical procedure will depend on the degree of liver impairment and the presence or absence of ascites. Morbidity and mortality will be greater in the Child's grade C than in a grade A patient. If an elective procedure is being considered, it is worth spending time and effort improving the patient's general condition, ascites, clotting and proteins. In all these procedures mortality is considerably less when they are done electively rather than as an emergency.

Devascularization/transection procedures

The original operations for direct ligation of bleeding oesophageal varices were the Borema/Crile and Milnes–Walker procedures. These involved a transthoracic approach to the lower oesophagus and, after division of the often massive perioesophageal vessels, suture of the intraoesophageal vessels after a longitudinal or transverse division of the muscular coat; they are hardly ever done today.

The Hassab procedure (Figure 17.12)

This procedure was invented in Egypt for the treatment of the large number of patients with schistosomiasis. Through an abdominal approach after splenectomy, the upper stomach and

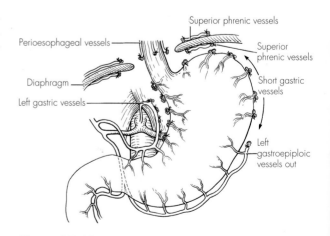

Figure 17.12
Hassab devascularization procedure.

Hassab[42] reported a low mortality and good long-term results, but it must be remembered that schistosomiasis (bilharzia) has a different pathology and natural history from cirrhosis.

The Sugiura procedure (Figure 17.13)

This Japanese operation[43] is a far more extensive procedure, involving abdominal and thoracic incisions, devascularization, splenectomy, truncal vagotomy and pyloroplasty and transection of the lower oesophagus. Sugiura reports excellent results with a remarkably low mortality for such an extensive procedure, but it has not become popular outside Japan.

Simple oesophageal transection

The invention of stapling devices has made this operation quicker and simpler. The concept of interrupting the intramural flow from abdomen to thorax was implicit in Tanner's[44] porta–azygous disconnection in which the upper stomach was divided and resutured by hand. Spence and Johnston[45] pioneered the stapling operation in which division and reanastomosis is done in one action (Figure 17.14). This is certainly the treatment of choice if an inexperienced surgeon has performed a laparotomy for bleeding without making the correct preoperative diagnosis, and it is also the simplest treatment in an emergency when sclerotherapy has failed, but it may not have the best long-term results in preventing recurrent varices. If it is performed in an emergency, the tamponade tube can be left down during the first part of the operation until the surgeon is ready to introduce the stapling gun.

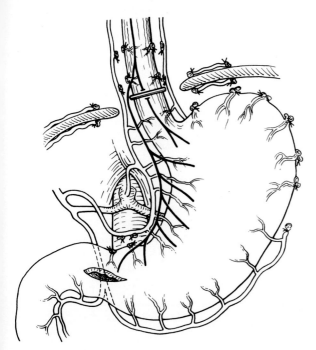

Figure 17.13
Sugiura procedure.

lower oesophagus were devascularized by ligating and dividing all the vessels close to the greater and lesser curves. (This is not easy as some of the veins are very dilated. Clips may be useful for the smaller vessels.) The oesophagus was not divided.

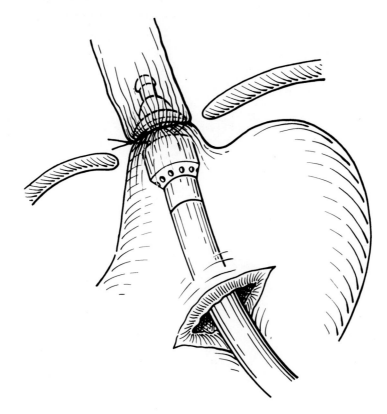

Figure 17.14
Oesophageal transection with stapling 'gun'. Adapted from Bailey and Love's Short Practice of Surgery. CV Mann, RCG Russell & NS Williams (eds), 22nd edn. Chapman & Hall Medical, p. 716, figure 45.24.

Technique The abdomen is opened through an upper midline incision with careful haemostasis of the dilated veins in the abdominal wall, especially around the umbilicus. After dividing the peritoneum over it, the lower oesophagus is mobilized, as for a truncal vagotomy, but this will mean ligating some large paraoesophageal veins which lie close to the oesophageal wall. Those well away may be left. Ideally, both vagal trunks should be preserved but at least one must be, otherwise there will be delayed gastric emptying. Once the lower oesophagus has been mobilized for several centimetres, an anterior gastrotomy is made in the anterior wall of the body of the stomach (high-pressure venous bleeding from the stomach wall may have to be controlled with suture ligation). The circular stapling device ('gun') is inserted into the oesophagus with its anvil well separated from the staple cartridge. Ideally, the 28–29 cm diameter cartridge should be used but the smaller (25 cm) is sometimes the only one that can be inserted without splitting the oesophagus. A silk ligature is tied around the oesophagus and tightened around the stem of the stapling device as low in the oesophagus as possible. It is important that the ligature really tightens the oesophagus and narrows it at this point so that the staples pass through the full thickness of the wall on both sides. It is obviously disastrous if the oesophagus is cut but not stapled! That is why the anvil and cartridge must be wide apart. The gun is then closed, fired and withdrawn. The doughnut must be inspected and, should it be incomplete, further full-thickness sutures must be inserted into the staple line to prevent haemorrhage and leakage (the staple line may be palpated from within the lumen by a finger introduced through the gastrotomy). Once haematosis is satisfactory, the gastrotomy is closed with two layers, special care being taken with haematosis. Closure of the abdominal wall must be thorough and meticulous to avoid leakage of ascitic fluid after the operation.

Modified devascularization/transection

In our unit we have modified and combined the operations to devascularize the upper stomach and lower oesophagus without splenectomy, followed by a transection without truncal vagotomy (Figure 17.15).[36] The lesser curve and oesophageal dissection is very similar to that during highly selective vagotomy, and it is important to dissect well the oesophagus (6 cm) to make sure of ligating and dividing the lower perforating veins. The large paraoesophageal veins are left to carry the blood to the azygous system. It is sometimes a difficult and tedious procedure and occasionally it is not possible, because of the risk of bleeding, to go far enough up the oesophagus. If the transection is too high up the oesophagus, varices will reform in the part below the transection line.

Complications These include occasional leakage from the staple line and stricture formation (this should be very rare if the medium-sized stapling head is used). These patients are susceptible to infection in the chest and in the abdominal cavity, and if there is ascites it accumulates after the operation (due to sodium retention) and may leak persistently from the wound. Even patients with no ascites before surgery may develop it afterwards

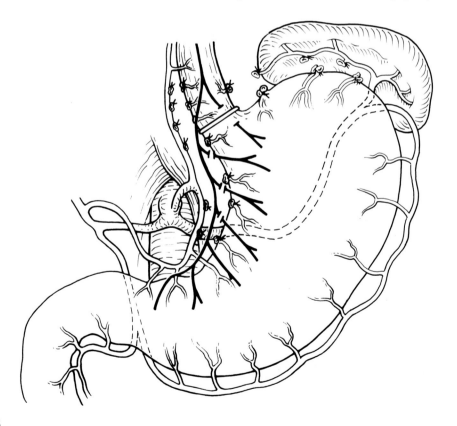

Figure 17.15
Combined devascularization/transection operation. (Adapted from Bailey and Love's Short Practice of Surgery. CV Mann, RCG Russell & NS Williams (eds), 22nd edn. Chapman & Hall Medical, p. 716, figure 45.24.)

and therefore spironolactone should be started before or immediately after operation. A very careful abdominal wall closure is therefore important. If varices reform some years later, they may be injected while still small and under low pressure.

Shunt operations

The aim of all shunt operations is to provide a large bypass between the portal and systemic venous systems so that the portal system is decompressed, thereby relieving pressure from the varices. If shunts remain patent, they are very effective in preventing bleeding from varices, but their main side-effect is portosystemic encephalopathy. The 'selective' distal splenorenal shunt of Warren was designed to decompress the portal system without stopping the portal flow to the liver. More recent evidence suggests that the shunt may not be as selective as was at first believed, and that, with time, encephalopathy also develops after this procedure. The different forms of shunt are classified in Table 17.5 and illustrated in Figure 17.16. The simplest operation that has stood the test of time is the end-to-side portacaval shunt and this probably has the best patency rate. All shunts have a risk of thrombosing, especially if the calibre of the vessels is small, but most stay patent for many years (Figure 17.17). In children under 10 years, shunts are contraindicated for this reason, but children have a remarkable ability to open up spontaneous shunts as they grow up.

Table 17.5   Types of portosystemic shunt procedures

Portacaval	–	End-to-side
	–	Side-to-side
Splenorenal	–	Proximal and splenectomy
	–	Distal
Mesocaval	–	H graft with vein or synthetic material
Gastrocaval	–	Left gastric vein to inferior vena cava

Technique of end-to-side portacaval shunt The abdomen is opened through a long right subcostal incision with the table tilted to the left. Great care must be taken to ligate the dilated veins in the abdominal wall and within the peritoneal cavity. The hepatic flexure of the colon is mobilized with care (small vessels that would normally just be diathermized in patients with portal hypertension may have to be ligated) and retracted downwards. The liver is retracted upwards after ligation and division of the round ligament and the falciform ligament. The duodenum is Kocherized and mobilized to the left to reveal the underlying vena cava, which is exposed by dividing the parietal peritoneum overlying it. It is cleared over its anterior two thirds throughout its length from the renal veins to its disappearance into the liver. The portal vein is identified above the pancreas and in the free border of the lesser omentum behind the common bile duct and it is cleared and mobilized throughout its length as far up into the porta hepatis as possible before it divides. The left gastric vein which joins it is often ligated and divided so that the portal vein can be moved downwards without tension towards the inferior vena cava (if the opening in the inferior vena cava is too anterior or to the

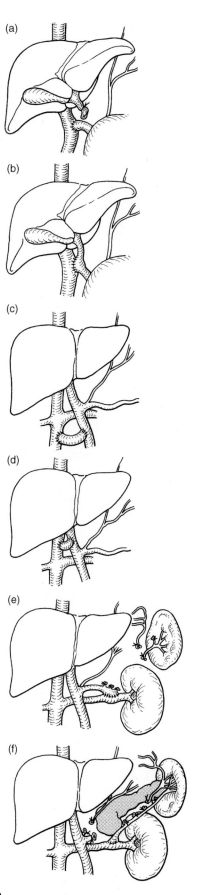

Figure 17.16

Different forms of portosystemic shunts. A, End-to-side portacaval; B, side-to-side portacaval; C, mesocaval H graft; D, portacaval H graft; E, standard splenorenal; F, distal splenorenal.

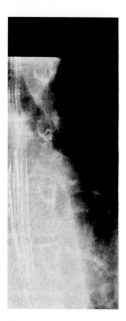
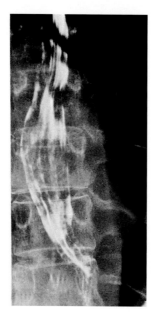

Figure 17.17
Venous phase of arteriogram showing patent splenorenal shunt after 16 years.

right, the portal vein is angulated just before its insertion, which can slow the flow and lead to thrombosis). The portal vein is ligated as high as possible and divided with the proximal end open and flow control with a gentle clamp such as a 'bull-dog'. A Satinsky clamp is placed on the left-hand side of the anterior wall of the vena cava, maintaining most of the flow in the inferior vena cava. An oval piece of the wall, exactly the same size as the cross-section of the portal vein, is excised and an end-to-side anastomosis performed with a continuous fine vascular suture. The portal vein and inferior vena cava are both flushed before the final stitches are inserted and then the clamps are removed. For the operative details of other types of shunts, specialist books on operative surgery should be consulted.

The present place of shunts in the management of oesophageal, as opposed to gastric, varices is small.[46] They are particularly indicated in patients with good liver function and an underlying disease with a relatively good prognosis, and in those who for social or other reasons are not able to come to hospital for regular checks, or do not live near emergency medical care, should they bleed. For years, Orloff[47] was a lone voice recommending emergency portacaval shunt. Cello and colleagues[48] have added evidence that, in experienced hands, a shunt is a viable alternative to many attempts at sclerotherapy. However, with the great reduction in the number of elective shunts, hands are becoming less experienced!

Transjugular intrahepatic portosystemic stent shunt (TIPSS)

This technique of shunting was introduced into clinical practice at the end of the 1980s,[49] although the idea and experimental work were considerably older.[50] The theoretical advantages were to reduce the mortality and morbidity of an open operation and

to produce a partial shunt that might reduce the risk of encephalopathy. The theoretical disadvantages were that the lumen was narrow with a potential for thrombosis and, unlike mesocaval and splenorenal shunts, it could not be used unless the portal vein was patent. (Recently attempts have been made to recanalize the portal vein by a transhepatic approach before placing the transjugular shunt).[51]

The early results were just as expected from open shunt surgery: in those groups of patients in which there was a low thrombosis rate, there was a relatively high risk of encephalopathy, and in those patients in whom the shunt thrombosed, there was little encephalopathy but a higher incidence of rebleeding. Whereas its safety has now been established in several studies, the indications are the same as for other shunt surgery,[52] which in many units are few. It might be argued that it would be indicated for bleeding gastric varices which are difficult to inject, but in this situation even open shunt alone is not enough: the varices must be ligated to control the immediate bleeding. A possible indication is intractable ascites[53] but the first controlled trial[54] has shed doubt on this. It is a rescue operation for uncontrollable oesophageal variceal bleeding in patients unfit for open surgery. It is a technically

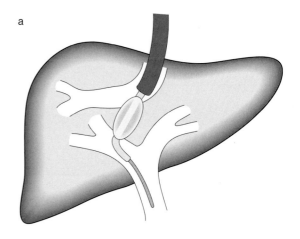

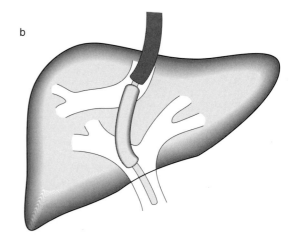

Figure 17.18
Transjugular intrahepatic portosystemic stent shunt. (a) Balloon dilatation of track, and (b) stent in position between right hepatic veins and right branch of portal vein.

demanding procedure and as the indications are few, but critical when they occur, only those in major referral centres are likely to obtain adequate experience. It may be useful as a 'bridge to transplantation' but there are not sufficient prospective randomized trial data to draw firm conclusions for any indication and it tends to be used for individual patients with special problems.[55]

Technique The patient is sedated and the catheter introduced via the right internal jugular vein into the right or middle hepatic vein. The needle is then advanced through the liver to a branch of the portal vein, which is identified by injecting contrast. The tract is then dilated with a balloon and an 8 or 10 mm metal stent is inserted (Figure 17.18).

CONCLUSION AND OVERALL RESULTS

The results of all types of treatment for bleeding oesophageal varices will depend on three factors:

1. How quickly the patients reach hospital.
2. The underlying liver disease.
3. The stage the disease has reached at presentation.

There is little doubt that survival from initial bleed has been improved by prompt and efficient sclerotherapy and that sclerotherapy improves the long-term survival when compared with no active treatment.

Future research will be directed towards pharmacological control of portal pressure, possibly with drugs that produce portal venous dilatation rather than mesenteric arterial constriction. However, prevention of the cirrhosis must be the ultimate aim and, although we know many of the major causes are preventable (alcohol, hepatitis B, bilharzia), a complex variety of economic, political and social factors have yet to be overcome.

REFERENCES

1. Vorobioff J, Groszmann RJ, Picabea E et al. Prognostic value of hepatic venous pressure gradient measurements in alcoholic cirrhosis: a 10-year prospective study. *Gastroenterology* 1996; **111:** 701–709.
2. Conn HO. The varix volcano connection. *Gastroenterology* 1980; **79:** 1133.
3. Butler H. The veins of the oesophagus. *Thorax* 1951; **6:** 276.
4. Kitano S, Terblanche J, Kahn D & Bornman PC. Venous anatomy of the lower oesophagus in portal hypertension: practical implications. *Br J Surg* 1986; **73:** 525.
5 Vianna A, Hayes PC, Moscoso G et al. Normal venous circulation of the gastroesophageal junction. A route to understanding varices. *Gastroenterology* 1987; **93:** 876.
6. Spence RA. The venous anatomy of the lower oesophagus in normal subjects and in patients with varices: an image analysis study. *Br J Surg* 1984; **71:** 739.
7. Hosking SW, Robinson P & Johnson AG. The effect of Valsalva's manoeuvre and hyoscinbutyl-bromide on the pressure gradient across the wall of oesophageal varices. *Gut* 1987; **28:** 1151.
8. Schiano TD, Adrain AL, Cassidy MJ et al. Use of high resolution endoluminal sonography to measure the radius and wall thickness of esophageal varices. *Gastrointest Endosc* 1996; **44:** 425–428.
9. Hosking SW, Doss W, El-Zeiny H, Robinson P, Barsoum M & Johnson AG. Pharmacological constriction of the lower oesophageal sphincter – a simple method of controlling variceal haemorrhage. *Gut* 1988; **19:** 1098.
10. Japanese Research Society for Portal Hypertension. The general rules for recording endoscopic findings on oesophageal varices. *Jpn J Surg* 1980; **10:** 84.
11. Beppu K, Inokuchi K, Koyanagi N et al. Prediction of variceal haemorrhage by esophageal endoscopy. *Gastrointest Endosc* 1981; **27:** 213.
12. Calès P, Zabotto B, Meskens C et al. Gastroesophageal endoscopic features in cirrhosis. *Gastroenterology* 1990; **98:** 156.
13. North Italian Endoscopic Club for the Study and Treatment of Oesophageal Varices. Prediction of the first variceal haemorrhage in patients with cirrhosis of the liver and esophageal varices: a prospective multicentre study. *N Engl J Med* 1988; **319:** 983.
14. Pugh RNH, Murray-Lyon IM, Dawson JL, Pietroni ML & Williams R. Transection of oesophagus for bleeding oesophageal varices. *Br J Surg* 1983; **60:** 646–649.
15. Conn HO, Lindenmuth WW, May CJ & Rambsy GR. Prophylactic portacaval anastomosis: a tale of two studies. *Medicine (Baltimore)* 1972; **51:** 27.
16. Paquet KJ. Prophylactic endoscopic sclerosing treatment of the oesophageal wall in varices – a prospective controlled randomised trial. *Endoscopy* 1982; **14:** 4.
17. Witzel L, Walbergs E & Merki I. Prophylactic endoscopic sclerotherapy of oesophageal varices: a prospective controlled study. *Lancet* 1985; **i:** 773
18. Koch H, Henning H, Grimm H & Soehendra N. Prophylactic sclerosing of esophageal varices – results of a prospective controlled trial. *Endoscopy* 1986; **18:** 40.
19. Gregory PB, Hartigan P, Amodeo D et al. Prophylactic sclerotherapy for esophageal varices in alcoholic liver disease: results of a VA cooperative randomized trial. *Gastroenterology* 1987; **92:** 1414A.
20. Santangelo WC, Dueno MI, Estes BL & Krejs GJ. Prophylactic sclerotherapy of large oesophageal varices. *N Engl J Med* 1988; **318:** 814.
21. Sauerbruch T, Wotzka R, Kopcke W et al. Prophylactic sclerotherapy before the first episode of variceal haemorrhage in patients with cirrhosis. *N Engl J Med* 1988; **319:** 8.
22. Piai G, Cipolletta L, Claar M et al. Prophylactic sclerotherapy of high-risk oesophageal varices: results of a multicentre prospective controlled trial. *Hepatology* 1988; **8:** 1495.
23. Triger DR, Smart HL, Hosking SW & Johnson AG. Prophylactic sclerotherapy for oesophageal varices: long term results of a single-centre trial. *Hepatology* 1991; **13:** 117–123.
24. Potzi R, Bauer P, Reichel W, Kerstan E, Renner F & Gangl A. Prophylactic endoscopic sclerotherapy of oesophageal varices in liver cirrhosis. A multicentre prospective controlled randomised trial in Vienna. *Gut* 1989; **30:** 873.
25. Editorial. Prophylactic sclerotherapy of oesophageal varices: is it justified? *Lancet* 1988; **i:** 1369.
26. Inokuchi K. Prophylactic portal non-decompression surgery in patients with oesophageal varices. *Ann Surg* 1984; **200:** 61.
27. Conn HO. Vasopressin and nitroglycerin in the treatment of bleeding varices: the bottom line. *Hepatology* 1986; **6:** 523.
28. Planas R, Quer JC, Boix J et al. A prospective randomised trial comparing somatostatin and sclerotherapy in the treatment of acute variceal bleeding. *Hepatology* 1994; **2:** 370–375.
29. Burroughs AK, Hamilton G, Phillips A, Mezzanotte G, McIntyre N & Hobbs KEF. A comparison of sclerotherapy with staple transection of the oesophagus for the emergency control of bleeding from oesophageal varices. *N Engl J Med* 1989; **321:** 857.
30. Rosemurgy AS, Goode SE, Zwiebel BR, Black TJ & Brady PG. A prospective trial of transjugular intrahepatic portasystemic stent shunts versus small-diameter prosthetic H-graft portacaval shunts in the treatment of bleeding varices. *Ann Surg* 1996; **224:** 378–384.
31. Terblanche J, Bornman PC, Kahn D et al. Failure of repeated injection sclerotherapy to improve long-term survival after oesophageal variceal bleeding: a five year prospective controlled clinical trial. *Lancet* 1983; **ii:** 1328.
32. Moreto M, Zaballa M, Ojembarrena E et al. Combined (short term plus long term) sclerotherapy versus short term only sclerotherapy: a randomised prospective trial. *Gut* 1994; **35:** 687–691.
33. Warren WD, Henderson JM, Millikan WJ et al. Distal splenorenal shunt versus endoscopic sclerotherapy for long term management of variceal bleeding: preliminary report on a prospective, randomised trial. *Ann Surg* 1986; **203:** 454.
34. Rikfers LF, Burnett DA, Volentine GD, Buchi KN & Cormier RA. Shunt surgery versus endoscopic sclerotherapy for long term treatment of variceal bleeding: early results of a randomised trial. *Ann Surg* 1987; **206:** 261.
35. Elsayed SS, Shiha G, Hamid M et al. Sclerotherapy versus sclerotherapy and propranolol in the prevention of rebleeding from oesophageal varices: a randomised study. *Gut* 1996; **38:** 770–774.

36. Triger DR, Johnson AG, Brazier JG et al. A prospective trial of endoscopic sclerotherapy versus oesophageal transection and gastric devascularization in the long term management of bleeding oesophageal varices. *Gut* 1992; **33:** 1553–1558.

37. Sanyal AJ, Freedman AM, Luketic VA, et al. Transjugular intrahepatic portosystemic shunts compared with endoscopic sclerotherapy for the prevention of recurrent variceal hemorrhage: a randomised controlled tial. *Ann Inter Med* 1997; **126:** 849–857.

38. Raia S, Da Silva LC, Gayotto LCC, Forster SC, Fukushima J & Strauss E. Portal hypertension in schistosomiasis: a long term follow-up of a randomised trial comparing three types of surgery. *Hepatology* 1994; **2:** 398–403.

39. Sarin SK, Nanda R, Sachdev G, Chari S, Anand BS & Broor SL. Intravariceal versus paravariceal sclerotherapy: a prospective, controlled, randomised trial. *Gut* 1987; **28:** 657.

40. Hosking SW, Robinson P & Johnson AG. The use of manometric assessment of varices in patients undergoing maintenance sclerotherapy. *Gastroenterology* 1987; **95:** 846.

41. Gimson AES, Ramage JK, Panos MZ et al. Randomised trial of variceal banding ligation versus injection sclerotherapy for bleeding oesophageal varices. *Lancet* 1993; **342:** 391–394.

42. Hassab MA. Nonshunt operations in portal hypertension without cirrhosis. *Surg Gynecol Obstet* 1970; **131:** 648.

43. Sugiura M & Futagawa S. Further evaluation of the Sugiura procedure in the treatment of oesophageal varices. *Arch Surg* 1977; **112:** 1317.

44. Tanner NC. Operative management of haematemesis and melaena. *Ann R Coll Surg Engl* 1958; **22:** 30.

45. Spence RA & Johnston·GW. Results in 100 consecutive patients with stapled oesophageal transection for varices. *Surg Gynecol Obstet* 1985; **160:** 323.

46. Deans GT, Spence RAJ & Johnston GW. A quarter of a century of portasystemic shunting for oesophageal varices. *J R Coll Surg Edinb* 1989; **34:** 37.

47. Orloff MJ, Bell RH Jr, Hyde PV & Skivolocki WP. Long term results of emergency portacaval shunt for bleeding oesophageal varices in unselected patients with alcoholic cirrhosis. *Ann Surg* 1980; **192:** 325.

48. Cello JP, Grendell JH, Crass RA, Weber TE & Trunkey DD. Endoscopic sclerotherapy versus portacaval shunt in patients with severe cirrhosis and acute variceal haemorrhage: long term follow-up. *N Engl J Med* 1987; **316:** 11.

49. La Berge JM, Ring EJ, Gordon RL et al. Creation of transjugular intrahepatic portosystemic stent-shunt procedure for variceal haemorrhage. *N Engl J Med* 1994; **3:** 165–174.

50. Rosch J, Hanafee WN & Snow H. Transjugular intrahepatic portacaval shunt: an experimental work. *Am J Surg* 1971; **121:** 588–592.

51. Ring EJ, La Berge JM, Gordon RL et al. Transjugular intrahepatic portasystemic shunts in patients with portal vein occlusion. *Radiology* 1993; **186:** 523–527.

52. Cabrera J, Maynar M, Granados R et al. Transjugular intrahepatic portosystemic shunt versus sclerotherapy in the elective treatment of variceal hemorrhage. *Gastroenterology* 1996, **110:** 832–839.

53. Ochs A, Haag K, Sellinger M et al. TIPS: efficacy and survival in 49 patients with refractory and 'untreatable' ascites. *Hepatology* 1993; **18:** 292A.

54. Lebrec D, Giuily N, Hadengue A et al. Transjugular intrahepatic portosystemic shunts: comparison with paracentesis in patients with cirrhosis and refractory ascites: a randomized trial. *J Hepatol* 1996, **25:** 135–144.

55. Rössle M. The transjugular intrahepatic portosystemic shunt. *J Hepatol* 1996; **25:** 224–231.

18

MISCELLANEOUS DISORDERS OF THE OESOPHAGUS

D Alderson

OESOPHAGEAL WEBS

True webs of the oesophagus are thought to occur in 1–8% of the population,[1] although the majority are asymptomatic. They may be congenital or acquired and are usually thin, semilunar membranes covered in mucosa, most commonly in the cervical portion of the oesophagus (Figure 18.1).

Congenital webs are extremely rare and represent failure of coalescence of the oesophageal vacuoles which normally leads to luminal patency. This occurs by about day 30 of embryological development and incomplete vocuolization, when severe, leads to oesophageal atresia. Webs are thought to represent the most minor form of the abnormality, persisting usually as thin, diaphanous membranes.[2] They usually occur in the mid-oesophagus and present in infancy or childhood.[3,4] Symptoms largely reflect the degree of luminal obstruction by the web. At the severe end of the scale, this can present as neonatal vomiting or regurgitation of undigested bile-free food in infancy, often in association with choking and aspiration.[4] Symptoms however, may be mild in childhood and some patients only seek relief of their dysphagia as adults.[5]

Acquired oesophageal webs may be associated with iron deficiency anaemia, glossitis and koilonychia, known as the Plummer–Vinson or Patterson Brown–Kelly syndrome.[6–8] The syndrome is rarely complete and some of the abnormalities may be secondary to nutritional problems as a result of the web. In this rare syndrome, dysphagia occurs secondary to the presence of a postcricoid web and some patients may have oropharyngeal leukoplakia, which may predispose them to an increased risk of carcinoma of the hypopharynx[9] (Figure 18.2). There may also be an association between oesophageal webs and epidermolysis bullosa.[10] In this condition, the oesophagus is extremely sensitive to trauma, which can result in damage and shedding of the mucosa, producing a web-like appearance. Webs have also been described in association with pemphigus and pemphigoid.[11,12]

The majority of webs, whether congenital or acquired, produce no symptoms at all and are chance findings during radiological evaluation of the oesophagus for other reasons.

Symptomatic webs cause obstruction and the degree of luminal obstruction is generally an indication of symptom severity.

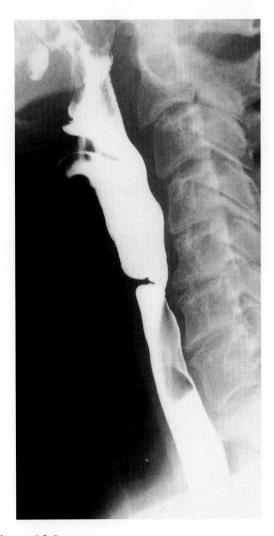

Figure 18.1

Lateral view during barium swallow of a semilunar cervical oesophageal web.

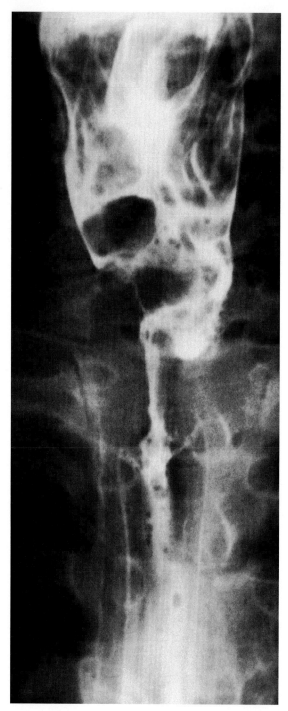

Figure 18.2
Hypopharyngeal carcinoma in a patient with Plummer–Vinson syndrome.

They are easily missed, both radiologically and particularly at flexible fibreoptic endoscopy. In the case of the latter, the endoscopist frequently ruptures the web unwittingly and in so doing, may alleviate the patient's symptoms. If this is not successful, then endoscopic dilatation using either a bougie or a balloon will produce web disruption.[13] Although operative excision has been described[14] there can be little justification for such an approach with modern endoscopic instrumentation.

SCHATZKI'S RING

Schatzki's ring was first described in 1953.[15] It occurs in the lower oesophagus, at the level of the squamocolumnar junction, nearly always in association with a sliding hiatus hernia. It does not, however, have a consistent relationship to the lower oesophageal sphincter. Unlike most oesophageal webs it is concentric. There is usually marked distortion of the muscularis mucosae, but not of the circular muscle of the oesophageal wall. The exact pathogenesis of the lesion remains uncertain, although there is a strong relationship with gastro-oesophageal reflux disease.[16,17] It has been suggested that the ring develops in response to reflux and acts as a physiological barrier to prevent pathological oesophageal acidification. It is noteworthy that patients with wide rings complain of reflux symptoms, whereas those with narrow openings, often complain only of dysphagia.[18]

The most frequent presenting symptom is an episode of acute oesophageal obstruction during a meal, with a large particle of food, such as piece of meat or bread. Many patients learn how to induce vomiting with upward dislodgement of the bolus allowing them to return to normal eating. The recurring nature of such events has generated the term 'episodic aphagia'.[19] About 20% of Schatzki rings are detected in asymptomatic individuals during barium swallow. Rings can, however, be difficult to identify, both radiologically and endoscopically. Cine-radiography of the oesophagus is the most reliable technique to demonstrate the presence of a ring, although tight rings are easily diagnosed by both radiology and endoscopy. Schatzki found rings of less than 12 mm in diameter invariably produced dysphagia for solids and those greater than 20 mm never produced obstructive symptoms.[20]

Asymptomatic rings require no treatment and patients with reflux symptoms simply require appropriate medical antireflux therapy. Rings which produce dysphagia can be dealt with by conventional dilatation using bougies or by balloon dilatation, followed by medical antireflux therapy. There should be little enthusiasm for surgery for obstructive symptoms alone. As long ago as 1963 it was obvious that intermittent dilatation was superior to surgical methods.[21] Conversely, the presence of a wide ring in a patient with significant reflux symptoms who might otherwise be considered a suitable candidate for antireflux surgery should not be viewed as a contra-indication to surgery.

OESOPHAGEAL INFECTIONS

The human oesophagus is relatively resistant to bacterial infection but fungal and viral infections do occur. They are particularly important in immunocompromised individuals.

The three most commonly encountered infections of the oesophagus in Western societies are herpetic oesophagitis, candidal oesophagitis and cytomegaloviral oesophagitis. Symptoms can vary from mild discomfort, to severe life-threatening clinical problems. Rarely, actinomycosis, mucormycosis, histoplasmosis and tuberculosis can affect the oesophagus, as does the protozoan *Trypanosoma cruzi* (see Chagas disease below).

Herpetic oesophagitis

This is caused by herpes simplex virus and this infection may be confused or coexist with candidiasis of the oesophagus or cytomegalovirus infection. The clinical presentation usually includes odynophagia, dysphagia and heartburn. There may be a history of a herpetic lesion on the lip, preceding the onset of oesophageal symptoms by several days. Examination of the oropharynx may be normal or may show vesicles in this region. The severity of mucosal involvement determines the radiological appearances. The condition is becoming increasingly well recognized in the immunocompromised host with leukaemia, lymphoma or following bone marrow transplantation.

The condition evolves in several phases, with initially a vesicular lesion, which is followed by the presence of sharply demarcated small ulcers with raised margins, typically in the middle and upper third of the oesophagus, which may have a grey or yellowish necrotic base. The mucosa surrounding the ulcer is erythematous. The ulcers ultimately enlarge and coalesce. Finally, there is a necrotic phase, during which the infected epithelium is diffusely involved, producing a generalized oesophagitis. The diagnosis is made on endoscopic biopsy, where there are typical cytopathic changes of viral replication. These are most marked at the margins of the herpetic ulcer, revealing multinucleate giant cells, with balloon degeneration of cells demonstrating basophilic nuclei, ground glass inclusions and chromatin margination. There are no cytoplasmic inclusions.

The differential diagnosis includes the other types of infectious oesophagitis, gastro-oesophageal reflux disease and in those patients who have undergone bone marrow transplantation, graft versus host disease. Treatment is with an appropriate antiviral agent, such as acyclovir.

Candidal oesophagitis

Candida can proliferate anywhere along the gastrointestinal tract and like herpetic infection, is seen increasingly frequently in immunosuppressed patients with organ transplants, or those undergoing cancer chemotherapy. Other predisposing causes include chronic illness such as diabetes mellitus, malignancy, long-term antibiotics and local tissue damage, for instance due to corrosive damage or irradiation.[22,23]

The presenting symptoms are usually again, odynophagia and dysphagia, but patients may present with weight loss, back pain and gastrointestinal bleeding. Barium studies are said to be normal in 20–80% of patients, but exudates, ulcers and strictures have all been identified by contrast radiology. Endoscopic examination is the procedure of choice. When early and mild, there are small patches of white exudate. These coalesce as the disease increases in severity, the underlying mucosa becoming increasingly erythematous with subsequent ulceration. Ultimately, the entire circumference of the oesophagus can become involved, with an underlying erythematous and extremely friable mucosa. This can bleed and if this mucosa should slough circumferentially, a stricture can develop. Diagnosis is established by oesophageal brushing, which demonstrates characteristic candidal mycelia.

Treatment in general requires dealing with the underlying cause such as discontinuation of immunosuppression, if feasible. Specific therapy conventionally involves the use of nystatin given by mouth, 100,000 units every 2 h. Very little is absorbed and there is no significant effect on the rest of the gastro-intestinal flora. An alternative drug, particularly where patients have not responded to nystatin, is ketoconazole 200 mg daily for 5 days.

Strictures can develop after severe candidal ulceration and are dealt with by dilatation in the same way as other benign oesophageal strictures.

Cytomegaloviral (CMV) oesophagitis

Primary CMV oesophagitis, tends to occur in immunosuppressed individuals, although it may occur secondarily to the gross epithelial damage which can occur in graft-versus-host disease.

In primary disease, the oesophageal mucosa has a characteristic appearance, with superficial erosions demonstrating a geographic serpiginous non-raised border. This distinguishes CMV from herpes virus infection. The diagnosis is established by biopsy and/or cytological brushings. The characteristic histological change involves a basophilic intranuclear inclusion, a clear halo surrounding the nucleus and the presence of multiple smaller intracytoplasmic inclusions.

All of the above infections can occur in graft-versus-host disease. This is most commonly seen with bone marrow transplantation and viral oesophagitis seems to occur at any time from two months to two years after bone marrow transplantation. The condition itself requires increased immunosuppression and it is important that this should therefore be properly distinguished from these unusual forms of oesophagitis, which require an entirely different therapeutic strategy.

Chagas' disease

Chagas' disease is confined to South American countries, especially Brazil, Argentina, Bolivia and Venezuela. The condition is caused by the protozoan *T. cruzi* involving insect vectors (Triatoma, Rheduviidae). The condition can be induced experimentally by inoculation of experimental animals with *T. cruzi*.

During the acute phase of illness, parasites penetrate the bloodstream and lymphatics reaching different tissues, but particularly the myocardium and smooth muscle. There is then a potentially long intermediate phase which is asymptomatic, and may last several years before a further chronic symptomatic phase occurs. Characteristically, patients develop cardiomyopathy and/or megaoesophagus.

Clinically, the oesophageal symptoms are similar to those seen in severe achalasia, with intermittent dysphagia initially which worsens as the oesophagus dilates to a point when dysphagia becomes total. There is pronounced destruction of both Auerbach's and Meissner's plexuses, which worsens as the oesophagus dilates.[24] The mechanism by which this destruction occurs is still debated.

The diagnosis is usually easily made by barium swallow, in association with appropriate immunological tests.

Since the neural destruction is permanent, there is no definitive treatment. In the early stages, when patients are symptomatic but still have a normal diameter oesophagus, the usual treatment is intermittent dilatation. When the oesophagus is dilated, but less than 7 cm in diameter, surgery is required. The most reliable procedure appears to be cardiomyectomy with fundoplication, which can provide excellent symptomatic relief in over 80% of patients.[25]

Once gross dilatation has occurred, there is no motor function at all in the oesophageal body, so that resection is required. Transhiatal oesophagectomy with a gastric replacement conduit is the most appropriate procedure.[26]

DRUG-INDUCED OESOPHAGITIS

A variety of drugs are known to cause oesophageal damage (Table 18.1). The problem seems to arise mainly in the elderly, in association with defective peristalsis or where a reflux-induced stricture is present. Swallowing tablets without a fluid bolus and ingestion late at night have also been cited as factors which can contribute to the problem.

Anti-inflammatory drugs, antibiotics and potassium chloride tablets are the two most common culprits and although drug

Table 18.1 Agents causing oesophagitis

Antibiotics
  Doxycycline
  Tetracycline
  Clindamycin
  Erythromycin
  Lincomycin
  Minocycline
  Oxytetracycline
  Penicillin
  Tinidazole
  Spiramycin
  Pivampicillin
Benzalkonium chloride
Emepromium bromide
Potassium chloride
Hydrochlorothiazide
Terolidine hydrochloride
Multivitamins
Ferrous sulphate, succinate
Alprenolol chloride
Quinidine
Ascorbic acid
Estramustine phosphate
Pantogar
Chloral hydrate
Phenobarbitone
Clinitest tablets
Steradent
Chemotherapeutic agents
Analgesics, anti-inflammatories
  Aspirin
  Indomethacin
  Phenylbutazone
  Tolectin

discontinuation will usually allow resolution of the inflammation, major complications can ensue including perforation, haemorrhage and death.[27]

With the more widespread use of combined chemotherapy and radiotherapy for oesophageal cancer, it is also evident that this combination can lead to oesophageal injury. Although radiation alone has long been recognized as a cause of damage, the addition of chemotherapy to low-dose irradiation can induce a clinically distinct form of oesophagitis, characterized by episodic inflammation occurring with each dose of chemotherapy.[28]

CORROSIVE INGESTION

Chemical burns to the pharynx, oesophagus and stomach still occur regularly, despite obvious warnings on virtually all common household cleaners and corrosives. Most accidental ingestions occur in children, where the ingestion of small alkaline batteries is also a common event. Attempted suicide by the ingestion of caustic agents is rare in the UK, in comparison to Eastern Europe and North America.

The severity of the damage to tissues depends on the type of agent swallowed, the concentration and amount, and the duration of tissue contact. Strong alkalis are relatively odourless and tasteless, which can account for their ingestion in children, as well as large volume deliberate ingestion by adults. Conversely, the offensive odour and bitter taste of strong acids, make them less likely to be ingested accidentally and ingested in smaller volume when taken deliberately. Alkaline agents cause liquefaction, dissolution of lipoproteins and collagen, saponification of fats, tissue dehydration and thrombosis of blood vessels with further degeneration and fibrous stricturing. Acid agents cause a coagulative necrosis with eschar formation and this coagulant may limit penetration to deeper layers. Nevertheless, the risk of stricture development in the oesophagus is much higher following acid ingestion than with alkalis. Acids also cause greater gastric damage than alkalis, due to the induction of pylorospasm and pooling of acid in the antrum.[29,30]

Involvement of all layers of the oesophagus may lead to perforation, mediastinitis and fistula formation.[31] Necrotic tissue begins to slough within a few days, to leave an ulcerated surface during which time secondary infection with bacteria or fungi can occur. An extensive review in North America indicated that alkaline ingestion was associated with about a 4% risk of stricture development and a 2% mortality, compared to acid ingestion with a 33% risk of stricture development and an 18% mortality.[32]

The patient's presenting symptoms and signs are notoriously unreliable in predicting the severity of injury. It is important to establish the nature and approximate amount of the caustic substance swallowed, the time elapsed since swallowing and whether it was a voluntary or accidental act. Indicators of a severe burn may be severe chest and epigastric pain, inability to swallow saliva, fever, tachycardia, shock-like syndrome, peritonitis, haematemesis, acidosis or evidence of coagulopathy. Acute supraglottic oedema may necessitate urgent tracheostomy.

Table 18.2 Classification of oesophageal burns

GRADE

0 Normal appearances, no endoscopic damage visible
1 Hyperaemia, oedema and superficial erosions (mucosal damage)
2 Ulceration (transmucosal involvement)
3 Deep ulceration, mediastinal pleural or peritoneal penetration
   (perioesophageal involvement)

Early fibreoptic examination is mandatory, to visualize the lesions and grade them (Table 18.2). A full examination of the oesophagus, stomach and duodenum should be undertaken with a thin endoscope, unless deep ulcers are encountered in the oesophagus, in association with extensive necrosis. The recognition of a grey or black eschar in such patients, is associated with a high risk of oesophageal perforation. A contrast swallow should be carried out if perforation is suspected clinically, but is not apparent on chest radiograph.

The immediate management of the patient should ensure that the airway is adequate, followed by intravenous fluids and analgesics. Unless there is an obvious perforation clinically, a chest radiograph should be performed, followed by endoscopy. If no burn is identified, the patient can be safely discharged. Those with oedema only, can resume normal eating immediately. With more severe injuries, it is probably appropriate to recommence oral feeding when patients can swallow saliva satisfactorily. Most centres advocate the use of antibiotics in such patients. There is no evidence that steroids have a beneficial effect, despite their widespread use in the past.[33-35] Patients with deep ulcers require nutritional support, either parenterally or via a feeding jejunostomy. Although lesions of lesser degree will usually heal in 3–4 weeks, those causing extensive mucosal necrosis will take up to 3 months to heal. During that time, regular endoscopy or barium swallow examinations should be carried out to assess stricture development. About 50% of patients with extensive mucosal necrosis will develop a significant stricture.

The role and timing of dilatation in the management of such strictures remains controversial. Most centres seem to time initial dilatations according to the severity of the burn, beginning as early as the third or fourth day or waiting until full re-epithelization has taken place.[36] Although repeat dilatation is acceptable in the short term, patients should not be committed to a protracted course of dilatations with generally unsatisfactory swallowing and surgery should be considered in patients who require regular dilatation more than three months after the injury.

Other than the need for emergency surgery to deal with perforation or bleeding, elective surgery should be deferred for at least three months, when the fibrotic phase is becoming established. Most patients who require surgical treatment have either multiple or long narrow strictures in the oesophagus, which necessitate oesophageal replacement. Because there is often associated gastric involvement in such individuals, colon is the preferred replacement conduit, although the stomach may be used when it is available and otherwise healthy.

However, it is generally believed that a colonic interposition gives the best long-term functional result, which is relevant as many such patients are young.

Considerable controversy still exists about the risk of developing cancer in the damaged oesophagus and stomach. The life-time risk is certainly less than 5%.[37-39] In consequence, some authors prefer to leave the oesophagus in situ, and use a bypass technique. If regular surveillance is undertaken, then such a policy seems justifiable as survival rates for cancer occurring in a damaged oesophagus are much higher than those occurring in the normal oesophagus.[40]

CROHN'S DISEASE OF THE OESOPHAGUS

Clinical involvement of the oesophagus by Crohn's disease is rare. Pathological evidence of Crohn's may, however, be present in 15–20% of patients without oesophageal symptoms.[41,42] Although dysphagia is the most common symptom, fistulation has been described.[43-45]

The diagnosis is established by either barium swallow or endoscopy and biopsy which reveal features similar to Crohn's disease elsewhere in the gastrointestinal tract (apthous and linear ulcers, cobblestone lesions, chronic erosions and areas of engorgement and granularity).[46]

A possible association exists between Crohn's disease involving the oesophagus and Behçet's syndrome.[47,48]

The rarity of oesophageal Crohn's disease means that most cases have been dealt with by methods traditionally used elsewhere in the gastrointestinal tract. Balloon dilatation of strictures and resection (for multiple intramural fistulous tracts) have both been described.[44,49]

AUTOIMMUNE DISEASES AND THE OESOPHAGUS

The oesophagus can be involved in all of the autoimmune conditions usually included under the heading of 'collagen vascular disorders'. These include systemic sclerosis, polymyositis, dermatomyositis, systemic lupus erythematosus and polyarteritis nodosa, although the condition of greatest relevance is systemic sclerosis (scleroderma).

Systemic sclerosis

This condition usually occurs in the third to fifth decade of life, is more common in women than in men and usually causes death from cardiac, renal or pulmonary involvement. The condition has characteristic cutaneous appearances with oedema, thickening and sclerosis of the skin, associated with subcutaneous calcinosis. Unlike some of the other collagen disorders, visceral involvement is unusual but the oesophagus is affected in up to 80% of cases.[50,51]

The predominant and specific pathological feature is smooth muscle atrophy, which is replaced by fibrous tissue. The striated muscle of the oesophagus is completely unaffected and it remains intact among the atrophied smooth muscle. Whether smooth muscle atrophy is the primary event or occurs secondary to neural degeneration remains unknown.

Whatever the precise pathogenesis of the condition, characteristically, oesophageal peristalsis becomes progressively impaired, until active transport of food or liquid into the stomach is lost. The lower oesophageal sphincter is affected, resulting in loss of the antireflux barrier. Patients have a range of symptoms related to their motility disturbance, ranging from mild to severe dysphagia with regurgitation and aspiration, as well as reflux symptoms related both to the lower oesophageal sphincter defect, as well as a defective peristaltic acid clearance mechanism. The incidence of stricture formation varies widely in reported series, between 2 and 48%.[52,53]

The diagnosis of oesophageal involvement in systemic sclerosis is usually made easily by contrast radiology. Reduced or absent peristalsis is evident and oesophagitis in association with free gastro-oesophageal reflux and stricture formation can both be recognized. Endoscopy is important in such individuals to correctly assess the extent of mucosal damage related to reflux.

Although oesophageal manometry provides the most precise information about the motor dysfunction in the oesophageal body and the extent of the defect in lower oesophageal sphincter function, the test is not required for the majority of patients. Similarly, although 24 h pH monitoring of the oesophagus is the most appropriate way to quantitate the extent of reflux, it is not required for most patients. A grading system, based on manometric criteria, to classify oesophageal involvement in this condition as mild, moderate and severe, was developed by Garrett in 1971.[54] The correlation between manometric findings, 24 h pH monitoring, oesophagoscopy and barium studies, is shown in Table 18.3.

The treatment of oesophageal problems in systemic sclerosis centres around the management of the reflux-associated complications. There are no drugs which specifically influence the oesophageal body motor defect and improve swallowing. The availability of potent acid suppressive therapy using a proton pump inhibitor has been effective and has undoubtedly reduced the need for surgical intervention. Stricture development in this condition is dealt with exactly as in other patients with reflux disease. Very few patients require antireflux surgery and selection of an appropriate group is difficult, due to the progressive nature of the oesophageal body motor defect. Clearly, as time goes by, what might begin as an effective surgical antireflux barrier, becomes a mechanical barrier to the weakening peristalsis. If antireflux surgery is required, one of the partial fundoplication procedures should be used to minimize the risks of dysphagia, which is generally greatest with 360° fundoplication.

Polymyositis, dermatomyositis

These disorders primarily affect skeletal muscle, although in the latter condition there are additional skin changes including erythema, sclerodactyly and telangiectasia. Up to 60% of patients will have difficulties with deglutition as a result of involvement of the pharyngeal constrictor mechanism and the cricopharyngeus muscle[55] and symptoms of aspiration are not uncommon. There may be some involvement of the smooth muscle in the lower two thirds of the oesophagus, but this is unusual.

Systemic lupus erythematosus

This clinical entity involves skin, joints and visceral organs, particularly kidneys, lungs, heart and the gastrointestinal tract. Oesophageal involvement is not common and is clinically similar to that seen in systemic sclerosis. The same treatment approaches are therefore indicated.

Polyarteritis nodosa and other connective tissue disorders

Polyarteritis nodosa and rheumatoid disease may be associated with motility disorders of the oesophagus but few patients have symptoms.[56-59] Dysphagia can be caused by rheumatoid changes of the cricoarytenoid joint and oesophageal stricture has been reported, particularly in the upper third of the oesophagus.[60] Dysphagia can also occur in Sjögren's syndrome, although this may be largely due to reduced secretion of saliva, leading to impaired deglutition.[61]

OESOPHAGEAL DIVERTICULA

Diverticula can occur anywhere in the oesophagus and are traditionally classified by their location, their origin as either congenital or acquired and if in the latter category, the proposed mechanism of formation (pulsion or traction).

Pulsion diverticula develop when high intraluminal pressure

Table 18.3 Classification of oesophageal involvement in scleroderma

DEGREE	MANOMETRY SWALLOW	PH MONITORING	OESOPHAGOSCOPY	BARIUM CINERADIOGRAPHY
I	Variability in the strength of contractions after swallowing	Normal	No visible mucosal damage	Delayed oesophageal transit
II	Feeble contractions occurring constantly after swallowing; LOS tone normal or reduced	Moderate to severe GOR	Oesophagitis I° to II°	Dilatation; impaired swallowing; air oesophagram
III	Entire smooth muscle portion of the oesophagus paralysed; LOS tone markedly reduced or lost	Severe GOR with extremely long duration in supine position/sleep	Circular erosive lesions III° peptic ulcers; stricture formation (IV°)	Ulcers; cardia wide open; barium reflux stenosis

Modified from Garrett et al.[54]

acts on a point in the oesophageal wall, distal to which there is a degree of relative obstruction, either structural or functional. Any symptoms which arise can be due either to the disorder which gives rise to the diverticulum or from the mechanical effects of the diverticulum itself. Traction diverticula are not really abnormalities of the oesophagus at all, but represent the effects of extrinsic pathology on the oesophageal wall. Tuberculous lymph nodes were historically cited as the principal cause of this type of diverticulum. It is clear with the reduction in tuberculosis that traction diverticula are extremely rare. Malignant mediastinal lymph nodes do not usually give rise to symptomatic traction diverticula.

Pharyngo-oesophageal diverticula represent the most common site. Although usually attributed to Zenker, the first description of this type of diverticulum was made by Ludlow in 1769.[62] They arise through the dehiscence of Killian, which is a potential posterior defect between the circular fibres of the cricopharyngeus muscle below and the oblique fibres of the inferior constrictor above.[63] This topic is covered in detail elsewhere (Chapter 7).

Although diverticula can occur at any level in the body of the oesophagus, they are most common in the lower half (Figure 18.3a,b). Proximal diverticula may have been more common in the past, in association with tuberculous lymph glands in the neck and a similar process may have accounted for many mid-thoracic diverticula. There is nevertheless, increasing evidence that most mid-thoracic diveriticula are of the pulsion type and probably reflect underlying disorders of oesophageal motility, in which normally coordinated peristaltic activity is inconsistent and where a degree of functional distal obstruction occurs, as in achalasia or diffuse oesophageal spasm.[64,65]

Epiphrenic or distal oesophageal diverticula usually develop from the right posterolateral border of the oesophagus, just above the diaphragm, but can arise in the abdominal segment from the anterolateral wall. Again, the pathogenesis seems to be similar to the mid-oesophageal types, with a high incidence of primary motor disturbance, which is confirmed on manometry, in association with conditions such as achalasia and diffuse oesophageal spasm.[66,67]

Clinical features

Symptoms largely reflect the degree to which the diverticulum itself produces pressure effects and the underlying motility disorder, which had led to the formation of the diverticulum. Most patients present with a combination of dysphagia and/or chest pain. Regurgitation and respiratory symptoms are unusual.

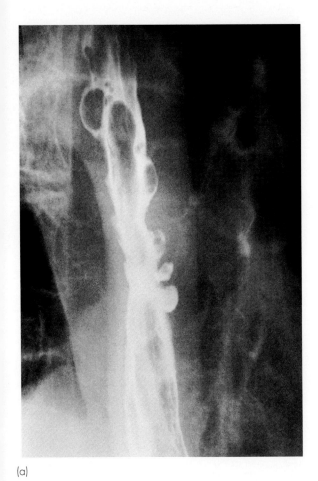

(a)

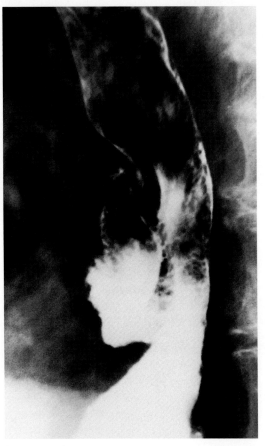

(b)

Figure 18.3

Multiple diverticula and a solitary diverticulum associated with ulceration

Diagnosis

Diverticula are best demonstrated by radiology but are often apparent on fibreoptic endoscopy. Because of the high incidence of underlying motor dysfunction, special tests such as manometry and pH monitoring, may be required to fully elucidate the nature of the underlying motor defect and exclude any symptom component due to pathological gastro-oesophageal reflux.

Treatment

When diverticula are small, treatment is largely directed towards the underlying motor disorder, rather than the diverticulum itself. This is particularly so in the case of mid-oesophageal diverticula, which rarely achieve great size. Epiphrenic diverticula on the other hand, may be large and require local treatment in their own right. Excision is appropriate for large diverticula, since they can become complicated by inflammation, fistula formation, neoplastic change and even spontaneous perforation.[68] The purpose of surgery is to correct the underlying pathophysiological disorder, as well as excision of the diverticulum. Three factors should be considered removal of the diverticulum with secure oesophageal closure, correction of distal obstruction by myotomy and the addition of an antireflux procedure as deemed appropriate. Diverticulectomy is probably best undertaken in conjunction with the appropriate associated procedures via a left thoracotomy, as advocated at The Mayo Clinic and by Belsey. Diverticulectomy in conjunction with oesophagomyotomy has produced consistently the best results.[66,69] The addition of a non-obstructive antireflux procedure, such as the Belsey Mark IV operation, in patients where the underlying disorder includes gastro-oesophageal reflux disease or if the myotomy should traverse the gastro-oesophageal junction, again seems appropriate. The procedure lends itself to a thoracoscopic approach with stapled closure of the diverticular neck. There are no reported series as yet, but as the open operation can be reproduced without compromise by a minimal access method, this ought to be the future treatment of choice.

Intramural pseudodiverticulosis of the oesophagus

This is a rare condition in which there are multiple small flask-shaped diverticula in the wall of the oesophagus (Figure 18.4). The condition was first described by Mendl et al. in 1960.[70] The aetiology remains obscure, although pathological studies indicate that there is abnormal dilatation of the ducts of the sub-mucosal oesophageal glands.[71-79] The condition usually presents in the fifth or sixth decade of life, with mild dysphagia, which seems to be progressive in about a third of cases. The diagnosis is usually established by barium swallow and there seems to be no clear oesophageal motor abnormality. There is no primary treatment for this condition. If there is associated reflux disease, then treatment is essentially for the complications of reflux, such as stricture formation, rather than pseudodiverticulosis. There have been reports of secondary infection,

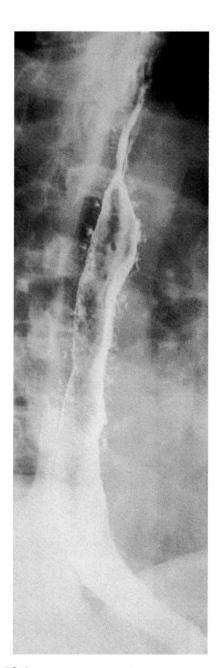

Figure 18.4
Oesophageal pseudodiverticulosis.

particularly with candida[77] and eradication of such organisms in proven cases seems appropriate.

OESOPHAGEAL CYSTS AND DUPLICATIONS

Cysts and duplications of the oesophagus are uncommon congenital lesions of mixed embryogenesis. They usually present in childhood and present diagnostic difficulties by being confused with benign oesophageal tumours or other mediastinal masses. Duplications of the gastrointestinal tract are rare congenital lesions with oesophageal duplication comprising 10–20% of all cases,[80,81] although this makes the oesophagus the second most common site for duplication, after the ileum.

The development of duplications and cysts is based on three embryological theories. The split notochord syndrome is based on the relationship of the notochord to the neural tube. It is implied that during separation of the notochord from the endoderm, a gap may appear in the notochord, which allows an endodermal diverticulum to develop from the foregut, which may herniate through or adhere to the neural tube, giving rise to a variety of abnormal endodermal remnants, such as cysts. Because they are attached to the notochord, they may impede the union of the vertebral bodies and hence there is a 5–15% incidence of vertebral column anomalies in patients with gastrointestinal duplications.[82] These duplications or congenital cysts are often referred to as posterior mediastinal cysts, enteric cysts or neuroenteric cysts. A second theory,[83] can be described as tracheobronchial foregut duplication, implying that a developmental error occurs during separation of the tracheobronchial bud from the foregut during fetal life. Incomplete separation results in a fistulous communication between the foregut and respiratory tree and if partial regression occurs during fetal life, a duplication with close relationship to the tracheobronchial tree may persist. Interestingly, these duplications may be lined by a ciliated epithelium and are not associated with vertebral abnormalities.

The third major theory is the mucosal disorder syndrome, thought to represent dysvacuolization[84] and diverticular outpouching of the mucosa. This is thought to be due to coalescence of an excess of residual gut vacuoles not used in the creation of the normal gastrointestinal tract but which persist and form intramural cysts and duplications.

Acquired cysts

These are discussed above under the heading of intramural pseudodiverticulosis, which can be considered as examples of multiple retention cysts. Small cysts can occur in the upper oesophagus which can displace the mucosa into the oesophageal lumen.[85]

MEDIASTINAL FIBROSIS

This is an uncommon condition which can accompany retroperitoneal fibrosis or occur in isolation.[86,87] As with retroperitoneal fibrosis, a variety of aetiological theories have been put forward although the majority of cases must be considered idiopathic. The characteristic clinical picture results in a variety of symptoms and signs related to organ encasement and entrapment, the most common of which is superior vena caval obstruction.[88] The condition can, however, be complicated by intractable left ventricular failure,[89,90] pulmonary hypertension,[91] oesophageal varices,[88,92] chylothorax,[93] constrictive pericarditis[90,94] and dysphagia.[87,95]

The diagnosis can be suspected on computed tomographic scanning and differentiation between this condition and malignancy is important. Mediastinoscopy is best avoided in patients with superior vena caval obstruction and thoracoscopy may be an appropriate method of assessing such patients and obtaining histological proof of the condition.

There is no effective medical therapy for this condition and drugs which impair collagen cross-linking or stimulate collagen breakdown (penicillamine, colchicine) do not seem to be effective. Oesophageal lysis is not really a feasible proposition and either a transpleural or subcutaneous conduit represents the only realistic method of alleviating severe dysphagia permanently. Because the condition usually produces pronounced cardiovascular disturbances, however, such major intervention is rarely appropriate.

VASCULAR ABNORMALITIES AFFECTING THE OESOPHAGUS

A number of vascular abnormalities can produce dysphagia although it should not be simply assumed that the presence of vascular indentation on the oesophagus as seen during barium radiology is necessarily the cause of symptoms. This is particularly true of the common indentations seen where the aortic arch crosses the oesophagus and the anomaly of the aberrant right subclavian artery said to be present in about 1% of subjects.

A number of congenital vascular anomalies can, however, produce dysphagia. The first account of this was probably made by Bayford in 1787. These vascular rings include double aortic arch, a right-sided arch with a ring produced by the ligamentum arteriosum, aberrant right subclavian artery, left subclavian artery with a right aortic arch and abnormalities of the origin of the brachiocephalic trunk and left common carotid artery.[95,97] These vascular rings are estimated to account for about 1% of congenital abnormalities of the heart and great vessels.

Acquired causes include aneurysm of the aorta, an enlarged left atrium, diffuse enlargement of the heart and pressure due to the left common carotid artery and even the vertebral artery.[98,99]

With the widespread availability of digital subtraction angiography, most of these lesions can be demonstrated without great difficulty nowadays. For most congenital abnormalities, although dysphagia may occur, respiratory symptoms and compression of the trachea are more common and usually the principal stimulus for surgical correction. Of the acquired lesions, many will occur in elderly patients and give rise to only mild dysphagia so that surgical correction of the underlying abnormality is not necessarily essential.

THE MALLORY–WEISS SYNDROME, INTRAMURAL RUPTURE AND INTRAMURAL HAEMATOMA

The syndrome in which haematemesis occurs as a result of a mucosal tear at or close to the gastro-oesophageal junction was first described in 1929.[100] In the classical history, forceful vomiting is followed by haematemesis, often with an antecedent history of considerable alcohol ingestion. In recent years, two variations of this injury have been recognized. With intramural haematoma, injury leads to bleeding into the wall of the oesophagus and the problem is particularly evident in patients with coagulation disorders.[101] Intramural rupture was first described as a spontaneous event by Marks and Keet in 1968.[102] There is no major overt blood loss but the patients characteristically have marked epigastric and/or retrosternal pain associated with odynophagia.[103] Intramural rupture usually presents with very similar symptoms, although the pain may be severe enough to suggest myocardial infarction, aortic dissection or complete oesophageal rupture.

The Mallory–Weiss syndrome is much more common in males than in females and accounts for 2–11% of endoscopic diagnoses as a cause of acute upper gastrointestinal haemorrhage.[104,105]

Although the original description of the Mallory–Weiss syndrome indicated that forceful vomiting led to mucosal lacerations at about the level of the gastro-oesophageal junction, usually precipitated by alcohol, it is now recognized that neither vomiting nor alcohol are necessary prerequisites for the development of these lesions. Tearing at this level can be induced by violent coughing, status asthmaticus, epileptic seizure or closed cardiac massage. The characteristic lesion is a longitudinal laceration of the mucosa extending deeply into the submucosa. The lacerations are nearly always single, although multiple lesions have been described. Although the condition is described as occurring at the gastro-oesophageal junction, the majority of lacerations do at least involve the stomach and/or the gastro-oesophageal junction. Isolated oesophageal lacerations are rare. It is noteworthy that many patients have other associated lesions in the upper gastrointestinal tract which might be associated with vomiting, including oesophagitis, gastritis, duodenitis and active peptic ulcer disease.[104-108] As indicated above, intramural haematoma may be particularly likely to occur in association with vomiting in patients with coagulation defects, such as elderly individuals on anticoagulant therapy. The haematoma can be extensive, reaching from the gastro-oesophageal junction to the carina.

The diagnosis of Mallory–Weiss syndrome is nearly always made on endoscopy and barium swallow is essentially unhelpful. In contrast, intramural rupture is best diagnosed by barium swallow, where the true and false lumens of the oesophagus give a double-barrelled appearance.[109] Intramural haematoma is usually diagnosed by endoscopy, although it would appear that the endoscopic findings are frequently misinterpreted as either neoplasia or a vascular lesion arising in the oesophageal wall. The smooth outline demonstrable by barium swallow may be more useful and computed tomography may also be valuable.[110]

Many Mallory–Weiss tears are associated with trivial haemorrhage and no resuscitation of the patient is necessary. With more severe bleeds, attention needs to be paid to the restoration of haemodynamic stability and in a small proportion of patients, haemorrhage may be prodigious and require intervention. Local injection with adrenaline is the most appropriate first-line procedure and if this fails, thermal endoscopic methods can be attempted or transcatheter embolization.[111,112] Surgery should be required in only a tiny proportion of cases and should involve a vertical gastrotomy which should not cross the gastro-oesophageal junction. The bleeding area can then be under-run and the gastrotomy closed. Neither intramural rupture nor haematoma require active intervention. Both conditions resolve spontaneously. Oral fluids should be restricted until the patient's symptoms have resolved which usually takes 7–14 days.[103]

REFERENCES

1. Clements JL, Cox GW, Torres WE & Weens HS. Cervical esophageal webs – a Roentgen-anatomic correlation: observations on the pharyngoesophagus. *AJR* 1974; **121:** 221–235.
2. Ladd WE. Congenital anomalies of the oesophagus. *Pediatrics* 1950; **6:** 9–19.
3. Bluestone CD, Kerry R & Sieber WK. Congenitial esophageal stenosis. *Laryngoscope* 1969; **79:** 1095–1104.
4. Liebman WM & Samloff IM. Congenital membranous stenosis of the mid esophagus. *Clin Pediatr* 1973; **12:** 660–662.
5. Longstetch DF, Wolochow DA & Tu RT. Double congenital mid esophageal webs in adults. *Dig Dis Sci* 1971; **24:** 162–165.
6. Patterson DR. A clinical type of dysphagia. *J Laryngol Rhinol Otol* 1919; **34:** 289–291.
7. Kelly AB. Spasm at the entrance of the oesophagus. *J Laryngol Rhinol Otol* 1919; **34:** 285–289.
8. Vinson DP. Hysterical dysphagia. *Minn Med* 1922; **5:** 107–108.
9. Wynder EL, Hultboig S, Jacobsson F & Bross IJ. Environmental factors in cancer of the upper alimentary tract. Swedish study with special reference to Plummer–Vinson (Patterson–Kelly) syndrome. *Cancer* 1957; **10:** 470–487.
10. Shearman DJC & Finlayson NDC. *Diseases of the Gastrointestinal Tract and Liver.* Edinburgh: Churchill Livingstone, 1982: 114.
11. Raque CJ, Stein KM & Samitz MH. Pemphigus vulgaris involving the esophagus. *Arch Dermatol* 1970; **102:** 371–373.
12. Benedict EV & Lever WE. Stenosis of the oesophagus in benign mucous membrane pemphigoid. *Ann Otol Rhinol Laryngol* 1952; **61:** 1120–1133.
13. Bremner CG. Benign strictures of the esophagus. *Curr Prob Surg* 1982; **19:** 475.
14. Ikard RW & Rosen ME. Mid esophageal web in adults. *Ann Thorac Surg* 1977; **24:** 355–358.
15. Schatzki R & Gary JE. Dysphagia due to diaphragm-like localised narrowing in the lower esophagus (lower oesophageal ring). *AJR* 1953; **70:** 911–922.
16. Postlethwait RW & Musser AW. Pathology of lower esophageal web. *Surg Gynecol Obstet* 1965; **120:** 571–575.
17. Vansant JH. Surgical significance of the lower esophageal ring. *Ann Surg* 1972; **175:** 733–739.
18. Postlethwait RW. *Surgery of the Esophagus.* New York: Appleton-Century-Crofts, 1979.
19. Postlethwait RW & Sealy WC. Experiences with the treatment of 59 patients with lower esophageal web. *Ann Surg* 1967; **165:** 786–796.
20. Schatzki R. The lower esophageal ring: long term follow-up of symptomatic and asymptomatic rings. *AJR* 1963; **90:** 805–810.
21. Wilkins EW Jr & Barlett MK. Surgical treatment of the lower esophageal ring. *New Engl J Med* 1963; **268:** 461–464.
22. Zguyer PB, Brunton FJ and Rooke HWP. Candidiasis of the esophagus. *Br J Radiol* 1971; **44:** 131–136.
23. Mathieson R & Dutta SK. Candida esophagitis. *Dig Dis Sci* 1983; **28:** 365–370.
24. Koberle F. Chagas' disease and Chagas' syndrome: the pathology of American trypanosomiasis. *Parasitology* 1968; **63:** 116–119.
25. Pinotti HW & Bettarello A. Chagasic mega-oesophagus. In: Jamieson GG (ed.) *Surgery of the Oesophagus.* Edinburgh: Churchill Livingstone, 1988: 471–481.
26. Pinotti HW. A new approach to the thoracic esophagus by the abdominal transdiaphragmatic route. *Langenbecks Arch Chir* 1983; **359:** 229–235.
27. Lewis JH. Gastrointestinal injury due to medicinal agents. *Am J Gastroenterol* 1986; **81:** 819–834.
28. Boal DKB, Neuberger PE & Teele RL. Esophagitis induced by combined radiation and adriamycin. *Am J Radiol* 1979; **132:** 567–570.
29. Kray H. Treatment of corrosive lesions of the esophagus. *Acta Otolaryngol* (Suppl) 1952; **102:** 1–49.
30. Zargar SA, Kochkar R, Naqi B et al. Ingestion of corrosive acids. Spectrum of injury to upper gastrointestinal tract and natural history. *Gastroenterology* 1989; **97:** 720–727.
31. Pense SC, Wood WJ, Stempel TK et al. Tracheoesophageal fistula secondary to muriatic acid ingestion. *Burns Including Thermal Injury* 1988; **14:** 35–38.
32. Tucker JA & Yarington CT. The treatment of caustic ingestion. *Otolaryngol Clin North Am* 1979; **12:** 343–350.
33. Ferguson MK, Migliore M, Staszak VM et al. Early evaluation and therapy for caustic esophageal injury. *Am J Surg* 1989; **157:** 116–120.

34. Sugawa C & Lucas CE. Caustic injury of the upper gastrointestinal tract in adults, a clinical and endoscopic study. *Surgery* 1989; **106:** 802–807.

35. Anderson KD, Rouse TM & Randolph JG. A controlled trial of corticosteroids in children with corrosive injury of the oesophagus. *N Engl Med J* 1990; **323:** 637–640.

36. Gorney J. Bougies for chemical esophageal burns. *N Engl J Med* 1971; **285:** 526.

37. Kiviranta UK. Corrosion carcinoma of the esophagus. *Ann Otolaryngol* 1952; **42:** 89.

38. Bigelow NB. Carcinoma of the esophagus developing at the site of stricture. *Cancer* 1953; **6:** 1159.

39. Ti TK. Esophageal resection with pharyngogastrostomy for corrosive strictures of the pharynx and esophagus. *Br J Surg* 1980; **67:** 798–800.

40. Cs'ikos M, Horv'ath O, Petri I et al. Late malignant transformation of chronic corrosive esophageal strictures. *Langenbecks Arch Chir* 1985; **365:** 231–238.

41. Gaucher P, Bigard MA, Begue JY, Laugros A, Regent D & Macinot C. Esophageal localization of Crohn's disease. *Nouv Presse Med* 1977; **6:** 1369–1372.

42. Cameron DJ. Upper and lower gastrointestinal endoscopy in children and adolescents with Crohn's disease: a prospective study. *J Gastroenterol Hepatol*, 1991; **6:** 355–358.

43. Freson M, Kottler RE & Wright JP Crohn's disease of the oesophagus. A case report. *S Afr Med J* 1984; **66:** 417–418.

44. Rowe PH, Taylor PR, Sladen GE & Owen WJ. Cricopharyngeal Crohn's disease. *Postgrad Med J* 1987; **63:** 1101–1102.

45. Steel A, Dyer NH & Matthews HR. Cervical Crohn's disease with oesophago-pulmonary fistula. *Postgrad Med J* 1988; **64:** 706–709.

46. Kurtz B, Steinhardt HJ & Malchow H. The radiological and endoscopic appearances of Crohn's disease of the upper gastro-intestinal tract. *ROFO Fortschr Geb Rontgenstr Nuklearmed* 1982; **136:** 124–128.

47. Jaeger K & Appel A. Crohn's proctocolitis with involvement of the esophagus and mouth. *Chirurg* 1979; **50:** 170–172.

48. Roge J. Behçet's syndrome and the digestive tract. *J Mal Vasc* 1988; **13:** 235–239.

49. Mannell A & Hamilton DG. Crohn's disease of the oesophagus: a case report. *Aust NZ J Surg* 1980; **50:** 303–308.

50. Treacy WL, Baggenstoss AH, Slocumb CN & Code CF. Scleroderma of the oesophagus: a correlation of histologic and physiologic findings. *Ann Intern Med* 1963; **59:** 351–356.

51. Saladin TA, French AB, Zartafonetis CJD & Pollard HM. Oesophageal motor abnormalities in scleroderma and related diseases. *Am J Dig Dis* 1966; **11:** 522–535.

52. Kemp Harper RA & Jackson DC. Progressive systemic sclerosis. *Br J Radiol* 1964; **38:** 825–834.

53. Henderson RD & Pearson FC. Surgical management of oesophageal scleroderma. *J Thorac Cardiovasc Surg* 1973; **66:** 686–691.

54. Garrett JM, Winkelmann RK, Schlegel JF & Code CF. Oesophageal deterioration in scleroderma. *Mayo Clin Proc* 1971; **46:** 92–96.

55. Jacob H, Berkowitz D, McDonald E, Bernstein LHG & Beneventano T. The oesophageal motility disorders of polymyositis. A prospective study. *Arch Intern Med* 1983; **143:** 2262–2264.

56. Turner R, Lipshutz W, Miller W, Rittenberg G, Schumacher HR & Cohen S. Oesophageal dysfunction in collagen disease. *Am J Med Sci* 1973; **265:** 191–199.

57. Tatelman M & Keech MK. Oesophageal motility in systemic lupus erythematosus, rheumatoid arthritis and scleroderma. *Radiology* 1966; **86:** 1041–1046.

58. Nishihai M, Asuba O & Homma N. Rheumatoid oesophageal disease. *Am J Gastroenterol* 1977; **67:** 29–33.

59. Sun DCN, Roth SH, Mitchell CS & Englund DW. Upper gastrointestinal disease in rheumatoid arthritis. *Am J Dig Dis* 1974; **19:** 405–410.

60. John V, Stirling AJ & Matthews HR. Rheumatoid stricture of the oesophagus. *BMJ* 1978; **i:** 479.

61. Tsianos EB, Chiras CD, Drosos AA & Moutsopoulos HM. Oesophageal dysfunction in patients with primary Sjogren's syndrome. *Ann Rheum Dis* 1985; **44:** 610–613.

62. Ludlow A. A case of obstructed deglutition from preternatural dilatation of and bag formed in the pharynx: observations and inquiries. *Soc Physicians (London)* 1769; **3:** 85–101.

63. Killian G. La boudre de l'oesophage. *Ann Mal Orielle Larynx* 1908; **34:** 1–52.

64. Kaye MD. Oesophageal motor dysfunction in patients with diverticula of the mid-thoracic oesophagus. *Thorax* 1974; **29:** 666–672.

65. Rivkin L, Bremner CG & Bremner CH. Pathophysiology of mid-oesophageal and epiphrenic diverticula of the oesophagus. *S Afr Med J* 1984; **66:** 127–129.

66. Debas HT, Payne WS, Cameron AJ & Carlson HC. Physiopathology of lower esophageal diverticulum and its implications for treatment. *Surg Gynecol Obstet* 1980; **151:** 593–600.

67. Evander A, Little AG, Ferguson MK et al. Diverticula of the mid and lower oesophagus: pathogenesis and surgical management. *World J Surg* 1986; **10:** 820–828.

68. Scully RE, Mark EJ & McNeely BU. Case records of the Massachusetts General Hospital (Case 32, 1982). *N Engl J Med* 1982; **307:** 426–433.

69. Belsey R. Functional disease of the esophagus. *J Thorac Cardiovasc Surg* 1969; **52:** 164–188.

70. Mendl K, McKay JM & Tanner CH. Intramural diverticulosis of the esophagus and Rokitanski–Aschoff sinuses in the gallbladder. *Br J Radiol* 1960; **33:** 496–501.

71. Lupovitch A & Tippins R. Esophageal intramural pseudo-diverticulosis. A disease of adnexal glands. *Radiology* 1974; **113:** 271–272.

72. Boyd RM, Bogoch A, Greig. JH & Trites EW. Esophageal intraluminal pseudodiverticulosis. *Radiology* 1974; **113:** 267–270.

73. Wightman AJA & Wright EA. Intramural oesophageal diverticulosis: a correlation of radiological and pathological findings. *Br J Radiol* 1974; **47:** 496–498.

74. Umlas J & Sakhuja R. The pathology of esophageal intramural pseudodiverticulosis. *Am J Clin Pathol* 1976; **65:** 314–320.

75. Castillo S, Aburashed A, Kimmelman J & Alexander LC. Diffuse intraluminal esophageal pseudo-diverticulosis: new cases and review. *Gastroenterology* 1977; **72:** 541–545.

76. Fromkes J, Thomas FB, Mekhijian H et al. Esophageal intramural pseudodiverticulosis. *Am J Dig Dis* 1977; **22:** 690–700.

77. Montgomery RD, Mendl K & Stephenson SF. Intramural diverticulosis of the oesophagus. *Thorax* 1975; **30:** 278–284.

78. Cho SR, Sanders MM, Turner MA et al. Esophageal intramural pseudodiverticulosis. *Gastrointest Radiol* 1981; **6:** 9–16.

79. Murney RE, Linne JH & Curtis J. High amplitude peristaltic contractions in a patient with esophageal intramural pseudo-diverticulosis. *Dig Dis Sci* 1983; **28:** 843–847.

80. Nehme AE & Rabiah F. Ciliated epithelial esophageal cyst: case report and review of the literature. *Am Surg* 1977; **43:** 114–118.

81. Whitaker JA, Deffenbaugh LD & Cooke AR. Esophageal duplication cyst. *Am J Gastroenterol* 1980; **73:** 329–332.

82. Bower RJ, Sieber WK & Kiesewetter WB. Alimentary tract duplications in children. *Ann Surg* 1978; **188:** 669–674.

83. Vaage S & Knutrud O. Congenital duplications of the alimentary tract with special regard to their embryogenesis. In: Rickam PP (ed.) *Progress in Pediatric Surgery*, Baltimore, 1974; 103–123.

84. Bremer JL. Diverticula and duplications of the intestinal tract. *Arch Pathol* 1944; **38:** 132–140.

85. Kahle M & Weber EG. Cysts of the esophagus. *Hepato-Gastroenterology* 1980; **27:** 372–376.

86. Barrett NR. Idiopathic mediastinal fibrosis. *Br J Surg* 1958; **46:** 207–218.

87. Hache L, Woolner LB & Bernatz PE. Idiopathic fibrous mediastinitis. *Dis Chest* 1962; **41:** 9–25.

88. Buckberg GD, Dilley RB & Longmire WP Jr. The protean manifestations of sclerosing fibrosis. *Surg Gynecol Obstet* 1966; **123:** 729–736.

89. Pang J, Vicary FR & Beck ER. Coexisting retroperitoneal and mediastinal fibrosis *Postgrad Med J* 1983; **59:** 450–451.

90. Pick RA, Joswig BC & Bloor CM. Recurrent cardiac constriction after pericardiectomy. *J Thorac Cardiovasc Surg* 1969; **144:** 2061–2062.

91. Arnett EN, Bacos JM, Macher AM et al. Fibrosing mediastinitis causing pulmonary arterial hypertension without pulmonary venous hypertension. *Am J Med* 1977; **632:** 634–643.

92. Partington PF. Diffuse idiopathic fibrosis. *Am J Surg* 1961; **101:** 239–244.

93. Bristo LD, Mandal AK, Oparah SS & Bauer HM. Bilateral chylothorax associated with sclerosing mediastinitis. *Int Surg* 1983; **68:** 273–275.

94. Hanley PC, Shub C & Lie JT. Constrictive pericarditis associated with combined idiopathic retroperitoneal and mediastinal fibrosis. *Mayo Clin Proc* 1984; **59:** 300–304.

95. Albrechtsen D & Nygaard K. Idopathic mediastinal fibrosis. *Acta Chir Scand* 1984; **147:** 219–222.

96. Tucker BL, Meyer BW, Lindesmith GG, Stiles QR & Jones JC. Congenital aortic vascular ring. *Arch Surg* 1969; **99:** 521–523.

97. Eklof D, Ekstrom G, Eriksson BD et al. Arterial anomalies causing compression of the trachea and/or the oesophagus. *Acta Paediatr Scand* 1971; **60:** 81–89.

98. Coppola ED. Dysphagia caused by elongation and tortuosity of the common carotid artery. *N Engl J Med* 1964; **270:** 572–574.

99. Vasquez MT, Garcia MAM, Wollrich FS & Maganda TC. Cervical dysphagia lusoria from vertebral arterial compression. *Arch Surg* 1983; **118:** 125–126.

100. Mallory GK & Weiss S. Haemorrhages from lacerations of the cardiac orifice of the stomach due to vomiting. *Ann J Med Sci* 1929; **178:** 506–515.

101. Shay SS, Berendon RA & Johnson LF. Oesophageal haematoma: four new cases, a review and proposed aetiology. *Dig Dis Sci* 1981; **26:** 1019–1024.

102. Marks IJ & Keet AD. Intramural rupture of the oesophagus. *BMJ* 1968; **iii:** 536–537.

103. Meulman N, Evans J & Watson A. Spontaneous intramural haematoma of the oesophagus: a report of three cases and a review of the literature. *Aust NZ J Surg* 1994; **64:** 190–193.

104. Knauer CN. Mallory–Weiss syndrome: characterisation of seventy-five Mallory–Weiss lacerations in five hundred and twenty-eight patients with upper gastrointestinal haemorrhage. *Gastroenterol* 1976; **71:** 5–8.

105. Michel L, Serrano A & Malt RA. Mallory–Weiss syndrome: evolution of diagnostic and therapeutic patterns over two decades. *Ann Surg* 1980; **192:** 716–721.

106. Atkinson M, Bottrill MB, Edwards AT, Mitchell WM Peet BG & Williams RE. Mucosal tears at the oesophago-gastric junction (the Mallory–Weiss Syndrome). *Gut* 1961; **2:** 1–11.

107. Degradi AE, Brodrick JT, Juler G et al. The Mallory–Weiss syndrome and lesion: a study of thirty cases. *Ann J Dig Dis* 1966; **11:** 710–721.

108. Bubrick MP, Lundeen IW, Onstade GR et al. Mallory–Weiss syndrome: analysis of fifty-nine cases. *Surgery* 1980; **88:** 400–405.

109. Lichter J & Borrie J. Intramural oesophageal abscess. *Br J Surg* 1965; **52:** 185–188.

110. Herbetko J & Brunton FJ. Oesophageal haematoma: report of three cases. *Clin Radiol* 1988; **39:** 462–463.

111. Carsen GM, Casarella WJ & Spiegel RM. Transcatheter embolization for treatment of Mallory–Weiss tears of the oesophago-gastric junction. *Radiology* 1978; **128:** 309–313.

112. Papp JP. Electrocoagulation of actively bleeding Mallory–Weiss tears. *Gastrointest Endosc* 1980; **26:** 128–130.

PART TWO

Stomach and Duodenum

edited by TV Taylor

19

ANATOMY OF THE STOMACH

TV Taylor

GROSS ANATOMY

The stomach, the most dilated part of the gastrointestinal tract, is a crescentic-shaped reservoir, lying between the oesophagus and the duodenum. Acting as a storage organ for ingested food, it initiates the process of digestion by liquefaction and then releases its contents into the duodenum in a precisely controlled manner. The stomach lies in the epigastric, umbilical and left hypochondrial regions of the abdomen, behind the anterior abdominal wall. Extending superiorly to occupy the undersurface of the left side of the diaphragm, it sweeps caudally and to the right, terminating just to the right of the midline at the level of the first lumbar vertebra. Its shape and position are modified by changes within itself and the surrounding viscera. When lying empty its internal volume is little more than 50 ml; when maximally distended in the adult, this volume increases to about 1500 ml by lengthening of the greater curvature and increase of the transverse diameter, while the inlet and outlet remain fixed in position.

Segments

The stomach is divided into five anatomical parts: cardia, fundus, body, antrum and pylorus (Figure 19.1). The cardia is a short segment immediately continuous with the oesophagus. The large dome-shaped fundus sweeps superiorly and to the left, creating the sharp angle of His* between its medial convexity and the intra-abdominal oesophagus. The body or corpus of the stomach lies immediately distal. It is the largest part of the stomach and, together with the fundus, the most distensible. Beyond the incisura angularis the stomach gradually narrows into its thicker walled antrum. The incisura angularis is often a sharp notch on the lesser curvature which marks the approximate junction of the cranial two-thirds and caudal one-third of the stomach. The outlet of the stomach is formed by the annular condensed muscular pylorus which continues into the duodenum.

Curvatures

The left border of the stomach is formed by the lesser curvature which extends between the cardiac and pyloric sphincters.

*Wilhelm His (1863–1934) was Professor of Anatomy in Leipzig, Basel, Göttingen and Berlin.

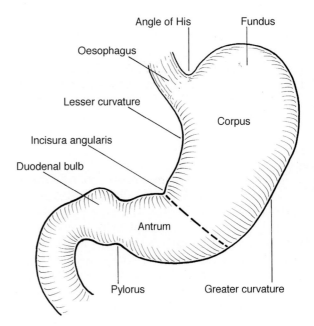

Figure 19.1
Anatomical regions of the stomach.

Along the lesser curvature runs the 'magenstrasse' (German: 'food road') of the stomach in which there is marked muscular condensation along its length. The greater curvature is directed along the right border of the stomach; it is distensible and 4–5 times the length of the lesser curvature. From the cardiac orifice of the stomach it sweeps as an arc backwards, superiorly and to the left, extending up to the fifth intercostal space at the level of the left nipple. It next sweeps downwards and forwards, again convexly, crossing the midline to end at the pylorus.

Orifices

The opening by which the oesophagus communicates with the stomach is the cardiac orifice. It is situated on the left of the median plane behind the seventh costal cartilage and at the level of the 11th thoracic vertebra. Its origin coincides with the lower end of the lower oesophageal sphincter and with an abrupt change in the mucosa from squamous to columnar. At the opening into the duodenum is the pyloric orifice, accurately marked by an external prepyloric vein on the serosa and by an internal heavy condensation of circular muscle forming the anatomical pyloric sphincter. This gateway to the duodenum is under a highly sophisticated system of neurological control, regulating food emptying and restricting undue duodenogastric reflux. The stomach has an anterior and a posterior surface lying between the curvatures, both freely mobile, and extending between the orifices, which themselves are fixed in position.

MACROSCOPIC STRUCTURE

The stomach is enclosed in a diaphanous layer of serosa or visceral peritoneum (Figure 19.2). This serosa is deficient only at the two curvatures, where it is continuous with the greater and lesser omenta on the respective curvatures, and at a point close to the cardiac orifice, where the stomach is contiguous with the undersurface of the diaphragm.

In view of its main function as an organ for the storage of food, the stomach has a thick muscular wall comprising three lattice-like layers of smooth muscle fibres: longitudinal, circular and oblique. The longitudinal fibres are the most superficial, continuing from the oesophagus along the whole length of the organ to the duodenum. They are best developed near the curvatures (particularly the lesser), and additional fibres originating in the body and antrum produce an antral condensation proximal to the pylorus. The middle, circular fibres encase the whole stomach, forming the thickest layer. These circular fibres are the most abundant distally and along the lesser curvature. With numerous interdigitations, however, they completely surround the whole stomach. The innermost layer of oblique fibres is thin, flimsy and in some areas deficient, as these fibres sweep down the organ, medially lying close to the lesser curvature and laterally lying almost horizontal. In contrast to the outer two layers, they are better developed proximally.

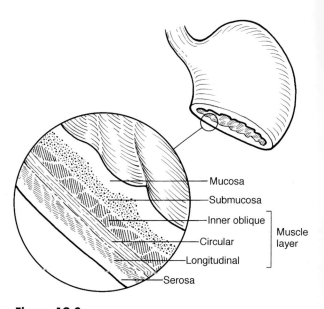

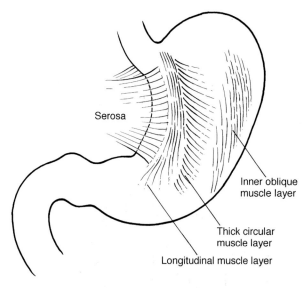

Figure 19.2
Peritoneal covering of the stomach.

Serosa

Inner oblique muscle layer

Thick circular muscle layer

Longitudinal muscle layer

Mucosa
Submucosa
Inner oblique
Circular
Longitudinal
Serosa
Muscle layer

Figure 19.3
Cross-section of mucosa and muscle layers at the level of the oesophagogastric junction.

The submucous coat consists of loose, areolar tissue, lying between and connecting the mucous and muscular layers.

The mucous membrane is a thick coat with a smooth velvety texture (Figure 19.3). Beginning abruptly at the oesophagogastric junction, in the upper part of the stomach it lies in numerous longitudinally disposed pink, glistening, tortuous folds or rugae, which diminish towards the antrum. Antral mucosa has a paler colour with fewer and less prominent rugae. When the stomach is distended, the folds tend to be obliterated. The mucosa is streaked with closely applied tenacious mucus (see Chapter 22).

ANATOMICAL RELATIONS

The cardiac end of the stomach is fixed to the diaphragm; the pylorus is attached, somewhat loosely, together with the duodenum and head of the pancreas to the posterior abdominal wall. The pylorus lies in the horizontal transpyloric plane, 2 cm to the right of the median plane and between the first and second lumbar vertebrae.

Anterosuperiorly to the stomach are the left lobe of the liver, which has a concave gastric impression, the diaphragm and the anterior abdominal wall. The diaphragm separates it from the left lung and pleura and the apex of the heart. Posteroinferiorly, the omental bursa intervening, is the 'stomach bed', formed by the crura of the diaphragm, the spleen, the left adrenal gland, the splenic vessels, the body and tail of the pancreas, the anterior surface of the left kidney, the left renal vein and artery, the splenic flexure of the colon, the fourth part of the duodenum and the proximal jejunum (Figure 19.4). Medially, the lesser curvature and lesser omentum are related to the undersurface of the left lobe of the liver. The omentum becomes attached to the liver, beneath which its free border surrounds the bile duct, hepatic artery and portal vein at the aditus to the lesser sac. Just behind the pylorus runs the common bile duct and the gastroduodenal artery, immediate

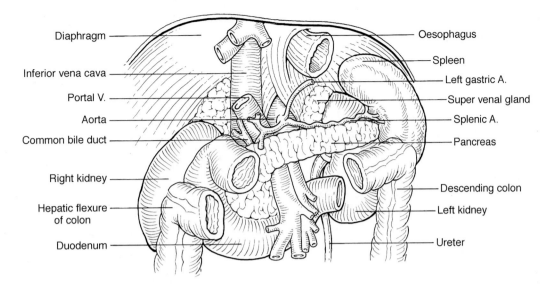

Figure 19.4
Anatomical relationship of organs and structures posterior to the body of the stomach.

posterior relations of which are the superior mesenteric and portal veins; behind these, in turn, runs the inferior vena cava.

The lesser omentum extends from the hepatic peritoneal attachments superiorly to the lesser curvature of the stomach inferomedially. In a slim subject the lesser omentum is extremely thin, flimsy and transparent; through it can be seen the body of the pancreas at the back of the lesser sac. The lesser omentum is permeated by vessels and lymphatics. Within the superior recess of the omental bursa lie the inferior vena cava and caudate lobe of the liver. From the greater curvature in an inferolateral direction extends the greater omentum – a large, mobile and dependent sheet of areolar and fatty tissue; its reflection runs over the transverse colon and on to the pancreas to form the inferior confines of the lesser sac. This omental bursa can be entered only through the foramen of Winslow (Jacob Benignus Winslow (1669–1760), a Danish anatomist who taught in Paris), the confines of which are: superiorly, the caudate lobe of the liver; posteriorly, the

inferior vena cava; inferiorly, the first part of the duodenum; and anteriorly, the portal vein, hepatic artery and common bile duct, which form its free border.

VASCULAR SUPPLY

The blood supply of the stomach is derived from four main arteries arising from the coeliac artery, which runs a short distance from the abdominal aorta before trifurcating into the left gastric, splenic and the common hepatic arteries. The next main arterial branch of the aorta is the superior mesenteric artery, which supplies the whole of the small and much of the large intestine; rarely the superior mesenteric artery arises in common with the coeliac trunk from the aorta (Figure 19.5).

About 50% of the rich gastric blood flow comes from the *left gastric artery*, the smallest branch of the coeliac trunk. This artery passes upwards and to the left behind the omental bursa, to the cardiac end of the stomach, where it gives off two

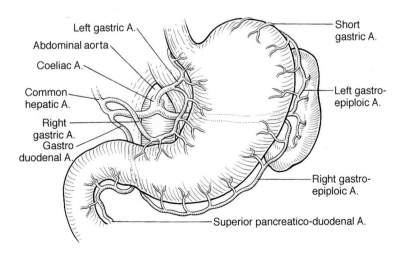

Figure 19.5
Arterial blood supply to the greater and lesser curves of the stomach.

or three oesophageal branches which ascend through the diaphramatic hiatus to anastomose with the oesophageal branches of the thoracic aorta. The artery then runs forwards and downwards along the lesser curvature of the stomach, to which it is closely applied, as far at least as the antrum. The artery gives off four to six branches which run subserosally along both the anterior and posterior walls of the stomach from the lesser curvature for a distance of 4–6 cm along the gastric walls. Here the vessels penetrate the muscular layers, ultimately to ramify widely in the mucosa, where arterioles provide blood along the core of the mucosal villi. At the level of the incisura angularis the left gastric artery anastomoses with the right gastric artery at a point where three or four closely applied branches run along the wall of the stomach to form the crow's foot.

The *right gastric artery* arises from the common hepatic artery above the superior portion of the first part of the duodenum; it runs within the lesser omentum to the pyloric end of the stomach. Passing along the lesser curvature, it gives off several branches to the anterior and posterior walls of the gastric antrum before it anastomoses with the left gastric artery.

The gastroduodenal artery has much clinical importance. Not only is it the vessel that bleeds as a result of deep penetration and erosion by a posterior duodenal ulcer, it also demarcates the posterior wall of the duodenal bulb during gastrectomy. It descends from the common hepatic artery between the superior part of the duodenum and the neck of the pancreas, lying close to a fixed line of peritoneal reflection from the posterior surface of the first centimetre of the duodenum. It normally lies behind and to the left of the common bile duct. At the inferior aspect of the first part of the duodenum it terminates by dividing into the right gastroepiploic and superior pancreaticoduodenal arteries. It supplies a number of small branches to the distal stomach and pancreas, which are easily damaged at gastrectomy. Occasionally this vessel arises from the superior mesenteric artery and more rarely from the right gastric artery.

The short gastric arteries supply the fundus of the stomach, arising from the splenic artery as it enters the lieno-renal ligament. These are delicate vessels which may be easily torn during vagotomy, repair of hiatus hernia, antireflux procedures or bariatric surgery.

The greater curvature of the stomach derives its blood supply from the right and left gastroepiploic arteries. The right gastroepiploic artery is the larger terminal branch of the gastro-duodenal artery. It skirts the right margin of the lesser sac and runs from right to left along the greater curvature of the stomach, giving off numerous small arcades to the stomach as it goes. These small branches run subserosally for a distance of 3–5 cm before penetrating the muscular layers and ultimately ramifying widely in the mucosa to anastomose with small branches of the other gastric vessels. It ends by anastomosing with the left gastroepiploic artery about two-thirds of the way down the greater curvature. The latter vessel arises from the splenic artery and runs along the greater curvature between peritoneal folds of the greater omentum, giving off gastric branches subserosally. The arcade formed by these epiploic vessels runs at a distance of about 2 cm from the greater curvature of the stomach. Thus all the blood supply of the stomach and the first part of the duodenum is derived from the coeliac axis, though vessels do anastomose with branches of the superior mesenteric artery, chiefly through the inferior pancreatico duodenal artery, its first branch.

The veins of the stomach accompany the arteries but ultimately drain into the portal and splenic veins. The splenic vein joins the superior mesenteric to form the portal vein at the neck of pancreas. Systemic veins draining the lower one-third of the oesophagus have collateral channels in the submucosal plexus at the gastro-oesophageal junction that communicate with the submucosal veins of the portal venous system draining the stomach. These are the veins that become widely dilated and varicose in portal hypertension.

LYMPHATIC DRAINAGE

The stomach has a rich lymphatic system. From a syncytium of tiny anastomosing lymphatics in the mucosa, the abundant lymph channels run with the blood vessels penetrating the muscular layers of the stomach. These channels drain into lymph nodes close to the curvatures of the stomach, usually within 3 cm – these are referred to as 'N$_1$ nodes'. Those in the region of the cardia communicate with channels from the oesophagus. The superior gastric nodes follow the vessels of the upper two-thirds of the lesser curvature along the left gastric artery. Those along the lower stomach drain into the hepatic and pyloric nodes. Vessels from the greater curvature run around the tail of the pancreas and close to the hilum of the spleen. Nodes more than 3 cm from the stomach are referred to as 'N$_2$ nodes', whereas those that lie along the posterior abdominal wall and para-aortic regions are called 'N$_3$ nodes'. Ultimately, gastric lymph drains into the thoracic duct together with the lymphatic plexus from the oesophagus, pancreas and duodenum.

INNERVATION

The stomach derives its innervation from the autonomic fibres of the vagus nerve (parasympathetic) and from some sympathetic nerves.

The vagus nerve is composed of motor and sensory fibres and has an extensive course and distribution through the neck, thorax and greater part of the abdomen. Cephalically the fibres of the vagus nerve are connected to three nuclei in the medulla oblongata. The dorsal nucleus is a mixed nucleus representing the fused general visceral efferent and visceral afferent columns. It lies in the central grey matter of the lower, closed part of the medulla oblongata. Efferent fibres are distributed to the involuntary muscle of the bronchi, heart, oesophagus and stomach and to the whole of the small intestine and proximal large intestine as far as the distal transverse colon. Lower down, the nucleus ambiguus gives origin to the efferent nerves that supply striated muscle. The lower part of the nucleus of the tractus solitarius receives those vagal fibres that are distributed through the internal laryngeal nerve, from the tongue, tonsil, palate and pharynx.

The rootlets of the nerve unite to form a flat cord, which passes below the flocculus of the cerebellum to the jugular foramen, through which it leaves the cranium. The nerve gives rise to a superior and an inferior ganglion, beyond which it passes vertically down in the neck between the internal jugular vein and internal carotid artery as far as the thyroid cartilage. The right nerve then continues through the thorax, giving off bronchial branches and uniting with filaments from the second third and fourth thoracic sympathetic ganglia to form the right posterior pulmonary plexus. This nerve next passes on to the oesophagus, forming part of the oesophageal plexus. The left nerve follows a similar course through the left side of the mediastinimum. Having given off the posterior bronchial branches, it receives filaments from the second, third and fourth thoracic sympathetic ganglia, which together form the left posterior pulmonary plexus. From this plexus branches run on to the oesophagus, where they form the anterior part of the oesophageal plexus. From the oesophageal plexus the anterior and posterior vagal trunks are formed, and these enter the abdomen through the oesophageal diaphragmatic hiatus (Figure 19.6)

The distribution of these nerves below the diaphragm frequently varies but, in general, the left vagus runs anteriorly and the right posteriorly. These nerves supply the gut with its parasympathetic innervation as far as the distal transverse colon, beyond which the parasympathetic supply is derived from the second, third and fourth sacral roots by way of the inferior mesenteric plexus.

Preganglionic sympathetic nerve fibres reach the coeliac and other preaortic ganglia through the thoracic splanchnic nerves arising between T5 and T12. From ganglia in the coeliac plexus, postganglionic fibres are distributed along the blood vessels to the gastric musculature and other viscera.

Some 90% of vagal fibres are afferent and, in addition, afferent sympathetic fibres from the stomach and small intestine pass through the coeliac and the thoracic splanchnic nerves.

The anterior vagus nerve enters the diaphragmatic hiatus closely applied to the lower 2.5 cm of oesophagus and beneath the peritoneum which is reflected from the lesser omentum, in front of the oesophagus and up on to the undersurface of the diaphragm. A single stout vagal trunk usually exists at this level, continuing vertically downwards to the oesophagogastric junction, where it spreads out in a spatulate configuration. Less commonly, two, three or even more anterior vagal trunks exist, always closely applied to the anterior oesophageal wall, or even embedded in its outer layer of longitudinal muscle fibres.

The spatulate expansion of vagal fibres gives off branches which, to the left, run across the oesophagogastric junction within a consistently placed fatty bundle surrounded by areolar tissue; those fibres to the right give off the hepatic branches. The hepatic branches of the anterior vagus are easily seen in a thin subject as they sweep across the lesser omentum underneath the left lobe of the liver to approach the porta hepatis. The main anterior vagus nerve then continues as the anterior nerve of Latarjet, superficially situated beneath the anterior peritoneal layer of the lesser omentum. It courses parallel to the edge of the lesser curvature. As it runs down the stomach it gives off numerous fine branches which run along the anterior gastric wall adherent to the undersurface of the serosa. These branches have no particular predilection to run with vessels along the wall of the stomach, and they rarely branch before penetrating the muscularis and ultimately ramifying widely within the gastric mucosa. The gastric branches of the nerve of Latarjet run superficial to the vessels along the lesser curvature.

The nerve of Latarjet commonly bifurcates or even trifurcates along its course down the stomach, often at quite a high level on the proximal stomach. The anterior nerve continues down to the antrum and pylorus, which it supplies, and an additional branch may run from the hepatic branches around the distal stomach and superficial to the gastroepiploic vessels to innervate the greater curvature. An additional branch which passes to the greater curvature is the so-called 'criminal nerve of Grassi' which branches high up from the anterior vagal trunk at the oesophageal level and extends across to the fundus, which it innervates. Failure to divide the latter two vagal branches is a cause of incomplete vagotomy of the parietal area of the stomach.

The terminal ramifications of the hepatic branches of the anterior vagus run down to innervate the proximal duodenum, gallbladder and part of the head of the pancreas.

The posterior vagus nerve trunk is usually thicker than the anterior nerve and runs at a distance of about 1 cm posterior to the oesophagus, buried in some loose areolar tissue. Sometimes more than one posterior trunk is present, and the nerve may be concealed behind the upper part of the right side of the diaphragm. At the level of the oesophagogastric junction the nerve gives off the large coeliac branches which run directly to the coeliac plexus of nerves. The continuation of the nerve approaches the stomach to become closely applied to the point at which the left gastric artery approaches the lesser curvature. The nerve then continues as the posterior nerve of Latarjet. It has a distribution along the posterior wall of the stomach that is a mirror image of the distribution of the

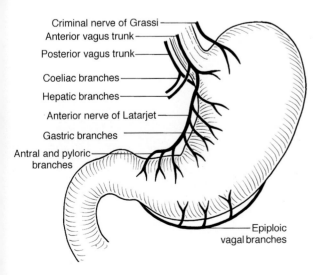

Figure 19.6
Innervation of the stomach.

anterior nerve along the anterior wall. The posterior nerve of Latarjet, however, does not always run along the whole length of the stomach, sometimes stopping at the proximal antrum or a little more distally. Like the anterior nerve, the posterior nerve of Latarjet may bifurcate or trifurcate at any level along the proximal or mid-stomach. The relationship to blood vessels borne by the gastric branches of the posterior nerve of Latarjet is identical to that of the anterior nerves.

The coeliac branches of the posterior vagus extend widely to innervate the small bowel, pancreas and proximal large bowel as far as the distal transverse colon.

The sympathetic innervation of the stomach comes from the thoracic splanchnic nerves. Preganglionic sympathetic nerve fibres run in the greater (T5–T9) and lesser (T10–T12) splanchnic nerves to reach the coeliac and other preaortic ganglia. The sensory gastric nerves pass through the coeliac and superior mesenteric plexuses and along the dorsal roots to the spinal cord. These sensory nerves are capable of reacting to stretch, ischaemia and chemical change.

MICROSCOPIC ANATOMY

In common with the rest of the alimentary tract, the stomach has four main layers or coats.

The serosa or visceral peritoneum comprises a single layer of mesothelial cells resting on a layer of loose areolar connective tissue. The three muscular layers, already described above, are separate layers of smooth muscle, the thickest of which is the circular muscle; this has its greatest concentration along the lesser curvature, and in the antrum and lower corpus. The layers are interconnected by transitional fascicles. The smooth muscle fibres are made up of discrete spindle-shaped cells. The pylorus is an anatomical sphincter at the gastric outlet consisting of a marked condensation of circular smooth muscle.

The gastric mucosa begins abruptly at the oesophagogastric junction, where the stratified squamous epithelium with underlying mucous cells changes to columnar epithelium. The mucosa of the fundus and body of the stomach contains the

acid-secreting or oxyntic cells and the chief cells, which secrete pepsin. In addition, mucous cells are present in this part of the stomach. The mucosal change at the oesophagogastric junction is easily apparent, the columnar mucosa being pinker and thicker and also being formed by numerous villous projections (between which lie deep crypts). Glands in the cardiac area of the stomach are few; some are tubular and some compound, racemose in type. Mucus-secreting glands and oxyntic and zymogenic cells are also sparse. The glands in the fundus and body are much more numerous and are simple tubular glands, two or more opening into a single duct, which is very short. The chief cells are small cuboidal cells containing coarse granules of pepsinogen. Oxyntic cells are larger and lie between the chief cells and the basement membrane. They are connected with the lumen of the gland by fine channels that pass between the chief cells. They are relatively sparse, protruding into the ducts in a beaded pattern, and are most numerous at the base of the ducts; they stain deeply with eosin. The antrum contains numerous gastrin-secreting or 'G' cells lying deep within the gastric pits and can be demonstrated by their ability to take up an immunofluorescent dye. Also in the antrum are mucous cells, which are indistinguishable from the goblet cells of the large intestine. In addition, there are a few argentaffin cells which take up silver stain when exposed to silver nitrate in the absence of a reducing agent.

The pyloric glands consist of two or three short convoluted tubes opening into a funnel-shaped duct, which occupies about two-thirds of the depth of the mucous membrane. Towards the outlet of the stomach epithelial cells are predominantly mucous in type, oxyntic cells being present but very sparse. A dense framework of connective and lymphoid tissue lies between the glands. The lymphoid tissue is collected into tiny masses which resemble the minute follicles of the intestine and are referred to as gastric lymphatic follicles. Deep to the glands of the mucous membrane is a thin stratum of involuntary muscle fibres, the muscularis mucosae; it consists of an inner circular and outer longitudinal layer. The circular fibres extend in strands between the glands, which empty in response to muscular contraction.

20

SECRETORY PHYSIOLOGY

MJ Hobsley

GASTRIC SECRETORY PHYSIOLOGY

Structure of gastric mucosa

The surface area of the gastric epithelium is greatly increased by repetitive folding: at the macroscopic level by the gastric rugae, then the invaginations called crypts which branch into about four gastric glands, and finally within the oxyntic cells themselves (see below). Altogether, the apparent surface area of the gastric epithelium is probably magnified several hundredfold. The surface epithelial cells secrete mucus and are ubiquitous within the stomach on the surface, i.e. in those parts of the stomach in direct contact with food; they also penetrate a short distance down the crypts (neck cells). The secretion of acid and enzymes takes place within the gastric glands: the acid from the parietal or oxyntic cells, the enzymes from chief cells. However, there are no parietal cells in and no acid secreted by the pyloric antral region of the stomach, roughly that part distal to the incisura or notch two-thirds of the way along the lesser curvature of the stomach. The boundary between body and antral regions is often indistinct in an individual, and very variable in its position in different individuals.

The oxyntic (parietal) cell

The word parietal means 'situated in the wall', and is therefore less apt than oxyntic, which means 'acid secreting'. Oxyntic cells bulge away from the lumen of the gastric glands[1] and are distributed particularly in the upper reaches of the glands. They are formed from progenitor cells in the neck region and travel gradually down the glands as they age.[2-4] It takes at least a year in the human to turn over the oxyntic cell population.[5] Oxyntic cells cannot divide; they cannot synthesize DNA.

In the resting cell, not much of the apical membrane directly abuts onto the lumen but a few secretory canaliculi invaginate the cell surface. There are many tubules or vesicles in the apical area and the cell abounds with large mitochondria, evidence of the excessive metabolic demands made when the cell is active.

When oxyntic cells are stimulated to secrete, the secretory canaliculi enlarge dramatically,[6] the apical membrane becomes greatly expanded and its microvilli lengthen considerably; there is in all a tenfold increase in surface area, made available by the diminution in size of the tubules and vesicles.[7-9] The tubules and vesicles do not seem to be in continuity, either functional or morphological, with the apical membrane when the cell is resting,[10,11] but continuity can be demonstrated when the cell has been stimulated[10,12] (Figure 20.1). Secretion of hydrochloric acid is dependent on these prior morphological changes, although the morphological changes can be induced without necessarily producing secretion.[9,13,14]

The oxyntic cells also secrete intrinsic factor (see later).

The chief cell

The chief cells constitute the majority of the cells lining the gastric glands of the body, and lie particularly in the basal regions of the glands, while the oxyntic cells lie nearer the surface of the stomach. Chief cells are responsible for most of the pepsinogen secreted by the stomach, although there is some pepsinogen in the glands of the fundic and pyloric regions, which contain no chief cells. Brunner's glands of the first half of the duodenum also contain pepsinogen, as do the mucous neck cells of the glands of the body. In normal mucosa, chief cells retain the ability to synthesize DNA and can replicate; however, in gastric mucosa regenerating after injury they can be produced by differentiation of immature neck cells.[15,16]

Pepsinogen is an inactive proenzyme, converted to the active enzyme pepsin by the acidity of gastric juice.[17,18] Below pH 6.5, pepsinogen itself is activated, and by a process of autocatalysis causes the breakdown of pepsinogen (c. 42 500 Da) to pepsin (c. 35 000 Da)[19,20] Pepsinogen is synthesized in the endoplasmic reticulum near the base of the cell and stored in concentrated form in secretory granules. When the gland is stimulated to secrete, pepsinogen is released from the granules and passes through the apical surface into the lumen.

Pepsinogen is not a single substance but a group that can be separated into at least seven components, Pg 1–7, by electrophoresis.[21-23] However, antigenically they can be divided into two groups, pepsinogen I and II (PG–I, PG–II) which respectively contain Pg 1–5 and Pg 6–7. The fundic glands contain both PG–I and PG–II, but the other gastroduodenal sites at which pepsinogen is found contain only PG–II.[24,25]

Pepsin is a proteolytic enzyme, with a pH optimum that

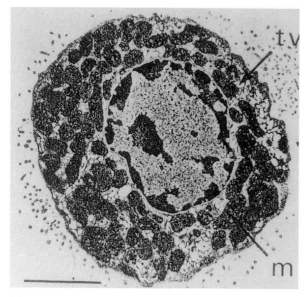

(a)

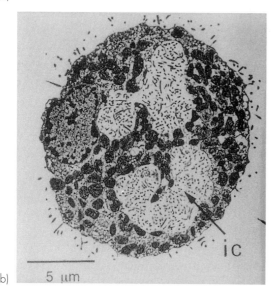

(b)   5 μm

Figure 20.1

(a) Isolated rat parietal cell in the resting state. The canalicular membrane is stored within the cytoplasm in the form of tubulovesicles (tv). Mitochondria (m) are abundant. (b) Rat parietal cell in the stimulated state. The canalicular membrane has now become much more prominent as the intracellular canaliculus (ic). (Reproduced from Lewin MJM. In Mignon M & Galmiche JP (eds) *Safe and Effective Control of Acid Secretion.* London: John Libbey, 1988: 5.)

varies with the substrate but is always acid (1.5–5.5).[22] It becomes denatured at alkaline pH and is therefore destroyed when it reaches the small intestine. Human pepsins are of the type known as endopeptidases: they attack several peptide linkings within the molecule but very few at the ends, so that peptides but not amino acids are formed.

Mucus-secreting cells

The cells secreting mucus line the whole length of the alimentary tract, including the salivary glands, pancreas and biliary

tract. In the stomach, the surface epithelial cells line the luminal surface, and they penetrate some distance into the crypts as the neck cells. The gastric mucus-secreting cells[26,27] are basically simple columnar epithelial cells in form; they contain a Golgi complex that is usually large and elaborate, with about ten membrane cisternae, and numerous vesicles and secretory granules in the cytoplasm. The rough endoplasmic reticulum is prominent and is concentrated in the basal and lateral cytoplasm. Mucin granules are stored immediately deep to the apical membrane.

Mucus occurs in three different sites: within the cells in the secretory granules; on the surface of the stomach wall as a tenacious insoluble gel; and within the lumen as a solution mixed with the other gastric contents. It would appear that the soluble form lubricates the passage of food and that the insoluble coat forms a protective layer to prevent the stomach from destroying itself by the proteolytic action of acid–pepsin (see Chapter 21).

Nine-tenths of mucus is water, containing electrolytes in similar concentrations to those in plasma. The main organic constituents are glycoproteins of very large molecular weights (exceeding 10^6 Da). These large molecules are slowly broken down by proteolysis to produce the soluble form. Synthesis of the protein core takes place in the rough endoplasmic reticulum of the oligosaccharide side-chains in the Golgi complex.[28,29]

Mucus-secreting cells proliferate by mitotic activity in the region of the neck of the crypt, and the new cells migrate up into the surface of the stomach wall. As they migrate, they gradually lose their ability to proliferate. The turnover rate of mucus-secreting cells is rapid: the whole gastric surface is replaced within 6 days.

G cells and other endocrine cells

The realization that the gut was an endocrinological organ stems from the discovery of secretin at the beginning of this century (p. 301). At first the evidence was basically morphological – the description that diffusely situated over the whole body were a family of specialized clear cells with particular staining characteristics with silver salts and close relationship to nerve endings – but it was Pearse[30] who added a functional common denominator when he realized their common property of processing amines to produce hormones (*a*mine *p*recursor *u*ptake and *d*ecarboxylation giving rise to the acronym APUD). Pearse's suggestion that all the APUD cells arose from the neural crest of the embryo has been confirmed for many but it is probably not true for the endocrine cells of the gut and pancreas. The close relationship between endocrine and nerve cells is emphasized by the fine structure of endocrine cells which contain granular vacuoles that resemble neurosecretor and synaptic vesicles, and by their production of neurosecretor and neurotransmitter-like substances.[31]

Endocrine cells are distributed throughout the gut and its related organs, but are concentrated more densely in certain areas, such as the gastric antrum. Some connect with the intestinal lumen via microvilli, which are thought to function as receptors, but others lie deeper, near the basement membrane.

Some have projections of cytoplasm that seem to bring them into close contact with neighbouring cells, an arrangement that has suggested that some of the effects of the agents secreted are exerted by local action rather than after diffuse carriage in the circulation – the concept of paracrine rather than endocrine action. These gut endocrine cells also contain electron-dense secretory granules in which the peptides they produce are stored.

A large number of empirical stains are used to demonstrate peptide-producing endocrine cells, but the most frequently used involve silver salts. The argentaffin reaction describes the ability of the cell to extract silver ions from the reagent and reduce them to metallic silver; the argyrophil reaction consists of a similar extraction of the silver ions, but the reduction to visible metallic silver requires a further reagent. However, the identification and categorization of the cells have been transformed by the use of immunocytochemistry. There are antibodies available for a number of general neuroendocrine markers, including neurone-specific enolase, the protein chromogranin and the so-called protein gene product 9.5, and of these markers it appears that chromogranin can be identified in the secretory granules of all cells of the diffuse neuroendocrine system.[32,33] There are also antibodies available not only to the specific peptides secreted but also to their precursor forms, so that it has become possible in certain cases to determine the topographical pathways of the elaboration of the hormone within the cell.[34]

G cells, the gastrin-secreting cell of the mucosa of the gastric antrum, are pear shaped, contain much cytoplasm (which is faintly granular and eosinophilic) and have a large round clear nucleus. They contain the typical secretory granules, and in many cells the ultrastructure of these is sufficiently typical as to allow the deduction that they contain gastrin. The first demonstration that the G cell is the source of (most) gastrin was by McGuigan.[35] The densest distribution of the antral G cells is in the area of the junction between the mucous neck cells and the mucoid cells of the antral mucosa and half way down the glands. The cells are usually in contact both with the basal membrane and with the lumen of the glands via microvilli.

Somatostatin (D) cells occur throughout the whole length of the gastrointestinal tract, and immunochemical methods have demonstrated somatostatin both in the D cells and in the nerves of the gut. A typical D cell has a pole that reaches the lumen and a basal cytoplasmic elongation in which transport of secretory granules has been demonstrated,[36] and the secretory granules are large (Figure 20.2).

Other gut endocrine cells, with their initial identifiers, secretory agents and zones of distribution, are given in Table 20.1. For more information on those produced mainly in the duodenum, see pp 309–311. The table includes some peptide messengers that seem only to be produced in neurones: they are included because they have important distributions in the enteric nerves and may have physiological functions related to the alimentary tract. The list is by no means exhaustive.

For completeness it should be mentioned that there are large numbers of gut endocrine cells that produce amines

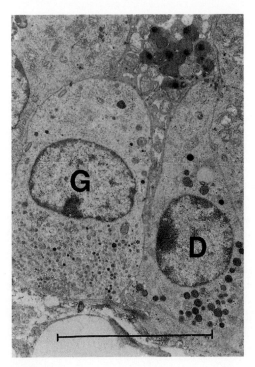

Figure 20.2

Gastrin-containing cell (G) with electron lucent and electron dense secretory granules in the basal half of the cell, and a somatostatin-containing cell (D) with larger electron dense granules. Bar=5 μm. (Reproduced with permission from Polak J. In *Handbook of Physiology*, sect. 6: The Gastrointestinal System, vol. iii: Neural and Endocrine Biology. Bethesda, MD: American Physiological Society, 1968: 77–87.

Table 20.1   Gut hormones (other than gastrin and somatostatin)

HORMONE	CELL	DISTRIBUTION	CHARACTERISTICS
Motilin	M	Duodenum, jejunum	Increases gastric motility
Secretin	S	**Duodenum,** jejunum	See p. 310
Gastric inhibitory polypeptide	K	**Duodenum,** jejunum	See p. 311
Cholecystokinin/ pancreozymin	I	Duodenum, jejunum, enteric nerves	See p. 310
Glucagon	A	Pancreas, gastric fundic A cells	Carbohydrate metabolism
Glicentin (enteroglucagon)	GLI	Ileum, large bowel, also in gastric A cells	Probably gut motility
Insulin		Pancreatic islet cells	Carbohydrate metabolism
Pancreatic polypeptide family: neuropeptide Y, peptide YY	PP	Pancreatic islet and exocrine tissue, colon	Uncertain
Vasoactive intestinal peptide		Neurones only, **gut,** CNS, urogenital tract	Vagal neurotransmission plus hormonal vasodilatation
Neurotensin		Neurones everywhere	Gut motility and blood flow +, etc.
Calcitonin gene related peptide		Neurones everywhere, **spinal cord, thyroid**	Unknown

rather than peptides as their hormonal products – the enterochromaffin cells with serotonin, the enterochromaffin-like cells that produce histamine.

Mechanism of secretion: acid

We are here concerned with the cellular mechanisms that result in the secretion by the oxyntic cell of hydrochloric acid-containing gastric juice, and with the electrolyte composition of the end-product.

Overview of cellular mechanisms

Recent technical advances using enzymatic digestion with collagenase have made it possible to isolate from gastric mucosa preparations of whole gastric glands,[37] of purified concentrates of individual cells such as the oxyntic cell,[38] and of subcellular elements of particular cells, e.g. microsomes.[39] Together with various indirect methods for measuring the secretion of acid[40-44] (these are necessary because when the cell secretes acid at the apical aspect it is also secreting bicarbonate ions at the base and neutralization rapidly occurs), these techniques have demonstrated the following scheme (Figure 20.3):

1. There are fundamental roles for ATP and the potassium ion. If the plasma membrane of oxyntic cells is made permeable by saponin, then the addition of ATP to the cell suspension

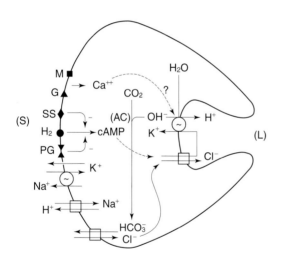

Figure 20.3

Mechanisms of gastric acid secretion: (L) is the luminal aspect, (S) the serosal aspect of the parietal cell. The H^+, K^+-ATPase pump (~) secretes H^+ into the lumen in exchange for K^+ which has reached the lumen in association with Cl^-. The OH^- ion split off the H^+ produces HCO_3^- (with the help of carbonic anhydrase, AC) and the HCO_3^- is expelled from the base of cell in exchange for Cl^-. The basement membrane includes a Na^+/H^+ exchanger and a Na^+, K^+-ATPase pump. M, muscarinic type (M_2) acetyl choline receptor; G, gastrin receptor; SS, somatostatin receptor; H_2, histamine H_2 receptor; PG, prostaglandin E_2 receptor. The second messengers with cAMP and Ca^{2+} are indicated. Note the inhibitory effects of somatostatin and prostaglandin E_2 on the production of cAMP. (Reproduced from Lewin MJM. In Mignon M & Galmiche JP (eds) Safe and Effective Control of Acid Secretion. London: John Libbey, 1988: 10.

stimulates the cells to secrete acid, but only if there are also K^+ ions present.[45]

2. The enzyme that produces the hydrogen ions from water, the 'gastric proton pump', is the H^+, K^+-ATPase, unique to the oxyntic cell and situated on the secretory membrane with a molecule of about 100 000 Da.[39,46-48]

3. Since hydrogen ion is excreted into the gastric lumen in exchange for a potassium ion, acid secretion depends on the presence of K^+ in the lumen and therefore on the prior secretion of K^+ into the lumen. While the mechanism for this prior K^+ secretion is unclear, it seems likely that it is linked to Cl^- secretion[49] and dependent on cyclic AMP (cAMP).[13]

4. There are numerous receptors sited at the basal membrane, each receptor being specific for one of the chemical agents that can affect the production of gastric acid. When the reagent triggers the receptor, a second messenger is produced that travels through the cell to the secretory locus. Oxyntic cell receptors fall into two groups according to whether they use calcium ions or cAMP as the second messenger. The first group includes the receptors for gastrin[50,51] and acetylcholine (the latter appears to be of the muscarinic M_2 type).[52-54] The second group, using cAMP, includes the histamine H_2 receptor,[43,55,56] somatostatin and prostaglandin E_2. The histamine H_2 receptor is positively coupled to adenylate cyclase and therefore when stimulated it increases cAMP production and so increases acid secretion,[57] while the somatostatin[58] and prostaglandin E_2 receptors are negatively coupled to adenylate cyclase and therefore act as inhibitors of gastric acid secretion.

5. The effects of agents that inhibit gastric secretion can be related to this scheme. Omeprazole inhibits the proton pump; somatostatin and prostaglandin analogues inhibit the H_2 receptor, but non-competitively and therefore only partially; while the H_2 antagonists such as cimetidine and ranitidine act competitively and therefore much more effectively. Pirenzepine, an M_1-muscarinic receptor, probably acts presynaptically because the local acetylcholine receptor is of the M_2 type.

6. At the basolateral membrane there are also HCO_3^-–Cl^- and Na^+–K^+ exchangers to complete the round of ionic transfers.

Electrolyte composition of gastric secretion

The quantitative assessment of human gastric acid secretion can yield helpful diagnostic and therapeutic information about patients with diseases of the upper gastrointestinal tract (see Chapter 21), but the maximum value can only be derived from such studies by taking into account some mathematical considerations in relation to the electrolyte concentrations in human gastric juice. The rest of this section applies only to human gastric juice.

Gastric secretion is not pure hydrochloric acid. All samples, whether basal or resulting from stimulation with various agonists in varying doses, contain potassium in the range 12–20 mmol/l. This is an interesting fact because the hydrogen ions in gastric juice are now known to result from their secretion in exchange for potassium that was already in the lumen (see previous section). When secretion is maximally stimulated, the juice is isotonic with plasma, after taking into account the space-occupying effect of the plasma proteins (Table 20.2). Raising the osmolality of the extracellular space with intravenous hypertonic sodium chloride produces a small depression of histamine-stimulated secretion, suggesting that solvent drag has an effect on the secretion process. However, alkalinizing the extracellular space with hypertonic sodium bicarbonate produces a much greater inhibitory effect (unpublished observations), presumably because the K^+, H^+-ATPase pump cannot cope with the accentuation of the already large hydrogen ion gradient between the extracellular space (which ultimately provides the bulk of the gastric juice; 40 nmol/l) and the juice itself (140 mmol/l).

In the circumstances of maximal gastric secretion, there is considerable evidence that the output of hydrogen ions is proportional to the number of oxyntic cells in the individual stomach, whether the relationship is explored in terms of actual cell counts[59] or of postulated correlates such as height, weight, lean body mass or total body potassium.[60] This fact suggests that, at least when maximally stimulated, each oxyntic cell produces a secretion containing the same concentration of hydrogen ion, and at the same rate.

At lower rates of secretion, the concentrations of hydrogen and chloride ions fall progressively as rate diminishes, the concentration of sodium rises, and the concentration of potassium remains constant. Until very low rates of water output are reached (approaching the basal level), however, there is a

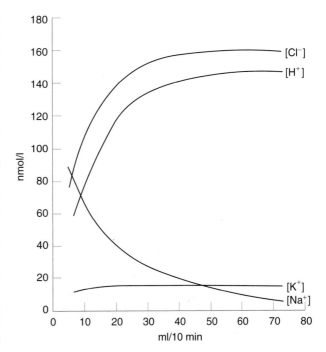

Figure 20.4
Relationship between rate of secretion of gastric juice and electrolyte concentrations. The curves are the smoothed results from over 1600 secretion studies in the author's files.

linear relationship between electrolyte outputs and volume rates of secretion (Figure 20.4). Over a very wide range of secretion rate, therefore, it appears that alterations in volume output reflect alterations in the rate of secretion of a gastric juice of constant electrolyte composition. Table 20.2 gives the details of this composition.

As the volume rate diminishes and the sodium ion concentration increases, the hydrogen ion concentration falls more quickly than the chloride ion concentration. These observations have suggested that some alkalinizing agent is present to a roughly constant effect over the whole range. There are two main theories about the nature of the alkalinizing tendency: back-diffusion (Teorell)[61] and two-component (Hollander).[62]

The back-diffusion theory suggests that after a pure solution of hydrochloric acid has been secreted, diffusion of hydrogen ions back into the mucosa takes place in exchange for bicarbonate ions. The two-component hypothesis postulates the existence of an alkaline component of gastric juice, secreted at a constant volume rate and with constant concentrations of its electrolytes, sodium, chloride and bicarbonate.

From most viewpoints, these two theories turn out to be mathematically identical in their effects on gastric juice, but the two-component theory is easier to visualize. Table 20.2 presents the available information on alkaline component. It has, however, been pointed out that occasional samples of gastric juice, obtained under maximal stimulation, exhibit the ionic concentrations of the hypothetical pure acid component of gastric juice.[63] This finding suggests that alkaline component and/or back-diffusion are not essential phenomena and could be common, but not ubiquitous, associations.

Table 20.2 Electrolyte concentrations of gastric price compared with plasma

Ion (mmol/l)	ACID COMPONENT (? PURE JUICE)	ALKALINE COMPONENT	PLASMA
H+	145	—	—
Na+	7	80	140
K+	17	17	4
Cl	170	92	90
HCO₃	—	8	25
Sum of ions (mmol/l)	339	197	259
Protein concentration (g/litre)	—	—	70
Sum of ions corrected for protein concentration (mmol/l)	339	—	364*

*This figure has been obtained by multiplying 259 by 1000/(1000 − 70) on the assumption that the specific gravity of plasma proteins approximates 1.0, and therefore that the volume of water in 1 litre of plasma is (1000 − 70) ml.

After allowing for plasma constituents of small molecular size and therefore significant osmotic contribution, e.g. urea, glucose, that do not appear in gastric juice it will appear that the acid component is practically isotonic.
From Gardham JRC & Hobsley M. *Clin Sci* 1970; **39:** 77.

One possible artefact is duodenogastric reflux, which with its ion mixture of mainly sodium chloride and sodium bicarbonate would constitute a suitable alkalinizing influence. There is evidence that reflux from beyond the pylorus can be quantified in terms of its sodium content, and the concept has grown of a duodenogastric reflux-corrected gastric juice, V_G[64] (and also of a pyloric loss-corrected gastric juice, using unabsorbable markers like phenol red, etc.). Swallowed saliva is another possible contender for apparent alkaline component, but so far no suitable marker has been found to enable its measurement in gastric juice. The use of V_G has enhanced the accuracy of conventional gastric secretion studies in a number of situations, including the correlation with stature and the effect of cigarette smoking,[65,66] the measurement of the adequacy of vagotomy[67] and the relationship of insulin- to histamine-stimulated secretion.[68]

Mechanism of secretion: pepsin

The basic pattern[17] is that a proenzyme, pepsinogen, is synthesized by the endoplasmic reticulum, concentrated and stored in secretory granules, and released into the lumen, where the low pH of the secreted hydrochloric acid converts pepsinogen into pepsin. The stimulators for pepsin release act at receptors located at the basolateral membrane.

There are several different receptors for stimuli on peptic cells. Acetylcholine stimulates pepsinogen secretion by chief cells, both in the intact animal[69] and in monolayer cultures.[70] Atropine inhibits the secretion, so muscarinic receptors are involved, but there is conflicting evidence as to whether they are of the M_1 type (strong inhibition by pirenzepine) or the M_2 type (weaker inhibition by pirenzepine). In the intact human, histamine undoubtedly seems to stimulate pepsinogen secretion,[69] but in models at the cellular level the link is much less clear cut; thiocyanate selectively inhibits acid[71] but not pepsinogen, while histamine stimulates acid but not pepsinogen. The explanation for these inconsistencies is unclear. There is a little evidence for β-adrenergic stimulation. Gastrin (and pentagastrin) certainly stimulates pepsinogen secretion in the intact animal, but since gastrin is inhibited by atropine[1] or H_2 antagonists,[72] one cannot be certain that it is acting directly on the chief cell. However, at the cellular level there is no doubt that cholecystokinin is a strong stimulator of pepsinogen secretion.[73] Secretin has been suggested to have a physiological role because in physiologically relevant concentrations it apparently stimulates pepsinogen secretion in the intact human.[74] Somatostatin inhibits pepsinogen secretion[75] resulting from many different stimuli.

The linkage between stimulus and secretion appears to involve at least two different pathways, one using cAMP as a mediator[71] and the other using calcium.[76] Adrenergic agents and secretin follow the first pathway, cholinergics and cholecystokinin peptides the second.

The release of pepsinogen is at least partly by the mechanism of exocytosis: the secretory granules disappear, fuse with the plasma membrane and with each other to form the so-called exocytotic figures, and are then released into the lumen.

However, it is likely that there is another release mechanism. When peptic stimulation commences there is a large release of pepsinogen first, with rapid depletion of the granules, but when that is complete there is a continued slower release[69] without the necessity, apparently, for the pepsinogen to be first organized into granules.

Mechanism of secretion: mucus

The main stimulatory pathway is cholinergic, acting via the vagus nerve or by the topical application of food or acetylcholine on the gastric mucous membrane.[77] Gastrin, cholecystokinin and secretin have all been implicated, but mostly only in animal experiments. However, secretin infusion in the human has been shown to produce an increase in the mucin content of gastric juice.[78]

Another important secretagogue of mucus is the prostaglandin family.[79] The most important seem to be the prostaglandin E-type analogues, and the action of the prostaglandins is both topical and intravenous. The prostaglandins stimulate an increase in mucus in the lumen, in the adherent gel (which increases in thickness) and in the rate of synthesis of mucin.

The protein core of mucin is elaborated on the rough endoplasmic reticulum while the oligosaccharide side-chains are synthesized in the Golgi complex. The mucin is concentrated and stored in tightly-packed granules beneath the apical membrane. In the absence of stimulation, granules are released intermittently from the apical surface and are replaced by new granules from the Golgi apparatus, the process being exocytotic.[27] When stimulated, the older cells expel a mass release of mucus. Finally, and rarely, mucus cells exfoliate.

Mechanism of secretion: intrinsic factor

Castle's intrinsic factor[80] a glycoprotein essential for the absorption of cyanocobalamin (vitamin B_{12}) in the terminal ileum, is made and secreted in the parietal cells of man and some animals, but in the peptic cells of others. The same agents that stimulate the parietal cell in man to secrete acid also stimulate the secretion of intrinsic factor. Vagotomy decreases intrinsic factor production, but omeprazole and atropine do not reduce it. Synthesis takes place in the rough endoplasmic reticulum, the IF is localized to the tubulovesicles and on stimulation there is rapid transfer to the microvilli and release. There are only small stores, so the secretion is short lived and has usually ceased by the time acid secretion is fully established.

VAGUS NERVE

Efferent connections

There are about 60 000 fibres in the vagus nerve below the diaphragm, and only 2000 of them are efferent.[81] They arise in the dorsal motor nucleus of the vagus nerve and the nucleus ambiguus and terminate in the millions of ganglia of the alimentary tract. After external denervation (vagotomy) there seems to be only a minor loss of gastric neurones[82] and often only a small or subtle loss of function. These are puzzling features of the enteric nervous system. Most of the ganglia can have no direct connection to the efferent fibres of the vagus.

Stimulation of the vagus results in the excitation of gastric secretion via the release of acetylcholine.[83] The effect is independent of the nature of the vagal stimulant, and is inhibited both by atropine and pirenzepine. Pepsin secretion is also stimulated by the vagus nerve via muscarinic pathways.

The effects of vagotomy are considered elsewhere (p. 474).

Afferent connections

The vast majority of the afferent vagal fibres in the abdominal vagal trunks probably carry signals concerned with the integration of the motor activity of the gut. However, there is good evidence that vagovagal long-loop reflexes are involved in the stimulation of gastric secretion, e.g. resulting from gastric distension[84] or hepatic glucose deprivation.[85] The central connection of these fibres is ultimately to the dorsal motor nucleus of the vagus nerve via the tractus solitarius and its nucleus.

Inhibitory factors

Among the efferent vagal fibres there are probably some that carry signals inhibiting gastric secretion. If appetite is suppressed by emotional factors or by suddenly ingesting food, then the appetite juice (see below, *Phases of Gastric Secretion and Physiological Regulation*) evoked by sham feeding is inhibited. There have been suggestions that the inhibitory fibres release a chemical, which has been named vagogastrone.[84]

GASTRIN

Gastrin stimulates gastric secretion by a hormonal mechanism, i.e. via the systemic venous blood. It acts synergistically with acetylcholine in central stimulation and is probably the principal or sole pathway for the stimulation of secretion by food.

Release of gastrin from the G cells in response to vagal excitation is dependent on the strength of the vagal signal.[85] The sole pathway for the vagal signal is via the antral fibres so that antral denervation abolishes the gastrin response.[86] On the other hand, if the antrum is left vagally innervated but the fundus denervated, the gastrin response to vagal stimulation is greatly increased.[87] It has been suggested that the fundus produces an inhibitor of gastrin release. Whatever the exact mechanism, it is a general truth that a high acid concentration in the antrum depresses the gastrin response to vagal stimulation, while a low acid concentration enhances it.

The vagus is not the only agent that stimulates gastrin release. The bombesin-like gastrin releasing peptide stimulates gastric acid and pepsin production via gastrin release: it is present in many neurones of the myenteric and mucosal plexuses. It appears that gastrin releasing peptide may be an important intermediary in the vagal release of gastrin, perhaps responsible for that part of the gastrin release that cannot be blocked with atropine.[88]

Finally, it should be pointed out that somatostatin inhibits gastrin release.

PHASES OF GASTRIC SECRETION AND PHYSIOLOGICAL REGULATION

An increase in the secretion of acid and pepsin is necessary in preparing for and digesting a meal, and it is important that at the end of the meal the secretory tap is turned off again. The physiological processes involved in regulation are many, complicated, delicate and beautifully balanced.

Basal secretion

Not all animals produce a basal secretion of acid and pepsin, but man does. Basal secretion is low in pepsin and in hydrogen ion and other electrolyte concentrations. It continues during sleep at the same rate as in the fasting awake subject. When trying to measure basal secretion in awake subjects it is necessary to allow a long time to ensure that the subject is properly at rest; secretion in the second half-hour is less than in the first half-hour.[89]

At the low rates of secretion in basal circumstances, measurements are particularly susceptible to errors produced by pyloric losses and duodenogastric reflux. Many statements in the literature made on the basis of studies in which such errors were not corrected are therefore suspect. Thus it is often claimed that basal secretion occurs as a result of vagal stimulation, but a complete surgical vagotomy does not abolish basal secretion, although it does usually reduce it to a minor extent. The true mechanism of basal secretion is unknown.[89]

Because of the small size of basal secretion, it is difficult to determine directly whether its magnitude is related to stature in the same way that maximal secretion is. Indirectly, however, it is likely that it is so related because there is a direct correlation between basal secretion and maximal secretion in individuals.[90]

Appetite juice (cephalic phase)

Gastric secretion is stimulated by the smell, sight and even thought of food. There is evidence that the last of these is the strongest stimulus. The response is reflex, as confirmed by Pavlov in his celebrated experiments on conditioned reflexes in dogs, and the effector arc is obliterated by vagotomy.[91] Twice as strong a stimulus of gastric secretion as the thought of food is sham feeding, i.e. the mouthing and mastication of food followed by its evacuation from the mouth without swallowing. Half as large again as the response to sham feeding is that to insulin-stimulated hypoglycaemia, a response that is also vagally mediated in that it is also abolished by vagotomy.[92] The effect of insulin is complex: at first it inhibits gastric secretion; only later does the stimulatory effect become manifest. For this reason, when insulin is injected intravenously to test the integrity of the vagal component of gastric juice stimulation, the 0.5–2 h period after the injection gives the most reproducible measure of vagal function.[93]

Low blood glucose itself is not the factor that stimulates the vagus, but rather glucose deprivation of cerebral tissue, a factor that can be achieved by injecting a non-metabolizable glucose analogue such as 2-deoxy-D-glucose. Such analogues produce a gastric secretory effect similar to that of insulin hypoglycaemia.

The fact that the vagal element of gastric secretory stimulation can be quantified by glucose deprivation does not mean that the normal stimulus for the secretion of appetite juice is hypoglycaemia. It is rare for blood glucose levels to fall to an extent that stimulates gastric secretion. Moreover, hunger (at least in dogs) cannot initiate appetite juice, nor can exogenous hyperglycaemia inhibit the secretory response to sham feeding.[94] The mechanism whereby olfactory, visual and cerebral stimuli produce vagal stimulation and hence the appetite juice remain entirely unknown.

Gastric phase

The gastric phase of gastric secretion refers to events that tend to increase gastric secretion once the food has reached the stomach. Almost the whole of the secretory response is due to the gastrin released from the G cells, each of which has one surface, covered with microvilli, that is exposed to the stomach lumen. The immediate stimulant to the G cell appears to be the mixture of peptones produced from protein in the food: the instillation of peptone solutions into the stomach in increasing doses produces corresponding stepwise elevations both of serum gastrin levels and of gastric secretion.[95] Although it seems clear that access to the cell is via its 'open' end, it is not known exactly what the chemical substances are that cause the cell to secrete or whether the final triggering occurs at the cell surface or in its interior. Luminal calcium ions and acetylcholine also stimulate the G cell, probably also via the same pathway.

Although this direct chemical action is the main route whereby food in the stomach stimulates gastric secretion, distension of the stomach has some effect, acting via vagal afferents and completion of the reflex arc, both directly via acetylcholine to the parietal cell and indirectly via gastrin release. The effect of distension is shown by the fact that non-nutrient solutions can produce a release of gastrin.[96]

The gastric phase of gastric secretion continues while food remains in the stomach to stimulate gastrin secretion, and is liable to continue to some extent even when the stomach has emptied the meal because of the so-called intestinal phase of gastric secretion. However, even during the gastric phase the seeds are being sewn that will stop gastric secretion (see below, *Inhibition of Gastric Secretion*).

A meal is as potent a stimulus of gastric hydrochloric acid secretion as is histamine or pentagastrin.[97]

Intestinal phase

Physiologists are divided nowadays as to whether one should refer to the time-hallowed concepts of appetite juice, gastric and intestinal as three separate phases of gastric secretion. For example, they point to the undoubted fact that central vagal stimulation results in gastrin release, and that any gastric secretory effect of chyme in the intestine is difficult to disentangle from the direct effect of any food that still remains in the stomach. With regard to the intestinal phase of gastric secretion, one is bound to say that the question of whether it exists at all is still open. Most of the evidence comes from research in animals, and there is conflicting evidence about whether the duodenum or the upper jejunum or both are involved, and about whether the mechanism is hormonal or neural.[98]

On the other hand, there is no doubt that there is an intestinal phase of inhibition of gastric secretion.

Inhibition of gastric secretion

This section is concerned with those agents and mechanisms that are known or strongly suspected to be involved in the physiological control of gastric secretion.

1. The cephalic phase is well named the appetite juice. Any environmental or emotional circumstance that reduces appetite also reduces or abolishes the appetite juice. Vagal inhibitory fibres and a 'vagogastrone' may be involved (p. 311). It has been suggested that somatostatin might fit the bill for vagogastrone: it is released during vagal stimulation by sham feeding[99] or insulin hypoglycaemia,[100] and inhibits all mechanisms of gastric secretion (see below).

2. The important inhibitory phenomenon of the gastric phase of gastric secretion is the effect of antral acidification. Acidifying the gastric content has been found to suppress the release of gastrin and the associated acid secretion,[101-103] with a meal, and with sham feeding.[104] The mechanism of this inhibition is unknown but candidates for the intermediary include somatostatin and the prostaglandins E.

3. While the first two phases of gastric secretion are mainly concerned with stimulation of the secretion, the intestinal phase is mainly concerned with stopping secretion. The stimuli triggering the inhibition of gastric secretion are the entry into the duodenum of acid, fat and hypertonic solutions; the mechanisms involved will be discussed below in the section on the duodenum.

Non-physiological inhibition

A host of stimuli and artificial situations are known or suspected to inhibit gastric secretion. They may be grouped as pharmacological, pathological and surgical and many of these factors or agents have been useful in elucidating the physiology of gastric secretion. One example has already been given, the hypoglycaemia-producing agents that mimic appetite juice. Other agents that are probably not involved in the normal physiological control of gastric secretion include epidermal growth factor, and various peptides such as calcitonin gene-related peptide, thyrotropin-releasing hormone and various opioids; some of these peptides act when injected into the brain. Gastritis reduces gastric secretion, possibly via the local release of interleukin-1, and infection of the antrum with *Helicobacter pylori* both destroys parietal cells and interferes with their ability to secrete acid. Surgeons perform vagotomy to destroy the appetite juice and this reduces pentagastrin- or histamine- or meal-stimulated gastric juice by a mechanism that is unclear, or else they reduce all types of gastric secretion by the removal of parietal cells in gastrectomy. Such non-physiological factors will find recognition in other chapters in this book.

PHYSIOLOGY OF THE DUODENUM

Duodenal secretions

The exocrine secretions of the duodenum are succus entericus and the secretions of Brunner's glands.

Succus entericus

This is the secretion derived from the intestinal glands lining the whole of the small intestine, including the duodenum. It is alkaline in reaction, with a pH of about 7.6, and in its electrolyte composition resembles a protein-poor plasma with a bicarbonate concentration of about 25 mmol/l and a sodium concentration of about 150 mmol/l but a potassium concentration of about 15 mmol/l, i.e. considerably higher than in plasma.[105] Little is known about its physiology because of the difficulty of collecting it separately from bile and pancreatic juices in the intact human, but indirect evidence suggests that it is produced at a rate in excess of 5 litres per 24 h and is mostly reabsorbed in the terminal ileum and in the colon. A very important constituent is enteropeptidase (enterokinase), an enzyme secreted from the membrane of the microvilli, and essential for the conversion of trypsinogen (the inactive precursor secreted by the pancreas) into trypsin, the form of the enzyme that is active in digesting protein.

Brunner's glands

The secretion of Brunner's glands is rich in mucus, alkaline, and serves a protective function in consequence of those properties. The control of secretion appears to be partly vagal and partly hormonal.

Bile and pancreatic secretions

The production of bile in the liver is a continuous process. The bile acid anions secreted into the canaliculi carry water with them by their osmotic force, and this constitutes the largest contribution to the volume of the bile;[106] however, some water also accompanies other solutes such as glutathione. Phospholipids and cholesterol are added to the bile by secretion from the canaliculi: the mechanism involved is unknown, but quantitatively related to the bile acids in the canaliculi. Small amounts of conjugates of fat-soluble substances such as bilirubin, vitamins and steroid hormones are secreted into the bile in the canaliculi; likewise, vesicles containing cholesterol and phospholipid. During the passage of the bile along the biliary tree, these vesicles become transformed by spontaneous physiochemical changes into the micelles[107] – the polarized nests of ions, each bearing both positive and negative charges, that form soluble complexes with calcium ions and are so important in fat absorption. Hepatic bile is modified by the addition of a bicarbonate-rich solution of electrolytes secreted by the hepatic and bile ducts. This modified bile is stored in the gall bladder, where it is concentrated by the absorption of sodium chloride and water through the activity of the mucosal cells of the gall bladder. Passage of the bile into the duodenum only occurs when the pressure in the biliary tree exceeds that exerted by the sphincter of Oddi. This happens when the limit of storage capacity in the system has been reached, or when the products of a meal enter the duodenum and stimulate contraction of the gall bladder.

Several mechanisms are involved. Vagal afferents from the duodenum stimulate an increased production of hepatic bile and an increased secretion of water and electrolytes, including bicarbonate, from the ductular cells. The hormone secretin is released from the S cells of the duodenal mucosa, and this also stimulates the duct cells to secrete bicarbonate. The hormone cholecystokinin/pancreozymin is also released from the appropriate duodenal cells and acts on the gall bladder to stimulate contraction.

There is argument about whether exocrine pancreatic secretion is produced under basal circumstances in man; if it is, the rate is very small. Stimulated secretion consists of enzymes and an aqueous solution of electrolytes. Food products in the duodenum act via vagal reflex arcs and via the release from the duodenal mucosa of the hormones secretin and cholecystokinin.[108] Secretin has its main effect on the stimulation of secretion of water and electrolytes, particularly bicarbonate; the vagus and cholecystokinin have almost no effect on water and electrolytes but stimulate the release of the pancreatic hormones amylase, lipase and trypsin.

In terms of acid–base balance, the electrolytes of stimulated pancreatic secretion are opposite in pattern to those of gastric secretion. Instead of the chloride of the anionic side of the electrolytes of gastric juice being constant in concentration over a wide range of secretion rates, and a shift in the balance between sodium and hydrogen ions increasing towards the dominance of acidity as the rate of secretion increases, in pancreatic juice it is the sodium (and potassium) concentrations that are relatively fixed; the anions chloride and bicarbonate vary reciprocally with bicarbonate, increasing as the rate of secretion rises. These contrasting patterns make for a delicate mechanism controlling the pH of the luminal contents of the duodenum. The more acidic the acid chyme reaching the duodenum, the greater the stimulus to the release of secretin and the more alkaline the pancreatic juice secreted. Thus the more acid the duodenal contents, the more rapidly are they first neutralized, then alkalinized so that the optimal pH for the action of the pancreatic enzymes is reached.

Hormonal factors

The duodenal mucosa contains a large number of species of physiologically active peptide hormones, many of which have already been mentioned. Their cells of origin have already been described (p. 302) but there will be some recapitulation here. This is a recent and rapidly expanding field, and any description is bound to become quickly out of date. Technical advances in the development of specific antibodies and histological staining techniques have permitted the parent cells to be identified, and the use of antibody assays has allowed the measurement of their concentrations in the circulation. It is important to appreciate that many of these peptides have not been assigned any physiological role, and that many act not as hormones (i.e. chemical messengers transmitted via the circulation to have their effects at distant sites) but as chalones (i.e. messengers that act by diffusion into neighbouring tissues only).

Secretin

Secretin, the first hormone to be discovered,[109] is a polypeptide composed of 27 amino acid residues and exists in only the one molecular form. In structure it resembles several other of the hormones of the gastrointestinal tract, e.g. gastric inhibitory polypeptide, glicentin, glucagon and vasoactive intestinal polypeptide (see below). The hormone is produced and stored in special S cells that lie deep in the mucosal glands of duodenum and jejunum.

The stimulus for the release of secretin is the presence in the duodenal lumen of acid and the products of the intragastric peptic breakdown of proteins. Secretin may have several target organs. There is no doubt that it acts on the duct cells of the pancreas, stimulating them to secrete an alkaline liquid rich in bicarbonate ions, and it is likely that it has a similar effect on the duct cells of the biliary tree. The mechanism involved in these actions appears to be via cAMP. It is also widely accepted that secretin is responsible for the inhibitory effect upon gastrin-stimulated (but not histamine-stimulated) gastric secretion that is known to be produced by the presence of acid in the duodenum. Thus secretin is usually thought of as an important element of the gastric inhibitory aspect of the intestinal phase of gastric secretion. However, no mechanism for such an action of secretin has been elucidated and there is no doubt that an apparent inhibitory effect of secretin on histamine-stimulated secretion has been shown to be due to duodenogastric reflux,[110] so that some workers doubt whether secretin is a physiological inhibitor of meal-stimulated gastric acid secretion.

Cholecystokinin/pancreozymin (CCK/PZ)

At first thought of as two separate hormones, it gradually became apparent that CCK and PZ were one and the same. Together with secretin, this is probably the most important of the duodenal/intestinal hormones. Like secretin, it has many important functions. Unlike secretin, it exists in several molecular forms called CCK-8, CCK-12, CCK-33, CCK-39 and CCK-58, where the number of each form refers to the number of amino acid residues. Each of these forms has a common terminal sequence of five amino acids, Gly-Trp-Met-Asp-Phe-NH$_2$), and it is not surprising that it shares many of its actions with gastrin, which has the same terminal segment.

The main cells of origin of CCK are in the duodenum and proximal small intestine, but it is also found in the brain and in the parasympathetic nerves to the distal small intestine and the large intestine. Under basal circumstances, the plasma contains all the molecular forms except CCK-8, which is thought to be the biologically active form. The stimuli to the release of CCK are the presence of acid[111] and of food products of digestion, fatty acids, peptides/peptones and amino acids within the lumen of the duodenum, and also distension of the gastric antrum. Recent evidence suggests that CCK is the all-important

link between gastric secretion and gastric emptying on the one hand, and bile and pancreatic secretion and delivery to the duodenum on the other.[112]

The actions of CCK affect not just the gall bladder and biliary duct system but also the pancreas. The gall bladder is stimulated to contract and the sphincter of Oddi to relax, thereby resulting in the discharge of bile into the duodenum. With regard to the pancreas, there is a stimulation of the secretion of enterokinase and of glucagon and a trophic effect on the exocrine pancreas in general. Less well documented effects are the inhibition of gastric and intestinal motility. There is also good evidence that CCK released by acid, fat and protein digests in the duodenum inhibits gastrin-stimulated gastric secretion,[113] therefore like secretin, it is a candidate for the negative aspect of the intestinal phase of gastric secretion. However, its mechanism of action remains unknown and it is also not certain whether the amount of CCK released by duodenal action is sufficient to have an inhibitory effect.

Gastrin releasing hormone

This hormone was originally called bombesin, a name derived from the frog from whose skin this polypeptide was first obtained. It is found in nerves throughout the digestive tract, but maximally in the antrum of the stomach and in the duodenum and upper small intestine. Its main function seems to be to translate vagal nerve stimulation into gastrin release by the G cells (p. 302).

Vasoactive intestinal peptide

Like gastrin releasing hormone this polypeptide containing 28 amino acids is found in the brain and the autonomic nervous system, including the nerves to the gut. It inhibits the effect of CCK that produces contraction of the gall bladder, and also inhibits gastric secretion, although again its physiological role is uncertain. Although vasoactive intestinal peptide is released by acid or fat in the duodenum, and has therefore been suggested to form part of the inhibitory aspect of the intestinal phase of gastric secretion, human studies have shown that exogenous vasoactive intestinal peptide does not inhibit gastric acid or plasma gastrin responses to a meal or to pentagastrin.[114] Perhaps its main function is to stimulate secretion by the intestine of water and electrolytes: oversecretion can produce the Werner–Morrison syndrome of watery diarrhoea.

Somatostatin

Somatostatin (SS) is a cyclic polypeptide containing 14 amino acid residues (SS-14) although it has also been described in a larger form (SS-28). It was originally isolated from the hypothalamus but has now been found to be very widely distributed in nerves and nerve cells in the central and peripheral nervous systems, and also in the S cells of the mucosa of the gastointestinal tract and of the pancreas. There is evidence that it is released from the duodenal S cells in response to the presence of fat or amino acids in the duodenal lumen. Since exogenous somatostatin has a profoundly inhibiting effect on all forms of gastric acid secretion, no matter what the stimulus to secretion,[115,116] and indeed also of pepsin and intrinsic factor secretion, it is not surprising that it, too, has been invoked as part of the inhibitory phase of intestinal gastric secretion. Unfortunately, it is not known whether this hypothesis is correct. Much of the difficulty is due to the fact that somatostatin probably acts mostly via a local effect on neighbouring cells – the so-called paracrine effect. It has been shown that S cells in the gastric mucosa are anatomically very close to parietal cells in the fundus and to G cells in the antrum, and even have processes that seem to extend to their neighbouring cells.[117] However, the effects of exogenous somatostatin are so diverse and strong that it is difficult not to believe but that it is physiologically important. Its other actions include the inhibition of gastrin release and the reduction of gastric mucosal blood flow, and indeed it probably inhibits the release of most of the other hormones of the gastrointestinal tract from their cell of origin.

Neurotensin

Neurotensin is a peptide containing 13 amino acid residues; it is found in the nerves of the gastrointestinal tract and in the N cells of the terminal ileum. Levels of neurotensin in the plasma increase within a few minutes of the start of a meal, so it is likely that the mechanism for its release involves the gastroduodenal region. In man it has been shown that oleic acid in the duodenal lumen stimulates the release of neurotensin, and that this agent suppresses meal- or gastrin-stimulated gastric secretion. However, this inhibition requires an intact vagal innervation of the stomach,[118,119] so neurotensin probably does not contribute to the physiological inhibitory component of the intestinal phase of gastric secretion.

Gastric inhibitory peptide

This is a large molecule containing 43 amino acid residues. It is produced in the K cells of the duodenum and upper jejunum, released in response to the presence of fat in the duodenal lumen, and was originally shown to suppress both gastrin- and histamine-stimulated secretion from vagally denervated (Heidenhain) gastric pouches in the dog. Further work has, however, demonstrated that exogenous gastric inhibitory peptide does not inhibit gastric secretion in humans and that fat inhibits gastric secretion equally well whether it is given into the duodenum or intravenously, and without any correlation with the magnitude of any related gastric inhibitory peptide release. It is unlikely to be involved in the intestinal phase of gastric secretion.

GASTRIC AND DUODENAL BLOOD FLOW

Anatomy

The anatomy of the arteries supplying the stomach and duodenum is described in Chapter 19. Briefly, for the stomach, the coeliac trunk gives rise to the hepatic, left gastric and splenic arteries, and a loop is formed along the greater curvature by the left gastroepiploic artery, a branch of the splenic artery, and the right gastroepiploic artery, a branch of the gastroduodenal

artery, which is itself a branch of the hepatic artery. A second loop is formed along the lesser curvature by the left gastric and the right gastric arteries, the latter being a branch of the hepatic artery. Branches are given off at intervals from these two loops, separately to the anterior and posterior surfaces of the stomach. The short gastric arteries arise from the splenic artery near the upper margin of the greater curvature, and supply the neighbouring fundic areas. There are also minor contributions from branches around the head and body of the pancreas. For the pancreas, the main supply to the head is from the gastroduodenal artery via its anterior and posterior superior pancreaticoduodenal branches, which anastomose around the head of the pancreas with the anterior and posterior inferior pancreaticoduodenal arteries arising from the superior mesenteric artery. Several short arteries also supply the body and tail from the splenic artery.

The main veins tend to follow the arteries and (greater curvature) empty into the splenic and superior mesenteric veins and thus to the portal vein, or (lesser curvature) directly into the portal vein via the right and left gastric veins.

Microanatomy

The arteries pierce the muscle coat of the stomach and presumably (though good studies of this region are lacking in man) give off muscular branches within this layer. There is a relative dearth of anastomoses between anterior wall and posterior wall vessels along the lesser curvature, and this may explain the phenomenon of necrosis of the lesser curve that sometimes follows proximal gastric vagotomy.

In the submucosa, the arteries anastomose with themselves to form primary arcades which then produce a second arcade of smaller anastomosing branches which finally run in the muscularis mucosae or just in the base of the mucosa. These vessels are the source of the mucosal arterioles that supply the mucosal capillaries. The mucosal capillaries run parallel with the gastric glands and therefore reach the luminal surface at right angles. There they form loops around the opening of the gastric glands and their blood drains into collecting veins. The venous system follows the pattern of the arteries. There are some communications between the mucosal capillaries.

Arteriovenous anastomoses have been described[120] in human gastric submucosa, but more recent studies seem to have refuted their existence.[121,122]

The arrangement in parallel of the muscular vascular bed and the mucosal/submucosal vascular bed permits alteration of the flow through one of the beds without that through the other necessarily following suit. The flow through the mucosa is dependent on the flow through the arteriolar submucosal network and can be decreased by constriction of the latter or increased by its dilatation.[123]

Gastric blood flow measurements

Total gastric blood flow in an animal can be measured by tying off all the veins draining the stomach except for one and collecting the effluent from that vein in a measured time. A less traumatic variation is to place a magnetic cuff (transducer) around the vein and measure the current produced in the cuff by the passage through its magnetic field of the charged particles (ions) in the blood: the current is proportional to the rate of flow.[124,125]

A large number of methods for the measurement of mucosal blood flow exist. It is, however, important to know that the aminopyrine method,[126] which until recently was the most popular, has now been shown to be unreliable.[127] Much work that has been done with aminopyrine is now waiting to be re-examined. Fractional extraction techniques assume that 30–60 seconds after the intravenous injection of an isotope, the fraction of the isotope within an organ is the same as the fraction of the cardiac output reaching that organ. A modification of this method is to inject microspheres labelled with an isotope, on the assumption that the spheres are halted when they reach blood vessels smaller in diameter than they are and that their distribution is proportional to the local blood flow. There is some evidence that these assumptions are not true in all circumstances.[128]

Newer and probably more reliable techniques include inert gas clearance and laser-Doppler velocimetry. The hydrogen gas clearance technique[129,130] is particularly useful, not only because it can be used in the conscious human but also because it is quantitative, in that it gives flow in units of millilitres per minute per 100 g. As hydrogen gas is breathed, it can be detected in the gastric mucosa by the current it produces in a platinum electrode held against the mucosa. When the breathing of hydrogen stops, its disappearance from the mucosa (which is a function of the mucosal blood flow) can be measured from the rate of diminution of the current. However, there are problems: pure hydrogen gas is explosive and breathing the pure gas produces severe hypoxia. The use of hydrogen–air mixtures may solve these problems. Laser-Doppler velocimetry is a promising technique that relies on the Doppler shift in wavelength of light scattered by moving red blood cells.[131]

CONTROL OF GASTRIC CIRCULATION

Nervous system

The influence of the nervous system on gastric mucosal blood flow was first noted by Beaumont[132] and his observations were extended by Wolf,[133] both workers seizing opportunities provided by a patient with an external gastric fistula. These were fundamentally important observations on gastric physiology and are classical studies. Certain emotional patterns, such as fear, depressed blood flow, as demonstrated by a pale, dry mucosa, while others increased blood flow, as demonstrated by engorgement.

In the modern era, experimental animal studies involving the implantation of electrodes into the brain have tended to suggest that stimulation of the posterior hypothalamus produces a reduction in gastric mucosal blood flow via the sympathetic route, while stimulation of the anterior hypothalamus increases flow by the vagal route.[134] These results were in dogs: subsequent studies of central stimulation in other species have not yielded such clear-cut results.

The sympathetic nerves to the stomach are adrenergic, and electrical stimulation of these nerves in animals leads to contraction of the arterioles[135] and reduction in both total[136] and mucosal[137] blood flow.

In numerous animal experiments, it has been conclusively shown that stimulation of the vagus causes dilatation of the gastric arterioles within a few seconds,[125] and this effect is not (despite an earlier suggestion to the contrary) secondary to the increased gastric secretion that is also produced, because the latter starts only after several minutes. Surgical vagotomy, at least in the short term (weeks), does reduce gastric mucosal blood flow as anticipated,[138] but there seems to be no permanent effect.[139]

In most studies relating the neural system to gastric blood flow there has in general been a parallelism between the directions in change in blood flow and in gastric acid secretion, but certainly no strict proportionality and occasionally not even parallelism.

Chemical agents

This term includes a wide variety of molecules: hormones, amines, prostaglandins and leukotrienes.

Gastrointestinal hormones

The increase in gastric mucosal blood flow produced by gastrin (or pentagastrin)[140] occurs at the same proportional rate as the concomitant increase in gastric secretion, and so it would appear that the increased blood flow may be secondary to the increased gastric secretion. This response is different to the effect of histamine (see below). In the dog, inhibition of pentagastrin-stimulated secretion by VIP and (separately) by secretin is similarly accompanied by a secondary fall in gastric mucosal blood flow.[141] Motilin[142] and neurotensin[143] behave in the same way. The effect of glucagon on gastric blood flow varies in different circumstances. Finally, somatostatin is particularly interesting in this context in that it can alter gastric mucosal blood flow independently of its inhibitory effect on secretion, even causing an increase in blood flow at the same time as secretion is reduced.[144,145]

Amines

The former widespread use of histamine as a reliable agonist for producing maximal gastric secretion in animals and man has led to considerable interest in its effects on the gastric circulation. By and large, the increase in gastric acid secretion is accompanied by an increase in gastric mucosal perfusion. However, there are many discrepancies in published reports. Reasons for the contradictions include: differences in dose and in the site of administration; the fact that histamine acts on two different kinds of receptor, H_1 and H_2, and that the agonists and inhibitors of these receptors are not always pure in their actions; differences in the species of experimental animal; and uncertainty about the physiological role of histamine in gastric secretion.[68] The subject has been reviewed elsewhere.[146]

The study of catecholamines has also been beset with experimental difficulties. The consensus position[146] is that adrenaline and noradrenaline both constrict the gastric arterioles via α receptors, but that a later escape occurs, mediated by β receptors.

Prostaglandins

The prostaglandins have paracrine properties, i.e. they act as chemical messengers but only over a limited range. Prostacyclin, PGI_2 is produced in large quantities in the walls of blood vessels and in other cells within the gastric mucosa. This and other prostaglandins increase gastric mucosal blood flow,[147,148] whereas aspirin and indomethacin, drugs which inhibit the enzyme cyclooxygenase that converts arachidonic acid into intermediaries on the way to prostaglandins, reduce resting gastric mucosal blood flow.[149] Despite increasing perfusion, the prostaglandins reduce gastric secretion,[150] a combination that may explain the cytoprotective properties of prostaglandins, i.e. their role in protecting the gastric mucosa against ulcerogenic agents.[129]

Leukotrienes

Leukotrienes are fatty acids containing 20 carbon atoms, formed from arachidonic acid by the enzyme lipo-oxygenase. Leukotriene C_4 produces severe venoconstriction in rat gastric submucosa[155] and could be implicated in the aetiology of gastric ulcer.

GASTRIC CIRCULATION PHYSIOLOGY AND PATHOLOGY

In animal studies, gastric blood flow increases with eating, mainly because of an increase in mucosal flow,[152] but it decreases with age.[153,154]

The relationships between gastric mucosal blood flow on the one hand, disruption of the mucosal barrier to acid back-diffusion and integrity of the mucosa (resistance to ulcerogenic agents) on the other, are subjects considered elsewhere in this book (pp 324–334).

REFERENCES

1. Helander HF. The cells of the gastric mucosa. *Int Rev Cytol* 1981; **70:** 217–289.
2. Coulton GR & Firth JA. Cytochemical evidence for functional zonation of parietal cells within the gastric glands of the mouse. *Histochem J* 1983; **15:** 1141–1150.
3. Helander HF & Sundell GW. Ultrastructure of inhibited parietal cells in the rat. *Gastroenterology* 1984; **87:** 1064–1071.
4. Jacobs DM & Sturtevant RP. Circadian ultrastructural changes in rat gastric parietal cells under altered feeding regimens: a morphometric study. *Anat Rec* 1982; **203:** 101–113.
5. Lipkin M. Proliferation and differentiation of gastrointestinal cells. *Physiol Rev* 1973; **53:** 891–915.
6. Golgi C. Sur la fine organisation des glandes peptiques des mammifères. *Arch Ital Biol* 1893; **19:** 448–453.
7. Helander HF & Hirschowitz BI. Quantitative ultrastructural studies on gastric parietal cells. *Gastroenterology* 1972; **63:** 951–961.
8. Ito S & Schofield GC. Studies on the depletion and accumulation of microvilli and changes in the tubulovesicular compartment of mouse parietal cells in relation to gastric acid secretion. *J Cell Biol* 1974; **63:** 364–382.
9. Zalewsky CA & Moody FG. Stereological analysis of the parietal cell during acid secretion and inhibition. *Gastroenterology* 1977; **73:** 66–74.
10. Forte JG, Black JA, Forte TM et al. Ultrastructural changes related to functional activity in gastric oxyntic cells. *Am J Physiol* 1981; **241:** G349–G358.
11. Forte TM & Forte JG. Definition of extracellular space in secreting and non-secreting cells. *J Cell Biol* 1970; **47:** 782–786.
12. Sedar AW. Uptake of peroxidase into the smooth-surfaced tubular system of the gastric acid-secreting cell. *J Cell Biol* 1969; **43:** 179–184.
13. Black JA, Forte TM & Forte JG. Inhibition of HC1 secretion and the effects of ultrastructure and electrical resistance in isolated piglet gastric mucosa. *Gastroenterology* 1981; **81:** 509–519.
14. Carlisle KS, Chew CS & Hersey SJ. Ultrastructural changes and cyclic AMP in frog gastric cells. *J Cell Biol* 1978; **76:** 31–42.
15. Lehy T, Zeitoun P, Dubrasquet P, Bonfils S, Dufougery F & Houdement JC. Etude histoclinique et ultrastructurale de la cicatrisation de l'ulcère de constrainte chez le rat. *Biol Gastroenterol* 1970; **2:** 107–124.
16. Matsuyama M & Suzuki H. Differentiation of immature mucus cells into parietal, argyrophil and chief cells in stomach grafts. *Science* 1970; **96:** 385.
17. Langley JN. On the histology and physiology of pepsin-forming glands. *Phil Trans R Soc Lond [Biol]* 1881; **172:** 664–711.
18. Langley JN & Edkins JS. Pepsinogen and pepsin. *J Physiol (Lond)* 1886; **7:** 371–415.
19. Kageyama T & Takahashi K. Isolation of an activation intermediate and determination of the aminoacid sequence of the activation segment of human pepsinogen A. *J Biochem (Tokyo)* 1980; **88:** 571–582.
20. Kay J & Dykes CW. The first cleavage site in pepsinogen activation. *Adv Exp Med Biol* 1976; **95:** 103–127.
21. Samloff IM. Slow-moving protease and the seven pepsinogens. Electrophoretic demonstration of the existence of eight proteolytic fractions in human gastric mucosa. *Gastroenterology* 1966; **57:** 659–669.
22. Samloff IM. Pepsinogens, pepsins and pepsin inhibitors. *Gastroenterology* 1971; **60:** 586–604.
23. Seijffers MJ, Turner MD, Miller LL & Segal HL. Human pepsinogens and pepsin. *Gastroenterology* 1965; **48:** 122–125.
24. Samloff IM. Cellular localization of group I pepsinogens in human gastric mucosa by immunofluorescence. *Gastroenterology* 1971; **61:** 185–188.
25. Samloff IM & Liebman WM. Radioimmunoassay of group I pepsinogens in serum. *Gastroenterology* 1984; **66:** 494–502.
26. Filipe MI. Mucins in the human gastrointestinal epithelium: a review. *Invest Cell Pathol* 1979; **2:** 195–216.
27. Neutra MR The functional ultrastructure of mucous cells. *Chest* 1982; **81** (Suppl.): 14S–19S.
28. Bennett G, Leblond CP & Haddad A. Migration of glycoprotein from the Golgi apparatus to the surface of various cell types as shown by radioautography after labelled fucose injection into rats. *J Cell Biol* 1974; **60:** 258–284.
29. Rambourg A, Hernandez W & Leblond CP. Detection of complex carbohydrates in the Golgi apparatus of rat cells. *J Cell Biol* 1969; **40:** 395–414.
30. Pearse AGE. The diffuse neuroendocrine system: historical review. In Ratzenhofer M, Hofler H & Walter GF (eds) *Interdisciplinary Neuroendocrinology*, Basel: Karger, 1984: 1–7.
31. Fujita T. Concept of paraneurons. *Arch Histol Jpn* 1977; **40:** Suppl. 1–12.
32. Wilson BS & Lloyd RV. Detection of chromogranin in neuroendocrine cells with a monoclonal antibody. *Am J Pathol* 1984; **115:** 458–468.
33. Varndell IM, Lloyd RV, Wilson BS & Polak JM. Ultrastructural localisation of chromogranin: a potential marker for the electron microscopic recognition of endocrine cell secretory granules. *Histochem J* 1985; **17:** 981–992.
34. Polak JM & Varndell IM (eds). *Immunolabelling for Electronmicroscopy*. Amsterdam: Elsevier, 1984.
35. McGuigan JE. Gastric mucosal intracellular localization of gastrin immunofluorescence. *Gastroenterology* 1968; **53:** 315–327.
36. Larsson L-I. Evidence of anterograde transport of secretory granules in processes of gastric paracrine (somatostatin) cells. *Histochemistry* 1984; **80:** 323–326.
37. Berglindh T. The mammalian gastric parietal cell in vitro. *Annu Rev Physiol* 1984; **46:** 377–392.
38. Lewin MJM, Cheret AM, Soumarmon A & Girodet J. Méthode pour l'isolement et le tri des cellules de la muquese fundique de rat. *Biol Gastroenterol (Paris)* 1974; **7:** 139–144.
39. Forte, JG, Forte GM & Saltman P. K+-stimulated phosphatase in microsomes isolated from gastric mucosa. *J. Cell Physiol* 1967; **69:** 293–304.

40. Berglindh T & Obrink KJ. Histamine as a physiological stimulant of gastric parietal cells. In Yellin T (ed) *Histamine Receptors*. New York: Spectrum, 1979: 35.

41. Berglindh T, Dibona DR, Ito S & Sachs G. Probes of parietal cell function. *Am J Physiol* 1980; **238:** G165–G176.

42. Davidson WD, Klein KL, Kurokawa K & Soll AH. Instantaneous and continuous measurement of ^{14}C-labeled substrate oxidation to $^{14}CO_2$ by minute tissue specimens: an ionization chamber method. *Metabolism* 1981; **30:** 596–600.

43. Berglindh T, Helander HF & Obrink KJ. Effects of secretagogues on oxygen consumption, aminopyrine accumulation and morphology in isolated gastric glands. *Acta Physiol Scand* 1976; **97:** 401–414.

44. Soll AH. Secretagogue stimulation of [^{14}C]aminopyrine accumulation by isolated canine parietal cells. *Am J Physiol* 1980; **238:** G366–G375.

45. Berglindh T, Dibona DR. Pace CS & Sachs G. ATP-dependence of H^+ secretion. *J Cell Biol* 1980; **85:** 392–401.

46. Ganser AL & Forte JG. K^+ stimulated ATPase in purified microsomes of bullfrog oxyntic cells. *Biochim Biophys Acta* 1973; **307:** 169–180.

47. Forte JG, Ganser AL, Beesley RC & Forte TM. Unique enzymes of purified microsomes from pig fundic mucosa. *Gastroenterology* 1975; **69:** 175 189.

48. Forte JG, Ganser AL & Ray TK. The K^+-stimulated ATPase from oxyntic glands of gastric mucosa. In Kaskebar DK, Sachs G & Rehm W (eds) *Gastric Hydrogen Ion Secretion*. New York: Marcel Dekker, 1976: 302.

49. Soumarmon A, Abastado M, Bonfils S & Lewin MJM. Cl– transport in gastric microsomes. *J Biol Chem* 1980; **255:** 11682–11687.

50. Lewin MJM, Soumarmon A, Bali JP et al. Interaction of ^3H-labelled synthetic human gastrin with rat gastric plasma membranes: evidence for the existence of biologically reactive gastrin receptor sites. *FEBS Lett* 1976; **66:** 168–172.

51. Soumarmon, Cheret AM & Lewin MJM. Localization of gastrin receptors in intact isolated and separated rat fundic cells. *Gastroenterology* 1977; **73:** 900–903.

52. Batzri S & Dyer J. Aminopyrine uptake by guinea pig gastric mucosal cells: mediation by cyclic AMP and interaction among secretagogues. *Biochim Biophys Acta* 1981; **675:** 416–426.

53. Berglindh T. Effects of common inhibitors of gastric acid secretion on secretagogue-induced respiration and aminopyrine accumulation in isolated gastric glands. *Biochim Biophys Acta* 1977; **464:** 217–233.

54. Ecknauer R, Dial E, Thompson WJ, Johnson LR & Rosenfeld GC. Isolated rat gastric parietal cells: cholinergic response and pharmacology. *Life Sci* 1981; **28:** 609–621.

55. Dial E, Thompson WJ & Rosenfeld GC. Isolated parietal cells: histamine response and pharmacology. *J. Pharmacol Exp Ther* 1981; **219:** 585–590.

56. Fellenius E, Elander B, Wallmark U et al. A micro-method for the study of acid secretory function in isolated human oxyntic glands from gastroscopic biopsies. *Clin Sci* 1983; **64:** 423–431.

57. Chew CS, Hersey SJ, Sachs G & Berglindh T. Histamine responsiveness of isolated gastric glands. *Am J Physiol* 1980; **238:** G312–G320.

58. Levine RA, Kohen KR, Schwartzel EH Jr & Ramsay CE. Prostaglandin E$_2$- histamine interactions on cAMP, cGMP, and acid production in isolated fundic glands. *Am J Physiol* 1982; **242:** G21–G26.

59. Card W & Marks I. The relationship between the acid output of the stomach following 'maximal' histamine stimulation and the parietal cell mass. *Clin Sci* 1960; **19:** 147–163.

60. Hassan MA & Hobsley M. The accurate assessment of maximal gastric secretion in control subjects and patients with duodenal ulcer. *Br J Surg* 1973; **58:** 171–179.

61. Teorell T. Electrolyte diffusion in relation to acidity regulation of gastric juice. *Gastroenterology* 1947; **9:** 425–443.

62. Hollander F. Studies in gastric secretion. IV. Variations in the chloride content of gastric juice and their significance. *J Biol Chem* 1932; **97:** 585–604.

63. Hobsley M & Whitfield PF. The electrolyte composition of pure gastric juice. *J. Physiol (Lond)* 1977; **271:** 57P–58P.

64. Hobsley M. Pyloric reflux; a modification of the two-component hypothesis of gastric secretion. *Clin Sci Mol Med* 1974; **47:** 131–144.

65. Whitfield PF & Hobsley M. Maximal gastric secretion in smokers and non-smokers with duodenal ulcer. *Br J Surg* 1985; **72:** 955–957.

66. Whitfield PF & Hobsley M. Comparison of maximal gastric secretion in smokers and non-smokers with and without duodenal ulcer. *Gut* 1987; **28:** 557–560.

67. Maybury NK, Russell RCG, Faber RG & Hobsley M. A new interpretation of the insulin test validated and then compared with the Burge test. *Br J Surg* 1977; **64:** 673–676.

68. Boulos PB, Faber RG, Whitfield PF, Parkin JV & Hobsley M. Relationship between insulin- and histamine-stimulated gastric secretion before and after vagotomy. *Gut* 1983; **24:** 549–556.

69. Hirschowitz BI. Secretion of pepsinogen. In Code CF (ed.) *Handbook of Physiology*, vol. 2, Alimentary Canal. Secretion. Washington, DC: American Physiological Society, 1967: 889–933.

70. Sanders MJ, Amirian DA, Ayalon A & Soll AH. Regulation of pepsinogen release from canine chief cells in primary monolayer culture. *Am J Physiol* 1983; **245:** G641–G646.

71. Hersey SJ, Miller M, May D & Norris SH. Lack of interaction between acid and pepsinogen secretion in isolated gastric glands. *Am J Physiol* 1983; **245:** G775–G779.

72. Hirschowitz BI & Gibson RG. Effect of cimetidine on stimulated gastric secretion and serum gastrin in the dog. *Am J Gastroenterol* 1978; **70:** 437–447.

73. Hersey SJ, May D & Schyberg D. Stimulation of pepsinogen release from isolated gastric glands by cholecystokinin-like peptides. *Am J Physiol* 1983; **244:** G192–G197.

74. Berstad A & Petersen H. Dose–response relationship of the effect of secretin on acid and pepsin secretion in man. *Scand J Gastroenterol* 1970; **5:** 647–654.

75. Barros D, Bloom SR & Baron JH. Inhibition by somatostatin (growth hormone release-inhibiting hormone, GH-RIH) of gastric acid and pepsin and G-cell release of gastrin. *Gut* 1978; **19:** 315–320.

76. Chew CS & Brown MR. Release of intracellular Ca and elevation of inositol triphosphate by secretagogues in parietal and chief cells isolated from rabbit gastric mucosa. *Biochim Biophys Acta* 1986; **888:** 116–125.

77. Florey H. Mucin and the protection of the body. *Proc R Soc Lond [Biol]* 1955; **143:** 147–158.

78. Andre C, Lambert R & Descos F. Stimulation of gastric mucous secretions in man by secretin. *Digestion* 1972; **7:** 284–293.

79. Domschke W, Domschke S, Hornig D & Demling L. Prostaglandin-stimulated gastric mucus secretion in man. *Acta Hepatogastroenterol* 1978; **25:** 292–294.

80. Castle WB. Observations on the etiologic relationship of achylia gastrica to pernicious anaemia. I. Effect of administration to patients with pernicious anaemia of contents of normal human stomach recovered after ingestion of beef muscle. *Am J Med Sci* 1929; **178:** 748–764.

81. Hoffman HH & Schnitzlein HN. The number of nerve fibres in the vagus nerve of man. *Anat Rec* 1961; **139:** 429–435.

82. Radke R, Stach W & Weiss R. Innervation of the gastric wall related to acid secretion: a light and electron microscopy study on rats, rabbits and guinea pigs. *Acta Biol Med Ger* 1980; **39:** 687–696.

83. Hirschowitz BI & Gibson RG. Cholinergic stimulation and suppression of gastric release in gastric fistula dogs. *Am J Physiol* 1978; **235:** E720–E725.

84. Grossman MI. Regulation of gastric acid secretion. In Johnson LR (ed.) *Physiology of the Gastrointestinal Tract*. New York: Raven Press, 1981: 659.

85. Hirschowitz BI. The vagus and gastric secretion. In Brooks FP & Evers PW (eds) *Nerves and the Gut*. Thorofare, NJ: Slack, 1977: 96.

86. Hirschowitz BI, Fong J & Molina E. Effects of pirenzepine and atropine on vagal and cholinergic gastric secretion and gastrin release and on heart rate in the dog. *J Pharmacol Exp Ther* 1983; **225:** 263–268.

87. Hirschowitz BI & Gibson RG. Augmented vagal release of antral gastrin by 2-deoxyglucose after fundic vagotomy in dogs. *Am J Physiol* 1979; **236:** E173–E179.

88. Holst JJ, Knuhsen S, Jensen SL et al. Interrelation of nerves and hormones in stomach and pancreas. *Scand J Gastroenterol* 1983; **82:** 85–99.

89. Faber RG & Hobsley M. Basal gastric secretion: reproducibility and relationship with duodenal ulcers. *Gut* 1977; **18:** 57–63.

90. Roxburgh JC. *The acute and chronic effects of cigarette smoking upon various aspects of gastric secretion*. MS thesis, University of London, 1989.

91. Athow AC, Lewin MR, Sewerniak AT & Clark CG. Gastric secretory response to modified sham feeding and insulin after vagotomy. *Br Surg* 1986; **73:** 132–135.

92. Maybury NK, Faber RG & Hobsley M. Post-vagotomy insulin test: improved predictability of ulcer recurrence after corrections for height and collection errors. *Gut* 1977; **18:** 449–456.

93. Faber RG, Russell RCG, Parkin JV, Whitfield P & Hobsley M. The predictive accuracy of the postvagotomy insulin test: a new interpretation. *Gut* 1975; **16:** 337–342.

94. Moore JG & Crespin F. Influence of glucose on cephalic–vagal-simulated gastric acid secretion in man. *Dig Dis Sci* 1980; **25:** 117–122.

95. Lam SK, Isenberg JI, Grossman MI, Lane WH & Walsh JH. Gastric acid secretion is abnormally sensitive to endogenous gastrin released after peptone test meals in duodenal ulcer patients. *J Clin Invest* 1980; **65:** 555–562.

96. Schiller LR, Walsh JH & Feldman M. Distension-induced gastrin release: effects of luminal acidification and intravenous atropine. *Gastroenterology* 1980; **78:** 912–917.

97. Fordtran JS & Walsh JH. Gastric acid secretion rate and buffer content of the stomach after eating: results in normal subjects and in patients with duodenal ulcer. *J Clin Invest* 1973; **52:** 645–657.

98. Hirschowitz BI. Neural and hormonal control of gastric secretion. In Schultz SG, Forte JG & Rauner BB. (eds) *Handbook of Physiology*, sec. 6: The Gastrointestinal System. Bethesda, MD: American Physiological Society, 1989: 127.

99. Konturek SJ, Kwiecien N, Obtulowicz W, Bielanski W, Oleksy J & Schally AV. Effects of somatostatin 14 and somatostatin 28 on plasma hormonal and gastric secretory response to cephalic and gastrointestinal stimulation in man. *Scand J Gastroenterol* 1985; **20:** 31–38.

100. Webb S, Levy I, Wass JA, Llorens A et al. Studies on the mechanisms of somatostatin release after insulin induced hypoglycaemia in man. *Clin Endocrinol* 1984; **21:** 667–675.

101. Konturek SJ, Biernat J & Oleksy J. Serum gastric and gastrin responses to meals at various pH levels in man. *Gut* 1974; **15:** 526–553.

102. Thompson JC & Swierczek JS. Acid and endocrine responses to meals varying in pH in normals and duodenal ulcer subjects. *Ann Surg* 1977; **186:** 541–548.

103. Walsh JH, Richardson CT & Fordtran JS. pH dependence of acid secretion and gastrin release in normal and ulcer patients. *J. Clin Invest* 1975; **55:** 462–468.

104. Feldman M & Walsh JH. Acid inhibition of sham feeding stimulated gastrin release and gastric acid secretion: effect of atropine. *Gastroenterology* 1980; **78:** 772–776.

105. Gamble JL. *Chemical Anatomy, Physiology and Pathology of the Extracellular Fluid.* Boston: Harvard University Press, 1964, 15.

106. Paumgartner G & Sauerbruch T. Secretion, composition and flow of bile. *Clin Gastroenterol* 1983; **12:** 3–23.

107. Somjen GJ & Gilat T. Contribution of vesicular and micellar carriers to cholesterol transport in human bile. *J Lipid Res* 1985; **26:** 699–704.

108. Debas HT & Grossman MI. Pure cholecystokinin: pancreatic protein and bicarbonate response. *Digestion* 1973; **9:** 469–481.

109. Bayliss WH & Starling EH. The mechanism of pancreatic secretion. *J Physiol (Lond)* 1902; **28:** 325–353.

110. Fiddian-Green RG, Parkin JV, Faber RG, Russell RCG, Whitfield PF & Hobsley M. The quantification in human gastric juice of duodenogastric reflux by sodium output and by bile-labelling using indocyanine green. *Klin Wochenschr* 1979; **57:** 815–824.

111. Chen YF, Chey WY, Chang T-M & Lee KY. Duodenal acidification releases cholecystokinin. *Am J Physiol* 1985; **249:** G29–G33.

112. Fried M, Erlacher URS, Schwizer W et al. Role of cholecystokinin in the regulation of gastric emptying and pancreatic enzyme secretion in humans. *Gastroenterology* 1991; **101:** 503–511.

113. Mayer EA, Elashoff J, Mutt V & Walsh JH. Reassessment of gastric inhibition by cholecyskinin and gastric inhibitory polypeptide in dogs. *Gastroenterology* 1982; **83:** 1047–1050.

114. Holm-Bentzen M, Christiansen J, Kirkegaard P, Olsen S, Petersen B & Fahrenkrug J. The effect of vasoactive intestinal polypeptide on meal-stimulated acid secretion in man. *Scand J Gastroenterol* 1983; **18:** 659–661.

115. Arnold R & Lankisch PG. Somatostatin and the gastrointestinal tract. *Clin Gastroenterol* 1980; **9:** 733–753.

116. Konturek SJ, Tasler J, Cieszkowski M, Coy DH & Schally AV. Effect of growth hormone release-inhibiting hormone on gastric secretion, mucosal blood flow and serum gastrin. *Gastroenterology* 1976; **70:** 737–741.

117. Larsson LI, Goltermann N, De Magistris L, Rehfeld J & Schwartz TW. Somatostatin cell processes as pathways for paracrine secretion. *Science* 1979; **205:** 1393–1395.

118. Kihl B & Olbe L. Fat inhibition of gastric acid secretion in duodenal ulcer patients before and after proximal gastric vagotomy. *Gut* 1980; **21:** 1056–1061.

119. Kihl B, Roekaeus A, Rosell S & Olbe L. Fat inhibition of gastric acid secretion in man and plasma concentration of neurotensin-like immunoreactivity. *Scand J Gastroenterol* 1981; **16:** 513–526.

120. Barlow TE, Bentley FH & Walder DN. Arteries, veins and arteriovenous anastomoses in the human stomach. *Surg Gynecol Obstet* 1951; **93:** 657–671.

121. Piasecki C. Observations on the submucous plexus and mucosal arteries of the dog's stomach and first part of the duodenum. *J Anat* 1975; **119:** 133–148.

122. Gannon B, Browning J, O'Brien P & Rogers P. Mucosal microvascular architecture of the fundus and body of the human stomach. *Gastroenterology* 1984; **86:** 866–875.

123. Guth PH & Smith E. Neural control of gastric mucosal blood flow in the rat. *Gastroenterology* 1975; **69:** 935–940.

124. Kolin A. Blood flow determination by electromagnetic method. *Med Phys* 1960; **3:** 141–155.

125. Jacobson ED, Eisenberg MM & Swan KG. Effects of histamine on gastric blood flow in conscious dogs. *Gastroenterology* 1966; **51:** 466–472.

126. Jacobson ED, Linford RH & Grossman MI. Gastric secretion in relation to mucosal blood flow studied by a clearance technique. *J Clin Invest* 1966; **45:** 1–13.

127. Leung FW, Guth PH, Scremin OU, Golanska EM & Kauffman GL Jr. Regional gastric mucosal blood flow measurements by hydrogen gas clearance in the anaesthetized rat and rabbit. *Gastroenterology* 1984; **87:** 28–36.

128. Greenway CV & Murthy VS. Effects of vasopressin and isoprenaline infusions on the distribution of blood flow in the intestine: criteria for the validity of microsphere studies. *Br J Pharmacol* 1972; **46:** 117–188.

129. Murakami M, Lam SK, Inada M & Miyake T. Pathophysiology and pathogenesis of acute gastric mucosal lesions after hypothermic restraint stress in rats. *Gastroenterology* 1985; **88:** 660–665.

130. Cheung LY & Sonnenschein LA. Measurements of regional gastric mucosal blood flow by hydrogen gas clearance. *Am J Surg* 1984; **147:** 32–37.

131. Saita H, Murakami M, Seki M & Miyake T. Evaluation of the measurement of gastric mucosal blood flow by laser Doppler velocimetry in rats. *Gastroenterology* 1984; **86:** 1228 (abstract).

132. Beaumont W. *Experiments and Observations on the Gastric Juice and the Physiology of Digestion.* New York: Dover, 1833.

133. Wolf S. Gastric function throughout one eventful year. In Wolf S (ed.) *The Stomach.* New York: Oxford University Press, 1965: 179.

134. Leonard AS, Long D, French LA, Peter ÉT & Wangensteen OH. Pendular pattern in gastric secretion and blood flow following hypothalamic stimulation: origin of stress ulcer? *Surgery* 1964; **56:** 109–120.

135. Schnitzlein HN. Regulation of blood flow through the stomach of the rat. *Anat Rec* 1957; **127:** 735–753.

136. Jansson G, Kampp M, Lundgren O & Martinson J. Studies on the circulation of the stomach. *Acta Physiol Scand Suppl* 1966; **277:** 91.

137. Blair EL, Grund ER, Reed JD, Sanders DJ, Sanger G & Shaw B. The effect of sympathetic nerve stimulation on serum gastrin, gastric acid secretion and mucosal blood flow responses to meat extract stimulation in anaesthetized cats. *J Physiol (Lond)* 1975; **253:** 493–504.

138. Mackie DB & Turner MD. Vagotomy and submucosal blood flow. *Arch Surg* 1971; **102:** 626–629.

139. Bell PRF & Shelley T. Gastric mucosal blood flow and acid secretion in conscious animals measured by heat flow. *Am J Dig Dis* 1968; **13:** 685–696.

140. Ivarsson LE, Darle N, Hulten L, Lindhagen J & Lundgren O. Gastric blood flow and distribution: the effect of pentagastrin in anesthetized cat and man as studied by an inert gas elimination method. *Scand J Gastroenterol* 1982; **17:** 1037–1048.

141. Konturek SJ, Dembinski A, Thor P & Krol R. Comparison of vasoactive peptide (VIP) and secretin in gastric secretion and mucosal blood flow. *Pfluegers Arch* 1976; **361:** 175–181.

142. Konturek SJ, Dembinski A, Krol R & Wunsch E. Effect of 13-NLE-motilin on gastric secretion, serum gastrin level and mucosal blood flow in dogs. *J Physiol (Lond)* 1977; **264:** 665–672.

143. Osumi Y, Nagasaka Y, Fu LH & Fujiwara M. Inhibition of gastric acid secretion and mucosal blood flow induced by intraventricularly applied neurotensin in rats. *Life Sci* 1978; **23:** 2275–2280.

144. Leung FW & Guth PH. Dissociated effects of somatostatin on gastric acid secretion and mucosal blood flow. *Am J Physiol* 1985; **248:** G337–G341.

145. Sonnenberg A & West C. Somatostatin reduces gastric blood flow in normal subjects but not in patients with cirrhosis of the liver. *Gut* 1983; **24:** 148–153.

146. Guth PH, Leung FW & Kauffman GL Jr. Physiology of gastric circulation. In Schultz SG, Wood JD, Rauner BB (eds) *Handbook of Physiology*, sect. 6, vol. 1. Bethesda, MD: American Physiological Society, 1989: 1371.

147. Whittle BJR, Boughton-Smith NK, Moncada S & Vane JR. Actions of prostacyclin (PGI$_2$) and its product 6-oxo-PGF$_1$ on the rat gastric mucosa in vivo and vitro. *Prostaglandins* 1978; **15:** 955–967.

148. Main IHM & Whittle BJR. Gastric mucosal blood flow during pentagastrin- and histamine-stimulated acid secretion in the rat. *Br J Pharmacol* 1973; **49:** 534–542.

149. Main IHM & Whittle BJR. Investigation of the vasodilator and antisecretory role of prostaglandins in the rat gastric mucosa by use of non-steroidal anti-inflammatory drugs. *Br J Pharmacol* 1975; **53:** 217–224.

150. Cheung LY & Lowry SF. Effects of intra-arterial infusion of prostaglandin E$_1$ on gastric secretion and blood flow. *Surgery* 1978; **83:** 699–704.

151. Whittle BJR, Oren-Wolman N & Guth PH. Gastric vasoconstrictor actions of leukotriene C4, PGF$_{2a}$, and a thromboxane mimetic U-46619 on the rat submucosal microcirculation in vivo. *Am J Physiol* 1985; **248:** G580–G586.

152. Bond JH, Prentiss RA & Levitt MD. The effects of feeding on blood flow to the stomach, small bowel and colon of the conscious dog. *J Lab Clin Med* 1979; **93:** 594–599.

153. Varga F & Csaky TZ. Changes in the blood supply of the gastrointestinal tract in rats with age. *Pfluegers Arch* 1976; **364:** 129–133.

154. Ballard KW, Paulsen M, Oren-Wolman N & Guth PH. Age-related changes in the gastric submucosal arterioles and gastric acid secretion. *Microvasc Res* 1983; **25:** 176–185.

21

MEASUREMENT OF GASTRIC SECRETORY AND MOTOR FUNCTION

S Holt

Ingested food and fluid is received and stored by accommodation in the fundus and body of the stomach. This food is mixed with gastric secretions, ground to a fine particulate suspension and emptied into the duodenum in a controlled manner. Gastric secretory testing is not assessed in routine clinical practice because there are few circumstances in which this test is of clinical relevance. In contrast, the assessment of gastric motor function is attaining increased use as the role of disturbed gastric motility is recognized as a cause of symptoms.

Gastric motor function is initiated by eating and coordinated by complex neurohormonal mechanisms resulting in regulated delivery of food to the duodenum. Coordination of contractions in the stomach is mediated by the flow of electrical activity that originates from a pacemaker high on the greater curvature. Experimental evidence suggests that the fundus controls the emptying of liquids and the antrum appears to be of importance in handling of solid food. This chapter provides an overview of clinical measurements of gastric motor and secretory function with special reference to the use of non-invasive isotopic methodology.

WHY MEASURE GASTRIC EMPTYING?

Gastric emptying rate measurement is finding a more general role in the investigation of patients with upper gastrointestinal symptoms. Studies of emptying have been useful in defining disordered gastric motor function in patients who have symptoms after gastric surgery or symptoms of gastric stasis in the presence of autonomic neuropathy or systemic disease. The confirmation of gastric incontinence in patients with dumping syndrome, after gastric resection, may be important in the planning of corrective surgery or drug therapy. In addition, the treatment of gastroparetic disorders with prokinetic drugs, such as metoclopramide, domperidone or cisapride, can be evaluated by sequential studies of gastric emptying rate. There are many causes of gastric stasis without mechanical obstruction of the stomach (Table 21.1).

Quantitation of gastric emptying rate has aided understanding of the physiology or pathophysiology of gastric motor function. Studies of the emptying of liquid and solid phases of a test meal provide indirect information about functions of the gastric antrum and integrated reflexes such as receptive relation of the stomach. The contribution of the rate of emptying of the stomach to the absorption rate of drugs has shed light on important drug absorption–motility interactions. Several techniques are available for the measurement of gastric emptying rate in humans but each possesses disadvantages or limitations (Table 21.2).

SCINTIGRAPHIC TECHNIQUES FOR GASTRIC EMPTYING RATE MEASUREMENT

External scintigraphic detection of a gamma-emitting isotope that has been incorporated into a test meal, using a rectilinear scanner[1,2] or a gamma camera,[3-5] has provided a generally accepted method for the non-invasive determination of gastric emptying rate in humans. Rectilinear scanners are obsolete and most measurements are now undertaken with a gamma camera. A series of scintigraphic measurements of intragastric radioactivity are made at intervals after the ingestion of a radio-labelled meal. Gastric emptying of liquid and solid components of the meal can be determined when each phase of the meal is labelled (Figure 21.1).

The gamma camera can be used for bilateral detection of intra-abdominal counts, thereby providing correction of changes in radiation attenuation due to difference in the depth of radioactivity.

Differences in measurements due to stomach movement are encountered with the subject in the supine and upright position and there are errors in measured emptying rates if unilateral

Table 21.1 Some causes of gastric stasis without mechanical obstruction

Allergies	Jejunal haematoma
Amputations	Ketoacidosis
Amyloidosis	Labyrinthic disorders
Anaemia (iron deficiency)	Lead poisoning
Anaesthesia	Malnutrition
Anorexia nervosa	Ménétrier's disease
Appendicitis	Menstruation
Biliary tract disease	Migraine
Brain tumours or injury	Multiple sclerosis
'Cast syndrome'	Muscular dystrophy
Childbirth	Myopathy
Chronic gastritis	Myotonic dystrophy
Diabetes	Pancreatitis
Drugs (various)	Paraplegia
Electrolyte imbalance	Peritonitis
Emotional disorders (various)	Pneumonia
Endocarditis	Poliomyelitis (bulbar)
Exercise	Polymyositis
Familial autonomic dysfunction	Pseudo-obstruction syndrome
Fractures (various)	Radiation sickness
Gastric carcinoma	Reflux oesophagitis
Gastric ulcer (type 1)	Retroperitoneal disease
Gastroenteritis	Sciatica
Head injury	Scleroderma
Hepatic coma	Sepsis (various sites)
Hepatitis	Spinal tuberculosis
Herniorrhaphy	Spondylolisthesis
Hypercalcaemia	Surgical procedures (various)
Hyperglycaemia	Tabes dorsalis
Hyperthyroidism	Tachygastria
Hypocalcaemia	Tuberculosis
Hypokalaemia	Typhoid fever
Hypothyroidism	Uraemia
Idiopathic gastroparesis	Vagotomy
Infiltrative disease of the gut	Viral-like infection
Irradiation	

produce results similar to those obtained with a gamma camera.[8,9]

In one study, Holt et al.[9] undertook simultaneous measurements of the gastric emptying rate of the solid and liquid phases of a dual isotopically labelled test meal using a gamma camera and a simple scintillation detector, similar to that used in a hand-held probe.[8] Results with this simple scanning apparatus were compared with simultaneous measurements made by a gamma camera. A dual labelled test meal was used to measure liquid and solid emptying simultaneously. Anterior and posterior scans were taken at intervals to 120 min using both a gamma camera and the scintillation probe. Good relative agreement between the methods was obtained for both solid phase and liquid phase data. The application of the simple probe technique provided a non-invasive and simple method for assessing solid and liquid phase gastric emptying by the human stomach.

A number of methods for the simultaneous measurement of the liquid and solid components of the test meal have been described.[2,5,10] Two isotopes of different energy are used for marking the liquid and solid phase of a test meal. A variety of isotopes have been incorporated into different test meals for the scintigraphic determination of gastric emptying rate. At present, technetium-99 m (^{99m}Tc), indium-113 m (^{113m}In) or indium-111 (^{111}In) are favoured because they give radioactive emissions that are suitable for scintigraphy and, in the amounts used, they provide a relatively small radiation dose. For the study of the emptying of the liquid component of a test meal technetium and indium are often used when attached to diethylenetriamine penta-acetic acid (DTPA).[2] In this chemical form these isotopes are not absorbed, they can be mixed thoroughly with the test fluid and they do not adsorb to gastric mucosa.[11]

The solid component of a test meal can be labelled as an inert particle such as plastic-coated filter paper[2] or as a physiological solid such as chicken liver.[12] Radiolabelled chicken liver can be prepared by injecting technetium-99m[12] or indium-113m colloid[13] into the wing vein of a live chicken. The chicken is

detection alone is used with a gamma camera.[6,7] In the absence of sophisticated nuclear medicine equipment, gastric emptying can be assessed using a single scintillation detector which may

Table 21.2 Methods for the assessment of gastric emptying rate in man

METHOD	NON-INVASIVE	RADIATION EXPOSURE	ACCURATE QUANTITATION	LIQUID AND SOLIDS STUDIED	ACCEPTABILITY FOR REPEATED USE
Radiology	+?	+	−	+?	−
Gastric aspiration	−	−	+	−	−
Duodenal aspiration	−	−	+	+	−
Scintigraphic techniques	+	+	+	+	+?
Ferromagnetic tracer	+	−	+	−	+
Absorption kinetics of model drugs	+?	−	−	−	+
Breath alcohol analysis	+	−	−	−	+
Ultrasonography	+	−	+?	−	+

Advantages and limitations are indicated + = yes, +? = yes with reservation, − = no.

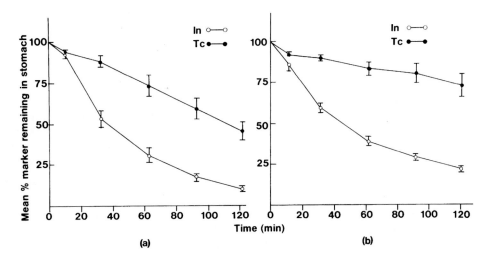

Figure 21.1

(a) and (b) Mean gastric emptying curves of solid (●) and liquid (○) emptying, derived from eight healthy volunteers. The solid phase of the meal consisted of ^{99m}Tc-labelled filter paper particles, coated with plastic, and the liquid was [^{113}In]DTPA. Solids empty in an approximate linear manner with time and liquids empty in an exponential manner. The curves in (a) are with a meal of low-energy density and those in (b) are with a meal of high-energy density. Emptying of the higher energy density meal is slower.

killed at 15–30 min after administration of the isotope. The animal's liver is then removed, cooked, diced into cubes and added to a test meal. Labelled chicken liver contains the tracer isotope in the Kupffer cells of the organ and there appears to be little dissociation of the isotope from the food during preparation of the test meal or the emptying studies.

Radiolabelled chicken liver empties from the stomach in a manner similar to small inert particles such as plastic-coated filter paper.[13] Alternative solid food markers include technetium sulphur colloid in whole eggs,[14] in vitro labelled chicken liver,[5] iodine labelled noodles[5] and the iodinated fibre α-methylcellulose.[16] The tagging of chicken liver in a live chicken produces a very high labelling efficiency with good in vitro and in vivo stability. In contrast, in vitro labelling of the chicken liver gives high labelling initially but within 1 hour one-third of the labelling dose of sulphur colloid may become dissociated.

Many of the contemporary methods of production of solid phase markers have overcome some of the problems inherent in earlier studies in which the isotope was not tightly bound to the solid phase of the meal. In some previous studies, elution of isotope may have led to uncertainty about what portion of the test meal had been labelled. By using isotopes with different gamma emission it is possible to quantitate simultaneously the solid and liquid emptying of a test meal by external scintiscanning.

If required, the quantitation of duodenogastric reflux can be undertaken at the same time as emptying rate measurements if two isotopes of different energy (one for assessing reflux and one for measuring emptying rate) are used. For example, the fate of intravenous [^{99m}Tc]iminiodiacetic acid (or related compounds) in the biliary tree and digestive tract can be observed by scintigraphy.[17] If duodenogastric reflux occurs, the isotope is seen in the stomach and the percentage of the total administered dose that has been refluxed into the stomach can be calculated. At the same time the patient can take a drink of

[^{113m}In]DPTA or [^{111}In]DPTA labelled liquid and gastric emptying can be monitored.

Since a wide variety of factors influence the measurement of gastric emptying,[6] the conditions of gastric emptying rate measurement should be standardized carefully. Several factors appear to be important for the accuracy of scintigraphic studies of gastric emptying. These factors include stability of radionuclide markers and high labelling efficiency, standardized meal composition and size (Figure 21.1), standard patient position during imaging, correction techniques for radionuclide decay and imaging protocol. Each of these items should receive close attention so that valid results from comparisons of gastric emptying rate measurements between control and patient groups or between sequential investigations in the same subject are obtained.

Reproducibility studies in normal subjects have shown variability in the day-to-day measurement of gastric emptying rates, which perhaps reflects the many factors that may influence this process.[2,18–21] The importance of correction techniques and their influence on errors during collimation has been emphasized.[6,7,22–24] If gastric emptying rate measurements are performed, a facility should generate control measurements in healthy, age-matched volunteers.

Radiolabelled food can be seen by scintigraphy to move anteriorly as it descends from the fundus into the antrum and this movement may increase anterior counts due to decreased tissue attenuation.[7] Christian et al.[22] have indicated that corrections for varying depth and attenuation are most important in studies using large meals in normal-sized or obese individuals. In the absence of dual heads for imaging it has been suggested that the patient can be imaged from in front and turned immediately to be imaged from behind and the geometric mean calculated for respective gastric regions of interest.[22] In earlier studies, Christian et al.[25] found that the average half emptying time for a 300 g meal can be overestimated by approximately

10% by anterior imaging alone, with the highest overestimate being 50%.

Gastric emptying data acquired by scintigraphy can be presented in a variety of ways and some methods of analysis may be more sensitive for detecting abnormalities in gastric emptying. Since gastric emptying of liquids occurs in an approximately exponential manner with time, liquid emptying can be expressed as a half-time or as the percentage of the isotope emptied by the stomach in a given time. Unfortunately, deviations from exponential and linear emptying curves are common (Figure 21.2). In contrast, solids empty from the stomach in a linear manner with time and results for solid emptying are best expressed as the amount emptied per unit time, or perhaps the percentage of isotope emptied per minute. Quantitation of an early emptying percentage (e.g. the amount of the liquid or solid phase of a test meal emptied in 10 or 15 minutes) is useful in defining problems with receptive relaxation (liquids) or gastric incontinence (liquids and solids). The importance of standardization for reporting gastric emptying data has been emphasized.[26] Mathematical models for analysis of gastric emptying data, such as power exponential analysis, do not add materially to clinical usage of the test. Although gastric emptying is often expressed as a half emptying time, this measurement describes only a limited area of the gastric emptying curve.

TESTS OF GASTRIC SECRETION

Three phases of gastric acid secretion have been recognized: cephalic, gastric and intestinal. In the first two phases, acid is 'switched on'; in the third it is 'turned off' (see Chapter 20). All these phases proceed simultaneously by complex interactions between neural and hormonal stimuli in the central nervous system, stomach and duodenum. The process of gastric acid secretion is integrated from the first perceptions of food to more than 1 hour postprandially.

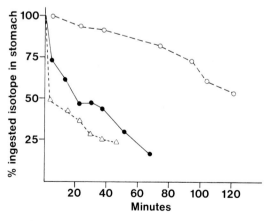

Figure 21.2
Abnormal patterns of gastric emptying curves in three individuals. Note the deviation from linear or exponential forms. In healthy individuals and in disease states deviations from linear and exponential emptying profiles are apparent in the three emptying curves.

The introduction of flexible orogastric tubes and aspiration techniques by Rehfuss[27] led to the fractional analysis approach. Over the ensuing 30–40 years many different test meals were introduced and chemical indicators were applied to measure gastric acidity.[28] Hollander[29] proposed the two-component hypothesis for gastric secretion after studies of the electrolyte content of gastric juice. Kay[30] put forward the concept of maximal stimulation of acid output, and Card and Marks[31] indicated the correlation between parietal cell mass and maximal acid secretion.

Although many academic physicians have built a research career on acid secretory studies, few clinical circumstances dictate the need for such testing (Table 21.3). There are basically three important gastric secretory function tests. These include basal, pentagastrin- and insulin-stimulated secretion, which all require orogastric intubation. Basal secretion is collected from a nasogastric tube as one 60-min or four 15-min aspirates. The volume, pH and titrable acid in the aspirate are measured and the reading is expressed in millimoles of hydrochloric acid per hour. The normal range for basal acid output (BAO) is 1–5 mmol/h but 4% of normal individuals may have a BAO of more than 10 mmol/h. The BAO is often high in the Zollinger–Ellison syndrome, and a ratio of basal acid output: maximal acid output of more than 60% suggests this diagnosis.

Maximal acid output (MAO) is the total acid output during the hour after maximal pentagastrin stimulation (pentagastrin 6 µg/kg sc) or during the peak hour after maximal betazole stimulation (betazole 40 µg/kg). More than 40 mmol/h of acid can be found in 40% of normal individuals. The peak acid output (PAO) is a measurement based on the two highest consecutive 15-min periods of acid output following stimulation. This value

Table 21.3 The limited clinical role of gastric acid secretory testing

CLINICALLY USEFUL CIRCUMSTANCE	NO CLINICAL RELEVANCE	CONTRAINDICATIONS
Diagnosis and management of (ZE) syndrome*	Routine peptic ulcer	Pyloric obstruction
Investigation of hypergastrinaemia, e.g. pernicious anaemia†	Surgical planning‡	Anatomic deformity of upper gastrointestinal tract
Severe recurrent peptic ulceration, e.g. ZE, postgastric surgery	Distinguish benign and malignant ulcer disease	Recurrent upper gastrointestinal bleeding

*Serum gastrin estimation and response to secretin is more accurate for the diagnosis of Zollinger–Ellison (ZE) syndrome.
†Serum B_{12} levels and a Schilling test are more sensitive and specific.
‡The estimation of acid output pre- or postoperatively cannot predict the likelihood of recurrent ulceration, though with a positive insulin test are more likely to get a recurrent ulcer after vagotomy.

is doubled to express the measurement in millimoles per hour. It has been noted that PAO will occur in 50% of cases in the interval from 15 to 45 min after maximal stimulation with a secretagogue. Other secretagogues have been used, e.g. intravenous histamine infusion, Histalog (1.7 mg/kg) and histamine acid phosphate (10 µg/kg). Pentagastrin has been particularly favoured because it has only minimal transitory side-effects in the dose of 0.6 µg/kg when given by intramuscular or subcutaneous injection.

The insulin test is based on the fact that hypoglycaemia is a potent stimulus to acid secretion and the major component of the stimulus is via the vagus nerve. Vagotomy will, therefore, abolish the secretory response to insulin-induced hypoglycaemia and the insulin test forms the basis of investigations which assess vagal integrity and, by inference, completeness of surgical vagotomy. In this test, venous blood (2 ml) is withdrawn at zero time and 0.2 units/kg of soluble insulin (preferably monocomponent) are injected through the same needle. Eight 15-min gastric aspirates are collected and venous blood is taken, for blood glucose estimation, at 30 and 45 minutes after the insulin infusion. An insulin test must be preceded by a basal 1-h collection and it may be followed by a pentagastrin stimulation test. During the insulin test careful patient observation should be maintained and concentrated dextrose (50 ml of 50% solution) should be available for injection in case the subject lapses into hypoglycaemic coma. There is considerable debate over the interpretation of a normal or abnormal insulin test. It is generally agreed that an incomplete vagotomy is likely to be present if the 2-h postinsulin acid output exceeds the 2-h basal output by more than 0.5 mmol/h or if the acid output is perceived to be greater than 2 mmol/h above the basal collection; alternatively, a rise of acid concentration of 20 mmol/l after insulin has been used, in the first hour to indicate an early response and in the second hour a late response.

In recent years it has become recognized increasingly that the rate of acid secretion in response to food has relevance to the studies of upper gastrointestinal disease. Early information on the secretory response of the stomach to food was obtained from experiments in laboratory animals with gastric pouches. Rune[32] estimated acid output in response to a solid meal, but this technique required arterial puncture in order to measure changes in arterial base.

Fordtran and Walsh[33] suggested a method for measuring gastric acid secretion in the presence of food in the human stomach. These workers assessed the acid secretory response to a meal consisting of steak, bread and butter by intragastric titration with sodium bicarbonate. Malagelada and colleagues[34] used a much more refined technique with both gastric and duodenal markers to measure gastric secretory responses without artificially maintaining the pH of the stomach at 5.5. This avoided the possibility of substantially altering perhaps both gastric acid secretion and serum gastrin levels. Using Fordtran's[33] technique, but substituting a meat extract (Oxo) for the steak meal, Taylor et al.[35] developed a novel test for gastric acid secretion in humans.

Tubeless gastric secretory tests have not been generally accepted and they have been regarded as strictly qualitative.

Dye tests and radiotelemetry cannot be recommended for routine clinical use because even in the assessment of achlorhydria false-positive and false-negative results are common. The dye tests (Diagnex Blue Test, Squibb) utilize a carboxylic cation exchange resin, the hydrogen ions of which have been replaced by those of an indicator's cation. After ingestion, the indicator cations are released from the resin by hydrogen ions if acid is present in the gastric secretion. The indicator cations which are released in the stomach are absorbed and excreted in the urine and their quantitation provides an indirect indication of gastric acidity.

In recent times, much interest has focused on the measurement of 24 h intragastric acidity using direct pH recordings. This interest has emerged during the research and development of several new antisecretory drugs. These techniques are used to investigate the effects of drugs on nocturnal and meal stimulated acid secretion. Several commercially available 24 h pH monitoring methods are available, where a pH electrode is placed in the gastric lumen and pH data are collected by an analogue solid-state recorder which can be interfaced with a computer to give a 24 h record of intragastric pH. The positioning of the electrode is very important for accurate intragastric pH measurements because pH in the stomach varies by location. Effective H^+ activity is measured and this can be converted into acid concentration by a correction factor (activity coefficient). To convert pH measurements accurately into concentration, precise measurements of Na^+ and K^+ in gastric aspirates are required, but in clinical use the sum of $Na^+ + K^+$ can be assumed to be about 50 mmol/l. Tables for conversion of electrode pH values to hydrogen ion concentration in gastric juice are available and should be corrected for temperature.

CONCENTRATION OF RADIOISOTOPES BY THE STOMACH: APPLICATIONS

Isotopic scanning of the stomach following the intravenous administration of ^{99m}Tc pertechnetate (TcO_4^-) has been proposed as a technique for estimating acid output but its reliability is in question. The concentration of TcO_4^- by the stomach has been investigated by many scientific groups. Herbert et al.[36] calculated a stomach uptake of TcO_4^- of 6% of the total administered dose at 5 h using a rectilinear scanner. Using similar methods, Irvine et al.[37] measured a gastric uptake of between 2.8 and 13.3% of the administered dose in six normal individuals at 1 h, and Harden et al.[38] derived figures of 2.4–11.4% in ten normal subjects at 1 h, with 1.3–5.5% at 20 min. The ability of TcO_4^- to localize in gastric mucosa has led to the use of this compound for the imaging of Meckel's diverticulum which may contain ectopic stomach epithelium,[39–47] the diagnosis of Barrett's epithelium in the oesophagus,[48,49] the location of intrathoracic gastrogenic cysts[50] and the detection of retained gastric antrum after surgery.[51] It has also been used to detect jejunal intussusception,[52] intestinal duplication,[53] perforation of the stomach,[54,55] neoplasia[56] and intestinal mucosal disease.[57]

There is considerable debate about the precise mechanism of handling of TcO_4^- by the stomach. The concept that the secretion of TcO_4^- by the parietal cell gains indirect support from studies that have demonstrated a correlation between acid output and pertechnetate clearance.[58-60] Premedication with the parietal cell agonist pentagastrin increases the uptake of TcO_4^- in the mouse stomach by 65%.[61] Sfakianakis et al.[62] demonstrated that pentagastrin will accelerate the accumulation of TcO_4^- in implanted vascularized patches of ectopic gastric mucosa, but the net effect of the secretagogue is a lowering of target to background ratio due to washout of the intraluminal activity with an associated increase in background activity.

To add to the controversy surrounding the cellular handling of TcO_4^-, there are a number of autoradiographic studies which have shown concentration of the isotope by gastric columnar mucous epithelium. These studies show such localization occurring in the dog,[63,64] the rat[65] and the mouse,[66] without a major degree of radioactivity in parietal or chief cells. Furthermore, tissue containing non-parietal cells, such as the gastric antrum, can be visualized at scintigraphy after administration of TcO_4^-.[51,60] Perhaps some of the most convincing evidence that the parietal cell does not exclusively concentrate TcO_4^- comes from studies in patients with pernicious anaemia, in whom the stomach may often be visualized by external scintigraphy.[37,52,65] Conflicting views about the mechanism of TcO_4^- concentration by stomach epithelium is not likely to be the result of different methods used in various studies but could relate to species difference.

Studies in humans[58,67] provide evidence of a relationship between gastric mucosal blood flow and TcO_4^- clearance. Bickel et al. reported that for a given level of secretory stimulation with betazole (histamine) there was a good relationship between the gastric clearance of TcO_4^-, aminopyrine or iodine and gastric secretion. Their method has been challenged by those scientists who do not accept the assumption that pertechnetate secretion is predominantly parietal with the non-parietal contribution being related to blood levels of the isotope in a 'passive' manner. Taylor et al.[59] have shown that TcO_4^- clearance by the rat stomach correlates with amino[^{14}C]pyrine and [^{3}H]quinine clearance under basal conditions. In separate experiments, Taylor et al.[67,68] compared gastric acid secretion and TcO_4^- clearance by the stomach and proposed that external scintiscanning of the stomach after intravenous TcO_4^- administration gives a useful semiquantitative measure of gastric acid secretion in a non-invasive manner.

CONCLUSION

Accurate measurements of gastric emptying rate can be achieved by scintigraphy. These tests are useful in managing patients with upper digestive symptoms of diverse cause. Gastric acid secretory testing has little role in clinical practice but remains important in the research of acid-related disease.

REFERENCES

1. Griffith GH, Owen GM, Kirkman S & Shields R. Measurement of rate of gastric emptying using chromium-51. *Lancet* 1966; **i:** 1244–1245.
2. Heading RC, Tothill P, McLoughlin GP & Shearman DJC. Gastric emptying rate of measurement in man: a double isotope scanning technique for simultaneous study of liquid and solid components of a meal. *Gastroenterology* 1976; **71:** 45–50.
3. Harvey RF, Brown NJG, Mackie DB, Keeling DH & Davies WT. Measurement of gastric emptying time with a gamma camera. *Lancet* 1970; **i:** 16–18.
4. Van Dam APM. The gamma camera in clinical evaluation of gastric emptying. *J Nucl Med* 1971; **110:** 371–374.
5. Malmud LS, Fisher RS, Knight LC & Rock E. Scintigraphic evaluation of gastric emptying. *Semin Nucl Med* 1982; **12:** 116–125.
6. Tothill P, McLoughlin GP & Heading RC. Techniques and errors in scintigraphic measurements of gastric emptying. *J Nucl Med* 1978; **19:** 256–261.
7. Tothill P, McLoughlin GP, Holt S & Heading RC. The effect of posture on errors in gastric emptying measurements. *Phys Med Biol* 1980; **25:** 6: 1071–1077.
8. Ostick DG, Green G, Howe K, Dymock IW & Cowley DJ. Simple clinical method of measuring gastric emptying of solid meals. *Gut* 1976; **17:** 189–191.
9. Holt S, Neal C, Colliver J & Guram M. Measurement of gastric emptying rate in humans: simplified, scanning method. *Dig Dis Sci* 1990; **35:** 1345–1351.
10. Moore JG, Christian PE & Coleman RE. Gastric emptying of varying meal weight and composition in man: evaluation of dual liquid and solid phase isotopic method. *Dig Dis Sci* 1981; **26:** 16–22.
11. Heading RC, Tothill P, Laidlaw AJ & Shearman DJC. An evaluation of 113 m indium DTPA chelate in the measurement of gastric emptying by scintiscanning. *Gut* 1971; **12:** 611–615.
12. Meyer JH, Macgregor IL, Gueller R, Martin P & Cavalieri R. ^{99m}Tc-tagged chicken liver as a marker of solid food in the human stomach. *Dig Dis* 1976; **21:** 296–304.
13. Holt S, Reid J, Taylor TV & Tothill P. Gastric emptying in solids in man. *Gut* 1982; **23:** 292–296.
14. MacGregor IL, Parent J & Meyer JH. Gastric emptying of liquid meals and pancreatic and biliary secretion after subtotal gastrectomy or truncal vagotomy and pyloroplasty in man. *Gastroenterology* 1977; **72:** 195–205.
15. Weiner K, Graham LS, Reedy T, Elashoff J & Meyer JH. Simultaneous gastric emptying of two solid foods. *Gastroenterology* 1981; **81:** 257–266.
16. Carlson GL. Radiolabelled fiber. A physiologic marker for gastric emptying and intestinal transit of solids. *Dig Dis Sci* 1980; **25:** 81–87.
17. Muhammed I, Holt S, McGloughlin GP & Taylor TV. Non-invasive estimation of duodenogastric reflux using technetium-99 m iminodiacetic acid. *Lancet* 1980; **ii:** 1162–1165.
18. Calderson M, Sonnemaker RE, Hersh T & Burdine JA. ^{99m}Tc-human albumin microspheres (HAM) for measuring the rate of gastric emptying. *Radiology* 1971; **101:** 371–374.
19. Chaudhuri TK. Use of ^{99m}Tc-DTPA for measuring gastric emptying time. *J Nucl Med* 1974; **15:** 391–395.
20. Sheiner HJ, Quinlan MF & Thompson IJ. Gastric motility and emptying in normal and post-vagotomy subjects. *Gut* 1980; **21:** 753.
21. Collins, PJ, Horowitz M, Cook DJ, Harding PE & Shearman DJC. Gastric emptying in normal subjects – a reproducible technique using a single scintillation camera and computer system. *Gut* 1983; **24:** 1117–1125.
22. Christian PE, Datz FL, Sorenson JA & Taylor A. Technical factors in gastric emptying studies. *J Nucl Med* 1983; **24:** 264–267.
23. Van Deventer G, Thomson J & Graha LS. Validations of corrections for errors in collimation on measuring gastric emptying of nuclide labelled meals. *J Nucl Med* 1983; **24:** 187–196.
24. Meyer JH, VanDeventer G & Graham LS. Error and corrections with scintigraphic measurement of gastric emptying of solid foods. *J Nucl Med* 1983; **24:** 197–203.
25. Christian PE, Moore JG & Sorenson JA. Meal size and gastric emptying. *J. Nucl Med* 1981; **22:** 831–832.
26. Elashoff JD, Reedy TJ & Meyer JH. Analysis of gastric emptying data. *Gastroenterology* 1982; **83:** 1306–1312.
27. Rehfuss ME. History of the development of gastric analysis procedures. In *Diseases of the Stomach* (1927). Cited by Hollander F & Penner A. History of gastric analysis. *Am J Dig Dis.* 1938; **5:** 739–743.
28. Hollander F & Penner A. History of gastric analysis. *Am J Dig Dis* 1938; **5:** 739–743.
29. Hollander 1932.
30. Kay AW. The effect of large doses of histamine on gastric secretion of HCl. *BMJ* 1953; **2:** 77–80.
31. Card WI & Marks IN. The relationship between acid output of the stomach following 'maximal' histamine stimulation and the parietal cell mass. *Clin Sci* 1960; **19:** 147–163.
32. Rune SJ. Comparison of the rates of gastric acid secretion in man after ingestion of food and after maximal stimulation with histamine. *Gut* 1966; **7:** 344.

33. Fordtran JS & Walsh JH. Gastric acid secretion rate and buffer content of the stomach after eating. *J Clin Invest* 1973; **52:** 645–657.

34. Malagelada JR, Longstreth GF, Summerskill WHJ & Go VLW. Measurement of gastric functions during digestion of ordinary solid meals in man. *Gastroenterology* 1976; **70:** 203–210.

35. Taylor TV, Elder JB, Ganguli PC & Gillespie IE. Comparison of an intragastric method of estimating acid output with the pentagastrin test in normal and duodenal ulcer subjects. *Gut* 1978; **19:** 865–869.

36. Herbert B, Kulke W & Shepherd RTH. The use of technetium 99m as a clinical tracer element. *Postgrad Med J* 1965; **41:** 656–662.

37. Irvine WJ, Stewart AG, McLoughlin GP & Tothill P. Appraisal of application of 99mTc in assessment of gastric function. *Lancet* 1967; **ii:** 648–653.

38. Harden R McG, Alexander WD & Kennedy I. Isotope uptake and scanning of stomach in man with 99mTc-pertechnetate. *Lancet* 1967; **i:** 1305–1309.

39. Jewett TC, Duszynski DO & Allen JE. The visualisation of Meckel's diverticulum with 99mTc pertechnetate. *Surgery* 1970; **68:** 567–571.

40. Kilpatrick AM & Aseron CA Jr. Radioisotope detection of Meckel's diverticulum causing acute rectal hemorrhage. *N Engl J Med* 1972; **287:** 563–566.

41. Rosenthal L, Henry JN, Murphy DA & Freeman LM. Radiopertechnetate imaging of the Meckel's diverticulum. *Radiology* 1972; **105:** 371–376.

42. Berquist TH, Nolan NG & Adson MA. Diagnosis of Meckel's diverticulum by radioisotope scanning. *Mayo Clin Proc* 1973; **48:** 98–103.

43. Geerken RG & Collin DB. 99mTc sodium pertechnetate scanning of the abdomen, a valuable tool for detection of Meckel's diverticulum. *Med Ann D* 1973; **42:** 556–561.

44. Jaros R, Schussheim A & Levy LM. Preoperative diagnosis of bleeding Meckel's diverticulum utilising 99mtechnetium pertechnetate scinti-imaging. *J Pediatr* 1973; **82:** 45–53.

45. Leoinadas JC & Germann DR. Technetium 99mpertechnetate imaging in diagnosis of Meckel's diverticulum. *Arch Dis Child* 1974; **49:** 21–28.

46. Wine CR, Nahrwold DL & Waldhusen JA. Role of the technetium scan in the diagnosis of Meckel's diverticulum. *J Pediatr Surg* 1974; **9:** 885–891.

47. Ho JE & Konieczny KE. The pertechnetate Tc99m scan: an aid in the evaluation of gastrointestinal bleeding. *Paediatrics* 1975; **66:** 34–39.

48. Berquist TH, Nolan NG, Carlson HC & Stephens DH. Diagnosis of Barrett's esophagus by pertechnetate scinitigraphy. *Mayo Clin Proc* 1973; **48:** 256–260.

49. Gordon F, Ramirez-Delgollado J, Munoz R, Cuaren A & Lauda L. Diagnosis of Barrett's esophagus with radioisotopes. *Am J Roentgenol Radium Ther Nucl Med* 1974; **121:** 716–721.

50. Mark R, Young L & Sutherland JB. Diagnosis of intrathoracic gastrogenic cyst using 99mTc pertechnetate. *Radiology* 1973; **109:** 137–142.

51. Chaudhuri TK, Chaudhuri TK & Safaie-Shirazi S. Radioisotope scan – a possible aid in differentiating retained gastric antrum from Zollinger–Ellison syndrome in patients with recurrent peptic ulcer. *Gastroenterology* 1973; **65:** 697–703.

52. Mikolajkow A & Chomicki OA. Scanning of the stomach with 99mTc. *Digestion* 1970; **3:** 357–361.

53. Hofmeyer NG. Stomach scanning after intravenous 99mTc administration; preliminary report. *S Afr Med J* 1967; **41:** 472–474.

54. Schwesinger WH, Croon RD & Habibian MR. Diagnosis of an enteric duplication with pertechnetate 99mTc scanning. *Ann Surg* 1975; **181:** 428–431.

55. Barkley RM, Munoz O & Parkey RW. Intestinal duplication detected with technetium 99m sodium pertechnetate imaging of the abdomen. *Dig Dis* 1977; **22:** 1122–1127.

56. Duszynski DO & Anthane R. Jejunal intussusception demonstrated by Tc99m pertechnetate and abdominal scanning. *Am J Roentgenol Radium Ther Nucl Med* 1970; **109:** 729–732.

57. Holt S, Ford MJ, Graham S & Heading RC. Abnormal gastric emptying in primary anorexia nervosa. *Br J Psychiatry* 1981; **139:** 550–552.

58. Bickel JG, Witten TA & Killian MK. Use of pertechnetate clearance in the study of gastric physiology. *Gastroenterology* 1972; **63:** 60–66.

59. Taylor TV, Pullen BR, Elder JB & Torrance B. Observations of gastric mucosal blood flow using 99mTc in rat and man. *Br J Surg* 1975; **62:** 788–791.

60. Wine CR, Nahrwold DL, Rose RC & Miller KS. Effect of histamine on technetium 99m excretion by the gastric mucosa. *Surgery* 1976; **80:** 591–594.

61. Khettery J, Eftmann E & Grand RJ. Effect of pentagastrin, histalog, glucagon, secretin, and perchlorate on the gastric handling of 99mTc-pertechnetate in mice. *Radiology* 1976; **120:** 629–631.

62. Sfakianakis GN, Anderson GF & King DR. The effect of gastrointestinal hormones on the pertechnetate imaging of ectopic gastric mucosa in experimental Meckel's diverticulum. *J Nucl Med* 1981; **22:** 678–683.

63. Marsden DS, Alexander C, Yeung P, Dunn A & Lazarevic B. Autoradiographic explanation for the uses of 99mTc in gastric scintiphotography. *J Nucl Med* 1973; **14:** 632 (abstract).

64. Priebe CJ, Marsden DS & Lazarevic B. The use of 99mtechnetium pertechnetate to detect transplanted gastric mucosa in the dog. *J Pediatr Surg* 1974; **9:** 605–613.

65. Bartelink A, Smeets EHJ, Hoedemaker Ph Y, Veeger WA, Worldring MG & Abels J. 99mTc in the examination of the stomach. In *Proceedings of the IXth International Congress on Internal Medicine*. Congress Series 137. Amsterdam: Excerpta Medica, 1966: 381–387.

66. Chaudhuri TK, Heading RC, Greenwald A & Chaudhuri TK. Measurement of gastric emptying time (GET) of solid meal using 99mTc-DTPA. *J Nucl Med* 1974; **15:** 483–488.

67. Taylor TV, Bone D & Torrance B. A non-invasive test of gastric function. *Br J Surg* 1977; **64:** 702–708.

68. Taylor TV. Non-invasive investigation of the upper gastrointestinal tract using technetium 99m. *Ann R Coll Surg Engl* 1979; **61:** 37–44.

22

GASTRIC MUCOSAL DEFENCE MECHANISMS

T Scratcherd

The gastrointestinal tract has defensive mechanisms which protect it from injury by both internal and external aggression. The process begins in the mouth where the exquisite senses of taste, touch and temperature allow the acceptance or rejection of substances according to their character and from the learning process of past experience. Some irritants pass the buccal mechanism and enter the stomach and are rejected by vomiting; others remain to cause damage to the mucosa. This chapter deals with those processes that combat or prevent damage to the gastroduodenal mucosa, these being either intrinsic or extrinsic in origin. Mucus plays an important role in this process and is the first part of the defensive mechanism.

MUCUS

Mucus is secreted by the surface cells of the gastroduodenal mucosa. Three phases may be recognized: the presecreted intracellular store which gives the stained epithelium its characteristic appearance: a viscous soluble mucus within the luminal content; and a water-insoluble transluscent gel which adheres to the epithelial surface and forms a continuous cover over the whole of the mucosa. When examined on unfixed specimens it has a thickness in humans that varies between 50 and 450 μm, with a mean thickness of about 180 μm[1] (Figure 22.1). Whereas the mucosal surface as well as the gastric pits are covered, mucus does not line the gastric glands and as yet there is no satisfactory explanation as to how the glands are protected from the action of acid and pepsin. The mucus that appears in the fluid of the lumen is mainly water-soluble and includes degraded mucus (subunit form) formed by the action of pepsin on the adherent gel. Mucus protects the mucosa from damage during the normal processes of digestion.

Rheological studies on isolated mucous gel and studies in vivo demonstrate that it has considerable stability.[3] Its structure remains unchanged after exposure to isotonic saline over 24 hours, to solutions varying from pH 1 to pH 8, to bile and to hypertonic solutions (2 M) of NaCl. It is highly resistant to mechanical disruption and it will flow and reseal over 30–120 minutes. It is these properties that allow mucous to maintain a continuous effective adherent cover over the mucosal surface, and its viscoelastic properties are ideal in protecting against mechanical damage by foodstuffs as they are being continually

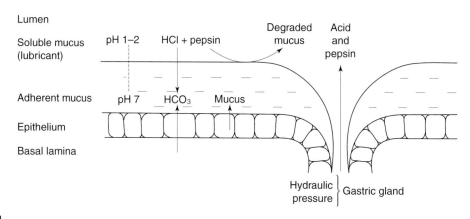

Figure 22.1
The mucus–bicarbonate barrier showing the adherent mucous layer and mechanisms that protect against acid and pepsin. (Reproduced from Allen et al.[2])

triturated by movements brought about by antral muscle contraction during mixing and gastric emptying. The adherent and the soluble mucus form a slimy lubricant which allows the easy passage, to and fro, of gastric chyme. Yet mucus remains strongly adherent to the mucosa. Mucus protects not only against these physical forces, but also against those chemical agents (acid and pepsin) that are designed to attack protein.

Mucin glycoprotein structure

Mucous glycoproteins are large molecules (2–45×10^6 molecular weight) made up of units (usually referred to as a subunit, with a molecular weight of 5×10^5), joined together by disulphide bridges.[4] Each subunit consists of a protein core to which are attached oligosaccharide side-chains. The latter are linked to the protein core by *O*-glycosidic bonds between *N*-acetylgalactosamine and serine or threonine. These side-chains, which may be branched, project from the protein core to produce a close packing so that the oligosaccharides form a sheath of carbohydrate around the protein backbone. The subunit has been likened to a bottlebrush, where the protein core is the wire and the carbohydrate chains represent the bristles (Figure 22.2).

The constituent sugars (up to 19 for gastric mucus) of the oligosaccharides are galactose, *N*-acetylgalactosamine, *N*-acetylglucosamine, fucose and sialic acid. Ester sulphate groups are also carried on the sugar chains, and these together with sialic acid give the chains a negative charge. The molar ratio of these sugars can vary in different regions of the gastrointestinal tract and in different species, and in some glycoproteins one or more of these sugars may be absent. Human mucous glycoproteins from all regions of the gastrointestinal tract have ABH antigens for the ABO blood group system. The presence of strong negatively charged groups on the carbohydrate side-chains results in molecular expansion and an increase in viscosity. A most important feature of the glycoproteins is the hydrophilic action of the carbohydrate side-chains. Water molecules are strongly attracted to the matrix formed by the side-chains and become trapped within the interstices of the gel, thus accounting for the fact that 95% of mucus is water.[4] Two structural regions are recognized in each subunit: a glyco-sylated region with closely packed carbohydrate, in which the protein backbone is buried and forms a protective sheath guarding it from proteolytic attack; and a non-glycosylated region where there are few carbohydrate chains attached. This latter state leaves the protein core exposed and accessible to attack by proteolytic enzymes such as pepsin. It is at these non-glycolysate sites of the protein core that the disulphide bridges join the subunits together to form the polymeric mucin structure.

The viscous and gel-forming properties of native mucus are lost if the mucous glycoprotein is dissociated into its subunits. Mucous gel only forms with polymeric mucin molecules created by covalent interactions at high concentrations. The nature of these interactions is unknown but it has been suggested that there is an interdigitation of the carbohydrate side-chains between adjacent mucin molecules or that a more specific lectin-type interaction occurs.[6] The precise chemical structure of these carbohydrate side-chains does not determine whether these molecules are able to form a gel. As noted above, although the composition of the terminal sugars varies according to secretor status gel formation is unaffected.

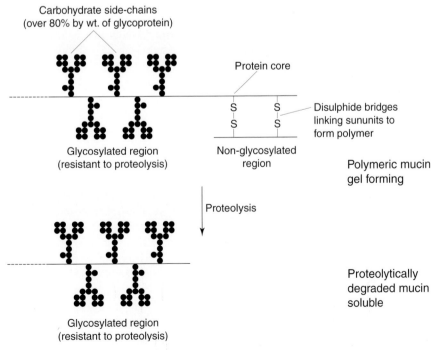

Figure 22.2

The structure of gastric mucin, showing the site of proteolysis associated with the breakdown of polymeric mucin.[5]

SECRETION OF BICARBONATE BY THE GASTRIC MUCOSA

Bicarbonate secretion is controlled by local, hormonal and neuronal factors. These have been investigated by inhibiting acid secretion with histamine H_2-receptor antagonists or by the H^+, K^+-ATPase inhibitor omeprazole, as they have been found not to inhibit fundic secretion of bicarbonate. This procedure allows bicarbonate to be collected and not dissipated as CO_2 in a reaction with simultaneously produced acid. Basal rates of HCO_3^- secretion vary from 0.3 to 1.0 μmol/cm^2 per hour, rates that are said to correspond to 2–10% of the maximum acid secretion in the same species. The secretory mechanisms of bicarbonate by the antrum and H^+-inhibited oxyntic area appear to be identical.[7] The process of bicarbonate secretion is largely active, because in in vitro preparations secretion is inhibited by anoxia or the addition to the organ bath of dinitrophenol or cyanide. Cellular mechanisms have been studied chiefly in amphibia, where precise control of the ionic environment may be maintained and where potential differences and ionic fluxes have been accurately measured. In such preparations *Rana temporaria* fundic mucosa requires luminal chloride to support bicarbonate secretion. As secretion is not associated with changes in transmembrane potential, an electroneutral Cl^-/HCO_3^- exchange at the luminal membrane has been proposed. Since carbonic anhydrase has been located in the apical cytoplasm, it has been suggested that some bicarbonate (<5%) is produced by hydration of CO_2 from cell metabolism, but it is largely concerned with maintaining cellular acid–base status. This view is supported by the observation that acetazolamide (a carbonic anhydrase inhibitor) inhibits secretion when administered into the lumen. There are some differences among the various species used, but the consensus of opinion is that bicarbonate enters the surface cell over the basolateral membrane via a sodium-dependent 4,4-diisothiocyano-2,2-disulphonate stilbene (DIDS)-sensitive mechanism and that the membrane contains a Na^+,K^+-ATPase. However, a precise description of cellular events cannot yet be given as there are many interspecies differences and there is a lack of adequate data.[7] Secretion in vitro can be stimulated by stable cholinergic drugs, dibutyryl cyclic GMP and some prostanoids. Cyclic GMP diesterase is also present in the surface mucosal cells where it is thought to be the intracellular messenger. A cholinergic mechanism appears to be important in vivo because bicarbonate secretion is stimulated by stable cholinergic drugs such as bethanecol.

Stimulation of the cut peripheral end of the cervical vagus nerve in the anaesthetized cat[8] increases acid secretion 6–10-fold and causes a modest increase in bicarbonate output from 20–60%. Duodenal bicarbonate increases further from 65 to 155%. Hexamethonium abolishes the effect and atropine reduces the response considerably but does not quite abolish it.[9] Basal bicarbonate secretion is unaffected by these drugs. The failure of atropine completely to abolish the effects of vagal stimulation suggests that a component of the response is non-cholinergic. Some of the prostaglandins ($PGF_{2\alpha}$ and synthetic analogues such as 16,16-dimethyl-PGE_2) are effective and

so is the hormone cholecystokinin, but histamine, secretin and pentagastrin are not. There is some evidence that neurotensin, pancreatic polypeptide and glucagon may stimulate bicarbonate secretion. The movements of other ions, either through the apical or basolateral membranes of the surface cell, have not been fully elucidated. Although sodium movements parallel those of bicarbonate into the lumen, the mere act of increasing luminal pH in the antrum increases mucosal permeability.[10,11] If this mechanism also applies to the oxyntic area, the manipulations necessary to determine bicarbonate secretion could themselves have an effect on the transport mechanisms. At the moment there are only sufficient data to give a sketchy description of secretory mechanisms.

GASTRIC BICARBONATE SECRETION IN HUMANS

Bicarbonate secretion in humans has been studied by inhibiting acid secretion with H_2-receptor antagonists. Physiological sodium chloride solutions were perfused at high rates through the stomach, and pH and $P\text{co}_2$ were measured with appropriate electrodes. The bicarbonate concentrations were calculated using the Henderson–Hasselbalch equation.[12] An alternative method depends on the assumptions made in the two-component model of gastric secretion (parietal and non-parietal secretions). A fixed relationship is assumed to exist between the osmolalities of parietal and non-parietal secretions and plasma.[13] Using the pH,$P\text{co}_2$ method the basal bicarbonate secretion has been estimated to be 236 ± 48,[14] 347 ± 100[15] and 366 ± 23 μmol/h[16] (mean ± SEM). The osmolality method gives much higher figures of 2600 ± 600 μmol/h, severalfold greater than the pH,$P\text{co}_2$ method.[13] Infusion of the stable choline ester, bethanecol, increased the output of bicarbonate. Reflex excitation of vagal efferents by sham feeding (chew and spit method) also increased bicarbonate output by about 70%, thus demonstrating that the mechanism in humans is similar to that in other animals, such as the cat, and is in part at least cholinergic. In line with this view was the observation that anticholinergic drugs inhibited about 90% of the response, leaving the residue to be secreted by some other mechanism.[16,17] The output of bicarbonate was found to be independent of gastric pH (pH 2–7) and therefore independent of acid secretion.[16] This latter finding has not been universal. Perfusion of acid through the gastric lumen has been shown to increase the bicarbonate output in humans,[18] from Heidenhain pouches in dogs[19] and from isolated gastric mucosa of amphibians.[20] Stimulation of the vagus nerve in the anaesthetized cat increased both acid and bicarbonate outputs, the bicarbonate response being slightly ahead of the acid. This phenomenon has been interpreted as a defensive mechanism, a preparatory event to combat possible acid damage.[21] When food reaches the stomach and the gastric phase begins, the stomach is distended. Graded inflation of a balloon in the corpus stimulates bicarbonate secretion, which is not abolished after proximal gastric vagotomy and therefore appears to be mediated through intramural plexuses.[16] Infusions of gastrin (G17) inhibit bicarbonate secretion, but this effect is dependent on an intact vagal innervation.[22]

After proximal gastric vagotomy the basal rate of bicarbonate secretion is increased by about 30%[23] and is reduced to preoperative levels by anticholinergics, but a year later this effect disappears. It has been claimed that proximal vagotomy is without effect on basal HCO_3^- secretion,[24] but it is important to note that it is increased in phase III of the motor migrating complex. It is not known whether this is due to the concomitant secretion of acid or to a neural mechanism acting simultaneously, which affects both motility and secretion. There are many unresolved questions relating to the interplay between the various stimuli in the physiological control of bicarbonate secretion, such as the acidity of the luminal content, vagal action and the gastrointestinal hormones.[25]

Secretion of bicarbonate by the duodenum

In species without Brunner's glands, such as the bullfrog, a high rate of bicarbonate secretion is maintained by the surface cells which decline distally.[26] The rate of alkalinization of a medium facing the duodenal mucosa is at about $1.0\ \mu mol/cm^2$ per hour, which is about 2–10 times that found in the antrum or fundus of this species. Studies using the short-circuited mucosa in an Ussing chamber have demonstrated that there is active transmucosal transport of bicarbonate and that this is about 60% of the total HCO_3^- secreted. Of the remainder, 35% is due to passive transport and 5% due to endogenous HCO_3 production. The active component is dependent on sodium in the serosal solution but not in the luminal solution and is inhibited by ouabain or frusemide when presented to the nutrient side. Secretion is independent of chloride. A model has been proposed in which HCO_3 enters the cell across the basolateral membrane coupled to Na^+ (cotransport), the movement obtaining energy from a high transmembrane sodium gradient. This gradient is kept intact by the outward movement of sodium from an oubain-sensitive $Na^+,K^+ATPase$ situated in the basolateral membrane. The bicarbonate then exits passively from the cell down an electrochemical gradient across the luminal membrane.[27] Stimulation can be brought about by prostaglandins and inhibited by cyclo-oxygenase inhibitors. Dibutyryl cAMP, gastric inhibitory polypetide and pancreatic glucagon stimulate, whereas acetazolamide inhibits this secretion.

SECRETION OF BICARBONATE IN THE INTACT ANIMAL

In both the anaesthetized and conscious animal, duodenal bicarbonate is secreted in response to prostaglandin E_2,[28-30] glucagon and gastric inhibitory peptide.[31] Vasoactive polypeptide (VIP) and carbachol are active in stimulating bicarbonate secretion in the rat. It is noteworthy that cholinergic drugs and VIP are also active bicarbonate stimulants of the cat, dog, rat and porcine pancreas[32,33] and secretion is effective in the proximal duodenum of the cat.[34] Acid in the duodenum of man releases both secretin and VIP.[35] Experiments on rat, cat, dog and humans clearly show that acid in the duodenal lumen increases bicarbonate secretion[29,36] and that the response is related to the acid concentration. Two stimulatory mechanisms

may be at work for at low pH (about 2) the effect was blocked by cyclo-oxygenase inhibitors, but at higher pH (5) these drugs were without effect. High acidities would therefore stimulate the production of prostaglandin synthesis, which has been confirmed for rat and human.[29,37] The release of a powerful humoral stimulant has been demonstrated in an experiment where two sheets of bullfrog mucosae (either from the fundus or duodenum) were mounted in parallel, with the nutrient surfaces bathed by a common solution. An acid solution of pH 2 was placed on the luminal side in the case of the fundus, and a solution of pH 4 in the case of the duodenum. Bicarbonate secretion occurred in the tissue that was exposed to less acid, whereas duodenal mucosae produced a humoral agent which stimulated bicarbonate secretion in parallel duodenal and fundic mucosae. Although stimulating bicarbonate secretion in fundic and antral tissue, the corresponding fundic mucosa did not stimulate the duodenum. Thus two different factors are involved in mediating the gastric and duodenal responses to intraluminal acid.[20] The autonomic nerves are also involved in the control of bicarbonate secretion. Electrical excitation of the vagus nerves stimulates mucosal bicarbonate output, which was only partially blocked by atropine but abolished by the ganglionic blocking agent hexamethonium. Thus both cholinergic and non-cholinergic control (possibly VIP)[21] as well as an adrenergic mechanism are effective in increasing bicarbonate output.

PROTECTIVE MECHANISMS

A most useful categorization of the forces that produce mucosal damage has been proposed by Allen and Garner,[38] who divide them into two groups, those produced by the body itself (endogenous aggressors) and those that man inflicts upon himself (exogenous aggressors):

- *Endogenous aggressors* – acid, pepsin, biliary reflux.
- *Exogenous aggressors* – Helicobacter pylori. ethanol, non-steroidal anti-inflammatory drugs (NSAIDs), hypertonic solutions, abrasions (mechanical damage).

Natural defence mechanisms have evolved against acid and pepsin and also against mechanical damage, which is a normal consequence of digestion. These defence mechanisms do little to fend off attack by some of the external aggressors.

MUCUS–BICARBONATE BARRIER

Protection against acid

The adherent mucus provides a stable layer but on its own does not provide a very effective barrier against hydrogen ions. It is a well-hydrated substance and only serves to reduce the rate of diffusion by a factor of about 4 when compared with the same thickness of fluid, so that equilibrium across the mucous layer would occur within a matter of minutes. Its effectiveness as a barrier to acid derives from the presence of bicarbonate ion, which is secreted into the adherent mucous layer by the surface epithelial cells beneath. The hydrogen ions from the lumen diffuse rapidly through the mucous gel layer and are neutralized by bicarbonate ions coming from the epithelial cells[39] (see Figure 22.1). The function of the mucus is to prevent dispersion and rapid neutralization of the bicarbonate mixing with a larger volume of acid gastric juice. Consequently a pH gradient exists between the lumen of the stomach and the surface of the epithelial cell, with a pH of about 2 on the luminal side and near neutrality at the epithelial surface. However, it has been calculated that the maximal amount of bicarbonate available is not sufficient to neutralize the H^+ when the luminal pH is 1.5.[4,39] This situation only occurs physiologically in the interdigestive periods. During the digestion of a meal, although the rate of acid secretion is highest initially, the acidity is low because of the high buffering capacity of the meal. As digestion proceeds and the stomach empties, the rate of acid secretion falls, but the acidity rises as the buffering capacity of the meal diminishes. Using the dog stomach wall in a chamber preparation it has been confirmed that there is a gradient of pH. At a luminal pH of 3.0 the average pH of mucus was 6.52, and at a luminal pH of 1.1 the gradient was completely eliminated. Further lowering of luminal pH to 1.0 caused an increase in the average maximum pH of mucus to 6.03, but simultaneously there was a significant drop in transmural potential difference which would indicate disruption of epithelial integrity. It has been suggested that the neutralization under these circumstances is due to an alternative source of bicarbonate, not directly from epithelial cells but from tissue fluid.[40] It has also been proposed that the secretory products from the oxyntic cell may be transported directly from the surface cells by capillaries. During acid secretion, for every hydrogen ion secreted into the lumen by the parietal cell, one hydroxyl group passes over the basolateral membrane into the blood to combine with CO_2 to form bicarbonate, a mechanism that could supply a ready source of bicarbonate.[41]

Protection against pepsin

The mucous gel is relatively resistant to penetration by enzymes such as pepsin, which have large molecular weights (32 000–40 000) and (because of their size) cannot diffuse through the adherent mucous layer and attack the underlying epithelial cells.[5] Thus the continuous adherent layer of mucus physically excludes the pepsin.

Instillation of acid alone into the pylorus-ligated rat stomach at pH 1 for a 2-hour period does not damage the adherent mucus or the mucosa, but if pepsin is added to the acid (1–2 mg/ml) there is a progressive disruption of the adherent mucus over the same time period associated with focal haemorrhages.[42] Since pepsin erodes the mucous layer by a proteolytic action at its surface (see Figure 22.1), its effectiveness as a barrier to peptic attack depends on the depth of the adherent mucus and the integrity of its structure. The loss of mucus by continuous hydrolysis and the release of degraded glycoprotein is made good by synthesis and secretion of new mucus by the surface epithelial cells, so maintaining the thickness of the barrier. A dynamic balance exists between secretion and digestion. Excess pepsin added to the stomach or excessive vagal stimulation by insulin-induced hypoglycaemia causes the

mucous layer to change from its normal translucent to a granular appearance with areas of discontinuity. At these points focal epithelial damage occurs, accompanied by bleeding. Under these circumstances there is an increase in the luminal mucin glycoprotein content.

The mucous barrier and peptic ulcer disease

The integrity of the mucous barrier is necessary for an effective protective function. Protection is reduced in both gastric and duodenal ulcer due to a poorer gel with loss of quality.[43] The reason for this loss is an increased rate of mucus degradation because of an increased aggressiveness of pepsin. In humans there are a number of pepsin types, of which pepsin 3 and pepsin 1 are the most important. Pepsin 3 is the major pepsin in humans, with pepsin 1 accounting for only about 3.6% of total peptic activity in non-ulcer controls. In patients with gastric ulcer and duodenal ulcer, pepsin 1 accounts for 23 and 16.5% of total peptic activity, respectively. Pepsin 1 is more mucolytic than pepsin 3, having about twice the activity at low pH, but the difference becomes more marked as the pH rises, so that at pH 4 pepsin 1 has four times the activity of pepsin 3. In addition, pepsin 1 has a potent collagenolytic action. Thus pepsin 1 digests mucus more effectively so that patients with peptic ulcer disease have an increased erosion of the mucous barrier.[44]

Recent observations relating to the gastric mucosal damaging effects of *H. pylori* are clearly important in influencing the damaging effect of acid-pepsin by back diffusion.

PROSTAGLANDINS

The prostaglandins produced by the gastrointestinal mucosa are involved both in physiological control mechanisms and in the maintenance of mucosal integrity. They also are used as therapeutic agents.

Biosynthesis of prostaglandins in the gastrointestinal tract

Endogenous prostaglandins are derived from the 20-carbon polyunsaturated fatty acids arachidonic, dihomo-γ-linolenic and eicosapentaenoic acid. The biosynthesis of cyclo-oxygenase and lipo-oxygenase eicosanoids from arachidonic acid is illustrated in Figure 22.3.

Arachidonic acid can be derived from the diet, by metabolic changes to dietary linolenic acid, or be cleaved from cell membranes by phospholipase A_2 in response to mechanical, pathological or pharmacological stimuli. Two metabolic pathways then diverge, one initiated by cyclo-oxygenase to form labile endoperoxides, and one influenced by lipo-oxygenase to form hydroperoxy intermediates (HETEs). The endoperoxides are then converted into prostacyclin, prostaglandins (PGE_2, $PGF_{2\alpha}$ and PGD_2) or thromboxane A_2, depending on the appropriate enzyme system in the tissue.[45,46]

The other arachidonic acid metabolites formed by the action of lipo-oxygenase arise from hydroperoxyeicosatetraenoic acids, which are converted into hydroxy derivatives (the HETEs) and into the leukotrienes (LTA_4, LTB_4, LTC_4 and LTD_4).

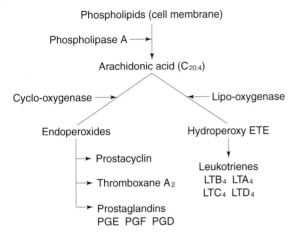

Figure 22.3
The biosynthesis of the prostaglandins and the leukotrienes.

The gastric mucosa can generate prostaglandins of the E type and also prostacyclin. The amounts formed vary according to the species, reflecting the differences in the distribution of cyclo-oxygenase and prostacyclin synthetase and probably also the experimental methods used in their estimation. The labile nature of many of the products and intermediates also makes absolute levels difficult to measure.[47,48]

Cellular sources

The gastric mucosa possesses the potential for generating prostanoids, but the precise cell source remains uncertain. Both parietal surface cells and the endothelial cells of the mucosal vasculature may have the capacity to generate prostanoids.[47,49] Enriched parietal cells from dog mucosa produce these in the following order: $PGF_{2\alpha} > PGE_2 >$ prostacyclin (measured as the metabolite 6-oxo-$PGFl_{1\alpha}$),[49] whereas rat gastric mucosa produces greater amounts of PGE_2 in parietal than non-parietal cells.

FUNCTION OF THE PROSTANOIDS

Antisecretory actions

Prostaglandins E_1 and E_2 have pronounced antisecretory effects, as demonstrated in dog, cat, rat and humans.[48] Prostanoid inhibition of acid secretion occurs with all the stimuli that excite gastric secretion, i.e. feeding, vagal stimulation, pentagastrin or histamine infusions. Prostaglandins are effective by intra-arterial or intravenous routes. Initial reports suggested that oral administration was ineffective, but this is not always the case.[50]

The advent of potent analogues has brought the prostanoids into the therapeutic arena. For example the methyl analogue of PGE_1 misoprostol is less easily metabolized, being resistant to inactivation by 15-hydroxy-prostaglandin dehydrogenase; it is also more potent and longer lasting in its effect. These analogues are effective both topically and parenterally. The use of the isolated parietal cell has been essential in the elucidation of the action of the prostaglandins. They exert their antisecretory action by specifically interfering with histamine activation of parietal cell function, thus inhibiting a catalytic subunit of adenylate cyclase and preventing the formation of cAMP (Figure 22.4).

Histamine stimulates the parietal cell through the produc-

tion of cAMP, first combining with a receptor (R_s) which is linked to the catalytic subunit of adenylate cyclase by guanine nucleotide binding protein (G_s) and causing the conversion of ATP into cAMP. Prostaglandins, on the other hand, combine with their specific receptor (R_i), which in its turn is coupled to an inhibitory guanine nucleotide binding protein (G_i), which blocks the production of cAMP by adenylate cyclase.[52] In concentrations required to inhibit acid secretion, PGE_2 and prostacyclin inhibit the intracellular rise in cAMP induced by histamine.[53] It has been shown that PGE_2 inhibits the histamine and the potentiated response to a combination of histamine and pentagastrin or histamine and carbachol, but when pentagastrin or carbachol were the only stimulants, no inhibition was observed.

In considering these events the physiological activation of the parietal cell has to be remembered.[54] It has three receptors: one each for gastrin, histamine and acetylcholine. Potentiation of the secretory response occurs when the cell is exposed to combinations of these agents. The potentiated response is greater than the sum of the individual responses. Histamine is probably being continuously secreted from some enterochromaffin-like cell, whereas gastrin and acetylcholine are phasically produced in response to a meal. With the histamine component blocked by G_i (the inhibitory GTP binding protein), acid secretion becomes inhibited.

Secretory function

It is now established that the prostaglandins have a secretory as well as an inhibitory function. They stimulate bicarbonate secretion into the surface layer of mucus and probably play an important role in maintaining the integrity of the surface cell layer.

Soluble mucus

Prostaglandins of the E series and their synthetic analogues increase the output of luminal mucus in the stomach. The magnitude of response varies between two- and fivefold stimulation. As the effect is independent of their inhibitory action on acid secretion, it has been suggested they act directly on the epithelial surface cell.[52] Whether this is a true stimulation is not yet clear, as it could be due to a 'washout' of soluble mucus associated with the surface layer, in turn brought about by bicarbonate secretion as the electrolyte flows through the gel.

Adherent mucus

There are significant increases in the adherent layer in gastric mucosa of the rat, *Rana temporaria* and humans on gastric instillation of 16,16-dimethyl PGE_2. Up to a threefold increase can be induced in a 2-hour period in the rat.

Biosynthesis of mucus

The protein core of the glycoprotein is synthesized by translation of mRNA in the rough endoplasmic reticulum, and the carbohydrate side-chains are added after transfer through the cell to the Golgi apparatus. Here *N*-acetylglycosamine becomes attached to the seryl or threonyl residues on the protein core,

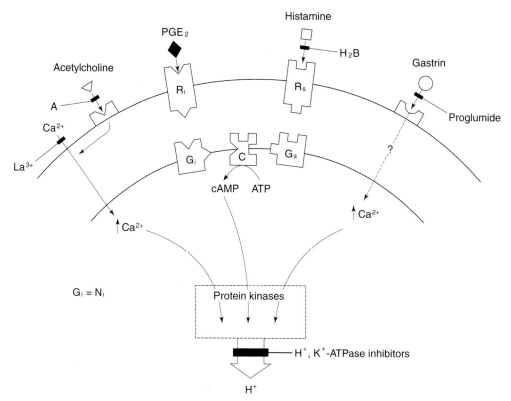

Figure 22.4

Activation of canine parietal cell. Receptors for acetylcholine, histamine and gastrin are indicated. These receptors are selectively inhibited by atropine (A), H_2 blockers (H_2B) and proglumide, respectively. Acetylcholine and gastrin are calcium dependent. Histamine acts through the adenylate cyclase system: a receptor R_s, the stimulatory guanine nucleotide binding protein, G_s, and the catalytic subunit, C. Prostaglandinns inhibit, via an inhibitory receptor, R_i, coupled to an inhibitory guanine nucleotide binding protein, G_i.[51]

followed by the stepwise addition of the sugars, one at a time, until the carbohydate chain is complete. Sialic acid and then ester sulphates are added. The glycoprotein is packaged in a compact state as membrane-bound granules which pass toward the luminal membrane of the epithelial cell. Prostaglandins stimulate the incorporation of precursors (amino acids and sugars) into mucous glycoproteins at doses less than the antisecretory dose.

Effects on the surface cell

When the synthetic analogue 15(R)-15-methyl-PGE_2 is given orally to humans over a 2-month period, there is an increase in the thickness of both antral and fundic surface cells. These changes cannot be explained by proliferative activity, but it appears that the prostanoid retards both senescence and exfoliation of cells. Similar results were obtained in rats, in which species, there was delayed elimination of thymidine from the mucosa, indicating a slowing of DNA turnover. Natural PGE_2 also produced tropic changes in rat mucosa not caused by the production of new cells as the mitotic index was reduced. Indomethacin had an antitropic effect, which suggests that endogenous prostanoids may participate in epithelial regeneration.[55-58] Prostaglandin E_2 can increase the thickness of the mucous gel and affect epithelial cell hydrophobicity and cellular restitution after injury.

Stimulus for prostaglandin secretion

The ability of the gastric mucosa to generate prostanoids would naturally lead to the conclusion that they are in some way related to physiological function, but there are difficulties in identifying the cells that produce and degrade them. The very rapid degradation of some of the prostanoids makes detection and quantification difficult. Animal experiments first suggested that luminal acid was the stimulus that caused local prostaglandin release, and this has been confirmed in man when acid instilled in the stomach increased luminal prostaglandin output and at the same time stimulated bicarbonate secretion.[18] The evidence suggests that PGE_1 is responsible for the bicarbonate secretion.[18] Since this response can be inhibited by indomethacin, it implies that prostaglandins are involved in regulation of basal secretion. Aggression to the mucosa will cause the release of prostanoids, but the link between stimulus and response has yet to be determined.

The vasoactive properties of prostaglandins

The prostanoids can increase or decrease mucosal blood, depending on experimental conditions. If there is a link between acid secretion and mucosal blood flow, then if acid secretion is inhibited, mucosal blood flow will fall. Prostanoids inhibit acid secretion, but the ratio of mucosal blood flow to acid secretion is increased. Thus if there is a line between secretion and blood flow (determined by metabolic demand) the prostanoids contribute to a vasodilator effect. Under resting conditions PGE$_2$ reduces vascular resistance and increases mucosal blood flow, whether applied topically or by intravenous or intra-arterial routes, demonstrating a direct vasodilator action. Microscopic visualization has confirmed this direct action by the observation that the submucosal arterioles are dilated and that there is an increase in red cell velocity in the mucosal capillaries and venules.[59] Prostacyclin also increases or decreases mucosal blood flow, depending on dose and whether the stomach is actively secreting acid or at rest; once again, the ratio of mucosal blood flow to acid secretion remain either unaltered or elevated.

GASTRIC BLOOD FLOW

The concept has long been accepted that gastric secretion and mucosal blood flow increase in parallel, and this is brought about largely by a redistribution of flow between mucosal and muscle layers.[60,61] However, this conclusion has been questioned largely on the grounds of methodology. Currently there is considerable debate about the validity of methods used to measure blood flow. It is out of place here to give a detailed critical analysis: the reader is thus referred to review articles by Guth and Leung[62] and Holm and Perry.[63] What is indisputable is that blood flow to the mucosa increases when a meal is taken.[64-67] What is also not in dispute is that the mucosal circulation can also be affected from higher centres, with hyperaemia (vasodilatation) or pallor (vasoconstriction) of the mucosal vessels occurring according to the psychological status (sadness or anger) of the individual.[66,67] In experimental animals electrical stimulation of the caudal hypothalamus causes a reduction in total gastric blood flow, whereas stimulation of the rostral hypothalamus increases it.[68] What is less certain is the distribution of blood flow between mucosal and muscle layers and between body and antrum, and what mechanisms bring about these changes. Claims have been made that: (1) acid secretion and mucosal blood flow are tightly linked; (2) mucosal flow can increase at the expense of the muscle circulation; (3) mucosal blood flow is a constant fraction (approximately 70–80%) of the total gastric blood flow; (4) blood flow may increase or decrease without affecting acid secretion; and (5) acid secretion may increase without affecting blood flow.[69-71] These divergent results reflect the different methodologies employed, with each of the several methods having advantages and disadvantages. They may also be based on assumptions that are only approximate, and the experiments have been performed under different conditions.

The principles that apply in general to blood flow through other tissues probably also apply to the stomach. Blood does not flow continuously through the capillaries but is intermittent (vasomotion). Flow is also determined by metabolic demand; in the fundic mucosa usage of oxygen is very high as the parietal cell concentrates hydrogen ions by a factor of 2.5 million. As evidence of this function, the parietal cell is very rich in

mitochondria, which occupy 30–40% of the cell volume. The very high oxygen consumption of the parietal cell requires a very high blood flow or very high oxygen extraction rate. The greater the metabolic demand for oxygen the shorter will be the time interval in the vasomotion phenomenon, until in periods of great oxygen usage flow will become continuous and recruitment of capillaries will occur.[72] If these conditions apply to the mucosal circulation, then under secretagogue stimulation (where gastric motility may hardly be affected) it will not be surprising that the proportion of the blood flow through the mucosa could increase in parallel with acid secretion. The reason is that it appears (from published diagrams of the gastric circulation) that the two circulations, mucosa and muscle, are mainly in parallel.[62] The flow through each would then depend on the intrinsic resistances to flow in each circulation.

What might happen to the gastric circulation under the physiological stimulus of a meal? In addition to the simple secretagogue stimulation described above, there would be different influences brought to bear on the two circulations. Gastric motility would increase, creating vasodilatation in muscle, and a reduction in resistance in this circuit would upset the previous balance between mucosa and muscle. There would also be an additional effect on vascular smooth muscle of both circulations as an increased vagal drive occurs, having direct effects through cholinergic mechanisms, possibly by presynaptic inhibition of sympathetic fibres[73] and indirect effects from the release of VIP. Electrical stimulation of the cut peripheral end of the vagus nerve to the stomach of the cat induces a rapid onset in vasodilatation with a time course too fast to have resulted from a metabolic demand from the parietal cell.[74] Sympathetic stimulation, on the other hand, results in a decrease in both mucosal and total blood flow. There does not seem to be unanimity concerning the link between acid secretion and mucosal blood flow. One view is that there is no simple relationship between acid secretion and mucosal blood flow,[63] whereas another paper claims that there is a linear correlation between increments in acid output and blood flow.[75] In the latter experiment inhibition of acid secretion by either cimetidine or omeprazole returned mucosal blood flow to baseline levels, which would suggest that metabolic demand is an important factor in the control mechanism. There would also be further influences from gastrointestinal hormones which affect secretion and motility, though the patterns of release, that occur during a meal have not yet been tested on blood flow.

The role of local circulatory control mechanisms in determining mucosal blood flow has been confirmed and extended using the Moody–Durbin chambered stomach flap preparation. This (externally denervated) preparation allows precise control of inflow (arterial) and outflow (venous) pressures to be maintained at predetermined levels. At the same time it measures mucosal and total blood flow and oxygen consumption with the mucosa in a basal and stimulated state.[76] A functional hyperaemia was observed in the mucosa when oxygen consumption was elevated and acid secretion was stimulated by pentagastrin. The increase in oxygen consumption occurred as a result of both an increase in oxygen extraction and an increase in delivery (mucosal blood flow). The functional hyperaemia was absent from the muscularis. Further evidence of metabolic control was furnished by the effects of occlusion of the arterial supply to the stomach flap before and after pentagastrin. On return of the circulation reactive hyperaemia occurred, the magnitude of which was a function of the duration of occlusion. However, a myogenic mechanism may also be operative, as elevation of the venous pressure to 20 mmHg caused mucosal vasoconstriction.[76]

Role of mucosal blood flow in mucosal protection

The integrity of the mucosal circulation is a major factor in the ability of the gastric mucosa to resist injury.[77] In the presence of satisfactory tissue perfusion injury is resisted, but when the blood flow is reduced there is an increased liability to damage.[78]

The presence of the enzyme cyclo-oxygenase in the mucosal lamina propria and in the blood vessels might suggest that prostaglandins are formed at these sites and have some part to play in the physiological control of mucosal blood flow. Prostaglandins act locally, and because they are metabolized rapidly they are often difficult to detect. The cyclo-oxygenase inhibitor indomethacin reduces resting mucosal blood flow by about 50% in both rat and man, suggesting that prostaglandins are, at least in part, responsible for the control of resting blood flow.[79,80] Intraluminal administration of PGE_1, PGE_2 and 16,16-dimethyl-PGE_2 increase mucosal blood flow, confirming that the effect of indomethacin is likely to be due to local depletion of prostaglandins.

Topical application of alcohol, indomethacin, leukotriene C_4 (LTC_4) or platelet activating factor all decrease mucosal blood flow and oxygenation with varying degrees of congestion. Under such ischaemic and congestive conditions, the addition of 0.2 mol/l HCl causes gastric bleeding and erosions.[77] The microvasculature is generally regarded as the primary target for ethanol-induced injury. Alcohol (100 ml 40%) will produce exfoliation of the surface epithelium, damage to the mucosal microvessels, extravasation of red cells and plasma and extensive oedema of the superficial lamina propria. It is recognized that some of the prostaglandins have a protective effect on the mucosa which is independent of their acid inhibitory action because it occurs at a dose which is lower than the inhibitory dose. Part of this action is due to their effects on the structure of the mucous barrier (see above) and on their ability to stimulate bicarbonate secretion, but it is more likely that the prostanoids act as vasodilators to promote blood flow through the superficial vascular bed, although this may be only part of a more general effect on the vascular endothelium. They cause ultrastructural changes in human capillaries which could be the basis of the protective mechanism.[81,82]

Severe stress is well known to cause mucosal lesions and is likely to have a circulatory basis, attributed to the opening of arteriovenous anastomoses,[83,84] but the existence of such anastomoses in the gastric mucosa has been denied by others.[85]

EXOGENOUS AGGRESSORS: ALCOHOL AND NSAIDS

The mucus–bicarbonate barrier offers little protection against these agents and it is readily permeated by them. They cause destruction of the epithelial cells, with vascular damage and haemorrhage in severe cases. In the case of damage by ethanol there is a massive release of gelatinous material, which is largely fibrin covered by a layer of mucus and containing

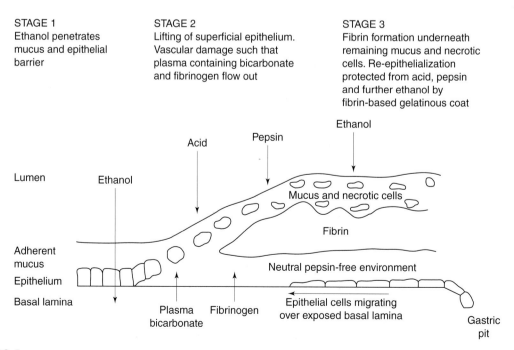

STAGE 1
Ethanol penetrates mucus and epithelial barrier

STAGE 2
Lifting of superficial epithelium. Vascular damage such that plasma containing bicarbonate and fibrinogen flow out

STAGE 3
Fibrin formation underneath remaining mucus and necrotic cells. Re-epithelialization protected from acid, pepsin and further ethanol by fibrin-based gelatinous coat

Figure 22.5
Mucosal response to acute ethanol injury and subsequent protection.[4]

necrotic cells. Its thickness is about ten times that of the adherent mucous layer. This coat is effective in protecting the underlying tissue from further attack by alcohol, and the bicarbonate rich exudate that accompanies it also provides protection against acid and pepsin. Under this protective umbrella re-epithelialization takes place from the gastric pits. Leukotrienes have been implicated, but at the moment this observation must be *sub judice* as the reports are conflicting.[86-88] The primary point of attack would seem to be the microvasculature, with the formation of intravascular platelet thrombi leading to vascular stasis and submucosal haemorrhage. The protective action of the prostaglandins would appear to be in maintaining blood flow (see Prostaglandins above). A summary of the pathophysiology of alcohol-induced injury is given in Figure 22.5. The damaging effect of *H. pylori* on the gastric mucosal is discussed in Chapter 26.

REFERENCES

1. Kerrs S, Allen A & Pearson JP. A simple method for measuring thickness of the mucus gel layer adherent to rat, frog and human gastric mucosa: influence of feeding, prostaglandin, *N*-acetylcysteine and other agents. *Clin Sci* 1982; **63:** 187–95.
2. Allen A, Hutton DA, Leonard AJ, Pearson JP & Sellers LA. The role of mucus in the protection of the gastroduodenal mucosa. *Scand J Gastroenterol* 1986; **21:** (Suppl. 125): 71–77.
3. Bell AE, Allen A, Morris ER & Ross-Murphy SB. Functional interactions of gastric mucus glycoprotein. *Int J Macromol* 1984; **6:** 309–315.
4. Sellars LA & Allen A. Mucus and gastroduodenal mucosal protection. In Rees WDW (ed.) *Advances in Peptic Ulcer Pathogenesis.* Lancaster: MTP Press, 1988: 121.
5. Allen A, Hunter AC, Leonard AJ, Pearson JP & Sellars LA. Peptic activity and the mucus-bicarbonate barrier. In Garner A & Whittle JR (eds) *Advances in Drug Therapy of Gastrointestinal Ulceration.* London: Wiley, 1989: 139.
6. Silbergerg A. Mucus glycoprotein, its biophysical and gel forming properties. In: *Mucus and Related Topics.* Cambridge, UK: Soc Exp Bio, 1989: 43–63.
7. Flemstrom G. Gastric and duodenal mucosal bicarbonate secretion. In Johnson LR (ed.) *Physiology of the Gastrointestinal Tract*, 2nd edn. New York: Raven Press, 1987: 1011–1129.
8. Nylander O, Flemstrom G, Delbro D & Fandriks L. Vagal influence on gastroduodenal HCO₃-secretion in the cat in vivo. *Am J Physiol* 1987; **252:** G522–528.
9. Konturek SJ, Bilski J, Tasler J & Laskiewicz J. Gut hormones in the stimulation of gastroduodenal alkaline secretion in conscious dogs. *Am J Physiol* 1985; **248:** G867–891.
10. Kauffman GL & Thompson MR. Titration of sodium channels in gastric mucosa. *Proc Natl Acad Sci USA* 1975; **72:** 3731–3734.
11. Bajaj SC, Spenney JG & Sachs G. Properties of the gastric antrum. III. Selectivity and modification of shunt conductance. *Gastroenterology* 1977; **72:** 72–77.
12. Forssell H & Olbe L. Continuous computerised determination of gastric bicarbonate secretion in man. *Scand J Gastroenterol* 1985; **20:** 767–774.
13. Feldman M. Gastric bicarbonate secretion in humans. Effect of pentagastrin, bethanecol, and 11,16, trimethyl prostaglandin E₂. *J Clin Invest* 1983; **72:** 295–303.
14. Gardam JR & Hobsley M. The electrolytes of alkaline human gastric juice. *Clin Sci* 1970; **39:** 77–87.
15. Rees WDW, Botham D & Turnberg LA. A demonstration of bicarbonate production by the normal human stomach in vivo. *Dig Dis Sci* 1982; **27:** 961–966.
16. Forssell H. Studies on gastric bicarbonate secretion in man. *Acta Chir Scand Suppl* 1987; **540:** 1–54.
17. Konturek SJ, Thor P, Bilski J, Tasler J & Cieszkowski M. Cephalic phase of gastroduodenal alkaline secretion. *Am J Physiol* 1987; **252:** G742–747.
18. Crampton JR, Gibbon LC & Rees WDW. Effect of luminal pH on the output of bicarbonate and PGE₂ by the normal human stomach. *Gut* 1987; **28:** 1291–1295.
19. Garner A & Hurst BC. Alkaline secretion by the canine Heidenhain pouch in response to exogenous acid, some gastrointestinal hormones and prostaglandin. In Gati T, Szollar LG & Ungvary G (eds) *Advances in Physiological Sciences, Nutrition, Digestion and Metabolism*, vol. 12. Oxford: Pergamon Press, 1981; 215.
20. Heylings JR, Garner A & Flemstrom G. Regulation of gastroduodenal HCO₃ transport by luminal acid in the frog in vitro. *Am J Physiol* 1984; **246:** G235–242.
21. Nylander O, Flemstrom G, Delbro D & Frandriks L. Vagal influences on gastroduodenal HCO₃ secretion in the cat in vivo. *Am J Physiol* 1987; **252:** G522–529.
22. Feldman M, Blair AJ & Richardson CT. Effect of proximal gastric vagotomy on calculated gastric HCO₃ and non-parietal volume secretion in man: studies during basal conditions and gastrin-17 infusion. *J Clin Invest* 1987; **79:** 1615–1620.
23. Forssell H & Olbe L. Effect of proximal gastric vagotomy on basal and vagally stimulated gastric bicarbonate secretion in duodenal ulcer patients. *Scand J Gastroenterol* 1987; **22:** 949–955.
24. Konturek SJ, Kwiecien N, Obtulowicz W et al. Vagal cholinergic control of gastric alkaline secretion in normal subjects and duodenal ulcer patients. *Gut* 1987; **28:** 739–744.
25. Allen A, Flemstrom G, Garner A & Kivilaakso. Gastro-duodenal mucosal protection. *Physiol Rev* 1993; **73:** 823–857.
26. Simson JNL, Merhav A & Silen W. Alkaline secretion by amphibian duodenum. I. General characteristics. *Am J Physiol* 1981; **240:** G401–408.
27. Simson JNL, Merhav A & Silen W. Alkaline secretion by amphibian duodenum. II. Short circuit current and Na⁺ and Cl⁻ fluxes. *Am J Physiol* 1981; **240:** G472–479.
28. Flemstrom G, Garner A, Nylander O, Hurst BC & Heylings JR. Surface epithelial HCO₃ transport by mammalian duodenum in vivo. *Am J Physiol* 1982; **243:** G348–358.
29. Isenberg JL, Smedfors B & Johansson C. Effect of graded doses of intraluminal H⁺, prostaglandin E₂, and inhibition of endogenous prostaglandin synthesis on proximal duodenal bicarbonate secretion in the unanesthetised rat. *Gastroenterology* 1985; **88:** 303–307.
30. Smeaton LA, Hirst BH, Allen A & Garner A. Gastric and duodenal bicarbonate transport in vivo. Influence of prostaglandins. *Am J Physiol* 1983; **245:** G751–759.
31. Hurst BC, Heylings JR, Nylander O, Uddiun KK, Garner A & Flemstrom G. Duodenal bicarbonate secretion in response to glucagon and related peptides. *Regul Pept* 1982; **4:** 367.
32. Scratcherd T, Case RM & Smith PA. A sensitive method for the biological assay of secretin and substances with 'secretin-like' activity in tissues and biological fluids. *Scand J Gastroenterol* 1975; **10:** 821–28.
33. Fahrenkrug J, Haglund U, Jodal M, Lundgren O, Olbe L & Schaffalitzky de Muckadell OB. Nervous release of vasoactive intestinal polypeptide in the gastrointestinal tract of cats: possible physiological implications. *J Physiol (Lond)* 1978; **284:** 291–305.
34. Case RM, Garner A & Uddin KK. Simultaneous determination of duodenal and pancreatic bicarbonate transport: differential effects of secretin and prostaglandin E₂ in the cat in vivo. *J Physiol (Lond)* 1984: **340:** 36P.
35. Bloom SR, Mitchell SJ, Greenberg GR et al. Release of VIP, secretin, motilin, after duodenal acidification in man. *Acta Hepatogastroenterol* 1978; **25:** 365.
36. Konturek SJ, Bilski J, Tasler J & Laskiewicz J. Gastroduodenal alkali response to acid and taurocholate in conscious dogs. *Am J Physiol* 1984; **247:** G149–154.
37. Aly A, Green K & Johansson C. Prostaglandin synthesis in the human gastrointestinal tract. *Scand J Gastroenterol* 1987; 22 (Suppl. 127): 35.
38. Allen A & Garner A. Mucus and bicarbonate secretion in the stomach and their possible roles in mucosal protection. *Gut* 1980; **21:** 249–262.
39. Williams SE & Turnberg LA. Demonstration of a pH gradient across mucus adherent to rabbit gastric mucosa: evidence for a 'mucus–bicarbonate' barrier. *Gut* 1981; **22:** 94–96.
40. Patronella CK, Vanek I & Bowen JC. In vitro measurement of gastric mucus pH in canines: effect of high luminal acidity and prostaglandin E₂. *Gastroenterology* 1988; **95:** 612–618.
41. Davies RE. Hydrochloric acid production by isolated gastric mucosa. *Biochem J* 1948; **42:** 609–618.
42. Leonard A & Allen A. Gastric mucosal damage by pepsin. *Gut* 1986; **27:** A1236.
43. Younan F, Pearson JP, Allen A & Venables CW. Gastric mucus degradation in vivo in peptic ulcer patients and the effects of vagotomy. In Chantler EN, Elder JB & Elstein M. (eds) *Mucus in Health and Disease.* New York: Plenum Press, 1982: 235.

44. Pearson JP, Ward R, Allen A, Roberts NW & Taylor WH. Mucus degradation by pepsin: comparison of mucolytic activity of human pepsin 1 and pepsin 3: implications in peptic ulceration. *Gut* 1986; **27:** 243.

45. Allen A, Garner A, Hunter AC & Keogh JP. The gastroduodenal mucus barrier and the place of the eicosanoids. In Hiller K (ed.) *Advances in Eicosanoids and the Gastrointestinal Tract.* Lancaster: MTP Press, 1988: 195.

46. Main IHM. Pharmacology of prostaglandins. *Postgrad Med J* 1988; **64** (Suppl. 1): 3–6.

47. Postius S, Ruoff H-J and Szelenyi I. Prostaglandin formation by isolated parietal cells and non-parietal cells of the rat. *Br J Pharmacol* 1985; **84:** 871–877.

48. Robert A, Nezamis JE & Phillips JP. Inhibition of gastric secretion by prostaglandin. *Am J Dig Dis* 1967; **12:** 1073–1076.

49. Skoglund ML, Gerber JG, Murphy RC & Nies AS. Prostaglandin production by intact isolated parietal cells. *Eur J Pharmacol* 1980; **66:** 148.

50. Befrits R & Johansson C. Oral PGE$_2$ inhibits gastric secretion in man. *Prostaglandins* 1985; **29:** 143–152.

51. Soll AII. Review. Antisecretory drugs: cellular mechanisms of action. *Aliment Pharmacol Ther* 1987; **1:** 77–89.

52. McQueen S, Hutton D, Allen A & Garner A. Gastric and duodenal surface mucus gel thickness in rat: effects of prostagladins and damaging agents. *Am J Physiol* 1983; **245:** G388–393.

53. Major JS & Scholes P. The localization of a histamine H$_2$-receptor adenylate cyclase system in canine parietal cells and its inhibition by prostaglandins. *Agents Actions* 78; **8:** 324–331.

54. Soll AH & Berglindh T. Physiology of gastric isolated glands and parietal cells. Receptors and effectors regulating function. In Johnson LR (ed.) *Physiology of the Gastrointestinal Tract,* 2nd edn. New York: Raven Press, 1987: 883–909.

55. Tytgat GNJ, Offerhaus GJA, van Minnen AJ, Everts V, Hensen-Logmans SC & Samoson G. Influence of oral 15(R)–15 methyl prostaglandin E$_2$ on human gastric mucosa. A light microscopic, cell kinetic and ultrastructural study. *Gastroenterology* 1986; **90:** 1111–1120.

56. Johansson C, Uribe A, Rubio C & Isenberg JL. Effect of oral prostaglandin E$_2$ on DNA turnover in gastric and intestinal epithelia of the rat. *Eur J Clin Invest* 1986; **16:** 509–514.

57. Uribe A, Johansson C & Rubio C. Cell proliferation of the rat gastrointestinal mucosa after treatment with E$_2$ prostaglandins and indomethacin. *Digestion* 1987; **36:** 238–245.

58. Svendsen LB, Jorgensen FS, Hart Hensen O, Johansen A, Horn T & Larsen JK. Influence of the prostaglandin E$_1$ analogue rioprostil on the human gastric mucosa. *Digestion* 1987; **37:** 29–34.

59. Holm-Rutili L & Obrink KJ. Effects of prostaglandin E$_1$ and gastric mucosal microcirculation and spontaneous acid secretion in the rat. In Allen A (ed.) *Mechanisms of Mucosal Protection in the Upper Gastrointestinal Tract.* New York: Raven Press, 1984: 279.

60. Jacobson ED, Linford RH & Grossman MI. Gastric secretion in relation to mucosal blood flow studied by a clearance technique. *J Clin Invest* 1966; **45:** 1–13.

61. Harper AA, Read JD & Smy J. Gastric blood flow in anesthetised cats. *J Physiol (Lond)* 1968; **194:** 795–807.

62. Guth PH & Leung FW. Physiology of the gastric circulation. In Johnson LR (ed.) *Physiology of the Gastrointestinal Tract.* New York: Raven Press, 1987; 1031–1053.

63. Holm L & Perry MA. The role of blood flow in gastric secretion. *Am J Physiol* 1988; **254:** G281–293.

64. Bond JH, Prentiss RA & Levitt MD. Effects of feeding on blood flow to the stomach, small bowel and colon of the conscious dog. *J Lab Clin Med* 1979; **93:** 594–599.

65. Semb BKH. Regional gastric flow changes after meal stimulation measured by the hydrogen gas clearance technique in the conscious cat. *Scand J Gastroenterol* 1982; **17:** 839–842.

66. Beaumont W. *Experiments and Observations on Gastric Juice and the Physiology of Digestion.* New York: Dover, 1833.

67. Wolf S. *The Stomach.* New York: Oxford University Press, 1965.

68. Leonard AS, Long D, French LA, Peter ET & Wagensteen OH. Pendular pattern in gastric secretion and blood flow following hypothalamic stimulation: origin of stress ulcer? *Surgery* 1964; **56:** 109–120.

69. Varo V, Dobronte Z & Sagi I. Interrelation between gastric blood flow and HCl secretion in dogs. *Acta Med Acad Sci Hung* 1978; **35:** 1–20.

70. Polanski DB, Shirazi SS & Coon D. Lack of correlation of gastric acid secretion and blood flow. *J Surg Res* 1979; **26:** 320–325.

71. Jacobsen ED. Effects of histamine, acetylcholine and norepinephrine on gastric vascular resistance. *Am J Physiol* 1963; **204:** 1013–1017.

72. Guyton AC. *Textbook of Medical Physiology.* Philadelphia: WB Saunders, 1986.

73. Van Hee RH & Vanhoutte PM. Cholinergic inhibition of adrenergic neurotransmission in the canine gastric artery. *Gastroenterology* 1978; **74:** 1266–1270.

74. Yano S, Fujiwara A, Ozaki Y & Harada M. Gastric blood flow responses to autonomic nerve stimulation and related pharmacological studies in rats. *J Pharm Pharmacol* 1983; **35:** 641–646.

75. Pique JM, Leung FW, Tan HW, Livingston E, Scremin OU & Guth PH. Gastric mucosal blood flow response to stimulation and inhibition of gastric acid secretion. *Gastroenterology* 1988; **95:** 642–650.

76. Kiel JW, Riedel GL & Shepherd AP. Local control of canine mucosal blood flow. *Gastroenterology* 1987; **93:** 1041–1053.

77. Sato N, Kawano S, Tsuji S & Kamada T. Microvascular basis of gastric mucosal protection. *J Clin Gastroenterol* 1988; **10** (Suppl. 1): S13–18.

78. Holm L. Gastric mucosal blood flow and mucosal protection. *J Clin Gastroenterol* 1988; **10** (Suppl. 1): S114–119.

79. Main IHM & Whittle BJR. Investigation of the vasodilator and antisecretory role of prostaglandins in the rat gastric mucosa by the use of non-steroidal anti-inflammatory drugs. *Br J Pharmacol* 1975; **53:** 217.

80. Konturek SJ, Kwiecien N, Obtulowicz et al. Effect of carprofen and indomethacin on gastric function, mucosal integrity and generation of prostaglandins in man. *Hepatogastroenterology* 1982; **29:** 267–270.

81. Tarnawski A, Stachura J, Gergely H & Hollander D. Microvascular endothelium: a major target for alcohol injury of the human gastric mucosa. Histochemical and ultrastructural study. *J Clin Gastroenterol* 1988; **10** (Suppl. 1): S53–64.

82. Tarnwawski A, Stachura J, Hollander D, Sarfeh IJ & Bogdal J. Cellular aspects of alcohol induced injury and prostglandin protection of the human gastric mucosa. Focus on the mucosal microvessels. *J Clin Gastroenterol* 1988; **10** (Suppl. 1): S35–45.

83. Katajima M, Otsuku S, Shimizu A et al. Impairment of gastric microcirculation in stress. *J Clin Gastroenterol* 1988; **10** (Suppl. 1): S120–128.

84. Barlow TE, Bentley FH & Walder DN. Arteries, veins and arteriovenous anastomoses in the human stomach. *Surg Gynecol Obstet* 1951; **93:** 657–671.

85. Gannon B, Browning J & O'Brien P. The microvascular architecture of rat stomach. *J Anat* 1982; **135:** 667–683.

86. Pihan G, Rogers C & Szabo S. Vascular injury in acute gastric mucosal damage. Mediatory role of leukotrienes. *Dig Dis Sci* 1988; **33:** 625–632.

87. Broughton-Smith NK & Whittle BJR. Failure of the inhibition of rat mucosal 5-lipogenase by novel acetohydroxamic acids to prevent ethanol-induced damage. *Br J Pharmacol* 1988; **95:** 155–162.

88. Fukuda T, Arakawa T & Kobayashi K. Roles for endogenous leukotrienes in damage caused by ethanol in isolated gastric cells. *J Clin Gastroenterol* 1988; **10** (Suppl. 1): S140–145.

23

RADIOLOGICAL INVESTIGATIONS

AR Wright
GM Fraser

In this chapter, the roles of the various radiological methods for the examination of the stomach and duodenum are discussed with reference to plain films, the barium meal, transabdominal ultrasonography, computed tomography, endoluminal ultrasonography, magnetic resonance imaging and angiography/interventional radiology.

PLAIN RADIOGRAPHY

In general, plain radiographs are of limited value in the investigation of the stomach and duodenum. A perforated duodenal or gastric ulcer will show free gas under the diaphragm in 70% of cases and this is better demonstrated on an erect chest radiograph than on an erect abdominal radiograph (Figure 23.1).[1] Foreign bodies in the stomach, if radiopaque, may be detected on an abdominal radiograph. Rarely, a fungating carcinoma of the stomach, particularly in the gastric fundus, may be seen protruding into the gastric air bubble. A characteristic filling defect in the gastric fundus can also be seen following a fundoplication procedure (Figure 23.2). Similarly, a large

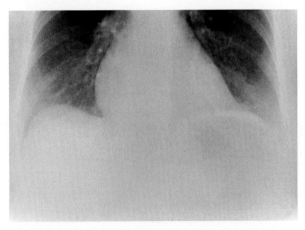

Figure 23.2
A lobulated filling defect is seen in the gastric fundal gas shadow due to a previous fundoplication.

gastric ulcer on the lesser curve of the stomach may occasionally be seen as a gas-filled structure protruding from the lumen. Pathological dilatation of the stomach, for which there are many causes, can be recognized on the plain film when the stomach is gas filled. Gas can be seen within the gastric wall in emphysematous gastritis.

BARIUM MEAL

The double-contrast barium meal is now the standard radiological method for examining the stomach and duodenum, and has virtually supplanted the single-contrast examination, which should only be used in specific clinical situations, or where patients are elderly and frail and unable to tolerate the manoeuvring on the screening table required for the double-contrast examination.

The principle underlying the double-contrast barium meal is to distend the lumen of the stomach and duodenum with gas and to coat the mucosa with barium. In this way the fine mucosal detail of the stomach and duodenum can be recognized (Figure 23.3).

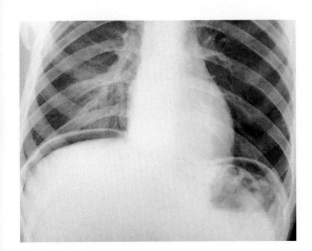

Figure 23.1
Erect chest radiograph. Free gas under the diaphragm in patient with perforated duodenal ulcer.

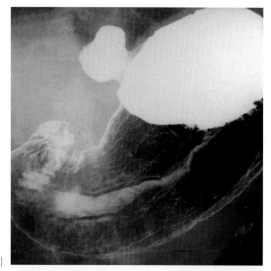

(a)

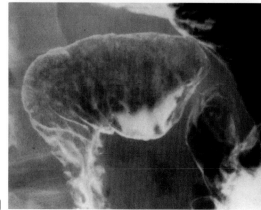

(b)

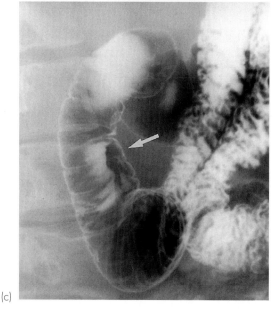

(c)

Figure 23.3

(a) Double-contrast barium meal showing the body of the
stomach and antrum. The mucosa is coated with barium and
the lumen of the stomach distended with air. Individual mucosal
folds are clearly visible. (b) The duodenal cap after injection of
20 mg i.v. Buscopan. The normal surface villous pattern is
clearly demonstrated. (c) The duodenal loop showing a
prominent ampulla (arrow).

Technique

The nature and purpose of the examination should always be
explained to the patient, who may be apprehensive. The examination is usually carried out in the morning and should be performed on an empty stomach. This means that the patient
should fast for at least 6 hours and preferably overnight.

The best results are obtained using a high density barium
(250% w/v).[2] Approximately 100–150 ml of this suspension are
given. In order to achieve adequate gaseous distension, proprietary effervescent tablets or powders are swallowed which will
rapidly release 400–500 ml of carbon dioxide into the stomach.

A better examination will result if the stomach and duodenum are hypotonic. This can be achieved by giving an intravenous injection of a smooth muscle relaxant such as 20 mg
hyoscine-*n*-butylbromide (Buscopan) or 0.2 mg glucagon. Both
are safe drugs, but Buscopan should be avoided in patients
with cardiac disease, and may precipitate glaucoma or urinary
retention in susceptible individuals. If Buscopan is given, the
patient should be warned that it may cause transient blurring
of near vision. Glucagon should be avoided in patients with
suspected phaeochromocytoma and in unstable diabetics, and
may rarely cause anaphylaxis.

A detailed account of the double-contrast barium meal technique is beyond the scope of this text, and those readers seeking further information are referred elsewhere.[3,4] In essence, the
patient is rotated to obtain optimal mucosal coating, with care
being taken to avoid filling of the duodenal loop early in the
examination, which may overlap, and partially obscure, the
barium-coated stomach, particularly the antrum. Spot films are
taken in different positions to show the various stomach and
duodenal areas in double contrast. Speed in performing the
examination is necessary to prevent flocculation of the barium
in the stomach.

The single-contrast examination may still be used if gastric
outlet, duodenal or upper jejunal obstruction is suspected. A
medium density (100% w/v) barium is preferable in this situation. In some patients, it may be impossible to perform a formal double-contrast series due to immobility or infirmity. In
these cases also, single contrast may be used.

Specific examination of the duodenum may be carried out if
the routine views of the duodenum obtained during the standard barium meal have not been adequate. This technique,
known as hypotonic duodenography, involves intubation of
the duodenum, followed by injection of air and barium down
the tube. An intravenous injection of smooth muscle relaxant is
given at the same time.

Water-soluble contrast media

Water-soluble contrast media are indicated instead of barium
when perforation is suspected, or to confirm or exclude anastamotic leakage postoperatively. This is because water-soluble
media are harmless when spilled into the peritoneal cavity,
whereas barium may produce a fibrotic reaction. Where there
is a risk of aspiration, non-ionic, low-osmolality agents are preferred as standard water-soluble agents may cause aspiration
pneumonia or pulmonary oedema if inhaled.[5]

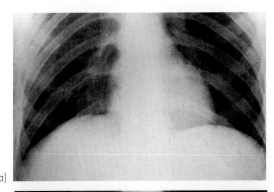

(a)

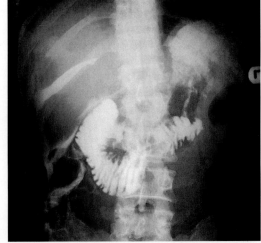

(b)

Figure 23.4
Perforated duodenal ulcer. (a) Chest radiograph does not show free gas under the diaphragm. (b) Same patient. Supine abdomen after 50 ml of gastrografin has been given orally. Extensive leakage of gastrografin from the perforated ulcer into the peritoneal cavity.

In a patient with a suspected perforated gastric or duodenal ulcer, 50 ml of a water-soluble contrast medium such as Gastrografin are given and the patient lies on the right side for 5 minutes. Plain abdominal radiographs and a chest radiograph are then taken. Where there is a perforation, either a leak of Gastrografin or free gas will be seen in 96% of patients (Figure 23.4). This technique has the added advantage that it may demonstrate stretching of the duodenal loop in acute pancreatitis, which may clinically mimic a perforation.[6] In cases of suspected anastamotic leakage, the patient should be rotated after ingesting the contrast medium to ensure that all leaks are detected.

Peptic ulcer disease and related conditions

Gastric ulcer and gastric erosions

Gastric ulcers occur most commonly in the middle-aged and elderly, and are seen most frequently in alcoholics, analgesic users and people from low socioeconomic groups. Gastric ulcers are typically found along the lesser gastric curve, and in the distal stomach, but can occur along the greater curve or in the fundus.

There are numerous radiological signs of benign gastric

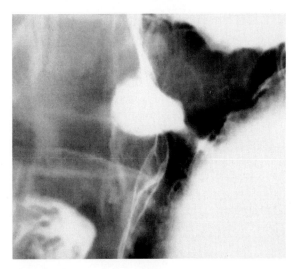

Figure 23.5
Profile view of benign gastric ulcer showing rounded, barium-filled ulcer crater projecting beyond the gastric lumen.

ulceration. In profile, the ulcer will be seen as a barium-filled projection, usually rounded, outside the gastric lumen, and the size of the lesion can be judged on this view (Figure 23.5). Gastric ulcers can be very large, and this usually implies benignity. A radiolucent mound representing oedema around the ulcer crater may be present, and this is generally symmetrical and well defined. Any evidence on profile views of undermining of the gastric mucosa or gastric wall tissues by the ulcer is a good sign of benignity.

When seen *en face*, the benign ulcer appears as a barium pool, again usually of round or oval contour. Oedema adjacent to the ulcer can be recognized as a halo of radiolucency around the neck of the ulcer crater (Figure 23.6).

A pattern of smooth, converging folds leading towards the

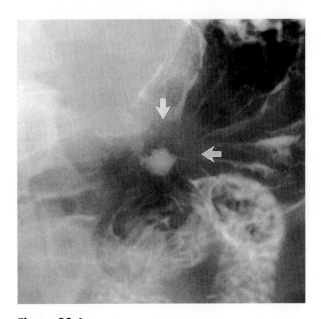

Figure 23.6
En face view of benign gastric ulcer showing central barium collection with surrounding halo of mucosal oedema (arrowed).

ulcer is often seen in the chronic or healing phase due to scarring in the ulcer base (Figure 23.7). Occasionally, an ulcer may heal with a linear scar or a simple depression. Significant deformity at the site of the healed ulcer is unusual.[7]

Since ulceration may also occur in relation to malignant lesions of the stomach, it is important to determine whether gastric ulcers detected during the barium meal are unequivocally benign, or whether they are indeterminate or definitely malignant. Ulcers in the latter two categories will require further investigation, usually with endoscopy, whereas radiologically benign lesions are followed radiologically to complete healing (which is itself a cogent sign of benignity). The radiological signs that allow discrimination between benign and malignant lesions are shown in Table 23.1

Gastritis

Although the diagnosis of gastritis, particularly if mild, is more likely to be made by the endoscopist than the radiologist, there are several recognized forms of gastritis that can be regularly detected radiologically. The term 'erosive gastritis' is used to refer to a form of gastritis characterized by multiple gastric erosions. Gastric erosions are encountered in alcoholics and analgesic users, as well as in patients with extensive trauma or other physiological stress. Erosions are small areas of ulceration without penetration of the muscularis mucosa, and are

Table 23.1 Radiological signs of benign versus malignant gastric ulcers

BENIGN	MALIGNANT
Projects beyond gastric lumen	Does not project – sits on mass
Smooth contour	Irregular contour
May be deep	Usually shallow
Symmetrical oedema mound	Adjacent tissues usually irregular, nodular or rigid
Undermining of adjacent tissues	No undermining
Smooth, converging folds	Nodular or irregular folds
Heals completely	Rarely heals completely

seen on barium studies as small bariums pools, which may be surrounded by a rim of oedema (Figure 23.8). The barium meal is a relatively insensitive method of detecting gastric erosions compared with endoscopy.[8] Antral gastritis is again usually an endoscopic diagnosis, consisting of antral mucosal inflammation, particularly in the prepyloric region, and associated with peptic ulcer disease and alcohol abuse. The radiological signs are unreliable, and consist of loss of distensibility of the antrum, thickened folds and erosions. Hypertrophic gastritis is recognized by thickening of gastric folds and enlargement and prominence of the normal surface pattern of the areae gastricae throughout the stomach. Hypertrophic gastritis is associated with peptic ulceration and gastric hypersecretion. Atrophic gastritis appears as a lack of the normal rugal folds, particularly in the region of the gastric fundus and greater curvature, as well as absence of the areae gastricae (Figure 23.9). There is an increased risk of malignancy in patients with atrophic gastritis, and careful evaluation is needed, especially if gastric ulceration is also present. In Ménétrier's disease, the gastric rugae are markedly hypertrophic, particularly in the proximal stomach and along the greater curvature. The hypertrophied folds can appear mass-like, and differentiation from tumour infiltration may require biopsy (Figure 23.10).[9]

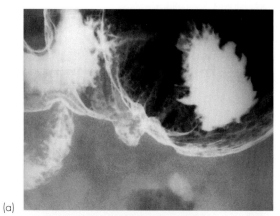

(a)

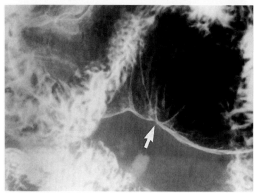

(b)

Figure 23.7
(a) Benign gastric ulcer on the greater curve of the body of the stomach. (b) Repeat barium meal after 2 months' therapy with H$_2$-receptor blockers. The ulcer has healed with scar formation (arrowed).

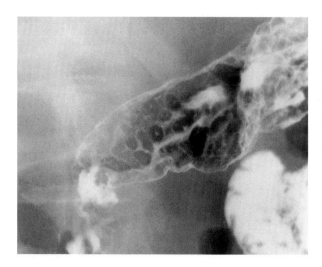

Figure 23.8
Multiple gastric erosions in the gastric antrum. Punctate barium pools are present, each surrounded by a rim of oedema.

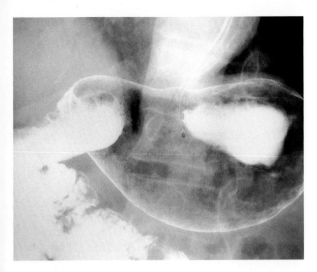

Figure 23.9
Atrophic gastritis with complete loss of the rugal folds and areae gastricae in the fundus and along the greater curve of the stomach.

Duodenal ulcer

This is the most frequently encountered disorder of the duodenum, and is well demonstrated with radiological techniques. Ulcer craters of the duodenal cap are seen on the double-contrast barium meal as well-defined constant pools of barium, usually surrounded by a rim of oedema or radiating mucosal folds (Figure 23.11). Where there has been previous ulceration, the duodenal cap may be scarred and distorted. In these cases, it can be difficult to exclude active ulceration on barium studies and endoscopy may be needed. Ulceration infrequently occurs in the postbulbar part of the duodenum, where it has a

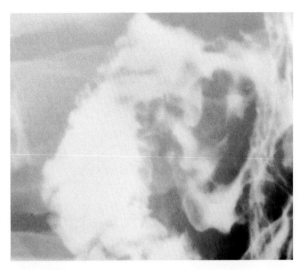

Figure 23.11
Acute ulcer in the duodenal cap. The barium-filled ulcer crater is surrounded by oedematous mucosa.

similar appearance to bulbar ulceration. Duodenal ulcers may be associated with haemorrhage, stenosis, perforation and penetration of adjacent organs.

The expression 'giant ulcer' refers to benign duodenal ulceration with a crater size in excess of 2 cm in diameter. The significance of this entity lies in the fact that it may be mistaken on barium studies for a diverticulum or the duodenal cap itself due to its size, and that there is a high incidence of complications, in particular haemorrhage.[10]

Other inflammatory conditions

Gastric Crohn's disease may be the sole manifestation of the disease, but more commonly is part of a more widespread involvement. In mild cases, the barium meal may reveal aphthous ulcers consisting of small erosions with a surrounding rim of oedema. This appearance is non-specific and is indistinguishable from ordinary gastric erosions (which may coexist in patients with Crohn's disease). In more advanced cases, thickening and distortion of the mucosal folds occur with ulceration. The gastric antrum and pyloric region are commonly affected, and there may be distortion and loss of the usual anatomical features of the distal stomach and proximal duodenum.[11] A similar appearance may be encountered in eosinophilic gastritis, as well as gastric tuberculosis and syphilis.

With Crohn's disease in the duodenum, aphthous ulceration may occur, and the proximal duodenum may become involved with extensive disease of the distal stomach, as stated above. Otherwise, duodenal Crohn's disease may appear similar to disease elsewhere in the small intestine with thickening of the valvulae conniventes, cobblestoning and stricture formation.

Following ingestion of caustic substances, particularly acids, a corrosive gastritis may occur. Initially the superficial mucosal and submucosal layers undergo necrosis, and in severe cases there may be necrosis of the full thickness of the stomach wall with perforation. In the chronic phase, there is usually fibrosis

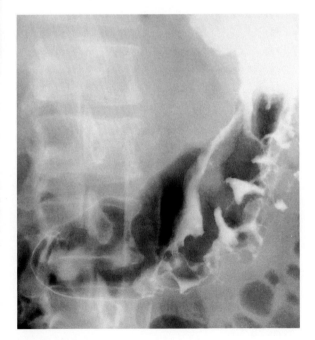

Figure 23.10
Ménétrier's disease. Massive hypertrophy of gastric rugae along the greater curve of the stomach.

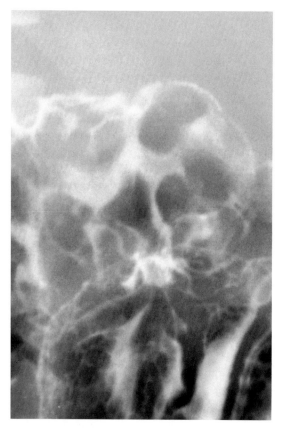

Figure 23.12
Brunner's gland hyperplasia in the duodenal cap. Multiple polypoid filling defects are present giving a cobblestone effect.

and contraction of the stomach. Radiological examination of the stomach in the acute phase should be carried out with care, and use of a water-soluble contrast medium should be considered due to the risk of perforation. Irregularity of the mucosal surface may be seen, and undermining of the mucosa by the contrast medium is a sign of mucosal sloughing. In chronic cases, barium is safe to use, and allows the degree of gastric contracture to be assessed.

In emphysematous gastritis, intramural gas is present, and this may be recognized initially on the plain film as a series of linear radiolucencies following the contour of the stomach wall. There are several causes for this rare disorder, including: infection with a gas-forming organism, usually occurring in diabetics; ingestion of caustic agents, where it is a sign of gastric wall necrosis; vascular compromise of the stomach wall; and intramural dissection of air following violent retching or in association with mediastinal or retroperitoneal emphysema.

Neoplastic diseases

Benign polypoid lesions of the stomach include hyperplastic polyps, adenomatous polyps, villous adenomas and carcinoid tumours. These tend to appear radiologically as polypoid lesions elsewhere in the gastrointestinal tract, namely radiolucent filling defects coated with barium. It can be difficult to distinguish the different types radiologically and biopsy may be required as adenomas and carcinoid have malignant potential.

Gastric leiomyomas and lipomas appear smooth and hemispherical with their epicentre in the gastric wall. The overlying mucosa is usually intact.

Benign duodenal neoplasms occur infrequently and include adenomas, lipomas, leiomyomas, neurogenic tumours and hamartomas. They are seen as filling defects on barium studies, and biopsy is usually required to exclude malignancy. In Brunner's gland hyperplasia, one or more polypoid lesions are seen in the duodenal cap, which may have a cobblestone appearance (Figure 23.12)

The most common malignant tumour of the stomach is primary carcinoma, which may have a number of different radiological presentations. Early gastric carcinoma (i.e. confined to the gastric mucosa) may simply cause a plaque-like or depressed abnormality accompanied by radiating mucosal folds on the barium meal (Figure 23.13). There may be nodularity of the folds or of the central lesion.

The radiological appearances of more advanced gastric carcinoma are typically those of an irregular mass lesion, often large, with an abrupt transition between normal and abnormal mucosa (Figure 23.14). Large, annular lesions in the gastric antrum may cause outlet obstruction.

Ulceration may be present on the surface of the lesion, and when the underlying carcinoma is small and markedly ulcerated, the ulcer may be mistaken for a benign lesion. Table 23.1 shows the radiological features that allow differentiation between benign and malignant ulcers. When ulceration occurs in association with a large mass, the diagnosis is usually obvious.

Linitis plastica is caused by a form of gastric carcinoma which infiltrates the stomach wall, stimulating a fibrotic reaction. In this variant, the mucosa is often intact, and there is little evidence of a mass lesion or ulceration. Radiologically, linitis plastica

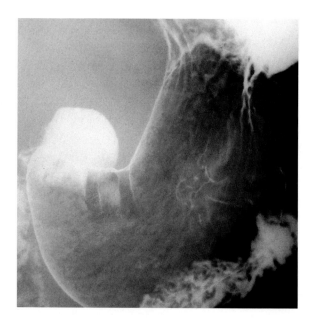

Figure 23.13
Early gastric cancer. Small depressed area in the body of the stomach surrounded by radiating mucosal folds, some showing slight nodularity.

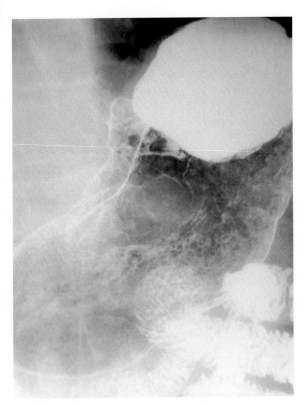

Figure 23.14
Advanced gastric carcinoma with large irregular mass arising from lesser curve of stomach.

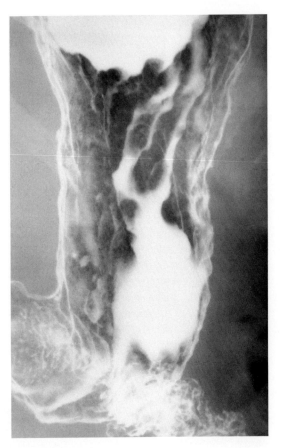

Figure 23.15
Primary gastric lymphoma. There is diffuse thickening of the wall of the gastric fundus and body with loss of distensibility, enlargement of rugal folds and relative preservation of the lumen.

appears as an indistensible stomach with reduction in the size of the gastric lumen, and often a smooth mucosal surface.

Primary gastric lymphoma is usually of non-Hodgkin's type and may produce a radiological picture indistinguishable from carcinoma. However, it often produces a diffuse thickening of large areas of the gastric wall with enlargement of the rugal folds and preservation of the lumen, and these features may suggest the diagnosis (Figure 23.15).[12]

Gastric leiomyosarcomas are similar in appearance on the barium meal to benign leiomyomas, albeit usually larger in size. As they are predominantly exophytic, they are often best appreciated with cross-sectional imaging such as computed tomography (CT).

Metastatic spread to the gastric wall is usually from breast, malignant melanoma and lung tumours as well as lymphoma. Melanoma and lymphoma metastases may produce a characteristic target lesion. Otherwise, metastatic lesions have relatively non-specific radiological features, resembling a polypoid or intramural lesion when small and progressing to appearances indistinguishable from carcinoma (Figure 23.16).

In general, malignant tumours of the duodenum are infrequent and are usually carcinomas involving either the papilla of Vater or the duodenum proper. Presenting symptoms may be variable, and depend on the exact site of the tumour. Barium studies show an irregular filling defect, often with ulceration, and there may be evidence of duodenal obstruction. Other malignant primary tumours of the duodenum include sarcomas and lymphomas.

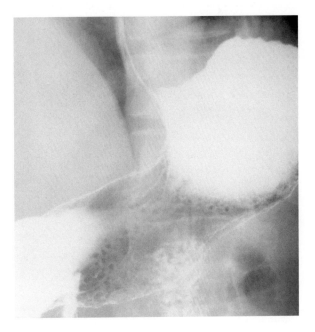

Figure 23.16
Multiple small polypoid filling defects due to metastatic spread to gastric wall from malignant melanoma.

The duodenum may also be the site of secondary neoplasia, either from direct spread from neighbouring organs, such as the pancreas, colon or right kidney, or metastatic disease from primary tumours in the breast, kidney, colon and malignant melanoma.

Miscellaneous conditions

Diverticula are relatively uncommon in the stomach and usually occur in the region of the gastric fundus. They are thought to be congenital in origin, and are usually asymptomatic and discovered as an incidental finding. As in the oesophagus, intramural diverticula occur rarely in the stomach, and are generally found along the distal greater curve. By contrast, duodenal diverticula are a common finding, being seen in up to 5% of barium studies. The majority arise from the concave wall of the duodenum, and may be in contact with or indent the pancreas (Figure 23.17). Most duodenal diverticula are asymptomatic, although problems can arise from retained food debris, bacterial overgrowth or the presence of heterotopic gastric or pancreatic tissue.

Intramural haematoma of the duodenum is most commonly seen with abdominal trauma, although it can occur due to a bleeding tendency. The presentation is usually one of abdominal pain with signs of duodenal obstruction. Barium studies may show narrowing due to annular thickening of the duodenal wall with proximal dilatation, and there may be thickening of the valvulae conniventes resulting from oedema. As discussed later, the diagnosis can be confirmed with CT or magnetic resonance imaging (MRI). This is an important diagnosis to make radiologically as conservative treatment is usually indicated.

The duodenum may also be ruptured following blunt trauma, and this is more likely to happen at the junction of the second and third parts where the duodenum crosses the spine.

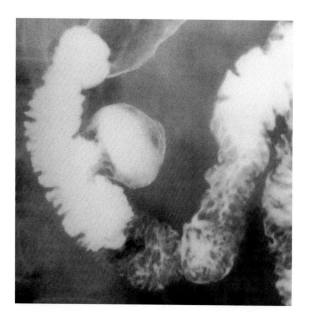

Figure 23.17
Large duodenal diverticulum arising from the concave border of the second part.

The plain radiographic signs are essentially those of retroperitoneal gas, such as outlining of the kidneys/psoas muscles, and may be subtle. In suspected cases, a contrast study using water-soluble media should be carried out if the plain films are unhelpful.

A relatively uncommon condition which is uniquely diagnosed by the barium meal is the superior mesenteric artery syndrome. This syndrome classically occurs in thin, rapidly growing adolescents and is characterized by abdominal pain and vomiting. At barium meal, the diagnostic features are dilatation of the second part of the duodenum with vigorous to-and-fro peristalsis and an abrupt cut-off in the third part of the duodenum.[13] When encountered in older patients, this syndrome may be caused by metastatic malignant glands in the root of the mesentery or a carcinoma of the body of the pancreas.[14]

The postoperative stomach

Radiological examination is commonly requested for the evaluation of the postoperative stomach. As there are many different gastric surgical procedures, it is important for the radiologist to be informed as accurately as possible of the nature of the surgery to allow optimization of the examination. In the immediate postoperative period, radiological assessment using water-soluble contrast media is often of value in the detection or exclusion of anastomotic leaks, sinus tracks and fistulas.

In cases of suspected recurrent anastomotic or jejunal ulceration, endoscopy is preferable to the barium meal because of difficulty in interpretation due to the distorted postsurgical anatomy. However, the double-contrast barium meal is capable of showing an ulcer crater in about 50% of cases, and indirect signs of ulceration in a further 30%.[15] For similar reasons, endoscopy may be preferable in suspected recurrent gastric carcinoma following surgery.

Radiological examination plays an important role in the follow-up of patients who have undergone banded gastroplasty for weight reduction. If the proximal pouch volume is greater than 50 ml or the outlet diameter greater than 10 mm the patient will fail to lose weight.[16]

Extrinsic displacement of the stomach

The barium meal may provide the initial evidence of an extrinsic abnormality as it is often the first examination requested in a patient with non-specific upper abdominal symptoms.[17] Displacement of the stomach from behind is best recognized from a lateral projection. Causes include pancreatitis, pancreatic tumours and pseudocysts, enlarged para-aortic nodes, left renal and adrenal masses and splenomegaly. An enlarged spleen may also push the stomach inferiorly and medially. Displacement by the liver is usually to the left, inferiorly and posteriorly. Patients found to have extrinsic compression of the stomach are best further evaluated using ultrasonography or CT.

Accuracy of the double-contrast barium meal

The accuracy of the double-contrast barium meal in detecting peptic ulceration and gastric cancer is, in some series, as high as 90–95%.[18] When compared with a third diagnostic method such as surgery or post-mortem examination, radiology and endoscopy are found to be equally accurate in the diagnosis of these two conditions.[19,20] In addition, Cotton and Shorvon[21] have carried out a multiseries analysis, comparing the accuracy of the double-contrast barium meal and endoscopy, which has suggested that the two techniques are equally accurate in the detection of gastric ulcers.

A confident radiological diagnosis that a gastric ulcer is benign is almost invariably correct.[22] However, to maintain such a degree of confidence in the accuracy of the barium meal the examination must be technically of a high standard. The ulcer crater and its surrounding mucosa must be clearly demonstrated both *en face* and in profile, and the ulcer must be followed to healing by serial barium radiology (see Figure 23.7). Moreover, the radiologist must be willing to classify a number of lesions as indeterminate. These require early endoscopy and biopsy.[23]

As stated previously, the double-contrast barium meal cannot be regarded as being as accurate as endoscopy in the detection of superficial mucosal lesions such as gastritis and duodenitis, the detection rate of these conditions being in the region of 50%.[8,24] On the other hand, the barium meal is more likely than endoscopy to demonstrate lesions in the distal duodenum and lesions compressing or displacing the stomach or duodenum.

Role versus endoscopy

Since both the double-contrast barium meal and fibreoptic upper gastrointestinal endoscopy are accurate diagnostic techniques, what factors should guide the clinician to choose one or the other? In making such a decision a knowledge of exactly what each examination involves is essential. Many doctors are unaware of the degree of co-operation required from the patient in order to obtain a satisfactory double-contrast barium meal and refer old, frail, demented and arthritic patients for barium meal examination in the mistaken belief that it is less traumatic for these patients than endoscopy. In a prospective study involving 96 patients who had both a double-contrast barium meal and endoscopy, Dooley et al.[25] found that it was the younger patients who experienced moderate or severe discomfort at endoscopy. On the other hand, patients over 55 years of age tended to prefer endoscopy as they found greater difficulty in retaining gas in the stomach and manoeuvring on the X-ray table compared with younger patients.

Most patients undergoing endoscopy prefer sedation and tolerate the examination better when sedated,[26] but this has the drawback that the patient is off work for the whole day and requires transport to and from the hospital. Furthermore, it has been shown that patients over 50 years of age tolerate endoscopy without sedation better than younger patients.[26] The double-contrast barium meal is performed without sedation and takes only a short period of the working day. It would therefore seem sensible to refer young patients, who are more likely to be working, for barium meal, and older patients, who are more likely to have suspected neoplastic lesions requiring

biopsy, for endoscopy. In this way the two examinations will be truly complementary and not competitive.

Safety and cost are other considerations which may influence the referring clinician. The estimated mortality rate of upper gastrointestinal endoscopy is in the order of 1 in 10,000–12,000 examinations,[18,27] and there is a higher risk of significant morbidity.[28,29] The barium meal, although very safe, is not without complications. Barium sulphate is itself an inert substance, but commercial barium preparations have various additives which may cause allergic reactions.[30] The commonly used smooth muscle relaxants, glucagon and Buscopan, also have side-effects, as mentioned previously. There is also the small risk involved in exposure to ionizing radiation during the procedure.

With regard to cost, there is probably little to choose between the two examinations to the National Health Service but the fee for endoscopy is significantly higher in the private sector, both in the UK and in the USA. Other considerations which may influence the choice of examination are waiting lists and local expertise.[27,28]

Laufer[31] has emphasized a most important practical point by showing that when a radiologist has achieved a good double-contrast examination and is confident of his or her diagnosis then there will be almost 100% correlation with endoscopy. However, when the radiologist is in doubt, an accuracy of only 75% can be expected. If a barium meal is negative and the patient remains symptomatic then endoscopy should be performed, especially if the radiologist was not confident of the diagnosis. In such cases abnormalities will be detected at endoscopy in approximately 5% of cases.[32] Equally importantly, if endoscopy has been performed as the primary investigation and no lesion has been detected despite clinical evidence to the contrary, then the clinician should not hesitate to request a double-contrast barium meal.

TRANSABDOMINAL ULTRASONOGRAPHY

Ultrasonography is not generally useful in the detection of gastric or duodenal pathology in adults due to the presence of intraluminal gas. Occasionally, however, an area of focal thickening may be identified in patients with gastric tumours, particularly in gastric lymphoma, where the wall thickening is often extensive. However, this is a non-specific sign and may also be seen in gastritis and peptic ulceration.[33]

Ultrasonographic examination may be used as an alternative to barium studies in the diagnosis of hypertrophic pyloric stenosis in the vomiting infant. The length of the hypertrophied pyloric muscle is measured, as well as the muscle thickness and overall transverse diameter of the pylorus. Length in excess of 2 cm and muscle thickness greater than 4 mm are accurate predictors of hypertrophic pyloric stenosis. A pylorus greater than 1.5 cm in overall diameter is also suggestive, although this measurement is less reliable (Figure 23.18).[34]

Ultrasonography may also be used as a method of assessing gastric emptying, the emptying time being determined by the measurement of changes in the cross-sectional area of the gastric antrum.[35]

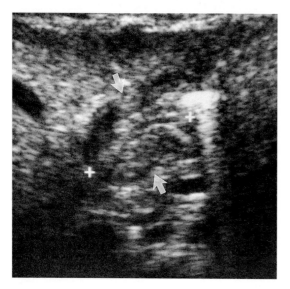

Figure 23.18

Transabdominal ultrasonographic scan showing elongated pylorus (arrowed). The hyperechoic area proximal to the pylorus is caused by gas in the gastric antrum. (Courtesy of Dr G.M.E. Hendry, Royal Hospital for Sick Children, Edinburgh.)

COMPUTED TOMOGRAPHY

The principal use of CT in this area is in the staging of gastric neoplasms, and the majority of patients having CT will have had the diagnosis made by other means. Occasionally, focal or diffuse thickening of the stomach will be seen in patients having upper abdominal CT for other reasons, and this may lead to suspicion of a gastric neoplasm. In order to avoid false-positive diagnoses, it is important to be aware that this appearance can be spurious if the stomach is poorly distended. In doubtful cases, additional contrast and/or gas-producing agents should be given, together with an intravenous smooth muscle relaxant, and the patient rescanned (Figure 23.19). Further information may be provided by decubitus scans. Provided that the stomach is well distended with contrast and/or gas, focal thickening of greater than 1 cm is regarded as abnormal, with the proviso that the wall thickness at the oesophagogastric junction and gastric antrum may be thicker than this in normal patients.[36]

Although CT is widely used to stage gastric cancer, its precise accuracy for this purpose still remains somewhat controversial. In order to stage correctly, CT must be able to give accurate information about extent of local disease, spread to adjacent organs, involvement of lymph nodes, peritoneal disease and distant metastases. Early reports suggested that it was reliable for predicting localized disease and assessing local and distant spread, and correlated closely with surgical findings.[36–38]

However, initial optimism was tempered in the light of later series. Kleinhaus and Militianu[39] found that CT had a staging accuracy of 72% overall in a group of 49 patients when compared with surgery, with a tendency to understage disease. Prediction of lymph node involvement and tumour spread to adjacent organs was unreliable. In another study of 37 patients, 61% of those deemed Stage I on CT criteria were found at

surgery to be Stage III/IV; and 50% of patients considered unresectable on CT were considered operable at surgery.[40] The series of Sussman et al.[41] reported on 75 patients, in whom 47% were incorrectly staged by CT. Patients were both understaged and overstaged, due mainly to difficulty in assessing tumour status in lymph nodes, and direct invasion of adjacent organs.

It is generally accepted that distant metastases are well demonstrated with CT. For lung metastases, CT is the most sensitive imaging modality, and liver metastases are also well shown by contrast-enhanced CT.[42]

Faced with such conflicting reports, it is clearly difficult to define the precise role and clinical utility of CT in gastric carcinoma staging. As with staging of oesophageal carcinoma, CT would appear to be most helpful in confirming advanced disease. Where CT shows limited disease, it would seem reasonable at the present time to confirm staging with laparotomy.

Technical refinements to CT scanners are likely to improve staging accuracy. Spiral-acquisition CT, for example, allows the

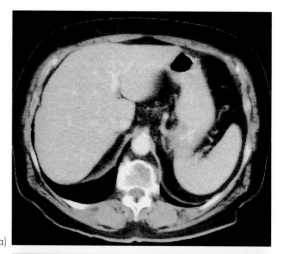

(a)

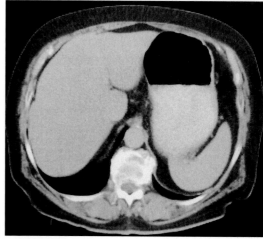

(b)

Figure 23.19

Upper abdominal CT scans in a patient with non-Hodgkin's lymphoma. (a) The stomach appears grossly thickened, raising the possibility of gastric involvement. (b) Same patient after intravenous injection of Buscopan and adequate distension of the stomach with oral contrast and gas. The stomach is seen to be of normal thickness.

upper abdomen to be scanned in a single breath-hold. Small lesions in the scanned volume are therefore less likely to be overlooked due to breathing artefact or slice misregistration.[43] Spiral-acquisition CT is the most accurate imaging modality for lung metastases,[44,45] and would be expected to have increased sensitivity for lymph nodes, and liver and peritoneal metastases, although specificity will not be improved.[46] Similarly, optimization of scanning technique may be of benefit. Some workers have advocated the use of low-density oral contrast media, such as water or oil emulsions, when staging gastric carcinoma.[47–49] When intravenous contrast is given as well, visualization of the primary tumour is improved, as is detection of liver metastases and nodal enlargement.[50] The authors routinely use a combination of oral water, intravenous contrast and spiral acquisition for this indication (Figure 23.20).

In cases of gastric lymphona, CT appearances of the local lesion may be similar to gastric carcinoma. However, diffuse wall thickening, extensive thickening (greater than 3 cm) and smooth or lobulated outer contour of the lesion with preservation of fat planes between the lesion and adjacent organs are said to be more in favour of lymphoma.[36,51] Moreover, the diagnosis may be suggested by CT signs of lymphoma elsewhere, such as splenomegaly or intra-abdominal lymph node enlargement in a typical distribution.

Gastric leiomyosarcoma typically appears on CT as a large mass, which is usually exophytic in location, and which may show calcification. Because of the tendency to grow outside the gastric lumen, leiomyosarcoma is often difficult to characterize on barium studies. There may be ulceration of the gastric mucosa overlying the tumour, and areas of necrosis are often seen within it (Figure 23.21).[36,52,53] Liver metastases and local spread to adjacent viscera are well shown by CT.

CT is of value in the assessment of primary tumours of the duodenum, although these are rare. It is also helpful in confirming the presence of an intramural mass in cases of duodenal

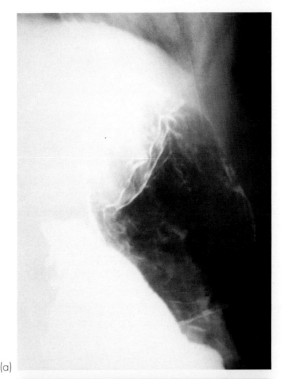
(a)

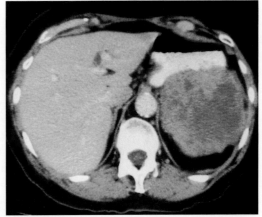
(b)

Figure 23.21
Gastric leiomyosarcoma. (a) Barium meal showing abnormal appearance and position of gastric fundus consistent with extrinsic compression. (b) CT scan with intravenous contrast. There is a large irregular exophytic mass arising from the posterior surface of the gastric fundus and displacing the stomach anteriorly. Areas of necrosis are seen within the mass.

intramural haematoma due to trauma or blood dyscrasias. However, MRI can confirm its haemorrhagic nature by virtue of its signal characteristics.

In general, the many pathological processes which can cause displacement and invasion of the stomach or duodenum from outside, such as hepatic, renal, splenic and pancreatic neoplasms and cysts, are well demonstrated on CT.

ENDOLUMINAL ULTRASONOGRAPHY

Endoluminal ultrasonography (EUS) is a relatively new technique which shows promise for gastric cancer staging. It has the potential to overcome some of the deficiencies of CT

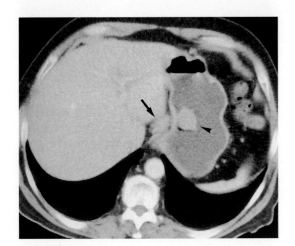

Figure 23.20
Gastric carcinoma staging CT scan using spiral acquisition, intravenous contrast and water as oral contrast. There is enhancement of the stomach wall with good visualization of the polypoid primary lesion (arrowhead). An enlarged coeliac node is seen adjacent to the lesser gastric curve (arrow).

because its strengths lie in assessment of degree of tumour penetration and local lymph node involvement. A high frequency ultrasound probe, typically 7.5–12 MHz, attached to an endoscope is passed into the water-filled gastric lumen. Assessment can be made of the local lesion, regional lymph nodes and the left hepatic lobe. The bulk of the right hepatic lobe and peritoneum is generally outside the range of the probe, which is limited to approximately 10 cm.

With EUS, five alternating hyper-/hypoechoic layers can be identified in the normal gastric wall: (1) hyperechoic – mucosa; (2) hypoechoic – deep mucosa; (3) hyperechoic – submucosa; (4) hypoechoic – muscularis propria; (5) hyperechoic – serosal interface. Gastric cancer is seen as a hypoechoic disruption of the layers, and the depth of penetration can be determined in relation to this. In T1 tumours (invasion as far as submucosa), disruption of the first three layers is seen; in T2 lesions (invasion of muscularis propria), four layers are disrupted; T3 tumours (invasion of serosa without involvement of adjacent structures) are shown as penetration through the fifth layer; and T4 lesions can be seen to invade adjacent structures. Using these criteria, EUS correlates with surgical/pathological tumour stage in up to 92% of cases, and is significantly better than CT.[54,55]

Detection of metastatic lymph nodes with EUS relies on ultrasonographic appearance rather than size alone. Involved nodes are characteristically hypoechoic, and well defined or rounded. Using these criteria in a series of 83 patients, Akahoshi et al.[56] were able to detect involved nodes in 83%, but poor sensitivity was encountered with small nodes in the region of 5 mm in diameter (seen mainly in patients with early gastric cancer). Botet et al.[55] found a 76% concordance in 50 patients between EUS and pathological staging of lymph nodes, a significantly better result than with CT (48%). In this study also, there was a tendency for EUS to understage lymph nodes. Tio et al.[54] reported 86% sensitivity for lymph node metastasis in a group of patients with gastric carcinoma. Specificity was poor, however, at 47%.

As EUS appears better suited to the local staging of gastric cancer, and CT is preferable for distal metastases, the two techniques may prove to be complementary, particularly with further technical refinements. However, reliable preoperative staging of gastric cancer with imaging remains a significant challenge.

MAGNETIC RESONANCE IMAGING

MRI is not well suited to examination of the stomach at the present time. The relatively low spatial resolution is a drawback, and the long acquisition times needed for conventional spin-echo imaging mean that patient movement, breathing and other physiological artefacts produce a degraded image. Gradient-echo sequences allow images to be obtained during a single breath-hold, but these sequences are prone to susceptibility artefact where there is an interface between bowel gas and fluid. This can result in effacement of adjacent structures, such as the stomach wall. Gastric tumours have been identified on MRI, but normally must be extensive before they can be

reliably demonstrated.[57] The same applies to lymph node enlargement in the upper abdomen.

In gastric cancer staging, MRI may be useful in the detection of liver metastases, and in differentiating haemangioma from metastases.[58–61] However, transabdominal ultrasonography and contrast-enhanced CT are usually preferred because of relatively low cost and increased versatility and availability.

Bowel wall haematomas have a characteristic evolving appearance on MRI due to magnetically-active haemoglobin degradation products.[62,63] This can be helpful in the diagnosis of duodenal haematoma when barium studies and CT are equivocal.

ANGIOGRAPHY AND INTERVENTIONAL RADIOLOGY

The main use of angiography in the investigation of the stomach and duodenum is in the detection of acute upper gastrointestinal haemorrhage. It is now widely accepted that a patient with acute upper gastrointestinal bleeding should be examined initially by endoscopy, which is widely available, well tolerated, often identifies the cause of haemorrhage and allows coagulation of the bleeding site. If the bleeding point has not been identified at endoscopy it can usually be detected by angiography, as long as the rate of bleeding exceeds 0.5 ml/min (Figure 23.22). Both the coeliac axis and the superior mesenteric artery should be selectively catheterized.[64] In some centres, radionuclide studies are carried out prior to angiography as they are said to be more sensitive for the detection of bleeding.[65] If positive, angiography is then carried out to determine the bleeding site.

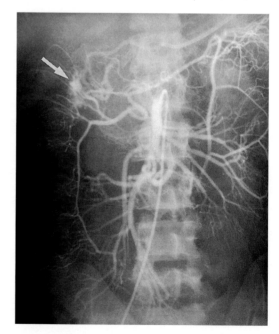

Figure 23.22
Bleeding postbulbar duodenal ulcer. Superior mesenteric arteriogram showing pooling of contrast in the duodenum (arrow) from a bleeding inferior pancreaticoduodenal artery. Bleeding ulcer confirmed at operation. (Courtesy of Dr D.C. Grieve.)

Once the site of haemorrhage has been identified, catheter techniques may be used for therapeutic purposes. Vasoconstrictor agents such as vasopressin, infused selectively into the vessel supplying the bleeding lesion, are usually effective in controlling haemorrhage. Alternatively, the vessel responsible for the bleed can be selectively embolized. A wide range of embolic agents is available, including gelatin sponge and steel coils. Embolization in the upper gastrointestinal tract can usually be carried out without risk of gut infarction due to the rich collateral blood supply. However, the risk is increased in patients with pre-existing vascular disease, or where previous surgery has disrupted collateral vessels.

Balloon dilatation of stenosed gastroduodenal and gastrojejunal anastamoses is now an established procedure.[66,67] In some series a combined endoscopic and radiological approach is used.[68] The inflated balloon exerts a radial force against the stricture without the longitudinal shearing force of bougienage. This, together with the use of guide wires, reduces the risk of perforation during dilatation.

Percutaneous gastrostomy and gastrojejunostomy performed under fluoroscopic control is a useful alternative to total parenteral nutrition in patients with an intact small bowel. It is a safe, technically easy and cost-effective technique for patients who are unable to take sufficient calories by mouth, and it is simpler and cheaper than surgical gastrostomy. Percutaneous gastrostomy is adequate for patients with oesophageal obstruction. Positioning the tube in the jejunum is preferable when reflux or aspiration is likely to occur.[69]

REFERENCES

1. Field S. The acute abdomen. In Sutton D (ed.) *Textbook of Radiology and Imaging*, 4th edn. Edinburgh and London: Churchill Livingstone, 1987: 929–957.
2. Montgomery DP, Clamp SE, De Dombal FT et al. A comparison of barium sulphate preparations used for the double-contrast barium meal. *Clin Radiol* 1982; **33:** 265–269.
3. Roberts GM. Barium meal technique. The normal stomach and duodenum. In Simpkins KC (ed.) *A Textbook of Radiological Diagnosis*, 5th edn. London: HK Lewis, 1988: 157–173.
4. Levine MS, Rubesin SE, Herlinger H & Laufer I. Double-contrast upper gastrointestinal examination: technique and interpretation. *Radiology* 1988; **168:** 593–602.
5. Bell KE, McKinstry CS & Mills JOM. Iopamidol in the diagnosis of suspected upper gastrointestinal perforation. *Clin Radiol* 1987; **38:** 165–168.
6. Fraser GM & Fraser ID. Gastrografin in perforated duodenal ulcer and acute pancreatitis. *Clin Radiol* 1974; **25:** 397–402.
7. Gelfand DW & Ott DJ. Gastric ulcer scars. *Radiology* 1981; **140:** 37–43.
8. Ott DJ, Gelfand DW, Wu WC & Kerr RM. Sensitivity of single- vs. double-contrast radiology in erosive gastritis. *AJR* 1982; **138:** 263–266.
9. Reese DF, Hodgson JR & Dockerty MB. Giant hypertrophy of the gastric mucosa (Ménétrier's disease): a correlation of the roentgenographic, pathologic and clinical findings. *AJR* 1962; **88:** 619–626.
10. Lumsden K, MacLarnon JC & Dawson J. Giant duodenal ulcer. *Gut* 1970; **11:** 592–599.
11. Cohen WN. Gastric involvement in Crohn's disease. *AJR* 1967; **101:** 425–430.
12. Menuck LS. Gastric lymphoma, a radiologic diagnosis. *Gastrointest Radiol* 1976; **1:** 157–161.
13. Lee CS & Mangla JC. Superior mesenteric artery compression syndrome. *Am J Gastroenterol* 1978; **70:** 141–150.
14. Anderson JR, Earnshaw PM & Fraser GM. Extrinsic compression of the third part of the duodenum. *Clin Radiol* 1982; **33:** 75–81.
15. Salter RH, Girdwood TG, Scott-Harden WG & Cole TP. Endoscopic and radiological assessment of recurrent ulceration after peptic ulcer surgery. *Br J Radiol* 1978; **51:** 257–259.

16. Grundy A, McFarland RJ, Gazet JC & Pilkington TRE. Radiological appearances following vertical banded gastroplasty. *Clin Radiol* 1985; **36:** 395–400.
17. Stephens DH, Sheedy PF & James EM. Neoplastic lesions. In Margulis AR & Burhenne HJ (eds) *Alimentary Tract Radiology*, 3rd edn. St Louis: CV Mosby, 1983: 1316–1356.
18. Gelfand DW, Ott DJ, Munitz HA & Chen YM. Radiology and endoscopy: a radiologic viewpoint. *Ann Intern Med* 1984; **101:** 550–552.
19. Gelfand DW & Ott DJ. Single- vs. double-contrast gastrointestinal studies: critical analysis of reported statistics. *AJR* 1981; **137:** 523–528.
20. Brown P, Salmon PR, Burwood RJ, Knox AJ, Glendinnen BG & Read AE. The endoscopic, radiological and surgical findings in chronic duodenal ulceration. *Scand J Gastroenterol* 1978; **13:** 557–560.
21. Cotton PB & Shorvon PJ. Analysis of endoscopy and radiography in the diagnosis, follow-up and treatment of peptic ulcer disease. *Clin Gastroenterol* 1984; **13:** 383–403.
22. Fraser GM. Peptic ulcer and gastritis. In Simpkins KC (ed.) *A Textbook of Radiological Diagnosis*, 5th edn. London: HK Lewis, 1988: 225–254.
23. Thompson G, Somers S & Stevenson GW. Benign gastric ulcer: a reliable radiologic diagnosis. *AJR* 1983; **141:** 331–333.
24. Kunstlinger FC, Thoeni RF, Grendell JH et al. The radiographic appearance of erosive duodenitis: a radiographic–endoscopic correlative study. *J Clin Gastroenterol* 1980; **2:** 205–211.
25. Dooley GP, Weiner JM & Larson AW. Endoscopy or radiography? – the patient's choice. Prospective comparative survey of patient acceptability of upper gastrointestinal endoscopy and radiography. *Am J Med* 1986; **80:** 203–207.
26. Cann PA & Kerrigan DD. Is routine sedation appropriate for upper gastrointestinal endoscopy (UGE)? *Gut* 1988; **29:** 1488–1489.
27. Colin-Jones DG. Endoscopy or radiology for upper gastrointestinal symptoms? *Lancet* 1986; **i:** 1022–1023.
28. Simpkins KC. What use is barium? *Clin Radiol* 1988; **39:** 469–473.
29. Meyers MA & Ghahremani GG. Complications of gastrointestinal fiberoptic endoscopy. *Gastrointest Radiol* 1977; **2:** 273–280.
30. Janower ML. Hypersensitivity reactions after barium studies of the upper and lower gastrointestinal tract. *Radiology* 1986; **161:** 139–140.
31. Laufer I. Assessment of the accuracy of double contrast gastroduodenal radiology. *Gastroenterology* 1976; **71:** 874–878.
32. Arfeen S, Salter RH and Girdwood TG. A negative double contrast barium meal – qualified reassurance. *Clin Radiol* 1987; **38:** 49–50.
33. Derchi LE, Biggi E, Neumaier CE & Cicio GR. Ultrasonographic appearances of gastric cancer. *Br J Radiol* 1983; **56:** 365–370.
34. Haller JO & Cohen HL. Hypertrophic pyloric stenosis: diagnosis using US. *Radiology* 1986; **161:** 335–339.
35. Bolondi L, Bortolotti M, Santi V, Calletti T, Gaiani S & Labò G. Measurement of gastric emptying time by real-time ultrasonography. *Gastroenterology* 1985; **89:** 752–759.
36. Balfe DM, Koehler RE, Karstaedt N, Stanley RJ & Sagel SS. Computed tomography of gastric neoplasms. *Radiology* 1981; **140:** 431–436.
37. Lee KR, Levine E, Moffat RE, Bigongiari LR & Hermreck AS. Computed tomographic staging of malignant gastric neoplasms. *Radiology* 1979; **133:** 151–155.
38. Moss AA, Schnyder P, Marks W & Margulis AR. Gastric adenocarcinoma: a comparison of the accuracy and economics of staging by computed tomography and surgery. *Gastroenterology* 1981; **80:** 45–50.
39. Kleinhaus U and Militianu D. Computed tomography in the preoperative evaluation of gastric carcinoma. *Gastrointest Radiol* 1988; **13:** 97–101.
40. Cook AO, Levine BA, Sirinek KR & Gaskill HV. Evaluation of gastric adenocarcinoma. Abdominal computed tomography does not replace celiotomy. *Arch Surg* 1986; **121:** 603–606.
41. Sussman SK, Halvorsen RA, Illescas FF et al. Gastric adenocarcinoma: CT versus surgical staging. *Radiology* 1988; **167:** 335–340.
42. Halvorsen RA and Thompson WM. Gastrointestinal cancer: diagnosis, staging and the follow-up role of imaging. *Semin Ultrasound CT MR* 1989; **10:** 467–480.
43. Kalender WA, Seissler W, Klotz E & Vock P. Spiral volumetric CT with single-breath-hold technique, continuous transport, and continuous scanner rotation. *Radiology* 1990; **176:** 181–183.
44. Remy-Jardin M, Remy J, Giraud F & Marquette C-H. Pulmonary nodules: detection with thick-section spiral CT versus conventional CT. *Radiology* 1993; **187:** 513–520.
45. Collie DA, Wright AR, Williams JR, Hashemi-Malayeri B, Stevenson AJM & Turnbull CM. Comparison of spiral-acquisition CT and conventional CT in the assessment of pulmonary metastatic disease. *Br J Radiol* 1994; **67:** 436–444.

46. Zeman RK, Fox SH, Silverman PM et al. Helical (spiral) CT of the abdomen. *AJR* 1993; **160:** 719–725.
47. Angellini G, Macarini L & Fratello A. Use of water as an oral contrast agent for CT study of the stomach. *AJR* 1987; **149:** 1084.
48. Raptopoulos V, Davis MA, Davidoff A et al. Fat-density oral contrast agent for abdominal CT. *Radiology* 1987; **164:** 653–656.
49. Baert AL, Roex L, Marchal G, Hermans P, Dewilde D & Wilms G. Computed tomography of the stomach with water as an oral contrast agent: technique and preliminary results. *J Comput Assist Tomogr* 1989; **13:** 633–636.
50. Minami M, Kawauchi N, Itai Y, Niki T & Sasaki Y. Gastric tumours: radiologic-pathologic correlation and accuracy of T staging with dynamic CT. *Radiology* 1992; **185:** 173–178.
51. Buy J-N and Moss AA. Computed tomography of gastric lymphoma. *AJR* 1982; **138:** 859–865.
52. Clark RA & Alexander ES. Computed tomography of gastrointestinal leiomyosarcoma. *Gastrointest Radiol* 1982; **7:** 127–129.
53. Scatarige JC, Fishman EK, Jones B, Cameron JL, Sanders RC & Siegelman SS. Gastric leiomyosarcoma: CT observations. *J Comput Assist Tomogr* 1985; **9:** 320–327.
54. Tio TL, Coene PPLO, Schouwink MH & Tytgat GNJ. Esophagogastric carcinoma: preoperative TNM classification with endosonography. *Radiology* 1989; **173:** 411–417.
55. Botet JF, Lightdale, CJ, Zauber AG et al. Preoperative staging of gastric cancer: comparison of endoscopic US and dynamic CT. *Radiology* 1991; **181:** 426–432.
56. Akahoshi K, Misawa T, Fujishima H, Chijiiwa Y & Nawata H. Regional lymph node metastasis in gastric cancer: evaluation with endoscopic US. *Radiology* 1992; **182:** 559–564.
57. Winkler ML, Hricak H & Higgins CB. MR imaging of diffusely infiltrating gastric carcinoma. *J Comput Assist Tomogr* 1987; **11:** 337–339.
58. Curati WL, Halevy A, Gibson RN, Carr DH, Blumgart LH & Steiner RE. Ultrasound, CT, and MRI comparison in primary and secondary tumours of the liver. *Gastrointest Radiol* 1988; **13:** 123–128.
59. Heiken JP, Weyman PJ, Lee JK et al. Detection of focal hepatic masses: prospective evaluation with CT, delayed CT, CT during arterial portography, and MR imaging. *Radiology* 1989; **171:** 47–51.
60. Rummeny E, Wernecke K, Saini S et al. Comparison between high field-strength MR imaging and CT for screening of hepatic metastases: a receiver operating characteristic analysis. *Radiology* 1992; **182:** 879–886.
61. Itai Y, Ohtomo K, Furui S, Yamauchi T, Minami M & Yashiro N. Noninvasive diagnosis of small cavernous haemangioma of the liver: advantage of MRI. *AJR* 1985; **145:** 1195–1199.
62. Martin B, Mulopulos GP & and Butler HE. MR imaging of intramural duodenal hematoma. *J Comput Assist Tomogr* 1986; **10:** 1042–1043.
63. Hahn PF, Stark DD, Vici L-G & Ferruci JT. Duodenal hematoma: the ring sign in MR imaging. *Radiology* 1986; **159:** 379–382.
64. Hemingway A & Allison D. Angiography in acute upper gastrointestinal bleeding. In Simpkins KC (ed.) *A Textbook of Radiological Diagnosis*, 5th edn. London: HK Lewis, 1988: 194–205.
65. Winzelberg GG, Froelich JW, McKusick KA & Strauss HW. Scintigraphic detection of gastrointestinal bleeding: a review of current methods. *Am J Gastroenterol* 1983; **78:** 324–327.
66. Hegedüs V & Raaschou HO. Radiologically guided dilatation of stenotic gastroduodenal anastomosis. *Gastrointest Radiol* 1986; **11:** 27–29.
67. Mishkin JD, Meranze SG, Burke DR, Stein EJ & McLean GK. Interventional radiologic treatment of complications following gastric bypass surgery for morbid obesity. *Gastrointest Radiol* 1988; **13:** 9–14.
68. Lindor KD, Ott BJ & Hughes RW. Balloon dilatation of upper digestive tract strictures. *Gastroenterology* 1985; **89:** 545–548.
69. Gray RR, St Louis EL & Grosman H. Percutaneous gastrostomy and gastrojejunostomy. *Br J Radiol* 1987; **60:** 1067–1070.

24

ENDOSCOPY OF THE STOMACH AND DUODENUM

CP Willoughby
KFR Schiller

Much of the ground relevant to endoscopy of the stomach and duodenum is covered in Chapter 3. It is therefore appropriate to refer the reader to that chapter, and to concentrate in this chapter on normal and abnormal appearances and on therapeutic procedures in the stomach and duodenum.

ENDOSCOPIC DIAGNOSIS IN THE STOMACH AND DUODENUM

There is a wide range of normal appearances in the stomach and duodenum which the trainee endoscopist must learn to recognize. Standard endoscopic atlases can be a useful source of information and reference.[1-3] In addition, there is an atlas available for use on CD-ROM.[4] Here it is only possible to mention a few of these appearances.

Normal variant appearances

The dentate or Z-line which represents the junction of squamous and columnar epithelium is highly variable in appearance. Normally occurring irregularities and mucosal islands can be confused with oesophagitis or with Barrett's epithelium.

Within the stomach, the rugae vary in prominence between individuals and also with the degree of gastric distension induced by air insufflation. They tend to be less marked in the antrum (Figure 24.1, see colour plate also), but large folds can occur in the prepyloric region, sometimes as sentinel folds leading to the site of duodenal ulcer (DU) or ulcer scar. Peristaltic activity is common in the distal stomach and takes the form of symmetrical contraction waves, occurring approximately every 20 seconds and propagating towards the pylorus.

The pylorus itself is normally relaxed and open except during peristalsis and appears as a ring diaphragm when traversed by an endoscope. Normally, there is no pyloric canal. The proximal duodenum (Figure 24.2, see colour plate also) tends to be rather smooth and bulb-like, with a velvety mucosal pattern reflecting the villous nature of the small bowel lining. A

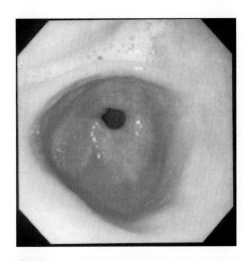

Figure 24.1
Normal gastric antrum and pylorus.

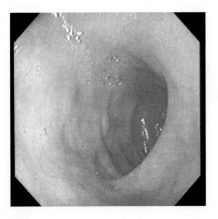

Figure 24.2
Normal proximal duodenum.

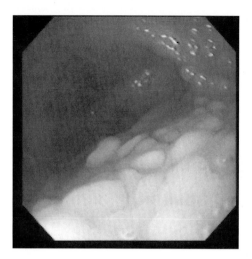

Figure 24.3
Polypoid appearance in the duodenal bulb.

polypoid appearance caused by ectopic gastric mucosa or hypertrophy of Brunner's glands is commonly observed (Figure 24.3, see colour plate also). As the superior duodenal fold is passed and the second part of the duodenum entered, the gross architecture of this area is typified by clearly visible circumferential folds or valvulae conniventes (Figure 24.4, see colour plate also). Between these, the papilla of Vater can sometimes be seen as a nipple-like structure at the cephalad end of a discrete longitudinal fold (Figure 24.5, see colour plate also) but is often better identified with a side-viewing instrument. Congenital periampullary diverticula are common, being found in about 5% of normal subjects.

In addition to the normal anatomical appearances, the endoscopist should be familiar with minor iatrogenic changes caused by the instrument itself. Small areas of mucosal redness are commonly seen in the apex of the bulb during withdrawal

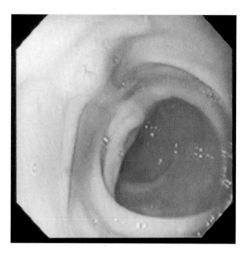

Figure 24.5
Normal duodenal papilla.

after the instrument has been passed into the second part of the duodenum. Similar appearances due to minor trauma are seen when a nasogastric tube has been *in situ* for some time. Areas of minor haemorrhage occur at the site of mucosal biopsies. Excessive suction can traumatize the gastric or duodenal mucosa causing typical round, often raised, areas of artefactual redness or frank petechial bleeding (Figure 24.6, see colour plate also).

Mucosal lesions

'Gastritis'

True superficial gastritis is variably recognizable at endoscopy, and there is a relatively poor correlation between the interpretation of visual and biopsy-derived histopathological appearances. Some endoscopists report 'gastritis' when they see a diffuse or spotty redness of the mucosa, most commonly in the gastric antrum. Antral redness may imply investigation for the presence of *Helicobacter pylori*, especially if found in association with duodenal ulcer disease. Shallow erosions may occur with mucosal redness in the antrum and body of the stomach, particularly in patients who have taken non-steroidal anti-inflammatory drugs

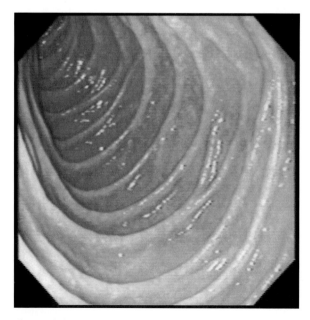

Figure 24.4
Normal second part of duodenum.

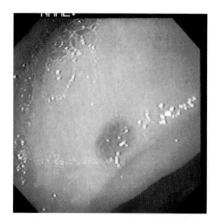

Figure 24.6
Suction artefact.

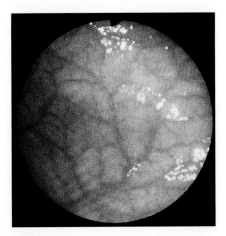

Figure 24.7
Gastric mucosal atrophy. (Reproduced, with permission, from Schiller KFR, Cochel R & Hunt RH. A Colour Atlas of Gastrointestinal Endoscopy. London: Chapman & Hall, 1986.)

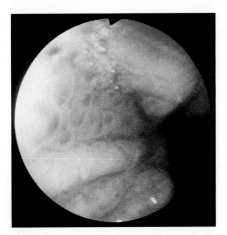

Figure 24.9
Rugal folds in portal gastropathy. (Reproduced, with permission, from Schiller KFR, Cochel R & Hunt RH. A Colour Atlas of Gastrointestinal Endoscopy. London: Chapman & Hall, 1986.)

(NSAIDs). 'Reflux' gastritis may occur due to duodenogastric alkaline reflux, particularly following previous gastric surgery.

Patchy or diffuse mucosal pallor in the stomach occurs in the presence of true atrophic gastritis, sometimes with associated intestinal metaplasia. In gastric atrophy (Figure 24.7, see colour plate also), the mucosa is obviously thinned and the vascular pattern exaggerated, giving rise to a somewhat 'colonic' appearance at endoscopy. Secondary dysplasia or carcinoma may develop in such areas.

It cannot be overemphasized that gastritis is a histopathological concept, and that the diagnosis of gastritis and its grading must be based on the interpretation of appearances in specimens submitted to a pathologist for assessment. The Sydney classification represents the most recent system.[5]

'Gastropathy'

Normal gastric rugae vary greatly in prominence. Markedly thickened and tortuous rugae occur in Ménètrier's disease (Figure 24.8, see colour plate also), but this is a much over-diagnosed condition, rarely seen in clinical practice.

Prominent 'beefy' gastric rugae with generalized or punctate erythema often occur in patients with chronic liver disease – the

so-called 'portal gastropathy',[6] also referred to as 'gastric measles' (Figure 24.9, see colour plate also). Biopsy specimens show inflammatory infiltration and a disproportionate degree of vascular ectasia. In the presence of these mucosal changes, profuse gastrointestinal bleeding may occur which responds poorly to standard medical management, though it may be reduced if the underlying portal hypertension is treated effectively.

Duodenitis

Non-specific patchy redness and swelling of the folds in the proximal duodenum is commonly referred to as 'duodenitis' by the endoscopist, although again, the correlation with histologically proven inflammation is not perfect. Small erosions and punctate erythema occasionally produce a salami-like appearance of the duodenal mucosa (Figure 24.10, see colour plate also), and larger erosions can also be found. Such patients may be asymptomatic but the condition is often present in patients with symptoms of 'non-ulcer dyspepsia', and may represent a phase in the natural history of duodenal ulcer disease proper.[7] The relevance of *H. pylori* to duodenitis is uncertain.

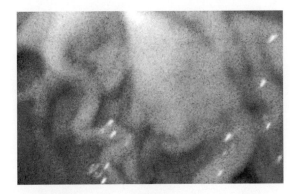

Figure 24.8
Ménètrier's disease. (Reproduced, with permission, from Schiller KFR, Cochel R & Hunt RH. A Colour Atlas of Gastrointestinal Endoscopy. London: Chapman & Hall, 1986.)

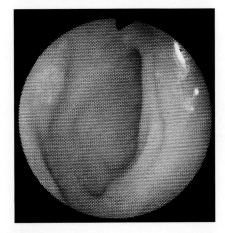

Figure 24.10
Salami-type duodenitis. (Reproduced, with permission, from Schiller KFR, Cochel R & Hunt RH. A Colour Atlas of Gastrointestinal Endoscopy. London: Chapman & Hall, 1986.)

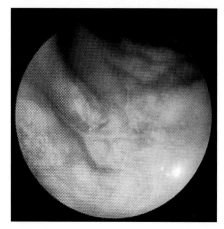

Figure 24.11
Sparsity of small bowel mucosal folds in coeliac disease
(illustrated by dye spray).(Reproduced, with permission, from
Schiller KFR, Cochel R & Hunt RH. A Colour Atlas of
Gastrointestinal Endoscopy. London: Chapman & Hall, 1986.)

Coeliac disease

In coeliac disease, the duodenal valvulae conniventes are often
much less prominent than usual (Figure 24.11, see colour plate
also). On close inspection, the duodenal mucosa may be
atrophic in appearance or show a mosaic pattern even without
dye spray enhancement. In patients with unexplained anaemia
or other features of possible malabsorption, it is always worth
taking at least four duodenal biopsy specimens to check for
villous atrophy. Appearances are as reliable as those obtained
from jejunal biopsies.[8]

Miscellaneous mucosal lesions

A wide variety of other mucosal abnormalities may occasionally
be detected at gastroduodenoscopy. Isolated angiomas (Figure
24.12, see colour plate also) are frequent, whereas profuse vascular anomalies are seen in hereditary haemorrhagic telangiectasia. Diffuse gastric vascular ectasia, particularly in the antrum,
has a characteristic appearance giving rise to the descriptive
term 'watermelon stomach' (Figure 24.13, see colour plate also).

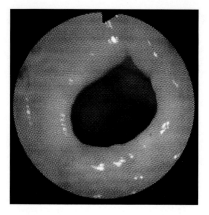

Figure 24.13
Diffuse vascular ectasia – 'watermelon stomach'.

In the proximal duodenum, small discrete pale nodules are
common, and may be due to heterotopic gastric mucosa or
hyperplasia of Brunner's glands. Accurate differentiation, if indeed
this is required, depends on examination of biopsy specimens.

Ulcerative lesions

Gastric and duodenal ulcer

Benign gastric ulcers (GUs) are most commonly found on the
lesser curve, or on the incisura or angulus, but may occur at
any site within the stomach. Multiple lesions are not uncommon. The typical benign GU has a well demarcated edge with
rugae radiating from the lip of the crater (Figure 24.14, see
colour plate also). In GUs which have bled recently, stigmata
of haemorrhage such as haematin spots in the basal slough or
visible vessels with or without continued bleeding may be present (Figure 24.15, see colour plate also). Giant GUs several
centimetres in diameter can occur especially in elderly patients,
but have the same visual attributes as smaller benign lesions.
During successful medical treatment, an ulcer diminishes progressively in width and depth, ultimately healing to a pale scar
often surrounded by radiating erythematous folds (Figure
24.16, see colour plate also), though fibrosis may be more

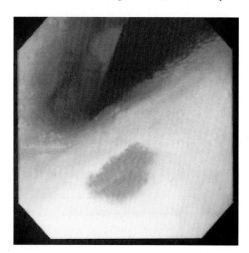

Figure 24.12
Gastric angioma seen on inversion view.

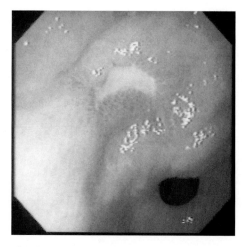

Figure 24.14
Benign gastric ulcer.

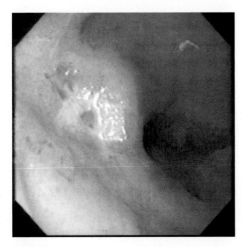

Figure 24.15
Gastric ulcer with visible vessel in its base.

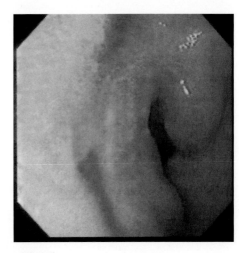

Figure 24.17
Duodenal ulcer.

extensive, leading to the formation of an 'hour-glass' stomach. DUs are almost invariably benign and most occur in the first few centimetres of the duodenum (Figure 24.17, see colour plate also). They vary greatly in size and shape and are often associated with inflammation and oedema of the surrounding mucosa. Multiple ulcers, particularly 'kissing' ulcers on the anterior and posterior duodenal walls are common. In the past, DUs have been characterized by cycles of healing and recurrence, with or without treatment, and this in turn has led to distortion and scarring of the proximal duodenum with the development of pseudodiverticula, resulting in the typical trefoil deformity of chronic duodenal ulcer disease seen on barium radiology. *H. pylori* eradication therapy, with the likelihood of less frequent ulcer recurrence after healing, may in the future reduce the incidence of such scarring.

Differentiation between benign and malignant gastric ulcer

A small proportion of apparently benign GUs are either frank carcinomas or contain small foci of cancer within them. Ulcer-

cancers tend to have somewhat beaded or irregular edges and are surrounded by radiating rigid mucosal folds which may stop short of the rim of the crater. Reliable differentiation between benign and malignant lesions requires histological examination by multiple biopsies; some gastroenterologists in addition take cytological smears. In most instances even where an apparently benign GU is diagnosed, a check endoscopy is performed after a standard course of medical treatment and further biopsies taken if healing appears incomplete.

Gastric carcinoma

Broadly speaking, a cancer of the stomach may present as a lump or solid lesion, as a flat, depressed or raised ulcerated lesion, or as a widely infiltrative mainly submucosal lesion (linitis plastica), or any combination of these forms.

The typical advanced gastric carcinoma takes the form of an irregular ulcer with rolled, everted edges, commonly in the prepyloric antrum or on the lesser curve (Figure 24.18, see colour plate also). Small satellite areas of ulceration may be seen where there is extensive neoplastic infiltration of gastric

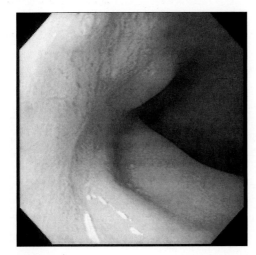

Figure 24.16
Ulcer scar in the duodenum.

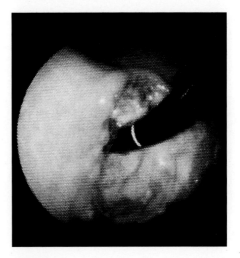

Figure 24.18
Ulcerating gastric carcinoma.

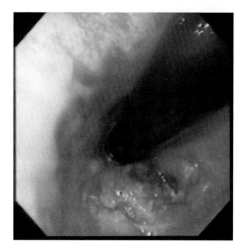

Figure 24.19
Stenosing cancer of the gastric cardia seen on inversion.

rugae. Stenosing lesions of the cardia (Figure 24.19, see colour plate also), originating in the lower oesophagus but more commonly in the stomach, may hinder or prevent passage of the endoscope into the stomach. Any resistance to the advance of the instrument through the oesophagogastric junction is a cause for concern and careful inspection of the lowest portion of the oesophagus, and of the cardia by an inversion manoeuvre, together with multiple biopsies from the local mucosa is important if a tumour is suspected. Prepyloric cancers often lead to structural or functional gastric outlet obstruction; the finding of a large volume of gastric contents with necrotic food debris, despite appropriate pre-endoscopy preparation, should lead to a careful assessment of the prepyloric region, with this possibility in mind. Gastric atony in the absence of outlet obstruction, for example, due to diabetes mellitus, may also cause food and fluid retention.

Unfortunately, in the UK, most gastric carcinomas are only diagnosed at a late stage when the prospect of a curative resection is very small. So-called early gastric cancers, i.e., tumours confined to the mucosa and submucosa, may be ulcerated,

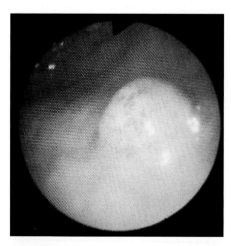

Figure 24.20
Early gastric cancer. (Reproduced, with permission, from Schiller KFR, Cochel R & Hunt RH. A Colour Atlas of Gastrointestinal Endoscopy. London: Chapman & Hall, 1986.)

plaque-like or slightly polypoid[9] (Figure 24.20, see colour plate also). When found, the chances of a successful excision are high, but the condition has no specific symptoms and, outside Japan, the proportion of such early lesions rarely exceeds 10%. The wider availability of 'fast-track' investigation or age-selected dyspeptic patients by direct access endoscopy services may in the future result in more gastric tumours being detected at an early stage. Furthermore, endoscopic snare resection of early gastric cancer using a saline cushion technique to separate the submucosa from the muscularis propria offers the prospect of curative treatment with minimal intervention.[10]

Lymphomas

Primary lymphomas account for less than 5% of all gastric malignant tumours. They occur most commonly in the body of the stomach and may be ulcerative, infiltrating or polypoid. Endoscopic and radiological differentiation from gastric carcinoma may be impossible, though lymphomatous ulcers are often shallower and more 'punched out' in appearance than GUs or carcinomatous ulcers; even histological examination of biopsy specimens is not always conclusive. There is currently a great deal of interest in so-called mucosa associated lymphoid tissue tumours (MALT tumours). These are low grade, B cell gastric lymphomas which may be promoted by *H. pylori* infection. Anti-*H. pylori* treatment has produced tumour regression in some instances.[11]

Periampullary carcinomas

Cancer of the ampulla of Vater is rare, with an incidence of about 0.3 per 100,000 population. The tumour has a much better prognosis than carcinoma of the head of the pancreas proper, and is more often potentially curable by resection. Adenocarcinomas may arise from the ampulla itself or from the adjacent duodenal or bile duct mucosa. Macroscopically, they may be ulcerative or stenosing. A careful examination of the second part of the duodenum is important to identify such growths in cases of unexplained upper gastrointestinal bleeding or jaundice, and visualization and biopsy of the area in question may be easier with a side-viewing duodenoscope.

Mass lesions

Mucosal lesions

Although as mentioned above, many gastric carcinomas form typical malignant ulcers, other carcinomas present endoscopically as florid, polypoid mucosal growths (Figure 24.21, see colour plate also) in the gastric body or antrum. Duodenal carcinoma is relatively rare and usually presents as an ulcerated polypoid lesion not easily confused with benign DU.

The commonest gastric polypoid lesion is the so-called regenerative polyp, though its pathogenesis is uncertain. These polyps are usually multiple, sessile and hemispherical with a diameter of 5 mm or less (Figure 24.22, see colour plate also). They have no malignant potential.

Isolated benign adenomas of the stomach (Figure 24.23, see colour plate also) are not uncommon and can usually be

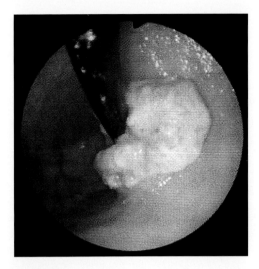

Figure 24.21
Polypoid gastric cancer. (Reproduced, with permission, from Schiller KFR, Cochel R & Hunt RH. A Colour Atlas of Gastrointestinal Endoscopy. London: Chapman & Hall, 1986.)

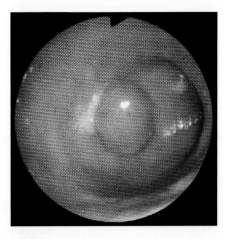

Figure 24.23
Pedunculated benign gastric adenoma. (Reproduced, with permission, from Schiller KFR, Cochel R & Hunt RH. A Colour Atlas of Gastrointestinal Endoscopy. London: Chapman & Hall, 1986.)

removed safely by snare polypectomy. Multiple gastric adenomas occur in cases of familial adenomatous polyposis (FAP),[12] although fundic gland hyperplasia is a more frequent and virtually universal gastric finding in patients with this condition. Duodenal polyposis is present in almost all patients with FAP and frank malignant change, especially in the periampullary area, often develops in time.

Other mucosal polypoid lesions are occasionally found at endoscopy in the stomach or duodenum. Hamartomatous small bowel polyps, as in the Peutz–Jeghers syndrome, are rare, and present with bleeding or obstructive symptoms; peroperative endoscopy can be helpful in management by minimizing the rate of enterotomy or of re-laparotomy.[13] Duodenal gastrinomas, as in the Zollinger–Ellison syndrome, are even rarer but have occasionally been diagnosed by endoscopy and biopsy.[14]

Submucosal lesions

The commonest gastric mass lesion of submucosal origin is the leiomyoma. These benign but potentially locally invasive

tumours are usually sessile and often ulcerate centrally to give a typical umbilicated appearance (Figure 24.24, see colour plate also). Bleeding can occur from the crater. The bulk of the tumour is frequently extragastric, with only a small portion visible in the stomach lumen. Routine biopsies usually only show normal overlying gastric mucosa, but occasionally a multiple biopsy technique, where further deep samples are taken from the base of an initial biopsy site, will show typical smooth muscle histology. Smooth muscle tumours are not suitable for snare polypectomy because of the likelihood of an extragastric component.

Other submucosal mass lesions such as lipomas are occasionally found in the stomach or duodenum at endoscopy, but the appearances are generally non-specific. Here again, standard biopsy techniques are unlikely to yield material other than of the overlying mucosa.

Infiltration of the submucosa of the stomach is typically due to the cancer variant, linitis plastica. Endoscopically this condition should be suspected if all or part of the stomach is poorly distensible and has rigid, aperistaltic, swollen and reddened rugae (Figure 24.25, see colour plate also). Biopsy specimens usually reveal a submucosal poorly differentiated

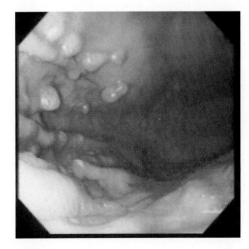

Figure 24.22
Regenerative polyps in the stomach.

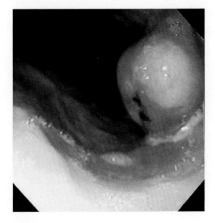

Figure 24.24
Gastric leiomyoma.

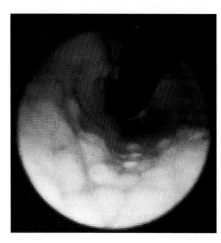

Figure 24.25
Linitis plastica. (Reproduced, with permission, from Schiller KFR, Cochel R & Hunt RH. A Colour Atlas of Gastrointestinal Endoscopy. London: Chapman & Hall, 1986.)

adenocarcinoma with variable degrees of mucosal infiltration. Similar endoscopic appearances may very rarely occur where infiltrating fibrotic processes such as systemic sclerosis or sarcoidosis involve the stomach.

Tumour infiltration of the duodenum is most commonly seen as a late feature of large carcinomas of the pancreatic head. The duodenal loop may at first be widened (a commonly reported radiological sign) and rendered 'stiff' in character. Later, luminal encroachment leads to stenosis or the appearance of obvious tumour tissue in the second part of the duodenum (Figure 24.26, see colour plate also). At this stage of the disease, palliative endoscopic stenting to relieve biliary obstruction may be technically impossible and a surgical bypass procedure with gastrojejunostomy is often preferable to avoid the sequelae of high intestinal obstruction.

THERAPEUTIC PROCEDURES

Endoscopic therapy in the main employs devices which are passed through the biopsy channel of the endoscope and whose positioning and action can therefore be directly observed by the endoscopist. Other types of therapy are merely endoscopy aided, e.g. percutaneous endoscopic gastrostomy.

Endoscopic treatment of gastroduodenal bleeding

This topic is covered in Chapter 38 but is discussed here in outline. Essentially, endoscopic control of bleeding from lesions in the stomach and duodenum has been most successfully achieved by the application of thermal energy (either by heater probe or laser), or by direct injection into the bleeding site.

Heater probe treatment is relatively cheap and effective. The success of the technique is operator dependent but in experienced hands may reduce the incidence of continued bleeding and of rebleeding after treatment[15-17] and possibly can also reduce the chances of surgical intervention and overall mortality.[18]

Alternatively, heat energy can be applied to bleeding points by an argon or neodymium-YAG laser. Although this mode of therapy is undoubtedly effective, particularly in cases of recurrent bleeding,[19] the equipment needed is very expensive and not widely available. Other cheaper methods of achieving haemostasis seem, in general, just as useful in cases of bleeding from peptic ulcers, although laser treatment may be particularly valuable in haemorrhage from telangiectases or other vascular anomalies[20,21] and in their prophylactic ablation.

An alternative method of arresting haemorrhage, particularly in peptic ulcers where a discrete bleeding point can be identified, is the local injection of adrenaline, alcohol or sclerosants such as ethanolamine. This technique is simple, quick and requires no special equipment other than endoscopic injection needles, but again may be significantly operator dependent in terms of success.[22] The use of single agents such as 1:10,000 adrenaline or absolute alcohol is as effective as adrenaline–sclerosant combinations.[23,24] Rarely, mucosal or even full thickness gastric necrosis has been described after such injection treatments.[25,26]

Removal of upper gastrointestinal polyps

Pedunculated mucosal polyps in the stomach or duodenum can be snared or excised with a wire diathermy loop in the same manner as the more commonly encountered colonic polyps. Sessile lesions should be approached with caution, as perforation of the gastric wall is a significant hazard. Snare excision of submucosal polypoid lesions such as leiomyomas should not be performed because of the unacceptable perforation risk. Small polyps can be removed by a 'hot biopsy' technique using special insulated forceps.

Dilatation of pyloric stenosis and narrowed stomata

Perendoscopic balloon dilatation can be used in cases of gastric outlet obstruction due either to peptic ulcer-associated pyloric stenosis or to postgastrectomy stricturing, with a long-term success rate of up to 70%.[27] In most series, balloon dilata-

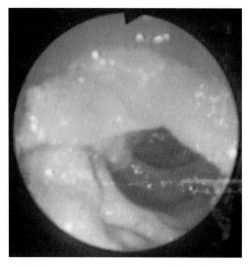

Figure 24.26
Duodenal involvement by pancreatic cancer.

tion is more successful in postoperative strictures than in pyloric fibrosis and scarring secondary to peptic ulceration.[28] The technique is essentially similar to balloon dilatation of oesophageal strictures.

Foreign body removal

Most small ingested foreign bodies will pass naturally through the gastrointestinal tract and intervention, either endoscopic or surgical, is only appropriate if there is a significant clinical problem or a high chance of complications. Endoscopic removal of foreign bodies is generally reserved for large objects which will clearly cause obstruction, for potentially toxic materials such as mercury batteries, or for other hazardous objects which may perforate the gut[29] (Figures 24.27 and 24.28, see colour plate also). A wide variety of specialized retrieval devices is available, e.g. rat-toothed forceps for grasping the milled edges of coins, but most foreign bodies can be dealt with using simple accessories such as snares, tripod forceps, or wire baskets. Overtube systems may be used to protect the oesophagus and to allow the easier manoeuvring of objects through the cardia, but have the disadvantage of making maintained gastric insufflation difficult or impossible. Where there is a risk of dropping a foreign body into the bronchial tree during retrieval and particularly in children, endoscopy under general anaesthesia with a protected airway may be advisable.

Laser therapy for tumours

The main use of palliative laser treatment in the gastrointestinal tract has to date been in the debulking of tumours in the oesophagus or colon and the maintenance of luminal patency.

In the stomach itself, laser energy can be employed to palliate tumours of the cardia and to preserve an adequate swallowing channel, but in general the technique is more successful in

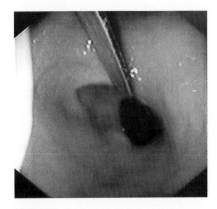

Figure 24.28
Spoon in the stomach – removed with a standard polypectomy snare.

dysphagic patients with growths in the more proximal oesophagus.[30] Gastric outlet obstruction by prepyloric tumours can be treated by laser debulking. Transfusion requirements may be reduced if laser therapy is used to ablate the surface of large bleeding gastric cancers.[31] There is evidence from a small series of patients that endoscopic laser irradiation may be an adequate curative procedure in at least some cases of early gastric cancer.[32]

Photodynamic therapy is an alternative mode of laser treatment applicable to gastrointestinal neoplasms. This technique employs an intravenously administered photosensitizer, usually a haematoporphyrin derivative, which is selectively retained in tumour tissue. Later activation of the sensitizer by exposure to a laser light of appropriate wavelength, transmitted endoscopically to the growth, results in local tissue destruction, probably by the release of singlet oxygen. Most experience to date has been gained in the palliative management of oesophageal tumours, where the results can be comparable to those achieved by neodymium-YAG laser treatment.[33-35] Experience with large gastric carcinomas is limited. Small tumours and early gastric cancers have been successfully eradicated using the technique,[36] although some authors have reported late recurrences. Skin photosensitization and phototoxicity are potential hazards of the procedure. It may find its main place as a relatively non-invasive therapy for small superficial gastric or periampullary tumours in elderly patients or those otherwise unfit for surgery.[37]

Percutaneous endoscopic gastroscopy

Feeding gastrostomy has been a source of medical interest since the classical physiological studies by Beaumont[38] on an accidentally created gastric stoma. Surgical gastrostomy has been used for many years for long-term enteral feeding in patients with mechanical obstruction to swallowing or, occasionally, swallowing problems due to chronic neurological disorders.

The first report of an endoscopically placed gastrostomy system appeared in 1980.[39] Since then, various such devices have been described which can either be inserted under endoscopic or radiological control and which may employ 'pull' or

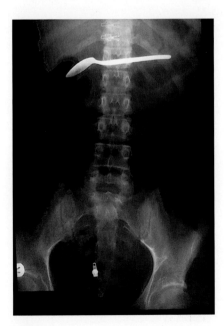

Figure 24.27
Radiograph of swallowed spoon in the stomach.

'push' techniques, the latter usually over a guide-wire inserted into the stomach.

Percutaneous endoscopic gastrostomy (PEG) is now established as a speedy, cheap, easy and relatively safe procedure, and has found a wide application in suitable patients with nutritional problems. In comparison with nasogastric tube feeding, endoscopic gastrostomy is generally better tolerated and cosmetically more acceptable.[40] Both short- and long-term enteral nutrition can usually be achieved safely and effectively.[41,42]

The indications for PEG are given in Table 24.1. In a patient who has sustained a major stroke with consequent impairment of swallowing, enteral feeding by nasogastric tube is usually indicated in the early acute phase. There is a debate as to whether PEG should be considered in the first few days when the prognosis in uncertain, or whether it should be reserved for patients whose general prognosis appears reasonable with a stabilization of the neurological state but who continue to have a severe disturbance of swallowing. In addition, PEG may sometimes reduce the risk of reflux and aspiration in subjects with chronic swallowing problems,[43] but in many cases, aspiration of oral secretions continues and respiratory problems are not totally avoided by using the technique.

Table 24.1 Possible indications for percutaneous endoscopic gastrostomy

1. Chronic neurological disease
   Cerebrovascular accidents
   Motorneurone disease
   Multiple sclerosis
2. Head and neck cancer
3. Obstructing oesophageal tumour
4. Multiple trauma necessitating long-term enteral feeding
5. Major oral surgery
6. Gastric decompression

PEG insertion is contraindicated in patients with significant coagulation disorders, with abdominal sepsis and in the presence of ascites, multiple adhesions or peritoneal malignancy. Failure of transillumination (see below) implies that abdominal puncture may be unsafe. Enteral nutritional support by this means in patients with anorexia nervosa is generally thought to be unhelpful.

Various prepacked and sterile implantation kits are commercially available, the gastrostomy tube being retained in situ either by a balloon or a 'bumper' disc in the stomach, and by some external fixation clip on the abdominal wall. Each system has its own advantages and disadvantages, and it is probably best for an operator to become familiar with one device in order to maximize success and minimize complications. A 'traction' insertion procedure is the most frequently used, and is now described briefly.

The patient is prepared for the procedure in same manner as for a standard diagnostic gastroscopy. Broad spectrum prophylactic antibiotics are sometimes given and may reduce the rate of peristomal skin infections.[44] With the subject in the left lateral

position, and lightly sedated, a routine OGD is performed to exclude significant pathology or gastric outlet obstruction. With the endoscope in situ, the patient is then turned into the supine position with careful attention to preservation of the airway and to oropharyngeal suction. The stomach is insufflated with air to appose its anterior aspect to the abdominal wall and transilluminated, the room being temporarily darkened, to confirm that a safe gastric puncture can be made. The high intensity transillumination feature of some modern video systems is particularly useful in this context. Digital pressure over the transilluminated area, which should ideally be well below the left coastal margin and away from the midline, can be seen endoscopically as a rounded indentation into the stomach and further localizes the potential gastrostomy site.

After the latter is marked on the skin, a second operator prepares the skin with a suitable antiseptic and surrounds the site with sterile drapes. Local anaesthetic is infiltrated into the skin and subcutaneous tissues and a small incision is made with a scalpel. While the endoscopist preserves the necessary gastric distension, the assistant punctures the stomach through the incision with a trocar and cannula, withdraws the former and passes one end of a strong thread through the cannula into the gastric lumen. This thread is grasped by the endoscopist using forceps or a snare and is drawn out of the patient's mouth as the gastroscope is removed; the other end of the thread is held firmly by the assistant. The gastrostomy tube is tied firmly to the thread protruding from the patient's mouth and pulled down the oesophagus by steady traction from the assistant (Figure 24.29). When the proximal end of the gastrostomy tube abuts onto the gastric cannula, the two are pulled out through the abdominal wall incision until the internal retention disc or flange of the tube lies against the stomach wall. The cannula is discarded and the tube fixed in position by a suitable face-plate, which must not, however, be applied too tightly. Enteral feeding via the gastrostomy can be started 10–12 h later.

The overall implantation success rate with this type of system is of the order of 95%[45] and the procedure usually only takes 10–20 min.

Procedure-related major complications are rare (less than 3%) but include bleeding and gastric perforation. Occasionally there are minor early complications, such as asymptomatic

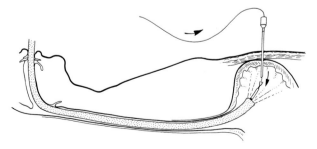

Figure 24.29
Procedure of percutaneous endoscopic gastrostomy. Adapted from Keighley MRB, Williams NS. *Surgery of the Anus, Rectum and Colon*, 2nd edn. p. 102. London: W.B. Saunders, 1999.

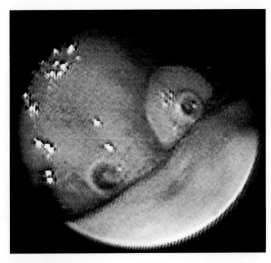

Figure 24.30
Epithelialized gastrostomy, with an adjacent second PEG.

pneumoperitoneum, wound infection and transient paralytic ileus. Late complications are not infrequent, the most common being mechanical failure of system components, or tube blockage.[45] Sometimes the internal flange of the feeding tube becomes epithelialized and therefore buried in the gastric wall; this occurs particularly if external fixation is excessively tight, either ab initio or as a result of inappropriate cleaning of the site.[46] If at a later stage it is impossible to remove such a buried and blocked tube, a second gastrostomy can be positioned beside it (Figure 24.30, see colour plate also). Ideally, where a tube has been removed or replaced, the old prosthesis should be recovered from the stomach by means of a snare; gastrostomy tubes have occasionally caused intestinal obstruction if allowed to migrate down the gut.[47,48] Tube replacement can be either by a repetition of the original procedure or by the use of a suitable 'button' device which is inserted through the established fistula tract of the initial gastrostomy. In a proportion of patients with recoverable swallowing problems, the gastrostomy tube can eventually be removed electively. However, long-term enteral feeding by this means is usually both safe and effective.

REFERENCES

1. Blackstone MO. *Endoscopic interpretation: normal and pathologic appearances of the gastrointestinal tract.* New York: Raven Press, 1984.
2. Silverstern FE & Tytgat GNJ. *Gastrointestinal Endoscopy,* 3rd edn. London: Mosley–Wolfe, 1997.
3. Schiller KFR, Cochel R & Hunt RH. *A colour atlas of gastrointestinal endoscopy.* London: Chapman & Hall, 1986.
4. Misiewicz JJ, Forbes A, Price A, Shorvon P, Triger D & Tytgat GNJ. *CD-Atlas of clinical gastroenterology.* Aylesford, UK: Times–Mirror International Publishers Ltd, 1994.
5. Misiewicz JJ, Tytgat GNJ, Goodwin CS et al. The Sydney System: a new classification of gastritis. In: *Working Party Reports; World Congress of Gastroenterology.* Sydney: Blackwell Scientific, 1990; 1.
6. McCormack TT, Sims J, Eyre-Brook I et al. Gastric lesions in portal hypertension: inflammatory gastritis or congestive gastropathy? *Gut* 1985; **26:** 1226.
7. Sircus W, Duodenitis: a clinical, endoscopic and histopathologic study. *Q J Med* 1985; **56:** 593.
8. Chadwick VS. Clinical investigation of patients with malabsorption and diarrhoea. In: Bouchier IAD, Allan RN, Hodgson HJE, Keighley MRB (eds) *Gastroenterology: clinical science and practice.* London: WB Saunders, 1993: 467.
9. Sakita T. Endoscopy in the diagnosis of early ulcer cancer. *Clin Gastroenterol* 1973; **2:** 345.
10. Tada M, Murakami A, Karita M, Yanai H & Okita K. Endoscopic resection of early gastric cancer. *Endoscopy* 1993; **25:** 445.
11. Wotherspoon AC, Doglioni C, Diss TC et al. Regression of low-grade B-cell gastric lymphoma of mucosa-associated lymphoid tissue type after eradication of *Helicobacter pylori. Lancet* 1993; **342:** 575.
12. Spigelman AD, Talbot IC, Williams CB, Domizio P & Phillips RKS. Upper gastrointestinal cancer in patients with familial adenomatous polyposis. *Lancet* 1989; **ii:** 783.
13. Spigelman AD, Thomson JPS & Phillips RKS. Towards decreasing the re-laparotomy rate in the Peutz–Jeghers syndrome: the role of per-operative small bowel endoscopy. *Br J Surg* 1990; **77:** 301.
14. Rolny P, Ekman R, Sjolund K, Wickbom G & Ohrn PG. Endoscopic diagnosis and treatment of duodenal gastrinoma. *Gastrointest Endosc.* 1990; **36:** 511.
15. O'Brien JD, Day SJ & Burnham WR. Controlled trial of bipolar probe in bleeding peptic ulcers. *Lancet* 1986; **i:** 464.
16. Lin HJ, Lee FY, Kang WM, Tsai YT, Lee SD & Lee CH. Heat probe thermocoagulation and pure alcohol injection in massive peptic ulcer haemorrhage: a prospective randomised controlled trial. *Gut* 1990; **31:** 753.
17. Jaramillo JL, Carmona C, Galvez C, de la Mata M & Mino G. Efficacy of the heater probe in peptic ulcer with a non-bleeding visible vessel. A controlled randomised study. *Gut* 1993; **34:** 1502.
18. Fullarton GM, Birnie CG, MacDonald A & Murray WR. The effect of introducing endoscopic therapy on surgery and mortality rates for peptic ulcer haemorrhage: a single centre analysis of 1125 cases. *Endoscopy* 1990; **22:** 110.
19. Marcon NE. Lasers in gastrointestinal haemorrhage. *Eur J Gastroenterol Hepatol* 1990; **2:** 94.
20. Naveau S, Aubert A, Poynard T & Chaput JC. Longterm results of treatment of vascular malformations of the gastrointestinal tract by neodymium-YAG laser photocoagulation. *Dis Dis Sci* 1990; **35:** 821.
21. Potamiano S, Carter CR & Anderson JR. Endoscopic laser treatment of diffuse gastric vascular ectasia. *Gut* 1994; **35:** 461.
22. Oxner RBG, Simmonds NJ, Gertner JG, Nightingale JMD & Burnham WR. Controlled trial of endoscopic injection treatment for bleeding from peptic ulcers with visible vessels. *Lancet* 1992; **339:** 966.
23. Rutgeerts P, Gevers AM, Hiele M, Broeckaert L & Vantrappen G. Endoscopic injection therapy to prevent rebleeding from peptic ulcers with a protruding vessel: a controlled comparative trial. *Gut* 1993; **34:** 348.
24. Choudari CP & Palmer KR. Endoscopic injection therapy for bleeding ulcers; a comparison of adrenaline alone with adrenaline plus ethanolamine oleate. *Gut* 1994; **35:** 608.
25. Loperfido S, Patelli G & La Torre L. Extensive necrosis of gastric mucosa following injection therapy of bleeding peptic ulcer. *Endoscopy* 1990; **22:** 285.
26. Chester JF & Hurley PR. Gastric necrosis: a complication of endoscopic sclerosis for bleeding peptic ulcer. *Endoscopy* 1990; **22:** 287.
27. Kozarek RA, Botoman VA & Patterson DJ. Longterm follow up in patients who have undergone balloon dilatation for gastric outlet obstruction. *Gastrointest Endosc* 1990; **36:** 558.
28. Kadota T, Hiraide H, Imai J & Tamakuma S. An easy and safe modified method of endoscopic balloon dilatation for postgastrectomy anastomotic stricture. *Surg Gyn Obstet* 1990; **170:** 445.
29. Schiller KFR & Forgacs IC. Foreign bodies in the upper gastrointestinal tract. In: Bennett JR & Hunt RH (eds) *Therapeutic endoscopy and radiology of the gut,* 2nd edn. London: Chapman & Hall, 1990: 91.
30. Krasner N. Palliative laser therapy for tumours of the gastrointestinal tract. *Ballière's Clin Gastroenterol* 1991; **5:** 37.
31. Barr H & Krasner N. Interstitial laser photocoagulation for treating bleeding gastric cancer. *BMJ* 1989; **299:** 659.
32. Yasuda K, Mizuma Y, Nakajima M & Kawai K. Endoscopic laser treatment for early gastric cancer. *Endoscopy* 1993; **25:** 451.
33. McCaughan JS, Hicks W, Laufman L, May E & Roach R. Palliation of oesophageal malignancy with photoradiation therapy. *Cancer* 1984; **54:** 2905.
34. McCaughan JS, Nims TA, Guy GT et al. Photodynamic therapy for esophageal tumours. *Gastrointest Endosc* 1990; **36:** 85.

35. Patrice T, Foultier MT, Yactayo S et al. Endoscopic photodynamic therapy with haematoporphyrin derivative for primary treatment of gastrointestinal neoplasms in inoperable patients. *Dis Dis Sci* 1990; **35:** 545.

36. Kato H, Kawaguchi M, Konaka C et al. Evaluation of photodynamic therapy in gastric cancers. *Lasers Med Sci* 1986; **1:** 67.

37. Ell C & Gossner L. Photodynamic therapy: its potential for the treatment of gastrointestinal malignancies and precancerous conditions. *Endoscopy* 1994; **26:** 262.

38. Beaumont W. *Experiments and observations on the gastric juice and the physiology of digestion.* Plattsburgh: FP Allen, 1833.

39. Gauderer MWL, Ponsky JL & Izant RJ. Gastrostomy without laparotomy: a percutaneous endoscopic technique. *J Paediatr Surg* 1980; **15:** 872.

40. Park RHR, Allison MC, Lang J et al. Randomised comparison of percutaneous endoscopic gastrostomy and nasogastric tube feeding in patients with persisting neurological dysphagia. *BMJ* 1992; **304:** 1406.

41. Wicks C, Gimson A, Vlavianos P et al. Assessment of the percutaneous endoscopic gastrostomy feeding tube as part of an integrated approach to enteral feeding. *Gut* 1992; **33:** 613.

42. Hull MA, Rawlings J, Murray FE et al. Audit of outcome of longterm enteral nutrition by percutaneous endoscopic gastrostomy. *Lancet* 1993; **341:** 869.

43. Cogan R & Weinryb J. Aspiration pneumonia in nursing home patients fed via gastrostomy tubes. *Am J Gastroenterol* 1989; **84:** 1509.

44. Jain NK, Larson DE, Schroeder KW et al. Does antibiotic prophylaxis reduce peristomal skin infection after endoscopic percutaneous gastrostomy: a prospective randomized clinical trial. *Gastrointest Endosc* 1986; **32:** 139.

45. Larson DE, Burton DE, Schroeder KW & Dimagno EP. Percutaneous endoscopic gastrostomy. Indications, success, complications and mortality in 314 consecutive patients. *Gastroenterology* 1987; **93:** 48.

46. Vautier G & Scott BB. Blocked gastrostomy tubes. *Lancet* 1994; **343:** 1105.

47. McGovern R, Barkin JS, Goldberg RI & Phillips RS. Duodenal obstruction: a complication of percutaneous endoscopic tube migration. *Am J Gastroenterol* 1990; **85:** 1037.

48. Berry DP & Vellacott KD. High jejunal obstruction: a complication of percutaneous endoscopic gastrostomy. *Br J Surg* 1992; **79:** 1171

25

GASTRITIS AND DUODENITIS

H Thompson

There has always been considerable confusion and controversy over the classification, aetiology and clinical significance of gastritis, duodenitis and acute gastroduodenal mucosal damage. Considerable efforts have been made to clarify these disorders in the human subject and in the experimental animal. Nevertheless, it is probable that there is still an overlap of aetiological mechanisms in histologically proven cases of chronic gastritis and chronic duodenitis. The various types of mucosal damage and inflammatory disorders of the stomach and duodenum are discussed in this chapter in the light of current knowledge up to the date of writing, but it must be acknowledged that further advances may improve our knowledge of the aetiology, clinical significance, complications and treatment of these various entities. A combination of endoscopic assessment, biopsy findings, clinical features, bacteriology and serological observations have been most rewarding in the investigation and the follow-up of gastroduodenal disease. The headings under which the spectrum of disease is discussed are not intended to represent a new classification because it is recognized that there is already a conflict between existing systems of classification.

GASTRITIS

Acute gastric mucosal injury

This entity includes acute haemorrhagic gastritis which is characterized by congestion, erosions, haemorrhagic changes, excess surface mucus and even acute ulcers in the gastric mucosa. It may be complicated by gastrointestinal haemorrhage with haematemesis or malaena and more rarely by perforation. The majority of cases are self-limiting but blood transfusion may be necessary and in life-threatening cases it may become necessary to introduce treatment with various drugs or to carry out gastrectomy. Gastric erosions are defects in the mucosa which are limited to the mucosa and do not penetrate the muscularis mucosae. Acute gastric ulcers, on the other hand, correspond to defects which penetrate through the muscularis mucosae into the submucosa or even more deeply with a risk of perforation. Aetiological factors have been identified in a significant proportion of cases.

Acute erosive gastritis due to drugs, alcohol or chemical agents

Non-steroidal anti-inflammatory drugs (NSAIDs)[1] and/or alcohol probably represent the chief offenders in this day and age. Salicylates, such as acetylsalicylic acid (aspirin), remain one of the most ulcerogenic agents with some studies showing peptic ulcer disease in up to 28% of patients taking them in high dose. Recent acetylsalicylic acid ingestion has been demonstrated in 51–58%[2] of cases of acute haemorrhagic gastritis complicated by gastrointestinal haemorrhage. An American study suggests that there is no increased risk of gastrointestinal bleeding if aspirin is taken on less than four days a week.[3] Alcohol appears to be synergistic; both salicylates and alcohol disrupt the gastric mucosal barrier and can be regarded as 'Barrier Breakers'. The incidence of upper gastrointestinal tract symptoms in patients taking aspirin ranges from 6 to 33% and includes nausea, vomiting, dyspepsia and epigastric burning. Gastric mucosal damage is most severe in the antral and prepyloric area (Figures 25.1–25.6) but erosions may also be clustered focally in the body of the stomach or near the greater curvature.[4] Soluble aspirin is much less dangerous. Most NSAIDs cause gastric mucosal damage through blockade of the enzyme cyclo-oxygenase with reduction in cytoprotective

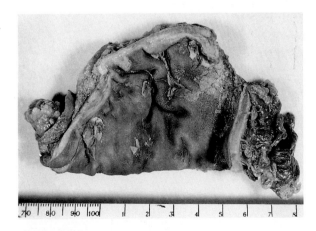

Figure 25.1
Acute erosive gastritis involving the antral and prepyloric area (H&E ×).

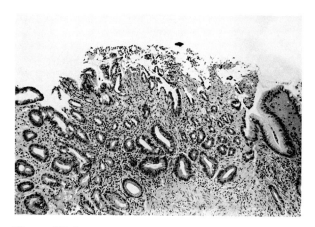

Figure 25.2
A superficial erosion in acute erosive gastritis (H&E ×).

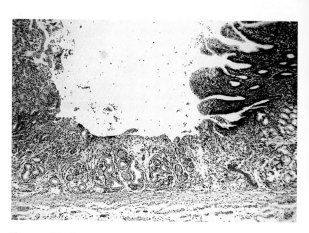

Figure 25.4
Healing erosion in acute erosive gastritis (H&E ×).

gastric prostaglandins. A wide variety of drugs act in a similar way including naproxen, piroxicam, indomethacin, ibuprofen, mefenamic acid, sulindac, tolmetin, fenoprofen, azapropazone, diflunisal, phenylbutazone, benorylate, flufenamic acid, ketoprofen, oxyphenbutazone, diclofenac, benoxaprofen, aminophenazone, penicillin, pyrazolone derivatives, rauwolfia, chloramphenicol, metamizol, clofibrate, ipanoic acid, feprazonum, fentiazac, indoprofen and antineoplastic cytotoxic agents. Other drugs which have been implicated in gastrointestinal haemorrhage include ethacrynic acid, potassium chloride, heparin and warfarin. Oral ferrous sulphate can also be injurious to the gastric mucosa.

The risk of gastrointestinal bleeding due to NSAIDs is predominant among older subjects over the age of 60[5,6] or 65[7]. The role of steroids, however, is much more controversial. One study[6] showed that corticosteroid treatment roughly doubled the incidence of haemorrhage from peptic ulcers. A number of controlled trials, however, have shown that steriods are not ulcerogenic or that there is only a weak association[8] particularly in patients with liver disease and there is no evidence that steroids cause gastritis.

Alcohol alone can precipitate acute erosive gastritis particularly the consumption of spirits on an empty stomach, but it must be remembered that heavy drinkers who indulge in binge

drinking of beer are also at risk. Gastric erosions have also been described after consumption of home brewed larger[9] contaminated by acetaldehyde and acetic acid. The natural course of acute erosive gastritis is that it will resolve spontaneously whether or not gastrointestinal haemorrhage has occurred as a complication. Patients with severe haemorrhagic gastritis can be treated with high dose sucralfate, ranitidine or omeprazole but uncontrollable bleeding may require gastrectomy as an emergency procedure. It has been suggested that pre-existing gastritis renders the gastric mucosa more susceptible to acute gastric mucosal damage but this is difficult to prove. Prostaglandins such as misoprostol have been recommended in recent publications for patients with crippling arthritis who require treatment with NSAIDs in order to protect them from gastrointestinal haemorrhage. Studies in human volunteers[10,11] confirm that prostaglandins reduce the number of haemorrhagic lesions in the gastric mucosa that occur following ingestion of a measured volume of alcohol. Cimetidine, ranitidine and sucralfate have also been recommended as prophylactic agents in circumstances where there is a risk of acute haemorrhagic gastritis or gastric erosions.

Acute corrosive gastritis or gastric necrosis can result from ingestion of corrosive agents such as caustic soda, bleach,

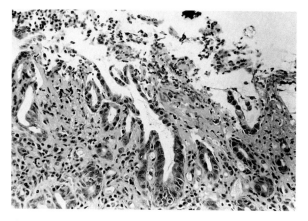

Figure 25.3
A superficial erosion in acute erosive gastritis (H&E ×).

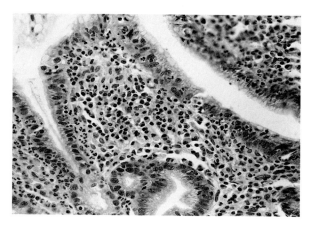

Figure 25.5
Neutrophils in lamina propria and in surface epithelium in acute erosive gastritis.

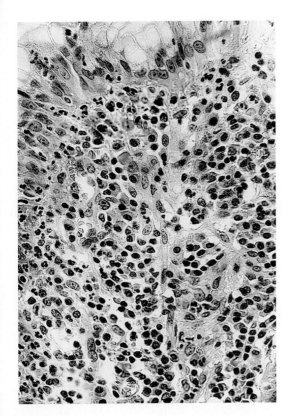

Figure 25.6
Neutrophils in lamina propria and in surface epithelium in acute erosive gastritis (H&E ×).

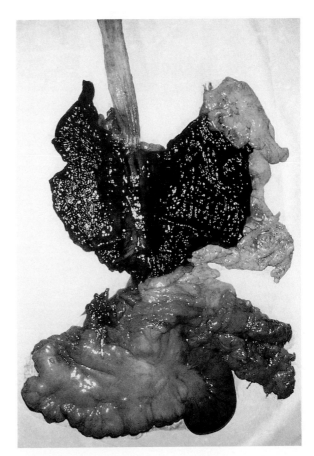

Figure 25.7
Cyanide poisoning showing gross black discolouration of the gastric mucosa. Discolouration is absent in some cases of cyanide poisoning (H&E ×).

disinfectants, lysol, phenol, cyanide (Figure 25.7), toxic chemicals etc. Accidental swallowing of fluids from unlabelled bottles may be responsible for this dangerous situation which may also be complicated by metabolic and toxic states. Perforation of the stomach or duodenum can also occur. Deliberate ingestion of such fluids, of course, may be a suicidal gesture with disastrous consequences. If the patient survives the acute state of corrosive poisoning and succumbs at a later stage the stomach may show the picture of linitus plastica appearance with a granulomatous histological reaction rather than malignant infiltration. Unfortunate individuals who have taken an overdose of barbiturates or aspirin may show erosive or corrosive gastritis at autopsy. Acute gastric necrosis has also been described in anorexia nervosa and bulimia[12] with a surgical mortality rate of 50–65% overall and a mortality of 100% without operation. Atony, muscular atrophy following starvation in anorexia nervosa, neurogenic paralysis due to malnutrition and questionable superior mesenteric artery syndrome may contribute to this complication. Necrosis occurs when intragastric pressure exceeds gastric venous pressure.

Acute erosive gastritis has also been attributed rarely to acute infection with *Helicobacter pylori* in children[13] and adults.[14-22] Self-inoculation of cultures of *H. pylori* was reported by Marshall et al.[14] Marshall developed symptoms of hunger on wakening, irritability, headache and bad breath. Few symptoms remained at the 14th day. Endoscopy did not reveal any gross abnormality but the histological appearances were those of acute erosive gastritis. Tinidazole treatment promoted resolution of the gastritis. Other cases[18] of self-inoculation have been recorded.

Review of a small epidemic of gastritis reported by Ramsey et al.[19] with hypochlorhydria, similar to a condition reported by Osler in 1920, revealed *H. pylori* in the gastric biopsies. The patients were volunteers taking part in a study involving multiple gastric intubations and the cause had been assumed to be viral at the time.

Salmeron et al.[20] described a case of acute purulent gastritis in a 28-year-old man due to *H. pylori* which was cured by erythromycin. Several reports draw attention to halitosis as a feature of acute gastritis due to *H. pylori*. Marshall has pointed out that in acute gastritis if *H. pylori* is not cleared then mild gastrointestinal disturbance may persist while the patient develops hypochlorhydria or achlorhydria over a period of 3–12 months. The inflammation in the body of the stomach regresses but the antropyloric region and duodenal bulb are still affected. Acid secretion returns. The possibility of peptic ulcer disease then depends on acid-peptic aggressive factors. Genetic factors, rate, volume or control of gastric acid secretion will determine whether a patient develops an ulcer. The gastritis in these cases subsides with or without treatment with antibiotics and/or bismuth. *H. pylori* is cleared in most of the cases following effective treatment but the infection may persist associated with chronic gastritis.

Haemorrhagic necrotic lesions have more recently been described in the fundus of the stomach as a complication of the haemolytic–uraemic syndrome,[23] which in some cases is due to gastrointestinal infection with Verocell-cytotoxin-producing *Escherichia coli* following ingestion of incompletely cooked contaminated meat. It is probable that gastric or duodenal lesions are the result of microthrombosis in vessels and that such lesions are ischaemic in type. Cytomegalovirus infection in immunodeficient patients can be associated with vasculitis. Acute erosive gastritis has been a rare complication of salmonella infection, yersiniasis, herpes simplex and other viral infections.

Certain infectious fevers have been implicated in the past as a rare cause of acute erosive gastritis. Diphtheria, for example, which fortunately is not a problem at the present time, was a recognized cause although it can be argued that the lesions were due to stress rather than to local gastric mucosal infection.

Stress lesions associated with acute haemorrhagic gastritis

Stress lesions (Figure 25.8), characterized as haemorrhagic erosions, are responsible for coffee ground vomit in very ill patients and they can cause serious or potentially fatal gastrointestinal haemorrhage; even when asymptomatic they may be a prominent feature at autopsy (Figure 25.9) with or without altered blood in the stomach or intestine. Predisposing factors are numerous and include pneumonia, sepsis, renal failure, cor pulmonale, congestive heart failure, burns, severe trauma, septicaemia, haemorrhagic states, multiple organ failure, major surgery, hypovolaemia, hypothermia, malignant disease and intensive treatment unit care. Multiple haemorrhagic erosions with or without acute ulcers measuring 2 cm or more in diameter in the gastric or duodenal mucosa are characteristic. Stress lesions characterized as ulcers in the duodenum as a complication of extensive burns are known as Curling's ulcers;

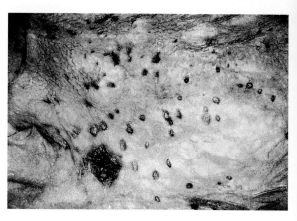

Figure 25.9

Stress lesions in the form of haemorrhagic erosions and acute ulcers discovered at autopsy in a patient with cirrhosis of the liver (×).

comparable ulcers can occur in the stomach or oesophagus. Ulcers complicating head injury or neurosurgery have been described as Cushing's ulcers. Congestion and oedema of the gastric mucosa are additional features. The lesion usually develops within six days of the clinical condition precipitating stress. Haemorrhagic erosions in the stomach and duodenum may be obscured by post-mortem autolysis and they may have undergone spontaneous healing if the patient has survived several days after gastrointestinal haemorrhage so that they are no longer identifiable at autopsy. There is a risk of perforation and peritonitis associated with stress ulceration of the stomach. Moody et al.[24] has drawn attention to stress lesions of the stomach in experimental animal studies. The aetiology is multifactorial and includes hypovolaemia, hypoperfusion of the gastric mucosa, focal mucosal ischaemia, impairment of defence mechanisms such as bicarbonate and mucin secretion, intramucosal buffering capacity, endogenous prostaglandin synthesis and in addition excessive hydrogen ion diffusion from the gastric lumen into the mucosa. Mucosal ischaemia resulting from systemic shock and hypotension weakens the mucosal barrier and allows back diffusion of acid through the damaged mucosal surface. Pre-existing chronic gastritis is said to make the mucosa more susceptible to acute stress lesions. Acute haemorrhagic gastritis in cirrhotic patients[25] has been attributed to endotoxaemia, congestion of the stomach due to portal hypertension and alcohol ingestion. The features of acute haemorrhagic gastritis can also be seen in disseminated intravascular coagulation, microthrombosis and purpura. Arteritis or necrotizing angiitis may also mimic acute haemorrhagic gastritis. Prophylactic treatment with H_2 blockers, such as cimetidine, and with sucralfate, which acts in a different way, protect seriously ill patients from developing lesions in the stomach and duodenum. Other agents which have been successfully used in prophylaxis include antacids, antimuscarinic drugs, somatostatin and vasoactive drugs such as vasopressin. The erosions which occur in certain infectious fevers are probably due to stress rather than to direct infection of the gastric mucosa.

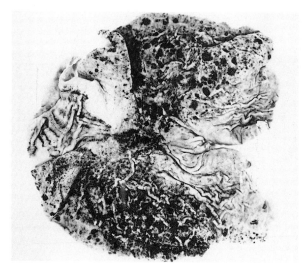

Figure 25.8

Stress lesions in the gastric mucosa with numerous haemorrhagic erosions (H&E ×).

Phlegmonous gastritis

This is a rare condition which is associated with suppurative inflammation of the stomach principally involving the submucosa.[26-28] It may be limited to the pyloric canal or it may be diffuse involving the entire stomach. The mucosa is often intact and the serosa is covered with fibrinous exudate. There is marked inflammatory hyperaemia. The haemolytic streptococcus is the organism that is most frequently involved, but other organisms have been isolated including staphylococci and *E. coli*. If gas-forming organisms are involved then emphysematous gastritis develops. Patients present with upper abdominal pain, nausea and vomiting and they are seriously ill with a risk of perforation. There is a high mortality rate but gastrectomy with antibiotic therapy is curative. A chronic form rarely develops with organization and fibrosis. Since the introduction of antibiotics this condition has become rarer still. Predisposing factors which have been cited include pre-existing gastritis, pharyngitis, puerperal sepsis and endocarditis.

Acute gastric lesions due to physical agents

Gastric freezing[29] using a balloon filled with ethyl alcohol was introduced for the treatment of chronic peptic ulcer around 1960 but this method of treatment has now been abandoned because of complications. Freezing induced superficial mucosal ulceration with necrosis which could extend down to the muscle coat. There was a risk of gastrointestinal haemorrhage or perforation with this procedure. Electrical damage associated with focal necrosis has also been described in the gastric mucosa due to the use of electrical probes[30] which have been introduced to arrest haemorrhage from bleeding vessels. Experimental studies in animals have been valuable in determining the appropriate electrical charge which can be used to stop bleeding without the risk of gastric necrosis and perforation. Irradiation of the stomach can lead to irradiation gastritis, acute gastric ulceration and chronic ulceration. This is extremely rare as a problem in clinical practice.

CHRONIC GASTRITIS

The classification of chronic gastritis is controversial and it is probable that there is an overlap in aetiological and histological features. Interest is focused on the role of *H. pylori*, duodenogastric reflux, autoimmune factors and environmental influences in the aetiology of gastritis.

Strickland and Mackay's[31] classification of Type A and Type B gastritis is now obsolete, but since the terms are still encountered in the literature it is important to understand that Type A gastritis corresponded to chronic atrophic gastritis and Type B represented chronic antral gastritis or multifocal environmental gastritis which was later classified as Type AB gastritis.

Helicobacter-associated chronic gastritis

It is generally accepted that this is the commonest variety of chronic gastritis which exists as chronic superficial gastritis or chronic atrophic gastritis predominantly involving the antral mucosa although it may extend up into the junctional and body

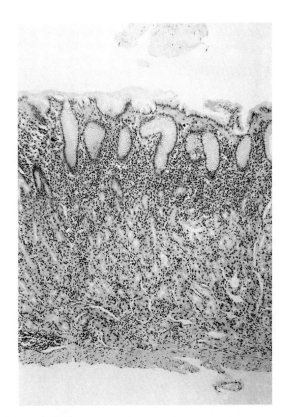

Figure 25.10
Chronic superficial gastritis in body of stomach (H&E ×).

mucosa or it may be multifocal. There is chronic inflammatory cellular infiltration of the lamina propria with a predominance of lymphocytes and plasma cells (Figures 25.10–25.13). Other inflammatory cells such as neutrophils and eosinophils participate according to the activity of the inflammatory process. Surface epithelium may be normal or regenerative in type and there may be foci of infiltration with neutrophils. Microscopic lesions resembling crypt abscesses are occasionally encountered. The condition may be described as active or quiescent according to the number of neutrophils present in the inflammatory infiltrate. Macroscopic or microscopic inflammatory

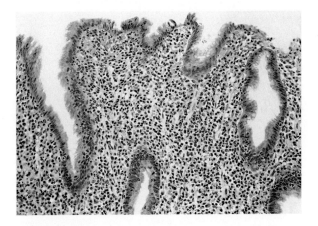

Figure 25.11
Active chronic superficial gastritis showing plasma cells and lymphocytes in the subepithelial and interfoveolar zones of the lamina propria with occasional neutrophils (H&E ×).

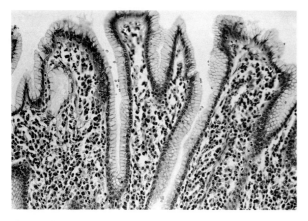

Figure 25.12
Quiescent chronic superficial gastritis with increased numbers of plasma cells and lymphocytes in subepithelial and interfoveolar zones of the lamina propria (H&E ×).

erosions are occasionally observed and again they may be multifocal.

Progression of gastritis is associated with the formation of lymph follicles, foci of inestinal metaplasia (Figure 25.14) and atrophy of mucin-secreting glands (Figures 25.15 and 25.16) representing chronic atrophic gastritis. Lymphoid hyperplasia can be a prominent feature and there is a very, very small risk that this could progress to low grade B cell lymphoma in the long term. Foci, islets and zones of intestinal metasplasia introduce a very, very small risk of gastric cancer arising from Type

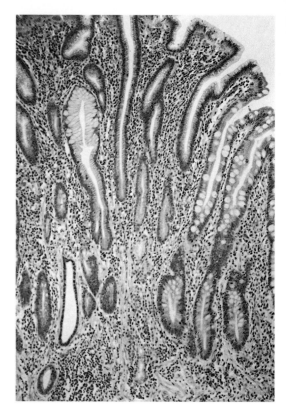

Figure 25.14
Type B gastritis involving the antral region showing a focus of intestinal metaplasia (H&E ×).

III intestinal metaplasia (formerly classified as Type 2B) in later years. Fibrosis can occur but it is not a prominent feature. There is no correlation with clinical symptoms although there may be some degree of hyperchlorhydria. Occasionally chronic superficial gastritis observed during pregnancy is associated with temporary achlorhydria.

About 90% of patients with chronic gastritis have evidence of *H. pylori* infection which can be confirmed by identification of the organism on the mucosal surface, by breath test or by serological tests. *H. pylori* is a curved, wavy or a seagull-shaped organism closely applied to the mucosal surface,

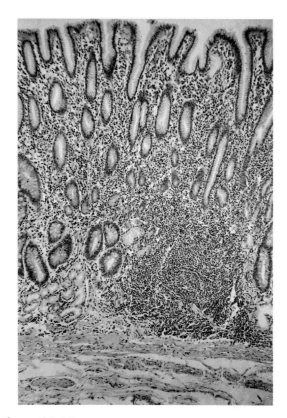

Figure 25.13
Type B gastritis involving antral region showing chronic inflammatory cellular infiltration and lymph follicles (H&E ×).

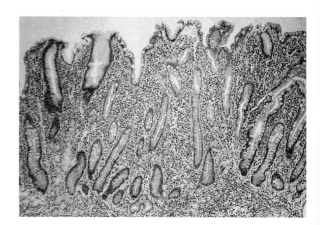

Figure 25.15
Type B gastritis involving pyloric region showing atrophy of mucin-secreting glands and intestinal metaplasia (H&E ×).

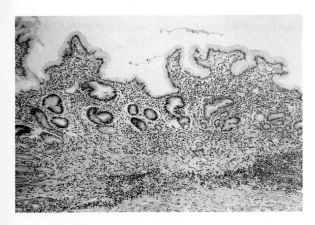

Figure 25.16
Type B gastritis involving pyloric region showing atrophy of mucin-secreting glands (H&E ×).

foveolae or necks of glands. Although they can be seen in a haematoxylin and eosin (H & E) preparation, other stains facilitate diagnosis, e.g. Giemsa, 1//2 Gram etc. The prevalence of *H. pylori* increases with age and its incidence is related to socioeconomic status. The populations of some countries have a high incidence of *H. pylori* at an early age. Differences in family structure, living standards, diet and culinary habits may contribute to early infection. Familial infection is known to occur in such circumstances. There is no conclusive evidence that alcohol has an aetiological role. However, the literature before the discovery of *H. pylori* suggests that the role of alcohol is controversial. Pitchumoni and Glass[32,33] showed a significant increase in antral gastritis in alcoholics. Parl et al.[34] found that chronic gastritis develops more frequently in alcoholic patients and evolves into chronic atrophic gastritis at an earlier age than in non-alcoholic subjects. Cheli et al.[35] on the other hand, found only a slight increase in antral gastritis in alcoholics and concluded, after reviewing the literature, that alcohol does not seem to have an important aetiological role in chronic gastritis, particularly in the gastric fundus. Roberts[36] describes gastric foveolar hyperplasia among alcoholic subjects.

Warren and Marshall[37] drew attention to the possible role of *H. pylori*[38] in the pathogenesis of gastritis. In a study by Price et al.[39] the organism was cultured from 69% of patients with peptic ulcer disease, 80% of patients with duodenal ulcer, 71% of gastric biopsies showing gastritis and only one from twelve normal biopsies. Scanning electron microscopy reveals the bacteria deep to the surface mucus layer. The observations support the hypothesis that *H. pylori* is aetiologically related to gastritis and peptic ulceration particularly duodenal ulcers. Dooley and Cohen[40] state that the aetiological role of *H. pylori* in Type B gastritis has been accepted. Treatment with bismuth plus antibiotics eradicates the infection with resolution, improvement in or diminished severity of the gastritis. The organisms have also been identified in foci of gastric metaplasia in the duodenum and it has been suggested that their presence in the duodenum can lead to the development of duodenal ulcer disease. Serum antibodies are present in a high proportion of those infected by

the organism. There is a high incidence of recovery of the organisms in patients with Type B antral gastritis and in duodenal ulcer disease. On the other hand, there is a low incidence of recovery of the organism in patients with pernicious anaemia. The organisms are located on the epithelial surface below the mucous layer and they can be identified by the Warthin–Starry silver stain (Figure 25.17), crystal violet, Giemsa, modified Gram stain, H & E and fluorescent staining with acridine orange. The organisms possess a powerful urease enzyme which is responsible for ammonia production. The bacteria are most numerous over tight junctions; microvilli are absent, sparse or rudimentary. There is frequently a neutrophil response with polymorphs emigrating through the epithelium but there is no evidence of penetration of the bacteria into the lamina propria. Therapeutic clearance of the organisms is followed by resolution of the gastritis or a decrease in the gastritis score. There is, however, a risk of relapse due to reinfection.

Peterson et al.[41] have pointed out in a study of 23 healthy volunteers that fundic *H. pylori* found in 14 of 23 biopsy specimens were frequently associated with histologically and endoscopically normal fundic mucosa whereas in the pyloric region there was a strong correlation between *H. pylori* and active superficial gastritis.

Although *H. pylori*-associated gastritis is frequently asymptomatic, one study[42] has drawn attention to *Helicobacter*-associated gastritis as a cause of abdominal pain in children. It is of interest that hypergastrinaemia apparently due to *H. pylori*, which has been cited as a possible factor in the genesis of duodenal ulcer, responds to antibiotics.[43] It is still not clear how the organism causes gastritis since the pathogenic mechanisms are controversial. However, there is a considerable amount of evidence[44] which supports an aetiological role. Another spiral organism which has been occasionally associated with gastritis is *Gastrospirillum hominis*[45,46] The incidence is around 0.3% with gastritis. Its role in the aetiology of gastritis is still unclear. Gastrin cell autoantibodies have been demonstrated in 16% of patients with antral gastritis using a highly sensitive avidin–biotin technique.[47] It has been suggested, therefore, that some cases of antral gastritis may have an autoimmune aetiology.

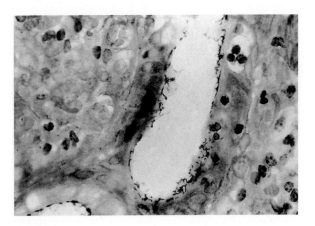

Figure 25.17
Helicobacter pylori (Warthin–Starry Silver stain ×).

Hypersecretory antral gastritis

This variety of chronic gastritis, delineated by Lambert[48] and Correa[49] is associated with duodenal ulcer. The histological features include chronic inflammatory cellular infiltration, lymph follicles, mucin depletion and foveolar hyperplasia. The pyloric glands are normal in number and there may be small foci of intestinal metaplasia. According to Correa this variety is not usually associated with *H. pylori* infection. Erosions can occur and it has been suggested that gastric mucosal damage and irritation are due to excess secretion of acid and pepsin overcoming the gastric mucosal barrier. Differentiation between *H. pylori*-associated chronic gastritis and hypersecretory gastritis is controversial since duodenal ulcer disease is associated with both varieties of gastritis. Wyatt and Dixon[50] and others claim a high incidence of *H. pylori* in chronic antral gastritis whereas Correa[49] claims a low incidence of the organism in hypersecretory gastritis. Another ill-defined variety of hypersecretory gastritis which has been described in the literature is hyperplastic hypersecretory gastritis which predominantly involves the gastric body mucosa. Its relationship to *H. pylori* infection and Ménétrier's disease is unknown.

Bile reflux gastritis, reactive gastritis, chemical gastritis

Dixon et al.[51] have drawn attention to new and different criteria for the diagnosis of bile reflux gastritis or chemical trauma to the gastric mucosa associated with bile reflux. The histological

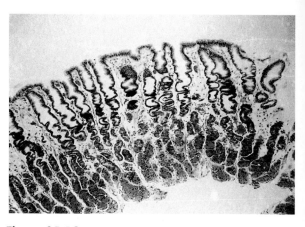

Figure 25.19
Foveolar hyperplasia in bile reflux gastritis; body of stomach (H&E ×).

features include foveolar hyperplasia (Figures 25.18 and 25.19), oedema, and smooth muscle fibres in the lamina propria, capillary congestion and a relative paucity of acute and chronic inflammatory cells. These features were found in association with raised intragastric bile acid concentrations and increased pH consistent with bile reflux. These features appear to be more reliable markers of reflux gastritis than those commonly used in other systems of classification, but it is not claimed that duodenogastric reflux is always accompanied by this picture. Increased numbers of chronic inflammatory cells due to multifactorial causation may also be found. Dixon et al.[51] have devised a scoring system for the assessment of bile reflux gastritis. It is also pointed out that severe foveolar hyperplasia without inflammatory cell response can be misinterpreted as premalignant dysplasia. Without doubt, foveolar hyperplasia is a very important marker for bile reflux as suggested by Mosimann et al.[52-54] and it can be misinterpreted as dysplasia by inexperienced observers.

O'Connor et al.[55] suggests that there are two grades of bile reflux gastritis, namely chronic superficial and atrophic gastritis. Emmanouilidis et al.[56] also claim that translucency of the surface epithelium, oedema of the upper portion of the lamina propria, decrease of parietal cells and predominant presence of neutral mucin in the cells in the surface epithelium and in the neck of the glands occur in bile reflux gastritis. Translucency of the epithelium has been described as the most characteristic lesion of the erythematous areas by Burbige et al.[57] Rubio and Slezak[58] also describe subnuclear vacuolization in foveolar epithelium as another histological marker for protracted duodenogastric reflux. Previous gastric surgery in the form of gastroenterostomy or gastrectomy is a risk factor for bile reflux gastritis. The diagnosis is established by inference since it is difficult to demonstrate abnormal recurrent bile reflux into the stomach. It is noteworthy that retrograde passage of duodenal contents into the stomach is normal during fasting and after feeding. Evidence for abnormal reflux is derived from direct sampling studies of gastric contents for bile acids and non-invasive techniques using a gamma camera to trace the passage of isotopes excreted in bile. Owing to continued gastric

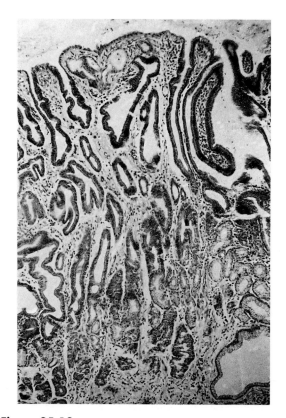

Figure 25.18
Foveolar hyperplasia in bile reflux gastritis; pyloric region (H&E ×).

emptying, bile does not normally accumulate in the stomach. Animal experiments indicate that bile and duodenal secretions can break the gastric mucosal barrier although histological studies show foveolar hyperplasia without the usual recognized features of gastritis assessed on the lamina propria cellular infiltrate. Surgical procedures incorporating fashioning of a Roux loop with a 25–40 cm limb minimizes the risk of bile reflux gastritis. It has previously been suggested that recurrent bile reflux into the stomach can lead to the development of erosions and gastric ulcer.

Multifocal environmental gastritis (Type AB, pangastritis, Type B, dietary)

This is very comparable with *Helicobacter*-associated gastritis or Type B gastritis and probably represents the same entity. There is a high incidence of this condition in less developed countries[59] and in Japan. The populations in these countries also have a high incidence of *H. pylori* infestation. The detection rate of *H. pylori* in patients attending for gastroscopy in Japan has been reported as 84%.[60] Furthermore, there is a recognized association between multifocal environmental gastritis and the intestinal variety of gastric carcinoma. The gastritis appears to begin as multiple small foci at the junction between the body and antral mucosa and spreads with the development of new lesions on the lesser curvature above and below this junction. Intestinal metaplasia is a prominent feature associated with atrophy of mucin-secreting glands. Foci of gastritis in the body mucosa show atrophy of parietal cell glands and pseudopyloric metaplasia. Gastric ulcer represents another complication and it may develop high up on the lesser curvature of the stomach.

Postgastrectomy gastritis

Biopsy studies following gastrectomy or gastroenterostomy have demonstrated that chronic atrophic gastritis frequently develops in the gastric remnant corresponding to the body of the stomach. Gastritis is most severe in the region of the anastomosis but there is a distinct loss of parietal cells throughout the body of the stomach. Postsurgical atrophy with loss of parietal and zymogenic cells is not associated with high serum gastrin or with circulating antibodies to parietal cells. Serum pepsinogen I (PG-I) concentration[61] falls with increasing severity of mucosal damage. On the other hand pepsinogen II (PG-II) levels are persistently raised. Fundic glands and chief cells which secrete PG-I and PG-II are gradually lost and they are replaced by metaplastic pseudopyloric glands which produce only PG-II. However, in mild atrophic gastritis PG-I concentration is raised, probably due to an increased rate of release of PG-I from a smaller chief cell mass. Reflux of enteric contents containing bile and pancreatic juice are believed to be important factors in the development of this type of gastritis. It is noteworthy that the majority of patients with duodenal ulcer harbour *H. pylori* before surgery, after surgery and reflux of bile the organism disappears from the mucosa in the majority of cases. The organism may, however, persist in a few cases. If a Roux loop has been constructed and bile has been diverted

from the stomach then *H. pylori* remains on the surface of the mucosa. The gastritis is associated with intestinal metaplasia and a recognized incidence of dysplasia and gastric cancer 15–30 years later. Bile vomiting due to alkaline reflux gastritis occurs in about 3% of postgastrectomy patients.[62] It is of note that bile diversion surgery does not arrest progression of gastritis, although it may relieve the distressing symptom of bile vomiting. Lipid islands or focal subepithelial collections of lipid-containing histiocytes resembling xanthoma are not infrequently encountered in patients who have been treated by gastrectomy or gastric surgery.

Varioliform gastritis, chronic verrucous gastritis, chronic lymphocytic gastritis

Varioliform or chronic verrucous gastritis[63,64] is diagnosed when endoscopic examination reveals multiple erosions longitudinally arranged along folds of the greater curvature and on the anterior and posterior walls of the antrum. Occasionally the erosions occur in the fundus and cardiac regions. The lesions have an unusual appearance consisting of small raised nodules with a central necrotic area. These erosions have also been described as aphthous ulcers. Histologically, the erosions are frequently associated with lymphocytic gastritis which is characterized by infiltration of gastric surface epithelium by T lymphocytes reminiscent of coeliac disease (Figure 25.20). Haot et al.[63] also reinvestigated the original Lyon series of varioliform gastritis. Of the original 90 cases, 35 patients were identified and their biopsies were reassessed. Lymphocytic gastritis was identified in 26 of these 35 cases. The baseline for diagnosis was 30 lymphocytes per 100 epithelial cells. Haot et al. concluded that there are two different types of clinical varioliform gastritis, one chronic and diffuse with lymphocytic infiltration and the other more acute and limited to the antrum. Dixon et al.[65] identified *H. pylori* infection in 41% of their cases of lymphocytic gastritis and considered that *H. pylori* could have an aetiological role. The numbers of lymphocytes per 100 epithelial cells was higher in this series than in Haot's series: 55.3 ± 10.5 (± SD) compared to control mean 3.7 ± 1.3. There was frequently a fall in the lymphocytic counts 6–22 weeks later:

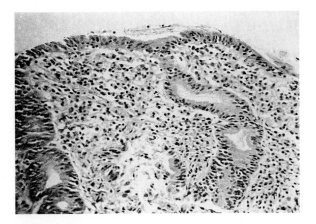

Figure 25.20
Varioliform or lymphocytic gastritis showing lymphocytes in the surface epithelium (H&E ×).

48.8 ± 28.8 per 100 epithelial cells. It is of notes that Steer,[66] in his studies of *H. pylori*, found that the number of intraepithelial lymphocytes was increased in association with peptic ulceration. Previous claims that varioliform gastritis was associated with numerous IgE cells in the lamina propria as suggested by Lambert et al.[67] and Andre et al.[68] have not been confirmed by Dixon. It would appear, therefore, that the majority of cases of varioliform gastritis correspond to lymphocytic gastritis, but a proportion can be classified as other types of gastritis. An allergic basis for varioliform gastritis has been suggested in some papers. Lesions may persist for long periods although healing has been reported after treatment with prednisolone.

Gastritis cystic polyposa (Gastritis cystica profunda)

This variety of gastritis is characterized by polyps and cysts accompanied by gastritis on the gastric side of the gastroenterostomy stoma or gastroduodenostomy opening. Ozenc et al.[69] described five patients who presented with abdominal pain, nausea and vomiting and gastrointestinal bleeding. Surgical intervention was carried out to relieve obstruction and prolapse and to rule out carcinoma. The disorder develops on average 9.5 (range 1–26) years after gastric surgery. A recent case has been described in a patient who had no antecedent gastric surgery although there was a history of gastric ulcer diathesis.[70] This variety of gastritis is related to the reflux of bile and intestinal secretions through the stoma into the adjacent stomach. Other authors describe dysplasia and malignant change complicating this variety of gastritis.

Chronic atrophic diffuse gastritis (also known as Type A gastritis)

This entity is characterized by chronic inflammatory cellular infiltration of the lamina propria in the body of the stomach associated with atrophy and disappearance of gastric glands containing parietal cells and zymogenic cells. There is extensive pseudopyloric gland metaplasia and usually widespread intestinal metaplasia (Figure 25.21). Lymph follicles are increased in number. This variety is associated with hypochlorhydria or achlorhydria according to the number of surviving parietal cells in the gastric glands. Small numbers of microscopic cysts may be present in the mucosa and submucosa. Serological studies show that antibodies to parietal cells and intrinsic factor are frequently present in the serum. If patients are followed-up for approximately 15 years many of them will develop pernicious anaemia. Low levels of PG-I and PG-II are present in blood and urine. Hypergastrinaemia occurs due to the presence of an intact antrum with G cells. Foci of intestinal metaplasia frequently show sulphomucin predominance representing Type III intestinal metaplasia. A fetal sulphoglycoprotein antigen related to blood antigens has been demonstrated in the gastric juice. Foci of dysplasia may appear as a premalignant complication and there is a distinct gastric cancer risk. The disease is most common in subjects of Scandinavia or Northern European extraction and there is an increased frequency in persons of blood group A who have

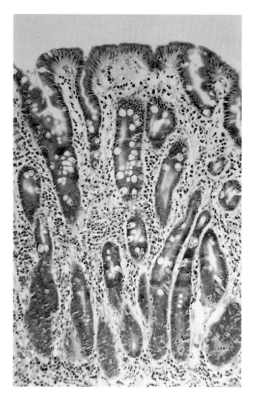

Figure 25.21
Chronic atrophic diffuse gastritis showing loss of parietal cell glands and intestinal metaplasia (H&E ×).

light blue eyes and prematurely grey hair. It is rare in other populations. It is probable that chronic superficial gastritis and multifocal environmental gastritis can progress over the years leading to chronic atrophic diffuse gastritis. Autoimmune and genetic factors appear to be involved in the aetiology.

Adult pernicious anaemia

Deficient secretion by parietal cells of intrinsic factor which binds dietary vitamin B_{12} making it absorbable leads to pernicious anaemia in adults. This is associated with atrophy of the parietal cell zymogenic cell glands and autoantibodies to parietal cells and intrinsic factor can be detected in the serum. Accordingly it is usually classified as an autoimmune disease. The loss of parietal cells and zymogenic cells is accompanied by pseudopyloric gland metaplasia and extensive intestinal metaplasia. Joske et al.[71] carried out a biopsy study of 100 cases and found complete gastric atrophy in 40 and residual parietal and zymogenic cells in the other 60. Microscopic cysts may be present in the mucosa. Atrophy of the mucosa is accompanied by atrophy of all coats of the stomach wall including muscle. Restoration of parietal cell glands has been reported following steroid therapy in a few cases. Hypergastrinaemia is present due to large numbers of G cells in the antral mucosa and there may also be hyperplasia of enterochromaffin-like (ECL) cells in the antral and body mucosa. Complement fixing antibodies against the microsomes of acid-secreting cells are present in a high proportion of patients and about 55–60% also have specific antibody against intrinsic factor. There is a possibility that in cases without demonstrable serum antibodies, these may be present as cell-bound antibodies in the mucosa of the small intestine or mononuclear cells. Serum antibodies to thyroid microsomes may be present and conversely patients with thyroid disease such as Hashimoto's disease and thyrotoxicosis may have gastric parietal cell antibodies. A genetic factor is involved in the aetiology and this may be recessive or dominant with incomplete expression in relatives. Chronic inflammatory cellular infiltration is frequently present and the features are indistinguishable from chronic atrophic diffuse gastritis or Type A gastritis. The pyloric region usually remains normal but it may show Type B gastritis or it may also be affected by atrophic gastritis. In a biopsy study of 86 patients with pernicious anaemia Flejou et al.[72] found a 36% incidence of antral gastritis associated with a low infestation of *H. pylori*, i.e. 6%. Rebiopsy of 25 of the patients five years later showed no change in the pattern of gastritis. They suggested that the antral gastritis that may accompany body gastritis in pernicious anaemia appears more likely to be an extension of primary Type A body gastritis (autoimmune) rather than a secondary Type B (chronic) gastritis and that the antrum, like the body of the stomach, may be resistant to colonization. In this series, only three of the 86 patients showed evidence of *H. pylori* in the body of the stomach. Other workers consider that the associated antral gastritis represents Type B or hypersecretory gastritis. It is noteworthy that in Northern Scandinavian countries infestation with the tapeworm *Diphyllobothrium latum* can lead to varying degrees of gastric atrophy, inflammatory changes and intestinal metaplasia comparable to the changes found in pernicious anaemia. Likewise the blood picture is that of megaloblastic anaemia. The tapeworm interferes with the vitamin B$_{12}$ intrinsic factor complex or prevents binding of vitamin B$_{12}$ with intrinsic factor.

Patients with pernicious anaemia have an increased risk of gastric cancer. Hyperplasia of ECL cells may lead to the development of single or multiple polypoid tumours which have been called microcarcinoids. These generally pursue a benign course but there is a small risk of malignancy and development of a typical carcinoid tumour. Approximately 20–30% of patients have other types of polyp.[73,74] One study also showed foci of dysplasia classified as moderate or severe degree in 11%.[74]

Gastric atrophy

In this condition the body of the stomach shows loss of parietal cell zymogenic glands and their substitution by pseudopyloric glands and zones or islets of intestinal metaplasia. Chronic inflammatory changes are absent or minimal in degree. The entity represents an end-stage or inactive stage of pernicious anaemia or chronic atrophic diffuse gastritis and does not imply any other aetiology.

Juvenile pernicious anaemia

There are three different syndromes:

1. The first is associated with gastric atrophy corresponding to the adult type and it occurs in later childhood and adolescence.

2. The second, referred to as 'true' juvenile pernicious anaema, is accompanied by a histologically normal gastric mucosa and deficiency of secretion of intrinsic factor by parietal cells from birth. Acid secretion is reduced but it returns to normal when vitamin B$_{12}$ therapy is given. If intrinsic factor is added to the diet then vitamin B$_{12}$ is absorbed in the normal way from the small bowel.

3. The third variety is described as Imerslund's syndrome. There is an abnormality in the intestinal absorption of the normal complex although intrinsic factor and vitamin B$_{12}$ intrinsic factor complex are combined normally. Levine and Allen[75] studied gastric biopsies from nine patients with juvenile pernicious anaemia using the immunoperoxidase technique and suggested that the term embraces a heterogeneous group of disorders which might be caused by the following mechanisms:

- Inadequate synthesis of intrinsic factor secretion;
- A block in intrinsic factor secretion;
- The secretion of an abnormal intrinsic factor that does not bind to cobalmin;
- The secretion of other abnormal intrinsic factors that could contain a number of other functional defects.

Granulomatous gastritis

There is a spectrum of disorders which can lead to granulomatous gastritis. These are discussed below.

Sarcoidosis

Gastric lesions due to sarcoidosis are of three main types. First, non-caseating giant cell systems may be scattered throughout the gastric mucosa without any gross macroscopic lesion. The granulomas are often discovered as incidental findings during endoscopy and biopsy. The clinical significance of these scattered lesions is small and the biological behaviour of the disease depends on involvement of other organs. Second, sarcoid granulomas can occur in association with chronic gastric ulcers. It is debatable whether they are a co-existent phenomena or whether they precipitate the development of a chronic gastric ulcer. The gastric ulcer is treated as an ordinary peptic ulcer. The third type of presentation is associated with a linitis plastica form of the disease involving the pyloric region or more diffusely involving the greater part of the stomach. There is extensive involvement of the gastric wall (Figure 25.22) with numerous non-caseating epithelioid cell follicles and Langhans' giant cells together with superficial ulceration. Round Schaumann bodies which show concentric lamination and calcification, asteroid bodies and calcium oxalate crystals may be identified in the cytoplasm of the giant cells. Wesenberg–Hamasaki bodies with an oval or needle-like configuration showing periodic–Schiff (PAS) positivity may be seen in a perivascular location. Slight fibrinoid necrosis may be present in the centre of the giant cell follicles. Sarcoid lesions also involve the gastric lymph nodes and granulomatous angiitis can also occur. This type of gastric sarcoidosis is very difficult to differentiate from the linitis plastica variety of carcinoma of

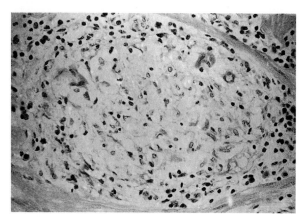

Figure 25.22
Sarcoidosis with sarcoid granuloma in muscle coat (H&F x)

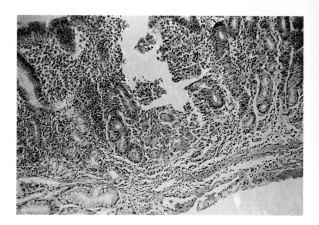

Figure 25.23
Crohn's disease. Random biopsy of gastric mucosa with granuloma in the base of the mucosa (H&E x).

the stomach. Biopsies may be difficult to interpret and may not exclude neoplasia since granulomas are rarely found in association with gastric cancer or gastric lymphoma. The clinical presentation may be of non-ulcer dyspepsia or gastric outlet obstruction and the symptoms, signs and endoscopic appearances may be indistinguishable from those of gastric cancer. Gastrectomy is not infrequently carried out on these patients and when the diagnosis has been clearly established, after excluding malignancy, steroid therapy can be introduced with excellent results.

Crohn's disease

Crohn's disease of the stomach, leading to the diffusely infiltrating linitis plastica appearance, is encountered rarely with thickening of the stomach wall, ulceration, sinuses, oedema and fibrosis. The majority of patients have active Crohn's disease in the ileum or colon, but Crohn's disease of the stomach can be a primary presenting feature. Crohn's disease of the stomach is usually continuous with Crohn's disease in the duodenum. Gastric involvement may be controlled with steroid therapy but if there is gastric outlet obstruction partial gastrectomy or gastroenterostomy may have to be carried out. Gastric and duodenal involvement can lead to non-ulcer dyspepsia.

Random biopsies of the stomach may unexpectedly show giant cell follicles in patients with Crohn's disease (Figure 25.23) of the ileum or colon. The lesions are incidental and do not lead to any gross abnormality. Tanaka et al.[76] describe minute endoscopic lesions of the stomach in 75% of patients with Crohn's disease observed over a period of 10 years. In this study epithelioid cell granulomas were found in the serial sections of 83% of cases. Jouin et al. in their study of 129 cases of Crohn's disease over a period of 12 years found involvement of the upper gastrointestinal tract in 28%. Granulomas were encountered in 16% of patients.

Foreign body granulomas

Food granulomas are not uncommon in association with active or healed peptic ulcers due to food particles such as insoluble vegetable material or cereal husks becoming embedded in the tissues. Sutures derived from previous gastric surgical procedures may also give rise to granulomas. Other agents which can induce granulomas include barium, beryllium, kaolin and the abrasive ingredients of toothpaste.

Tuberculosis

Gastric involvement is extremely rare and may take the form of caseating granulomas or ulcers. Identification of acid-fast bacilli is essential for diagnosis.

Syphilis

Gastric lesions in secondary and tertiary syphilis are rare. Antral lesions can occur in secondary syphilis. Ultimately the lesions may become fibrotic. Spirochaetes can be demonstrated in the lesions.

Histoplasmosis

Granulomas, with or without necrosis, contain the organism which can be identified using PAS or Grocott silver stain.

Other rare infections

Granulomatous lesions have also been described in association with phycomycosis, paracoccidioidomycosis, anisakiasis and mycobacterial infections particularly in patients with the acquired immune deficiency syndrome (AIDS).

Isolated granulomatous gastritis

In some cases of granulomatous gastritis there is no obvious cause and the aetiology is therefore regarded as idiopathic. Some of these cases show thickening of the antrum and prepyloric region leading to gastric outlet obstruction. Gastric or duodenal ulcers may also be present. Granulomas can also occur in the gastric lymph nodes.

Other rare granulomatous disorders

Granulomatous lesions have also been described in chronic granulomatous disease of childhood, Wegener's granulomatosis, allergic granulomatosis and vasculitis. Sarcoid-type granulomas can also be associated with malignant tumours such as carcinoma and lymphoma distributed in the stomach wall and lymph nodes.

Eosinophilic gastritis

This uncommon condition affects children and young adults who frequently have a history of asthma or allergy. There is diffuse thickening of part of the stomach. The antrum and pylorus are the areas usually affected. On endoscopic examination the features may resemble carcinoma, the mucosa being red and oedematous with erosions. There is extensive infiltration with eosinophils.[78-80] Various types have been described, for example: mucosal, which behaves like other inflammatory disorders; submucosal, which can lead to obstruction; serosal, which can be associated with eosinophilic peritonitis; and systemic, which can be associated with involvement of other abdominal and distant organs. Perforation is a rare complication. Patients may also suffer from asthma. Serum IgE levels frequently correlate with the severity of the disease and peripheral eosinophilia is encountered in a high proportion of cases. There may be a therapeutic response to steroid therapy; occasional cases have been treated by surgical resection. Parasitic or worm infestation can also lead to an eosinophilic infiltration. Examples include anisakiasis from herring worm larvae, sarcocystic cysts from contaminated meat, hookworm disease, oesophagostomiasis and angiostrongyliasis.

Inflammatory fibroid polyp

(Eosinophilic granuloma, gastric fibroma with eosinophilic infiltration, gastric submucosal granuloma, polypoid eosinophilic gastritis and inflammatory pseudotumour).

This is a polypoid lesion which may be ulcerated. Histologically it consists of granulation tissue or fibrovascular tissue with a variable eosinophilic infiltrate. It involves the submucosa and mucosa. There is no evidence of blood eosinophilia and its relationship to eosinophilic gastritis is dubious. It probably represents a reparative type granulation tissue nodule.

Ménètrier's disease (hyperplastic gastropathy)

This condition, which is more common in men, is associated with thickening of the gastric mucosa and rugae accompanied by cystic dilatation of glands with mucin.[81] The four features which identify this entity are large gastric mucosal folds, low or less commonly normal gastric acid secretion, increased gastric protein loss and characteristic histology. There is also foveolar hyperplasia, atrophy of the fundic glands and pseudopyloric metaplasia. Groups of glands and cysts may penetrate through the muscularis mucosa into the submucosa. Ming[82] has classified this disease into mucous cell hyperplasia, glandular cell hyperplasia or mixed mucous glandular cell hyperplasia varieties. There may be associated protein-losing gastroenteropathy and hypochlorhydria. Chronic superficial gastritis may be superimposed. It represents a spectrum of clinical, endoscopic and histological features. Schindler's disease[83] occupies the other end of the spectrum corresponding to Ming's glandular cell type characterized by large mucosal folds, normal or high gastric acid secretion, normal protein metabolism and parietal and chief cell hyperplasia with a relative or absolute reduction in mucous cells. There is some evidence that Schindler's disease may progress to Ménètrier's disease and then go on to atrophic gastritis. Spontaneous retrogression of both entities has been recorded. Ménètrier's disease has been cited as a premalignant disorder with an incidence of cancer in 10–13% of cases but a more realistic assessment is around 5%. The cancer association is still controversial. The condition can occur in adults or children. An association with cytomegalic inclusion body disease has recently been described in children. Familial disease[84] is rare.

Opportunistic infections

Partial gastric outlet obstruction associated with an inflamed pyloric ring has been encountered due to cryptosporidiosis in patients with AIDS.[85] Cytomegalovirus has also been cited as a cause of gastritis with erosions in AIDS[86] and renal transplant cases.[87] Fungal infections such as candidiasis, aspergillosis or mucormycosis can give rise to erosive lesions in the gastric mucosa especially in immunocompromised patients at autopsy. Fungi, especially candida, are not infrequently found in gastric ulcer craters. *Giardia lamblia* may be identified on the mucosal surface in patients with giardiasis.

Other types of gastritis

Some workers refer to zonal gastritis surrounding a chronic gastric ulcer. Variable inflammatory and regenerative epithelial changes are encountered.

Etat mammelonné refers to a mamillated or finely nodular state of the gastric mucosa which may represent finely nodular hyperplasia of the parietal cell glands or chronic gastritis with alternating areas of foveolar hyperplasia and glandular atrophy.

Another confusing entity is the occurrence of non-neoplastic fundic gland cystic polyps. These can occur as part of the familial polyposis coli syndrome or Gardner's syndrome but more commonly they are idiopathic and cause difficulty in classification. Eidt and Stolte[88] suggest that they are of reversible functional secretory genesis rather than being hamartomatous. There is an association with colorectal adenomas and adenocarcinomas.

Collagenous gastritis is characterized by a focal, narrow subepithelial band of collagen comparable to that encountered in collagenous colitis and in some cases of adult coeliac disease. It may represent a response to a dietary antigen and in rare cases it may be associated with coeliac disease.

Immunodeficiency gastritis is encountered in 40% of patients with hypogammaglobulinaemia who are subject to repeated bacterial infections. It exists as a pangastritis and there is an absence of plasma cells. Achlorhydria is common and it is established that these patients have a high incidence of gastric cancer.

Rugal hyperplastic gastritis or gastropathy comprises various ill-defined entities with enlarged rugal folds. The histological diagnosis in such cases embraces Ménètrier's disease, Zollinger–Ellison syndrome, lymphoma, carcinoma, peptic ulcer disease, postoperative gastritis, granulomatous disease and gastric varices.

The Zollinger–Ellison syndrome is associated with hyperplasia of the parietal cell glands. In itself it is not a gastritis. Biopsy and parietal cell counts can consolidate the diagnosis.

Congestive gastropathy (Portazgastropathy)

This term has been applied to cases of so-called gastritis associated with portal hypertension[89] of various aetiologies. Dilated and tortuous submucosal veins and vascular ectasia in the mucosa are prominent features. Patients with severe or persisting gastropathy are prone to clinically significant haemorrhage. Corbishley et al.[90] have pointed out that endoscopic biopsy cannot be used to diagnose this disorder or assess its management. Foster et al.[91] emphasizes that the degree of capillary dilatation is unrelated to histological gastritis. In their series 9 of 23 patients had reflux gastritis and 3 of 23 had evidence of *H. pylori* infestation.

DIAGNOSIS OF GASTRITIS

Accurate diagnosis can only be based on clear endoscopic anatomical location of the biopsy sites. Ideally multiple biopsies from the antral and body mucosa are essential for assessment combined with information on endoscopic appearances, clinical features, serology and bacteriology but it is recommended that two biopsies from the antral mucosa and two biopsies from the body mucosa are sufficient for the Sidney classification system.

H. pylori is easily identified in Giemsa preparations as a possible aetiological agent. The location of inflammatory cellular infiltration, i.e. superficial or diffuse, the presence of erosions, neutrophils, regenerative epithelial changes, foveolar hyperplasia, the state of the glands and secretory cells, the presence of intestinal metaplasia, etc. can all be assessed and taken into consideration in order to arrive at a clinopathological interpretation. Chronic atrophic diffuse gastritis and pernicious anaemia in the body of the stomach can be confirmed by carefully selected gastric biopsies. Serial gastric biopsies are also of considerable value in confirming the diagnosis and assessing progression and response to treatment.

Surgical resection specimens

The majority of specimens are derived from partial gastrectomy procedures. It is possible to assess gastritis in the antral region and in the junctional zone between the antrum and body of the stomach. A limited zone of body mucosa may be included in the specimen according to whether it is a simple antrectomy or an extended gastrectomy.

Total gastrectomy specimens provide an excellent opportunity to assess gastritis but most of the specimens have been resected for advanced gastric cancer with extensive superficial or deep ulceration which makes interpretation difficult. Occasionally total gastrectomy is carried out for early gastric cancer and more detailed assessment of gastritis is possible.

Surgical resection of the body of the stomach is very uncommon but provides an opportunity to assess the body mucosa and cardiac mucosa. Resection of cardiac mucosa and part of the body mucosa may be carried out for the treatment of carcinoma of the cardia or lower oesophagus. Again, there is a limited opportunity to investigate gastritis.

Local wedge resection of ulcer craters or small gastric cancers has limited value in the assessment of gastritis although the presence of intestinal metaplasia may be informative.

DUODENITIS

Duodenitis is an equally controversial subject in respect of classification and aetiology.

ACUTE MUCOSAL INJURY AND STRESS LESIONS

Acute erosive gastritis may extend into the duodenum in patients who have taken NSAIDs or other injurious agents. It is noteworthy that cimetidine has been cited as a rare cause of duodenal erosion.[92] Stress lesions and haemorrhagic erosions can also occur in the duodenum. Curling's ulcer is a well recognized complication of burns and Cushing's ulcers can occur in neurosurgical patients or those with head injury. Corrosive agents which damage the stomach may also enter the duodenum and cause mucosal necrosis. Opportunistic infections such as cytomegalic inclusion body disease can also affect the duodenal mucosa, particularly in renal transplant patients.

CHRONIC DUODENITIS

Whitehead et al.[93] has classified duodenitis as slight, moderate or severe. Slight duodenitis has a normal architecture, normal surface epithelium and an increased number of lymphocytes and plasma cells. In moderate duodenitis, the surface epithelium is abnormal, occasionally deformed with shortened villi and focal gastric metaplasia. In severe duodenitis, there is erosion of the surface epithelium, marked inflammatory change, deformed villi and extensive gastric metaplasia. Jenkins et al.[94] more recently, have modified this grading system into slight duodenitis with oedema of the lamina propria, appreciable lymphocytic plasma cell response, intraepithelial polymorphs and gastric metaplasia and into severe duodenitis with appreciable polymorph reaction, villous atrophy and decreased lymphocytic and plasma cell response. There are, of course, other varieties of duodenitis which will be discussed briefly later. The diganosis of duodenitis is assisted by identification of neutrophils migrating through the surface epithelium (Figure 25.24) of the duodenal mucosa and infiltrating the lamina propria. Acute inflammatory erosions with leucocytic exudate streaming out of the mucosa are also encountered in duodenitis (Figures 25.25 and 25.26) and these may be an obvious feature during endoscopy. Regenerative epithelial changes are frequently present on the mucosal surface. Morphometric studies have been carried out to assess the numbers of chronic inflammatory cells, particularly plasma cells (Figures 25.27 and 25.28) in the lamina propria. Hasan et al.[95] and Scott et al.[96] have shown that increased numbers of plasma cells are present

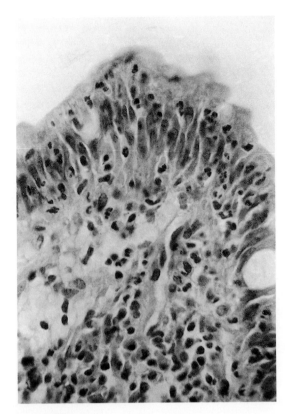

Figure 25.24
Duodenitis showing neutrophils emigrating through surface epithelium (H&E ×).

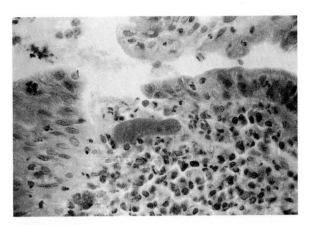

Figure 25.26
Minute inflammatory erosion in duodenitis (H&E ×).

in duodenitis. Brunner's glands are usually unaffected but nodular hyperplasia has been described in patients with renal transplants and those in renal failure. Brunner's glands may be destroyed in the vicinity of ulcer scars. Gastric glands with mucin-secreting cells are present in the majority of cases but parietal cells may also be present. Islets and zones of gastric epithelium in the duodenum may be infested with *H. pylori*.

Duodenitis has been incriminated as a cause of non-ulcer dyspepsia. In a series of cases of non-erosive and erosive gastritis studied by Sircus[97] 81.7% developed one or more duodenal ulcers sooner or later. Erosive duodenitis *per se* is an

uncommon cause of continuing disability and non-erosive duodenitis gives rise to dyspepsia extremely rarely. There is a sevenfold increase in the incidence of duodenitis in the relatives of those with duodenal ulcer disease. Treatment of the duodenal ulcers with cimetidine resulted in healing in 68.5% but resolution of duodenitis was observed in only 28.1%. Duodenal ulcer without duodenitis at any time was only seen in 8.2% and duodenitis without an ulcer at any time in 18.3% of cases. Marshall[17] suggests that duodenitis represents antral-type gastritis occurring in genetically susceptible individuals where the gastrointestinal junction lies not at the pylorus but in the duodenal bulb and that it is related to persistent

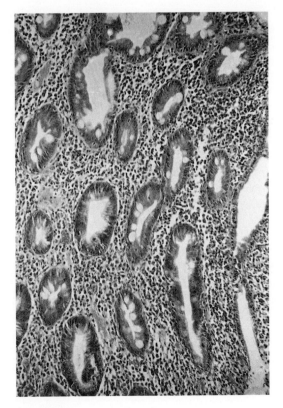

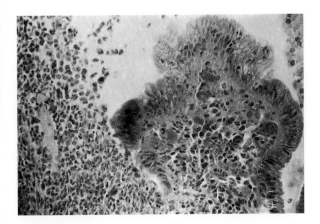

Figure 25.25
Inflammatory erosion in duodenitis with gastric metaplasia at the edge (H&E ×).

Figure 25.27
Duodenitis showing chronic inflammatory cellular infiltration of the lamina propria (H&E ×).

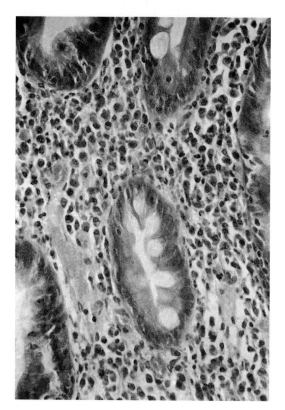

Figure 25.28
Duodenitis showing infiltration of the lamina propria with plasma cells and lymphocytes (H&E ×).

Helicobacter infection. Contradictory views have also been expressed. It is relevant to note that variable isolation rates for *H. pylori* have been reported in non-ulcer dyspepsia and the general impression is that there is insufficient evidence to incriminate it, in contrast to duodenal ulcer disease.

Cheli[98] investigated 38 cases of chronic duodenitis and found that basal hydrochloric acid secretion was normal in 39%, hypochlorhydria was present in 29% and hyperchlor-hydria in 32%. Maximal acid output was normal in 71%, decreased in 19% and increased in 10%. Moreover, fasting serum gastrin was also within normal limits. Cheli concluded that acid-peptic disease is not aetiopathogenic in the causation of most cases of chronic duodenitis. Erosive bulbitis is characterized by hyperchlorhydria but only rare cases of chronic duodenitis are accompanied by severe hypochlorhydria Cheli proposed that the term bulbitis should be used for the endoscopic picture of congestion and erosions involving the proximal duodenum and duodenal bulb associated with hypochlorhydria and he suggested that chronic duodenitis should be regarded as a different entity unconnected with acid peptic disease. Jenkins[94] on the other hand concluded that severe duodenitis appeared to be of clinical importance in relation to peptic ulceration. Carrick et al.[99] discussed the significance of functioning gastric metaplasia in ulcerogenesis. Surprisingly Congo red staining of the duodenal bulb revealed that functioning endogenous acid-producing tissue could be found most often at the edges of duodenal ulcers and also occasionally in non-ulcer subjects. Their study identified duodenal infection with *H. pylori* as the strongest risk factor for development of duodenal ulceration. The finding of endogenous acid production around the edges of duodenal ulcers suggests an active role for parietal cells in the duodenum. The authors postulate a synergistic role for duodenal *H. pylori* and endogenous acid production in the development of duodenal ulceration. Shousha[100] studied duodenal biopsy specimens from 80 patients with chronic renal failure. Chronic duodenitis was present in 59% but only 9% showed evidence of active inflammation. Gastric metaplasia was present in 62.5% yet *H. pylori* was identified in only two patients (2.5%). It is suggested that the duodenal environment in patients with chronic renal failure remains hostile to the growth of these organisms, despite the presence of gastric metaplasia. Interpretation is further obscured by the fact that congenital gastric heterotopia can occur in the duodenum without *Helicobacter* infestation. Lessels and Martin[101] assessed the incidence of gastric heterotopia in the population as 2% in patients without duodenal ulcer disease. The incidence of non-ulcer dyspepsia in the population has been assessed as 3% of 502 routine endoscopies.

PSEUDOMELANOSIS DUODENI

This condition was first described in 1976. It may be complicated by gastrointestinal bleeding. Endoscopic study may show erosions and a non-eroded background mucosa with a peculiar diffuse peppered appearance corresponding to numerous tiny black spots. Pounder et al.[102] performed electron probe X-ray analysis in one case and identified the pigment as iron sulphide. The condition may complicate chronic renal failure which was present in seven of nine cases reported by Kang et al.[103] who also suggested that the pigment is derived from iron absorbed from the lumen. Follow-up examination in one case has demonstrated that the condition is reversible.[104]

OTHER VARIETIES OF DUODENITIS

Adult coeliac disease

Total, subtotal or partial villous atrophy occurs in adult coeliac disease and dermatitis herpetiformis associated with chronic inflammatory cellular infiltration of the lamina propria with plasma cells, lymphocytes, eosinophils and histiocytes. Surface epithelium is more cuboidal and more cellular than normal with an increased number of T lymphocytes (theliocytes). There is also crypt hyperplasia and the features may be indistinguishable from duodenitis although neutrophils are not usually present in significant numbers. Certain viral infections in children which cause gastroenteritis can give rise to duodeno-jejunal abnormalities resembling coeliac disease.

Alpha chain disease and immunoproliferative small intestinal disease

In alpha heavy chain disease the lamina propria is packed with plasma cells which contain alpha chain immunoglobulin. The mucosa may be villous, convoluted or flat with normal columnar enterocytes. Serum IgA is considerably elevated in the majority of patients. The disease is encountered predominantly in males aged 10–30 years in Mediterranean countries, Iran, Iraq and South Africa among the low socioeconomic status groups. There is a high incidence of B cell malignant lymphoma in these patients although treatment with tetracyclines may lead to temporary improvement in their clinical status. The symptomatology includes chronic diarrhoea, weight loss and abdominal pain. Malabsorption and steatorrhoea are frequently present.

Crohn's disease

Foci of ulceration, chronic inflammatory cellular infiltration, villous abnormalities, neutrophils, epithelial regenerative changes and granulomas can occur in Crohn's disease and the features may mimic duodenitis.

Whipple's disease

Numerous foamy PAS-positive macrophages are located in the lamina propria in this disorder. The diagnosis can be confirmed by electron microscopic identification of the bacilli responsible for this infection. Dilatation of lacteals is an additional feature and there may be chronic inflammatory changes and even erosions in the mucosa with or without neutrophils. Granulomas have also been described.

Cytomegalic inclusion body disease

This viral infection with inclusion bodies is not uncommonly found in renal transplant cases and in patients with AIDS.

Mycobacterial infection

Vazquez-Iglesias et al.[105] described a case of mycobacterial infection (*Mycobacterium avium intracellulare*) of the duodenium in a patient with AIDS simulating Whipple's disease.

Parasitic disease

Giardia lamblia infestation is easily recognized by the identification of the parasites on the surface of the mucosa. If few parasites are present then the diagnosis is much more difficult. Inflammatory changes are not a prominent feature. Strongyloidiasis may be encountered, particularly in patients with AIDS, with the worms or larvae embedded in the mucosa, glands or even submucosa. There may be associated inflammatory changes. Hookworm infestation is rare in the UK but it can occur in other parts of the world. Rarely, the parasites are identified attached to the duodenal mucosa.

Other rare disorders

Abetalipoproteinaemia (acanthocytosis) can be identified in children with foamy vacuolation of enterocytes covering the upper two thirds of the villi. The vacuoles contain neutral fat which can be demonstrated in frozen sections. Congenital lymphangiectasis rarely involves the duodenum in young children. Hypogammaglobulinaemia may be associated with duodenal and jejunal mucosal changes resembling coeliac disease. Patients with the Zollinger–Ellison syndrome and those who have had a gastrectomy may show partial villous atrophy in duodenal biopsies. Patients suffering from tropical sprue or

AIDS may show villous abnormalities which may be difficult to differentiate from coeliac disease. Certain cytotoxic drugs, e.g. methotrexate, can also induce villous abnormalities.

INTERPRETATION OF DUODENAL BIOPSIES

The anatomical site of biopsies is clearly important. Erosive bulbitis involves the duodenal bulb with or without an associated duodenal ulcer. If an ulcer crater or scar is evident on endoscopy this information should be communicated to the histopathologist since the duodenitis is usually associated with the peptic ulcer. Multiple biopsies from the first, second or even third part of the duodenum are clearly important in the interpretation of chronic duodenitis. A diagnosis of adult coeliac disease and enteropathy associated with dermatitis herpetiformis can be established from biopsies of the second or third part of the duodenum. Parasites and inclusion bodies can be clearly identified in biopsy material. There is sometimes difficulty in deciding whether biopsies have come from the duodenum or stomach and the experience of the endoscopist is a critical factor. Dissecting microscopy is valuable for the assessment of villous architecture if the biopsies are sufficiently large for correct orientation.

REFERENCES

1. Roth SH & Bennett RE. Non-steroidal anti-inflammatory drug gastropathy – recognition and response. *Arch Intern Med* 1987; **147:** 2093–2100.
2. Langman MJS. Epidemiological evidence of the association of aspirin and acute gastrointestinal bleeding. *Gut* 1970; **11:** 627–634.
3. Levy M. Aspirin use in patients with major upper gastrointestinal bleeding and peptic ulcer disease. *N Engl J Med* 1974; **290:** 1158–1162.
4. Levine MJ, Verstandig A & Laufer I. Serpiginous gastric erosions caused by aspirin and other non-steroidal anti-inflammatory drugs. *AJR* 1986; **146:** 31–34.
5. Faulkner G, Prichard P, Somerville K & Langman MJS. Aspirin and bleeding peptic ulcers in the elderly. *BMJ* 1988; **297:** 1311–1313.
6. Henry DA, Johnston A, Dobson A & Duggan J. Fatal peptic ulcer complications and the use of non-steroidal anti-inflammatory drugs, aspirin and corticosteroids. *BMJ* 1987; **295:** 1227–1229.
7. Collier DStJ & Pain JA. Non-steroidal anti-inflammatory drugs and peptic ulcer perforation. *Gut* 1985; **26:** 359–363.
8. Consumers' Association. Do corticosteroids cause peptic ulcers? *Drug Ther Bull*, 1987; **25:** 41–43.
9. O'Keane M, Smith S & Goldberg A. Gastric erosions caused by home-brewed lager. *Lancet* 1971; **2:** 795–797.
10. Agrawal NM, Godiwala T, Arimura A & Dajani EZ. Cytoprotection by a synthetic prostaglandin against ethanol-induced gastric mucosal damage. *Gastrointest Endosc* 1986; **32:** 67–70.
11. Tarnawski A, Hollander D, Stachura J, Klimczyk B, Mach T & Bogdal J. Prostaglandin protection of the human gastric mucosa against alcohol-induced injury: endoscopic, histologic, and functional assessment. *Scand J Gastroenterol* 1986; **21** (Suppl 125): 165–169.
12. Abdu RA, Garritano D & Culver O. Acute gastric necrosis in anorexia nervosa and bulimia: two case reports. *Arch Surg* 1987; **122:** 830–832.
13. Barbosa A, Queiroz DM, Mendes EN, Rocha GA, Carvalho AS & Roquette MLV. *Campylobacter pylori* associated acute gastritis in a child. *J Clin Pathol* 1989; **42,** 779 (letter).
14. Marshall BJ, Armstrong JA, McGechie DG & Glancy RJ. Attempt to fulfil Koch's postulates for pyloric *Campylobacter*. *Med J Aust* 1985; **142:** 436–439.
15. Marshall BJ, McGechie DB, Rogers PA & Glancy RJ. Pyloric *Campylobacter* infection and gastroduodenal disease. *Med J Aust* 1985; **142:** 439–445.
16. Editorial. Pyloric *Campylobacter* finds a volunteer. *Lancet* 1985; **i:** 1021–1022.
17. Marshall BJ. The *Campylobacter pylori* story. *Scand J Gastroenterol* 1988; **23** (Suppl 146): 58–66.

18. Morris A & Nicholson G. Ingestion of *Campylobacter pylori* causes gastritis and raised fasting gastric pH. *Am J Gastroenterol* 1987; **82:** 192–199.

19. Ramsey EJ, Carey KV, Peterson WL et al. Epidemic gastritis with hypochlorhydria. *Gastroenterology* 1979; **76:** 1449–1457.

20. Salmeron M, Desplaces N, Lavergne A & Houdart R. *Campylobacter*-like organisms and acute purulent gastritis. *Lancet* 1986; **ii:** 975–986 (letter).

21. Graham DY, Alpert LC, Lacey Smith J & Yoshimura HH. Iatrogenic *Campylobacter pylori* infection is a cause of epidemic achlorhydria. *Am J Gastroenterol* 1988; **83:** 974–980.

22. Frommer DJ, Carrick J, Lee A & Hazell SL. Acute presentation of *C. pylori* gastritis. *Am J Gastroenterol* 1988; **83:** 1168–1171.

23. Garo B, Geier B, Le Guillow M et al. Necrose gastro-duodenale an cours d'un syndrome hemolytique et uremique de l'adulte. *Gastroenterol Clin Biol* 1988; **12:** 401.

24. Moody FG, Cheung LY, Simons MA & Zalewsky C. Stress and the acute gastric mucosal lesion. *Am J Dig Dis* 1976; **21:** 148–154.

25. Shibayama Y. An experimental study into the cause of acute haemorrhagic gastritis in cirrhosis. *J Pathol* 1986; **149:** 307–313.

26. Starr A & Wilson JM. Phlegmonous gastritis. *Ann Surg* 1957; **145:** 88–93.

27. Eliason EL & Wright VWM. Phlegmonous gastritis. *Surg Clin North Am* 1938; **18:** 1553–1564.

28. Pritchard JE & McRoberts JW. Phlegmonous gastritis. *Can Med Assoc J* 1931; **25:** 183–187.

29. Peter ET, Bernstein EF, Sosin H, Madsen AJ, Walder AI & Wangensteen OH. Technique of gastric freezing in the treatment of duodenal ulcer. *JAMA* 1962; **181:** 760–764.

30. Morris DL, Brearley S, Thompson H & Keighley MRK. A comparison of the efficacy and depth of gastric wall injury with 3.2 and 2.3 mm bipolar probes in canine arterial haemorrhage. *Gastrointest Endosc* 1985; **31:** 361–363.

31. Strickland RG & Mackay IR. A re-appraisal of the nature and significance of chronic atrophic gastritis. *Am J Dig Dis* 1973; **18:** 426–440.

32. Pitchumoni CS & Glass GBJ. Alcohol injury to gastrointestinal mucosa. In Glass GBJ (ed.) *Progress in Gastroenterology* Vol. 3. New York: Grune & Stratton, 1977; 717.

33. Pitchumoni CS & Glass GBJ. Patterns of gastritis in alcoholics. *Biol Gastroenterol* 1976; **9:** 11–16.

34. Parl FF, Lev R, Thomas E & Pitchumoni CS. Histologic and morphometric study of chronic gastritis in alcoholic patients. *Hum Pathol* 1979; **10:** 45–56.

35. Cheli R, Persasso A & Giacosa A. *Gastritis*. London: Springer, 1987: 82–83.

36. Roberts DM. Chronic gastritis, alcohol and non-ulcer dyspepsia. *Gut* 1972; **13:** 768–774.

37. Warren JR & Marshall BJ. Unidentified curved bacilli on gastric epithelium in active chronic gastritis. *Lancet* 1983; **i:** 1273–1275.

38. Editorial. *Campylobacter pylori* becomes *Helicobacter pylori*. *Lancet* 1989; **ii:** 1019–1020.

39. Price AB, Levi J, Dolby JM et al. *Campylobacter pyloridis* in peptic ulcer disease: microbiology, pathology and scanning electron microscopy. *Gut* 1985; **26:** 1183–1188.

40. Dooley CO & Cohen H. The clinical significance of *Campylobacter pylori*. *Ann Intern Med* 1988; **108:** 70–79.

41. Peterson WL, Lee E & Feldman M. Relationship between *Campylobacter pylori* and gastritis in healthy humans after administration of placebo or indomethacin. *Gastroenterology* 1988; **95:** 1185–1197.

42. Mahony MJ, Wyatt JI & Littlewood JM. *Campylobacter pylori* gastritis. *Arch Dis Child* 1988; **63:** 654–655.

43. Levi S, Dollery CT, Bloom SR et al. *Campylobacter pylori*, duodenal ulcer disease and gastrin. *BMJ* 1989; **299:** 1093–1094.

44. Collins JSA, Hamilton PW, Watt PCH, Sloan JM & Love AHG. Superficial gastritis and *Campylobacter pylori* in dyspeptic patients – a quantitative study using computer-linked image analysis. *J Pathol* 1989; **158:** 303–310.

45. Editorial. *Gastrospirillum hominis*. *Lancet* 1989; **ii:** 252–253.

46. McNulty CAM, Dent JC, Curry A et al. New spiral bacterium in gastric mucosa. *J Clin Pathol* 1989; **42:** 585–591.

47. Uibo RM & Krohn KJE. Demonstration of gastrin cell auto-antibodies in antral gastritis with avidin–biotin complex antibody technique. *Clin Exp Immunol* 1984; **58:** 341–347.

48. Lambert R. Chronic gastritis. *Digestion* 1972; **7:** 83–126.

49. Correa P. Chronic gastritis (non-specific). In Whitehead R (ed.) *Gastrointestinal and Oesophageal Pathology*. New York: Churchill Livingstone, 1989: 402–420.

50. Wyatt JI & Dixon MF. Chronic gastritis – a pathogenetic approach. *J Pathol* 1988; **154:** 113–124.

51. Dixon MF, O'Connor HJ, Axon ATR, King RFJG & Johnston D. Reflux gastritis: distinct histopathological entity? *J Clin Pathol* 1986; **39:** 524–530.

52. Mosimann R, Loup P, Fontolliet C & Mosimann F. Post-operative reflux gastritis. Results of surgical treatment. *Scand J Gastroenterol* 1981; **16** (Suppl 67): 237–239.

53. Mosimann F, Sorgi M, Wolverson RL et al. Gastric histology and its relationship to enterogastric reflux after duodenal ulcer surgery. *Scand J Gastroenterol* 1984; **19** (Suppl 92): 142–144.

54. Mosimann F, Donovan IA, Thompson H, Fielding JWL, Harding LK & Alexander-Williams J. Screening procedure for identifying patients after gastric operations at high risk of developing premalignant histological changes. *World J Surg* 1985; **9:** 606–611.

55. O'Connor HJ, Wyatt JI, Dixon MF & Axon ATR. Campylobacter-like organisms and reflux gastritis. *J Clin Pathol* 1986; **39:** 531–534.

56. Emmanouilidis A, Nicolopoulou-Stamati P & Manousos O. The histological pattern of bile gastritis. *Gastrointest Endosc* 1984; **30:** 179–182.

57. Burbige EJ, French SW, Tarder G & Belber JP. Correlation between gross appearance and histologic findings in the post-operative stomach. *Gastrointest Endosc* 1979; **25:** 3–5.

58. Rubio CA & Slezak P. Foveolar cell vacuolisation in operated stomachs. *Am J Surg Pathol* 1988; **12:** 773–776.

59. Correa P. Multifocal environmental gastritis. In Whitehead R. (ed.) *Gastrointestinal and Oesophageal Pathology*. Edinburgh: Churchill Livingstone, 1989: 410–416.

60. Editorial. Campylobacters in Ottawa. *Lancet* 1985; **ii:** 135–136.

61. Sipponen P, Samloff IM, Saukkonen M & Varis K. Serum pepsinogens I and II and gastric mucosal histology after partial gastrectomy. *Gut* 1985; **26:** 1179–1182.

62. Ritchie WP. Alkaline reflux gastritis: a critical appraisal. *Gut* 1984; **25:** 975–987.

63. Haot J, Hamichi L, Wallez L & Mainguet P. Lymphocytic gastritis: a newly described entity: a retrospective endoscopic and histological study. *Gut* 1988; **29:** 1258–1264.

64. Haot J, Berger F, Andre C, Moulinier B, Mainguet P & Lambert R. Lymphocytic gastritis versus varioliform gastritis. A historical series revisited. *J Pathol* 1989; **158:** 19–22.

65. Dixon MF, Wyatt JI, Burke DA & Rathbone BJ. Lymphocytic gastritis – relationship to *Campylobacter pylori* infection. *J Pathol* 1988; **154:** 125–132.

66. Steer HW. The gastro-duodenal epithelium in peptic ulceration. *J Pathol* 1985; **146:** 355–362.

67. Lambert R, Andre C, Moulinier B & Bugnon B. Diffuse varioliform gastritis. *Digestion* 1978; **17:** 159–167.

68. Andre C, Gillon J, Moulinier B, Martin A & Fargier MC. Randomised placebo-controlled double blind trial of two dosages of sodium cromoglycate in treatment of varioliform gastritis: comparison with cimetidine. *Gut* 1982; **23:** 348–352.

69. Ozenc A, Ruacan S & Aran O. Gastritis cystic polyposa. *Arch Surg* 1988; **123:** 372–373.

70. Fonde EC & Rodning CB. Gastritis cystica profunda. *Am J Gastroenterol* 1986; **81:** 459–464.

71. Joske RA, Finckh ES & Wood IJ. Gastric biopsy. *Q J Med* 1955; **24:** 269–294.

72. Flejou JF, Bahame P, Smith AC, Stockbrugger RW, Rode J & Price AB. Pernicious anaemia and Campylobacter-like organisms: is the gastric antrum resistant to colonisation? *Gut*, 1989; **30:** 60–64.

73. Elsborg L, Andersen D, Myhre-Jensen O & Bastrup-Madsen P. Gastric mucosal polyps in pernicious anaemia. *Scand J Gastroenterol* 1977; **12:** 49–52.

74. Stockbrugger RW, Menon GG, Beilby JOW, Mason RR & Cotton PB. Gastroscopic screening in 80 patients with pernicious anaemia. *Gut* 1983; **24:** 1141–1147.

75. Levine JS & Allen RH. Intrinsic factor within parietal cells of patients with juvenile pernicious anaemia. A retrospective immunohistochemical study. *Gastroenterology* 1985; **88:** 1132–1136.

76. Tanaka M, Kimura K, Sakai H, Yoshida Y & Saito K. Long-term follow-up for minute gastro-duodenal lesions in Crohn's disease. *Gastrointest Endosc* 1986; **32:** 206–209.

77. Jouin H, Baumann R, Abbas A, Duclos B, Weill-bousson M & Weill JP. Upper digestive tract involvement is frequent in Crohn's disease. *Gastroenterol Clin Biol* 1986; **10:** 549–553.

78. Whitington PF & Whitington GL. Eosinophilic gastroenteropathy in childhood. *J Pediatr Gastroenterol Nutr* 1988; **7**: 379–385.
79. Blackshaw AJ & Levison AD. Eosinophilic infiltrates of the gastrointestinal tract. *J Clin Pathol* 1986; **39**: 1–7.
80. Lucas S. Eosinophilic gastroenteritis. *J Clin Pathol* 1986; **39**: 696 (letter).
81. Simson JNL. Hyperplastic gastropathy. *BMJ* 1985; **291**: 1298–1299.
82. Ming SC. Tumours of the oesophagus and stomach. *Washington DC: Armed Forces Institute of Pathology*, 1973; Fascicle 7, 115–119 and 153–154.
83. Lawson HH. Primary giant mucosal folds. *S Afr J Surg* 1975; **13**: 33–42.
84. Larson B, Tarp U & Kristensen E. Familial giant hypertrophic gastritis (Ménètrier's disease). *Gut* 1987; **28**: 1517–1521.
85. Garone MA, Winston BJ & Lewis JH. Cryptosporidiosis of the stomach. *Am J Gastroenterol* 1986; **81**: 465–470.
86. Balthazar EJ, Megibon AJ & Hulnick DH. Cytomegalovirus oesophagitis and gastritis in AIDS. *AJR* 1985; **144**: 1201–1204.
87. Cohen EB, Komorowski RA, Kauffman HM & Adams M. Unexpectedly high incidence of cytomegalovirus infection in apparent peptic ulcers in renal transplant recipients. *Surgery* 1985; **97**: 606–612.
88. Eidt S & Stolte M. Gastric glandular cysts – investigations into the genesis and relationship to colorectal epithelial tumours. *Z Gastroenterol* 1989; **27**: 212–217.
89. McCormack TT, Sims J, Eyre-Brook I et al. Gastric lesions in portal hypertension: inflammatory gastritis or congestive gastropathy? *Gut* 1985; **26**: 1226–1232.
90. Corbishley CM, Saverymuttu SH & Maxwell JD. Use of endoscopic biopsy for diagnosing congestive gastropathy. *J Clin Pathol* 1988; **41**: 1187–1190.
91. Foster FN, Wyatt JI, Bullimore DW & Losowsky MS. Gastric mucosa in patients with portal hypertension: prevalence of capillary dilatation and *Campylobacter pylori*. *J Clin Pathol* 1989; **42**: 919–921.
92. Al Nakib B. Duodenal erosions during cimetidine therapy. *Lancet* 1979; **i**: 607(letter).
93. Whitehead R, Roca M, Meikle DD, Skinner J & Truelove SC. The histological classification of duodenitis in fibreoptic biopsy specimens. *Digestion* 1975; **13**: 129–136.
94. Jenkins D, Goodall A, Gillet FR & Scott BB. Defining duodenitis: quantitative histological study of the mucosal responses and their correlations. *J Clin Pathol* 1985; **38**: 1119–1126.
95. Hasan M, Hay F, Sircus W & Ferguson A. Nature of the inflammatory cell infiltrate in duodenitis. *J Clin Pathol* 1983; **36**: 280–288.
96. Scott BB, Goodall A, Stephenson P & Jenkins D. Duodenal bulb plasma cells in duodenitis and duodenal ulceration. *Gut* 1985; **26**: 1032–1037.
97. Sircus W. Duodenitis: a clinical, endoscopic and histopathologic study. *Q J Med* 1985; **56**: 593–600.
98. Cheli R. Is duodenitis always a peptic disease. *Am J Gastroenterol* 1985; **80**: 442–444.
99. Carrick J, Lee A, Hazell S, Ralston M & Daskalopoulos G. *Campylobacter pylori*, duodenal ulcer and gastric metaplasia: possible role of functional heterotopic tissue in ulcerogenesis. *Gut*, 1989; **30**: 790–797.
100. Shousha S. Gastric metaplasia and *Campylobacter pylori* infection of duodenum in patients with chronic renal failure. *J Clin Pathol* **42**: 348–351.
101. Lessels AM & Martin DF. Heterotopic gastric mucosa in the duodenum. *J Clin Pathol* 1982; **35**: 591–595.
102. Pounder DJ, Ghadially FN, Mukherjee TM et al. Ultrastructure and electron probe X-ray analysis of the pigment in melanosis duodeni. *J Submicrosc Cytol* 1982; **14**: 389–400.
103. Kang JY, Wu AYT, Chia JLS, Wee A, Sutherland IH & Hori R. Clinical and ultrastructural studies in duodenal pseudomelanosis. *Gut* 1987; **28**: 1673–1681.
104. Yamase H, Norris M & Gillies C. Pseudomelanosis duodeni: a clinicopathologic entity. *Gastrointest Endosc* 1985; **31**: 83–86.
105. Vazquez-Iglesias JL, Yanez J, Durana J & Arnal F. Infection by *Mycobacterium avium intracellulare* in AIDS: endoscopic duodenal appearance mimicking Whipple's disease. *Endoscopy* 1988; **20**: 279–280.

26

PATHOLOGY OF GASTRIC AND DUODENAL ULCER

GY Saleh
RM Genta

Discontinuities in the mucosal lining of the gastrointestinal tract can be divided into *erosions* and *ulcers*. An erosion is a circumscribed superficial loss of mucosa that does not penetrate the muscularis mucosae. An ulcer, in contrast, consists of a circumscribed loss of substance that reaches into the muscularis mucosae and involves the submucosa and possibly deeper layers. These histological definitions, however, cannot be directly translated into nosological entities because erosions may evolve into ulcerations. Furthermore, endoscopic observation, an essential component in the description of many conditions, is often not capable of discriminating between an erosion and a shallow ulceration.[1]

This chapter reviews the pathological features of gastroduodenal erosions, peptic ulcer disease and ulcers associated with the use of non-steroidal anti-inflammatory drugs (NSAIDs). In addition there is an outline of the role of the pathological examination in the work-up of patients with gastroduodenal ulcers.

ACUTE EROSIONS AND ULCERS

Gastric erosions are acute lesions which may be associated with a wide variety of aetiopathogenetic mechanisms, including burns, trauma, sepsis, major surgery, NSAID administration, or excessive alcohol intake.[2-4] The common pathogenetic denominator of these clinical settings is believed to be reduced mucosal blood flow, which may be precipitated either by systemic hypotension (as in shock) or by local events triggered by interference with regulation of vascular mediators (such as in the case of NSAID ingestion). Ischaemia, in turn, results in a disruption of cytoprotective mechanisms leading to peptic/acid damage to the mucosa.[5]

Regardless of the aetiology, the macroscopic and histological appearance of erosions is similar: they are frequently multiple and involve preferentially the antrum, but they may be also found in the corpus. Individual lesions are usually smaller than 0.5 cm and endoscopically are well delineated, shallow and haemorrhagic. Microscopically, the surface epithelium is lost and replaced by a layer of fibrin mixed with polymorphonuclear cells and cellular debris (Figure 26.1, see colour plate also). The damage is limited to the mucosal epithelium, which includes the surface layer as well as the underlying glands. When the pathogenetic insult subsides, these lesions are repaired by simple re-epithelialization, without the formation of fibrosis or scar; thus, the *restitutio ad integrum* is complete.

In some circumstances, erosions may fail to heal and evolve into ulcers, with loss of tissue beyond the muscularis mucosae. Acute stress ulcers are usually multiple, measure more than 0.5 cm, and exhibit well-delineated craters of variable depth. In the ulcer bed there is usually fibrin mixed with an inflammatory exudate and necrotic debris; because these ulcers often bleed profusely, blood clots frequently fill the crater.[6] There is an abrupt transition between the necrotic edges of the ulcer and the adjacent mucosa. The surrounding mucosa may be

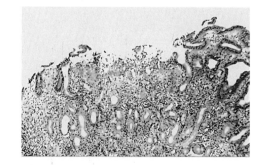

Figure 26.1

Antral erosion. The tissue loss is limited to the epithelium. There is a fibrinopurulent exudate in the area of the eroded surface. A mixed inflammatory infiltrate is visible in the lamina propria immediately subjacent to the erosion (haematoxylin and eosin, ×100).

entirely normal, unless the patient has previously existing chronic gastritis or duodenitis.

PEPTIC ULCER DISEASE

Peptic ulcers are chronic, most often solitary lesions that occur at any level of the gastrointestinal tract exposed to the action of acid–peptic juices. In descending order of frequency, ulcers occur in the duodenum, the stomach, the distal oesophageal mucosa, the margins of a gastrectomy and heterotopic gastric mucosa.[7] Approximately 98% of peptic ulcers occur in the stomach and duodenum, with a ratio of about 1:4.

Pathogenesis

Helicobacter pylori infection is the major cause of peptic ulcer not associated with the use of NSAIDs or with the Zollinger–Ellison syndrome.[8] This organism has been detected in the stomach of virtually all patients with duodenal ulcer and in more than 90% of gastric ulcer patients who were not NSAID users. Cure of *H. pylori* infection in these patients facilitates the cure of peptic ulcer and essentially prevents its recurrence, an event which occurs within 1 year in more than 80% of patients treated with acid-inhibiting therapy alone.[9]

Pathology

In the stomach the vast majority of peptic ulcers occur on the lesser curvature in the antrum, in an area close to the incisura angularis. Gastric ulcers occurring on the greater curvature and in other parts of the stomach, such as the fundus, are much more likely to be associated with chronic use of NSAIDs than with *H. pylori* gastritis. In the duodenum, peptic ulcers most commonly occur in the first part, either on the anterior or posterior walls.[1,6] When they occur at both sites simultaneously, they are known as kissing ulcers.

Peptic ulcers are usually sharply demarcated from the surrounding mucosa, which is generally slightly reddened, oedematous and elevated around the margins of the lesion. They are usually relatively small, measuring between 0.5 and 2.0 cm in diameter. Some patients have very large ulcers measuring more than 3.0 cm in diameter. Such ulcers have been defined as giant ulcers; the distinction is relevant because they may be misdiagnosed endoscopically as malignant.[10] The ulcer walls are perpendicular and limit a crater of variable depth, which may perforate the wall and penetrate into the adjacent structures, most commonly the pancreas. The base of the crater is grey–tan and may contain necrotic debris mixed with blood or appear clean, showing a white–grey rim of fibrous tissue. The mucosa surrounding ulcers appears grossly normal, unless an ulcer is complicated by extensive fibrosis. In the stomach, particularly in the antrum, rugal folds often appear to radiate from the ulcer crater. This feature, considered useful in differentiating benign ulcers from ulcerating malignant tumours, is either missing or greatly attenuated in benign gastric ulcer arising in an atrophic stomach.

Microscopically, the mucosa immediately surrounding the ulcer shows chronic active inflammation (Figure 26.2, see colour plate also). Regenerative changes with large cells

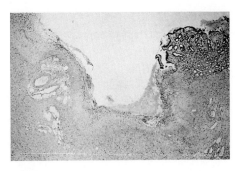

Figure 26.2
Peptic ulcer. The edges of the crater are sharply demarcated and the centre contains a small amount of fibrinopurulent exudate. There is a band of inflammatory infiltrate around the bed of the ulcer; in the lower portions fibrous tissue is beginning to form (haematoxylin and eosin, ×40).

exhibiting bizarre nuclei and frequent mitoses are so widespread that, when small samples of such areas are examined in biopsy specimens, the histological diagnosis of dysplasia or even cancer is occasionally entertained (Figure 26.3, see colour plate also). However, in regeneration there is usually evidence of surface maturation, mitotic activity is confined to the deeper foveolar regions, and nuclei have more even chromatin, thin nuclear membrane and are more uniform in appearance.[11] In contrast, the appearance of dysplasia is essentially that of an adenoma, with marked cytological abnormalities, hyperchromatic enlarged nuclei, loss of surface maturation and cytoplasmic basophilia due to mucin depletion. These distinctions, however, can be treacherous and, quite appropriately, an old pathologists' adage warns: 'never diagnose cancer within three glands from an ulcer'. Underneath the regenerative epithelium there is granulation tissue with a prominent mixed cellular infiltrate. More centrally, there is an area of necrosis with inflammatory cells, fibrin, debris and sometimes micro-organisms; this represents the active ulcer, i.e. the area of gastric or duodenal wall that is actually being destroyed. Fibrosis, the result of healing of the ulcer at its edges, forms a rim extending from around the crater to beneath the epithelium into the

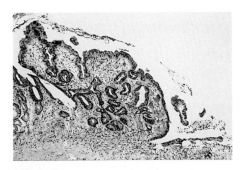

Figure 26.3
High-power photomicrograph of an edge of the ulcer depicted in Figure 26.2. The epithelial cells adjacent to the necrotic border show regenerative activity (large nuclei and increased nucleus : cytoplasm ratio). In contrast to dysplastic or neoplastic cells, however, they remain arranged in an orderly fashion and the nuclear chromatin is fine (haematoxylin and eosin, ×100).

surrounding connective and muscular tissues. Depending on the age of the ulcer and the number of previous recurrences, the fibrous component may be small enough to escape detection in the examination of an endoscopic biopsy specimen, or large and hard enough to mimic the gross appearance and the consistency of a malignant tumour. A lymphoid infiltrate, often arranged in lymphoid fol-licles, is usually found around the ulcer edges; rarely, the infiltrate may be so severe as to mimic malignant lymphoma of the stomach.[12] Below the necrotic base of an ulcer, vessels show prominent inflammation and some degree of arteritis obliterans is often found. When disrupted by the ulcerative process, these arteries bleed into the ulcer, and the magnitude of the haemorrhage depends of the size of the damaged vessels.

Duodenal ulcers are usually accompanied by duodenitis and gastric metaplasia of the duodenal surface epithelium. This is characterized by the replacement of enterocytes and goblet cells by tall columnar cells containing apical mucin of the gastric (neutral) type. These patches of metaplastic epithelium, the extent of which appears to be directly proportional to the degree of hyperacidity, are often colonized by H. pylori and exhibit the same type of surface cell disruption seen in the stomach. It has been postulated that this damage to the metaplastic duodenal epithelium is the mechanism that initiates the appearance of a peptic ulcer in the duodenum.[8]

Complications

The most common complications of peptic ulcer disease in order of frequency are haemorrhage, penetration with or without perforation and obstruction. Approximately one-third of patients experience one of these complications at some point during the course of their disease; ulcers most commonly associated with complications are those located in the pyloric channel and in the postbulbar duodenum. Bleeding occurs when an ulcer erodes into a vessel. Perforation results when the ulcer erodes through the serosa of the viscus. The search for perforation in a resected stomach or duodenum often requires careful handling and examination of the ulcer. The actual perforation may be barely visible and is often obscured by the presence of coagulated blood, fibrin and other debris.[13,14] Examination of the serosa in the vicinity of the ulcer will invariably reveal severe acute inflammation.

An ulcer may burrow in an area where the stomach or the duodenum are in intimate contact with a solid organ such as pancreas or liver. In such cases, the ulcer continues its penetration beyond the wall of the viscus and invades the parenchyma of the organ, where it usually elicits a dramatic inflammatory response, followed by fibrous build-up that clinically and radiographically may mimic a tumour. The examination of such specimens is often complicated because it is rarely possible to separate the portion of gastrointestinal tract from the penetrated organ, to which it becomes fused into a hard fibrous mass. Rarely, the perforation occurs in the vicinity of another hollow structure, like a small intestinal loop, the transverse colon or the gall bladder, followed by formation of a fistula. Gastric outlet obstruction is the clinical syndrome resulting from the distortion

and narrowing of the pyloric area caused by fibrosis, oedema or smooth muscle spasm. It occurs almost exclusively in patients with a long-standing peptic ulcer of the pyloric channel or the duodenum. Surgical repair or various techniques of pyloric dilatation are often necessary because medical management of the obstruction is usually unsuccessful.[15]

OTHER CAUSES OF ULCERS

Both benign and malignant tumours may produce gastric mucosal ulcerations. Ulcers originating on gastric or duodenal stromal tumours are readily recognized because they are usually located on a mass protruding into the gastric cavity or the duodenal lumen.

Malignant ulcers originate most often in adenocarcinomas.[16] They are usually solitary, their shape may be irregular and their edges are frequently heaped up. Ulcers associated with malignant lymphomas are often flat or only slightly elevated, multiple and may attain a very large size (up to 10–12 cm in diameter).[17]

Immunocompetent patients rarely develop infectious ulcers. However, in immunocompromised subjects cytomegalovirus and, rarely, histoplasmosis may cause gastric ulcers. In these patients, duodenal ulcers and erosions may be due to cytomegalovirus, histoplasmosis, cryptosporidiosis and infection with *Mycobacterium avium intracellulare*.[18]

ROLE OF THE PATHOLOGIST IN THE EVALUATION OF GASTRODUODENAL ULCER

The pathological evaluation of gastroduodenal ulcers may involve the examination of biopsy or resection specimens. Biopsies are generally obtained to determine the aetiology of the ulcer. Most commonly this involves excluding malignancy (carcinoma or lymphoma), but occasionally the question of an infectious aetiology is raised. To ensure optimal yield from the histological examination, it is recommended that between four and eight adequate biopsy specimens be obtained from the margins of the ulcer. Except for one representative specimen from the base of the ulcer (which may be useful for detecting infectious organisms), necrotic areas should be avoided. Furthermore, sampling from the apparently intact gastric mucosa (in both gastric and duodenal ulcer) is imperative to demonstrate H. pylori because this organism is difficult to visualize in the immediate vicinity of ulcers. It is further recommended that large forceps be used whenever possible, that each biopsy be placed in a separate formalin container, and that an attempt be made at accurate on-edge orientation on the processed specimens in the histopathological laboratory rather than on the fresh biopsies.

Specimens resected for the treatment of duodenal ulcers usually consist of a portion of the gastric antrum and segments of the vagus nerves. Since the pathology requisition form often states 'bleeding ulcer', or simply 'ulcer', the examining pathologist may be mystified by the absence of an ulcer in the specimen. To avoid confusion and unnecessary delays in the diagnosis, pathologists should be fully informed about the nature of these specimens. When a segment of the stomach is resected for a gastric ulcer, the question of malignancy often arises and frozen section consultation is frequently requested. Adequate sampling of the margins is necessary to establish the benign or malignant nature of the ulcer. Following these guidelines will maximize the contribution of pathology to the diagnosis and management of these patients.

REFERENCES

1. Graham DY. Peptic diseases of the stomach and duodenum. In Sivak MV Jr (ed.) *Gastroenterologic Endoscopy.* Philadelphia: WB Saunders, 1987: 431–453.
2. Chamberlain CE. Acute hemorrhagic gastritis. *Gastroenterol Clin North Am* 1993; **22:** 843–873.
3. Brown TH, Davidson PF & Larson GM. Acute gastritis occurring within 24 hours of severe head injury. *Gastrointest Endosc* 1989; **35:** 37–40.
4. Allison MC, Howatson AG, Torrance C et al. Gastrointestinal damage associated with the use of non-steroidal anti-inflammatory drugs. *N Engl J Med* 1992; **327:** 749–754.
5. Silen W. Gastric mucosal defense and repair. In Johnson LR (ed.) *Physiology of the Gastrointestinal Tract,* 2nd edn. New York: Raven Press, 1987: 1055–1069.
6. Goldman H. Stress ulcer and chronic peptic ulcer disease. In Ming SC & Goldman H (eds) *Pathology of the Gastrointestinal Tract.* Philadelphia: WB Saunders, 1992: 517–536.
7. Grossman MI. Peptic ulcer: definition and epidemiology. In Rotter J, Samloff IM & Rimoin DL (eds) *The Genetics and Heterogeneity of Common Gastrointestinal Disorders.* New York; Academic Press, 1980: 19–29.
8. Dixon M. Acid, ulcers, and *H. pylori. Lancet* 1993; **342:** 384–385.
9. Graham DY. Treatment of peptic ulcers caused by *Helicobacter pylori. N Engl J Med* 1993; **328:** 349–350.
10. Lumsden K, MacLarnon JC & Dawson J. Giant duodenal ulcer. *Gut* 1970; **1:** 592–599.
11. Lechago J. Histopathology of peptic ulcer. In Brooks FP, Cohen S & Soloway RD (eds.) *Peptic Ulcer Disease.* New York: Churchill Livingstone, 1985: 31–44.
12. Genta RM, Hamner HW & Graham DY. Gastric lymphoid follicles in *Helicobacter pylori* infection: frequency, distribution, and response to triple therapy. *Hum Pathol* 1993; **24:** 577–583.
13. Kozoll DD & Meyer KA. Symptoms and signs in the prognosis of gastroduodenal ulcers. An analysis of 1904 cases of acute perforated gastroduodenal ulcers. *Arch Surg* 1961; **82:** 528–539.
14. Norris JR & Hubrich WS. The incidence and clinical features of penetration in peptic ulceration. *JAMA* 1961; **178:** 386–390.
15. Graham DY. Ulcer complications and their nonoperative treatment. In Sleisenger MH & Fordtran JS (eds.) *Gastrointestinal Disease,* 5th edn. Philadelphia: WB Saunders, 1993: 698–712.
16. Correa P. Pathology of gastric cancer. *Clin Oncol* 1984; **3:** 251–257.
17. Brooks JJ & Enterline HT. Primary gastric lymphoma. A clinicopathologic study of 58 cases with long-term follow-up and literature review. *Cancer* 1983; **51:** 701–711.
18. Goodgame RW, Genta RM, Go MF & Graham DY. Infectious gastritis. In Surawicz C & Owen RL (eds) *Gastrointestinal and Hepatic Infections.* Philadelphia: WB Saunders, 1994: 47–72.

27

EPIDEMIOLOGY OF PEPTIC ULCERATION

DG Maxton
JP Miller

Epidemiology is the study of the distribution and determinants of disease and injury in human populations. There are therefore two aspects, one descriptive identifying populations with high and low frequencies of a particular disease and the other analytical which attempts to determine the reason for the unequal distribution. In the case of peptic ulcer disease, the hope is that epidemiological studies will lead to clues to the cause of the condition.[1] This approach implies that information obtained from population studies applies to individuals within that and other populations. This assumption may not be valid in a disease, such as peptic ulceration, where the same clinical syndrome may have different aetiological factors in different individuals. The reasons for a particular person within a group developing a peptic ulcer are probably complex and include genetic, environmental and psychological factors. However, epidemiological studies may be able to identify important determinants leading to increased frequency within groups if not in individuals. The difficulties are compounded for peptic ulceration because background incidence over time, environmental factors, diagnostic accuracy and treatments which alter the natural history of the disorder may all be changing simultaneously. As a result, valid comparisons of studies performed at different times or places may not be possible.

It is difficult to determine the incidence and prevalence of peptic ulceration in large populations.[2] The main measures of disease frequency used are (1) mortality rates, (2) post-mortem studies, (3) complication rates particularly ulcer perforation, (4) hospital admission or diagnosis rates, (4) general practitioner or primary care referrals, (5) self-reported disease frequency, (6) questionnaire and interview surveys, often a combination of case finding and hospital referral in small or closed communities and (7) case-control studies. All these methods have their limitations. Mortality rates based on death certification may be inaccurate and more importantly may not reflect ulcer frequency in the overall population in a chronic disease from which relatively few people die. Mortality studies have been criticized as being as much a measure of the age distribution of the population with ulcer and the quality of medical care as of ulcer incidence.[3] Data can be corrected for the age distribution of the at-risk population but quality of health care is more difficult to assess.

Post-mortem studies are also probably not representative of the overall population but of a selected group of hospital patients with a bias towards the specialist interest of the staff of the institution involved. In retrospective post-mortem studies involving multiple pathologists it is difficult to ascertain how assiduously evidence of peptic ulceration was sought, whereas in prospective studies overreporting may occur especially with respect to gastric or duodenal scarring. A potential advantage claimed for such studies is that a combination of active ulceration and scarring might reflect life-time prevalence. This supposes that all active ulcers heal to leave discernible scars which is probably incorrect.

Statistics of ulcer perforation may be more secure and therefore offer a better measure of overall ulcer frequency. Most patients with this complication are treated surgically in hospital. Although a number do die unreported at home, if this proportion remained constant comparisons over time would still be accurate. However, only a minority of ulcer patients suffer this complication. This proportion is claimed to be fixed relative to the total ulcer population[4] but this is largely an assumption since the size of the total ulcer population is unknown. Reported perforation rates vary from 6 to 11%,[3,5-7] and perforation may be becoming more frequent, especially in elderly women.[8] Nevertheless data on ulcer perforation, especially before 1950, remain an important source of information. Bleeding is less reliable as the cause may not be peptic ulceration, although in more recent studies only cases with ulceration confirmed by endoscopy are usually included.

Hospital admission rates for peptic ulceration are well

documented especially in Western countries. Not all countries, however, provide comprehensive health care facilities to the entire population and admission statistics may not reflect the situation in the community. Few data sources of this type can distinguish 'new' from 'old' ulcer cases or even re-admission of the same patient. Further, some studies sample only a proportion of admissions, often 10%. Hospital admission data are also prone to change with trends in medical treatment, particularly for uncomplicated ulceration. Thus, before the advent of effective drug therapy, it was common to admit ulcer patients for a 'milk drip' regimen and bed rest. A fall in admissions may not, therefore reflect decreased ulcer frequency but rather the demise of this form of therapy.

General practitioner (or Office) and self-reported studies of illness or work absence are often available from Government Social Security files. However, it is often impossible to decide from these sources how secure the diagnosis of peptic ulcer is, as the level of investigation is unknown. Dyspepsia is a non-specific complaint and patients with typical symptoms may not necessarily have an ulcer. Questionnaire and community survey data must carry the same qualification. Case-control studies are used particularly to investigate environmental factors in the pathogenesis of peptic ulcer. However, few studies control for more than age, sex, smoking and possibly socioeconomic grouping. In a disease where environmental factors may be multiple more sophisticated control data and larger groups may be necessary.

Major changes have occurred in the procedures available for the diagnosis of peptic ulceration in the last 40 years. Before routine radiological examination with barium meal, duodenal and gastric ulceration could not be distinguished outside surgical or post-mortem studies. With barium meal, examination of the duodenum can be difficult and discrimination between active ulceration and scarring or evidence of past inflammation is unreliable. The introduction of upper gastrointestinal endoscopy has allowed much more accurate diagnosis of significant disease, both acute ulcers and scarring, in both stomach and duodenum but comparisons between studies using different techniques may not be valid. Neither technique is suitable for epidemiological assessment of large populations.

Environmental factors probably play a large part in the pathogenesis of peptic ulcer and in its variable frequency. These temporal and geographical fluctuations should facilitate identification of causative factors. However, few would disagree that the last 150 years have produced and are still producing marked changes in the environment, working practices, social habits and diet. Against this changing social background it is difficult to define a fixed base for comparison. A complicating factor is the tendency of possible environmental factors to interact and vary together. Thus smoking, alcohol use, hygiene levels, diet, occupation and low socioeconomic status, all putative factors in the pathogenesis of peptic ulcer, may all be correlated with each other. It is the aim of the epidemiologist to tease apart these separate factors, within the clear limitations of the study design and data sets available.

DEFINITIONS, ANATOMY AND PATHOLOGY

Peptic ulcers arise in mucosa which is bathed in gastric juice, usually containing hydrochloric acid and pepsin. Typically the ulcers are either gastric (between the cardia and the pylorus) or duodenal (usually in the duodenal bulb). Ulcers may occur at other sites, however, including the lower oesophagus, the postbulbar duodenum (commonly in hypersecretory states), the jejunum (in relation to gastroenterostomy stomas), and in Meckel's diverticulum when acid-secreting heterotopic gastric mucosa is present. All epidemiological studies refer to the common gastric and duodenal ulceration.

An ulcer is a break in the gastrointestinal epithelium and underlying mucosa deep enough to breach the muscularis muscosae. It may be round, oval or linear. Erosions are generally smaller and more superficial leaving the muscularis mucosae intact. The distinction between a small superficial ulcer and an erosion may not be easy at endoscopy. It is widely assumed that an erosion must be a necessary stage in the development and healing of an ulcer. This need only be so if all ulcers begin with a breach in the epithelium rather than damage to deeper layers of the mucosa. There is little doubt that many erosions heal without ever becoming ulcers.

HISTORICAL TRENDS IN ULCER DISEASE

Numerous authors have pointed out that there have been dramatic changes in the characteristics of peptic ulceration over the last 150 years.[9-13] The traditional view is that in the latter half of the nineteenth century, peptic ulceration was a relatively rare disorder of the stomach in young women, commonly around 20–25 years old. These cases were usually of acute gastric ulcers near the cardia and were diagnosed at post-mortem having caused death usually from perforation. The available data up to 1940 have been reviewed by Ivy[14] and Jennings.[15] Both point out that before 1900 duodenal ulcer was comparatively rare compared with gastric ulcer. By the first quarter of the twentieth century post-mortem data suggested that duodenal and gastric ulcer incidence had reached approximate parity.[14] However, other contemporary investigators reported that duodenal ulcer was being seen in clinical practice much more frequently than gastric ulcer, with ratios of between 14:1 and 5:1 for duodenal:gastric ulcer quoted.[14] At the same time, peptic ulceration was also becoming a disease of men rather than women, a male to female ratio of 4:1 being recorded.[14,15]

Ulcer perforation rates continued to increase in the first half of this century reaching a peak in the 1950s in the UK.[3] A similar trend was reported from Scandinavia and Germany. Data from insurance companies, the Army and general practitioners confirmed a reducing frequency of cases of ulceration, both complicated and uncomplicated, after 1950.[3,16-18] Doll[19] also noted a reduction in British mortality from gastric ulcer during the 1950s. Other European countries did not always show the same trends. In Switzerland, for example, age-adjusted death rates from gastric ulcer showed a progressive fall between 1921 and 1980 in both men and women.[20] In contrast mortality rates from duodenal ulcer rose during the same period.[20]

Data have been much more plentiful in the last 40 years. It is widely believed that the frequency of peptic ulcer has declined during this period, at least in Western Europe and the USA. Thus in the USA between 1962 and 1978 gastric and duodenal ulcer mortality rates decreased by 58 and 68%, respectively.[21] National figures from the USA also recorded a fall of around 30% in peptic ulcer hospitalization rates during the 1970s.[21-24] The fall was proportionally more for duodenal ulcer than gastric ulcer with one study claiming that admissions for gastric ulcer had not changed significantly over that time.[22] Most of the decline occurred in uncomplicated cases which might reflect altered treatment practices rather than prevalence.

Further evidence that the changes in ulcer frequency are genuine comes from the decline in peptic ulcer surgery. Elective surgery for uncomplicated peptic ulceration at the Mayo Clinic fell from 49/100 000 population per year in 1956–1960 to 6/100 000 in 1982–1985.[25] The decline was greatest in men with duodenal ulcer. Interestingly, the incidence of emergency operations remained constant at 10/100 000 per year.[25] This observation is difficult to explain as the criteria for elective operation were claimed not to have changed significantly over the study period. It is possible that the presentation of peptic ulcer disease altered with complicated disease representing a greater proportion of cases. A similar surgical study from Seattle conducted between 1966 and 1975 also noted a decline in elective surgery for duodenal ulcer and in surgery for duodenal ulcer perforation.[26] The results of neither of these studies could be explained by a change in population, or surgical or medical treatment practice.

American office records confirm a trend for reduced consultation rates for peptic ulceration.[27,28] The decline was most marked in men with duodenal ulcer declining from 43.0/1000 in 1958–1960 to 9.3/1000 in 1981–1984.[28] Consultation rates declined in women with duodenal ulcer from 19.9/1000 to 7.5/1000 over the same period. In contrast, only a modest fall in physician visits for gastric ulcer was observed in men and in women the rates rose.[28] Cimetidine therapy was introduced into the US in late 1977 and may have speeded the later decline in consultation rates but the overall trends were observed before this date.

Broadly similar trends to those observed in the USA have been seen in Great Britain.[29] Hospital admissions for peptic ulcer in England and Wales fell between 1958 and 1977.[30] The observation was also recorded in Scotland as continuing between 1975 and 1990.[31] This was true for both perforated and non-perforated gastric and duodenal ulcers. The trend tended to be greater for gastric than duodenal ulcers and was most apparent in those aged under 45 years. The principal exception was elderly women in whom a 145% rise in perforated duodenal ulcer occurred between 1958 and 1982.[8] In comparison perforated gastric ulcers were only 20% more common over the same period. Comparable data from Scotland, however, showed a doubling of perforated gastric and duodenal in women aged over 65.[8,31] The perforation rates in those over 75 may be even higher. Further evidence of the decline in duodenal ulcer cases comes from doctors themselves. Claims by doctors for medical sickness benefit under this diagnosis declined steadily between 1947 and 1965.[17]

Some of these time trends have been seen in other areas of the world. Swedish surgical data confirm a marked fall in elective surgical procedures between 1956 and 1986, with a 50% drop in emergency operations.[32] The increased incidence of gastric ulcer in elderly women has been confirmed in New Zealand and Germany.[33,34] However, in Copenhagen, Denmark between 1963 and 1968 the annual incidence of both gastric and duodenal ulcer did not vary significantly nor did the perforation rate.[35] In contrast, in northern Norway the last 40 years have seen an increasing incidence of peptic ulcer.[36]

Reports from outside Western Europe and North America show markedly differing trends. In Japan, although a 'Westernized Country' the incidence of gastric ulcer exceeds that of duodenal ulcer in most of the country.[37] Age-adjusted death rates for both types of ulcer have been declining slowly over the last 30 years but the point prevalence rates appear to be stable over the 10 years from 1974 to 1983.[37] Possibly of more interest are the relatively scanty data from the developing world or less-industralized countries. Duodenal ulcer is rare in the rural black population of South Africa.[38,39] However, although ulcer rates have been declining in the West an increasing number of urban black South Africans in Johannesburg have been admitted with duodenal ulcer.[39] The incidence also seems to be rising in young black Zimbabweans.[40] Similarly, during 1970–1980 peptic ulcer admissions and perforations increased in Hong Kong by 21 and 71%, respectively, the trends being most significant for duodenal ulcer.[41] These latter findings cannot be explained by changes in population or altered medical practice.

It seems certain, therefore, that the pattern of peptic ulceration has changed very significantly over the last 100 years in Western Europe and North America. For example, it has been calculated that perforated gastric ulcers in young men now occur with between a quarter and a tenth of their previous frequency.[30] However, an explanation for the large rise in the incidence of duodenal ulceration, especially in men, over the first half of the twentieth century, and its subsequent wane is required. The most plausible hypothesis was suggested by Susser and Stein,[42] who believe that the data are consistent with a 'cohort' or 'generation' effect. Thus individuals would acquire their risk of ulcer disease at a relatively early age and this would persist for life. In other words an individual's risk of developing ulcer disease would relate to the year of birth rather than age. Generations born between 1870 and 1900 are suggested to be at increased risk of peptic ulceration for whatever reason.[43-45]

The cohort phenomenon is apparent in ulcer mortality data for both gastric and duodenal ulcer from England and Wales and from several other European Countries.[43,44] The effect was further confirmed in the mortality data for gastric ulcer in men and women from West Germany, Italy, Scotland, Denmark, France, Spain, the Republic of Ireland, Switzerland and the Netherlands.[20,43] Similar trends are probably apparent in data from 11 other European Countries. Superimposed on the cohort phenomenon for men with gastric and duodenal ulceration in Italy and the Netherlands was a period effect in which death rates increased in all age groups between 1941 and

Table 27.1 Incidence of duodenal ulcer

AUTHOR(S)	DATE	CASES/1000 PER YEAR		LOCATION	TYPE OF STUDY	PERIOD
		MEN	WOMEN			
Pulvertaft[5]	1959	2.15	0.62	York, UK	Hospital referrals (+ autopsy)	1952–1957
Litton and Murdoch[48]	1963	5.42	1.28	South-west Scotland	Hospital referrals	1957–1959
Dunlop[49]	1968	4.28	1.26	Central Scotland	Hospital referrals	1962
Monson and MacMahon[50]	1969	2.89	1.50	Massachusetts	Postal survey	–
Bonnevie[51]	1975	1.83	0.84	Copenhagen, Denmark	Hospital referrals	1963–1968
Hugh et al.[52]	1984	3.8	3.8	Australia	Health statistics	1981
Kaier et al.[53]	1985	3.1	1.5	Faroe Islands	Hospital survey	1981–1983

1950.[43] The hypothesis is further supported by data from Harvard graduates in the USA showing an increased risk of gastric ulcer for those born around 1855 and of duodenal ulcer for those born around 1885.[45]

The factors producing these cohort effects are unknown. The changes are unlikely to result from changes in clinical management or diagnostic coding which would affect all age groups at the same time. The changes are too rapid to be explained by genetic factors and environmental factors appear likely. One possibility is the rate of infection with the bacterium *Helicobacter pylori*. This does not mean, however, that other environmental influences cannot be a superimposed on the background cohort effect. Thus the increased frequency of ulcer perforation observed recently in elderly women may be due to a new factor possibly non-steroidal anti-inflammatory drugs (NSAIDs).

The importance of the time trends and cohort effect in peptic ulcer is that they will influence all epidemiological studies of the disease. Thus differences in incidence rates, sex ratios and age characteristics of patients with peptic ulcer determined at different times or places may not be readily interpretable. Any postulated environmental factor or factors should preferably explain these trends.

INCIDENCE AND PREVALENCE

Ulcer frequency can be defined in terms of incidence, that is the number of new cases of ulcer during a study period, or prevalence, the proportion of subjects in a given population with an ulcer at a particular time. Prevalence can further be divided into disease frequency in a population at a specific

point in time (point prevalence) and that over a specified time (period prevalence). One year and lifetime prevalence are examples of period prevalence rates. Particular characteristics of the natural history of ulcer disease mean that measures of both incidence and prevalence should be used cautiously. Peptic ulcer is a relapsing and remitting disease. Incidence rates reported in the literature may have more to do with when the ulcer was first diagnosed and therefore reflect local diagnostic facilities or case finding than when the ulcer first occurred in any individual. Some studies use the history of onset of first symptoms to offset this factor but patient memories prove fallible when checked against medical records.[46]

Prevalence rates will be affected not only by the frequency of disease, but also its duration. Thus if a given number of individuals suffer from peptic ulcer but for longer, the period prevalence for active disease over a short time will increase. Another consideration pertinent to both measures is the frequency of silent or asymptomatic ulceration.[47] Such ulcers may remain undetected in all except post-mortem studies, unless individuals without symptoms are investigated. All these factors, in addition to the influence of background trends, age structure of the population under investigation and the limitations of trial methodology, need to be taken into consideration when interpreting data on ulcer frequency.

Annual incidence

Tables 27.1 and 27.2 show the annual incidence of duodenal and gastric ulcer from a selection of studies in the western world over the last 40 years. About 2–3 men/1000 per year develop a duodenal ulcer and a third to a half that number of

Table 27.2 Incidence of gastric ulcer

AUTHOR(S)	DATE	CASES/1000 PER YEAR		LOCATION	TYPE OF STUDY	PERIOD
		MEN	WOMEN			
Pulvertaft[5]	1959	0.53	0.31	York, UK	Hospital referrals (+ autopsy)	1952–1957
Litton and Murdoch[48]	1963	0.55	0.32	South-west Scotland	Hospital referrals	1957–1959
Dunlop[49]	1968	0.61	0.28	Central Scotland	Hospital referrals	1962
Monson and MacMahon[50]	1969	0.35	—	Massachusetts	Postal survey	—
Bonnevie[35]	1975	0.33	0.30	Copenhagen, Denmark	Hospital referrals	1963–1968
Hugh et al.[52]	1984	0.7	0.7	Australia	Health statistics	1981
Kaier et al.[53]	1985	1.3	0.7	Faroe Islands	Hospital survey	1981–1983

women. Gastric ulcer is less common, with 0.5 men/1000 per year afflicted and rather less women. Prepyloric ulcer was about half as common as that in the body and fundus of the stomach.[54] Up to 20–30% of patients with gastric ulcer are reported to have a duodenal ulcer as well.[54,55] For example, in Copenhagen the annual incidence for gastric ulcer alone was 0.31/1000 but 0.44/1000 if patients with both duodenal and gastric ulcer were included.[51] Clearly these figures are only population averages and the incidence of ulceration will vary with age and time.

Prevalence

Based on National Health Interview Survey data, the 1-year period prevalence of self-reported peptic ulcer in the USA was 1.7–1.9% between 1961 and 1981.[11] However, it has been argued that the best measure of prevalence of peptic ulcer is the rate in subjects having autopsies for an unrelated cause of death. On this criterion point prevalence rates for active peptic ulceration, both gastric and duodenal, were 4.3% for men and 1.8% for women in Leeds between 1930 and 1949.[56] A similar Dutch study, however, found incidental chronic gastric ulcers in 5.5% and 4.3% of men and women, respectively.[57] The comparable figures for duodenal ulcer were higher at 7.9% and 4.5%.[57] However, it may not be valid to exclude deaths from peptic ulcer from the statistics. In addition the patients coming to hospital post-mortem may not represent the community at large and in particular are likely to be biased towards an older age group.

Few studies have thoroughly investigated asymptomatic patients to attempt a true point prevalence. However, Ihamaki et al.[58] studied 358 control individuals in Finland as part of an endoscopic study of gastric mucosa in families with gastric carcinoma. There was a point prevalence for duodenal ulcer of 14/1000 and 3/1000 for gastric ulcer. In Japan a radiological screening service of industrial employees reported an overall prevalence for gastric ulcer of 1.4% and 0.8% for duodenal ulcer.[59] However, the population screened were bank and industrial employees and therefore unlikely to be representative of the community as a whole. A more recent prevalence study offered endoscopy to subjects with dyspepsia and to healthy matched controls in a small community (2027 eligible individuals) in north Norway. The point prevalence was 1.8% for both gastric and duodenal ulcer in men and 1.4% for gastric and 2.9% for duodenal in women in those with symptoms.[60] Added to this was a further substantial 0.6% prevalence of asymptomatic peptic ulceration in men and 1.4% in women.

Lifetime prevalence

It is frequently stated that 10% of individuals will suffer from peptic ulceration during the course of their lifetime. Relatively few populations have been studied, however, and the situation may well vary in different races, environments and particularly in studies performed at different times. Moreover, figures collected in middle-aged living individuals can only increase as they continue to age. Thus in male Massachusetts physicians self-reported lifetime prevalence rates for duodenal ulcer rose

progressively with age from 3.3% in 25–34 year olds to 11.7% in those over 75 years.[50] Figures for gastric ulcer also increased from 0.22% at 25–34 years to reach a maximum of 2.7% in those aged 65–74 years. On the assumption that few will develop new ulcers when aged over 75, this suggests a lifetime prevalence for peptic ulceration of around 14% for men in this socioeconomic group. Clearly this self-reported study could not take into account asymptomatic ulcers. The same criticism could be levelled at the survey of 41 457 randomly selected adults in the US in 1989.[61] Although 10% reported that a physician had diagnosed peptic ulcer disease diagnostic method must vary. Some individuals will subsequently develop ulcer disease.

Ihamaki et al.[58] did endoscope asymptomatic individuals in his study of gastric cancer families. Lifetime prevalence combining both sexes for peptic ulceration as a whole was estimated to be 5.9% based on the presence of an active peptic ulcer, a scarred stomach or duodenum or a history of ulcer surgery.[58] These data must be treated with caution as numbers were very small. For example, only one active gastric and five active duodenal ulcers were found in the entire study group. In addition the figure obtained is almost certainly an underestimate of lifetime prevalence as the mean patient age was only 46 years and prolonged follow-up could only lead to an increase. Bernersen and colleagues[60] in Sorreisa, northern Norway estimated the lifetime prevalence of symptomatic peptic ulceration to be 6.2% in men and 2.7% in women with a ratio of duodenal:gastric ulceration of 3.2:1 and 1.3:1 for men and women, respectively.

Post-mortem studies have the potential to provide information about the cumulative frequency of chronic peptic ulceration because scarring from previous ulceration may be detected as well as active disease and evidence of ulcer surgery. In young people, however, peptic ulcer is rarely fatal and it may not be safe to assume that the proportion of ulcers and scars in patients coming to post-mortem is the same as that in the remainder of the population. Moreover, ulcers may heal without apparent scarring so post-mortem studies may underestimate the proportion of people who have at some time had ulcer disease. Generally, however, post-mortem studies have shown higher lifetime prevalences than clinical studies.

Watkinson[56] reported in 1960 the results of two post-mortem studies. One was very carefully performed in Leeds, England between 1930 and 1949 by a single pathologist, Professor Matthew Stewart, and covered 88% of the hospital deaths (more than 13 000 examinations) over that period. An overall incidence of ulceration in men of 21.1% was recorded, 9.9% chronic active ulcers, 8.5% chronic inactive ulcer or scarring (including previous ulcer surgery) and 2.7% acute ulceration.[56] Corresponding figures for women were a total of 11% with peptic disease with 3.4% active, 6.2% inactive and 2.2% acute ulceration. The acute group is small but may represent a terminal event immediately preceding death rather than a predisposition to peptic ulcer during life. In this survey 11.6% of men had evidence of duodenal ulcer either currently or at some previous time and 3.9% evidence of gastric ulcer. Women had a lower lifetime prevalence, 4.8% for duodenal ulcer and 2.8% for gastric ulcer. A small number had both ulcer types and figures include ulcer related deaths but exclude acute lesions.

Watkinson[56] also gives details of a similar study conducted nationally at 18 separate locations in the UK. Figures are somewhat lower with a lifetime prevalence of peptic ulcer of 15.2% in men and 9.7% in women. Evidence of duodenal ulcer was found in only 5.3% of men nationally rather than the 11.6% recorded in Leeds, when corrected for the differing age profile. However, gastric ulcer prevalence was similar. The differences between these studies may be partly the result of alterations in disease incidence over the time between the dates of each investigation but most probably also reflects the care taken to inspect the specimens for scarring.

A Dutch study reported an overall incidence of peptic ulceration at post-mortem, reflecting lifetime prevalence, at 24.3% between 1940 and 1959.[57] Undoubtedly, some of the findings represented acute terminal erosions. Nevertheless, excluding ulcer related deaths, 17.6% of men and 10.0% of women had evidence of chronic peptic ulceration. In Malmo, Sweden an impressive 88% of all, not just hospital, deaths came to post-mortem during the year 1969.[62] Total frequency of peptic ulcer disease was 17.9%, 20.9% in men and 14.7% in women. In this region gastric ulcer as evidenced by active lesions and scars was more common than duodenal ulcer, occurring in 10.7% and 5.5%, respectively. This difference may reflect local geographical variation.

The truly important measure of ulcer prevalence may be the percentage of patients in a population with its spectrum of ages who have the ulcer diathesis and therefore might require medical treatment. Clearly this is changing as background trends alter and depends on the age and socioeconomic profile of the population. New environmental factors may intervene. Nevertheless the Sorreisa study from Norway, taking into account asymptomatic ulceration and combining active ulceration and duodenal scarring, estimated that 10.5% of men and 9.5% of women in their population had peptic ulcer disease either active or in remission.[60] A 'best guess', therefore, does indeed suggest that around 10% of a Western population have peptic ulcer disease either gastric or duodenal and symptomatic or silent. Lifetime prevalence figures may therefore need to be revised upwards to include asymptomatic individuals if these findings are confirmed.

SEX DIFFERENCES

The prevalence of peptic ulcer differs between the sexes.[3,63] However, the exact nature of the relationship of ulcer disease to gender has altered significantly over time and is continuing to change. In general, it is true to say that over the last 100 years peptic ulcer has been more common in men than women.[63] This was not always the case, for in the nineteenth century peptic ulcer and gastric ulcer in particular was very much a disease of young women.[14,15] However, the explosion in peptic ulcer disease since the turn of the century has predominantly affected men rather than women leading to a male preponderance in most reports. The scale of the increased

male susceptibility to ulcer disease is variable but some studies are shown in Table 27.3. It is important to bear in mind the date and methodology in each report because historical trends may profoundly influence the sex ratio of ulcer disease.

Table 27.3 Sex differences in ulcer frequency

AUTHOR(S)	DATE	LOCATION	MALE : FEMALE RATIO	
			DUODENAL	GASTRIC
Pulvertaft[5]	1959	York, UK	3.5 : 1	1.7 : 1
Dunlop[49]	1968	Central Scotland	3.4 : 1	2.2 : 1
Monson and MacMahon[50]	1969	Massachusetts	1.9 : 1	—
Vogt and Johnson[27]	1980	Portland, Oregon	3.7 : 1	1.4 : 1*
Sonnenberg[28]	1987	USA	1.2 : 1	0.9 : 1†
Bernersen et al.[60]	1990	Sorreisa, Norway	2.0 : 1	0.9 : 1

*Figures for 1973.
†Figures for 1981–1984.

Peptic ulcer incidence (gastric and duodenal ulcers were not separately reported) found at post-mortem in Philadelphia over the years 1920–1932 was 2.0% for men and 1.5% for women.[14] In the subsequent 5 years (1933–1937), at the same hospital the frequency had risen to 4.1% for men and 2.2% for women, an overall male : female ratio in both studies of approximately 2 : 1.[14] A similar study from Cook County Hospital, Chicago covering 1929–1936 gave ulcer incidence rates at post-mortem (including scarring) of 5.9% for men and 2.9% for women, again a ratio of 2 : 1 male over female.[14] British data from the Leeds necropsy study between 1930 and 1949 did distinguish gastric from duodenal ulceration. The 'best estimate' of duodenal ulcer frequency from that study, excluding ulcer-related deaths, was 9.6% for men and 4.4% for women, a ratio of around 2 : 1.[56] The figures for gastric ulcer were much closer, 2.9% in males and 2.3% in females. However, cases coming to post-mortem for non-ulcer-related deaths will clearly represent an older age group and therefore lag behind the sex ratio in the community if that is not stable. The sex ratio in the community may alter if the background secular trends affect the sexes to different extents. Support that this might be so comes from reports from the USA of clinical studies suggesting male : female ratios of 5.5 : 1 and 4 : 1 during the same time period as post-mortem data a ratio of only 2 : 1.[14]

Ulcer complications probably provide data about a more representative age sample of the whole ulcer disease population although it should be remembered that men and women with ulcer disease are not necessarily equally prone to develop complications. Data on ulcer perforation rates are available from the west of Scotland over a continuous period from 1924 to 1973.[64–67] Throughout the 50 years of the survey there have always been more males than females, but the male : female ratio for ulcer perforation has steadily fallen. Combining both duodenal and gastric ulcer perforations for the period 1924–33 the male : female ratio was 19 : 1, falling to 12 : 1 between 1944 and 1953, and finally to 4 : 1 between 1964 and 1973. The data for both types of ulcer are shown in Table 27.4. The most striking change is the fall in male predominance for duodenal ulcer perforation from a male : female ratio of 21 : 1 in 1924–43 to

Table 27.4 Male : female ratio of ulcer perforation in the West of Scotland 1924–1973 (references 64–67)

PERIOD	OVERALL MALE : FEMALE RATIO	MALE : FEMALE RATIO DUODENAL	GASTRIC
1924–1933	19:1	21:1	8.7:1
1934–1943	18:1	21:1	8.7:1
1944–1953	12:1	14:1	3.5:1
1954–1963	6:1	7:1	1.8:1
1964–1973	4:1	4.4:1	1.7:1*

*Figures to 1970 only.

4.4:1 in 1970. Male : female ratios for gastric ulcer perforations also fell over the same period from 8.7:1 to only 1.7:1. Confirmation of these figures has come from other studies. For example, Truelove[68] reported that at the Radcliffe Infirmary, Oxford during the period 1938–1951, 388 men were treated for perforated duodenal ulcer but only 20 women, a ratio of nearly 20:1. In Bergen, Norway, the male : female ratio of perforated peptic ulcer fell from 10:1 to 1.5:1 between 1935 and 1990.[69] It is conceivable that men with ulcers have a greater tendency to perforation which may lead to the high relative perforation ratios. Thus, the sex ratio for total ulcer incidence, including perforation and other presentations, in York between 1952 and 1957 was only 3.2:1 male to female for duodenal ulcer and 1.6:1 for gastric ulcer.[5] The sex ratio of the total perforation rate in York over the same period was 9.5:1 male to female.[4] However, the tendency for men to develop duodenal ulcers, which have a greater chance of presenting as an acute perforation, rather than gastric ulcers may explain part of this difference.

In the last 30 years the male ascendency in ulcer disease has tended to decline. This is supported by data from a variety of epidemiological and clinical studies. In 1962 in Central Scotland the male : female ratio for all duodenal ulcers was 3.1:1 and 1.9:1 for gastric ulcer.[49] These findings are similar to those in York and south-west Scotland at the same period[4,5,48] but the male dominance is much less than in the perforation figures from a neighbouring area of Scotland.[65] Elective ulcer surgery at the Mayo Clinic declined between 1956–1960 and 1981–1985 from 67 to 7 operations per 100 000 person-years in men and from 35 to 5 in women.[25] The male : female ratio thus fell from 1.9:1 to 1.3:1 over the period. On the other hand emergency ulcer surgery was performed 5.8 times more frequently in men than women in 1956–1960 but by 1981–1985 emergency operations in men were only 1.3 times the female rate[25] suggesting that not only was the relative tendency of men to have ulcer disease decreasing but also the susceptibility of men with ulcer disease to develop complications. These figures include both ulcer types. The greatest decline was in elective operations for duodenal ulcer in men, less for men and women with gastric ulcer and least for women with duodenal ulcer. These findings largely predated the introduction of the H_2 receptor antagonists as potent drug therapy for ulcer disease.

Other sources of data show the same trend with the sex difference declining over time. In the USA the male to female ratio for self-reported peptic ulcer recorded by the National Health Interview Survey decreased from 2.8:1 in 1958 to 1:1 in 1981.[63] This decrease in sex ratio appeared to be due both to a decline in male and an increase in female rates. However, hospital out-patient attendances for peptic ulcer between 1967 and 1973 fell for both men and women. The male : female ratio remained stable at 3.7:1 for duodenal ulcer and 1.5:1 for gastric ulcer[27] but the period covered was only 6 years. Also in the USA the male : female ratio in hospital admission rates for duodenal ulcer fell from 2.2 in 1965 to 1.8 in 1981.[63] In fact, age-adjusted hospitalization rates fell for both sexes but the rate of decline was faster in men thus reducing the sex difference. The male to female ratio for gastric ulcer hospital admissions fell from 1.5:1 to 1.1:1 between 1965 and 1981. Gastric ulcer hospitalization rates were generally more stable than for duodenal ulcer but the ratio has altered due to a moderate decrease in male rates accompanied by a slight increase in female rates.

These trends have been confirmed in the UK by figures on hospital admissions from the years 1958–1977.[30] Non-perforated duodenal ulcer requiring hospital admission occurred in 3.8 times as many men as women in 1958 but by 1977 the ratio had fallen to 2.8:1. Admissions with this diagnosis fell in both sexes but, as in the USA, more profoundly in men. The male : female ratio for non-perforated gastric ulcers also fell from 1.9:1 to 1.3:1 over the same period, again predominantly due to falling rates in males. Similar overall trends were apparent for perforated ulcers with the exception of elderly women in whom an increase in perforated duodenal ulcer was recorded.[30]

Mortality rates are available for a large number of Western countries. Age-adjusted death rates in 19 European countries have been averaged over a period of 30–60 years up to about 1980.[43] In all these countries mortality rates for both duodenal and gastric ulcer were greater in men than women although the exact ratio varied between countries. However, this male excess in mortality rate is also changing. The male : female ratio for age-adjusted duodenal ulcer death rate in the USA dropped from 5.4:1 in 1950 to 2.3:1 in 1980.[63] The corresponding sex ratio for gastric ulcer deaths fell over the same period from 4.0:1 to 1.8:1.[63] Mortality figures from the Federal Republic of Germany also showed a declining male : female ratio for both duodenal and gastric ulcer-related deaths.[34] For duodenal ulcer, males outnumbered females 7.1:1 in 1952 and this fell to 1.7:1 in 1980. The change here was mostly due to a fourfold rise in women dying from duodenal ulcer complications. Male : female gastric ulcer mortality was 4.2:1 in 1952 and 1.2:1 in 1980, due both to a fall in disease frequency in men and an increase in women.[34]

In the Western world the sex ratio of peptic ulcer disease has been profoundly influenced by the historical trends in ulcer frequency. The high incidence of peptic ulcer in the twentieth century appears to have affected the sexes unequally. Duodenal ulcer became a disease of men, especially before 1950, leading to a particularly high male : female ratio. This male preponderance has begun to decline in Europe and America mostly due to a dramatic decline in duodenal ulcer frequency in men. The differences between the sexes in gastric ulcer disease was never as marked as for duodenal ulcer. Nevertheless, here too the sex difference has declined over the years since 1950 and now has almost reached parity at least in the USA. The change has been brought about by a stable or even increasing number of women developing gastric ulceration while the rate in men has declined.

The situation may still be changing. Ulcer perforations have been increasing in women over the age of 65 years in the UK leading to a decrease in the male : female ratio.[8] In 1958–1962 the male : female ratios for duodenal and gastric ulcer perforation in the over 65s in England and Wales was 5.4 : 1 and 2.8 : 1, respectively, corrected for population. Corresponding figures for 1978–1982 were 1.9 : 1 and 1.1 : 1. The changes in the ratio for duodenal ulcer was partly due to a modest 13% decline in the rate for men but mainly reflects an increase of 145% in perforations in women over 65 years. Gastric ulcer perforation rates increased by 20% in women and decreased by 51% in men in this age group.[8] Similar trends were present in data from Scotland.[8] This increase in perforation rates in elderly women, at a time when ulcer disease generally appears to be decreasing in frequency, suggests another factor is operating in this age group. The most likely candidate would appear to be NSAIDs.

Ulcer prevalence in the community, including past and asymptomatic disease, was assessed in north Norway in 1987.[60] The overall ulcer prevalence was 10.5% in men and 9.5% in women, a ratio close to unity. The male : female ratio was 2.0 : 1 for duodenal ulcer and 0.9 : 1 for gastric ulcer. However, it should be remembered that this was a relatively small study of 2027 patients in perhaps an atypical geographical area. It would be fair to say that the sex ratio at present still seems to favour men in duodenal ulcer disease, perhaps by around 2 : 1 but the sex ratio in gastric ulcer is tending towards unity or even to an excess in women in the more elderly age groups.

There are important exceptions to these generalizations. The trends relate only to industrialized westernized countries. In the less-developed areas of the world the sex ratio resembles that in Europe in the 1930s with males far exceeding females in ulcer frequency. A review of the sex ratio of duodenal ulcer in India, for example, calculated a mean male : female ratio in 11 reported series of 17.6 : 1 with a range of 9 : 1 to 33 : 1.[70] Similarly, in areas of high incidence in Black Africa the mean male preponderance in 18 studies was 9 : 1 males over females.[38] Again the range was wide from 2.1 : 1 to 30 : 1. In developing countries men may tend to come to hospital more readily than women but this factor is unlikely to be the whole explanation. Even in the developed world local factors can distort the the sex ratio. A particular example is the high incidence of peptic ulcer disease in women in eastern Australia, first noticed in 1943 and continuing into the 1970s.[71] This phenomenon was probably related to heavy aspirin ingestion among women in the area which was not so prevalent among men in the same district.

Nevertheless almost all studies of ulcer frequency in the twentieth century, both gastric and duodenal, have found a male preponderance of some degree. The reasons for the relative protection of women are not clear. Healthy female controls were reported to have a slightly lower peak acid output than males but this was not corrected for the lower weight of the female subjects.[72] Food-stimulated acid secretion as a percentage of peak acid output did not vary between the sexes although the serum gastrin level was 2–3 times higher in women.[73] These findings were interpretated as showing an insensitivity of the parietal cell to gastrin in women.[72] No changes were found in different phases of the menstrual cycle.[73] A more recent study included both controls and patients with duodenal ulcer. In controls maximal and basal acid output was again lower in females but this difference disappeared when corrected for body weight.[74] Male patients with duodenal ulcer had significantly higher maximal acid output than females with the disease even when corrected for weight. Basal acid output corrected for weight tended to be higher in males with duodenal ulcer but did not reach significance. Pepsinogen I levels, but not pepsinogen II nor the ratio of the two, were also significantly higher in healthy men than women and in one of two groups of patients with duodenal ulceration.[74] More studies are required to investigate whether differences in acid secretion underlie the male susceptibility to peptic ulcer disease.

Another possibility is that female hormones protect against ulcer disease in some way and there is support for this hypothesis. Female sex was the most important single factor identified by multiple linear regression analysis to improve duodenal ulcer healing.[75] Peptic ulcer is almost unknown during pregnancy and sufferers often have symptomatic respite during and after pregnancy.[76,77] These observations led Truelove[68] to perform a clinical trial of stilboestrol in men with chronic duodenal ulcer. The therapy was successful, healing 50% of ulcers compared with 10% on placebo, but at the expense of unacceptable side-effects. Oestrogen deficiency might contribute to the susceptibility of elderly women to the ulcerogenic effects of NSAIDs. Against this, however, female sex did not protect against ulcer perforation in the nineteenth century.

It is possible that other factors linked to ulcer disease are not equally divided between the sexes. Smokers have a higher prevalence of peptic ulcer than non-smokers and this is true for women as well as men.[78] Moreover the habit is more common in men and was particularly so 50 years ago when the male : female sex ratio was greatest. The epidemiology of cigarette smoking in the UK, however, does not support a causal link.[44] Overall ulcer incidence and mortality in both men and women have decreased in the last 30 years, particularly in men and the younger age groups of both sexes.[30,44] In contrast, cigarette smoking has been constant in men and has increased in young women over this period.[44] Other factors, such as stress or diet, alone or in combination, may afflict the sexes to different extents. It appears that in the Western world women are beginning to achieve equality with men in ulcer frequency.

AGE

To determine accurately the relationship between age and peptic ulcer would appear to be simple but in practice it is deceptively difficult. In a relapsing and remitting disease the age at diagnosis or development of a complication may not coincide with the age at which symptoms and therefore the first clinical attack of ulceration began. Thus, age at diagnosis may relate more to access to health care and particularly to availability of diagnostic procedures. Age of initial symptom onset may be a better estimate of when the first ulcer occurred in an individual but human memory in this regard is notoriously fallible and moreover ulceration may be asymptomatic. Further it is difficult to separate an effect of ageing itself from other epidemiological factors which affect differing age groups to varying extents. Thus an increased frequency of peptic ulceration in patients aged 60–70 years, say, may be due to a degenerative effect of ageing, an environmental factor to which that age group is particularly exposed or to an increased prevalence related to birth cohort, i.e. a generational effect. As birth cohorts born around 1880–1890 had the greatest susceptibility to ulcer disease,[43] and each succeeding cohort since then has had a gradually falling prevalence, one might expect the mean age of ulcer patients to be increasing due to this factor.

The mean age of patients with peptic ulcer is indeed increasing although other influences may play a role in the phenomenon. For example, on the west coast of Scotland mean age of perforated peptic ulcer in males increased from 43.9 years in the period 1924–1943 to 54.9 years in 1964–1973.[66] The mean age in females was consistently lower but showed the same tendency to increase with time, rising from 40.9 years in 1924–1943 to 48.1 years in 1964–1973. In Norway median age of peptic ulcer perforation rose from 38 to 60 years between 1935 and 1990.[69] Median age of perforation in women also increased from 55 to 69 years over the same time.[69] Clearly, these observations must be seen against the background of an ageing population in Western Countries but they do appear to be real.[79] However, the population with peptic ulcer appears to be ageing out of proportion to this factor. Between 1970 and 1978 the percentage of persons aged over 60 years in the overall population of the USA rose from 14 to 15%, but the proportion of over 60s admitted to hospital for duodenal ulcer increased from 27% to 36% and for gastric ulcer from 40% to 48%.[22]

Evidence from the UK also suggests that the number of young patients with complicated duodenal ulceration is falling, a 62% reduction being seen between 1958–1962 and 1978–1982 in men aged 15–44 years.[8] However, over the same period the decline was less in men aged over 65, only 13%, thereby increasing the relative representation of this age group. For women the situation, at least in the UK, is different again. Between the same dates admissions for perforated duodenal ulcer of women aged 15–44 years in England and Wales fell by 36%, but increased by 145% in those over 65 years.[8] Perforated gastric ulcer showed similar trends over the 20 years of the study. In men, the overall decline was 66%, but 86% in those aged 15–44 years and only 51% in those over 65 years. In women, perforated gastric ulcer admissions rose overall by 11% between 1958 and 1982.[8] This increase again disproportionately affected the older population. Whereas perforated gastric ulceration declined in frequency in those aged 15–44 years, it increased by 20% in those over 65 years.

These observations suggest the changes in age-related incidence, at least in women, are not due to a birth cohort effect. Such an influence should lead to gradually decreasing ulcer frequency over time, albeit possibly biased to the younger age groups depending on the relative magnitude of the effect. A more likely explanation is that a new ulcerogenic factor is active in elderly women. Cigarette consumption does not explain the results because the proportion of women smokers aged over 65 years fell slightly over the same period although those that did smoke consumed a greater number of cigarettes each week.[8] NSAID ingestion for arthritic and other conditions by elderly women in particular would appear a more likely candidate.[8]

Data on mortality from ulcer complications is probably misleading as an index of ulcer prevalence when related to age, because deaths from ulcer disease are likely to be concentrated in the elderly who have other medical problems and are therefore less likely to survive the episode. Nevertheless, death rates from peptic ulcer have generally fallen in recent years in the USA but the fall has been least in those aged 65 or over.[22] Age-specific death rates in the UK between 1958 and 1983 have actually risen in women over 65 years old for both duodenal and gastric ulcer while falling in men of the same age.[8] This further confirms the trend for ulcer patients now both to be older and more likely to be female than in the past.

The current age profile of the ulcer population is difficult to determine. Peptic ulcer occurs in all age groups but is rare below the age of 20. Duodenal ulcer in children is well recognized but between 1960 and 1985 only 110 cases were collected in Newcastle, UK in children under 15 years.[80] Mean age at diagnosis was 11.6 years but symptoms were present in almost half before the age of 10 years and in 15% under 6 years of age. Boys are more commonly affected than girls, a male:female ratio of 3.8:1 being recorded. Increased awareness that peptic ulcer exists in this age group and the availability of diagnostic endoscopy may lead to more cases in children being recognized.[81]

In adults, clearly the longer one lives the greater likelihood each individual has of developing peptic ulceration. Thus in male Massachusetts physicians questioned in 1967, the lifetime prevalence of duodenal ulcer rose from 3.3% in those aged 25–34 years to 11.9% in those over 75 years.[50] The greatest increase occurred between the groups aged 35–44 and 45–54 years, the prevalence rising from 3.6% in the former to 9.3% in the latter. In gastric ulcer the lifetime prevalence also generally increased with age but the largest increase occurred later at about the age of 65 years.[50] Estimated incidence rates of duodenal ulcer (the number of newly diagnosed cases per 1000 male doctors per year) therefore progressively rose with age to peak in those aged 55–64 years and then decline slightly. Gastric ulcer incidence also increased with age peaking later in those aged 65–74 years.

Two studies of ulcer incidence in south-west Scotland and the Faroe Islands conducted in 1958 and 1981, respectively, also showed a peak incidence of duodenal ulcer in men aged 50–59 years.[48,53] The observation of a mid-life peak in ulcer incidence was also present in men with gastric ulcer at the same age in the Faroes but occurred 10 years later in the 60–69 decade in Scotland. Too few women with peptic ulcer were seen in the Scottish study to make a judgement but the paper from the Faroes reported that, in contrast to men, female duodenal and gastric ulcer incidence tended to increase gradually with age although there was a low incidence for both types of ulcer in the 40–49-year-old group.[53] Data from central Scotland also identified a peak of duodenal ulcer incidence in men at age 30–50 and later in gastric ulcer at 60–69 years.[49] Numbers were small in women but showed identical trends.

Other studies, however, have shown an increasing incidence of new cases of peptic ulcer in both men and women as they age. Thus the age-specific incidence of ulcer perforation in Glasgow in 1961 rose with increasing age for both males and females although because of the age structure of the population the greatest number occurred in the 50–54 year age group.[65] A similar relationship of increasing frequency of ulcer perforations with age was reported from Oxford between 1957 and 1963.[6] However, it is not clear in either study that the perforation occurred during the first attack of ulcer disease. A propensity to perforate related to age might, therefore, produce the same result. New diagnoses of ulcer disease, both complicated and uncomplicated, in Copenhagen County between 1963 and 1968 were observed to rise with age in both men and women and in both gastric and duodenal ulcer.[35,51]

A more recent study investigated the incidence of peptic ulcer disease in Gothenberg, Sweden in 1985.[82] As one might expect the number of active peptic ulcers per 1000 inhabitants increased with age, except in those over 80 years. This presumably reflects cumulative lifetime prevalence to ulcer disease. However, in 454 patients the diagnosis of peptic ulcer was made for the first time during the year of the study. The age at first diagnosis per 1000 inhabitants for all cases of peptic ulcer is shown in Figure 27.1. There was a clear tendency for the incidence of peptic ulcer to increase with age, both overall and in men and women. In the 122 male subjects with duodenal ulcer the incidence per 1000 inhabitants rose with age except in those over 75 years (Figure 27.2). The peak incidence was therefore 70–75 years. There were fewer new

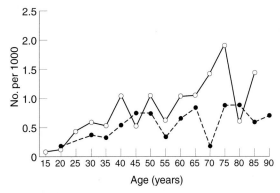

Figure 27.2
Age at first diagnosis of duodenal ulcer per 1000 inhabitants in Gothenberg, Sweden, 1985. O, Men (n = 122); ●, Women (n = 81). (Reproduced with permission from Schöön et al.[82])

female patients with duodenal ulcer (only 81 cases), and the trends were less clear cut. However, incidence rose until age 50 then appeared to plateau. Age-adjusted incidence of new gastric ulcer patients (46 men, 71 women) also generally increased with age in both sexes to 75 years but then decreased in the very elderly (Figure 27.3). It would seem, therefore, that an individual's chance of developing a new peptic ulcer, either gastric or duodenal, increases with age but possibly falls slightly after reaching 75 years. Probably, as might be expected, the chance of dying as a result of a peptic ulcer complication rises markedly with advancing years.

There are significant variations within these overall trends of increasing ulcer incidence with age. Gastric ulcer incidence seems to show a generally smooth increase with age in both men and women. Duodenal ulcer incidence, on the other hand, appears to rise rapidly between the ages of 30 and 40 years in men and between 40 and 50 years in women, rising more slowly in older age groups of both sexes. The disproportionate increase in elderly women with ulcer complications has already been mentioned.

As with all epidemiological data in peptic ulcer disease extrapolation from one place and period to another may not

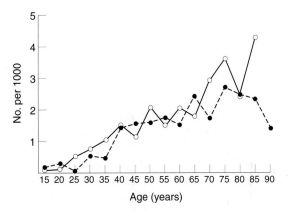

Figure 27.1
Age at first diagnosis of peptic (duodenal and gastric) ulcer per 1000 inhabitants in Gothenberg, Sweden, 1985. O, Men (n = 227); ●, women (n = 227). (Reproduced with permission from Schöön et al.[82])

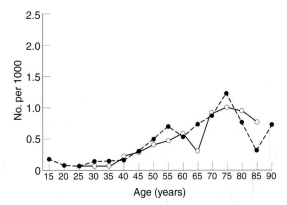

Figure 27.3
Age at first diagnosis of gastric ulcer per 1000 inhabitants in Gothenberg, Sweden, 1985. O, Men (n = 46); ●, women (n = 71). (Reproduced with permission from Schöön et al.[82])

be possible. Mean age of duodenal ulcer patients in India appears to be somewhat younger at 30–40 years than in the developed world.[70] This may reflect the different patterns of ulcer disease in less-developed countries. A study from Singapore has reported racial differences in the age of symptom onset.[83] Ethnic Chinese living in Singapore have a higher prevalence of duodenal ulcer than Malays.[84] The mean age of symptom onset in Chinese is 33.7 years, significantly younger than the 43.6 recorded in the Malay population.[83] Indeed it has been suggested that there are major differences in patients with duodenal ulcer according to age of disease onset.[85,86] Patients with an onset under the age of 30 years are more likely to have a positive family history and a history of gastrointestinal haemorrhage than those with late onset. Children with duodenal ulcer are also likely to have a family history of ulcer disease.[80]

GEOGRAPHICAL VARIATION

Peptic ulceration occurs worldwide but with large variations in its frequency in different locations. In the less-developed world, where disease is generally less well documented, duodenal ulcer is much more common than gastric ulcer and most studies from these areas reflect this preponderance. Thus, whereas the duodenal : gastric ulcer ratio in the UK is 2–4 : 1 that in India is around 19 : 1 and in high incidence areas in Africa it is around 33 : 1.[38,70] The characteristics of duodenal ulceration seen in developing countries may also be different with a tendency to fibrosis and pyloric stenosis rather than the perforation and haemorrhage seen in the West.[38,70]

Nevertheless, in both Africa and India there are areas of high and low incidence of peptic ulceration and these observations have been the subject of excellent reviews.[38,70] High prevalence areas in black African populations south of the Sahara include the West Coast, particularly Nigeria, Ghana and the Cameroons, together with Northern Tanzania and Ethiopia.[38,40] The greatest prevalence of all seems to be the Nile–Congo watershed of Rwanda, Burundi and eastern Zaire. For example, in one hospital in Burundi 79% of all major surgery was for peptic ulcer.[38] Low prevalence areas include most of rural South Africa, Mozambique and Kenya. Similar major differences are apparent in peptic ulcer prevalence within the Indian subcontinent. Hospital admissions rates for peptic ulceration in high incidence areas such as eastern India and southern India below Bombay exceed those found in other regions of the country by a factor of ten. Relatively low incidence areas for peptic ulcer are in the north and the Punjab.[38]

In most European countries and the USA, duodenal ulcer is now only about 2–4 times as frequent as gastric ulcer.[3] The variation in this ratio between different European countries does not show any clear cut relationship to geography.[87] Exceptions to this rule are northern Norway and Arctic areas which seem to have less duodenal and more gastric ulcer disease, so the ratio between the two may be close to unity.[36,53] Lately, however, this difference appears to be less marked with a ratio of 1.7 : 1 in favour of duodenal disease resembling the rest of Europe.[88] Southern Norway does correspond to the rest of Europe with duodenal ulcer the more common disease.[36] Japan also has a particular high incidence of gastic ulcer with a gastric : duodenal ulcer ratio of up to 5 : 1.[37,87]

However, within these large-scale geographical variations there are marked local regional differences. In the UK, for instance, the incidence of gastric ulcer perforation is relatively uniform but the duodenal ulcer perforation rate is four times higher in Scotland than in England and Wales.[29] The differing pattern between northern and southern Norway has already been mentioned and variation in ulcer frequency also occurs between the islands of Japan.[37] Gastric ulceration predominates in the large northern island of Hokkaido whereas an excess of duodenal ulcer is found in Okinawa in the south. Widely differing rates of ulcer frequency have been recorded between Australian states. Gastric ulcers were diagnosed four times more often in New South Wales than in Victoria for example.[52] This finding may be due to local environmental factors such as high analgesic drug intake.

In both India and Africa, there are isolated low incidence areas adjacent to or within high incidence regions. Examples of this phenomenon are the low incidence in part of eastern Nigeria and the rarity of duodenal ulcer in Kond tribesmen in Orissa, eastern India, in contrast to other groups in the state.[38,70,89] Genetic or racial susceptibility is a possible explanation of the markedly contrasting geographical frequency of peptic ulcer but an environmental factor or factors, such as diet, could also be operating. Very localized regional differences in ulcer incidence in similar racial groups are more likely to be explained by the superimposition of a locally acting environmental factor, either ulcerogenic or protective, on the background epidemiological pattern.

DIET

Differences in diet are obvious potential environmental mediators for the geographical and local variations in ulcer frequency.[90] Dietary factors could either predispose to ulceration or protect against the disease. In India the high incidence in the south corresponds to the major rice-eating areas.[89,91] In contrast, the incidence is low in northern India, particularly the Punjab, where the staple food is unrefined wheat eaten in chapattis.[89] The Kond tribes of Orissa, who exhibit low frequency of ulcer disease in an otherwise high frequency area, also have a diet based on cereal rather than rice.[89] A higher prevalence of peptic ulcer was also found in rice-eating areas of southern China compared to the cereal-eating north but the differences were less marked than in India.[92] These observations have led to speculation that dietary fibre may be protective in some way either directly or by stimulating mastication or salivary flow.[90] Support for a protective role for dietary fibre has come from the demonstration that the relapse rate of duodenal ulcer over 5 years in Bombay was reduced from 80% in a group maintained on a rice-based diet to 14% in those converted to an unrefined wheat 'Punjabi' diet.[93] The results are impressive, but only 21 patients were followed in each group. Chinese customs mean less bran is used in bread making which may explain the smaller difference in ulcer disease between rice and cereal-eating ares.[92] Reports from Norway also suggested benefit from a high-fibre diet in preventing duodenal ulcer relapse.[94] Of duodenal ulcer patients on a low-fibre diet 80% relapsed in 6 months compared with 45% on a high-fibre intake. Pretreatment of rats with a Punjabi diet also appeared to protect them against stomach ulcers after pyloric ligation further strengthening the hypothesis.[95] The animal experiments could not, however, be specific about which dietary factors in the Punjabi diet were protective.

Against the dietary fibre theory is the observation from Norway that fibre intake did not influence acute ulcer healing of either gastric or duodenal ulcers.[94] Moreover, the close correlation between ulcer prevalence and fibre intake evident in India is not observed in Africa.[89] In the UK the fall in duodenal ulcer frequency preceded changes in dietary fibre intake in the general population.[90] A case-control study of 78 patients in Nottingham could not identify any association between high total fibre or cereal intake and protection from duodenal ulceration.[96] However, the relative risk of developing an ulcer tended to be reduced with a high vegetable fibre intake although the number of patients studied was small. Fibre intake may not be equally significant with respect to ulcer disease in all areas.

The twentieth century has been characterized by immense changes in dietary habits in Western Europe and the USA. Analysis of the pronounced historical changes in ulcer frequency in both regions has led to suggestions that the increase in ulcer disease in the first half of the century was due to the introduction of refined carbohydrate foods. The subsequent fall has further been correlated with an increasing consumption of vegetable oils, rich in polyunsaturated essential fatty acids.[97] In particular, vegetable oils contain high levels of linoleic acid, the precursor of prostaglandins found in gastroduodenal mucosa, which are believed to promote mucosal protection and accelerate repair.[97]

These theories have gained a little support. The Nottingham case-control study did suggest that a low refined sugar intake was protective even when the confounding effects of smoking, social class, obesity and energy intake were taken into account.[96] Any protective role of linoleic acid (an ω–6 fatty acid derived mainly from plants) would be less apparent in fish-eating communities where the diet is relatively rich in ω–3 fatty acids (e.g. eicosapentaenoic) found in marine oils. This might explain, at least in part, the high incidence of gastric ulcer found in Japan and the Arctic.[36,37] In addition, linoleic acid intake assessed by composition of subcutaneous adipose tissue has recently been reported to be reduced in patients with duodenal ulcer compared with controls.[98]

There is no good evidence from population studies that bland diets are protective in peptic ulcer disease nor that increased spice consumption is an important predisposing factor. The geographical variability in India particularly may simply reflect generalized malnutrition or protein and vitamin deficiencies. The hypothesis that diet is responsible for the marked geographical and historical trends in ulcer frequency is attractive. However, there is at present a paucity of rigorously controlled trials to substantiate the competing claims of different dietary factors, and of diet overall, with respect to other important environmental ulcerogens.

RACIAL FACTORS

Investigation of the degree to which racial groups, as opposed to individuals within them, are susceptible to peptic ulceration is hampered by the marked cultural differences between ethnic groups. This may be compounded by differences in social class between racial groups, for example between Whites and non-Whites in the USA.[99] Thus the prevalence of peptic ulcer among the three main racial groups sharing the small island of Singapore is greatest in Chinese, less in Indians and least in Malays.[83,84] Although geography and climate are clearly the same for all, other important environmental factors such as diet, smoking habits and socioeconomic profile will be specific to each race so the observation does not prove a genetic racial predisposition. Indeed there may be support for the concept that environmental factors are more important in the finding of a diminishing difference in ulcer frequency between Chinese and Malay over the last three decades.[83,84]

The classic experiments to discriminate between genetic and environmental factors in other disease areas have studied migrant populations. Indian communities originally from high incidence areas on the subcontinent have tended to retain their predisposition to peptic ulceration when living in other countries, for example Malaysia, Fiji and South Africa.[70] However these migrant communities may retain their own dietary and social customs even in foreign countries or have had insufficient time to become assimilated into the host nation. Further, migrant workers from southern Europe in the former West Germany have a higher ulcer frequency than that found in either German residents or their own native country.[87] Indochinese migrants to Australia also have a high prevalence of duodenal ulcer although the increase is not seen in other ethnic groups.[100] However, migrant workers are likely to be in the lower socioeconomic groups and also have substantial stress levels. Interpretation of these data is difficult.

SOCIOECONOMIC GROUP AND OCCUPATION

The influence of socioeconomic group or occupation on ulcer prevalence may be altering over time. The accepted pattern has been that gastric ulceration is more common in lower as against higher social classes and the opposite relationship exists for duodenal ulcer.[3,101] However, birth cohort data suggest that the increase in frequency of gastric ulceration, as measured by death rates, affected the higher before the lower social orders.[2] Duodenal ulcer frequency followed this trend with a rising wave of disease affecting upper class men born before 1870 and with the lower classes showing higher rates after this.[2] Gastric ulcer trends therefore appear to lead those for duodenal ulceration. These statistics are based solely on men and reflect death rates which might be influenced by access to health care.[3]

Standardized mortality ratios (SMR) are available for

England and Wales from 1921–1923 and 1959–1963. In both periods, gastric ulcer deaths have been consistently more frequent in those in unskilled occupations.[3] In 1921–23 more deaths were recorded from duodenal ulcer than would be expected in social classes I and II (SMR = 133).[3] However, 40 years later the trend had reversed to resemble gastric ulcer with social class I (SMR = 70) and II (SMR = 84) relatively protected from death from duodenal ulcer and an excess in Social Class V (SMR = 136).[3] Data from the USA from 1950 confirm the finding of an excess of deaths from ulcer, both gastric and duodenal, concentrated in the lower socioeconomic groups.[3]

Studies in living patients show generally similar trends. In 1951 Doll et al.[102] suggested that social status had no influence on the incidence of duodenal ulcer, but gastric ulcers were more common in the semiskilled. The General Register Office (England and Wales), confirmed this observation in 1956 giving a mean annual incidence per 1000 for gastric ulcer in social classes I and II of 0.34, for class III 0.60, and classes IV and V 0.92 confirming this trend.[5] Corresponding results for duodenal ulcer were 2.08, 2.26 and 3.13, respectively.[5]

Figures for the single city of York also show a significantly higher incidence of duodenal ulcer in the lower social classes.[5] Between 1957 and 1959 the incidence of peptic ulcer in a predominantly rural area of south-west Scotland was recorded and correlated with social class.[48] The increased prevalence of gastric ulcer in unskilled men was again apparent and duodenal ulcer was also more common in the same group. Thus, 94 cases of duodenal ulcer would have been expected in social classes I and II but only 54 were observed. Conversely, in social classes IV and V 294 cases were observed and only 170 expected.[48] These findings were confirmed from Stirling, central Scotland for both men and women except that social class III was also observed to have a low ulcer risk.[49]

Social class or socioeconomic grouping covers a multitude of other potentially confounding variables relating to housing, access to health care, diet, alcohol intake and smoking. This last factor is particularly important as cigarette smoking is known to be associated with increased risk of peptic ulceration. An American study recorded smoking habit and used highest educational attainment, divided into elementary, high school or college, as a rough estimate of socioeconomic group.[78] A history of peptic ulceration was greatest in subjects who had only completed elementary school and least in college graduates. Those who had intermediate educational attainment and only completed high school had an incidence of peptic ulcer history between the other two groups.[78] The findings were similar in both smokers and non-smokers and apparent in both men and women. At the present time, both duodenal and gastric ulcer seem to have a predilection for the lower socioeconomic groups with poor educational attainment, possibly due to associated environmental factors.[103]

Occupation largely determines social class or socioeconomic group. It is possible that certain jobs may predispose to ulceration and explain the differences in prevalence between socioeconomic groups. Generally jobs which could predispose to peptic ulceration might be regarded as 'stressful' and also be associated with smoking and alcohol abuse or perhaps attract certain personality types.[2] Agricultural workers have a low duodenal ulcer prevalence, reflected by both low morbidity and mortality.[48,102] Foremen and executives in Great Britain are reported to have high rates of duodenal ulcer, although in the USA higher rates of peptic ulcer were found in foremen alone and not executives.[2,104] Executives would largely fall into social classes I and II and generally these groups, as discussed above, have low ulcer prevalence. It is difficult to reconcile these findings. Shift workers are more likely to have ulceration than those working regular hours.[59] However, presumably shift workers are also more likely to have semiskilled or unskilled jobs. Low employment status has been identified as a factor in gastric ulcer development in addition to non-daytime working.[105] Occupational differences may be accentuated in Blacks living in South Africa. A total of 105 patients with duodenal ulcer in Johannesburg were compared with matched and unmatched hospital controls. Men with duodenal ulcer were significantly better educated than those in either of the control groups, and were therefore more likely to occupy professional, technical and clerical positions.[39] No differences were observed in the few women studied.

These findings have been contested from elsewhere in South Africa, albeit in a predominantly Indian rather than African patient group.[106] Indian males with duodenal ulcer were more likely to be in a lower category of work authority and therefore feel 'powerlessness' and under more stress than other hospital patients of the same race.[106] The patients with duodenal ulcer, however, had improved on their father's occupational status.[106] It is extremely difficult to categorize authority, prestige and 'powerlessness' and therefore these findings must be treated with caution. These findings in a less-developed country suggest greater prevalence in educated people, at least in Africans, a pattern that was characteristic of Western countries 60–80 years ago.

URBANIZATION

In the UK, residence in an urban rather than a rural area has been observed to increase the risk of developing both gastric and duodenal ulceration. Duodenal ulcers were 2.43 and 2.03 times more common in men and women, respectively, living in the small town of Dumfries, Scotland than the surrounding countryside.[48] Corresponding town/country ratios for gastric ulcer were 2.84 for men and 2.12 for women.[48] In addition, perforated peptic ulcer was twice as common in Oxford City than in rural Oxfordshire.[6] The ratio of duodenal ulcer in the city of York to that in the adjacent countryside was 2.1:1 in 1952 although curiously had fallen to 1.3:1 only 4 years later.[5] Duodenal ulcer is rarely reported for rural Africa and India, but is appearing in increasing frequency in urban areas.[38,39,70]

The historical trends in ulcer disease, the birth cohort effect and the lower prevalence in rural areas led Susser and Stein[42] to suggest that peptic ulceration and duodenal ulcer in particular, may be a disease of an 'early phase of urbanization'. The recent Western trend for decreased ulcer frequency where urbanization has been established for some time, coupled with the rising ulcer rates in Hong Kong and the less developed world where living in cities is relatively new, would tend to support this theory. It would also neatly explain the birth cohort data from America and Great Britain.

The major difficulty is the lack of specificity about the nature of the factor or factors involved. It is clear that the factor providing the change associated with early urbanization must be environmental because the changes are too rapid to be genetic.[107] Susser and Stein[42] themselves suggest that early urbanization was particularly stressful but later city dwellers have adapted more readily to their surroundings.

This hypothesis is obviously difficult to confirm or refute. Sonnenberg et al.[108] have drawn attention to the parallels between declining peptic ulcer mortality and specific occupational factors. Since 1900, occupation has progressively switched from heavy manual 'blue collar' jobs to sedentary 'white collar' professions. In addition the work hours and conditions have progressively improved so that occupational workload or occupational energy expenditure has decreased mirroring peptic ulcer incidence. They suggest a causal relationship between these two observations. The higher frequency of ulcer disease in lower socioeconomic groups engaged in energy-intensive manual labour would tend to support this theory. However, the evidence must be regarded as circumstantial for the twentieth century has seen many changes in diet, social habits, smoking and stress. Even in 1985–1986 after adjustment for age, sex, smoking and social class, physical activity at work was still associated with duodenal ulcer in a study in Nottingham, England.[109] The relative risk of developing duodenal ulceration for moderate and high physical activity compared with sedentary work was 1.3 and 3.6 respectively.[109]

If it is correct that early urbanization predisposes to peptic ulceration in some way then the current polarization towards the cities in less-developed countries might produce another epidemic of ulcer disease, mitigated only by the effective new therapeutic agents available.

SEASONAL VARIATION

There is a general impression that peptic ulcer tends to occur during the spring and autumn months.[11,110] This was originally suggested by Ivy[14] on the basis of the marked fall in ulcer mortality recorded in the summer months from 1938–1943. Mortality appeared to be at its lowest in July and August. This trend is also apparent from other data.[111] Admissions to 166 Veterans Administration Hospitals throughout the USA during 1963–1968 again showed a fall in June, July and August.[112] These findings included uncomplicated duodenal ulcer admissions as well as perforations and haemorrhage. Hospital admission data for peptic ulceration in the entire USA between 1970 and 1980 also showed a decrease in the summer (or increase in the winter) the changes representing a variation of plus or minus 10% of the mean level.[11]

This pattern of a summer deficit in ulcer frequency is the most consistent in the literature. Incidence of ulcer perforation in Glasgow has shown the same pattern, being maximal in January for the 20 years between 1954 and 1973.[66] Indeed, there was a marked increase between 22 December and 4

January, tentatively explained by local festivities over Christmas and the New Year.[7] Gastrointestinal haemorrhage also shows a similar seasonal pattern in both London and the USA.[113,114] This trend for reduced bleeding in the months of July and August holds for both duodenal and gastric ulcer.[113] A prospective study of 50 patients with ulcer disease (41 with duodenal ulcer) recorded seasonal changes.[115] Over a follow-up period of up to 5 years, patients underwent endoscopy on average 5–6 times per year. Abdominal pain and endoscopically demonstrated ulcer rates were again lowest in August, but also fell in December which is not a frequent observation. It should also be pointed out that several smaller studies have been unable to confirm this seasonal variation.[11]

Several factors suggest the trend is indeed real. It occurs in both gastric and duodenal ulcers, but not other causes of gastrointestinal haemorrhage. The low ulcer admission rate in August cannot be explained by low overall admission rate since it was still apparent when compared with a control disease, essential hypertension.

The most obvious explanation is that the diminished frequency of ulcer manifestations is related to the holiday period either artefactually by physician or patient taking holidays outside the region or due to reduced patient stress levels. An alternative is that the observation is related to warm weather and a single southern hemisphere study reported reduced ulcer admissions in January, the warm month in that part of the world.[116] Against this, however, no correlation was found between environmental ambient temperature and the frequency of gastrointestinal haemorrhage in either the UK or USA.[112,113]

SMOKING AND ALCOHOL

Smoking

There seems to be little doubt that cigarette smokers have an increased frequency of peptic ulceration. Studies have shown an increased prevalence of smoking in patients with peptic ulcer and conversely an increased prevalence of peptic ulcer in smokers.[2,11,78,117–120] Criticisms of early investigations were that objective confirmation of ulceration was seldom recorded but reliance placed on questionnaires, and gastric and duodenal ulcers were not distinguished. An argument advanced against a causal relationship was the lack of a dose–response relationship correlating ulcer frequency with number of cigarettes smoked. All these objections have now been met.

An endoscopic survey recorded 11.9% of smokers with gastric ulcer against 4.6% of non-smokers.[121] Equivalent figures for duodenal ulcer were 12.8 and 6.1%. A Scandinavian case–control study also recorded higher rates of smoking in patients with peptic ulcer, particularly in duodenal disease, than in control groups.[117] The relative risk for smoking varied with consumption up to 2.1 for gastric ulcer and 3.7 for duodenal ulcer and was broadly similar for men and women. Further, the finding of delayed healing and more frequent relapse of both duodenal and gastric ulcer in smokers strengthens the association.[75,122,123] If it is accepted that a relationship exists between smoking and peptic ulceration then this will influence other possible associations. Thus coffee and alcohol consumption, stress and socioeconomic group, for instance, are all variables interacting with smoking and this should be borne in mind when interpreting data on other environmental factors.

Alcohol

The increased frequency of peptic ulceration in hepatic cirrhosis has led to the belief that alcohol is 'bad' for ulcers.[124,125] In fact, short of the extreme of alcoholic cirrhosis there is little evidence for this view and indeed possibly some that a moderate alcohol intake is protective.[126] A history of peptic ulcer was given in 15.6% of white men who smoked but did not drink compared to 12.1% who also smoked but drank over three alcoholic drinks per day.[78] Similar trends for reduced ulcer frequency in subjects who regularly consumed alcohol occurred in non-smoking men and both smoking and non-smoking women.[78] In a Scandinavian case–control study, the number of alcohol users, but possibly not abusers, with ulcers was again significantly lower than the control group.[117] This finding was consistent both for patients with duodenal and gastric ulcer. In addition, linear regression analysis identified moderate alcohol intake as an independent factor promoting acute ulcer healing, although not preventing relapse.[75] A prospective study in Hawaiian men also failed to implicate alcohol as a risk factor for ulceration.[127] The evidence to date would suggest that moderate alcohol intake can be allowed to peptic ulcer patients and may even be beneficial. Moderate alcohol consumption is not proven to be a risk factor for either gastric or duodenal ulceration.

Other dietary factors

Coffee drinking was also postulated to be a factor associated with an increased risk of developing peptic ulcer later in life.[120] Coffee drinking is, of course, related to cigarette consumption and this may explain the original observation.[78] Two further studies have not shown evidence that coffee, independent of smoking, is a risk factor for ulceration.[78,117] Soft drink consumption is also said to be higher in those who will develop peptic ulceration in the future but this remains controversial.[120] A relationship has also been suggested between body build and ulcer, but this association was refuted in subsequent trials.[78,118] Milk and fruit consumption have not shown an association with peptic ulcer.[127]

DRUG INGESTION

Steroids

There is a widespread but anecdotal dogma among practising clinicians linking corticosteroid treatment with increased risk of peptic ulceration. This belief appears to originate in early reports, when steroids first came into use, of ulcer development or exacerbation by the drugs.[128] The difficulty is that the overall incidence of peptic ulcer in patients on treatment with steroids or adrenocorticotrophic hormone is low and therefore prospective or case–control studies are difficult. This problem is the same with other drug treatments. As a result the technique of

using combined data or meta-analysis of side-effects reported in different studies has been used, but without reaching a consensus. Conn and Blitzer[128] combined 42 studies with a total of 5331 patients. Overall, 0.8% of 2346 control patients developed peptic ulceration compared with 1.3% treated with steroids. This difference is not significant. The studies were then divided into those of double-blind design and those that were not. In the double-blind studies peptic ulcers were reported in 1.0% of control patients and 1.4% of steroid-treated patients.

In non-double-blind studies, only 0.4% of control patients were recorded as having peptic ulcer compared to 1.1% in the steroid treatment group. Neither difference is statistically significant, and the finding may reflect a tendency to diagnose more peptic ulceration if patients are known to be taking steroids. The authors concluded that no association existed between corticosteroid therapy and peptic ulceration in general. However, a significant increased incidence of ulceration occurred if duration of steroid therapy exceeded 30 days or a total dose of more than 1000 mg of prednisolone was given.[128]

This view remained controversial primarily because very few patients in the combined trials actually developed ulceration, only 56 of 5331. These ulcer cases were spread between 18 of 2346 control patients and 38 of 2985 treated with steroids. There is a clear trend to increased ulcer frequency with steroid treatment and the small number of ulcers gives a strong possibility of a type II statistical error, that is the erroneous negative reporting of a true association because of insufficient numbers. This point was taken up by Messer et al.[129] who expanded the analysis to include 71 controlled clinical trials with 5961 patients. Of 3064 steroid-treated patients, 55 (1.8%) had ulcers compared with 23 (0.8%) of 2897 controls. This is statistically significant and represents a relative risk of 2.3. An increased risk of gastrointestinal bleeding also occurred in the steroid-treated group.[129] Although it is true to say that the difference was not so apparent in the double-blind as in the open studies, all the trends were in favour of increased ulceration with steroid treatment even in low dosage. In general the later meta-analysis is to be preferred and it appears likely that there is an increased frequency of peptic ulceration with steroids increased by prolonged and/or high-dose treatment. The relative risk is around 2–3-fold and probably lower than many physicians believe.

Case–control studies have generally not found a significantly increased risk of peptic ulcer complications in patients receiving oral corticosteroids.[130–131] The situation is complicated by the possibility that the underlying medical condition may predispose to ulceration and also many patients on oral steroids are taking other medication including NSAIDs.[131] Two case–control studies using community-based control populations have failed to show an increased rate of peptic ulcer complications.[130–131] Indeed one suggested a reduced relative risk for steroid therapy at 0.4 but patient numbers in both studies were small.[130] In another hospital-based investigation of life-threatening ulcer complications only four of 295 patients were taking prednisolone alone compared with 141 patients prescribed NSAIDs, suggesting steroid ingestion is not an important factor in the vast majority of ulcer complications.[132]

A different approach to corticosteroid risk reviewed past drug prescription as recorded by a medical insurance programme in patients admitted with upper gastrointestinal bleeding.[133] Over 100 000 patients were eligible and 16 of 4265 exposed to steroids were admitted with bleeding. After adjustment for confounding variables a modest relative risk value of 1.4 was calculated.[133] The study did not take into account duration of therapy or dosage. Taken overall the evidence would suggest an increased risk of peptic ulceration or its complications with corticosteroid therapy probably related to dose levels but the risk is probably less than commonly supposed.

Aspirin

It is 50 years since aspirin was associated with acute gastric mucosal lesions, but there is still controversy over the exact nature of the risk. Much of the data linking aspirin ingestion with peptic, and particularly gastric ulceration is based on case–control studies, and the methodological design has been criticized. Indeed, the first of these reports did not use control groups at all and many subsequent studies used hospital controls. This may not be appropriate as patients may be taking aspirin for other reasons and community controls should be preferred. All such studies have the problem of recall bias. There are particular problems with defining the relationship with aspirin.

Aspirin is a widely available over-the-counter medication, often taken as a compound preparation and is frequently taken as a general analgesic or panacea for many conditions. It is difficult, therefore, to separate chronic aspirin users where the drug might have caused ulceration from those who took it because of pain or other symptoms after the ulcer disease began. This factor would exaggerate the possible risk of aspirin ingestion. A way round this problem is to use paracetamol as a control analgesic to determine an additional risk for aspirin ingestion. It may also be important to separate habitual chronic 'heavy' users from light intermittent acute ingestion. An additional possibility, especially as much published data relate to peptic ulcer complications, is that aspirin use may predispose not to ulceration but to the risk of bleeding or perforation.

In the early 1960s, Billington[134] pointed out a rising incidence and mortality rate for gastric ulcers in young women in Australia at a time when peptic ulceration rates were falling in other parts of the developed world. The change was particularly marked in Queensland and New South Wales and it was suggested that the cause was an exogenous ulcerogenic factor. The possible connection with aspirin ingestion was made in a series of 78 patients with chronic gastric ulcer reported from this area of whom 57 took this drug.[135] Aspirin consumption in the population of the area was high possibly because, taken as a compound preparation with phenacetin and caffeine, it had a reputation as a mild stimulant, though chronic headache was the most commonly recorded indication for its use.

For a 4-year period beginning in 1962, 118 patients from this area of Australia with perforated peptic ulcers were studied.[136] Of the 24 women in whom a drug history was available 75% took aspirin regularly. In 62.5% the drug usage was heavy,

that is at least two doses daily for 6 months prior to admission. Of the male patients 28% also admitted 'heavy' aspirin use.[136] An excess of gastric perforations was observed in those of both sexes with heavy aspirin ingestion as opposed to pyloric and duodenal perforations seen in those without this factor.[136] Analysis of gastrointestinal haemorrhage data from the same unit confirmed the increased frequency of gastric ulceration in patients taking more than two doses of aspirin per day.[137] Further support for this association came from a study of 295 patients with uncomplicated peptic ulceration.[71] A total of 55% of patients (67% of women and 44% of men) were heavy aspirin users. Aspirin ingestion in the women seemed particularly associated with gastric ulceration, 52 of 61 patients regularly taking the drug.[71] No association with duodenal ulceration was found. None of these studies included a control group.

Gillies and Skyring,[138] however, compared 150 patients with peptic ulceration (100 gastric ulcer, 50 duodenal ulcer) with age- and sex-matched hospital controls. Overall, 57% with gastric ulcer took aspirin daily compared with 22% in the controls, a highly significant difference. Patients with gastric ulcer also took aspirin in larger doses and for longer. No relationship with duodenal ulcer was observed. The increased aspirin intake of gastric ulcer patients was also apparent when compared with community controls.[139] However, this study did not distinguish between those patients in whom aspirin had exacerbated known peptic ulcer disease and those with new lesions.

This point was addressed by the Boston Collaborative Drug Surveillance Program which investigated aspirin use in both upper gastrointestinal haemorrhage and uncomplicated peptic ulcer excluding those patients known to have predisposing conditions.[140] Predisposing conditions included past diagnosis of upper gastrointestinal disease.[140] In the 25 000 admissions surveyed, regular (4 or more days per week) aspirin ingestion was significantly associated with major upper gastrointestinal bleeding compared with hospital controls (16% versus 6.9%, respectively) if haemorrhage from duodenal ulceration was excluded. The site of the bleeding, however, was not well investigated in these patients and many probably did not have gastric ulcers, but rather gastritis or gastric erosions. In those bleeding from duodenal ulceration, there was a trend for regular aspirin consumption compared with controls (11.6% vs 6.9%) but this did not reach significance.[140] Regular aspirin use was also significantly more frequent in uncomplicated gastric ulcer than in controls (19% vs 6.9%) but not in duodenal ulcer (7.9% vs. 6.9%). The study failed to show a correlation between light aspirin use, less than 4 days per week, and hospital admissions for bleeding or peptic ulceration.

Another American study suggested relative risk levels for gastrointestinal haemorrhage of 15.0 for heavy aspirin use taken within 1 week before bleeding and 5.6 for occasional use including within a week of bleeding.[141] For aspirin discontinued at least 1 week earlier, the relative risk was 1.6. These estimates seem very high and may not distinguish between aspirin taken for symptoms related to peptic disease and other non-gastrointestinal indications. This question has been addressed in a British study of gastrointestinal haemorrhage using community-based controls and using paracetamol as an analgesic control which has similar availability and indications as aspirin but which is not believed to be ulcerogenic.[142] A total of 346 matched pairs were involved and both aspirin and paracetamol ingestion were significantly increased in the patients with haemorrhage. The relative risk for aspirin exposure in the 2 days before admission was 4.8 compared to 2.1 for paracetamol.[142] This excess risk for aspirin over paracetamol extended for analgesics taken up to 2 weeks before bleeding, and was greatest for duodenal ulcer. A Dutch case–control study also suggested a relative risk for haemorrhage of 2.2 for aspirin users.[130]

Additional evidence for the ulcerogenic effect of aspirin has come from controlled trials in the cardiovascular field. The Aspirin Myocardial Infarct Study (AIMS) used 1 g aspirin daily to attempt to prevent a further myocardial infarct in 4524 patients. Symptoms suggestive of peptic ulcer or gastritis occurred in 23.7% of the aspirin group and 14.9% receiving placebo.[143] Frank upper gastrointestinal bleeding was observed in 3.3% of the patients receiving aspirin, slightly more than the 2.0% incidence in those taking placebo.[143] Another attempt to reduce mortality in myocardial infarct survivors by randomizing to either 1.5 g aspirin per day or anticoagulants resulted in 77 'critical' gastrointestinal events in the 651 patients taking aspirin over a mean of 29 months.[144] Of the patients taking aspirin, 22 (3%) patients confirmed peptic ulceration compared with 6 (1%) on oral anticoagulants.[144]

The evidence of an association between uncomplicated peptic ulceration and aspirin usage appears strongest for gastric ulcer in young to middle-aged women. However, aspirin use also increased the risk of gastrointestinal bleeding from both duodenal and gastric ulcers. The available figures suggest an approximate doubling of risk for haemorrhage with an attributable risk of 25–45/100 000 users per year.[142]

Non-aspirin non-steroidal anti-inflammatory drugs

Non-steroidal anti-inflammatory drugs (NSAIDs) have become one of the most widely prescribed groups of drugs in clinical practice. Reports of adverse events are frequent with NSAIDs and a large amount of data now associates NSAIDs with upper gastrointestinal side-effects. Much of this evidence has been reviewed by Langman.[145]

Isolated spontaneous reports to regulatory agencies have an inherent difficulty with under-reporting and probably less than 10% of adverse events are recorded. Adverse events observed during clinical trials often have the advantage of occurring during double-blind, placebo-controlled studies so that the chances of identifying those which are actually due to the drug in question are increased. However, side-effects from NSAIDs are generally infrequent in the context of the large number of prescriptions written. A meta-analysis combining 100 trials of NSAIDs reported proven ulceration in two of 821 patients given a variety of NSAIDs compared to none in 758 placebo controls.[145] Haemorrhage occurred in 24 of 1157 taking NSAIDs against 8 of 1103 on placebo. Abdominal pain and dyspepsia

was also more common in patients taking NSAIDS. It is difficult to determine from these combined trials how thoroughly ulcers were sought or even the degree of bleeding.

Retrospective case–control studies are a much more common way of studying this problem. However, recall bias may occur and careful control matching is required. Data generated from hospital notes or general practitioner letters or records must be regarded as unreliable because recording of NSAID usage is variable and possibly more likely if it is believed to be relevant to the immediate clinical problem. Nevertheless, Duggan and colleagues[146] in Australia conducted a case–control study of 180 patients with peptic ulcer (95 gastric : 85 duodenal) diagnosed at endoscopy and hospital controls, matched for age, sex and social class. Gastric ulcer was significantly associated with NSAID ingestion with a relative risk of 5.0. No increased risk was found for uncomplicated duodenal ulcer.[146] This association of NSAIDs with uncomplicated gastric ulcer, was confirmed in other Australian studies.[147,148] Duodenal ulcer was not studied. In the UK, Clinch and colleagues[149] investigated previous NSAID intake in an elderly population with upper gastrointestinal symptoms undergoing endoscopy. A highly significant association between peptic ulceration with antecedent NSAID use was found, although data collection may not have been complete.

Data are more plentiful on ulcer complications. Bartle et al.[150] in Canada found the percentage of patients with upper gastrointestinal haemorrhage taking a non-aspirin NSAID was 23.2% compared with 6.5% in controls, a significant difference. However, the control population was a strange mixture of medical inpatients and hospital visitors. In Nottingham, UK a study of bleeding peptic ulcers concentrated on those aged over 60 and believed to be at greatest risk for NSAID use and ulcer complications.[151] Both hospital and community controls were available for comparison. A total of 230 matched patients were investigated and a highly significant increased frequency of NSAID use was observed in patients with peptic ulcer over both sets of controls. The increased risk was apparent for both gastric and duodenal ulcers and men and women. The overall relative risks for ulcer cases to be non-aspirin NSAID takers over controls were 3.8 and 2.7 compared with hospital and community controls, respectively.[151] A case–control study from Holland of 161 patients with bleeding ulcer and matched hospital controls confirmed the association with NSAIDS but suggested a higher relative risk of 7.4.[130] NSAID usage was associated with bleeding gastric and duodenal ulcers in women but only reached statistical significance in men for duodenal ulceration.[130]

Perforation and bleeding data have been combined as 'life-threatening complications' in a British surgical study of 235 ulcer patients which included sudden deaths at home.[132] A total of 141 patients (60%) were taking a NSAID compared with 123 of 1246 (9.9%) of a hospital control group. However, the control group was not matched. The mortality in patients with an ulcer complication associated with NSAID was twice that of patients with no such drug history. However, patients on NSAIDS were older and had other medical conditions. The study also observed that a life-threatening emergency was the first sign of an ulcer in 58% of patients taking a NSAID.[132] A predilection for producing early complications or silent ulcers may explain the lack of association between NSAID ingestion and uncomplicated ulceration in some studies.

A third British study retrospectively recorded NSAID ingestion in 269 patients with perforated peptic ulcer and in 269 age- and sex-matched controls.[152] In those aged over 65 years, there was a highly significant association between NSAID intake and ulcer perforation. This association was not present in younger patients. The finding appears stronger for patients with perforated gastric ulcer of whom 44% were NSAID users compared with 32% of patients with duodenal ulcer. The authors drew attention to circumstantial evidence of increasing frequency of ulcer perforation in their district and the rising number of NSAID prescriptions issued nationally.[152]

The association between increasing presciption of NSAIDs and rising incidence of ulcer complications has been challenged by data from Puget Sound, Washington State.[153] Between 1977 and 1983 admissions for perforated peptic ulcer remained stable at around nine per year, while NSAID prescriptions increased fourfold. The relative rate of NSAID users being admitted with perforated ulcer over non-NSAID users was only 1.6 when adjusted for age.[153] This study had the advantage that NSAID usage was defined by prescription records not patient recall, but numbers were small. A similar study in Saskatchewan, Canada also detected no significant risk except in women over 75 years and those with a previous ulcer history.[154] However, in Michigan and Minnesota 47 136 NSAID-exposed patients were compared with 44 638 who had not taken this group of drugs and a small increase in relative risk of bleeding of 1.5 was found in NSAID users after correction for confounding variables.[133] Of 122 cases who died from peptic ulcer complications between 1976 and 1984, 34% had filed a prescription for a NSAID in the previous 30 days compared with 11% of 3897 population controls.[133] This suggests a relative risk for fatal complications of 4.7. The excess of peptic ulcer complications was confirmed in a retrospective study of 103 954 elderly Tennessee patients. Four times more current NSAID users than non-users required hospital admission for ulcer complications, with the risk particularly high for those given a prescription in the last month.[155] The fact that the risk of NSAID-induced complication is dose related rising with higher dosage is persuasive evidence that the association is causal.[155,156] Risk may vary with particular drug within the group.[155,156]

The evidence points to an association between NSAID use and particularly the development of peptic ulcer complications. This appears to have its greatest impact in those aged over 65 years. Seen from the population standpoint it has been suggested that in the UK a serious complication occurs once in every 30 000 prescriptions for NSAIDs in those under 60 years of age and once with every 3000 above this age.[157] These figures, and those from the USA, suggest approximately two cases of haemorrhage for every 11 000 patient-months of NSAID treatment.[145] Individual risk is clearly low, but NSAID use may still be responsible for at least 200 deaths per year in the UK given their widespread usage.[151] Cockel[158] has even argued that up to 90% of total ulcer deaths (4000 annually) may be due to this factor as both NSAID use and fatal ulcer complications are concentrated in the elderly and unfit.

ASSOCIATED DISEASES

With common conditions such as peptic ulceration it is easy for spurious associations to be noted. These false associations occur for several reasons which have been the subject of reviews.[159,160] Particular problems are referral bias and detection bias.[159] Referral bias leads to patients with a particular, or more than one, disease coming to medical attention at different rates. This factor alone will lead to spurious associations as patients with two diseases, for example both arthritis and peptic ulcer, may attend medical practitioners for either condition and be investigated.[159] As a result the chances of detecting either disease is enhanced and a false association observed. In detection bias the intensity of search for other pathology varies between diseases. It is currently routine to endoscope patients with chronic renal failure awaiting transplantation and as a result asymptomatic ulcer disease is frequently detected. Without similar investigation of the control group the observed association may be artificial. In addition, it has been pointed out that patients with multiple pathology are more likely to be admitted to hospital and false associations will be noted if non-hospitalized controls are used.[159] Further, many potentially important accessory features such as social class distribution or smoking habit are often ignored.[160] It is of note that the smallest surveys in any disease produce the highest prevalence of peptic ulcer and therefore strongest disease associations.[160]

In a survey of the literature then available Langman and Cooke[160] concluded that peptic ulcer is unusually frequent in chronic renal failure and possibly so in hyperparathyroidism, liver cirrhosis, cardiovascular disease (except hypertension) and chronic respiratory disease. No compelling evidence was found for association with other general medical or gastrointestinal diseases. Possible negative associations identifying conditions with a reduced incidence seem limited to pernicious anaemia with histamine-fast achlorhydria and possibly hypoadrenalism.[160]

A very high frequency of ulcer, mainly duodenal, has been found in patients in chronic renal failure receiving haemodialysis or following renal transplantation.[160] Outside of these forms of treatment the evidence that chronic uraemia predisposes to peptic ulceration appears weak.[160]

In two surveys of patients and doctors in general practice greater than expected coexistence of coronary heart disease and chronic bronchitis was found in patients with duodenal ulcer.[161,162] The relative risk for each condition was around 2.0. Chronic pulmonary disease was also found at post-mortem to occur with greater than expected frequency in patients with peptic ulceration.[57] The association of cardiovascular disease has been strengthened by other reports of associations between peptic ulceration with aortic aneurysm and aortic calcification.[160,163] Hypertension, however, has been reported to have a negative association with peptic ulcer at least in middle-aged men.[164]

Sonnenberg,[165] in an analysis of almost 2.5 million residents of West Germany who were accepted for medical rehabilitation on the basis of doctor certification, could find no association between duodenal ulcer and 'hypertensive diseases', that is either ischaemic heart disease or cerebrovascular disease. Gastric ulcer was significantly associated with ischaemic heart disease alone.[165] However, the ratio of observed to expected incidence, although statistically significant, was only 1.1. This might be explained by the presence of another independent factor common to both diseases of which smoking seems the most likely candidate.

Smoking might also underline any association between peptic ulceration and chronic pulmonary disease as a significant causal factor for both diseases. Data are controversial on whether the association of peptic ulcer with lung disease can be entirely attributed to smoking or whether the lung disease itself is an additional independent factor. The German rehabilitation data could not associate chronic obstructive pulmonary disease or asthma with either type of peptic ulcer.[165] An Australian study compared ventilatory function in 27 gastric ulcer and 29 duodenal ulcer patients with 56 age- and sex-matched controls.[166] Care was taken to match body build and socioeconomic group. Vital capacity and forced expiratory volume in 1 second were significantly reduced in both smokers and non-smokers with gastric ulcer when compared with controls. No significant differences were observed between patients with duodenal ulcer and controls.[166] These results suggest that a ventilatory function defect is present in patients with gastric ulcer not attributable to smoking alone. A prospective study of 5933 Hawaiian men of Japanese ancestry also found a forced expiratory volume in 1 second of 94% of predicted at baseline examination in those who developed a peptic ulcer over the following 20 years.[167] However, after correction for the effect of smoking no independent correlation with peptic ulcer was found.[167]

In hepatic cirrhosis an increased frequency of peptic ulceration has been recorded particularly if a portacaval anastomosis has been formed.[124,125,165] A British series has put the overall prevalence in 290 cirrhotics at 11.3% with no difference between males and females nor between those with alcoholic and non-alcoholic aetiology.[125] However, this figure and the 14.3% quoted for peptic ulceration in hyperparathyroidism is not greatly different from the total ulcer prevalence in the community.[160] The prevalence of peptic ulcer, predominantly duodenal ulcer, has been reported to be reduced in diabetes mellitus, possibly due to autonomic neuropathy.[168,169] There is an increased frequency of peptic ulceration in rheumatoid arthritis but this may relate to drug treatment.[160]

Another possible way of investigating the association of common medical conditions with peptic ulceration is the analysis of survival after peptic ulcer surgery. It is generally recognized that there is an increased late mortality after curative peptic ulcer surgery, the effect beginning 12–20 years postoperatively,[170,172] although not apparent in all studies.[173] The reduced survival found in most studies is quite small, 4 years or 92% relative survival rate.[171,172] However, the excess mortality is almost totally related to smoking-associated disease particularly bronchial carcinoma, mostly in men.[170,172] There was no

increase and possibly a decrease in death from cerebrovascular and ischaemic heart disease.[172,173] These findings suggest the association of peptic ulceration with chronic pulmonary disease, hypertension and atherosclerosis is not strong.

PSYCHOLOGICAL FACTORS

Anecdotal evidence has long associated psychological stress in the aetiology of peptic ulceration. Within this concept are two broad but related aspects. Peptic ulcer patients may be exposed to more life stress than unaffected individuals or alternatively may have a 'personality-type' which predisposes to the disease. The former possibility has been investigated in several studies.[174,176] In neither chronic gastric nor duodenal ulcer patients could an increase in frequency of stressful life events in the 2 years prior to ulcer diagnosis or relapse be demonstrated over controls in the community.[174,175] Another study of 49 men with peptic ulcer confirmed no increase in the number of stressful life events over both healthy male controls and patients with renal stones or gallstones.[176]

The question of a 'personality-type', predisposing to ulcer production is more difficult. This has been investigated prospectively. Paffenbarger et al.[120] correlated the psychological traits, both self- and physician assessed, recorded in 26 954 students while at Harvard University or the University of Pennsylvania with those who developed peptic ulceration over the next 35 years. None of the 10 recorded traits which included nervousness and feelings of persecution distinguished the 487 ex-students with ulceration from the remainder.[107] However, a case–control study comparing 163 ex-students, again from Harvard, who had died of peptic ulceration and 163 age- and sex-matched controls suggested that, while at university, the group that later developed ulcer complained of more somatic symptoms such as palpitation and sleeplessness.[177] This finding might suggest a difference in life experience or basic personality.

Prospective studies using data collected before disease onset must be preferable to retrospective studies where recall bias may be operating. Nevertheless when 132 peptic ulcer patients were matched with the same number of population controls and asked an exhaustive list of personal, employment and personality details, no differences could be found in relation to psychiatric morbidity, type A personality, personal worries or the demands of work.[178] In contrast, 181 gastric ulcer sufferers in a similar study were found to display personality differences from the normal population.[179] Traits of tough mindedness, anxiety and submissiveness were found to be characteristic of gastric ulcer patients. These findings are difficult to interpret as some of the personality features appear to be contradictory. It was speculated that this represented 'internal conflict', and predisposed to ulceration.[179]

Another study confirmed abnormal personality traits in ulcer patients but no one type was found consistently.[176] Excessive dependency, hypochondriasis and low ego strength were the best discriminators.[176] A cohort study of 50-year-old patients observed for two decades identified no abnormal personality traits prior to developing peptic ulcer but differences after the diagnosis.[180] This suggests that any personality trait is a consequence of the disease rather than the cause of it. Another possibility that should be noted is that either stress or personality differences may not predispose to ulcer formation, but make certain individuals more likely to seek medical advice, that is they exhibit 'learned illness behaviour'.

It is clear that stress, either acute or chronic and personality have complex interactions and a single simple ulcer personality type has not been identified. More recent research has tended to accept that no increase in frequency of stressful life events occurs in ulcer patients, but investigated whether the same stress is perceived differently from control individuals.[176,181,182] Patients with duodenal ulcer did not perceive the hypothetical effect that 81 potential life events would have on them more strongly than controls.[182] However, patients with ulcer have been reported to perceive real problems more negatively.[183] More sophisticated techniques of identifying the degree and effect of stress have suggested that chronic stress of over 6 months duration involving marked goal frustration were significantly and independently associated with the onset and relapse of duodenal ulcers.[181] Patients who perceived themselves as stressed were 1.8 times more likely to develop a peptic ulcer compared with non-stressed individuals according to a survey of 4511 US adults.[184] An individuals perception and response to stress rather than the stressor itself may be the crucial factor.

The same effects were found with acute stress, but only if it constituted severe immediate threat.[181] This finding might relate to the peak of ulcer perforation found during the acute stress of wartime bombing. The relationship between stress, psychological factors and peptic ulceration, at present rather weak and confused, may become clearer with better assessment of the effects of both stress and personality. No particular ulcer-prone personality type has so far been identified.

GENETIC FACTORS

Genetic factors have long been assumed to be important in peptic ulceration because of the familial clustering of cases. A positive family history of ulcer disease is found in 20–50% of patients with peptic ulcer compared with only 5–15% of controls.[185,186] More accurate assessment of the degree of increased prevalence in families has been provided by study of all relatives of ulcer patients. Doll and Buch[186] reported a frequency of ulcer disease 2–3 times greater in first-degree relatives of patients with peptic ulcer than in relatives of controls or in the general population. The relative risk for relatives of patients with gastric ulcer was 1.8 compared with relatives of controls and 2.6 for relatives of patients with duodenal ulcer. This tendency for ulcer cases to run in families has been been amply confirmed.[187,188]

Doll and Kellock[189] in a further study went on to demonstrate that peptic ulcer in relatives of gastric ulcer sufferers tended to be gastric ulcers and conversely relatives of patients with duodenal ulcer tended to have duodenal ulcers. Indeed, almost the entire excess of peptic ulcer in relatives of patients with ulcer was due to an increased rate of ulceration at the same site as the patient. This clear tendency for ulcer site to be concordant was very highly significant and was independent of sex, generational effect or social class.[189]

The finding of separate inheritance of gastric and duodenal ulcer was subsequently confirmed by Monson.[187] Doll and Kellock[189] suggested that the predisposition to develop combined gastric and duodenal ulcer was also inherited separately from isolated ulceration at either site. Thus four of 18 relatives of patients with combined gastric and duodenal ulceration also had both types of ulcer whereas combined ulcers occurred in only two of 111 relatives of patients with isolated gastric or duodenal ulcers. However, the numbers are too small for a definite conclusion.

Familial aggregation of peptic ulcer might, of course, be the result of environmental rather than genetic factors. Twin studies have shown concordance for peptic ulceration is greater in identical (monozygotic) than in fraternal (dizygotic) pairs.[185] In a thorough Danish study published in 1972 both individuals were affected in 53% of identical twin pairs compared with only 36% for fraternal twins.[185,190] These findings, although reporting higher concordance rates than previous studies imply that ulcer disease is not entirely genetically determined as concordance did not reach 100% in identical twins. However, they do suggest that a large part of familial aggregation may be genetically determined. These family studies have been admirably reviewed by Rotter.[185] It is noteworthy that again ulcer site was usually concordant within twin pairs supporting the genetic differentiation of gastric and duodenal ulcers.

Genetic markers have been extensively investigated to determine potential associations with peptic ulcer disease. Probably the best documented, with consistent reports running into the hundreds, is the association with ABO blood groups.[185] Aird and colleagues[191] in 1954 noted that 74.6% of patients with peptic ulcer were blood group O compared to only 68.5% of controls, a highly statistically significant increased prevalence. The increased risk for individuals with blood group O is not great at about 30–40% over all other groups.

The relationship of blood group O to peptic ulcer seems to be particularly strong for duodenal ulcer and patients with combined duodenal and gastric ulcers. On the other hand isolated gastric ulcers can be divided into two types depending on blood group association. Johnson et al.[192] reported that gastric ulcers of the body of the stomach, that is proximal to the gastric angulus, do not show an association with blood group O but rather a modest excess of group A. Patients with pre-pyloric ulcers, distal to the angulus, on the other hand behaved like those with duodenal ulcers with a relative frequency of blood group O of 1.58:1 recorded over other blood groups.[192] However, a study in Prague, Czechoslovakia could find no association between gastric ulceration and blood group although site was not taken into account.[193] Blood group O has also been reported by several investigators to predispose to ulcer complications, particularly bleeding, although curiously not to surgical intervention.[193,194]

The pathophysiological basis of the association of peptic ulcer with blood group remains unclear. Langman and Doll[194] suggested the association was related to the predisposition of ulcer patients with blood group O to bleed and hence seek medical attention. This cannot be the entire explanation as the association is still apparent even when patients with bleeding are excluded.[185] Another hypothesis links blood group O to acid hypersecretion, as defined by maximal acid output and serum pepsinogen I, and thereby to duodenal and prepyloric ulceration.[195] However, a literature review concluded no consistent relationship had been delineated.[185] Indeed more recent work has suggested blood group O is only associated with duodenal ulcer patients who present over the age of 30 and who do not show acid hypersecretion[86,192] but other studies do not confirm this.[83]

Peptic ulcer has also been associated with the inherited ability of some people to secrete their ABO blood group substances into body fluids, particularly saliva but also gastric juice.[185,196,197] Individuals with this ability (secretors) or inabilty (non-secretors) inherit the property independent of ABO blood group. People with blood group O may or may not secrete a non-group specific H-substance antigen and therefore can also be defined as secretors or non-secretors. H-substance can also be secreted by individuals of A, B and AB blood types. Non-secretors of whatever ABO blood group are 40–80% more likely to have a duodenal ulcer than secretors.[185,196] The association is also apparent for gastric ulcers although the increased incidence in non-secretors is less at 20–40%.[185,196]

The risks for ABO blood group and ABH secretion ability are independent and therefore multiplicative.[185] Individuals who are both blood group O and non-secretor are therefore calculated to be at a 2.5-fold increased risk of developing a duodenal ulcer.[185] Non-secretors have been reported to come to operation more often than secretors, although there is no difference in frequency of bleeding.[194] The reason for this observation is obscure as is the mechanism underlying the increased ulcer risk. An effect on duodenal and gastric defence perhaps via mucus has been suggested but is still speculative.[194,195]

The mucosal lining of the stomach contains four types of aspartic proteinases that are distinguishable immunologically and have the ability to hydrolyse proteins at acid pH. Two of these are pepsinogens, pepsinogen I and pepsinogen II, and two are cathepsins, slow-moving proteinase and cathepsin D.[198] Pepsinogen I has been extensively studied as it is found only in the chief and mucus neck cells of the gastric fundus and levels can be measured in the serum.[199] As a quantitative relationship is believed to exist between gastric chief and parietal cells, elevated serum pepsinogen I levels have been considered to identify individuals with an increased parietal cell mass.[198] Further twin studies have suggested that serum pepsinogen I levels may be genetically determined allowing its use as a genetic marker in ulcer disease.[200]

Samloff et al.[199] compared serum pepsinogen I levels in 924 subjects, including 300 healthy controls, 389 hospital controls, seven patients with Zollinger–Ellison syndrome and 77 patients with duodenal ulcer. The 'normal' range was wide, but almost two-thirds (64%) of duodenal ulcer sufferers had serum levels of pepsinogen I above the upper limit. Serum pepsinogen I levels were grossly raised in Zollinger–Ellison syndrome. In the small number of patients with combined gastric and duodenal ulcers or prepyloric gastric ulcers approximately half had high pepsinogen I values, but elevated serum levels were found in only 21% of the remaining patients with gastric ulcer. Two further observations were made in this study.[199] Women were consistently found to have lower serum pepsinogen I levels than men of the same age. In addition, the distribution of serum pepsinogen I was bimodal in patients with duodenal ulcer disease but unimodal in both groups of controls.[199] This finding suggests that patients with duodenal ulcer might be separable into two populations according to pepsinogen I levels. If, as proposed, a high serum pepsinogen I correlates with increased parietal cell mass and therefore excess acid output, these two populations may have different pathophysiological mechanisms underlying their disease.[199]

Serum pepsinogens I and II have also been found in a prospective study to identify individuals with a risk of developing ulcer disease, both duodenal and gastric.[201,202] In a large cohort of Hawaiian men followed for 14 years, 115 developed a gastric ulcer and 47 a duodenal ulcer.[202] In comparison to the control group, premorbid serum pepsinogens I and II were significantly higher in patients who subsequently developed ulcer disease.[202] Serum pepsinogen I was highest in duodenal ulcer cases whereas pepsinogen II was highest in gastric ulcer. A low pepsinogen I/pepsinogen II ratio was particularly associated with gastric ulceration. Individuals with this pattern were 10 times more likely to develop a gastric rather than a duodenal ulcer.[202]

Studies of families with a history of ulcer disease has allowed Rotter and colleagues[200] to identify two large kindreds in whom an elevated serum pepsinogen I segregated between generations as an autosomal dominant trait. Further, 10 of 11 patients with clinical duodenal ulcer disease in these families had hyperpepsinogenaemia. The single discrepant individual had had a partial gastrectomy which will lower serum pepsinogen levels. However, eight family members had high serum pepsinogen I values without apparent ulcer disease.[200] An elevated serum pepsinogen I may therefore identify some, but not all, patients with duodenal ulcer in particular. This may be especially true when there is a strong family history of ulcer disease, so that serum pepsinogen I may be valuable as a genetic marker for a proportion of ulcer disease patients.[185]

There is evidence which suggests that *Helicobacter pylori* infection contributes at least in part to the hyperpepsinogenaemia found in peptic ulceration.[203,204] The data linking hyperpepsinogenaemia and duodenal ulceration will have to be re-examined in the light of this new evidence.

Peptic ulcer has been associated with a number of other inherited genetic markers. These include rhesus positivity, ability to taste phenylthiourea, alpha-1-antitrypsin deficiency, HLA-B5 and glucose-6-phosphatase deficiency. The data have been reviewed by Rotter[185] but in general the associations are weak and based on a small number of reports. Probably the best documented is rhesus positivity but the relative risk ascribed to this marker is only 1.1:1. Further, the relationship of peptic ulcer with phenylthiourea taste sensitivity could not be demonstrated in one report despite a study design with substantial power to detect at least a twofold difference in incidence.[205] This again suggests that the relationship of ulcer disease with this genetic factor is weak. All these associations together cannot account for more than a tiny proportion of peptic ulcer disease and moreover give no clue to an underlying mechanism of ulcer production.

An alternative to identifying inherited genetic markers is to separate on the basis of phenotypic differences. In the case of ulcer disease this would manifest as differences in clinical presentation, complications or disease course. Lam and Ong[85] studying a Chinese population in Hong Kong divided patients according to the age of onset of symptoms. Those subjects whose symptoms began before the age of 20 years (early onset) reported a significantly stronger family history of dyspepsia than those with symptoms beginning after 30 years of age (late onset). A positive family history is also often found in children with duodenal ulcer.[80] Lam and Ong[85] found an excess of blood group O only in the late-onset patients whereas A,B and AB subjects predominated in the younger ulcer patients. Blood group distribution in the early onset group was similar to controls. Clinical presentation also varied between groups. Gastrointestinal haemorrhage was the predominant complication in the early onset group despite the lack of predominance of blood group O individuals who have a tendency to bleed. In contrast, ulcers in the late onset patients had an increased rate of perforation and were more often multiple or led to pyloric stenosis.[85]

Kang[83] has confirmed many of these findings in Singapore. In his series, patients with duodenal ulcer with symptom onset during the first three decades were more likely to be men, to have a family history of dyspepsia and to have had a gastrointestinal haemorrhage than patients presenting later. Maximal acid output was also higher in the early-onset patients. The mean increase was around 22%, 28.4 mmol/h versus 23.5 mmol/h in early and late groups, respectively. Early-onset patients with gastric ulceration were also more likely to be men than those presenting later, but the two groups were similar with respect to family history of dyspepsia, history of gastrointestinal bleeding and gastric acid output.[83]

Lam et al.[86] have also proposed dividing the duodenal ulcer population into two subgroups, but in more than one way. Separated on the basis of age, early onset patients (symptoms beginning under age 30) were confirmed to have an excess of men, more gastrointestinal bleeding, no significant blood group O predominance and more acid hypersecretors than a later onset group. These findings are consistent in both Chinese living in Hong Kong and a Scottish population in Edinburgh.[86] However, in the Scottish patients familial late-onset duodenal ulcers with acid hypersecretion formed another distinct subgroup.

As separation on the basis of symptoms before 30 years of age is clearly arbitrary, the authors also distinguished patient groups on the criteria of maximum acid secretory capacity, corrected for body weight. Two subgroups again emerged.[86] The first was composed of patients with a stimulated acid output within the normal range, who had an increased likelihood of gastrointestinal haemorrhage, perforation and being blood group O, whose peak age of onset fell in the fourth decade and who did not usually have a family history of ulcer disease.

In contrast, acid hypersecretors (defined as a stimulated maximal acid output greater than 2 standard deviations above the mean) with duodenal ulcer were predominantly blood groups A, B and AB, tended to have an early age of onset (in the third decade) and a strong family history of peptic ulcer disease.[86] The prevalence of a family history again suggests genetic factors are influencing ulcer disease at least in this latter group of duodenal ulcer subjects.

The separation of duodenal ulcer patients by maximal acid output introduces the concept that duodenal ulcer patients might be distinguishable by physiological testing of subclinical markers which in turn may be genetically determined. However, it is quite possible that acquired factors, such as *H. pylori* infection, might influence gastric acid output.[206] Acid secretory capacity and elevated pepsinogen I levels have already been mentioned as possible discriminatory properties, but an exaggerated serum gastrin response to a meal, increased sensitivity of acid stimulation to gastrin, impaired inhibition of gastrin and acid secretion by gastric acid or antral distension and an increased rate of gastric emptying have all been reported in some patients with duodenal ulcer.[185] However, it must be clearly emphasized that none of these abnormalities is found in all ulcer patients.

Study of the genetics of peptic ulcer disease is particularly difficult in a condition in which environmental factors are probably important and few reliable or easily measurable subclinical genetic markers are available. The failure to demonstrate a consistent abnormality, either clinically or subclinically, in all patients and the epidemiological pattern of the disease means the bulk of peptic ulcer disease cannot be explained by a single Mendelian genetic defect.

There are two current hypotheses to explain the genetics of ulcer disease. The first is polygenic inheritance.[185] This concept suggests the hereditary component of a disease reflects the combined contribution of many genes, resulting in a continuum of genetic predisposition to the illness. Clinical disease would thus depend on the presence of a sufficient number of these genes, probably in association with environmental factors, to push each individual case beyond a 'threshold'. The alternative hypothesis is that of genetic heterogeneity.[185,207] This theory implies that a clinical disorder is, in reality, a group of distinct diseases with a variety of aetiologies and pathophysiological mechanisms, both genetic and non-genetic, which result in a similar clinical syndrome.

Rotter has argued convincingly that genetic heterogeneity probably underlies peptic ulcer disease particularly duodenal ulceration.[185,207] The evidence for this assertion is based on several well-documented findings. The separate inheritance of gastric and duodenal ulcer has long been recognized.[189] Within duodenal ulceration arbitrary division on the basis of age of symptom onset still distinguishes broad patient groups with and without a positive family history and characterized by an abnormal physiological marker in excess acid secretion.[83,86] Other subclinical physiological markers such as rapid gastric emptying or altered gastrin response to a meal may be important properties of other subgroups.[185] These findings would suggest or at least are consistent with separate inheritance.

Further powerful evidence in favour of genetic hetero-geneity is the observation of a bimodal distribution of serum pepsinogen I in patients with duodenal ulcer which is not apparent in control populations suggesting a subpopulation with genetically determined elevated levels.[199] Particularly important in the support for genetic heterogeneity is the small number of distinct but rare inherited clinical syndromes with peptic ulceration as a prominent feature. These are multiple endocrine adenomatosis type I (including Zollinger–Ellison), systemic mastocytosis and the recently described tremor–nystagmus–ulcer syndrome.[185] Family studies have also identi-fied two ulcer kindreds with autosomal dominant hyper-pepsinogenaemia.[200] The point is not lost that all these patients with a clear genetic predisposition to ulceration would, before the description of specific syndromes, have been incorporated into the mass of peptic ulcer disease. On the basis of these findings Rotter[185] has suggested a genetic classification of peptic ulcer as shown in Table 27.5. Although this must be regarded as tentative at present, the separation of peptic ulcer on genetic and physiological criteria is begin-ning to be attempted.

Table 27.5 Genetic classification of peptic ulcer (proposed by Rotter)

I. Peptic ulcer associated with rare genetic syndromes
   A. Multiple endocrine adenomatosis I
   B. Systemic mastocytosis
   C. Tremor–nystagmus–ulcer syndrome
II. Gastric ulcer
III. Combined gastric and duodenal ulcer
IV. Hyperpepsinogenaemic I duodenal ulcer
   A. Without postprandial hypergastrinaemia
   B. With postprandial hypergastrinaemia
V. Normopepsinogenaemic I duodenal ulcer
   A. Without rapid gastric emptying
   B. With rapid gastric emptying
VI. Childhood duodenal ulcer
VII. (Immunological form of duodenal ulcer)
VII. Peptic ulcer associated with other chronic diseases
   A. Peptic ulcer and chronic lung disease
   B. Duodenal ulcer and renal stones
   C. (Duodenal ulcer and coronary artery disease)

The more tentative entities are indicated in brackets (see Rotter[185]).

Genetic heterogeneity and polygenic inheritance are not mutually exclusive and within the various heterogeneous forms of ulcer disease some may prove to be polygenic in origin. Nevertheless, the mucopolysaccharidoses, hyperlipidaemia and even diabetes mellitus all previously thought to be either a sin-gle disease or display polygenic inheritance are now believed to be examples of genetically heterogeneous conditions. The genetic features of peptic ulceration can also be explained most readily on this basis although environmental factors, possibly interacting with genetic predisposition, are likely to be of particular importance in determining who develops clinical disease.

HELICOBACTER PYLORI

The association between chronic gastritis and peptic ulceration has been known for some time.[208–211] However, the isolation in 1983 by Marshall and Warren[212] of curved bacteria from gastric antral biopsies of patients with chronic antral gastritis and pep-tic ulcer has suggested an important new factor in the patho-genesis of both conditions.[213,214] The organism identified is a microaerophilic Gram-negative spiral-shaped bacterium which is found beneath the mucus on the surface of gastric epithelial cells. It is not found on small bowel mucosa or areas of intesti-nal metaplasia within the stomach. The bacterium is able to move within the gastric mucus and clusters around intercellular junctions, protected from the acidic environment by a powerful urease enzyme which produces ammonia from urea, and by bicarbonate secreted into the mucus layer by the underlying gastric epithelium. The bacterium was originally designated a 'Campylobacter-like organism' and successively called *Campylobacter pyloridis* and *C. pylori*. Several structural fea-tures not present in other *Campylobacter* species have led to its reclassification in a new genus as *Helicobacter pylori*.[215]

The strongest case for a pathological role for *H. pylori* is in gastritis.[216,217] Type A gastritis is the autoimmune form linked to pernicious anaemia, occurring mainly in the fundus of the stomach and not strongly associated with *H. pylori* carriage. Type B gastritis, however, is found predominantly in the antrum of the stomach and histologically the mucosa is inflamed and infiltrated with plasma cells, lymphocytes and often neutrophils. Between 80 and 100% of patients, including children, with histologically proven chronic active Type B gas-tritis, have *H. pylori* present in the gastric mucosa.[217–221] This observation has been repeated on numerous occasions and appears to be true regardless of geographical location or racial group.[217] Conversely *H. pylori* is rarely present in entirely nor-mal stomachs.[216,218] Two normal volunteers deliberately ingested live *H. pylori* and both developed gastritis.[222,223] In one case the illness was self-limiting but in the other a persistent gastritis developed from which *H. pylori* could be isolated.

Although *H. pylori* is therefore widely regarded as causal of type B chronic gastritis, the organism's relationship to peptic ulcer disease is less clear. Around 80% of patients with gastric ulceration have an associated chronic antral gastritis in which *H. pylori* can be demonstrated.[224,225] However, this does not nec-essarily mean that *H. pylori* is a contributory cause in gastric ulceration as it has been suggested that the bacterium might colonize damaged epithelium secondarily. There is none the less evidence that eradication of *H. pylori* may reduce relapse rates in gastric ulceration.[226–228] There are fewer trials of *H. pylori* eradication in gastric compared to duodenal ulceration but reviews confirm the observation.[228] NSAID-use may be an independent aetiological factor, especially in *H. pylori* negative cases.

The evidence is more compelling in duodenal ulceration. Reviews combining multiple publications report 86–100% of duodenal ulcer patients as having *H. pylori*-associated chronic antral gastritis.[220,228,229] *H. pylori* has also been identified in areas of gastric metaplasia in the duodenum, usually associated with duodenitis, which may help to clarify the role of an organism associated with gastric epithelium in the pathogenesis of duodenal ulcer formation.[230] Indeed in a survey of 137 subjects, 90 with active or inactive duodenal ulcer disease and 47 normals, the presence of duodenal infection with *H. pylori* conferred a 51 times greater risk of duodenal ulceration.[231] *H. pylori* infection in the gastric antrum increased the likelihood of duodenal ulceration only 7.6-fold.[231] The close link between *H. pylori* infection and peptic ulceration, both gastric and particularly duodenal, has been repeated many times and must now be regarded as true.[228] However, the observed association between *H. pylori* and duodenal ulceration might, again in principle, merely reflect bacterial superinfection of damaged mucosa, particularly areas of gastric metaplasia in the duodenum produced by excess luminal acid. A direct cause–effect relationship between *H. pylori* colonization and ulcer disease has not been strictly proven.[232]

Evidence for an aetiological role for *H. pylori* in duodenal ulcer disease comes from the demonstration that eradication of the organism alters the natural history of the disease by reducing ulcer relapse rate. Before *H. pylori* was identified it had been observed that the one-year recurrence rates for duodenal ulcers healed with bismuth-containing compounds was approximately 55% compared with around 85% for ulcers healed with H₂-receptor antagonists. Bismuth-containing compounds have subsequently been shown to suppress and in some cases eradicate *H. pylori* infection suggesting *H. pylori* status influences duodenal ulcer relapse.[234]

This important point has now been investigated in numerous studies.[228] Coghlan and colleagues[234] healed acute duodenal ulcers with either cimetidine or colloidal bismuth and assessed *H. pylori* status at endoscopy at the end of treatment. Without maintenance treatment, 19 of 24 (79%) who were *H. pylori* positive at the end of active treatment suffered an endoscopically confirmed relapse within 1 year compared to only four of the 15 (27%) who were *H. pylori* negative.[234] However, assessment of *H. pylori* status close to the end of active treatment may be misleading because infection may be suppressed rather than eradicated. Indeed three of the four patients reported by Coghlan et al. as relapses although initially *H. pylori* negative had gastritis and evidence of infection at the time of ulcer recurrence. Marshall et al.[235] randomized duodenal ulcer patients into four different treatment regimens including antibiotics aimed at eradicating *H. pylori*. *H. pylori* status was determined 2 weeks after the end of treatment and no maintenance treatment given. When *H. pylori* was cleared at this time the 12-month relapse rate was 21% (5 of 24) compared to 84% (37 of 44) when *H. pylori* infection persisted, a highly significant (P < 0.0001) difference. The study also observed that *H. pylori* status influenced acute ulcer healing. Only 61% of acute ulcers healed when *H. pylori* was not eradicated compared with a 92% healing rate when it was (P < 0.001).[235]

Rauws and Tytgat[236] chose to study only patients with severe duodenal ulcer disease, that is breakthrough ulceration on maintenance H₂-receptor antagonists or frequent relapse off such treatment. All patients were *H. pylori* positive before treatment and they were given a 4-week course of colloidal bismuth either alone or with two antibiotics, metronidazole and amoxycillin, in an attempt to eradicate *H. pylori* infection. *H. pylori* status was determined after a further 4 weeks of treatment with ranitidine 150 mg daily alone. Of the 38 patients who completed the study with healed ulcers 17 were *H. pylori* negative a month after active treatment.[236] All but two of the patients in whom the infection was eradicated had received 'triple therapy' with colloidal bismuth and both antibiotics. During one year of follow-up none of the 17 *H. pylori*-negative subjects relapsed compared with 17 of the 21 (81%) with persistent infection. Nine patients whose ulcer disease recurred and who had remained positive for *H. pylori* were subsequently given 'triple therapy'. *H. pylori* was eradicated in seven and no ulcer relapses occurred in these individuals over the next 12 months.[236]

A similar study from New South Wales, Australia also targeted recurrent or resistant duodenal ulcer disease which had failed to respond to or relapsed after H₂-receptor antagonist treatment.[237] A total of 78 patients received 4 weeks of H₂-receptor antagonists followed by 'triple therapy' (colloidal bismuth subcitrate, tetracycline and metronidazole) over the following 4 weeks. *H. pylori* status was assessed after a further month without treatment. Ulcers healed in all 78 and *H. pylori* was eradicated in 75 (96%). At 1 year follow-up 73 patients were available for re-endoscopy of whom 71 remained *H. pylori* negative and free of duodenal ulceration. The two *H. pylori*-positive subjects had endoscopic duodenitis but no ulcer. At 2 years follow-up 57 patients were re-endoscoped and all remained free of infection and ulceration. Of 34 subjects evaluated at 3 years 33 also had neither reinfection nor ulceration and the same was true for all 15 patients followed for 4 years.[237] Other studies have confirmed that eradication of *H. pylori* infection appears to reduce the risk of duodenal ulcer relapse even in aggressive and recurrent disease or those with complications.[238–240] The same observation has been made in at least 15 well-conducted clinical trials involving over 1000 patients and the evidence mounts almost daily.[228] This remains the strongest evidence that *H. pylori* is important in the pathogenesis of duodenal ulceration and alters the natural history of the disease.

Demonstration of increased risk of developing an ulcer with increased density of *H. pylori* infection, that is a biological gradient in the association would support a cause–effect relationship. Khulusi et al.[241] showed that in *H. pylori*-infected patients the mean density of the organism was seven times greater in the antrum in those with a duodenal ulcer compared with those without an ulcer. They further suggested that there may be a critical value of infection density below which duodenal ulceration is not found. Alam et al.[242] also reported that duodenal but not gastric ulcers were associated with increased *H. pylori* infection density. These observations together with the varying virulence of *H. pylori* strains may explain why relatively few patients infected with the organism develop ulcer disease.

If the role of *H. pylori* in peptic ulcer disease is confirmed as causal, the epidemiology of the infection in the community will clearly be pertinent. In epidemiological surveys indirect methods, rather than endoscopy and histology, are used to identify those with *H. pylori* infection. Commonly these are either serological tests assessing serum IgG antibodies to *H. pylori* or urea breath tests utilizing the ability of the organism's urease enzyme to break down urea.[243,244] It is generally assumed that the presence of anti-*H. pylori* antibodies indicates active infection with the organism which it is believed rarely clears spontaneously once established.[245,246] This view has been challenged in a Swiss study where only 24 of 49 healthy people with anti-*H. pylori* antibodies had evidence of active colonization as assessed by a positive urea breath test.[247] This might suggest a more dynamic process with significant spontaneous eradication over time but confirmation is needed. In 441 of 490 asymptomatic individuals studied in Houston, Texas the results of serological and urea breath testing were concordant.[248] In only around 9% (44 of 490) was there positive serological testing with a negative urea breath test.[248]

In initial evaluations of serological testing a close relationship was established between the presence of serum antibodies, histological gastritis and the culture of the organism from gastric mucus.[245,246] At present it is not known whether infections may be spontaneously cleared as in one volunteer who deliberately ingested the organism.[223]

H. pylori infection is found worldwide. However, most data on its epidemiology infection relate to Westernized relatively developed countries and are almost certainly not applicable to other regions or ethnic groups. In Western societies the overall prevalence of the infection in the community has been estimated at between 20 and 60%.[243,246,248–252] All studies have shown the prevalence rates to be heavily age dependent.[252] Infection is rare in children in developed societies. In Newcastle, England, less than 1% of children under 5 years are seropositive for *H. pylori* IgG and less than 6% show evidence of infection between the ages of 5 and 16 years.[253] In Finland 4.6% of 3-year olds tested in 1980 were seropositive.[254] Similarly only 5% of French children have *H. pylori* antibodies by the age of 10 years.[255] Jones et al.[246] in Manchester, England found serum antibodies in only 10 of 260 (4%) control individuals under 20 years of age. A higher prevalence was reported from Edinburgh, Scotland with 11% of 7 year olds seropositive for *H. pylori*.[256]

Over the age of 20 there is an increasing prevalence of *H. pylori* infection in asymptomatic subjects. Seropositivity rates were estimated in Manchester to be 19% between the ages of 21 and 30 rising to plateau at 49% in those aged over 60 years.[246] Very similar levels were reported from Leeds with 50% of those over 50 infected.[243] Investigation of 749 randomly selected men from Caerphilly, South Wales demonstrated the prevalence of positive *H. pylori* antibodies rising sharply in middle age from 29.3% in those aged 30–34 years to over 60% in those aged 45 and over.[251] In the elderly rates were even higher with 75% of men aged 70–75 years seropositive.[251]

These observations have been repeated elsewhere in developed societies. In a Finnish study of healthy blood donors the prevalence of infection in those over 50 years was also over 50%.[250] In the USA, prevalence rates of *H. pylori* antibody among 485 asymptomatic volunteers also rose progressively

from around 30% at age 25, to 55% at age 55 and to 80% at 75 years.[248] This trend has been a consistent finding in previous North American studies.[249,257] Increasing *H. pylori* prevalence with age has now been reported in populations from all major continents in the world.[255]

In developing countries the association of *H. pylori* with chronic gastritis and peptic ulcer remains very strong but the epidemiological pattern of asymptomatic disease is different. Prevalence still rises with age but infection as evidenced by *H. pylori* antibody seroconversion occurs more frequently and at a younger age. Thus, 17.5% of children in Thailand have antibodies by the age of 9 and in Gambia, West Africa 15% of babies are seropositive by 20 months and 46% by 60 months.[258,259] Below the age of 10 years around 50% of children in the Ivory Coast and Algeria have *H. pylori* antibodies, a level not reached in Western societies until 45–50 years of age.[255] Infection rates in poor Brazilian children increased progressively from 16.4% in those aged 1 month to 2 years to 64.3% in 15–18 year olds. This latter figure is above the overall population prevalence in many developed countries.[260] However, 9-year-old children in rural Colombia are almost all (87%) infected so *H. pylori* carriage may become universal in some societies.[261] In a small study Graham et al.[262] found *H. pylori* infection rates in 20–29 year olds to be 21, 67, 33 and 46% for those from the USA, China, Mexico and India, respectively. The difference between the USA and China was confirmed in a larger survey of the same age group.[263] Rates in older adults may be even higher with prevalences of 80–90% found in asymptomatic individuals in West Africa and Algeria.[255] This observation was confirmed in Hyderabad, India where the prevalence of *H. pylori* infection in an asymptomatic population of lower socioeconomic class was over 80% by the age of 20 years.[264] A notable exception to this trend is the Australian Aborigines who have a very low rate of both *H. pylori* infection and peptic ulcer.[265]

Other reports from South America,[252,266] Africa[255,267,268] and the USA[248,252,269] have shown a similarly high prevalence of *H. pylori* antibodies among poor population groups and in economically deprived areas. It is tempting to suggest that differences in prevalence relate to standards of hygiene and other socioeconomic conditions, such as poor housing and large family size. However, as with epidemiological factors associated with peptic ulcer, it is difficult to seperate diet, social habits and socioeconomic conditions from geographical and genetic factors. Nevertheless, the frequency of *H. pylori* infection is significantly higher in Blacks (70%) than Whites (34%) occupying the same metropolitan area of the USA.[248] This difference remains after adjustment for age, gender, educational level, income and tobacco and alcohol consumption. There were significant inverse correlations between both income and educational attainment and *H. pylori* infection, prevalence being lower in better educated high-income groups in both white and black populations.[248] Similarly in the UK, *H. pylori* infection in Welsh men was lowest in social classes I and II, intermediate in class III and highest in groups IV and V.[251] The differences were most marked for the youngest age group. Between the ages of 30 and 34 the prevalence rate for social classes IV and V

(57.9%) is five times the rate in classes I and II (11.1%). Evidence for an association between low socioeconomic circumstances and therefore poor housing conditions with overcrowding is accumulating. Patel et al.[256] observed that independent risk factors for *H. pylori* infection in children in Edinburgh, Scotland were single parent family status, crowded homes and living in rented-housing estates, all factors likely to correlate with low income. Median family income was also a strong predictor of seropositivity among US Army recruits even after controlling for the effect of race.[270] In a retrospective analysis of 471 male factory workers in Stoke, England subjects were twice as likely to have *H. pylori* infection if during childhood their home was crowded or they regularly shared a bed.[271] Galpin et al.[272] confirmed this association and also suggested that indoor toilet facilities in childhood correlated with *H. pylori* infection rates. However, the association of seropositivity with other measures of poor childhood hygiene, particularly a fixed hot water supply and indoor bathroom and toilet was not confirmed in another British study.[273] Similar findings have been made in the USA among Black and Hispanic populations where high *H. pylori* infection rates correlated with poor childhood conditions as judged by family income and occupation.[274]

Socioeconomic factors are also important in less-developed countries. In Korea an inverse relationship between economic factors and *H. pylori* infection was demonstrated. Thus, 12% of children from affluent homes were seropositive compared with 41% among the lowest socioeconomic group.[275] However, the study could not define the particular economic or hygiene measure responsible for the result.

Racial reports are conflicting and especially difficult to separate from cultural and socioeconomic factors. Native American Indians are over-represented in the group of children with *H. pylori*-associated ulcer disease in Vancouver, Canada.[276] Differences in peptic ulcer frequency have been shown among the three main racial groups in Singapore.[277] Although *H. pylori* infection rates are similar in Chinese, Malay and Indian patients who have peptic ulceration, racial differences in *H. pylori* colonization rates in the community might still contribute to the differences in peptic ulcer frequency between the three ethnic groups. Vietnamese immigrants to Australia living in better economic conditions have a lower infection rate than controls in Vietnam itself.[100] This suggests that racial factors are not as important as environment in determining infection rates.

The details of the mode of transmission of *H. pylori* are still unclear. Organisms very closely related to *H. pylori* have been isolated from the stomachs of primates[278,279] and although related bacteria have been cultured from the stomachs of other animals these generally appear to be of different *Helicobacter* species.[280,281] Nevertheless, some *H. pylori* isolated from pigs are genotypically identical to those found in humans.[282] In addition abattoir workers with direct contact with animal carcasses have an increased carriage of *H. pylori* antibodies[283] although reduced seropositivity is not found in populations which do not eat pork or beef.[255,284] Overall it appears unlikely that *H. pylori* infection in humans is a zoonosis and more likely that transmission is from a human reservoir. The method of spread of infection is also uncertain. *H. pylori* can survive in water and

chilled foods and both have been suggested as possible routes of infection.[285,286] At least in poor communities in South America childhood *H. pylori* infection appears to be associated with poor external water sources.[287] Another study from the same area again implicated stream water as a potential vehicle for *H. pylori* transmission and also eating raw vegetables.[261] The possibility of multiple transmission pathways especially in children must be considered.[288] *H. pylori* has been transmitted between patients via serial endoscopy and biopsy.[289] All patients were infected by an identical strain making a common source very likely.[289] It is difficult to imagine that this represents a frequent method of spread in the community.

Direct spread of *H. pylori* from person to person in the community appears a more plausible explanation and is supported by indirect evidence. Antibody prevalence is increased above the rate in the general population in individuals resident in closed societies, for example, prisons, psychiatric units and orphanages.[290–292] Gastroenterologists, who are often in daily contact with gastric secretions, have seropositivity rates substantially higher than an age-matched control group.[293,294] Endoscopy assistants, however, have no excess of *H. pylori* carriage.[295,296] In addition there have been anecdotal reports of 'epidemics' of *H. pylori* infection.[297]

Several studies have investigated the frequency of *H. pylori* carriage in the families of infected children. In Toronto, Canada *H. pylori* antibody was detected in 25 of 34 (73.5%) parents of colonized children, but in only 8 of 33 (24.2%) parents of non-colonized children.[298] Of 22 siblings of infected children, 18 (81.8%) had specific antibodies to the organism compared with only 5 of 37 (13.5%) controls. Data from Italy also suggest higher rates of *H. pylori* carriage in parents and siblings of children with peptic ulcer associated with *H. pylori* compared with relatives of children with *H. pylori*-negative peptic ulcer.[299] The intrafamilial clustering of *H. pylori* infection observed may be explained by person to person spread within the family especially as young children may have fewer outside contacts than adults. However, food and water sources are likely to be common to all family members and might also explain the observation. Spouses of patients infected by *H. pylori* have also been investigated for increased infection rates. Of 54 partners of *H. pylori*-positive duodenal ulcer patients 42 (78%) were also harbouring the infection compared with only two (20%) of 10 with *H. pylori*-negative ulceration.[300] Further in eight of 18 couples the infecting strain was identical as measured by rRNA gene patterns. Parente et al.[301] confirmed a higher rate of *H. pylori* seropositivity in spouses of duodenal ulcer patients. It is noteworthy that positivity rate increased with time of cohabitation. However, at least two other studies[302,303] have not found a higher infection rate in spouses of *H. pylori*-positive patients although the index cases did not have ulceration so the infectivity and virulence of the organism may have been less. Using adult index cases positive for *H. pylori*, Jones et al.[304] also found a low level of antibody prevalence in household contacts; in fact, the levels were similar to the general population.

It is generally suggested that a major period of acquisition of *H. pylori* infection is in childhood. The mode of spread is probably oral–oral possibly via water and from a human source. Viable *H. pylori* have not been recovered from the faeces of infected subjects but the plethora of other bacteria would make detection extremely difficult. An alternative approach is to use the polymerase chain reaction to detect minute amounts of *H. pylori* DNA in stool.[305] Reports suggest the organism may be present in saliva or dental plaque, at least in some cases.[306] The exact mode of spread, however, remains to be determined. If most infection occurred in childhood and persisted lifelong a neat explanation would be provided for the 'cohort effect' of increasing seroprevalence with age and the similar effect seen in peptic ulcer epidemiology. Certainly in developing countries with high prevalence rates at the ages of 15–20 years infection must occur in childhood. Early infection in developed countries is supported by studies correlating childhood living conditions with seropositivity. However *H. pylori* prevalence in asymptomatic 1–5 year olds admitted for routine surgery in Belgium was only 6.2%.[307] In Scotland, 11% of those aged 11 years were infected.[256] A Finnish study investigated the same children at 3-yearly intervals.[254] During the follow-up period from 3 to 12 years of age the seropositivity rate increased from 4.6 to 5.7%.[308] The annual seroconversion rate in these children was only 0.3%, similar to the estimated adult rate based on reinfection after successful eradication.[308,309]

Infection must occur in adult life to explain the high prevalence in gastroenterologists, institutionalized individuals and spouses of ulcer patients. An annual rate of adult acquisition of 0.5% over 50 years would result in 25% of the population infected at age 70 years and explain a large proportion of the prevalence at that age. It appears likely that a peak of infection occurs in early childhood especially in developing countries and is added to at a small but appreciable rate throughout adolescence and adult life. Improvements in personal and public health and hygiene are probably acting to reduce the infection rate at all ages including early childhood, thereby depleting the cohort of infected patients susceptible to ulcer disease in later life.

H. pylori appears to be implicated in the pathogenesis of gastritis but whether it is the cause of peptic ulcer disease remains controversial. The considerable protection against relapse of duodenal ulcer afforded by its eradication argues strongly for a pathogenetic role for the organism in this disease. The epidemiological observations of *H. pylori* infection are similar to those of peptic ulcer itself and it would be tempting to explain the entire pattern of ulcer disease on this basis. The increasing prevalence of infection with age might explain the rise in peptic ulcer this century, the 'cohort effect' relating to birthdate and the current decline in ulcer disease as infection rates fall. The association of socioeconomic factors, particularly hygiene and overcrowding with *H. pylori* carriage would also fit many of the epidemiological observations on peptic ulcer disease. *H. pylori* infection also affects serum pepsinogen levels and this together with cross-infection may explain the intrafamilial clustering of ulcer disease.[310,311]

However, other factors known to influence ulcer disease do not correspond to the epidemiological pattern of *H. pylori*. Several studies have shown no association between cigarette smoking and *H. pylori* carriage.[248,312] The increased incidence of peptic ulcer in men is also not generally apparent or too small to explain the excess of male peptic ulcer cases.[248,263,313] Alcohol and NSAID use do not predispose to *H. pylori* carriage.[248,252] Geographical factors are not easily explained solely on *H. pylori* infection rates. In some parts of Africa *H. pylori* infection is almost universal over 20 years of age and yet peptic ulcer rates as determined by hospital admissions for complications vary over the continent and are, in many cases, less than in developed countries with lower infection levels. This 'African Enigma' remains although reduced virulence of the bacterium, nutritional or immunological factors related to infection in early childhood have been postulated. Even in Western societies around 50% of middle-aged adults have been colonized by the organism yet only a minority will develop frank peptic ulceration.

Duodenal and gastric ulceration are clearly multifactorial disorders. It would be simplistic to expect close parallels between *H. pylori* infection and ulcer disease epidemiologically when other processes such as the development of gastric metaplasia within the duodenum may be essential before a patient with *H. pylori* infection can develop a duodenal ulcer. Other factors, such as smoking, diet or genetic predisposition, may interact with each other and possibly *H. pylori* to produce a breach in the mucosa of the upper gastrointestinal tract. The relative importance of each aspect in the production of a common final entity manifest as peptic ulceration may be as individual as the patient. The work suggesting that eradication of *H. pylori* affords major protection against relapse of peptic ulcer and alters the natural history of the disease implies, however, that infection with the organism is a factor of comparable importance to acid in the pathogenesis of this disorder.

REFERENCES

1. Kurata JH. Ulcer epidemiology. An overview and proposed research framework. *Gastroenterology* 1989; **96**: 569.
2. Susser M. Causes of peptic ulcer. A selective epidemiological review. *J Chronic Dis* 1967; **20**: 435.
3. Langman MJS. Peptic ulcer. In *The Epidemiology of Chronic Digestive Disease*. London: Edward Arnold, 1979: 9.
4. Pulvertaft CN. Comments on the incidence and natural history of gastric and duodenal ulcer. *Postgrad Med J* 1968; **44**: 597.
5. Pulvertaft CN. Peptic ulcer in town and country. *Br J. Prev Soc Med* 1959; **13**: 131.
6. Sanders R. Incidence of perforated duodenal and gastric ulcer in Oxford. *Gut* 1967; **8**: 58.
7. Billington BP. Gastric ulcer: age, sex and a curious retrogression. *Aust Ann Med* 1960; **9**: 11.
8. Walt R, Katschinsky B, Logan R, Ashley J & Langman M. Rising frequency of ulcer perforation in elderly people in the United Kingdom. *Lancet* 1986; **i**: 489.
9. Mendeloff AI. What has been happening to duodenal ulcer? *Gastroenterology* 1974; **67**: 1020.
10. Watkinson G. Epidemiological aspects of peptic ulcer disease. *Top Gastroenterol* 1979; **7**: 3.
11. Kurata JH & Haile BM. Epidemiology of peptic ulcer disease. *Clin Gastroenterol* 1984; **13**: 289.
12. Lam SK. Pathogenesis and pathophysiology of duodenal ulcer. *Clin Gastroenterol* 1984; **13**: 447.
13. Langman MJS. What is happening to peptic ulcer? *BMJ* 1982; **1**: 1063.
14. Ivy AC. The problem of peptic ulcer. *JAMA* 1946; **132**: 1053.
15. Jennings D. Perforated peptic ulcer: changes in age-incidence and sex distribution in the last 150 years. *Lancet* 1940; **i**: 395.
16. Sonnenberg A. Disability pensions due to peptic ulcer in Germany between 1953 and 1983. *Am J Epidemiol* 1985; **122**: 106.

17. Meade TW, Arie THD, Brewis M, Bond DJ & Morris JN. Recent history of ischaemic heart disease and duodenal ulcer in doctors. *BMJ* 1968; **2**: 701.
18. Taylor P. Sickness absence: facts and misconceptions. *J R Coll Physicians Lond* 1974; **8**: 315.
19. Doll R. In Avery Jones F (ed.) *Modern Trends in Gastroenterology.* London: 1952.
20. Sonnenberg A. Occurrence of a cohort phenomenon in peptic ulcer morbidity from Switzerland. *Gastroenterology* 1984; **86**: 398.
21. Kurata JH, Elashoff JD, Haile BM & Honda GD. A reappraisal of time trends in ulcer disease: factors related to changes in ulcer hospitalization and mortality rates. *Am J Public Health* 1983; **79**: 1066.
22. Elashoff JD & Grossman MI. Trends in hospital admission and death rates for peptic ulcer in the United States from 1970 to 1978. *Gastroenterology* 1980; **78**: 280.
23. Bloom BS. Cross-national changes in the effects of peptic ulcer disease. *Ann Intern Med* 1991; **114**: 558.
24. Kurata JH, Honda GD & Frankl H. Hospitalization and mortality rates for peptic ulcers: a comparison of a large health maintenance organisation and United States data. *Gastroenterology* 1982; **83**: 1008.
25. Gustavsson S, Kelly KA, Melton JC & Zinsmeister AR. Trends in peptic ulcer surgery: a population based study in Rochester, Minnesota, 1956–85. *Gastroenterology* 1988; **94**: 688.
26. Smith MP. Decline in duodenal ulcer surgery. *JAMA* 1977; **237**: 987.
27. Vogt TM & Johnson RE. Recent changes in the incidence of duodenal and gastric ulcer. *Am J Epidemiol* 1980; **111**: 713.
28. Sonnenberg A. Changes in physician visits for gastric and duodenal ulcer in the United States during 1958–1984 as shown by the National Disease and Therapeutic Index (NDTI). *Dig Dis Sci* 1987; **32**: 1.
29. Brown RC, Langman MJS & Lambert PM. Hospital admissions for peptic ulcer during 1958–72. *BMJ* 1976; **1**: 35.
30. Coggon D, Lambert P & Langman MJS. 20 years of hospital admissions for peptic ulcer in England and Wales. *Lancet* 1981; **i**: 1302.
31. Jibril SA, Redpath A & McIntyre DMC. Changing pattern of admission and operation for duodenal ulcer in Scotland. *Br J Surg* 1994; **81**: 87–89.
32. Gustavsson S & Nyren O. Time trends in peptic ulcer surgery, 1956 to 1986. A nationwide survey in Sweden. *Ann Surg* 1989; **210**: 704.
33. Lee SP. Rising female predominance in incidence of gastric ulcer. *BMJ* 1982; **285**: 853.
34. Sonnenberg A & Fritsch A. Changing mortality of peptic ulcer disease in Germany. *Gastroenterology* 1983; **84**: 1553.
35. Bonnevie O. The incidence of duodenal ulcer in Copenhagen County. *Scand J Gastroenterol* 1975; **10**: 385.
36. Ostensen H, Burhol PG, Bonnevie O & Bolz KD. Changes in the pattern of peptic ulcer disease in the northern part of Norway between 1946 and 1981. *Scand J Gastroenterol* 1982; **17**: 1073.
37. Kawai K, Shirakawa K, Misaki F, Hayoshi K & Watanabe Y. Natural history and epidemiological studies of peptic ulcer disease in Japan. *Gastroenterology* 1989; **96**: 581.
38. Tovey FI & Tunstall M. Duodenal ulcer in black populations in Africa south of the Sahara. *Gut* 1975; **16**: 564.
39. Segal I, Dubb AA, Leonard OT, Solomon A, Sottomayor MC & Zwane EM. Duodenal ulcer and working-class mobility in an African population in South Africa. *BMJ* 1978; **1**: 469.
40. Gangaidzo I, Kure C, Mason P, Sitma J & Gwanzura L. Prospective endoscopic study of duodenal ulcer in Zimbabwean Blacks. *Central Afr J Med* 1992; **38**: 397.
41. Koo J, Ngan YK & Lam SK. Trends in hospital admission, perforation, and mortality of peptic ulcer in Hong Kong from 1970 to 1980. *Gastroenterology* 1983; **84**: 1558.
42. Susser M & Stein Z. Civilisation and peptic ulcer. *Lancet* 1962; **i**: 115.
43. Sonnenberg A, Muller H & Pace F. Birth-cohort analysis of peptic ulcer mortality in Europe. *J Chronic Dis* 1985; **38**: 309.
44. Sonnenberg A. Smoking and mortality from peptic ulcer in the United Kingdom. *Gut* 1986; **27**: 1369.
45. Polednak AP. Peptic ulcer mortality in men born in 1850–99. *Lancet* 1973; **ii**: 970.
46. Weir RD & Backett EM. Studies of the epidemiology of peptic ulcer in a rural community: prevalence and natural history of dyspepsia and peptic ulcer. *Gut* 1968; **9**: 75.
47. Pounder RE. Silent peptic ulceration: deadly silence or golden silence. *Gastroenterology* 1989; **96**: 626.
48. Litton A & Murdoch WR. Peptic ulcer in South-West Scotland. *Gut* 1963; **4**: 360.
49. Dunlop JM. Peptic ulcer in Central Scotland. *Scott Med J* 1968; **13**: 192.
50. Monson RR & MacMahon B. Peptic ulcer in Massachusetts physicians. *N Engl J Med* 1969; **281**: 11.
51. Bonnevie O. The incidence of gastric ulcer in Copenhagen County. *Scand J Gastroenterol* 1975; **10**: 231.
52. Hugh TB, Coleman MJ, McNamara ME, Norman JR & Howell C. Epidemiology of peptic ulcer in Australia. *Med J Aust* 1984; **141**: 81.
53. Kaier T, Roin J, Djuurhuus J, Dahl S & Bonnevie O. Epidemiological aspects of peptic ulcer disease in the Faroe Islands. *Scand J Gastroenterol* 1985; **20**: 1157.
54. Mountford RA, Brown P, Salmon PR, Alvarenga C, Neumann CS & Read AE. Gastric cancer detection in gastric ulcer disease. *Gut* 1980; **21**: 9.
55. Baron JH. An assessment of the augmented histamine test in the diagnosis of peptic ulcer. *Gut* 1963; **4**: 243.
56. Watkinson G. The incidence of chronic peptic ulcer found at necropsy. *Gut* 1960; **1**: 14.
57. Levij IS & De La Fuente AA. A post-mortem study of gastric and duodenal peptic lesions. *Gut* 1963; **4**: 349.
58. Ihamaki T, Varis K & Siurala M. Morphological, functional and immunological state of the gastric mucosa in gastric carcinoma families. *Scand J Gastroenterol* 1979; **14**: 801.
59. Segawa K, Nakazawa S, Tsukamoto Y et al. Peptic ulcer is prevalent among shift workers. *Dig Dis Sci* 1987; **32**: 449.
60. Bernersen B, Johnsen R, Straume B, Burhol PG, Jenssen TG & Stakkevold PA. Towards a true prevalence of peptic ulcer: the Sorreisa gastrointestinal disorder study. *Gut* 1990; **31**: 989.
61. Sonnenberg A & Everhart JE. The prevalence of self-reported peptic ulcer in the United States. *Am J Public Health* 1996; **86**: 200.
62. Lindstrom CG. Gastric and duodenal peptic ulcer disease in a well-defined population. A prospective necropsy study in Malmö, Sweden. *Scand J Gastroenterol* 1978; **13**: 139.
63. Kurata JH, Haile BM & Elashoff JD. Sex differences in peptic ulcer disease. *Gastroenterology* 1985; **88**: 96.
64. Illingworth CFW, Scott LDW & Jamieson RA. Acute perforated peptic ulcer frequency and incidence in the West of Scotland. *BMJ* 1944; **2**: 617.
65. McKay C. Perforated peptic ulcer in the West of Scotland: a survey of 5343 cases during 1954–63. *BMJ* 1966; **1**: 701.
66. McKay C. Prevalence of peptic ulcer and its complications. *Scott Med J* 1977; **22**: 288.
67. Jamieson RA. Acute perforated peptic ulcer. Frequency and incidence in the West of Scotland. *BMJ* 1955; **2**: 222.
68. Truelove SC. Stilboestrol, phenobarbitone and diet in chronic duodenal ulcer. *BMJ* 1960; **2**: 559.
69. Svanes C, Salvesen H, Stangel and L, Svanes K & Soreide O. Perforated peptic ulcer over 56 years: time trends in patients and disease characteristics. *Gut* 1993; **34**: 1666.
70. Tovey F. Peptic ulcer in India and Bangladesh. *Gut* 1979; **20**: 329.
71. Chapman BL & Duggan JM. Aspirin and uncomplicated peptic ulcer. *Gut* 1969; **10**: 443.
72. Grossman MI, Kirsner JB & Gillespie JE. Basal and histalog-stimulated gastric secretion in control subjects and in patients with peptic ulcer or gastric cancer. *Gastroenterology* 1963; **45**: 14.
73. Feldman M, Richardson CT & Walsh JH. Sex-related differences in gastrin release and parietal cell sensitivity to gastrin in healthy human beings. *J Clin Invest* 1983; **71**: 715.
74. Feldman M, Richardson CT, Lam SK & Samloff IM. Comparison of gastric acid secretion rates and serum pepsinogen I and II concentrations in occidental and oriental duodenal ulcer patients. *Gastroenterology* 1988; **95**: 630.
75. Sonnenberg A, Muller-Lissner SA, Vogel E et al. Predictors of duodenal ulcer healing and relapse. *Gastroenterology* 1981; **81**: 1061.
76. Francis HH & Smellie JH, General diseases in pregnancy – 2. *BMJ* 1964; **1**: 955.
77. Vessey MP, Villard-Mackintosh L & Painter R. Oral contraceptives and pregnancy in relation to peptic ulcer. *Contraception* 1992; **46**: 349.
78. Freidman GD, Siegelaub AB & Seltzer CC. Cigarettes, alcohol, coffee and peptic ulcer. *N Eng J Med* 1974; **290**: 460.
79. Sonnenberg A. Temporal trends and geographical variations of peptic ulcer disease. *Aliment Pharm Ther* 1995; **9** Suppl 2: 3.
80. Murphy MS, Eastham EJ, Jimenez M, Nelson R & Jackson RH. Duodenal ulceration: review of 110 cases. *Arch Dis Child* 1987; **62**: 554.
81. Editorial. Duodenal ulcers in childhood. *Lancet* 1987; **ii**: 891.
82. Schöön IM, Mellstrom D, Oden A & Ytterberg BO. Incidence of peptic ulcer disease in Gothenberg, 1985. *BMJ* 1987; **299**: 1131.

83. Kang JY. Age of onset of symptoms in duodenal and gastric ulcer. *Gut* 1990; **31**: 854.

84. Kang JY. Peptic ulcer surgery in Singapore, with particular reference to racial differences in incidence. *Aust N Z J Med* 1985; **15**: 604.

85. Lam SK & Ong GB. Duodenal ulcers: early and late onset. *Gut* 1976; **17**: 169.

86. Lam SK, Koo J & Sircus W. Early and late-onset duodenal ulcer in Chinese and Scots. *Scand J Gastroenterol* 1983; **18**: 651.

87. Sonnenberg A. Geographic and temporal variations in the occurrence of peptic ulcer disease. *Scand J Gastroenterol* 1985; **20**(Suppl. 110): 11.

88. Eriksen BO, Garpestad OK, Sondena H & Burmol PG. Peptic ulcer patterns in Artic Norway. *J Clin Gastroenterol* 1995; **20**: 100.

89. Tovey FI, Jayaraj AP, Lewin MR & Clark CG. Diet: its role in the genesis of peptic ulceration. *Dig Dis* 1989; **7**: 309.

90. Editorial. Diet and peptic ulcer. *Lancet* 1987; **ii**: 80.

91. Malhotra SL. Peptic ulcer in India and its aetiology. *Gut* 1964; **5**: 412.

92. Tovey FI. Duodenal ulcer in China. *J Gastroenterol Hepatol* 1992; **7**: 427.

93. Malhotra SL. A comparison of unrefined wheat and rice diets in the management of duodenal ulcer. *Postgrad Med J* 1978; **54**: 6.

94. Rydning A, Berstad A, Aadland E & Odegaard B. Prophylactic effect of dietary fibre in duodenal ulcer disease. *Lancet* 1982; **ii**: 736.

95. Jayaraj AP, Tovey FI & Clark CG. Possible dietary protective factors in relation to the distribution of duodenal ulcer in India and Bangladesh. *Gut* 1980; **21**: 1068.

96. Katschinski BD, Logan RFA, Edmond M & Langman MJS. Duodenal ulcer and refined carbohydrate intake: a case–control study assessing dietary fibre and refined sugar intake. *Gut* 1990; **31**: 993.

97. Hollander D & Tarnawski A. Dietary essential fatty acids and the decline in peptic ulcer: a hypothesis. *Gut* 1986; **27**: 239.

98. Grant HW, Palmer KR, Riermesma RR & Oliver MF. Duodenal ulcer is associated with low dietary linoleic acid intake. *Gut* 1990; **31**: 997.

99. Kurata JH & Haile BM. Racial differences in peptic ulcer disease: fact or myth? *Gastroenterology* 1982; **83**: 166.

100. Kolt SD, Kronborg IJ & Yeomans ND. High prevalence of duodenal ulcer in Indochinese immigrants attending an Australian university hospital. *J Gastroenterol Hepatol* 1993; **8**: 128.

101. Hunt RH & Milton-Thompson GJ. The epidemiology and pathogenesis of gastric ulcer. *Front Gastrointest Res* 1980; **6**: 57.

102. Doll R, Jones FA & Buckatzsch MM. Occupational factors in the aetiology of gastric and duodenal ulcers. *Spec Rep Ser Med Res Counc* 1951; **276**: 7.

103. Levenstein S, Kaplan GA & Smith M. Sociodemographic characteristics, life stresses and peptic ulcer. A prospective study. *J Clin Gastroenterol* 1995; **21**: 185–192.

104. Dunn JP & Cobb S. Frequency of peptic ulcer among executives, craftsman and foremen. *J Occup Med* 1962; **4**: 343.

105. Tuchsen F, Jeppesen HJ & Bach E. Employment status, non-daytime work and gastric ulcer in men. *Int J Epidemiol* 1994; **23**: 365.

106. Moshal MG, Schlemmer L & Naidoo NK. Social mobility in African patients with duodenal ulcers. *BMJ* 1978; **2**: 1788.

107. Segal I. The trauma of the urban experience. *J R Coll Physicians Lond* 1988; **22**: 45.

108. Sonnenberg A, Sonnenberg GS & Wirths W. Historic changes of occupational work load and mortality from peptic ulcer in Germany. *J Occup Med* 1987; **28**: 756.

109. Katschinsky BD, Logan RFA, Edmond M & Langman MJS. Physical activity at work and duodenal ulcer risk. *Gut* 1991; **32**: 983.

110. Sonnenberg A, Wasserman IH & Jacobsen SJ. Monthly variation of hospital admission and mortality of peptic ulcer disease: a reappraisal of ulcer periodicity. *Gastroenterology* 1992; **103**: 1192.

111. Bendahan J, Gilboa S, Paran H et al. Seasonal pattern in the incidence of bleeding caused by peptic ulcer in Israel. *Am J Gastroenterol* 1992; **87**: 733.

112. Hall WH, Read RC, Mesard L, Lee LE & Robinette CD. The calendar and duodenal ulcer. *Gastroenterology* 1972; **62**: 1120.

113. Langman MJS. The seasonal incidence of bleeding from the upper gastro-intestinal tract. *Gut* 1964; **5**: 142.

114. William Beaumont Society, US Army. Seasonal incidence of upper gastrointestinal tract bleeding. *JAMA* 1968; **198**: 184.

115. Gibinski K, Rybicka J, Nowak A & Czarnecka K. Seasonal occurrence of abdominal pain and endoscopic findings in patients with gastric and duodenal ulcer disease. *Scand J Gastroenterol* 1982; **17**: 481.

116. Linn HW. Analysis of peptic ulcer in South Australia based on study of 1027 case reports. *Med J Aust* 1946; **2**: 649.

117. Ostensen H, Gudmundsen TE, Ostensen M, Burhol PG & Bonnevie O. Smoking, alcohol, coffee and familial factors. Any association with peptic ulcer disease? *Scand J Gastroenterol* 1985; **20**: 1227.

118. Monson RR. Cigarette smoking and body form in peptic ulcer. *Gastroenterology* 1970; **58**: 337.

119. Doll R & Peto R. Mortality in relation to smoking: 20 years observations on male British doctors. *BMJ* 1976; **2**: 1525.

120. Paffenbarger RS, Wing AL & Hyde RT. Chronic disease in former college students. *Am J Epidemiol* 1974; **100**: 307.

121. Ainley CC, Forgacs IC, Keeling PWN & Thompson RPH. Outpatient endoscopic survey of smoking and peptic ulcer. *Gut* 1986; **27**: 648.

122. Lam SK & Koo J. Accurate prediction of duodenal ulcer healing rate by discriminant analysis. *Gastroenterology* 1983; **85**: 403.

123. Sontag S, Graham DY, Belsito A et al. Cimetidine, cigarette smoking and recurrence of duodenal ulcer. *N Engl J Med* 1984; **311**: 689.

124. Tabaqchali S & Dawson AM. Peptic ulcer and gastric secretion in patients with liver disease. *Gut* 1964; **5**: 417.

125. Chen LS, Lin MC, Huang SJ et al. Prevalence of gastric ulcer in cirrhotic patients and its relation to portal hypertension. *J Gastroenterol Hepatol* 1996; **11**: 59.

126. Chou SP. An examination of the alcohol consumption and peptic ulcer association – results of a national survey. *Alc Clin Exp Res* 1994; **18**: 149.

127. Kato I, Nomura AM, Stemmermann GN & Chyou PH. A prospective study of gastric and duodenal ulcer and its relation to smoking, alcohol and diet. *Am J Epidemiol* 1992; **135**: 521.

128. Conn HO & Blitzer BL. Non-association of adrenocorticosteroid therapy and peptic ulcer. *N Engl J Med* 1976; **294**: 473.

129. Messer J, Reitman D, Sacks HS, Smith H & Chalmers TC. Association of adrenocorticosteroid therapy and peptic ulcer disease. *N Engl J Med* 1983; **309**: 21.

130. Holvoet J, Terriere L, Van Hee W, Verbist L, Fierens E & Hautekeete ML. Relation of upper gastrointestinal bleeding to non-steroidal anti-inflammatory drugs and aspirin: a case control study. *Gut* 1991; **32**: 730.

131. Piper JM, Ray WA, Daugherty MS & Griffin MR. Corticosteroid use and peptic ulcer disease: role of non-steroidal anti-inflammatory drugs. *Ann Intern Med* 1991; **114**: 735.

132. Armstrong CP & Blower AL. Non-steroidal anti-inflammatory drugs and life threatening complications of peptic ulceration. *Gut* 1987; **28**: 527.

133. Carson JL, Strom BL, Soper KA, Werst SL & Morse ML. The association of non-steroidal anti-inflammatory drugs with upper gastrointestinal tract bleeding. *Arch Intern Med* 1987; **147**: 85.

134. Billington BP. Observations from New South Wales on the changing incidence of gastric ulcer in Australia. *Gut* 1965; **6**: 121.

135. Douglas RA & Johnston ED. Aspirin and chronic gastric ulcer. *Med J Aust* 1961; **2**: 893.

136. Duggan JM. Aspirin ingestion and perforated peptic ulcer. *Gut* 1972; **13**: 631.

137. Duggan JM. Aspirin in chronic gastric ulcer: an Australian experience. *Gut* 1976; **17**: 378.

138. Gillies MA & Skyring A. Gastric ulcer, duodenal ulcer and gastric carcinoma: a case–control study of certain social and environmental factors. *Med J Aust* 1968; **2**: 1132.

139. Gillies MA & Skyring A. Gastric and duodenal ulcer. The association between aspirin ingestion, smoking and family history of ulcer. *Med J Aust* 1969; **2**: 280.

140. Levy M. Aspirin use in patients with major upper gastrointestinal bleeding and peptic ulcer disease. *N Engl J Med* 1974; **290**: 1158.

141. Levy M, Miller DR, Kaufmann DW et al. Major upper gastrointestinal tract bleeding. Relation to the use of aspirin and other non-narcotic analgesics. *Arch Intern Med* 1988; **148**: 281.

142. Coggon D, Langman MJS & Spiegelhalter D. Aspirin, paracetamol and haematemesis and melaena. *Gut* 1982; **23**: 340.

143. Aspirin Myocardial Infarction Study Research Group. A randomized, controlled trial of aspirin in persons recovering from myocardial infarction. *JAMA* 1980; **243**: 661.

144. The EPSIM Research Group. A controlled comparison of aspirin and oral anticoagulants in prevention of death after myocardial infarction. *N Engl J Med* 1982; **307**: 701.

145. Langman MJS. Epidemiologic evidence on the association between peptic ulceration and anti-inflammatory drug use. *Gastroenterology* 1989; **96**: 640.

146. Duggan JM, Dobson AJ, Johnson H & Fahey P. Peptic ulcer and non-steroidal anti-inflammatory agents. *Gut* 1986; **27**: 929.

147. Piper DW, McIntosh JH, Ariotti DE, Fenton BH & McLennan R.

Analgesic ingestion and chronic peptic ulcer. *Gastroenterology* 1981; **80**: 427.

148. McIntosh JH, Byth K & Piper DW. Environmental factors in aetiology of chronic gastric ulcer: a case–control study of exposure variables before the first symptoms. *Gut* 1985; **26**: 789.

149. Clinch D, Banerjee AK, Ostick G et al. Non-steroidal anti-inflammatory drugs and gastrointestinal adverse effects. *J R Coll Physicians Lond* 1983; **17**: 228.

150. Bartle WR, Gupta AK & Lazor J. Non-steroidal anti-inflammatory drugs and gastrointestinal bleeding. *Arch Intern Med* 1986; **146**: 2365.

151. Somerville K, Faulkner G & Langman M. Non-steroidal anti-inflammatory drugs and bleeding peptic ulcer. *Lancet* 1986; **i**: 462.

152. Collier D St J & Pain LA. Non-steroidal anti-inflammatory drugs and peptic ulcer perforation. *Gut* 1985; **26**: 359.

153. Jick SS, Perera DR, Walker AM & Jick H. Non-steroidal anti-inflammatory drugs and hospital admission for perforated peptic ulcer. *Lancet* 1987; **ii**: 380.

154. Guess HA, West R, Strand LM et al. Fatal upper gastrointestinal haemorrhage or perforation among users and non-users of non-steroidal anti-inflammatory drugs in Saskatchewan, Canada. *J Clin Epidemiol* 1988; **41**: 35.

155. Smalley WE, Ray WA, Daugherty SR & Griffin MR. Non-steroidal anti-inflammatory drugs and the incidence of hospitalizations for peptic ulcer disease in elderly persons. *Am J Epidemiol* 1995; **141**: 539.

156. Carson JL, Strom BL, Morse ML et al. The relative gastrointestinal toxicity of the non-steroidal anti-inflammatory drugs. *Arch Intern Med* 1987; **147**: 1054.

157. Langman MJS. The changing face of peptic ulceration. *Scand J Gastroenterol* 1987; **22**(Suppl. 136), 37.

158. Cockel R. NSAIDs: should every prescription carry a government health warning? *Gut* 1987; **28**: 515.

159. Donaldson RM. Factors complicating observed associations between peptic ulcer and other diseases. *Gastroenterology* 1975; **68**: 1608.

160. Langman MJS & Cooke AR. Gastric and duodenal ulcer and their associated diseases. *Lancet* 1976; **i**: 680.

161. Fry J. Peptic ulcer: a profile. *BMJ* 1964; **2**: 809.

162. Monson RR. Duodenal ulcer as a second disease. *Gastroenterology* 1970; **59**: 712.

163. Jones AW, Kirk RS & Bloor K. The association between aneurysm of the abdominal aorta and peptic ulceration. *Gut* 1970; **11**: 679.

164. Medalie JH, Kahn HA, Neufeld HN, Riss E, Goldbourt V & Oron D. Association between blood pressure and peptic ulcer incidence. *Lancet* 1970; **ii**: 1225.

165. Sonnenberg A. Concordant occurrence of gastric and hypertensive diseases. *Gastroenterology* 1988; **95**: 42.

166. Kellow JE, Tao Z & Piper DW. Ventilatory function in chronic peptic ulcer. *Gastroenterology* 1986; **91**: 590.

167. Stemmermann GN, Marcus EB, Buist AS & McLean CJ. Relative impact of smoking and reduced pulmonary function on peptic ulcer risk. *Gastroenterology* 1989; **96**: 1419.

168. Dotevall G. Incidence of peptic ulcer in diabetes mellitus. *Acta Med Scand* 1959; **164**: 463.

169. Hosking DJ, Moody F, Stewart IM & Atkinson M. Vagal impairment of gastric secretion in diabetic autonomic neuropathy. *BMJ* 1975; **1**: 588.

170. McLean Ross AH, Smith MA, Anderson JR & Small WP. Late mortality after surgery for peptic ulcer. *N Engl J Med* 1982; **307**: 519.

171. Lundegardh G, Holmberg L & Krusemo UB. Long-term survival in patients operated on for benign peptic ulcer disease. *Br J Surg* 1991; **78**: 234.

172. Tersmette AC, Offerhaus JA, Giardello FM et al. Long-term prognosis after partial gastrectomy for benign conditions. *Gastroenterology* 1991; **101**: 148.

173. Lee S, Iida M, Yao T, Shindo S, Fujishima M & Okabe H. Long-term follow-up of 2529 patients with gastric and duodenal ulcer; survival rate and causes of death. *Gastroenterology* 1988; **94**: 381.

174. Piper DW, McIntosh JH, Ariotti DE, Calogiuri JV, Brown RW & Shy CM. Life events and chronic duodenal ulcer: a case control study. *Gut* 1981; **22**: 1011.

175. Thomas J, Greig M & Piper DW. Chronic gastric ulcer and life events. *Gastroenterology* 1980; **78**: 905.

176. Feldman M, Walker P, Green JL & Weingarden K. Life events stress and psychological factors in men with peptic ulcer disease. *Gastroenterology* 1986; **91**: 1370.

177. Polednak AP. Some early characteristics of peptic ulcer decedents. *Gastroenterology* 1974; **67**: 1094.

178. Adami H-O, Bergstrom R, Nyren O et al. Is duodenal ulcer really a psychosomatic disease? A population based case–control study. *Scand J Gastroenterol* 1987; **22**: 889.

179. Alp MH, Court JM & Grant AK. Personality pattern and emotional stress in the genesis of gastric ulcer. *Gut* 1970; **11**: 773.

180. Jess P. Personality pattern in peptic ulcer disease: a cohort study. *J Internal Med* 1994; **236**: 271.

181. Ellard K, Beaurepaire J, Jones M, Piper D & Tennant C. Acute and chronic stress in duodenal ulcer disease. *Gastroenterology* 1990; **99**: 1628.

182. McIntosh JH, Nasiry RW, McNeil D, Coates C, Mitchell H & Piper DW. Perception of life event stress in patients with chronic duodenal ulcer. *Scand J Gastroenterol* 1985; **20**: 563.

183. Walker P, Luther J, Samloff IM & Feldman M. Life events stress and psychosocial factors in men with peptic ulcer disease. *Gastroenterology* 1988; **94**: 323.

184. Anda RF, Williamson DF, Eslobedo LG et al. Self-perceived stress and the risk of peptic ulcer disease. *Arch Intern Med* 1992; **152**: 829.

185. Rotter JI. The genetics of peptic ulcer. In Rotter JI, Samloff IM & Rinoin DL (eds) *Genetics and Heterogeneity of Common Gastrointestinal Disorders*. London: Academic Press, 1980: 3.

186. Doll R & Buch J. Hereditary factors in peptic ulcer. *Ann Eugen* 1950; **15**: 135.

187. Monson RR. Familial factors in peptic ulcer, the occurrence of ulcer in relatives. *Am J Epidemiol* 1970; **91**: 453.

188. Kubickova Z & Vesely KT. The value of investigation of the incidence of peptic ulcer in families of patients with duodenal ulcer. *J Med Genet* 1972; **9**: 38.

189. Doll R & Kellock TD. The separate inheritance of gastric and duodenal ulcers. *Ann Eugen* 1951; **16**: 231.

190. Gotlieb-Jensen K. *Peptic Ulcer: Genetic and Epidemiological Aspects Based on Twin Studies*. Copenhagen: Munksgaard, 1972.

191. Aird I, Bentall HH, Mehigan JA & Fraser Roberts JA. The blood groups in relation to peptic ulceration and carcinoma of colon, rectum, breast and bronchus. *BMJ* 1954; **2**: 315.

192. Johnson HD, Love AHG, Rogers NC & Wyatt AP. Gastric ulcers, blood groups and acid secretion. *Gut* 1964; **5**: 402.

193. Veseley KT, Kubickova Z & Dvorakova M. Clinical data and characteristics differentiating types of peptic ulcer. *Gut* 1968; **9**: 57.

194. Langman MJS & Doll R. ABO blood group and secretor status in relation to clinical characteristics of peptic ulcer. *Gut* 1965; 6: 270.

195. Hanley WB. Hereditary aspects of duodenal ulceration: serum pepsinogen level in relation to ABO blood groups and salivary ABH secretor status. *BMJ* 1964; **1**: 936.

196. Doll R, Drane H & Newell AC. Secretion of blood group substances in duodenal, gastric and stomal ulcer, gastric carcinoma and diabetes mellitus. *Gut* 1961; **2**: 352.

197. Clarke CA, Edwards JW, Haddock DRW, Howel-Evans AW, McConnell RB & Sheppard PM. ABO blood groups and secretor character in duodenal ulcer. *BMJ* 1956; **2**: 725.

198. Samloff IM. Peptic ulcer. The many proteinases of aggression. *Gastroenterology* 1989; **96**: 586.

199. Samloff IM, Liebman WM & Panitch NM. Serum group I pepsinogens by radioimmunoassay in control subjects and patients with peptic ulcer. *Gastroenterology* 1975; **69**: 83.

200. Rotter JI, Sones JQ, Samloff IM et al. Duodenal ulcer disease associated with elevated serum pepsinogen I. *N Engl J Med* 1979; **300**: 63.

201. Samloff IM & Taggart RT. Pepsinogens, pepsins and peptic ulcer. *Clin Invest Med* 1987; **10**: 215.

202. Nomura A. Elevated serum pepsinogen I and II levels differ as risk factors for duodenal ulcer and gastric ulcer. *Gastroenterology* 1986; **90**: 570.

203. Fraser AG, Prewett EJ, Pounder RE & Samloff IM. Twenty-four hour hyperpepsinogenaemia in helicobacter-positive subjects is abolished by eradication of the infection. *Gut* 1992; **33**: S3.

204. Veenendaal RA, Biemond I, Pena AS, Van Duijn, Kreuning J & Lamers CBHW. Influence of age and helicobacter infection on serum pepsinogens in healthy blood transfusion donors. *Gut* 1992, **33**: 452–455.

205. Li Z-L, McIntosh JH, Byth K, Stuckey B, Steil D & Piper DW. Phenylthiocarbamide taste sensitivity in chronic peptic ulcer. *Gastroenterology* 1990; **99**: 66.

206. Levi S, Beardshall K, Haddad G, Playford R, Ghosh P & Calam J. *Campylobacter pylori* and duodenal ulcer: the gastrin link. *Lancet* 1989; **i**: 1167.

207. Rotter JI & Rimoin DL. Peptic ulcer disease: a heterogenous group of disorders? *Gastroenterology* 1977; **73**: 604.

208. Gear MWL, Truelove SC & Whitehead R. Gastric ulcer and gastritis. *Gut* 1971; **12**; 639.

209. Delaney JP, Cheng JW, Butler BA & Ritchie WP. Gastric ulcer and regurgitation gastritis. *Gut* 1970; **11**: 715.

210. Steer HW & Colin-Jones DG. Mucosal changes in gastric ulceration and their response to carbenoxolone sodium. *Gut* 1975; **16**: 590.

211. Magus HA, Gastritis. In Jones FA (ed.) *Modern Trends in Gastroenterology.* London: Butterworth, 1952: 323.

212. Marshall BJ & Warren JR. Unidentified curved bacilli in the stomach of patients with gastritis and paptic ulceration. *Lancet* 1984; **i**: 1311.

213. Editorial. Spirals and ulcers. Lancet 1984; **i**: 1336.

214. Petersen WL. *Helicobacter pylori* and peptic ulcer disease. *N Engl J Med* 1991; **324**: 1043.

215. Editorial. *Campylobacter pylori* becomes *Helicobacter pylori*. *Lancet* 1989; **ii**: 1019.

216. Langenberg M-L, Tytgat GNJ, Schipper MEI, Reitra PJ & Zanen HC. Campylobacter-like organisms in the stomach of patients and healthy individuals. *Lancet* 1984; **i**: 1348.

217. Wyatt JI. The role of *Campylobacter pylori* in the pathogenesis of peptic ulcer disease. *Scand J Gastroenterol* 1989; **24**(Suppl. 157): 7.

218. Mahony MJ, Wyatt JI & Littlewood JM. *Campylobacter pylori* gastritis. *Arch Dis Child* 1988; **63**: 654.

219. Drumm B, Sherman P, Cutz E & Karmali M. Association of *Campylobacter pylori* in the gastric mucosa with antral gastritis in children. *N Engl J Med* 1987; **316**: 1557.

220. Rauws EAJ, Langenberg W, Houthoff HJ, Zanen HC, Tytgat GNS. *Campylobacter pyloridis*-associated chronic active antral gastritis. *Gastroenterology* 1988; **94**: 33.

221. O'Connor HJ, Dixon MF, Wyatt JI, Axon ATR, Dewer EP & Johnson D. *Campylobacter pylori* and peptic ulcer disease. *Lancet* 1987; **ii**: 633.

222. Morris A & Nicholson G. Ingestion of *Campylobacter pyloridis* causes gastritis and raised fasting gastric pH. *Am J Gastroenterol* 1987; **82**: 192.

223. Marshall BJ, Armstrong JA, McGechie DB & Glancy RJ. Attempt, to fulfil Koch's postulates for *Campylobacter pylori*. *Med J Aust* 1985; **142**: 436.

224. Marshall BJ, McGechie DB, Rogers PA & Glancy RJ. Pyloric Campylobacter infection and gastrointestinal disease. *Med J Aust* 1985; **142**: 439.

225. Dixon MF. *Campylobacter pylori* and chronic gastritis. In Rathbone BJ & Heatley RV (eds) *Campylobacter pylori and Gastroduodenal Disease.* Oxford: Blackwell, 1989.

226. Graham DY, Lew GM, Klein PD et al. Results of treatment of *Helicobacter pylori* infection on the recurrence of gastric or duodenal ulcers: a randomised single-blind, single centre study. *Gastroenterology* 1993; 100: A74.

227. Tatsuta M, Ishikawa H, Iishi H, Okuda S & Yokota Y. Reduction of gastric ulcer recurrence after suppression of *Helicobacter pylori* by cefixine. *Gut* 1990; **31**: 973.

228. Rauws EAS & Tytgat GN. *Helicobacter pylori* in duodenal and gastric ulcer disease. *Ballieres Clin Gastroenterol* 1995; **9**: 529.

229. Wyatt JI. *Campylobacter pylori*, duodenitis and duodenal ulceration. In Rathbone BJ & Heatley RV (eds) *Campylobacter pylori and Gastroduodenal Disease.* Oxford: Blackwell, 1989: 117.

230. Wyatt JI, Rathbone BJ, Dixon MF & Heatley RV. *Campylobacter pylori* and acid induced gastric metaplasia in the pathogenesis of duodenitis. *J Clin Pathol* 1987; **40**: 841.

231. Carrick J, Lee A, Hazell S, Ralston M & Daskalopoulos G. *Campylobacter pylori*, duodenal ulcer and gastric metaplasia: possible role of functional heterotopic tissue in ulcerogenesis. *Gut* 1989; **30**: 790.

232. Moss S & Calam J. *Helicobacter pylori* and peptic ulcers: the present position. *Gut* 1992; **33**: 289.

233. Martin DF, May SJ, Tweedle DEF, Hollanders D, Ravenscroft MM & Miller JP. Differences in relapse rates of duodenal ulcer after healing with cimetidine or tripotassium dicitrato bismuthate. *Lancet* 1981; **i**: 7.

234. Coghlan JG, Gilligan D, Humphries H et al. *Campylobacter pylori* and recurrence of duodenal ulcers: a 12 month follow up study. *Lancet* 1987; **ii**: 1109.

235. Marshall BJ, Goodwin CS, Warren JR et al. Prospective double-blind trial of duodenal ulcer relapse after eradication of *Campylobacter pylori*. *Lancet* 1988; **ii**: 1437.

236. Rauws EAJ & Tytgat GNJ. Cure of duodenal ulcer associated with eradication of *Helicobacter pylori*. *Lancet* 1990; **335**: 1233.

237. George LL, Borody T, Andrews P et al. Cure of duodenal ulcer after eradication of *Helicobacter pylori*. *Med J Aust* 1990; **153**: 145.

238. Lambert JR, Borromeo M, Korman MG, Hansky J & Eaves ER. Effect of colloidal bismuth (De-Nol) on healing and relapse of duodenal ulcers: role of *Campylobacter pyloridis*. *Gastroenterology* 1987; **92**: A1489.

239. Smith AC. Duodenal ulcer disease. What role does *Campylobacter pylori* play? *Scand J Gastroenterol* 1989; **24** (Suppl. 160): 14.

240. Graham DY, Hepps KS, Ramirez FE et al. Treatment of *Helicobacter pylori* reduces the rate of rebleeding in peptic ulcer disease. *Scand J Gastroenterol* 1993; **28**: 939.

241. Khulusi S, Mendall MA, Patel P et al. *Helicobacter pylori* infection density and gastric inflammation in duodenal ulcer and non-ulcer subjects. *Gut* 1995; **37**: 319.

242. Alam K, Schubert TT, Bologna SD & Ma CK. Increased density of *Helicobacter pylori* on antral biopsy is associated with severity of acute and chronic inflammation and likelihood of duodenal ulceration. *Am J Gastroenterol* 1992; **87**: 423.

243. Wyatt JI & Rathbone BJ. The role of serology in the diagnosis of *Campylobacter pylori* infection. *Scand J Gastroenterol* 1989; **24** (Suppl. 160): 27.

244. Graham DY, Klein PD, Evans DJ et al. *Campylobacter pylori* detected non-invasively by the ¹³C-urea breath test. *Lancet* 1987; **i**: 1174.

245. Marshall BJ, McGechie DB, Francis GJ & Utley PJ. Pyloric Campylobacter serology. *Lancet* 1984; **ii**: 281.

246. Jones DM, Eldridge J, Fox AJ, Sethi P & Whorwell PJ. Antibody to the gastric campylobacter-like organism (*Campylobacter pyloridis*): clinical correlations and distribution in the normal population. *J Med Microbiol* 1986; **22**: 57.

247. Meyer B, Werth B, Beglinger C et al. *Helicobacter pylori* infection in healthy people: a dynamic process? *Gut* 1991; **32**: 347.

248. Graham DY, Malaty HM, Evans DG, Evans DJ, Klein PD & Adam E. Epidemiology of *Helicobacter pylori* in an asymptomatic population in the United States. *Gastroenterology* 1991; **100**: 1495.

249. Dooley CP, Fitzgibbons P, Cohen H, Appleman MD, Perez G & Blaser MJ. Prevalence and distribution of *Campylobacter pylori* in an asymptomatic population. *Gastroenterology* 1988; **94**: A102.

250. Siurala M, Sipponen P & Kekki M. *Campylobacter pylori* in a sample of Finnish population: relations to morphology and functions of the gastric mucosa. *Gut* 1988; **29**: 909.

251. Sitos F, Forman D, Yarnell JWG et al. *Helicobacter pylori* infection rates in relation to age and social class in a population of Welsh men. *Gut* 1991; **32**: 25.

252. Feldman RA. Prevention of *Helicobacter pylori* infection. *Bailliares Clin Gastroenterol* 1995; **9**: 447.

253. Thomas JE, Eastham EJ, Elliott TSJ, Dobson CM & Berkeley D. The prevalaence of *C. pylori* infection in childhood and its relation to symptoms. *Gut* 1988; **29**: A707.

254. Ashorn M, Maki M, Hllstrom M et al. *Helicobacter pylori* infection in Finnish children and adolescents. *Scand J Gastroenterol* 1955; **30**: 876–879.

255. Megraud F, Brassens-Rabbe MP, Denis F, Belbouri A & Hoa DQ. Seroepidemiology of *Campylobacter pylori* in various populations. *J Clin Microbiol* 1989; **27**: 1870.

256. Patel P, Mendall MA, Khulusi S, Northfield TC, Strachan DP. *Helicobacter pylori* infection in childhood: risk factors and effect on growth. *B Med J* 1994; **309**: 1119.

257. Perez-Perez GI, Dworkin BM, Chodos JE & Blaser MJ. *Campylobacter pylori* antibodies in humans. *Ann Intern Med* 1988; **109**: 11.

258. Guillermo I, Perez-Perez GI, Taylor GN et al. Seroprevalence of *Helicobacter pylori* infections in Thailand. *J Infect Dis* 1990; **161**: 1237.

259. Sullivan PB, Thomas JE, Wight DGD et al. *Helicobacter pylori* in Gambian children with chronic diarrhoea and malnutrition. *Arch Dis Child* 1990; **65**: 189.

260. Oliveira AM, Queiroz DM, Rocha GA & Medes EN. Seroprevalence of *Helicobacter pylori* infection in children of low socioeconomic level in Belo Horizonte, Brazil. *Am J Gastroenterol* 1994; **89**: 2201.

261. Goodman KJ, Correa P, Tengana Aux HJ et al. *Helicobacter pylori* in the Colombian Andes. *Am J Epidemiol* 1996; **144**: 290.

262. Graham DY, Klein PD, Opekun AR et al. Epidemiology of *Campylobacter pylori* infection: ethnic considerations. *Scand J Gastroenterol* 1988; **23** (Suppl. 142): 9.

263. Graham DY, Klein PD, Opekun AR & Boulton TW. Effect of age on the frequency of active *Campylobacter pylori* infection diagnosed by the ¹³C urea breath test in normal subjects and patients with peptic ulcer disease. *J Infect Dis* 1988; **157**: 777.

264. Graham DY, Adam E, Reddy GT et al. Seroepidemiology of *Helicobacter pylori* infection in India. *Dig Dis Sci* 1991; **36**: 1084.

265. Dwyer B, Kaldor J, Tee W & Raios K. The prevalence of *Campylobacter pylori* in human populations. In Rathbone BJ & Heatley RV (eds) *Campylobacter pylori and Gastroduodenal Disease.* Oxford: Blackwell Scientific, 1989: 190–196.

266. Klein PD, Graham DY, Opekun AR et al. High prevalence of *Campylobacter pylori* (CP) infection in poor and rich Peruvian children determined by ¹³C breath test. *Gastroenterology* 1989; **96**: A260.

267. Lachlan GW, Gilmour HM & Jass JJ, *Campylobacter pylori* in Central Africa. *BMJ* 1988; **296**: 66.

268. Rouvroy D, Bogaerts J, Nsengiumwa O, Omar M, Versailles L & Haot J. *Campylobacter pylori*, gastritis, and peptic ulcer disease in Central Africa. *BMJ* 1987; **295**: 1174.

269. Dehasa M, Dooley CP, Cohen H, Fitzgibbons P, Perez-Perez GI & Blaser MJ. High prevalence of *Campylobacter pylori* (CP) in an asymptomatic Hispanic population. *Gastroenterology* 1989; **96**: A115.

270. Smoak BJ, Kelley PW, Taylor DN. Seroprevalence of *Helicobacter pylori* infections in a cohort of US Army recruits. *Am J Epidermol* 1994; **139**: 513.

271. Webb PM, Knight T, Greaves S et al. Relation between infection with *Helicobacter pylori* and living conditions in childhood. *B M J* 1994; **308**: 750.

272. Galpin OP, Whittaker CJ & Dubiez AJ. *Helicobacter pylori* infection and overcrowding in childhood. *Lancet* 1992; **339**: 619.

273. Mendall MA, Goggin PM, Molineaux N et al. Childhood living conditions and *Helicobacter pylori* seropositivity in adult life. *Lancet* 1992; **339**: 896.

274. Malaty HM & Graham DY. Importance of childhood socioeconomic status on the current prevalence of *H. pylori* infection. *Gut* 1994; **35**: 742.

275. Malaty HM, Kim JG, Kim SD & Graham DY. Prevalence of *Helicobacter pylori* infection in Korean children. *Am J Epidemiol* 1996; **143**: 257.

276. Hassall E & Dimmick JE. Unique features of *Helicobacter pylori* disease in children. *Dig Dis Sci* 1991; **36**: 417.

277. Kang JY, Wee A, Math MV et al. *Helicobacter pylori* and gastritis in patients with peptic ulcer and non-ulcer dyspepsia: ethnic differences in Singapore. *Gut* 1990; **31**: 850.

278. Curry A, Jones DM & Eldridge J. Spiral organisms in the baboon stomach. *Lancet* 1987; **ii**: 634.

279. Baskerville A & Newell DG. Naturally occurring chronic gastritis and *C. pylori* infection in the rhesus monkey: a potential model for gastritis in man. *Gut* 1988; **19**: 465.

280. Fox SG, Correa P, Taylor NS et al. *Helicobacter mustelae*-associated gastritis in ferrets: an animal model of *Helicobacter pylori* gastritis in humans. *Gastroenterology* 1990; **99**: 352.

281. Lee A, Hazell SL, O'Rourke J & Kouprach S. Isolation of a spiral-shaped bacterium from the cat stomach. *Infect Immun* 1988; **56**: 2843.

282. Jones DM & Eldridge J. Gastric Campylobacter-like organisms (GCLO) from man ('*C. pyloridis*') compared with GLCO strains from the pig, baboon and ferret. In *Proceedings of the Fourth International Workshop on Campylobacter Infections*, Gothenburg, 1987.

283. Vaira D, D'Anastasio C, Holton J et al. *Campylobacter pylori* in abbatoir workers. Is it a zoonosis? *Lancet* 1988; **ii**: 725.

284. Hopkins RJ, Russell RG, O'Donnoghue JM, Wasserman SS, Lefkowitz A & Morris JG. Seroprevalence of *Helicobacter pylori* in Seventh-day Adventists and other groups in Maryland. *Arch Intern Med* 1990; **150**: 2347.

285. Klein PD. *Helicobacter pylori* is a waterborne disease in Peruvian children. *Gastroenterology* 1990; **98**: A69.

286. Park CE & Stankiewicz ZK. Survival of *Campylobacter pylori* in food and water. In *Abstracts of the 87th Annual Meeting of the American Society for Microbiology*, Washington, DC; 1987: 275.

287. Klein PD. Gastrointestinal Physiology Working Group, Graham DY et al. Water source as risk factor for *Helicobacter* infection in Peruvian children. *Lancet* 1991; **337**: 1503.

288. Neale KR & Logan RP. The epidemiology and transmission of *Helicobacter pylori* infection in children. *Aliment Pharm Ther* 1995; **9** Suppl 2: 77.

289. Langenberg W, Rauws EAJ, Oudbier JH & Tytgat GNJ. Patient-to-patient transmission of *Campylobacter pylori* infection by fibreoptic gastroduodenoscopy and biopsy. *J Infect Dis* 1990; **161**: 507.

290. Reiff A, Jacobs E & Kist M. Seroepidemiological study of the immune response to *Campylobacter pylori* in potential risk groups. *Eur J Clin Microbiol Infect Dis* 1989; **8**: 592.

291. Lambert JR, Lin SK, Nicholson L et al. High prevalence of *H. pylori* antibodies in institutionalised adults. *Gastroenterology* 1990; **98**: A74

292. Lambert JR, Lin SK, Sievert W et al. High prevalence of *Helicobacter pylori* antibodies in an institutionalised population. *Am J Gastroenterol*, 1995; **90**: 2167.

293. Mitchell HM, Lee A & Carrick J. Increased incidence of *Campylobacter pylori* infection in gastroenterologists: further evidence to support person-to-person transmission of *C. pylori*. *Scand J Gastroenterol* 1989; **24**: 396.

294. Su YC, Wang WM, Chen LT et al. High seroprevalence of IgG against *Helicobacter pylori* amongst endoscopists in Taiwan. *Dig Dis Sci* 1996; **41**: 1571.

295. Rawles JW, Harris ML, Paull G et al. Antibody to *Campylobacter pyloridis* in endoscopy personnel, patients and controls. *Gastroenterology* 1987; **92**: A1589.

296. Lin SK, Lambert SR, Schembri MA, Nicholson L & Korman MG. *Helicobacter pylori* prevalence in endoscopy and medical staff. *J Gastroenterol Hepatol* 1994; **9**: 319.

297. Pardo-Mindan FJ, Joly M, Robledo C, Sola J & Valerdiz S. Duodenal ulcer 'epidemic' in a pathology department. *Lancet* 1989; **i**: 153.

298. Drumm B, Perez-Perez GI, Blaser MJ & Sherman PM. Intra-familial clustering of *Helicobacter pylori* infection. *N Engl J Med* 1990; **322**: 359.

299. Oderda G, Vaira D, Holton J et al. *Helicobacter pylori* in children with peptic ulcer and their families. *Dig Dis Sci* 1991; **36**: 572.

300. Georgopoulos SD, Mentis AF, Spiliadis CA et al. *Helicobacter pylori* infection in spouses of patients with duodenal ulcer and comparison of ribsonal RNA gene patterns. *Gut* 1996; **39**: 634.

301. Parente F, Maconi G, Sangaletti O et al. Prevalence of *Helicobacter pylori* infection and related gastroduodenal lesions in spouses of *Helicobacter pylori* positive duodenal ulcer patients. *Gut* 1996; **39**: 629.

302. Perez-Perez GI, Witkin SS, Decker MD & Blaser MJ. Seroprevalence of *Helicobacter pylori* infection in couples. *J Clin Microbiol* 1991; **29**: 642.

303. Alam K, Cutler A & Schubert T. Prevalence of *Helicobacter pylori* in spouses of infected patients. *Gastroenterology* 1993; **104**: A31.

304. Jones DM, Eldridge J & Whorwell PJ. Antibodies to *Campylobacter pyloridis* in household contacts of infected patients. *BMJ* 1987; **294**: 615.

305. Ho SA, Dixon MF, Wyatt JI & Quirke P. The molecular diagnosis of *Helicobacter pylori*. In Miller JP & Bell GD (eds) *Progress in Gastroenterology: Helicobacter pylori and Other Insights.* Wells Medical, 1991: 17.

306. Krajden S, Fuksa M, Anderson J et al. Examination of human stomach biopsies, saliva and dental plaque for *Campylobacter pylori*. *J Clin Microbiol*, 1989; **27**: 1397.

307. Blecker U, Lanciers S, Hauser B & Vandenplas Y. The prevalence of *Helicobacter pylori* positivity in a symptom-free population aged 1–40 years. *J Clin Epidemiol* 1994; **47**: 1095.

308. Parsonnet J. The incidence of *Helicobacter pylori* infection. *Aliment Pharm Ther* 1995; **9** Suppl 2: 45.

309. Cullen DJ, Collins BJ, Christiansen K et al. When is *Helicobacter pylori* infection acquired? *Gut* 1993; **34**: 1681.

310. Drumm B, Perez-Perez GI, Blaser MJ & Sherman PM. Intrafamilial clustering of *Helicobacter pylori* infection. *N Eng J Med* 1990; **322**: 359.

311. Bamford KB, Bickley J, Collins IS et al. *Helicobacter pylori*: comparisons of DNA fingerprints provides evidence for intrafamilial infection. *Gut* 1993; **34**: 1348.

312. Maxton DG, Srivastanva ED, Whorwell PJ & Jones DM. Do non-steroidal anti-inflammatory drugs or smoking predispose to *Helicobacter pylori* infection? *Postgrad Med J* 1990; **66**: 717.

313. Replogle ML, Glaser SL, Miatt RA & Parsonnet J. Biologic sex as a risk factor for *Helicobacter pylori* infection in healthy young adults. *Am J Epidemiol*, 1995; **142**: 856.

28

CHRONIC GASTRIC ULCER

PE Donahue

Chronic gastric ulceration remains a serious problem, with an incidence and complication rate which has remained remarkably constant for the past 50 years. Unfortunately, the potential of modern databases for the evaluation of large groups of patients with respect to treatment and long-term complications has largely not been realized. Analysis of the gastric ulcer problem has been limited to isolated groups of patients, followed for different periods and using different markers of outcome.

INCIDENCE

Chronic gastric ulcer is a disease which has many possible cofactors, and which presents in a variety of ways. The precise incidence of gastric ulcer has varied considerably during the past century, for reasons which are unclear to us; similarly, the incidence of elective treatment of ulcer has declined during the past 40 years. Prior to the twentieth century, duodenal ulcer was rarely mentioned, whereas gastric ulcer was not an infrequent occurrence. For example, perforated ulcers began to be recognized during the eighteenth century, with half of these noted in young women who had acute gastric ulcers as the pathological event.[1]

Interestingly, perforation of juxtapyloric ulcers is a more modern phenomenon, recorded first at the beginning of the twentieth century. The death rate for patients with perforated ulcer reached a plateau in the 1950s, with a steady decline since that time. Gastric ulcer mortality began to decline before the decline in duodenal ulcer mortality; for some reason the death rate for patients with gastric ulcer began to decline approximately 5 years before that for those with duodenal ulcer. Whether duodenal and gastric ulcers are diseases of urbanization is a question that defies convenient explanation, but the fact remains for interpretation, providing a fascinating opportunity for epidemiologists to analyse potential risk factors (Table 28.1).

The trend for declining death rates has continued during the past two decades for all types of peptic ulcer, although the decline is most marked for duodenal ulcers; this statement is based on data from hospital admissions, surgical procedures, and deaths from ulcers.[2-7] In the USA, the mortality for gastric

Table 28.1 Risk factors for gastric ulcer

Healed (previous) ulcer
Chronic gastritis
Non-steroidal anti-inflammatory drug or steroid treatment
Helicobacter infection
Deformed pylorus

ulcer as well as duodenal ulcer is now in the range of $1.0/10^5$ for men as well as women.[8] In Great Britain, although there has been no change in the number of perforated ulcers as a cause of death, there has been a noticeable decrease in hospital admissions for ulcer in young patients only; death rates from gastric ulcer were similar for men and women in 1985 ($20/10^5$). This figure represents a fall in the rate for men and an increase in that for women.[9] In the USA there has been a similar decrease in the number of patients who require surgical intervention for peptic ulcer disease. In California, for example, there is an interesting correlation between an increased number of endoscopic procedures performed between 1975 and 1980 and a 37% decrease in the number of operations. After the introduction of H_2 blockers for routine treatment of peptic ulcers, the number of operations decreased by 90% (1981–1985), and both endoscopic procedures and expenditure decreased (by 40% respectively).[10]

Mortality from peptic ulcer has another interesting relationship, described by Sonnenberg,[8] who analysed the year of birth versus the mortality rate for the 100 years between 1850 and 1950. In his analysis, there was a birth cohort effect, namely that the mortality for a group of patients was more closely related to the year of their birth than to the year of their death. This in turn suggests that environmental factors influenced the onset of the ulcer disease, and that these factors were similar for all individuals born during a given period. The highest mortality for peptic ulcer occurred in those born around the turn of the century, and decreased in all subsequent generations. In the same report, Sonnenberg documents the rise in mortality rates for older patients, a rise which continued through 1975. Another aspect of the problem is illustrated by a report from Sweden, where an encouraging decline in the rate of elective operation (to $6.0/10^5$) is offset by a persistent incidence of emergency operations $(12/10^5)$.[11]

Although the decreases noted in mortality and incidence are welcomed by all, the subset of patients who suffer complications from peptic ulcer continues to pose a challenge to clinical management. The number of patients who require emergency intervention has remained steady, even increasing in incidence in older patients, in whom associated diseases of cardiac and pulmonary systems are present. Whether these older individuals represent a cohort at increased risk because of when they were born becomes irrelevant to the team of physicians and surgeons who must care for them; instead, the clinician is faced with the more typical problems of disease management – determination of aetiology, appropriate medical treatment of the ulcer, and recognition/treatment of those complications which require surgical intervention.

Although the incidence of surgical intervention for gastric ulcer has decreased, there has not been a corresponding decrease in the number of patients who require emergency operation. In Helsinki, for example, the rate of elective operation for gastric ulcer decreased from 9.4 to $3.1/10^5$ individuals, and for duodenal ulcer from 15.5 to $6.7/10^5$ individuals. However, the annual incidence of emergency surgery for haemorrhage and perforation has increased, varying from 7.2 to $10.5/10^5$ individuals, but the mean age of patients undergoing surgery has also increased.[11]

TYPES OF GASTRIC ULCER

Big, giant, kissing, prepyloric, channel, stress-related, acute, chronic, healed, antral, mucosal, full-thickness, types I–IV – all of these terms describe ulcers which occur in the stomach. None of these terms completely describes the pathogenesis of a gastric ulcer, since the aetiology of ulcers remains unclear. If we knew precisely how ulcers occur, then we might devise more effective preventive measures, or our treatments would be more genuinely curative. Instead, we are at a primitive, descriptive stage of knowledge, in which the location of an ulcer or the common circumstance which attends its appearance must be substituted for true understanding of its pathogenesis. As the following paragraphs develop aspects of ulcers of the stomach, it will be clear that we know many details which are potentially of great help in forming a treatment plan, and which offer a reasonable guarantee that the problem can be 'managed' effectively. Let us continue to strive for a better understanding of the mechanisms which cause these lesions, and hopefully to achieve the goal of *preventing* ulcers rather than treating their complications.

Classification of gastric ulcers based on location: types I–IV

The subdivision of gastric ulcers based on location has been fruitful in the sense that a rational basis for pathogenesis and treatment can be based upon it. Johnson[12,13] proposed a division of gastric ulcer into three sites in his reports of 1957 and 1965: type I – gastric ulcers located on the lesser curve of the stomach, at the incisura angularis: type II – gastric ulcers found in the presence of a duodenal ulcer or scarred pylorus; type III – prepyloric gastric ulcers, or ulcers in the pyloric channel. These are distinguished from some of the less dramatic forms of mucosal disease, such as gastritis, and acute gastric mucosal lesions.

Csendes et al.[14] have proposed the recognition of the type IV gastric ulcer as a definite entity, based on the high incidence of this lesion in their clinic in Santiago. As many as 27% of the gastric ulcers treated in their clinic were in the 'high' location.

A remaining question, and one which does not as yet have a good answer, is how to categorize the acute gastric mucosal lesion. These lesions, often multiple, found in conjunction with sepsis, shock, trauma and major injuries of the head and extremities, are not generally thought of as having a relation to chronic ulceration. On the other hand, they arise in some of the same circumstances as chronic ulcers, and cause surgical complications of haemorrhage and perforation in a few patients, especially those who take non-steroidal anti-inflammatory drugs (NSAIDs). As discussed below, there are some signs that these lesions and their relation to chronic ulcer deserves re-evaluation.

PATHOGENESIS

Mucosal factors

There are many particular aspects of mucosal structure and function, innervation and blood supply and paracrine, endocrine and hormonal factors that affect mucosal function. The only way to address these multiple factors is to mention salient findings which have shed light on part of the 'ulcer' problem, while at the same time admitting that the disease is essentially undefined in its particular causation. A fair statement of the present is that we are phenomenologists, grasping at possible factors in each patient, yet unsure of which aspects of the equation deserve the most emphasis at a given time.

Location

The site of the ulcer is of great interest. Mucosal junctions, that is the boundary of the corpus and antrum, of the antrum and duodenum, and the region of the squamocolumnar junction, have been noted to be the site of ulcers in most cases. Peptic ulcer of the oesophagus occurs immediately proximal to the mucosal oesophagogastric junction; peptic ulcer of the duodenum occurs just distal to the mucosal gastroduodenal junction; peptic ulcer of the stomach occurs just distal to the boundary of the corpus and antrum. The variable location of this boundary among different stomachs (4–12 cm proximal to the pylorus on the lesser curvature and 5–10 cm proximal to the pylorus on the greater curvature) determines whether the ulcer is proximal (high) or distal (low).[15] This location factor is referred to as the 'rule of Oi' and should be kept in mind when mucosal factors are considered; precisely what it is about the antral mucosa which sets the stage for ulceration is unknown, but perhaps a combination of blood supply and innervation as well as intrinsic mucosal defences (adaptive cytoprotection) are responsible.[16]

Innervation

Innervation of the stomach and adaptive cytoprotection are important considerations, and our knowledge of these has increased since the early 1980s. Prior to 1980, traditional views of sympathetic and parasympathetic nerves were predominant and it was thought that vagal factors included mainly cholinergic nerves, and sympathetic nerves only adrenergic neurotransmitters. Since then, our understanding of the complexity of neural pathways and neurotransmitters within these pathways has expanded dramatically. It is now clear that peptides, hormones and the entire family of ganglionic and peripheral neurotransmitters are involved in the transmission of messages to mucosal structures. The role of direct innervation is poorly understood, especially in the light of several studies showing that only relatively few of the ganglia in the myenteric plexus appear to have discrete connections with the brain. A number of studies have shown that neural peptides affect gastrointestinal motility, acid secretion and the development of experimental gastroduodenal ulcers.[17]

However, increased knowledge of specific peptides and transmitters has not resulted in a more coherent view of the problem of ulcers from the clinical standpoint; this point is of added significance with respect to gastric ulcers because they will be recognized with greater frequency as the population ages.

There are some new aspects of motor innervation that have become apparent in our studies of gastric efferent vagus nerve innervation. When we tried to explain physiological evidence of efferent nerve function (acid secretion) on the greater curve of the stomach,[18] we employed retrograde axonal tracing to define a set of previously undefined nerves which traverse the neurovascular pedicles of the greater curve. In the rat and the ferret we found that the gastroepiploic nerves, the short gastric nerves and the posterior gastric nerves have efferent vagus nerve fibres.[19-21] Further, when exploring the routes by which these nerves reach the brainstem, we discovered that the right gastroepiploic nerves (in the rat) actually traversed the pylorus.[21] Later, when the optimal surgical treatment of type II gastric ulcers is discussed, the possible relevance of this factor will be highlighted.

Efferent nerves to the stomach have long been the focus of experimental and clinical studies, but these nerves and their function cannot explain the genesis of gastric lesions; available evidence suggests that gastric acid is an essential cofactor, but that is hardly a new idea because the 'no acid, no ulcer' statement has been made since the beginning of the twentieth century. The current focus of most studies of the stomach and its ulceration have concentrated on mucosal factors and local factors which influence mucosal destruction, proliferation and protection.

Since the advent of techniques for selective obliteration of afferent nerves, either singly or throughout the body, there has been renewed interest in attempting to define the role which *afferent* nerves play in gastric function. The work of Holzer et al.[22,23] in Graz has been especially helpful in introducing the concept that the afferent nerves mediate local defence mechanisms, and that animals without afferent nerve function have a greater propensity for the development of mucosal lesions. Of note, studies to date have investigated acute mucosal ulceration (type III ulcers) and do not yet address the deep chronic ulcers that account for much gastric pathology. Nerve tracing techniques have also been applied to the afferent vagus nerve pathways to the stomach and have shown that there is an ipsilateral organization to these nerves; that is, the nerves to the anterior gastric wall appear to be almost completely separate from those which supply the posterior gastric wall.[24,25] In a parallel study we have shown further that selective ablation of the afferent vagus nerves on the right or on the left side exerted a protective effect on the gastric mucosa supplied by that nerve.[26] Whereas these findings show some variance with other studies of afferent nerves, they are supported by the results of the companion axonal tracing of afferent nerves. Many of the studies in the literature have not shown, in a rigorous way, that afferent nerves were truly blocked, and we believe that the true nature of afferent nerve–mucosa interaction can only be defined if this important variable is controlled in individual experiments.

Do the afferent nerves mediate local protection or adaptive cytoprotection? The answer to this question is not fully known at present.

Adaptive cytoprotection

Adaptive cytoprotection is the term used to describe the protective effect of mild gastric irritants on the gastric mucosa; this effect is found when the mild irritant (e.g. 25% alcohol, 2 mol/l NaCl) is given before the application of a harsh irritant (e.g. 100% alcohol). Mild irritants have been shown to increase mucosal blood flow, and there is evidence that harsh irritants cause little or no damage when mucosal blood flow is high.[27] A report by Svanes et al.[28] used an ingenious method to determine whether blood flow alone was the critical factor in mediating the protective response: the blood flow in the coeliac artery was reduced by 60%, as determined by Doppler ultrasound flowmetry. In the cats in this study, decreased blood flow eliminated the protective effect of prior exposure to a mild irritant. Further, there was a highly significant correlation between mucosal blood flow and the presence of deep mucosal lesions.

In addition to blood flow, other mucosal factors provide protection to the mucosa; possibly the effect of blood flow is always to provide a pre-existing defence mechanism with the energy and renewable supplies required for further function. Mucus and bicarbonate are factors which occur in the mucosa and which are thought to participate in the protective response.

When the mucous coat is damaged or diminished by low secretion rates, the stomach is at greater risk of injury. Aspirin, ethanol, bile salts or steroids can inhibit secretion, whereas acid, prostaglandins and other factors can stimulate secretion of mucus. Mucus alone, however, is inadequate to prevent the mucosa from luminal acid; bicarbonate secretion is thought to be an important cofactor in the protection of the gastric wall, possibly acting most efficiently in the so-called 'unstirred' layer at the mucus–mucosa interface.[27]

Work from Philadelphia utilized topical anaesthetics to obliterate the effect of afferent nerves on adaptive cytoprotection, and found that bile salt injury was not prevented in the presence of afferent blockade with topical lignocaine. The authors concluded that production of mucus was not the critical factor but that interference with prostaglandin synthesis or release was responsible for the observed results.[29]

Blood flow

High mucosal blood flow has been implicated as an important factor in protective responses in the stomach, as referred to above by Holzer et al. and by other workers. Prostaglandins of the E, A and I series have been shown to be gastric mucosal vasodilators, but there is no agreement regarding the importance of prostaglandins in adaptive cytoprotection.[29]

Growth factor

Epidermal growth factor (EGF) has a potent trophic action on the cells of the gastrointestinal tract. The major source of EGF which is amenable to experimental manipulation is the salivary gland; removal of the sublingual–submandibular salivary gland complex in rats results in a decrease in mucosal growth, mucosal integrity and loss of protection against ulcerogenic drugs. In rats undergoing water restraint stress, for example, addition of preliminary sialadenectomy results in a twofold increase in the number of lesions. Further, these animals were less protected by exogenous EGF or prostaglandin therapy than animals with intact salivary glands.[30] The effect of EGF is possibly mediated by changes in the rate of DNA synthesis and epithelial proliferation, as shown by the original report of Takeuchi and Johnson.[31] Another effect of EGF is the stimulation of mucosal prostaglandin E_2 synthesis; it is possible that the effect of sialadenectomy on stress ulceration is due in part to reduced prostaglandin formation in the gastric mucosa. In the study by Konturek et al.,[30] referred to above, there was some residual prostaglandin synthesis in the gastric mucosa, and it was possible to aggravate the effect of stress by adding indomethacin to further reduce the amount of mucosal prostaglandin. One hypothesis of the precise relationship of EGF and prostaglandins is that both are involved in the maintenance of gastric mucosal blood flow; this was first proposed by Muramatsu et al.[32] in 1985.

Bile reflux

Consideration of the role of bile reflux in promoting gastric ulcer has been productive because it provides a unifying concept for several of the major factors which affect gastric ulcer. For example, mucosal and antral motility factors can both be interpreted in the light of aggravation by bile and duodenal content; in all of this discussion, bile reflux is used as a phrase to equate with enterogastric reflux, and with full awareness that factors other than bile may irritate the gastric mucosa.

The observations by du Plessis[33] and Lawson[34] on the relation of bile reflux and gastric ulcers has been very useful; in addition to stimulating productive studies for more than two decades, they also reinforced the recommendations of those who suggested that the best way to approach the majority of the 'postgastrectomy' syndromes was not to perform 95% of the resections (which could be avoided by employing other procedures). Since these studies were performed, the focus of investigations has concentrated on more discrete components of the gastric wall. Some of the factors now being evaluated, such as infection of the gastric mucosa, had yet to be described.

Chronic gastritis – *Helicobacter pylori* infection

There is substantial evidence that chronic gastritis is a risk factor for the eventual development of ulcer disease, as confirmed in a study by Sipponen et al.[35] In 454 consecutive patients, 11% of 321 with gastritis in the biopsy specimens developed ulcers, compared with 0.8% of the patients in whom gastritis was not present at the initial biopsy. The highest incidence of ulcerogenesis was in middle-aged men, 41–60 years old, who had chronic antral gastritis or chronic gastritis of the corpus and antrum; the cumulative 10-year risk of ulcer was low when the antrum and corpus were normal. This study is of extreme interest in the light of discoveries about chronic bacterial infection of the gastric and duodenal mucosa, and provides further evidence that gastritis and duodenitis cannot be ignored as significant pathologic entities.

As discussed in previous chapters, *H. pylori* is associated with gastritis and/or gastroduodenal ulceration; the medical community is increasingly aware of this association, following the initial report in 1983. Since that time, a number of investigators have confirmed the association, including a report in which Koch's postulates were confirmed with respect to this agent.[36,37] In another recent study utilizing germ-free mice, Lee and colleagues[38] in Boston have shown conclusively that bacterial colonization can cause the histological picture of active chronic gastritis in a small animal model. Although the association of this bacterial agent with gastritis and ulcer is now generally accepted, it is by no means clear what attempt should be made to control or eradicate this agent, and exactly what role it plays in the pathogenesis of pathological lesions. For example, whereas most patients with gastritis have *Helicobacter* infections, and there is a strong correlation of this infection with gastritis, there are exceptions. Braverman et al.[39] in Israel reported on 147 patients: 24% of those with gastritis did not have evidence of infection; conversely, 11% of those without gastritis were positive for *Helicobacter*. There may be other cofactors which need to be identified and the presence of *Helicobacter* may not be an all or none phenomenon. A recent study provides some evidence about one way in which infection could remain quiescent for some time.

Until recently, *Helicobacter* infection was thought to be a surface phenomenon; however, a report by Wyle et al.[40] suggests otherwise. Patients with gastric ulcer in their clinic had a 48% incidence of infection, and those with chronic gastritis had *H. pylori* in the lower portion of the gastric mucosa. When these cells were examined by transmission electron microscopy, the bacteria were found in two types of association: closely adherent to the surface, or actually invading the cells of the mucosa. These latter bacteria appeared to be either intact or in the process of disintegration.[40]

Previous ulcer: a specific risk?

The possibility that the mere presence of a chronic ulcer is a separate risk factor for recurrence is of interest, and has recently gained support with an elegant experimental study in rats. When acetic acid-induced ulcers were followed at intervals of 2 weeks to 4 months, the findings suggested that healing did not return to a normal pattern. Instead, the mucosa was thinner than normal (25–45% reduction), with increased connective tissue. Another change observed was that the mucosa showed dilatation of gastric glands and a reduction in the microvascular network. If these alterations result in an altered nutrient supply or microcirculation, then mucosal defences might be impaired, predisposing to ulcer recurrence.[41] Another consideration which will be mentioned subsequently is the possibility that gastric motility is adversely affected by the presence of an ulcer, especially one in a critical location. When we examined the pyloric ring of patients with pyloric thickening, for example, we found a distinct band of fibrosis within the sphincter; the prevailing view of many surgeons is that pyloric thickening is a result of oedema and acute ulcer reaction, and that healing of the ulcer allows the return of normal function. Perhaps a severely deformed pylorus is never able to return to a normal pattern of function.[42]

Non-steroidal anti-inflammatory drug treatment

The widespread use of NSAIDs in the treatment of arthritic conditions, especially in elderly patients, has been associated with a specific risk of gastric ulcer. Possible explanations include the inhibition of mucosal defence mechanisms, especially prostaglandin production.

Another effect of these drugs is the inhibition of the proliferation of mucosal cells from the periphery of the ulcer, as shown by Levi et al.[43] In gastric ulcer, there was a marked difference in the regeneration index at the ulcer edge in those subjects not receiving NSAIDs; the index was derived from a mitosis index in glands at the edge of the ulcer. In rats with cryoprobe-induced ulcers, the deficiency in mitotic index and healing was also noted when a NSAID (indomethacin) was employed, which was reversed by the prostaglandin E_1 analogue misoprostol.[43] This is another possible mechanism for the association of NSAIDs and gastric ulcer.

The magnitude of the problem associated with aspirin therapy is provided by the work of Kurata and Abbey,[6] who analysed 4524 subjects in the Aspirin Myocardial Infarction Study. In males, the risk of hospitalization for duodenal ulcer was 10.7 times higher in those taking aspirin (1.0 g/day). The adjusted relative risk for gastric ulcer was 9.1; due to the small numbers of females in the study, the risk for women was not calculated. For the group as a whole, the risk of hospitalization for peptic ulceration was 7.7 times higher than the expected rate.[6] A similar conclusion that NSAID treatment increases the risk of ulcer morbidity is shown by Griffin et al.,[44] who demonstrated, in a case–control study, that NSAID use carried a relative risk of 4.0 for ulcer bleeding and death, and that deaths were equally distributed between gastric and duodenal ulcers. The risk of bleeding was greater than perforation, but 25% of patients had both bleeding and perforation. Of concern, 11% of the population studied were taking NSAID therapy. Finally, Armstrong and Whitelaw,[45] in a recent autopsy study of undiagnosed peptic ulcer complications, found that 81 of 153 patients dying of such complications were taking anti-inflammatory drugs. Clearly the risk of these widely used compounds is underestimated both by physicians and their patients.

COMPLICATIONS

The problems which bring patients to the attention of physicians and surgeons are one or more of the following: pain, bleeding, perforation or obstruction of the gastric outlet. These complications need not exist independently; and frequently coexist.

Bleeding

No single complication of an ulcer commands the attention of the medical community as does massive bleeding. As mentioned above, the incidence of bleeding has probably not decreased in recent years, although the number of patients requiring emergency operation has definitely decreased, largely due to the advent of effective endoscopic haemostatic techniques.

When an ulcer bleeds, the patient's subsequent course is almost entirely dependent on the location and size of the ulcer, as well as particular attributes of the bleeding site. For example, the presence of a visible vessel in the ulcer base or the presence of a clot on the surface of the ulcer is a distinct risk factor for rebleeding. An ulcer which is actively bleeding at the time of initial endoscopy has an 80% chance of continued or recurrent bleeding,[46] whereas the visible vessel rebleeds in about 50% of cases.[47,48]

Endoscopic Doppler studies provide another insight regarding recurrence rates in gastric ulcer, as shown by Lunde and Kvernebo[49] of Oslo. Patients with ulcers at the lesser curvature of the corpus were found to have decreased blood blow in the ulcer bed compared with the ulcer margin. The low flow rates at the site of the ulcer persisted at 4 months, despite healing of the ulcer in 14 of 15 of the patients studied. Perhaps the submucosa and ulcer base never fully recover the normal pattern of blood flow, explaining the potential for recurrent ulcers in the same general area. This is one of several studies which indicate that the healing of an ulcer crater does not imply that complete structural and functional normality has been re-established in the locus of the ulcer, and that further study should be devoted to discovering the reasons why a 'normal' environment does not occur after healing of an ulcer.

Perhaps the most important concept to keep in mind is that the incidence of bleeding from peptic ulcer has remained stable, as shown by the report of Kurata and Corboy;[50] approximately 8% of gastric ulcers and 15% of duodenal ulcers continue to be complicated by haemorrhage.

Perforation

Perforation of ulcers is a traditional benchmark of ulcer incidence, as alluded to previously, because the presence of a perforation is usually not subject to misinterpretation. The mortality of perforated ulcers has not changed appreciably in recent years, although the average age and number of associated conditions has changed. The report of Gunshefski et al.,[51] is typical, in that the mean age of perforated ulcer patients was 61 years, the mortality was 24%, and 44% of the patients were taking ulcerogenic drugs (either NSAIDs or steroids). The site of the perforation was in the gastric body in 18%, and in the pyloric region in 20% of these individuals.[51] An association between medication and ulcer complications is a recurring theme at the present time, and the message that we must be alert to ulcer complications in patients of this type is particularly apposite. Furthermore, many patients have a delay in diagnosis, or are too sick at the time of diagnosis to undergo a definitive procedure, as shown by the fact that only 38% of patients did so.

When considering the possibility of perforation, one should be aware of its sometimes subtle presentation. A report from St Louis describes four additional patients to the previously described 104 patients who had gastrocolic fistula as a result of benign gastric ulcer. A surprising factor in 75% of patients reported during a 10-year period was the use of NSAIDs or steroidal anti-inflammatory drugs; there was also a high percentage of young female patients. When patients present with weight loss, diarrhoea and faecal vomiting, this complication should be suspected, even though the clinical team may be preoccupied with the management of pain, bleeding or the question of perforated viscus.[52] This report suggests a change in the pathogenesis of gastrocolic fistula, which was previously found as a result of recurrent ulcer disease in patients who had undergone a retrocolic gastrojejunostomy with incomplete (or without) vagotomy.

Obstruction

Blockage of the gastric outlet by ulcer disease has a wide range of expression, ranging from complete obstruction with a pinhole aperture in the distal stomach to that of a chronically scarred and dysfunctional gastric outlet. Perhaps we have been too lenient in identifying those patients with diseased, but not completely obstructing lesions, especially when due to juxtapyloric (type II) ulcers. Perhaps there are criteria which would make the clinical diagnosis of obstruction easier, making it more convenient for physicians and surgeons to identify those patients who will benefit from treatment directed towards a physiological problem at the gastric outlet.

In the past it was not difficult to identify the patient who required resection or bypass of the gastric outlet. This approach was reserved for individuals with weight loss, obvious enlargement of the stomach, and near complete obstruction as judged endoscopically. With smaller calibre flexible endoscopes, it is now possible to negotiate even a severely deformed pyloric ring, and endoscope passage alone does not exclude the presence of a diseased pyloric ring.

A report by Lu and Schulze-Delrieu[53] from Iowa City is of interest in this regard. These investigators report that the use of a double-contrast radiographic technique can identify changes in the configuration and movements of the gastroduodenal junction which result from peptic ulcer disease involving the proximal and distal pyloric muscle loops. During a 4-year period, 50 cases of pyloric ulcer were studied; in 18, the ulcers maintained a consistent location with respect to the muscles of the pylorus, leading to many strange deformities of the gastric outlet, including pseudodiverticula and reversal of the pyloric angulation. The most common site for peptic lesions in the pyloric segment was the protuberance of the lesser curvature called the pyloric torus; this resulted in radiographic evidence of increased duodenogastric reflux. Pyloric closure was further impaired in this setting because the mucosa no longer prolapsed into the gastric outlet as it normally does. One-third of patients had reflux oesophagitis in addition to pyloric disease.[53] Perhaps these abnormalities of the pyloric ring can explain a number of problems, such as the propensity for recurrence which pyloric ulcers display, especially when treated by medical therapy alone or by highly selective vagotomy without pyloroplasty. Perhaps the inclusion of 'form and function pyloroplasty' by Holle et al.[54] in their earlier reports explains some of their success in the treatment of ulcers near the pyloric ring.

Malignancy

The question of whether a benign ulcer can become malignant is one which has been answered in the negative sense by several recent reports. It would seem that a malignant lesion can manifest itself by the presence of an ulcer in its surface. Furthermore, it is possible for a malignant gastric ulcer to heal while the patient receives standard medical treatment; this factor underscores the necessity for multiple biopsies of an ulcer during the acute phase, as well as biopsies of the healed ulcer scar, which occasionally reveal the presence of carcinoma.

Lee et al.[55] reviewed 2529 patients with peptic ulcer treated between 1963 and 1975 and followed for 9–23 years. A total of 38 patients subsequently died of cancer, including nine in whom the site of the cancer coincided with the previously diagnosed gastric ulcer. Although these cancers were related to the original ulcer, the number of deaths from gastric cancer in patients with gastric ulcer was significantly lower than that expected using age- and sex-matched death rates in the general population in Fukuoka.[55] Another study of the relationship between gastric ulcer and cancer was reported by Hole et al.[56] who studied 13 000 autopsies in a single hospital over a 20-year period and reported a prospective 1-year study of 7000 autopsies in 17 centres. In both studies, a lower than expected incidence of gastric cancer was found in subjects with pathological evidence of active or previous gastric and duodenal ulcer. Although a statistical association between lung cancer and gastric ulcer was found, there was no increased risk of gastric carcinoma in patients with gastric ulcer.[56] Another recent study has confirmed this finding, namely that, in general, the only excess mortality observed in patients after gastric resection was accounted for by men and the use of tobacco products.[57] In 2663 patients in Amsterdam who had undergone gastrectomy between 1931 and 1960, postoperative mortality was noted to be increased by the 12-year interval. When risk ratios for specific causes of death were obtained, both men and women had increased rates for cancer of the lung; cancer of the stomach was observed slightly more than predicted by the model (observed/expected: 1.6 and 3.2 for men and women, respectively, with gastric ulcer; and 0.8 and 1.0 for men and women, respectively, with duodenal ulcer). The authors note that we must be cognizant that this potential problem is still of concern because there are still many patients with recurrence of ulcer disease, despite the advent of non-resectional approaches for duodenal ulcer.

Although the incidence of cancer is low in patients with gastric ulcer, there are indicators seen on biopsy which can predict the eventual appearance of gastric cancer, and which can be a guide to individual patient management. Lansdown et al.[58] in Leeds identified 40 patients with an initial histological diagnosis of gastric epithelial dysplasia; of these, 20 were considered to have true dysplasia on further analysis, 13 of whom had 'high-grade' dysplasia. Of these 13, 85% developed gastric cancer within 15 months; when operated upon, the patients usually had early cancer, and none had lymph node metastases. It would appear that a diagnosis of high-grade dysplasia is an indication for radical surgical treatment, all other factors being equal.

MEDICAL TREATMENT

Medical treatments include one or several of the medications (Table 28.2) which have been shown to accelerate or promote ulcer healing.

Table 28.2 Pharmacological agents for treatment of gastric ulcer

THERAPEUTIC CLASS	TARGET
Antacids	Gastric acid
H$_2$-receptor antagonists	Gastric acid
Anticholinergics	Gastric acid
Tricyclics	Gastric acid
Substituted benzimidazoles	Gastric acid
Prostaglandins	Gastric acid, cytoprotection, blood flow
Sulphated disaccharides	Base of ulcer, protect growth factor
Colloidal bismuth	Growth factor, ulcer base bacteria, H$^+$ diffusion
Liquorice extracts	Mucous and secretory cells

Histamine H$_2$-receptor antagonists

Following the original report from Chicago, that the use of a histamine receptor antagonist (H$_2$ site) accelerated the rate of gastric ulcer healing, there have been numerous reports that the rate of healing is influenced by the use of this drug. Recently there have been several prospective trials comparing the use of H$_2$ blockers with omeprazole. In all these studies the healing rate for ulcers is similar with both agents, although omeprazole has a statistically significant advantage.[60] The advantage is usually quite clear when the H$_2$ blocker is compared with placebo; when compared with an agent with therapeutic effects, there is usually a less clear-cut difference. There are, furthermore, failures in every treatment group, reinforcing the need to consider surgical treatment at some point to prevent the development of serious complications, a concept described previously by Littman and Hanscom[60] of Chicago.

Omeprazole

Omeprazole, designed to interfere with the proton pump mechanism in the oxyntic cells, is the latest and perhaps the only molecular-based treatment to be employed for gastric ulcer. Exposure to gastric acid inactivates omeprazole, so the drug has been formulated in pH-sensitive granules which release omeprazole only when the pH is above 6.0; with this formulation the bioavailability of omeprazole is about 50%. This drug has unparalleled efficacy in the treatment of peptic ulcer. Sixteen randomized, controlled trials of omeprazole and H$_2$-receptor blockers have shown an advantage in favour of omeprazole of −2 to +30% after 2 weeks for duodenal ulcer; at 4 weeks the advantage was smaller but still significant (20 mg omeprazole and 300 mg ranitidine). For patients with resistant ulcers, a dose of 40 mg/day of omeprazole is usually effective, but recurrence rates after discontinuation of the drug are comparable with those observed when H$_2$ blockers are discontinued.[61] Patients with gastric ulcers also heal in 86–96% of cases, including patients with ulcers of the corpus, antrum and prepyloric areas; again a treatment advantage has been observed for omeprazole versus H$_2$-receptor antagonist therapy. For patients with relapse of gastric ulcer, omeprazole at 40 mg/day appears to be more effective than H$_2$-receptor antagonists, but it would appear that there are many instances in which a surgical option should be employed rather than depending on continued medical therapy.

The possibility of side-effects and toxicity deserve mention when long-term treatment with new drugs is considered. The main concern of omeprazole treatment has been whether hypergastrinaemia (hypergastrinaemia and carcinoid treatment have been reported in rats treated with omeprazole) would pose a specific risk. In humans, the increase in plasma gastrin is usually on the order of 2–4-fold, although tenfold increases have been reported. Short-term treatment with omeprazole seems to be safe, whereas long-term treatment may cause hyperplasia of enterochromaffin-like cells and possibly carcinoid tumours;[62] further definition of the precise risk must await long-term studies. In the interim, a prudent suggestion has been made, namely the use of shorter periods of omeprazole treatment, for example for 3 days of each week.[63] The concept of prophylactic long-term medical treatment has been found to be one which has definite advantages and which has found wide acceptance in the medical community.

The duration of prophylactic or maintenance therapy is an important practical problem. The report of Pym et al.[64] of 311 patients with healed ulcers is of interest, in that patients received either nocturnal cimetidine or placebo for 3 years.

The cimetidine was cost-effective for the first 2 years of treatment, but was not found to be of benefit during the third year. The cimetidine effect was seen in gastric ulcers (which predominated in this study) as well as in duodenal ulcers. This fact is not surprising in light of the previous report of Sontag, from Chicago, which identified a definite therapeutic role for cimetidine in the treatment of gastric ulcer.[68] Although maintenance cimetidine is effective, even in a once-daily bedtime dose, the use of this agent does not prevent subsequent problems arising from gastric ulcer. The major advantage of maintenance therapy is an increase in healing rate compared with placebo, and a greater incidence of freedom from both daytime and nocturnal pain. One report describes 76% ulcer-healing with cimetidine treatment versus 55% in placebo-treated controls; the freedom from pain was 77%/89% (daytime/nighttime) with cimetidine versus 67%/74% in placebo-treated controls.[65] This report and others are usually focused on the short-term responses of patients to treatment and do not answer some of the questions about the need for surgical treatment in patients who do not achieve prompt healing or who suffer recurrence of their ulcer in the follow-up period. Increasingly, the choice of a surgical alternative is reserved for those individuals who have a frank surgical complication, such as perforation or bleeding, as discussed elsewhere.

Antacids

Antacid therapy is more effective than placebo in controlling gastric ulcer, and comparable to H_2-blocker therapy, although ulcer healing is protracted with antacid treatment (average 2 weeks longer). Until recently, the mechanism of action of antacids has been thought to relate to neutralization of acid and its deleterious effects on the mucosa. However, these compounds, especially those containing aluminium hydroxide, increase the production of prostanoids and sulphhydryl-containing compounds. When patients with gastric ulcer were given high-dose co-magaldrox (Maalox TC) therapy, cultured biopsy specimens exhibited this property, suggesting that stimulation of endogenous prostaglandin is one of the effects of these agents.[66]

Prostaglandin analogues

With the introduction of a prostaglandin E_1 analogue, a new variable has been introduced into the compound equation of drugs used to treat gastric lesions. Originally approved for the prevention of the gastric ulcers associated with NSAID treatment, these agents are used for a variety of disease conditions.[67] At present, however, there is no clear advantage to the use of these drugs, even for their stated purpose. When analysed for their success in healing ulcers, the results are much less clear than with H_2 blockers; rates of healing range from 39 to 54%, making it clear that these are not the agents of choice for the initial treatment of gastric ulcer.[68]

Sucralfate

Sucralfate is an agent with unique actions in protecting the gastric mucosa, and is used for both treatment and prevention of ulcers in the stomach. A recent report illustrates the type of

result achieved with sucralfate when compared to ranitidine for acute gastric ulcer. At 12 weeks, over 80% of patients were healed with either treatment. When sucralfate versus placebo was utilized for maintenance therapy, there was a significant advantage for the sucralfate group in terms of recurrence rates: by 12 months, 55% of the placebo group and 32% of the sucralfate group had had a recurrence. This is certainly of interest, but the high recurrence rate in both groups underscores the chronicity of gastric ulcers, especially in patients with recurrent ulcer, or pyloric stenosis.[69]

Bismuth compounds

Bismuth compounds have a number of effects on the gastric mucosa, including cytoprotection and an anti-infective action against *Helicobacter*. In the European trials, colloidal bismuth subcitrate or subsalicylate have been employed, and the results of treatment have shown efficacy comparable with H_2 blockers or sucralfate for the healing of ulcers. Unfortunately, some of the early trials encountered problems with absorption of the heavy metal bismuth, resulting in a disastrous neuropathy in a large number of French patients. Other reports of toxicity were reported from Australia and elsewhere, leading to caution in introducing this drug into the USA. Since the toxicity has not been reported recently, there is probably little risk at present; however, because approximately 0.2% of an ingested dose is absorbed, the current suggestion is that courses of bismuth therapy should not be longer than 6–8 weeks, with a rest period of 6–8 weeks before resumption of treatment. Unsupervised therapy with this agent is not recommended.[70]

The mechanism of action of bismuth compounds is complex; among the effects which have been verified are the following: binding with mucus and glycoproteins, binding of pepsin and binding of EGF to the ulcer base. Also, the back-diffusion of hydrogen ions is retarded, and *Helicobacter* species are destroyed by bismuth citrate.[71,72] This drug is possibly one of the most effective compounds that can be used for ulceration, and it will certainly receive continued attention in the future.

Antibiotics

These have been used singly, or more recently in combination. When a single antibiotic (cefixime 100 mg/week for 2 weeks) was combined with cimetidine (800 mg/day) and compared with cimetidine alone for the treatment of ulcer with proven *H. pylori* infection, there was a short-term eradication of bacteria as well as a lower recurrence rate at 12 weeks in the antibiotic group; recurrent ulcer rates, however, were similar in both groups by 24 weeks,[73] suggesting several possible explanations. Triple therapy comprising colloidal bismuth, metronidazole and either tetracycline or amoxycillin has been reported to have high rates of healing and low relapse rates. This is discussed in greater detail in Chapter 29.

SURGICAL TREATMENT

There is little consensus between experienced surgeons about the 'ideal' operation for gastric ulcer, despite wide experience with diverse operations over the past 100 years. The lack of consensus is not really surprising, given the limited data available for the analysis of late results. Ultimately, the choice of operation seems to be dictated by the early experience and preferences of the training programme during which techniques of gastrectomy were first learned. A monograph by Wangensteen and Wangensteen[74] reviews the rich history of operative approaches for gastric lesions and illustrates the simultaneous development of techniques which allowed treatment of both malignant and benign lesions. Many of the lessons of the past century still deserve review, as the problems with which we are confronted still employ many of the principles discovered during the 'golden' age of surgery encompassed during the lives of the Professors Wangensteen.

When discussing certain treatment options for gastric ulcer the 'location-based' classification is of real value because it allows individualization of treatment depending on the type of lesion. Since type II and type III ulcers are thought to be partially due to hypersecretion of acid, optimal treatment of these lesions will include vagotomy (truncal, selective, highly selective or extended highly selective).

Type I gastric ulcer

The most effective treatment for this lesion is surgical removal of the distal stomach, usually encompassing the extent of the ulcer in the resection. In practical terms, a 50% resection must be performed, either alone or in conjunction with a truncal vagotomy. When we perform a 50% resection in this way, it is suggested that vagotomy should not be performed unless there is some evidence that a previous duodenal ulcer existed, or there is some pre-existing deformity of the pylorus. The practical benefits of having intact vagi are several, most important being the avoidance of hypomotility and the preservation of receptive accommodation function in the proximal stomach.

With regard to technique of gastric resection I prefer the Billroth I procedure (Figures 28.1–28.4), but there are many surgeons who employ the Billroth II successfully. Both procedures have their advocates, and experienced surgeons know that there is very little objective evidence to support the superiority

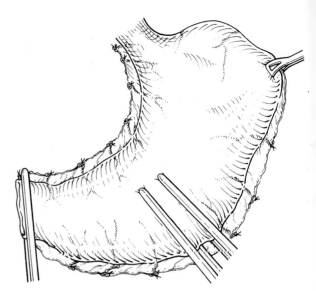

Figure 28.2
Billroth I procedure   The Payr clamp is applied to include 5.0 cm of the gastric wall; then, when the anastomosis is performed, the size of the gastric orifice will approximate to the size of the duodenal orifice. After cutting along the distal edge of the Payr clamp, a TA-90 (4.8 mm staple) stapling device is placed to complete the resection of the gastric tissue.

of either procedure. The essential part of the procedure is that approximately 50% of the stomach should be removed, including all the diseased antral mucosa, and that there should be no postoperative complication.

Billroth I gastrectomy

In 1881 Theodor Billroth performed the first successful partial gastrectomy for a patient with carcinoma of the antrum. The

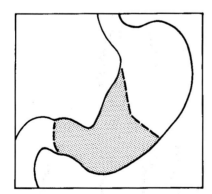

Figure 28.1
Billroth I procedure   The 'rule of thumb' for gastric resection is that 50% of the stomach will be removed. The inclusion of a tongue-like piece of lesser curvature ensures that the extension of the gastric antrum in this area will be removed.

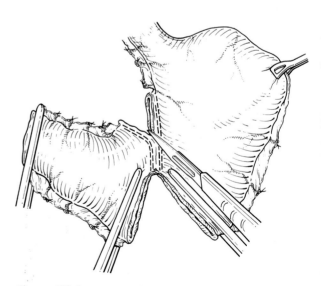

Figure 28.3
Billroth I procedure   As the left gastric artery has been ligated prior to this step, there is little difficulty in completing this portion of the operation. To ensure that the pathology has been adequately resected, the specimen is opened in the operating room.

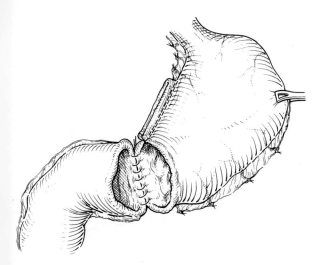

Figure 28.4

Billroth I procedure Gastroduodenal anastomosis requires a
two-layer (outer non-absorbable or absorbable, inner layer
absorbable) anastomosis to prevent bleeding or leakage
postoperatively. The posterior wall outer layer is placed first,
and we believe that a 'perfect' anastomosis requires seven
posterior wall sutures. After completing this anastomosis, an
'angle of sorrows' stitch is placed at the junction of the anterior
wall–posterior wall–duodenum. This precise point is at risk of
leakage due to poor blood supply.

techniques of gastric resection since that time have not
changed dramatically, although there are numerous modifications in the details of reconstruction of intestinal continuity.
When the gastric remnant is sewn to the duodenum, the
stomach can be closed completely, with the anastomosis
between the anterior or posterior gastric wall of the duodenum
as proposed by Kutscha-Lissberg or Kocher. Another approach
is to close the duodenal stump completely, suturing the gastric
remnant to the end of the stomach, as von Haberer and Finney
and Winkelbauer proposed in the 1920s. Others, notably
Schoemaker in 1911, proposed that a tubularization of the gastric remnant be performed to allow complete excision of the
gastric antrum, which sometimes extends cephalad along the
lesser curve of the stomach. As alluded to previously, the concept of complete removal of the antrum has won substantial
support, and today most surgeons include this manoeuvre in
the performance of a gastric resection. The specific details of
the procedure are best shown in a surgical atlas, and the
description by Siewert and Castrup[75] is both comprehensive
and illustrative.

Billroth II gastrectomy[76]

The direct anastomosis between the gastric remnant and the
duodenum is technically easy in most cases, and preferred by
many surgeons. The essential part of this procedure is the
avoidance of an afferent limb which is too long, and the avoidance of either acute or chronic afferent loop problems. There
may be a greater tendency towards gastric atrophic mucosal
disease following this procedure.

Between 1918 and 1923 Kelling and Madlener proposed

that gastric ulcers might be treated successfully by removing
the distal stomach, leaving an ulcer base in situ in the proximal stomach. The attraction of this approach is based on the
well-known hazards of performing a resection of this portion
of the stomach, notably leakage at the suture line and peritonitis. All would agree that total gastrectomy should be
avoided for this type of lesion, and most concur that lesser
operations, such as vagotomy and drainage, wedge excision
of the ulcer, or drainage alone have not been generally successful (although there are reports of positive outcomes in the
literature). In an era when the advantages of modern surgical treatment were largely unavailable, there was a role for
this type of treatment.[77] However, alternatives such as the
Pauchet procedure, or the rotation gastrectomy provide a
practical alternative to the Kelling–Madlener approach
(Figures 28.5–28.8).[78]

Operative procedures for bleeding and perforation

Oversewing the bleeding vessel or perforation combined with
vagotomy and pyloroplasty is not the optimal treatment for
gastric ulcer but is reserved for specific complications, or for
the treatment of unstable patients who cannot tolerate a more
physiologically demanding operation. When combined with
excision of the ulcer base, the operation is more attractive, and
has been effective in some circumstances. However, vagotomy
and pyloroplasty do not address the basic problem of diffuse
mucosal disease nearly as well as gastric resection.

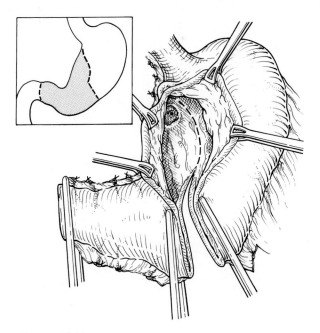

Figure 28.5

Pauchet procedure The gastric resection is planned with
reference to palpable pathology in the gastric wall. If there is
any doubt about the exact location of the lesion, an endoscope
can be inserted into the stomach. Usually, palpation alone, in
the area of sentinel nodes, will reveal the site of the ulcer
lesion.

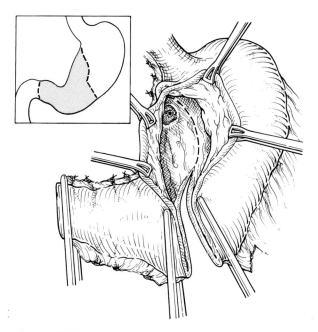

Figure 28.6

Pauchet procedure The anterior wall of the excision is a 'freehand' cut, which is made with appropriate attention to haemostasis as the stomach is opened. If the ulcer is on the posterior wall, then more of the lesser wall should be preserved; this goal is accomplished by having the line of excision very close to the lesser curve. The posterior line of excision is then executed, to include the ulcer in its entirety if at all possible.

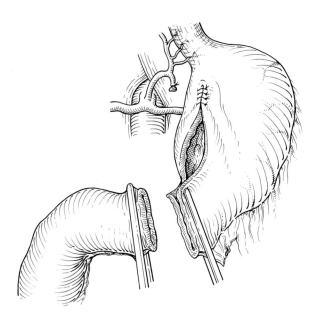

Figure 28.7

Pauchet procedure Suture approximation of the lesser curve is begun at the proximal portion of the resection before the remnant is removed from its posterior attachments; traction is thus maintained on the lesser curvature of the stomach, and accurate suture placement is achieved. At this point, even when the ulcer is located posteriorly, the appearance of the anastomosis is that of a 'normal' case.

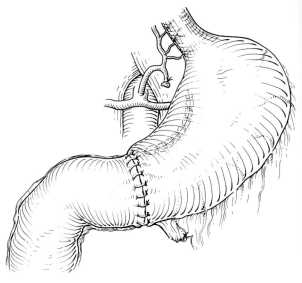

Figure 28.8

Pauchet procedure When the anastomosis is complete, and the Payr clamp is released, the stomach appears to rotate because the new lesser curve may be situated more or less anteriorly or posteriorly (more of the posterior or anterior wall, respectively, remains in situ).

Type II and type III gastric ulcer

If the patient has a type II ('combined') gastric ulcer or pyloric channel ulcer, then a vagotomy and pyloroplasty makes more sense from the perspective that hyperacidity is thought to be prominent in these patients. However, in general terms truncal vagotomy for gastric ulcer is complicated by a higher recurrence rate than gastric resection, and introduces the possibility of gastric atony and increased duodenogastric reflux postoperatively; on balance, these factors are best avoided.

Highly selective vagotomy (HSV); extended HSV

This procedure is best reserved for type II and type III gastric ulcers, although on occasion a type I gastric ulcer is amenable to this conservative surgical approach.

Technique: extended proximal gastric vagotomy The essence of this procedure is division of preganglionic vagal efferents in six of the seven possible pathways to the gastric wall (Figures 28.9–28.14). As a result of our clinical and experimental studies, we believe that the standard proximal gastric vagotomy fails to achieve the desired level of denervation of the parietal cell mass.

The seven possible routes of ingress of preganglionic vagal efferents are the perioesophageal space (for 5–6 cm proximal to the gastroesophageal junction) (site 1), the lesser curve of the corpus (Site 2), the 'heel' of the crow's foot (site 3), the gastropancreatic fold (site 4), the proximal greater curve opposite the short gastric vessels (site 5), the left gastroepiploic pedicle (site 6), and the right gastroepiploic pedicle (site 7). Extended proximal selective vagotomy divides efferent

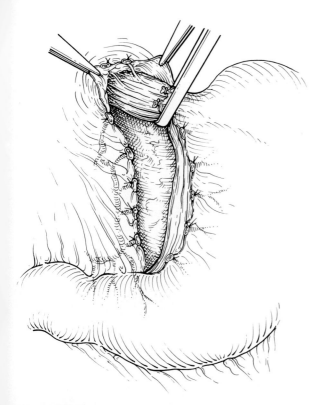

Figure 28.9

Extended highly selective vagotomy Dissection of the lesser
curve of the stomach, as shown, results in division of both the
vagal and sympathetic nerve branches and the blood vessels
which supply the proximal lesser curve of the stomach.
Dissection begins proximal to the crow's foot, and proceeds
toward the oesophagus. After incision and elevation of the
gastric attachments of the phreno-oesophageal ligament (shown
elevated by two forceps), the perioesophageal space becomes
evident. This potential space is 'developed' by blunt dissection
along the oesophageal wall; it is traversed by neurovascular
elements entering from either the right side, or closely applied
to the posterior and left lateral margin of the oesophagus.

vagus nerve fibres in areas 1, 2, 3, 4, 6 and 7; site 5 is spared
so that blood supply to the proximal stomach will be
preserved.

We have found that there is a persistent pattern of acid
secretion along the greater curvature of the stomach which is
eliminated by division of the nerves to the greater curvature;
this observation is based on use of the endoscopic Congo red
test. These areas of the stomach are in locations which have
been noted to be difficult to denervate when the intraoperative
pH test has been used. In addition, our own work has shown
that these areas do contain preganglionic vagal fibres which
can be traced back to the dorsal motor nucleus of the vagus
nerve.

Performing the endoscopic Congo red test (Table 28.3) The test is
ideally performed when the dissection is almost complete to
allow the few intact vagal fibres to give visible proof of the
effect of prior surgical dissection. The operator can ascertain
the precise margin of the antral–corpal junction. Also, if there
is evidence of persistent secretion along the greater curvature

Table 28.3 Intraoperative performance of the
endoscopic Congo red test

1. Discontinue anticholinergic/H_2 blockers 24 hours before surgery
2. Request that anaesthestist avoids anticholinergic premedication
3. Prepare endoscope and solutions; check air/water/suction
   (a) Endoscope – ask biomedical engineer to check for stray currents
   (b) Fill 500 ml basins: one with NaCl, one with 0.5% $NaHCO_3$
   (c) Add 3.0 g Congo red powder to the bicarbonate
   (d) Have a size 14–16 nasogastric tube and a 50 ml irrigating syringe ready
4. Give pentagastrin (6 µg/kg) s.c. 15–20 minutes before test
5. Place endoscope and light source at head of table; remove to endoscope with three rubber bands 5 cm apart (nasogastric tube will facilitate rapid irrigation and aspiration of solution)
6. Insert endoscope; anaesthestist may help with laryngoscope; pass scope into stomach under direct vision and assess whether lavage (saline) necessary to remove debris/mucus
7. Have gastroesophageal junction tethered with a catheter to minimize risk of aspiration of acidic solution; place a lap pad in right gutter to prevent air migration downstream
8. Inject 200 ml 0.5% bicarbonate – Congo red solution via nasogastric tube; entire stomach now must have a red/black coating. Aspirate stomach via nasogastric tube and `plug' the tube. Begin observation (timed)
9. *Positive findings:* blackened areas are seen within 2 minutes (the red-to-black colour change occurs as the pH falls below 3.0); in contrast, denervated areas secrete acid slowly enough to delay the colour change for 8–10 minutes
   (a) If test ++: note area of positivity and search for intact nerve fibres before repeating test.
   (b) If entire stomach is black within 2 minutes (including denervated area) repeat lavage with a 2.0% bicarbonate – Congo red mixture – remember the goal is to show a differential rate of secretion between innervated and denervated mucosa, and the final $NaHCO_3$ concentration is not critical

at this point, there will be less question about the existence of
secretory fibres from the gastroepiploic nerves (see below).
The test is performed after stimulating the parietal cells with
pentagastrin (6 µg/kg s.c.) or by Histalog injection (50 mg s.c.);
these secretagogues counteract the depressant effects of anaesthetics on acid secretion and are given at least 15 minutes
before the performance of the test. When a positive result is
encountered during the test, the surgeon can immediately perform additional dissection in the area with presumably intact
vagal fibres and repeat the test to confirm that the rapid acid
secretion in that area has disappeared.[18]

Vagotomy of the parietal cell mass is then continued by
completing the dissection along the distal lesser curve at the
crow's foot and by dividing the right and left gastroepiploic
nerves. We refer to division of the 'heel' of the crow's foot as a
way to ensure that any small nerve branches to the distal corpus are divided; this 'heel' consists of the tissue in a 2×2 cm
area located between the anterior and posterior nerves of
Latarjet just proximal to the crow's foot. Finally, the lesser curvature of the stomach is sutured to reapproximate the anterior
and posterior margins of the lesser omentum; this 'serorrhaphy'
has proven value in preventing reinnervation of the stomach
with preganglionic vagal efferents following highly selective
vagotomy.[79]

The type of drainage procedure employed for type II or

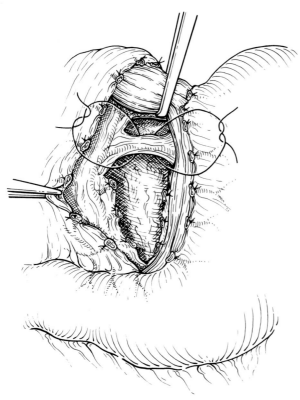

Figure 28.10

Extended highly selective vagotomy The posterior leaf of the lesser omentum becomes continuous with two structures near the oesophagogastric junction: the gastropancreatic fold and the meso-oesophagus. After ligation of the clamps, the operator employs blunt dissection with fingertips to separate areolar connections between these two structures. Figure 28.11 reveals the appearance of the gastropancreatic fold after these manoeuvres.

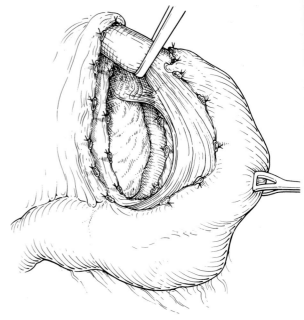

Figure 28.11

Extended highly selective vagotomy The lesser curve of the stomach is seen from the patient's right side. Note the gastropancreatic fold, which is composed of peritoneal reflections between the pancreas and posterior gastric wall. This fold is traversed by the posterior gastric artery and is accompanied by a preganglionic branch of the vagus nerve supplying the posterior gastric wall. The fold is divided until the spleen is seen; next, 5.0 cm of the distal oesophagus is bared, completing the proximal dissection.

type III ulcers is partly determined by the experience of the surgeon. I have used anterior pylorectomy as well as a variety of drainage procedures in the past, and favour this procedure (Figures 28.15 and 28.16) over alternatives.

Type IV gastric ulcer

The high gastric ulcer can be effectively removed by a conservative distal resection which is somewhat similar to the rotation gastrectomy alluded to previously. When removing a high lesion, it may be necessary to have the tongue of lesser curvature extend into the distal gastroesophageal junction. In such a case, the use of a Roux-en-Y jejunal limb offers a convenient way to both preserve and reconstruct the gastric remnant. In all cases, total gastrectomy is the last choice of operation for a benign condition.

RECURRENT ULCER DISEASE (See Chapter 34)

When a recurrent ulcer is discovered after previous surgical treatment, the general approach to the patient must include three possible explanations: a new problem, unrelated to the previous treatment; the primary problem, expressing itself

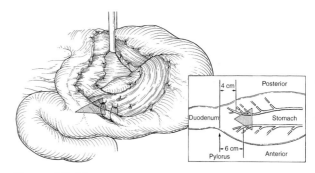

Figure 28.12

Extended highly selective vagotomy In this view the stomach has been 'turned' clockwise on its longitudinal axis, allowing the surgeon to view the lesser curve directly. The lesser curve is displayed as shown, and the insertion of the anterior and posterior nerves of Latarjet is clearly seen. The tissue between the terminal branches of the anterior and posterior nerves of Latarjet (shaded) can now be safely dissected, including any recurrent branches extending towards the corpus. The shaded area between the terminal branches of the crow's foot is termed the 'instep' of the crow's foot. *Inset* The relationships of the anterior and posterior nerves of Latarjet are shown; note that terminal branches of the anterior nerve enter the antrum approximately 2.0 cm proximal to the terminal branches of the posterior nerve.

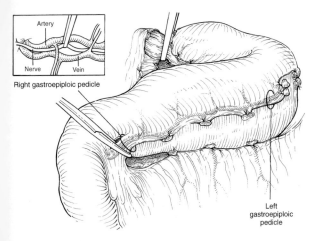

Figure 28.13

Extended highly selective vagotomy   The greater curve is shown after division of the left gastroepiploic pedicle, with the clamp exposing the right gastroepiploic pedicle. It is frequently possible to divide the right gastroepiploic nerve alone, sparing the right gastroepiploic artery and vein; these vessels must be spared if previous splenctomy has been performed.
Inset   The major right gastroepiploic nerve is found between the gastroepiploic artery and nerve. To ensure that accessory nerve branches are divided, the omentum between the colon and the greater curve of the stomach is completely divided.

again despite therapy; or a specific complication of the previous operation. As stated previously, this situation is one which requires the insight and experience of a trained surgeon

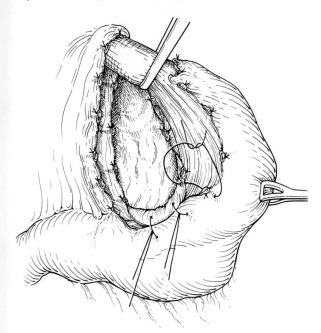

Figure 28.14

Extended highly selective vagotomy   The final operative manoeuvre which is performed is the reapproximation of the serosa of the anterior and posterior gastric walls at the completion of dissection. The aims of the reperitonealizing the lesser curve include the prevention of leakage from the lesser curve if inadvertent injury has occurred, and prevention or retardation of regrowth of vagus nerve fibres.

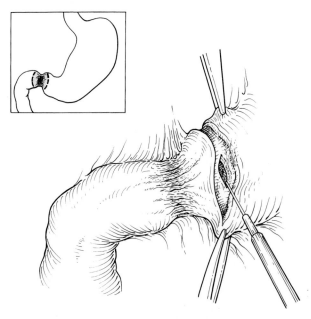

Figure 28.15

Anterior pylorectomy   The palpable scar at the gastric outlet is defined by light application of the needle-tip diathermy apparatus. It is helpful to plan and define the extent of scar excision before opening the duodenum because landmarks are easily lost once the lumen is opened. A needle-tipped coagulator is ideal for opening the two layers separately; the seromuscular coat has few blood vessels, whereas the mucosal layer is more richly vascularized. Individual vessels are coagulated as they are encountered.

because many of the possible problems may not be recognized by a practitioner who is not well versed in the possible complications of surgical treatment.[80] If a type I gastric ulcer recurs, the answer will usually be found in the extent of gastric resection. When type II and type III ulcers recur, there is usually a deficiency of the vagotomy component of the primary operation, and an attempt should be made to define the completeness of the original vaogotomy. If a highly selective vagotomy was performed, then every attempt should be made to review the technique of vagotomy because there are well-defined portions of the operative technique which are commonly neglected. When a type IV ulcer recurs, the extent of the gastric resection may have been insufficient or a stagnant gastric remnant may have been created by the original operation.

Since the multiplicity of treatments referred to above can be employed for recurrent ulcers, the once-held view that recurrent ulcers are surgical lesions has been modified. Each of the ulcer lesions must be evaluated on its own merits, in the light of potential aggravating factors, and several possible medical alternatives must be considered. It is only when the recurrent ulcer presents as a surgical emergency that the surgical alternative must be employed, and it in these circumstances that the approach described above will be most effective.

NEW TREATMENTS

There is some hope that chronic ulcers can be healed (or encouraged to heal) in the future by the use of techniques

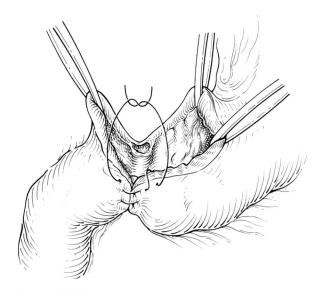

Figure 28.16

Anterior pylorectomy   After complete excision of the scarified anterior pyloric ring, the lumen of the stomach and the duodenum are clearly seen. The ends of the severed pyloric muscle are apparent at the superior and inferior portion of the dissection. Before suturing the duodenum and stomach, digital exploration of the second portion of the duodenum is performed to discover occult stenosis. Disparity of lumen size between the stomach and duodenum is addressed as shown: two 'bites' of gastric tissue for every one of duodenum are taken, beginning the moment that a disparity is noted. In this way, an anastomosis can be easily fashioned with a gastric lumen twice as large as the duodenal lumen.

which address the root pathology of the gastric ulcer lesion. As the discussion above has highlighted, the term gastric ulcer encompasses a variety of acute and chronic lesions, and the chronic lesions have variable factors that influence their course. As a result, the discussion of new techniques unfortunately reflects the current state of medical science: a blank slate, awaiting the insights and discoveries of the future. Will endoscopic techniques, such as laser, be able to 'change the soil' in which the ulcer grows? Can we do something specific which will alter the healing potential of the gastric wall? Will genetic engineering show us ways to enhance natural healing, as can now be done experimentally?

There are many opportunities for future achievements which will have a positive effect on this common and complicated disease entity, and we all await their development.

REFERENCES

1. Susser M & Stein Z. Civilisation and peptic ulcer. *Lancet* 1962; **i:** 115–119.
2. Rudick J. Gastric ulcer. In Nyhus LM & Wastell C (eds) *Surgery of the Stomach and Duodenum*, 4th edn. Boston: Little Brown, 1986: 243–261.
3. Coggon D, Lambert P & Langman MJS. 20 years of hospital admissions for peptic ulcer in England and Wales. *Lancet* 1981: **i:** 1302–1304.
4. Wylie CM. The complex wane of peptic ulcer. I. Recent national trends in deaths and hospital care in the United States. *J Clin Gastroenterol* 1981; **3:** 327–332.
5. Elashoff JD & Grossman MI. Trends in hospital admissions and death rates for peptic ulcer in the United States from 1970 to 1078. *Gastroenterology* 1975; **68:** 280–285.
6. Kurata JH & Abbey DE. The effect of chronic aspirin use on duodenal and gastric ulcer hospitalizations. *J Clin Gastroenterol* 1990; **12:** 260–266.
7. Sonnenberg A. Geographic and temporal variations in the occurrence of peptic ulcer disease. *Scand J Gastroenterol* 1985; **20** (Suppl. 110): 11–24.
8. Sonnenberg A. Factors which influence the incidence and course of peptic ulcer. *Scand J Gastroenterol* 1988; **23** (Suppl. 155): 119–140.
9. Bloom BS, Fendrick AM & Ramsey SD. Changes in peptic ulcer and gastritis/duodenitis in Great Britain, 1970–1985. *J Clin Gastroenterol* 1990; **12:** 100–108.
10. Bloom BS, Fox NA & Jacobs J. Patterns of care and expenditures by California Medicaid for peptic ulcer and other acid-related disorders. *J Clin Gastroenterol* 1989; **11:** 615–620.
11. Paimela H, Tuomp PK, Perakyl T, Saario I, Hockerstedt K & Kivilaakso E. Peptic ulcer surgery during the H₂-receptor antagonist era: a population-based epidemiological study of ulcer surgery in Helsinki from 1972 to 1987. *Br J Surg* 1991; **78:** 28–31.
12. Johnson HD. Etiology and classification of gastric ulcers. *Gastroenterology* 1957; **33:** 121–127.
13. Johnson HD. Gastric ulcer: classification, blood group characteristics, secretion patterns and pathogenesis. *Ann Surg* 1965; **162:** 996–1002.
14. Csendes A, Braghetto I & Smok G. Type IV gastric ulcer: a new hypothesis. *Surgery* 1987; **101:** 361–366.
15. Griffith CA. Anatomy. In Nyhus LM & Harkins HN (eds) *Surgery of the Stomach and Duodenum*, 2nd edn. Boston: Little Brown, 1969: 25–52.
16. Oi M & Oshida K. The association of esophageal, gastric, and duodenal ulcers. *Gastroenterology* 1959; **36:** 57–68.
17. Hernandez DE. Neurobiology of brain-gut interactions. Implications for ulcer disease. *Dig Dis Sci* 1989; **34:** 1809–1816.
18. Donahue PE, Bombeck CT, Yoshida J et al. The endoscopic Congo red test during proximal gastric vagotomy. *Am J Surg* 1987; **153:** 249–255.
19. Donahue PE, Yoshida J, Polley EH & Nyhus LM. Preganglionic vagus nerve fibers also enter the greater curvature of the stomach in rats and ferrets. *Gastroenterology* 1988; **94:** 1292–1294.
20. Yoshida J, Polley E, Nyhus LM & Donahue PE. Brainstem topography of vagus nerve to the greater curvature of the stomach. *J Surg Res* 1989; **46:** 60–69.
21. Yoshida J, Polley EH, Nyhus LM & Donahue PE. Pyloroplasty divides vagus nerve fibers to the greater curve of the stomach: an axonal tracing study. *Ann Surg* 1988; **208:** 708–713.
22. Holzer P & Sametz W. Gastric mucosal protection against ulcerogenic factors in the rat mediated by capsaicin-sensitive afferent neurons. *Gastroenterology* 1986; **91:** 975–981.
23. Holzer P, Pabst MA, Lippe ITh et al. Afferent nerve-mediated protection against deep mucosal damage in the rat stomach. *Gastroenterology* 1990; **98:** 838–848.
24. Donahue PE, Sugitani A & Nyhus LM. Selective gastric afferent nerve blockade with capsaicin: facilitated by ipsilateral vagus innervation in rat. *Res Surg* 1991; **3:** 24–28.
25. Sugitani A, Donahue PE, Doyle MD, Anan K & Nyhus LM. The ipsilateral organization of the afferent nerves to the stomach. *J Surg Res* 1993; **54:** 212–221.
26. Sugitani A, Donahue PE, Doyle MD, Newson BL & Nyhus LM. Inhibition of afferent vagus nerves decreases gastric stress lesions. *Am Surg* 1992; **58:** 699–704.
27. Miller TA. Gastroduodenal mucosal defense: factors responsible for the ability of the stomach and duodenum to resist injury. *Surgery* 1988; **103:** 389–397.
28. Svanes K, Gislason H, Guttu K, Herfjord JK, Fevang J & Gronbech JE. Role of blood flow in adaptive protection of the cat gastric mucosa. *Gastroenterology* 1991; **100:** 1249–1258.
29. Mercer DW, Ritchie WP Jr & Dempsey DT. Do sensory neurons mediate adaptive cytoprotection of gastric mucosa against bile acid injury? *Am J Surg* 1992; **163:** 12–18.
30. Konturek PK, Brzozowski T, Konturek SJ & Dembinski A. Role of epidermal growth factor, prostaglandin, and sulfydryl radicals in stress-induced gastric lesions. *Gastroenterology* 1990; **99:** 1607–1615.
31. Takeuchi K & Johnson LR. Pentagastrin protects against stress ulcerations. *Gastroenterology* 1979; **76:** 327–334.
32. Muramatsu I, Hollenberg MD & Lederis K. Vascular actions of epidermal growth factor–urogastrone: possible relation to prostaglandin production. *Can J Physiol Pharmacol* 1985; **63:** 994–999.
33. du Plessis DJ. The importance of the pyloric antrum in peptic ulceration. *S Afr J Surg* 1963; **1:** 3–11.
34. Lawson HH. The reversibility of postgastrectomy alkaline gastritis by a Roux-en-Y loop. *Br J Surg* 1972; **59:** 13–17.

35. Sipponen P, Varis K, Fraki O, Korri UM, Seppala K & Siurala M. Cumulative 10-year risk of symptomatic dudodenal and gastric ulcer in patients with or without chronic gastritis. A clinical follow-up study of 454 patients. *Scand J Gastroenterol* 1990; **25:** 966–973.
36. Marshall BJ, Armstrong JA, McGechie DB & Glancy RJ. Attempt to fulfill Koch's postulates for pyloric *Campylobacter. Med J Aust* 1985; **142:** 436–439.
37. Morris A & Nicholson G. Ingestion of *Campylobacter pyloridis* causes gastritis and raised fasting gastric pH. *Am J Gastroenterol* 1987; **82:** 192–199.
38. Lee A, Fox JG, Otto G & Murphy J. A small animal model of human *Helicobacter pylori* active chronic gastritis. *Gastroenterology* 1990; **99:** 1315–1323.
39. Braverman DZ, Rudensky B, Dollbergg L et al. *Campylobacter pylori* in Israel: prospective study of prevalence and epidemiology. *Isr J Med Sci* 1990; **26:** 434–438.
40. Wyle FA, Tarnawski A, Schulman D & Dabros W. Evidence for gastric mucosal cell invasion by *C. pylori:* an ultrastructural study. *J Clin Gastroenterol* 1990; **12** (Suppl. 1): S92–S98.
41. Tarnawski A, Hollander D, Krause WJ, Dabros W, Stachura J & Gergely H. 'Healed' experimental gastric ulcers remain histologically and ultrastructurally abnormal. *J Clin Gastroenterol* 1990 **12** (Suppl. 1): S139–S147.
42. Donahue PE, Richter HM, Liu KJM & Nyhus LM. Thickened pylorus in prepyloric or channel ulcers: edema or fibrosis. *Am J Surg* 1991.
43. Levi S, Goodlad RA, Lee CY et al. Inhibitory effect of non-steroidal anti-inflammatory drugs on mucosal cell proliferation associated with gastric ulcer healing. *Lancet* 1990; **336:** 840–843.
44. Griffin MR, Ray WA & Schaffner W. Non-steroidal anti-inflammatory drug use and death from peptic ulcer in elderly patients. *Ann Intern Med* 1988; **109:** 359–363.
45. Armstrong CP & Whitelaw S. Death from undiagnosed peptic ulcer complications: a continuing challenge. *Br J Surg* 1988; **75:** 1112–1114.
46. Wara P. Endoscopic prediction of major rebleeding: a prospective study of stigmata of hemorrhage in bleeding ulcer. *Gastroenterology* 1985; **88:** 1209–1214.
47. Griffith WJ, Neumann DA & Welsh JD. The visible vessel as an indicator of uncontrolled or recurrent gastrointestinal hemorrhage. *N Engl J Med* 1979: **300:** 1411–1413.
48. Storey DW, Bown SG, Swain CP et al. Endoscopic prediction of recurrent bleeding in peptic ulcers. *N Engl J Med* 1981; **305:** 915–917.
49. Lunde OC & Kvernebo K. Gastric blood flow in patients with gastric ulcer measured by endoscopic laser Doppler flowmetry. *Scand J Gastroenterol* 1988; **23:** 546–550.
50. Kurata JH & Corboy EG. Hemorrhage due to peptic ulcer: current trends. *J Clin Gastroenterol* 1988; **10:** 259–268.
51. Gunshefski L, Flancbaum L & Brolin RE. Changing patterns in perforated peptic ulcer disease. *Am Surg* 1990; **56:** 270–274.
52. Soybel DI, Kestenberg A, Brunt EM & Becker JM. Gastrocolic fistula as a complication of benign gastric ulcer: report of four cases and update of the literature. *Br J Surg* 1989; **6:** 1298–1300.
53. Lu CC & Schulze-Delrieu K. Pyloric deformation from peptic disease. Radiographic evidence for incompetence rather than obstruction. *Dig Dis Sci* 1990; **35:** 1459–1467.
54. Holle GE, Frey KW, Thieme Ch & Holle FK. Recurrence of peptic ulcer after selective proximal vagotomy and pyloroplasty in relation to changes in clinical signs and symptoms between 1969 and 1983. *Surg Gynecol Obstet* 1988; **167:** 271–281.
55. Lee S, Iida M, Yao T, Shindo S, Okabe H & Fujishima M. Long-term follow-up of 2529 patients reveals gastric ulcers rarely become malignant. *Dig Dis Sci* 1990; **35:** 763–768.
56. Hole DJ, Quigley EM, Gillis CR & Watkinson G. Peptic ulcer and cancer: an examination of the relationship between chronic peptic ulcer and gastric carcinoma. *Scand J Gastroenterol* 1987; **22:** 17–23.
57. Tersmette AC, Johan G, Offerhaus A et al. Long-term results after partial gastrectomy for benign conditions. *Gastroenterology* 1991; **101:** 148–153.
58. Lansdown M, Quirke P, Dixon MF, Axon AT & Johnston D. High grade dysplasia of the gastric mucosa: a marker for gastric carcinoma. *Gut* 1990; **31:** 977–983.
59. Cooperative Study Group. Double blind comparative study of omeprazole and ranitidine in patients with duodenal and gastric ulcer: a multi-centre trial. *Gut* 1990; **31:** 653–656.
60. Littman A & Hanscom DH. The course of recurrent ulcer. *Gastroenterology* 1971; **61:** 592–654.
61. Maton PN. Omeprazole. *N Engl J Med* 1991; **324:** 965–976.
62. Creutzfeldt W, Lamberts R, Stockmann F & Brunner G. Quantitiative studies of gastric endocrine cells in patients receiving long-term treatment with omeprazole. *Scand J Gastroenterol Suppl* 1989; **166:** 122–128.
63. Hewsen EG, Yeomans MD, Angus PW. et al. Effect of 'weekend therapy' with omeprazole on basal and stimulated acid secretion and fasting plasma gastrin in duodenal ulcer patients. *Gut* 1988; **29:** 1715–1720.
64. Pym B, Sandstad J, Seville P, Buth K, Middleton WR & Piper DW. Cost-effectiveness of cimetidine maintenance therapy in chronic gastric and duodenal ulcer. *Gastroenterology* 1990; **99:** 27–35.
65. Frank WO, Young M, Palmer RH, Karlstadt R, Rockhold F & Mounce W. Once-daily bedtime dosing regimen of cimetidine in the treatment of gastric ulcer. *Clin Ther* 1989; **11:** 595–603.
66. Gasbarrini G, Andreone P, Baraldini M, Cursaro C & Micaletti E. Antacids in gastric ulcer treatment: evidence of cytoprotection. *Scand J Gastroenterol* Suppl 1990; **174:** 44–47.
67. Feldman M. Prostaglandins and gastric ulcers: from seminal vesicle to misoprostol (Cytotec). *Am J Med Sci* 1990; **300:** 116–132.
68. Walt RP. Prostaglandins and peptic ulcer therapy. *Scand J Gastroenterol* Suppl 1990; **174:** 29–36.
69. Blum AL, Bethge H, Bode JC et al. Sucralfate in the treatment and prevention of gastric ulcer: multi-centre double blind placebo controlled study. *Gut* 1990; **31:** 825–830.
70. Gorbach SL. Bismuth therapy in gastrointestinal disease. *Gastroenterology* 1990; **99:** 863–875.
71. Wagstaff AJ, Benfield Pl & Monk JP. Colloidal bismuth subcitrate. A review of its pharmacodynamic and pharmacokinetic properties and its therapeutic use in peptic ulcer disease. *Drugs* 1988; **36:** 121–248.
72. Tytgat GNJ. Colloidal bismuth subcitrate: a review. *Digestion* 1987; **37** (Suppl. 2): 31–41.
73. Tatsuta M, Ishikawa H, Iishi H, Okuda S & Yokota Y. Reduction of gastric ulcer recurrence rate after suppression of *Helicobacter pylori* by cefixime. *Gut* 1990; **31:** 973–976.
74. Wangensteen OH & Wangensteen SD. History of gastric surgery: glimpses into its early and more recent past. In Nyhus LM & Wastell C (eds) *Surgery of the Stomach and Duodenum,* 3rd edn. Boston: Little Brown, 1977: 3–39.
75. Siewert JR & Castrup HJ. Billroth I Gastrectomy. In Nyhus LM and Baker RJ (eds) *Mastery of Surgery.* Boston: Little Brown, 1984: 494–500.
76. Hoerr SO & Steiger E. Billroth II Gastrectomy. In Nyhus LM & Baker RJ (eds) *Mastery of Surgery.* Boston: Little Brown, 1984: 501–514.
77. Nyhus LM. Gastric ulcer. In Harkins HN & Nyhus LM (eds) *Surgery of the Stomach and Duodenum,* 2nd edn. Boston: Little Brown, 1969: 203–225.
78. Donahue PE & Nyhus LM. Surgical excision of gastric ulcers near the gastroesophageal junction. *Surg Gynecol Obstet* 1982; **155:** 85–88.
79. Yoshida J, Polley EH, Nyhus LM & Donahue PE. Serorrhaphy prevents gastric reinnervation after proximal gastric vagotomy. *Surg Forum* 1988; **39:** 132–133.
80. Donahue PE & Sugitani A. Gastrointestinal endoscopy and general surgical practice: surgical endoscopy versus surgeon endoscopists. *Am Surg* 1991; **57:** 330–333.
81. Donahue PE & Nyhus LM. Exposure of the periesophageal space. *Surg Gynecol Obstet* 1981; **152:** 218–220.

29

CHRONIC DUODENAL ULCER

DG Colin-Jones
DY Graham

Dramatic advances in our understanding of the causes of peptic ulceration have had a major impact on management. The ability to assign causative roles to *Helicobacter pylori* and non-steroidal anti-inflammatory drug (NSAID) use in peptic ulcer disease and proof that successful therapy of *H. pylori* infection cures peptic ulcer disease have led to a reassessment of the indications for surgery and the type of surgery performed. The amount of elective surgery performed in the management of peptic ulcer disease has dramatically declined and we shall soon see the day when surgeons with great technical skill in peptic ulcer disease surgery will be rare. This may happen just as it did when chest surgeons were no longer needed for the management of patients with chronic pulmonary infections (Figure 29.1, see colour plate also).

Until recently cure of peptic ulcer disease required surgery. That option often substituted new problems associated with gastrectomy or truncal vagotomy for ulcer disease. With it came an alliteration of undesirable Ds: diarrhoea, dumping, duodenogastric reflux, dysphagia, dyspepsia and death.

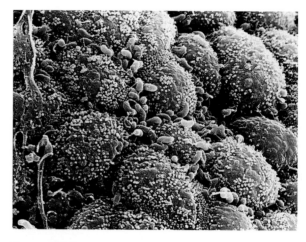

Figure 29.2
Helicobacter pylori. Scanning electron micrograph showing the spiral organisms concentrated between the mucosal cells. The rough cellular surface is due to microvilli. (Courtesy Mr H.W. Steer.)

Recently it has become evident that peptic ulcer disease can be cured with medical therapy. The change in our thinking is a direct result of recent studies linking gastritis and peptic ulcer disease to an infection with the bacterium, *Helicobacter pylori*[1,2] (Figure 29.2) For decades it was known that peptic ulcer occurred in association with gastritis. The discovery that successful treatment of *H. pylori* infection led to healing of gastritis suggested that it might also cure gastritis-associated peptic ulcer disease. That hypothesis is now, to some extent, proven and has resulted in new approaches to the management of patients with peptic ulcer.

INCIDENCE

The rise and fall of duodenal ulceration has been a remarkable feature of the prevalence of the disease over the last century.[3,4] The epidemiology of ulcer disease is discussed in detail in Chapter 27, but in any discussion on the aetiology of chronic duodenal ulcer, note must be taken of what was probably a low prevalence of duodenal ulcer in the last century, with a

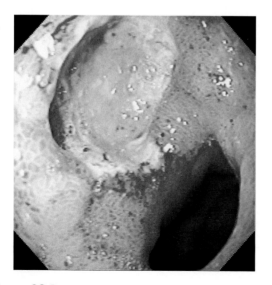

Figure 29.1
Duodenal ulcer. A deep crater can be seen on this endoscopic photograph.

rapid rise in the first half of this century and then subsequently a steady fall,[4,5] at least in the western world. This pattern is, however, not true for all groups since the fall in prevalence of duodenal ulcer has plateaued for elderly men and is rising for elderly women.[6] In the western world the prevalence of duodenal ulceration reaches a peak in middle life, in the late 40s and early 50s. This is similar in Japan but is probably different from the third world where, in India and Africa, the peak prevalence probably occurs 10 years earlier.[7] Earlier epidemiological studies were bedevilled by a number of difficulties, especially that of accurate diagnosis. History-taking is quite inadequate, picking up a large number of cases of non-ulcer dyspepsia, and giving a falsely high figure. A barium meal is relatively inaccurate because it cannot distinguish scarring from active ulceration, so endoscopy, which unfortunately is invasive, is the only method by which a really accurate prevalence can be determined. However, data are now available from India, Japan and Scandinavia. Khuroo et al.[8] sent a questionnaire to a randomly selected population of 2763 adults of whom 239 had dyspeptic symptoms, and they were able to endoscope 80% of them. In contrast to earlier studies these workers then randomly selected for endoscopy 177 individuals from the remaining population who had no dyspeptic symptoms. They found a point prevalence of peptic ulcer disease to be 4.7%, with a lifetime prevalence of 11.2%. In their community duodenal ulcers were 17 times more common than gastric and were more common in men. There seemed to be no relationship between peptic ulcer and socioeconomic status. In Japan,[9] the peak incidence for duodenal ulcer in men is 35–45 years of age, about 10 years earlier than in women and with only a slight fall from the peak with advancing age. In Gothenburg[10] a one year review of all cases of peptic ulceration diagnosed by a barium meal or endoscopy (active craters only) showed a 1.5:1 male to female ratio for duodenal ulcer and a peak incidence over the age of 60 years for both sexes, about 1.5 cases per thousand population. In a small Norwegian community a survey followed by upper gastrointestinal endoscopy in 309 dyspeptics and 310 controls,[11] found the prevalence of dyspepsia was 30% in men and that for peptic ulcer was 8.7%; figures for women were slightly lower (24% and 5.2%, respectively). It has been suggested that duodenal ulcer disease 'burns itself out' after a number of years. This view is not universally held and for many patients the disease is a chronic one, remitting and recurring.[12]

AETIOLOGY

Classical teaching explains duodenal ulceration in terms of an imbalance between aggressive forces (acid and pepsin) and defensive forces (mucus and the mucosa) within the duodenal cap (Figure 29.3). The belief that acid is the most crucial factor leading to duodenal ulcers – a belief which formed the foundation for major gastric surgery – can no longer be sustained. Many factors contribute to the development and natural history of chronic duodenal ulceration, not all of which are known, but the discovery of an associated infection with *H. pylori* has proved to be of critical importance resulting in major changes in management.

Helicobacter pylori

H. pylori is a Gram-negative microaerophilic bacterium whose natural niche is the human stomach (Figure 29.2). *H. pylori* infection may be the most common infection worldwide. The magnitude of the morbidity associated with this infection is only now becoming recognized. For example, about one in six infected individuals develop peptic ulcer. In addition, a proportion of those infected may eventually develop gastric carcinoma. *H. pylori* infection precedes development of peptic ulcers and is not simply a secondary invader.[13]

The old aphorism, 'no acid, no ulcer', seems to hold true for duodenal ulceration, and now to that could be added a new aphorism, 'no *Helicobacter pylori*, no duodenal ulcer', for this

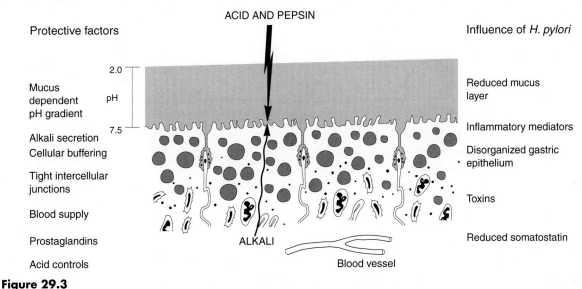

Figure 29.3
Schematic representation of the mucosal barrier. Acid and pepsin threaten the integrity of the epithelium which has its defence system. This balance is disturbed in the presence of *Helicobacter pylori*.

recently discovered spiral bacterium has been found in almost all cases of duodenal ulcer, which are not associated with non-steroidal anti-inflammatory drugs (NSAIDs), and this holds true around the world. Although the presence of these organisms has been reported sporadically for most of the twentieth century and indeed Gram-negative bacteria were found in close relation to 80% of gastric ulcers in 1975,[14] it was in 1983 that the organism was first cultured in Australia by Marshall and Warren.[15] Subsequent to this there has been an explosion of interest in this organism.

It is now generally accepted that *H. pylori* is the major cause of peptic ulcer disease. Thus, peptic ulcer has changed from being a manifestation of abnormal regulation of acid secretion to one manifestation of a bacterial infection. The link between peptic ulcer and gastritis was established more than 40 years ago and has been confirmed repeatedly. The discovery that *H. pylori* was also the major cause of gastritis begged the question of whether cure of the infection would heal both the gastritis and peptic ulcer disease. Many hundreds of studies have now been reported and the results have been consistent: cure of *H. pylori* infection will heal ulcers,[16] virtually eliminate recurrence[17,18] and improve gastritis.[19] This marked change in outcome has proved true for both gastric and duodenal disease as well as for ulcers complicated by bleeding.[20]

The pathogenesis of peptic ulcer in relation to *H. pylori* is still unclear. There is an increased prevalence of cytotoxin production in those patients with a duodenal ulcer when compared with those who have only gastritis,[21] and there is an increase in acid secretion in infected individuals which regresses slowly after eradication;[22,23] however, most individuals with *H. pylori* infection do not develop ulcer disease. The risk of ulcer disease is about one in six. The fact that most infected individuals do not develop peptic ulcer is not unusual for an infectious disease, depending on virulence factors in the organism and the host response.[24] For example, streptococcal infections are associated with many different outcomes such as pharyngitis, asymptomatic carrier state, rheumatic fever, scarlet fever, cellulitis, and necrotizing fasciitis. *H. pylori* is a pathogen as it is always associated with histological gastritis which is most often asymptomatic but may lead to gastric atrophy, gastric carcinoma, primary gastric MALTOMA (MALT – mucosal associated lymphoid tissue), or ulcer disease.[25]

The frequency of *H. pylori* infection is high in the general population but has been falling in Western populations coincidental with improvements in standards of living and sanitation. *H. pylori* is a curious organism by virtue of remarkable specialization with an apparent 'requirement' for gastric epithelium. It can be found throughout the stomach and in the duodenal bulb associated with metaplastic gastric epithelium. *H. pylori* may be detected by a variety of methods. It can be seen histologically using special stains such as the Warthin–Starry or Giemsa stains. It is easily seen on electron microscopy but it can only be reliably cultured from endoscopic biopsies as it does not thrive in the acid environment of the gastric lumen. It is now possible to detect the presence of this organism with a high level of certainty,[26] using a variety of tests, both invasive and non-invasive. It is often life-long and thus a simple sero-

logical test for the presence of anti-*H. pylori* IgG is often the quickest and simplest method of identifying whether *H. pylori* infection is present. Other options include the urea breath test, which is a simple, non-invasive test based on the fact that *H. pylori* contains abundant urease. Administration of labelled urea results in the rapid appearance of labelled carbon dioxide in the breath. Urea breath tests are available using radioactive ^{14}C as well as stable ^{13}C. Alternatively, at endoscopy gastric mucosal biopsies can be obtained for documenting the presence of the organism by histological demonstration of typical acute or chronic gastritis and the organism. A mucosal biopsy can also be placed in an indicator medium to detect the presence of urease activity (e.g. CLO test, Delta West Pty Ltd, Bentley, Western Australia). Culture and sensitivity is generally not needed for successful treatment of the infection.

The infection initially proved to be difficult to cure. It was subsequently recognized that, like tuberculosis, a combination of several antimicrobials lead to cure in most patients. The best combination is not yet known[27] but there are a number of protocols that will cure the infection in the vast majority of cases (see Chapter 30). Reinfection has proved to be rare in the western world (e.g. approximately 0.5% per year) such that cure of the infection leads to cure of peptic ulcer. When antimicrobial resistance is suspected it is useful to culture the organism and obtain antibiotic sensitivities before choosing a treatment regimen.

Genetic aspects

The changing incidence of duodenal ulcers, with a dramatic rise in the early part of the century and subsequently a steady fall in the majority of communities, indicates that the environment exerts a major effect. The main factor is now thought to be *H. pylori* infection. Currently we are unable to distinguish whether host or bacterial factors are the more important. Host factors are suggested by studies on genetic markers such as blood group substances. Although there is an increased incidence of ulcers in people of blood group O who do not secrete their blood group substances into body fluids, the risk of having a duodenal ulcer is increased only by the order of 25–30%.[28] Some of the strongest evidence of a genetic influence was suggested by studies on serum pepsinogens, especially hyperpepsinogenaemia 1, which appeared to be inherited as an autosomal dominant and is associated with increased liability to duodenal ulceration.[29,30] Recently, it has become apparent that increased serum pepsinogen I was actually an epiphenomenon and a reflection of *H. pylori* infection.[31] However, genetic influences may play a role in susceptibility to *H. pylori* infection.[32] There is no specific HLA group which is associated with duodenal ulcer. We anticipate that the eventual outcome will be to find important host and bacterial factors that may act alone or in concert to lead to peptic ulcer disease.

Socioeconomic factors

With the changing prevalence of duodenal ulceration there has also been – as far as can be judged on incomplete data – a change in the distribution of ulcer disease, which used to be found in the higher socioeconomic classes but currently is found more frequently in working classes.[3] The reasons for this are uncertain but smoking and diet could be important.

Diet

The influence of eating on gastric function is well known. Since dietary indiscretion can produce symptoms, in the lay person's mind it is self-evident that diet has an important aetiological relationship with ulcers. Initial studies completely failed to confirm this long-held view, but most of these studies looked at the influence of different diets on acid secretion – which was very little.[33] Then the emphasis gradually began to change. The differing prevalence of ulcer disease in India correlated with the different diets, and Tovey and his colleagues using an experimental ulcer model demonstrated lipid-soluble protective substances.[34] It is possible that these protective substances are linoleic and linolenic acid, which have been shown to exert a protective effect experimentally, probably by metabolism to prostaglandins. This might be the explanation for the reduction in gastric acid secretion in volunteers on a diet containing high levels of linoleic acid.[35] There is no evidence that diet increases the likelihood of healing an ulcer, but it may reduce the relapse rate – a high fibre diet being helpful in this regard.[36] A high fibre diet contains linoleic acid and one of the explanations for the falling incidence of peptic ulcer disease has been postulated as being due to the rise in unrefined foods in recent years.[37] Buffering of gastric contents might be relevant, either through the type of food eaten or by the intragastric buffering effect of greater salivary flow produced in response to chewing unrefined food compared with less salivary flow with cooked foods.[38] The impact of H. pylori has relegated dietary factors, but these are still important; they have been reviewed by Tovey et al.[39]

Herpes simplex virus

Some patients with duodenal ulcer have higher levels of circulating antibodies to Herpes simplex type 1 than a control group and levels rise with ulcer relapse. It has been suggested that infection with Herpes simplex is an important environmental ulcerogen.[40] Evidence for this hypothesis is extremely limited, and a controlled trial has failed to show that the relapse rate for duodenal ulcer reduced by acyclovir.[41]

Smoking

Smoking has been firmly established as an adverse factor in ulcer disease,[42] increasing the incidence of duodenal ulcer, and probably its mortality. The effect of smoking on acid secretion is debated but it seems to cause no change in basal acid output, whereas chronic smoking has been associated with a raised stimulated acid output.[43,44] Healing is reduced or delayed in smokers,[45] but the therapeutic gain from the use of H$_2$ receptor antagonists is similar to that of non-smokers – duodenal ulcers in smokers do badly on placebo.[42] This adverse effect of smoking is reversible since relapse after healing is probably reduced if the individual can stop smoking.[46] The suppression of acid and pepsin secretion with treatment such as ranitidine

may be less successful if patients smoke (especially at night), than if they do not smoke over the same period.[47] It is possible that this poorer suppression contributes to delayed healing of the ulcer. Interestingly the adverse effect of smoking on ulcer healing with H$_2$ receptor antagonists may not be found with mucosal protective drugs such as sucralfate,[48] which suggests a deleterious mucosal action by smoking, through an unknown mechanism. After the H. pylori infection has been cured, smoking is no longer a risk factor.[49,50]

Stress

To most patients stress is an important factor in ulcer disease, but in fact the relationship between stress and duodenal ulcer disease has never been proved. The classic studies by Beaumont and later Wolf[51] appeared to demonstrate changes in gastric mucosal appearance and secretion at times of stress. More recently gastric hypersecretion has been reported in two subjects with gastric and prepyloric ulcers[52] who were undergoing periods of extreme stress, with a steady reduction back to normal in their acid secretion (both basal and peak) as they recovered from the stress. Stress has been reported to influence acid secretion, with a rise in basal acid output in 12 volunteers subjected to 4 days of tough physical exercise, but no increase in peak output was found.[53] Hypnotherapy has been shown to modulate gastric acid secretion, increasing basal output markedly when good food was contemplated, and reducing it when deeply relaxed.[54] Furthermore, hypnotherapy has been found to reduce the relapse rate of DU previously healed with ranitidine from 100% to 53%.[55] Stress is ubiquitous and of minor clinical importance in peptic ulcer disease.

Acid secretion

Increased acid secretion is widely held to be central to the development of duodenal ulcer, yet, although there is an increase both in basal acid secretion and stimulated acid secretion in response to pentagastrin there is a considerable overlap with the normal population.[56] However, we now know that many 'normal' controls would have been infected with H. pylori which has been shown to increase acid secretion, both basal and stimulated.[22] Careful studies have shown that acid output during the day when eating normally is elevated in patients with duodenal ulcer compared with healthy controls.[57] This increased secretion is associated with an increase in the parietal cell mass, and the parietal cells are probably more sensitive to stimuli.[58] The increased parietal cell sensitivity has now been shown to be reversible and is due to inflammatory cell mediators secreted in response to the H. pylori infection. Similarly, a reversible increased parietal cell sensitivity (left shift in the dose–reponse curve) to intravenously administered gastrin releasing peptide (GRP) has been demonstrated. Overnight secretion is higher in patients with duodenal ulcer than in controls (although there is considerable individual variation), so that the intragastric pH is acidic throughout the 24 hours except for the temporary buffering effect of a meal (Figure 29.4). Nocturnal acidity can be abolished by an H$_2$ receptor antagonist given as a single dose at bed-time, thus

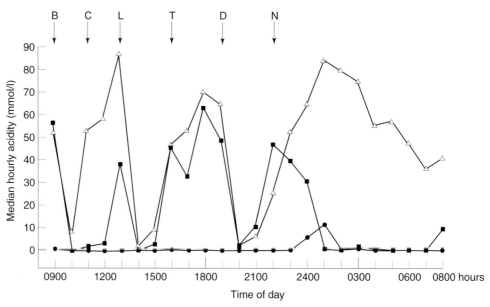

Figure 29.4

Intragastric acidity monitored over 24 hours can be influenced by H$_2$ receptor antagonists, especially overnight. The buffering effect of food is clearly seen. The reduction of acid is much greater with omeprazole. (Reproduced with permission from Lanzon-Miller et al.[59])

stimulating interest in single night-time dosage as treatment for duodenal ulcer[59] (Figure 29.4). This increased secretion is related to the state of the ulcer, being higher when the ulcer crater is present than when healed,[60] but curiously, the intraduodenal bulb pH is not different from controls when the crater has healed, and is lower when the ulcer is in remission.[61] However, measurement of the intrabulb pH is technically difficult and, furthermore, it does not measure the crucial factor, namely the duration and degree of acid load at the vulnerable point on the surface of the duodenal mucosa. An increase in vagal drive has been postulated and supported by an increased response to sham feeding in patients with duodenal ulcer compared with controls and patients with gastric ulcer,[62] but evidence for this is weak (see below). Drugs acting on the mucosa and which have no effect on gastric secretion can heal about 70% of duodenal ulcer, so clearly factors other than just gastric secretion are required for an ulcer to develop. None the less there is good evidence that acid, as well as *H. pylori*, is essential in the pathogenesis of a duodenal ulcer and that a peak acid secretion of at least 15 mmol/h is needed for an individual to develop a duodenal ulcer.

Pepsins

Because pepsin tends to follow acid secretion, and is appreciably more difficult to measure than acid, for many years pepsin has tended to be neglected. None the less, pepsin has powerful proteolytic activity and is capable of breaking down protein and mucus in an acid environment. It is therefore potentially damaging to the gastric epithelium. Pepsins are derived from pepsinogens as a result of the action of acid, the pepsinogens being stored in peptic cells. The pepsinogens have now been classified into four different types which can be measured in the serum: pepsinogen 1, pepsinogen 2, and cathepsins E and

D (formerly known as slow-moving proteinases). Serum pepsinogen is raised in just over half of duodenal ulcer subjects.[63] It has been shown to correlate with the acid secretory capacity of the stomach and is probably related to *H. pylori* infection (see under genetic aspects). However, when secreted and converted to the active pepsin, the situation is more complex, with at least seven distinct pepsins having been described,[64] each with a different pH at which it shows peak activity. Pepsin-1 seems to be particularly resistant to alkaline degradation and is the pepsin which tends to be elevated in duodenal ulcer disease. There is appreciable elevation of serum pepsinogens-1 and -2 in association with superficial gastritis which is related to *H. pylori* infection. Pepsin in gastric juice is strongly correlated with acid secretion and may not suppress with an H$_2$ receptor antagonist.[65] There appears to be no relationship between the level of pepsin secretion and disease activity,[66] but colloidal bismuth reduces the output of pepsin in duodenal ulcer without affecting acid secretion, suggesting that there may be a role for pepsin in duodenal ulcer disease.[67] Unfortunately, pepsin is degraded when frozen which invalidates any study where batch measurements are made after freezing,[68,69] not only making it difficult to study pepsin but also making interpretation of some earlier studies less certain.

Hormonal regulation of gastric acid

In the rare Zollinger–Ellison syndrome there is hypergastrinaemia which produces intractable ulcer disease through enormous gastric hypersecretion. Without treatment this carries a high mortality because of ulcer complications (see Chapter 36). Gastrin not only stimulates acid secretion, but also has a trophic effect on the gastric mucosa. Gastrin levels in duodenal ulcer are within the normal range, well below those usually found in the Zollinger–Ellison syndrome, but in the typical patient with duodenal ulcer it appears that the basal plasma gastrin levels are not appropriately reduced by a low intragastric pH, suggesting a deficient negative feedback mechanism. A number of abnormalities in gastrin secretion have been found in patients with peptic ulcer including exaggerated meal stimulated gastric secretion, exaggerated gastrin release to gastrin releasing peptide (GRP), a left shift in the dose–response curve for acid secretion in response to an infusion of GRP, and a failure of plasma gastrin levels to fall appropriately with a low gastric pH. All of these abnormalities have now been shown to be reversible and a consequence of the inflammation that accompanies *H. pylori* infection.[70] This abnormal autoregulation is of great interest. It has been suggested that deficient somatostatin release from the D cells within the gastric antrum is involved[71] since somatostatin plays a key role in regulation of gastrin secretion by a local paracrine action, being stimulated by a low antral pH to exert a restraining influence on the G cells.[70] However, it has been speculated that *H. pylori*, which preferentially colonizes the gastric antrum, interferes with the feedback mechanism by producing ammonia deep to the mucus layer and in close proximity to the surface cells of the antrum thereby influencing pH at the mucosal surface.[72] Reduction in fasting gastrin levels followed eradication of the organism. Neurohumoral control of gastric secretion is complex; for example, GRP stimulates gastrin release but also stimulates pepsin secretion perhaps as a mediator for the vagus.[73] Basal levels of pancreatic polypeptide (PP) are raised in duodenal ulcer, but respond normally to a meal; PP is under the control of the vagus.[74]

Vagal drive

Dragstedt[75] proposed that the increased basal acid secretion found in many of his patients was due to increased vagal activity. Based on this he proposed vagotomy as a treatment for these patients. Although basal acid output is diminished by vagotomy this does not prove that the original hypersecretion was due to increased vagal tone since vagotomy reduces acid secretion in response to all stimulants. A possible way of testing to see if increased vagal drive[62] is responsible for acid hypersecretion could be to undertake sham feeding, which augments gastric secretion by activating efferent vagal pathways to the stomach. It has been argued that if increased vagal activity in the resting state were the cause of that basal hypersecretion in patients with duodenal ulcer, they might be expected to secrete little or no additional acid in response to sham feeding. This has been tested and a small minority of patients – 4 out of 29[76] and 9 out of 28[77] – failed to augment acid secretion in response to sham feeding. Normal subjects do increase their response with sham feeding,[76] so it would suggest that increased vagal drive is part of the duodenal ulcer disease process for a small number of duodenal ulcer patients only. However, vagal tone might be expected to increase pepsin secretion more significantly in these patients but this was not found.[78] Moreover, it has been found that the response to sham feeding in active duodenal ulcer patients was very similar to controls, with a small and short-lived rise in acid

secretion, whereas the inactive ulcer patients showed a gradual but sustained rise over 1 hour.[78] The increased vagal drive concept is probably flawed; *H. pylori* rules.

Mucosal resistance

Whereas the aggressive actions of acid and pepsin are necessary for an ulcer to develop, the abilities of the duodenum to neutralize the acid and of the mucosa to resist autodigestion are also crucial, but much more complex and not so well understood.

Neutralizing gastric acid

The intraluminal pH of the duodenum rises abruptly in the duodenal cap owing to effective neutralization, chiefly by alkaline secretions from bile, pancreas and Brunner's glands. This effect seems to be less marked in patients with duodenal ulcer in remission.[61] Isolated duodenal mucosa secretes alkali at about twice the rate of basal gastric alkali secretion, with extracellular bicarbonate being the major source of transported alkali.[79] Control of this alkaline secretion is incompletely understood but it seems to be influenced by the vagus and linked by reflexes to intraluminal pH.[80]

Mucus

The mucus gel layer provides an ideal means of maintaining a pH gradient and containing the bicarbonate in close proximity to the mucosal cells. It is a combination of both the mucus layer and the bicarbonate which allows for mucosal protection (Figure 29.3). This mucus/bicarbonate barrier is very effective in protecting the mucosa from damaging acidity, with an excellent correlation between the extent of damage to the villi by luminal acid and the magnitude of bicarbonate secretion by the surface epithelial cells in the rabbit duodenum.[81] Overall, in duodenal ulcer it appears that the duodenal bicarbonate response to an acid load is defective, so that an abnormal duodenal pH gradient in response to luminal acid has been demonstrated. Thus patients with duodenal ulcer fail to maintain a neutral pH adjacent to the mucosal cells when challenged by luminal acidity,[82] but this alone is unlikely to account for the persistence of a focal ulcer – other factors seem likely to contribute.

Mucosal cell protection

The cells of the duodenal cap need both to be able to resist injury by acid and pepsin and also to repair themselves in the event of the pH dropping at the cell surface. Superficial damage causes disruption and exfoliation of the surface cells, but if it is without damage to deeper mucosal cells it is very promptly repaired by migration of cells from the deeper layers of the mucosa (restitution). Prostaglandins are actively involved in the protection of the mucosa by several mechanisms. They stimulate the secretion of mucus and bicarbonate to increase protection of the duodenal mucosa.[83] Prostaglandins also influence mucosal blood flow.[84] Because of these properties, deficiency of mucosal prostaglandins would be a very plausible explanation for poor duodenal mucosal defence in duodenal ulcer, and this has been reported.[85] Synthetic prostaglandins increase the healing rate of duodenal ulcers, but whether this is by virtue of their cytoprotective properties or by their ability to reduce acid secretion is not yet known. Prostaglandins are derived from the essential fatty acids, arachidonic and linoleic acids. This may be the mechanism by which changes in dietary habits in this century have led to changing prevalence of ulcer disease.[37]

Gastric metaplasia

Gastric metaplasia is invariable in duodenal ulcer, with patches of gastric type mucus cells interspersed between absorptive and goblet cells of the duodenal villi. It is an acquired change. The cells have the staining characteristics of gastric mucus and are the areas infected by *H. pylori* in the duodenum. There is a strong correlation with duodenitis and duodenal ulcer.[25]

Anatomical factors

The duodenal bulb in duodenal ulcer is structurally and functionally different from that of the normal individual, it is often smaller, scarred, has a higher proportion of its surface covered in non-villous mucosa, and may well have abnormal motility. No explanation has yet been found to account for the localized ulceration. If it were simply a case of gastric hypersecretion one would expect, for example, the whole wall of the duodenal cap to be ulcerated rather than a discrete area. Various suggestions have been made, such as a jet of acid abutting onto the ulcer site as it leaves the stomach through the pylorus.[86] Of particular interest is the gastric metaplasia which surrounds the duodenal ulcer and is the preferential site of ulceration.[87,88] Gastric metaplasia is thought to be the result of any form of mucosal injury, be it local trauma or acid hypersecretion.[89] Whether the ulcer is related to reduced mucosal resistance at the site of metaplasia or localized secretion of acid within the cap is uncertain, but functioning parietal cells have been demonstrated adjacent to the edge of an ulcer crater originating in areas of gastric metaplasia.[88] An alternative hypothesis is that there is localized increase in mucosal susceptibility to acid attack owing to local autoimmune reactions analogous to those seen in the thyroid gland.[90] Localized ischaemia has been suggested as a factor leading to ulcer formation but there is still uncertainty about its importance.[86,91]

Epidermal growth factor

Epidermal growth factor (EGF), a polypeptide, is secreted in saliva and by other mucous membranes and appears to stimulate healing of breaches in the epithelium. It is found in salivary glands and Brunner's glands, and has been shown to be secreted in the urine where it has been identified as being identical to urogastrone.[92] EGF has both acid inhibitory and mucosal protective effects but which is pre-eminent in ulcer healing is not yet known.[91] EGF has locally active properties as removal of salivary glands slows the healing of gastric ulcers.[93] This is not without interest, as in India a diet requiring chewing with consequent increased salivary flow is associated with a lower prevalence of duodenal ulcer.[38]

Non-steroidal anti-inflammatory drugs (NSAIDs) (See Chapter 30)

There is now convincing evidence that the taking of NSAIDs is associated with an increased frequency of gastrointestinal haemorrhage and perforation from peptic ulceration, with some NSAIDs carrying a higher risk than others.[94] However, an association between NSAID taking and uncomplicated duodenal ulcer is uncertain.[95] In careful case-controlled studies it has been shown that about one-third of admissions for gastrointestinal haemorrhage may be as a consequence of taking an NSAID.[96] Ulcer perforation also appears to be associated with NSAID-taking as there is a rising frequency of ulcer perforation in the UK, especially in the elderly, in whom there has been a dramatic rise in prescriptions for NSAIDs.[97] The elderly seem to be at special risk from NSAIDs.[98] Interaction between NSAIDs and *H. pylori* may be important but is not yet resolved.[99] NSAID ulcer is suspected by a history of NSAID use and negative tests for *H. pylori* infection. Both *H. pylori* infection and NSAID use are common and in many patients both possible aetiologies are present. The modern approach to ulcer therapy and prevention is upon causation. *H. pylori* is now regarded as the most common cause of peptic ulcer, irrespective of whether the ulcer is in the stomach or duodenal bulb.[100,101] NSAID use is the second most common cause. NSAID use, either overt or covert, accounts for a sizeable proportion of gastric ulcer.[102,103]

Failure of healing

The cells in the duodenum migrate from the crypts to the tips of the villi. With a rapid cell turnover swift healing is possible. Indeed, traumatic breaches of the duodenal mucosa heal rapidly, often within hours, partly from proliferation of cells at the edge of the lesion and partly from restitution (increased migration of cells to repair the defect). Cellular proliferation can be inhibited by chalones released from nearby cells or stimulated by EGF; in addition a protein, fibronectin, binds to cell surfaces and collagen thus encouraging migration of cells into the slough of the ulcer base – such complex interactions at the ulcer base are little understood.[91] Vascular supply is important in healing and it has been found that oxygen saturation at the margin of an active duodenal ulcer may be low, which is a predictor of poor ulcer healing.[104] If a duodenal ulcer fails to heal, covert ingestion of NSAIDs should be considered.

Motility

About a third of patients with duodenal ulcer may empty their stomachs more swiftly than controls, but only 10% have both acid hypersecretion and increased speed of gastric emptying.[105] So few of these patients are likely to have a substantially raised duodenal acid load, although in some there may be a reduction in retrograde duodenal contractions which mix the gastric acid swiftly with alkaline secretions of the duodenum.[106] Motility disorders do not appear to be important in the aetiology of most cases of duodenal ulcer.

Conclusion

Full elucidation of the causes of duodenal ulcer disease is a long way from being achieved but infection with *H. pylori* is clearly of critical importance. The end point of the disease process is an ulcer crater which does not heal or keeps recurring. This may be due to local mucosal/healing factors, or to the acid load at the mucosal surface. Infection with *H. pylori* affects both aspects by increasing acid secretion and causing mucosal inflammation, the latter resulting in impaired resistance and reduced healing properties. *H. pylori* infection accounts for 95% of duodenal ulcer with two smaller subgroups: those associated with NSAIDs, and those in whom no cause can be found. More needs to be known about the factors which lead to ulceration in some people infected with *H. pylori* whereas not in others – the importance of toxin production is probably crucial. *H. pylori* plays an enabling role allowing other factors which of themselves would seldom lead to ulceration to have a major adverse effect. In some cases of duodenal ulcer the significant adverse factor might possibly be raised acid output (cause unknown as yet), in others it might be smoking (again, the mechanism is unknown but probably involves mucosal defences) whereas in others poor diet, ingestion of NSAIDs or congenital influences are the additional adverse factors. So, currently in clinical practice it is best to consider that most chronic duodenal ulcer have one cause, namely, *H. pylori* infection; but the infection is a necessary factor for most ulcers, sometimes causing an ulcer as a single factor, whilst in other individuals it enables one or more of a number of other adverse extrinsic and intrinsic factors to have an aetiological influence. Eradication of *H. pylori* is achievable in the majority of duodenal ulcer sufferers and offers the exciting prospect of cure of their disease.

PATHOLOGY

There is a spectrum of inflammatory changes which may occur in the duodenal cap, from minor inflammatory cell infiltrate which is not visible to the endoscopist, to deep ulceration (Figure 29.5a). Ulceration of the epithelium of the duodenal cap may be very superficial, without complete penetration through the mucosa, when it is then classified as an erosion. These are often multiple and are associated with duodenal ulcer disease. Two main types of peptic ulcer are recognized: acute ulcers which destroy the mucosa but do not usually extend deeper than the submucosa, and chronic ulcers which, as the term implies, are associated with more chronic inflammation, fibrosis, and may penetrate deeply into the muscularis propria.

Acute duodenal ulcers tend to develop under conditions of stress, for example, after severe burns (Curling's ulcer), septic shock, or after intracranial trauma or surgery (Cushing's ulcer). They may also be associated with ingestion of anti-inflammatory drugs. The ulcers occur almost invariably in the proximal duodenum and as they are relatively superficial, usually heal with minimal scarring.

Chronic duodenal ulcers are found in the duodenal cap, with only about 3% being postbulbar, and about three-quarters

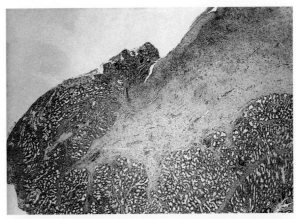

(a)

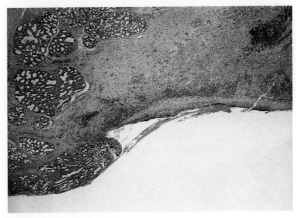

(b)

Figure 29.5a,b
Sections through a deep duodenal ulcer, penetrating through the mucosa, with slough and debris on the surface, with fibrinoid necrosis and, underneath, organizing granulation and fibrous tissue. (Courtesy of Dr Margaret Jeffreys.)

are less than 3 cm across. An ulcer in the second part of the duodenum or beyond strongly suggests the Zollinger–Ellison syndrome. A chronic ulcer has a clearly defined edge, being a penetrating lesion containing slough and debris and surrounded by an oedematous mucosa (Figure 29.5b), often with associated duodenitis and duodenal erosions. The base of a chronic ulcer is formed by fibrous tissue within a damaged muscularis or thickened serosa. The ulcer surface contains a layer of polymorphonuclear cells, many of which are damaged by peptic digestion. There is some fibrinoid necrosis which often stains intensely eosinophilic, and beneath this is an organizing zone of granulation tissue with the active deposition of fibrous tissue. Deeper still there is usually mature fibrous tissue. Any artery incorporated into this base usually shows endarteritis obliterans unless it is an acute ulcer. A variety of inflammatory cells may be seen. These inflammatory cells, especially the neutrophils, may extend into the surrounding epithelium including the villi. Of particular importance are foci of gastric metaplasia in the villous epithelium.[88] These are of importance because they will be colonized by *H. pylori* in the majority of cases of duodenal ulcer. Gastric metaplasia is particularly widespread in duodenal ulcer disease but may be found in the normal population where there is no history or evidence of duodenal ulceration. In controls the gastric metaplasia is minor, very localized and forms a small part of the surface area of the duodenum. In duodenal ulcer disease gastric metaplasia may involve more than a third of the mucosa of the duodenal cap.[87,88] Healing results in scarring with fibrous tissue beneath an abnormal mucosa.

CLINICAL FEATURES OF UNCOMPLICATED DUODENAL ULCER

Duodenal ulcers may present in a wide variety of ways and variable symptoms, often making diagnosis difficult.[107] The typical duodenal ulcer story is of epigastric pain, sometimes radiating into the back or into the lower chest, coming on intermittently, particularly if the patient has missed a meal. The pain may wake the patient at night and if relief is obtained by antacids or something to eat, there is a very high probability of an active duodenal ulcer.[108] The pain may be described as burning or gnawing. Although a small meal may bring relief, a large meal may well aggravate. Vomiting may occur and if it does this often gives temporary relief. The attacks of pain occur periodically and as the ulcer relapses it will cause recurrent attacks of pain over several days or weeks and may then remit leaving minimal dyspeptic symptoms until the next relapse.[109] These relapses vary enormously in their frequency from one relapse in, say, two or three years[110] to almost continuous symptoms with no more than a few days with freedom from symptoms in the untreated state. It is very important to remember this range of severity when considering treatment (see below). Because of the benefit from small meals and milk, patients typically gain weight. The old story of a duodenal ulcer occurring in the rising young executive no longer applies, nowadays the patient is typically male, a smoker, middle aged and with a long dyspeptic history. Sometimes the patient may present with a complication such as haemorrhage or perforation with virtually no warning symptoms at all.[111] This particularly tends to occur in the elderly patient and more especially so in someone who is taking anti-inflammatory drugs. The reason for this is not fully understood, although clearly the analgesic effect of the NSAIDs is bound to diminish awareness of pain.

When taking a history from a patient with suspected duodenal ulceration it is important to obtain a clear history not only of the location of the pain but also when it tends to occur, and relieving factors, such as antacids and small meals, and aggravating factors. Of particular importance is waking at night, which should always make the doctor consider an organic disorder such as duodenal ulcer or cholelithiasis. Heartburn is a common associated symptom which may well be difficult to distinguish from simple reflux oesophagitis. Waterbrash (a sudden flooding of the mouth with saliva) is a vagally mediated reflex which suggests mucosal damage within the oesophagus, stomach or duodenum and should alert the doctor to the likelihood of an organic disorder, or a reaction to a gastric irritant such as excess alcohol. If the patient vomits, almost invariably this gives good relief from the immediate symptoms and indeed the patient may want to go back and complete his

meal. There is rarely any change in bowel habit unless the patient is taking excessive quantities of magnesium-containing antacids, when diarrhoea may follow. The Zollinger–Ellison syndrome is, however, often associated not only with peptic ulceration but also with diarrhoea and malabsorption and should be considered very strongly in a patient presenting with both typical ulcer symptoms and diarrhoea. Smoking is an important risk factor and a positive family history should be sought.

When examining the patient the doctor should ask him to point to the location of the pain. In ulcer disease the patient will point with one or two fingers, whereas a patient with a functional gut disorder will tend to rub the flat of his hand across the whole of the upper abdomen. There may be epigastric tenderness which if over the aorta is of no diagnostic significance but elsewhere may be a useful clue. The Glasgow group have developed a system for weighting different symptoms which point towards a duodenal ulcer.[108] A previous history of having had a diagnosis of an ulcer in the past was found to be a useful discriminator, and particularly valuable in the Glasgow experience was being woken at night with relief being achieved by having something to eat or an antacid.

INVESTIGATIONS

Endoscopy

Upper gastrointestinal endoscopy (oesophagogastroduodenoscopy) (Figure 29.1) is more accurate than radiology in diagnosing duodenal ulceration because it has the facility for distinguishing scarring from a previous, healed ulcer from active ulceration.[112] It is therefore the investigation of choice for suspected duodenal ulcer disease. Interpretation of the endoscopic findings is easier if the patient is not on any healing treatment and is either in, or has just recently had, a relapse. Ulcer-like symptoms but no lesion seen in the duodenum would suggest that the patient has ulcer-like dyspepsia (see below). It has recently been shown that ulcers wax and wane and may not always be symptomatic. The more often a patient is endoscoped, the more likely it is that an ulcer crater will be present, albeit that the patient may be unaware that the ulcer has recurred[113] (Figure 29.6). Endoscopy during an active phase is particularly important if a previous examination has shown duodenitis. Erythematous duodenitis is probably not associated with symptoms, whereas erosive duodenitis (Figure 29.7, see colour plate also) is probably part of duodenal ulcer disease.[114] Before embarking on any long-term treatment, and especially before embarking on surgery, it is important to establish that the patient has true duodenal ulcer disease by undertaking the examination during an active phase of ulcer-like pain. The use of videoendoscopy, polaroid cameras, and video tapes now enable the endoscopist to answer the major criticism levelled at the technique, namely that there is no documentation of visual appearances and one is totally dependent on the opinion of the endoscopist. Obtaining antral tissue by biopsy is of real importance to determine whether or not there is an infection with *H. pylori*. The biopsy can be used in a urease-dependent test, or cultured and antibiotic sensitivities

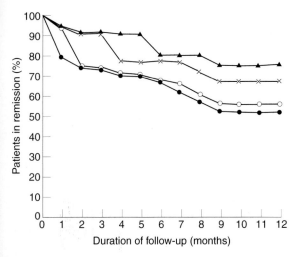

Figure 29.6
Duodenal ulcer relapse is often silent but may be detected at endoscopy. Boyd et al.[113] have demonstrated that the more frequently a patient is endoscoped, regardless of symptoms, the more frequently a recurrent ulcer will be found. Intervals between endoscopic examination of asymptomatic patients: ●, 1 month; ○, 2 months; ×, 4 months; Δ, 6 months. (Reproduced with permission from Boyd et al.[113])

obtained. Since no patient with duodenal ulcer should have surgery until their *H. pylori* status has been determined and the organism eradicated, this is an important part of the endoscopic investigation.

Radiology

A double-contrast barium meal in which the stomach is distended with air is superior to a single contrast barium meal, but still may miss duodenal ulcers and have difficulty in interpreting the appearances of the duodenal cap; when there is scarring it is very difficult to distinguish the deformity from active ulceration. It is, therefore, not the first line investigation,[115] but has the great advantage of being able to document

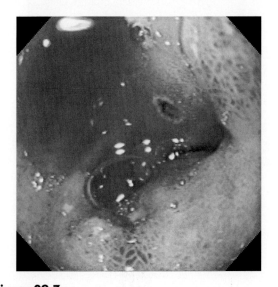

Figure 29.7
Erosive duodenitis as part of duodenal ulcer disease.

what is seen and to observe motility and gastric emptying.[116] It therefore has merit in assessing the functional appearances of the pylorus and duodenal cap, so as to ensure that there is no hold-up to the passage of food which might require surgery. Some surgeons therefore require a barium meal to be administered before undertaking a highly selective vagotomy, to ensure that there is no fibrotic stenosis of the pylorus/duodenum which would render the result of a highly selective vagotomy unsatisfactory.

Acid studies

There is no longer any need for acid secretion studies for diagnostic purposes. The accuracy of endoscopy and double contrast radiology make this investigation completely unnecessary. The major indication for acid secretion studies is research. For example, when undertaking controlled trials of different forms of vagotomy as treatment of duodenal ulcer disease it is vital to know how successful the vagotomy has been.[117] Use of tests such as a pentagastrin test, insulin/Hollander test, or sham feeding after vagotomy (in one of its forms) may be regarded as reasonable to assess the completeness of vagotomy. These tests are no more than a useful prognostic indicator when considering the likelihood of recurrent ulcer after surgery.[118] At present there is no convincing evidence that adjusting the type of operation for a duodenal ulcer according to acid secretion has any particular advantage.

When Zollinger–Ellison syndrome is suspected, overnight acid secretion or prolonged basal acid secretion followed by a standard pentagastrin test should be undertaken as well as the fasting serum gastrin.

Serum gastrin

Fasting serum gastrin should be measured before surgery in all cases of duodenal ulcer when off all acid-suppressing treatment in order to exclude overt Zollinger–Ellison syndrome. Gastrin levels do not need to be measured in every case of duodenal ulcer, only the resistant cases, although a single fasting gastrin may miss some cases of the Zollinger–Ellison syndrome. If it is found to be elevated then there is a place for undertaking acid secretion studies, particularly looking at the basal to stimulated acid output ratio (which is raised in Zollinger–Ellison syndrome) or the overnight acid secretion. If the raised serum gastrin and a raised acid secretion suggest Zollinger–Ellison syndrome then a secretin test should be undertaken to look for an inappropriate rise in the serum gastrin, which would be highly suggestive of a gastrinoma.[119] A low acid output with a raised serum gastrin suggests gastric atrophy or drug therapy rather than Zollinger–Ellison syndrome.

Intractability

Intractability was recently equated with clinically severe disease such that it recurs frequently and symptomatically despite maintenance therapy with antisecretory drugs (e.g. H_2-receptor antagonists), development of ulcer complications despite ongoing maintenance antisecretory therapy, or failure to heal despite prolonged therapy with an effective dose of acid pump inhibitor. The introduction of H_2-receptor antagonists resulted in intractability becoming an infrequent indication for surgery. Development of acid pump inhibitors, better understanding of the causes of ulcer disease and recognition that treatment of *H. pylori* infection could cure the most common form of ulcer, have almost eliminated intractability as an indication for surgery. It has also become increasingly recognized that covert NSAID use is responsible for ulcers being resistant to healing.[120] Successful treatment of the *H. pylori* infection and exclusion of NSAID use should be ascertained before declaring an ulcer intractable. A rare patient with a poorly healing gastric ulcer in a stomach with gastritis may still require surgery to exclude cancer.

COMPLICATIONS

The major danger from a duodenal ulcer is the occurrence of a complication, which is often life-threatening (Figure 29.8). However, it has recently been shown that elimination of *H. pylori* not only cures the ulcer in the short to medium term, but appears to eliminate complications also.[20,121–127]

Haemorrhage

Haemorrhage from peptic ulcer remains a common problem. Bleeding is typically self-limited, and the patient can generally be managed conservatively. The widespread availability of endoscopic haemostasis has further reduced the need for life-saving surgical intervention[128] but there is no evidence that medications of any sort affect the outcome of bleeding. Patients who have bled from peptic ulcer are at an increased risk of having additional episodes of haemorrhage. Although it has now been shown that chronic maintenance therapy with H_2 receptor antagonists will markedly reduce this risk[129–133] (Figure 29.8), two studies have shown that cure of *H. pylori* infection eliminated the risk of future bleeding (no ulcer, no complications), at least in the short term.[20,134] Thus, patients

who have bled should be investigated for *H. pylori* status and for NSAID use. If *H. pylori* infection is present, it should be treated; maintenance H_2-receptor antagonist therapy should not be discontinued until one is confident that the infection has been cured. If the patient was receiving NSAIDs (including aspirin) such medications should be prohibited in the future. If this is not an option because of severe arthritis, co-therapy with misoprostol (200 μg b.i.d. or t.i.d.) or ranitidine should be prescribed. Maintenance therapy with an H_2-receptor antagonist is recommended only if the patient cannot tolerate misoprostol and the ulcer was duodenal in location.

Perforation (Figure 29.9, see colour plate also)

Perforation is a complication of peptic ulcer disease and both the perforation and the underlying disease must be considered when planning long-term treatment. The primary issue remains the question of which operation is optimal for a specific patient. A randomized trial comparing non-operative treatment with careful observation revealed similar outcome, and the decision

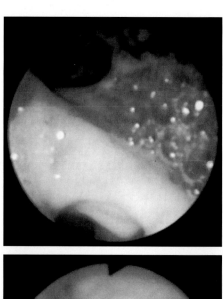

(a)

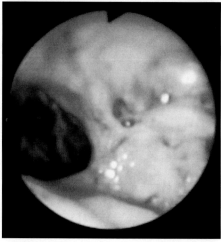

(b)

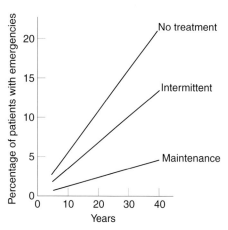

Figure 29.8
Mathematical model, based on data in the literature, to indicate the likelihood of a medical emergency arising from a peptic ulcer while the patient is on no treatment, intermittent H_2 receptor antagonist treatment, and continuous maintenance therapy. (Reproduced, with permission, from Sonnenberg.[137])

Figure 29.9
(a) Endoscopic picture of a perforation (dark area, top) above the lumen: the perforation was posterior and had been sealed off. (b) Endoscopic picture of the perforation (same patient as in a) showing a visible vessel (at 2 o'clock). The patient presented with severe pain and a major haemorrhage.

not to operate may be based on the age and clinical condition of the patient.[135] Current evidence suggests that simple closure of the perforation and proximal selective gastric vagotomy or seromyotomy is the preferred operation.[128] The long-term plan for a patient who survived the perforation and is ready to be discharged from the hospital depends on whether the patient received a definitive ulcer operation, had simple closure of the perforation, was managed with conservative medical therapy, or whether the perforation was a complication of concomitant NSAID use. In general, *H. pylori* status should be determined and, if present, the infection should be eradicated. As removal of *H. pylori* infection cures peptic ulcer disease it is presumed that it will also prevent this complication although, this hypothesis has not yet been studied. Even if the patient received a definitive ulcer operation, *H. pylori* should be eradicated if present. As with bleeding, if the perforation is possibly related to NSAID use then further use should be prohibited unless the patient requires such therapy. For these patients, misprostol or acid-suppressing prophylaxis is recommended.

Penetration

The incidence of penetration is unknown because penetration can only be diagnosed reliably at surgery, by autopsy, when a biopsy of an ulcer reveals liver or pancreatic tissue, or when there is a fistulous communication evident between the stomach or intestine and adjacent structure, such as the biliary tree or colon. Data from surgical series reveal that penetration is identified in approximately 20% of patients who required surgery for their peptic ulcer disease. Patients with penetrating ulcer have clinically severe peptic ulcer disease and present as having 'intractable' ulcer disease.

Obstruction

Approximately 2% of all patients with ulcer develop outlet obstruction; 90% are caused by previous or coexistent duodenal or channel ulcers. Active ulcer is present in more than 75% of cases. Inflammatory swelling surrounding the ulcer, muscular spasm, associated with nearby ulcer, or cicatricial narrowing with fibrosis are the factors responsible for the obstruction. Conservative medical management with decompression of the obstructed stomach, correction of fluid, electrolytes, and acid–base abnormalities, plus intravenous H_2-receptor antagonists are the mainstay of initial resuscitation and therapy. Two events have occurred to reduce to some extent, the need for surgery of obstruction: endoscopic balloon dilatation and treatment of the *H. pylori* infection. Intraoperative dilatation of the stenotic segment combined with highly selective vagotomy is often successful in the long-term management of patients with pyloric stenosis. One would presume that the combination of therapy that cures the disease (*H. pylori* therapy) and endoscopic dilatation of the pyloric ring should be equally effective. Our approach to these patients is resuscitation followed by balloon dilatation of the pylorus, vigorous antisecretory therapy (e.g. omeprazole 40–60 mg daily) followed by treatment of the *H. pylori* infection.[128] For those in whom the therapy is not successful, one should consider missed cancer.

DIFFERENTIAL DIAGNOSIS

Recurrent symptoms

The typical symptoms of a duodenal ulcer are diagnostic, unfortunately these are found in only a minority of such patients and therefore the differential diagnosis is wide. The most common diagnosis mimicking duodenal ulcer pain is **non-ulcer dyspepsia**. This has recently been broken down into several categories and defined as upper abdominal or lower retrosternal pain thought to originate from the upper gastrointestinal tract where no focal cause can be found.[136] Table 29.1 lists the major symptoms which suggest non-ulcer dyspepsia. The category of ulcer-like dyspepsia is a particularly difficult one to separate from actual duodenal ulceration and cannot readily be made unless an endoscopy has been done when the patient is symptomatic and off treatment. The problem is further compounded by the uncertainty over the clinical significance of duodenitis. This matter has not been fully resolved but at the present time it seems most likely that in erythematous duodenitis (that is to say patchy areas of erythema on the surface of folds within the duodenal cap but without any erosion) is an incidental finding

Table 29.1 Symptoms suggesting non-ulcer dyspepsia

General	Patient remains well
	Weight steady
	A 'worrier'
Reflux-like dyspepsia	Retrosternal discomfort
	Especially:
	On stooping
	After large meals
	On lying flat
	Burning retrosternal discomfort
	Temporary relief from antacids
	Severity is cyclical
	Recent weight gain
Motility-type dyspepsia	Abdominal distension
	Hungry but premature satiety
	Epigastric heaviness or fullness
	Variable and multiple food intolerances
	Often difficult to reproduce
	Pain is diffuse – often several pains – not at night
	Nausea prominent
	Associated features of the irritable bowel
	If vomits, 'cannot face food'
	Not episodic – tends to be continuous
Ulcer-like dyspepsia	Intermittent epigastric pain
	Better for small meals
	Woken at night
	Relief from antacids
	Finger-pointing sign
	Seldom vomiting
Air swallowing	Repeated belching, but no relief of symptoms
	Distension
	Nausea
	Often at the same time each day (e.g. after evening meal)
	Worse with stress

and not associated with any symptoms and does not indicate predisposition towards duodenal ulceration. On the other hand erosive duodenitis (that is to say patchy areas of erythema and often oedema with small, often multiple, shallow areas of erosion) probably does cause symptoms and may often be a part of duodenal ulcer disease.[98] The *H. pylori* status of the patient should be determined.

The dysmotility type of dyspepsia is usually easier to distinguish from duodenal ulceration because of the symptoms of bloating, premature satiety and nausea. There is a marked overlap between dysmotility-like dyspepsia and irritable bowel syndrome. As many patients with duodenal ulcer disease have reflux symptoms, it can at times be very difficult to distinguish between gastro-oesophageal reflux disease (increased reflux of gastric contents into the lower oesophagus, with or without visible oesophagitis) as an isolated diagnosis from that associated with an ulcer. Severe or persisting symptoms and relapse after a course of treatment warrant further investigation to separate these two and endoscopy is the investigation of choice. Table 29.2 lists the major symptoms and features suggesting an organic cause for the pain.

Abdominal pain and dyspepsia due to gallstones must

Table 29.2 Factors suggesting the need for early investigation

Age greater than approximately 45 years
Weight loss
Anaemia
Being woken at night
Radiation of pain into the back
Periodicity
Smoking
Taking non-steroidal anti-inflammatory drugs
A past history of a peptic ulcer or hiatus hernia
Vomiting
Pointing to the location of pain with a finger as it is relatively localized

always be considered in a patient presenting with a possible ulcer. Typical biliary colic with severe pain waking the patient, spreading through into the back and developing into an excruciating pain with vomiting and then subsequently with a temporary development of jaundice needs no distinction from duodenal ulcer pain. However, many patients experience more minor symptoms than this, for example discomfort after eating a large meal, especially if fatty, and if it does occasionally wake them at night, as an ulcer can, gallstones should be considered, and an ultrasound undertaken.

Chronic pancreatitis can be extremely difficult to diagnose, especially in its early stages. The symptoms can wax and wane just as in duodenal ulcer disease, the pain is often epigastric going through to the back. It may be made worse by very large meals but tends to be more persistent pain, dragging the patient down rather than clearing completely as often happens in the course of duodenal ulcer pain. Not only is it difficult to diagnose clinically but it is also difficult to diagnose on investigation as ultrasound has a very low sensitivity and especially in the early stages before calcification has occurred in the gland,

both ultrasound, computed tomography scanning and endoscopic pancreatography can miss minor changes. It is very important to look for risk factors such as gallstones and alcohol when considering pancreatitis as the cause of pain.

Mesenteric ischaemia is probably underdiagnosed, occurring in the older patient who is usually a smoker, and often starting insidiously with a non-specific postprandial abdominal pain. As the symptoms progress so the pain increases in frequency and severity and often weight loss occurs, sometimes with malabsorption. Almost invariably, investigation for peptic ulcer disease has to be undertaken, especially as angiography is a highly invasive procedure.

Duodenal ulcers may be silent, especially in the elderly and those taking NSAIDs,[111] so patients presenting with evidence of gastrointestinal bleeding or anaemia need to be investigated by oesophagogastroduodenoscopy despite absence of symptoms. A drug history sometimes provides a vital clue.

Acute and severe symptoms

Patients presenting for the first time with peptic ulcer or with an exacerbation of their ulcer disease may mimic an acute abdomen. Indeed a complication of a peptic ulcer, such as a contained perforation, may have taken place. The differential diagnosis here includes acute pancreatitis, acute peritonitis of any cause, cholecystitis and biliary colic, acute exacerbation of inflammatory bowel disease, and even an acute infective gastroenteritis due to an organism such as *Campylobacter jejuni* needs to be considered. Mesenteric infarction may also mimic a complicated peptic ulcer (see Chapter 34).

REFERENCES

1. Graham DY. *Helicobacter pylori*: its epidemiology and its role in duodenal ulcer disease. *J Gastroenterol Hepatol* 1991; **6**: 105–113.
2. Dixon MF. *Helicobacter pylori* and peptic ulceration: histopathological aspects. *J Gastroenterol Hepatol* 1991; **6**: 125–130.
3. Langman MJS. Aetiology of peptic ulcer. In Misiewicz JJ, Pounder RE & Venables CW (eds) *Diseases of the Gut and Pancreas* 2nd edn. Oxford: Blackwell Scientific Publications, 1994.
4. Kurata JH. Ulcer epidemiology: an overview and proposed research framework. *Gastroenterology* 1989; **96**: 569–580.
5. Bonnevie O. Peptic ulcer in Denmark. *Scand J Gastroenterol* 1980; **15**: 163–174.
6. Walt R, Katschinski B, Logan R, Ashley J & Langman M. Rising frequency of ulcer perforation in elderly people in the United Kingdom. *Lancet* 1986; **i**: 489–492.
7. Tovey FI. Peptic ulcer in India and Bangladesh. *Gut* 1979; **20**: 329–347.
8. Khuroo MS, Mahajan R, Zargar SA, Javid G & Munshi S. Prevalence of peptic ulcer in India: an endoscopic and epidemiological study in urban Kashmir. *Gut* 1989; **30**: 930–934.
9. Kawai K, Shirikawa K, Misaki F, Hayashi K & Watanabe Y. Natural history and epidemiologic studies of peptic ulcer disease in Japan. *Gastroenterology* 1989; **96**: 581–585.
10. Schoón I-M, Mellstróm D, Odán A & Ytterberg B-O. Incidence of peptic ulcer disease in Gothenburg 1985. *BMJ* 1989; **299**: 1131–1134.
11. Bernersen B, Johnsen R & Straume B. Non-ulcer dyspepsia and peptic ulcer: the distribution in a population and their relation to risk factors. *Gut* 1996; **38**: 822–825.
12. Malliwah JA, Tabaqchali M, Watson J & Venables CW. Audit of the outcome of peptic ulcer disease diagnosed 10 to 20 years previously. *Gut* 1996; **38**: 912–915.
13. Sipponen P, Varis K, Fraki O, Korri UM, Seppala K & Siurala M. Cumulative 10-year risk of symptomatic duodenal and gastric ulcer in patients with or without chronic gastritis. A clinical follow-up study of 454 outpatients. *Scand J Gastroenterol* 1990; **25**: 966–973.

14. Steer HW & Colin-Jones DG. Mucosal changes in gastric ulceration and their response to carbenoxolone sodium. *Gut* 1975; **16**: 590–597.
15. Marshall BJ & Warren JR. Unidentified curved bacilli in the stomach of patients with gastritis and peptic ulceration. *Lancet* 1984; **1**: 1311–1315.
16. Hosking SW, Ling TKW, Man Yee Yung et al. Randomised controlled trial of short term treatment to eradicate *Helicobacter pylori* in patients with duodenal ulcer. *BMJ* 1992; **302**: 502–504
17. Hopkins RJ, Girardi LS & Turney EA. Relationship between *Helicobacter pylori* eradication and reduced duodenal and gastric ulcer recurrence: a review. *Gastroenterology* 1996; **110**: 1244–1252.
18. Forbes G, Glaser M, Cullen DJE et al. Duodenal ulcer treated with *Helicobacter pylori* eradication: seven year follow-up. *Lancet* 1994; **29**: 258–260.
19. Witteman EM, Mravunac M, Becx MJ et al. Improvement of gastric inflammation and resolution of epithelial damage one year after eradication of *Helicobacter pylori*. *J Clin Pathol* 1995; **48**: 250–256.
20. Labenz J & Borsch G. Role of *Helicobacter pylori* eradication in the prevention of peptic ulcer bleeding relapse. *Digestion* 1994; **55**: 19–23.
21. Tee W, Lambert JR & Dwyer B. Cytotoxin production by *Helicobacter pylori* from patients with upper gastrointestinal tract disease. *J Clin Microbiol* 1995; **33**: 1203–1205.
22. el-Omar EM, Penman ID, Ardill JE, Chittajallu RS, Howie C & McColl KE. *Helicobacter pylori* infection and abnormalities of acid secretion in patients with duodenal ulcer disease. *Gastroenterology* 1995; **109**: 681–691.
23. Harris AW, Gummett PA, Misiewicz JJ & Baron JH. Eradication of *Helicobacter pylori* in patients with duodenal ulcer lowers basal and peak acid outputs to gastrin releasing peptide and pentagastrin. *Gut* 1996; **38**: 663–667.
24. Go MF & Graham DY. How does *Helicobacter pylori* cause duodenal ulcer disease: the bug, the host, or both? *J Gastroenterol Hepatol* 1994; **9** suppl. 1: S8–10.
25. Tytgat GN & Dixon MF. Role of *Helicobacter pylori* in the pathogenesis of peptic ulcer disease. In Hunt RH (ed.) *Proton Pump Inhibitors and Acid-related Disorders*. Osaka: Adis International 1994; 79–97.
26. Rathbone BJ & Heatley RV (eds) *Campylobacter pylori and Gastroduodenal Disease*. Oxford; Blackwell Scientific Publications, 1989.
27. Tytgat GN. Review article: treatments that impact favourably upon the eradication of *Helicobacter pylori* and ulcer recurrence. *Aliment Pharmacol Ther* 1994; **8**: 359–368.
28. Clarke CA, Edwards JW, Haddock DRW, Howel Evans AW & McConnell PB. ABO blood groups and secretor character in duodenal ulcer. *BMJ* 1956; **2**: 725–731.
29. Samloff IM, Liebman WM & Panitch NM. Serum group I pepsinogen by radioimmunoassay in control subjects and patients with peptic ulcer. *Gastroenterology* 1975; **69**: 83–90.
30. Samloff IM. Peptic ulcer: the many proteinases of aggression. *Gastroenterology* 1989; **96**: 586–595.
31. Graham DY, Opekun AR, Lew GM & Malfertheiner P. Is serum pepsinogen I a genetic marker for duodenal ulcer or a surrogate marker for *Helicobacter pylori* infection? (Abstract) *Gastroenterology* 1990; **98**: A53.
32. Malaty HM & Graham DY. Importance of childhood socioeconomic status on the current prevalence of *Helicobacter pylori* infection. Gut 1994; **35**: 742–745.
33. Lennard-Jones LE, Fletcher J & Shaw DG. Effect of different foods on the acidity of the gastric contents in patients with duodenal ulcer. Part III: Effect of altering the proportions of protein and carbohydrate. *Gut* 1968; **9**: 177–182.
34. Jayaraj AP, Tovey FI & Clark CG. Possible dietary protective factor in relation to the distribution of duodenal ulcer in India and Bangladesh. *Gut* 1980; **21**: 1068–1076.
35. Grant HW, Palmer KR, Kelly RW & Wilson NH. Dietary linoleic acid, gastric acid, and prostaglandin secretion. *Gastroenterology* 1988; **94**: 955–959.
36. Rydning A & Berstad A. Dietary fibre and peptic ulcer. *Scand J Gastroenterol* 1986; **21**: 1–5.
37. Hollander D & Tarnawski A. Dietary essential fatty acids and the decline in peptic ulcer disease – a hypothesis. *Gut* 1986; **27**: 239–242.
38. Malhotra SL. New approaches to the pathogenesis of peptic ulcer based on the protective action of saliva. *Am J Dig Dis* 1970; **15**: 489–496.
39. Tovey FI, Jayaraj AP, Lewin MR & Clark CG. Diet: Its role in the genesis of peptic ulceration. *Dig Dis* 1989; **7**: 309–323.

40. Rune SJ & Vestergaard BF. IgA antibodies to herpes simplex virus type I in duodenal juice and saliva from patients with peptic ulcer and non-ulcer controls. *Scand J Gastroenterol* 1984; **19**: 81–84.
41. Rune SJ, Linde J, Bonnevie O et al. Acyclovir in the prevention of duodenal ulcer recurrence. *Gut* 1990; **31**: 151–152.
42. Chiverton SG & Hunt RH. Smoking and duodenal ulcer disease. *J Clin Gastroenterol* 1989 **11** (Suppl 1): S29–S33.
43. Parente F, Lazzaroni M, Sangaletti O, Baroni S & Bianchi Porro G. Cigarette smoking, gastric acid secretion and serum pepsinogen I concentrations in duodenal ulcer patients. *Gut* 1985; **26**: 1327–1332.
44. Whitfield PF & Hobsley M. Comparison of maximal gastric secretion in smokers and non-smokers with and without duodenal ulcer. *Gut* 1987; **28**: 557–560.
45. Korman MG, Shaw RG, Hansky J & Schmidt GT. Influence of smoking on healing rate of duodenal ulcer in response to cimetidine or high-dose antacid. *Gastroenterology* 1981; **80**: 1451–1453.
46. Hull DH & Beale PJ. Cigarette smoking and duodenal ulcer. *Gut* 1985; **26**: 1333–1337.
47. Boyd EJS, Wilson JA & Wormsley KG. Smoking impairs therapeutic gastric inhibition. *Lancet* 1983; **i**: 95–97.
48. Lam SK, Hui WY, Lau WY et al. Sucralfate over comes adverse effect of cigarette smoking on duodenal ulcer healing and prolongs subsequent remission. *Gastroenterology* 1987; **92**: 1192–1201.
49. Graham DY, Lew GM, Klein PD et al. Effect of treatment of *Helicobacter pylori* infection on the long-term recurrence of gastric or duodenal ulcer. A randomized, controlled study. *Ann Intern Med* 1992; **116**: 705–708.
50. Borody TJ, George LL, Brandl A, Andrews P, Jankiewicz E & Ostapowicz N. Smoking does not contribute to duodenal ulcer relapse after *Helicobacter pylori* eradication. *Am J Gastroenterol* 1992; **87**: 1390–1393.
51. Wolf S. The psyche and the stomach. *Gastroenterology* 1981; **80**: 605–614.
52. Peters MN & Richardson C. Stressful life events, acid hypersecretion and ulcer disease. *Gastroenterology* 1983; **84**: 114–119.
53. Øktedalen O, Guldvog I, Opstad PK, Berstad A, Gedde-Dahl D & Jorde R. The effect of physical stress on gastric secretion and pancreatic polypeptide levels in man. *Scand J Gastroenterol* 1984; **19**: 770–778.
54. Klein KB & Spiegel D. Modulation of gastric acid secretion by hypnosis. *Gastroenterology* 1989; **96**: 1383–1387.
55. Colgan SM, Faragher EB & Whorwell PJ. Controlled trial of hypnotherapy in relapse prevention of duodenal ulceration. *Lancet* 1988; **i**: 1299–1300.
56. Baron JH. *Clinical Tests of Gastric Secretion: History, Methodology and Interpretation*. London; Macmillan, 1978.
57. Feldman M & Richardson CT. Total 24 hour gastric acid secretion in patients with duodenal ulcer: comparison with normal subjects and effects of cimetidine and parietal cell vagotomy. *Gastroenterology* 1986; **90**: 540–544.
58. Feldman M. Neural and hormonal factors in peptic ulcer disease. *J Clin Gastroenterol* 1981; **3** (suppl.2): 51–56.
59. Lanzon-Miller S, Pounder R, Hamilton M et al. Twenty-four hour intragastric acidity and plasma gastrin concentration before and during treatment with either ranitidine or omeprazole. *Aliment Pharmacol Ther* 1987; **1**: 239–251.
60. Achord JL. Gastric pepsin and acid secretion in patients with acute and healed duodenal ulcer. *Gastroenterology* 1981; **81**: 15–18.
61. Kerrigan DD, Read NW, Taylor ME, Houghton LA & Johnson AG. Duodenal bulb acidity and the natural history of duodenal ulceration. *Lancet* 1989; **2**: 61–63.
62. Skoubo-Kristensen E. Sham feeding-pentagastrin test in healthy subjects and peptic ulcer patients. *Scand J Gastroenterol* 1984; **19**: 461–466.
63. Venables CW. Mucus, pepsin and peptic ulcer. *Gut* 1986; **27**: 233–238.
64. Walker V & Taylor WH. Pepsin I secretion in chronic peptic ulceration. *Gut* 1980; **21**: 766–771.
65. Deakin M, Glenny HP, Ramage JG, Burland WL & Williams JG. Large single daily dose of histamine H₂ receptor antagonist for duodenal ulcer. How much and when? A clinical pharmacological study. *Gut* 1987; **28**: 566–572.
66. Cargill JM, Peden N, Saunders JHB & Wormsley KG. Very long term treatment of peptic ulcer with cimetidine. *Lancet* 1978; **ii**: 1113–1115.
67. Baron JH, Barr J, Batten J, Sidebotham R & Spencer J. Acid, pepsin, and mucus secretion in patients with gastric and duodenal ulcer before and after colloidal bismuth subcitrate (DeNol). *Gut* 1986; **27**: 486–490.
68. Burget DW, DeGara CJ & Hunt RH. Instability of pepsin in stored gastric juice – cause for concern? *Gut* 1984; **25**: A1153.

69. Deakin M, Ramage J, Paul A, Gray SP, Billings J & Williams JG. Don't freeze pepsin! *JR Nav Med Serv* 1985; **71**: 96–97.

70. Lamers CBHW. Hormonal regulation of gastric acid in peptic ulcer disease. *Scand J Gastroenterol* 1988; **23** (suppl 146): 5–10.

71. Harty RF, Maico DG & McGuigan JE. Antral release of gastrin and somatostatin in duodenal ulcer and control subjects. *Gut* 1986; **27**: 652–658.

72. Levi S, Beardshall K, Haddad G, Playford R, Ghosh P & Calam J. *Campylobacter pylori* and duodenal ulcers: the gastrin link. *Lancet* 1989; **1**: 1167–1168.

73. Skak-Nielsen T, Holst JJ & Nielsen OV. Role of gastrin-releasing peptide in the neural control of pepsinogen secretion from the pig-stomach. *Gastroenterology* 1988; **95**: 1216–1220.

74. Schwartz TW, Stadil F, Chance RE, Rehfeld JF, Larson L-I & Moon N. Pancreatic-polypeptide response to food in duodenal-ulcer patients before and after vagotomy. *Lancet* 1976; **i**: 1102–1105.

75. Dragstedt LR. A concept of the aetiology of gastric and duodenal ulcers. *Gastroenterology* 1956; **30**: 208–220.

76. Feldman M, Richardson CT & Fordtran JS. Effect of sham feeding on gastric acid secretion in healthy subjects and duodenal ulcer patients: evidence for increased basal vagal tone in some ulcer patients. *Gastroenterology* 1980; **79**: 796–800.

77. Kohn A, Annibale B, Suriano G, Severi C, Spinella S & Delle Fave G. Gastric acid and pancreatic polypeptide responses to modified sham feeding: indication of an increased basal vagal tone in a subgroup of duodenal ulcer patients. *Gut* 1985; **26**: 776–782.

78. Sandvik A, Kaul BK, Waldum H & Petersen H. Gastric acid and pepsin secretion in response to modified sham feeding in active and inactive duodenal ulcer disease. *Scand J Gastroenterol* 1985; **20**: 602–606.

79. Flemstrom G & Garner A. Gastroduodenal HCO$_3$ transport: characteristics and proposed role in acidity and mucosal protection. *Am J Physiol* 1982; **242** (Gastrointest Liver Physiol 5) G183–G193.

80. Forsell J, Stenquist B & Olbe· L. Vagal stimulation of human gastric bicarbonate secretion. *Gastroenterology* 1985; **89**: 581–586.

81. Wenzl E, Feli W, Starlinger M & Schiessel R. Alkaline secretion. A protective mechanism against acid injury in rabbit duodenum. *Gastroenterology* 1987; **92**: 709–715.

82. Isenberg JI, Selling JA & Koss MA. Impaired proximal duodenal mucosal bicarbonate secretion in patients with duodenal ulcer. *N Engl J Med* 1987; **316**: 374–379.

83. Isenberg JI, Hogan DL, Koss MA & Selling JA. Human duodenal mucosal bicarbonate secretion. Evidence for basal secretion and stimulation by hydrochloric acid and a synthetic prostaglandin E1 analog. *Gastroenterology* 1986; **91**: 370–378.

84. Leung FW, Itoh M, Hirabayashi K & Guth PM. Role of blood flow in gastic and duodenal mucosal injury in the rat. *Gastroenterology* 1985; **88**: 281–289.

85. Smith CL & Hillier K. Duodenal mucosa synthesis of prostaglandins in duodenal ulcer disease. *Gut* 1985; **26**: 237–240.

86. Kirk RM. Does the jet of acid emerging through the pylorus determine the site of duodenal bulbar ulcers? *BMJ*, 1975; **3**: 629–630.

87. Marshall BJ, Goodwin CS, Warren JR et al. Prospective double-blind trial of duodenal ulcer relapse after eradication of *Campylobacter pylori*. *Lancet* 1988; **ii**: 1437–1442.

88. Carrick J, Lee A, Hazell S, Ralston M & Daskalopoulos G. *Campylobacter pylori*, duodenal ulcer, and gastric metaplasia: possible role of functional heterotopic tissue in ulcerogenesis. *Gut* 1989; **30**: 790–797.

89. Graham D. *Campylobacter pylori* and peptic ulcer disease. *Gastroenterology* 1989; **96**: 615–625

90. Kirk RM. Could chronic peptic ulcers be localised areas of acid susceptibility generated by autoimmunity? *Lancet* 1986; **i**: 772–775.

91. Wormsley KG. Aetiology of ulcers. In Piper DW (ed.) *Clinical Gastroenterology*, vol.2/Number 3. London; Bailliere Tindall, 1988.

92. Gregory H. Isolation and structure of urogastrone and its relationship to epidermal growth factor. *Nature* 1975; **257**: 325–327.

93. Olsen PS, Poulsen SS, Therkelsen K & Nexø E. Effect of sialoadenectomy and synthetic human urogastrone on healing of chronic gastric ulcers in rats. *Gut* 1986; **27**: 1443–1449.

94. Henry DH, Lim LL-Y, Gardia Rodgriguez A et al. Variability in risk of gastrointestinal complications with individual non-steroidal anti-inflammatory drugs: results of a collaborative meta-analysis. *BMJ* 1996; **312**: 1563–1566.

95. Hawkey CJ. Non-steroidal anti-inflammatory drugs and peptic ulcers. *BMJ* 1990; **300**: 278–284.

96. Coggon D, Langman MJS & Spiegelhalter D. Aspirin, paracetamol, and haematemesis and melaena. *Gut* 1982; **23**: 340–344.

97. Somerville K, Faulkner G & Langman MJS. Non-steroidal anti-inflammatory drugs and bleeding peptic ulcer. *Lancet* 1986; **i**: 462–464.

98. Griffin MR, Ray WA & Schaffner W. Nonsteroidal anti-inflammatory drug use and death from peptic ulcer in elderly persons. *Ann Intern Med* 1988; **109**: 359–363.

99. Taha AS, Sturrock RD & Russell RI. Mucosal erosions in longterm non-steroidal anti-inflammatory drug users: predisposition to ulceration and relation to *Helicobacter pylori*. *Gut* 1995; **36**: 334–336.

100. Borody TJ, Brandl S, Andrews P, Jankiewicz E & Ostapowicz N. *Helicobacter pylori*-negative gastric ulcer. *Am J Gastroenterol* 1992; **87**: 1403–1406.

101. Borody TJ, George LL, Brandl S et al. *Helicobacter pylori*-negative duodenal ulcer. *Am J Gastroenterol* 1991; **86**: 1154–1157.

102. Soll AH. Gastric, duodenal, and stress ulcer. In: Sleisinger M Fordtran J (eds) *Gastrointestinal Disease*. Philadelphia: WB Saunders, 1993; 580–679.

103. Graham DY. Prevention of gastroduodenal injury induced by chronic nonsteroidal anti-inflammatory drug therapy. Gastroenterology 1989; **96**: 675–681.

104. Leung FW, Tallos EG, VanDeventer GM & Guth PH. Reduction in the index of oxygen saturation at the margin of an active duodenal ulcer predicts poor healing. *Gastroenterology* 1987; **92**: 1502.

105. Barbara L, Corinaldesi R & Stanghellini V. Aggressive vs. defensive factors in the pathogenesis of peptic ulcer disease. In: Bianchi Porro G & Bardham KD (eds) *Topics in Peptic Ulcer Disease*. Verona: Cortina International, 1987.

106. Borgström S & Arborelius M Jr. Duodenal motility pattern in duodenal ulcer disease. *Scand J Gastroenterol* 1978; **13**: 349–352.

107. Talley NJ, McNeil D & Piper DW. Discriminant value of dyspeptic symptoms: a study of the clinical presentation of 221 patients with dyspepsia of unknown cause, peptic ulceration, and cholelithiasis. *Gut* 1987; **28**: 40–46.

108. Crean GP, McCormack A, Spiegelhalter DJ, Knill-Jones RP & Holden RJ. An attempt to distinguish between non-ulcer dyspepsia and peptic ulcer. In: Rees WDW (ed.) *Peptic Ulcer Disease. Proceedings of the Seventh BSG-SKF international Workshop.* Welwyn Garden City: Smith Kline & French, 1987.

109. Bennett JR, Colin-Jones DG, Dyer N, Lee PWR & Smith P. *Practical Problems in Gastroenterology.* London: Martin Dunitz, 1986.

110. Frederiksen H-JB, Matzen P, Madsen P et al. Spontaneous healing of duodenal ulcers. *Scand J Gastroenterol* 1984; **19**: 417–421.

111. Armstrong CP & Blower AL. Non-steroidal anti-inflammatory drugs and life threatening complications of peptic ulceration. *Gut* 1987; **28**: 527–532.

112. Dooley CP, Larson AW, Stace NH et al. Double contrast barium meal and upper gastrointestinal endoscopy. A comparative study. *Ann Intern Med* 1984; **101**: 538–545.

113. Boyd EJS, Penston JG, Johnston DA & Wormsley KG. Does maintenance therapy keep duodenal ulcers healed? *Lancet* 1988; **i**: 1324–1327.

114. Sircus W. Duodenitis: a clinical, endoscopic and histopathologic study. *Q J Med* 1985; **56**: 593–600.

115. Cotton PB & Shorvon PJ. Analysis of endoscopy and radiography in the diagnosis follow-up and treatment of peptic ulcer disease. *Clin Gastroenterol* 1984; **13**: 383–403.

116. Colin-Jones DG. Endoscopy or radiology for upper gastrointestinal symptoms? *Lancet* 1986; **i**: 1022–1023.

117. Primrose JN, Axon ATR & Johnston D. Highly selective vagotomy and duodenal ulcers that fail to respond to H$_2$ receptor antagonists. *BMJ* 1988; **296**: 1031–1035.

118. Graffner H & Lindell G. Increased ulcer relapse rate after PCV in smokers. *World J Surg* 1988; **12**: 277–279.

119. Frucht H, Howard JM, Slaff JI et al. Secretin and calcium provocative tests in the Zollinger–Ellison syndrome: a prospective study. *Ann Intern Med* 1989; **111**: 713–722.

120. Perrault J, Fleming CR & Dozois RR. Surreptitious use of salicylates: a cause of chronic recurrent gastroduodenal ulcers. *Mayo Clin Proc* 1988; **63**: 337–342.

121. George LL, Borody TJ, Andrews P et al. Cure of duodenal ulcer after eradication of *Helicobacter pylori*. *Med J Aust* 1990; **153**: 145–149.

122. Rauws EA & Tytgat GN. Cure of duodenal ulcer associated with eradication of *Helicobacter pylori*. *Lancet* 1990; **335**: 1233–1235.

123. Borody T, Andrews P, Manusco N, Jankiewicz E & Brandl S. *Helicobacter pylori* reinfection 4 years post-eradication. *Lancet* 1992; **339**: 1295 (letter).

124. Borody TJ, Cole P, Noonon S et al. Recurrence of duodenal ulcer and *Campylobacter pylori* infection after eradication. *Med J Aust* 1989; **151**: 431–435.

125. Marshall BJ, Goodwin CS, Warren JR et al. Prospective double-blind trial of duodenal ulcer relapse after eradication of *Campylobacter pylori*. *Lancet* 1988; **ii**: 1437–1442.

126. Coghlan JG, Gilligan D, Humphries H et al. *Campylobacter pylori* and recurrence of duodenal ulcers – a 12-month follow-up study. *Lancet* 1987; **ii**: 1109–1111.

127. Hentschel E, Brandstatter G, Dragosics B et al. Effect of ranitidine and amoxycillin plus metronidazole on the eradication of *Helicobacter pylori* and the recurrence of duodenal ulcer. *N Engl J Med* 1993; **328**: 308–312.

128. Graham DY. Ulcer complications and their nonoperative treatment. In Sleisinger M & Fordtran J (eds) *Gastrointestinal Disease*. Philadelphia: WB Saunders, 1993: 698–712.

129. Penston JG & Wormsley KG. Asymptomatic duodenal ulcers occurring during maintenance treatment with ranitidine. *Aliment Pharmacol Ther* 1990; **4**: 569–576.

130. Penston JG & Wormsley KG. Review article. Maintenance treatment with H₂-receptor antagonists for peptic ulcer disease. *Aliment Pharmacol Ther* 1992; **6**: 3–29.

131. Penston JG & Wormsley KG. Nine years of maintenance treatment with ranitidine for patients with duodenal ulcer disease. *Aliment Pharmacol Ther* 1992; **6**: 629–645.

132. Penston JG & Wormsley KG. Long-term mainenance treatment of gastric ulcers with ranitidine. *Aliment Pharmacol Ther* 1990; **4**: 339–355.

133. Van Deventer GM, Elashoff JD, Reedy TJ, Schneidman D & Walsh JH. A randomized study of maintenance therapy with ranitidine to prevent the recurrence of duodenal ulcer. *N Engl J Med* 1989; **320**: 1113–1119.

134. Graham DY, Hepps KS, Ramirez FC, Lew GM & Saeed ZA. Treatment of *H. pylori* reduces the rate of rebleeding in peptic ulcer disease. *Scand J Gastroenterol* 1993; **28**: 939–942.

135. Crofts TJ, Park KG, Steele RJ, Chung SS & Li AK. A randomized trial of nonoperative treatment for perforated peptic ulcer. *N Engl J Med* 1989; **320**: 970–973.

136. Colin-Jones DG et al. Management of dyspepsia: report of a working party. *Lancet* 1988; **i**: 576–579.

137. Sonnenberg A. Comparison of different strategies for treatment of duodenal ulcers. *BMJ* 1985; **290**: 1185–1187.

30

MEDICAL MANAGEMENT OF DUODENAL ULCER DISEASE

MA Quine
G Moody
DG Colin-Jones

INTRODUCTION

The medical management of duodenal ulcer disease has been revolutionized by the discovery of the bacterium *Helicobacter pylori*. Eradication of this bacterium has turned a common chronic clinical problem into one that can be cured by a week's course of tablets. Treatment of active disease is now only one aspect of management: eradication to prevent relapse in those patients known to have a past history of duodenal ulcer disease, particularly those with complications, is also important. It is imperative that as many patients as possible benefit from eradication of this organism as eradication has displaced acid-suppressing therapy as the first line treatment. There is also the added advantage that the patient may be protected against gastric carcinoma and coronary heart disease as there is some evidence that *H. pylori* is implicated in these two pathologies.[1-4]

However, a small minority of ulcers in the duodenum do not appear to be related to the bacterium. Acid suppression continues to have its place in medical treatment and the advent of proton pump inhibitors has contributed to the improvement in healing times for peptic ulceration. Although short eradication courses for *H. pylori* are often all that is required for the management of uncomplicated acute duodenal ulceration, the few *H. pylori*-negative ulcers demand further consideration and possible investigation. Has the ulcer been caused by non-steroidal anti-inflammatory drugs (NSAIDs) does the ulceration represent Crohn's disease or is it the result of a Zollinger–Ellison syndrome? In these patients acid suppression will continue to play a large part either for the control of disease or for the prevention of relapse. In addition, in those patients with complicated duodenal ulceration (e.g. bleeding ulcers), effective acid suppression is extremely important in maintaining healing while confirmation of eradication of the organism is carried out.

HELICOBACTER PYLORI-POSITIVE ULCER DISEASE

Once *H. pylori* has been detected in a patient with duodenal ulcer disease, eradication of the organism alone will heal an uncomplicated ulcer and prevent relapse in well over 90% of cases.[5-7] Indeed in some studies the recurrence rate has been zero so that patients certainly in these studies, can be thought of as cured.[2] This is now the most important aspect of the medical management of peptic ulcer disease and will be discussed first.

Eradication of *H. pylori*

It is now thought to be unnecessary to heal the ulcer before eradication. Presumably the concept that we should heal the ulcer first is a relic from the time when eradication of *H. pylori* was only considered in those patients who had resistant ulcers. Successful eradication heals a higher percentage of ulcers than acid suppression alone (using H_2 blockers),[8] so it would seem inappropriate to delay effective treatment for a less effective one. Studies have also shown that some eradication regimes are less successful if given to patients who have already been on proton pump inhibitors for a period of time: in some way the organism becomes tolerant of the antibiotics in this situation.[9]

There are now very many different regimens for the treatment of *H. pylori*, but the two main types used are dual or triple therapies, given for one or two weeks. Monotherapy is not sufficient. Although resistance to colloidal bismuth subcitrate does not develop, and although the incidence of relapse after a healing dose of bismuth is lower than after cimetidine, eradication rates are less than 10%. Eradication of the bacterium is difficult mainly because it lives beneath the adherent layer of mucus and penetration of antimicrobials into this area is poor; eradication regimes therefore require two or more drugs to maximize the chances of success. There are now many studies comparing various regimes and eradication rates for some of the more effective treatments are around 90%. However, there are two important factors which dictate the success of the individual regime outside the research environment. First, compliance is an important consideration; some of the courses of treatment include up to 18 tablets a day. Simple regimes may be more effective solely because they contain fewer tablets. Courses of antibiotics that produce minimal side-effects and early symptom relief are also more likely to be completed.[10] Secondly, different strains of the bacterium may be more or less resistant to the antibiotics used, and this may vary from district to district.[11]

Dual therapy

The dual therapies include the use of bismuth plus an imidazole, furazolidone or oxacillin and these give eradication rates of around 70%. The alternative dual regimen, which is more widely known, is the combination of omeprazole, 20 mg bd (or 40 mg od) with amoxycillin 1 g bd (or 500 mg qds), for two weeks. This became popular because it had a low side-effect profile and appeared to be associated with a good compliance record (which may have explained in part some of its success). However, studies comparing its eradication rates have varied enormously from less than 30% to 90%.[12,13] The latter rates have only been produced in Germany, and this may be relevant as perhaps geographical variations may affect the success of different treatments. Overall eradication rates are lower with dual therapies than with triple therapies which at the present time are the most effective way of treating *H. pylori*.

Triple therapy

Eradication rates are consistently high with the use of three drugs in combination. The simplest regimes are the most suitable for patients outside studies (those that are twice daily rather than three or even four times daily), as compliance is probably one of the most important factors dictating the chances of successful eradication.[10] The therapy which has gained wide acceptance in the UK is the combination of an acid-suppressing drug with two antibiotics. This makes a lot of sense as most antibiotics work better when the pH is higher than the acidic environment of the stomach. The usual approach is to combine omeprazole with two of the following: clarithromycin, metronidazole (or tinidazole in place of metronidazole) and amoxycillin. There are some variations in the doses, and in the length of treatment used (one or two weeks), but the common ones used, at the time of writing, are given in Table 30.1.

A proton pump inhibitor (twice daily dose), with two antibiotics is the treatment currently favoured by the authors. The choice of antibiotic depends on local factors such as bacterial resistance and cost. Metronidazole resistance varies widely from district to district around the UK. In some parts of London it is as high as 65% whereas in other London districts it is only 34%.[14] Outside London (within the UK), resistance is probably

Table 30.1 Various standard regimens for *H. pylori*

| THERAPY | ERADICATION RATE (%) | | COST(£)[a] |
	OVERALL	METRONIDAZOLE RESISTANT	
Dual therapy			
2/52 – O 40 mg od, A 500 mg qds	28		38.71
2/52 – O 40 mg bd, A 1 g bd	88		74.16
2/52–O 40 mg od, A 500 mg tds	48		37.89
Triple therapy			
2/52–CBS 120 mg qds, T 500 mg qds, M 400 mg tds.	63	33	18.29
2/52–O 40 mg od, A 500 mg tds, M 400 mg tds	90	76	39.71
2/52 –. R 300 mg od, A 500 mg tds, M 400 mg tds	75	50	17.06
1/52–O 40 mg od, A 500 mg tds, M 400 mg tds	91	88	19.85
1/52–O 40 mg od, C 250 mg tds, M 400 mg tds	86	56	35.49

[a] Cost are calculated from Mims 1996 and the Drug tariff 1996. O, omeprazole; A, amoxycillin; M, metronidazole; C, clarithromycin; R, ranitidine; CBS, colloidal bismuth sub.

not as clinically significant as it was first thought to be, although failure to eradicate after a first course of treatment, which included metronidazole would then usually be followed by a course which did not include this drug. As yet there is no evidence to suggest that *H. pylori* is ever resistant to amoxycillin.

The use of omeprazole, amoxycillin (or metronidazole) and clarithromycin for 7–10 days has recently been shown to give rates of 95–96%[15] and this is likely to replace the proton pump inhibitor, amoxycillin and metronidazole regimen as first-line therapy.

Once the eradication course has been completed it is not clear whether the patient should be continued on acid suppression or not. Before *H. pylori* eradication, of course, clinicians became used to prescribing a healing course of 4–8 weeks of treatment with an H_2 blocker or equivalent. It appears that it is probably not necessary to continue treatment in the uncomplicated ulcer but of course the clinician may be guided by patients' symptoms.[16] In the case of complicated ulcers, patients should continue on treatment to reduce the risk of further complications until eradication has been confirmed (see below).

Confirming eradication

Uncomplicated duodenal ulcer disease

It is open to debate as to whether it is necessary to prove that *H. pylori* has been eradicated in those patients presenting with uncomplicated duodenal ulcers.[17,18] All those patients that have become asymptomatic following dual or triple therapy can be assumed to be cured unless they have recurrent or continued symptoms.

The reinfection rate of *H. pylori* in the adult population is less than 1% per year (some studies have shown that the rate of acquisition is as low as 0.3–0.5% per patient year[19,20]) so for practical purposes, continued or recurrent symptoms represent failure to eradicate the bacterium rather than a second infection. There are a number of methods that can be used for detecting continued infection: rebiopsy at gastroscopy, urea breath tests or serological blood tests. These are discussed in turn. Of course if the original diagnosis was not in doubt then it is unnecessary to repeat the gastroscopy just to retest for *H. pylori*. Urea breath tests or blood tests showing falling titres of *H. pylori* antibodies provide an excellent method for confirming or refuting eradication without having to expose the patient to a second invasive procedure (which is also an unnecessary expense).

Biopsy detection of *H. pylori* If there has been doubt about the original diagnosis (or perhaps if it has been difficult to distinguish between the relative importance of two concurrent pathologies on the patient's symptoms) then it may be appropriate to repeat the endoscopy. This would then provide the clinician with the opportunity to take a second biopsy for *H. pylori* detection. Biopsies could also be taken for culture to obtain antibiotic sensitivities to increase the chances of successful eradication following the next course of treatment. The second gastroscopy and biopsy should be deferred for at least four weeks after the completion of the eradication course to reduce the chances of a falsely negative result in the case of patients with a partially treated, suppressed infection.

In general *H. pylori* is found in highest concentrations in the gastric antrum. Biopsy of this area, 1–2 cm from the pyloric ring, therefore gives the highest chance of diagnosing infection. Biopsy material can either be sent to the histology department or used with the test kits that are now widely available on most endoscopy units. The organism appears curved or 'S' shaped and is seen on simple Giemsa staining. However, biopsy urease tests are quick, cheap and simple to perform in the endoscopy unit and are now well accepted as an accurate determinant of *H. pylori* status; sensitivity rates are reported at 92–95%. The biopsy urease test relies on the urease of *H. pylori* which digests urea to produce carbon dioxide and ammonia, which subsequently reacts with water to produce an alkali. This then turns the colour of the pH indicator in the gel from yellow to red giving a positive result.

$$NH_2\text{-}CO\text{-}NH_2 + H_2O \xrightarrow{\textit{H. pylori} \text{ urease}} CO_2 + 2NH_3$$

$$NH_3 + H_2O \rightarrow NH_4^+ + OH^-$$

One or two biopsy specimens are taken and pushed firmly into the gel. The slide is then resealed and kept warm (30–40°C) for two hours and then at room temperature for up to 24 hours during which time the gel will turn pink (in the case of the standard CLO test kit), if *H. pylori* is present. For practical purposes the gel usually turns pink within a couple of hours though the kit should be kept for up to 24 hours to avoid missing those that take longer to react.

Sensitivity Though biopsy testing for *H. pylori* has a greater than 90% sensitivity, there are two situations where a false negative may occur (particularly in those patients who are being retested for the organism). First, the distribution of the bacterium is uneven. In addition, gastric atrophy, which follows chronic *H. pylori* gastritis or partial gastrectomy, may further reduce the numbers of *H. pylori* present because bacterial growth is slowed up in a hypoacidic environment. For this reason taking two or three biopsies may decrease the false negative rate due to sampling errors. All biopsies should then be sent for histology or put in the same urease test kit. A second reason for a false negative result may be because the patient is on acid suppressants. Proton pump inhibitors have a direct antibacterial effect on the organism without being effective eradicators on their own and this partial suppression may lead to a negative result. Interestingly, these drugs also cause the organism to migrate from the antrum into the body or even fundus of the stomach: biopsy of these areas for histology or urease testing may detect the bacterium when an antral biopsy has been negative.[21] For this reason it is good practice to take specimens from the body or even fundus as well as the antrum (which can then all be placed in the gel or sent to the laboratory) to increase the chances of an accurate result.

Specificity Specificity of the CLO test is around 97% when performed correctly. False positives can occur if the patient has gastric atrophy. In this situation the patient's gastric juices are less acidic and allow other bacteria to colonize the stomach, such as *Proteus* and *Klebsiella* spp. which also produce ureases albeit in smaller quantities. If this is suspected it may be advisable to send specimens for histology.

The bacterium can also be detected by bacteriological culture. This demands the speedy transport of the biopsy in broth or transport medium to the laboratory as, rather strangely, it dies in gastric acid. This method is lengthy and laborious – bacteria take at least 3 days to grow and may not become apparent for 6–7 days – but culture of the organism does have its place in those patients who have failed eradication and are thought to have a resistant organism. Bacteriological testing can then be carried out to assess which antibiotics may be effective.

Urea breath tests The urea breath test is an effective way of detecting the organism without the need for further gastroscopy and is therefore readily acceptable to the patient. It is also based on the activity of the enzyme urease. The patient drinks a liquid urea meal which contains a labelled carbon atom: either a weakly radioactive ^{14}C or a stable non-radioactive isotope ^{13}C. The urea is broken down by the bacterial urease in the stomach to produce ammonia and labelled carbon dioxide which is detected in the patients breath (Figure 30.1).

The cheaper option at the present time is to use ^{14}C. This can be measured at most hospitals using a normal scintillation counter though because it is radioactive it has to be closely

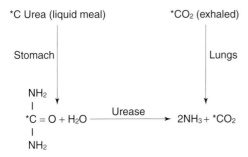

Figure 30.1
The simplified urea breath test.

monitored and is therefore not suitable for pregnant women or young children. ^{13}C is safe for general use but its measurement requires a mass spectrometer which is usually only available in specialist centres, so that the sample may have to be sent away for analysis.

There are currently a number of kits on the market which all differ slightly in their protocol but all have a sensitivity and specificity of over 97% and 95%, respectively, it is an extremely accurate method for detecting *H. pylori*.

Serological tests Antibodies to *H. pylori* circulate in the serum and can be detected, in most cases, for up to a minimum of six months after eradication of the organism. During this time the titres will usually fall to half their original level so that for practical purposes, at six months, the antibodies will be either undetectable or present in low concentrations, though in some patients antibodies may persist for longer. For this reason these tests are less useful in confirming eradication because they cannot be performed for at least this period after treatment. Again there are many different kits available commercially; most have sensitivities and specificities of over 80%, though their accuracy depends very much on the population used to validate the assay. One practical point to bear in mind is that there appears to be an increased prevalence of false negative serology in the elderly population. This might be because the elderly generally produce less antibodies or perhaps because they have an increased risk of atrophic gastritis which in turn might decrease the exposure of the immune system to the antigens of *H. pylori*.

Current controversies in management

Many clinicians are now happy to make the diagnosis of a duodenal ulcer on the grounds of the history alone in a patient who is young, i.e. under the age of 45 years. The chance of such a patient who has a clear history which does not contain any sinister features, having an underlying malignancy is remote. It is the authors' practice to perform serological testing to detect the presence of *H. pylori*, and then to treat empirically with eradication therapy. This means that some patients who would have had normal endoscopies but who are *H. pylori* positive will be given treatment: in a small number of these patients, the treatment will produce side-effects. There is also the theoretical risk that this policy will increase the chances of drug resistance. However, for the busy district

general hospital, this rationale eases the burden on the endoscopy unit, and may of course protect the patient from future gastric carcinoma even if it does not relieve symptoms in the short term.[22] If the original pathology was wrongly attributed, the patient is likely to represent to the general practitioner or hospital doctor, especially if the situation is explained when treatment is offered. A flow chart summarizing the management of uncomplicated duodenal ulcer is given in Figure 30.2.

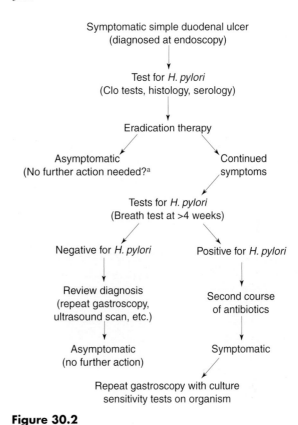

Figure 30.2
Management of uncomplicated duodenal ulcer disease. [a] No further action at this stage is controversial (see text).

Complicated duodenal ulcer disease

By contrast it would also seem logical that in those patients who had experienced complications from their duodenal disease (such as bleeding or outflow obstruction), formal attempts should be made to ensure that eradication has been successful before maintenance drugs such as proton pump inhibitors are discontinued. In fact, studies show that in those patients presenting with bleeding duodenal ulcers successful eradication has been associated with vastly decreased rebleeding rates compared with those in whom *H. pylori* was not eradicated.[23,24] It remains to be seen whether similar successes can be obtained with ulcers complicated by perforation though one study[25] suggests that this is not the case and that ulcers that perforate may represent a different disease, e.g. ulcers caused by NSAIDs.

A flow chart summarizing the management of complicated duodenal ulcer is given in Figure 30.3.

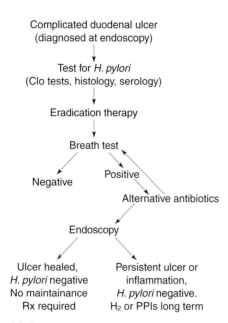

Complicated duodenal ulcer
(diagnosed at endoscopy)

↓

Test for *H. pylori*
(Clo tests, histology, serology)

↓

Eradication therapy

↓

Breath test

Negative ← → Positive

Positive → Alternative antibiotics

↓

Endoscopy

Ulcer healed, *H. pylori* negative No maintainance Rx required

Persistent ulcer or inflammation, *H. pylori* negative. H₂ or PPIs long term

Figure 30.3
Management of complicated duodenal ulcer disease.

Past history of ulcer disease

Because peptic ulcer disease is so common, clinicians often see patients who have a past history of peptic ulcer disease though they may be currently asymptomatic. In these patients it is simple to send blood for serology; if patients are found to be positive for *H. pylori* it would seem sensible to prescribe eradication therapy, especially in those patients who have a past history of ulcer-related complications.

Gastric ulcer disease

Although *H. pylori* is probably responsible for a smaller proportion of gastric ulcers than duodenal ulcers it is important that the infection be checked for and treated in all patients found to have a gastric ulcer. *H. pylori* is found in 58–94% of such patients[26,27] and Graham et al.[28] reported 2-year relapse rates of 13% after eradication of the organism compared with 74% in patients who had been given acid supression alone. One practical problem in patients with gastric ulcers and *H. pylori* is that these patients tend to have extensive gastric atrophy increasing the chances of a false negative urease biopsy test. For this reason multiple specimens should be taken. Other methods for detecting the organism such as serology or breath tests may be necessary before it is assumed that the patient does not have the infection. Similarly as with patients with duodenal ulcer, it is of benefit to use the eradication therapy at the start of the treatment for a gastric ulcer as one study has shown that healing rates are higher when the bacterium has been eliminated.[29] Also, as in duodenal ulcer patients, the risk of rebleeding from a gastric ulcer is reduced by eradication.[23]

HELICOBACTER PYLORI-NEGATIVE ULCER DISEASE

What of patients who do not appear to have this notable organism present? A small number of patients (less than 5%)

have been shown to have *H. pylori*-negative duodenal ulcer disease. However, before patients are treated in the more traditional manner with the various drugs which will be discussed at length below, two possibilities must be considered. First, was the test for *H. pylori* falsely negative? Sampling errors as mentioned earlier may have occurred, perhaps insufficient biopsy material was selected. Is the patient on acid suppressants, and if so were biopsies taken from high in the stomach. In fact ideally, acid suppressants particularly proton pump inhibitors should be stopped for not less than two weeks before the endoscopy because of the chances of the infection being suppressed. Of course this has advantages in other ways: the pathology is more likely to be revealed with the patient off maintenance treatment. Any single antibiotic can decrease the numbers of bacteria present; is the patient on a course of antibacterials for pathology unrelated to the dyspepsia? For this reason all antibiotics should be stopped for at least one month before testing for *H. pylori*. If there is doubt about these possibilities after a patient has been shown to have a *H. pylori*-negative duodenal ulcer then it would be worth considering serological blood testing to provide further evidence about the patient's *H. pylori* status.

The second possibility is whether the ulceration has been caused by NSAIDs or underlying pathology, namely a Zollinger–Ellison syndrome or Crohn's disease. A clear history for NSAIDs or aspirin (prescribed or self-medication) must be sought and a gastrin level performed in cases when particularly extensive disease has been found; gastrin levels should be measured when the patient is not taking proton pump inhibitors. The clinician should check for Zollinger–Ellison syndrome where there is history of diarrhoea accompanying the dyspepsia. Crohn's disease may be diagnosed histologically, though this may require a second gastroscopy.

If this is not the case and the patient has benign *H. pylori*-negative ulcer disease then the management continues with the drugs that are described in turn below.

Acid suppression

Most agents in peptic ulcer disease are aimed at reducing acid secretion, the percentage and duration of acid supression is directly related to healing of peptic ulcers. Conventional doses of H₂ receptor antagonists achieve acid supression for 9–12 hours compared to 18 hours for conventional doses of proton pump inhibitors (Figure 30.4). However, without eradication of associated underlying *H. pylori* relapse is almost inevitable.

There are several classes of acid supressing drugs.

Histamine 2 receptor antagonists Basal and lateral membranes of parietal cells have three main receptors; acetylcholine, histamine and gastrin. There may also be an opiate receptor because nalmetine (an opiate receptor antagonist) has also been shown to inhibit acid secretion too.[30] H₂ receptor antagonists are competitive antagonists at the receptor site.

Proton pump inhibitors Hydrogen, potassium-ATPase, the proton pump, is the final common pathway for secretion of acid. The inhibiton of the pump therefore produces a more reliable

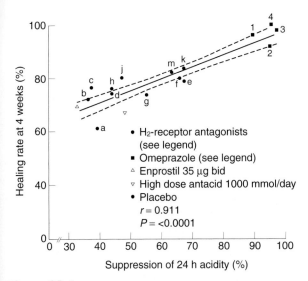

Figure 30.4
Regression line and 95% confidence limits for the relationship
between suppression of 24 h intragastric acidity and
proportion of duodenal ulcers healed after 4 weeks for a
variety of antisecretory drugs. H_2 receptor antagonist dosage
regimens: a, cimetidine 200 mg qid; b, cimetidine 400 mg
bid; c, oxmetidine 400 mg bid; d, cimetidine 300 mg qid;
e, ranitidine 150 mg bid; f, cimetidine 600 mg bid;
g, cimetidine 200 mg tid + 400 mg nocte; h, ranitidine
150 mg nocte; j, cimetidine 800 mg nocte; k, ranitidine
300 mg nocte; m, famotidine 40 mg nocte. Omeprazole
dosage regimens: 1, 20 mg once daily; 2, 30 mg once daily;
3, 40 mg once daily; 4, 60 mg once daily.

and profound inhibition of acid secretion than blockade of any
of the surface receptors.

H_2 receptor antagonists

These were a major breakthrough in the treatment of peptic
ulcer disease in the 1970s. Cimetidine was the first to be introduced in 1977 and had healing rates for duodenal ulcers
approaching 95% after 8 weeks' treatment. Cimetidine inhibits
gastric acid secretion in response to histamine, pentagastrin,
vagal stimulation and food as well as inhibiting nocturnal acid
secretion. It is well absorbed from the small intestine, reaches
peak levels after 1–2 h and has a half-life of 2 h. It is a competitive inhibitor at the parietal cell and so only achieves partial suppression of acid when food is eaten.

A single night-time dose of 800 mg of cimetidine gives identical healing rates as 400 mg twice daily and will probably
increase patient compliance.[31,32] Healing rates also progressively
increase with duration of treatment. Thus healing rates at 2
weeks with 300 mg, qid are 39.8%, at 4 weeks with 400 mg bd
are 72.1%, at 6 weeks at 400 mg bd are 79.3% and at 8 weeks
on 400 mg, bd are 92.9% (Table 30.2).[33]

Once healing has been achieved there will be a minority of
patients who will need treatment to prevent symptoms or complications and to this end maintenance treatment was developed which usually consisted of nocturnal therapy with half
the healing dose (that is 400 mg nocte of cimetidine).
Fortunately relapse on maintenance treatment seems associated

Table 30.2 Healing rates for duodenal ulcers after 2,
4, 6 and 8 weeks of treatment with H_2 receptor antagonists

DRUG	DOSE	NO. WEEKS	HEALING RATE (%)
Cimetidine	300 mg qid	2	39.8
Cimetidine	400 mg bd	4	72.1
Cimetidine	400 mg bd	6	79.3
Cimetidine	400 mg bd	8	92.9
Ranitidine	150 mg bd	2	59.5
Ranitidine	150 mg bd	4	79.0
Ranitidine	150 mg bd	6	85.9
Ranitidine	150 mg bd	8	94.0

Adapted from Chiverton et al.[34]

with a low complication rate so that it is safe to take treatment
even if the ulcer does recur.[35]

Ranitidine is a more potent H_2 receptor antagonist launched
some 5 years after cimetidine and has marginally better healing
rates than cimetidine. The healing rates again increase as duration of therapy increases; at 2 weeks on 150 mg bd 59.5% of
ulcers are healed, at 4 weeks 72.1% are healed, at 6 weeks
85.9% are healed and at 8 weeks 94.0% are healed (Table
30.2).[33]

Maintenance treatment with 150 mg can be given after the
evening meal and will supress acid response to eating well into
the night.[36,37] Healing rates for gastric ulcers with H_2 receptor
antagonists follow a similar pattern but in general take slightly
longer to heal (see Table 30.3).[38]

Famotidine and nizatidine are two other less commonly used
H_2 receptor antagonists. The half-life of famotidine is slightly
longer than the other H_2 receptor antagonists and its duration of
action is 30% longer. However, both drugs have similar efficacy
to ranitidine and cimetidine with a similar side-effect profile
although famotidine is weakly negatively inotropic.

The side-effect profile of H_2 receptor antagonists is very
good, diarrhoea, headache and dizziness being the most frequently reported adverse effects. Gynaecomastia and impotence are rarely reported side-effects of therapy secondary to
antiandrogen effects. However, ranitidine, unlike cimetidine,
does not significantly interfere with the cytochrome $P450$ system which leads to a slightly better side-effect profile, particularly in the elderly.

Table 30.3 Healing rates for gastric ulcers at 4, 6, 8
and 12 weeks of treatment by H_2 receptor antagonists

DRUG	DOSE	NO. WEEKS	HEALING RATE (%)
Cimetidine	400 mg bd	4	69.7
Cimetidine	400 mg bd	6	73.4
Cimetidine	400 mg bd	10	88.5
Cimetidine	400 mg bd	12	93.9
Ranitidine	150 mg bd	4	62.9
Ranitidine	150 mg bd	6	85.9
Ranitidine	150 mg bd	8	90.8
Ranitidine	150 mg bd	12	92.6

Adapted from Freston and Biancho Porro.[39]

Anticholinergic drugs

These drugs were developed to block the muscarinic effects of acetylcholine and thereby reduce gastric acid secretion. However, the side-effect profile (blurred vision, dry mouth and constipation) was too great even with the more selective M_1 antimuscarinic drugs (pirenzepine). Thus widespread use has never occurred and will not with the advent of proton pump inhibitors.

Prostaglandin analogues

Prostaglandins have several effects on the gastrointestinal tract:

1. Inhibition of gastric acid secretion via blockade of cAMP and possibly also by a neural mechanism. They also stimulate HCO_3 ion secretion by gastric and duodenal mucosa;

2. Cytoprotection of gastric mucosa;

3. Stimulation of smooth muscle.

Although they have theoretical advantages they are not widely used in clinical practice because healing rates with high doses are not as effective as H_2 receptor antagonists. Diarrhoea is a well recorded side-effect and there are concerns over long-term use regarding the risk of gastric mucosal hyperplasia.[40] Its main use in clinical practice appears to be as prophylaxis in patients on NSAIDs, indeed two studies from the USA have reported a significantly reduced incidence of gastric ulcers in patients taking NSAIDs.[40,42]

Substituted benzimidazoles (proton pump inhibitors)

Proton pump inhibitors act by blocking H^+,K^+-ATPase, the final common pathway for gastric acid secretion.[43] It is well absorbed from the small intestine, is weakly basic and has a half-life of 40 min but despite this it inhibits acid secretion for longer with a mean decrease in intragastric acidity of around 80%.[44] Proton pump inhibitors decrease 24 h acid secretion by more than 90% compared to 50–80% with recommended doses of H_2 receptor antagonists.

Omeprazole was the first proton pump inhibitor to be licensed for the treatment of peptic ulcer disease. It has been shown to be superior to H_2 receptor antagonists in both the healing of ulcers and in symptom relief. The 90% healing rate at 4 weeks with omeprazole is similar to that achieved at 8 weeks with standard doses of H_2 receptor antagonists. It is also more effective than ranitidine 150 mg bd at healing gastric ulcers despite concurrent NSAID therapy.[45,46] Ulcer relapse rates are similar for both H_2 receptor antagonists and proton pump inhibitors. Omeprazole is well tolerated and has a similar side-effect profile to H_2 receptor antagonists and a small effect on the cytochrome $P450$ enzymes which may influence the bioavailability of warfarin, phenytoin, diazepam and prednisolone.[47]

Lansoprazole was the second proton pump inhibitor to be marketed and has a similar mode of action to omeprazole but is 25% more potent in humans.[48] It heals approximately 90% of duodenal ulcers at 4 weeks and 30 mg of lansoprazole may be superior to 20 mg of omeprazole in healing both duodenal and gastric ulcers.[49] It also has less effect on cytochrome $P450$ enzymes but otherwise its tolerance is similar to omeprazole.

Pantoprazole, which has recently been launched, is the newest proton pump inhibitor and current data suggest that it has similar efficacy to both omeprazole and lansoprazole.

The same rules for maintenance treatment did apply to proton pump inhibitors but since the advent of *H. pylori* the approach has somewhat changed and is discussed in more detail below. There are still concerns about the long-term use of proton pump inhibitors but others perceive their safety profile as encouraging.[50,51] Proton pump inhibitors cause profound hypochlorhydria in most patients with a consequently raised serum gastrin. In rats cases of gastric enterochromaffin-like cell carcinoids have been reported which are thought to be secondary to the trophic effects of gastrin. However, the serum gastrin levels in patients on 20 mg of omeprazole are considerably lower than in patients with pernicious anaemia.[52] A recent study by Kuipers et al.[53] however, did show that atrophic gastritis develops in patients who are *H. pylori* positive and on long-term proton pump inhibitors thus emphasizing the need to eradicate the infection in those needing maintenance treatment.

Antacids

These decrease gastric acidity thereby increasing gastric and duodenal pH. Pepsin activity is almost abolished at a pH equal to or greater than 4.0. The effects of antacids are dependent on gastric emptying and are longest lived 1–3 hours after a meal compared to on an empty stomach. Suspensions are more effective than tablet preparations. They can be divided as follows.

1. Alginate antacids – a raft is formed by the action of acid on bicarbonate mixed with alginate and thus neutralizing it. This is meant to be more effective in gastro-oesophageal reflux but less so in duodenal ulcer disease.

2. Neutralizing antacids – these contain alkaline salts of magnesium and/or aluminium which directly neutralize acid. However, there may also be an effect on prostaglandin production in the mucosa leading to improved mucosal defence.

Other compounds

Sucralfate

This is an aluminium salt of sucrose octosulphate. It is not absorbed and is thought to act by a mucosal protective effect by stimulating the local production of prostaglandins.[54] It may also act by becoming a viscous, gel-like substance which improves the barrier against acid and pepsin attack at the base of an ulcer, binding for up to 6 h after ingestion.[54] There are few data on long-term use of this compound but some concern has been raised regarding the absorption of aluminium and Alzheimer's disease.

Colloidal bismuth

There are several preparations available, the most commonly used being colloidal bismuth subcitrate. This has several modes of action including chelation of protein in the ulcer base, stimulation of local prostaglandin production and an anti-*H. pylori* effect. However, the role of this preparation in eradication regimes was surpassed by proton pump inhibitors because of the unpleasant nature of the compound although there has been interest in a bismuth ranitidine preparation.

General measures in the treatment of acute peptic ulcer disease

Factors which adversely effect healing of ulcers include the following.

1. Smoking – smoking increases the incidence of duodenal ulceration and reduces the healing rate for active treatment. A meta-analysis concluded that there is a smaller percentage of duodenal ulcers successfully healed in smokers.[55]

2. NSAIDs – ingestion of aspirin and related compounds causes direct damage to the gastric mucosa and will impair healing with standard doses of antacids.

3. Alcohol – alcohol is both a stimulus to acid secretion and a gastric irritant. However, the are too many compounding factors in most studies in view of the strong association of smoking with alcohol to draw any strong conclusions.

4. Diet has little role in the treatment of peptic ulcer disease. Most physicians urge a normal healthy high fibre diet.

About 95% of duodenal and 80% of gastric ulcers are associated with *H. pylori* and treatment should be directed at eradicating the organism which will allow healing to occur. Once this has been established few patients will require maintenance treatment. For patients who have complicated ulcers, that is bleeding, stenosis or perforation, it is imperative to establish that eradication is complete as they too may not need maintenance treatment although this is still disputed by some.

MAINTENANCE TREATMENT IN PEPTIC ULCER DISEASE

Patients who relapse or who have complicated peptic ulcer disease may need maintenance treatment. Patients with complicated disease should have their *H. pylori* status re-checked to ascertain eradication either by means of a breath test or repeat biopsy. Once eradication has been established this substantially reduces the risk of further complications and re-infection rates are less than 1% per year. Maintenance treatment may be necessary for patients who are negative for the organism or who relapse after eradication and this should be with the lowest dose of either a H_2 receptor antagonist or proton pump inhibitor that keeps symptoms and complications under control. Less than 10% of duodenal ulcers fail to heal after standard treatment. Factors which influence this include smoking, NSAIDs and severe comorbid disease (cardiopulmonary disease).

There are a number of studies confirming that long-term maintenance with cimetidine is safe with few adverse effects, with events initially reported by as many as 8% in the first year reducing to 1% after 4 years.[56] This is also true of ranitidine.[35]

NSAID-associated gastric ulcers will heal satisfactorily with proton pump inhibitors, H_2 receptor antagonists or misoprostol if the NSAID is stopped. If it must be continued then a higher dose of proton pump inhibitor is usually required. One study of 40 mg of omeprazole showed 81% and 95% of gastric ulcers were healed at 4 and 8 weeks, respectively compared to 52% and 82% with 20 mg of omeprazole at 4 and 8 weeks, respectively.[45] There is now increasing evidence that misoprostol can be used to prevent both duodenal and gastric ulcers in high risk patients on NSAIDs.[44]

MEDICAL OR SURGICAL TREATMENT

Long-term healing with eradication of *H. pylori* has radically reduced the need for surgery. Gastric acid secretion can now be controlled successfully in many patients with peptic ulcer disease and thus the decision when or whether to refer for surgery has become infrequent and must be approached with great care. Those patients who develop complicated disease are straightforward as are the patients who fail to respond to medical treatment. Young patients who do not wish to take lifelong treatment should probably be referred for surgery or encouraged to comply with treatment as complications maybe life-threatening.

The only indications for surgery now are:

1. *H. pylori*-positive persistent duodenal ulcer and failed eradication despite repeated courses with assessment of *H. pylori* sensitivities;

2. *H. pylori*-negative persistent duodenal ulcer with poor control of symptoms with proton pump inhibitors and H_2 receptor antagonists;

3. Complicated NSAID-associated ulcer where the NSAID cannot be stopped;

4. *H. pylori*-negative complicated duodenal ulcer. This may have been negative from the start or the complication may have occurred despite successful eradication of *H. pylori*.

REFERENCES

1. Forman D, Newwell DG, Fullerton F et al. Association between infection with *Helicobacter pylori* and risk of gastric cancer: evidence from a prospective investigation. *BMJ* 1991; **302:** 1302–1305.
2. Parsonnet J, Friedman GD, Vandersteen DP et al. *Helicobacter pylori* infection and the risk of gastric carcinoma. *N Engl J Med* 1991; **325:** 1127–1131.
3. Nomura A, Stemmermann, GN, Chyou PH et al. *Helicobacter pylori* infection and gastric carcinoma among the Japanese Americans in Hawaii. *N Engl J Med* 1991; **325:** 1132–1136.
4. Patel P, Mendell MA, Carrington D et al. Association of *Helicobacter pylori* and *Chlamydia* pneumonia infection with coronary heart disease and cardiovascular risk factors. *BMJ* 1995; **311:** 711–714.
5. Rauws EA & Tytgat GN. Cure of duodenal ulcer associated with eradication of *Helicobacter pylori*. *Lancet* 1990; **335:** 1233–1235.
6. El-Omar E, Penman I, Doman CA, Ardill JES & McColl KEL. Eradicating *Helicobacter pylori* infection lowers gastrin mediated acid secretion by two thirds in patients with duodenal ulcer. *Gut* 1993; **34:** 1060–1065.
7. Tytgat GNJ. Review article. Treatments that impact favourably upon the eradication of *H. pylori* and ulcer recurrence. *Aliment Pharmacol Ther* 1994; **8:** 359–368.
8. Marshall BJ, Goodwin CS, Warren JR et al. Prospective double blind trial of duodenal relapse after eradication of *Campylobacter pylori*. *Lancet* 1988; **ii:** 1437–1442.

9. Labenz J, Leverkus F & Borsh G. Omeprazole plus amoxycillin for the cure of *Helicobacter pylori* infection: factors affecting treatment success. *Scand Gastroenterol* 1994; **29:** 1070–1075.

10. Graham DY, Lew GM, Malaty HM et al. Factors influencing the eradication of *Helicobacter pylori* with triple therapy. *Gastroenterology* 1992; **102:** 493–496.

11. Owen RJ, Bell GD, Desai M et al. Biotype and molecular fingerprints of metronidazole resistant strains of *Helicobacter pylori* from antral gastric mucosa. *J Med Microbiol* 1993; **38:** 6–12.

12. Logan RPH, Rubio MA & Gummett PA. Omeprazole and amoxycillin suspension for *Helicobacter pylori* (abstract). *Irish J Med Sci* 1992; **161**(suppl): 16.

13. Labenz J, Stolte M, Domain C et al. Omeprazole or clarithromycin for eradication of Hp in DU disease(abstract). *Acta Gastroenterol Belg* 1993; **56**(suppl 131): 139.

14. Logan RP, Gummett PA, Misiewicz JJ et al. One week's anti *Helicobacter pylori* treatment for duodenal ulcer. *Gut* 1994; **35:** 15–18.

15. Lerang F, Moum B, Haug JB et al. *Gastroenterology* 1996; **110:** A173.

16. Hosking SW, Ling TK, Yung MY et al. Randomised controlled trial of short term treatment to eradicate *Helicobacter pylori* in patients with duodenal ulcer. *BMJ* 1992; **305:** 502–504.

17. Reilly TG & Walt RP. Testing to check success of treatment to eradicate *Helicobacter pylori*. Routine testing is necessary. *BMJ* 1996; **312:** 1362.

18. Bodger K & Heatley RV. Testing to check the success of treatment to eradicate *H. pylori*. Patients' well being should not be risked for marginal cost savings. *BMJ* 1996; **312:** 1361–1362.

19. Parsonnet J, Blaser MJ, Perz GI et al. Symptoms and risk factors of *Helicobacter pylori* infection in a cohort of epidemiologists. *Gastroenterology* 1992; **102:** 41–46.

20. Kuipers EJ, Pena AS, Van Kemp G et al. Seroconversion for *Helicobacter pylori*. Lancet 1993; **342:** 328–331.

21. Logan RPH, Walker MM, Misiewicz JJ et al. Changes in the intragastric distribution of *Helicobacter pylori* during treatment with omeprazole. *Gut* 1995; **36:** 12–16.

22. Briggs A, Schulper MJ, Logan RPH, Aldous J, Ramsay ME & Baron JH. Cost effectiveness for eradication of *Helicobacter pylori* in the management of dyspeptic patients under 45 years of age. *BMJ* 1996; **312:** 1321–1325.

23. Labenz J & Borsch G. Role of *Helicobacter pylori* eradication in the prevention of peptic ulcer bleeding relapse. *Digestion* 1994; **55:** 19–23.

24. Graham DY, Hepps KS, Ramirez FC et al. Treatment of *Helicobacter pylori* reduces the rate of rebleeding in peptic ulcer disease. *Scand J Gastroenterol* 1993; **28:** 939–942.

25. Reinbach DH, Cruickshank G & McColl KE. Acute perforated duodenal ulcer is not associated with *Helicobacter pylori* infection. *Gut* 1993; **34:** 1344–1347.

26. Marshall BJ & Warren JR. Unidentified curved bacilli in the stomach of patients with gastritis and peptic ulceration. *Lancet* 1984; **i:** 1311–1315.

27. Lambert JR & Lin SK. Prevalence/disease correlates of *H. pylori*. In Hunt RH & Tytgat GNJ (eds) *Helicobacter pylori: Basic Mechanisms to Clinical Care*. Dordrecht: Kluwer, 1994: 95–112.

28. Graham DY, Lew GM, Klein PD et al. Effect of treatment of *Helicobacter pylori* infection on the long term recurrence of gastric or duodenal ulcer. A randomised, controlled study. *Ann Intern Med* 1992; **116:** 705–708.

29. Labenz J & Borsch G. Evidence for the essential role of *Helicobacter pylori* in gastric ulcer disease. *Gut* 1994; **35:** 19–22.

30. Feldman M, Moore L & Walsh JH. Effect of oral nalmetene, an opiate receptor antagonist, on mean stimulation of gastric acid secretion and serum gastrin concentration in man. *Regul Pept* 1985; **11:** 245–249.

31. Thomas JM & Misiewicz G. Histamine H_2 receptor antagonists in the short and longterm treatment of duodenal ulcers. *Clin Gastroenterol* 1984; **13:** 50–54.

32. Christenson E, Juhl E & Tygstrup N. Treatment of duodenal ulcers. Randomised clinical trial of a decade, (1964–74). *Gastroenterology* 1977; **73:** 1170–1175.

33. Pounder RE, Williams JG, Hunt RH, Vincent SH, Milton-Thompson GJ & Misiewicz JJ. The effects of oral cimetidine on food stimulated gastric acid secretion and 24 hour intragastric acidity. In Burland WL & Simkins MA (eds) *Cimetidine: Proceedings of the Second International Symposium on Histamine H_2 Receptor Antagonists*, Amsterdam: Excerpta Medica, 1977.

34. Chiverton SG & Hunt RH. Medical regimes in short and longterm ulcer management. *Ballière's Clin Gastroenterol* 1988; **2:** 655–676.

35. Boyd EJS, Wilson JA & Wormsley KG. Safety of maintenance treatment of duodenal ulcer with ranitidine. *Scand J Gastroenterol* 1984; **19:** 394–400.

36. Merki H, Witzel L, Harre K, Scheurle E & Neumann J. Single dose treatment with H_2 receptor antagonists: is bedtime administration too late. *Gut* 1987; **27:** 451–454.

37. Ireland A, Colin-Jones DG, Gear P & Golding PL. Ranitidine 150 mg twice daily versus 300 mg nightly in the treatment of duodenal ulcers. *Lancet* 1984; **ii:** 274–276.

38. Freston JW. Overview of medical therapy of peptic ulcer disease. *Gastroenterol Clin North Am* 1990; 121–140.

39. Freston JW & Biancho Porro G. Medical treatment of acute peptic ulcer disease. In *Proton Pump Inhibitors and Acid Related Disorders*, Osaka: Adis International, 1994: 101–117.

40. Herting RL & Nissen CH. Overview of misoprostol clinical effects. *Dig Dis Sci* 1986; **31:** 54–59.

41. Graham DY, White RH & Moreland LW. Duodenal and gastric ulcer prevention with misoprostol in arthritis patients taking NSAIDs. *Ann Intern Med* 1993; **119:** 257–262.

42. Jaszewski R, Graham DY, Strommat SC et al. Treatment of NSAID induced gastric ulcers with misprostol. A double blind multi centred study. *Dig Dis Sci* 1992; **37:** 1820–1824.

43. Walan A. Omeprazole. *Ballieres Clin Gastroenterol* 1988; **2:** 629–33.

44. Naesdal J, Bodeman G & Walan A. Effect of omeprazole: a substituted benzimidazole, on 24 hour intragastric acidity in patients with peptic ulcer disease. *Scand J Gastroenterol* 1984; **19:** 916–919.

45. Walan A, Bader JP, Classen M et al. Effect of omeprazole and ranitidine on ulcer healing and relapse rates in patients with benign gastric ulcers. *N Engl J Med* 1989; **320:** 69–77.

46. Bardhan KD, Bianchi Porro G, Bose K et al. A comparison of two different doses of ompeprazole versus ranitidine in the treatment of duodenal ulcers. *J Clin Gastroenterol* 1986; **8:** 40–44.

47. Rodriguez D & Freston JW. The effect of proton pump inhibitors on cytochrome P450 metabolism. In Giuli, Tytgat G et al. (eds) *The Oesophageal Mucosa*, Amsterdam: Elsever, in press.

48. Tomlan KG, Sanders SW, Buchi KR et al. Gastric pH levels after 15 mg and 30 mg of lansoprasole and 20 mg of omeprazole. *Gastroenterology* 1994; **106:** A107.

49. Petite JP, Slama J-L, Lich H et al. Comparison du lansoprsole (30 mg) et de l'omeprazole (20 mg) dans le traitment de l'ulcere duodenal. *Gastroenterol Clin Biol* 1993; **17:** 334–340.

50. Colin-Jones DG. Safety of lansoprasole. *Alimen Pharmacol Ther* 1993; **7**(suppl): 56–60.

51. Brunner G, Creutzfeldt W, Harle U et al. Efficacy and safety of longterm treatment with omeprazole in patients with acid related disease resistant to ranitidine. *Scand J Gastroenterol* 1989; **3**(suppl): 72–76.

52. Carlsson E, Larsson H, Mattsson H et al. Pharmacology and toxicology of omeprazole – with special reference to effect on gastric mucosa. *Scand J Gastroenterol* 1986; **21**(Suppl 118): 31–35.

53. Kuipers EJ, Lundell L, Klinkenberg-Knol EC et al. Atrophic gastritis and *Helicobacter pylori* infection in patients with reflux oesophagitis treated with omeprazole or fundoplication. *N Engl J Med* 1996; **334:** 1018–1022.

54. Lam SK, Lau WY, Lai CL et al. Efficacy of sucralfate in corpus, pre-pyloric and duodenal ulcer associated gastric ulcers. A double blind, placebo controlled study. *Am J Med* 1985; **79**(suppl): 24–31.

55. Sontag S, Graham DY, Belsito A et al. Cimetidine, cigarette smoking and recurrence of duodenal ulcers. *N Engl J Med* 1984; **311:** 689–693.

56. Bardhan KD, Hunter JO, Miller JP et al. Antacid maintenance therapy in the prevention of duodenal ulcer relapse. *Gut* 1988; **29:** 1748–1754.

31

NON-STEROIDAL ANTI-INFLAMMATORY DRUGS AND GASTRODUODENAL INJURY

S Holt
TV Taylor

Non-steroidal anti-inflammatory drugs (NSAIDs) lead all other medications in terms of their reported prevalence of serious side-effects.[1,2] Their most common side-effect is injury to the gastric or duodenal mucosa with resulting inflammation and/or peptic ulceration. In addition, it has been increasingly recognized that NSAIDs are a common cause of renal and hepatic toxicity, especially in the elderly.[3,4] Many studies have pointed to a recent increase in the number of prescriptions for NSAIDs and there has been an expontential rise in over-the-counter use of these drugs.

About 1–2% of the population of the USA and Great Britain may be daily NSAID users (Figure 31.1). Epidemiological investigations have repeatedly drawn attention to the association of NSAID use and the presentation of life-threatening complications of peptic ulcer. More recently, NSAID use has been shown to be associated with lower gastrointestinal bleeding.[5] Endoscopic abnormalities are common in patients receiving NSAIDs, often manifested by clinically silent prepyloric erosions, mucosal haemorrhages and peptic ulceration.[5]

Much interest has focused on the pattern of use of NSAIDs and evidence has accumulated that they may sometimes be inappropriately prescribed, especially where analgesia could be obtained without the need for an ulcerogenic medication. Patients appeared to be poorly educated about the potential complications of NSAIDs, and the circumstances are compounded by the fact that NSAID-associated complicated peptic disease may often present in an unheralded manner.

EPIDEMIOLOGY

Many attempts have been made to look at the relative risk properties of certain NSAIDs for the causation of gastroduo-

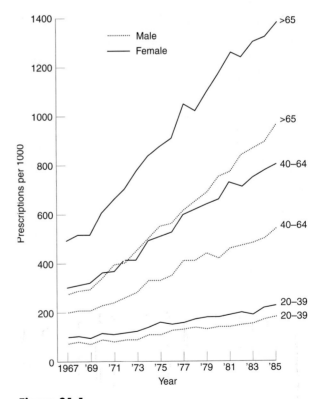

Figure 31.1
Age-specific prescription rates for men and women receiving NSAIDs (excludes preparations sold 'over the counter').
(Source: Medical Data Index (Intercontinental Medical Statistics Ltd).

denal injury.[5] Overall, there is little credible evidence to suggest that one NSAID is less ulcerogenic than another, although newer substituted or modified NSAID molecules have been developed which show some promise of inducing less gastrointestinal mucosal damage (Table 31.1). Meta-analysis has been used to attempt to stratify the risk of individual drugs for the causation of serious gastrointestinal complications but no specific NSAID is risk free. Claims that one NSAID is safer than another based on studies of microbleeding from the gastrointestinal tract are to be viewed with suspicion because there is little evidence of a correlation of these measures with ulcero-genesis. For the purposes of this discussion, salicylate and related compounds are considered to be examples of NSAIDs because these drugs have similar metabolic actions and side-effects to classic NSAIDs. There is some evidence that side-effects from the following commonly used NSAIDs occur with an increasing degree of frequency (in the order that they are listed): ibuprofen, diflunisal, fenoprofen, naproxen, sulindac and tolmetin.[1,2]

Case–control endoscopic studies have shown that up to three-quarters of patients taking NSAIDs can have significant endoscopic lesions, including but not limited to gastric erythema, erosions and varying degrees of peptic ulcerations.[6,7] Formerly, benign gastric ulcer disease was encountered on the lesser curvature of the stomach but such ulceration at this location has been recognized as a 'disappearing disease'. Benign gastric ulceration is now seen infrequently and, if present, it

---

Table 31.1 Classification of NSAIDs.

Propionic acids
Fenoprofen (fenoprofen, Nalfon)
Flurbiprofen (Ansaid)
Ibuprofen (ibuprofen, Motrin, Ibu-Tab, Rufen, Aches-N-Pain, Advil, Genpril, Haltran, Ibuprin, Medipren, Midol 200, Motrin I.B., Nuprin, Pamprin-IB, Trendar)
Ketoprofen (Orudis)
Naproxen (Naprosyn)
Naproxen sodium (Anaprox, Anaprox DS)

Oxicams
Piroxicam (Feldene)

Phenylacetic Acids
Diclofenac sodium (Voltaren)

Salicylates
Aspirin
Choline magnesium trisalicylate (Trilisate)
Diflunisal (Dolobid)
Salsalate (Salflex, Salsitab, Arthra-G, Mono-Gesic, Disalcid)

Indoles
Indomethacin (indomethacin, Indameth, Indocin, Indo-Lemmon, Indomethacin SR)
Sulindac (Clinoril)
Tolmetin sodium (Tolectin, Tolectin DS, Tolectin 600)

Fenamates
Meclofenamate (meclofenamate, Meclodium, Meclomen)
Mefenamic acid (Ponstel)

Naphthylalkanones
Nabumetone (Relafan)

Modified from *Drug Facts and Comparisons*, 44th edn. St Louis: Lippincott, 1990: 1016.

---

tends to be associated with lower socioeconomic status, often in the presence of substance abuse. In contrast, superficial or chronic gastric ulceration is being found increasingly in the antrum of the stomach, especially in elderly subjects receiving NSAIDs.[1]

It is important to recognize that gastroduodenal injury occurs in the patient taking NSAIDs often in the absence of symptoms and many studies have demonstrated a mismatch between endoscopic findings and the presence of upper gastrointestinal complaints.[1] Endoscopic studies in asymptomatic patients receiving NSAIDs have revealed duodenal lesions in approximately up to one-quarter of subjects and gastric lesions in approximately three-quarters of NSAID recipients.[1] It is noteworthy that these studies have been extended to patients taking enteric coated preparations and gastric or duodenal mucosal lesions can be expected in more than half of individuals receiving these allegedly safer, coated medications.[8]

Data have accrued which indicate that NSAID use has changed the pattern and clinical picture of the presentation of complicated peptic ulcer disease. Several studies have shown that more than half of patients who present with a life-threatening complicated peptic ulcer disease, such as haemorrhage or perforation, are taking NSAIDs.[9–14] Calculation of the odds ratio and statistical interpretation of the data from each of these studies indicate that this association is highly significant and probably causal.[1]

Studies in both the UK and the USA have shown that, regardless of geographic region, NSAID use is to be encountered in approximately 60% of patients presenting with haemorrhage or perforation of peptic ulcer.[9–14] Follow-up of these patients who presented with haemorrhage and perforation revealed that many individuals were elderly and continued to take the medication, in some cases for questionable indications.[14] Examination of the reason why the patient was taking NSAIDs before the presentation with complicated peptic ulcer revealed that, in at least 50% of circumstances, either a non-ulcerogenic medication could have been used or NSAID use was deemed unnecessary.[14]

Over-the-counter NSAID use is as likely to be associated with complications of peptic ulcer disease as is prescription use. These data imply that secondary prevention may be important. Both patient and physician education in terms of the magnitude of the public health problem posed by the adverse affects of NSAIDs is required. Identification of the patient's risk of gastroduodenal injury and intervention by the switching of NSAIDs with non-ulcerogenic drugs may be much more important for impacting the problem than applying prophylactic pharmacological therapy for NSAID-induced gastroduodenal injury.[1]

It has been pointed out that the mortality from peptic ulcer disease remains stubbornly high, especially in the elderly. It is possible that the use of NSAIDs in the elderly may well account for much of this persistent mortality.[13] However, patients taking NSAIDs often have multisystem disease coincidental with advanced age. By their very nature, these patients represent a high-risk group for medical or surgical intervention.[13]

MECHANISM OF MUCOSAL DAMAGE BY NSAIDs

Non-steroidal anti-inflammatory drugs break the gastric mucosal barrier, with the result that hydrogen ions diffuse backwards into the mucosa and initiate an inflammatory process which can cause a breach in the epithelial lining of the upper gastrointestinal tract.[15-19] Coincidental with this occurrence is a change in transmucosal potential difference and elevation in the sodium concentration of the gastric luminal content.[15-19] It is clear that NSAIDs inhibit cyclo-oxygenase, thereby interfering with the conversion of arachidonic acid into endoperoxides.[15-19] Experimental evidence suggests that NSAIDs interfere with mucosal defences by a direct toxic mechanism, in addition to any effects that they may exert on prostaglandin metabolism.

Prostaglandins exert a general protective effect in the gastrointestinal tract and interference with their synthetic pathway will tend to impair mucosal integrity.[19] Prostaglandins promote mucosal protection and contribute to repair of the lining of the gastrointestinal tract by a variety of mechanisms.[19] The mucosal protective features of prostaglandins include stimulation of bicarbonate secretion, stimulation of mucus synthesis, enhancement of mucous gel thickness, increase in hydrophobicity of gastric mucosa, enhancement of mucosal blood flow, stimulation of sodium-active transport and inhibition of acid secretion.[15-19] Injury to the gastric or duodenal mucosa is known to stimulate prostaglandin production as a homeostatic process.

The role of prostaglandins in the promotion of the integrity of the gastroduodenal mucosa has led to the use of synthetic prostaglandins, such as enprostil or misoprostol, in the prophylactic treatment of NSAID-induced injury.[20-23] Synthetic prostaglandins and their analogues appear to be protective against NSAID injury only when used in amounts that exert an antisecretory effect on gastric acid production.[20-23] In fact, there is little evidence that the 'cytoprotective' properties of synthetic prostaglandin drugs, such as enprostil or misoprostol, have much to do with their therapeutic effects in NSAID-induced injury. The bulk of the effect of these drugs appears to be attributable to their ability to reduce acid secretion.

The dose of synthetic prostaglandins required to reduce acid secretion is relatively high and therefore troublesome adverse effects are noted when prostaglandins are used in therapeutic doses for the treatment or prophylaxis of NSAID-induced gastroduodenal injury. Although the effects of prostaglandins in antisecretory doses have been described as adverse effects, many of these effects are predictable consequences of the systemic administration of a prostaglandin. They include prominent abdominal pain and diarrhoea.[20-23] The prevalence of abdominal pain and diarrhoea in patients receiving misoprostol is such that about one-third of recipients may have to cease taking prophylaxis with effective prophylactic doses of prostaglandin analogues because of these troublesome adverse effects.

MANAGEMENT OF NSAID-INDUCED GASTRODUODENAL INJURY

Synthetic analogues of naturally occurring prostaglandin E_1, such as misoprostol and enprostil, have found a role in the prophylaxis of NSAID-induced gastroduodenal injury.[23] Misoprostol and enprostil differ from naturally occurring prostaglandin E_1 in that these modified molecules have a much longer half-life and, after oral administration, they are metabolized to a free acidic form of the drug which is pharmacologically active. These drugs produce a dose-related effect on gastric secretory activity. The mechanisms whereby synthetic prostaglandin analogues may reduce gastric acid secretion remain somewhat poorly defined, but it is suggested that they exert an effect on a receptor site on the basolateral cell membrane of the parietal cell and perhaps exert direct intracellular effects on microtubular formation within the parietal cell. Some studies have indicated that synthetic analogues of prostaglandin may reduce gastric secretion by acting on the site of coupling between histamine receptors and adenyl cyclase.

Misoprostol has been shown, in controlled clinical trials, to be effective for the prophylaxis of NSAID-induced gastric mucosal injury.[23] Large multicentre clinical trials in the USA have shown that misoprostol can prevent NSAID-induced gastric ulcer in patients with arthritis and these synthetic prostaglandins do not appear to affect the course of arthritic disease. However, compared with placebo, misoprostol does not achieve a significant difference in the relief of epigastric pain that can be attributed to NSAID use. It is of note that some of the dyspeptic symptoms induced by NSAIDs may be relieved fortuitously by the analgesic effect of the NSAID.[21-23]

The direct effect of prostaglandins on the smooth muscle of the gastrointestinal tract accounts for the relatively high frequency of dose-related adverse effects that are seen with these drugs. Therapeutic doses of misoprostol (200 µg q.i.d.) result in diarrhoea in between 15 and 30% of patients.[23] Diarrhoea is less often encountered at the 100 µg q.i.d. dosage regimen, but the drug may not be quite as effective in prophylaxis when used in this smaller dose. Recent data have questioned the overall efficacy of misoprostol as a cytoprotective, prophylactic agent for NSAID injury to the gastroduodenum, but, in general, clinical trials of H_2-receptor antagonists or sucralfate in standard therapeutic doses have not shown a beneficial prophylactic effect of these agents in the management of NSAID-induced gastric ulcer. However, controlled clinical trials have shown that H_2-receptor antagonists and proton pump inhibitors are effective in the prophylaxis of duodenal injury induced by NSAIDs.[24-26]

More recently, acid suppression has been reinvestigated as the basis for treatment for NSAID-related peptic ulcer disease. Patients with NSAID-induced peptic ulceration differ from the general pool of ulcer patients in terms of their age and sex distribution and in terms of the anatomical location of their ulcers (Table 31.2). Although *Helicobacter pylori* is not believed to play a major role in NSAID-associated gastritis, duodenitis or peptic ulceration, the *H pylori* status of a patient with ulceration, especially duodenal ulceration, should be assessed. In the event that *H pylori* is present in the patient with duodenal ulcer, appropriate eradication therapy should be used, primarily to reduce the risk of recurrence of the ulcer even in the presence of NSAID use.

Table 31.2 Comparison between features of classic peptic ulcer disease and NSAID-induced gastroscopy.

FACTOR	CLASSIC PEPTIC ULCER DISEASE	NSAID GASTROPATHY
Location	Duodenal	Antral, prepyloric
Aetiology	Unknown	NSAID-associated, reduction of, mucosal, prostaglandins PGE$_2$)
H. pylori	Positive (80%)	Negative (80%)
Sex	Male	Female
Age group	Younger	Older
Management	H$_2$ blockers, sucralfate, proton pump, inhibitors, antacids	Misoprostol, H$_2$ blockers, sucralfate, ?antacids, proton, pump inhibitors

Modified from Holt and Saleeby.[1]

NSAID-induced gastroduodenal injury is related to the back diffusion of hydrogen ions, and, in simplistic terms, if hydrogen ions are not available for back diffusion then mucosal injury may not occur. It should be noted that the treatment of NSAID-induced gastroduodenal injury is quite a separate circumstance from prophylaxis.[27] The H$_2$-receptor antagonists and proton pump inhibitors are effective in healing many gastric and duodenal ulcers in patients on NSAIDs, even when NSAID therapy is continued.[27] Similar observations have been made in relationship to sucralfate. Large multicentre trials comparing proton pump inhibition with H$_2$-receptor antagonists in the treatment of gastric ulcer, which included patients taking NSAIDs, demonstrated a therapeutic benefit for ulcer healing of omeprazole 20 or 40 mg daily in comparison to ranitidine 300 mg daily.[28] This statistically significant benefit from the use of proton pump inhibition is attributed to the more profound reduction of acid secretion that is seen with proton pump inhibitors.[27,28] This raises the issue that perhaps adjusted, higher doses of H$_2$-receptor antagonists may be useful in the management of NSAID-induced gastroduodenal injury. This notion has been supported in recent studies.[27]

The over-riding issue is how to treat a patient with peptic ulcer who is taking an NSAID. The first important step is to review the indication for the NSAID and if possible stop the drug.[27] Since frank misuse of NSAIDs is common, then this is more often possible than the clinician might have initially supposed. If there is a good indication to continue the NSAID, then the ulcer can be healed using an H$_2$-receptor antagonist, or perhaps a proton pump inhibitor, with some indication that proton pump inhibition may result in more rapid healing.[28] In the event that the patient needs to continue NSAID treatment, then if the ulcer is duodenal, prophylaxis can be undertaken by the prescription of a standard dose of an H$_2$-receptor antagonist, whereas if the ulcer is gastric then a synthetic prostaglandin analogue such as misoprostol is to be preferred.[27] Proton pump inhibitors cannot be recommended for maintenance or long-term therapy of NSAID-associated inflammation or ulceration until unresolved safety concerns are addressed and efficacy is reproducibly validated.

The role of surgery

Surgical intervention plays a major role in the treatment of NSAID-associated complicated peptic ulcer and standard operative intervention for haemorrhage or perforation is recommended. High morbidity and mortality can be anticipated in series of patients with NSAID-associated ulcer complications by virtue of the patient's age and the common occurrence of coexisting disease. Life-threatening complications of peptic ulcer occur often without warning in the NSAID user and patients taking NSAIDs may have a mild coagulopathy because these drugs interfere with platelet function.

There may be an uncommon circumstance that requires elective surgery for peptic ulcer disease where a definite need to continue NSAID therapy is encountered in the *H pylori*-negative patient who has failed prophylactic or active and optimal medical treatment for peptic ulcer.

CONCLUSION

The prevalence of NSAID-induced injury to the gastroduodenal mucosa is particularly troublesome, especially in the elderly.[1] In a study of approximately 100 000 Medicaid recipients over the age of 65 years in the USA, death from peptic ulcer was associated with NSAIDs in 34% of the patients compared with control subjects, of whom only 11% received NSAIDs.[29] Scheiman et al.[30] in a recent review of NSAID-induced peptic ulceration have drawn attention to important risk factors for NSAID-associated peptic ulceration; these include age greater than 60 years, a prior history of ulcer disease and concomitant corticosteroid use. Other possible risk factors are female sex, *H pylori* infection and cigarette smoking. Patients who consume high doses of NSAIDs or indulge in multiple NSAID or concomitant aspirin use appear to be at particular risk for NSAID-induced ulcer disease. It would appear that more judicious prescribing of NSAIDs is required, with perhaps more patient and physician education. Contemporary data reinforce the need for more patient education, especially in view of the availability of these drugs as over-the-counter medication.[31]

The problem of adverse effects of NSAIDs could be impacted by secondary preventive efforts where high-risk patients are identified and simple intervention with cessation of NSAIDs are undertaken. It would appear that secondary preventive efforts offer a much more cost-effective option for the reduction of the prevalence of NSAID-induced gastroduodenal injury than does prophylactic pharmacotherapy.

For the future an important goal must be the development of an NSAID which does not irritate the gastric mucosa. There are currently 16 500 deaths per annum in the United States directly attributable to NSAIDs. It is possible that with the recent introduction of the drug Celebrax (Pfizer) the problem may have been resolved.

REFERENCES

1. Holt S & Saleeby G. Gastric mucosal injury induced by nonsteroidal anti-inflammatory drugs (NSAIDS). *South Med J* 1990; **84:** 355–360.
2. Rossi AD, Hsu JP & Falch GA Ulcerogenicity of piroxicam: an analysis of spontaneously reported data. *BMJ* 1987; **294:** 147–150.

3. Dunn MJ, Simonson M, Davidson EW et al. Nonsteroidal anti-inflammatory drugs and renal function. *J Clin Pharmacol* 1988; **28:** 524–529.

4. Lewis JH. Hepatic toxicity of nonsteroidal anti-inflammatory drugs. *Clin Pharmacol* 1984; **3:** 128.

5. Holt S, Irshad M, Howlen CW & Maneiro M. Nonsteroidal anti-inflammatory drugs and lower gastrointestinal bleeding. *Dig Dis Sci* 1993; **38:** 1619–1623.

6. Larki EN, Smith JL, Lidsky MD et al. Gastroduodenal mucosa and dyspeptic symptoms in arthritic patients during chronic nonsteroidal anti-inflammatory drug use. *Am J Gastroenterol* 1987; **82:** 1153–1158.

7. Silvoso GR, Ivey KS, Butt JH et al. Incidence of gastric lesions in patients with rheumatic disease on chronic aspirin therapy. *Ann Intern Med* 1979; **91:** 517–520.

8. Jaszewski R. Frequency of gastroduodenal lesions in asymptomatic patients on chronic aspirin or nonsteroidal anti-inflammatory drug therapy. *J Clin Gastroenterol* 1990; **12:** 10–13.

9. Armstrong CP & Blower AL. Nonsteroidal anti-inflammatory drugs and life-threatening complications of peptic ulceration. *Gut* 1987; **28:** 527–532.

10. Somerville K, Faulkner G & Langman M. Nonsteroidal anti-inflammatory drugs and bleeding peptic ulcer. *Lancet* 1986; **i:** 462–464.

11. Griffin MR, Ray WA & Schaffner W. Nonsteroidal anti-inflammatory drug use and death from peptic ulcer in elderly persons. *Ann Intern Med* 1988; **109:** 359–363.

12. Permutt RP & Cello JP. Duodenal ulcer disease in the hospitalized elderly patient. *Dig Dis Sci* 1982; **27:** 1–6.

13. Pounder R. Silent peptic ulceration: deadly silence or golden silence? *Gastroenterology* 1989; **96** (Suppl.): 626–631.

14. Saleeby G & Holt S. Why do patients with life-threatening complications of peptic ulcer take nonsteroidal anti-inflammatory drugs? *Am J Gastroenterol* 1990; **85:** 1294 (abstract).

15. Rees WDW & Turnberg LA. Mechanisms of gastric mucosal protection a role for the mucus–bicarbonate barrier. *Clin Sci* 1982; **62:** 343–348.

16. Domschke W, Domschke S, Hornig D et al. Prostaglandin-stimulated gastric mucus secretion in many. *Acta Hepatogastroenterol* 1978; **25:** 292–294.

17. Kivilaakso E & Flemstrom G. Surface pH gradient and prostaglandin cytoprotection in gastroduodenal mucosa. In Allen A, Flemstrom G, Garner A et al (eds) *Mechanism of Gastric Mucosal Protection in the Upper Gastrointestinal Tract.* New York: Raven Press, 1984: 227–232.

18. Lichtenberger LM, Richards JE & Hills BA. Effect of 16,16-dimethyl prostaglandin E₂ on the surface hydrophobicity of aspirin-treated canine gastric mucosa. *Gastroenterology* 1985; **88:** 308–314.

19. Vane JR. Inhibition of prostaglandin synthesis as a mechanism of action for aspirin-like drugs. *Nature* 1971; **231:** 232–235.

20. Kaufman GL, Whittle BJR, Aures D et al. Effects of prostacyclin and a stable analogue, 6-PG, on gastric secretion, mucosal blood flow, and blood pressure in conscious dogs. *Gastroenterology* 1979; **77:** 1301–1306.

21. Chaudhury TK & Jacobson ED. Prostaglandin: cytoprotein of gastric mucosa. *Gastroenterology* 1978; **74:** 59–63.

22. Hawkey CJ & Rampton DS. Prostaglandins and the gastrointestinal mucosa: are they important in its function, disease or treatment? *Gastroenterology* 1985; **89:** 1162–1188.

23. Graham DY, Agrawal N & Roth SH. Prevention of NSAID-induced gastric ulcer with misoprostol: multicentre, double-blind placebo-controlled trial. *Lancet* 1988; **ii:** 1277–1280.

24. Roth SH, Bennett RE, Mitchell CS et al. Cimetidine therapy in nonsteroidal anti-inflammatory drug gastropathy. *Arch Intern Med* 1987; **147:** 1798–1801.

25. Caldwell JR, Roth SH, Wu WL et al. Sucralfate treatment of nonsteroidal anti-inflammatory drug-induced gastrointestinal and mucosal damage. *Am J Med* 1987; **83** (Suppl. 3B): 74–82.

26. Greb WH, Von Schrader HW, Cerlek S et al. Endoscopic studies of nabumetone in patients with rheumatoid arthritis: a comparative endoscopic and histologic evaluation. *Am J Med* 1987; **83** (Suppl. 4B): 19–24.

27. Howden CW, Saleeby G, Holt L & Holt S. Follow-up of patients with NSAID-related complicated peptic ulcer disease (CPUD). *Am J Gastroenterol* 1991; **86:** 1313.

28. Walan A, Bader JP, Classen M et al. Effects of omeprazole and ranitidine on ulcer healing and relapse rates in patients with benign gastric ulcer. *N Engl J Med* 1989; **320:** 69–75.

29. Holt S, Holt, S, Saleeby G & Todd M. Gastroduodenal injury from non-steroidal anti-inflammatory drugs: risk management issues. *Gastroenterol Nurs* 1991; **14:** 124–126.

30. Scheiman JM et al. NSAID-induced peptic ulcer disease: pathogenesis, risk factors, and management. *Dig Dis* 1994; **12:** 210.

31. Holt, S. Over-the-counter histamine H₂-receptor antagonists. How will they affect the treatment of acid-related diseases? *Drugs* 1994; **47:** 1–11.

32

ANTISECRETORY DRUGS: CONTEMPORARY ISSUES

S Holt
TV Taylor

The 1980s and 1990s have witnessed a counter-revolution in the treatment of acid-related disease. Formerly, discussions or comparisons of gastric surgical techniques were as common as comparisons of the safety and efficacy of H_2-receptor antagonists (H_2RAs) for the treatment of peptic ulcer. At present, in the area of acid-related disease, the use of proton pump inhibitors and the treatment of *Helicobacter pylori* are the foci of attention. As the second millennium approaches, the recognition of the infectious aetiology of peptic ulcer disease and the advent of agents that produce prolonged, profound reduction of acid secretion have created new horizons for the management of acid-related disease. The development of H_2RAs with enhanced molar potency and the use of proton pump inhibitors are significant therapeutic advances.[1,2] The use of these more potent drugs reinforces the recognition that more profound reduction of gastric acid may enhance efficacy of treatment in terms of accelerated healing and relief of symptoms of acid-related disease.[1,2]

The objectives of this chapter are to analyse contemporary concerns about antisecretory drugs in common clinical usage and assist in the development of clinical concepts for the management of acid-related disease.

NEOHISTORICAL PERSPECTIVES AND CHANGING TRENDS

The protagonists of the use of proton pump inhibitors for the first line treatment of acid-related disease have been beleaguered by unresolved safety concerns about these drugs, and perhaps a failure to acknowledge that H_2RAs alone afford effective therapy for large numbers of patients with acid-related disease.[1,2] The general safety of H_2RAs appears to be well established, with a few residual and specific concerns.[3] Furthermore, it is appearing increasingly likely that proton pump inhibitors are also very safe, even in the long term. The pharmacological properties of H_2RAs are such that the Food

and Drug Administration in the USA and several regulatory agencies in Europe have approved them for use as over-the-counter (OTC) medications, without prescription.[3]

All therapeutic decisions in Western societies are being heavily influenced by cost containment and health care reform. Modern medical practice is increasingly determined by outcome measurements. The trends in managed care organizations are towards disease state management. Clinical protocols for the management of peptic ulcer disease continue to evolve, but in addition to conventional antisecretory interventions, treatment decisions for duodenal ulcer will become influenced by the presence or absence of *H. pylori* in the gastric antrum. Disease state management protocols are ideally suited to pharmacological interventions in acid-related disease, where outcomes are related to drug efficacy and compliance. Ulcer disease management strategies developed by collaborative research among clinicians, pharmaceutical companies and pharmacy benefit management organizations are rapidly gaining acceptance.

OVER-THE-COUNTER H_2RAs

The effect of changes in health care organization will play a major role in the use of antisecretory drugs and the OTC availability of H_2RAs may significantly affect the overall management of acid-related disease in clinical practice.[3]

In 1989, the Danish regulatory authorities approved the use of H_2RA as OTC medications. Other European countries and the USA have followed this lead in rapid succession. Following this switch, cumulative postmarketing surveillance studies have not shown any major effects of OTC H_2RAs on acid-related disease. In particular, evidence of incomplete ulcer healing with increased relapse rates, more complicating peptic ulcer or adverse drug effects have not surfaced as problems.[3] The utilization of OTC H_2RAs in the face of increasing recognition of the importance of *H. pylori* in acid-related disease remains underexplored and special studies of high-risk groups, such as users of non-steroidal anti-inflammatory drugs (NSAIDs), are required.[4,5] At the time of writing, all commercially available H_2RAs are candidates for the switch to OTC status, but the H_2RA with the superior safety profile that is first to gain assent for use is likely to be the most widely used agent.

CLINICAL EFFICACY OF H₂RAs

Many studies have indicated therapeutic equivalence among H_2RAs but available H_2RAs have important differences in chemical structure and activity (Table 32.1). These structural differences transmit into different pharmacological and therapeutic activities, making the selection of one agent perhaps more desirable in certain types of acid-related disease or in a specific clinical circumstance. Discussions about the clinical efficacy of H_2RAs or comparisons among available H_2RAs in terms of therapeutic benefit can be dismissed by the recognition that those available are essentially therapeutically equivalent when used in standard therapeutic dosages. Commercially sponsored studies that compare non-equipotent doses of antisecretory drugs are predictable in their outcome and they are hardly worthy of much consideration.

Table 32.1   Chemical structure of H_2RAs

DRUGS	RING STRUCTURE	SIDE-CHAIN (R)	THERAPEUTIC DOSE (MG/DAY)
Histamine		$CH_2CH_2NH_2$	—
Cimetidine		$CH_2SCH_2CH_2NHCNCH_3$ $\parallel$ $N-C\equiv N$	800–1200
Ranitidine		$CH_2SCH_2CH_2NHCNCH_3$ $\parallel$ $CHNO_2$	300
Nizatidine		$CH_2SCH_2CH_2NHCNHCH_3$ $\parallel$ $CHNO_2$	300
Famotidine		$CH_2SCH_2CH_2CNH_2$ $\parallel$ NSO_2NH_2	40
Roxatidine		$OCH_2CH_2CH_2NHCCH_2OCCH_3$ $\parallel$ $\parallel$ O O	150

Nizatidine combines the ring structure of famotidine with the side-chain of ranitidine. Roxatidine is a piperidine derivative with a double ring structure. The heterocyclic five-membered rings (furan of ranitidine, imidazole of cimetidine and thiazole of nizatidine and famotidine) are replaced by a phenyl ring in roxatidine acetate.

STRUCTURE–ACTIVITY FEATURES OF H₂RAS

Famotidine differs from the earlier H_2RAs in having a thiazole ring structure with two side-chains which result in hydrophilicity and higher affinity for the H_2 receptor (Table 32.1). The guanidinothiazole moiety, when substituted in H_2RA molecules, confers the properties of increased molar potency for the reduction of acid secretion compared with other H_2RAs.[6] To achieve an equipotent antisecretory effect, less famotidine is required compared with other H_2RAs. Famotidine is the most potent H_2RA,[6] approximately eight times more potent than cimetidine. The mode of action of antisecretory drugs are summarized in Figure 32.1.

Nizatidine has a thiazole ring but a lower receptor affinity than famotidine because the aminoethyl moiety of nizatidine differs in receptor affinity from the guanidine configuration of famotidine.[6] However, the thiazole structure of famotidine and nizatidine determines the lack of ability of these drugs to bind to the cytochrome P_{450} drug metabolizing enzyme system in the liver, such that cytochrome P_{450}-dependent drug interactions do not occur with famotidine or nizatidine.[6] In contrast, cimetidine and ranitidine bind cytochrome P_{450} enzymes and they have a potential for drug interactions mediated by this mechanism. Proton pump inhibitors are much more effective than H_2RAs in reducing gastric acidity but they bind with various isozymes of cytochrome P_{450}.[1,2]

Some differences are apparent in the pharmacokinetics of the various H_2RAs (Table 32.2). Cimetidine, ranitidine and famotidine dosages should be reduced in patients with impaired renal function but more severe renal compromise is required before a reduction in dosage of famotidine is required, compared with cimetidine or ranitidine.

Overall, H_2RAs have been shown to have therapeutic equivalence by healing about 80–95% of peptic ulcer disease within an 8-week period. The time to relief of symptoms and time to ulcer healing have been recognized to be functions of the potency with which an agent reduces acid secretion (Figure 32.2). Putative advantages in terms of accelerated healing or symptom relief have been seen with more potent acid suppressing agents such as proton pump inhibitors.[1,2] However, for patients with peptic ulcer who are *H. pylori* positive the first-line treatment should be eradication of the organism.

H_2RAs are particularly suited as parenteral agents for the reduction of gastric acid in the prophylaxis of stress-induced mucosal disease, especially in the patient in the intensive care unit.[7] H_2RAs sharply increase pH values in the stomach when given intravenously. Concomitant use of bronchodilators, antiarrhythmic agents or anticoagulant drugs with cimetidine should be avoided, or at least closely monitored, because of the possibility of clinically significant drug interactions.[6]

The recognition that reflux oesophagitis requires an overall greater degree of acid suppression for healing and symptom relief than gastric or duodenal ulcer disease has led to a particular clinical niche for proton pump inhibitors in the treatment of gastrooesophageal reflux disease.[1,2,8] H_2RAs may

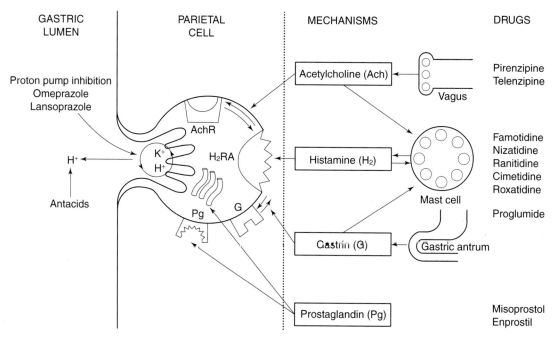

Figure 32.1

Parietal cell and secretagogue mechanisms. H_2RAs remain the mainstay of pharmacological control of acid secretion. Proton pump inhibition is achieved by irreversible blockage of the high-energy dependent H^+,K^+-ATPase enzyme system located on the apical membrane of the parietal cell.

be effective in the treatment of moderate gastro-oesophageal reflux disease especially if they are used in divided or in higher doses.[2,8]

DRUG INTERACTIONS WITH H_2RAs

Drug absorption interactions that are dependent on pH changes and altered pH-dependent dissociation of orally administered drugs can occur with all antisecretory drugs.[6] The rate of absorption of bioavailability of all H_2RAs may be affected by concomitant antacid use in some circumstances, but these changes are not considered to be of clinical significance.

Available H_2RAs do not materially affect the rate of absorption of concomitantly administered drugs because they have no clinically significant effects on gastric emptying rate in humans.[9] Drug interactions with H_2RAs as a consequence of altered biodistribution or elimination are reported rarely and the main drug interactions described with H_2RAs are caused by the inhibition of the hepatic metabolism of concurrently administered drugs[6] (Figure 32.3).

Cimetidine binds the cytochrome P_{450} enzyme systems, attaching the oxygen binding ligand[6] (see Figure 32.2). Ranitidine may bind cytochrome P_{450} enzymes, especially at higher dosage, and it shares the potential of cimetidine for

Table 32.2 Differences between H_2RAS

VARIABLE	RANITIDINE	NIZATIDINE	FAMOTIDINE	CIMETIDINE	ROXATIDINE
Relative potency	4–10	4–10	20–50	1	2–5
Standard oral dose	300 mg o.d. 150 mg b.i.d.	300 mg o.d. 150 mg b.i.d.	40 mg o.d. 20 mg b.i.d.	800 mg o.d. 400 mg b.i.d.	150 mg o.d.
Chemical ring	Furan	Thiazole	Thiazole	Imidazole	Piperidine, double ring
Bioavailability (%)	50–60	70	37–45	60–70	Rapid metabolism (M-1 M-4 metabolites) 90
Time to peak after oral dose (h)	1–3	0.5–3	1–3	1–2	1–3
Elimination half-life (h)	2–3	1–2	2.5–3.5	2	2
Cytochrome P_{450} binding affinities[a]	Weak	None	None	Strong	Weak

Famotidine is the most potent H_2RA with the longest duration of action.
[a]Famotidine and nizatidine do not bind cytochrome P_{450} drug metabolizing enzyme systems.

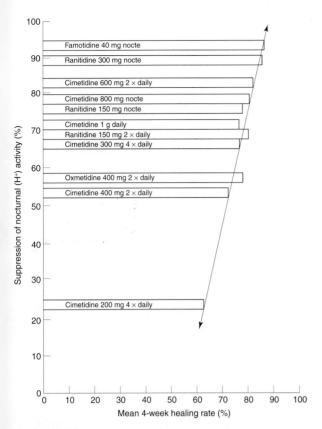

Figure 32.2
A significant correlation exists between potency of suppression of nocturnal intragastric acidity and healing rates of duodenal ulcer. The data in this figure are replotted from meta-analysis studies. The histograms show healing rates with different regimens of H_2RAs for the healing of duodenal ulcer show therapeutic equivalence.

drug interactions with a wide variety of different drugs that are metabolized by cytochrome P_{450}.[6] However, drug interactions with ranitidine, mediated through the cytochrome P_{450} enzyme system, appear to be much less common but less predictable than those encountered with cimetidine.[6]

Drug interactions with H_2RAs are summarized in Table 32.3. Cimetidine is known to impair the elimination of a variety of drugs that are metabolized by the liver, including warfarin, nicoumalone or phenindione, diazepam, phenytoin, chlor-methiazole, chlordiazepoxide, theophylline and antipyrine.[6] Cimetidine can also compromise amidopyrine demethylation and metoprolol elimination (Table 32.3). Each of these effects is mediated by the binding of cimetidine to cytochrome P_{450} enzymes. Although the affinity of ranitidine for cytochrome P_{450} isozymes is lower than that of cimetidine, drug interactions have been noted between ranitidine and benzodiazepines, fentanyl, metoprolol, midazolam and warfarin (Table 32.3). Clinically significant adverse effects with cimetidine or ranitidine have been noted as a result of drug interactions with warfarin, midazolam and other compounds. Roxatidine has been shown to have no clinically significant effect on diazepam, propanolol or antipyrine elimination but it may bind cytochrome P_{450} enzymes and has a potential for

drug interaction, which may become apparent with more widespread use of the drug.

An important, but debated, drug interaction with H_2RAs is the repeated observation that cimetidine, ranitidine and nizatidine may cause enhancement of alcohol absorption. Some studies have shown an increase in peak blood alcohol concentrations and an increase in the absolute bioavailability of ethanol during treatment with H_2RAs and acute alcohol intake.[10] It is believed that certain H_2RAs may interact with selected isozyme fractions of gastric alcohol dehydrogenase that may be responsible for significant first pass metabolism of ethanol by the stomach.[10] Unlike cimetidine, ranitidine or nizatidine, it appears that famotidine may not interact with alcohol in this manner.[11]

Alcohol consumption or abuse appears to be an important determinant of dyspepsia and H_2RAs are frequently taken by patients who consume alcohol.[10,11] This putative alcohol–H_2RA interaction although questioned, had raised medicolegal and clinical concerns, especially in relation to the availability of H_2RAs as OTC medications in the USA. In addition, complex factors determine ethanol pharmacokinetics. These factors may not have been taken into account completely in studies where no effects of H_2RAs on ethanol absorption have been noted.[11]

ADVERSE EFFECTS OF H_2RAs

Extensive postmarketing surveillance data that have been obtained from the clinical or research use of H_2RAs indicate that these drugs are well tolerated, with an overall occurrence of side-effects of the order of 2–3%.[6] However, H_2RAs are the most frequently prescribed drugs, on a worldwide basis, and even an infrequent side-effect is of clinical concern. Adverse effects of H_2RAs on all body systems have been described but many of these reports are anecdotal or involve single case reports. These adverse effects of H_2RAs are often examples of reversible toxicity and difficulty is often encountered in attributing the adverse event directly to the prescribed drug.[6]

Sporadic reports of central nervous system toxicity have been noted with H_2RAs, including headache, speech disorder, hallucinations, somnolence, restlessness and mental confusion. Mental confusion has been reported with some consistency with the use of cimetidine or ranitidine, especially in the elderly.[6] Such reports have usually involved parenteral dosing with these H_2RAs, especially in patients with coexisting cerebrovascular, hepatic or renal disease. Vigilance is required with the use of H_2RAs, especially ranitidine or cimetidine, in elderly patients at risk. This is important in patients who have significant multisystem illness with hepatic or renal failure.

Cimetidine and ranitidine may affect certain aspects of endocrine function but roxatidine, nizatidine and famotidine are not believed to exert these effects.[6] Cimetidine is antiandrogenic and it displaces dihydrotestosterone competitively from androgen binding sites. Cimetidine and ranitidine may stimulate serum prolactin levels and cause occasional impotence or breast tenderness, but some reports have produced conflicting data about the antiandrogenic effects of H_2RAs.[6]

Several adverse cardiovascular events have been variously

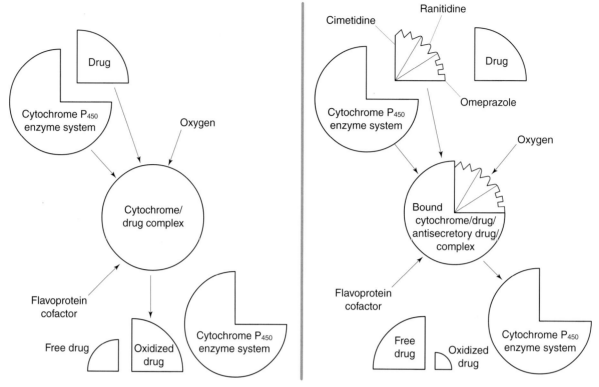

Figure 32.3

Potential interaction of cimetidine, ranitidine and omeprazole with cytochrome P$_{450}$. Omeprazole binds a different cytochrome P$_{450}$ isozyme group from cimetidine. Ranitidine binds weakly to cytochrome P$_{450}$ enzymes. These interactions result in interference with the metabolism of certain other drugs (see Table 32.3).

ascribed to H$_2$RAs but there is difficulty in implicating these drugs as a direct cause of many of these side-effects.[12] Patients with cardiovascular disease may receive H$_2$RAs frequently for coexisting acid–peptic disorders. Certain risk factors for the alleged cardiovascular effects of H$_2$RAs have been identified, including severe concomitant cardiovascular disease, the use of antiarrhythmic drugs with H$_2$RA–drug interaction potential (e.g. lignocaine), and rapid bolus administration of H$_2$RAs, especially cimetidine. Decreased systolic blood pressure has been noted in patients receiving large intravenous doses of cimetidine, ranitidine and famotidine.[6,12]

No evidence appears to exist that one H$_2$RA is any safer than another for use in the patient with cardiovascular disease, except perhaps for the recommendation of avoidance of high-dose bolus injections of H$_2$RAs in individuals with severe cardiac or other systemic illness.[6,12] Haematological problems have been reported with H$_2$RAs, including neutropenia, thrombocytopenia, haemolytic anaemia and rarely agranulocytosis or pancytopenia.[6] Clinically insignificant increases in serum creatinine have been noted due to cimetidine administration in some studies, as a consequence of the ability of cimetidine to compete with the tubular secretion of creatinine. Several H$_2$RAs have been reported to cause rare cases of interstitial nephritis and some disproportionate dosage adjustments of H$_2$RAs are necessary in cases of renal failure. It is notable that many of these adverse effects have not been noted with famotidine or nizatidine, even when these drugs are used at high doses.[6,13]

All available H$_2$RAs can cause elevations of hepatic transaminase enzymes but documented cases of acute hepatic injury are uncommon.[6] Ranitidine, when administered intravenously, causes a dose-dependent increase in hepatic enzyme levels and the prevalence of hepatic toxicity may be higher with this compound than with the other H$_2$RAs.[14] Increases in serum bile acids with hyperbilirubinaemia and mild abnormality of levels of serum transaminase enzymes have been reported with cimetidine, perhaps implying an ability of this drug to affect bile secretion.[14]

Although uncommon, clinical hepatitis with cimetidine and ranitidine may be associated variably with fever or rash that recurs on challenge with these drugs. These findings suggest an allergic mechanism of hepatotoxicity in some cases.[14] Cases of cholestatic jaundice have been reported with cimetidine and ranitidine. An acute cholestatic syndrome with rash and hypereosinophilia has been well documented with ranitidine. Furthermore, ranitidine has been associated with the possible causation of granulomatous hepatitis. Although reports of liver toxicity appear to be less with roxatidine, nizatidine and famotidine, more patient-years of experience have been gained with cimetidine and ranitidine.[14]

CARCINOGENICITY OF ANTISECRETORY DRUGS

In hypochlorhydria unrelated to drug therapy, such as following gastric surgery, in pernicious anaemia or in chronic

Table 32.3 Drug interactions with H_2RAs

CLASS DRUGS	RANITIDINE	CIMETIDINE	POTENTIAL OUTCOME OF CYTOCHROME P_{450} INTERACTION
Antiarrhythmics			
Encainide	—	*	—
Flecainide	—	*	—
Lignocaine	—	*	Lignocaine toxicity
Quinidine	—	—	—
Anticoagulants			
Dicoumarol	—	—	—
Warfarin	*	*	Prolonged bleeding time
Antidepressants (tricyclic)			Prolonged bleeding time
Amitriptyline	—	*	—
Amoxapine	—	*	Anticholinergic effects (dry mouth, decreased gastric emptying)
Doxepin	—	*	—
Imipramine	—	*	—
Nortriptyline	—	*	Orthostatic hypotension
Antidiabetic agents			
Glipizide	*	—	Hypoglycaemia
Glibenclamide	*	—	—
Tolbutamide	—	—	Sedation, drowsiness, fatigue
Benzodiazepines			
Alprazolam	—	*	Bradycardia, hypotension
Chlordiazepoxide	—	—	—
Diazepam	*	*	—
Chlordiazepoxide	—	*	—
Diazepam	—	*	—
Flurazepam	—	*	—
Midazolam	*	*	Decreased heart rate
Triazolam	—	*	—
β-Adrenergic blockers			CNS and respiratory depression
Labetalol	—	*	—
Metoprolol	*	*	—
Propranolol	*	*	—
Calcium channel blockers			Theophylline toxicity (headache, palpitations, dizziness, nausea, hypotension, tachycardia, seizures)
Diltiazem	*	*	—
Nifedipine	*	*	—
Verapamil	—	*	—
Other			—
Carbamazepine	—	*	—
Cyclosporine	*	*	—
Digitoxin	—	*	Decreased heart rate
Fluorouracil	—	*	—
Meperidine	—	*	CNS and respiratory depression
Metronidazole	—	*	—
Phenobarbitone	—	*	—
Phenytoin	—	*	—
Theophylline	*	*	Theophylline toxicity (headache, palpitations, dizziness, nausea, hypotension, tachycardia, seizures)

Potential interactions between cimetidine or ranitidine and a variety of drugs are possible due to interaction of these H_2RAs with cytochrome P_{450} enzyme systems that metabolize drugs in the liver. Famotidine and nizatidine do not interact with cytochrome P_{450}. Roxatidine is a weak substrate for cytochrome P_{450} and it may have unknown drug interactions mediated by cytochrome P_{450} which may only become apparent with more widespread use of the drug. Not all potential drug interactions are known to be of clinical significance.

gastritis, there is a circumstance of potential production and absorption of N-nitroso compounds which has been proposed as a risk for gastric cancer. Bacterial overgrowth may occur at high intragastric pH, with the reduction of dietary nitrate to nitrite and the subsequent formation of N-nitroso compounds, which are proven carcinogens. This theory is controversial. A further factor which may be important in the promotion of carcinogenesis is the hypergastrinaemia which follows acid secretory inhibition and this may lead to gastric endocrine neoplasia, but has not been noted in humans. Drugs which reduce acid secretion by more than about 50% produce a marked rise in serum gastrin levels.[15] Gastrin stimulates both acid secretion and gastric mucosal cell growth. The most prominent growth promoting effect of gastrin on the gastric mucosa is the self-replication of endocrine-enterochromaffin-like cells in the oxyntic mucosa.[1,2] Surveillance studies of patients taking H$_2$RAs or proton pump inhibitors have generally produced reassuring evidence that these drugs are unlikely to pose any significant risk of gastric neoplasia.[3]

Several reasons have been suggested as the cause of the increasing incidence and risk of gastric cancer with hyposecretion of acid, and much attention has been focused on the powerful proton pump inhibitor, omeprazole, as a potential carcinogen.[15,17] Omeprazole and lansoprazole, the most effective secretory inhibitory drugs, have not yet gained universal acceptance as first line therapy for acid-related disease in Western society.[1,2] Their use, however, provides the most effective form of drug therapy for controlling the symptoms of gastro-oesophageal reflux disease, the most common cause of dyspepsia.[1,2]

Standard toxicological studies in animals have shown that omeprazole is not mutagenic, but indirect carcinogenicity is manifest by locally invasive gastric carcinoid neoplasia in the rat and can be attributed to drug-induced hypergastrinaemia.[15] It has been found that in certain rat species orally administered omeprazole resulted in enhanced incorporation of tritiated thymidine into pronase digests of gastric mucosa, raising an issue that the drug was genotoxic.[16] However, the demonstration of the suppressibility of this uptake by arresting cell division with hydroxyurea implied that the proposed assay may not have been a valid measure of genotoxicity.[16] It is remotely conceivable that a small amount of thymidine uptake in the assay could have occurred as a result of unscheduled DNA synthesis[15,16] and matters remain unresolved. More importantly, in humans, no evidence of an increased incidence of carcinoid-like gastric neoplasia has been demonstrated. Far less attention has yet been directed towards the potential promotion of extragastric, gastrin-dependent neoplasia of the pancreas, small intestine or colon,[1,2] especially in humans.

The avidity with which omeprazole binds isozyme fractions of cytochrome P$_{450}$ is similar to that exhibited by cimetidine, such that drug interaction potential exists.[1] Omeprazole inhibits the metabolism of anticoagulants (warfarin), anticonvulsants (phenytoin) and benzodiazepines (diazepam).[1,2] There is as yet little evidence that these potential interactions are clinically relevant.[1,2] Lansoprazole may be subject to many of the concerns that have been expressed about omeprazole. To date, despite increasingly widespread usage over the past decade, no evidence of an increased incidence of gastric malignancy has been attributed to omeprazole.

CONCLUSION

Short-term, potent reduction of acid secretion with antisecretory drugs remains an effective and apparently safe means of managing the majority of acid-related disease, for which, in recent times, surgery has played an ever decreasing role. It remains to be seen whether or not less invasive surgical techniques, such as laparoscopic vagotomy, will restore the balance. Currently, however, the first line management of *H. pylori*-related peptic ulcer disease is to eradicate the microorganism.

REFERENCES

1. Holt S & Howden CW. Omeprazole: overview and opinion. *Dig Dis Sci* 1991; **36**: 385–393.
2. Holt S. Proton-pump inhibition for acid-related disease. *South Med J* 1991; **84**: 1078–1079.
3. Holt S. Over the counter H$_2$ receptor antagonists. How will they affect the treatment of acid-related diseases? *Drugs* 1994; **47**: 1–11.
4. Holt S & Saleeby G. Gastric mucosal injury induced by anti-inflammatory drugs (NSAIDs). *South Med J* 1991; **84**: 355–360.
5. Holt L, Holt S, Saleeby G & Tood M. Gastroduodenal injury from nonsteroidal anti-inflammatory drugs: risk management issues. *Gastroenterol Nurs* 1991; **14**: 124–126.
6. Schunack W. What are the differences between H$_2$-receptor antagonists? *Aliment Pharmacol Ther* 1987; **1**(Suppl. 1): 493s–503s.
7. Freston JW. Safety perspectives on parenteral H$_2$-receptor antagonist. *Am J Med* 1987; **83**(Suppl. 6A): 58–67.
8. Sontag SJ, Hirschowitz BI, Holt S et al. Two doses omeprazole versus placebo in symptomatic erosive esophagitis: the US multicenter study. *Gastroenterology* 1992; **102**: 109–118.
9. Holt S, Heading RC, Taylor TV, Tothill P & Forrest JA. Is gastric emptying abnormal in duodenal ulcer? *Dig Dis Sci* 1985; **31**: 685–692.
10. Holt S. On: Alcohol and H$_2$-receptor antagonists: over the counter, under the table? *Am J Gastroenterol* 1991; **86**: 113–116.
11. Guram M, Howden CW & Holt S. Increased blood alcohol levels with some H$_2$-receptor antagonists. *J Pharm Med* 1991; **1**: 275–279.
12. Salmon P, Darrag HA, Fitzgerald D, Lamb R, Kenny M & Hirata Y. Lack of effect of famotidine on cardiac performance assessed by noninvasive hemodynamic measurements. *Eur J Clin Pharm* 1989; **36**(Suppl.): A–136.
13. Humphries TJ. Famotidine: a notable lack of drug interactions. *Scand J Gastroenterol* 1987; **22**(Suppl. 134): 55–60.
14. Souza Lima MA. Hepatitis associated with ranitidine. *Ann Intern Med* 1984; **101**: 207–208.
15. Holt S, Powers RE & Howden CW. Antisecretory therapy and genotoxicity. *Dig Dis Sci* 1991; **36**: 545–547.
16. Holt S, Zhu ZH & Powers RE. Observations on a proposed measure of genotoxicity in rat gastric mucosa. *Gastroenterology* 1991; **101**: 650–656.
17. Wormsley KG. Assessing the safety of drugs for the long-term treatment of peptic ulcers. *Gut* 1984; **25**: 1416–1423.

33

SURGICAL TREATMENT OF CHRONIC DUODENAL ULCER

TV Taylor

EPIDEMIOLOGY IN RELATION TO MORTALITY

Throughout the nineteenth century, duodenal ulcer was a rare disease. With the turn of the century there came a massive increase in the prevalence of the disorder and consequently in complications and fatalities. In 1946, Ivy[1] estimated that 10% of the American male population would have a duodenal ulcer before the age of 65 years. Since the late 1950s there has been a steady decline in the overall prevalence of the condition, when expressed in terms of hospital admissions, outpatient attendances and time lost from work as a result of this disorder. This decline long preceded the introduction of the first effective ulcer-healing drugs, the H_2-receptor antagonists.[2] Numerous studies of the occurrence of new cases of duodenal ulcer in specific populations reported decreases of 40–50% between the 1950s and 1970s.[3] The decline in the number of hospital admissions for problems associated with peptic ulcer in the USA is shown in Figure 33.1. Exact figures on the incidence of the disorder are difficult to obtain because of the fluctuating nature of the disease, a lack of precise diagnostic methods prior to widespread use of endoscopy in the early 1970s, the number of asymptomatic ulcers and the number of patients who purchase over-the-counter antacids to relieve ulcer dyspepsia without presenting to a doctor. Perhaps surprisingly, and despite the massive use of H_2-receptor antagonists in recent years, there has been an increase in ulcer-associated mortality in England, Wales, Finland and other European countries. According to the Registrar General's figures for England and Wales there are approximately 4500 ulcer-related deaths per year, about the same number as from cancer of the pancreas and oesophagus (Figure 33.2). There is, however, one fundamental difference between deaths from peptic ulcer and those from the above and other solid tumour malignancies, that is that many of the ulcer-associated deaths are potentially preventable, whereas there is no likelihood, in the near future, of a significant reduction occurring in the number of deaths from these malignancies. Figures 33.3–33.5 show the increase which has occurred in recent years in specific ulcer-associated deaths, which has been most significant in elderly females. A possible explanation for this phenomenon is the marked increase in use of non-steroidal anti-inflammatory drugs (NSAIDs) which has occurred recently (Figure 33.6). Other possibilities which may be considered relevant include the increased incidence of colonization of the stomach and duodenum by *Helicobacter pylori* and the marked reduction which has occurred in elective peptic ulcer surgery.

PATHOGENESIS IN RELATION TO THE USE OF NSAIDs

There is now little doubt that duodenal ulcers can occur with significantly increased incidence following treatment with NSAIDs. In the UK in 1985, 22 million prescriptions were given

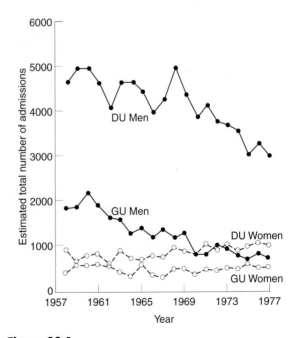

Figure 33.1

Decline in hospital admissions for duodenal (DU) and gastric (GU) ulcer in the USA.

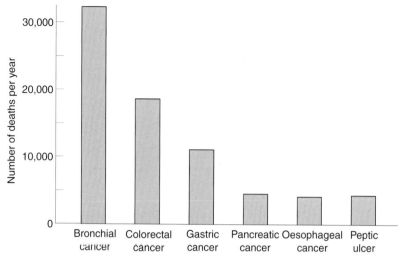

Figure 33.2
Mortality from peptic ulceration and the major malignancies in England and Wales.

for these drugs, and an even larger volume was sold over the counter. The age-specific prescription rates for NSAIDs have increased exponentially in recent years, particularly in females over the age of 65 years, and this may be the cause of increased mortality from peptic ulcer disease. In the USA, 44 million prescriptions were given for NSAIDs in 1985 and these were responsible for 21% of all adverse drug reports to the US Food and Drug Administration.

The worldwide market for NSAIDs is worth at least $US 2 billion per year, and it has been estimated in the USA that at least half of the cost of using these drugs in individual patients is related to treating their side-effects within the gastrointestinal tract. NSAIDs may cause gastritis, acute erosions, gastric ulcer, prepyloric ulcer, duodenal ulcer, small intestinal erosions and even large bowel hemorrhage. Gastric mucosal damage induced by NSAIDS was first demonstrated in 1938. It has been shown that gastric ulcers occur in up to 20% of patients taking NSAIDs for 3 months, and duodenal ulcer in about 8% at 3 months.

It is difficult to obtain exact figures for the risk of bleeding in patients on NSAIDs as the results reported in different series have varied widely. In addition, there is little correlation between endoscopic findings and dyspeptic symptoms in those taking NSAIDs, and many ulcers may be asymptomatic, possibly as a result of the analgesic effect of these drugs. It has been estimated from meta-analysis of pooled data that the relative risk for gastroduodenal damage due to aspirin and nonsteroidals is about four times that in the control population, and that the mortality risk for NSAIDs is about 7.5 times that in age- and sex-matched controls. The risk associated with the taking of paracetamol is less than with other NSAIDs. Complications increase with increasing age. It was estimated by Pounder in 1989[i] that 76% of patients taking long-term

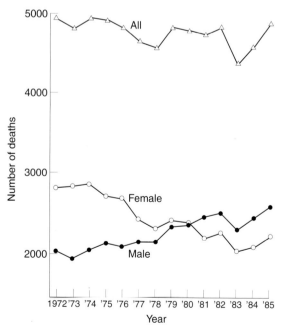

Figure 33.3
Standardized death rate from peptic ulceration in England and Wales 1972–1985, based on 1985 population figure. (Source: Office of Population and Census Survey.)

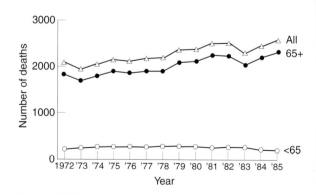

Figure 33.4
Standardized death rate from peptic ulceration in England and Wales, 1972–1985 (females). (Source: Office of Population and Census survey.)

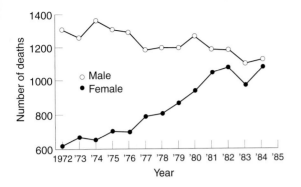

Figure 33.5
Mortality from duodenal ulceration in England and Wales, 1972–1985. (Source: Office of Population and Census survey.)

aspirin for rheumatic disease had gastric erythema, 40% had gastric erosions and 17% had chronic gastric ulcers, compared with an incidence of 5% gastric erythema and 1% of gastric ulceration in controls. Even patients taking low-dose aspirin in the prophylaxis of coronary artery disease have been shown to have a remarkably increased risk of gastrointestinal haemorrhage. Hudson and colleagues[5] in 1991 looked at the effect of low-dose aspirin on the gastric mucosa and found that a dose of 300 mg per day induced more damage than a smaller dose of 75 mg, but when enteric-coated aspirin was given in a dose

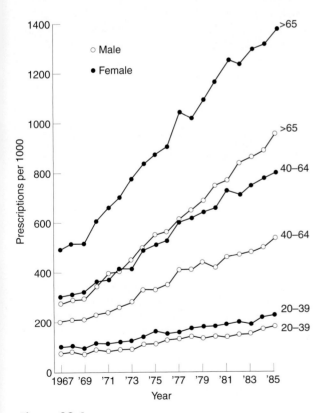

Figure 33.6
Age-specific prescriptions for non-steroidal anti-inflammatory drugs (NSAIDs) in England and Wales over recent years. (Source: Medical Data Index (Intercontinental Medical Statistics Ltd.)

of 300 mg the risk of gastric damage was least. In addition to damaging the stomach, NSAIDs can cause bleeding from the small intestine, where small intestinal diaphragmatic strictures similar to those encountered in Crohn's disease may develop. It is unlikely that *H. pylori* plays a major role in the mechanism of non-steroidal-induced gastric damage.

Saleeby and colleagues[6] in 1991 showed that many patients were being treated with NSAIDs inappropriately, and that these could be stopped without the patients' joint or other underlying problems deteriorating. Clearly, better education of the public could lead to a reduced ingestion of these drugs. There is no evidence that the ulcers produced by NSAIDs differ in any way from peptic ulcers developing in patients not taking these agents. There is, however, a marked difference in the risk of adverse gastrointestinal side-effects occurring with different agents, and these have been estimated to vary from 1.23 per ten prescriptions with meclofamate to 6.52 per ten prescriptions with piroxicam. It has been shown that the majority of gastrointestinal side-effects induced by NSAIDs occur within 3 months of taking the drug, and that there is a substantial decline in the risk within 1 month of stopping treatment.

PATHOGENESIS IN RELATION TO *H. PYLORI*

The problem with all secretory inhibitory drugs, including the H_2-receptor antagonists and omeprazole, is that whilst they are capable of healing ulcers, in the vast majority of cases relapse rates are extremely high within 1–2 months of starting therapy. Stopping any of these drugs results in a return of acid and pepsin secretion to pretreatment levels within a matter of days. Even after continuing the drug for 2 or more years the patient still has an intact vagus, parietal cell and G-cell mass, thus secretion is fundamentally unimpaired. Recurrence rates on complete cessation of drug therapy with the above treatment reached 90% at 1 year, and, even using maintenance therapy in the recommended doses of 400 mg of cimetidine and 150 mg of ranitidine per day, recurrence rates approximated to 2.5% per month, 30% per year. Some years ago it was noted that the period to relapse following effective treatment with the bismuth-containing preparation De-Nol was prolonged when compared with the H_2-receptor antagonists. This work has been substantiated and it now appears that if the organism *H. pylori* can be eradicated by a combination of De-Nol with two appropriate antibiotics then relapse of the ulcer, in the short-term at least, may be very uncommon. Experience with the use of triple therapy consisting of De-Nol and two antibiotics is increasing and consistently reduced incidences of ulcer relapse have been reported. Leading workers in the field, such as Tytgat in Amsterdam and Graham in Houston (see Chapters 29 and 30), have experienced that eradication of the organism results in a prolonged ulcer-free period, and there is only a low incidence of recolonization of the stomach with *H. pylori* at 1 year. Such efficacious medication in the long term goes some considerable way in emphasizing the importance of *H. pylori* in the pathogenesis of peptic ulceration. Even if it is not the main aetiological factor, clearly the organism would appear to play a very important role, as evidenced by the low relapse rate which follows eradication of *Helicobacter*. The fact remains, however, that before the very recent work on prolonged ulcer healing by eradication of *H. pylori*, the only way to heal an ulcer and prevent it from recurring in the long term was by some form of acid-reducing surgery, of which we have a century of experience.

The story surrounding observations on the organism *H. pylori* and its possible relationship with peptic ulcer disease is intriguing. Before the beginning of the twentieth century, bacterial infection was implicated in the aetiology and pathogenesis of peptic ulceration, commonly described organisms in relation to the ulcer crater being staphylococci and streptococci. With more sophisticated methods of measuring acid and pepsin secretion and the recognition of several gastrointestinal hormones, the focus of research shifted to hyperacidity as the major, if not the only, aetiological factor in peptic ulceration. Strategies based on this assumption virtually monopolized the approach of investigators to this problem until the 1980s.

In 1975 Steer and Colin-Jones[7] reported Gram-negative bacteria in close association with the ulcers of about 80% of patients with gastric ulcer, but absent from six subjects with a normal mucosa. They cultured *Pseudomonas aeruginosa* from biopsy specimens. In retrospect it is very likely that what they saw microscopically were *Helicobacter*-like organisms, but they cultured pseudomonas which had contaminated their endoscopes. In 1983, much interest was generated when Warren and Marshall[8] found curved or spiral 'campylobacter-like' organisms in endoscopic antral mucosal biopsies from patients with gastritis and peptic ulceration (Figure 33.7). It was suggested then that these bacteria might be the cause of gastritis and peptic ulcers and it was rapidly shown by many other workers from all over the world that these organisms were commonly present in patients with gastritis and ulceration. Koch's third and fourth postulates demand that innoculation with the micro-organism should produce the disease in a susceptible individual and that micro-organisms should then be found in the diseased areas. In an attempt to fulfil these postulates Marshall and Warren[9] showed that the ingestion of 10^9 colony forming units of campylobacter-like organisms led to an acute and painful inflammatory reaction in previously normal gastric mucosa. Further evidence linking campylobacter-like organisms with acute gastritis came with an outbreak of hypochlorhydric gastritis in 17 of 37 volunteers who had undergone gastric secretion studies in which a pH electrode that had not been adequately sterilized between experiments was used.

It has now become clear that these organisms have been overlooked for some considerable time. Although they resemble bacteria of the genus *Campylobacter*, they do not fit morphologically with any known species. They have 4–6 unipolar sheathed flagella, unlike the single unsheathed flagellum of most *Campylobacter* species. This led to a change of nomenclature in 1989 to *Helicobacter pylori*; before that the name had been changed from *Campylobacter pyloridis*.[10,11]

The close contact of these organisms with inflamed gastric-type epithelium below the mucosal layer, their occasional phagocytosis by polymorphonuclear leucocytes and their absence from normal mucosa suggest that they are aetiologically related to gastritis. Their ability to adhere to cell membranes seems a further step towards proving their pathogenecity. Also, eradication of the organisms leads to disappearance of these changes.[12-17]

The epidemiology of the organism has not yet been evaluated fully. Its prevalence varies with age, race, geographic location and associated disease states such as non-ulcer dyspepsia and gastric or duodenal ulceration. Overall the organism is present in about 20% of the asymptomatic population, 60–70% of patients with non-ulcer dyspepsia, 70–90% of patients with gastric ulcer and 80–100% of patients with duodenal ulcer.

H. pylori is sensitive in vitro to a number of antibiotics, including β-lactams, macrolides, tetracycline, clarithromycin and metronidazole. However, in vitro sensitivity does not parallel in vivo efficacy in eradicating the micro-organisms. Bacterial resistence to amoxycillin, colloidal bismuth subcitrate and metronidazole, in combination, does not appear to be a problem. It would appear that a 2-week course of triple therapy is capable of eradicating the organism from the majority of patients with helicobacter-associated gastritis or ulceration and that, once eradicated, reinfection is uncommon, at least within 1–2 years (Chapter 29). It clearly needs to be determined in the next few years whether or not such therapy is optimal in the treatment of peptic ulceration and whether it should be used as a first-line mode of therapy, prior to the use of acid-inhibiting drugs, such as the H_2-receptor antagonists or omeprazole. If this turns out to be the case then there may be an even smaller role for elective surgery in the management of chronic peptic ulceration.[18]

HISTORY OF ULCER SURGERY

William Beaumont (1785–1853), a US Army Doctor, treated and observed for some 8 years a Canadian named Alexis St Martin, who had been wounded at close range on 6 June 1822, by a shot in the stomach. He was left with a gastric fistula through which a large area of gastric mucous membrane could

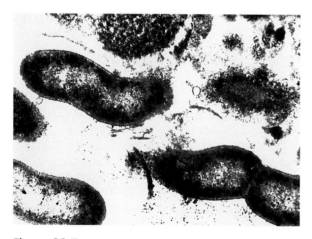

Figure 33.7
The organism *Helicobacter pylori*.

be seen. Beaumont studied the gastric mucosa of Alexis, and carried out experiments on the gastric juice. The studies formed the subject of a book *Experiments and Observations on the Gastric Juice and the Physiology of Digestion*, in 1833.[19] The influence of the patient's state of mind on the gastric mucosa was impressive, anger turning the mucous membrane red! These experiments were repeated over a century later by Wolff and Wolff,[20] who studied an experimental subject, 'Tom', with a gastric fistula similar to that of Alexis St Martin. The experiments described by Beaumont and Wolff and Wolff are classic and do much to show the effect of emotion and the sympathetic nervous system on the gastric mucosa.

Surgery for duodenal ulcer was initiated over a century ago to overcome mechanical obstruction to the pyloric outlet. Gastroenterostomy for an obstructing cancer was described by Anton Wolfler,[21] one of Billroth's assistants, in 1881. This procedure was first performed for duodenal ulcer in 1892 by Eugene Doyen of Paris. Moynihan of Leeds[22] and the Mayo brothers[23] developed international reputations largely on the strength of their ability to perform gastroenterostomy for duodenal ulcer with a mortality of 1% or less in large numbers of patients (500 and 2000 respectively) by the time of World War I. Over a 20-year period at the start of the twentieth century, abdominal surgery had been revolutionized, largely as a result of the important observations in the field of antisepsis by Semmelweis and Lister.[24] Indeed, when in 1881 Billroth[25] performed the first partial gastrectomy for gastric cancer he became a convert to surgical antisepsis. He performed his classic operation on Teresa Heller, using a somewhat loose application of the principles of antisepsis enunciated by Lister. As early as 21 November 1881, Rydiger[26] became the first to perform an operation like a Billroth I for gastric ulcer. His patient, a 30-year-old woman, had suffered for 3 years from gastrointestinal bleeding. After this operation she went home cured, and after bearing five children, was still healthy a quarter of a century later.

Vagotomy

A scientific basis for vagotomy was propounded by Ivan Pavlov[27] who was awarded the Nobel prize in 1904 for an elegant piece of work in which he showed that division of the vagi abolished the cephalic phase of gastric secretion. The presence of the antral hormone, gastrin, was demonstrated by John Edkins in 1906, and in 1963 the Liverpool physiologist, R A Gregory, was able to confirm the former scientist's findings and to isolate gastrin.[28] The aphorism 'no acid, no ulcer' was enunciated by Schwartz[29] in 1910, and holds true to the present day, despite current heated debate over the role of *H. pylori*.

In 1925, Bircher[30] described a type of selective vagotomy of the gastric fundus. In 1922 André Latarjet[31] performed an operation resembling a selective vagotomy in 24 patients, six of whom had duodenal ulcer; he had previously described that vagotomy produced gastric stasis, so he added a gastroenterostomy to all of these procedures. It was not until 1943, however, that vagotomy became established as an operation for duodenal ulcer by Dragsted and Owens.[32] Initially they performed a

supradiaphragmatic truncal vagotomy alone, but like Latarjet discovered that an accompanying gastrojejunostomy was necessary to relieve the bloating, distension and possible gastric ulceration that accrued as a result of delayed gastric emptying. Truncal vagotomy accompanied with a drainage procedure, either pyloroplasty or gastrojejunostomy, became the most commonly performed operation for chronic dudodenal ulcer in Great Britain, and has remained so to the present day. Truncal vagotomy results in approximately a 65% reduction in maximal acid output; removal of the G-cell-containing antrum is followed by a similar reduction. The combination of truncal vagotomy with antrectomy results in approximately 95% reduction in acid secretion. In a careful follow-up study of 589 patients operated on for duodenal ulcer, Pollock[33] showed in 1952 that neostomal ulcer was observed in only 2%.

Drainage procedures

The necessity for a drainage procedure when performing truncal vagotomy had been confirmed by many workers in the 1950s and 1960s. The Heineke–Mikulicz pyloroplasty was first performed in 1886, and in 1887 Mikulicz reported the case of a female factory worker aged 17 for whom he did a pyloroplasty for a bleeding duodenal ulcer. A deep crater extending 2 cm into the pancreas was present at operation.

Gastrojejunostomy

Gastrojejunostomy alone has been shown to be an unsatisfactory procedure for duodenal ulcer from as early as 1925, when Lewisohn[34] reported a 34% incidence of neostomal ulcer after gastrojejunostomy at the New York Mount Sinai Hospital. In 1930, Judd and Hazeltine[35] reported a technique of pylorplasty and concomitant excision of duodenal ulcer, stating that satisfactory results could be obtained in 90% of patients; however high recurrence rates were soon reported. Gastrojejunostomy was used by Dragsted[36] to complement truncal vagotomy, and became widely used until Weinberg et al.[37] in 1956, described a favourable report of vagotomy and pyloroplasty with an 8% incidence of recurrence.

Billroth I gastrectomy

Between the 1920s and 1960s, gastric resection was also widely used for chronic duodenal ulcer. However, in 1939 one of the keenest exponents of Billroth I operation for duodenal ulcer, Hans van Haberer, abandoned the procedure, finding that neostomal ulcer complicated the operation with an unexpectedly high frequency. Ordahl et al.[38] in Boston, and Goligher et al[39] in Leeds, in the mid-1950s, reported an approximately 20% incidence of neostomal ulcer in patients with duodenal ulcer treated by Billroth I resection. However, vagotomy plus antrectomy, as developed by H Harkins, has been widely used and remains probably the most effective way of preventing recurrent ulceration, albeit at the cost of significant postoperative sequelae.

Billroth II gastrectomy

Even after the more radical degree of gastric resection achieved in performing a Billroth II procedure, recurrence rates as high as 24% at 10 years have been reported in 1965 by Scott, from the Vanderbilt Clinic. With the advent of increasing use of vagotomy, by the mid-1960s few surgeons were still performing gastric resection alone for chronic duodenal ulcer.

Antral exclusion

The operation of antral exclusion was devised in 1895 by Eiselsberg[40] for advanced gastric cancer. This procedure was associated with a tremendous increase in acid–pepsin secretion. Dragsted and his associates,[41] in 1951, showed an extremely high incidence of recurrent stomal ulceration, the reason being that when the G cells are taken out of circuit from the main gastrointestinal tract, inhibitory factors are prevented from reducing the outpouring of gastrin from these cells, and consequently hypergastrinaemia increases acid–pepsin secretion, resulting in stomal ulceration.

Selective vagotomy

Selective vagotomy was introduced by Franksson[42] and Jackson[43] in the late 1940s, in the hope that, by preserving the hepatic branches of the anterior vagus and coeliac branches of the posterior vagus, the incidence of postvagotomy diarrhoea and dumping could be reduced. As the nerves of Latarjet, which continue from the main vagal trunks after the hepatic and coeliac branches are given off, are completely divided, then the antrum is also denervated, thus necessitating some form of drainage procedure. Selective vagotomy with a drainage procedure was shown to be a reliable method of denervating the acid-secreting part of the stomach, and, at the same time, of reducing the incidence of postvagotomy diarrhoea, but the procedure was never widely adopted. This was because, firstly, many surgeons could not see the advantages of preserving the hepatic and coeliac branches, and secondly, soon after the procedure was developed, and before it became more widely used, highly selective vagotomy was developed and surgeons employing denervation of the stomach in the treatment of peptic ulceration tended to polarize between either truncal vagotomy and one of its associated procedures, or the more recent highly selective vagotomy.

Highly selective vagotomy

The ultimate in conservative division of the gastric vagi, hence the alternative terms 'proximal gastric vagotomy' and 'parietal cell vagotomy', restricts denervation to the acid–pepsin-secreting part of the stomach, the fundus and corpus. The parietal cell area of the stomach is wholly denervated by this procedure, whilst at the same time the innervation of the antrum and pylorus is completely preserved. Antral innervation is maintained by the careful preservation of the nerves of Latarjet, which run along the anterior and posterior walls of the lesser curvature of the stomach and are frequently multiple, fanning from the continuation of the main vagus nerves as they run along the lesser curvature. The hepatic branches of the anterior vagus and the coeliac branches of the posterior vagus are thus preserved and hence the innervation of the hepatobiliary system, pancreas and the whole of the small bowel is maintained.

The operation was promulgated to overcome three of the major side-effects of the more radical forms of the vagotomy: diarrhoea, dumping and duodenogastric reflux with bilious vomiting. These complications are unpredictable and frequently incurable. The concept of proximal gastric vagotomy originated in experimental work carried out by Griffith and Harkins in 1957.[44] It is possible that Latarjet himself was performing a procedure not too dissimilar from this, back in the 1920s, but Holle introduced the technique in man in 1967, although he performed a drainage procedure with it, usually a pyloroplasty. It was felt that the use of this drainage procedure was unnecessary and that the effects may be deleterious so that Johnston and Wilkinson[45] in Leeds, and Amdrup and Jensen[46] in Copenhagen performed the operation without a drainage procedure in 1970. Short-term results showed no evidence of impaired motor function of the stomach so that gastric drainage was not carried out by the vast majority of the investigators using this procedure. These early workers showed that complete parietal cell denervation could be achieved by this technique, at least in the short term. A disadvantage of the operation is, however, that it is unquestionably more tedious to perform than truncal vagotomy and drainage, and complete parietal cell denervation may not always be achieved by the less experienced operator. Argument existed in the early days of the performance of this procedure about the preservation of the vagally innervated antrum, which when kept in continuity seemed to offer the potential, at least theoretically, of further protection. The operation has now been shown to be very safe, with a low incidence of dumping and diarrhoea, the former being virtually abolished; some longer-term studies have, however, shown disturbingly high incidences of late recurrent ulceration.[47–63]

Anterior lesser curve seromyotomy with posterior truncal vagotomy

As a modification of highly selective vagotomy, anterior lesser curve seromyotomy with posterior truncal vagotomy was introduced by the author in 1979. The arguments in favour of the performance of this alternative pylorus-preserving technique were: firstly, technical simplicity; secondly, the confident performance of complete parietal cell denervation of the posterior wall of the stomach; and, thirdly, the elimination of the small potential risk of ischaemic necrosis of the lesser curvature of the stomach. The low incidence of dumping and diarrhoea associated with highly selective vagotomy is also maintained when performing this alternative procedure.[64–68]

INDICATIONS FOR SURGERY IN PEPTIC ULCER DISEASE

Elective operation for duodenal ulcer was one of the most common procedures performed by the general surgeon until the 1980s. Indeed, Moynihan in 1928, maintained that all patients with a duodenal ulcer should undergo surgical treatment. Now, very few surgeons regularly operate on patients with uncomplicated ulcer disease. There remain, however, indications for performing elective ulcer surgery under certain circumstances. It was shown by Pulvertaft, in 1968, that on reaching the age of 50 years both male and female patients have a 25% risk of significant ulcer haemorrhage within the next decade of their lives. The corresponding figures for risk of perforation over the decade between the ages of 50 and 60 years are 9% for males and 7% for females. These incidences increase with each subsequent decade therafter. The overall mortality for upper gastrointestinal bleeding remains today, as it has throughout the twentieth century, at around 10%, and the mortality for ulcer perforation is at least 10%.[18] These complications give rise to the overall mortality for peptic ulceration of 4500 per year in England and Wales. These figures may change, however, with successful eradication of *H. pylori*, and future data are awaited with interest.

If progress is to be made towards reducing this mortality, then ulcers in those patients who are at risk of developing these complications must be healed and healing must be maintained in the long term. Apart from the potential which the long-term eradication of *H. pylori* may show, at present the only established way of maintaining ulcer healing is by ulcer surgery. The more aggressive this surgery, in terms of acid reduction, the more likely is the ulcer to remain healed but at the price of some undesirable and often incurable side-effects such as dumping and diarrhoea. The more conservative the surgery, the less likely the patient is to have undesirable side-effects. However, there is an unacceptably high incidence of ulcer recurrence with the more conservative forms of surgery. Today we need to revise radically our overall indications for elective ulcer surgery in the light of the ever-increasing array of effective drug therapy available to us. However, some indications remain.

INDICATIONS FOR ELECTIVE ULCER SURGERY

Intractable pain

Intractable pain, often producing loss of sleep and social and economic dislocation, used to be the major indication for elective ulcer surgery. Now, most patients achieve symptomatic relief within days of beginning a course of either an H_2-receptor antagonist or omeprazole. Those 5–10% of patients whose pain is not relieved by these powerful drugs may not be helped by surgery. In these refractory patients, the diagnosis must be challenged and evidence sought for a second pathology such as chronic pancreatitis or Zollinger–Ellison syndrome. Further endoscopy is required for these patients in order to establish the presence of ulceration, and, in addition, this is one of the few indications for carrying out tests of acid secretion in response to a pentagastrin stimulus. If a pentagastrin test shows a high basal acid output and a high peak acid output with a low ratio of peak output to basal output, then serum gastrin estimations should be carried out and computed tomography of the upper abdomen performed to look for a gastrinoma. It remains important to advise heavy smokers or drinkers to curtail these habits. Whilst smoking is not a cause of peptic ulceration, it undoubtedly contributes to morbidity and there is a very definite and proven association between cigarette smoking and duodenal ulcer disease. It may well be that reduced smoking habits in the male population in this country have contributed in some way towards the decline in the overall prevalence of the disorder, and conversely that increased tobacco consumption in females may be related to their rising mortality rates.

For those whose pain is alleviated by drug therapy and whose ulcers subsequently heal, the question of duration of medication arises. The H_2-receptor antagonists are very safe drugs to use, even in the long term, and, despite anxieties about omeprazole, there has been no case of gastric cancer or carcinoid after ten years use of this drug in patients in Holland. In view of the almost inevitable ulcer recurrence after stopping potent acid secretory inhibitors, the question of long-term maintenance or full-dose continuous therapy remains pertinent. Despite the extensive use of these drugs over the past decade, ulcer mortality remains high and the high incidence of relapse following cessation of these drugs remains a problem.[18] Of deaths from ulcer complications, 95% occur in patients over the age of 55 years. The mean age of death for males is 69 years and for females is 72 years.

Elective ulcer surgery has the potential to reduce ulcer mortality by maintaining ulcer healing in the long term. In a large study from Edinburgh in which mortality was assessed in patients undergoing surgery for peptic ulcer, no patient who had previously undergone peptic ulcer surgery developed a fatal ulcer-associated complication.[69] The same is true of most large studies, which show that, whereas ulcer recurrence occurs, often in undesirably large numbers after ulcer surgery, the number of perforations and significant bleeding episodes subsequent to surgery are few. Although the potential for recurrence of ulceration remains in some patients after peptic ulcer surgery, perhaps the aggression of the ulcer is reduced, and with it the potential to bleed or perforate.

If, therefore, a policy were employed whereby those patients with an aggressive ulcer diathesis at the age of 50 underwent surgical treatment, then many deaths in later years might be prevented. An aggressive ulcer diathesis implies those ulcers in *H. pylori*-negative patients which recur rapidly after cessation of H_2-receptor antagonists, or those in whom these drugs fail to control symptoms completely or to heal the ulcer within 2 months. This strategy should prevent these patients from developing complications which carry a 10% mortality later in life. Clearly, not all complications of ulceration in the elderly could be prevented by such a strategy because many patients present with a complication from a hitherto asymptomatic ulcer, and this is particularly true of those who are treated with NSAIDs. However, close scrutiny of mortality rates in those with a well-established ulcer diathesis gives room for optimism. If we consider a cohort of 1000 patients with an aggressive ulcer diathesis by the age of 50 years, from Pulvertaft's figures, over the next decade 250 will bleed and 75% of these, who are treated conservatively, will rebleed, giving rise to a mortality for bleeding of 10% (43 deaths) over a decade.[18] The corresponding figures for ulcer perforation over the same decade would give rise to nine deaths (9% incidence and 10% mortality). Thus 52 of the 1000 patients in whom no permanent acid reduction was achieved might die. What of the mortality of elective peptic ulcer surgery? In 1975 Johnston estimated that the mortality for highly selective vagotomy was 0.3% in 5000 patients, and the mortality for anterior lesser curve seromyotomy and posterior truncal vagotomy is 0.16%.[67] Thus, if these patients were treated electively by highly selective vagotomy or lesser curve seromyotomy at the age of 50 years, where an ulcer diathesis had become well established, there would be only two deaths in a series of 1000 patients, which represents a massive potential reduction in mortality from peptic ulcer in those with a chronic well-established ulcer diathesis. Both of these procedures can be performed laparoscopically. Clearly the above argument could not be applied to all patients with duodenal ulcer. Some have ulcers which remain asymptomatic up to the time that either perforation or major haemorrhage occurs. In others, the ulcer diathesis begins late in life, sometimes symptoms being present for the first time at or beyond the age of 50. Having conceded the above, however, the majority of patients with chronic peptic ulcers which have the potential to bleed or perforate develop symptoms before the age of 50 years. Once such an ulcer diathesis is established, there is a high incidence of relapse and recurrence, the rate of which increases with increasing age, as indeed does the likelihood of a potentially fatal complication. Now that anterior lesser curve seromyotomy with posterior truncal vagotomy or highly selective vagotomy can be performed endoscopically, however, the surgical argument could once more gain strength.

It could be recommended, therefore, that those subjects with a well-established ulcer diathesis who frequently relapse after cessation of treatment by H$_2$-receptor antagonists and after a course of therapy to eliminate *H. pylori* should be considered for elective ulcer surgery, particularly if they are approaching the age of 50 years. Only in this way can ulcer complications be potentially prevented and the mortality reduced. At the present time there is no evidence that the new medical methods of treating ulcers are reducing mortality in fact it is still increasing.

Gastric outlet stenosis

Aggressive duodenal ulceration with the formation of dense fibrous tissue in the region of the ulcer may give rise to stenosis of the first part of the duodenum just beyond the pylorus.[70] This produces dilatation of the stomach with hypertrophy of the gastric musculature and an increase in acid output, thus increasing the aggression of the process of ulceration. The condition is suspected clinically from the history of postprandial vomiting,[71] often of large volume, and occasionally the vomitus may contain undigested food residue of meals which were eaten 2–3 days previously. Weight loss is common and abdominal examination reveals a succession splash in the epigastrium or left hypochondrium long after the last meal was taken.[72-77] In the patient with a very thin abdomen peristalsis of the small intestine may be visible. A 3–4-day trial of fasting, nasogastric suction, fluid and electrolyte replacement and parenteral H$_2$-receptor antagonist therapy should differentiate transient obstruction caused by acute inflammation and oedema from chronic cicatricial obstruction which requires surgical correction. Endoscopy will also

indicate the presence of narrowing; when the normal end-viewing gastroscope will not pass into the duodenum, significant stenosis is present. Sometimes the narrowing may be so severe that a guide wire passed along the endoscopic biopsy channel may not pass through the stricture.

Endoscopy should always be carried out as it enables the important differentiation to be made between benign and malignant causes of gastric outlet obstruction. In the presence of raised mucosal irregularities, with active ulceration of the mucosal tissue, biopsies should always be taken to exclude a small prepyloric carcinoma.

Quantitation of the degree of gastric outlet obstruction can be acquired by radioisotope scanning. A liquid- and solid-phase marker used simultaneously to label a meal, such as cornflakes, porridge, hamburgers or omelettes, can estimate independently liquid- and solid-phase gastric emptying. Liquid meals commonly have a $T_{1/2}$ emptying time of 10–15 minutes, whereas solid components empty more slowly, normally having a $T_{1/2}$ of about 45 minutes. In the presence of marked pyloric stenosis, little or no emptying may be seen in the first 1–2 hours of the examination. Barium meal examination also gives the radiologist an indication of the presence of significant pyloric stenosis when the barium fails to empty from the stomach; in addition, a rather beaked appearance of the column of barium leaving the stomach further supports such a diagnosis.

It is possible, in the presence of mild to moderate pyloric stenosis, where there is a predominance of oedema rather than frank fibrosis, to dilate the gastric outlet endoscopically using a balloon dilator passed over a guide wire. This procedure is feasible when dilatation is not too difficult, but there is a risk of perforation of the duodenum, which usually coincides with the site of the ulcer crater. There is also a significant risk of recurrence of the stenosis following endoscopic dilatation alone. In general, a significant degree of pyloric stenosis remains a firm indication for operative treatment of this condition.[78] The operation of choice is proximal gastric vagotomy or anterior lesser curve seromyotomy and posterior truncal vagotomy, either of which should be performed with a small distal posterior gastroenterostomy or pyloroplasty.[79,80]

Penetration

A posterior duodenal ulcer may penetrate into the pancreas or posterior abdominal wall. There may be abscess formation or complete erosion of the back of the duodenum, the base of the ulcer comprising the head of the pancreas, covered by a layer of necrotic debris. Under these circumstances, healing is much more difficult to achieve with drug therapy. It may also be difficult to exclude underlying pancreatic disease as a cause of the problem rather than peptic ulceration *per se*. If there is no delay in gastric emptying, the operation of choice is a pylorus-preserving vagotomy with biopsy of any inflammatory mass which may exist in the region of the pancreas.

Perforation

The development of acute peritonitis due to free perforation of a duodenal ulcer is usually regarded as an absolute indication for surgery.[81,82] Around the turn of the century, non-operative intervention resulted almost inevitably in death, although conservative therapy with nasogastric aspiration, analgesia, H_2-receptor antagonists and antibiotics has been shown to be remarkably successful in recent years.[83,84] Although one would not advocate such a conservative approach as the first-line treatment of perforation, it may be used for those, who, by virtue of coexisting medical conditions, are regarded as a major risk for anaesthesia and operation, or for moribund patients presenting in irreversible shock, where surgical therapy is associated with a mortality in excess of 50%. Surgical management here is emergency laparotomy and either simple oversew of the perforation or the addition of an acid-reducing procedure[85-88] (see Chapter 34).

The mortality from perforation is at least 10%, as many of these patients have coexisting medical conditions, which are exacerbated by peritonitis and general anaesthesia.

Haemorrhage

Bleeding from an ulcer may be an indication for either elective or emergency surgery. Recurrent episodes of persistent low-grade bleeding may be an indication for surgery, particularly in elderly patients who present with recurrent anaemia despite the use of H_2-receptor antagonists. Those who have once bled run the risk of rebleeding in about 75% of cases over a subsequent 5-year period. The mortality from a major haemorrhage is about 10%, or higher in those over the age of 65 years. Thus, two distinct haemorrhagic episodes could be regarded as an indication for elective peptic ulcer surgery, particularly if the patient is over the age of 50 years. Acute bleeding is today the most common indication for duodenal ulcer surgery, which for active and persistent bleeding should be carried out as an emergency procedure (see Chapter 38). Patients who are bleeding are assessed from the point of view of length of duodenal ulcer history, previous episodes of bleeding, degree of shock, extent of transfusion and coexisting medical state. No hard and fast rules have generally been accepted for surgical intervention.[89-91] Clearly, the more blood that is transfused, the greater the haemodynamic and clotting problems that exist when the operation is finally performed. On the other hand, early surgery may submit to operation many who would otherwise settle spontaneously. Hunt, by carrying out an aggressive policy of admission to an intensive care unit and the performance of emergency surgery after a 4-unit blood transfusion, showed that mortality could be reduced from 9.5 to 2.7% in three consecutive 3-year periods.[92-94] However, a similar study carried out by an haematemesis management team in Glasgow failed to produce such a reduction in mortality.[95] The patient who is at risk from further haemorrhage can, to some extent, be predicted by endoscopy, which must always be performed to identify the site of bleeding and to exclude the presence of varices.[96] The presence of fresh bleeding, fresh thrombus or a visible vessel identifies the patient who is at risk of further bleeding.[97] In one large study, 28 of 289 patients had a visible vessel. All experienced recurrent bleeding and in four patients it was uncontrollable.[98] Of those patients without a visible

vessel, 75% had a single bleeding episode. Both similar and conflicting results have been reported by others. Most surgeons feel, however, that such a visible vessel is an indication for surgery.[99]

A number of therapeutic options now exist whereby an endoscopic procedure may arrest the haemorrhage. These include the use of monopolar and bipolar electrodes, heater probes, laser and the injection of substances such as adrenaline, saline or a sclerosing agent in and around the ulcer (see Chapter 24). Most of these methods are effective in achieving short-term arrest of haemorrhage in a high proportion of patients, although rebleeding rates are high and none of these methods has as yet been shown to reduce ulcer mortality significantly. Of the above, probably the best is the injection of adrenaline. A further simple new method introduced by the author is that of isolated duodenal tamponade[100] (Figure 33.8). The bulb-like shape of the first part of the duodenum, where 95% of duodenal ulcers occur, is created proximally by the heavy condensation of circular muscle which makes up the pyloric sphincter, and distally by a natural anatomical narrowing and abrupt 90° angulation. The volume of the balloon used in this device is about 30 ml, its maximum radius is 2.5 cm and the radius of the relatively rigid and indistensible pyloric sphincter is about 1 cm. These anatomical contours make the duodenal bulb suitable for impaction within it of the balloon, which can accurately and predictably exert pressure on its walls. The balloon has been designed in order to produce tamponade on the walls of the duodenal bulb. It surrounds a central tube which is flexible, but non-compressible when the balloon is inflated, thus maintaining gastrointestinal continuity between the stomach and second part of the duodenum. The device is passed over the distal 7 cm of a conventional flexible end-viewing gastroduodenoscope to abut against a ring-like backstop. Inflation is possible by means of a 70 cm fine tube which runs along the length of the endoscope; its other end is attached by means of a three-way tap to a pressure recording manometer. In use, the gastroduodenoscope and deflated balloon are inserted through the pylorus and into the duodenal cap. The bleeding ulcer is identified in the usual way and the presence of active bleeding or a visible vessel can be appreciated by advancing the tip of the endoscope just into the second part of the duodenum. The balloon is inflated to fill the duodenal bulb completely and the endoscope is then withdrawn, leaving the balloon inflated and impacted in the duodenal bulb, producing tamponade within its walls. Once the balloon is inflated, traction applied to the endoscope results in disconnection of the endoscope from the balloon, as the latter cannot be withdrawn through the dense muscle of the pyloric sphincter. Intestinal continuity is maintained when the balloon is inflated because the reinforced central tube is non-collapsible. The balloon can be inserted in as little as 3 minutes and, in the author's experience, haemorrhage has always been arrested. It is then left in place, inflated overnight. The device is entirely disposable and no expensive back-up facilities are required. It can be inserted immediately the patient is endoscoped, either in the accident and emergency department, the endoscopy suite or on the ward. No skills additional to those

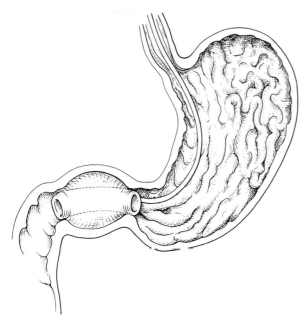

Figure 33.8
A duodenal tamponade balloon used for arresting
haemorrhage from a duodenal ulcer.

of performing adequate endoscopic examination of the duodenum are required to apply this device, which is extremely
simple and safe to insert. The patency of the central tube
maintains intestinal continuity, which is likely to prevent the
hypersecretory affects associated with complete gastric outlet
obstruction.

Although such endoscopic techniques and devices hold
promise in arresting haemorrhage from duodenal ulcer, surgery
remains the only definitive way in which long-term security
can be obtained, by combining an acid-reducing operation
with oversew of the bleeding ulcer. The operation of choice is
a pylorus-preserving vagotomy with oversew of the bleeding
point in the ulcer crater. Either polydioxanone (PDS) or a
totally non-absorbable suture material should be used for this
purpose; the duodenum is opened longitudinally, distal to the
pylorus, and closed transversely, the pylorus remaining intact.

IS THERE A ROLE FOR ENDOSCOPIC ULCER SURGERY IN THE FUTURE?

It is possible that the development of endoscopic techniques
may in the future give rise to a greater role for surgery in the
treatment of chronic duodenal ulceration. Laparoscopic cholecystectomy has rapidly become the treatment of choice for
symptomatic gallstones. Laparoscopic techniques are also
being developed for use elsewhere in the gastrointestinal tract,
even in aiding colonic or oesophageal resection. Carrying out
the operation of anterior lesser curve seromyotomy with posterior truncal vagotomy employing a laparoscope and a laser has
also been shown to be possible. The posterior vagus nerve
trunk can be identified and divided laparoscopically; the gastric
branches of the anterior nerve of Latarjet can be divided using
a laser as they run along the anterior gastric wall close to the
lesser curvature before penetrating the seromuscular layer of

the stomach. Alternatively a sliver of lesser curvature can be
removed by a stapling technique. Highly selective and truncal
vagotomy have also been achieved endoscopically. Such procedures are being carried out although there is, as yet, no
report of their long-term efficacy in the surgical literature.
However, these may be techniques which, like laparoscopic
cholecystectomy, become more widely employed in the future;
they have the advantage of short hospital stay and early return
to work. The role of and enthusiasm for laparoscopic techniques in ulcer surgery will depend again on the long-term
efficacy of *H. pylori* eradication therapy.

SURGICAL TECHNIQUES

Anatomy relating to highly selective vagotomy

The disposition of the vagal fibres in relation to the lower
oesophagus, gastro-oesophageal junction and lesser curvature
has been discussed previously, but there are several points
worthy of emphasis here. The anterior vagus nerve is closely
applied to the anterior oesophageal wall and, having given off
the hepatic branches, it becomes splayed, in a spatulate fashion, at the gastro-oesophageal junction (Figure 33.9). Here it
gives branches to the gastric fundus before continuing along
the lesser curvature of the stomach. Along the gastric lesser
curvature, branches pass from the nerve or nerves of Latarjet to
innervate the parietal cell mass. These branches run superficial
to the serosa of the stomach, to which they are closely adherent. They pass superficial to, and have no particular predilection to run with, the vasculature from the left gastric vessels.
About one-third of the distance along the wall of the stomach
the nerves penetrate the serosa and musculature to ramify and
form a complete, complex submucosal syncitium before innervating the parietal cells[68] (Figure 33.10).

Both the anterior and posterior nerves of Latarjet are often
multiple, two or three divisions of the vagus running down in
the lesser omentum to the antrum and lying 1–2 cm from the

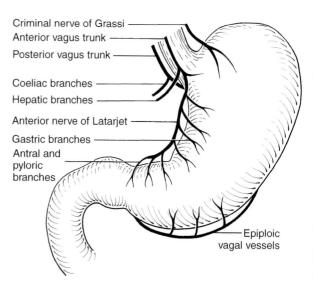

Criminal nerve of Grassi
Anterior vagus trunk
Posterior vagus trunk

Coeliac branches
Hepatic branches

Anterior nerve of Latarjet

Gastric branches
Antral and
pyloric
branches

Epiploic
vagal vessels

Figure 33.9
The vagus nerve trunks.

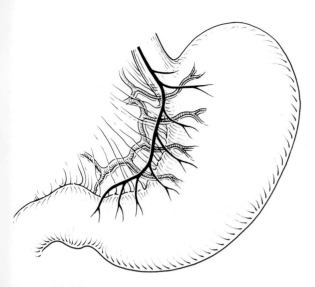

Figure 33.10
Anatomical relationship between blood vessels and nerves along the gastric lesser curvature.

lesser curvature. At the 'crow's foot', which corresponds approximately to the incisura, the terminal fibres of the nerve spread out across the anterior and posterior antral walls. These are the fibres which must be preserved in this operation.

Operative technique of highly selective vagotomy

Meticulous care of fine detail is required in achieving adequate denervation of the parietal cell mass at this operation. Good access to the proximal stomach and distal oesophagus is essential. A long upper midline incision extending from the tip of the xiphoid, skirting the umbilicus and extending 2–3 cm below gives the best exposure. A sternum-lifting hook retractor, similar to that described by Goligher, is useful (Figure 33.11). This is attached by a chain to an anaesthetist's square headframe, so as to exert considerable traction on the lower sternum, thus lifting it and allowing better access to the distal oesophagus and cardia of the stomach.

The dissection begins with the incision of the peritoneum over the distal oesophagus as it is reflected from the diaphragm on to the viscera. The index and middle fingers of the operator are gently insinuated round the distal oesophagus, which is carefully mobilized over the lower 8 cm or so. A soft rubber sling placed around the lower oesophagus may be helpful at this point. The anterior vagus nerve trunk is mobilized next and a fine sling is placed around it (Figure 33.12).

The posterior nerve is now identified before the operator returns to the anterior nerve at its lower end. The posterior trunk lies some distance, usually 1–2 cm, behind the distal oesophagus, and is more easily separated from adjacent fatty tissues than is the anterior trunk. This nerve is usually larger than the anterior and may be multiple, two or occasionally three trunks being present. Mobilization over a distance of about 8 cm of distal oesophagus is carried out and a fine sling is placed around it. In carrying out the mobilization of the vagal trunks the surgeon may find it helpful to divide the triangular ligament over the left lobe of the liver and thus separate this from the diaphgram.

If more than one anterior nerve trunk exists, the main one can be identified as that with the spatulate spread of fibres at the gastro-oesophageal junction. This is the nerve which gives off the hepatic branches, which can usually quite easily be seen spreading across in the direction of the porta hepatis. Smaller subsidiary nerves are divided. The slings around the nerve trunks are used gently to retract the trunks to the patient's right and the lower 8–10 cm of distal oesophagus is meticulously cleared of any residual vagal fibres which can be seen running downwards beside the longitudinal muscle fibres. These nerves are elevated with a nerve hook and diathermized. A constant anatomical feature at this point of the dissection is a fatty bundle of areolar tissue which crosses the

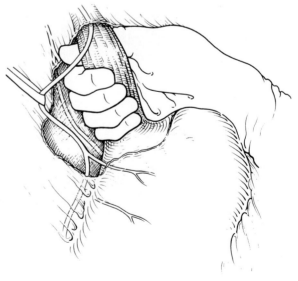

Figure 33.12
Mobilization of the vagal trunks. The anterior trunk is closely applied to the anterior oesophageal wall. The posterior trunk lies in the loose fatty and areolar tissue about 2 cm behind the posterior oesophageal wall.

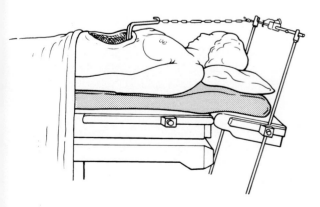

Figure 33.11
Positioning of the patient on the operating table, showing the use of the sternal retractor.

oesophagogastric junction anteriorly. The bundle contains many nerve fibres spreading across to fan out on the fundus of the stomach. It is the author's practice to divide this structure between Lahey forceps.

A window is next made in the lesser omentum, which is largely avascular, to allow access to the lesser sac of the peritoneum. The dissection and division of the branches of the nerves of Latarjet as they run across on to the serosa of the stomach is next begun. The nerves of Latarjet may bifurcate or even trifurcate quite high along the lesser curvature, but the major branch always terminates as a 'crow's foot' close to the incisura angularis of the stomach.

Detachment of the anterior leaf of vessels and nerves should begin just above the terminal two branches of the 'crow's foot', 6 cm from the pyloric ring (Figure 33.13). With the nerve of Latarjet clearly in view, the vessels and nerves of the anterior leaf are clamped and divided close to the lesser curvature so as not to damage the main nerve. Fine mosquito-type artery forceps are useful for this purpose. Fine ligatures, for example 3/0 Vicryl are suitable for this process, rather than clips which tend to become detached by catching on swabs. The use of diathermy should always be kept to an absolute minimum. The dissection proceeds proximally and extends on to the lesser curvature itself, high on the wall of the stomach (Figure 33.14). By taking small bites of tissue, it is possible to progress to the level of the distal oesophagus at the point where the fibrofatty bundle was divided, all branches of the nerve of Latarjet from the parietal cell area of the stomach thus having been disconnected.

In the intermediate tissue between the anterior and posterior vagus nerves there is some loose connective tissue containing a

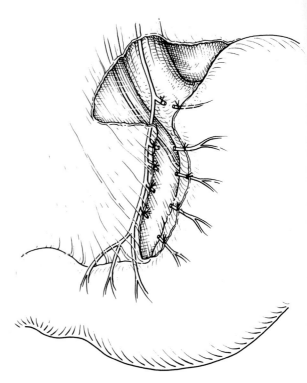

Figure 33.14
The completed anterior leaf of the highly selective vagotomy showing preservation of the nerve of latarjet and the antral innervation.

few blood vessels. These vessels, which are end-arteries, should be clipped, divided and tied, care being taken not to pick up the gastric wall musculature itself. Some filmy adhesions often exist between the stomach and the anterior wall of the pancreas; these should be divided. The posterior nerve of Latarjet can be closely inspected if the stomach is lifted anteriorly and viewed through a window in the lesser curvature.

Staying close in the dissection to the stomach, the posterior leaf of lesser omentum is next dissected clear. Beginning again 6 cm from the pylorus, the dissection proceeds proximally with care being taken to pick out only small bites of tissue and to stay close to the lesser curvature without actually picking up the gastric wall itself. Tying ligatures on the gastric wall, thus picking up some gastric tissue, and excessive use of diathermy are the main factors that render the patient vulnerable to the major technical complication of this procedure, namely ischaemic necrosis of the lesser curvature of the stomach. Conversely, straying too far from the lesser curvature renders the posterior nerve or nerves of Latarjet vulnerable to damage, so precise attention to detail is required and only small amounts of tissue should be picked up with each bite.

It is of major importance to continue the dissection of the lesser curvature up to the oesophagogastric junction. (Figure 33.15) The operator's right hand should eventually pass round this junction to reveal that the lesser omentum containing the anterior and posterior nerves of Latarjet is completely separated from the lesser curvature. When this has been achieved, all the nerve fibres running to the lesser curvature from the continuation of the remaining vagal trunks will have been

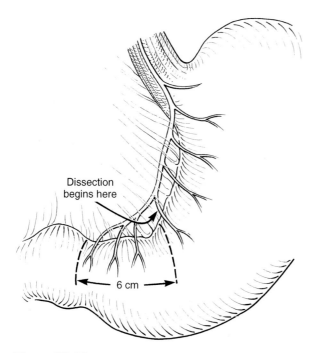

Dissection begins here

6 cm

Figure 33.13
The point of initiating the dissection along the anterior lesser curvature. This is classically at the site of the crow's foot 6 cm from the pylorus.

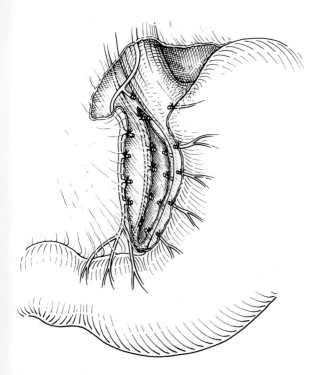

Figure 33.15
The completed highly selective vagotomy.

divided; thus vagotomy of the proximal part of the stomach, the most difficult part of the operation, must be complete.

Attention must now be paid to the distal extent of vagal denervation. Clearly this is an area where insufficient dissection may lead to incomplete vagotomy and more extensive dissection may denervate the essential motor nerves to the antrum. The exact delineation between the parietal area of the stomach and the alkaline antrum can be accurately determined by using the Grassi test, in which a pH probe is applied to the gastric mucosa after an infusion of pentagastrin.[101] This test and the Congo red test[102–106] are based on the fact that denervated parietal cells are less sensitive to circulating pentagastrin than innervated cells. The gastric mucosa is cleansed through a small gastrostomy and a probe is used to map out the mucosal pH during the intravenous infusion of 6 μg/kg per hour of pentagastrin. A pH below 5 indicates residual innervation. Under these circumstances Congo red has also been used to delineate the corpus–antrum junction, which is detected by colour changes. Using this test the exact area of the residual innervation can be detected and subsequently dennervated.

These intraoperative tests for the completeness of vagotomy add considerably to the tedium of the operation. Their value remains contentious, but they have a role in training the vagotomist to achieve adequate denervation of the stomach. Training surgeons to perform this and other more complex gastric operations is becoming an increasing problem in modern surgery, where, with the development of better drug therapy for peptic ulcer and related diseases, few elective vagotomies are being performed anywhere in the Western world.

Nyhus and Donohue[107] have recently shown that dividing the gastroepiploic vessels on the greater curvature of the stomach

at the antrum–corpus junction may lead to more complete denervation of the stomach, as a branch of the vagus can sweep round the pyloric region and run up from the distal stomach to the acid-secreting area. Division of the gastroepiploic vessels close to the greater curvature at this point can lead to more adequate parietal cell denervation and consequently to a reduction in the incidence of recurrent ulcer.

Before completing the operation some surgeons invaginate the lesser curvature of the stomach by suturing the anterior to the posterior gastric wall, thus minimizing any potential risk of perforation due to ischaemic necrosis of the stomach.

Complications of highly selective vagotomy

Lesser curve necrosis is specific to this operation and occurs in a small percentage of cases during the first postoperative week. The perforation may occur anywhere from the oesophagogastric junction down to the incisura angularis and may range in size from less than 1 cm to a 5–6 cm large defect.[108] The condition may occur in about 1% of proximal gastric vagotomies, and is undeniably operator dependent. The technical points of excessive use of diathermy and ligature or clamping of the lesser curvature have already been made. In addition, renal insufficiency, hypertension and generalized atherosclerosis may contribute to this problem.[110] Kennedy and colleagues [109] have pointed out that all three of their patients who, in a series of over 400 cases, developed ischaemic necrosis of the lesser curvature had undergone a combination of proximal gastric vagotomy and fundoplication, whilst in 367 cases treated by proximal gastric vagotomy alone none developed necrosis. In view of this link, and the incidence of 'gas bloat' which follows Nissen fundoplication, it is possible that marked gastric dilatation predisposes to the problem. An alternative hypothesis is that division of the short gastric vessels as well as those on the lesser curvature renders the blood supply to the latter inadequate. In view of this important finding the two operations should not be combined.

The classic features of ischaemic necrosis are epigastric pain, which may be referred to the shoulder-tip or back, shock and generalized peritonitis. Free gas is usually present, lying beneath the diaphragm. Expeditious surgical treatment is required to close the defect. Extensive and delayed perforation may require treatment by gastric resection. Of 19 cases reported in the world literature,[108,109] nine died, confirming the serious nature of this complication.

Holle started performing conservative ulcer surgery in 1964, when he performed proximal gastric vagotomy with pyloroplasty. His own observations led him to believe that a delay in gastric emptying occurred following proximal gastric vagotomy alone.[111–117] The whole question of the mechanism of gastric emptying after highly selective vagotomy remains controversial. Holle, however, maintains that there is significant cicatricial stenosis in about 20% of patients undergoing duodenal ulcer surgery, and 80% have some degree of narrowing; he has added a pyloroplasty in over 1500 patients undergoing proximal gastric vagotomy for duodenal ulcer. Preoperative gastric emptying, assessed by a semisolid meal marked with 300 μl of [^{99m}Tc]DTPA, was delayed in 65%, and when the test was repeated postoperatively, 22% had accelerated emptying, which was severe in 5%. Sixty per cent of his patients had a negative insulin response. The long-term results of this study have been reported as good, with a 4.3% incidence of unsatisfactory results. With increasingly high incidences of recurrent ulceration being reported after highly selective vagotomy without pyloroplasty, perhaps more attention should be given to the contributions of Holle.[118-120]

Anterior lesser curve seromyotomy with posterior truncal vagotomy

Ten years of experience with proximal gastric vagotomy showed that the operation had largely overcome the major problems associated with truncal vagotomy, namely dumping and diarrhoea. The incidence of these complications was less than 1% with the pylorus-preserving procedure. Although Holle felt that pyloroplasty should always be performed with a highly selective vagotomy, the principal protagonists of the procedure, Amdrup and Johnston, were directly opposed to this view because they felt that the performance of the pyloroplasty negated the whole thesis underlying the pylorus-preserving procedure. Holle, however, still did not experience a significant incidence of dumping and diarrhoea and, as late recurrence rates have progressively risen following highly selective vagotomy, he may ultimately be proven to have been correct, in that, by assisting gastric emptying and by not significantly increasing the incidence of dumping and diarrhoea after highly selective vagotomy, pyloroplasty may just prove to be a useful adjunct to the procedure.

The technical precision required to perform an adequate highly selective vagotomy and the somewhat tedious nature of the procedure soon took its toll. Many surgeons never attempted the procedure on these technical grounds, despite its physiological advantages. Many of those who did so were clearly unable to achieve a satisfactory degree of parietal cell denervation and thus had high recurrence rates at an early stage after the procedure, making it perhaps more suitable for the highly skilled specialist. The few vagotomies that are now practised throughout the world further emphasize the nature of the problem of training surgeons adequately to perform this difficult operation.

It was for the above reasons, and because of the risk of ischaemic necrosis, which, though rare, is potentially fatal and totally unpredictable, that lesser curve seromyotomy was developed.[45,64-66]

Anatomical considerations were again of paramount importance in developing this procedure. There are three points of fundamental importance in considering the anatomy of those branches of the nerve of Latarjet which pass along the anterior and posterior walls of the stomach to innervate the parietal cell mass. First, there is no particular predilection for these nerves to run with blood vessels along the lesser curvature of the stomach. Second, as pointed out by Mitchell, the nerves can be traced for some distance beneath the serous coat of the stomach

before they penetrate the gastric musculature; and, third, the vagus branches always run superficial to and more obliquely than the blood vessels along the lesser curvature of the stomach.

Myotomy of the pylorus and the distal oesophagus are safe surgical procedures which have been established for most of the twentieth century; seromyotomy of the lesser curvature of the stomach was first investigated in the dog.[97] Applying the above anatomical considerations to denervating the parietal cell mass, branches of the nerve of Latarjet are divided by seromyotomy as they run initially closely applied to the serosa. Division of the longitudinal and circular muscle fibres produces wide separation of the divided nerve bundles. After myotomy in the dog, there was a marked shift to the right of the dose-response curve and a profound inhibition of pepsin output in response to pentagastrin stimulation (0.375–6 μg/kg per hour i.v.) The insulin response (0.2 units/kg) was almost completely abolished. Secretory inhibition after lesser curve myotomy in the dog was similar to that produced by highly selective vagotomy. These results gave an anatomical and physiological basis for the performance of the procedure in the man.

Initially in man, the seromyotomy was performed along both anterior and posterior walls of the stomach. In the first study published on this technique, 25 patients with chronic duodenal ulcer were treated. The operation was found to be technically relatively easy to perform without risk of damage to the nerve of Latarjet or ischaemic necrosis of the lesser curvature. Secretory inhibition was identical to that achieved with conventional highly selective vagotomy. After performing some of these procedures, the author decided to modify the operation and carry out anterior lesser curve seromyotomy with posterior truncal vagotomy. The reasons for this were that, on technical grounds, it seemed easier to provide a more reliable method of denervating the posterior wall of the stomach as this is the most difficult area to denervate using either conventional highly selective vagotomy or posterior seromyotomy. Also, by totally denervating the posterior wall of the stomach, any problems that might have arisen as a result of the incomplete denervation of the posterior wall at either the antrum–corpus junction or the more proximal stomach were overcome. Experience showed that the addition of posterior truncal vagotomy to anterior lesser curve seromyotomy did not apparently increase the incidence of diarrhoea when compared with highly selective vagotomy, and dumping did not occur. The antral musculature after this operation derives its innervation from the 'crow's foot' branches of the anterior nerve of Latarjet. It has been shown that, by stimulating these nerves, motor contraction of the antrum is propagated from the anterior gastric wall to the posterior through intramural vagovagal arcs, the integrity of which is maintained irrespective of the division of the posterior nerve trunk. Gastric motility problems with this procedure, which preserves the pylorus, seemed no greater than after conventional highly selective vagotomy.

Technical details

The exposure is similar to that described for highly selective vagotomy.

The presence of ulceration is confirmed and the pylorus is inspected for the presence of stenosis; pyloric stenosis is, of course, a contraindication to this and other pylorus-preserving procedures unless it is judged on palpation to be mild, when the pylorus can be digitally dilated through a small gastrotomy. The left lobe of the liver may or may not be mobilized, in accordance with the preference of the surgeon. The peritoneum overlying the distal oesophagus is incised transversely at the level of the hiatus above the hepatic branches of the anterior vagus nerve. The peritoneum is gently pushed superiorly to expose the hiatus and the anterior surface of the oesophagus. The index and middle fingers of the surgeon's hand are now passed around the distal oesophagus, spreading these fingers into a position of alternating abduction and adduction so as gently to burrow through the attenuating soft areolar tissues surrounding the oesophagus. When these exploring fingers reach the medial side of the oesophagus a window is made through the anterior sheath of peritoneum so as to complete the circumferential dissection. By spreading the fingers more widely posteriorly and using a gauze swab on a holder anteriorly the oesophagus can be mobilized easily over a distance of about 7 cm (Figure 33.16).

At this point in the dissection the anterior vagus nerve will become apparent. Occasionally there may be more than one anterior nerve. The posterior nerve is next identified by sweeping the index finger widely round the posterior aspect of the oesophagus, when the nerve will be identified about two fingers' breadth behind and on the medial side of the lower posterior oesophageal wall. The posterior nerve, which tends to be a larger structure than the anterior, should be mobilized over a distance of approximately 6–7 cm by blunt digital dissection. This nerve can be multiple and great care should be exercised by the surgeon to ascertain that all of the vagal trunks have been identified. The posterior nerve trunk or trunks are now divided and a length of about 2–3 cm of nerve is excised.

Directing attention to the anterior nerve, this must be carefully preserved. It is dissected gently from the anterior oesophageal wall and placed beneath a slim rubber sling which is used to retract the trunk medially away from the oesophagus. Where more than one anterior trunk exists, these supplementary structures should be divided, preserving only the single main nerve with its characteristic spatulate lower end. By retracting the anterior nerve away from the oesophageal wall, this latter structure should be examined most carefully for any residual nerve fibres. These are capable of reaching the pareital cell area by an intramuscular course from the lower oesophagus and need to be identified and divided. This is best achieved by gently placing the oesophagus under tension and by using a nerve hook, elevating the nerve and diathermizing it. The lower 6–7 cm of the oesophagus is thus cleared of any nerves, apart from the single, carefully preserved, anterior vagus trunk.

Crossing the oesophagogastric junction anteriorly is a constantly placed fibrofatty areolar bundle which contains vagal fibres passing from the anterior nerve to the fundus of the stomach. This structure is next divided and ligated, exposing beneath it the anterior oesophagogastric junction where the serosa stops on the upper gastric extremity (Figure 33.17).

The lower part of the dissection is next begun by starting, as for highly selective vagotomy, about 6 cm proximal to the pylorus. The arguments discussed about the selection of the lower point of the dissection in performing a highly selective vagotomy are identical to those which are relevant here. Suffice it to say that the author begins his dissection at about 6 cm from the pylorus, usually just proximal to the lower branch of the 'crow's foot'. Unlike in highly selective vagotomy, where the dissection of nerves and vessels takes place

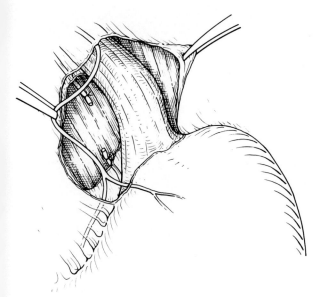

Figure 33.16
Anterior lesser curve seromyotomy and posterior trunkal vagotomy. Division of the posterior vagus nerve and removal of a length of vagus is shown.

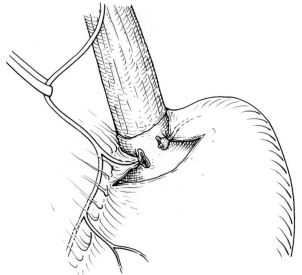

Figure 33.17
Ligation and division of the areolar tissue crossing the oesophago-gastric junction anteriorly. This fatty pad always contains some vagal nerve fibres.

immediately along the edge of the lesser curvature, here it begins some 1 cm along the wall of the stomach. The serosa is cut by blunt-nosed scissors, which are insinuated gently beneath the circular muscle layer of the stomach, and the submucosal plane is easily identified. The deeper circular and oblique muscle fibres are dissected off the submucosa with ease, for these layers separate easily once an appropriate plane has been found (Figure 33.18).

This dissection proceeds proximally, staying about 1 cm from the lesser curvature. As blood vessels are identified, they are clamped, divided and ligated and there are usually 4–6 such vessels which need dividing proximal to the completed dissection of the 'crow's foot'. As the dissection proceeds proximally, the circular muscle fibres thin out considerably but there remains, on the whole, little attenuation between the muscular and submucous tissues, making the dissection easy to perform by the gentle spread of the tips of the blunt-nosed scissors and then division of the 'freed up' seromuscular layers (Figure 33.19).

Just proximal to the oesophagogastric junction, already exposed by division of the fibrofatty bundle, the dissection moves laterally to end at the point of the oesophagogastric junction exposed by the division of the transversely running fibrofatty bundle referred to above. It is very important not to continue the dissection into the oesophageal musculature for the lower oesophageal sphincter must remain completely intact in order to prevent gastro-oesophageal reflux (Figure 33.20).

Completion of the lesser curve seromyotomy leads to wide separation of the seromuscular edges. The submucosa can be seen pouting through this defect and the surgeon is easily

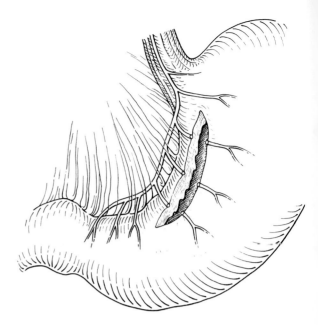

Figure 33.19
Progression of the anterior seromyotomy.

convinced that he has divided the anterior branches of the nerve of Latarjet which run across the stomach in the subserosal plane. The defect thus created by the seromyotomy along the lesser curvature is now sutured employing a method of 'overlap repair'. The lesser curve serosa is tacked across the other side of the defect using a continuous absorbable suture so as to prevent the possibility of reinnervation by sprouting (Figure 33.21). There is no evidence that sprouting nerve fibres can penetrate the seromuscular layer, which they would be required to do before reaching the underlying mucosa with its parietal cell mass. Closure of this defect completes the operation and the abdomen is closed with absorbable suture material.

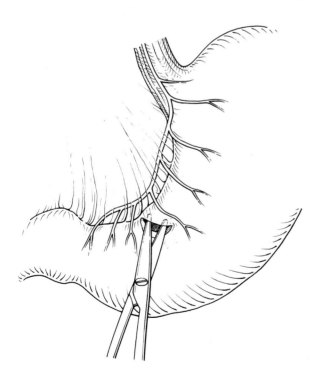

Figure 33.18
The anterior lesser curve seromyotomy is begun 6 cm proximal to the pylorus and about 1 cm lateral to the edge of the gastric lesser curvature.

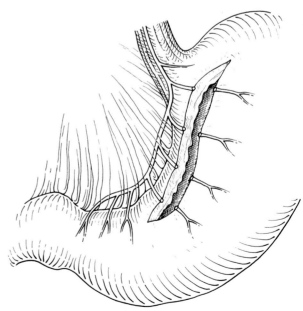

Figure 33.20
The completed anterior lesser curve seromyotomy.

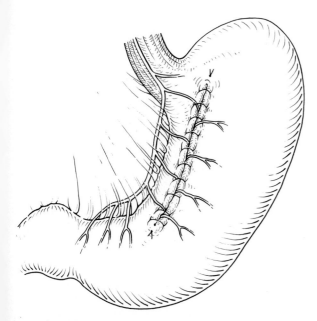

Figure 33.21
The overlap repair is performed to reinforce the defect created by the seromyotomy and to prevent nerve regeneration by sprouting of the divided vagi down to the denuded mucosa.

It is usual to leave a nasogastric tube in place for 48 hours, although acute gastric dilatation has not been reported after this operation. Equally, there has been no reported case of ischaemic necrosis of the lesser curvature. Significant gastric stasis occurs in about 2% of cases; dumping has not been encountered but the incidence of diarrhoea is about 2%. The author does not routinely use peroperative testing for the completeness of vagotomy, having been assured by numerous postoperative insulin tests that the parietal cell mass is usually completely denervated. As with all forms of vagotomy, there is a significant change in insulin status from negative to positive after the first year or so following the operation. The mortality for this operation is extremely low, probably lower than for any other type of vagotomy, because the risk of ischaemic necrosis of the lesser curvature has been overcome.

Anterior highly selective vagotomy and posterior truncal vagotomy

Hill and Barker,[121] in 1978, first performed this procedure and reported good results in a small number of patients. It differs from lesser curve seromyotomy in that the anterior dissection in their operation is a classic highly selective vagotomy, the plane of dissection being close to the lesser curvature.

Laparoscopic lesser curve seromyotomy with posterior truncal vagotomy

The recent surge of enthusiasm for minimally invasive procedures has extended sufficiently to demonstrate the feasibility of this operation. The principles are exactly the same as in the open operation, except that the dissection can be achieved through portals employing laparoscopic equipment. The oesophagus can be mobilized and the posterior vagus nerve

identified and divided. The anterior vagus nerve is preserved, although it is difficult to achieve the oesophageal clearance described above in the open operation. By a meticulous dissection with scissors, clips and diathermy or laser, the lesser curve dissection can be achieved. Alternatively a sliver of lesser curvature may be excised using a laparoscopic GA60 stapler. One of the great advantages of the laparoscopic procedure is that only an overnight stay is required, and postoperative mobilization of the patient is as rapid as after laparoscopic cholecystectomy. No long-term results have as yet been reported, but the minimally invasive nature of the procedure may go some way to promoting elective ulcer surgery to compete with the ever increasing array of drugs which effectively heal ulcers, at least in the short term.

It has also been shown that truncal vagotomy and highly selective vagotomy can be performed laparoscopically.

CLINICAL RESULTS OF SURGERY FOR DUODENAL ULCER

Gastrojejunostomy

Gastrojejunostomy alone was used in the treatment of chronic duodenal ulcer for half a century. Diversion of ulcerogenic gastric contents from the duodenum resulted in healing of the duodenal ulcer, but with an unacceptably high recurrence rate of stomach ulceration, in some series approaching 50%. It was shown, however, that if this procedure was performed only in those with duodenal ulcer whose levels of acid secretion were at the lower end of the spectrum, the results were quite good and recurrence rates of less than 10% were reported. Side-effects such as dumping and diarrhoea, in the absence of an accompanying vagotomy, were few, and the operation was extremely safe to perform. The overall high recurrence rates, however, precluded the further use of this procedure when performed alone in the treatment of duodenal ulcer.[122]

Gastric resection

Recurrent ulceration is much less of a problem with gastric resection than gastrojejunostomy, but the mortality is higher and the morbidity is significant. Early complications of Billroth I and Billroth II gastrectomy for chronic duodenal ulcer include haemorrhage and leakage from the suture line and stomal obstruction. The closed duodenal stump of a Polya gastrectomy is particularly prone to leak if meticulous care has not been exercised in closing the divided duodenum. Pancreatitis is also a complication of Polya gastrectomy. Internal herniation of loops of jejunum into the supracolic compartment of the peritoneal cavity through a mesenteric defect and jejunal volvulus may produce intestinal obstruction.

If major haemorrhage follows gastric resection this is usually reactionary in nature, with bleeding occurring from the suture line. The diagnosis can be confirmed endoscopically and reoperation may be necessary. Stomal obstruction occurred in only 11 patients of a series of 1774 who had gastric resection performed.[123] Abscess formation in the region of the stoma may be responsible for this, and the omentum becomes firmly fixed to the site of leakage along the anastomotic line. The overall result is oedema and obstruction which may not settle with conservative treatment. A swallow with a water-soluble contrast medium (Gastrografin) and the use of endoscopy are helpful in determining the cause of obstruction.

A leaking duodenal stump presents with high swinging pyrexia, tenderness, guarding and sometimes features of generalized peritonitis. Small leaks may become localized and present as subphrenic abscesses. If peritonitis develops, reoperation is mandatory. It is normally impossible to resuture the leaking stump itself; if it is achieved, further leakage is common. The situation may be salvaged by inserting a Foley-type balloon catheter into the duodenum and closing the stump around it. A duodenal fistula is formed which closes spontaneously following removal of the catheter after 12–14 days. Mortality from this complication remains high. Leakage may occur from the Billroth I anastomosis, particularly at the lesser curve aspect of the gastroduodenal anastomosis; the gastrojejunal anastomosis rarely leaks after Billroth II procedures.

Recurrence of ulceration is a greater problem following partial gastric resection without a vagotomy, rates of between 2 and 15% having been recorded over periods of follow-up ranging from 1 to 10 years.[124,125] These rates are probably underestimates as most studies of gastric resection without vagotomy were reported before the days of routine use of the fibreoptic endoscope.

Long-term nutritional sequelae may complicate gastric resection, manifesting as loss of weight, anaemia, hypoalbuminaemia and hypocalcaemia.[126,127] Tuberculosis may occur in association with nutritional problems.

The major postgastrectomy sequelae are dumping, diarrhoea, duodenogastric reflux and bilious vomiting.[128,129] Severe dumping occurs in about 3% of patients following gastric resection but tends to improve spontaneously with time. Diarrhoea is not common in the absence of vagotomy, but malabsorption of carbohydrates, fats and proteins may ensue and subclinical conditions such as lactose deficiency and coeliac disease may be highlighted by the gastrectomy.

Throughout the history of peptic ulcer surgery, a major reservation of surgeons to the performance of gastric resection has been the increased postoperative mortality associated with it. This mortality has decreased in recent years, and indeed Goligher et al.[130] reported no mortality following gastric resection in the large Leeds–York trial. Additionally in this trial the results of gastrectomy were hardly inferior to vagotomy. Suffice it to say, however, that the changing emphasis and practice in peptic ulcer therapy has left no role for elective gastric resection without vagotomy.

Truncal vagotomy

The overall mortality for truncal vagotomy and drainage was shown by Cox, in over 8000 cases, to be 0.8%. Adding antrectomy to a truncal vagotomy, rather than performing a drainage procedure, approximately doubles the mortality. Whether a pyloroplasty or a gastrojejunostomy is used as the drainage procedure does not affect the mortality.

Recurrent ulceration occurs in about 7% of cases in the long

term. This is almost invariably due to incomplete vagotomy. The inexperienced surgeon is particularly prone to overlooking the posterior vagus nerve trunk, or, when it is multiple, one of the trunks. Completing the vagotomy in these circumstances should be adequate treatment because, after a complete truncal vagotomy, in the absence of delayed gastric emptying and the rare Zollinger–Ellison syndrome, further recurrent ulcer is rare. The incidence of recurrence thus varies with the experience of the operator. Today, however, surgeons in training receive little exposure to vagotomy, and when the procedure is required one might expect to encounter less adequate vagotomies in the future.

The major problems following truncal vagotomy and drainage are dumping and diarrhoea. Rapid early gastric emptying is the major cause of this, accounting for about 90% of cases. The rare hypoglycaemic variety of dumping occurs in about 10%. The clinical effects of weakness, light headedness, palpitations, sweating and vertigo can be quite disabling. Dumping tends to improve with time after operation, but surprisingly it can occasionally develop for the first time some years later.

Diarrhoea also can be significantly disabling in about 3% of patients, who develop severe urgency, lower abdominal colic and sometimes incontinence of watery fluid. It tends to follow meals and is much more likely to occur and to be severe when cholecystectomy has been added to vagotomy.[131] Severely incapacitated patients may have up to 20 bowel actions per day.[132,133] The cause remains poorly defined. It is probably related to the rate of gastric emptying, the handling of bile acids by the gut and possibly to colonic motility disorders following parasympathetic denervation of the cranial but not the sacral outflow. Malabsorption and bacterial colonization of the proximal small bowel are thought perhaps to be factors.[134–137]

Duodenogastric reflux of bile may be a problem following any type of drainage procedure and leads to gastritis with bilious vomiting. If severe, a Roux-en-Y diversion may be necessary.

Dysphagia occurs after about 2% of vagotomies of all types. It may relate to denervation of the lower oesophageal sphincter, although ordinarily vagotomy does not have a measurable effect on oesophageal manometry. The condition may persist for 2–3 months but almost always resolves spontaneously without residual problems. Gastro-oesophageal reflux may occasionally complicate vagotomy and the acid-reducing effect of vagotomy has not been observed to be helpful in alleviating the symptoms associated with this problem. The major problem associated with the side-effects of dumping and diarrhoea is that, for the small percentage of patients who develop these, they are unpredictable and virtually untreatable. On the whole, those who go on to further gastric surgery have a disappointing result from this.

Selective gastric vagotomy

The concept of selective gastric vagotomy was introduced independently by Jackson[43] and Franksson[42] in 1948, the objective being to reduce the incidence of dumping and diarrhoea by preserving the integrity of the extragastric vagi through the anterior hepatic and posterior coeliac branches of the main trunks. Complete gastric parasympathetic denervation occurs, as a result of which a drainage procedure or antrectomy is required.[138,139] Few large series have been reported in the literature but there is little doubt that, despite the necessity for a drainage procedure, dumping and diarrhoea are uncommon, though they sometimes occur in a mild form. Recurrent ulcer rates have also been low following this procedure, for it has been argued that the technical performance of this operation is more likely to result in a complete gastric vagotomy than any other form of vagotomy. Acid tests would tend to support this. The operation also seems to be safe, Kennedy having reported no deaths in his series of 350. Perhaps selective vagotomy has not been given an adequate test and possibly it should have received greater recognition and been employed more widely.[140-145] It was surpassed, at least by proximal gastric vagotomy. In terms of the elimination of dumping and diarrhoea, surgeons were happier with this latter procedure, but the high incidence of recurrent ulceration now being reported after highly selective vagotomy has put something of a question mark over its long-term future. The other factor which led to the expression of some reservation in adopting selective gastric vagotomy was the more difficult nature of the technical procedure involved. From the evidence available, one can certainly say that selective vagotomy, particularly when combined with a suprapyloric antrectomy, is a procedure which, as stated by Griffiths, 'meets the old requirement of low recurrence and the new requirement of no dumping', albeit not as effectively as parietal cell vagotomy.

Vagotomy and antrectomy

By virtue of dividing the vagi and removing the G-cell mass, this operation produces a reduction in maximal acid output of 90% or more compared with the 65% reduction which follows vagotomy or antrectomy alone. Consequently, this combined procedure remains the most effective long-term assault on the ulcer and recurrence rates are low, invariably less than 2%.[146-150]

Such efficacy in ulcer treatment is achieved at the cost of increased perioperative mortality and complications. Mortality rates in large series vary from 0.6% to 2.7%.[151-155] Most impressively, Herrington and Sawyers have reported 3771 patients treated in Nashville, with a mortality of 1.5%. This series included 32% with a history of bleeding, 14% with gastric outflow obstruction and 3% who underwent operation for free perforation. The follow-up was excellent and only 1% of patients developed a recurrent ulcer, and a further 5% had unsatisfactory results overall. Dumping occurred in 25%, being severe in 1%. Diarrhoea was experienced by 15%, compared with 3% following selective gastric vagotomy, but this was only severe in 1%.[150] Approximately 3–4% experienced alkaline reflux gastritis, which is probably less of a problem when the antrum has been resected than after vagotomy and pyloroplasty. The low mortality is particularly impressive when one considers that most deaths occurred in patients undergoing emergency surgery to control massive bleeding and in elderly patients with coexisting vascular and renal disease. The morbidity for any type of surgery performed in the emergency situation for uncontrollable bleeding or perforation is at least 10%, and often 25% or more. The cause of recurrent ulcers, which occurred in only 0.5% of cases, was either incomplete vagotomy or a functioning endocrine tumour. Only two recurrent ulcers occurred out of the whole series of 3771 patients, where vagotomy was shown to be incomplete. All recurrences occurred within 2 years, in contrast to many later recurrences which follow proximal gastric vagotomy. Recurrence is much less common after both truncal vagotomy and selective vagotomy with antrectomy than after vagotomy and pyloroplasty.[151]

Highly selective vagotomy

Throughout the 1970s and early 1980s, many large series of cases were reported following highly selective vagotomy. Initial enthusiasm has now become tempered with scepticism or frank concern as a result of escalating levels of recurrent peptic ulceration. The Copenhagen group[46] reported ulcer recurrence rates of 30% or more and the surprising feature has been the steady escalation of recurrences with increasing time after the operation. Such observations seem unique to this procedure. Recurrence after all other forms of vagotomy, if it does occur, tends to do so within 2 years of the time of the operation and is directly attributable to incomplete vagotomy. An argument has been expressed in favour of reinnervation of the stomach, as a result of nerve sprouting, being responsible for increasing levels of acid secretion and thereby recurrence.[156] There is no doubt that reinnervation, as expressed in terms of increasing acid output with time in response to an insulin stimulus, does occur. Following truncal vagotomy, some 50% of patients who were initially found in the early postoperative period to be insulin negative will revert to a positive status after about 1 year. After highly selective vagotomy this incidence is higher; indeed, the vast majority of, if not all, patients will revert to an insulin positive-status with time. Following truncal vagotomy, nerve sprouting would have to occur from the oesophageal level. After proximal gastric vagotomy, if nerve sprouting was responsible, it would conceivably take place from both the oesophagus and the innervated antrum. The latter might be expected to be more likely to occur in view of the much larger surface area and more approximate site to the parietal cell mass.[157] If this process of reinnervation was responsible for the recurrent ulcers that occur after proximal gastric vagotomy, why then do ulcers go on recurring for up to at least 18 years after operation? Any process of reinnervation by sprouting would be likely to be complete by well before 2 years from the time of the operation. Hancock et al.[158] found a significant reduction in the peak acid output in response to insulin when highly selective vagotomy was combined with a rotation gastropexy, which was thought to prevent vagal regeneration. Joffe and Bapat[159] have carried out elegant studies in the rat following proximal gastric vagotomy, in which they have shown on electron microscopy that reinnervation does seem to occur. It has been suggested that this reinnervation does not occur as a result of ingrowth from the antrum but represents a completely new set of parasympathetic nerves innervating the stomach.[160] It is possible that other factors could be responsible. Hormone levels have been studied of gastrin in particular, but no evidence has been produced of any consistently identifiable abnormality of hormone secretion in these patients. It is also difficult to implicate *H. pylori* as the cause because there is nothing in the sequence of events which take place over the operation and subsequent years which might influence helicobacter status.

The other possibility is that recurrences might relate in some way to the absence of a drainage procedure. Holle and colleagues[161,162] have not reported the high incidence of late ulcer recurrence that follows proximal gastric vagotomy without drainage. Their reasons for performing pyloroplasty are to compensate for any reduction in antropyloric gastric motor function that may occur as a result of proximal gastric denervation. They argue that, by adding a pyloroplasty, inherent post-prandial antral contractility can be lowered without impairment of gastric emptying. They stated that this protective treatment is indispensible for the maintainance of adequate motility. They may indeed be right, and if there is no significant price to pay for the pylorplasty in terms of increased dumping and diarrhoea, then the reduced incidence of recurrent ulcer which follows the addition of a pyloroplasty is easily justified.

Three factors contribute together to produce dumping and diarrhoea: division of the hepatic branches of the anterior vagus; division of the coeliac branches of the posterior vagus; and the drainage procedure. It has been shown that selective gastric vagotomy when combined with pyloroplasty is accompanied by a low incidence of dumping and diarrhoea. In addition, dumping and diarrhoea are very uncommon after a drainage procedure without a form of vagotomy. When the posterior vagus nerve is divided, but the hepatic branches of the anterior vagus and pylorus are preserved, as in the operation of anterior lesser curve seromyotomy and posterior truncal vagotomy, the incidence of dumping and diarrhoea has been consistently shown to be extremely low. Thus, usually at least two of these three factors are needed for the patient to be at risk of dumping and diarrhoea, and when all three factors are present, as after truncal vagotomy and pyloroplasty, the incidence is much higher. It is likely, therefore, that adding pyloroplasty to highly selective vagotomy will not produce a significant problem with dumping and diarrhoea, and this indeed seems to be the case. The major argument in favour of highly selective vagotomy in the treatment of chronic duodenal ulcer remains the low incidence of the untreatable side-effects of dumping and diarrhoea, and these represent the present-day criteria which are applied to the success of an operation because recurrent ulceration can be coped with, at least in the short term, by suitable medical therapy.

CLINICAL TRIALS IN THE TREATMENT OF DUODENAL ULCER

Because of the high recurrence rates when H_2-receptor antagonist therapy is ceased, it is becoming clear that clinicians and patients have to decide between long-term drug treatment,

often using full therapeutic doses, or operation in the *H. pylori* negative patient. Prospective controlled long-term trials of elective surgery against medical treatment are therefore important, but few exist. Harling et al.[163] reported a controlled trial of 86 duodenal ulcer patients with severe symptoms who were randomized to full-dose cimetidine plus maintenance therapy for 1 year, or parietal cell vagotomy, and followed for a mean of 57 months. In the cimetidine group only 12% remained free of symptoms during the follow-up period, and 35% had operations for recurrent symptoms, while 53% had regular medical treatment. The overall recurrence rate after parietal cell vagotomy was rather high, at 17%, and the final Visick grading was 75% excellent or good; the authors concluded that operation was the treatment of choice in patients with a history of severe symptoms from peptic ulceration and rapid recurrence after medical treatment.

Graffner and his colleagues[164] analysed the results of 405 consecutive parietal cell vagotomies over 10 years and confirmed that:

1. Recurrences occurred earlier in patients with pyloric and pre-pyloric ulcers.

2. The post-operative peak acid output to pentagastrin was higher in those who developed recurrent duodenal ulcer than in those who did not.

3. The recurrence rate depended upon surgical expertise.

4. Over half the recurrent ulcers were successfully treated medically.

Anderson[165] reported that long-term medical treatment and surgery were equally acceptable options for most patients, but he pointed out that, in Denmark, operation was cheaper for the patient in the long term. He also made the point that, in these days of powerful ulcer-healing drugs, recurrent ulceration may no longer be the main criterion of success of surgery. Lack of side-effects, in particular the incurables (dumping and diarrhoea), are now more important because recurrence of ulceration often responds to a further course of H_2-receptor antagonists. In France, Bader[166] advocated a sequential strategy where the indications for drug treatment and operation were different. Surgery only became an option when an ulcer had healed and rapidly relapsed on repeated occasions.

The debate about the most appropriate treatment of uncomplicated duodenal ulceration has continued over recent years. However, one message that has come across strongly is that if surgery is indicated, then highly selective vagotomy or pylorus-preserving vagotomy is the operation of choice because it is associated with minimal morbidity and virtually no mortality. The somewhat high ulcer recurrence rate after highly selective vagotomy is, however, of some concern. It is still only 25 years since these operations were first described. By the mid 1980s recurrence rates in those long-term studies following highly selective vagotomy were creeping up, and in the studies of Herrington et al.,[167] Stael von Holstein et al.,[168] Enskog et al.,[169] Marceau et al.[170] and Paimela et al.,[171] they averaged 9.2, 18, 13.8, 12 and 16%, respectively. The variable incidence of recurrence is due in part to differing surgical technique and experience, and seniority does not necessarily guarantee success. In a study reported by Enskog et al, the individual senior surgeon had an ulcer recurrence rate of 54% in a series of 24 operations. Undoubtedly, highly selective vagotomy is an operation which must be learnt from an experienced vagotomist in the operating theatre rather than from a textbook in the library.

In selecting patients for peptic ulcer surgery some emphasis should clearly be placed on the identification of the group or groups of patients who may do badly. Primrose and colleagues[172] were able to link poor results of both medical and surgical treatment with smoking habits. Several papers have reported poor results following highly selective vagotomy when the ulcer was pyloric or prepyloric; Jordan and Thornby[173] noted recurrence rates after highly selective vagotomy of 6 and 21% for duodenal and pyloric or prepyloric ulcers, respectively, while Muller et al.[174] noted recurrence rates of 14 and 35% for the same conditions. Muller suggested that the addition of a drainage procedure to highly selective vagotomy would be beneficial when treating pyloric canal ulcers. Heberer and Teichman[175] stated that pyloric and prepyloric ulcers should no longer be treated by highly selective vagotomy. Jordan and Thornby[173] stated that when selective vagotomy and antrectomy and highly selective vagotomy were compared prospectively, the recurrence rate was significantly reduced after selective vagotomy and antrectomy (2.2 versus 10.1%). However, if the pyloric ulcers were excluded, no significant difference in ulcer recurrence could be demonstrated between the two groups. Primrose and colleagues[172] found that patients whose ulcers were refractory to treatment with H_2-receptor antagonists had a higher ulcer recurrence rate after highly selective vagotomy than did patients who responded well to H_2-receptor antagonists. However, no such association was found by Goodman and colleagues[176] in a study of similar size, although a high proportion of non-responders remained symptomatic without ulcer recurrence; 50% of ulcer recurrences in this study occurred in patients taking NSAIDs.

A comparison of the effects of placebo, ranitidine and highly selective vagotomy on 24-hour ambulatory intragastric pH in patients with duodenal ulcer was reported by Rogers et al.[177] Twenty patients with endoscopically confirmed chronic duodenal ulcers who had been referred for surgical treatment were studied when taking either placebo or ranitidine 300 mg at night, and again 4–13 weeks after highly selective vagotomy. Indeed, there was little difference in noctural pH between the two treatments, but the day-time pH was lower in the medically treated group.

The important question of whether greater degrees of gastric denervation would achieve better results was assessed in a trial comparing highly selective vagotomy with extended highly selective vagotomy in duodenal ulcer patients.[178] In those with extended highly selective vagotomy a greater degree of dissection was carried on down the lesser curvature, and also the gastroepiploic nerves were sectioned. Both groups were well matched but no differences were found in reduction in maximal acid output or basal secretion at 3 years after operation, and no significant difference existed clinically between the two

groups. All of these surgeons were highly experienced, having performed at least 500 highly selective vagotomies before undertaking the study, and clearly the extended procedure offered no advantage in their hands. In a study in which anterior lesser curve seromyotomy with posterior truncal vagotomy was compared with proximal gastric vagotomy in 91 patients at 3 years, there was no significant difference in ulcer recurrence rates, postoperative peak acid output reduction, postoperative complications or patient satisfaction.[179] The authors pointed out, however, that anterior lesser curve seromyotomy with posterior truncal vagotomy was performed in a signifcantly shorter time and with fewer difficulties than was the conventional highly selective gastric denervation procedure. Modifications of this technique, using an argon laser at open operation, have now been described, and laser lesser curve superficial seromyotomy has been carried out endoscopically.

Holle[180], in a series of over 1200 duodenal ulcer patients, examined the cause for recurrence. They found that inadequate vagotomy, or sometimes incomplete drainage, accounted for 80% of the recurrences. They calculated that 6.3% of duodenal ulcer patients had recurrent ulcers after highly selective vagotomy and pyloroplasty, a figure lower than most series where no pyloroplasty had been added. Graffner and colleagues[181] put forward the hypothesis that increased ulcer relapse rates after parietal cell vagotomy were related to smoking habits of patients, 24% recurrence being found amongst smokers compared with 7% in non-smokers. Siriwardena and Gunn[182] pointed out that, in their hands, anterior lesser curve seromyotomy and posterior truncal vagotomy for chronic duodenal ulcer compared favourably with traditional highly selective vagotomy at 5 years.

LAPAROSCOPIC VAGOTOMY: AN OPERATION FOR THE 1990s?

Is there any role for elective peptic ulcer surgery in the 1990s? Contemporary surgical gastroenterologists must have posed this question and many medical peers must have dismissed elective surgical treatment to the history books. The latter view has had a most profound effect, for how many of today's gastroenterologists refer cases for surgery? Their argument is at first sight a good one. Virtually all chronic peptic ulcers will succumb to the powerful H_2-receptor antagonists cimetidine, ranitidine or famotidine.[183] The occasional resistant ulcer will thereafter almost inevitably heal with omeprazole.[184] Using acid secretory inhibition to heal ulcers, great strides have been made since the introduction of the H_2-receptor antagonists. A problem arises, however, in maintaining ulcer healing. Stopping a 2-month course of any of the above drugs results in recurrence rates of up to 90% at 1 year.[185] Even long-term low-dose maintenance therapy has a recurrence rate of 2.5% per month,[4] or 30% per year.

Since the early 1980s there has been no reduction in ulcer-associated mortality in England and Wales despite vast investment in the H_2-receptor antagonists.[18] The number of deaths from peptic ulcers, nearly 4500 per year, is as high as that from oesophageal or pancreatic cancers in these countries.[186] Indeed, ulcer mortality is rising, year by year, particularly in the elderly female.[187] Moreover, this increase is occurring at a time when the overall prevalence of the disorder is estimated to be declining. What is the reason for this?

The rise cannot be attributed to increased rates of colonization or virulence of *H. pylori*, although detailed studies of the natural history of different strains of the organism bear further investigation. It has been suggested that some strains of the organism are more pathogenic or ulcerogenic than others.[188] It is possible, though unlikely, that a particular strain is more virulent in terms of producing ulcer perforation or bleeding, particularly in the elderly female. A more likely explanation relates to the increasing use of NSAIDs, particularly in the elderly. Over 22 million prescriptions for these drugs are dispensed annually in the UK.[189] This figure does not allow for the even greater volume sold over the counter. Even the use of ultra-low-dose aspirin (75 mg/day) in the prophylaxis of coronary artery disease is a significant risk factor for ulcer bleeding.[190] In a study, within 3 months of taking NSAIDs, 17% of the patients developed ulcers, 40% developed gastric erosions and over 70% developed gastric erythema.[191] These drugs are, however, potent in the relief of 'rheumatic' pain and may alleviate unexplained abdominal pain in the elderly. If further proof of their irritant effect was needed, merely stopping the drug frequently results in alleviation of dyspepsia and healing of the ulcers. These drugs are probably the major cause of the rise in ulcer-associated mortality which we are witnessing and this is unrelated to *H. pylori* infection.

Another factor, equally difficult to assess in absolute terms, may be the dramatic reduction in the use of peptic ulcer surgery since the early 1980s.[18] Throughout the Western world there has been an approximately 80% reduction in the performance of elective definitive acid-reducing operations over this time. This may have played a role in the increased mortality because definitive acid reduction results in long-term, if not permanent, ulcer healing. The ulcers which do recur after surgery rarely perforate or bleed because acid secretion has been reduced and the ulcer diathesis blunted. McLean Ross et al., in a long-term (15 years) follow-up of 779 patients who had undergone acid-reducing surgery, showed that although mortality was high from smoking-related diseases none died from peptic ulceration[192] Indeed, many of these patients must have been taking NSAIDs! It would seem, therefore, that a potential exists for reducing the ulcer-associated mortality by permanent reduction in acid secretion.

Mortality and morbidity associated with peptic ulcer surgery has declined due to the development of pylorus-preserving vagotomy and abandonment of gastric antral resection. Perioperative mortality for highly selective vagotomy and for anterior lesser curve seromyotomy are as low as 0.3%[69] and 0.16%[193], respectively. Importantly, dumping and diarrhoea, resulting largely from destruction or bypass of the pylorus, has been overcome; 'gastrojejunostomy is a disease, pyloroplasty is an incurable disease'.

The open operative procedures carry short-term morbidity and an economic burden due entirely to a long abdominal incision, in contrast to the rapid recovery made when, for example, cholecystectomy is performed laparoscopically. Few would now question that laparoscopic cholecystectomy is here to stay. Both conventional highly selective vagotomy and lesser curve seromyotomy with posterior truncal vagotomy can now be performed through the laparoscope. Feasibility, however, is not the hallmark of justification for the widespread adoption of these techniques. So far, only a handful of studies exist in the literature and these are largely animal based.[45,194,195] Not only do they confirm the feasibility of the laparoscopic technique but it has also been shown that acid inhibition of the order of 'open' vagotomy can be achieved. One study compared truncal vagotomy, highly selective vagotomy and anterior lesser curve seromyotomy and posterior truncal vagotomy in 20 pigs.[196] The anterior lesser curve seromyotomy and posterior truncal vagotomy was found to be technically the most feasible and may well lend itself to the use of a laser. If laparoscopic vagotomy is to be encouraged then only highly selective or anterior curve seromyotomy with posterior truncal vagotomy can be considered, in view of the necessity to eliminate the incurables of dumping and diarrhoea. Katkhouda has now performed anterior seromyotomy with posterior truncal vagotomy in 80 patients with excellent short-term clinical results. (personal communication). Few long-term studies have yet been published and it will take several years to assess their safety and long-term rates of recurrent ulceration.

For the first time in many years, the surgeon, when treating peptic ulcers, may have a cost advantage. These laparoscopic techniques may provide permanent acid inhibition to safe levels for the cost of 2 hours of operating time, 2 days in the hospital and a short convalescence thereafter. The cost of 10 years maintenance therapy of cimetidine (400 mg) and ranitidine (150 mg) is £1200 and £1800, respectively.[197] A problem germane to the strategy of employing laparoscopic vagotomy will undoubtedly be that of training surgeons to perform the technique properly and safely. Lack of appropriate surgical skills could allow potentially serious problems, such as ischaemic necrosis of the lesser curve, to occur after highly selective vagotomy. Surveillance for the emergence of such possibly life-threatening complications must be mandatory. If these procedures can be performed with skill, safety and precision, as appears to be the case, then they may have an important role in reducing the considerable mortality of peptic ulceration that still exists.

The presence of most peptic ulcers today has been associated with *H. pylori* infection and eradication of the infection usually results in healing of the ulcer. Reinfection rates are not yet completely and accurately known but appear to be low. Under these circumstances, there is little place for elective peptic ulcer surgery unless the ulcer proves to be resistant to triple therapy. The number of such resistant ulcers is low, therefore the need for elective peptic ulcer surgery has been dramatically reduced. NSAID-related ulcers, however, are unrelated to *H. pylori* infection and require a different therapeutic strategy. For ulcer perforation and some patients with bleeding ulcers surgery is still required. The surgeon will therefore be required to have a knowledge of the operative techniques described herein and must gain as much experience of their performance as is possible under the above circumstances.

Where the ulcer occurs in the absence of *H. pylori* infection the most likely cause relates to the ingestion of NSAIDs. Long-term H_2-receptor antagonists may be necessary but may not always be effective or the patient may not be compliant. Under such circumstances ulcer surgery should be performed.

REFERENCES

1. Ivy AC. The problem of peptic ulcer. *JAMA* 1946; **132**: 1053–1059.
2. Langman MJS. What is happening to peptic ulcer? *BMJ* 1982; **184**: 1063–1064.
3. Mendeloff AI. What has been happening to duodenal ulcer? Gastroenterology 1974; **76**: 1020–1022.
4. Pounder R. Duodenal ulcers that are difficult to heal. *BMJ* 1989; **297**: 1560–1561.
5. Hudson N, Everitt S, Edwards T & Hawkey CJ. Elevation of gastric mucosal leukotriene B$_4$ levels in patients on longstanding NSAID therapy. *Gastroenterology* 1991; **100**: A86.
6. Saleeby G, Holt L & Holt S. Pattern and prevalence of NSAIDs use in complicated peptic ulcer disease. *Gastroenterology* 1991; **100**: A17.
7. Steer HW & Colin-Jones DG. Mucosal changes in gastric ulceration and their response to carbenoxolone sodium. *Gut* 1975; **16**: 590–597.
8. Warren JR & Marshall B. Unidentified curved bacilli on gastric epithelium in active chronic gastritis. *Lancet* 1983; **i**: 1273–1275.
9. Marshall BJ & Warren JR Unidentified curved bacilli in the stomach of patients with gastritis and peptic ulceration. *Lancet* 1984; **i**: 1311–1314.
10. Marshall BJ Barrett LJ, Prakash C, McCallum RW & Guerrant RL. Urea protects *Helicobacter* (*Campylobacter*) *pylori* from the bactericidal effect of acid. *Gastroenterology* 1990; **99**: 697–702.
11. Tytgat GNJ, Axon ATR, Dixon MF, Graham DY, Lee A & Marshall BJ *Helicobacter pylori*: causal agent in peptic ulcer disease? In Working Party Reports, *World Congresses of Gastroenterology*, 26–31 August 1990. Oxford: Blackwell, 1990: 36–45.
12. Cave DR & Vargas M Effect of a *Campylobacter pylori* protein on acid secretion by parietal cells. *Lancet* 1989; **ii**: 187–189.
13. Malfertheiner P & Ditschuneit H. Pathogenic mechanisms of *H. pylori*. In Malfertheiner P & Ditschuneit H (eds) *Helicobacter pylori, Gastritis and Peptic Ulcer*. Berlin: Springer, 1990: 63–127.
14. Hunt RH. *Campylobacter pylori* and spontaneous hypochlorhydria. In Rathbone, BJ & Heatley, RV (eds) *Campylobacter pylori and Gastroduodenal Disease*. Oxford: Blackwell, 1989: 176–184.
15. Misiewicz JJ, Tytgat GNJ, Goodwin CS et al. The Sydney system: a new classification of gastritis. In Working Party Reports, *World Congresses of Gastroenterology*, 26–31 August 1990. Oxford: Blackwell, 1990: 1–10.
16. Dwyer B, Kaldor J, Tee W & Raios K. The prevalence of *Campylobacyter pylori* in human populations. In Rathbone, BJ & Heatley, R.V. (eds) *Campylobacter pylori and Gastroduodenal Disease*. Oxford: Blackwell, 1989: 190–196.
17. Wyatt JI. *Campylobacter pylori*, duodenitis and duodenal ulceration. In Rathbone, BJ & Heatley, RB (eds) *Campylobacter pylori and Gastroduodenal Disease*. Oxford: Blackwell, 1989: 117–124.
18. Taylor TV. Deaths from peptic ulceration. *BMJ* 1985; **291**: 653–655.
19. Beaumont W. *Experiments and Observations on the Gastric Juice and the Physiology of Digestion*. Plattsburgh, NY: FP Allen, 1833.
20. Wolff S & Wolff HG. *Human Gastric Function, an Experimental Study of a Man and his Stomach*. London: Oxford University Press, 1943.
21. Wolfler A. Gastroenterostomine. *Zentrabl Chir* 1883; **8**: 705–710.
22. Moynihan BGA. Observations upon the treatment of chronic diseases of the stomach. *Surg Gynecol Obstet* 1908; **6**: 4–11.
23. Mayo WJ. A study of gastric and duodenal ulcers with special reference to their surgical cure. *Surg Gynecol Obstet* 1908; **6**: 600–606.
24. Lister J. *The Collected Papers of Joseph Baron Lister*, 1867, vol. 2. Oxford: Clarendon Press, 1909.
25. Billroth T. Offenes Schreiber and Hern, L. Wittelshöfer, *Wien Med Wochenschr* 1881; **31**: 161.
26. Rydiger L. Die erste magen Resection beim Magengeschwür. *Berl Lus Wochenschr* 1882; **19**: 39.
27. Pavlov IP. *The Work of the Digestive Glands*. London: Griffin, 1902.
28. Gregory RA & Tracey HJ. Constitution and properties of two gastrins extract from hog antral mucosa. *J Physiol (Lond)* 1963; **169**: 18.
29. Schwartz K. Uber penetrierande magen und jejunal geschwür. *Beitr Klin Chrf* 1910; **67**: 96–99.
30. Bircher E. *Die Technik der Magenchirurgie*. Stuttgart: Enke, 1925: 20–25.
31. Latarjet A. Resection des nerfs de l'estomac. Technique opératoire. Résultats cliniques. *Bull Acad Natl Med (Paris)* 1922; **87**: 681–686.
32. Dragstedt LR & Owens FM. Supradiaphragmatic section of the vagus nerves in the treatment of duodenal ulcer. *Proc Soc Exp Biol Med* 1943; **53**: 152–156.
33. Pollock AG. Vagotomy in the treatment of peptic ulcer. *Lancet* 1952; **ii**: 795–798.
34. Lewisohn R. The frequency of gastrojejunal ulcers. *Surg Gynecol Obstet* 1925; **40**: 70–74.
35. Judd ES & Hazeltine ME. The results of operations for excision of the duodenum. *Ann Surg* 1930; **92**: 563–565.
36. Dragstedt LR. Acid ulcer. *Ann Surg* 1936; **62**: 118–122.
37. Weinberg JA Stempien SJ & Movius HJ. Vagotomy and pyloroplasty in the treatment of duodenal ulcer. *Am J Surg* 1956; **92**: 202–206.
38. Ordahl NB, Ross RP & Baker DV. The failure of partial gastrectomy with gastroduodenostomy in the treatment of duodenal ulcer. *Surgery* 1955; **38**: 158–161.
39. Goligher JC, Moir PJ & Rigley JH. Billroth I and polya gastrectomy operations for duodenal ulcer, a comparison. *Lancet* 1956; **ii**: 220–222.
40. Eiselsberg A. Uber ausschaltun inoperabler pylorus strikturen nebst bemerkungen uber die jejunostomie. *Arch Klin Chir* 1895; **50**: 919–922.
41. Dragstedt LR, Oberhelman HA & Smiktt CA. Experimental hyperfunction of the gastric antrum with ulcer formation. *Ann Surg* 1951; **134**: 332–336.
42. Franksson C. Selective abdominal vagotomy. *Acta Chir Scand* 1948; **96**: 409–412.
43. Jackson, RG. Anatomic study of the vagus nerves with a technique of transabdonminal selective gastric vagus resection. *Arch Surg* 1948; **57**: 333–335.
44. Griffith CA & Harkins HN. Partial gastric vagotomy: an experimental study. *Gastroenterology* 1957; **32**: 96–102.
45. Johnston D & Wilkinson AR. Highly selective vagotomy without a drainage procedure for duodenal ulcer. *Br J Surg* 1970; **57**: 289–292.
46. Amdrup E & Jensen HE. Selective vagotomy of the parietal cell mass preserving innervation of the undrained antrum. *Gastroenterology* 1970; **59**: 522–525.
47. ordan PH Jr. Parietal cell vagotomy without drainage for treatment of duodenal ulcer. *Arch Surg* 1976; **111**: 370–374.
48. Liavag I & Roland M. A seven-year follow-up of proximal gastric vagotomy: clinical results. *Scand J Gastroenterol* 1979; **14**: 49–52.
49. Madsen P & Kronborg O. Recurrent ulcer 5½–8 years after highly selective vagotomy without drainage and selective vagotomy with pyloroplasty. *Scand J Gastroenterol* 1980; **15**: 193–199.
50. Hallenbeck G, Gleysteen JC Aldrete JS et al. Proximal gastric vagotomy. Effects of two operative techniques on clinical and gastric secretory results. *Ann Surg* 1976; **184**: 435–437.
51. Nilsell K. Five- to nine-year results of selective proximal vagotomy with or without pyloroplasty for duodenal ulcer. *Acta Chir Scand* 1979; **145**: 251–256.
52. Storey DW, Boulos PB, Ward MWN and Clark CG. Proximal gastric vagotomy after 5 years. *Gut* 1981; **22**: 702–706.
53. Siebert R & Muller C. Proximal-gastriche Vagotomie: eine Zwischenbalanz. *Chirurg* 1981; **152**: 511–515.
54. Stoddard CJ, Duthie HL & Johnston AG. The four- to eight-year results of the Sheffield trial of elective duodenal ulcer surgery: highly selective or truncal vagotomy. *Br J Surg* 1974; **71**: 779–782.
55. Koffman CG, Hay DJ, Ganguli PC et al. Randomized trial of elective highly selective or truncal vagotomy in chronic duodenal ulceration. *Br J Surg* 1983; **70**: 41–44.
56. Hoffman J, Jensen HE, Poulsen PE et al. Prospective controlled vagotomy trial for duodenal ulcer: results after five years. *Br J Surg* 1984; **73**: 583–587.
57. deMiguel J. Recurrence after proximal gastric vagotomy without drainage for duodenal ulcer: a 3- to 6-year follow-up. *Br J Surg* 1977; **64**: 473–476.
58. Amdrup E, Anderson D & Hestrup N. The Aarhus County vagotomy trial. 1. An interim report on primary results and incidence of sequelae following parietal cell vagotomy and selective vagotomy in 148 patients. *World J Surg* 1978; **2**: 85–89.
59. Fraser AG, Brunt PW & Matheson NA. A comparison of highly selective vagotomy with truncal vagotomy and pyloroplasty: one surgeon's results after five years. *Br J Surg* 1983; **70**: 485–489.

60. Jordan PH Jr. An interim report on parietal cell vagotomy versus selective vagotomy and antrectomy for treatment of duodenal ulcer. *Ann Surg* 1979; **189**: 643–647.

61. Jensen HE & Amdrup I. Follow-up of 100 patients 5 to 8 years after parietal cell vagotomy. *World J Surg* 1978; **2**: 525–529.

62. Holst-Christensen J, Jonsen OH & Kronberg O. Recurrent ulcer after proximal gastric vagotomy for duodenal and prepyloric ulcer. *Br J Surg* 1977; **64**: 42–45.

63. Kronberg O, Jorgensen PM & Holst-Christensen J. Influence of different techniques of proximal gastric vagotomy upon risk of recurrent duodenal ulcer and gastric acid secretion. *Acta Chir Scand* 1977; **143**: 53–55.

64. Taylor TV. Lesser curve superficial seromyotomy: an operation for duodenal ulcer. *Br J Surg* 1979; **66**: 733–737.

65. Walker WS & Taylor TV. A modification to the technique of lesser curve seromyotomy. *Ann R Coll Surg Engl* 1982; **64**: 123–124.

66. Taylor TV, Gunn AR, MacLeod DAD et al. Anterior lesser curve seromyotomy and posterior truncal vagotomy in the treatment of chronic duodenal ulcer. *Lancet* 1982; **ii**: 846–848.

67. Taylor TV, Gunn AA, MacLeod DAD et al. Mortality and morbidity after anterior lesser curve seromyotomy with posterior truncal vagotomy for duodenal ulcer. *Br J Surg* 1985; **72**: 950–951.

68. Taylor TV. Lesser curve myotomy in the dog: an experimental study. *Ann Surg* 1980; **191**: 414–418.

69. McLean Ross AH, Smith AA, Anderson JR & Small WP. Late mortality after surgery for peptic ulcer. *New Engl J Med* 1982; **307**: 519–522.

70. Balaint JA & Spence S. Pyloric stenosis. *BMJ* 1959; **1**: 890–892.

71. Ellis H. Pyloric stenosis due to duodenal ulceration. In Wastell C (ed.) *Chronic Duodenal Ulcer.* London: Butterworth, 1974: 251.

72. Howe CT & LeQuesne LP. Pyloric stenosis: the metabolic effects. *Br J Surg* 1964; **51**: 923–926.

73. Hurst AF & Steward MJ. *Gastric and Duodenal Ulcer.* London: Oxford University Press, 1929.

74. Johnston D. A new look at vagotomy. In Nyhus LM (ed.) *Surgery Annual.* New York: Appleton-Century-Crofts, 1974: 125.

75. Keynes WM. Simple and complicated hypertrophic stenosis in the adult. *Gut* 1965; **6**: 240–244.

76. Kozoll DD & Meyer KA. Obstructing gastroduodenal ulcers. *Arch Surg* 1964; **88**: 793–796.

77. Kozoll DD & Meyer KA. Obstructing gastroduodenal ulcer: symptoms and signs. *Arch Surg* 1964; **89**: 491–494.

78. Rachlin L. Vagotomy and Heineke–Mikulicz pyloroplasty in the treatment of pyloric stenosis. *Am Surg* 1970; **36**: 251–255.

79. Kreel L & Ellix H. Pyloric stenosis in adults: a clinical and radiological study of 100 consecutive patients. *Gut* 1965; **6**: 253.

80. White CM, Harding LK, Keighley MRB et al. Gastric emptying after treatment of stenosis secondary to duodenal ulceration by proximal gastric vagotomy and duodenoplasty or pyloric dilatation. *Gut* 1978; **19**: 783–785.

81. Finney, JT. Perforating ulcer of the stomach. *Ann Surg* 1900; **32**: 1–6.

82. Adler J, Ingram D & Hause T. Perforated peptic ulcer: a seasonal disease? *Aust NZ J Surg* 1984; **54**: 59–64.

83. Boey J, Wong J & Ong GB. A prospective study of operative risk factors in perforated duodenal ulcers. *Ann Surg* 1982; **195**: 265–267.

84. Booth RAD & Williams JA. Mortality of perforated duodenal ulcer treated by simple suture. *Br J Surg* 1971; **58**: 42–44.

85. Kay PH, Moore KTH & Clark RG. The treatment of perforated duodenal ulcer. *Br J Surg* 1978; **65**: 801–804.

86. Coggon A, Lambert P & Langman MJS. 20 years of hospital admission for peptic ulcer in England and Wales. *Lancet* 1981; **i**: 1302.

87. Cohen MM. Treatment and mortality of perforated peptic ulcer: a survey of 852 cases. *Can Med Assoc J* 1971; **105**: 263–266.

88. Johnston D, Lyndon PJ, Smith RB & Humphrey CS. Highly selective vagotomy without a drainage procedure in the treatment of haemorrhage, perforation and pyloric stenosis due to peptic ulcer. *Br J Surg* 1973; **60**: 790–797.

89. MacLeod IA & Mills PR. Factors identifying the probability of further hemorrhage after acute upper gastrointestinal hemorrhage. *Br J Surg* 1982; **69**: 256–258.

90. Cutler JA & Mendeloff AI. Upper gastrointestinal bleeding; nature and magnitude of the problem in U.S. *Dig Dis Sci* 1981; **26** (Suppl): 90–96.

91. Himal HS, Watson WG, Jones CW, Miller L & Maclean LD. The management of upper gastrointestinal hemorrhage. *Ann Surg* 1974; **179**: 489–493.

92. Hunt PS. Surgical management of bleeding chronic peptic ulcer. A 10-year prospective study. *Ann Surg* 1984; **199**: 44–50.

93. Silverstein FE, Gilbert DA, Tedesco FJ, Buenger NK & Persing J. The national ASGE survey on upper gastrointestinal bleeding. I. Study design and baseline data. *Gastrointest Endosc* 1981; **27**: 73–79.

94. Macleod IA, Mills PR, MacKenzie JF, Joffe SN, Russell RI & Carter DC. Neodymium YAG photocoagulation for a major hemorrhage from peptic ulcers and single vessels: a single-blind controlled study. *BMJ* 1983; **286**: 345–348.

95. Allan R & Dykes R. A study of the factors influencing mortality rates from gastrointestinal hemorrhage. *Q J Med* 1976; **45**: 533–550.

96. Donahue PE & Nyhus LM. Massive upper gastrointestinal hemorrhage. In Nyhus, LM & Westell, C (eds) *Surgery of Stomach and Duodenum* Boston: Little Brown, 1977: 421–456.

97. Schiller KFR, Truelove SC & Williams DG. Hematemesis and melena, with special references to factors influencing the outcome. *BMJ* 1970; **2**: 7–14.

98. Graham DY. Limited value of early endoscopy in the management of acute upper gastrointestinal bleeding, prospective controlled trial. *Am J Surg* 1980; **140**: 284–290.

99. Hunt PS. Surgical management of bleeding chronic peptic ulcer. A ten-year prospective study. *Ann Surg* 1984; **199**: 44–50.

100. Taylor TV. Isolated duodenal tamponade for the treatment of bleeding duodenal ulcer. *Lancet* 1988; **i**: 911–912.

101. Grassi G. The technique of proximal selective vagotomy. *Chir Gastroenterol* 1971; **5**: 399–404.

102. Jensen HE, Kragelund E & Amdrup E. Intraoperative studies of the stomach (leucomethylene blue staining of the vagus, intragastric determination of pH, and Congo red staining of the mucosa). *Chir Gastroenterol* 1971; **15**: 30–34.

103. Grassi G & Orecchia C. A comparison of the intraoperative tests of completeness of vagal section. *Surgery* 1974; **75**: 13–18.

104. Ahonen J, Hoepfner-Hallikainen D, Inberg M & Scheinin TM. The value of corpus - antrum border determinations in highly selective vagotomy. *Br J Surg* 1979; **66**: 35–38.

105. Kusakari K, Nyhus L, Gillison E. et al. An endoscopic test for completeness of vagotomy. *Arch Surg* 1979; **105**: 386–390.

106. Salk RP, Greenberg AG, Farris JM et al. The practicability of the Congo red test, or is your vagotomy complete? *Am J Surg* 1976; **132**: 144–146.

107. Nyhus LM and Donohue PE Cited in Nyhus LM & Wastell C (eds) *Surgery of the Upper Gastrointestinal Tract.* 1994.

108. Schwobel M, Uhlschmid G & Largiader F. Uber die Pathogenese der Mangenwandnekrose nach selective-proximaler Vagotomie. *Chirurg* 1981; **52**: 328–332.

109. Kennedy T, Magill P, Johnston GW et al. Proximal gastric vagotomy, fundoplication and lesser curve necrosis. *BMJ* 1979; **1**: 1455–1457.

110. Taylor TV & Pearson KW. Recurrent ulcer after vagotomy. *Lancet* 1976; **ii**: 1303.

111. Holle F. Form- und funktionsgerechte operation, Eine grundsatz moderner Ulcuschirurgie. *Langenbecks Arch Chir* 1965; **308**: 205–233.

112. Holle F, Holle GE, Klempa J, Lissner J & Welsh KH. Form und funktionsgerechte chirurgie des Gastroduodenalulcus (508 Falle). *Ergeb Chir Orthop* 1970; **54**: 1–44.

113. Holle F. *Spezielle Magenchirurgie.* Heidelberg: Springer, 1968: 486–496.

114. Holle F. Effect of proximal gastric resection (fundectomy) on gastric secretion and motility. In Holle, F. & Andersson, S. (eds) *Vagotomy – Latest Advances.* Heidelberg: Springer, 1974: 65–67.

115. Holle F. Randomized study: SPV with versus without pyloroplasty. In Holle, F. & Andersson, S. (eds) *Vagotomy – Latest Advances.* Heidelberg: Springer, 1974: 182–183.

116. Holle GE & Reiser SB. Effect of selective proximal vagotomy without and with pyloroplasty on gastroduodenal motility. *Am J Dig Sci* 1985; **36**: 773–777.

117. Wilbur BG & Kelly KA. Effect of proximal gastric, complete gastric and truncal vagotomy on canine gastric electric activity, motility and emptying. *Ann Surg* 1973; **178**: 295–303.

118. Emoas S & Fernstrom M. Prospective, randomized trial of selective proximal vagotomy with pyloroplasty and selective proximal vagotomy with and without pyloroplasty in the treatment of duodenal, pyloric and prepyloric ulcers. *Am J Surg* 1985; **149**: 236–243.

119. Holle GE, Auerback Y, Hock H & Holle F. Changes of cell population in the antrum after selective proximal vagotomy and pyloroplasty in gastro-duodenal ulcer. *Surg Gynecol Obstet* 1985; **160**: 211–219.

120. Holle GE, Buck R, Pradayrol L, Wunsch E & Holle F. Behavior of somatostatin-immunoreactive cells in the gastric mucosa before and after selective proximal vagotomy and pyloroplasty in treatment of gastric and duodenal ulcers. *Gastroenterology* 1985; **89**: 736–745.

121. Hill GL & Barker MCJ. Anterior highly selective vagotomy with posterior truncal vagotomy: a simple technique for denervating the parietal cell mass. *Br J Surg* 1978; **65**: 702–705.

122. Grimson KS. Surgical procedures for peptic ulcer: critique of committee report. *Gastroenterology* 1953; **24**: 275–280.

123. Cehen AM & Ottinger LW. Delayed gastric emptying following gastrectomy. *Ann Surg* 1976; **184**: 689–696.

124. Postlethwait RW & Dillon ML. Gastric resection for duodenal ulcer. *Surgery* 1971; **69**: 829–831.

125. Postlethwait RW. Five year follow-up results of operations for duodenal ulcer. *Surg Gynecol Obstet* 1973; **137**: 387–392.

126. Welch CE & Ellis DS. Physiology of the surgically altered stomach. *Annu Rev Med* 1961; **12**: 19–38.

127. Fischer AB. Twenty-five years after Billroth II gastrectomy for duodenal ulcer. *World J Surg* 1984; **8**: 293–302.

128. Fenger, HJ. Clinical and experimental studies of dumping disposition: a method of preoperative evaluation of individual dumping disposition. *Acta Chir Scand [Suppl]* 1967: 371.

129. Chaimoff C & Dintsman M. The longer-term fare of patients with dumping syndrome. *Arch Surg* 1972; **105**: 554–556.

130. Goligher JC, Pulvertaft CN & de Dombal FT. Five to eight year results of Leeds York controlled trial of elective ulcer surgery for duodenal ulcer. *BMJ* 1968; **2**: 781–784.

131. Taylor TV, Lambert ME, Qureshi S & Torrance HB. Should cholecystectomy be combined with vagotomy and pyloroplasty? *Lancet* 1978; **i**: 295–298.

132. Ballinger WF. The extra gastric effects of vagotomy. *Surg Clin North Am* 1961; **46**: 455–463.

133. Ballinger WF. Postvagotomy changes in the small intestine. *Am J Surg* 1967; **114**: 382–386.

134. Browning GC, Cuchin KA & MacKay C. Small bowel flora and bowel habits studied at intervals following vagotomy drainage. *Br J Surg* 1972; **59**: 908–910.

135. Gray HMW. A cuase of intestinal obstruction after gastroenterostomy. *Lancet* 1904; **ii**: 526–528.

136. Hammer JM, Seay TH, Johnston RL et al. The effect of antiperistaltic bowel segments on intestinal emptying time. *Arch Surg* 1959; **79**: 537–539.

137. Barrett CR Jr & Holt TR. Postgastrectomy blind loop syndrome: megablastic anemia secondary to malabsorption of folic acid. *Am J Med* 1966; **41**: 629–635.

138. Amdrup BM & Griffith CA. Selective vagotomy of the parietal cell mass. I. With preservation of the innervated antrum and pylorus. *Ann Surg* 1969; **170**: 207–210.

139. Amdrup BM & Griffith CA. Selective vagotomy of the parietal cell mass. II. With suprapyloric mucosal antrectomy and suprapyloric antral resection. *Ann Surg* 1969; **170**: 215–220.

140. Griffith CA. Long-term results of selective vagotomy plus pyloroplasty: 12 to 17 year follow-up. *Am J Surg* 1980; **139**: 608–612.

141. Griffith CA. Gastric vagotomy vs total abdominal vagotomy. *Arch Surg* 1960; **81**: 891–895.

142. Griffith CA. Selective gastric vagotomy. *West J Surg Obstet Gynecol* 1962; **70**: 107 (part I), 195 (part II).

143. Griffith CA. Completeness of gastric vagotomy by the selective technic. *Am J Dig Dis* 1967; **12**: 333–338.

144. Griffith CA. Significant functions of the hepatic and celiac vagi. *Am J Surg* 1969; **118**: 251–255.

145. Griffith CA. Selective vagotomy plus suprapyloric antrectomy with and without pylorotomy for duodenal ulcer. *Ann Surg* 1974; **179**: 516–519.

146. Sawyers JL, Herrington JL Jr & Burney DP. Proximal gastric vagotomy compared with vagotomy and antrectomy and selective gastric vagotomy and pyloroplasty. *Ann Surg*, 1977; **186**: 510–515.

147. Sawyers JL, Scott HW Jr, Edwards WH et al. Comparative studies of the clinical effects of truncal and selective gastric vagotomy. *Am J Surg* 1968; **115**: 165–169.

148. Harkins HN, Schmitz EJ, Harper HP et al. A combined physiologic operation for peptic ulcer. *West J Surg* 1953; **61**: 316–321.

149. Harkins HN, Griffith CA & Nyhus LM. The revised 'combined operation' with selective gastric vagotomy. *Am Surg* 1967; **33**: 510–516.

150. Jordan PH Jr & Condon RE. A prospective evaluation of vagotomy pyloroplasty, vagotomy/antrectomy for the treatment of duodenal ulcer. *Ann Surg* 1970; **172**: 547–553.

151. Palumbo LT & Sharpe WS. Distal antrectomy with vagotomy for duodenal ulcer: results in 611 patients. *Ann Surg* 1975; **182**: 610–615.

152. Wolf JS, Bell CC Jr & Zimbert YH. Analysis of 10 years experience with surgery for peptic ulcer disease. *Am Surg* 1972; **38**: 187–193.

153. Hubert JP Jr, Kierman PD & Bearhs OH. Truncal vagotomy and antral resection in the treatment of duodenal ulcer. *Mayo Clin Proc* 1980; **55**: 19–24.

154. Herrington JL Jr, Sawyers JL, & Scott HW Jr. A 25-year experience with vagotomy–antrectomy. *Arch Surg* 1973; **106**: 469–474.

155. Herrington JL Jr. Truncal vagotomy with antrectomy. Symposium on peptic ulcer disease, 1976. *Surg Clin North Am* 1976; **56**: 1335.

156. Joffe SN, Crochet A & Doyle D. Morphological and functional evidence of reinnervation of the gastric parietal cell mass after parietal cell vagotomy. *Am J Surg* 1982; **143**: 80–84.

157. Faxen A. Parietal cell vagotomy and selective vagotomy with pyloroplasty. *Scand J Gastroenterol* 1978; **13**: 7–13.

158. Hancock DM, Sankar MY, Old JM et al. The combination of proximal gastric vagotomy with a rotational gastropexy for duodenal ulcer. *Br J Surg* 1978; **65**: 706–710.

159. Joffe SN & Bapat RD. The temporary effect of proximal gastric vagotomy on experimental duodenal ulcers and gastric secretion. *Br J Surg* 1979; **66**: 234–239.

160. MacLeod RS & Cohen Z. Highly selective vagotomy and truncal vagotomy and pyloroplasty for duodenal ulcer: a clinical review. *Can J Surg* 1979; **22**: 113–118.

161. Holle FK & Holle GE. Selective vagotomy and pyloroplasty. In Scott HW & Sawyers JL (eds) *Surgery of the Stomach, Duodenum and Small Intestine*. Oxford: Blackwell, 1990.

162. Reiser SB & Holle GE. Motor and electrical activity of the gastroduodenal junction before and after submucosal pyloroplasty in the dog. *World J Surg* 1982; **6**: 231–234.

163. Harling H, Balsley I & Bentzen E. Parietal cell vagotomy or cimetidine maintenance therapy for duodenal ulcer? *Scand J Gastroenterol* 1985; **20**: 747–750.

164. Graffner HO, Liedberg GF & Oscarson JEA. Parietal cell vagotomy in the surgical treatment of chronic duodenal, pyloric and prepyloric ulcer disease. *Int Surg* 1985; **70**: 139–144.

165. Anderson D. Prevention of ulcer recurrence: medical vs surgical treatment. The surgeon's view. *Scand J Gastroenterol* 1985; **20** (Suppl.110): 89–92.

166. Bader JP. The surgical treatment of peptic ulcer disease: a physician's view. *Dig Dis Sci* 1985; **30** (Suppl): 52S–54S.

167. Herrington JL Jr, Davidson J III, & Shumway SJ. Proximal gastric vagotomy: follow-up of 109 patients for 6–13 years. *Ann Surg* 1986; **204**: 108–113.

168. Stael von Holstein C, Graffner H & Oscarson J. One hundred patients ten years after parietal cell vagotomy. *Br J Surg* 1987; **74**: 101–103.

169. Enskog L, Rydberg B, Adamai HO, Enander LK & Ingvar C. Clinical results 1–10 years after highly selective vagotomy in 306 patients with prepyloric and duodenal ulcer disease. *Br J Surg* 1986; **73**: 357–360.

170. Marceau P, Bourque RA, Piche P, Biron S & Potvin M. Long-term results of hyperselective vagotomy for duodenal ulcer. *Can J Surg* 1986; **29**: 421–423.

171. Paimela H, Hallikainen D, Ahonen J, Hockerstedt K, Palmu A & Scheinin TM. The prognostic significance of radiologically determined gastric emptying time before proximal gastric vagotomy. *Acta Chir Scand* 1986; **152**: 611–615.

172. Primrose JN, Axon ATR & Johnson D. Highly selective vagotomy and duodenal ulcers that fail to respond to H_2-receptor antagonists. *BMJ* 1988; **206**: 1031–1035.

173. Jordan PH & Thornby J. Should it be parietal cell vagotomy or selective vagotomy–antrectomy for treatment of duodenal ulcer? A progress report. *Ann Surg* 1987; **205**: 572–587.

174. Muller C, Liebermann-Meffert D & Allgower M. Pyloric and prepyloric ulcers. *World J Surg* 1987; **11**: 339–344.

175. Heberer G & Teichmann RK. Recurrence after proximal gastric vagotomy for gastric, pyloric, and prepyloric ulcers. *World J Surg* 1987; **11**: 283–288.

176. Goodman AJ, Kerrigan DD & Johnson AG. Effect of the pre-operative response to H_2 receptor antagonists on the outcome of highly selective vagotomy for duodenal ulcer. *Br J Surg* 1987; **74**: 897–899.

177. Rogers PN, Murray WR, Shaw R & Barr S. Surgical management of bleeding gastric ulcer. *Br J Surg* 1988; **75**: 16–17.

178. Braghetto I, Csendes A, Lazo M et al. A prospective randomized study comparing highly selective vagotomy and extended highly selective vagotomy in patients with duodenal ulcer. *Am J Surg* 1988; **155**: 443–446.

179. Oostvogel HJM & van Vroonhoven THJMV. Anterior lesser curve seromyotomy with posterior truncal vagotomy versus proximal gastric vagotomy. *Br J Surg* 1988; **75**: 121–124.

180. Holle F. Adequate selective proximal vagotomy with pyloroplasty as nonresective surgery for peptic ulcer disease: a 20 year review. *Int Surg* 1983; **68**: 295–298.

181. Graffner H & Lindell G. Increased ulcer relapse rate after PCV in smokers. *World J Surg* 1988; **12**: 277–281.

182. Siriwardena AK & Gunn AA. Anterior lesser curve seromyotomy and posterior truncal vagotomy for chronic duodenal ulcer: the results at five years. *Br J Surg* 1988; **75**: 866–869.

183. Bauerfeind P, Koelz HR & Blum AL. Ulcer treatment: regimens and duration of inhibition of acid secretion: How long to dose. *Scand J Gastroenterol* 1988; **23** (Suppl. 153): 23–32.

184. Bardhan KD. Omeprazole in the management of refractory duodenal ulcer. *Scand J Gastroenterol* 1989; **24** (Suppl. 168): 63–73.

185. Rubin R. Medical treatment of peptic ulcer disease. *Med Clin North Am* 1991; **75**: 981–998.

186. Pounder RE. Model of medical treatment for duodenal ulcer. *Lancet* 1981; **i**: 29–30.

187. *Mortality Statistics (General): Review of the Registrar General on Deaths in England and Wales.* London: HMSO, 1990: Series DH1 No. 24: 32.

188. Katschinski BD & Logan R. Changes in birth-cohort pattern of peptic ulcer mortality in England and Wales. *Postgrad Med J* 1991; **67**: 825–828.

189. Crabtree JE, Taylor JD, Wyatt JI et al. Mucosal IgA recognition of *Helicobacter pylori* 120 kDa protein, peptic ulceration and gastric pathology. *Lancet* 1991; **338**: 332–335.

190. Walt R, Logan R, Katschinski BD, Ashley J & Langman M. Rising frequency of ulcer perforations in elderly people in the United Kingdom. *Lancet* 1986; **i**: 489–492.

191. Naschitz JE, Yeshurun D, Odeh M et al. Overt gastrointestinal bleeding in the course of chronic aspirin administration for secondary prevention of arterial occlusive disease. *Am J Gastroenterol* 1990; **85**: 408–410.

192. Silvoso GR, Ivey KJ, Butt JH, Lockard OO, Holt SD & Sisk C. Incidence of gastric lesions in patients with rheumatic disease on chronic aspirin therapy. *Ann Intern Med* 1979; **91**: 517–520.

193. Johnston D. Operative mortality and postoperative morbidity of highly selective vagotomy. *BMJ* 1975; **4**: 545–547.

194. Shapiro S, Gordon L, Dayhkovsky L, Grundfest W & Chandra M. Development of laparoscopic anterior seromyotomy and right posterior truncal vagotomy for ulcer prophylaxis. *J Laparoendosc Surg* 1991; **1**: 277–286.

195. Voeller GR, Pridgen WL & Mangiante EC. Laparoscopic posterior truncal vagotomy and anterior seromyotomy: a pig model. *J Laparoendosc Surg* 1991; **1**: 375–379.

196. Hunter JG, Becker JM, Lee RG, Christian PE & Dixon JA. Anterior lesser curvature laser seromyotomy with posterior truncal vagotomy: a potential treatment of peptic ulcer disease. *Br J Surg* 1989; **76**: 949–952.

197. British Medical Association and The Pharmaceutical Press. *British National Formulary.* London: British Medical Association and The Pharmaceutical Press, 1992: No.24: 31–34.

34

COMPLICATIONS OF PEPTIC ULCER AND THEIR MANAGEMENT

PC Bornman
SM Graham
JP Dunn

In view of the marked decline in elective surgery for peptic ulcer disease since the 1970s, surgeons are now mostly confronted with the complications of the disease. Although modern medical therapy has had a major impact on hospital admissions for elective surgery, the operation rate for complications has not been noticeably affected and mortality is increasing. Most patients who present with complications have not been on prior medical therapy. Additionally an increasing number of elderly patients are now seen with analgesic-induced ulcer complications. The management of these patients is more complex and has led to modification of previously established treatment practices. Risk stratification has now been more clearly defined and lesser surgical procedures and endoscopic techniques have been developed to accommodate this high risk group.

This chapter addresses contemporary management of perforation, penetration, stenosis and haemorrhage.

PEPTIC ULCER PERFORATION

Historical perspective

Perforated peptic ulcer has been recorded as far back as the seventeenth century. One of the earliest accounts is by Madame de La Fayette of the fatal illness of her royal mistress, Princess Henrietta Ann, Duchess of Orleans, daughter of King Charles I of England and wife of Philip, brother of Louis XIV, King of France.[1] In 1729 the surgeon Christopher Rawlinson[2] gave a vivid description before the Royal Society of Physicians of a case with a perforated ulcer involving the upper stomach 'wide enough to contain the end of one's finger'.

Perforated duodenal ulcer was described somewhat later by Hamberger in 1747[3] and was followed by numerous isolated case reports over the ensuing 100 years. In 1843 Edward Crisp[4] reported on 50 cases and gave a description of the clinical course. The first reviews of the literature were published by Brinton[5] (1856), Muller[6] (1860) and Krauss[7] (1865).

Until the end of the nineteenth century perforated peptic ulcer was regarded as a uniformly fatal disease although during the eighteenth century there were a few case reports of patients who survived with spontaneous gastric fistulas. In 1876 Leube[8] a well-known and respected gastroenterologist, summed up the nihilistic attitudes of the medical fraternity by suggesting euthanasia as the only humane form of treatment for these unfortunate patients. This pessimism prompted clinicians to give surgery a chance.[9] Mikulicz[10] was the first to attempt suturing of a perforated gastric ulcer in 1880 but the patient died. It was not until 1892 that the first successful operation was carried out by Heussner for a perforated gastric ulcer.[11]

The evolution in the management of perforated peptic ulcer over the last century has been influenced by many factors, including the development of modern anaesthesia, the introduction of antibiotics and surgical trends in the treatment of uncomplicated peptic ulcers, particularly in recent times with the advent of *Helicobacter pylori* eradication therapy.

Epidemiology

The statistics on perforated peptic ulcer seem to be more reliable than those reported on uncomplicated ulcers, because of the acute presentation and need for surgery. It has also been suggested that the statistics faithfully reflect changes in chronic ulcer disease.[9,12] Yet there are marked geographical differences, worldwide, within the same country[13] and even in neighbouring areas.[14]

A detailed review of the epidemiology of peptic ulcer and the factors that might influence the prevalence of the disease is discussed elsewhere in this book. Reference will be made to pertinent trends in hospital admissions, age, gender ratio and factors that possibly influence the statistics.

Hospital admissions

In Western countries repeated surveys of well-defined population groups, such as in the West of Scotland,[15-18] showed a steady increase in the incidence of perforated peptic ulcer until the early 1950s and thereafter a gradual decline until the early 1970s. The same trend was also noted in Oxford Hospitals[14] where the incidence of perforated peptic ulcer was 14/100,000 in 1959 and only 7/100,000 in 1963. This reduction was mainly due to a decline in duodenal ulcer perforations. A similar decline was also observed in another survey in the same area over an 18-year period (1965–82) with the exception that the ratio of perforated duodenal and gastric ulcers has remained unchanged.[19] Hospital admissions for perforated ulcers in the USA between 1970 and 1978, however, have remained constant at approximately 10/100,000 admissions.[20]

It has been suggested that the introduction of H$_2$-receptor antagonists, in Europe and the USA in the late 1970s was responsible for a further drop in the incidence of perforated peptic ulcer.[21,22] There are, however, no detailed epidemiological studies available to substantiate this claim. In fact, when the admission rates in two district health regions in Trent and Rotherham (UK) were correlated during periods before and after the introduction of H$_2$-receptor antagonists, overall admission rates for perforations did not change appreciably.[23]

Whereas the incidence of peptic ulcer and its complications is declining in Western Europe and the USA, the opposite is true in Hong Kong.[24] Over a 10-year period (1970–1980) admissions for uncomplicated and complicated ulcers increased substantially, particularly in men over the age of 60 years. Of further interest was the finding that the male:female ratio has remained the same at 6:1.

In developing countries such as South Africa, the incidence of perforation among Blacks (which was an almost unknown disease during the first half of the century) has risen sharply. During the period 1973–1976 admissions for perforations have become as common as those for Whites in central Johannesburg.[25] It will be interesting to observe whether similar trends occur in other developing countries.

Gender ratio

The changes in the sex ratio in patients with perforated peptic ulcer are of particular interest. In England during the nineteenth century it was predominantly a disease of women. Country practitioners found perforated gastric ulcers in young women, which 'swept away beautiful and healthy creatures within a few hours'.[9] Many of these ulcers occurred near the oesophagogastric junction. These young women were reported in the Lancet of 1837–1838 as being typically unmarried and suffering from 'irregularity of the uterine function'.

A reversal in the gender ratio occurred soon after the turn of the century, when it became a disease which affected almost exclusively young men. One exception was a report from South Australia during World War II of an epidemic of gastric

ulcer perforations among women.[12] No clear explanation could be found for this phenomenon but there was a suspicion that analgesic abuse may have played an important role. Trauma, direct or indirect by strenuous labour has also been implicated during the industrial period[26] as well as stress during World War II[27] and civil unrest in Belfast.[28]

The most noticeable change in the epidemiology of perforated peptic ulcer in the last two decades is the marked increase in the number of women, in particular elderly females, with duodenal[19,29] and prepyloric ulcer perforation.[30] This, together with the fall in incidence in young men has markedly altered the sex ratio.[29] The study from Nottingham has also shown a similar trend for gastric ulcer[29] during the period 1958–1982. Although case–control studies are still lacking, there is little doubt that the use and abuse of non-steroidal anti-inflammatory drugs (NSAIDs) for musculoskeletal disorders can largely account for the increased incidence in elderly patients.[19,29,30]

Mortality trends and risk factors

Mortality figures have dropped precipitously since the beginning of the twentieth century. In 1901 Moynihan[31] reported a surgical mortality rate of 91% in 45 cases, whereas 7 years later he reported a figure of 34%.[32] In reviewing collected series totalling 15,340 cases between 1930 and 1940, DeBakey[33] found the operative mortality to be approximately 23%. More recent surveys of overall mortality have shown improvement in the overall prognosis. Devitt and Taylor[34] in 1967 calculated a mortality figure of 20% whereas Palmer[35] (1972), Johnston[36] (1980) and Boey et al.[37] (1987) documented figures of 11.2, 7 and 5.3%, respectively. However, even in recent times, mortality figures vary greatly and are determined to a large extent by the proportion of poor risk patients in a particular study. Most deaths occur in patients over the age of 60 years who also suffer from concomitant disease. Reports quoting operative mortality alone can be misleading and in this respect several studies[38-41] have shown that the death rate is almost doubled if moribund patients are included. Moreover, in an appreciable number of patients perforations go unnoticed and are only identified at post mortem.[42]

Risk factors

Age, concurrent medical illness, shock and delayed treatment

It has been recognized for some time that old age, concurrent medical illness, shock[43-45] and delay in treatment are the most important prognostic factors in perforated peptic ulcer. Perforations occurring while patients are in hospital for other conditions are also associated with a prohibitive mortality.[38,40,41]

The risk stratification in perforated duodenal ulcers has now been carefully studied in prospective series by the Hong Kong group.[37,46] In the first series,[46] operative risk factors were studied in 213 consecutive patients who underwent emergency surgery for perforated duodenal ulcer. A total of 45 complications developed in 27 patients (13%) including nine (4%) who died. Twenty-two patients experienced cardiorespiratory complications, renal failure occurred in four, wound and intra-abdominal abscess in ten, gastrointestinal bleeding in five, and there were four miscellaneous complications. By using a stepwise discriminant analysis it was calculated that serious concurrent medical disease, shock on admission (blood pressure <100 mmHg) and long-standing perforation of more than 48 hours were the most important independent risk factors that significantly contributed to mortality. Old age, extensive peritoneal contamination and a short history of prior ulcer symptoms (less than 6 months) appeared to be related to mortality but only through the above factors. Interestingly, the degree of peritoneal soiling *per se* did not affect the outcome of these patients. These observations were validated in a further prospective study by the same group[37] on 259 consecutive patients except for the finding that perforation of more than 24 hours was also an independent risk factor. All 16 deaths could be predicted. Mortality increased exponentially with number of risk factors.

A retrospective series on 284 patients admitted to the surgical units of the Royal Devon and Exeter Hospitals[47] concurred to a large extent with the studies by Boey et al.[37,46] although preoperative shock was a significant independent prognostic factor only in patients over the age of 70 years. Also delayed presentation was not significant. However, these patients were older (mean age 70 years) when compared with the Hong Kong series (mean age 51 years) and NSAIDs were used by no fewer than 43% of their patients. These factors may account for the higher overall mortality (26%) in this study. The mortality in patients with gastric ulcers (mostly elderly females) was appreciably higher (41%) when compared with those with duodenal ulcer perforation (26%).

In both studies medical illness was not stratified according to a severity of disease classification such as the APACHE II scoring system.[48] Shock was not clearly defined and no distinction was made between hypovolaemic and septicaemic shock. These shortcomings may be responsible for the low specificity achieved in these two studies. Of those predicted to die in both the UK and Hong Kong studies over half survived. Despite this, old age, major medical illness, shock and long-standing perforation[49] (Table 34.1) should continue to alert the surgeon.

Ulcer site and chronicity

The prognosis of gastric ulcer perforation is less favourable than that of duodenal ulcer (Table 34.2); also the higher the

Table 34.1 Mortality and time interval from perforation to operation

AUTHORS	DATE	<12 HOURS		>12 HOURS	
		n	MORTALITY	n	MORTALITY
Heslop et al.[53]	1952	89	7 (7.8)	9	2 (22)
Mickel and Morrison[51]	1952	298	12 (4)	81	21 (26)
Jones and Doll[50]	1953	261	5 (2)	37	5 (13.5)
Schmitz et al.[54]	1953	79	3 (3.8)	24	3 (12.5)
Reimer[55]	1967	184	15 (8)	51	15 (29.4)
Nemanich and Nioloff[41]	1970	54	4 (7.4)	25	5 (20)
Mattingly and Griffin[52]	1980	48	1 (2.1)	76	11 (14.5)

Values in parentheses are percentages.

Table 34.2 Mortality related to site of perforation

AUTHOR	DATE	n	DUODENAL		GASTRIC	
			n	MORTALITY	n	MORTALITY
Jones and Doll[50]	1953	651	529	42 (8)	122	27 (22)
Kozoll and Meyer[56]	1960	1638	992	123 (12.4)	646	130 (20.2)
Hardy et al.[57]	1961	198	172	6 (3.5)	26	13 (50)
MacKay[17]	1966	5221	4795	497 (10.4)	426	111 (26.1)
Reimer[55]	1967	86	67	8 (12)	19	7 (37)
Sanders[14]	1967	213	173	25 (14.5)	40	15 (37.5)
Donaldson and Jarrett[58]	1970	462	395	52 (13)	67	15 (22)
Cohen[39]	1971	838	746	117 (15.7)	92	36 (39.1)
Watkins et al.[19]	1984	166	149	17 (11.4)	17	4 (23.5)
Irvin[17]	1989	265	214	44 (20.5)	51	14 (27.4)

Values in parentheses are percentages.

ulcer on the stomach the poorer the prognosis.[56] Although earlier reports[59–62] have documented a higher mortality in patients with chronic ulcers, more recent data show that deaths occur more frequently with perforation of acute ulcers. Most of these patients are elderly and use NSAIDS.[47]

Associated haemorrhage

Associated haemorrhage, although uncommon, has serious prognostic implications (Table 34.3). Some patients may present with simultaneous haemorrhage and perforation whereas others bleed during the early postoperative period. The bleeding usually comes from an associated posterior ulcer, which in some cases may be due to a stress response to sepsis.[36]

Table 34.3 Mortality related to haemorrhage following patch closure

AUTHORS	DATE	n	INCIDENCE	MORTALITY
Jones and Doll[50]	1953	ns	40	12 (30)
Rogers[44]	1960	187	ns (14)	ns (60)
Krippaehne et al.[45]	1964	82	5 (6.1)	5 (100)
Nemanich and Nicoloff[41]	1970	104	16 (15)	9 (56)
MacDonough and Foster[63]	1972	187	14 (7.5)	3 (21)
Griffen and Organ[64]	1976	122	2 (1.6)	2 (100)
Playforth and McMahon[65]	1978	161	3 (1.8)	1 (33.3)
Stabile et al.[67]	1979	70	8 (11.4)	4 (50)
Wara et al.[66]	1983	56	1 (1.8)	1 (100)

Values in parentheses are percentages.
ns, not stated.

Pathology

Definitions

There is a problem with the nomenclature of the pathology of perforations. A clear distinction is not always made between *free perforation, confined perforation* and *penetration*. In some reports[38] free perforation is referred to as acute perforation, whereas penetration is called chronic perforation. Terminology should therefore be standardized and, to avoid confusion, descriptions must be based on pathological principles rather than on clinical grounds. The distinction between perforation and penetration should be based on whether there is egress of bowel content into the peritoneal cavity at some stage.

Free perforation should be defined as the extension of an ulcer through all the layers of the gastrointestinal tract with spillage of luminal content into the peritoneal space. This almost exclusively occurs with anterior lying duodenal and gastric ulcers into the greater sac and rarely from posterior gastric ulcers in the lesser sac.

Confined ulcer perforation is initially free but is sealed early with a fibrinous exudate covered by omentum, or more commonly by the undersurface of the liver. A residual walled-off collection may develop in relation to the perforation site, the so-called 'formes frustes' ulcer described by Singer and Vaughan[68] or 'sealed gaspocket' alluded to by Feldman.[69]

Penetration is more commonly associated with posterior lying ulcers of the duodenum and stomach. The pathogenesis is different from a confined perforation in that at no stage is there escape of bowel content into the peritoneal cavity. This is avoided by the inflammatory reaction and dense fibrous adhesions which develop pari passu with the process of penetration. These have been described by Haubrich et al.[70] as 'mural ulcers' when the muscular layer is penetrated, 'fibrous adhesion' with full-thickness penetration and 'confined perforation' when an adjacent organ is penetrated (Figure 34.1). Mural ulcers, however, are not strictly penetrating because the serosa is not breached.

Ulcer site

Although there is considerable variation in reported series on the site of perforation, most occur in the duodenal bulb.[35] This probably reflects the more common occurrence of duodenal ulcer rather than a greater propensity to perforate. Factors such as NSAID abuse may determine the prevalence of the ulcer site. In an analysis of 194 patients where the ulcer site was correlated with drug consumption, Jorgensen[30] found a strong association of analgesic abuse with prepyloric ulcer perforation, an observation which was also made earlier by others.[72,73] Duggan[74] observed in Australia in the early 1960s an association between chronic analgesic abuse and perforation of ulcers in the body of the stomach.

Most free perforations of the duodenum are situated on the anterior or superior aspect of the bulb. A proximal posterior duodenal ulcer may rarely leak into the lesser sac.[35] Posterior perforation of gastric ulcer has been observed in 13% of cases by Palmer[35] but a survey by Feldman[75] could not confirm this high incidence. In the earlier literature multiple perforations have been described in about 4% of cases.[33] This high incidence may be attributed to the inclusion of stress ulcers, which were more commonly encountered in the past.

'Kissing' (anterior and posterior) ulcers or confluent 'saddle' ulcers are important variations to recognize.[67] There is an increased risk of bleeding from posterior lying ulcers, whereas the 'saddle' variant may give rise to technical difficulties with simple closure, or pose problems in the management of the duodenal stump when a resection is required.[76] It is not possible to determine the true incidence of 'kissing' ulcers in the series of simple closure, but it is noteworthy that Lowdon[77] found no fewer than 20 cases in his series of 51 patients who underwent gastrectomy.

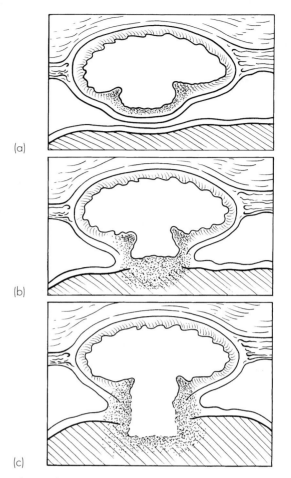

(a)

(b)

(c)

Figure 34.1

Degrees of penetration by peptic ulcer: (a) mural ulcer; (b) fibrous adhesion; and (c) confined perforation. (Reproduced with permission from Norris and Haubrich.)[71]

Acute and chronic ulcer

There is ongoing controversy as to whether a distinction can be made between so-called acute and chronic ulcers on macroscopic and microscopic appearances. According to Gilmour[59] the stomach or duodenal wall in acute ulcers is pink or red and mobile, and the perforation is small. In chronic ulcers the hole tends to be larger and there is more fibrosis and deformity. There may be adhesions between the ulcer area and neighbouring viscera, or penetration into the liver or pancreas. By using these criteria he could demonstrate a good correlation between the macroscopic appearance of the ulcer and the duration of ulcer dyspepsia. There are situations, however, where the distinction between acute and chronic ulcers is difficult particularly with long-standing perforation with associated oedema of the bowel wall and surrounding tissue.

Reports on the correlation between ulcer history and histological changes of the ulcer have been conflicting. In one of the original studies by Lowdon[77] differentiation was made between chronic and acute ulcers on the basis of the presence or absence of subserous fibrosis and obliterative endarteritis. A good correlation was found between histological changes and length of dyspepsia. This concept has been challenged by workers from Cape Town,[78] who showed fibrotic changes in all biopsies taken from the edge of the ulcer at the time of perforation. These findings concurred with those of Nuboer,[79] who noted changes of chronic ulcer in all cases undergoing gastrectomy for perforated ulcer.

The importance of both macroscopic and microscopic appearances of the ulcer in predicting the long-term outcome of patients after patch closure has not been studied. Correlating these with the duration of peptic ulcer disease might help to define the natural history more accurately.

Peritonitis

The free leakage of the gastric and duodenal content into the peritoneal cavity causes a severe chemical peritonitis which is usually sterile for the first 6–12 h (Table 34.4). The chemical irritation of bile and pancreatic and gastric juice is largely responsible for the severe hypovolaemic shock seen in delayed cases and results from massive sequestration of fluid and plasma into the peritoneal cavity.[57] A detailed study by Cope and his associates[85] on 24 patients with perforated peptic ulcer showed a rapid depletion of the extracellular fluid compartment and a reduced urine output with resultant haemoconcentration.

Table 34.4 Cultures from the peritoneal cavity taken at the time of surgery

AUTHORS	DATE	n	POSITIVE CULTURES	PREDOMINANT ORGANISMS
Turner[38]	1951	146	59 (40.4)	Streptococcus viridans, non-haemolytic Streptococcus
Hardy et al.[57]	1961	65	18 (27.7)	Streptococcus (non-haem/anaerobic) Staphylococcus
Hamilton and Harbrecht[82]	1967	74	44 (59.4)	(20 virulent)
Mark[80]	1969	64	22 (34.3)	
Wagensteen et al.[83]	1972	34	22 (64.7)	
Creco and Cahow[81]	1974	105	48 (45.7)	Staphylococcus, Streptococcus
Mattingly and Griffin[52]	1980	ns	ns(44)	
Boey et al.[84]	1982	143	48 (33.6)	Candida albicans, Escherichia coli, Pseudomonas, Streptococcus, Staphylococcus

Values in parentheses are percentages. ns, not stated.

In most reports the incidence of positive cultures (Table 34.5) and septic complications[50,81] increases with time. However, in one prospective study this was of clinical and prognostic importance only after 48 hours and in the presence of gross peritoneal soiling.[84] Of interest, though, was the finding that the organisms cultured from postoperative septic foci often differed from those cultured at the time of perforation.[83,84] The routine use of antibiotics may be responsible for these discrepancies and for the low incidence (4.3%) of septic complications in the study from Hong Kong.[84]

The organisms most commonly cultured during the early stages of perforation are streptococci and staphylococci which presumably come from the oral cavity.[81,84] Gram-negative bacteria supervene in delayed cases[51] with ileus and these are mostly

Table 34.5 Relation of intraperitoneal bacterial contamination with time interval between perforation and surgery

AUTHORS	DATE	POSITIVE CULTURE (%)				
		<6 h	7–12 h	13–24 h	25–48 h	49–96 h
Turner[38]	1951	26	58	23	58	
Hamilton and Harbrecht[82]	1967	36	—	—	—	20
Creco and Cahow[81]	1974	22	30	63	90	86
Mattingly and Griffin[52]	1980					
All cultures		25	26	50	37	78
Gram-negative organisms		—	22	37	43	57

responsible for the postoperative septic complications. *Candida albicans* has also been cultured but was not responsible for infections in the studies by Mark[80] and Boey et al.[84]

Clinical presentation and diagnosis

Events preceding perforation

Absence of ulcer history is noted in up to 25% of cases.[35] Some patients will give only a vague history of 'indigestion', for which they have taken proprietary medicines without consulting their physician. About half the patients will give a definite history of ulcer disease, including previous complication such as haemorrhage or perforation. Figures, however, vary depending on the population served by a particular institution. A history of dyspepsia is often absent in the elderly whereas younger patients tend to have a more chronic history.

Some patients experience acute exacerbation of their ulcer symptoms prior to the perforation. Turner[38] found that 44% of 185 patients developed increasing abdominal symptoms between 1 day and 2 weeks before the event. The most consistent 'risk factors' are excessive alcohol intake and dietary indiscretion[26,38,54,62] although the association remains tenuous. Physical exertion and trauma have also been implicated by some[16,38] but this could not be confirmed by others.[26]

Reports relating perforation to the time of day and week differ widely. In Scotland[16,86] patients perforate mostly in the late afternoon on Friday and Saturday and least often on Sunday and Monday. Across the Atlantic 27 of 100 patients in New York[87] perforated at night while in bed. Turner,[38] reporting from a different area in New York could not find any correlation with time.

The notion that most perforations happen during spring and autumn has not been substantiated by a number of reports. A review in 1940 by DeBakey[33] did not show any significant seasonal trends whereas MacKay[86] and Hendry et al.[88] showed that in Scotland more perforations occur in the winter. This was also the case in New York[38] and California.[80] It is interesting to speculate whether the increased use of analgesics and other medication for viral and chest infections during winter months might have been responsible for some of these trends. Although interesting, these findings are not clinically relevant.

Clinical presentation

There are few intra-abdominal catastrophies that can equal the dramatic presentation of a perforated peptic ulcer. The onset is marked by sudden onset of severe epigastric pain, which in some patients leads to collapse. Patients can usually tell the exact time and place when it occurred. The pain is initially located in the epigastrium but soon spreads throughout the abdomen. Shoulder-tip pain due to diaphragmatic irritation has been recorded in 23% in a collected series by DeBakey,[33] and Schmitz et al.[54] reported a 28% incidence. Nausea and vomiting are present in about half of the cases.

Another characteristic during the early stages of perforation is prostration. The patient has an anxious, haggard and pale expression with perspiration of the brow and temples and is peripherally shut down. One of the most consistent physical findings with free perforation is generalized, board-like rigidity of the abdomen. Moynihan's[89] description cannot be improved upon: 'every part offers the most inflexible opposition to pressure, the rigidity is obdurate, persistent, and unyielding'.

The pulse rate and temperature are usually normal in the beginning and most patients are not obviously shocked during the early stage. In untreated cases pain intensity subsides with time and the patient's condition appears somewhat improved. Excessive amounts of gas and fluid (bowel content and fluid sequestration) may accumulate if the perforation has not sealed off at an early stage. This gives rise to a distended and often tympanitic abdomen with associated ileus. The intense peritonitic signs usually diminish at this stage and a popping sign, described by Lui[90] may be elicited (a pop heard when testing for rebound tenderness). At this stage signs of hypovolaemic shock will be present and the temperature will start to rise. The patient rapidly becomes moribund and septicaemia may supervene.

Atypical presentations

A perforation may be occult in the chronically ill, immunosuppressed or otherwise debilitated patient. An appreciable number of cases are also diagnosed at post mortem.[42] The signs of a free perforation may rapidly subside if there is early sealing. In some, the diagnosis may be confused with acute cholecystitis or appendicitis when the leakage is sealed off in the right upper quadrant or tracks along the right paracolic gutter. It may also mimic acute pancreatitis or rarely a pseudocyst when there is posterior perforation into the lesser sac.

Special investigations

Radiology

An erect radiograph of the chest is the most important examination for detecting air under the diaphragm (Figure 34.2). Supine and erect radiographs of the abdomen are also commonly performed to exclude other causes of acute abdominal pain. An important additional or alternative view is the left lateral decubitus, i.e. the patient lying on the left side for 10 minutes (allowing the air to rise) and the radiograph taken with a horizontal beam. In the chest radiograph free air is seen beneath either dome of the diaphragm but in the decubitus view it rises to the lateral surface of the liver (Figure 34.3). The decubitus view is particulary useful for patients who are unable to stand or sit and there is also less chance of confusing

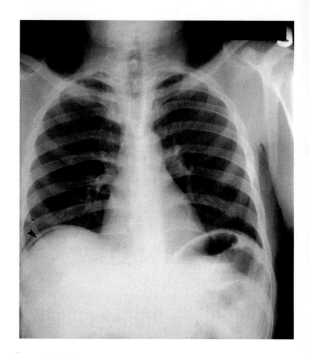

Figure 34.2
Erect chest radiograph demonstrating free air under the right dome of the diaphragm.

free air with bowel gas. With careful technique very small quantities of air may be detected.[91]

The supine view of the abdomen may also reveal free intraperitoneal air if this is abundant and if other views are not available. It may reveal the Rigler double-wall sign,[92] in which the gas on both sides of the wall highlights the serosal surface of the small bowel. The incidence of pneumoperitoneum in perforated peptic ulcer varies but taking advantage of the above techniques it should be possible to detect free air in over 70% of cases (Table 34.6). The introduction of additional air into the stomach via a nasogastric tube has been used in the past to increase chances of detecting free air[33,91] but the advisability of this manoeuvre should be questioned.

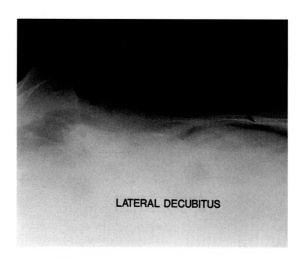

LATERAL DECUBITUS

Figure 34.3
Left lateral decubitus view demonstrating free air lying over the lateral surface of the liver.

Table 34.6 Incidence of free peritoneal air on plain radiograph

AUTHORS	DATE	n	FREE AIR
DeBakey[33a]	1940	1267	879 (69.4)
Mickel and Morrison[51]	1952	312	232 (74.4)
Stabins[93]	1953	128	93 (72.6)
Hardy et al.[57]	1961	206	124 (60.2)
Mark[80]	1969	41	36 (87.8)
Palmer[55a]	1972	2031	1515 (74.6)
Nemanich and Nicoloff[41]	1972	98	67 (68.4)
Donovan et al.[76]	1979	60	50 (83.3)
Mattingly and Griffin[52]	1980	124	82 (66.1)

Values in parentheses are percentages. [a]Collected series

It must be emphasized that the absence of free air in the peritoneal cavity does not exclude the diagnosis of perforated peptic ulcer nor is a pneumoperitoneum pathognomonic of the condition. It has been suggested that the time lapse between the perforation and taking of the radiograph may influence the diagnostic yield. In one study[80] more than 50% of the negative radiographs were taken within 6 hours of the event. Mickel and Morrison[51] found an incidence of only 30% in patients who presented within the first 3 hours and in all patients who were seen after 7 hours, whereas Mattingly and Griffin[52] found 66% had free air on admission and only 42% after 48 hours. However, the study by Nemanich and Nicoloff[41] time was not an important factor, suggesting that other aspects such as the site and size of the ulcer may be important in determining the presence of free air. Early sealing of the ulcer may result in a localized walled-off gas pocket in the subhepatic space, giving rise to the so-called 'formes frustes' type of perforation[68] (Figure 34.4).

Other causes of free air include perforation of small and large bowel, complicated cases of acute appendicitis and subphrenic abscess. Large bowel perforation is the second most common cause of free air in the peritoneal cavity and like perforated peptic ulcer, may give rise to massive pneumoperitoneum. A subphrenic abscess is capped by a gas pocket.[94] On plain radiography this can usually be distinguished from free air because the air-fluid level will not shift to another part of the abdomen with positioning.

The absence of free air should not be construed as evidence that the perforation has sealed. In this situation it would be advisable to carry out contrast studies, particularly when there is doubt about the diagnosis or when a conservative management policy is considered. A water-soluble medium, such as gastrografin, may actually show the presence and site of perforation or may demonstrate an ulcer crater (Figure 34.5). It must be remembered that many perforations are sealed off at the time of admission,[95] and in this situation a small acute ulcer can be easily missed with dilute contrast media.

Biochemistry and haematology

Raised serum amylase due to absorption from the peritoneal cavity has been recorded with variable frequency from 13[51] to

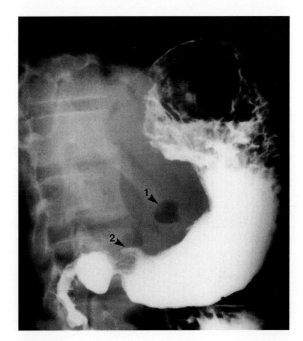

Figure 34.4
Early sealing of the ulcer leading to a localized walled-off gas pocket in the subhepatic space (arrow 1). In addition a 'double pylorus' demonstrated due to a 'penetrating' ulcer (arrow 2).

45%.[96] In most instances the level is seldom in the range seen with acute pancreatitis. In a comprehensive review Rogers[96] found levels in excess of 600 Somogyi units in less than 2% of cases. Similar findings were also reported in later studies.[45,57,80,97] The highest serum amylase levels were found in those cases with large perforations, marked fluid spillage and delayed presentation.

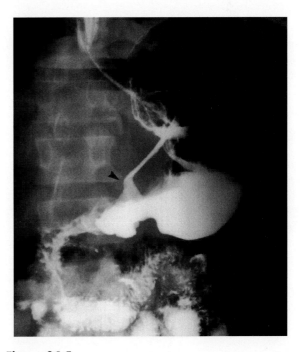

Figure 34.5
Contrast study demonstrating a prepyloric perforation.

A raised haematocrit is an indication of marked fluid loss into the peritoneal cavity and is seen in delayed cases with hypovolaemic shock.[57] Hypovolaemia may also give rise to a raised urea and electrolyte disturbances.

Management

Resuscitation

The initial resuscitation consists of establishing an intravenous line, the administration of analgesics and antibiotics and the placement of a nasogastric tube. Proper resuscitation is time well spent before definitive treatment is instituted.

Shocked patients may require large volumes of standard replacement fluids. Fresh frozen plasma and whole blood are given for cases with existing anaemia, coagulopathy or associated bleeding. In this situation, and in elderly patients, it is advisable to monitor fluid administration by a central venous line. A urinary catheter is mandatory. Opiates should be given for severe pain preferably through a controlled infusion system for more effective and safe administration.

A three-dose (perioperative) regimen of broad-spectrum antibiotics is given for perforations of short duration (6–12 h).[84] With more long-standing cases anaerobic coverage is also recommended.[52] Further antibiotic treatment may be governed by cultures taken at the time of surgery, although this is debatable because the organisms from septic foci often differ from those taken at the time of the perforation.[81,83,84]

The placement of a nasogastric tube forms an essential part of the initial management and its effectiveness has been proven by those who champion non-operative conservative treatment.[60,98] To achieve maximum benefit it is important that the tube is positioned correctly in the body/fundus area of the stomach which, in the supine position, is the most dependent part. X-ray screening should be used if there is any doubt about the correct position. Emptying of the stomach helps to minimize further spillage and is often followed by marked relief of the pain[60] usually within 2–3 hours.[99] Taylor and Warren[60] advise the initial use of a wide-bore tube to ensure complete emptying, but this would seem unnecessary unless the stomach contains large amounts of undigested food.

Emergency treatment of the perforation

Duodenal and pyloric channel ulcers The definitive treatment of perforated peptic ulcer has remained a controversial subject ever since the first report of successful simple closure by Mikulicz[10] in 1880. During the first half of the twentieth century treatment policies have varied from conservative treatment without surgery[61,98–101] to emergency gastrectomy.[77,79,102,103] The trends in management have been influenced by improved supportive measures (i.e. intravenous fluids and antibiotics), modern anaesthesia, the evolution of peptic ulcer surgery and, in more recent times, the advent of effective antiulcer drug therapy, in particular *Helicobacter pylori* eradication.

The literature on the three basic treatment strategies, namely non-operative conservative treatment, simple closure and immediate definitive surgery, is vast. Unfortunately, meaningful comparisons are limited by the shortcomings of predominantly retrospective studies. The conclusions in many of these studies are often based on bias rather than science.

Conservative non-operative treatment Conservative non-operative treatment by aspiration of the stomach was first used by Wagensteen[98] and was used exclusively for moribund patients too ill to withstand operation. The high morbidity and mortality (20%) of surgery during World War II, mostly from postoperative respiratory complications stimulated a number of workers to employ conservative non-operative therapy routinely.[53,60,100,101] Their premise was that ulcers frequently seal spontaneously and that routine nasogastric suction would aid this. In the 1950s Taylor and Warren,[60] Seeley and Campbell,[100] Heslop et al.[53] and Elliott and Lang[99] achieved remarkably low mortality figures (Table 34.7). Surgery was avoided in the majority of cases and there were few errors in diagnosis. These good results were attributed to careful adherence to the treatment protocol. This included effective gastric decompression, close observation and prompt surgical intervention in patients who continued to swallow air or who deteriorated.[60] Taylor and Warren were the first to draw attention to the marked difference in prognosis between acute ulcers (dyspepsia history of less than 3 months) and chronic ulcers. In their 1956 report[60] the mortality figure for chronic ulcers was 14% whereas no deaths occurred among 47 cases with acute ulcers. Of the 22 cases who required operative intervention, 21 were in the chronic ulcer group. On this basis they recommended conservative treatment only in patients with acute ulcers, a policy which was also followed by others.[76] Similar observations were also made in a more recent series by Kay et al. (1978),[61] in which no deaths occurred in the acute group of 26 patients. However, the reoperation rate was 24% and there were two subphrenic abscesses. In the chronic group three of 38 patients died and there was an alarming 63% reoperation rate with three fatalities.

Despite the earlier encouraging reports, non-operative treatment has not gained widespread acceptance. There are several

Table 34.7 Conservative non-operative treatment of perforated duodenal ulcer

AUTHORS	DATE	n	COMPLICATIONS	MORTALITY TOTAL	MORTALITY RELATED
Heslop et al.[53]	1952	104	13 (12.5)	9 (8.6)	5 (4.8)
Seeley and Campbell[101]	1956	139	ns ns	7 (5.2)	—
Taylor and Warren[60]	1956	93	10 (10.7)	11 (11.8)	4[b] (4.3)
Taylor[100a]	1957	1102	ns ns	57 (5.2)	25[b] (2.3)
Elliott and Lane[99]	1959	149	8 (5.4)	2 (1.3)	1 (0.7)
Keane et al.[104]	1988	42	2 (4.8)	1 (2.4)	1 (2.4)
Cocks et al.[106]	1989	93	6 (6.4)	4 (4)	3[b] (3.2)
Crofts et al.[105]	1989	40	6 (15)	2 (5)	0 (0)

Values in parentheses are percentages.
Related complications and mortality = reperforation, haemorrhage, gastric outlet obstruction, intraperitoneal sepsis bowel obstruction/ileus.
ns, not stated.
[a]Collected series.
[b]Excluding moribund patients.

possible reasons. First, since World War II safer anaesthesia and improved antibiotics have reduced surgical mortality. Secondly, patient selection and constant observation are difficult. Thirdly, there is always the risk of misdiagnosis in which conservative therapy would be inappropriate.[53] Therefore, in most centres conservatism is now reserved for moribund patients or those with localized perforation.

Some more recent studies, however, have again drawn attention to this form of treatment by reaffirming the good results of earlier reports (Table 34.7). In the first ever prospective randomized study, Crofts et al.[105] showed similar results when surgery and conservative treatment were compared in 83 consecutive patients studied at the Prince of Wales Hospital, Hong Kong. The operations performed in the surgical group were simple omental patch repair,[24] vagotomy and pyloroplasty[15] and Polya gastrectomy.[4] Eleven patients in the non-surgical group had no improvement during the first 12 hours of conservative treatment and were operated on. There were two deaths in each treatment group. The morbidity in the two groups was also similar, although there were more intra-abdominal abscesses in the conservative group. An important and somewhat disappointing finding was that elderly patients responded poorly to non-operative treatment. Six of nine patients over the age of 70 years eventually required emergency surgery for continued leakage. Nevertheless, this study confirms earlier reports[53,60,99,101] that conservative treatment with meticulous observation is safe and surgery can be avoided in the majority of cases.

In Melbourne, conservative management in one unit was compared with simple closure in another during the same period.[106] The non-operative group had lower mortality (6 versus 13%), shorter hospitalization and equivalent morbidity. In contrast to the findings of Taylor and Warren[60] and Kay et al.[61] chronic ulcer patients did not do worse.

The role of conservative non-operative treatment of perforated peptic ulcer deserves re-evaluation, particularly with the availability of potent antiulcer drug therapy. It is conceivable that this may become a more acceptable treatment choice in modern surgical units.

Surgical treatment Most of the controversy surrounding the management of perforated duodenal ulcer revolves around the choice between simple closure and immediate definitive surgery. There are three fundamental aspects by which these treatment options should be judged. First, the immediate outcome must be examined, in particular the mortality related to the specific treatment. Second, the natural history of the ulcer after simple closure must be weighed against potential postoperative sequelae of definitive ulcer surgery and third, the ability to prevent ulcer recurrence with *H. pylori*.

Comparison of the morbidity and mortality of these treatment options has been bedevilled by the lack of planned treatment protocols in retrospective studies, the selection of simple closure for high-risk patients and operations being carried out by surgeons with different levels of expertise. This is clearly reflected by a survey done by DeBakey[33] in a period in which where general anaesthesia was still regarded as

unsafe. In collected series of 11,284 cases mortality figures were lower for gastrectomy (13%) than for simple closure (26%). Indeed, several of the earlier reports from Europe, where resection has enjoyed its greatest popularity, achieved mortality figures of well below 10%.[107-109] Yet it is clear from these and later studies[110-124] that definitive surgery can be safely performed in centres with the necessary expertise.[46] In prospective studies comparing simple closure with definitive operation, mortality figures are similar[66,115-117] and therefore do not strongly support either option.[125]

The debate concerning the long-term outcome after these operations is more difficult to evaluate. Those in favour of a definitive operation at the time of the perforation or as a staged procedure 6–12 weeks after simple closure argue that 50–80% of patients with a past history of dyspepsia (Tables 34.8 and 34.9) will experience further ulcer symptoms. As many as 57% may require further surgery.[133] Definitive acute surgery reduces ulcer recurrence and its complications as effectively as elective ulcer surgery. The long-term side-effects are seldom incapacitating, particularly with highly selective vagotomy.

The conservative camp also has strong arguments which may become more convincing with the availability of modern drug therapy.

● Although risk factors for mortality have been more accurately defined, the selection of patients for definitive surgery is still difficult. In the controlled trial by Wara et al.[66] there were two deaths in patients after highly selective vagotomy; these patients, because of errors in judgement, should not have been included for randomization.

● Fewer elective operations are now carried out worldwide. Consequently, experienced surgeons, especially those competent in highly selective vagotomy, are not always available.

● The argument that definitive surgery in patients with chronic ulcers avoids immediate and late ulcer-related complications and deaths is not well founded (Tables 34.8 and 34.9). These problems may become even further reduced with careful follow-up and modern medical therapy.[140] Furthermore, complications occur with similar frequency in acute ulcers which are often excluded from definitive surgery.[139]

● The selection of patients for definitive surgery based on a history of preoperative dyspepsia is far from ideal. In the first instance, it is well recognized that a reliable history is not easily obtainable from distressed patients. There is also no uniform agreement on what length of ulcer dyspepsia can be termed chronic. Suggestions include 1 month,[113,141] 3 months (Table 34.9), 6 months,[40,41] 1 year,[49] and even 5 years;[63] 3 months has been used most commonly but there remains much inconsistency (Table 34.9). Based on this criterion 50–80% of patients will be submitted to an unnecessary definitive operation. The macroscopic appearance of the ulcer at the time of the perforation has also been disappointing in predicting intractability. In a study by King and

Table 34.8 Natural history of perforated duodenal ulcer after patch closure

AUTHORS	DATE	n	FOLLOW-UP (YEARS)	TOTAL RECURRENCE	LATE COMPLICATIONS[a]	LATE MORTALITY[a] (%)
Illingworth et al.[126]	1946	773	1–5	ns (70)	ns (20)	1.6
Tovee[127]	1951	78	5–20 'up to 20'	52 (67)	8 (10)	ns
Turner[38]	1951	143	50% >5	108 (76)	37 (26)	5
Stabins[93]	1953	167	6 months–20 years	109 (65)	38 (23)	ns
Harbrecht and Hamilton[128]	1960	146	ns	109 (75)	5 (3)	1
Hadfield and Watkin[112]	1964	69	ns	35 (51)	3 (4)	4
Nemanich and Nicoloff[41]	1970	60	1.5–14.5	37 (62)	8 (13)	ns
Creco and Capow[81]	1974	111	>5	61 (55)	9 (8)	ns
Jordan et al.[110]	1974	63	6.7	46 (73)	16 (25)	ns
Gray and Roberts[113]	1976	59	6 months–6 years	11[b] (19)	3 (5)	2
Playforth and McMahon[65]	1978	132	26 months	63 (48)	10 (8)	4

Values in parentheses are percentages.
[a] Ulcer related (haemorrhage and reperforation).
[b] Surgery.
ns, not stated.

Ross[137] only 18 of 53 patients in whom ulcers were intraoperatively assessed as chronic subsequently came to definitive surgery.

The subject has been further clouded by the seemingly different behaviour of ulcers after simple closure. A number of workers[40,83,114,116,131] could not confirm a difference in the natural history after simple closure between so-called acute and chronic ulcers. Moreover, the more aggressive ulcer diathesis seen in young males under 30 years old) in Hong Kong[142] could not be confirmed by a study in Cape Town.[139] Creco and Cahow[81] again found that 65% of recurrences occurred among older males (40–60 years) whereas others[49,137,139,143] have not observed any difference with regard to age or sex. Some of the discrepancies may be explained by the diligence of the follow-up studies (the routine use of endoscopy) and differences in the threshold for referral for surgery. Whatever the reasons, individual centres should be cautious in formulating treatment policies based on data from different geographical areas. A flexible policy should, therefore, be adopted based on local experience, available expertise and facilities.

Simple closure with omental patch (patch closure) has remained the treatment of choice for the majority of patients with perforated duodenal ulcer. This is clearly reflected in recent surveys carried out in England and the USA. A reply from a questionnaire sent to 274 consultant general surgeons in England revealed that simple closure with or without H_2-receptor antagonists was the preferred treatment.[144]

Table 34.9 Natural history of perforated ulcer after patch closure: ulcer recurrence in acute (<3 months dyspepsia) and chronic (>3 months dyspepsia) ulcers, and late complications and deaths

AUTHORS	DATE	n	FOLLOW-UP (YEARS)	RECURRENCE TOTAL	ACUTE (%)	CHRONIC (%)	SUBSEQUENT DEFINITIVE SURGERY TOTAL	ACUTE (%)	CHRONIC (%)	LATE COMPLICATIONS HAEM.	PERF.	TOTAL	ULCER DEATHS
Dean et al.[129]	1962	170	8–10	122 (72)	38	81	68 (40)	14	47	12	11	23 (13)	2
Cassel[130]	1969	224	10	—	—	—	81 (36)	20	44	13	9	22 (10)	ns
Rees et al.[131]	1970	107	ns	91 (85)	94	82	56 (52)	42	57	12	6	18 (17)	ns
McDonough and Foster[63]	1972	120	ns	47 (39)	22	53	44[b] (31)	ns	ns	3	—	3 (2)	ns
Skovgaard[132]	1977	156	3–23	111 (71)	12	87	75 (48)	—	—	—	—	14 (9)	0
Drury et al.[133]	1978	50	1–48 months	26 (52)	14	67	11 (22)	0	31	—	2	2 (4)	ns
Kay et al.[61]	1978	57	>2	ns (—)	—	—	13 (23)	13	30	2	2	4 (7)	ns
Baekgaard et al.[134]	1979	80	6–18	36 (45)	28	35	35 (44)	—	—	ns	ns	ns	ns
Dark and MacArthur[135]	1983	187	± 5 years	ns (ns)	—	—	54 (29)	6	38	—	15	15 (8)	ns
Tanphiphat et al.[114]	1985	27	12–80 months	14 (52)	80	68	9 (33)	40	32	4	—	4 (15)	ns
Ceneviva et al.[116]	1986	38	7	22 (58)	50	62	9 (24)	14	29	2	—	2 (5)	0
Gillen et al.[136]	1986	88	acute 17.5 months chronic 27.4 months	ns (—)	—	—	54 (61)	21	57	2	3	5 (6)	0
Boey and Wong[138]	1987	393	7	— (—)	52[a]	75[a]	ns	—	—	29	9	38 (10)	0
King and Ross[137]	1987	86	5–12	39 (45)	37	51	21 (24)	6	37	—	2	2 (2)	2
Bornman et al.[139]	1990	113	± 43 months	48 (43)	32	55	21 (19)	15	21	1	4	5 (4)	0

Values in parentheses are percentages.
ns, not stated.
[a] Cumulative recurrence rate.
[b] 44 of 139 patients.

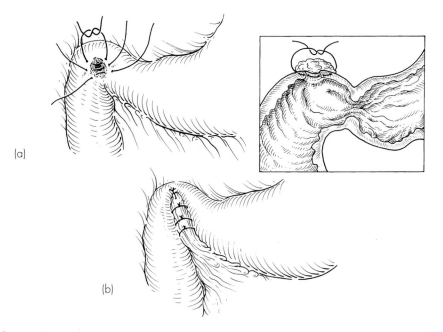

Figure 34.6
(a, b) Three absorbable seromuscular sutures are tied over an omental pedicel graft with an additional apex stitch.

Its simplicity and safety even in less experienced hands has been the major reason for the continued popularity of this procedure. Most surgeons still subscribe to the basic philosophy expressed by Graham[145] in 1937: 'We have no responsiblity for such patients but to save their lives. Any procedure which aims to do more than this can quite justifiably be considered meddlesome surgery. We have no responsibilities during the surgery to carry out any procedure designed to cure the patient of his original duodenal ulcer.'

Although the technique of closure has varied somewhat during its development it is now generally accepted that the use of an omental patch popularized by Graham[145] is the most effective and safe method of closure. Three seromuscular absorbable sutures are placed at the top, in the middle and at the bottom of the perforation and gently tied over an omental pedicle graft. An additional suture to fix the apex of the omentum is also useful (Figure 34.6). This technique allows easy closure of most perforated duodenal ulcers, even in the presence of severe oedema or fibrosis. When for some reason the omentum cannot be used, the falciform ligament is an alternative.[146] The laparoscopic approach has been increasingly used for simple closure with seemingly similar results to the open

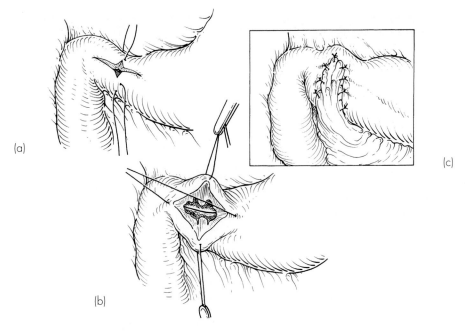

Figure 34.7
(a–c) Weinberg pyloroplasty with one layer interrupted closure covered with omental pedicel graft.

506 UPPER DIGESTIVE SURGERY

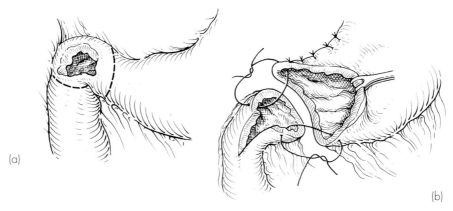

Figure 34.8

(a,b) Horsley slit for large anterior duodenal ulcer perforation.

approach. The efficacy of peritoneal clearance in the presence of gross contamination by gastric content, however, still needs to be determined.

Today with fibreoptic endoscopy, biopsy of the ulcer should be discouraged especially when closure is compromised. Difficulty in closure may be encountered in the presence of large perforations of acute ulcers, such as those induced by NSAIDs. In this situation some form of pyloroplasty should be used. Complete mobilization of the duodenum will facilitate this and an omental graft can be added (Figure 34.7). A vagotomy is unnecessary in this situation. Antrectomy should be considered in the rare case of large perforations where neither simple closure nor pyloroplasty are deemed safe. In most instances a Billroth I anastomosis can be safely performed, since the posterior wall of the duodenal cap is usually not involved. With large perforations the Horsley slit technique[147] (Figure 34.8) will ensure a safe and adequate stoma.

The overall *postoperative morbidity* after patch closure aver-

ages 16% (0–42%) (Table 34.10). It is important to note, however, that only about one-quarter of these complications are directly related to the ulcer. Half of the deaths in the series were due to systemic causes in patients with intercurrent illness (Table 34.10). Some patients die of overwhelming sepsis. Reperforation may be a factor but the incidence is unknown. Concurrent haemorrhage and postoperative bleeding remain the most lethal ulcer-related complications (Table 34.3). A history of recent gastrointestinal haemorrhage should compel the surgeon to consider a definitive operation. The mortality rate for simple closure is remarkably low especially as in most series this operation is also done in the most severely compromised patients.

One of the main concerns after patch closure alone is the risk of further life-threatening ulcer related complications (haemorrhage or reperforation). Although earlier series have reported an incidence of about 20%[93,139] more recent data (Tables 34.8 and 34.9) with few exceptions,[110,114,131] have shown

Table 34.10 Morbidity and mortality after patch closure

AUTHORS	DATE	n	MORBIDITY				MORTALITY			
			ALL CASES	ABDOMINAL[a]	ULCER RELATED[b]	SYSTEMIC	OVERALL	ULCER COMPLICATIONS	SEPSIS	SYSTEMIC
Hamilton and Harbrecht[82]	1967	44	13 (29.5)	6	3	4	4 (9.1)	2	0	2
Mark[80]	1969	52	7 (13.5)	6	0	1	7 (13.5)	0	4	3
Nemanich and Nicoloff[71]	1970	79	13 (16.3)	9	3	1	9 (11.4)	3	2	4
Rees et al.[131]	1970	97	14 (14.4)	1	9	4	10 (10.3)	3	0	7
Wagensteen[83]	1972	87	4 (4.5)	0	2	2	2 (2.2)	0	0	2
McDonough and Foster[63]	1972	187	9 (4.8)	4	5	0	19 (10.2)	6	4	9
Griffen and Organ[64]	1976	122	16 (13.1)	2	3	ns	8 (6.5)	3	2	3
Gray and Roberts[113]	1976	77	24 (31.1)	6	6	12	10 (13)	2	0	8
Skovgaard[182]	1977	249	48 (19.3)	28	6	14	23 (9.2)	2	12	9
Playforth and McMahon[65]	1978	161	29 (10)	13	6	10	8 (4.8)	3	0	5
Kay et al.[61]	1978	57	5 (9)	1	1	3	4 (7)	1	0	3
Sirinek et al.[62]	1981	60	25 (41.6)	4	3	18	10 (16.6)	0	ns	10
Heuman et al.[49]	1983	77	20 (26)	12	3	10	5 (6.5)	2	3	0
Total		1349	232 (17.2)	92 (6.8)	50 (3.7)	79	119 (8.8)	27	27	65

Values in parentheses are percentages.

ns, not stated.

[a]Abdominal, intra-abdominal sepsis, would infection and dehiscence, bowel obstruction.

[b]Ulcer related, rebleeding, reperforation, gastric outlet obstruction.

figures of well below 10%. Reports on deaths related to these complications remain sporadic (Tables 34.8 and 34.9), and occur during the first 2 years. Although uncomplicated ulcer disease has a recurrence rate of 80% within 1 year after stopping treatment,[148,149] the natural history of perforated duodenal ulcer appears to run a more benign course.[139] This difference is difficult to explain as the incidence of H. pylori would seem to be similar to that documented in uncomplicated ulcer disease.[150] Nevertheless, a strong case can be made for H. pylori eradication therapy on discharge to be followed by a endoscopy after 6 weeks to confirm ulcer healing and successful eradication therapy.

Until recently before data on H. pylori became available *definitive surgery* enjoyed support in some academic centres with an interest in the disease and has evolved from resection with or without vagotomy, to vagotomy and drainage and more recently patch closure with highly selective vagotomy. As stated earlier mortality figures for definitive procedures, when restricted to good-risk patients, do not differ from patch closure (Tables 34.11 and 34.12). The fear of developing mediastinitis with the dissection during vagotomy is unfounded and breakdown of suture lines is an uncommon event.

Despite the good results achieved with resection by pioneers in this field[103,107–110] vagotomy and drainage and highly selective vagotomy are now most commonly performed. Vagotomy and drainage remains attractive by virtue of its technical simplicity.[61,112,114,119,120] It is the operation of choice for those cases with associated haemorrhage or stenosis. Overall results after vagotomy and drainage are remarkably good, at least in the short to medium term (Tables 34.11 and 34.12).

Table 34.11 Immediate and long-term outcome of operations for perforated duodenal ulcer: patch closure, gastrectomy, vagotomy and antrectomy and vagotomy and drainage

AUTHORS	DATE	OPERATION	n	OP. MORBIDITY TOTAL	RELATED	OP. MORBIDITY TOTAL	RELATED	n	PERIOD (YEARS)	VISICK 1 AND 2	RECURRENCE TOTAL	SURGERY
Cooley et al.[103]	1955	Closure	70	ns	ns	6 (9)	5	7	ns	ns		
		Gastrectomy	112	ns	ns	5 (4)	1	1	ns	ns		
Hadfield and Watkin[112]	1964	Closure	107	ns	—	31 (29)	ns	69	2–5	49	35 (51)	ns
		V&D	61	14 (23)	1 (2)	3 (5)	1 (2)	39	1.5–4	90	ns	ns
Hamilton and Harbrecht[82]	1967	Closure	44	13 (30)	3 (7)	4 (9)	2 (5)	40	1.5	23	ns	25 (63)
		V & D 30										
		V & A 6	36	1 (3)	0	0	—	32	ns	85	1 (3)	0
Cohen[39]	1971	Closure	687	ns	ns	54 (8)	ns	ns	ns			
		Gastrectomy	22	ns	ns	3 (14)	ns	ns	ns			
Wagensteen et al.[83]	1972	Closure	89	ns	—	2 (2)	—	84	6–20	20	—	58 (69)
		V & D and										
		Gastrectomy	37	ns	—	ns	—	37	6–20	94	—	ns
Jordan et al.[110]	1974	Closure	306	63 (21)	ns	32 (10)	ns	63	6–7	27	46 (73)	22	35
(DU and GU)		Gastrectomy	327	43 (13)	ns	7 (2)	ns	144	5.2	87	10 (7)	ns
		V & A	208	40 (19)	ns	5 (2)	ns	53	4.2	91	0	
Gray and Roberts[113]	1976	Closure	77	22 (28)	2 (3)	10 (13)	2 (3)	59	0.5–6	43	—	11 (18)
		V & D	99	29 (29)	4 (4)	1 (1)	1 (1)	70	0.5–6	81	3 (4)	ns
Griffen and Organ[64]	1976	Closure	122	ns	—	8 (7)	3 (2)	122	ns		59 (48)	ns
		V & A	52	ns	—	5 (10)	1 (2)	52	ns	ns	ns	
Jordan and Korompai[111]	1976	Closure	40	ns	—	8 (20)	2 (5)	28	4	53	ns	14 (50)
								49	4.2	90	—	3 (6)
								55	4	93	1 (2)	0
Kay et al.[61]	1978	Closure	57	9 (16)	0	4 (7)	0	57	>2	ns	ns	13 (23)
		V & D	48	3 (6)	0	3 (6)	0	48	>2	ns	ns	5 (10)
Kirkpatrick and Bouwman[40]	1980	Closure	137	ns	—	9 (7)	2 (2)	67	1.5	ns	39 (85)	17 (25)
		V & D	32	ns	—	0	0	ns	ns			
		V & A	15	ns	—	3 (20)	1 (7)	ns	ns			
Mattingly and Griffin[52]	1980	Closure	64	— (25)	—	9 (14)	ns	ns	ns			
		V & D	50	— (12)	—	2 (4)	ns	ns	ns			
		V & A	6	— (17)	—	1 (17)	ns	ns	ns			
Watkins et al.[19]	1984	Closure	94	ns	—	10 (11)	ns	ns	ns	—	—	—
		V & D	58	ns	—	2 (3)	ns	ns	ns	—	—	—
		Gastrectomy	5	ns	—	2 (40)	ns	ns	ns	—	—	—
Tanphiphat et al.[114]	1985	Closure[a]	33	7 (21)	—	0	0	27	1–1.5	30	14 (52)	9 (33)
		V & D	32	7 (22)	1 (3)	0	0	26	1–1.5	81	3 (12)	ns
Irvin[17]	1989	Closure	78	23 (29)	3 (4)	32 (41)	3 (4)	ns	ns	—	—	—
		V & D	159	24 (15)	4 (3)	27 (17)	4 (3)	ns	ns	—	—	—

Values in parentheses are percentages.
DU, duodenal ulcer; GU, gastric ulcer; V & A, vagotomy and antrectomy; V & D, vagotomy and drainage; ns, not stated.
[a]Randomized studies.

Table 34.12 Immediate and long-term outcome of operations for perforated duodenal ulcer: patch closure, vagotomy and drainage and highly selective vagotomy

AUTHORS	DATE	OPERATION	n	OP. MORBIDITY TOTAL	RELATED	OP. MORBIDITY TOTAL	RELATED	n	LONG-TERM FOLLOW UP PERIOD (YEARS) n	VISICKS 1 AND 2 (%)	RECURRENCE TOT n	RECURRENCE SURGERY (%)	CUMULATIVE % RECURRENCE FREE %	PERIOD
Hinshaw et al.[118]	1968	V & D	180	11 (6)	1 (1)	2 (1)	0	ns						
Kahn and Ralston[119]	1970	V & D	81	24 (30)	2 (3)	0	—	78	0.5–3.5	85	1 (1)	1 (1)	—	—
Johnston et al.[120]	1973	HSV	5	0	0	0	—	ns	—	—	—	—	—	—
Jordan et al.[121]	1976	HSV	25	1 (4)	—	0	—	22	0.5–4	100	0	0	—	—
Sawyers and Herrington[122]	1977	HSV	21	3 (14)	0	—	—	20	0.5–3.5	100	0	0	—	—
Johnston[36]	1980	HSV	38	0	0	0	—	ns	—	—	—	—	—	—
									mean					
Boey et al.[115] (Chronic/DU)	1982	Closure[a]	35	0	0	0	0	0	35	40 months	57	—	37	40 months
		V&D[a]	32	0	0	0	0	0	32	40 months	90	—	88	40 months
		HSV[a]	34	0	0	0	0	0	34	40 months	97	—	96	40 months
Jordan[123]	1982	HSV	60	2 (3)	0	0	—	49>2 years	1–8	98	1 (2)		—	—
									median					
Wara et al.[66]	1983	Closure[a]	56	13 (23)	1 (2)	3 (5)	1 (2)	45	4	80	8 (18)	—	71	8 years
		HSV[a]	67	20 (30)	3 (5)	3 (5)	1 (2)	61	4	84	8 (13)	—	79	8 years
Ceneviva et al.[116]	1986	Closure	41	0	0	3 (7)	0	38	1–7	37	22 (58)	9 (24)	± for %41	7 years
		HSV	38	0	0	0	0	38	1–7	95	2 (5)	1 (3)	± for %96	7 years
Choi et al.[124]	1986	HSV	93	6 (6)	1 (1)	0	—	93	21 months	97	3 (3)		—	—
Boey et al.[117] (acute DU)	1988	Closure[a]	41	3 (7)	2 (5)	0	0	41	25	66	14 (34)	6 (15)	63	3 years
		HSV[a]	37	4 (11)	2 (5)	0	0	37	25	92	3 (8)	1 (3)	89	3 years

Values in parentheses are percentages.
DU, duodenal ulcer; V & D, vagotomy and drainage; HSV, highly selective vagotomy; ns, not stated.
[a]Controlled studies.

Highly selective vagotomy and patch closure has proved to be the safest of the definitive operations with only three deaths (all from one centre) being reported in a collective series of 312 cases (Table 34.12). Two prospective studies from Hong Kong have shown highly selective vagotomy superior in chronic ulcers to patch closure and vagotomy–drainage[115] and, in acute ulcers, to patch closure.[117] Similar conclusions were drawn from another controlled study by Ceneviva et al.[116] from Sao Paulo. The controlled series from Wara et al.[66] however, is less convincing especially with respect to recurrence rate.

Gastric ulcer About 20% of perforated peptic ulcers are confined to the stomach where they occur equally in males and females.[35,151,152] When compared to duodenal ulcers, more elderly patients with associated medical illnesses are affected. Most of the perforations occur on the anterior wall of the stomach and the majority of these are located in the antrum and body along the lesser curve.[33,56,153] Ulcers which perforate posteriorly or near the cardia are rare. Free leakage into the lesser sac has been estimated to occur in only 1%.[75]

As with duodenal ulcer perforation, arguments about the surgical management of perforated gastric ulcer revolve around the choice between patch closure and immediate gastrectomy. The case for definitive surgery has always been stronger for gastric than duodenal ulcers. There is about a 6% chance of missing a gastric carcinoma.[152,154,155] Patch closure is believed to be attended by more ulcer-related complications in the immediate postoperative period. Furthermore, gastrectomy may be easier for those perforations situated on the lesser curve. There

is also the perception that side-effects of gastrectomy for gastric ulcers are seen less commonly than after vagotomy and drainage or vagotomy and antrectomy for duodenal ulcer disease. Despite this notion, patch closure has remained by far the most commonly performed operation (Tables 34.13 and 34.14). A comparison of the morbidity and mortality of patch closure and definitive surgery is again limited by the selection in most series of patch closure for high-risk patients in most series. Nevertheless, it is noteworthy that the mortality figures, with few exceptions,[153,155] are lower after gastrectomy (Table 34.13).

Table 34.13 Mortality of gastric ulcer according to surgical treatment

AUTHORS	DATE	PATCH CLOSURE TOTAL	MORTALITY	GASTRECTOMY TOTAL	MORTALITY
Gall and Talbot[156]	1964	96	7(7.3)	14	3(21.4)
Donaldson and Jarrett[58]	1970	40	8(20)	15	0
Rees and Thorbjarnarson[159]	1973	37	9(24.5)	3	1(33.3)
Collier and Pain[157]	1985	45	11(24.4)	7	0
Wilson-MacDonald et al.[154]	1985	17	4(24)	6	0
Shein et al.[158]	1986	11	3(27.2)	20	3(15)
McGee and Sawyers[152]	1987	51	15(29.4)	27	4(14.8)
Lanng et al.[153]	1988	246	53(21.5)	41	10(24.3)
Hewitt et al.[155]	1990	94	10[a](10.6)	40	3(7.5)

Values in parentheses are percentages.
[a]Four deaths due to ulcer-related complications.

Table 34.14 Morbidity of gastric ulcer according to surgical treatment

AUTHORS	DATE	PATCH CLOSURE		GASTRECTOMY	
		TOTAL	RELATED MORBIDITY	TOTAL	RELATED MORBIDITY
Collier and Pain[157]	1985	45	2(4.4)	4	3(75)
Wilson-MacDonald et al.[154]	1985	17	1(5.8)	6	0
Schein et al.[158]	1986	11	2(18.2)	20	0
McGee and Sawyers[152]	1987	51	18(35.5)	27	2(7.4)
Lanng et al.[153]	1988	246	30(12.2)	41	6(14.6)
Hewitt et al.[155]	1990	94	7(7.4)	40	5(12.5)

It would seem that gastrectomy is preferable particularly for large perforations[157] and those closely associated with the lesser curve. High lesser curve and posterior wall ulcers can usually be managed by the Pauchet manoeuvre (Figure 34.9)[160–162] making total gastrectomy rarely indicated. Patch closure is preferable for small prepyloric perforations and those in poor risk patients. Carcinoma should be excluded intraoperatively or postoperatively with routine follow-up endoscopy. Although not as clearly documented the natural history of gastric ulcer after patch closure appears to be similar to that of duodenal ulcer.[58,152,153] The association between *H. pylori* and gastric ulcers is less well defined, particularly in those who present with a perforation. It is predicted that as with duodenal ulcers, a more conservative surgical approach will be adopted in the future in those patients who tests positive for *H. pylori*.

Summary

Perforated peptic ulcer remains one of the most common complications of peptic ulcer disease. While in Western countries the incidence has not changed appreciably, some developing countries have seen a sharp increase. The most noticeable epidemiological change is the marked increase of perforation among elderly patients. This can probably be accounted for by the use and abuse of NSAIDs for a variety of disorders. Although overall mortality has fallen to approximately 10% since the beginning of the twentieth century there has been no further improvement since the 1960s. This reflects the greater proportion of high-risk elderly patients presenting with this complication.

In most patients the clinical presentation is dramatic with generalized peritonitis and free air under the diaphragm on radiological examination. However, perforations can easily be missed in the chronically ill, immunosuppressed or otherwise debilitated patient. The initial treatment consist of analgesia, the correction of hypovolaemic shock, decompression of the stomach and antibiotics. Proper resuscitation is essential before definitive treatment is instituted. Risk stratification in perforated peptic ulcer has now been defined with more accurately. Old age, major medical illness shock, long-standing perforations

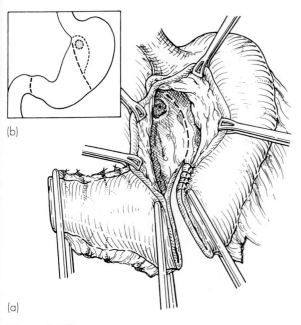
(a)
(b)

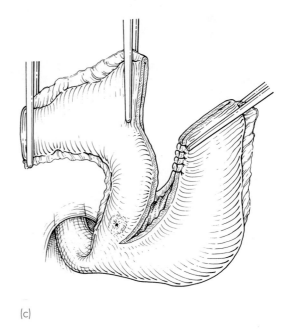
(c)

Figure 34.9

Pauchet manoeuvre. (a) Duodenum divided between two crushing clamps. Payr clamps are placed horizontally across the stomach at the antrum/body junction. (b) Piecemeal excision of lesser curve followed by a running haemostatic suture. Proportionately more anterior wall is left for fashioning of upper portion of lesser curve. (c) Excision of ulcer is facilitated by lifting the stomach upwards and keeping the excision strictly to the margin of the ulcer. Ligation of the left gastric artery is best carried out at this stage.

and associated haemorrhage all have serious prognostic implications.

The operative treatment of perforated duodenal ulcer has remained controversial. Patch closure by virtue of its simplicity has remained the emergency operation of choice in most centres, whereas definitive operations are confined to academic units with an interest in this condition. In the final analysis there is not much difference in the ultimate outcome after these two treatment strategies. The selection of patients for definitive surgery, however, remains problematic. There are as yet no reliable indicators of aggressive ulcer diathesis. A history of more than three months dyspepsia has been used most commonly in selecting patients for immediate definitive surgery. However, studies on the natural history after simple closure have shown that only about a third of such patients will eventually require a definitive operation. Although highly selective vagotomy has overcome many of the problems of the other definitive operations, the technical expertise required is no longer available. The efficacy of modern medical therapy and in particular *H. pylori* eradication in the long-term management of peptic ulcer has strengthened the case for patch closure and selective non-operative treatment.

A stage has now been reached where, except for technical reasons, definitive surgery can no longer be justified for duodenal or gastric ulcers.

PENETRATION

Introduction

Penetration as a clinical entity is less well defined. Consequently its true incidence is hard to determine from the literature. Most of the information comes from surgical series in the 1950s and 1960s when gastrectomy was the most commonly performed operation for peptic ulcer disease. The most widely quoted figures come from studies by Cassel et al.,[163] Haubrich et al.[70] and Norris and Haubrich[71] which report incidences ranging from 20 to 50%. Today most penetrating ulcers can be healed with modern medical therapy and therefore rarely come to urgent surgery.

Pathology

As stated before, a penetrating ulcer is one which erodes through the full thickness of the bowel wall without leakage into the peritoneal cavity. Most of these ulcers are situated on the posterior wall of the duodenum and stomach and frequently involve the pancreas. In Norris and Haubrich's[71] series of 169 cases of penetration the pancreas was affected in 96. The other structures involved were the gastrohepatic omentum,[30] biliary tract,[21] greater omentum,[13] mesocolon[11] and colon[5] Penetration was more commonly encountered in duodenal than gastric ulcers. In a more recent study by Jensen et al.[164] penetration was present in no fewer than 38% of high gastric ulcers.

Clinical presentation

Most patients with penetrating ulcers will have long-standing symptoms. In Cassel et al's[163] series 69% had ulcer dyspepsia

for five years or longer and whereas Haubrich et al.[70] found an average interval of 12 years.

The symptoms have been well documented in earlier reports.[70,71,163] The most common feature is pain radiating to the back which usually indicates penetration into the pancreas. A change in the typical diurnal rhythm, location, spread or intensity of the pain and resistance to standard medical therapy are also common. Associated haemorrhage (34%) and gastric stasis (26%) were reported in one series but did not occur more often than in patients with uncomplicated ulcers.[70] However, all these features may be present in non-penetrating ulcers.[70,71]

Barium contrast studies poorly discriminate penetrating from non-penetrating ulcers;[70,163] deformity is the same and depth of the ulcer is difficult to judge because of surrounding oedema. Very large ulcers can be completely missed and interpreted as a normal duodenal cap. Fistulous communication with the biliary system will show up as free air in the biliary tree on plain abdominal radiographs[165,166] and in about half the cases the diagnosis is confirmed by reflux of barium into the bile ducts.[167]

Endoscopy also has limitations in those cases where the base is obscured by necrotic slough. In the case of fistulas a slit-like opening may be visualized in the ulcer base.[168] Endoscopic retrograde cholangiopancreatography has aided the diagnosis and management of these fistulas particularly when the ulcer is post bulbar. Their precise anatomy, and evidence of biliary stricture, can now be defined and in rare instances a simultaneous pancreatic fistula may be demonstrated.[169]

Management

Most penetrating ulcers can now be treated safely and effectively with *H. pylori* eradication therapy. Accurate figures for healing rates are not available but with drug therapy complete disappearance of massive ulcers has been documented.[170] Penetration should, therefore, not be regarded in its own right as an indication for surgery. When surgery is contemplated, prior intensive medical treatment and, in some cases, hospitalization is advisable to facilitate the operation.

Surgical strategy

Anterior and posterior penetrating ulcers situated in the body of the stomach seldom pose technical problems and can be freed from the liver or pancreas by using blunt dissection. However, posterior penetrating duodenal ulcers and those situated on the superior border of the duodenum or prepyloric region may cause difficulties in managing the duodenal stump. Structures in the porta hepatis are also at risk. In most instances problems with handling the duodenal stump can be overcome by using the inferior edge of the ulcer crater for the posterior anastomosis and an anterior Horsley slit to ensure an adequate Billroth I anastomosis (Figure 34.10). Alternatively the duodenal stump can be closed by a number of techniques (Figures 34.11 and 34.12) when a Billroth II anastomosis is performed. A vagotomy should always accompany the above procedures. For the less experienced surgeon a vagotomy and

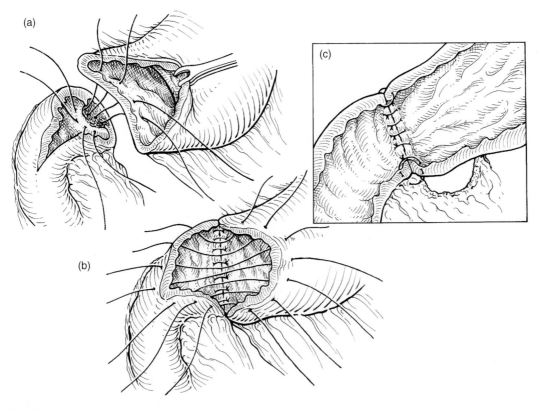

Figure 34.10
(a–c) Horsley slit and placement of sutures to inferior edge of ulcer crater.

Finney pyloroplasty (Figure 34.13), Jaboulay gastroduodenostomy (Figure 34.14) or gastroenterostomy will avoid hazardous dissection and the risk of being confronted with a difficult duodenal stump closure.

Problems may arise in cases with biliary and/or pancreatic fistula into the ulcer base. In this situation a vagotomy and drainage would be the safest option.[169] If an unsuspected fistula is found at surgery, the ulcer base must be kept in continuity with the gastrointestinal tract which can be achieved by a variety of manoeuvres (Figures 34.15 and 34.16). Hepaticojejunostomy is recommended for the rare case of biliary obstruction.

STENOSIS

Incidence

Reports on the incidence of gastric outlet obstruction vary considerably. Kozoll and Meyer[171] surveyed the series of peptic

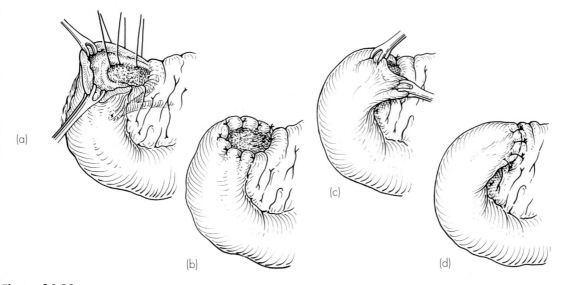

Figure 34.11
(a–d) Nissen technique of closing duodenal stump.

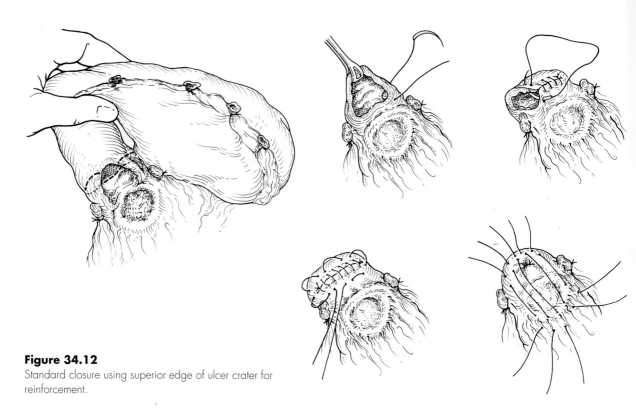

Figure 34.12
Standard closure using superior edge of ulcer crater for reinforcement.

ulceration up to 1964 and found that 2–23% of cases presented with obstruction. Their own study of 8451 patients admitted with peptic ulcer between 1936 and 1955 yielded 885 cases (11%) of obstruction. More recently, Jaffin and Kaye[172] reported this complication in 55 of 1185 peptic ulcer admissions, an incidence of approximately 5%. Overall, the surgeon can expect to encounter this problem in one in every 10–20 peptic ulcer admissions.

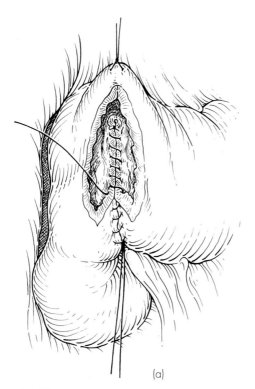

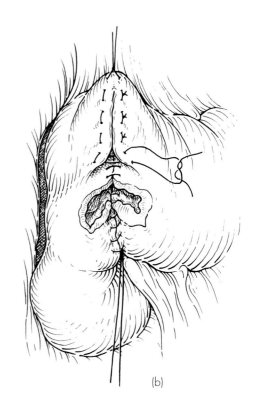

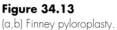

(a)

(b)

Figure 34.13
(a,b) Finney pyloroplasty.

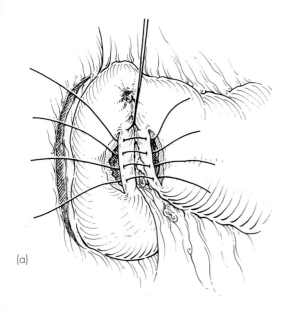

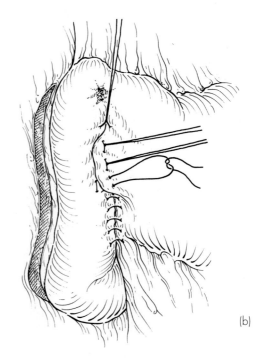

Figure 34.14
(a,b) Jaboulay gastroduodenostomy.

Pathology

The major pathological features which predispose to luminal narrowing include active ulceration with associated inflammation and the development of fibrosis.[173] There is some evidence that gastric emptying is additionally impaired in diabetics[174,175] particularly those with a peripheral neuropathy[176] who may be prone to this complication on an autonomic basis.

Obstruction to gastric outflow is most commonly caused by duodenal ulcer, prepyloric ulcer and pyloric channel ulcer. Gastric outlet obstruction is usually attributed to 'pyloric' stenosis but the obstruction is, in fact, most often in the duodenum.[177-179] In 95% of 502 operations for pyloroduodenal obstruction the lesion was duodenal.[180] Postbulbar duodenal ulcers are far less common but remain important in that 40–50% are associated with stricture.[181]

Lesser curve gastric ulcer only rarely produces obstruction if

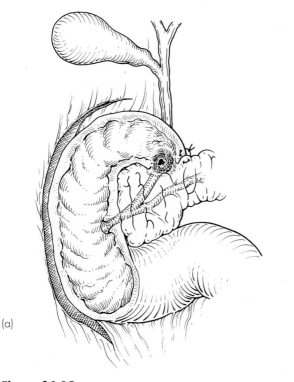

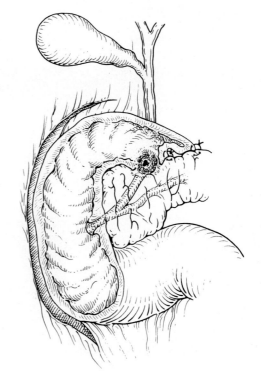

Figure 34.15
(a,b) Closure of duodenal stump in continuity with duodenal lumen.

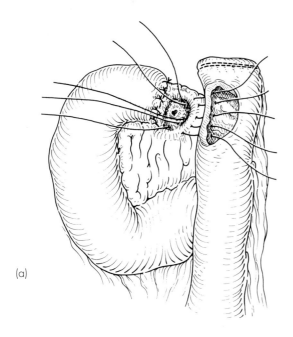

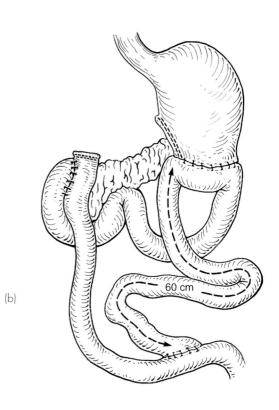

Figure 34.16
(a,b) Roux-en-Y 'ulcer'-jejunostomy for drainage of biliary and/or pancreatic fistula.

scarring and reaction are sufficient to create an 'opposite incisura' causing the 'hourglass' or bilocular stomach deformity.[94] Severe shortening of the lesser curve due to scarring may also produce delayed emptying and outlet obstruction. The pylorus, which is uninvolved, is pulled up while the greater curve forms a sump[182,183] the so-called 'tea-pot' stomach (Figure 34.17).

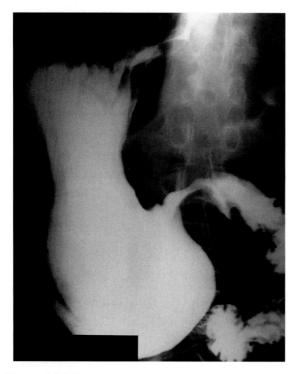

Figure 34.17
Tea-pot deformity due to severe shortening of the lesser curve causing a sump effect on the greater curve.

Clinical presentation

The obstructed stomach has been defined by the late Sir James Walton of the London Hospital as 'the stomach you can hear, the stomach you can see, and stomach you can feel'.[183] As such, the diagnosis is often clinically obvious, especially if there is accompanying weight loss. However, the affected group of patients typically has a long history of peptic ulcer disease of ten years or more[173] and past complications. In a number of studies haemorrhage, perforation or stenosis had previously occurred in up to 50%.[172,184–186] Patients tend to be older than other ulcer patients[187] with mean ages ranging from 52[188] to 60 years.[172] This may lead to diagnostic difficulties, especially in the elderly who present with intermittent vomiting and emaciation.[189] Confusion with functional disorders such as anorexia nervosa has also been reported.[190]

Three phases are evident in the clinical course of obstruction. The onset is often insidious with loss of appetite as the only early symptom. A change in the character of the pain is sometimes evident, becoming more postprandial and cramp-like in nature. In this 'compensated phase' gastric emptying is maintained by muscular hypertrophy.[179] Belching and induced vomiting are often present. Eventually the stomach decompensates (phase two) with atony and distension.[179] Vomiting becomes less frequent but more copious. The vomitus consists of unchanged food consumed some time before, and is characteristically free of bile. The patient complains of foul taste and halitosis. If untreated there is progression to dehydration and metabolic derangement with shock and prostration as the third phase. Physical examination reveals epigastric distension, succussion splash and visible peristalsis progressing from left to right. Depending on the chronicity and severity of the obstruction features of dehydration, anaemia and emaciation are present. Tetany, convulsions and eventually coma are evident in only the most advanced cases.

Fluid electrolyte and acid–base derangements

The immediate hazards to the patient with an obstructed stomach are dehydration, electrolyte disturbance and acid–base imbalance. The classic metabolic derangement is hypochloraemic hypokalaemic alkalosis. As gastric juice is chloride (Cl^-)-rich (140 mmol/l) there is significant loss of Cl^- in the vomitus, coupled with hydrogen H^+. Consequently the serum becomes hypochloraemic with the anion balance maintained by a rising bicarbonate (HCO_3^-). Early on this HCO_3^- is lost in compensatory fashion in the urine. As sodium (Na^+) is lost both in the vomitus and in the urine accompanying the HCO_3^-, it becomes urgently conserved at the renal tubule with HCO_3^- at the expense of the H^+ and potassium (K^+) cations. Thus compensation for the alkalosis falters as a paradoxical acid urine is produced. Similarly the hypokalaemia is accentuated and K^+ is replaced at the intracellular level by H^+. This promotes intracellular acidosis and extracellular alkalosis which decreases the concentration of ionized calcium (although total calcium concentration remains constant) and may lead to tetany.

Diagnostic tests

It must be emphasized that special investigations are deferred until the patient is resuscitated and the stomach decompressed. Although the diagnosis of obstruction can usually be readily reached, a wide differential of causes other than peptic ulceration exists. These include carcinoma of the stomach, gastric sarcoma and lymphoma, carcinoma of the pancreas, ampulla or duodenum, adult hypertrophic pyloric stenosis, and annular pancreas.[185]

Tests of gastric emptying

Apart from historical, clinical and radiological criteria, specific tests of emptying to confirm obstruction have been used. The saline load test[191] is judged positive if more than 400 ml of saline is retained by the stomach 30 minutes after 750 ml is instilled. However, this does not necessarily correlate with emptying of solid food. Other criteria include ≥200 ml overnight residue, ≥60% retention of administered barium after 4 hours[172,185,192], and radionuclide scanning of the emptying of various ^{99m}Tc-labelled foods.[193] All these tests are of limited practical value when operations incorporating drainage or resection are planned. They may assume importance in the detection of subclinical obstruction if highly selective vagotomy is contemplated.

Barium studies

Erect plain abdominal radiographs are useful in demonstrating a large gastric outline, a 'fuzzy fluid level'[194] and a paucity of distal duodenal and small bowel gas. Barium studies are generally advocated to help outline the cause, degree and point of obstruction. Kreel and Ellis[195] have studied this in 100 consecutive patients and describe three layers formed by air, gastric juice and barium in the erect position. However, there is a trend away from barium studies towards endoscopy as the sole investigation.[196] Indeed, barium can make gastroscopy difficult or impossible and should be deferred until after endoscopy if additional information is required.

Endoscopy

This has become the investigation of choice in gastric outlet obstruction after fluid resuscitation and nasogastric drainage have been instituted. The advantages are perceived as follows: (1) the need for clearing the stomach of barium preoperatively is obviated; (2) it may assist in gastric decompression especially when combined with lavage; (3) benign causes may be distinguished from malignant and biopsies may be taken; (4) more precise information on the nature of the obstructing process is gathered (e.g. acute inflammation versus scarring and fibrosis); (5) it facilitates immediate therapeutic possibilities such as placement of feeding tubes and dilatation of the stricture. Limitations include the fact that food residue may impair the examination and an impassable pyloric region may hide duodenal disease.

Management

Conservative treatment

Corrections of fluid electrolyte and acid–base balance The key to the treatment of the metabolic abnormalities is to give isotonic saline which will expand the extracellular fluid volume, increase renal blood flow, and allow conservation of Cl^- and excretion of HCO_3^-. Once adequate renal function is demonstrated judicious potassium supplementation is started. In the severely depleted patient the volume of replacement must be judged according to serum and urinary electrolytes, the calculated deficit and, if necessary, central venous pressure and arterial blood gas estimations. Overzealous replacement should be avoided and half the Na^+ deficit should be replaced in the first 24 hours. With correction of the salt deficit alkalosis will resolve.

Nutritional support The patient with gastric outlet obstruction may be nutritionally depleted at the time of presentation. The surgeon must decide whether to embark on surgery with the knowledge that the patient will likely be eating again within 4 or 5 days[179] or whether the malnutrition presents such a hazard to wound healing and recovery that a period of preoperative alimentation is justified. There is a lack of controlled clinical data to help in decision making. In general, nutritional support is indicated if a patient has been or will be nutritionally deprived for more than two weeks. Assessment of the degree of malnutrition is difficult without the aid of sophisticated techniques, but Hill[197] has outlined simple 'bedside' criteria: recent weight loss, depressed mood and activity and poor grip strength. Enteral feeding is preferable and can now be accomplished with endoscopic placement of a nasojejunal fine-bore feeding tube under fluoroscopic control. If this is unsuccessful, then intravenous hyperalimentation is indicated.

Decompression of the stomach Nasogastric decompression is an essential part of early treatment. It helps to prevent vomiting, to disrupt the distension–secretion cycle and to monitor ongoing losses. At the same time the removal of gastric acid may contribute to the reduction of inflammation and further relieve obstruction. Effective decompression can usually be achieved by simple drainage. Encouragement of clear fluid oral intake, however, assists in lavage and adds to patient comfort. If this fails, more active lavage is achieved through a wide-bore tube.

There are no clear guidelines as to how long one should continue nasogastric drainage. Equally uncertain is whether the length of preoperative drainage correlates with eventual outcome. Weiland et al.[192] found decompression necessary for an average of four days, before further surgical decisions could be taken. Smale et al.[175] found that 9% of 44 patients drained for more than three days preoperatively had delayed gastric emptying postoperatively, compared with 22% of 32 patients drained for less time. However, a variety of operations was used and the difference was not significant. This lack of clear definition is indicative of the potentially reversible nature of the obstruction.

Drug treatment In the obstructed state the mainstay of pharmacological treatment is intravenous H_2-receptor antagonists. The rationale for such antiulcer therapy is to heal any associated active ulceration which may be contributing to the obstruction. If normal gastric emptying resumes, standard medical treatment can be resumed.

Surgical treatment

Indications and timing Surgery for benign gastric outlet obstruction is rarely if ever an emergency. Operation is not normally considered before 72 hours as 40–60% of cases may improve during this period.[171,192,198] This is especially true for those with active ulceration. On the other hand up to 94% will eventually require surgery in the short or long term.[172,192] Therefore, undue delay may not be warranted if a history of chronicity or previous complication is elicited. The ultimate clinical judgement will be influenced by the patient's age and general medical status.

Choice of operation The choice of operation for obstructing duodenal, prepyloric or pyloric channel ulcers is truncal vagotomy combined with pyloroplasty, gastroenterostomy or antrectomy. Highly selective (proximal gastric or parietal cell) vagotomy combined with duodenoplasty, pyloroplasty or stricture dilatation may also be considered for obstructing duodenal ulcer. As with surgery for uncomplicated peptic ulcer, controversy surrounds the approach to gastric outlet obstruction with each operation having its advocates.

Truncal vagotomy and pyloroplasty has proved to be both safe and effective surgery for gastric outlet obstruction.[192,199–203] A recent study from the Mayo Clinic[204] showed that truncal vagotomy and drainage, when compared with highly selective vagotomy and drainage, had slightly more postoperative atony (8% versus 3%) and fewer 'good or excellent' results at three years (74% versus 86%). Neither difference was significant however.

Any of the described pyloroplasties can be used for drainage, each of which may have a particular advantage in a given situation. Although the Heineke–Mikulicz or Weinberg pyloroplasties (Figure 34.7) are applicable in most cases, when there is marked scarring or distortion the Finney (Figure 34.13) or Jaboulay (Figure 34.14) procedures and gastroenterostomy are technically easier.[173] The Finney technique incorporates a greater length of normal wall proximally and distally. Gastroenterostomy and the Jaboulay gastroduodenostomy have the additional advantage of avoiding the scarred region altogether. Both the Finney and the Jaboulay operations provide drainage superior to the Weinberg procedure in one study.[205]

Vagotomy and *antrectomy* is still advocated by many especially in the USA.[206] Herrington reported 3771 of these procedures in which outlet obstruction was the indication in 14%. Overall, excellent or good results were obtained in 94% of cases, and mortality fell to less than 1% in the latter part of the collected series. With technical modifications, problems with the duodenum can be overcome and in most instances a Billroth I anastomosis can be performed. Useful manoeuvres are the Horsley slit procedure (Figure 34.10) and an end-to-side anastomosis to the second part of the duodenum (Figure 34.18). If this is not possible the duodenum is closed and a Billroth II anastomosis performed. Despite theoretical advantages over drainage procedures (i.e. lower ulcer recurrence

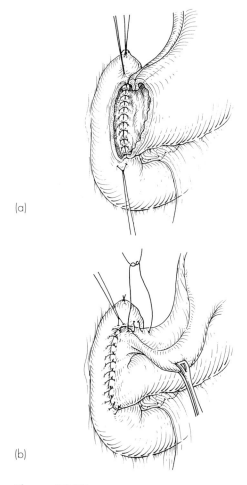

(a)

(b)

Figure 34.18
(a,b) End-to-side gastroduodenostomy.

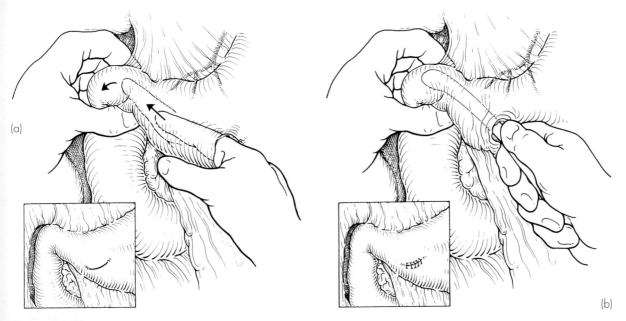

Figure 34.19
Dilatation of stenosis: (a) with index finger; (b) with hegar dilator (20 mm).

rate and improved drainage) vagotomy and antrectomy did not prove superior to vagotomy and pyloroplasty in two studies.[192,207]

In the rare instance of gastric ulcer producing obstruction (3% of Ellis's 225 cases)[179] the time honoured Billroth I partial gastrectomy is the procedure of choice.[208]

Highly selective vagotomy (HSV) and dilation of the outlet through a gastrotomy has been one approach to obstructing duodenal ulcer (Figure 34.19). This was initially enthusiastically reported by Johnston's group in Leeds in 1973[119] and again in 1976.[209] There were no recurrences in 23 cases but follow-up was short (mean 24 months). This group was compared in an uncontrolled manner with 23 contemporary patients undergoing truncal vagotomy and drainage. Excellent or good results were obtained in 96% of the former patients and 74% of the latter.

As previously noted the point of obstruction is frequently 'postpyloric'.[177,178] This makes *HSV* and *simple duodenoplasty* (Figure 34.20) an attractive possibility which has been used with success by Kennedy[178] in 25 patients. It avoids the not uncommon risk of perforation during dilatation.[132,209-211] He reports no morbidity, mortality or recurrence but with a maximum follow-up of only 30 months. Further series have used either dilatation or duodenoplasty with HSV (Table 36.15). Although early reports were encouraging,[120,178,188,209,212] some subsequent studies with longer follow-up revealed recurrence rates of 16–18%.[211-214] The Lahey Clinic group[211] found only 58% of their 19 patients achieved Visick's grade 1 or 2 and have abandoned HSV and dilatation.

HSV combined with pyloroplasty has also been employed in obstructing peptic ulcer disease. Lunde's 78 patients were followed for a mean of 90 months and 93% achieved Visick's ratings of 1 or 2. Only one symptomatic recurrence occurred, compared with 11% in their large series of 716 HSVs without

drainage.[179] Of these recurrences 50% were gastric ulcers, possibly implicating stasis as the causative factor. When pyloroplasty was added to HSV this group found a lowered maximal acid output, as did the Aarhus County Vagotomy Trial Group.[216] Donahue et al.[186] used HSV and drainage (mainly pyloroplasty) in 37 obstructed patients and encountered no recurrence. There were three mild cases of dumping. The superiority of this more demanding and time-consuming operation over truncal vagotomy and pyloroplasty has yet to be proved.

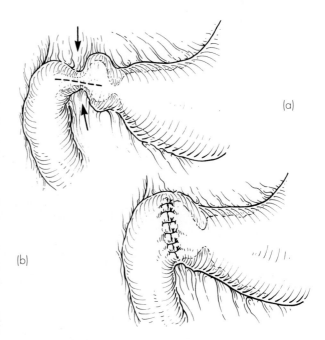

Figure 34.20
(a,b) Duodenoplasty performed by longitudinal incision (± 2 cm) with one layer transverse closure.

Table 34.15 HSV and dilatation/duodenoplasty

AUTHORS	DATE	CASES n	TECH	DIAM (mm)	FOLLOW-UP (MONTHS)	MORT	COMPL (n)	VISICK 1 AND 2 (%)	ULC REC (%)
Johnston et al.[120]	1973	15	D	14	>12	0	4 P	100	0
McMahon et al.[209]	1976	23	D	16	24	0	4 P 2 S	96	0
Kennedy[178]	1976	25	Pl	ns	≤30	0	0	ns	0
Delaney[188]	1978	11	D	15	18	0	0	ns	0
White et al.[212]	1978	7 5	D Pl	4–6	ns	0	2 S	ns	0
Dunn et al.[210]	1981	15	D	20	54	0	2 P	93	7
Ferraz et al.[213]	1981	11	D	14	14–46	0	3 S	67	18
Gorey et al.[214]	1984	44 18	D Pl	7–8	24–156	0	9 R 1 R	88	16 0
Rossi et al.[211]	1986	19	D	15	60–120	0	3 P	58	16
Hooks et al.[196]	1986	14 6	D	14–20	≤60	0	0	89	10
Barroso et al.[215]	1986	43	Pl	ns	96	0	0	ns	5

Tech, technique; D, dilatation; Pl, duodenoplasty; Diam, dilatation diameter (average); Mort, early postoperative mortality; Compl, complications; Ulc rec, ulcer recurrence rate; ns, not stated; P, perforation; S, stasis; R, recurrence/stenosis.

Endoscopic techniques

In the early 1980s successful endoscopic oesophageal dilatation with low pressure balloon catheters was reported.[217] The theoretical advantage was that a balloon provides an even radial pressure as opposed to the shearing effect of longitudinal dilatation.[218,219] This technique has now been extended to cases of benign gastric outlet obstruction.[220-231] At first a guide-wire was placed under direct vision through the stricture and advanced distally with fluoroscopic control. The endoscope was removed and a balloon catheter advanced over the wire. The scope was either replaced alongside the dilator[220] or left out,[222] and the balloon was inflated with contrast medium. Dilatation was monitored radiologically and sometimes with a pressure gauge[222] until 'waisting' of the balloon disappeared. The position of the balloon was maintained for 30–60 s[220-223] and repeated if necessary.

The main technical problem with the method was traversing a tight stenosis with the guide-wire without intragastric looping. Taylor[227] sought to solve this by developing a balloon device which fits over the end of a paediatric size gastroduodenoscope but tighter stenoses still required prior dilatation with the guide-wire technique.

More recently 'through-the-scope' 180 cm polyethylene dilators have been developed with 2 cm balloons of 8–18 mm diameter ('Rigiflex' Microvasive Inc, USA). These require a 2.8 mm biopsy channel (Figure 34.21). The latest refinement is a central lumen so that use of a guide-wire can be incorporated for very difficult strictures. Initial reports[223,224,226] claim success rates of 83–92%. 'Through-the-scope' balloon dilators have overcome many of the problems with the guide-wire technique. They offer ease of placement, visual monitoring of dilatation and immediate direct assessment of the result and avoid the need for X-ray screening.

Most authors recommend a balloon diameter of 15 mm on

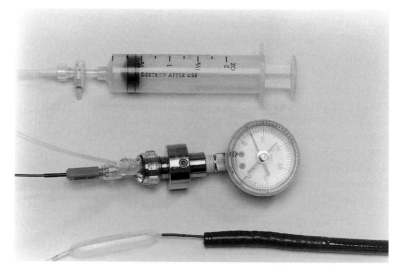

Figure 34.21
Rigiflex dilators (Microvasive Inc, USA) with pressure gauge used through wide channel (2.8 mm) gastroscope.

the basis that symptoms typically occur with a pyloric canal diameter of less than 10 mm[120,188,228] and that perforation rates of up to 27%[120,209] have been reported in dilatations to 20 mm intraoperatively.

Endoscopic-assisted dilatation of peptic gastric outlet obstruction is innovative and appears relatively safe and effective, at least in the short term (Table 34.16). Combined with ongoing medical treatment, it may gain acceptance in the relief of this condition and avoid early surgery in many. With repeated dilatations operation may be avoided altogether in high-risk groups, an approach analogous to treating oesophageal stenosis.

The role of endoscopic dilatation as a preoperative adjunct to highly selective vagotomy has not been established. Theroretically it may avoid either a drainage procedure or operative dilatation through a gastrotomy. Further postoperative dilatation would also be possible. However, long-term data are needed to assign its place next to surgical management.

Summary

As a complication of peptic ulceration, gastric outlet obstruction is less common and its presentation is less dramatic than haemorrhage or perforation. It nevertheless requires special attention to the correction of specific fluid, electrolyte and acid–base problems. In addition the need and timing of pre and postoperative nutritional support must be addressed. In allowing direct assessment and tissue biopsy, fibreoptic endoscopy has superseded contrast radiology and indirect methods in the evaluation of gastric outlet obstruction.

Vagotomy and drainage has enjoyed a deserved popularity in treatment of obstructing duodenal ulcer. The advantage of highly selective vagotomy over truncal vagotomy in this setting has not as yet been proved. Operative dilatation combined with highly selective vagotomy has become unpopular partly because of the risk of restenosis. No one operation is clearly superior and until controlled data are available a flexible surgical approach must be maintained.

Endoscopic dilatation is an alternative treatment for obstruction but does not alter the ulcer diathesis and as such remains adjunctive to medical or surgical acid reduction. Whether *H. pylori* eradication therapy will change the natural history of pyloric and duodenal stenosis associated with ulcer disease remains to be seen. As surgical services are presented with older and sicker candidates we must critically analyse our surgical options and remain open to non-operative solutions.

HAEMORRHAGE

Introduction

Two of the principal causes of upper gastrointestinal haemorrhage are gastric and duodenal ulcer. This section begins by briefly reviewing the clinical assessment, acute management and diagnostic evaluation of the patient presenting with upper gastrointestinal haemorrhage. Having established peptic ulcer as the source of bleeding, the indications for surgery are outlined with special attention to clinical and endoscopic prognostic factors. The evolution of modern surgical strategy follows with emphasis on the two major operative approaches: gastric resection and truncal vagotomy, pyloroplasty and underrunning. Lastly, the place of more conservative surgery and endoscopic methods of haemostasis is discussed.

Clinical assessment

Acute upper gastrointestinal haemorrhage (UGIH) is a common cause of emergency admissions to large community hospitals and is associated with an overall mortality of 5–10%.[232] Therefore, the presence of any of the signs of UGIH demands urgent attention with rapid resuscitation and early diagnosis being of prime importance. Haematemesis, either fresh or altered, and melaena are the hallmarks UGIH. In rare cases, massive UGIH can present as red blood per rectum, but this is a more common manifestation of lower gastrointestinal bleeding.

The immediate management of UGIH consists of taking an

Table 34.16 Endoscopic balloon dilatation of peptic gastric outlet obstruction

AUTHORS	DATE	n	FOLLOW-UP (MONTHS)	TYPE	DIAM (mm)	DIL (n)	SUC (%)	COMPL
Benjamin et al.[220]	1984	6	5–14	Guide-wire	10–15	1	83	0
Lindor et al.[221a]	1985	6	15	Guide-wire	12–20	1	87	0
Hogan et al.[222]	1986	9	7.5	Guide-wire	15–20	1.5	100	0
Craig and Gillespie[223]	1988	13	10	Thruscope	15	1.9	92	0
Griffin et al.[224]	1989	25	9	Thruscope	15	ns	83	0
Schmudderich et al.[226]	1989	9	7	Thruscope	15–18	2.5	89	0
DiSario et al.[229]	1994	30	15	Thruscope	6–15	2(1–4)	80	2[b]
Misra and Dwivedi[230]	1996	14	27 median	Thruscope	15–18	(1–3)	78	0
Lau et al.[231]	1996	41	39 median	Thruscope	12–20	—	51	4

Diam, dilatation diameter; dil, dilatations; suc, balloon diameter successfully achieved; Compl, complications; ns, not stated.
[a]Includes some non-peptic lesions.
[b]Perforation.

adequate history, performing a clinical examination and initiating resuscitative measures. In patients with severe haemorrhage priority must be given to resuscitation. When the patient's condition has been stabilized, diagnostic investigations can be undertaken and definitive treatment started. Depending on geography, one can expect peptic ulcer disease to account for approximately 30–50% of UGIH[233–246] (Table 34.17).

Table 34.17 Peptic ulcer as a percentage of upper gastrointestinal haemorrhage[a]

AUTHORS	DATE	(n)	TOTAL (%)	GU (%)	DU (%)
Palmer[233]	1969	1400	40	12	28
Schiller et al.[234]	1970	2149	44	15	29
Johnston et al.[235]	1973	817	54	8	46
Hellers and Ihre[236]	1975	157	52	18	34
Sereda et al.[237]	1977	513	37	9	28
Foster et al.[238]	1978	277	37	16	21
Silverstein et al.[239]	1981	2097	45	22	23
MacLeod and Mills[240]	1982	309	44	17	27
Harris and Heap[241]	1982	269	47	21	26
Vellacott et al.[242]	1982	1730	52	23	29
van Stiegmann et al.[243]	1983	1750	52	28	24
Hunt[244]	1984	1316	48	14	34
Rofe et al.[245]	1985	201	31	14	17
Clason et al.[246]	1986	326	52	16	36

DU, duodenal ulcer; GU, gastric ulcer.
[a]Cotemporary studies indicate peptic ulcer accounts for 31–54% of hospital admission for upper gastrointestinal haemorrhage. Duodenal ulcer (17–46%) is more prevalent than gastric ulcers (8–28%) in most series.

History and clinical examination

Although a carefully taken history may disclose the source of haemorrhage, it should be appreciated that one-third of patients bleeding from peptic ulcer will have no history of dyspepsia. Conversely, 40% of patients with dyspepsia will be bleeding from other lesions.[247] Several aspects of the clinical history, however, are important in identifying those patients at risk of dying from bleeding peptic ulcer. These include patients over 60 years of age and those with a medical history of cardiac, pulmonary, hepatic or renal disease.[232]

The clinical examination is directed at making an accurate assessment of the degree of haemodynamic disturbance and the patient's general status. Major haemorrhage is usually associated with the clinical findings of shock: hypotension (systolic BP <100 mm/Hg), tachypnoea, pallor, perspiration, rapid pulse (>100 beats/min), mental status changes and poor peripheral perfusion. Younger patients have a far greater capacity to compensate for haemorrhage and the clinical findings may be more subtle. Orthostatic manoeuvres may be helpful in eliciting intravascular volume depletion in these cases.

The general assessment is also of great importance. Attention must be given to cardiac, respiratory and renal problems as these will have considerable impact on prognosis and further management. Blood must be obtained for a full blood count, clotting profile, serum urea and electrolytes, and cross-matching of blood. Chest radiograph and electrocardiography are mandatory.

Resuscitation and general treatment

Ideally all elderly and unstable patients with UGIH should be admitted to a specialized multidisciplinary unit. Volume resuscitation is the cornerstone of treatment. Unless initial losses are fully replaced, determination of further bleeding is difficult and may lead to inappropriate intervention. Fluid should be given through large-bore intravenous catheters. In shocked patients, a central venous line and a urinary catheter are essential.

Those patients who do not respond to resuscitation demand urgent intervention to control haemorrhage. Failure to recognize this group and efforts to persist with prolonged resuscitation or multiple investigations carry a high morbidity and mortality. There is no evidence that antiulcer drugs, either intravenous or oral, reduce the incidence of further haemorrhage and their use should merely be seen as the start of definitive therapy.[248,249]

Diagnostic investigations

Endoscopy has become the procedure of choice to localize the source of UGIH since Palmer,[233] in 1969, provided clinical evidence of its superiority to barium studies. Barium studies are generally used when endoscopy is unavailable or fails to disclose a source of bleeding. As a last resort, selective visceral arteriography[250] can be used if the bleeding site is still elusive.

Most endoscopic series consistently identify the bleeding site in over 90% of cases.[251–262] Interestingly, several prospective, randomized trials[253,254,263–266] have not shown early endoscopic diagnosis to decrease the overall morbidity and mortality in patients with upper gastrointestinal bleeding. This, however, does not diminish the value of emergency endoscopy as the information obtained directly influences subsequent management. Previous studies have not made full use of the predictive value of endoscopic stigmata with regard to bleeding. More recently, therapeutic possiblities have also extended the role of endoscopy.

Prognositic factors and indications for operation

Historical perspective

Mikulicz[267] is credited with performing the first successful operation for gastric haemorrhage in 1887. Ten years later, dismayed by the high morbidity and mortality attended by surgery, he wrote 'it can never be prophesied with certainty in any individual case if haemorrhage is really of sufficient danger to justify surgical interference, so that one should always wait and see whether the bleeding will not be arrested by medical treatment'. This philosophy dominated the approach to peptic ulcer haemorrhage over the next 50 years. As Witts[268] observed in 1937: 'Patients with recurrent bleeding are the only ones of whom we can feel certain that they are likely to die if treated medically. Up to date we have had even more reason to feel certain that they are likely to die if treated surgically.'

In the face of this pessimism several determined surgeons rose to challenge the doctrinaire medical approach to ulcer haemorrhage. Noting that delay in definitive surgical therapy carried a high morbidity and mortality[269-271] Finsterer[272-274] in Europe, Balfour,[275] Allen and Benedict[276] in the USA and Gordon-Taylor[277,278] in the UK recommended that all patients with bleeding ulcers be taken to theatre within 48 hours. Using this aggressive approach Finsterer[273] and Gordon-Taylor[277-279] demonstrated substantial reductions in mortality for patients undergoing early surgery. The chief contribution of these pioneers was in emphasizing time as the critical factor in avoiding the failures of protracted medical therapy.

Yet, it was clear that most patients with peptic ulcer haemorrhage would settle on conservative therapy[269,280-282] and that no more than one-third of this group[283-286] would have further haemorrhage. With the increasing use of intravenous resuscitation[287] and other advances, it became evident that better discrimination was needed to avoid early operation on patients who otherwise might have settled with supportive therapy.

Clinical prognostic factors

In 1948, Hoerr et al.[288] and Dunphy and Hoerr[282] proposed selection criteria for surgery based on the rate of haemorrhage and its effect on the circulation. The authors suggested that operation should be performed when the circulation could not be stabilized after 2 l of blood or if transfusion of 500 ml was required every 8 hours in those who initially responded to resuscitation. In general these principles have remained the cornerstone for intervention.

Others have sought clinical factors, other than haemodynamic, to identify patients at risk for further bleeding or death. Table 34.18 indicates, duration of dyspepsia, a history of previous haemorrhage and the sex of the patient have not been reliable guides of prognosis. In fact, some have shown that a first haemorrhage and an absent or limited history of ulcer symptoms are worse indices than multiple previous bleeds or chronic ulcer dyspepsia.[234,235,297,299,301,303-305] The importance of the manifestation of haemorrhage (melaena, haematemesis or both) has also been equivocal.[280,299,304] Old age has long been held as a poor prognostic factor (Table 34.19), yet when carefully scrutinized, the presence of intercurrent disease seems to have a more significant influence on outcome than chronological age alone.[284,295,296,299,301,305-309] It is also evident that a gastric ulcer generally carries a worse prognosis than a duodenal ulcer. The basis for this seems to be that gastric ulcer patients are older and have more intercurrent disease.[234]

The presence of shock at the time of admission has emerged as a valuable predictor of rebleeding, need for surgery and mortality. Initially emphasized by Hoerr[288] and Dunphy and Hoerr[282] others have verified its predictive value in heterogeneous populations of upper gastrointestinal bleeding.[234,237,240,246,298,310] Similar conclusions have been reached in studies concerned with the specific problem of peptic ulcer haemorrhage.[237,243,311,312]

Table 34.18 Mortality for prognostic factors in massive peptic ulcer haemorrhage[a]

AUTHORS	DATE	SITE (%)		SEX (%)		PRIOR BLEED	DURATION OF DYSPEPSIA
		GU	DU	M	F		
Cullinan and Price[269]	1932	ns	ns	21	9	+	–
Welch and Yunich[281]	1940	35	6	11	8	–	–
Bohrer[289]	1940	24	14	19	17	ns	ns
Lewin and Truelove[290]	1949	ns	ns	20	16	–	–
Welch[284]	1949	22	11	ns	ns	–	ns
Amendola[291]	1949	ns	ns	ns	ns	ns	ns
Lewison[292]	1950	ns	ns	ns	ns	–	ns
Ferguson and Wyman[293]	1951	37	10	22	9	–	–
Fraenkel and Truelove[285]	1955	ns	ns	6	4	–	ns
Jones[294]	1956	16	8	8	6	–	ns
Snyder and Berne[295]	1957	36	13	20	12	–	–
Ward-McQuaid et al.[286]	1960	10	9	8	4	ns	ns
Coghill and Willcox[297]	1960	20	8	15	7	–	–
Foster et al.[296]	1963	24	28	ns	ns	ns	ns
Tanner[298]	1964	ns	ns	ns	ns	ns	ns
Hamilton et al.[299]	1965	ns	ns	ns	ns	–	–
Schiller et al.[234]	1970	9	6	6	7	ns	ns
Johnston et al.[235]	1973	17	7	ns	ns	ns	ns
Sereda et al.[237]	1977	19	6	ns	ns	ns	ns
Himal et al.[300]	1978	9	1	ns	ns	ns	ns
Silverstein et al.[301]	1981	8	7	ns	ns	ns	–
Vellacott et al.[242]	1982	13	10	ns	ns	ns	ns
van Stiegmann et al.[243]	1983	6	4	ns	ns	+	–
Morris et al.[302]	1984	ns	ns	ns	ns	+	ns
Hunt[244]	1984	9	4	ns	ns	ns	ns

DU, duodenal ulcer; GU, gastric ulcer.
+, denotes a positive correlation.
–, denotes a negative correlation.
ns, not stated.
[a]Mortality is related to ulcer site (GU vs DU), sex (M vs F), history of prior upper gastrointestinal bleed and duration of dyspepsia. Whereas sex, prior bleed and duration of dyspepsia have little prognostic value, a GU is more lethal than a DU.

Although age over 60 years, intercurrent illness and shock on admission are useful prognostic guides, no single parameter exists which allows precision in selecting patients for urgent surgery. The widespread application of fibreoptic endoscopy has produced a new set of prognostic factors: the endoscopic stigmata of recent haemorrhage (SRH). Subsequently, many centres have critically evaluated the accuracy of SRH in predicting outcome.

Endoscopic prognostic factors

Bleeding from ulcers that pulsate is bad news.

Hippocrates[313]

Although Hippocrates recognized the more ominous aspects of ulcer appearance, it was Foster et al.[238] who first proposed that certain endoscopic stigmata of recent haemorrhage (SRH) have prognostic value. He defined endoscopic stigmata as (1) fresh bleeding, (2) fresh or altered blood clot or black slough adherent to the lesion, (3) a vessel protruding from the base or margin of an ulcer. Of patients with ulcer-bearing stigmata, 53%

Table 34.19 Age as a risk factor for death in peptic ulcer haemorrhage

		AGE			
		<50 YEARS		>50 YEARS	
		PATIENTS	MORTALITY	PATIENTS	MORTALITY
AUTHORS	DATE	(n)	(%)	(n)	(%)
Welch and Yunich[281]	1940	75	1	50	20
Lewin and Truelove[290]	1949	92	6	116	28
Welch[284]	1949	ns	6	ns	23
Lewison[292]	1950	150	5	68	12
Ferguson and Wyman[293]	1951	51	6	106	24
Fraenkel and Truelove[285]	1955	135	0	242	9
Coghill and Willcox[297]	1960	106	1	229	19
Tanner[298]	1964	ns	1	ns	14
van Stiegmann et al.[243]	1983	ns	1	ns	8
		<60 YEARS		>60 YEARS	
		PATIENTS	MORTALITY	PATIENTS	MORTALITY
		(n)	(%)	(n)	(%)
Jones[294]	1956	1110	3	654	22
Snyder and Berne[295]	1957	39	8	34	29
Ward-McQuaid et al.[286]	1960	152	1	248	14
Foster et al.[296]	1963	40	12	90	35
Hamilton et al.[299]	1965	ns	3	ns	16
Morris et al.[302]	1984	42	0	100	10
Hunt[241]	1984	325	3	308	9

ns, not stated.

required surgery for further bleeding compared to only 3% in those without stigmata.

Most subsequent series[241,312,314-317] corroborate Foster's findings and show an increased risk of bleeding and need for surgery in patients with stigmata when compared to those with a clean ulcer base (Table 34.20). Two studies,[240,318] however, found SRH to have limited prognostic utility. Nonetheless, the incidence of rebleeding in the presence of stigmata ranged from 16%[315] to 53%[319] whereas bleeding recurred in less than 10% of ulcers without stigmata.

The prognostic accuracy for specific SRH varies considerably

Table 34.20 Endoscopic stigmata and percentage rebleeding

AUTHORS	DATE	(n)	STIGMATA YES	REBLEED (%)	STIGMATA NO	REBLEED (%)
Foster et al.[238]	1978	89	60	42 (53)	29	3 (3)
Harris and Heap[241]	1982	126	96	27 (17)	30	7 (7)
Macleod and Mills[240]	1982	136	74	40	62	35
Bornman et al.[315]	1985	177	98	16	79	5
Brearley et al.[316]	1985	72	43	51 (39)	29	10 (3)
Brearley et al.[319]	1987	278	116	53	162	8
Hunt[312]	1987	336	209	35 (26)	127	7 (5)
Chang-Chien et al.[317]	1988	193	156	18 (15)	37	0 (0)

Values in parentheses indicate the percentage of the total number of patients requiring operation for rebleeding.

(Table 34.21). Whereas all patients with a visible vessel in Griffith et al.[314] series rebled, others[312,320] found a visible vessel to predict further haemorrhage in 32–56% of cases. One study[317] found no rebleeding with a visible vessel. Active bleeding predicted further haemorrhage with an accuracy of 32–44%[312,317] whereas rebleeding occurred in 8–30% of cases associated with clot.[312,314,315,317,320,321] Blackspot or stain was associated with no increased risk of rebleeding.[315,321]

Several series have observed an increased mortality related to specific SRH.[316,320] Storey et al.[320] noted that all of the deaths were associated with a visible vessel (15%). In Brearley et al's[316] study, no patient without stigmata died, whereas mortality was 20% for active bleeding, 17% for visible vessel, 10% for clot and 0 for stain. Wara,[318] however, found little significant correlation between stigmata and mortality. The Forrest classification proposed in 1974[260] remains a useful indicator of risk of rebleeding, the need for surgery and mortality.[322]

It would appear that many of the disparities seen in these studies can be accounted for by the following factors. (1) The timing of endoscopy and whether the ulcer base was washed were widely variable and both would certainly influence the incidence and nature of detected stigmata. (2) There was a lack of standardization of nomenclature for stigmata. (3) The criteria for diagnosing rebleeding and the indications for surgery were inconsistent.

Nevertheless, it seems that certain categories of stigmata, especially active bleeding, visible vessel and clot are relevant indices of an unstable and potentially life-threatening situation and that such findings merit careful observation. Just as importantly the absence of stigmata indicates a group of patients who can be followed in a less stringent manner.[323] Moreover, it has now also been recognized that patients with blackspots can be included in this low-risk group.

Although the presence of shock on admission or endoscopic stigmata may in their own right predict rebleeding, the relationship is not strong enough to justify a pre-emptive operative policy. However, as has been shown in one study,[315] that the combination of shock and major stigmata may make a more compelling case for surgery.

Indications for and timing of surgery

Although imperfect, the aforementioned clinical and endoscopic signs do anticipate the risk of rebleeding and mortality and have allowed some definition of patients who may benefit from early surgical therapy. The timing of surgical intervention has long been debated by those who advocate and those who question planned early surgery. The issue is whether an aggressive surgical approach reduces the mortality associated with rebleeding. A number of recent retrospective studies have specifically addressed this contentious aspect of management.

Himal et al.[300] found a decrease in mortality after adopting an aggressive diagnostic and early surgical approach for bleeding gastric ulcer and high risk patients with duodenal ulcers. Hunt et al.[324,325] also observed a decline in mortality for bleeding peptic ulcer after adopting a policy of early endoscopy and surgery. They operated on all patients over 50 years who were

Table 34.21   Endoscopic stigmata and percentage rebleeding

AUTHORS	DATE	n	NONE (%)	BLACKSPOT (%)	CLOT (%)	VESSEL (%)	ACTIVE (%)
Griffiths et al.[314]	1979	157	ns	25[a]		100(75)	ns
Storey et al.[320]	1981	47	0	8[a](8)		56(50)	ns
Bornman et al.[315]	1985	98	5	0	25	50	ns
Wara[318]	1985	53	ns	ns	ns	32	ns
Beckley and Casebow[321]	1986	49	ns	ns	0	30	44
Hunt[312]	1987	209	7(5)	30[a](22)		38(46)	44(32)
Chang-Chien et al.[317]	1988	156	0	ns	16	0	32

[a]Denotes values where clot and blackspot were grouped together.
Values in parentheses indicate the percentage of patients requiring operation for haemorrhage.
ns, not stated.

shocked on admission and in those with recurrent or continued bleeding requiring more than five units of blood. In 1984 he reaffirmed this with long-term, prospective data.[244]

However, others are less persuaded by an early aggressive surgical approach. The Nottingham group has been most vocal in this regard. In 1979, Dronfield et al.[326] compared the mortality rates from peptic ulcer haemorrhage at two hospitals with different operation policies. Neither overall mortality rate (18% vs 13%) nor the postoperative mortality (20% vs 20%) were significantly different. In a subsequent report, Vellacott et al.[242] further questioned the value of early surgery as no change in overall mortality was noted at the same time that operative rates fell. The authors suggested that the value of an early aggressive surgical policy did not save more lives. However, a planned operative strategy was not in place.

Only three prospective randomized studies have addressed the question of optimal timing of operation for bleeding peptic ulcer. Read et al.[327] in 1965, evaluated immediate operation versus nonoperative management, followed, if necessary, by delayed operation for rebleeding. In 59 patients demonstrated to be bleeding massively from peptic ulcer, all deaths occurred after delayed operation (30%) and all were over 50 years of age.

Morris et al.[302] randomized 142 patients after stratification for age (over and under 60 years) and site of ulcer (duodenal versus gastric), to early surgical or expectant management. They employed comprehensive haemodynamic, endoscopic and historic criteria for entry into the early surgical group. In the expectant management group surgery was only undertaken after large blood loss (up to 16 units in 72 h). No patients under 60 with duodenal ulcer died. The overall mortality in patients over 60 years was 7% for early surgery versus 43% for late surgery. For duodenal ulcer, mortality was similar in both the early (7%) and the delayed (9%) group. The major difference was seen in gastric ulcer mortality (early 0, delayed 24%). The authors recommended an aggressive surgical approach in patients over 60 years, especially with gastric ulcer. One must appreciate that the liberal tranfusion policy in the expectant group and the rather aggressive inclusion criteria in the early surgery group may have been responsible for the equivocal results in the other arms of this study.

The opposite conclusion was drawn in a randomized trial from Barcelona.[328] Early surgical therapy and expectant management were compared in 69 patients over 50 years of age whose duodenal ulcers were endoscopically at low risk for rebleeding (active, non-arterial bleeding or evidence of recent haemorrhage in the absence of a visible vessel). Mortality was five times higher (14% versus 3%) in the early surgery group suggesting that an aggressive surgical approach in patients with low-risk endoscopic stigmata may indeed be harmful.

The vexing question of early versus delayed surgery has not been satisfactorily answered. The entry criteria for such a study remain difficult to define accurately. While age over 50 years, shock and important endoscopic stigmata qualify, many of these patients have serious associated medical illness. Thus a surgical trial under these circumstances raises ethical concerns. Likewise, the exclusion of such patients makes it difficult to gather adequate numbers to mount a definitive investigation. None the less, a sufficient database exists to justify certain conditions for surgical intervention. Guidelines based on these principles are outlined in Table 34.22.

Surgery

Once a decision has been made to operate on a patient with peptic ulcer haemorrhage, the next important choice is which surgical procedure to undertake. The operative strategy is

Table 34.22   Indications for surgery in peptic ulcer haemorrhage

Absolute indications
Exsanguinating haemorrhage
Arterial spurter with shock

Strong indications
Shock requiring more than four units of blood for resuscitation
Rebleed with shock
Rebleed requiring more than three units of blood over 24 hours
Major endoscopic stigmata (active bleeding, visible vessel, clot)

Relative indications
Less severe rebleed
Chronic ulcer diathesis meriting surgery

dictated to some extent by the location of the ulcer. Operative choice, however, is ultimately influenced by the haemodynamic and medical condition of the patient. The renowned Viennese surgeon Hans Finsterer[274] elegantly stated in 1939: 'The main purpose of operative treatment in the presence of acute haemorrhage is reliable haemostasis, the question of permanent cure of the ulcer being of secondary importance'. In spite of the enormous strides made in anaesthesia, pharmacology and intensive care, this policy is as true today as it was more than half a century ago. With this important concept in mind, this section discusses the evolution of surgery for peptic ulcer haemorrhage, the principal operations employed today and the rationale for their use.

Choice of operation

For one century, surgeons have been participants in the management of peptic ulcer haemorrhage. In the last 50 years much debate has centred on defining the proper operation for bleeding gastric and duodenal ulcer. As no prospective randomized studies have addressed this question, much of our understanding and decision making is based on prejudice or empiricism.

Billroth I gastrectomy was the dominant operation for both gastric and duodenal ulcer haemorrhage until the first report of vagotomy for bleeding in the 1950s.[292] Although gastrectomy was highly effective in arresting haemorrhage and controlling ulcer diathesis, it was associated with a considerable morbidity and mortality (Table 34.23). Vagotomy, pyloroplasty and underrunning (VP & U) was developed as a potentially less morbid and more physiological alternative.[335,336]

The techniques for Billroth I gastrectomy and vagotomy and pyloroplasty are illustrated elsewhere in this text. Figure 34.22(a) depicts the standard technique of suture control of a bleeding posterior duodenal ulcer through a longitudinal pyloroduodenotomy.[337] The ulcer is underrun with multiple, deep figure-of-eight sutures. An alternative is the circumferential three-vessel ligation described by Berne and Rosoff[338] in

which deep, simple ligatures are placed above and below the ulcer to control the gastroduodenal artery. A third central horizontal mattress suture is placed to secure both the arterial perforation and any collaterals which may communicate in this region (Figure 34.22 b,c).

Despite dissenting voices,[339] many centres actively investigated this simplified and seemingly safer approach to peptic ulcer haemorrhage with encouraging results (Table 34.24). Subsequently, numerous comparative studies helped to define the most appropriate roles for gastrectomy and VP & U in peptic ulcer haemorrhage. Relevant studies are listed in Table 34.25. Although the range of mortality is similar for both operations (gastrectomy 6–36%, VP & U 0–30%), 10 studies favour VP & U, two studies support gastrectomy and five are equivocal. Importantly, seven studies show a mortality rate of greater than 20% for gastrectomy as opposed to only two studies for VP & U. On the other hand, significant postoperative rebleeding appears to be somewhat lower for gastrectomy (0–10%) than for VP & U.

Table 34.23 Results of gastric resection for massive peptic ulcer haemorrhage

AUTHORS	DATE	n	MORT (%)	MORT DU (%)	MORT GU (%)
Finsterer[274]	1939	71	4	ns	ns
Walters and Cleveland[283]	1941	79	10	7	12
Welch[284]	1949	45	9	ns	ns
Lewison[292]	1950	56	7	ns	ns
Jones[294]	1956	82	25	36	14
Stewart et al.[329]	1956	155	13	8	18
Ward-McQuaid et al.[286]	1960	82	15	18	11
Large[330]	1960	64	14	20	6
Darin et al.[331]	1961	120	23	31	19
Brooks and Eraklis[332]	1964	75	21	20	22
Cocks et al.[333]	1972	367	17	ns	ns
Inberg and Linna[334]	1975	120	8	ns	ns

Mort, mortality; DU, duodenal ulcer; GU, gastric ulcer; ns, not stated.

Table 34.24 Results of vagotomy, pyloroplasty and ligation for duodenal ulcer haemorrhage

AUTHORS	DATE	n	MORTALITY (%)	REBLEED (%)
Weinberg[340]	1961	47	2	4
Dorton[341]	1961	47	0	0
Farris and Smith[342]	1967	100	6	8
Snyder and Stellar[343]	1968	131	17	10
Klingensmith and Oles[344]	1968	42	0	ns
Vogel[345]	1972	45	7	4
Jensen and Guldberg[346]	1974	92	8	15
Brooks et al.[347]	1975	78	11	8

ns, not stated.

When mortality is correlated with both the type of operation and site of ulcer (Table 34.26) it appears that VP & U is as good as or better than gastric resection for bleeding duodenal ulcer. With regard to gastric ulcer, three studies support gastric resection and three indicate VP & U as a safer alternative.

In the elderly, four reports[243,334,353,355] have shown VP & U to be a safer option for both gastric[243,334] and duodenal ulcer.[356,358] However, two[356,358] have found no difference in mortality for either operation in older age groups.

Surprisingly, a prospective, randomized comparison of gastric resection with VP & U has never been undertaken. As such, a clear, scientific basis for surgical decision making is lacking. Nevertheless, the accumulated retrospective experience seems to present reasonable circumstances for the use of both gastric resection and VP & U (Table 34.27). In all cases of bleeding duodenal ulcer, VP & U of the ulcer should be performed. In fit patients with bleeding gastric ulcer, a Billroth I gastrectomy is the most definitive procedure. There is evidence that VP & U should be considered in high risk patients or for difficult high-lying ulcers. It is important to note, however, that there are centres, especially in the USA,[337,353,355,356,358] that prefer vagotomy and antrectomy for healthy patients with bleeding

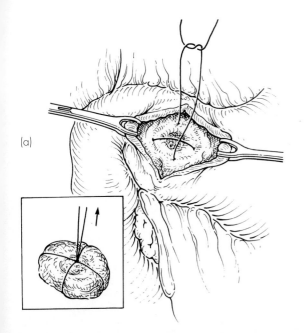

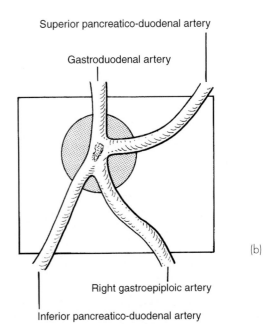

Superior pancreatico-duodenal artery

Gastroduodenal artery

Right gastroepiploic artery

Inferior pancreatico-duodenal artery

Figure 34.22

(a) Standard figure-of-eight suture ligation of a posterior bleeding duodenal ulcer. (b) The gastroduodenal artery complex identifying the gastroduodenal (GD), transverse pancreatic (TP), superior pancreaticoduodenal (SPD), and right gastroepiploic (RGE) vessels. (c) Method of achieving 'three vessel' circumferential ligation with superior and inferior horizontal mattress sutures and a central 'U' stitch.

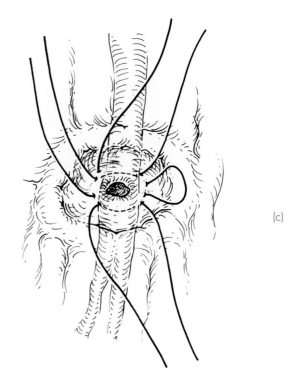

duodenal ulcer. In the final analysis, factors such as the experience of the operator and the ability of the patient to withstand a lengthy operation are important elements in surgical decision making.

Surgical alternatives

In 1977 Johnston[359] reported no deaths and no reoperations for rebleeding in 26 patients who had highly selective vagotomy, duodenotomy and under-running for bleeding duodenal ulcer and HSV with gastrotomy and under-running for bleeding gastric ulcer. However, this series represented a selective cohort that did not fall into a high-risk category. Bambach et al.[354] used HSV and under-running with no mortality in twelve cases. Despite excellent results it is not clear from this small database whether these more demanding techniques are safer or more effective than truncal vagotomy in the setting of peptic ulcer haemorrhage.

Endoscopic treatment

In recent years an increasing number of endoscopic techniques have been developed for the treatment of bleeding peptic ulcer (Table 34.28). Although laser photocoagulation has been applied extensively in numerous controlled trials,[360–370] a few have demonstrated a reduction in urgent surgery for rebleeding and mortality.[371] In many trials there has been a high exclusion rate either due to technical deficiencies or restricted access to the target.[360–363,368]

The dry, monopolar electrode has reduced the rebleeding and surgery rate in two controlled trials.[372,373] A randomized trial of the liquid monopolar electrode decreased rebleeding and urgent surgery in patients with a visible vessel but not in patients with active bleeding.[374] Only one controlled, trial of the 7 French multipolar electrode[375] showed a decrease in rebleeding in the treated group (17% vs 33%) but this had no impact on emergency operations or mortality. One controlled study using a 10 French multipolar probe[376] demonstrated a reduction in rebleeding, surgery, transfusion and hospital stay for ulcers with non-bleeding, visible vessels treated with electrocautery.

Several, uncontrolled trials of heater probes suggest a high

Table 34.25 Comparison of gastric resection versus vagotomy, pyloroplasty and under-running for peptic ulcer haemorrhage

| AUTHORS | DATE | GASTRECTOMY | | | VP & U | | |
		n	MORTALITY (%)	REBLEED (%)	n	MORTALITY (%)	REBLEED (%)
Akin and Sullivan[348]	1963	20	10	0	20	15	15
Foster et al.[349]	1965	77	28	8	77	10	7
Carruthers et al.[350]	1967	51	18	3	48	2	10
Feltis and Harit[351]	1967	36	14	5	14	14	0
Hampson et al.[352]	1968	176	6	ns	13	8	ns
Jones et al.[304]	1973	51	29	ns	17	6	ns
Inberg and Linna et al.[334]	1975	120	8	ns	23	9	ns
Buckingham and Remine[353]	1975	29	14	ns	32	9	ns
Bambach et al.[354]	1976	21	14	0	71	0	6
Stone et al.[355]	1978	109	6	ns	18	6	ns
Dronfield et al.[326]	1979	42	26	ns	68	16	ns
Vellacott et al.[242]	1982	ns	23	ns	ns	10	ns
Wara et al.[305]	1983	52	36	4	86	22	17
van Stiegmann et al.[243]	1983	100	13	4	69	7	6
Morris et al.[302]	1984	12	33	ns	44	9	ns
Welch et al.[356]	1986	178	22	ns	47	30	ns
Hunt[311]	1986	76	13	10	71	11	18

VP & U, vagotomy, pyloroplasty and under-running; ns, not stated.

(up to 95%)[377] success rate in controlling ulcer haemorrhage.[377-380] In the only prospective, controlled study,[381] the heater probe reduced the rebleeding and operative rate in accessible bleeding ulcers with high risk stigmata. However, poor success was seen for high, lesser curve ulcers which highlights a limitation of this technique.

Injection sclerotherapy, by virtue of its simplicity and availability has become the most widely used method of endoscopic control of bleeding peptic ulcers.

Adrenaline (1:10 000) alone[382] and in combination with sclerosants (polidocanol, ethanolamine oleate) significantly reduced the incidence of rebleeding and surgery.[383-386]. Alcohol injections alone achieved the same results in two fully published trials.[387-388]

In a meta-analysis of 30 randomized controlled trials evaluating the various types of haemostatic endoscopic treatments

by Cook et al.[371] rebleeding rate and need for emergency surgery and mortality were significantly reduced when all studies were combined. Although rebleeding rate and need for emergency surgery were significantly reduced with all three endoscopic techniques (thermal-contact devices, laser treatment and injection therapy), the reduction in overall mortality rate only reached statistical significance in the laser-treated group. However, in all three groups the mortality was significantly reduced in patients with high-risk non-bleeding visible vessels.

It is vital for the surgeon, the ultimate provider of haemostasis, to be familiar with therapeutic endoscopy as the approach to ulcer haemorrhage evolves. Present information indicates that endoscopic haemostasis will play an important initial role in patients who are at high risk for rebleeding and surgery. It is apparent that the potential exists to lower the rate of urgent

Table 34.26 Mortality for gastric resection versus vagotomy, pyloroplasty and under-running for gastric and duodenal ulcer haemorrhage

| AUTHORS | DATE | DUODENAL | | | GASTRIC | | |
		n	GASTR (%)	VP&U (%)	n	GASTR (%)	VP&U (%)
Foster et al.[349]	1965	95	32	10	59	24	11
Carruthers et al.[350]	1967	79	16	2	20	20	2
Hampson et al.[352]	1968	140	7	8	50	2	11
Buckingham and Remine[353]	1975	61	14	9	0	ns	ns
Dronfield et al.[326]	1975	69	44	12	41	21	50
Inberg and Linna[334]	1975	68	9	9	71	7	ns
Stone et al.[355]	1978	128	6	6	0	ns	ns
Brolin and Stremple[357]	1982	24	8	8	13	22	25
van Stiegmann et al.[243]	1983	81	24	9	88	11	0
Hunt[311]	1984	148	9	8	68	16	ns

Gastr, gastrectomy; VP&U, vagotomy, pyloroplasty and under-running; ns, not stated.

Table 34.27 An algorithm for the selection of an operation in peptic ulcer haemorrhage

ULCER	GOOD RISK	POOR RISK
Duodenal	Truncal vagotomy	Truncal vagotomy
	Pyloroduodenotomy	Pyloroduodenotomy
	Under-running of vessel	Under-running of vessel
	Pyloroplasty	Pyloroplasty
Gastric	Billroth I gastrectomy	Gastrotomy
		Under-running of ulcer
		Truncal vagotomy
		Pyloroplasty

operation and perhaps reduce the number of complications and deaths. Simplicity, safety and economy of administration should be the most important guides in choosing an endoscopic method of haemostasis. In this regard, injection sclerotherapy seems to best fulfil these requirements.

Summary

The patient presenting with evidence of upper gastrointestinal haemorrhage requires swift attention directed at resuscitation and diagnosis. Ideally all such patients should be cared for by a dedicated team of physicians, surgeons and nurses in a setting that allows for close observation and a planned approach. Up to one-third of initially stable patients will have further haemorrhage and most of the mortality resides in this group. Although there is no reliable way of forecasting who will rebleed, the presence of shock on admission and the endoscopic findings of active arterial bleeding, a visible vessel and clot define patients who should be carefully monitored. Likewise, the absence of shock and lack of significant endoscopic stigmata usually indicate a benign course.

Table 34.28 Techniques of endoscopic haemostasis

Injection
Absolute alcohol
Polidocanol
Adrenaline

Thermal
Laser photocoagulation
Electrocautery
   dry monopolar
   liquid monopolar
   multipolar
Heater probe

Other
Protocoagulants
   cryoprecipitate
   thrombin
Haemostatics
   microcrystalline collagen
Tissue adhesives
   trifluoroisopropyl-cyanoacrylate
Mechanical
   balloon
   clips

There are no absolute guidelines for surgical intervention in bleeding peptic ulcer. The decision to intervene, the timing of intervention and the choice of technique remain problematic. Current knowledge would indicate that early intervention should be recommended in elderly patients who are at risk for rebleeding. However, the presence of associated medical illness often compounds decision making.

Surgery has been the most definitive treatment for peptic ulcer haemorrhage but the safe and successful application of therapeutic endoscopy has given impetus to its use as first line therapy. When surgery is necessary, vagotomy, pyloroplasty and under-running of the ulcer has been the treatment of choice for duodenal ulcer in good-risk patients and Billroth I gastrectomy for gastric ulcer in good-risk patients.

These conventional operations for *H. pylori*-related ulcers complicated by bleedings have been reappraised with the significant reduction of ulcer recurrence and bleeding after successful eradication therapy.[389] For most patients, unless there are technical difficulties, under-running of the bleeding site would suffice, thus avoiding the postgastrectomy sequelae of definitive operations.

REFERENCES

1. Malloch A. *An Early Record of Perforating Duodenal Ulcer, Contributions to Medical and Biological Research*. Dedicated to Sir William Osler, New York: Paul B Hoeber, 1919; **1**: 137.
2. Rawlinson C. A preternatural perforation found in the upper part of the stomach. With the symptoms it produced, *Philadelphia Trans R Soc* 1727–28; **35**: 361.
3. Power D'A. Haller and Some Begone Observations in Pathology. *Med Rec* 1925; **122**: 415.
4. Crisp E. Cases of perforation of the stomach with deductions therefrom relative to the character and treatment of that lesion *Lancet* 1843; **ii**: 639.
5. Brinton W. An ulcer of the stomach. *Br For Med Chir Rev* 1856; **17**: 159.
6. Müller L. *Das corrosive Geschwür im Magen und Darmkanal (Ulcus Ventriculi perforans Chronicum rotundum) und dessen Behandling.* Erlangen: Enke, 1860.
7. Krauss J. *Das perforierende Geschwür im Duodenum.* Berlin: Hirschwald, 1865.
8. Leube WO. *Ziemssen Cyclopedia of the Practice of Medicine VII.* New York: William Wood, 1876: 192.
9. Jennings D. Perforated peptic ulcer. *Lancet* 1940; **238**: 395.
10. Mikulicz J. Über laparotomie bei Magen-und Darmperforation. *Samml Klin Vortr* 1885; **3**(Chirurgie 83): 2307.
11. Kriege H. Ein Fau von einem frei in die Bauchhöhle perforierten Magengeschwür Laparotomie, Naht der Perforations-stelle, Heilung, *Berl Klin Wochenschr* 1892; **29**: 1244.
12. Billington BP. The Australian gastric ulcer change: further observations. *Med J Aust* 1960; **2**: 19.
13. Brown RC, Langman MJS & Lambert PM. Hospital admissions for peptic ulcer during 1958–72. *BMJ* 1976; **1**: 35.
14. Sanders R. Incidence of perforated duodenal and gastric ulcer in Oxford. *Gut* 1967; **8**: 58.
15. Illingworth CFW, Scott LDW & Jamieson RA. Acute perforated peptic ulcer: frequency and incidence in the West of Scotland. *BMJ* 1944; **2**: 617, 655.
16. Jamieson RA. Acute perforated peptic ulcer: frequency and incidence in the west of Scotland. *BMJ* 1955; **2**: 222.
17. MacKay C. Perforated peptic ulcer in the west of Scotland: a survey of 5343 cases during 1954–63. *BMJ* 1966; **1**: 701.
18. MacKay C. Prevalence of peptic ulcer and its complications. *Scot Med J* 1977; **22**: 288.
19. Watkins RM, Dennison AR & Collin J. What happened to perforated peptic ulcer? *Br J Surg* 1984; **71**: 774.
20. Elashoff JD & Grossman MI. Trends in hospital death rates for peptic ulcer in the United States from 1970–1978. *Gastroenterology* 1980; **78**: 280.

21. Horisberger B. A review of the epidemiological development of peptic ulcer and an evaluation of duodenal ulcers in the Federal Republic of Germany before and after cimetidine. In Cuyler AJ & Horisberger B (eds) *Economic and Medical Evaluation of Health Care Technologies.* Berlin: Springer, 1983; 213.

22. Jönsson B. A review of the macro-economic evaluation of cimetidine. In Culyer AJ & Horisberger B (eds) *Economic and Medical Evaluation of Health Care Technologies.* Berlin: Springer, 1983; 243.

23. Bardhan KD, Cust G, Hinchliffe RFC, Williamson FM, Lyon C & Bose K. Changing pattern of admissions and operations for duodenal ulcer. *Br J Surg* 1989; **76**: 230.

24. Koo J, Ngan YK & Lam SK. Trends in hospital admissions, perforation and mortality of peptic ulcer in Hong Kong from 1970 to 1980. *Gastroenterology* 1983; **84**: 1558.

25. Cooke SAR. Perforated duodenal ulcer in the black population of central Johannesburg. *Br J Surg* 1977; **64**: 791.

26. Crohn BB, Rouse MO & Smith HW. The relationship of trauma to the perforation of peptic ulcer. *Gastroenterology* 1946; **7**: 456.

27. Steward DN & Winser DM de R. Perforated peptic ulcer during the period of heavy air raids. *Lancet* 1944; **i**: 14.

28. Compton SA, Cooper NK, Clyde RJ, Collins JSA & Friel CM. Perforated peptic ulcer and the civil disturbances in Belfast 1967–1974. *Ulster Med J* 1976; **45**: 205.

29. Walt R, Katschinski B, Logan R, Ashley J & Langman M. Rising frequency of ulcer perforation in elderly people in the United Kingdom. *Lancet* 1986; **i**: 489.

30. Jorgensen TG. Drug consumption before perforation of peptic ulcer. *Br J Surg* 1977; **64**: 247.

31. Moynihan BGA. On duodenal ulcer and its surgical treatment. *Lancet* 1901; **ii**: 1656.

32. Moynihan BGA. An address on gastroenterostomy and after. *BMJ* 1908; **i**: 1092.

33. DeBakey M. Acute perforated gastroduodenal ulceration: a statistical analysis and review of the literature. *Surgery* 1940; **8**: 1028.

34. Devitt JE & Taylor GA. Perforated peptic ulcer. *Can Med Assoc J* 1967; **96**: 519.

35. Palmer ED. Perforation of gastroduodenal ulcer. *Arch Intern Med* 1972; **130**: 957.

36. Johnston D. Treatment of peptic ulcer and its complications. In S Taylor (ed.) *Recent Advances in Surgery* No 10, Chap. 16, London: Churchill Livingston, 1980: 335.

37. Boey J, Choi SKY, Alagaratnam TT & Poon A. Risk stratification in perforated duodenal ulcers. A prospective validation of predictive factors, *Ann Surg* 1987; **205**: 22.

38. Turner FP. Acute perforations of stomach, duodenum, and jejunum. *Surg Gynecol Obstet* 1951; **92**: 281.

39. Cohen MM. Treatment and mortality of perforated peptic ulcer: A survey of 852 cases. *Can Med Assoc J* 1971; **105**: 263.

40. Kirkpatrick JR & Bouwman DL. Logical solution to the perforated ulcer, controversy. *Surg Gynecol Obstet* 1980; **150**: 683–6.

41. Nemanich GJ & Nicoloff DM. Perforated duodenal ulcer: long-term follow-up. *Surgery* 1970; **67**: 727.

42. Armstrong CP & Whitelaw S. Death from undiagnosed peptic ulcer complications: a continuing challenge *Br J Surg* 1988; **75**: 1112.

43. Reynolds PR, Cantor MO & Stebbins C. Effect of shock upon the mortality rate of perforated peptic ulcer. *Am J Dig Dis* 1950; **17**: 365.

44. Rogers FA. Factors affecting the mortality from acute gastroduodenal perforation. *Surg Gynecol Obstet* 1960; **111**: 771.

45. Krippaehne WW, Fletcher WS & Dunphy JE. Acute perforation of duodenal and gastric ulcer. *Arch Surg* 1964; **88**: 874.

46. Boey J & Wong J. A prospective study of operative risk factors in perforated duodenal ulcer. *Ann Surg* 1982; **195**: 265.

47. Irvin TT. Mortality and perforated peptic ulcer: a case for risk stratification in elderly patients. *Br J Surg* 1989; **76**: 215.

48. Knaus WA, Draper EA & Wagner DP. Apache II: a severity of disease classification system. *Crit Care Med* 1985; **13**: 818.

49. Heuman R, Larsson J & Norrby S. Perforated duodenal ulcer – long-term results following simple closure. *Acta Chir Scand* 1983; **149**: 77.

50. Jones FA & Doll R. Treatment and prognosis of acute perforated peptic ulcer *BMJ* 1953; **1**: 122.

51. Mickel S & Morrison WR. Acute perforated peptic ulcer. Criteria for operation and analysis of 500 cases. *N Engl J Med* 1952; **247**: 119.

52. Mattingly SS & Griffin WO. Factors influencing morbidity and mortality in perforated duodenal ulcer. *Surg* 1980; **46**: 61.

53. Heslop TS, Bullough AS & Brun C. The treatment of perforated peptic ulcer. A comparison of two parallel unselected series. *Br J Surg* 1952; **40**: 52.

54. Schmitz EJ, Harkins HN, Olson HL, Moore HG & Merendino KA. Perforated peptic ulcer: a study of 136 cases in County Hospital. *Ann Surg* 1953; **138**: 689.

55. Reimer J. Perforating gastric versus duodenal ulcers. Primary resection versus suture: an analysis of two 15 year series. *Acta Chir Scand* 1967; **133**: 381.

56. Kozoll DD & Meyer KA. General factors influencing the incidence and mortality of acute perforated gastro-duodenal ulcers. *Surg Gynecol Obstet* 1960; **111**: 607.

57. Hardy JD, Walker GR & Conn JH. Perforated peptic ulcer; an analysis of 206 consecutive cases with emphasis on pathophysiology changes and deaths. *Ann Surg* 1961; **153**: 911.

58. Donaldson GA & Jarrett F. Perforated gastroduodenal ulcer disease at the Massachusetts General Hospital from 1952–1970. *Ann J Surg* 1970; **120**: 306.

59. Gilmour J. Prognosis and treatment in acute perforated peptic ulcer. A review of 206 cases. *Lancet* 1953; **i**: 870.

60. Taylor H & Warren RP. Perforated acute and chronic peptic ulcer. Conservative treatment. *Lancet* 1956; **i**: 397.

61. Kay PH, Moore KTH & Clark RG. The treatment of perforated duodenal ulcer. *Br J Surg* 1978; **65**: 801.

62. Sirinek KR, Levine BA, Schwesinger WH & Aust JB. Simple closure of perforated peptic ulcer. Still an effective procedure for patients with delay in treatment. *Arch Surg* 1981; **116**: 591.

63. McDonough JM & Foster JH. Factors influencing prognosis in perforated peptic ulcer. *Am J Surg* 1972; **123**: 411.

64. Griffen GE & Organ CH. The natural history of the perforated duodenal ulcer treated by suture plication. *Ann Surg* 1976; **183**: 382.

65. Playforth MJ & McMohan MJ. The indications of simple closure of perforated duodenal ulcer. *Br J Surg* 1978; **65**: 699.

66. Wara P, Kristensen ES, Sorensen FH et al. The value of parietal cell vagotomy compared to simple closure in an elective approach to perforated duodenal ulcer. *Acta Chir Scand* 1983; **149**: 585.

67. Stabile BE, Hardy HJ & Passaro E. 'Kissing' duodenal ulcers. *Arch Surg* 1979; **114**: 1153.

68. Singer HA & Vaughan RT. The 'Formes Frustes' type of perforated peptic ulcer. *Surg Gynecol Obstet* 1930; **50**: 10.

69. Feldman M. Perforation of peptic ulcer. A roentgenologic consideration of the various forms and uncommon types of perforation. *Radiology* 1950; **55**: 217.

70. Haubrich WS, Roth JLA & Bockus HL. The clinical significance of penetration and confined perforation in peptic ulcer disease. *Gastroenterology* 1953; **25**: 173.

71. Norris JR & Haubrich WS. The incidence and clinical features of penetration in peptic ulceration *JAMA* 1961; **178**: 386.

72. Christensen E. Perforeret ulcers efter butazolidin behandling. *Ugeskr Laeger* 1954; **116**: 1646.

73. Cameron AJ. Aspirin intake in patients with peptic ulcer. *Gastroenterology* 1973; **64**: 705.

74. Duggan JM. Aspirin ingestion and perforated peptic ulcer. *Gut* 1972; **13**: 631.

75. Feldman M. Peptic ulcer perforation into the lesser peritoneal sac. A statistical study of 57 collected cases. *Am J Dig Dis* 1950; **17**: 333.

76. Donovan AG, Vinson TL, Maulsby GO & Gewin JR. Selective treatment of duodenal ulcer with perforation. *Ann Surg* 1979; **189**: 627.

77. Lowdon AGR. The treatment of acute perforated peptic ulcer by primary partial gastrectomy. *Lancet* 1952; **262**: 1270.

78. Dent DM, Bank S & Louw JH. Perforated duodenal ulcer: is the distinction between acute and chronic valid? *S Afr Med J* 1977; **51**: 529.

79. Nuboer JF. Primary partial gastrectomy for perforated ulcer. *Lancet* 1951; **ii**: 952.

80. Mark JBD. Factors influencing the treatment of perforated duodenal ulcer. *Surg Gynecol Obstet* 1969; **129**: 325.

81. Creco RS & Cahow CE. Alternatives in the management of acute perforated duodenal ulcer. *Am J Surg* 1974; **127**: 109.

82. Hamilton JE & Harbrecht PJ. Growing indications for vagotomy in perforated peptic ulcer. *Surg Gynecol Obstet* 1967; **124**: 61.

83. Wagensteen SL, Wray RC & Goldon GT. Perforated duodenal ulcer. *Am J Surg* 1972; **123**: 538.

84. Boey J, Wong J & Ong GB. Bacteria and septic complications in patients with perforated duodenal ulcers. *Am J Surg* 1982; **143**: 635.

85. Cope O, Hopkirk JF & Wight A. Metabolic derangements imperiling the perforated ulcer patient. *Arch Surg* 1955; **71**: 669.

86. Mackay C. Deaths from perforated peptic ulcer. A survey of 633 cases in the West of Scotland. *Scand J Gastroenterol* 1966; **1**: 299.

87. Moore FD, Peete WPJ, Richardson JE, Erskine JM, Brooks JR & Rogers H. The effect of definitive surgery on duodenal ulcer disease. A comparative study of surgical and non-surgical management in 997 cases. *Ann Surg* 1950; **132**: 652.

88. Hendry WS, Valerio D & Kyle J. Perforated peptic ulcer in North and East Scotland. *J R Coll Surg Edin* 1984; **29**: 69.

89. Moynihan BGA. *Address on Surgical Subjects. Philadelphia*: WB Saunders, 1928.

90. Lui AHF. An unusual sign in perforated peptic ulcer. *Am J Surg* 1957; **93**: 876.

91. Miller RE & Nelson SW. The roentgenologic demonstration of tiny amounts of free intraperitoneal gas: experimental and clinical studies. *Am J Roentgenol Radium Ther Nucl Med* 1971; **112**: 574.

92. Rigler LG. Spontaneous pneumoperitoneum: a roentgenologic sign found in the supine position. *Radiology* 1941; **37**: 604.

93. Stabins SJ. The aftermath of perforated duodenal ulcer. *Surgery* 1953; **34**: 614.

94. Petol D & Hollander D. Complications of peptic ulcer disease. In Haubrich WS, Kalser M, Roth JLA & Schaffner F *Backus Gastroenterology* 4th edn. Philadelphia: WB Saunders, 1985: 1155.

95. Berne CJ & Rosoff C Sr. Acute perfortion of peptic ulcer. In Nyhus LM & Wastell C (eds) *Surgery of the Stomach and Duodenum* 4th edn. Boston: Little Brown, 1986; 457.

96. Rogers FA. Elevated serum amylase. A review and an analysis of findings in 1000 cases of perforated peptic ulcer. *Ann Surg* 1961; **138**: 228.

97. Maynard A de L, Froix CJL & Oropeza G. Gastroduodenal perforation. With conclusions on the role of definitive surgery. *Arch Surg* 1968; **97**: 96.

98. Wagensteen OH. Non-operative treatment of localised perforation of the duodenum. *Minn Med* 1935; **18**: 477.

99. Elliott JC & Lane JD. Perforated peptic ulcer treatment by the non-operative method. *Am J Dig Dis* 1959; **4**: 950.

100. Taylor H. Guest lecture. The non-surgical treatment of perforated peptic ulcer. *Gastroenterology* 1957; **33**: 353.

101. Seeley SF & Campbell D. Non-operative treatment of perforated peptic ulcer, a further report. *Int Abst Surg* 1956; **102**: 435.

102. Von Harberer H. Zur therapie akuter Geschwursperforationen des Magens und duodenums in die freie Bauchhole. *Wien Klin Wochenschr* 1919; **32**: 413.

103. Cooley DA, Jordon GL, Brockman L & De Bakey ME. Gastrectomy in acute gastroduodenal perforation: Analysis of 112 cases. *Ann Surg* 1955; **141**: 840.

104. Keane TE, Dillon B, Afdhal NH & Cormack CJ. Conservative management of perforated duodenal ulcer. *Br J Surg* 1988; **75**: 583.

105. Crofts TJ, Park KGM, Steele RJC, Chung SSC & Li AKC. A randomised trial of non-operative treatment for perforated peptic ulcer. *N Engl J Med* 1989; **320**: 970.

106. Cocks JR, Kernutt RH, Sinclair GWG, Dawsons, JH McL & Hong BH. Perforated peptic ulcer: a deliberative approach. *Aust NZ J Surg* 1989; **59**: 379.

107. Mülleder A and Neuberger J. Zur Resektion beim perforierten. Magen-Duodenal ulcus. *Wien Klin Wochenschr* 1923; **36**: 743.

108. Odelberg A. Primary resection of the stomach in perforated gastric and duodenal ulcers. *Acta Chir Scand* 1972; **62**: 159.

109. Judine S. Etude sur les ulceres gastriques et duodenaux perfores. *J Int Chir* 1939; **4**: 219.

110. Jordan GL, De Bakey ME & Duncan JM. Surgical management of perforated peptic ulcer. *Ann Surg* 1974; **179**: 682.

111. Jordan PH Jr & Korompai FL. Evolvement of a new treatment for perforated duodenal ulcer. *Surg Gynecol Obstet* 1976; **142**: 391.

112. Hadfield JIH & Watkin DFL. Vagotomy in the treatment of perforated duodenal ulcer. *BMJ* 1964; **2**: 12.

113. Gray JG & Roberts AK. Definitive emergency treatment of perforated duodenal ulcer. *Surg Gynecol Obstet* 1976; **143**: 890.

114. Tanphiphat C, Tanprayoon J & Na Thalang A. Surgical treatment of perforated duodenal ulcer: a prospective trial between simple closure and definitive surgery. *Br J Surg* 1985; **72**: 370.

115. Boey J, Lee NW, Koo J, Lam PHM, Wong J & Ong GB. Immediate definitive surgery for perforated duodenal ulcers. *Ann Surg* 1982; **196**: 338.

116. Ceneviva R, de Castro e Silva O, Castelfranchi PL, Modena JPJ & Santos RF. Simple suture with or without proximal gastric vagotomy for perforated duodenal ulcer. *Br J Surg* 1986; **73**: 427.

117. Boey J, Branicki FJ, Alagaratnam TT et al. Proximal gastric vagotomy. The preferred operation for perforations in acute duodenal ulcer. *Ann Surg* 1988; **208**: 169.

118. Hinshaw DB, Pierandozzi JS, Thomas RJ & Carter R. Vagotomy and pyloroplasy for perforated duodenal ulcer. Observations on 180 cases. *Am J Surg* 1968; **115**: 173.

119. Kahn IH & Ralston GF. Perforated duodenal ulcer treated by vagotomy and drainage. *J R Coll Surg Edin* 1970; **15**: 41.

120. Johnston D, Lyndon PJ, Smith PB & Humphrey CS. Highly selective vagotomy without drainage procedure in the treatment of haemorrhage, perforation and pyloric stenosis due to peptic ulcer. *Br J Surg* 1973; **60**: 790.

121. Jordan PH, Hedenstedt S, Korompai FL & Lundquest G. Vagotomy of the fundic gland area of the stomach without drainage. *Am J Surg* 1976; **131**: 523.

122. Sawyers J & Herrington JL. Perforated duodenal ulcer management by proximal gastric vagotomy and suture plication. *Ann Surg* 1977; **185**: 656.

123. Jordan PH. Proximal gastric vagotomy without drainage for treatment of perforated duodenal ulcer. *Gastroenterology* 1982; **83**: 179.

124. Choi S, Alagaratnam TT & Wong J. Proximal gastric vagotomy in emergency peptic ulcer perforation. *Surg Gyaecol Obstet* 1986; **163**: 531.

125. Editorial. Perforated peptic ulcer. *Lancet* 1980; **ii**: 896.

126. Illingworth CFG, Scott LDW & Jamieson RA. Progress after perforated peptic ulcer *BMJ* 1946; **1**: 787.

127. Tovee EB. Late results of surgery in perforated duodenal ulcer. *Arch Surg* 1951; **63**: 408.

128. Harbrecht JP & Hamilton JE. Re-appraisal of simple suture of acute perforated peptic ulcer: indications for definitve operation. *Ann Surg* 1960; **152**: 1044.

129. Dean ACB, Clark CG & Sinclair-Gieben AH. The late prognosis of perforated duodenal ulcer. *Gut* 1962; **3**: 60.

130. Cassel P. The prognosis of the perforated acute duodenal ulcer. *Gut* 1969; **10**: 572.

131. Rees JR, Swan KG & Thorbjarnarson B. Perforated duodenal ulcer. *Am J Surg* 1970; **120**: 775.

132. Skovgaard S. Late results of perforated duodenal ulcer treated by simple closure. *World J Surg* 1977; **1**: 521.

133. Drury JK, McKay AJ, Hutchison JSF & Joffe SN. Natural history of perforated duodenal ulcers treated by suture closure. *Lancet* 1978; **ii**: 749.

134. Baekgaard N, Lawaetz O & Poulsen PE. Simple closure or definitive surgery for perforated duodenal ulcer. *Scan J Gastroenterol* 1979; **14**: 17.

135. Dark JH & MacArthur K. Perforated peptic ulcer in South West Scotland 1966–1980. *J R Coll Surg Edinb* 1983; **28**: 19.

136. Gillen P, Ryan W, Peel AIG et al. Duodenal ulcer perforation: the effect of H₂ antagonists? *Ann R Coll Surg Engl* 1986; **68**: 240.

137. King PM & Ross AH McL. Perforated duodenal ulcer: long-term results of omental patch closure. *J R Coll Surg Edinb* 1987; **32**: 79.

138. Boey J & Wong J. Perforated duodenal ulcer. *World J Surg* 1987; **11**: 319.

139. Bornman PC, Theodorou NA, Jefferey PC et al. Simple closure of perforated duodenal ulcer: a prospective evaluation of a conservative management policy. *Br J Surg* 1990; **77**: 73.

140. Simpson CJ, Lamont G, MacDonald I & Smith IS. Effect of cimetidine on prognosis after simple closure of perforated duodenal ulcer. *Br J Surg* 1987; **73**: 104.

141. Mason MC, Brennan TG & Giles GR. Acid secretion in patients with a perforated duodenal ulcer. *Scand J Gastroenterol* 1973; **8**: 421.

142. Boey J, Lee NW, Wong J & Ong GB. Perforations in acute duodenal ulcers. *Surg Gynecol Obstet* 1982; **155**: 193.

143. Jarret F & Donaldson GA. The ulcer diathesis in perforated duodenal ulcer disease: experience with 252 patients during a twenty-five year period. *Am J Surg* 1972; **123**: 406.

144. Stringer MD & Cameron AEP. Surgeons attitudes to the operative management of duodenal ulcer perforation and haemorrhage. *Ann R Coll Surg Engl* 1988; **70**: 220.

145. Graham RR. The treatment of perforated duodenal ulcer. *Surg Gynecol Obstet* 1937; **64**: 235.

146. Waterhouse G. Use of the falciform ligament in closure of perforated duodenal ulcer. In O'Leary JP & Woltering EA (eds) *Techniques of Surgeons*. New York: Wiley, 1985; 87.

147. Horsley JS. *Surgery of the Stomach and Small Intestine*, Chap 10, New York: Appleton, 1926.

148. Marks IN, Wright JP, Lucke W & Girdwood AH. *Scand J Gastroenterol* 1983; **18**(Suppl 83): 53–56.

149. Boyd EJJ, Wilson JA & Wormsley KG. In Misiewicz JJ & Wood JR (eds) *Recurrent Ulceration: in Ranitidine Therapeutic Advances*. Amsterdam: Experta Medica, 1984; **14**: 42.

150. Sebastain M. Prem Chandrau VP, Elashaal YIM & Sim AJW. *Helicobacter pylori* infection in perforated peptic ulcer disease. *Br J Surg* 1995; **82**: 360–362.

151. Kurata JH, Haile BM & Elashoff JD. Sex differences in peptic ulcer disease *Gastroenterology* 1985; **88**: 96.

152. McGee GS & Sawyers JL. Perforated gastric ulcers. A plea for management by primary gastric resection. *Arch Surg* 1987; **122**: 555.

153. Langg C, Hansen CP, Christensen A et al. Perforated gastric ulcer. *Br J Surg* 1988; **75**: 758.

154. Wilson-MacDondald J, Mortensen NJ McC & Williamson RCN. Perforated gastric ulcer. *Postgrad Med J* 1985; **61**: 217.

155. Hewitt P, Krige JEJ & Bornman PC. Perforated gastric ulcer – a comparison between simple closure and immediate gastrectomy. *Am Surg* 1993; **59**: 669–673.

156. Gall WJ and Talbot CH. Perforated gastric ulcer *Br J Surg* 1964; **51**: 500.

157. Collier St J & Pain JA. Perforated gastric ulcer. A reappraisal of the role for biopsy and oversewing. *J R Coll Surg Edinb* 1985; **30**: 26.

158. Schein M, Saadia R, Jamieson J & Decker GAG. Perforated gastric ulcers. A retrospective study of 32 patients. *Ann Surg* 1986; **52**: 551.

159. Rees J & Thorbjarnarson B. Perforated gastric ulcer. *Am J Surg* 1973; **126**: 93.

160. Pauchet, V. *La Practique Chirurgicale Illustrèe* Vol. 7. Paris: Librairie Octave Doin 1924: 71.

161. Lewis A & Qvist G. Operative treatment of high gastric ulcer with special reference to Pauchet's method. *Br J Surg* 1972; **51**: 1.

162. Donahue PE & Nyhus LM. Surgical excision of gastric ulcers near the gastro-oesophageal junction. *Surg Gynecol Obstet* 1982; **155**: 85.

163. Cassel C, Ruffine JM & Bone FC. The clinical features of walled off perforated peptic ulcer. An analysis of 100 cases. *South Med J* 1951; **44**: 1021.

164. Jensen H-E, Hoffman J & Wille-Jorgensen P. High gastric ulcer. *World J Surg* 1987; **11**: 325.

165. Kourias BG & Chouliaris A. Spontaneous, gastrointestinal biliary fistula complicating duodenal ulcer. *Surg Gynecol Obstet* 1964; **119**: 1013.

166. Lewis EA & Bohrer SP. Choledocho-duodenal fistula complicating chronic duodenal ulcer in Nigerians. *Gut* 1969; **10**: 146.

167. Garland LH & Brown JM. Roentgen diagnosis of spontaneous internal biliary fistula especially those involving the common duct. *Radiology* 1947; **38**: 152.

168. Fellor ER, Warshaw AL & Schapiro RH. Observations of management of choledocho-duodenal fistula due to penetrating peptic ulcer. *Gastroenterology* 1980; **78**: 126.

169. Aitken RJ, Bornman PC & Dent DM. Choledocho-pancreato-duodenal fistula caused by duodenal ulceration. *S Afr Med J* 1986; **69**: 707.

170. Jaszewski R, Cane SA & Cid AA. Giant duodenal ulcers. Successful healing with medical therapy. *Dig Dis Sci* 1983; **28**: 486.

171. Kozoll DD & Meyer KA. Obstructing gastroduodenal ulcer. *Arch Surg* 1964; **88**: 793.

172. Jaffin BW & Kaye MD. The prognosis of gastric outlet obstruction. *Ann Surg* 1985; **201**: 176.

173. Hermann RE. Obstructing duodenal ulcer. *Surg Clin N Am* 1976; **56**: 1403.

174. Feldman M & Schiller LR. Disorders of gastrointestinal motility associated with diabetes mellitus. *Ann Intern Med* 1983; **98**: 378–384.

175. Smale BF, Copeland JG & Reber HA. Delayed gastric emptying after operation for obstructing peptic ulcer disease: the influence of cimetidine. *Surgery* 1984; **96**: 592.

176. Loo FD, Palmer DW, Soergel KH, Kalbfleisch JH & Wood GM. Gastric emptying in patients with diabetes mellitus. *Gastroenterology* 1984; **86**: 485.

177. Kirk RM. The size of the pyloro-duodenal canal, its relation to the cause and treatment of peptic ulcer. *Proc R Soc Med* 1970; **63**: 944.

178. Kennedy T. Duodenoplasty with proximal gastric vagotomy. *Ann Coll Surg Engl* 1976; **58**: 144.

179. Ellis H. Pyloric stenosis complicating duodenal ulceration. *World J Surg* 1987; **11**: 315.

180. Herrington JL, Sawyers JL & Scott HW. A 25 year experience with vagotomy antrectomy. *Arch Surg* 1973; **106**: 469.

181. Scott HW, Sawyers JL, Gobble WG & Herrington JL. Definitive surgical treatment in duodenal ulcer disease. *Curr Probl Surg* 1968; **10**: 1.

182. Hinds SJ & Harper RAK. Shortening of the lesser curvature in gastric ulcer. *Br J Radiol* 1952; **25**: 451.

183. Ellis H. Pyloric stenosis In: Nyhus LM & Wastell C (eds) *Surgery of the Stomach and Duodenum*, 4th edn Boston: Little, Brown, 1986: 475.

184. Moodly FG, Cornell GN & Beal JM. Pyloric obstruction complicating peptic ulcer. *Arch Surg* 1962; **84**: 462.

185. Goldstein H, Janin M, Schapiro M & Boyle J. Gastric retention associated with gastroduodenal disease – a study of 217 cases. *Am J Dig Dis* 1966; **11**: 887.

186. Donahue PE, Yoshida J, Richter HM, Liu K, Bombeck T & Nyhus LM. Proximal gastric vagotomy with drainage for obstructing duodenal ulcer. *Surgery* 1988; **104**: 757.

187. Lunde O-C, Liavag I & Roland M. Proximal gastric vagotomy and pyloroplasty for duodenal ulcer with pyloric stenosis: a thirteen-year experience. *World J Surg* 1985; **9**: 165.

188. Delaney P. Preoperative grading of pyloric stenosis: a long term clinical and radiological follow-up of patients with severe pyloric stenosis treated by highly selective vagotomy and dilatation of the stricture. *Br J Surg* 1978; **65**: 157.

189. Phillips SL & Burns GP. Acute abdominal disease in the aged. *Med Clin North Am* 1988; **72**: 1213.

190. Lee S, Wing YK, Chow CC, Chung S & Yung C. Gastric outlet obstruction masquerading as anorexia nervosa. *J Clin Psychiatr* 1989; **50**: 184.

191. Goldstein H & Boyle JD. The saline load test: a bedside evaluation of gastric retention. *Gastroenterology* 1965; **49**: 375.

192. Weiland D, Dunn DH, Humphrey EW & Schwartz ML. Gastric outlet obstruction in peptic ulcer disease: an indication for surgery. *Am J Surg* 1982; **143**: 90.

193. Chandhuri TK. Use of ^{99m} Tc-DPTA for measuring gastric emptying time. *J Nucl Med* 1974; **15**: 391.

194. Caruso RD and Berk RN. The fuzzy fluid level sign. *Radiology* 1971; **98**: 369.

195. Kreel L and Ellis H. Pyloric stenosis in adults: a clinical and radiological study of 100 consecutive patients. *Gut* 1965; **6**: 253.

196. Hooks VH, Bowden TA, Mansberger AR & Sisley JF. Highly selective vagotomy with dilatation or duodenoplasty. *Ann Surg* 1986; **203**: 545.

197. Hill GL. Leading article: surgical nutrition – time for some clinical common sense. *Br J Surg* 1988; **75**: 729.

198. Brown CH. Duodenal ulcer complicated by obstruction: results of medical treatment. *Am J Dig Dis* 1959; **4**: 940.

199. Smith GK. Post-vagotomy atony. *Arch Surg* 1964; **88**: 872.

200. Ellis H, Starer F, Venables CW & Ware CC. Clinical and radiological study of vagotomy and gastric drainage in the treatment of pyloric stenosis due to duodenal ulceration. *Gut* 1966; **7**: 671.

201. Rachlin L. Vagotomy and Heineke–Mikulicz pyloroplasty in the treatment of pyloric stenosis. *Am Surg* 1970; **36**: 251.

202. Davis NP & Williams JA. Duodenal ulcer stenosis with gastric dilatation: treatment by vagotomy and pyloroplasty. *Am J Surg* 1971; **121**: 260.

203. De Matteis RA & Hermann RE. Vagotomy and drainage for obstructing duodenal ulcers. *Am J Surg* 1974; **127**: 237.

204. Hom S, Sarr MG, Kelly KA & Hench V. Postoperative gastric atony after vagotomy for obstructing peptic ulcer. *Am J Surg* 1989; **157**: 282.

205. Fry WJ & Thompson NW. Vagotomy and pylorplasty for duodenal ulcer. *Surg Clin North Am* 1966; **46**: 359.

206. Herrington JL. Truncal vagotomy with antrectomy – 1976. *Surg Clin North Am* 1976; **56**: 1335.

207. Sawyers JL & Scott HW. Selective gastric vagotomy with antrectomy or pyloroplasty. *Ann Surg* 1971; **174**: 541.

208. Siewert JR & Hölscher AH. Billroth I gastrectomy. In: Nyhus LM & Wastell C (eds) *Surgery of the Stomach and Duodenum*, 4th edn, Boston: Little, Brown, 1986: 263.

209. McMahon MJ, Greenall MJ, Johnston D & Goligher JC. Highly selective vagotomy plus dilatation of the stenosis compared with truncal vagotomy and drainage in the treatment of pyloric stenosis secondary to duodenal ulceration. *Gut* 1976; **17**: 471.

210. Dunn DC, Thomas WEG & Hunter JO. Highly selective vagotomy and pyloric dilatation for duodenal ulcer with stenosis. *Br J Surg* 1981; **68**: 194.

211. Rossi RL, Dral PF, Georgi B, Braasch JW & Shea JA. A five to ten year follow-up study of parietal cell vagotomy. *Surg Gynecol Obstet* 1986; **162**: 301.

212. White CM, Harding LK, Keighley MRB, Dorricott NJ & Alexander-Williams J. Gastric emptying after treatment of stenosis secondary to duodenal ulceration by proximal gastric vagotomy and duodenoplasty or pyloric dilatation. *Gut* 1978; **19**: 783.

213. Ferraz EM, Filho HA, Bacelar TS et al. Proximal gastric vagotomy in stenosed or perforated duodenal ulcer. *Br J Surg* 1981; **68**: 452.

214. Gorey TF, Lennon F & Hefferman SJ. Highly selective vagotomy in duodenal ulceration and its complications: a 12-year review. *Ann Surg* 1984; **200**: 181.

215. Barroso FL, Ornellas-Filho A, Saboya CJ et al. Duodenoplasty and proximal gastric vagotomy in peptic stenosis: experience with 43 cases. *Arch Surg* 1986; **121**: 1021.

216. Andersen D, Hostrup H & Amdrup E. The Aarhus County vagotomy trial. 11. An interim report on reduction in acid secretion and ulcer recurrence rate following parietal cell vagotomy and selective gastric vagotomy. *World J Surg* 1978; **2**: 91.

217. Kollath J, Starck E & Vittorio P. Dilatation of esophageal stenosis by balloon catheter. *Cardiovasc Intervent Radiol* 1984; **7**: 35.

218. Siegel JH & Yatto RP. Hydrostatic balloon catheters: a new dimension of therapeutic endoscopy. *Endoscopy* 1984; **16**: 213.

219. Gotberg S, Afzelius LE & Hambraens G. Balloon catheter dilatation of strictures in the upper digestive tract. *Radiology* 1982; **22**: 479.

220. Benjamin SB, Glass RL, Cattan EL & Miller WB. Preliminary experience with balloon dilatation of the pylorus. *Gastrointest Endosc* 1984; **30**: 93.

221. Lindor KD, Ott BJ & Hughes RW. Balloon dilatation of upper digestive tract strictures. *Gastroenterology* 1985; **89**: 545.

222. Hogan RB, Hamilton JK & Polter DE. Preliminary experience with hydrostatic balloon dilatation of gastric outlet obstruction. *Gastrointest Endosc* 1986; **32**: 228.

223. Craig PI & Gillespie PE. Through the endoscope balloon dilatation of benign gastric outlet obstruction. *BMJ* 1988; **297**: 396.

224. Griffin SM, Chung SC, Leung JW & Li AK. Peptic pyloric stenosis treated by endoscopic balloon dilatation. *Br J Surg* 1989; **76**: 1147.

225. Kozarekh RA. Hydrostatic balloon dilatation of gastrointestinal stenosis: a national survey. *Gastrointest Endosc* 1986; **32**: 15.

226. Schmudderich W, Harloff M & Riemann JF. Through-the-scope balloon dilatation of benign pyloric stenoses. *Endoscopy* 1989; **21**: 7.

227. Taylor TV. Experience with a pyloric dilator in patients with delayed gastric emptying. *J R Coll Surg Edinb* 1987; **32**: 239.

228. Dworken HJ & Roth HP. Pyloric obstruction associated with peptic ulcer. *JAMA* 1962; **180**: 1007.

229. DiSaria JA, Fennerty MB, Tietze CC et al. Endoscopic balloon dilation for ulcer-induced gastric outlet obstruction. *Am J Gastroenterol* 1994; **89**: 868–871.

230. Misra SP & Dwivedi M. Long-term follow-up of patients undergoing balloon dilation for benign stenoses. *Endoscopy* 1996; **28**: 552–554.

231. Lau JYW, Chung SCS, Sung JJY et al. Through-the-scope balloon dilation for pyloric stenosis: long-term results. *Gastrointest Endosc* 1996; **43**: 98–101.

232. Bornman PC & Theodorou NA. Management of acute upper gastrointestinal haemorrhage. *Cont Med Educ* 1985; **3**: 49.

233. Palmer ED. The vigorous diagnostic approach to upper gastrointestinal tract haemorrhage. *JAMA* 1969; **207**: 1477.

234. Schiller KFR, Truelove SC & Williams DG. Haematemesis and melaena, with special reference to factors influencing the outcome. *BMJ* 1970; **2**: 7.

235. Johnston SJ, Jones PF, Kyle J & Needham CD. Epidemiology and course of gastrointestinal haemorrhage in North East Scotland. *BMJ* 1973; **3**: 655.

236. Hellers G & Ihre I. Impact of change to early diagnosis and surgery in major upper gastrointestinal bleeding. *Lancet* 1975; **2**: 1250.

237. Sereda S, Lamont I & Hunt P. The experience of a haematemesis and melaena unit. A review of the first 513 consecutive admissions. *Med J Aust* 1977; **1**: 362.

238. Foster DN, Miliszewski KJA & Losowsky MS. Stigmata of recent haemorrhage in diagnosis and prognosis of upper gastrointestinal bleeding. *BMJ* 1978; **1**: 1173.

239. Silverstein FE, Gilbert DA, Tedesco FJ, Buenger NK & Persing J. The national ASGE survey on upper gastrointestinal bleeding I. Study design and baseline data. *Gastrointest Endosc* 1981; **27**: 73.

240. Macleod IA & Mills PR. Factors identifying the probability of further haemorrhage after upper gastrointestinal haemorrhage. *Br J Surg* 1982; **69**: 256.

241. Harris DCH & Heap TR. Significance of signs of recent haemorrhage at endoscopy. *Med J Aust* 1982; **2**: 35.

242. Vellacott DK, Dronfield MW, Atkinson M & Langman MJS. Comparison of surgical and medical management of bleeding peptic ulcers. *BMJ* 1982; **284**: 548.

243. Van Stiegmann G, Bornman PC, Terblanche J & Marks IN. Bleeding peptic ulcer with special reference to high-risk groups of patients. *Surg Gastroenterol* 1983; **2**: 245.

244. Hunt PS. Surgical management of bleeding chronic peptic ulcer. A 10 year prospective study. *Ann Surg* 1984; **199**: 44.

245. Rofe SB, Duggan JM, Smith ER & Thursby CJ. Conservative treatment of gastrointestinal haemorrhage. *Gut* 1985; **26**: 481.

246. Clason AE, Macleod DAD & Elton PA. Clinical factors in the prediction of further haemorrhage or mortality in acute upper gastrointestinal haemorrhage. *Br J Surg* 1986; **73**: 985.

247. Novis BH, Clain J, Barbezat G & Bank S. Urgent fibreoptic panendoscopy in upper gastrointestinal haemorrhage. *S Afr Med J* 1976; **50**: 93.

248. Langman MJS. Upper gastrointestinal bleeding: the trials of trials. *Gut* 1985; **26**: 217.

249. Kolkman JJ & Meuwissen SGM. A review on treatment of bleeding peptic ulcer: a collaborative task of gastroenterologist and surgeon. *Scand J Gastroenterol* 1996; **31**(Suppl 218): 16–25.

250. Baum S, Athanasoulis CA, Waltman AC & Ring EJ. Gastrointestinal haemorrhage; angiographic diagnosis and control. *Adv Surg* 1973; **7**: 95.

251. Hoare AM. Comparative study between endoscopy and radiology in acute upper gastrointestinal haemorrhage. *BMJ* 1975; **1**: 27.

252. Sugawa C, Werner MH, Hayes DF, Lucas CE & Walt AJ. Early endoscopy. A guide to therapy for acute haemorrhage in the upper gastrointestinal tract. *Arch Surg* 1973; **107**: 133.

253. Keller RT & Logan GM. Comparison of emergent endoscopy and upper gastrointestinal series radiography in acute upper gastrointestinal haemorrhage *Gut* 1976; **17**: 180.

254. Morris DW, Levine GM, Soloway RD, Miller WT & Marin GA. Prospective randomized study of diagnosis and outcome in acute upper gastrointestinal bleeding: endoscopy versus conventional radiography. *Am J Dig Dis* 1975; **20**: 1103.

255. Katon RM & Smith FW. Panendoscopy in the early diagnosis of acute upper gastrointestinal bleeding. *Gastroenterology* 1973; **65**: 728.

256. Dronfield MW, McIllmurray MB, Ferguson R, Atkinson M & Langman MJS. A prospective randomized study of endoscopy and radiology in acute upper gastrointestinal tract bleeding. *Lancet* 1977; **i**: 1167.

257. Dronfield MW, Langman MJS & Atkinson M. Outcome of endoscopy and barium radiography for acute upper gastrointestinal bleeding: controlled trials in 1037 patients. *BMJ* 1982; **284**: 545.

258. Cotton PB, Rosenberg MT, Waldram RPL & Axon ATR. Early endoscopy of esophagus, stomach and duodenal bulb in patients with haematemesis and melaena. *BMJ* 1973; **2**: 505.

259. Cotton PB. Endoscopy versus radiology in acute upper gastrointestinal bleeding. *Lancet* 1977; **i**: 1367.

260. Forrest JAH, Finlayson NDC & Shearman DJC. Endoscopy in gastrointestinal bleeding. *Lancet* 1974; **ii**: 394.

261. Villar HV, Fender HR, Watson LC & Thompson JC. Emergency diagnosis of upper gastrointestinal bleeding by fibreoptic endoscopy. *Ann Surg* 1977; **185**: 367.

262. Winans CS. Emergency upper gastrointestinal endoscopy: does haste make waste? *Am J Dig Dis* 1977; **22**: 536.

263. Graham DY. Limited value of early endoscopy in the management of acute upper gastrointestinal bleeding. *Am J Surg* 1980; **140**: 284.

264. Sandlow LJ, Becker GH, Spellberg MA et al. A prospective randomized study of the management of upper gastrointestinal hemorrhage. *Am J Gastroenterol* 1974; **61**: 282.

265. Allan R & Dykes P. A comparison of routine and selective endoscopy in the management of acute gastrointestinal hemorrhage. *Gastrointest Endosc* 1974; **20**: 154.

266. Peterson WL, Barnett CC, Smith HJ, Allen MH & Corbett DB. Routine early endoscopy in upper gastrointestinal bleeding. A randomized controlled study. *N Engl J Med* 1981; **304**: 925.

267. Mikulicz J. *Mitt Grenzgeb Med Chir* 1897; **2**: 184.

268. Witts LJ. Haematemesis and melaena. *BMJ* 1937; **1**: 847.

269. Cullinan ER & Price RK. Haematemesis following peptic ulceration. Prognosis and treatment. *St Bart's Hosp Rep* 1932; **65**: 185.

270. Chiesman WE. Mortality of severe haemorrhage from peptic ulcers. *Lancet* 1934; **i**: 572.

271. Gordon-Taylor G. Haematemesis. *Lancet* 1934; **i**: 572.

272. Finsterer H. Surgical therapy of acute profuse gastric and duodenal haemorrhages. *Wien Klin Wochenschr* 1931; **44**: 1125.

273. Finsterer H. Operative treatment of severe gastric haemorrhage of ulcer origin. A reply to critics. *Lancet* 1936; **ii**: 303.

274. Finsterer H. Surgical treatment of acute profuse gastric haemorrhages. *Surg Gynecol Obstet* 1939; **69**: 291.

275. Balfour DC. The surgical treatment of haemorrhagic duodenal ulcer. *Ann Surg* 1932; **96**: 581.

276. Allen AW & Benedict EB. Acute massive haemorrhage from duodenal ulcer. *Ann Surg* 1933; **98**: 736.

277. Gordon-Taylor G. Attitude of surgery in haematemesis. *Lancet* 1935; **ii**: 811.

278. Gordon-Taylor G. The problem of bleeding peptic ulcer. *Br J Surg* 1937; **25**: 403.

279. Gordon-Taylor G. The present position of surgery in the treatment of bleeding peptic ulcer. *Br J Surg* 1946; **33**: 336.

280. Jones FA. Haematemesis and melaena with special reference to bleeding peptic ulcer. *BMJ* 1947; **2**: 441.

281. Welch CS & Yunich AM. The problem for surgery in the treatment of massive hemorrhage of ulcer origin. *Surg Gynecol Obstet* 1940; **70**: 662.

282. Dunphy JE & Hoerr SO. The indication for emergency operation in severe hemorrhage from gastric or duodenal ulcer. *Surgery* 1948; **24**: 231.

283. Walters W & Cleveland WH. Results of partial gastrectomy for bleeding duodenal, gastric and gastrojejunal ulcer. *Ann Surg* 1941; **114**: 481.

284. Welch CE. Treatment of acute, massive gastroduodenal haemorrhage. *JAMA* 1949; **141**: 1113.

285. Fraenkel GJ and Truelove SC. Haematemesis with special reference to peptic ulcer. *BMJ* 1955; **1**: 999.

286. Ward-McQuaid JN, Pease JC, McEwen-Smith A & Twort RJ. Surgery in bleeding peptic ulcer. *Gut* 1960; **1**: 258.

287. Marriott HL & Kekwick A. Continuous drip blood transfusion. *Lancet* 1935; **i**: 977.

288. Hoerr SO, Dunphy JE & Grays S. Place of surgery in emergency treatment of upper gastrointestinal haemorrhage. *Surg Gynecol Obstet* 1948; **87**: 338.

289. Bohrer JV. Massive gastric hemorrhage: with special reference to peptic ulcer. *Ann Surg* 1941; **114**: 510.

290. Lewin DC & Truelove SC. Haematemesis with special reference to chronic peptic ulcer. *BMJ* 1949; **1**: 383.

291. Amendola FH. The management of massive gastroduodenal hemorrhage. *Ann Surg* 1949; **129**: 47.

292. Lewison EF. Bleeding peptic ulcer. *Int Abst Surg* 1950; **90**: 1.

293. Ferguson DA & Wyman AL. Bleeding peptic ulcer. *Lancet* 1951; **i**: 814.

294. Jones FA. Haematemesis and melaena with special reference to causation and to factors influencing the mortality from bleeding peptic ulcers. *Gastroenterology* 1956; **30**: 166.

295. Snyder EN & Berne CJ. Management of massive hemorrhage from peptic ulcer. *Am J Surg* 1957; **94**: 368.

296. Foster JH, Hickok DF & Dunphy JE. Factors influencing mortality following emergency operation for massive upper gastrointestinal hemorrhage. *Surg Gynecol Obstet* 1963; **117**: 257.

297. Cogill NF & Willcox RG. Factors in the prognosis of bleeding chronic gastric and duodenal ulcers. *Q J Med* 1960; **29**: 575.

298. Tanner NC. The diagnosis and management of massive haematemesis. *Br J Surg* 1964; **51**: 754.

299. Hamilton JL, Harbrecht PJ, Robbins RE & Noland JC. The behaviour and management of major acute bleeding from peptic ulcers. *Surg Gynecol Obstet* 1965; **121**: 545.

300. Himal HS, Perrault C & Mzabi R. Upper gastrointestinal haemorrhage: aggressive management decreases mortality. *Surgery* 1978; **84**: 448.

301. Silverstein FE, Gilbert M, Tedesco FJ, Buenger NK & Persing J. The national ASGE survey on upper gastrointestinal bleeding 2. Clinical prognostic factors. *Gastrointest Endosc* 1981; **27**: 80.

302. Morris DL, Hawker PC, Brearley S, Simms M, Dykes PW & Keighley MRB. Optimal timing of operation for bleeding peptic ulcer: prospective randomized trial. *BMJ* 1984; **288**: 1277.

303. Jensen HE, Amdrup E, Christiansen P et al. Bleeding gastric ulcer. Surgical and non-surgical treatment of 225 patients. *Scand J Gastroenterol* 1972; **7**: 535.

304. Jones PF, Johnston SJ, McEwan AB, Kyle J & Needham CD. Further haemorrhage after admission to hospital for gastrointestinal haemorrhage. *BMJ* 1973; **3**: 660.

305. Wara P, Berg V & Amdrup E. Factors influencing mortality in patients with bleeding ulcers. Review of 7 years experience preceding therapeutic endoscopy. *Acta Chir Scand* 1983; **149**: 775.

306. Heuer GJ. The surgical aspects of hemorrhage from peptic ulcer. *N Engl J Med* 1946; **235**: 777.

307. Mitty WF, Breen EJ, Wallace R & Grace WJ. Factors influencing mortality in bleeding peptic ulcers. *Am J Dig Dis* 1961; **6**: 389.

308. Andersen D, Klebe JG & Nielsen A. Evaluation of the prognostic significance of various factors in massive ulcer haemorrhage. *Scand J Gastroenterol* 1968; **3**: 537.

309. Thorne FL & Nyhus LM. Treatment of massive upper gastrointestinal hemorrhage. *Am Surg* 1965; **31**: 413.

310. Northfield TC. Factors predisposing to recurrent haemorrhage after acute gastrointestinal bleeding. *BMJ* 1971; **1**: 26.

311. Hunt PS. Bleeding ulcer: timing and technique in surgical management. *Aust NZ J Surg* 1986; **56**: 25.

312. Hunt PS. Bleeding gastroduodenal ulcers: selection of patients for surgery. *World J Surg* 1987; **11**: 289.

313. Hippocrates. *Aphorisms*, sect. 7, no. 21.

314. Griffiths WJ, Neumann DA & Welsh JD. The visible vessel as an indicator of uncontrolled or recurrent gastrointestinal hemorrhage. *N Engl J Med* 1979; **300**: 1411.

315. Bornman PC, Theodorou NA, Shuttleworth RD, Essel HP & Marks IN. Importance of hypovolaemic shock and endoscopic signs in predicting recurrent haemorrhage from peptic ulceration: a prospective evaluation. *BMJ* 1985; **291**: 245.

316. Brearley S, Morris DL, Hawker PC, Dykes PW & Keighley MRB. Prediction of mortality at endoscopy in bleeding peptic ulcer disease. *Endoscopy* 1985; **17**: 173.

317. Chang-Chien C, Wu C, Chen P et al. Different implications of stigmata of recent hemorrhage in gastric and duodenal ulcers. *Dig Dis Sci* 1988; **33**: 400.

318. Wara P. Endoscopy prediction of major rebleeding – a prospective study of stigmata of haemorrhage in bleeding ulcer. *Gastroenterology* 1985; **88**: 1209.

319. Brearley S, Hawker PC, Morris DL, Dykes PW & Keigley MRB. Selection of patients for surgery following peptic ulcer haemorrhage. *Br J Surg* 1987; **74**: 893.

320. Storey DW, Bown SG Swain CP, Salmon PR, Kirkham JS & Northfield TC. Endoscopic prediction of recurrent bleeding in peptic ulcers. *N Engl J Med* 1981; **305**: 915.

321. Beckley DE & Casebow MP. Prediction of rebleeding from peptic ulcer experience with an endoscopic Doppler device. *Gut* 1986; **27**: 96.

322. Laine J & Peterson WL. Bleeding peptic ulcer. *New Engl J Med* 1994; **331**: 717–727.

323. Longstreth GF & Feitelberg SP. Outpatients care of selected patients with acute non-variceal upper gastrointestinal haemorrhage. *Lancet* 1995; **345**: 108–111.

324. Hunt PS, Korman MG, Hansky J, Marshall RD, Peck GS & McCann WJ. Bleeding duodenal ulcer: reduction in mortality with a planned approach. *Br J Surg* 1979; **66**: 633.

325. Hunt PS, Hansky J & Korman MG. Mortality in patients with haematemesis and melaena: a prospective study. *BMJ* 1979; **1**: 1238.

326. Dronfield MW, Atkinson M & Langman MJS. Effect of different operation policies on mortality from bleeding peptic ulcer. *Lancet* 1979; **i**: 1126.

327. Read RC, Hueble HC & Thal AP. Randomized study of massive bleeding from peptic ulceration. *Ann Surg* 1965; **162**: 561.

328. Saperas E, Pique JM, Perez Ayuso R, Bordas JM, Teres J & Pera C. Conservative management of bleeding duodenal ulcer without a visible vessel: prospective randomized trial. *Br J Surg* 1987; **74**: 784.

329. Stewart JD, Cosgriff JH & Gray JG. Experiences with the treatment of acutely massively bleeding peptic ulcer by blood replacement and gastric resection. *Surg Gynecol Obstet* 1956; **103**: 409.

330. Large JM. Gastroduodenal haemorrhage as a surgical emergency. *BMJ* 1960; **1**: 932.

331. Darin JC, Polacek MA & Ellison EH. Surgical mortality of massive hemorrhage from peptic ulcer. *Arch Surg* 1961; **83**: 71.

332. Brooks JR & Eraklis AJ. Factors affecting the mortality from peptic ulcer. The bleeding ulcer and ulcer in the aged. *N Engl J Med* 1964; **271**: 803.

333. Cocks JR, Desmond AM, Swynnerton BF & Tanner NC. Partial gastrectomy for haemorrhage. *Gut* 1972; **13**: 331.

334. Inberg MV & Linna MI. Massive haemorrhage from gastroduodenal ulcer. *Acta Chir Scand* 1975; **141**: 664.

335. Smith GK & Farris JM. Rationale of vagotomy and pyloroplasty in management of bleeding duodenal ulcer. *JAMA* 1958; **166**: 878.

336. Westland JC, Movius HJ & Weinberg JA. Emergency surgical treatment of the severely bleeding duodenal ulcer. *Surgery* 1958; **43**: 897.

337. Herrington JL & Davidson J. Bleeding gastroduodenal ulcers: choice of operations. *World J Surg* 1987; **11**: 304.

338. Berne CJ & Rosoff L. Peptic ulcer perforation of the gastroduodenal artery complex: clinical features and operative control. *Ann Surg* 1969; **169**: 141.

339. Editorial. *Yearbook of General Surgery*. Chicago: *Year Book*, 1958–1959: 390.

340. Weinberg JA. Treatment of the massively bleeding duodenal ulcer by ligation, pyloroplasty and vagotomy. *Am J Surg* 1961; **102**: 158.

341. Dorton HE. Vagotomy pyloroplasty and suture – a safe and effective remedy for the duodenal ulcer that bleeds. A progress report on 100 consecutive cases. *Ann Surg* 1961; **153**: 378.

342. Farris JM & Smith GK. Appraisal of the long-term results of vagotomy and pyloroplasty in 100 patients with bleeding duodenal ulcer. *Ann Surg* 1967; **166**: 630.

343. Snyder EN & Stellar CA. Results from emergency surgery for massively bleeding duodenal ulcer. *Am J Surg* 1968; **116**: 170.

344. Klingensmith W & Oles P. Vagotomy and pyloroplasty for massively bleeding duodenal and gastric ulcers. *Am J Surg* 1968; **116**: 759.

345. Vogel TT. Critical issues in gastroduodenal haemorrhage: The role of vagotomy and pyloroplasty. *Ann Surg* 1972; **176**: 144.

346. Jensen HE & Guldberg O. Selective vagotomy and drainage for bleeding duodenal ulcer. *Acta Chir Scand* 1974; **140**: 406.

347. Brooks JR, Kia D & Membreno AA. Truncal vagotomy and pyloroplasty for duodenal ulcer. *Arch Surg* 1975; **110**: 822.

348. Akin JM & Sullivan MB. Pyloroplasty and vagotomy: Compromise procedure for control of acute peptic ulcer haemorrhage. *Surgery* 1963; **54**: 587.

349. Foster JH, Hickok DF & Dunphy JE. Changing concepts in the surgical treatment of massive gastroduodenal haemorrhage. *Ann Surg* 1965; **161**: 968.

350. Carruthers RK, Giles GR, Clark CG & Goligher JC. Conservative surgery for bleeding peptic ulcer. *BMJ* 1967; **1**: 80.

351. Feltis JM & Hamit HF. The surgical management of acute bleeding from peptic ulcers. *Surgery* 1967; **62**: 988.

352. Hampson LG, Mulder DS, Elias GL & Palmer JD. The emergency surgical treatment of massively bleeding peptic ulcer. *Arch Surg* 1968; **97**: 450.

353. Buckingham JM & Remine WH. Results of emergency surgical management of hemorrhagic duodenal ulcer. *Mayo Clin Proc* 1975; **50**: 223.

354. Bambach CP, Coupland AE & Cumberland VH. Haematemesis and melaena: Surgical management. *Aust NZ J Surg* 1976; **46**: 107.

355. Stone AM, Stein T, McCarthy K & Wise L. Surgery for bleeding duodenal ulcer. *Am J Surg* 1978; **136**: 206.

356. Welch CE, Rodkey GV & Gryska PVR. A thousand operations for ulcer disease. *Ann Surg* 1986; **204**: 454.

357. Brolin RE & Stremple JF. Emergency operation for upper gastrointestinal hemorrhage. *Am J Surg* 1982; **48**: 302.

358. Chang FC, Drake JE & Farha GJ. Massive upper gastrointestinal hemorrhage in the elderly. *Am J Surg* 1977; **134**: 721.

359. Johnston D. Division and repair of the sphincteric mechanism at the gastric outlet in emergency operations for bleeding peptic ulcer. A new technique for use in combination with suture ligation of the bleeding point and highly selective vagotomy. *Ann Surg* 1977; **186**: 723.

360. Swain CP, Bown SG, Storey DW, Kirkham JS, Northfield TC & Salmon PR. Controlled trial of argon laser photocoagulation in bleeding peptic ulcer. *Lancet* 1981; **ii**: 1313.

361. Vallon AG, Cotton PB, Laurence BH, Miro JRA & Oses JCS. Randomized trial of endoscopic argon laser photocoagulation in bleeding peptic ulcer. *Gut* 1981; **22**: 228.

362. Swain CP, Kirkham JS, Salmon PR, Brown SG & Northfield TC. Controlled trial of Nd YAG laser photocoagulation in bleeding peptic ulcers. *Lancet* 1986; **i**: 1113.

363. Jensen DM, Machicado GA, Tapia JI & Elashoff J. Controlled trial of endoscopic argon laser for severe ulcer haemorrhage. *Gastroenterology* 1984; **86**: 1125.

364. Escourrou J, Fretinos J, Bommelaer G & Edward R. Prospective randomised study of YAG photocoagulation in gastrointestinal bleeding. In Atsumi K & Nimsakul N (eds) *Proceedings of laser Tokyo '81*. Tokyo: Inter Group Corp, 1981: 5–30.

365. Rutgeerts P, van Trappen G, Broeckhaert L et al. Controlled trial of YAG laser treatment of upper digestive haemorrhage. *Gastroenterology* 1982; **83**: 410.

366. MacLeod IA, Mills PR, MacKenzie JF, Joffe SN, Russel RI & Carter DC. Neodymium yttrium aluminum garnet laser photocoagulation for major haemorrhage from peptic ulcer and single vessels: a single blind controlled study. *BMJ* 1983; **286**: 345.

367. Brown SG. Controlled studies of laser therapy for haemorrhage from peptic ulcers. *Acta Endosc* 1985; **15**: 1.

368. Krejs GJ, Little KH, Westergaard H, Hamilton JK, Spady DK & Potter DE. Laser photocoagulation for the treatment of acute peptic ulcer bleeding. *N Engl J Med* 1987; **316**: 1618.

369. Trudeau W, Siepler JK, Ross K, Cornich D & Prindiville T. Endoscopic neodymium YAG laser photocoagulation of bleeding ulcers with visible vessels. *Gastrointest Endosc* 1985; **31**: 138.

370. Matthewson K, Swain CP, Bland M, Kirkham JS, Brown SG & Northfield TC. Randomized comparison of Na YAG, heater probe and no endoscopic therapy for bleeding peptic ulcer. *Gastroenterology* 1990; **98**: 1239–1244.

371. Cook DJ, Guyatt GH, Salena BJ & Laine LA. Endoscopic therapy for acute non-variceal upper gastrointestinal haemorrhage. A meta-analysis. *Gastroenterology* 1992; **102**: 139–148.

372. Papp JP. Endoscopic electrocoagulation in the management of upper gastrointestinal bleeding. *Surg Clin North Am* 1982; **62**: 797.

373. Moreto M, Zaballa M, Ibanez S, Setein F & Figa M. Efficacy of monopolar electrocoagulation in the treatment of bleeding gastric ulcer. *Endoscopy* 1987; **19**: 54.

374. Freitas D, Donato A & Monteiro JG. Controlled trial of liquid monopolar electrocoagulation in bleeding peptic ulcers. *Am J Gastroenterol* 1985; **80**: 853.

375. O'Brien JD, Day SJ & Burnham WR. Controlled trial of small bipolar probe in bleeding peptic ulcers. *Lancet* 1986; **i**: 464.

376. Laine L. Multipolar electrocoagulation for the treatment of ulcers with non-bleeding visible vessels: a prospective, controlled trial. *Gastroenterology* 1988; **94**: A246.

377. Lin HJ, Tsai YT, Lee SD et al. Heater probe in massive peptic ulcer hemorrhage and shock. *J Clin Gastroenterol* 1988; **10**: 623.

378. Storey DW. Endoscopic control of peptic ulcer haemorrhage using the 'heater probe'. *Gut* 1983; **24**: A967.

379. Johnston JH, Sones JQ, Lang BW & Posey EL. Comparison of heater probe and YAG laser in endoscopic treatment of major bleeding from peptic ulcers. *Gastrointest Endosc* 1985; **31**: 175.

380. Shorvon PJ, Leung JWC & Cotton PB. Preliminary clinical experience with the heater probe at endoscopy in acute upper gastrointestinal bleeding. *Gastrointest Endosc* 1985; **31**: 364.

381. Fullarton GM, Birnie GG, Macdonald A & Murray WR. Controlled trial of heater probe treatment in bleeding peptic ulcers. *Br J Surg* 1989; **76**: 541.

382. Chung SCS, Leung JWC, Steele RJC, Crofts TJ & Li AKC. Endoscopic injection of adrenaline for actively bleeding ulcers: a randomized trial. *BMJ* 1988; **296**: 1631.

383. Panes J, Viver J, Forne M, Garcia-Olivares E, Marco C & Garau J. Controlled trial of endoscopic sclerosis in bleeding peptic ulcers. *Lancet* 1987; **ii**: 1292.

384. Rajgopal C & Palmer KR. Endoscopic injection sclerosis: effective treatment for bleeding peptic ulcer *Gut* 1991; **32**: 727–729.

385. Balanzo J, Sainz S, Such J et al. Endoscopic hemostasis by local injection of epinephrine and polidocanal in bleeding ulcers. A prospective randomized trial. *Endoscopy* 1988; **20**: 289–291.

386. Oxner RBG, Simmonds NJ, Gertner DJ, Nightingale JMD & Burnham WR. Controlled trial of endoscopic injection treatment for bleeding peptic ulcers with visible vessels. *Lancet* 1992; **339**: 966–968.

387. Pascu O, Draghici A & Acalovschi I. The effect of endoscopic hemostasis with alcohol on the mortality rate of non variceal upper gastrointestinal hemorrhage. A randomized prospective survey. *Endoscopy* 1989; **21**: 53–55.

388. Lazo MD, Andrade R, Medina MC, Garcia-Fernandez G, Sanchez-Cantos AM & Franquelo E. Effect of injection sclerosis with alcohol on the rebleeding rate of gastroduodenal peptic ulcers with non-bleeding visible vessels: a prospective controlled trial. *Am J Gastroenterol* 1992; **87**: 843–846.

389. Laine LA. *Helicobacter pylori* and complicated ulcer disease. *Am J Med* 1996; **100**: 52S.

35

COMPLICATIONS OF PEPTIC ULCER SURGERY

HE Jensen

EARLY COMPLICATIONS

Bleeding

Postoperative bleeding immediately after gastric surgery may be either intraperitoneal, from the ulcer or from the anastomosis.

Intraperitoneal bleeding may occur from a little tear in the capsule of the spleen. Bleeding may sometimes occur from the gastrocolic ligament after gastric resection or from the lesser omentum after parietal cell vagotomy; retractor lesions of the liver and bleeding from the omentum are occasionally seen. It should be mentioned that bleeding via an intraperitoneal drain seldom reflects the seriousness of an intraperitoneal bleed.

Postoperative bleeding may occur after failure to control the bleeding from an ulcer at operation. In our primary series[1] of patients operated for bleeding duodenal ulcer, 16% rebled and 8% came to surgery for the second time. We found that this complication occurred most often for surgeons with limited experience in the technique of ulcer transfixion. The most common cause was that the sutures were too superficial and had not been placed deeply beneath the ulcer. With increasing experience this complication diminishes. Another fact to consider is that the bleeding site might not have been found at operation. One should also consider defects in the coagulation system after multiple blood transfusions and treatment should be directed toward this. Gastroscopy immediately after gastric surgery may be dangerous because of the effect of distension on suture lines. In most cases the view at gastroscopy will be poor and the investigation will have neither diagnostic nor therapeutic value.

A bleeding artery in the line of the anastomosis will have a greater tendency to stop bleeding spontaneously than an artery bleeding from an ulcer crater which is surrounded by fibrotic tissue. A 'wait and see' policy will often be disastrous and early reoperation should always be considered as this will be less traumatic then massive bleeding and multiple transfusions.

The difficult duodenal stump

Prophylaxis

The problem of closure of a difficult duodenal stump after gastrectomy is less often confronted by surgeons today than in the past. In cases where the duodenum is the seat of severe fibrosis, oedema and ulceration in elective operations for duodenal ulcer it is important not to approach the organ and to stay out of the region by performing a vagotomy with or without a drainage procedure, which will usually be a gastroenterostomy. However, conditions such as recurrent ulceration or ulcer perforation may compel the surgeon to dissect around the duodenum, which will risk damage to the pancreas and common bile duct.

At elective surgery the surgeon can choose between several alternatives where the cuff of the duodenal stump is not long enough to provide secure closure.

A two-stage gastrectomy can be performed with prepyloric transection of the antrum, with or without stripping of the mucosa of the retained antrum. About 8–12 weeks later a second operation is performed, by which time the primary ulcer has healed and before the patient has had the opportunity of developing a gastroduodenal ulcer recurrence. This second operation to resect the retained antrum is easily performed as the duodenum is, at this time, no longer oedematous and fragile. The operation was first described by McKitteich and coworkers in 1944 but since then there have only been sporadic reports of its use in the literature.[2] It is, however, a useful method of obviating duodenal complications.

The use of a catheter duodenostomy has been advocated from various centres.[3-8] This method provides an effective low-pressure drainage for pancreatic juice and bile. Various different catheters have been recommended in the literature. The important point, however, is to close the duodenal cuff securely around the catheter with interrupted seromuscular sutures. The closure is then covered with omentum and checked for watertightness. In the postoperative period electrolyte imbalance may occur, especially of potassium and sodium, but this is seldom a great problem. After 2–3 weeks fistulography should be performed to ensure that the catheter is correctly positioned and that there is no leakage from the duodenum. Thereafter, the drain can be slowly withdrawn and secretions will gradually diminish and change character from bile to pus. Once the fistula channel is established the drain can be gradually removed by withdrawing it 2–3 cm at a time every few days.

Other technical approaches have also been used. The duodenal stump can be closed by sewing a small bowel loop over the defect. A Roux-en-Y loop has been used on the basis that such an anastomosis does not require the same mobilization as a primary closure of the duodenal stump. Appel[9] has taken the afferent loop of a Billroth II reconstruction and anastomosed it end-to-side in two layers to the duodenal stump. He reports an uncomplicated postoperative course in 11 patients.

Finally, it is possible to protect the closure of a duodenal stump by inserting a T tube through a Witzel-type fistula in the second or third portion of the duodenum or by placing a nasogastric tube far down in the afferent loop. The tube is placed on permanent suction for about a week.

Leakage

It is important that the diagnosis of duodenal stump blow-out is made early. Larsen and Foreman[10] reported a mortality of 85% for patients in whom an early diagnosis was not made. They emphasize that pain and tenderness localized to the right upper quadrant are constant findings and a persistent high fever is also a common feature.

In a series of 1992 patients who had undergone a partial gastrectomy for duodenal ulcer in the period 1936–1959 it was found[11] that the incidence of duodenal stump leakage fell from nearly 9 to 3%. One of seven patients died. A leaking duodenal stump was the most common serious complication after resection for duodenal ulcer. In a further review[12] it was found that leakage occurred within 5–21 days after surgery (mean 10 days). The patients in this review presented with high fever, leucocytosis and abdominal pain but pleural effusion and jaundice were also seen as presenting signs.

Ultrasonography and/or computed tomography (CT) will frequently reveal a fluid collection in the right upper quadrant before evidence of a pleural effusion or jaundice develops. If untreated, these patients will usually develop a diffuse peritonitis with fatal outcome. Adequate closure of the duodenal stump is dependent on the surgeon's experience.

In acute surgery with perforation of a giant duodenal ulcer, or sometimes in the case of a duodenal ulcer bleeding from the gastroduodenal artery in the posterior wall of the duodenum which is uncontrolled by a suture ligation, a duodenostomy may be a desirable procedure. An alternative is an approach whereby one continues to dissect the duodenum beyond the ulcer until a 2 cm collar of duodenal wall is achieved, with subsequent closure in two layers. The problem usually lies in the posterior duodenal wall, while the anterior wall is frequently normal in length and tensile strength. The location of the ulcer should be established by invagination of the anterior wall or examination through the duodenal stump. The surgeon should be sure of the location of the papilla of Vater so as not to compromise this by sutures. If a single layer closure is the only possibility, use of a linear stapler might be a safer solution, although this has never been proven in large series of patients.

Ischaemic necrosis

There are some reports in the literature of ischaemic necrosis of the gastric remnant following subtotal gastrectomy.[13-17] This problem may arise if all four major arteries are ligated and may occur after high subtotal gastrectomy where the fundic area is then supplied only by the left phrenic artery. Sometimes this artery is not large enough to supply the remnant adequately. In a small percentage of patients this vessel arises from the left gastric artery. In cases where the left gastric artery is ligated and the splenic artery is ligated proximal to the vasa brevia it has been shown in experimental studies in dogs[16] that there is a high risk of necrosis, especially of the greater curvature. This may even occur if the splenic artery is divided within the hilus of the spleen. Generally necrosis is rare because of the rich intramural vascular plexus of the stomach. The risk of necrosis should also be considered after parietal cell vagotomy or selective vagotomy where accidental damage to the spleen has necessitated splenectomy. If splenectomy is indicated this should be done with preservation of the vasa brevia. These conditions therefore indicate a conservative approach to lesions of the spleen.

The diagnosis of ischaemic necrosis is usually made upon about the fourth postoperative day when the gastric aspirate becomes evil smelling and contains old blood. At this point the patient is usually septic, with signs of an intra-abdominal catastrophy. The surgical management of this condition is total gastrectomy. In a few of these desperate cases we have chosen to obviate a reconstruction by closing the distal oesophagus and constructing a proximal oesophagostomy in the neck and a feeding jejunostomy. Some months later oesophagojejunal continuity may be established.

Gastric retention

Delayed gastric emptying is a well-known problem after all types of gastric surgery. A nasogastric tube is traditionally used for a few days after vagotomy and drainage and also after gastric resection. It does not seem necessary after parietal cell vagotomy. In 5–10% of cases gastric emptying will be compromised and the patient develops a large gastric aspirate. The causes are many and include technical mishaps, anastomotic leakage, postoperative pancreatitis, oedema of a narrow gastroduodenostomy, electrolyte disturbances and obstruction of the efferent loop. A barium meal will confirm the diagnosis. Sometimes only a small amount of barium will pass into the small intestine. The treatment should, in the first instance, be conservative with nasogastric suction and adequate fluid and electrolyte replacement. If there is bile in the gastric aspirate an obstruction distal to the anastomosis should be suspected and the patient reoperated upon. We place the patient in a semisitting position to prevent stagnation of secretion in the fundus of the stomach. Stimulation of motor function with drugs such as metoclopramide and domperidone might be helpful, although there is a lack of proof for this and their value is often limited in the immediate postoperative period.

If the patient still has a large gastric aspirate 10–12 days after operation success may be achieved in some cases by merely removing the nasogastric tube and giving the patient solid food to eat – from the simple principle that the stomach thereby has the opportunity to contract around some normal food. If this is unsuccessful it is recommended that the conservative approach with nasogastric suction and parenteral nutrition is continued, sometimes for many weeks.

If reoperation has to be performed the author's approach has been to undertake a high gastric resection with a Billroth II reconstruction.

Dragstedt et al.[18] demonstrated that truncal vagotomy without a drainage procedure was accompanied by significant gastric retention in 7% of patients. It has subsequently become routine to add a drainage procedure to selective gastric vagotomy and truncal vagotomy. One may, however, question this figure because some of these truncal vagotomies were done transthoracically without knowledge of conditions surrounding the pylorus. We are therefore faced with the problem that not all patients need a drainage operation after selective gastric vagotomy or truncal vagotomy. It is, however, impossible to preselect in which patient the drainage operation will be superfluous. It should be added that there is evidence that the drainage procedure is only necessary for a short period after selective vagotomy and truncal vagotomy. The duration of this period is variable and has not been fully documented. However, it is well established that a gastroenterostomy may be dismantled or the pylorus reconstructed after a pyloroplasty for severe dumping and/or diarrhoea without the patient developing gastric retention. This will be discussed later.

In a review of 37 patients[19] who all developed a severe gastric retention after Roux-en-Y diversion for alkaline reflux gastritis, all underwent further gastric resection to improve gastric emptying and 27 responded well, while ten underwent a third operation such as total gastrectomy. This is in agreement with the experience of others[20-22] and stresses the necessity of reducing the gastric remnant to about 10% in order to achieve satisfactory gastric emptying. Even this extent of resection may not be satisfactory as a motility problem may develop in the Roux jejunal interposition. The freeing of adhesions around the stomach and anastomosis is totally without value.

Postoperative pancreatitis

Injuries to the major pancreatic duct after resection for duodenal ulceration have been reported in the world literature. Injury of the duct of Santorini is, however, a rare phenomenon but may cause chronic recurrent pancreatitis. Postoperative pancreatitis may also occur after dissection around the duodenum or after traumatic mobilization of the tail of the pancreas. Most classically this complication is seen as a result of a lesion to the distal end of the tail of the pancreas during splenectomy. Pancreatitis demonstrated by an elevated serum amylase sometimes occurs without obvious reasons. Postoperative pancreatitis may appear with different grades of severity from a transient asymptomatic rise in amylase to a fulminant pancreatitis with leakage of pancreatic juice into the peritoneum and possible destruction of surrounding anastomosis.

The diagnosis of postoperative pancreatitis is primarily made by means of a raised serum amylase together with systemic signs and symptoms. The transient mild rise in the serum amylase level hardly requires any attention but in cases of doubt investigations should be undertaken (as with other forms of acute pancreatitis): for example, ultrasonography or CT, chest X-ray and measurement of blood gases.

Signs of postoperative pancreatitis should further lead one to suspect an anastomotic leakage, especially from the duodenal stump. The treatment of postoperative pancreatitis is primarily conservative, possibly supplemented with some form of intraperitoneal drainage.

Postoperative diarrhoea

The suspicion of a technical error in the formation of a gastroileostomy should be raised if the resection is immediately followed by persistent diarrhoea containing undigested food.[23,24] The situation is soon complicated by malnutrition, dehydration, hypoproteinaemia and weight loss. Early diagnosis and reoperation to establish a gastrojejunostomy is essential. The only differential diagnosis is that of a gastrojejunocolic fistula but signs and symptoms of this condition will usually present later than those of a gastroileostomy.

However, if the gastroileostomy is performed without gastric resection the pylorus may function normally and a major portion of the food may pass through the duodenum; such patients will develop few, if any, symptoms.[23]

Perioperative mortality

Table 35.1 gives a review of mortality for six different operative procedures for duodenal ulcer published in *Data Analysis for*

Table 35.1 Weighted mean operative mortality rates

	TOTALS		WEIGHTED MEAN(%)	SE (%)	95% CI (%)
	PATIENTS FOLLOWED	STUDIES			
Resections	1700	5	2.044	0.92	0.24 – 3.84
Truncal vagotomy with drainage	2871	22	0.44	0.14	0.16 – 0.72
Selective gastric vagotomy with drainage	1060	10	0.46	0.26	0.04 – 0.97
Resection plus vagotomy	1466	10	0.36	0.18	.003 – 0.72
Proximal gastric vagotomy with drainage	344	7	0.85	0.61	0.36 – 2.05
Proximal gastric vagotomy without drainage	13.145	44	0.20	0.05	0.11 – 0.29

From Chalmers[25] with permission of the publishers.

Clinical Medicine.[25] It is a meta-analysis which includes large patient series. This clearly shows that resections are associated with a higher mortality than are vagotomy procedures; half the deaths in the resected patients resulted from complications due to problems with the duodenal stump.

This material should be treated with caution, however, because the resections were performed during an earlier period than the vagotomies. It is interesting to know that in ten reports dealing with resection plus vagotomy in 1466 patients the mortality was less than after resection alone. On the contrary, one might say that there is no basis for the belief that mortality is increased when a vagotomy is added to a resection.

LATE COMPLICATIONS

Early dumping

Humphrey et al.[26] compared truncal vagotomy plus drainage, selective gastric vagotomy plus drainage and highly selective vagotomy without drainage and found a 20–32% incidence of mild to moderate dumping and a 0–2% incidence of severe dumping 1 year after surgery in patients who had undergone a drainage procedure. Where no drainage procedure was performed the incidence of dumping was the same as in control patients. Hoffmann et al.[27] made the same comparison 11–15 years after surgery and drew the same conclusions. They found, however, that severe dumping was more frequent after selective gastric vagotomy and drainage than after truncal vagotomy and drainage. The reason for this was not apparent. The feeling of faintness might be so severe in 2–3% of cases that the patient needs to lie down for 15–20 minutes immediately after the intake of food. Over the years, much research has been carried out with a view to better understanding the syndrome. Although much has been elucidated, we do not yet know why only some patients and not all develop symptoms, nor are we able to predict which patients will develop dumping. Rapid gastric emptying plays an important role. Smout et al.[28] studied gastric emptying after Billroth II resections in symptomatic and asymptomatic patients. All these patients had an increased rate of emptying of a semisolid meal in the first 5 minutes but the percentage of the meal remaining in the stomach was significantly less in symptomatic patients and a positive correlation was found between the initial emptying rate of semisolid and nausea, vomiting and vasomotor symptoms.

The dumping syndrome is described as a symptom complex with an intestinal component hyperperistalsis, epigastric discomfort, bloating, fullness, cramps, nausea and vomiting and a vasomotor component producing weakness, dizziness, pallor vertigo and the need to lie down, palpitations, sweating, tachycardia and increased peripheral blood flow, often followed by diarrhoea.

Large volumes of hypertonic fluid draw further fluid into the lumen of the bowel which distends the bowel and diminishes blood volume. It is known that plasma concentrations of several gut hormones are elevated in patients with the dumping syndrome but it is not known whether this is a primary or secondary phenomenon.[29]

The diagnosis is usually made clinically but may be confirmed by provocation tests, e.g. with 150–200 ml 50% glucose solution.[30] Such tests should be used especially if operative treatment for dumping is being considered. The treatment of dumping is dietary in the first instance, which means avoiding sugar, heavy meals and drinking during meals. It is especially important to inform the patients about those foods which have a high carbohydrate content, e.g. milk, chocolate. It is the author's impression that suggesting the patient drinks a large glass of water 5–10 minutes before a large meal is a simple tip that can ameliorate a later dumping attack. The idea is that the blood volume is increased before an attack of dumping. However, this observation is only anecdotal.

It has been shown[29,31] that the use of drugs such as somatostatin and antiserotonin can abort attacks, even with oral administration, but this is unlikely to become widespread in clinical practice, partly because of the short half-life of the drugs and partly because of the cost.

Surgical correction of dumping may rarely be considered and involves either dismantling of a gastrojejunostomy or reconstruction of the pylorus.

Late dumping

These symptoms are rather similar to the symptoms of early dumping. In particular, a feeling of faintness may appear after eating in a small percentage of patients who have undergone gastric resection or vagotomy with a drainage procedure. After oral intake of 50 g glucose the serum glucose concentration rises to significantly higher levels in all patients who do not have an intact pylorus than it does in controls. The same applies to serum insulin concentration. After 2–3 hours the glucose concentration falls to a little below the fasting levels and it is probably this hypoglycaemia which is the cause of the patients' symptoms. It is possible that gastrointestinal inhibitory peptide plays a role by stimulating the pancreatic β cells to secrete large amounts of insulin or by inhibiting glucagon release.

There is no simple explanation for the reactive hypoglycaemia but the rapid gastric emptying and a rapid absorption probably play a role. As a rule the diagnosis is made from the obvious symptoms, which disappear when sugar is eaten. In cases of doubt blood sugar concentration can be measured during an attack. This may, if necessary, be supplemented with a glucose tolerance test.

Diarrhoea

Diarrhoea after gastric surgery is of two main types. Episodic diarrhoea is seen mostly after truncal vagotomy where the patient has sudden attacks of urgent diarrhoea. This is sometimes so severe that the patient is incontinent. The second type is continuous diarrhoea where rapid gastric emptying and rapid intestinal transit play an important role, possibly in combination with malabsorption. Intestinal blind loop syndrome is also mentioned as a possible cause. The frequency and severity of diarrhoea has been studied in many centres. Raimes et al.[32] compared a group of 102 men 10 years after truncal vagotomy with a control group of cimetidine-treated patients and found that 11% of the patients who had undergone vagotomy had continuous diarrhoea and a further 22% suffered a single attack each week; 24% were dissatisfied with their symptoms and 8% found that the diarrhoea seriously affected their lives. The figures for the cimetidine-treated patients were significantly lower. Hoffmann et al.[27] found that severe diarrhoea was still a problem 13–16 years after truncal vagotomy and selective gastric vagotomy in 10 and 12% of patients, respectively. It is not always the case that dumping and diarrhoea diminish with the passage of time. Siim et al.[33] compared the situation 10 years after selective gastric vagotomy and drainage with that 5 years later in the same patients and found no improvement in their symptoms. Perhaps surprisingly some patients develop these problems *de novo* some years after their surgery.

The cause of the episodic form of diarrhoea after truncal vagotomy has been naturally blamed on the parasympathetic denervation of the gall bladder, small bowel and proximal colon. It is, however, not entirely clear why this diarrhoea should occur only sporadically and it is for this reason that medical treatment has made no great contribution to the problem. Taylor found that the addition of a cholecystectomy to a truncal vagotomy increased both the frequency and the severity of the diarrhoea. Condon et al.[34] found, however, that cholestyramine was effective in six patients. They suggested that the cause of postvagotomy diarrhoea is distension of the gall bladder, which suddenly empties itself so that a large volume of bile salts pass unabsorbed from the small bowel, thereafter affecting the colon. Cuschieri[35] found that the results with bile salt binding agents were disappointing in the long term and he introduced a 10 cm long distal onlay reversed ilial graft, with good results in six of seven patients.

The combination of truncal vagotomy with cholecystectomy results in an increased incidence of postvagotomy diarrhoea and bile reflux gastritis.[36] There is no evidence of an increased incidence of dumping syndrome, vomiting, symptomatic gastric statsis or recurrent peptic ulceration. The performance of the two operations, either synchronously or metachronously, is liable to produce the syndrome. This syndrome may be due to reflux of bile, which continuously trickles into the duodenum after cholecystectomy, through an incompetent gastric outlet (bile reflux gastritis); and the dumping of bile, which lies unbuffered in the small bowel lumen, onto the colonic mucosa; this bile may be of altered chemical composition after truncal vagotomy (postvagotomy diarrhoea).[37] The condition may respond, at least in part, to treatment with bile acid binding agents such as cholestyramine or aluminium hydroxide.[38] Alternative therapies are reconstruction of the pylorus or the insertion of a reversed peristaltic intestinal loop.

In patients with continuous diarrhoea investigations should be directed towards the possibility of malabsorption, which can be corrected.

Gastro-oesophageal reflux

Oesophagitis after gastric surgery may be related to changes in the gastro-oesophageal sphincter or in gastric emptying. The incidence depends of the type of gastric surgery but is probably highest after vagotomy and is severe in 1–2% of patients.

The symptoms are heartburn and dysphagia, which are due to the reflux of acid, bile or both of these into the oesophagus.

If acid reflux is the cause, medical treatment with H_2-receptor antagonists or omeprazole is usually very successful.

If the symptoms are due to bile reflux it is much more difficult to manage these patients medically and surgery should be considered. A Nissen fundoplication is probably the most popular operation. Whether one should add a fundoplication when performing a parietal cell vagotomy has long been a matter for discussion. A fundoplication procedure has been recommended for those patients in whom reflux is both objectively and subjectively evident. Lower oesophageal sphincter pressure was studied and gastro-oesophageal reflux determined before and after parietal cell vagotomy.[39] The lower oesophageal sphincter was not impaired in patients without gastro-oesophageal reflux so the routine addition of an antireflux procedure could not be recommended.

Duodenogastric reflux

Postoperative reflux gastritis occurs after any operation that destroys or bypasses the pylorus and is commonly found after a Billroth II reconstruction.

Mackie et al.[40] used a scintigraphic technique to study 35 controls and 55 patients treated by vagotomy and gastrectomy. Reflux occurred in 20% of normal subjects, with the highest activity 15 minutes after drinking milk and clearance within an hour. Reflux was more frequent after gastric surgery. The amount of reflux was similar in asymptomatic patients and in patients with bile vomiting. Asymptomatic patients, however, evacuated the stomach similarly to the normals, whereas bile vomiters showed a significant gastric retention of the refluxed material, with a peak at 25–30 minutes.

In most cases the symptoms appear without any evidence of mechanical obstruction. The patients complain of postprandial nausea, pain in the epigastrium and vomiting fluid which often contains bile. Gastroscopy shows a firey red mucosa, oedema and friability. Erosions are also sometimes seen.

The incidence of *Helicobacter pylori* has been studied in patients who have had gastric surgery and in unoperated ulcer patients.[41] It was found that the incidence of infection with *H. pylori* was similar after parietal cell vagotomy and in unoperated ulcer patients but was significantly lower after both Billroth I and Billroth II gastrectomies and vagotomy and drainage procedures. They also found that the absence of *H. pylori* correlated strongly with high reflux scales and increased bile acid concentrations in the stomach. The authors suggested that reflux may disrupt the mucous area and thereby destroy the *H. pylori* organisms beneath it.

A current long-term follow-up study of selective gastric vagotomy and pyloroplasty from our institution (S. Meisner, personal communication 1989) has, however, not confirmed that *H. pylori* is eliminated after this operation. It was found that half the patients had *H. pylori* in the stomach.

The medical treatment of this condition is aimed at supporting the stomach's mucosal resistance (sucralfate) or increasing the motility of the gastric remnant (metoclopramide). Either or both of these drugs have given only temporary relief and surgical correction is often indicated.

After a Billroth II reconstruction the afferent loop may be divided close to the gastric anastomosis and reanastomosed end-to-side to the efferent loop 50 cm distal to the gastric anastomosis. A Henley isoperistaltic jejunal loop measuring 25–30 cm may be interposed between the stomach and the duodenum. Another possibility is to dismantle the gastroduodenal anastomosis and to replace it with a Roux-en-Y anastomosis. Both procedures seem to give good results.[42] After pyloroplasty it is possible to reconstruct the pyloric ring, even after several years, and in a case of a gastrojejunostomy the operation of choice is to dismantle this anastomosis.

Bilious vomiting

Bilious vomiting after Billroth II resections has often been described as the afferent loop syndrome. The incidence is 2–3%. Vomiting of pure bile, 30–60 minutes after meals, is the most important symptom. Before vomiting, the patients complain of fullness, which increases to colicky pain. After vomiting the symptoms usually disappear. The phenomenon occurs periodically with intervals of up to several days. The most common explanation for this is intermittent obstruction of an afferent loop, which might be too long. The radiological findings are usually a slow gastric emptying time without visible passage of contrast into the afferent loop.

For many years the surgical treatment has been to construct an anastomosis between the afferent and efferent loops (Braun anastomosis) but the author prefers to convert a Billroth II reconstruction to a Roux-en-Y with an end-to-side anastomosis between the afferent and efferent loops, 50 cm distal to the gastrojejunostomy.

Dysphagia

Some patients complain of dysphagia immediately after parietal cell vagotomy but this symptom disappears spontaneously after 2–3 weeks. Although radiological examination of the oesophagus in these patients presents a rather alarming picture, with stenosis and proximal dilatation, they do not require further investigation or treatment.

Significant dysphagia may occur as a result of gastro-oesophageal reflux where the continous irritation causes fibrosis and finally stenosis. The latter complication can usually be prevented by effective medical treatment against reflux. Stenosis is best managed by endoscopic dilatation in combination with treatment of the underlying causes. If dysphagia occurs after gastric surgery (especially after total gastrectomy) where there is no evidence of reflux, one should consider the possibility of an anastomotic stenosis, possibly as a result of an anastomotic leakage. The latter should be excluded by radiological examination before dilatation is begun.

Weight loss

Fischer[43] made a study of 1025 patients 22–30 years after they had undergone a Billroth II resection for duodenal ulcer; 423

patients were traced. The changes in body weight of 299 patients are shown in Figure 35.1 and give a very varied picture of postoperative weight changes. In fact, 45% of the patients increased their weight and 48% lost weight. About 11% lost more than 10 kg. Only 7% showed no change in weight. Body weight changes were not related to dumping, diarrhoea, pain or vomiting or to the patients' own opinion of the operative results. It is possible that low calorie intake due to the reduced gastric capacity is the main cause for weight loss but there is a possibility that malabsorption, nitrogen loss and pancreatic dysfunction also play a role. It has not been possible to find any relationship between body weight changes and the serum albumin concentrations in patients who had undergone a Billroth II resection several years earlier.

Anaemia

In a study of 766 patients who had undergone Billroth II resection, performed 22–30 years previously, it was found that 51 (7%) developed anaemia.[43] As in other studies, iron deficiency was the most common cause. The incidence was 11%. No patients had vitamin B_{12} or folic acid deficiency.

There are probably several causes for the iron deficiency: inadequate intake, malabsorption or occult blood loss. While folic acid deficiency is caused by poor intake, vitamin B_{12} deficiency is mainly due to intrinsic factor deficiency resulting from gastric mucosal atrophy.

The diagnosis is confirmed by a low serum iron, a high serum transferrin or a microcytic anaemia. The serum folate and serum cobalamin should be measured. Macrocytic anaemia is so rare after gastric resection that in our opinion prophylactic therapy is not justified. Iron deficiency is, in contrast, more common. In most parts of the Western world diet is so variable and so many foods have iron supplements that

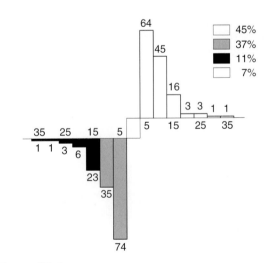

Figure 35.1

Body weight changes in 299 patients who had undergone a previous Billroth II resection. Columns indicate the number of patients in 5 kg groups. Forty-five per cent showed an increase in weight, 37% lost up to 10 kg, 11% lost more than 10 kg and 7% showed no change in weight. (Reproduced with permission from Fischer.[43])

further prophylactic therapy is not usually warranted. To date, iron deficiency and macrocytic anaemia have not been demonstrated after truncal or selective vagotomy and drainage or after parietal cell vagotomy.[33]

Bone disease

It has been known for many years that osteomalacia may appear in some patients after gastric resection, especially in elderly women. Osteomalacia is the most commonly reported bone disease after gastric surgery but osteoporosis or a combination of both may occur.

The aetiology remains unclear but malabsorption of vitamin D and/or calcium, decreased intake or rapid transit time are currently thought to be the most likely causes.[44] In patients with bone disease the mean phosphate concentration, alkaline phosphate level and serum albumin were all significantly different from those of a control group.

Tovey et al.[45] followed a series of patients continously as a screening procedure. They found that serum alkaline phosphatase estimation was the most useful single parameter: in patients with a rise, particularly a moderate one, bone disease should be suspected. If other causes are excluded a bone biopsy should be performed. Another possibility is to give the patient two calcium and vitamin D tablets four times a day prophylactically. A fall of the serum alkaline phosphatase to normal levels can be regarded as a sign of osteomalacia and occurred in 6.5% out of 227 patients.

In a study of 42 patients 5–7 years after gastric surgery it was concluded that there were no significant disturbances in bone mineral metabolism compared with controls.[46] Another study of 50 patients 3–4 years after gastrectomy came to the same conclusions.[47] It should be noted, however, that these two studies dealt mainly with middle-aged working men and that the observation time was relatively short. The incidence of metabolic bone disease is difficult to estimate in long-term follow-up studies as many patients reach an age where senile osteoporosis is common.

Cholelithiasis

The incidence of gallstone disease after antrectomy, with or without vagotomy, has been studied.[48] It was found that, 5 years after surgery, 18% of patients who had undergone a gastrectomy had developed gallstones. The figure was 30% when truncal vagotomy had been added and 12% if the vagotomy was selective. Truncal vagotomy has been shown to produce dilatation of the gall bladder. This dilatation is significantly greater than in non-operated duodenal ulcer patients and those after selective gastric vagotomy or parietal cell vagotomy.[49] It seems to be a result of denervation of the gall bladder. The contractility of the gall bladder is, however, unimpaired, probably because contraction is due to the release of cholecystokinin. Experimental studies have shown a diminution of bile flow and a change in the composition of bile which makes it more lithogenic. All these factors lead to a higher incidence of gallstones after truncal vagotomy. So far this has not been documented after other types of operation, especially selective gastric vagotomy and parietal cell vagotomy.

Jejunogastric intussusception

Retrograde intragastric intussusception is an extremely rare condition, appearing in the literature as sporadic case reports. It is usually a chronic recurrent intussusception with symptoms of recurrent discomfort in the epigastrium. If the obstruction is complete vomiting may supervene.

Acute intussusception may also occur, the patient presenting with acute colicky epigastric pain followed by vomiting and later haematemesis. The diagnosis is confirmed by a standard barium meal, where it is obvious that the jejunum is in the stomach. The treatment is surgical, with release of the intussusception and resection of the involved small bowel, were necessary, followed by a reconstruction of the Roux-en-Y type.

Metabolic neuropathy

Peripheral neuropathy is due to vitamin B_{12} deficiency after total gastrectomy, and after partial gastrectomy where there is atrophy of the mucosa of the gastric remnant.

The symptoms are weakness, tiredness and paraesthesia. Numbness and tingling of the extremities may also be present. The symptoms occur as a result of an unrecognized pernicious anaemia and may be regarded as a late stage of this disease.

When the diagnosis is confirmed by blood tests, treatment should be with vitamin B_{12}, whereupon the symptoms will disappear.

Gastric stump cancer

The development of cancer in the gastric remnant after gastrectomy might be a result of reflux of bile and pancreatic juice, a decreased acid secretion or a change in the bacterial composition allowing nitrate-reducing micro-organisms to develop. Nitrosamines are thought to be carcinogenic.

Since the first case of carcinoma of the gastric remnant was described by Balfour in 1922, it has been debated whether gastric resection increases the risk of gastric cancer in the stomach. In some studies it has been documented that the incidence is more or less as expected, whereas in others the risk was found to be increased.

The development of gastric cancer usually occurs between 15 and 30 years after the gastric resection. The tendency increases with the duration of observation. In an analysis the possible benefits of regular endoscopic screening by a Markov type of decision in a hypothetical cohort study was carried out. It was found that life expectancy would increase by 8–9 months or that 6.4 years of life would be gained per 100 endoscopies performed.[50] It was concluded that endoscopic screening would be beneficial only if there was a high expected frequency of gastric cancer.

From a review[51] of many studies it seems clear that the incidence is very variable and is related to methodology and to the interval between operation and the follow-up study. In the presence of achlorhydria numerous mucosal abnormalities have been described, such as active superficial gastritis, chronic atrophic gastritis, intestinal metaplasia, dysplasia, carcinoma in situ, early gastric cancer and gastric carcinoma. From a previous publication,[52] it was found that the number of patients with carcinoma of the gastric remnant expressed as a percentage of the total number of patients who had gastric surgery for peptic ulcer varied from 0.4 to 8.9%, and that the longer the exposure to hypochlorhydria the greater the risk involved.

Several authors have estimated the risk of the development of stump cancer by comparisons of the observed incidence of stump cancer with the expected incidence. Most of the reports show no significant differences between the observed and the expected number of cancers, suggesting that if there is a risk of development of carcinoma of the gastric stump it is not much greater than that in the normal population. Of interest is the fact that gastric cancer most commonly develops in the antrum which is retained after vagotomy. However, it has not yet been possible to demonstrate that there is a higher risk of developing carcinoma of the stomach up to 25 years after vagotomy for duodenal ulcer; the amount of clinical material investigated is not as large as that for gastric resection.

In a study of 4466 ulcer patients who had undergone gastric surgery between 1940 and 1960 it was demonstrated that in patients with duodenal ulcer the risk of death from gastric cancer was less in each 5-year period for the first 20 postoperative years.[53] However, 20 years or more after the operation there was a 3.7-fold increased risk. Thus a decreased risk in the first 20 years is subsequently reversed. In patients with gastric ulcer there was a threefold risk of death from gastric cancer for the first 20 years after the operation.

Fischer et al.[54] studied 1000 patients after Billroth II resections 20–30 years after surgery: 196 underwent gastroscopy and biopsy and not a single case of gastric cancer was found. Gastroscopy was repeated 5 years later in 72 patients and the number of biopsies was doubled to 16. In four patients one of the 16 biopsies showed early gastric cancer but the risk was still not as high as expected. The study demonstrates that the incidence of cancer increases with duration of observation and that it is necessary to take numerous biopsies, even from macroscopically normal mucosa, in order to verify potential development of cancer. Most authors agree that the incidence of cancer is sufficiently low to make routine gastroscopic screening unjustified.

RECONSTRUCTIVE GASTRIC SURGERY

At the time when gastric resection was undertaken in a large number of patients and when surgeons were well acquainted with the sequelae, it was natural to attempt reconstructions which could possibly prevent such complications as dumping and diarrhoea. Interest centred mainly on whether the food should pass through the duodenum (Billroth I) or through a gastrojejunostomy (Billroth II). No sure conclusion was forthcoming. No prospective randomized studies have been able to show any definite difference between the side-effects of Billroth I and Billroth II gastrectomies.

Other directions were also investigated, such as changing the size of the anastomosis or constructing a Hofmeister retrocolic gastroenterostomy. It has become apparent that the incidence of side-effects is the same after gastric resection as after pyloric bypass operations or destruction of the pylorus.

Pylorus-preserving gastrectomy

The first report of the successful clinical application of suprapyloric gastrectomy was published by Maki et al.[55] Descriptions of segmental resections of different types with and without vagotomy have been published but none of those involved an antrectomy of the same extent as that performed by Maki. He described his technique in recognition of the fact that there is a close correlation between the dumping syndrome and the destruction of the pyloric ring. Experimental studies based on action potentials, intraluminal pressure and emptying examinations demonstrated that the gesture transection should be performed at a maximum of 1.5 cm proximal to the pyloric ring. The first report, based on 31 cases, was promising and there was a normal pyloric sphincteric function and normal gastric emptying which eliminated dumping. These preliminary results were confirmed in a further study.[56] A follow-up study 1–9 years after surgery also showed excellent results,[57] whereas a study of 47 patients 2–7 years after the operation found that three patients had required a second operation because of retention and five developed a recurrent ulcer in the antral segment. It was concluded that the results did not seem superior to a Billroth I resection.[58] One may, however, question whether this conclusion is reasonable when based on small series.

Another possibility is to combine suprapyloric resection with selective gastric vagotomy.[59] In a pilot study of 20 patients no dumping occurred but one-third of the patients complained of mild to moderate stasis. Our limited experience showed that a successful result could be achieved if a retained antrum was no bigger than about 1 cm. If the antral stump was larger, problems developed. Pylorus-preserving gastrectomy never achieved any great popularity. This is probably somewhat unjust when one considers that patients were completely free of dumping and diarrhoea.

Closure of gastrojejunostomy

After vagotomy and gastrojejunostomy it is possible to improve the complications of severe diarrhoea, dumping and/or bile vomiting. Green et al.[60] reported the results of dismantling a gastrojejunostomy in 19 patients. During surgery it was confirmed that the lumen of the pylorus was adequate. No retention was observed either immediately after operation or 6 years later. About half the patients were completely relieved of their symptoms and another half improved. One patient developed no benefit. The best results were obtained for bile vomiting. The same experience was reported[61] with nine patients.

These results suggest that if a drainage procedure is considered after truncal or selective vagotomy it should be a gastrojejunostomy which leaves the pylorus untouched because any side-effects that then occur will be more easily correctable.

Furthermore, there are no documented advantages of pyloroplasty over gastroenterostomy.[62]

Reconstruction of the pylorus

There are few reports in the literature of pyloric reconstruction for severe postvagotomy diarrhoea and dumping. The series consist of rather few patients[63,64] but the general conclusion is that reconstruction is justified in most of those in whom late vasomotor dumping has been resistant to medical treatment (small meals, low in carbohydrate and high in fat and protein). Reconstruction of the pylorus will not generally be considered during the first year after surgery and certainly not before it has become evident that dietary treatment is unsuccessful. At the other extreme it has been shown that a reconstruction is possible up to 12 years after the primary operation if it is still possible to identify the pyloric ring. The procedure is relatively simple. Stay sutures are placed exactly in the centre of the pyloroplasty, which is opened along the suture line and resutured longitudinally with exact apposition of the pyloric ring.

Most patients are examined clinically and their gastric emptying studied by barium meal or by radioisotope scanning. After surgery an improvement in the patient's symptoms may be documented by showing that the transit time has returned to normal; many gain weight. A few patients do not seem to benefit from the operation. The symptoms of gastric outlet obstruction do not seem to be a major problem even after truncal vagotomy. It is, however, still doubtful that operation offers any relief to patients with explosive diarrhoea, which may be more a result of the vagotomy than of destruction of the pyloric function.

We reported[65] the difficulties encountered with closure of Jaboulay gastroduodenostomies. Eight patients underwent direct suture of the opening via a gastrotomy but the suture line broke down again within 9 months and the patients' symptoms returned. In two cases where the anastomosis was formally dismantled and the defects in the duodenum and stomach closed separately both patients developed severe postoperative complications. This experience and our experience with reoperations for recurrent ulcers after vagotomy and Jaboulay gastroenterostomies has led us to abandon this drainage procedure which has no superiority over a gastrojejunostomy.

Jejunal interposition

In the past the surgical armamentarium contained a series of operative procedures which were entirely useless, for example the conversion of a Billroth II to a Billroth I anastomosis or vice versa reducing the size of the stomal outlet or increasing the gastric remnant. In the past 20–25 years other procedures have been used. A 20–30 cm isoperistaltic segment of jejunum interposed between the stomach and the duodenum gave unsatisfactory results in most cases when used for dumping or diarrhoea.

A double limb pouch has been used. Each limb measured 10–12 cm and the limbs were anastomosed to each other to produce a large single receptacle where one segment was isoperistaltic and the other one antiperistaltic. The procedure was, however, abandoned because of unsatisfactory results in about half the patients.

The most popular form of reconstruction has been with a short (approximately 8 cm) antiperistaltic segment interposed between the gastric remnant and the duodenum. Excellent results were reported in 26 of 28 patients and it was maintained that bile reflux was not a problem.[66]

Reoperation for dumping and diarrhoea has never been a common procedure and now that the operative treatment of ulcer disease has diminished markedly, especially with regard to resective procedures, such reparative operations will probably gradually be regarded as historic curiosities.

The indication for jejunal interposition has been severe incapacitating diarrhoea where investigations have shown an extremely rapid small bowel transit time. A jejunal segment of 10–12 cm taken from 100 cm distal to the ligament of Treitz was reversed. Excellent results were reported in 7 of 10 patients.[67] No stasis or obstruction occurred. Cuschieri[35] has introduced a distal onlay reversed ileal graft of 10 cm with promising results but further documentation of this method is required from other sources.

Surgery for bile reflux gastritis

Severe bile reflux gastritis is a good indication for reconstructive surgery and it is seldom that such an operation is unsuccessful. Severe symptoms might indicate surgery after one or more attempts at medical treatment have given only temporary relief. In most cases gastroscopy will have demonstrated a severely inflamed and irritated gastric mucosa with small erosions, oedema and a tendency to bleeding.

The corrective procedure will obviously depend on the primary operation. It might be a reconstruction of the pylorus, dismantling of a gastroenterostomy and conversion of a Billroth I resection to a Billroth II procedure which would include a re-resection of the stomach and a Roux-en-Y anastomosis. Another possibility is the interposition of an isoperistaltic jejunal loop measuring 30 cm which will prevent bile reflux to the gastric remnant. If the primary reconstruction was a Billroth II procedure the efferent loop of about 30 cm can be used for interposition between the stomach and the duodenum. The afferent loop is disconnected at the gastrojejunostomy and anastomosed to the jejunum. It would probably be simpler to convert the gastroenterostomy to a Roux-en-Y anastomosis by dividing the afferent loop close to the stomach and performing an end-to-side anastomosis between the afferent and the efferent loop 50 cm distal to the stomach. Histology of the stomach was studied before and after diversion of bile in 33 patients.[68] There was no difference in the degree of gastritis, atrophy or intestinal metaplasia 10 months after the second operation. Only the incidence of dysplasia was improved significantly after a Roux-en-Y reconstruction.

Surgery for delayed gastric emptying

A slow rate of gastric emptying may be found after all gastric operations but is most marked after truncal vagotomy and drainage. Patients complain of epigastric pain, nausea, vomiting and weight loss. The diagnosis is made when a normal barium meal is significantly retained in the stomach after 4 hours. Food contrast examinations would appear to be more physiological but have not yet been standardized. Endoscopy may show gastritis because of bile reflux or frequently because of retention of undigested food. Occasionally a bezoar might be seen. The primary treatment is medical with a liquid diet; if the retention is due to a recurrent ulcer an H_2-receptor antagonist or omeprazole may be used. If conservative treatment does not improve the retention after 2–3 weeks, surgical treatment is indicated and reconstruction will depend on the nature of the primary operation and the cause of the retention. In most cases, however, one will probably end up with a high Billroth II resection and a Roux-en-Y anastomosis. The latter produces satisfactory results in three out of four patients.[69] One might, however, find a mechanical cause, e.g. a stenotic pyloroplasty or gastroenterostomy, which can be corrected directly. If a patient develops symptoms of gastric retention many years after a successful gastric resection one should obviously investigate possible causes of the condition, for example recurrent ulceration, carcinoma of the stomach or pancreatic disease.

REFERENCES

1. Jensen HE & Madsen OG. Selective vagotomy and drainage for bleeding duodenal ulcer. *Acta Chir Scand* 1974; **140:** 406–409.
2. Hoffmann J & Jensen H-E. Two-stage gastrectomy for the difficult duodenal stump. *JR Coll Surg Edinb* 1987; **32:** 13–14.
3. Pearson SC, Mackenzie RJ & Ross T. The use of catheter duodenostomy in gastric resection for duodenal ulcer. *Am J Surg* 1963; **106:** 194–205.
4. Mayfield RC & Abramson PD. The use of catheter duodenostomy in subtotal gastrectomy. *Am J Surg* 1955; **90:** 998–1001.
5. Austen WG & Baue AE. Catheter duodenostomy for the difficult duodenum. *Ann Surg* 1964; **160:** 781–787.
6. Lamphier TA & Crooker C. Catheter duodenostomy for the difficult duodenal stump. *South Med J* 1968; **61:** 751–757.
7. Griffen WO. Whither goest the duodenal stump blowout? *Arch Surg* 1973; **107:** 11.
8. Hjortrup A, Bulet O, Jensen FU & Bredesen J. Duodenal blow-out after gastric resection. *Res Surg* 1989; **1:** 57–59.
9. Appel A. Safe closure of the difficult duodenal stump. *Surg Gynecol Obstet* 1986; **163:** 73–74.
10. Larsen BB & Foreman RC. Syndrome of the leaking duodenal stump. *Arch Surg* 1951; **63:** 480–485.
11. Harvey HD. Complications in hospital following partial gastrectomy for peptic ulcer, 1936 to 1959. *Surgery* 1963; **117:** 211–221.
12. Welch CE & Rodkey GV. The surgeon at work. A method of management of the duodenal stump after gastrectomy. *Surg Gynecol Obstet* 1954; **98:** 376–379.
13. Rutter AG. Ischemic necrosis of the stomach following subtotal gastrectomy. *Lancet* 1953; **ii:** 1021–1022.
14. Jackson PP. Ischemic necrosis of the proximal gastric remnant following subtotal gastrectomy. *Ann Surg* 1959; **150:** 1071–1074.
15. Thompson NW. Ischemic necrosis of proximal gastric remnant following subtotal gastrectomy. *Surgery* 1963; **54:** 434–440.
16. Kilgare TL, Don Turner M & Hardy JD. Clinical and experimental ischemia of the gastric remnant. *Surg Gynecol Obstet* 1964; **18:** 1312–1316.
17. Schein M & Saadia R. Postoperative gastric ischaemia. *Br J Surg* 1989; **76:** 844–848.
18. Dragstedt LR, Harper PV, Tovee EB & Woodward ER. Section of the vagus nerves to the stomach in the treatment of peptic ulcer. *Ann Surg* 1947; **126:** 687–708.
19. Hocking MP, Vogel SB, Falasca CA & Woodward ER. Delayed gastric emptying of liquids and solids following Roux-en-Y biliary diversion. *Ann Surg* 1981; **194:** 494–501.
20. Hinder RA, Esser J & DeMeester TR. Management of gastric emptying disorders following the Roux-en-Y procedure. *Surgery* 1988; **104:** 765–772.
21. Eckhauser FE, Knol JA, Raper SA & Guice KS. Completion gastrectomy for postsurgical gastroparesis syndrome. *Ann Surg* 1988; **208:** 345–353.
22. Karlstrom L & Kelly KA. Roux-Y gastrectomy for chronic gastric atony. *Am J Surg* 1989; **157:** 44–49.
23. Ritter SA. Gastroileostomy with realignment and recovery. Report of a case. *J Int Coll Surg* 1958; **29:** 155–159.
24. Michels AG, Brown CH & Crile G. Surgical error of gastroileostomy. Report of six cases. *Am J Surg* 1951; **83:** 191–197.
25. Chalmers TC. *Data Analysis for Clinical Medicine. The Quantitative Approach to Patient Care in Gastroenterology.* Rome: International University Press, 1988: 101–144.
26. Humphrey CS, Johnston D, Walker BE, Pulvertaft CN & Goligher JC. Incidence of dumping after truncal and selective vagotomy with pyloroplasty and highly selective vagotomy without drainage procedure. *BMJ* 1972; **3:** 785–788.
27. Hoffmann J, Jensen H-E, Christiansen J, Olesen A, Loud FB & Hauch O. Prospective controlled vagotomy trial for duodenal ulcer. *Ann Surg* 1989; **209:** 40–45.
28. Smout AJPM, Akkermans LMA, Roelofs JMM, Pasma FG, Oei HY & Wittebol P. Gastric emptying and postprandial symptoms after Billroth II resection. *Surgery* 1987; **101:** 27–34.
29. Primrose JN & Johnston D. Somatostatin analogue SMS 201–995 (octreotide) as a possible solution to the dumping syndrome after gastrectomy or vagotomy. *Br J Surg* 1989; **76:** 140–144.
30. Linehan IP, Weiman J & Hobsley M. The 15-minute dumping provocation test. *Br J Surg* 1986; **73:** 810–812.
31. Reasbeck PG & Van Rij AM. The effect of somatostatin on dumping after gastric surgery: a preliminary report. *Surgery* 1986; **99:** 462–467.
32. Raimes SA, Smirniotis V, Wheldon EJ, Venables CW & Johnston IDA. Postvagotomy diarrhoea put into perspective. *Lancet* 1986; **ii:** 851–853.
33. Siim C, Lublin HKF & Jensen H-E. Selective gastric vagotomy and drainage for duodenal ulcer. A 10–13 years follow-up study. *Ann Surg* 1981; **194:** 687–691.
34. Condon JR, Robinson V, Suleman MI, Fan VS & McKeown MD. The cause and treatment of postvagotomy diarrhoea. *Br J Surg* 1975; **62:** 309–312.
35. Cuschieri A. Surgical management of severe intractable postvagotomy diarrhoea. *Br J Surg* 1986; **73:** 981–984.
36. Taylor TV, Lambert ME & Torrance HB. Should cholecystectomy be combined with vagotomy and pyloroplasty? *Lancet* 1978; **1,** 295–298.
37. Taylor TV. The postvagotomy and cholecystectomy syndrome. *Annals of Surgery,* 1981; **194,** 625–629.
38. Taylor TV, Lambert ME & Torrance HB. Value of bile acid binding agents in postvagotomy diarrhoea. *Lancet,* 1978; **1,** 635–636.
39. Ottignon Y, Pellisier E, Blum D et al. The effects of highly selective vagotomy on lower esophageal sphincter function (French). *Gastroenterol Clin Biol* 1989; **13:** 250–254.
40. Mackie C, Hulks G & Cuschieri A. Enterogastric reflux and gastric clearance of refluxate in normal subjects and in patients with and without bile vomiting following peptic ulcer surgery. *Ann Surg* 1986; **204:** 537–542.
41. O'Connor HJ, Dixon MF, Wyatt JI et al. Effect of duodenal ulcer surgery and enterogastric reflux on *Campylobacter pyloridis. Lancet* 1986; **ii:** 1178–1181.
42. Sousa JES, Troncon LEA, Andrade JI & Ceneviva R. Comparison between Henley jejunal interposition and Roux-en-Y anastomosis as concerns enterogastric biliary reflux levels. *Ann Surg* 1988; **208:** 597–600.
43. Fischer AB. Twenty-five years after Billroth II gastrectomy for duodenal ulcer. *World J Surg* 1984; **8:** 293–302.
44. Klein KB, Orwoll ES, Lieberman DA, Meier DE, McClung MR & Parfitt AM. Metabolic bone disease in asymptomatic men after partial gastrectomy with Billroth II anastomosis. *Gastroenterology* 1987; **92:** 608–616.
45. Tovey FI, Karamanolis DG, Godfrey J & Clark CG. Screening for early post-gastrectomy osteomalacia. *Practitioner* 1987; **231:** 817–822.
46. Hoikka V, Alhava EM, Savolainen K, Karjalainen P & Parviainen M. The effect of partial gastrectomy on bone mineral metabolism. *Scand J Gastroenterol* 1982; **17:** 257.
47. Pääkkönen M, Alhava EM & Karjalainen P. Bone mineral and intestinal absorption after partial gastrectomy. *Scand J Gastroenterol* 1982; **17:** 369–372.
48. Rehnberg O & Haglund U. Gallstone disease following antrectomy and

gastroduodenostomy with or without vagatomy. *Ann Surg* 1985; **201:** 315–318.

49. Parkin GJS, Smith RB & Johnston D. Gallbladder volume and contractility after truncal, selective and highly selective (parietal-cell) vagotomy in man. *Ann Surg* 1973; **178:** 581–586.

50. Sonnenberg A. Endoscopic screening for gastric stump cancer – would it be beneficial? *Gastroenterology* 1984; **87:** 489–495.

51. Clark CG, Fresini A & Gledhill T. Cancer following gastric surgery. *Br J Surg* 1985; **72:** 591–594.

52. Clark CG, Ward MWN, McDonald AM & Tovey FI. The incidence of gastric stump cancer. *World J Surg* 1983; **7:** 236–240.

53. Caygill CPJ, Hill MJ, Kirkhamm JS & Northfield TC. Mortality from gastric cancer following gastric surgery for peptic ulcer. *Lancet* 1986; **ii:** 929–931.

54. Fischer AB, Græm N & Jensen OM. Risk of gastric cancer after Billroth II resection for duodenal ulcer. *Br J Surg* 983; 70: 552–554.

55. Maki T, Shiratori T, Hatafuku T & Sugawara K. Pylorus-preserving gastrectomy as an improved operation for gastric ulcer. *Surgery* 1967; **61:** 838–845.

56. Liavåg I, Roland M & Broch A. Gastric function after pylorus-preserving resection for gastric ulcer. *Acta Chir Scand* 1972; **138:** 511–516.

57. Sekine T, Sato T, Maki T & Shiratori T. Pylorus-preserving gastrectomy for gastric ulcer – one- to nine-year follow-up study. *Surgery* 1975; **77:** 92–99.

58. Teigan T, Liavåg I & Roland M. Pylorus preserving gastric resection for gastric ulcer. A 5–7-year follow-up. *Acta Chir Scand* 1978; **144:** 249–253.

59. Griffith CA. Selective gastric vagotomy plus suprapyloric antrectomy. In Nyhns LM & Baker RJ (eds) *Mastery of Surgery.* Boston: Little Brown, 1987: 535–541.

60. Green R, Spencer A & Kennedy T. Closure of gastrojejunostomy for the relief of post-vagotomy symptoms. *Br J Surg* 1978; **65:** 161–163.

61. McMahon MJ, Johnston D, Hill GL & Goligher JC. Treatment of severe side effects after vagotomy and gastroenterostomy without pyloroplasty. *BMJ* 1978; **1:** 7–8.

62. Kennedy T, Johnston GW, Love AHG, Connell AM & Spencer EFA. Pyloroplasty versus gastrojejunostomy. *Br J Surg* 1973; **60:** 949–953.

63. Frederiksen H-JB, Johansen TS & Christiansen PM. Postvagotomy diarrhoea and dumping treated with reconstruction of the pylorus. *Scand J Gastroenterol* 1980; **15:** 245–248.

64. Cheadle WG, Baker PR & Cuschieri A. Pyloric reconstruction for severe vasomotor dumping after vagotomy and pyloroplasty. *Ann Surg* 1985; **202:** 568–572.

65. Hoffmann J, Fischer A & Jensen H-E. Unsuccessful experience with closure of Jaboulay gastroduodenostomies in the treatment of post-vagotomy dumping and diarrhea. *Ann Surg* 1983; **198:** 142–145.

66. Sawyers JL & Lynwood Herrington J. Superiority of antiperistaltic jejunal segments in management of severe dumping syndrome. *Ann Surg* 1973; **178:** 311–321.

67. Herrington JL & Sawyers JL. Remedial operations. In Nyhus LM & Wastell C (eds) *Surgery of the Stomach and Duodenum*, 3rd edn. Boston: Little Brown, 1977: 537–569.

68. Watt PCH, Sloan JM, Spencer A & Kennedy TL. Histology of the postoperative stomach before and after diversion of bile. *BMJ* 1983; **287:** 1410–1412.

69. Vogel SB & Woodward ER. The surgical treatment of chronic gastric atony following Roux-Y diversion for alkaline reflux gastritis. *Ann Surg* 1989; **209:** 756–763.

36

THE ZOLLINGER–ELLISON SYNDROME AND ENDOCRINE DISORDERS AFFECTING THE STOMACH

TJ Howard
E Passaro

INTRODUCTION

This chapter presents a novel approach to the localization and surgical excision of gastrinomas based on a theoretical construct of their development. This construct has been formulated by the assimilation and synthesis of clinical data and new information on the biological characteristics of these tumours. Through the utilization of this construct, we anticipate that both the surgical and conceptual approach to gastrinoma will change.

Historically, tumours of the endocrine pancreas first became clinically important after insulin was identified and characterized by Banting and Best in 1922.[1] Soon after the discovery of this hormone a prediction was made that a tumour of pancreatic β cells would be found, and its clinical manifestations would be the result of an overproduction of insulin.[2] This prediction was realized shortly thereafter when the first patient with an insulin-producing tumour was identified.[3] Over the ensuing years, collective clinical experience with insulinomas showed them to be small solitary tumours, contained within a well-defined capsule, intrapancreatic in location, and readily curable by simple excision.[4] As a result of their initial identification and the physiological importance of insulin, insulinomas became the clinical paradigm by which all subsequent islet cell tumours were evaluated.

Gastrinoma, the second islet cell tumour of the pancreas, was not identified until 22 years later. Unlike insulinomas, however, affected patients did not suffer from symptoms of hypoglycaemia but were found to have severe peptic ulcer disease. The observation that some islet cell tumours were associated with peptic ulcer disease had been reported as early as

1946[5-7] but the significance of this association remained unrecognized until 1955, when Zollinger and Ellison presented their landmark paper.[8] In this paper they postulated that an unrecognized hormone was being elaborated by these tumours and was causing the severe peptic ulcer disease. It was not until 6 years later that the isolation and characterization of the hormone gastrin from tumour extracts confirmed their theory.[9] When originally described, these tumours were termed non-β islet cell tumours to distinguish them from the previously described insulinomas. After the identification of gastrin in tumour extracts, these tumours became known as gastrinomas.[10] As clinical experience with gastrinomas grew, it became increasingly apparent that they did not fit the clinical paradigm of islet cell tumours derived from initial experience with insulinomas. Gastrinomas were often found to be multiple, located in extrapancreatic areas, and found within the duodenum and peripancreatic lymph nodes. As a result of these observations and their variance with the prevailing paradigm of insulinomas, gastrinomas were thought to be highly malignant lesions with a low probability for surgical cure.[11,12] It is against this backdrop that we will investigate the current treatment concepts and develop a systematic approach toward the evaluation and management of patients with gastrinoma.

CLINICAL FEATURES

Although the exact incidence of gastrinoma is unknown, it may be the most common of the pancreatic endocrine tumours. In a little more than a decade since its original description, Ellison and Wilson had compiled a registry of over 1000 cases. As a general guide to clinical frequency, reports of clinical series in the last decade are more numerous for gastrinoma than insulinoma. These tumours may not be frequent but they are not rare either, especially to physicians dealing with gastrointestinal disorders and particularly peptic ulcer disease. Some estimates suggest that they may occur in up to 0.1% of all patients with duodenal ulcer disease.[11] There is no racial or geographic predilection for these tumours, however most series show a slight male preponderance (65%). The peak onset of symptoms is between the third and fifth decades of life, although gastrinomas have been reported in the very young and very old.[13,14]

The most common presenting symptom is abdominal pain.[15] This pain is typically epigastric in location, burning in nature, and invariably associated with peptic ulceration. In most patients diarrhoea is common and may be the sole presenting symptom in up to 20% of patients.[16] Because these symptoms are non-specific, their average duration is approximately 5 years before the diagnosis of gastrinoma is made.[17]

Since the introduction of the gastrin radioimmunoassay (RIA) in 1970, patients have been diagnosed earlier and as a result, their initial clinical presentation has also changed[17-19] (Table 36.1). Prior to its availability, 80% of patients were diagnosed after a serious ulcer complication (bleeding, obstruction, perforation) and most had at least one previous ulcer operation. In contrast, after the introduction of the gastrin assay only 20% of patients had a serious ulcer complication and only 30% had a previous ulcer operation.[17] It is our impression that patients with gastrinomas are currently presenting with more chronic indolent symptoms of intractability rather than with acute ulcer complications such as bleeding or perforation.

Table 36.1 Comparison between the clinical presentations of patients with gastrinoma diagnosed in the pre-RIA and post-RIA periods.[17]

	PRE-RIA (*n* = 25)	POST-RIA (*n* = 35)
Duration of symptoms (>5 years)	57	60
Ulcer complications[a]	80	20
Ulcer operations	80	30

[a]Bleeding, obstruction or perforation.

The diagnosis of gastrinoma should be considered in any patient with a peptic ulcer not responding to conventional medical therapy or in those with an ulcer complication following a standard ulcer operation (vagotomy and antrectomy, vagotomy and pyloroplasty or highly selective vagotomy). In these patients the serum gastrin analysis has the highest diagnostic yield. Serum gastrin assay on all patients with peptic ulcer disease is unwarranted and not cost-effective.

AETIOLOGY

The endocrine pancreas is a complex organ which includes the islets of Langerhans plus a number of intrapancreatic extra-islet endocrine cells.[20,21] Although gastrinomas are found both in and about the pancreas, the identification of a specific cellular precursor capable of secreting gastrin in the adult human pancreas has not occurred.[22] Although some studies have shown that gastrin is produced in pancreatic islet δ cells along with somatostatin,[23,24] others have been unable to substantiate these findings.[25,26] There is currently no definitive evidence that a gastrin-secreting endocrine cell is present within the adult human pancreas. Furthermore, even those endocrine cells known to occur within pancreatic islets, such as the α, β, δ, PP cells, have an ontogeny which remains unclear.[27-30] The inability to address these fundamental questions has limited our understanding of pancreatic endocrine tumours in general and gastrinomas in particular. For gastrinomas, knowing the ontogeny of their cellular precursor may provide insight into their unique characteristics that distinguish them from insulinomas, particularly with regard to their intra-abdominal location, occurrence as multiple tumours and location within lymph nodes.

Although the cytological development of pancreatic islets is poorly understood, the morphological development of the gland as a whole is well known.[31] The mammalian pancreas develops from two distinct embryological sources: a ventral pancreatic bud and a dorsal pancreatic bud (Figure 36.1). The dorsal bud develops as an endodermal outpouching on the mesenteric border of the primitive gut just distal to the developing stomach in the area of the duodenum. The ventral bud develops concurrently as a similar outpouching on the opposite wall (antimesenteric border) of the primitive gut. These two buds remain separate and distinct entities until approximately

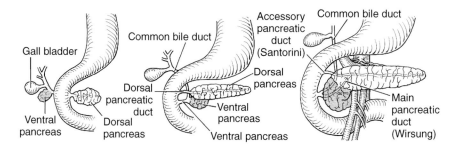

Figure 36.1
Embryological development of the pancreas. (a) The pancreas develops from two distinct buds: a dorsal and a ventral pancreatic bud. (b) At approximately 6 weeks of gestation complex morphological changes occur which cause the ventral pancreatic bud to migrate clockwise around the duodenum to lie in a dorsal position in the pancreatic head. (c) In the adult gland, the posterior pancreatic head and uncinate process are derived from the ventral pancreatic bud.

the 6th week of gestation, at which time complex morphological events occur which cause the ventral pancreatic bud to rotate 180° clockwise (dorsally) around the primitive duodenum to become the posterior pancreatic head and uncinate process (Figure 36.1). Anatomical evidence for these events has been the identification of a fine connective tissue plane which separates the posterior pancreatic head and uncinate process (ventral bud derivative) from the remaining pancreas (dorsal bud derivative).[32] In our experience, the majority of gastrinomas are located anatomically on the right side of the abdomen in an area called the gastrinoma triangle (Figure 36.2). This triangle is defined anatomically as the junction of the cystic duct and common duct superiorly, the second and third portions of the duodenum inferiorly, and the junction of the neck and body of the pancreas medially.[33] Topographically, this area (gastrinoma triangle) coincides with the path of the ventral pancreatic bud during its dorsal migration around the duodenum to become the posterior pancreatic head and uncinate process.

If one combines these two pieces of information it seem reasonable to hypothesize that the majority of sporadic gastrinomas are derived embryologically from cells in the ventral pancreatic bud. In support of this hypothesis, we found that cells producing pancreatic polypeptide (PP), a 36-amino acid hormone derived exclusively from the ventral pancreatic bud,[34,35] were identified in 78% (7 of 9) of gastrinomas found around the head of the pancreas (ventral bud derivation).[36] Conversely, no PP producing cells (0/5) were identified in gastrinoma localized to the body or tail of the pancreas (dorsal bud derivation). We then investigated a collective experience of pancreatic endocrine tumours (insulinomas, glucagonomas, somatostatinomas, and (PPomas) which correspond to endocrine cell types (α, β, δ, PP) found in normal pancreatic

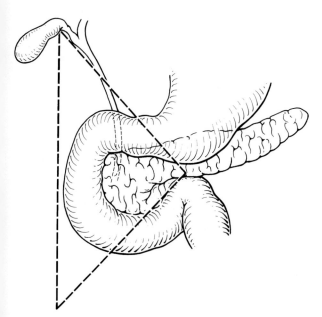

Figure 36.2

Gastrinoma triangle, defined as the junction of the cystic duct and common bile duct superiorly, the second and third portions of the duodenum inferiorly, and the neck and body of the pancreas medially.

islets.[37] Analysis of this group of tumours revealed that for insulinoma, glucagonoma, and PPoma, their topographical distribution within the abdomen paralleled that predicted based on the topographical distribution of their corresponding endocrine cells in the adult human pancreas. In this study, the distribution of 165 gastrinomas correlated closely with that of PPomas, a tumour associated with an endocrine cell derived exclusively from the ventral pancreatic bud. This theory of ventral bud derivation is appealing for several reasons; not only is it useful clinically in conceptualizing the intra-abdominal location of the majority of gastrin producing tumours, but it is also helpful in understanding the occurrence of benign tumour within lymph nodes and the presence of extrapancreatic tumours.

Gastrinomas are found within lymph nodes in approximately 40% of cases. Historically, these tumours have been considered to be metastatic disease from a primary tumour within the pancreas.[15] A number of observations, however, have challenged this interpretation. Many investigators have noted that tumours within lymph nodes (with or without an identifiable primary) can be resected for long-term cure (Table 36.2).[38–41] We have shown that the survival of patients with tumour in lymph nodes is no different from those patients who, for example, have an isolated pancreatic or duodenal tumour or in whom a tumour has never been found (Figure 36.3).[42] These findings are in marked contrast to patients with gastrinoma tumours in the liver.[42,43] Pathologists studying gastrinomas found within lymph nodes have identified certain histological features (dense capsule, cystic changes, hyalinized stroma) which suggest that these tumours resemble ectopic inclusions within lymph nodes (i.e. nodal tumours), rather than metastatic disease.[44] Furthermore, heterotopic pancreatic tissue has been identified in peripancreatic lymph nodes,[45] and chromogranin-positive cells (neuroendocrine differentiation) have been found in regional peripancreatic lymph nodes.[46] Using the ventral bud theory, it seems possible that gastrin-producing (gastrinoma) precursor cells from the migrating ventral pancreatic bud become ectopically located within lymph node tissue (embryonic rests) which later develop into gastrinomas within lymph nodes. Similarly, the occurrence of extrapancreatic tumours (outside the pancreatic substance) but within the gastrinoma triangle (area of ventral bud migration) can be explained by a similar mechanism.

In summary, both the clinical and pathological characteristics of gastrinomas are best explained by a theory of ventral pancreatic bud derivation. This theory not only provides insight into the ontogeny of gastrinomas but is also a useful construct to assist the surgeon in identifying tumours at operation and excising them for cure.

INVESTIGATION

Historically, the Zollinger–Ellison syndrome was diagnosed by identifying gastric acid hypersecretion in patients with ulcer disease. The two most useful techniques for quantitating excess acid were the basal secretory rate,[47] and the ratio of basal to maximally stimulated acid secretion.[48] Basal acid outputs that

Table 36.2 Compilation of retrospective cases of lymph node removal resulting in long-term cure

REFERENCE	n	NO. OF LYMPH NODES	ANATOMICAL LOCATION	PRIMARY TUMOUR	FOLLOW-UP (MONTHS)
Thompson et al.[39]	4	1	Peripancreatic	ND	72
	5	1	Peripancreatic	ND	24
Bornman et al.[41]	2	1	Uncinate	ND	60
	3	1	Ligament of Treitz	Yes	43
Delcore et al.[38]	—	1	Peripancreatic	ND	317
	—	1	Peripancreatic	ND	99
	—	1	Pancreatic neck	ND	24
Stabile and Passaro[42]	—	1	Peripancreatic	ND	99
	—	3	Peripancreatic	ND	72
	—	2	Peripancreatic	Yes	94
Friesen[116]	—	1	—	ND	36
	—	1	—	ND	216
	—	1	—	Yes	36
	—	2	—	Yes	72

ND, not detected.

exceeded 15 mmol/h in unoperated patients or 5 mmol/h in patients who had had an ulcer operation or a basal to maximal acid output ratio (BAO:MAO) greater than 0.6 were considered diagnostic.[48] These tests had minor problems, such as technical difficulties in performing them correctly and the fact that they were unpleasant for the patient. The major drawback, however, was their lack of sensitivity and specificity in discriminating between patients with gastrinomas and those with ordinary peptic ulcer disease.[49–51]

The development of the gastrin RIA in 1973 allowed the direct measurement of the peptide hormone elaborated by the tumour.[52] As expected, most patients with gastrinomas were found to have raised fasting serum gastrin level.[53] However, as experience with the gastrin RIA grew, it became apparent that fasting serum gastrin levels were not specific for gastrinoma and were found to be elevated with other diseases (Table 36.3). Furthermore, some patients with gastrinoma had normal serum gastrin concentrations and serum gastrin levels in individual patients were found to fluctuate widely from day to day. For these reasons, an elevated random serum gastrin level in the appropriate clinical setting is suggestive but not diagnostic of a gastrinoma.[54]

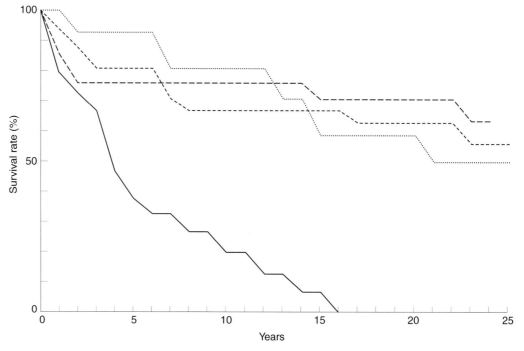

Figure 36.3
Life table analysis of survival curve for patients with gastrinoma who were followed for 25 years. ·······, No tumour found (n =10); ------, lymph node (n =16); – – – – –, pancreatic/duodenal (n = 14); ———, hepatic (n = 15; P < 0.05).

Table 36.3 Disease states associated with hypergastrinaemia

Increased gastric acid production
    Zollinger–Ellison syndrome
    Antral G-cell hyperfunction
    Antral G-cell hyperplasia
    Gastric outlet obstruction
    Retained excluded gastric antrum syndrome (REAS)
    Renal failure
    Short gut syndrome
Normal or decreased acid production
    Pernicious anaemia
    Chronic gastritis
    Vagotomy
    Gastric malignancy

Fortunately, provocative tests were soon discovered. It was found that the intravenous administration of secretin, calcium or bombesin can cause a gastrinoma to release gastrin.[55-57] In addition, the specificity of these agents in releasing gastrin only from tumour cells provided excellent discrimination between patients with gastrinoma and those with other forms of hypergastrinaemia. The secretin stimulation test, due to its excellent sensitivity, specificity and ease of administration, has become the provocative test of choice for diagnosis.[58,59]

As a test, 2 units/kg body weight of secretin (Kabi) is administered by rapid (bolus) intravenous infusion. Blood samples for gastrin assay are taken at 5 minutes before the intravenous secretin dose (basal) and then 1, 2, 5, 10, 20 and 30 minutes thereafter (stimulated).[48] A rapid increase in serum gastrin of greater than 200 pg/ml over basal level has become the standard criterion for making the diagnosis.[60]

There are two diseases that it is particularly important to distinguish from gastrinoma: retained excluded gastric antrum syndrome (REAS) and primary G-cell hyperplasia (Table 36.4). The retained gastric antrum syndrome is a rare condition. These patients have undergone a partial gastrectomy and Billroth II reconstruction in which antral mucosa, containing gastrin-producing G cells, remains in the proximal duodenal stump that has now become the afferent limb of the gastro-intestinal tract reconstruction.[61] Because these antral G cells are excluded from the acid stream, the normal inhibitory effect of a lowered intraluminal pH on gastrin release is lost. This results in persistent hypergastrinaemia and acid hypersecretion.[48] The clinical presentation of these patients is very similar to that of patients with gastrinoma. They have persistent ulcer disease refractory to standard medical therapy, with gastric acid hypersecretion and

hypergastrinaemia. These patients are distinguished from those with gastrinoma by always having a previous ulcer operation with Billroth II reconstruction, and by not responding to intravenous secretin.[62] Unlike a gastrin-producing tumour, the retained antral mucosa does not release gastrin when secretin is given.

Primary antral G-cell hyperplasia is also a rare syndrome which produces hypergastrinaemia.[63] This hypergastrinaemia and the resulting gastric acid hypersecretion occurs as a consequence of an increased number of gastrin-producing G cells (hyperplasia) in the gastric antrum. These patients are distinguished from those with gastrinoma on the basis of two clinical tests. In patients with primary G-cell hyperplasia, there is a marked rise in serum gastrin concentration following direct stimulation of the increased G-cell mass in the antrum by a test meal. Patients with gastrinoma do not have this increase.[48] In addition, patients with antral G-cell hyperplasia do not have an increase in serum gastrin level after the administration of intravenous secretin.[60] Antral G-cell hyperplasia is conclusively diagnosed by endoscopy and antral biopsy, which reveals the characteristic G-cell hyperplasia. The treatment of this syndrome is antrectomy, which results in a decreased serum gastrin concentration and cure of the disease.

Before the introduction of the gastrin RIA, an upper gastrointestinal barium examination was helpful in diagnosing the Zollinger–Ellison syndrome.[64] The findings were quite characteristic as the hypersecretory state produced increased gastric juice, seen on initial flow of barium into the stomach.[65] There were also large gastric rugal folds, particularly in the body and fundus of the stomach, which reflected the massive parietal cell hyperplasia which occurred as a consequence of persistent gastrin stimulation.[64] Dilatation of the duodenum and proximal jejunum with oedematous mucosal folds was also occasionally seen.[66] A flocculated granular appearance to the barium, produced by the low intraluminal pH, was noted. Ulcers found in unusual locations, such as the distal duodenum or proximal jejunum, were highly suggestive of the Zollinger–Ellison syndrome but currently these findings are extremely rare. It should be emphasized that, because patients are being diagnosed earlier in the course of their disease as a result of the gastrin RIA and provocative tests, these classic radiological findings in the upper gastrointestinal tract are much less common. Radiographic imaging techniques have therefore shifted from use as diagnostic aids to the preoperative localization of tumours (Table 36.5).

Abdominal ultrasonography, one of the first modalities used

Table 36.4 Diagnostic tests in the differentiation of gastrinoma from retained excluded antrum syndrome (REAS) and primary G-cell hyperplasia (PGCH)

TEST	GASTRINOMA	REAS	PGCH
Fasting hypergastrinaemia	+++	+++	+
Basal acid output	++	++	+
Secretin stimulation test	+++	−	−
Test meal	−	−	+++

Table 36.5 Sensitivity and specificity of radiographic imaging techniques used for the localization of gastrinomas

| TECHNIQUE | HEPATIC METASTASES | | PRIMARY TUMOUR | |
	SENSITIVITY (%)	SPECIFICITY (%)	SENSITIVITY (%)	SPECIFICITY (%)
Ultrasonography	14	—	21	92
Computed tomography	72	98	59	95
Angiography	86	100	68	94
Portal venous sampling	—	—	73	33

for gastrinoma localization, detected pancreatic tumours in only 14–28% of patients.[67,68] Recent studies have substantiated this low sensitivity. Abdominal wall thickness, air within the gastrointestinal tract and other technical factors have limited the usefulness of this technique.[68] Ultrasonography may be more useful intraoperatively as an adjunct to the manual palpation of the pancreas.[69,70] Intraoperative ultrasonography may be helpful, not only for identifying small intrapancreatic tumours but also in delineating a relationship of such tumours to the pancreatic duct and major vascular structures.[70]

Computed tomography (CT) was initially reported to be unreliable in the preoperative localization of gastrinomas.[71,72] However, newer generation CT scanners with improved spatial resolution and the development of rapid (bolus) intravenous contrast administration have improved the imaging sensitivity markedly.[73] Currently, gastrinomas are identified preoperatively by CT in 40–59% of cases.[73,74] CT has proven to be particularly useful for the preoperative detection of hepatic tumours. When used solely for this purpose, the sensitivity of CT increases to 62% and its specificity increases to 98%.[74] In certain situations selective angiography of the pancreas is a useful technique for demonstrating the presence of gastrinomas. Although initial series and individual case reports indicated a great deal of success with this technique,[75,76] the results from other series were less encouraging.[77,78] In the largest, most well-controlled study to date, Maton et al.[79] reported a sensitivity of 68% and specificity of 94% for extrahepatic gastrinomas and a sensitivity of 86% and specificity of 100% for hepatic gastrinomas.

Percutaneous transhepatic portal venous sampling (PVS) was recently introduced for the preoperative localization of gastrinomas and other tumours that secrete endocrine products. Its basis is the selective catheterization and blood sampling of different venous branches draining the pancreas. One looks for an increase or 'step up' in serum gastrin concentration. A moderate increase (>100 mg/dl) suggests the presence of a gastrinoma in the area of the pancreas drained by the venous branch. Success rates of 73–90% have been reported using PVS.[80,81] Unfortunately there are two major drawbacks which limit the usefulness of PVS for preoperative localization of gastrinomas. One is the high degree of technical competence and standardization that is needed in order to obtain meaningful results from this difficult technique.[81] The second is the low specificity (33% in the series from the NIH) of this technique, with the majority of false-positive results occurring in the region of the pancreatic head.[68] As has been discussed previously, this is the region (gastrinoma triangle) in which the great majority of pancreatic tumours are likely to be found. Consequently, we feel that, at its current level of development, it is unlikely that PVS offers any advantage over a careful intra-abdominal exploration.

Endoscopic ultrasonography (EUS) is a powerful tool to localize small pancreatic endocrine tumours. In one collaborative multi-institutional study, EUS was able to localize 32 of 39 pancreatic endocrine tumours (82% sensitivity) and among 19 control patients without tumours, EUS was negative in 18 (95% specificity).[82] In some institutions, EUS is not only capable of imaging the pancreas, but has also been effective in identifying

tumours within the duodenal wall and peripancreatic lymph nodes, areas traditionally difficult to image by any radiographic technique.[83]

The most recent, and potentially the most powerful imaging technique for preoperative localization of pancreatic endocrine tumours is octreotide scintigraphy. This technique involves injection of an indium-labelled probe ((^{111}In-DTPA-D-Phe1)-octreotide) which binds to somatostatin receptor-positive endocrine tumours, and the distribution of this isotope–receptor binding is visualized with a gamma camera.[84] Octreoscan scintigraphy provides improved preoperative localization, particularly of extrapancreatic and lymph node gastrinomas, compared to all other currently available imaging techniques.[85,86]

CURRENT TREATMENT CONCEPTS

Up to 30% of patients with gastrinoma have multiple endocrine neoplasia type I (MEN–I) syndrome.[87] These patients develop hyperplasia and/or tumour formation in several endocrine glands, including the pituitary, parathyroid and pancreas.[88] Patients with the MEN-I syndrome can usually be identified by a family history of parathyroid or pituitary tumours. Screening tests for hyperparathyroidism are also useful in identifying this subgroup of patients as they often develop hyperparathyroidism before the development of symptoms from their pancreatic endocrine tumour.[89] In patients with the MEN syndrome and gastrinomas, parathyroid hyperplasia is the most common (88%) associated endocrine abnormality.[78,89,90] In those patients without a suggestive family history or clinical evidence of hyperparathyroidism in whom the diagnosis of MEN-I is still suspected, we have found the serum prolactin level to be another sensitive test to aid in the establishment of the diagnosis of MEN-I syndrome.[91] Prolactin-secreting pituitary adenomas are found in 16–65% of patients.[78,89,90] Although not classically described as a component of the MEN-I syndrome, adrenal medullary involvement (phaeochromocytomas) has been noted in 9–19% of patients with a gastrinoma and the MEN-I syndrome.[78,90,92]

The clinical importance of identifying patients with gastrinoma who have the MEN I syndrome cannot be overemphasized as the effectiveness of surgical exploration for cure in this group of patients is controversial.[93,94] Based on histological observations,[95] PVS sampling data[96] and reported surgical experiences,[42,89,97,98] patients with the MEN-I syndrome have multiple, small duodenal and pancreatic tumours as well as islet cell hyperplasia. Both surgical and autopsy data suggest that whereas the duodenal and lymph node tumours in patients with the MEN I syndrome display gastrin immunoreactivity, the endocrine tumours found within the pancreas of these patients do not.[93,99] These observations imply that an aggressive attack on the duodenal and lymph node tumour in patients with MEN I may result in a higher surgical cure rate.[99] A recent prospective trial to address this issue studied ten patients with MEN I and the Zollinger–Ellison syndrome, all of whom were operated on for complete tumour removal, focusing primarily on small duodenal tumours and peripancreatic lymph nodes.[94] Despite an exhaustive and diligent search with multiple tumour excisions by experienced endocrine surgeons, no patient in this series had a long-term biochemical cure.[94] Total pancreatectomy has been done in a select subset of patients in whom pancreatic gastrinomas were considered malignant and had caused a high morbidity and mortality within the patients' immediate families.[100] Although the results from this small series of patients are good, total pancreatectomy cannot be generally adopted as a treatment modality for gastrinomas in most patients with the MEN-I syndrome because of the significant morbidity and mortality associated with this procedure. The ultimate role of surgical exploration and tumour resection in patients with MEN I and the Zollinger–Ellison syndrome remains unclear. Until the surgical approach can be more clearly defined, aggressive treatment of the peptic ulcer disease remains the primary focus of therapy in these patients.[11]

Despite the limitations of tumour resection for cure, surgical intervention in patients with the MEN-I syndrome is often helpful when directed at tumours which develop in the associated endocrine glands outside the pancreas. For example, in those patients with parathyroid hyperplasia and hyperparathyroidism, early parathyroidectomy can facilitate the control of gastric acid hypersecretion and increase the responsiveness of these patients to antisecretory medications.[101] Likewise, the removal of an associated prolactinoma by trans-sphenoidal hypophysectomy is occasionally useful in relieving visual symptoms that are caused by its compression of the optic chiasm.

Patients with gastrinoma and hepatic metastases should currently be treated medically. Apart from a few isolated reports in the literature, patients with hepatic metastases die from tumour progression with little chance for curative resection.[42,97,98,101] An interesting study investigating the efficacy of aggressive surgical debulking and metastatic tumour removal in this group of patients has been carried out at the National Institute of Health in Bethesda, Maryland.[102] Complete surgical resection of all identifiable tumour and postoperative chemotherapy with streptozotocin, doxorubicin and fluorouracil was the treatment protocol used. Complete resection of all identifiable tumour was possible in four of five cases attempted. In the four patients resected, there was a significant decrease in the amount of antisecretory medication needed to control their symptoms, and three of the four patients have no detectable tumour on follow-up. Two of the four patients are clinically and biochemically cured, with a normal fasting gastrin level and negative provocative tests at 14 and 32 months, respectively. Although these initial results are encouraging, further evaluation will be needed before this approach can be routinely adopted.

Systemic chemotherapy using streptozotocin and 5-fluorouracil, with or without doxorubicin, has been reported to be effective in decreasing the size of metastatic tumour in 50–70% of patients evaluated.[103,104] Octreotide (Sandostatin, Sandoz Pharmaceuticals, East Hanover, NJ) is a synthetic octapeptide with a structure and activity similar to somatostatin but a significantly longer half-life (90 minutes) and duration of action (8 hours).[105] Experimental work in animals showed inhibition of endocrine cell tumour growth in these systems through an, as yet, unknown mechanism.[106,107] This groundwork led to

experimental trials in humans where an analysis of several studies and case reports at an NIH conference supported this antiproliferative effect on endocrine tumour growth.[108] In a subgroup of 68 patients with gastreoenteropancreatic (GEP) tumours followed for at least 3 months, partial tumour regression was observed in 4.4%, stable disease was identified in 50%, and tumour progression was seen in 45%.[109] Unfortunately, this modest response rate in metastatic disease decreases over time. Caution must be exercised in interpreting these results as they are early reports which are small, lack consistent protocols and dosages, and suffer from insufficient follow-up. In addition to chemotherapy, hepatic artery embolization, hormonal therapy and treatment with interferon-α have also been advocated as effective treatments for controlling metastatic disease based on the results from preliminary reports.[110-112] Further trials are needed before the exact role of these therapies for widespread disease is known.

Clearly there is currently no good therapy for patients with hepatic metastases or for the rare patient with widely metastatic disease (bone, skin). Therefore, we would recommend that patients with hepatic metastases should not be operated on for tumour excision. The advent of improved radiographic imaging techniques, such as CT and angiography, have increased the sensitivity of the detection of patients with hepatic metastases preoperatively. Once they have been identified, a liver biopsy for tissue diagnosis is made and these patients are offered the option of entering into a specific chemotherapeutic protocol or are treated with standard medical therapy aimed at controlling their peptic ulcer disease.

SURGICAL TREATMENT

As with most other endocrine tumours, the ideal treatment of gastrinoma is surgical excision for cure.[11,92] Surgical cure in gastrinoma is defined as resection of all tumour such that the patient is eugastrinaemic, has a negative secretin stimulation test, requires no antisecretory medications and has no tumour recurrence on long-term follow-up. Surgical cure rates for gastrinoma were historically reported to be in the range 2–5%.[12,18,48,51,53,92] These data were generated from the results of early retrospective series and encompassed all patients with the diagnosis of gastrinoma. As a result, these values represent gross (overall) cure rates, which included both those patients with MEN-I syndrome and those with hepatic metastases, who we now know to be unlikely candidates for curative resection. Perhaps a more meaningful cure rate would be one which is derived from those patients with the more common sporadic gastrinoma who are candidates for curative resection. By utilizing this patient population (candidates for cure), several recent retrospective series have reported a collective cure rate of 30%.[17,97,113,114] Based on our recent experience, we feel that prospectively this cure rate may be much higher.[115]

All patients with sporadic gastrinoma without evidence of hepatic metastases should be offered surgical exploration for tumour excision and cure. There are several recent advances which have made a major impact on our ability to operate on patients with gastrinoma for cure. They are improved patient selection, knowledge of tumour location and detailed information of the natural history of gastrinoma within lymph nodes.

As mentioned above, there are two subgroups of patients with gastrinoma who are unlikely to be cured by current surgical techniques: patients with hepatic metastases and patients with the MEN-I syndrome without localized, identifiable tumour. Both of these groups can be accurately identified preoperatively, spared an unnecessary laparotomy and treated by other therapeutic options, such as those outlined above.

It was previously held that the identification of a gastrinoma at operation was difficult, being successful in only 41–90% of reported cases, depending on the surgeon's experience.[116,117] Currently it appears that the majority of tumours identified are small, extrapancreatic in location and occult within lymph nodes (Table 36.6). Gastrinomas are located predominantly in a discrete anatomical area within the abdomen (the gastrinoma triangle). In our own experience with 78 tumours, 88% were located in this area.[33] It should be emphasized, however, that this experience is not unique. In a recent review of 165 tumours from the surgical literature, we found that 75% were located within the gastrinoma triangle.[37] Of particular interest is the fact that, of those tumours which are most difficult to locate (i.e. extrapancreatic/extraintestinal and occult within lymph nodes), all were located within the triangle. These data suggest that, even in the absence of positive radiographic imaging, up to 90% of identified gastrinomas can be found by careful surgical exploration in a specific intra-abdominal location.

Lymph node "metastases" are identified in approximately 40% of patients with gastrinoma. As has been mentioned previously, the clinical course of these patients is benign.[38,42] Patients with tumour in lymph nodes do not go on to develop hepatic metastases or widespread disease, and their overall life expectancy is no different from those patients in whom a

tumour has never been found. Based on these clinical observations and the benign pathological appearance of these tumours, we suggest that patients with tumour within lymph nodes are candidates for abdominal exploration and attempts at curative resection.

Our current approach is to offer abdominal exploration in selected patients after a course of medical therapy arbitrarily set at 1 year. This allows us time to assess the patient's response to histamine H_2-receptor antagonists as well as their compliance with a strict medical regimen. This information is important intraoperatively when a decision needs to be made concerning a total gastrectomy.

Since approximately 75–90% of tumours and virtually all occult tumours are found in the gastrinoma triangle, the exploration is specifically directed at that area. Beginning at the superior aspect of the triangle, the cystic duct and common duct are identified and the portahepatis is carefully examined. All lymph nodes found in this area are removed and submitted for frozen section. The lesser sac is then widely opened by detaching the gastric omentum from the transverse colon outside the gastroepiploic arcades. The head of the gland is completely mobilized using a generous Kocher manoeuvre (Figure 36.4). By incising the retroperitoneum along the inferior margin of the pancreas, access is gained to the avascular plane lying dorsal to the gland and the body and tail of the gland can be thoroughly examined. Using direct visualization and bimanual palpation, the entire pancreas and duodenum are carefully examined and all palpable masses are meticulously excised and submitted for frozen section histological examination. All regional lymph nodes found within the triangle are excised and submitted for frozen section histology (Figure 36.5). Ultrasonography may be useful intraoperatively as an adjunct to manual palpation for the localization of small intrapancreatic tumours.[118] Again we emphasize that tumours within the pancreatic substance are relatively uncommon, being found in less than 10% of patients in our own series. If no tumour is found in the area of the gastrinoma triangle, the greater and lesser omenta are systematically searched. The splenic hilum, coeliac root and root of the mesentery are also explored for tumour. The duodenum down to the ligament of Treitz are inspected by operative endoscopic transillumination and carefully palpated for evidence of small duodenal adenomas.[119]

In those patients in whom a duodenal wall adenoma is suspected, exploration is performed through a longitudinal pyloroduodenotomy. The entire duodenal wall is thoroughly examined by palpation between the index finger intramurally and the thumb extramurally. If a lesion is discovered, it is excised with a full-thickness margin of normal duodenum. In most instances the longitudinal pyloroduodenotomy is reconstructed anatomically unless a total gastrectomy is also carried out.

The majority of tumours can be enucleated or excised locally. Rarely, in patients who are appropriate operative candidates with an otherwise curable tumour located deep in the head of the pancreas or duodenum which cannot be adequately excised locally, a pancreaticoduodenectomy of the Whipple type is performed.[120]

Table 36.6 Operative findings based on the collective analysis of 165 tumours in 155 patients from the surgical literature[37]

FINDING	%
Tumour location	
Peripancreatic	29
Duodenum	15
Pancreas	
Head	35
Body	8
Tail	13
No. of tumours found	
1	65
2	18
3	11
>3	5
Disease outside the pancreas	
Hepatic	17
Lymph node	28
Tumour size	
Mean:	2.9 cm
Range:	0.3–15 cm

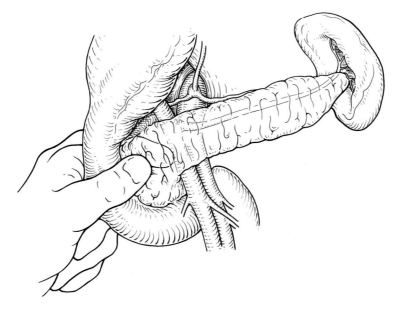

Figure 36.4
Manual intraoperative palpation of the pancreatic head after a generous Kocher manuoeuvre has freed up the posterior pancreatic head and duodenum from their dorsal attachments.

One caveat that we have learned from our own experience is that when gastrinomas are found they are usually identified early in the operative exploration, commonly within the first hour. Conversely, we have found that continued exploration after 2–3 hours does not seem to improve the likelihood of tumour identification and simply increases the risk of complications from the surgical procedure. In those patients in whom a tumour cannot be identified or who are found to have hepatic metastases intraoperatively, precluding curative resection, the decision is made as to whether or not to perform a total gastrectomy.

The role for total gastrectomy in treating patients with gastrinoma has changed rapidly since the introduction of the histamine H_2-receptor antagonists. Currently, the use of a total gastrectomy is limited to those patients who are refractory to maximal drug therapy or are non-compliant with their medical regimen. Although parietal cell vagotomy has been shown to be effective initially in the treatment of patients with gastrinoma,[117] the possibility that medication requirements will increase over time, uncertainty of the recurrence rates, and the subsequent difficulty in performing a total gastrectomy for those patients who are treatment failures argue against its routine use.

The technique that we use for total gastrectomy is similar to that described by Zollinger and Zollinger in their surgical atlas.[121] The stomach is removed and the continuity of the gut is restored by means of end-to-end or end-to-side retrocolic Roux-en-Y oesophagojejunostomy. An end-to-side oesophagojejunostomy with distal jejunojejunostomy (Braun procedure) should not be used because of the high incidence of postoperative alkaline oesophageal reflux.[122]

When performing a total gastrectomy in patients with gastrinoma, a few technical points bear emphasis. If the duodenum is diseased or thickly scarred it should be closed with sutures instead of staples.[78] In these instances, when the integrity of the duodenal closure is questioned, the use of an indwelling duodenal catheter is strongly advised.[123] The isolated jejunal limb which is used for Roux-en-Y reconstruction should be more than 45 cm in length to prevent bile reflux into the oesophagus.

Based on early studies, before the effective medical control of acid hypersecretion, the reported operative mortality for total gastrectomy in patients with gastrinoma was 15%.[15] More recently, however, with the introduction of histamine H_2-receptor antagonists, the mortality rate for total gastrectomy in patients with gastrinoma is 5–6%. If one excludes those patients operated on emergently, the operative mortality drops to 2.4%.[78]

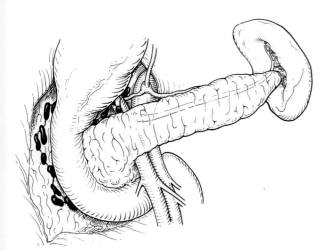

Figure 36.5
Location of peripancreatic lymph nodes around the head of the pancreas where the great majority of occult gastrinomas are found.

We have reported the results of surgical exploration in 15 patients who were operated on prospectively for cure.[115] Two of the patients had MEN type I syndrome and two patients had hepatic metastases and thus were excluded from the study. All 11 patients with sporadic gastrinoma underwent exploration with the sole intent of tumour localization and removal for cure. Of those 11 patients, tumour was found in ten (91%). Three patients had tumours located in the pancreatic head, three in the duodenum, and four were in extrapancreatic extraintestinal locations. All tumours identified were within the gastrinoma triangle, and all were easily excised without a pancreatic resection. Multiple tumours were found in 40% of patients, and there was lymph node involvement in 64%. Nine of 11 patients (82%) have been cured (eugastrinaemic, asymptomatic of antisecretory medications, and do not respond to secretin stimulation) after a median follow-up of 15 months (Table 36.7). Based on these initial results, we suspect the cure rate for gastrinoma excision prospectively, in appropriate candidates, is much higher than previously appreciated.

Table 36.7 Biochemical analysis of 11 patients in the authors' own series in which gastrinoma excision for cure was attempted

PATIENT	PREOP. SERUM GASTRIN (pg/ml)	POSTOP SERUM GASTRIN (pg/ml)	POSTOP SECRETIN TEST	FOLLOW-UP (MONTHS)
1	3858	84	–	78
2	176	74	–	43
3	1100	99	–	21
4	196	55	–	18
5	1568	88	–	17
6	190	46	–	15
7	3131	434	+	13
8	2605	95	–	13
9	1428	74	–	12
10	5494	63	–	8
11	1100	875	+	1

MEDICAL TREATMENT

The control of acid hypersecretion, diarrhoea and ulcer symptoms is the main goal of medical therapy in the treatment of patients with gastrinoma. The medical control of acid hypersecretion also plays an essential role in the preoperative preparation and perioperative management of patients who undergo exploration and gastrinoma excision for cure. Adequate control of gastric acid hypersecretion has been achieved with a number of drugs, including cimetidine,[104,124] ranitidine,[125] famotidine[126,127] and omeprazole.[128,129] Patients with gastrinoma typically require a large amount of medication for adequate control of their acid hypersecretion. For example, the mean dose of cimetidine currently given to patients in one large series was 4.6 g/day, with some patients requiring up to 10 g/day for adequate acid control.[48] Equivalently large doses of medication have been required in patients treated with ranitidine, famotidine and omeprazole.[125,126,129] In addition to these large initial dosages, increasing dosage requirements necessitating frequent medication adjustments are needed over time. Most patients require an increase in the dosage of their medication at least twice a year.[125–127] For those drugs which have short half-lives, such as cimetidine and ranitidine, the addition of an anticholinergic agent is usually required for optimal therapeutic effect.[124]

In all patients treated medically, strict criteria for the objective assessment of a reduction in gastric hypersecretion must be followed.[130] One reliable criterion that has been used is a reduction in the amount of the gastric acid produced to less than 10 mmol/h in patients with intact stomachs, and a reduction to less than 5 mmol/h in patients with previous acid-reducing operations.[131] Frequent endoscopy (every 6–12 months) and gastric acid analysis is essential in this patient population as the subjective assessment of symptoms is often misleading.[132] We found that the majority of medical treatment failures in our own practice were uncovered by routine endoscopy. These patients had persistent or recurrent ulceration despite treatment with an H_2-receptor antagonist which alleviated their symptoms. Histamine H_2-receptor antagonists are particularly effective in alleviating symptoms but are less effective in controlling mucosal damage and ulcer formation.

Despite the initial success of histamine H_2-receptor antagonists, it has been our experience, and that of others, that the long-term failure rates of cimetidine can be as high as 50%.[133–135] In addition, with the large doses of cimetidine required, up to 50% of men will develop impotence, gynaecomastia or breast tenderness due to the antiandrogenic effects of this drug.[136] Although ranitidine, famotidine and omeprazole lack this antiandrogenic side-effect, failure rates as high as 40% for ranitidine and 7.5% for omeprazole have been reported.[137] Omeprazole, an H^+, K^+-ATPase inhibitor, has been heralded as the drug of choice for patients with gastrinoma. This was due primarily to initial studies which showed its potency, long duration of action (greater than 48 h) and effectiveness at a constant dose over a prolonged period of time.[128,129] Despite early reports of two patients found to have carcinoid tumours of the stomach after long-term antisecretory treatment with omeprazole,[138] these initial concerns have not been borne out during long-term use.[139] Lansoprazole, a new substituted benzimidazole H^+ K^+-ATPase inhibitor, is as effective in both the short- and long-term management of patients with the Zollinger–Ellison syndrome as omeprazole.[140]

SUMMARY

The clinical presentation and conceptual paradigm of gastrinoma has changed markedly since its original description by Zollinger and Ellison in 1955. The gastrin RIA has allowed for the early diagnosis of patients with gastrinoma. As a result, tumours are currently found to be smaller, frequently extrapancreatic/extraintestinal in location, occult within lymph nodes and located predominantly within the gastrinoma triangle. The intra-abdominal location and clinical characteristics of gastrinomas (right side of the abdomen, extrapancreatic, occult within lymph nodes) are best explained by a theoretical construct of derivation from the ventral pancreatic bud. From the recent advances in diagnosis and localization of gastrinomas, we anticipate that surgical cure rates in the future will be much higher than has previously been appreciated.

REFERENCES

1. Banting FG & Best CH. The internal secretion of the pancreas. *J Lab Clin Med* 1922; **7**: 251–266.
2. Harris S. Hyperinsulinism and dysinsulinism. *JAMA* 1924; **83**: 729–733.
3. Wilder RM, Allan FN, Power MH & Robertson HE. Carcinoma of the islands of the pancreas. Hyperinsulinism and hypoglycemia. *JAMA* 1927; **89**: 348–355.
4. Kaplin EL, Arganini M & Kang S-J. Diagnosis and treatment of hypolycemic disorders. *Surg Clin North Am* 1987; **67**: 395–410.
5. Seiler S & Zinninger MM. Massive islet cell tumor of the pancreas without hypoglycemia. *Surg Gynecol Obstet* 1946; **82**: 301–305.
6. Brown CH, Neville WE & Hazard JB. Islet cell adenoma without hypoglycemia causing duodenal obstruction. *Surgery* 1950; **27**: 616–619.
7. Forty R & Barrett GM. Peptic ulceration of the third part of the duodenum associated with islet cell tumors. *Br J Surg* 1952; **40**: 60–63.
8. Zollinger RM & Ellison EH. Primary peptic ulceration of the jejunum associated with islet cell tumors of the pancreas. *Ann Surg* 1955; **142**: 709–728.
9. Gregory RA, Tracy HJ, Fench JM & Sircus N. Extraction of a gastrin-like substance from a pancreatic tumor in a case of Zollinger–Ellison syndrome. *Lancet* 1960; **i**: 1045.
10. Grossman MI. Gastrointestinal hormones: some thoughts about clinical applications. *Scand J Gastroenterol* 1972; **7**: 97–104.
11. Wolfe MM & Jensen RT. Zollinger–Ellison syndrome: current concepts in diagnosis and management. *N Engl J Med* 1987; **317**: 1200–1209.
12. McCarthy DM. The place of surgery in the Zollinger–Ellison syndrome. *N Engl J Med* 1980; **302**: 1344–1347.
13. Ellison EH & Wilson SD. Ulcerogenic tumor of the pancreas. *Proc Clin Cancer* 1967; **3**: 225–244.
14. Wilson SD. The role of surgery in children with the Zollinger–Ellison syndrome. *Surgery* 1982; **92**: 682–692.
15. Ellison EH & Wilson SD. The Zollinger–Ellison syndrome: reappraisal and evaluation of 260 registered cases. *Ann Surg* 1964; **160**: 512–530.
16. Isenberg JI, Walsh JH & Grossman MI. Zollinger–Ellison syndrome. *Gastroenterology* 1973; **65**: 140–165.
17. Ellison EC, Carey LC, Sparks J et al. Early surgical treatment of gastrinoma. *Am J Med* 1987; **82**(5B): 17–21.
18. Deveney CW, Deveney KS & Way LW. The Zollinger–Ellison syndrome 23 years later. *Ann Surg* 1978; **188**: 384–393.
19. McCarthy DM. Zollinger–Ellison syndrome. *Annu Rev Med* 1982; **33**: 197–215.
20. Deconinck JF. The ultrastructure of the human pancreatic islet. *Diabetologia* 1971; **7**: 266–282.
21. Larsson LI & Sunder F. Pancreatic polypeptide a postulated new hormone. *Diabetologia* 1976; **12**: 211–226.
22. Gregory RA, Grossman MI, Tracey HJ & Bentley PH. Nature of the gastric secretagogue in the Zollinger–Ellison tumors. *Lancet* 1967; **ii**: 543–544.
23. Erlandsen SL & Hegre OD. Pancreatic islet cell hormone distribution of cell types in the islet and evidence for the presence of somatostatin and gastrin within the D cells. *J Histochem Cytochem* 1976; **24**: 883–897.
24. Polak JM. A growth-hormone release-inhibiting hormone in gastrointestinal and pancreatic D cells. *Lancet* 1975; **i**: 1220–1222.
25. Creutzfield W. Pancreatic endocrine tumors – the riddle of their origin and hormone secretion. *Isr J Med Sci* 1975; **11**: 762–775.
26. Lofstra F. Are gastrin cells present in mammalian pancreatic islets? *Diabetologia* 1974; **10**: 291–297.
27. Robb P. The development of the islets of Langerhans in the human fetus. *QJ Exp Physiol* 1961; **46**: 335–343.
28. Pusyrev AA. The formation of endocrine cells in the human pancreas from epithelium of acini and ducts. *Arkh Anat Histol Embryol* 1979; **1**: 20–25.
29. Pearse AGE. The cytochemical and ultrastructure of polypeptide-hormone producing cells of the APUD series and embryologic, physiologic, and pathologic implications of the concept. *J Histochem Cytochem* 1969; **17**: 303–312.
30. Teitelman G. Transformation of catecholaminergic precursors into glucagon cells in mouse embryonic pancreas. *Proc Natl Acad Sci* 1976; **78**: 5225–5229.
31. Pictet RL, Clark WR, Williams HR & Rutter JW. An ultrastructural analysis of the developing embryonic pancreas. *J Dev Biol* 1972; **29**: 436–467.
32. Malaisse-Lagae F, Stefan Y, Cox J, Perrelet A & Orci L. Identification of a lobe in the adult human pancreas rich in pancreatic polypeptide. *Diabetologia* 1979; **17**: 361–365.
33. Stabile BE, Morrow DJ & Passaro E Jr. The gastrinoma triangle: operative implications. *Am J Surg* 1984; **147**: 25–31.
34. Alumets J, Håkanson R & Sundler F. Ontogeny of endocrine cells in the porcine gut and pancreas: an immunocytochemical study. *Gastroenterology* 1983; **85**: 1359–1372.
35. Orci L, Baetens D, Ravazzola V, Stefan Y & Malaisse-Lagae F. Pancreatic polypeptide and glucagon: nonrandom distribution in pancreatic islets. *Life Sci* 1976; **19**: 1811–1816.
36. Howard TJ, Sawicki M, Lewin KJ et al. Pancreatic polypeptide immunoreactivity in sporadic gastrinoma: relationship to intraabdominal location. *Pancreas* 1995; **11**: 350–356.
37. Howard TJ, Stabile BE, Zinner MJ, Chang S, Bhagavan BS & Passaro E Jr. Anatomic distribution of pancreatic endocrine tumors. *Am J Surg* 1990; **159**: 258–264.
38. Delcore R, Cheung LY & Friesen SR. Outcome of lymph node involvement in patients with Zollinger–Ellison syndrome. *Ann Surg* 1988; **208**: 291–298.
39. Thompson NW, Vinik AI, Eckhauser FE & Strodel WE. Extrapancreatic gastrinomas. *Surgery* 1985; **98**: 113–120.
40. Wolfe MM, Alexander RW & McGuigan JE. Extrapancreatic, extraintestinal gastrinoma: effective treatment by surgery. *N Engl J Med* 1982; **306**: 1533–1536.
41. Bornman PC, Marks IN, Mee AS & Price S. Favourable response to conservative surgery for extrapancreatic gastrinoma with lymph node metastases. *Br J Surg* 1987; **74**: 198–201.
42. Stabile BE & Passaro E Jr. Benign and malignant gastrinoma. *Am J Surg* 1985; **149**: 144–150.
43. Weber HE, Venzon DJ, Lin J-T et al. Determinants of metastatic rate and survival in patients with Zollinger–Ellison syndrome: a prospective long-term study. *Gastroenterology* 1995; **108**: 1637–1649.
44. Bhagavan BS, Slavin RE, Goldberg J & Rao RN. Ectopic gastrinoma and Zollinger–Ellison syndrome. *Hum Pathol* 1986; **17**: 584–592.
45. Murayama H, Kikuchi M, Imai T, Yamamoto Y & Iwata Y. A case of heterotopic pancreas in lymph node. *Virchows Arch* 1978; **377**: 175–179.
46. Perrier ND, Batts KP, Thompson GB, Grant CS & Plummer TB. An immunohistochemical survey for neuroendocrine cells in regional pancreatic lymph nodes: a plausible explanation for primary nodal gastrinomas? *Surgery* 1995; **118**: 957–966.
47. Aoyagi T & Summerskill WHJ. Gastric secretion with ulcerogenic islet cell tumor: importance of basal acid output. *Arch Intern Med* 1966; **117**: 667–672.
48. Jensen RT, Gardener JD, Raufman JP et al. Zollinger–Ellison syndrome: current concepts and management. *Ann Intern Med* 1983; **98**: 59–75.
49. Kaye MD, Rhodes J & Beck P. Gastric secretion in duodenal ulcers with particular reference to the diagnosis of Zollinger–Ellison syndrome. *Gastroenterology* 1970; **58**: 476–481.
50. Regan PT & Malagelada JR. A reappraisal of clinical, roentgenologic, and endoscopic features of the Zollinger–Ellison syndrome. *Mayo Clin Proc* 1978; **53**: 19–23.
51. Thompson JC, Reeder DD, Villar HV & Fender HR. Natural history and experience with diagnosis and treatment of the Zollinger–Ellison syndrome. *Surg Gynecol Obstet* 1975; **140**: 721–739.
52. McGuigan JE & Grieder MH. Immunochemical measurement of elevated levels of gastrin in the serum of patients with pancreatic tumors of the Zollinger–Ellison variety. *N Engl J Med* 1968; **278**: 1308–1313.
53. Stage JG & Stadil F. The clinical diagnosis of the Zollinger–Ellison syndrome. *Scand J Gastroenterol* 1979; **14**(Suppl 53): 79–91.
54. Walsh JH & Grossman MI. Gastrin. *N Engl J Med* 1975; **292**: 1324–1334, 1377–1384.
55. Isenberg JI, Walsh JH, Passaro E Jr et al. Unusual effect of secretion on serum gastrin, serum calcium and gastric acid secretion in a patient with suspected Zollinger–Ellison syndrome. *Gastroenterology* 1972; **62**: 626–629.
56. Passaro E Jr, Basso N & Walsh JH. Calcium challenge in the Zollinger–Ellison syndrome. *Surgery* 1972; **72**: 1–5.
57. Basso N, Lezoche E, Materia A, Passaro E Jr & Speranza V. Studies with bombesin in the Zollinger–Ellison syndrome. *Br J Surg* 1981; **68**: 97–100.

58. Ippoliti AF. Zollinger–Ellison syndrome provocative diagnostic tests. *Ann Intern Med* 1977; **87:** 787–788.

59. Lamers CBHW & Van Tongeren JHM. Comparative study of the value of the calcium, secretin, and meal stimulated increase in serum gastrin to the diagnosis of the Zollinger–Ellison syndrome. *Gut* 1977; **18:** 128–134.

60. McGuigan JE & Wolfe MM. Secretin injection test in the diagnosis of gastrinoma. *Gastroenterology* 1980; **79:** 1324–1331.

61. Van Heerden JA, Bernatz PE & Rovelstad RA. The retained antrum clinical considerations. *Mayo Clin Proc* 1971; **46:** 25–27.

62. Korman MG, Scott DF, Hansky J & Wilson H. Hypergastrinemia due to excluded gastric antrum: a proposed method for differentiation from the Zollinger–Ellison syndrome. *Aust N Z J Med* 1972; **3:** 266–271.

63. Friesen SR & Tomita J. Pseudo-Zollinger–Ellison syndrome: hypergastrinemia, hyperchlorhydria without tumor. *Ann Surg* 1981; **194:** 481–493.

64. Zboralske FW & Amberg JR. Detection of the Zollinger–Ellison syndrome: the radiologist's responsibility. *A J R* 1968; **104:** 529–543.

65. Cope V & Warwick F. The role of radiology in the detection of endocrine tumors of the gastrointestinal tract. *Clin Gastroenterol* 1974; **3:** 621–625.

66. Weber JM, Lewis S & Heasley KH. Observation on small bowel pattern associated with Zollinger-Ellison syndrome. *Am J Roentgenol Radium Ther Nucl Med* 1959; **82:** 973–977.

67. Hancke S. Localization of hormone-producing gastrointestinal tumor by ultrasonic scanning. *Scand J Gastroenterol* 1979; **14**(Suppl 53):115–116.

68. Franker DL & Norton JA. Localization and resection of insulinomas and gastrinomas. *JAMA* 1988; **259:** 3601–3605.

69. Klotter HJ, Ruckert K, Kummerle F & Rothmund M. The use of intraoperative sonography for endocrine tumors of the pancreas. *World J Surg* 1987; **11:** 635–641.

70. Cromack DT, Norton JA, Sigel B et al. The use of high resolution intraoperative ultrasound to localize gastrinomas: an initial report of a prospective study. *World J Surg* 1987; **11:** 648–653.

71. Dunnick NR, Doppman JL, Mills SR & McCarthy DM. Computed tomographic detection of nonbeta pancreatic islet cell tumors. *Radiology* 1980; **135:** 117–120.

72. Dangaard-Pedersen K & Stage JG. CT scanning in patients with the Zollinger–Ellison syndrome and carcinoid syndrome. *Scand J Gastroenterol* 1979; **14:** 117–122.

73. Stark DD, Moss AA, Goldberg HI & Deveney CW. CT of pancreatic islet cell tumors. *Radiology* 1984; **150:** 491–494.

74. Wank SA, Doppman JL, Miller DL et al. Prospective study of the ability of computed axial tomography to localize gastrinoma in patients with Zollinger–Ellison syndrome. *Gastroenterology* 1987; **92:** 905–912.

75. Mortiz M, Kahn PC, Callow AD et al. Unusual clinical manifestations and angiographic findings in a patient with the Zollinger–Ellison syndrome. *Ann Intern Med* 1969; **71:** 1133–1140.

76. Clemett AR & Park WM. Arteriographic demonstration of pancreatic tumor in the Zollinger–Ellison syndrome. *Radiology* 1967; **88:** 32–34.

77. Mills SR Doppman JL, Dunnick NR & McCarthy DM. Evaluation of angiography in Zollinger–Ellison syndrome. *Radiology* 1979; **131:** 317–320.

78. Thompson JC, Lewis BG, Weiner I & Townsend CM. The role of surgery in the Zollinger–Ellison syndrome. *Ann Surg* 1982; **197:** 594–607.

79. Maton PN, Miller DL, Doppman JL et al. Role of selective angiography in the management of patients with Zollinger–Ellison syndrome. *Gastroenterology* 1987; **92:** 913–918.

80. Cherner JA, Doppman JL, Norton JA et al. Selective venous sampling for gastrin to localize gastrinomas. *Ann Intern Med* 1986; **105:** 841–847.

81. Roche A, Raisonnier A & Gillon Savouret MC. Pancreatic venous sampling and arteriography in localizing insulinomas and gastrinomas: procedure and results in 55 cases. *Radiology* 1982; **145:** 621–627.

82. Rösch T, Lightdale CJ, Botet JF et al. Localization of pancreatic endocrine tumors by endoscopic ultrasonography. *N Engl J Med* 1992; **326:** 1721–1726.

83. Lightdale CJ, Botet JF, Woodruff JM & Brennan MF. Localization of endocrine tumors of the pancreas with endoscopic ultrasonography. *Cancer* 1991; **68:** 1815–1820.

84. Zimmer T, Liehr RM, Stötzel U et al. Endoscopic ultrasound (EUS) and somatostatin-receptor-scintigraphy (SRS) for the localization of insulinomas and gastrinomas (abstr.) *Gastroenterology* 1994; **106:** A331.

85. Kvols LK, Brown ML. O'Conner et al. Evaluation of radiolabeled somatostatin analog (e.g. 123I-octreotide) in the detection and localization of carcinoid and islet cell tumors. *Radiology* 1993; **187:** 129–33.

86. Cadiot G, Lebtalin R, Savda L et al. Preoperative detection of duodenal gastrinomas and peripancreatic lymph nodes by somatostatin receptor scintigraphy. *Gastroenterology* 1996; **111:** 845–854.

87. Fox PS, Hoffmann JW, Wilson SD & DeCosse JJ. Surgical management of the Zollinger–Ellison syndrome. *Surg Clin North Am* 1974; **54:** 395–407.

88. Harrison TS & Thompson NW. Multiple endocrine adenomatosis, I and II *Curr Probl Surg* 1975; 1–51.

89. Van Heerden JA, Smith SL & Miller LJ. Management of the Zollinger–Ellison syndrome in patients with multiple endocrine neoplasia type I. *Surgery* 1986; **100:** 971–976.

90. Ballard HS, Frame B & Hartock RJ. Familial multiple endocrine adenoma peptic ulcer complex. *Medicine* 1964; **43:** 481–512.

91. Stabile BE, Passaro E Jr & Carlson HE. Elevated serum prolactin level in the Zollinger–Ellison syndrome. *Arch Surg* 1981; **116:** 449–453.

92. Zollinger RM, Ellison EC, Fabri PJ, Johnson J, Sparks J & Carey LC. Primary peptic ulcerations of the jejunum associated with islet cell tumours: twenty-five year appraisal. *Ann Surg* 1980; **192:** 422–430.

93. Donow C, Pipeleers-Marichal M, Schroder S, Stamm B, Heitz PU & Klopell G. Surgical pathology of gastrinoma: site, size, multicentricity, association with multiple endocrine neoplasia type I, and malignancy. *Cancer* 1991; **68:** 1329–334.

94. MacFarlane MP, Fraker DL, Alexander R, Norton JA, Lubensky I & Jensen RT. Prospective study of surgical resection of duodenal and pancreatic gastrinomas in multiple endocrine neoplasia type I. *Surgery* 1995; **118:** 973–980.

95. Thompson NW, Lloyd RV, Nishiyama RH et al. MEN I pancreas: a histologic and immunohistochemical study. *World J Surg* 1984; **8:** 561–575.

96. Glowniak JV, Shapiro B, Vinik AI, Glaser B, Thompson NW & Cho KJ. Percutaneous transhepatic venous sampling of gastrin. Value in sporadic and familial islet-cell tumors and G-cell hyperfunction. *N Engl J Med* 1982; **307:** 293–297.

97. Norton JA, Doppman JL, Collen MJ et al. Prospective study of gastrinoma localization and resection in patients with Zollinger–Ellison syndrome. *Ann Surg* 1986; **204:** 468–479.

98. Deveney CW, Deveney KE, Stark D, Moss A, Stein S & Way LW. Resection of gastrinomas. *Ann Surg* 1983; **198:** 546–53.

99. Pipeleers-Marichal M, Somers G, Willems G et al. Gastrinomas in the duodenum of patients with multiple endocrine neoplasia type I and the Zollinger–Ellison syndrome. *N Engl J Med* 1990; **322:** 723–727.

100. Tisell LE, Ahlman H, Jansson S & Grimelius L. Total pancreatectomy in the MEN-I syndrome. *Br J Surg* 1988; **75:** 154–157.

101. Norton JA, Cornelius MJ, Doppman JL, Maton PN, Gardner JD & Jensen RT. Effect of parathyroidectomy in patients with hyperparathyroidism, Zollinger–Ellison syndrome, and multiple endocrine neoplasia type I: a prospective study. *Surgery* 1987; **102:** 958–966.

102. Norton JA, Sugarbaker PH, Doppman JD et al. Aggressive resection of metastatic disease in selected patients with malignant gastrinoma. *Ann Surg* 1986; **203:** 352–359.

103. Moertel CG, Hanley JA & Johnson LA. Streptozotocin alone compared with streptozotocin plus fluorouracil in the treatment of advanced islet cell carcinoma. *N Engl J Med* 1980; **303:** 1189–1194.

104. Zollinger RM, Ellison EC, O'Dorisio T & Sparks J. Thirty years' experience with gastrinoma. *World J Surg* 1984; **8:** 427–435.

105. Reichlin S. Somatostatin. *N Engl J Med* 1983; **309:** 1495–1501.

106. Pless J, Bauer W, Briner U & Doepfner W. Chemistry and pharmacology of SMS 201–995, a long-acting octreopetide analogue of somatostatin. *Scand J Gastroenterol* 1986; **119** (Suppl): 54–64.

107. Lamberts SWJ, Reubi J-C, Uiterlinden P et al. Studies on the mechanism of action of the inhibitory effect of the somatostatin analog SMS 201–995 on the growth of the prolactin/adrenocorticotropin-secreting pituitary tumor 7315a. *Endocrinology* 1986; **118:** 2188–2194.

108. Gorden PO, Comi RJ, Maton PN & Go VL. Somatostatin and somatostatin analoque (SMS 201–995) in treatment of hormone-secreting tumors of the pituitary and gastrointestinal tract and non-neoplastic disease of the gut. *Ann Intern Med* 1989; **110:** 35–50.

109. Trautmann ME, Neuhaus C, Lenze H et al. The role of somastostatin analogues in the treatment of enocrine gastrointestinal tumors. *Digestion* 1993; **54** (Suppl 1) 72–75.

110. Carrasco CH, Chuang VP & Wallace S. Apudoma metastatic to the liver: treatment with hepatic artery embolization. *Radiology* 1983; **149:** 79–83.

111. Shepherd JJ & Senator GB. Regression of liver metastases in patients with gastrin–secretin tumor treated with SMS 201–995. *Lancet* 1986; **ii:** 574.

112. Erickson B, Oberg K, Alm G et al. Treatment of malignant endocrine pancreatic tumours with human leukocyte interferon. *Lancet* 1986; **ii:** 1307–1309.
113. Malagelada JR, Edis AJ, Adson MA, Van Heerden JA & Go VLW. Medical and surgical options in the management of patients with gastrinoma. *Gastroenterology* 1983; **84:** 1524–1532.
114. Vogel SB, Wolfe MM, McGuigan JE, Hawkins IF, Howard RJ & Woodward ER. Localization and resection of gastrinomas in Zollinger–Ellison syndrome. *Ann Surg* 1987; **205:** 550–556.
115. Howard TJ, Zinner MJ, Stabile BE & Passaro E Jr. Gastrinoma excision for cure: a prospective analysis. *Ann Surg* 1990; **211:** 9–14.
116. Friesen SR. Treatment of the Zollinger–Ellison syndrome – a twenty-five year assessment. *Am J Surg* 1982; **143:** 331–338.
117. Richardson CT, Peters MN, Feldman M et al. Treatment of Zollinger–Ellison syndrome with exploratory laparotomy, proximal gastric vagotomy, and H$_2$-receptor antagonists. *Gastroenterology* 1985; **89:** 357–367.
118. Norton JA, Cromack DT, Shawker TH et al. Intraoperative ultrasonographic localization of islet cell tumors: a prospective comparison to palpation. *Ann Surg* 1988; **207:** 160–168.
119. Frucht H, Norton JA, London JF et al. Detection of duodenal gastrinomas by operative endoscopic transillumination, a prospective study. *Gastroenterology* 1990; **99:** 1622–1627.
120. Oberhelman HA. Excisional therapy for ulcerogenic tumors of the duodenum. *Arch Surg* 1972; **104:** 447–453.
121. Zollinger RM & Zollinger RM Jr. *Atlas of Surgical Operations*, vol II. New York: MacMillan, 1967.
122. Morrow DJ & Passaro E Jr. Alkaline reflux esophagitis after total gastrectomy. *Am J Surg* 1976; **132:** 287–291.
123. Passaro E Jr & Bircoll M. Internal duodenal decompression. *J Surg Res* 1972; **13:** 97–101.
124. McCarthy DM. Report on the United States experience with cimetidine in the Zollinger–Ellison syndrome and other hypersecretory states. *Gastroenterology* 1978; **74:** 453–458.
125. Collen MJ, Howard JM, McArthur KE et al. Comparison of ranititdine and cimetidine in the treatment of gastric hypersecretion. *Ann Intern Med* 1984; **100:** 52–58.
126. Howard JM, Chremos AN, Collen MJ et al. Famotidine, a new, potent, long-acting histamine H$_2$-receptor antagonist: comparison with cimetidine and ranitidine in the treatment of Zollinger–Ellison syndrome. *Gastroenterology* 1985; **88:** 1026–1033.
127. Vinayek R, Howard JM, Maton PN et al. Famotidine in the therapy of gastric hypersecretory states. *Am J Med* 1986; **81** (Suppl 4B): 49–59.
128. Lamers CBHW, Lind T, Moberg S, Jansen JBMJ & Olbe L. Omeprazole in Zollinger–Ellison syndrome. *N Engl J Med* 1984; **310:** 758–761.
129. Frucht H, Maton PN & Jensen RT. Use of omeprazole in patients with Zollinger–Ellison syndrome. *Dig Dis Sci* 1991; **36:** 394–404.
130. Jensen RT. Basis for failure of cimetidine in patients with Zollinger–Ellison syndrome. *Dig Dis Sci* 1984; **29:** 363–366.
131. Maton PN, Frucht H, Vinayek R, Wand SA, Gardner JD & Jensen RT. Medical management of patients with Zollinger–Ellison syndrome who have had previous gastric surgery: a prospective study. *Gastroenterology* 1988; **94:** 294–299.
132. Raufman JP, Collins SM, Pandol SJ et al. Reliability of symptoms in assessing control of gastric acid secretion in patients with Zollinger–Ellison syndrome. *Gastroenterology* 1983; **84:** 108–113.
133. Bonfils S Mignon M & Gratton J. Cimetidine treatment of acute and chronic Zollinger–Ellison syndrome. *World J Surg* 1979; **3:** 597–604.
134. Deveney CW, Stein S & Way LW. Cimetidine in the treatment of Zollinger–Ellison syndrome. *Am J Surg* 1983; **146:** 116–123.
135. Stabile BE, Ippoliti AF, Walsh JH & Passaro E Jr. Failure of histamine H$_2$-receptor antagonist therapy in Zollinger–Ellison syndrome. *Am J Surg* 1983; **145:** 17–23.
136. Jensen RT, Collen MJ, Pandol SJ et al. Cimetidine-induced impotence and breast changes in patients with gastric hypersecretory states. *N Engl J Med* 1983; **308:** 883–887.
137. Lloyd-Davies KA, Rutgersson K & Lovell S. Omeprazole in Zollinger–Ellison syndrome: four year international study. *Gastroenterology* 1986; **90:** 1523 (abstract).
138. Lehy T, Mignon M, Cadiot G et al. Gastric endocrine cell behavior in Zollinger–Ellison patients upon long-term potent antisecretory treatment. *Gastroenterology* 1989; **96:** 1029–1040.
139. Maton PN, Binayek R, Frucht H et al. Long-term efficacy and safety of omeprazole in patients with Zollinger–Ellison syndrome: a prospective study. *Gastroenterology* 1989; **97:** 827–836.
140. Metz DC, Pisegna JR, Ringham GL et al. Prospective study of efficacy and safety of lansoprazole in Zollinger–Ellison syndrome. *Dig Dis Sci* 1993; **38:** 245–256.

37

TUMOURS OF THE STOMACH

JWL Fielding

BENIGN TUMOURS

Gastric polyps

A gastric polyp is a discrete protrusion into the lumen of the stomach and the final diagnosis can only be made on the basis of histological examination of the excised lesion. Gastric polyps are uncommon, with an incidence of about 0.4% in autopsy series. Most are diagnosed radiologically or endoscopically, the latter method being more accurate and capable of detecting smaller lesions.

Although most polyps are discovered during investigation of symptomatic patients, it is uncertain whether these lesions are responsible for non-specific symptoms such as nausea, abdominal pain or other dyspeptic symptoms. Gastrointestinal bleeding from an ulcerated polyp or obstructive symptoms from a pedunculated antral polyp prolapsing through the pylorus may be the only symptoms that can be definitely ascribed to a gastric polyp. Approximately 85% of patients with gastric polyps have achlorhydria. An increased incidence is found in patients with atrophic gastritis, pernicious anaemia and gastric cancer. Hyperplastic polyps have been described adjacent to the gastroenterostomy following gastric resection.

Polyps may be classified as hyperplastic, adenomatous or metaplastic. Hyperplastic polyps, also referred to as regenerative or inflammatory polyps, are most commonly seen in the stomach, representing over 75% of all such lesions. Polyps are usually solitary and small (less than 2 cm), either sessile or pedunculated. Microscopically, these polyps consist of branching or elongated and hyperplastic glands which may be markedly dilated or cystic. Bundles of smooth muscle fibres from invaginated muscularis mucosa are often observed in the polyp. These glandular changes merge with normal epithelium and it may be difficult to distinguish a sharp margin for the polyp. The interstitium usually contains a lymphocytic infiltrate of varying degree. Since hyperplastic polyps are a reactionary change of normal mucosa, they are not true neoplasms and are therefore not capable of malignant degeneration.

Adenomatous polyps represent the second most common type of polyp. These are sessile or pedunculated and are more likely to be found in the antrum. These adenomas can adopt a villous, tubulovillous or purely tubular pattern. Microscopically,

there is an abrupt change between the adenomatous epithelium and the normal glandular epithelium. These polyps appear to be true neoplasms, with glands composed of poorly-differentiated cells with large hypochromic nuclei and frequent mitotic figures.

Because an adenoma is a true neoplasm, it has the potential to undergo malignant degeneration. The incidence of malignant change in adenomatous polyps has been reported as up to 75%.[1] Malignant potential appears to be related to size, with larger adenomas, particularly those greater than 2 cm, having a greater potential. Other suggestive evidence includes the observation that benign adenomatous polyps are occasionally found at the margin of gastric cancers. In addition, adenomatous polyps are frequently found coincidentally with a carcinoma. These findings support the malignant potential of adenomatous polyps, but as Ming concluded, an adenomatous polyp is not a frequent precursor of gastric cancer but is an important one.

Polyposis syndromes

Gastric polyps have been reported in many of the polyposis syndromes. They are more commonly recognized in Gardner's familial polyposis coli and Peutz–Jeghers syndromes. In the Gardner syndrome, an autosomal dominant disease, adenomatous polyps have been encountered. As yet, no instance of adenocarcinoma of the stomach developing from such polyps has been documented. In the Peutz–Jeghers syndrome, polyps of the stomach have been reported in as many as 25% of cases. Gastric carcinoma has been observed in people with this syndrome but it is unlikely that this develops from the polyp.

Smooth muscle tumours

Smooth muscle tumours of the alimentary tract are uncommon. They comprise about 1% of all gastrointestinal tract tumours. The stomach is, however, the most common site of these gastrointestinal tract tumours, about 45% of the lesions of the gastrointestinal tract occurring in the stomach.[2]

Leiomyomas account for 55–60% of all benign gastric tumours; 75% are found in patients between the ages of 30 and 70 years, and the male to female ratio is equal. There are no pathognomonic symptoms of gastric leiomyomas. The most common presenting symptom is haemorrhage. Less frequent presenting symptoms are pain, discomfort, a palpable mass, weight loss, weakness and peptic ulcer symptoms; 5% have no symptoms. Most are diagnosed either endoscopically or by barium studies. At endoscopy a small submucosal swelling is noted and on barium study a well-defined rounded filling defect is usually seen. The mucosal folds end sharply at the edge of the tumour and at the apex, which usually denotes ulceration.

On microscopic examination, the muscle fibres are arranged in walls or pallisades. There is usually a thin pseudocapsule. For symptomatic gastroleiomyomas, the treatment of choice is surgical removal of the tumour. Neither total gastrectomy nor simple biopsy is recommended. Simple excision with a wedge or sleeve resection is usually adequate. The extent of the operation largely depends on the size of the lesion. It may be necessary, on occasions, to undertake a subtotal gastrectomy. Tumour recurrence following excision is exceptionally rare.

GASTRIC CANCER

Epidemiology

Gastric cancer is one of the more common causes of death from malignant disease. In the *United Nations Demographic*

Table 37.1 Causes of death for most recent year available for 57 countries

MALIGNANCY	NUMBER
Stomach neoplasms	192 972
Colon and rectum	212 006
Lung	386 135
Breast	139 865
Cervix uteri	29 940
Leukaemia	66 232
Other malignant neoplasms	901 471

Source: *United Nations Demographic Year Book* 3.

Year Book,[3] which looked at the cause of death from malignant disease, gastric cancer resulted in 192 972 deaths (Table 37.1). There are wide international variations in incidence. It is common in Japan, South America and Eastern Europe. It occurs with intermediate frequency in Western Europe and is relatively uncommon in the USA (Table 37.2).[4] Five volumes of *Cancer in Five Continents* have now been published giving incidence rates obtained from Cancer Registries in various parts of the world at 5-year intervals. Median rates for males and

Table 37.2 Age-standardized and cumulative incidence rates for cancer of the stomach

	WORLD		TRUNCATED		0–64 YEARS		0–74 YEARS	
	MALE	FEMALE	MALE	FEMALE	MALE	FEMALE	MALE	FEMALE
Brazil, Fortaleza	44.6	16.7	58.9	22.8	2.39	0.90	5.46	2.05
Brazil, Recife	29.9	8.6	36.5	13.8	1.47	0.53	3.68	0.95
Brazil, Porto Alegre	30.7	12.4	34.1	9.1	1.40	0.37	—	—
Brazil, Sao Paulo	53.6	25.1	66.4	30.0	2.70	1.21	—	—
Colombia, Cali	49.6	26.3	56.7	28.6	2.38	1.17	5.23	2.74
Costa Rica	58.8	25.2	62.7	31.8	2.59	1.29	7.02	2.97
Martinique	25.3	10.9	34.2	12.0	1.41	0.49	2.93	1.42
Netherlands Antilles	19.1	7.1	14.8	6.5	0.62	0.26	2.29	0.75
Puerto Rico	17.6	8.6	16.7	9.4	0.71	0.38	2.01	0.97
Canada	13.2	5.9	14.5	6.4	0.60	0.26	1.52	0.64
Canada, Alberta	11.8	4.8	12.2	4.9	0.51	0.21	1.40	0.50
Canada, Brit. Col.	11.9	5.0	12.6	5.1	0.52	0.21	1.36	0.53
Canada, Manitoba	14.0	5.8	14.2	5.3	0.59	0.22	1.59	0.60
Canada, Mar. Provs.	13.5	5.6	16.5	6.1	0.69	0.25	1.51	0.62
Canada, New Brun.	16.7	6.3	19.5	6.1	0.81	0.24	1.88	0.70
Canada, Nova Scotia	11.1	5.1	14.0	6.2	0.59	0.26	1.26	0.57
Canada, PEI	12.7	5.3	17.5	5.7	0.74	0.22	1.21	0.48
Canada, Newfoundland	25.3	10.7	27.1	11.8	1.13	0.48	2.99	1.29
Canada, N W T & Yuk.	5.3	2.8	7.6	—	0.27	—	0.88	0.43
Canada, Ontario	11.5	5.5	13.3	5.9	0.55	0.24	1.29	0.58
Canada, Quebec	15.3	6.7	16.1	7.4	0.67	0.31	1.79	0.77
Canada, Saskatchewan	11.7	4.8	12.2	6.6	0.49	0.26	1.33	0.47
USA, Alameda: White	10.7	4.2	12.8	4.2	0.54	0.17	1.31	0.42
Black	16.7	7.1	18.5	9.9	0.79	0.43	1.89	0.77
USA, Bay Area: White	10.4	4.8	10.9	5.1	0.46	0.21	1.22	0.51
Black	19.1	6.0	22.8	7.3	0.96	0.30	2.23	0.63
Chinese	9.1	5.4	11.4	7.7	0.46	0.31	1.15	0.56
Filipino	4.1	2.5	2.9	4.6	0.11	0.19	0.55	0.35
Japanese	24.3	10.8	29.5	11.2	1.18	0.49	2.71	1.02
USA, Los Angeles: White	8.6	4.0	9.8	4.5	0.40	0.19	1.00	0.43
Latino	14.7	6.7	14.9	7.2	0.63	0.30	1.76	0.69
Black	15.6	6.4	17.7	7.0	0.72	0.29	1.81	0.77
Japanese	25.5	11.4	24.1	19.6	1.03	0.77	2.70	1.09
Chinese	14.0	8.7	22.7	13.1	0.96	0.54	1.46	0.91

Table 37.2 *contd*

	WORLD		TRUNCATED		0–64 YEARS		0–74 YEARS	
	MALE	FEMALE	MALE	FEMALE	MALE	FEMALE	MALE	FEMALE
Filipino	4.7	2.6	6.6	—	0.26	0.02	0.64	0.35
Korean	44.8	18.6	44.2	25.4	1.80	1.00	7.76	2.18
USA, Connecticut: White	10.8	4.3	11.5	4.5	0.48	0.18	1.29	0.47
Black	19.4	9.1	22.0	11.3	0.91	0.48	2.25	1.13
USA, Atlanta: White	6.1	3.1	6.8	3.2	0.27	0.14	0.74	0.38
Black	15.8	5.5	23.0	8.1	0.94	0.33	1.88	0.60
USA, Iowa	6.8	3.0	7.7	3.2	0.32	0.13	0.76	0.32
USA, New Orleans: White	7.3	3.2	8.1	4.5	0.34	0.18	0.83	0.37
Black	17.5	8.3	21.6	10.6	0.91	0.46	2.20	0.83
USA, Detroit: White	10.2	4.2	10.8	4.4	0.45	0.18	1.15	0.45
Black	16.9	6.8	22.6	7.7	0.94	0.31	1.97	0.79
USA, New Mexico: Hisp.	15.7	8.3	18.4	7.3	0.77	0.30	1.79	0.97
Other White	6.3	3.1	7.8	2.8	0.32	0.11	0.75	0.34
Amerind.	17.9	10.8	23.3	11.7	0.90	0.42	1.84	1.14
USA, New York City	12.4	6.3	13.8	6.8	0.57	0.28	1.41	0.70
USA, N Y S (less City)	9.4	4.4	10.5	4.5	0.44	0.18	1.05	0.48
USA, Utah	6.3	3.1	7.6	3.4	0.31	0.14	0.71	0.31
USA, Seattle	8.0	3.3	9.0	3.7	0.37	0.15	0.91	0.35
China, Shanghai	58.3	24.6	71.7	32.2	3.02	1.31	7.36	2.96
China, Tianjin	36.4	15.0	42.6	19.3	1.83	0.79	4.66	1.85
Hong Kong	19.2	9.6	23.6	12.7	0.99	0.51	2.45	1.06
India, Bangalore	12.6	7.1	18.5	11.5	0.75	0.45	1.50	0.73
India, Bombay	8.9	6.0	9.9	7.4	0.41	0.31	0.77	0.57
India, Madras	13.7	6.7	21.5	13.7	0.85	0.53	1.58	0.69
India, Nagpur	7.8	6.7	14.0	11.6	0.56	0.47	0.85	0.80
India, Poona	10.5	6.3	13.9	10.9	0.57	0.43	1.31	0.70
Israel: All Jews	16.2	9.3	16.1	9.4	0.67	0.38	1.82	1.05
Born Israel	12.4	6.9	10.3	6.6	0.42	0.24	1.40	0.79
Born Eur. Amer.	18.3	10.3	17.4	10.3	0.76	0.44	1.98	1.14
Born Afr. Asia	12.3	7.2	15.3	8.0	0.63	0.32	1.49	0.87
Non-Jews	7.9	4.9	9.7	4.0	0.38	0.14	0.95	0.63
Japan, Hiroshima	79.9	35.8	107.6	53.5	4.41	2.13	9.75	4.26
Japan, Miyagi	79.6	36.0	111.8	50.5	4.56	2.03	9.73	4.16
Urban	79.2	35.7	112.8	47.5	4.60	1.92	9.64	4.06
Rural	80.1	36.6	110.5	54.5	4.51	2.17	9.82	4.29
Japan, Nagasaki	82.0	36.1	117.2	49.7	4.73	1.98	9.98	4.03
Japan, Osaka	76.9	35.9	93.9	48.1	3.87	1.90	9.11	4.03
Kuwait: Kuwaitis	3.7	1.6	4.1	2.0	0.16	0.07	0.34	0.24
Non-Kuwaitis	8.7	3.9	8.2	3.2	0.36	0.12	1.03	0.53
Philippines, Rizal	9.4	6.7	12.3	8.0	0.51	0.33	1.11	0.72
Singapore: Chinese	37.3	15.4	48.2	18.9	2.02	0.76	4.61	1.81
Malay	9.4	6.8	9.4	11.4	0.36	0.48	1.25	0.83
Indian	15.5	16.6	20.0	16.5	0.83	0.71	2.18	1.85
Czech Rep., Slovakia	31.7	14.5	39.0	15.9	1.63	0.66	3.90	1.71
Urban	29.9	15.8	30.9	16.4	1.29	0.67	3.52	1.86
Rural	32.0	14.3	40.1	15.8	1.68	0.66	3.95	1.70
Denmark	14.3	6.7	14.1	7.0	0.58	0.28	1.56	0.66
Finland	24.6	12.9	25.7	13.7	1.07	0.55	2.81	1.37
France, Bas-Rhin	15.5	7.4	18.8	7.7	0.78	0.33	1.93	0.88
France, Calvados	15.8	8.1	19.8	8.6	0.81	0.36	2.00	0.94
Urban	15.2	7.9	20.5	9.0	0.85	0.36	1.81	0.93
Rural	16.9	8.6	18.8	8.2	0.75	0.35	2.30	0.96
France, Doubs	15.2	6.7	17.7	7.8	0.74	0.32	1.82	0.82
Urban	16.4	6.9	20.1	9.1	0.84	0.38	1.84	0.82
Rural	13.1	6.4	13.4	5.2	0.55	0.21	1.76	0.81
France, Isère	11.5	5.4	11.0	4.7	0.46	0.20	1.39	0.61
Germany, Hamburg	23.7	11.7	29.3	13.4	1.23	0.55	2.60	1.27
Germany, Saarland	23.6	12.1	25.7	12.0	1.06	0.50	2.69	1.24
Urban	24.5	12.0	25.8	11.5	1.07	0.47	2.90	1.27
Rural	21.4	11.5	22.4	12.0	0.91	0.51	2.38	1.18
Germany (former GDR)	25.2	12.3	28.7	13.6	1.19	0.56	3.12	1.42
Hungary, Szabolcs	32.4	12.8	45.6	17.8	1.91	0.73	4.09	1.54
Urban	32.6	16.1	44.5	18.3	1.88	0.74	3.74	1.70

Table 37.2 *contd*

	WORLD		TRUNCATED		0–64 YEARS		0–74 YEARS	
	MALE	FEMALE	MALE	FEMALE	MALE	FEMALE	MALE	FEMALE
Rural	32.5	11.9	46.1	17.8	1.92	0.73	4.19	1.50
Hungary, Vas	31.4	12.1	36.9	12.0	1.54	0.51	3.90	1.58
Iceland	31.4	14.0	34.4	13.8	1.44	0.59	3.69	1.59
Ireland, Southern	12.4	4.2	15.4	2.9	0.61	0.13	1.37	0.53
Italy, Varese	39.0	17.1	38.6	14.5	1.60	0.59	4.48	1.81
Italy, Parma	44.0	19.9	49.9	19.8	2.06	0.82	5.19	2.06
Italy, Ragusa	19.8	8.4	17.4	3.9	0.72	0.16	2.28	0.69
Neth., Eindhoven	20.7	9.5	24.3	10.1	1.00	0.42	2.48	1.07
Norway	18.1	9.2	18.4	9.7	0.76	0.39	2.11	0.99
Urban	18.5	9.3	18.3	9.9	0.76	0.41	2.18	1.01
Rural	17.8	9.1	18.5	9.5	0.76	0.38	2.06	0.98
Poland, Cracow City	32.9	13.4	39.1	15.2	1.65	0.63	3.99	1.59
Poland, Nowy Sacz	43.7	17.0	60.3	21.1	2.53	0.87	5.64	2.08
Poland, Warsaw City	23.2	8.9	25.6	9.8	1.07	0.40	2.78	0.97
Romania, County Cluj	34.2	13.6	43.3	16.6	1.82	0.67	4.24	1.72
Urban	32.6	12.6	40.2	14.0	1.71	0.56	3.97	1.55
Rural	35.7	14.5	47.2	19.4	1.95	0.80	4.53	1.90
Slovenia	34.9	15.1	41.1	17.3	1.69	0.71	4.35	1.73
Spain, Tarragona	16.9	7.8	19.8	7.9	0.80	0.33	1.89	0.77
Spain, Navarra	31.6	13.5	38.7	12.8	1.52	0.51	3.75	1.42
Spain, Zaragoza	20.8	10.4	21.3	6.7	0.87	0.28	2.10	1.02
Sweden	15.0	7.5	13.8	7.7	0.58	0.31	1.70	0.80
Switzerland, Basel	19.6	8.1	21.3	8.6	0.86	0.33	1.91	0.79
Switzerland, Geneva	13.5	6.3	16.2	5.1	0.71	0.21	1.54	0.67
Switzerland, Neuchâtel	17.9	6.8	12.1	6.1	0.48	0.26	2.08	0.75
Switzerland, Vaud	15.2	5.0	16.4	4.0	0.67	0.16	1.74	0.47
Urban	14.3	6.2	14.4	6.2	0.61	0.25	1.52	0.67
Rural	15.8	4.3	17.6	2.7	0.72	0.11	1.86	0.34
Switzerland, Zurich	14.8	6.6	16.7	7.4	0.69	0.31	1.72	0.74
UK, England & Wales	18.5	7.8	18.7	7.1	0.79	0.30	2.23	0.85
Urban	18.9	8.0	19.3	7.3	0.81	0.30	2.33	0.90
Rural	15.0	6.4	14.4	6.0	0.61	0.25	1.83	0.70
UK, Birmingham	20.3	8.4	21.6	8.2	0.91	0.34	2.48	0.93
UK, North Western	22.0	9.8	22.8	8.7	0.96	0.36	2.71	1.07
UK, Oxford	20.2	7.8	22.5	6.8	0.95	0.28	2.37	0.82
UK, South Thames	15.7	6.6	15.2	6.0	0.64	0.25	1.91	0.72
UK, South Western	16.8	6.8	16.5	5.9	0.71	0.25	2.05	0.73
UK, Trent	20.4	8.7	19.4	7.4	0.82	0.31	2.46	0.95
UK, Mersey	21.8	9.9	21.0	9.0	0.88	0.37	2.70	1.13
UK, Scotland	20.4	9.6	23.2	9.1	0.96	0.38	2.45	1.08
UK, East Scotland	22.0	10.1	27.6	9.8	1.15	0.38	2.68	1.06
UK, North Scotland	14.7	6.2	18.2	6.2	0.78	0.26	1.91	0.75
UK, N.E. Scotland	17.5	8.2	19.5	8.2	0.78	0.32	1.85	0.95
UK, S.E. Scotland	19.6	9.7	23.2	10.0	0.97	0.42	2.38	1.13
UK, West Scotland	21.7	10.0	23.6	9.1	0.98	0.38	2.60	1.12
Australia, Cap. Terr.	15.0	6.4	13.7	4.1	0.58	0.17	1.65	0.59
Australia, NSW	12.9	5.9	13.0	6.2	0.54	0.25	1.47	0.61
Urban	13.6	6.2	13.7	6.8	0.56	0.27	1.56	0.64
Rural	10.9	5.0	10.7	4.3	0.45	0.18	1.23	0.48
Australia, Queensland	13.0	4.7	11.1	4.2	0.46	0.16	1.45	0.56
Australia, South	13.1	5.7	14.1	5.3	0.58	0.22	1.50	0.57
Australia, Tasmania	12.6	4.8	12.3	3.2	0.51	0.14	1.56	0.54
Australia, Victoria	14.8	6.2	16.7	6.6	0.69	0.27	1.73	0.69
Australia, West	15.1	5.0	15.7	5.0	0.64	0.22	1.72	0.56
New Zealand: Maori	29.8	19.7	34.3	32.6	1.47	1.25	4.15	2.37
Non-Maori	13.7	6.0	14.1	5.6	0.59	0.22	1.59	0.63
Pac. Poly. Isl.	33.6	15.1	26.4	20.9	1.19	0.85	4.05	1.92
Hawaii: White	11.8	6.0	10.6	4.9	0.44	0.20	1.28	0.63
Japanese	28.4	14.1	28.3	15.9	1.15	0.62	2.92	1.47
Hawaiian	31.2	14.9	35.9	19.6	1.49	0.77	3.57	1.79
Filipino	6.8	4.6	7.8	8.8	0.31	0.36	0.63	0.36
Chinese	11.2	6.7	12.2	11.0	0.49	0.42	1.15	0.56

females from each volume show an initial slight increase, followed by a steady fall (Table 37.3). The highest rates for stomach cancer have always been those of Japan. Next are South America, Iceland and Eastern Europe. This international data is available from a limited number of countries and as this disease is common in less affluent societies, from which data is less readily available, these figures probably underestimate its significance.

Table 37.3 Age-standardized incidence rates (per 100 000) for stomach cancer

| RATE | VOLUME NUMBER OF *CANCER INCIDENCE IN FIVE CONTINENTS* | | | | |
	I	II	III	IV	V
Median					
Males	26.5	26.8	21.2	19.1	16.2
Females	12.8	13.8	10.0	9.2	6.9
Highest					
Males	95.5	95.3	91.4	100.2	82.0
	Miyagi	Miyagi	Osaka	Nagasaki	Nagasaki
Females	47.7	45.7	48.3	51.0	35.9
	Miyagi	Okayoma	Okayoma	Nagasaki	Osaka
Lowest					
Males	2.3	7.9	7.2	3.7	3.7
	Uganda	El Paso (Latin)	Nigeria	Dakar	Kuwait
Females	0.9	1.5	2.5	2.0	1.6
	Uganda	Hawaii (Filipino)	El Paso (other white)	Dakar	Kuwait

In addition to international variations, the incidence varies within regions of the country. In the UK, areas of high incidence include Wales, Scotland and the Midlands. A close examination of these areas demonstrates that the incidence was high in South Wales (33.5/100 000 men and 22.3/100 000 women) and Stoke on Trent (45.1/100 000 men and 29.6/100 000 women).

In many areas of the world, the incidence has decreased. In the USA the annual stomach cancer mortality rate decreased from 28.8/100 000 in 1930 to 13/100 000 in 1955.[5] In Japan, the mortality rate has declined from 82.6/100 000 in 1963 to 58/100,000 in 1976.[6] Similarly, in the UK the mortality rate decreased from 33/100 000 in 1940 to 23.4/100 000 in 1978.

The West Midlands Regional Cancer Registry studied 31716 cases over the period 1957–1981.[7] The age-standardized incidence per 100 000 for the whole period was 17.23. Initially, there was a slight increase from 17.42 to 19.22 during the quinquennium 1962–1966 but this had fallen to 15.30/100 000 by 1977–1981. These patterns in age-standardized annual incidence rates are the same in both males and females (Figure 37.1).

The incidence is approximately twice as high in males as in females. Gastric cancer develops in some patients under 30 years of age, but the highest incidence occurs in those over the age of 60 (Figure 37.2); the majority of cases occur between 60 and 80 (Figure 37.3).

Aetiology

Heredity

The variation of incidence in different areas suggests either genetic or environmental factors may be important. A study of Japanese migrants to Hawaii demonstrated that the incidence of gastric cancer among the Issei (first generation Japanese) is similar to that in Japan; the incidence among the Nisei (second generation Japanese) is significantly lower, but still remains higher than that of the USA Whites.[8] This alteration may be attributed to environmental factors, but since the incidence is not that of the local population, it leaves open the question of genetic influence. Dublin and Marks[9] found insured persons with a family history of gastric cancer had a subsequent gastric cancer mortality of about one-third greater than other insured persons, and Videbaek and Mosbech[10] reported an incidence of stomach cancer four times greater among the relatives of 302 cancer patients when compared with similar controls. Several reports have shown an increase in persons of blood group A.[11]

Occupation and socioeconomic grouping

The existence of a relationship between social class and gastric cancer is well established. In the USA, Denmark and Great Britain it has been demonstrated that the incidence is higher

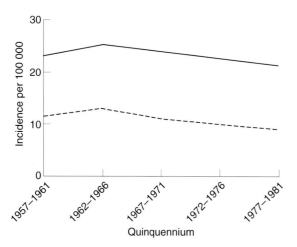

Figure 37.1
Age-standardized annual incidence rates per 100 000 by quinquennium and sex. —, Males; ----, females.

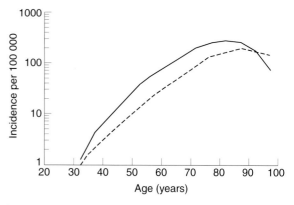

Figure 37.2
Incidence rates by age and sex. —, Males; ----, females.

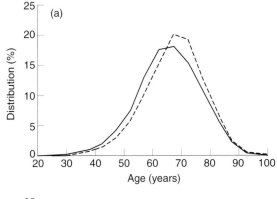

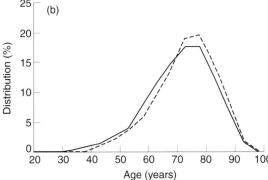

Figure 37.3
Distribution by age, sex (a, males; b, females) and decennium
(—, 1962–1971; ----, 1972–1981).

among social classes III–V.[5,12] The incidence is highest in social class III, particularly in those undertaking heavy work, and Stukonis and Doll[12] postulated that this group would eat more and therefore be exposed to more carcinogens in the diet. Among heavy workers, coal miners had the highest incidence. Thus, the important factor may be occupational, rather than dietary. This view gained support from the lower mortality recorded among farm workers. Craven et al.,[13] demonstrated a significantly higher incidence among miners in Wales (79/100 000) and the incidence is also high in urban as opposed to rural areas.[14]

The West Midlands Regional Cancer Registry has looked at 26 orders in the occupational classification. A comparison has been made between male cases of stomach cancer and male cases of all sites of cancer recorded in the Registry (1977–1984). Stomach cancer cases (Table 37.4) are significantly in excess in several groups, particularly in miners and quarrymen, glass and ceramic makers, furnace, forge and foundry workers, warehousemen, storekeepers and packers and labourers. The use of a more detailed occupational classification than these orders shows that male stomach cancer cases exceed in proportion all male Registry cases for underground coal miners and postmen, and mail sorters.

Smoking

The evidence of an association between cigarette smoking and stomach cancer is not clearly established but there is evidence of a positive association. Hammond and Horne[15] and Hirayama[6]

reported correlation with cigarette smoking. The relative risk of stomach cancer in males was 1.47 and in females 1.25 and, although this was much lower than the risk for lung cancer (4.13 in males and 2.10 in females), the absolute magnitude of excess deaths per 100 000 among daily cigarette smokers was similar for gastric cancer to that for lung cancer: 6.42 and 6.48 in males and 19.6 and 17.4 in females, respectively.

Dietary factors

The importance of diet in gastric cancer remains unclear. In the USA, the intake of beef, milk, citrus fruits and green vegetables has increased, and that of potatoes decreased.[5] In Japan, the striking change in the incidence of gastric cancer has been associated with changes in diet. The consumption of milk products increased 28-fold from 1949 to 1978; there has been a significant relationship with the increase in fatty foods and vitamin A, and the intake of yellow–green vegetables.[6]

Nitrates, nitrites and nitrosamines

There is much interest in the role of nitrates and associated compounds in the aetiology of gastric cancer. Many animals have been challenged with N-nitroso compounds and none have proved resistant, so it is likely that they may be implicated in human carcinogenesis. N-nitroso compounds may be produced from nitrates and nitrites taken in the diet. Epidemiological studies have investigated the possible source of nitrates and nitrites and their significance in the relationship to gastric carcinoma. Dietary nitrites come from three main sources: green and root vegetables, cured meat products and drinking water. Hill et al.[16] reported an association between high water nitrate concentration and gastric cancer in Worksop, and Haenszel et al.[17] demonstrated that Japanese drinking water often contained high nitrate levels in areas of high incidence, but in areas of low incidence the water was from municipal supplies with low nitrate levels. Hill[18] suggested that nitrates could be converted into N-nitroso compounds in many groups at high risk for gastric cancer. Cigarettes contain preformed N-nitroso compounds, oxides of nitrogen and cyanide, which are detoxified to thiocyanide (a catalyst of N-nitrosation reaction), which is secreted in saliva and so reaches the stomach with food. The atmosphere in coal mines is known to be rich in oxides of nitrogen. Gastric hypochlorhydria is found in chronic atrophic gastritis (pernicious anaemia and postoperatively), resulting in ideal conditions for bacterial production of N-nitroso compounds. The stomach, normally sterile, has significant bacterial colonization when the pH exceeds 4.[19]

Correa et al.,[20] in 1975, postulated a model for gastric cancer epidemiology. The histopathological sequence in gastric carcinogenesis is outlined in Figure 37.4. There have subsequently been a number of studies which have shown no correlation with N-nitroso compound concentration and have emphasized that such compounds are produced in greater amounts in the acid stomach. If this is so, then there should be a correlation in high-risk populations between nitrite intake and gastric cancer risk, and this has been claimed in many studies, none of which

Table 37.4 Male patients: distribution by occupation (1977–1980)

OCCUPATION	STOMACH CANCER (%)	ALL REGISTRY CASES (%)	PROPORTIONATE REGISTRATION RATIO (%)
Farmers, foresters, fishermen	4.5	4.7	96
Miners and quarrymen	5.0	4.0	125*
Gas, coke and chemical makers	0.5	0.5	100
Glass and ceramics makers	1.6	1.2	133*
Furnace, forge, foundry workers, etc.	3.7	3.0	123*
Electrical and electronic workers	2.0	2.0	100
Engineering and allied trade workers	20.1	22.1	91*
Woodworkers	2.0	2.0	100
Leatherworkers	0.2	0.3	67
Textile workers	0.2	0.4	50
Clothing workers	0.1	0.3	33
Food, drink and tobacco workers	1.7	1.6	106
Paper and printing workers	0.4	0.6	67
Makers of other products	1.2	1.3	92
Construction workers	4.3	4.0	108
Painters and decorators	1.8	1.9	95
Drivers of stationary engines, etc.	2.5	2.1	119
Labourers	10.9	9.6	114*
Transport and communications workers	7.7	7.0	110
Warehousemen, storekeepers, packers	5.3	4.4	120*
Clerical workers	4.4	5.0	88
Sales workers	4.8	5.3	91
Service, sport and recreation workers	5.6	5.3	106
Administration and managers	4.7	5.5	85
Professional	4.6	5.6	82*
Armed forces	0.2	0.3	67
	100.0	100.0	
Total specified	2816	32 042	
Not known	329	9822	
Total	3145	41 864	

*

is entirely convincing alone, but when taken together suggest a relationship.[21–23]

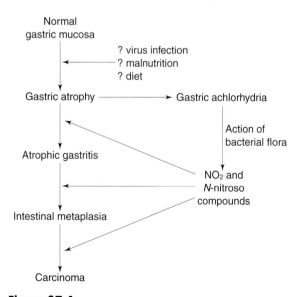

Figure 37.4
Histological sequence in gastric carcinogenesis postulated by Correa et al. (1975).

Soil type

The effect of trace elements has been known for some time. There have been positive associations between gastric cancer and organic matter, zinc, cobalt and chromium, but no definite associations for iron, vanadium, nickel, titanium and lead in England and Wales. Study has demonstrated an increased incidence of stomach cancer associated with sea clay, peat and reclaimed soils, and a lower than average incidence with river clay and ordinary sandy soils.[24,25]

H pylori

Recently there has been considerable interesting research into the significance of *Helicobacter pylori* infection. It is now considered that this organism is an important factor in the development of gastric cancer that is associated with the development of chronic atrophic gastritis and subsequent progression to malignancy.

Premalignant conditions and lesions of the stomach

A premalignant condition is a clinical state associated with a significantly increased risk of cancer. A precancerous lesion is a histopathological epithelial abnormality in which gastric cancer is more likely to occur than in normal mucosa.

Predisposing conditions

These include pernicious anaemia, hypogammaglobulinaemia and postoperative stomach. In pernicious anaemia, there is a threefold risk of cancer; in hypogammaglobulinaemia there is a 50-fold increase. Both these conditions are associated with gastric achlorhydria and atrophic gastritis, and it is these premalignant lesions which are associated with the development of malignancy. Gastric surgery for benign conditions predisposes to gastric carcinogenesis. After resection, there is an increased risk of developing gastric cancer which appears 10–15 years after the resection.[26] This appears to be a 3–4-fold increase and, as yet, has only been consistently reported following gastric resection. There is only one series which suggests that the risk may be increased following vagotomy and pyloroplasty.[27]

Premalignant lesions

Polyps A gastric polyp is a benign lesion originating from the gastric mucosa. Gastric polyps may be classified as focal hyperplasia, hyperplasiogenic polyps, adenomas and gastric polyposis. The most common are the hyperplasiogenic polyps but all are indistinguishable from the rare adenomatous polyp, in which malignancy rates of up to 75% have been reported.[1]

Chronic atrophic gastritis Chronic gastritis is frequently found in association with gastric cancer but whether it is precancerous is debatable. Freisen et al.[28] reported that 94% of superficial cancers were found in areas of gastritis and, in addition, carcinomas are found in 10% of cases with chronic gastritis and metaplasia.[29] The debate is clarified if chronic gastritis is related to its aetiology using the classification described by Correa[30]:

- Autoimmune chronic gastritis
- Hypersecretory chronic gastritis
- Environmental chronic gastritis.

Autoimmune chronic gastritis Complete atrophy, the end-result of chronic atrophic gastritis, has been recognized as a classical component of pernicious anaemia. The lesion characteristically involves the body and fundus diffusely, leaving the antrum intact. This type of gastritis increases in prevelance and severity with age, and is more common in males than females. Not all patients with this type of gastritis have overt pernicious anaemia, but a significant proportion will develop it.31 Intestinal metaplasia commonly accompanies this form of gastritis and since metaplasia is positively associated with gastric cancer, and is subject to dysplastic transformation, this type of gastritis assumes a high risk of developing a carcinoma, which is characteristically located in the body.

Hypersecretory chronic gastritis This is often found in association with duodenal or gastric ulceration. If there is an associated duodenal ulcer, the gastritis is confined to the antrum, and if the ulcer is in the stomach, the gastritis involves the antrum but will extend in association with the site of the ulcer.[32,33] Histologically, it is characterized by distortion of the glandular epithelium, but no significant intestinal metaplasia is found. This type of gastritis is associated with excessive secretion of hydrochloric acid and increased pepsin. There is no association between this gastritis and the development of malignancy.

Environmental gastritis This is prevalent in certain parts of the world, the geographical distribution coinciding with areas of high incidence of gastric cancer of the intestinal type. It is now recognized that these two syndromes are part of the same complex. The changes in gastric mucosa occur early in life, usually by the age of 20–25 years.[34] Among populations with a low incidence of gastric cancer, chronic gastritis is found in less than 20%, but this increases to 70% or more in high-incidence areas. This form of gastritis also has a characteristic pathology. It is multifocal, involving both antrum and body, and the early stages appear on the lesser curve and below the junction of the antrum and body. Initially, these are small foci, but as they enlarge they become confluent and may involve large areas of the body and antrum. Histologically, the milder lesions show the characteristic changes of acute gastritis, with a dense inflammatory exudate in the upper lamina propria. As it progresses, atrophy of the mucosa develops due to progressive loss of gastric glands, subsequent regeneration occurs, and the mucosa is replaced by intestinal-type mucosa. This phenomenon constitutes intestinal metaplasia of gastric mucosa. Some patients develop dysplastic changes which may progress to invasive adenocarcinoma of the intestinal type.

Migrants who live their first decade in a high-risk environment and move to a low-risk country display a cancer risk similar to that of the country of origin. Their descendants, however, have a much lower risk.[8] The incidence of chronic gastritis is certainly higher in the premigration countries, such as Japan, than it is in the postmigration countries, such as the USA.[35]

Intestinal metaplasia Intestinal metaplasia was a final step in the development of gastric cancer in the proposed pathway of Correa. This lesion is characterized by metaplastic changes occurring in the gastric epithelium. It has now been divided into three groups, according to histological and histochemical criteria.[36]

Type 1 This is the complete type, resembling normal small intestine. Mucin histochemistry reveals mainly O- and N-acetyl sialomucins.

Type 2 This is the incomplete metaplasia where goblet cells are found in association with columnar cells and occasional Paneth cells. The mucins are mainly neutral sialomucins.

Type 3 This resembles hyperplastic colonic mucosa and secretes sulphomucins. It is this type of intestinal metaplasia which is considered to be premalignant. The evidence for premalignant potential comes from a number of studies which have shown a higher proportion of patients with gastric cancer who have mucosa with sulphamucin-secreting intestinal metaplasia than is present in patients with benign gastric or duodenal ulcers.[37]

Dysplasia This is marked by atypical glandular formation, pleomorphic nuclei and increased mitoses. It is usually, but not invariably, associated with metaplastic gastric epithelium. There is little doubt that gastric dysplasia represents an advanced stage in the carcinogenic pathway.

Problems arise in the interpretation of the grade of dysplasia in histological sections. It is difficult for pathologists to discriminate between mild dysplasia and regenerative changes, and also moderate from severe dysplasia. This is a basis on which dysplasia is classified at present, i.e. into mild, moderate and severe. It is the severe dysplasia that is of greatest significance. In these cases, Farinati et al.[38] showed that 72% had a carcinoma or rapidly went on to develop one.

Pathogenesis of gastric cancer

The histopathological sequence postulated by Correa et al.[20] is still relevant to the development of gastric cancer. However, Lauren's[39] histopathological classification of established cancers (into diffuse and intestinal) highlights some of the problems with Correa's postulates. The lack of gastritis in diffuse lesions makes the relationship unclear. It may be that dysplasia is the important feature, as this can occur in foveolar epithelium as well as intestinal metaplasia and it may be the common pre-malignant mucosal change.[40] It is also noteworthy that the genetic factors, particularly family aggregations of gastric cancer and the increased incidence in blood group A, are confined to the diffuse type of gastric carcinoma. Thus, there is evidence to support two pathways for the development of gastric cancer, both of which have an identifiable association with other aetiological factors.

Pathology

Early gastric cancer

The Japanese have clearly demonstrated the importance of the early detection of gastric cancer. Of particular importance is 'early' gastric cancer, which is a lesion in which the depth of invasion of the primary tumour is limited histologically to the mucosa and submucosa of the stomach. This is irrespective of the presence or absence of lymph node metastases, which may be present in up to 15% of these early lesions. This latter feature detracts considerably from using this term in the formal staging of gastric cancer. However, it is of value in assessing macroscopically lesions which are endoscopically apparent.

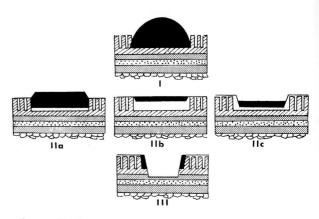

Figure 37.5
Macroscopic classification of early gastric cancer.

Both endoscopists and pathologists use the macroscopic classification of early gastric cancers, as shown in Figure 37.5.

Staging

The most appropriate staging system for gastric cancer is the TNM system. This is based on clinicopathological information and incorporates the concept of both 'early' and 'advanced' gastric cancer. The early gastric cancer is that in which the disease is confined to the mucosa and submucosa without lymph node metastases (stage 1). Advanced gastric cancer is all other stages of disease and includes the early gastric cancers with lymph node metastases. The staging system, as used in the Birmingham Cancer Registry series, is illustrated in Table 37.5. The feature of relevance to the primary is the specific depth of penetration, which is graded on a scale of T1–4, (Figure 37.6).

Lymph nodes are categorized into groups or tiers. These relate to the site of the primary tumour and are described as N1, N2 and N3 (Figure 37.7 and Table 37.6).

Any metastatic disease outside these descriptions of the primary and lymph node tiers are considered to be distant metastases.

Advanced gastric cancer

Any gastric cancer that has invaded as far as the muscularis mucosa (T3) is classified as an advanced lesion. Bormann classified morphological descriptions of these lesions into four types (Figure 37.8):

Table 37.5 Clinicopathological staging of gastric cancer

CLINICAL		MUCOSA T1	SUBMUCOSA T1	MUSCULARIS T2	SEROSA T3–4	LOCAL NODES N0–2	DISTANT METASTASES M
I	Curative resection[a]	+	±	−	−	−	−
II	Curative resection	+	+	+	±	−	−
III	Curative resection	+	±	±	±	+	−
IVa	Palliative resection[a,b]	+	±	±	±	±	±
IVb	No resection	+	±	±	±	±	±

[a]A curative resection is defined as a surgical resection with no macroscopic disease remaining.
[b]A palliative resection is defined as a surgical resection with macroscopic disease remaining.

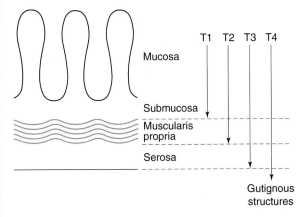

Figure 37.6
Depth of penetration of the primary lesion.

I   Fungating type of carcinoma

II Carcinomatous ulcer without infiltration of the surrounding mucosa

III Carcinomatous ulcer with infiltration of the surrounding mucosa

IV A diffuse infiltrating carcinoma.

These accommodate the other commonly used classification of (1) polypoidal, (2) ulcerating, (3) stenosing and (4) linitus plastica (leather-bottle stomach).

Microscpic features of gastric cancer

There are marked variations in the structure of gastric adeno-carcinomas. This is not only apparent between different tumours, but there is a heterogeneity within an individual tumour. Not surprisingly, a number of different classifications have been proposed for gastric cancer. Adenocarcinoma

Table 37.6   Lymph node groups for gastric cancer

SITE OF PRIMARY LESION	N1 NODES	N2 NODES
Upper third (Figure 37.7 left)	Left cardiac Right cardiac Lesser curvature Greater curvature	Supra- and infrapyloric Left gastric Common hepatic Splenic artery Splenic hilus Coeliac axis
Middle third (Figure 37.7 middle)	Right cardiac Lesser curvature Greater curvature Supra- and infrapyloric	Splenic artery Splenic hilus Left cardiac Left gastric Common hepatic Coeliac axis
Lower third (Figure 37.7 right)	Lesser curvature Greater curvature Supra- and infrapyloric	Right cardiac Left gastric Common hepatic Coeliac axis

N3 nodes: hepatoduodenal ligament, posterior aspect of pancreas, root of mesentery, diaphragmatic, paraoesophageal

N4 nodes: middle colic, para-aortic nodes

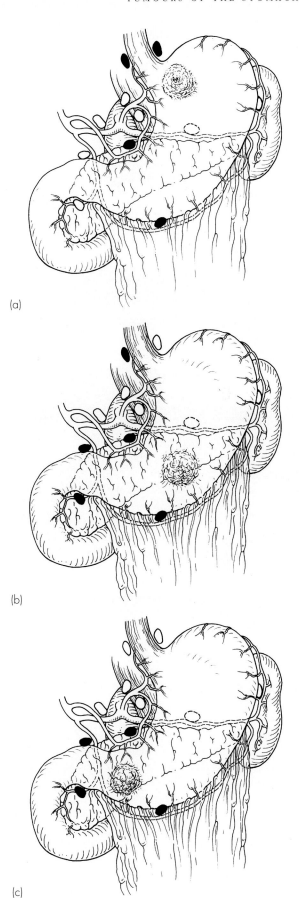

(a)

(b)

(c)

Figure 37.7
Lymph node groups (●, N1; ○, N2) for gastric cancer.

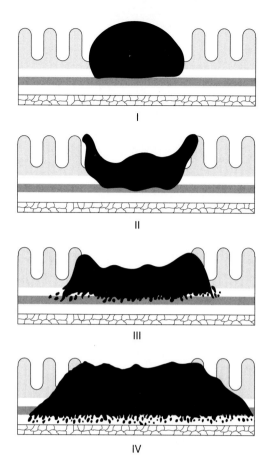

Figure 37.8
Bormann classification of advanced gastric cancer.

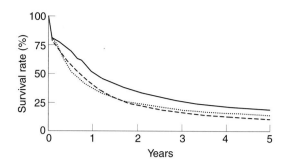

Figure 37.9
Resected cases 1972–1981. Annual age adjusted survival rates by differentiation. —, well differentiated; ----, poorly differentiated; ---- ----, anaplastic.

remains the most common histological lesion. In the West Midlands Cancer Registry Study, histology was available on 16 740 of 31 716 cases: 96.1% were classified as adenocarcinomas, 1.4% lymphomas, 0.1% carcinoids and 0.6% sarcomas. The rest were malignant tumours of an unspecified type. Various histological classifications have been derived to describe the adenocarcinomas.

Differentiation Adenocarcinomas can be classified simply by their differentiation into well-, moderately-, poorly-differentiated or anaplastic carcinomas. The separation of lesions into well or moderately differentiated has proved difficult, so commonly these two are combined, leaving three types of gastric carcinoma: well-differentiated, poorly-differentiated and anaplastic. For the period 1972–1981 at the West Midlands Cancer Registry, it has been possible to classify adenocarcinomas by degree of differentiation: 1632 were well differentiated, 2314 were poorly differentiated and 985 were anaplastic. The differentiation was not specified in 2618. The 5-year survival for these groups was 14.3, 8.1, 5.8 and 5.9%, respectively. Because of the heterogeneity of tumours, the most accurate influence of this on prognosis is established from the resected cases where 1161 were well differentiated, 1581 were poorly differentiated and 387 were anaplastic, the 5-year survival being 19.4, 11.4 and 14.4%, respectively (Figure 37.9). There is also a correlation between stage and differentiation, the anaplastic lesion being more common with the advanced

lesions, and early disease more frequently being a well-differentiated lesion (Figure 37.10).

Lauren classification This has been widely used in epidemiological studies and is based on the pathological examination of operative specimens collected at the University of Turku, Finland, between 1945 and 1976.[39] Gastric carcinomas are allocated to two main groups: the intestinal type and the diffuse type (Figure 37.11).

The intestinal type of carcinoma has a glandular structure with a papillary or solid area and is made up of large pleomorphic cells with variably shaped and hyperchromatic nuclei, often in mitosis. Polarized columnar cells with a well-developed brush border are observed lining glandular lamina. The diffuse type of carcinoma is composed of separate single or small clusters of cells. Occasionally, an aggregated appearance is present but, even then, the cells are only closely connected to each other. Glandular structure is uncommon and individual cells are small and uniform with indistinct cytoplasm and regular, often pyknotic, nuclei with infrequent mitoses. Mucin secretion is always present and is usually extensive throughout the tumour.

The mode of growth in these two types of tumour varies. The intestinal carcinomas are well defined and show considerable variation in different parts. There is often a profuse inflammatory cell infiltrate. The diffuse carcinomas have a more uniform structure, are not so well defined, and are characterized by a wider spread in the mucosa.

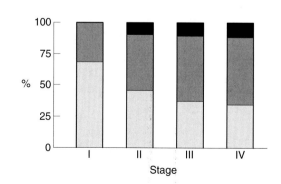

Figure 37.10
Resected cases 1972–1981. Distribution by stage and differentiation.

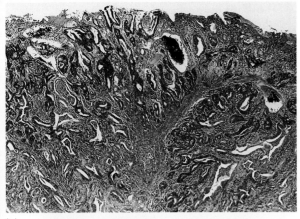

(a)

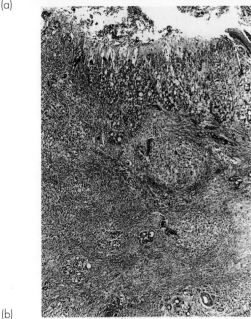

(b)

Figure 37.11

(a) Intestinal gastric cancer. (b) Diffuse gastric cancer.

In Lauren's series, 60% were polypoidal or fungating, 25% excavated and 15% infiltrating. The corresponding figures for diffuse carcinomas were 31, 26 and 43%, respectively. Intestinal metaplasia was found more commonly in association with the intestinal group. In this series, 53% of all tumours were classified as intestinal, 33% diffuse and 14% unclassified because of their atypical or poorly-differentiated structure. The prognosis was improved in the intestinal group compared with the diffuse group: the 3-year survival in 153 patients with curative treatment was 43% in those with intestinal-type tumours and 35% in the group with diffuse tumours.

World Health Organization (WHO) classification Oota[42] typed gastric adenocarcinomas according to their predominant component: evolving papillary, tubular, mucinous and signet-ring cell types. The papillary adenocarcinomas are composed of finger-like epithelial processes with fibrous cores. Tubular adenocarcinomas consist of branching glands embedded in, or surrounded by, fibrous stroma. In the mucinous adenocarcinomas, large amounts of mucin are present and this is often visible in the gross specimen. Signet-ring cell carcinomas are made up of isolated tumour cells with large amounts of intracellular mucin and considerable fibrosis.

Ming classification Ming[43] based his classification on a study of 171 gastric carcinomas. Tumours were classified into expanding (67%) and infiltrative (33%) types. The expanding lesion was characterized by tumour cells growing *en masse* and by expansion resulting in the formation of discrete tumour nodules. The infiltrative type penetrated individually and widely, eventually resulting in a diffuse involvement of the stomach. This classification emphasizes the biological behaviour as manifest by growth patterns. Both types show varying degrees of cell maturation but glandular structure was more common in the expanding carcinomas. There was some correlation with the two types of gross appearance. Among the expanding type, the tumour was fungating in 63%, ulcerated in 20%, polypoid in 10%, superficial in 4% and diffuse in 3%. With the infiltrative type, the carcinoma was diffuse in 68%, ulcerated in 27% and fungated in 5%. In the expanding tumours, there was intestinal metaplasia in the adjacent mucosa and in the intraglandular carcinoma dysplasia of metaplastic glands was frequent. In the infiltrative carcinomas these features were rarely seen.

Mulligan and Rember classification[44] This was the result of analysis of 297 gastric adenocarcinomas between 1927 and 1973. Carcinomas were allocated into three groups: (1) mucous cell carcinoma, (2) pylorocardiac gland cell carcinoma, and (3) intestinal cell carcinoma. The specific feature of this classification was the recognition of pylorocardiac gland cell carcinomas as a distinct group. These tumours are well demarcated and fungate into the lumen of the stomach. Microscopically, glands of varying size are lined by stratified or singly oriented cylindrical cells.

Merits of different classifications The simple classification by differentiation is the most frequently used and does give information relating to prognosis and a correlation with stage of disease. However, the most useful of the descriptive classifications is that described by Lauren. This correlates with epidemiological findings, can be related to possible aetiological factors, and is of prognostic value. However, for the present, it is wise to apply the WHO and Ming classifications in addition to the Lauren, as none of these classifications are entirely reproducible, nor are absolute prognostic indicators, nor do they relate to aetiology and histogenesis of cancer.

Anatomical distribution of the primary tumour

The stomach may be divided into certain anatomical areas (Figure 37.12). These are classically described as: the cardia, which represents the area at the gastro-oesophageal junction and is lined by mucus-secreting epithelium; the body, which is the area of the stomach with large mucosal folds and extends from the cardia to the incisura; and the pyloric antrum, the area of the stomach with a flat mucosa that extends from the incisura to the pylorus. The body of the stomach is associated with acid production, the antrum with

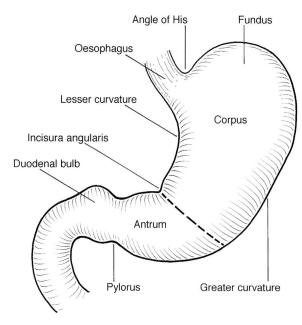

Figure 37.12
Anatomical areas of stomach.

the secretion of gastrin. Thus these anatomical areas are important in terms of the physiology of the stomach. Other descriptive sites include the lesser curve, the greater curve, the anterior wall and the posterior wall. Traditionally, the distribution of carcinomas has been described using a combination of these two classifications. The pyloric antrum has always been the most frequent site of adenocarcinoma of the stomach. Although this still pertains, there has been a significant increase in the incidence of lesions found at the cardia. During the period 1957–1961, 11.3% of tumours were sited at the cardia. This had increased to 21.2% by 1977–1981. Throughout this period antral lesions remained the most common; in 1957, 45.9% of tumours were located there. This decreased to 33% in 1977–1981 (Figure 37.13).

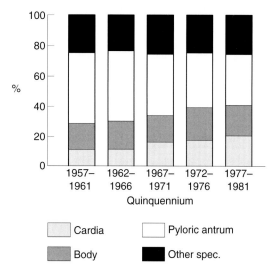

Figure 37.13
Distribution by site and quinquennium.

Methods of spread

In 1932, Carnett and Howell[45] described the mechanism of dissemination from gastric cancers as:

1. Direct extension into the pancreas, hepatic and splenic pedicles, abdominal wall, oesophagus, colon, duodenum and gall bladder.
2. Lymphatic embolization.
3. Lymphatic permeation.
4. Bloodstream embolism.
5. Transplantation, commonly causing bronchial and ovarian carcinomatosis.

Gastric carcinomas spread by direct extension into the duodenum and oesophagus and it is not true, as was once believed, that the pylorus is the limit of spread. Coller et al.[46] demonstrated microscopic duodenal involvement in 26.4% of cases, and this was confirmed in 1949 by Zinniger and Collins,[47] who demonstrated that 30% of lesions within 5 cm of the pylorus invaded the duodenum. The staging systems for gastric cancer give a clear indication as to the patterns of spread. In most Western countries, a similar distribution will be found as is seen in the West Midlands of Britain. Those with tumours confined to the stomach or stomach bed are staged as I–III. The proportion of patients who are node negative and in stage I or II has not altered significantly over a 25-year period. Similarly, the proportion with positive lymph nodes, but suitable for curative resection, has remained between 11% and 13.7%. The majority, however, still present with metastatic disease as a result of widespread lymphatic embolization or permeation, bloodstream embolism to the liver and more distant sites, and transplantation.

Clinical features

All patients with gastric cancer will have symptoms, and yet the diagnosis is commonly made when the disease is advanced. The difficulty for the physician is to differentiate between the symptoms of benign upper gastrointestinal disorders and those of a malignant tumour.

Men have gastric cancer more commonly than women. The highest incidence occurs between the ages of 55 and 65 years. The sex and age distribution are the same in both advanced and early gastric cancers.

Particularly relevant to the detection of early gastric cancer is an analysis of the first symptoms of disease. Swynnerton and Truelove[48] studied 371 patients presenting to the Radcliffe Infirmary, Oxford, and Lundh et al.[49] studied 901 patients in a European co-operative study. Table 37.7 represents the type of first symptom that these patients experienced. Swynnerton and Truelove made a detailed study of early dyspeptic symptoms in 251 patients, and 21.1% of these symptoms were mild (vague abdominal discomfort, fullness, belching, regurgitation), 26.3% had typical ulcer-type pain, 14.7% had pain after meals unrelieved by food or alkalis, 11.6% had a long history of vague dyspepsia, 18.7% had continuous pain and 7.6% projectile vomiting.

Table 37.7   Early symptoms of gastric cancer

SYMPTOMS	RADCLIFFE[11a] (N = 371)	EUROPE[7a] (N = 901)	WEST MIDLANDS[1] (N = 86)[1,c]
Gastrointestinal (dyspepsia, vomiting, abdominal pain, epigastric pain, indigestion, dysphagia, haematemesis, melaena)	310 (83.6)	678 (75.2)	71 (82.5)
Constitutional (weight loss, anaemia, weakness, lassitude, fever)	51 (13.7)	187 (20.8)	11 (12.8)
Other	10 (2.7)	36 (4.0)	4 (4.7)

Values in parentheses are percentages.
[a]First symptom.
[b]Symptoms at presentation of 'early' gastric cancer.
[c]Includes four patients whose symptoms were not known.

By the time the patient is admitted to hospital, the clinical features of the advanced lesion have changed from those at the time of the first symptom. The most striking feature is that 78.4% of all patients have lost weight by this time, compared with only 18.9% of patients with early gastric cancer.[50] Similar findings were reported by Green et al.[51] from their direct comparisons of early with advanced lesions. Weight loss was significantly less common in patients with early gastric cancer, and there was a significantly higher incidence of previous peptic ulceration. Two patients with early gastric cancer treated with cimetidine noted marked symptomatic improvement. It is always worth stressing that dyspepsia is a symptom and not a diagnosis, and that no patient over 40 years of age complaining of dyspepsia for the first time should be treated until a definite diagnosis has been established.

It is apparent that early gastric cancers produce symptoms. In the Japanese mass screening programmes, 50% of patients with early gastric carcinomas had symptoms.[52] The precise nature of symptoms is often related to the macroscopic type of early gastric cancer, ulcer-type symptoms being produced by type III lesions.

The types of symptom that can be attributed to gastric cancer are illustrated in Figure 37.14, which demonstrates the symptoms seen in the Cancer Registry patients at the time of presentation, being assessed either as a single or a combination of symptoms. Pain, either epigastric or abdominal, was most frequent as a single symptom. Weight loss and vomiting were frequently recorded when one or more symptoms were present. The data from the Cancer Registry also demonstrates that the median duration of recorded symptoms was frequently less than 5 months. Indigestion, particularly when it was the only symptom, was present for almost twice as long as the others (Figure 37.15).

In addition to these specific gastric-related symptoms, patients may present with manifestations of advanced malignancy. These can be specific and relate to the presence of metastatic disease.

Lymph node metastases Patients may present with palpable lymph nodes, the most classical of these being a node in the posterior triangle, the result of a retrograde lymphatic spread (Virchow's node).

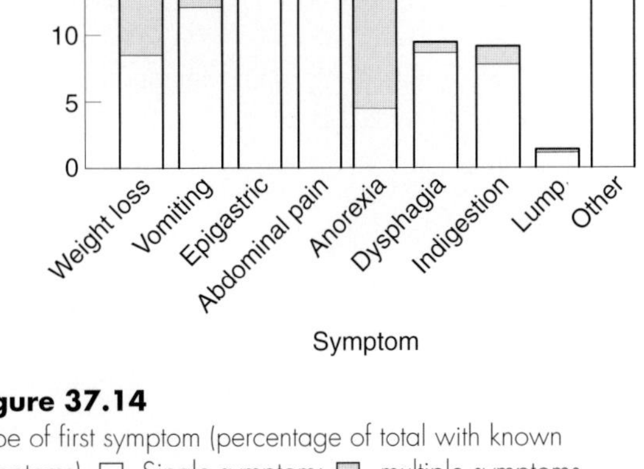

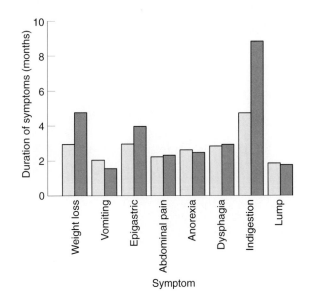

Figure 37.14
Type of first symptom (percentage of total with known symptoms). ☐, Single symptom; ▨, multiple symptoms.

Figure 37.15
Median duration by type of symptom. ■, Single symptom; ☐, one or more symptoms.

Blood-borne spread A classic site for blood-borne spread from gastric primaries is the liver. As a result the patient may present with features of hepatomegaly and jaundice. Other more distant sites in which metastases occasionally occur are lung and bone.

Transperitoneal spread As a result of transperitoneal spread to the ovary (Krukenberg tumours), patients may present with a pelvic mass. Peritoneal seedlings can occur and may produce ascites with associated abdominal distension.

Non-malignant manifestations of malignancy These are common features associated with any malignancy and include non-specific signs and symptoms of anaemia, anorexia and weight loss.

Investigations

The established methods of investigation of the upper gastrointestinal tract are radiology and fibreoptic endoscopy. These are complementary investigations and should not be considered mutually exclusive.

Barium meal

The only barium meal examination capable of diagnosing early gastric cancer is a double-contrast study, preferably facilitated by induction of hypotonia (Figure 37.16). This should not be considered technically adequate if the areae gastricae have not been demonstrated. A conventional single-contrast barium meal can give no grounds for reassurance in a symptomatic patient.

Fibreoptic endoscopy

The fibreoptic endoscope permits macroscopic assessment of the gastric mucosa and enables biopsies and direct brush cytology to be obtained. After macroscopic assessment of the lesion,

at least 6–8 biopsies should be taken.[53] If there is an ulcer, the area of greatest positive yield is its edge. Repeat endoscopy and biopsy may be necessary to establish the diagnosis, especially if there is radiological and endoscopic suspicion of malignancy, or if a benign gastric lesion fails to heal completely or fails to remain healed. In addition, a biopsy should always be taken from the healed area at review. Accuracy can be further increased by brushing all suspicious lesions for cytological examination. Using radiology and endoscopy in combination, the accuracy of diagnosis of gastric cancer is 98%.[54]

Gastric mucosal dyes have been used to assist endoscopists in the detection of lesions. A technique originated in Japan was first described in 1972.[55] This test improves the sensitivity of endoscopy in diagnosing early lesions and involves spraying the gastric mucosa with either a 0.3% solution of indigocarmine or a 0.2% solution of methylene blue. Endoscopic features of early gastric malignancy that the dye highlights are mucosal disruption, clubbing, confluence or convergence of mucosal folds and shallow ulcers with irregular margins. Congo red is a solution which changes from red to blue when in contact with acid-secreting mucosa and this is a useful technique for improving the sensitivity of endoscopic diagnosis.[56] The adminstration of mucus-dissolving agents such as chymotrypsin in addition to the dye (methylene or toluidine blue before gastroscopy) has been recommended. This allows in vivo staining of abnormal lesions (malignant or benign ulceration) instead of the indiscriminate staining of normal and abnormal mucosa that is seen with spraying at gastroscopy.[57]

Barium meal or endoscopy?

All the available data demonstrate that gastroscopy is the best investigation for the diagnosis of dyspepsia. The sensitivity of

(a)

Figure 37.16
Barium meal studies of (a) early and (b) advanced gastric cancers.

(b)

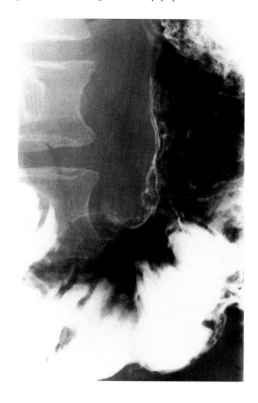

gastroscopy is 92% compared with 54% for a barium meal. The specificity of gastroscopy is 100% compared with 91% for a barium meal. In addition, the clinical outcome is affected significantly more often by gastroscopy. Gastroscopy will reveal a positive finding in 32% of patients who have a barium meal reported as normal.[58]

The advantages of a barium meal are its undisputed lower morbidity and mortality and its presumed acceptability by patients. In the West Midlands study, 2659 patients were investigated by endoscopy and there was no morbidity or mortality.[59] The compliance rate among patients offered endoscopy was 91%. This suggests that most patients find gastroscopy an acceptable procedure. This is supported by a study in which 96 patients had both gastroscopy and a barium meal and were asked to answer a questionnaire within 24 hours of the tests. There were no significant differences between the two groups but there was a tendency for gastroscopy to be the preferred investigation, and more patients were willing to have a repeat gastroscopy than to have a repeat barium meal. A double-contrast barium meal needs to be the first investigation in only a selected group of patients. Many clinicians would probably consider that a barium meal should be the initial investigation in patients who have dysphagia. In patients who have not had a preliminary barium meal demonstrating the cause of the dysphagia, there is a documented risk of perforation by the endoscope. Radiology gives information concerning the motility of the oesophagus, the site of obstruction and evidence of achalasia; dysphagia should be considered a discriminative symptom. A barium meal should also be considered in patients with persistent dyspepsia in whom the results of the endoscopy and ultrasonographic investigation of the liver and biliary tract are normal. Submucosal lesions of the stomach may be apparent in this group of patients.

Endoscopic ultrasonography

The advent of electronic miniaturization of ultrasonographic devices, such that they can be incorporated into the endoscope, allows anatomical definition of the upper gastrointestinal tract and surrounding organs. The superior resolution is achieved by using higher frequencies (7.5–10 MHz) than those used for percutaneous ultrasonography, as the endoscopic probe is closer to the target organ. This technique, which has the ability to resolve the layers of the gastric wall and to define a group of intramucosal or submucosal tumours, may be valuable in identifying those that can be treated endoscopically or for assessing resectability of oesophagogastric malignancies.[60]

Staging of gastric cancer by investigation

The initial investigations are directed towards establishing a histological diagnosis. It is then necessary to stage the tumour in order to define the most appropriate therapy. The initial site of metastatic disease in gastric cancer is invariably intraperitoneal and many patients will have advanced disease at presentation. In order to develop stage-appropriate therapy, it is valuable to assess patients preoperatively. Various investigations have been evaluated to try to provide information concerning the extent of

the primary lesion and the presence of metastatic disease. Simple radiology in the form of straight abdominal and chest radiographs are limited in their ability to demonstrate disease. A chest radiograph can be important in detecting pulmonary metastases but this is a very late feature in the progression of this disease. Computed tomography (CT) may be the most valuable of these investigations.[61] Forty-five patients with proven advanced gastric cancer were studied preoperatively and their findings compared with those of laparotomy. The accuracy of CT in detecting local infiltration into the pancreas, liver, transverse mesocolon and transverse colon was 95, 91, 97 and 93%, respectively. Lymph node enlargement was accurately predicted at the coeliac axis and para-aortic nodes in 88 and 91%, respectively. The presence of liver metastases was accurately predicted in 97%. Using the combined criteria of a large tumour and three-organ involvement on preoperative CT, there was an accurate correlation with the inability to resect the tumour at surgery.

Other investigations

Angiography does not give accurate information relating to the size, type or operability of gastric lesions.[62] Abnormalities in liver function tests may predict unresectability of the primary lesion in 76–89% of instances and, if three of four liver function tests are significantly elevated, radical resection is usually contraindicated.[63] Radioisotope liver scans have a high percentage of false-positive results and are not a reliable method of demonstrating metastatic disease. Scanning with antibodies has been used in an attempt to increase the sensitivity of isotope scanning. However, this has not been proven to increase the sensitivity significantly.[64]

Laparoscopy

Laparoscopy allows direct visual assessment of the peritoneal cavity. In a series[65] of 26 patients with primary gastric cancer, laparoscopy predicted that 20 had local disease and six had advanced disease. In subsequent operations in those with expected local disease, 15 had radical resections and five had palliative procedures. In the six patients with laparoscopically advanced disease, four were unresectable, one had a resection and one patient had a bypass procedure. Similarly, Gross and colleagues[66] studied 46 patients with gastric cancer and considered 19 to be free from metastatic disease and 27 to have disease too extensive for palliative resection. At operation, 16 of those with limited disease underwent resection. However, two patients had infiltration posteriorly, which was unresectable. Despite these false negatives, which were due to disease in sites inaccessible to the laparoscope, it was suggested that unnecessary laparotomy was avoided and that the minimal morbidity supported the use of this technique in unfit patients.

Surgical treatment

An operation is the only effective treatment of adenocarcinoma of the stomach – no patient should be denied its possible benefit. Although investigations may give an indication of stage, most patients need a laparotomy. Laparotomy should only be excluded in a terminal stage of disease or if the patient is otherwise unfit for operation. This general principle of operative assessment must be accepted for all patients because the most effective palliation is also achieved by surgical intervention. The aim of the 'stage-appropriate' operation for gastric cancer must be to apply a treatment designed for maximum survival time while allowing the patients to enjoy an optimal quality of life.

Preoperative assessment

The diagnosis of gastric cancer is established by radiology and endoscopy, the latter providing histological confirmation of cancer. Preoperative investigation should include a full haematological and biochemical screen (haemoglobin level, white cell count, erythrocyte sedimentation rate, urea and electrolyte levels, and liver function tests), chest radiograph and assessments of the cardiovascular system. Many patients are malnourished: hyperalimentation should be considered for them. The effect of preoperative feeding in patients 15% below their ideal body weight may be of value.[67] In a controlled trial, malnourished patients received hyperalimentation for 3 weeks preoperatively; among the 13 patients having total gastrectomy, three of the six controls (patients not given preoperative hyperalimentation) had an anastomotic dehiscence, compared with none of the seven patients who received hyperalimentation.

Preoperative preparation

Gastrectomy is a major operation with a significant mortality, particularly in the elderly. The general condition of the patient must be optimum at the time of operation. Particular attention should be paid to nutrition and to the state of the cardiovascular and respiratory systems. Prophylaxis against deep venous thrombosis should be started preoperatively, with both subcutaneous heparin (5000 units 2–3 times a day) and compression stockings.

The role of prophylactic antibiotics in reducing wound infection and anastomotic dehiscence has not been proved conclusively because there have been few controlled studies. The stomach of a normal individual is usually sterile. However, in patients with either gastric ulcers or carcinomas, there is significant colonization of the gastric contents; this is more common when the pH of the stomach is above 4.[19] There was a higher risk of wound sepsis in patients with a high pH, all of whom had heavily contaminated gastric juice. The most common organisms isolated from gastric juice that were subsequently found in wound infections were *Streptococcus viridans*, *Str. faecalis*, *Escherichia coli*, *Clostridium* species, *Bacteroides* species, *Haemophilus* and *Staphylococcus albus*. Thus, prophylactic broad-spectrum antibiotics should be used, starting preoperatively.

Principles of surgical treatment

The most appropriate operation for gastric cancer must be considered in relation to the known pattern of spread of the disease, the known pattern of recurrence following resection, whether the extent of the resection influences long-term survival, the postoperative mortality, and the effects of the reconstructive procedure on long-term morbidity.

Gastrectomy and lymphadenectomy

In 1932, Carnett and Howell[45] described the mechanism of dissemination from gastric cancers as:

1. Direct extension into the pancreas, hepatic and splenic pedicles, abdominal wall, oesophagus, colon, duodenum and gall bladder
2. Lymphatic embolization
3. Lymphatic permeation
4. Bloodstream embolism
5. Transplantation, commonly causing bronchial and ovarian carcinomatosis.

Gastric carcinomas may spread by direct extension into the duodenum and oesophagus, and it is not true that the pylorus is the limit of spread. Thus, the extent of the gastrectomy must take into account the site of the growth, and in distal lesions the surgeon should remove a significant proportion of duodenum. Similar attention must be paid to lesions at the cardia, achieving at least 5 cm clearance. Frozen section and scrape cytology from the edge of the resected specimen during the operation establishes that microscopic clearance has been achieved. Residual microscopic resection-line disease has now been established as a factor influencing survival. The British Stomach Cancer Group[68] reported that 22% of 390 patients entered into a study of adjuvant chemotherapy had microscopic resection-line disease; in this group of patients the survival was significantly worse than those with clear resection lines.

Lymph node metastases are common. The Japanese Research Society for Gastric Cancer has designated first (N1), second (N2), third (N3) and fourth (N4) tiers of nodes likely to be involved according to the location of the main lesion (Tables 25–27; Figures 25–4). They have defined groups whose involvement indicates increasing advancement of disease.[69] Gastrectomies are defined as R1, R2 and R3 resections, according to the extent of lymphadenectomy (e.g. an R1 resection excised N1 nodes). The degree of involvement of these tiers and the extent of surgical lymphadenectomy influences survival. The corrected 5-year survival rate for N1 involvement is 38.5%, for N2 involvement 22.8%, for N3 involvement 11.1% and for N4 involvement 8.5%. The corrected 5-year survival rate following R0 resections is 26%, R1 42.4%, R2 49.5% and R3 40%. This suggests that an R2 resection is associated with the best survival results and that an R3 resection need be considered only for those with N2 involvement, if the resections can be achieved with an acceptable postoperative mortality. Certainly, in Japan, the extension of the lymphadenectomy has not been associated with an increase in postoperative mortality.

The observed pattern of recurrence of gastric carcinoma after resection has important implications for surgical therapy.

Recurrence is in the gastric remnant in 10–15%[70] and this has been used as an argument for routine total gastrectomy (total gastrectomy *en principe*). The 5-year survival rate following total gastrectomy *en principe* is 42.1%, compared with 38.5% for subtotal resections for distal lesions. In the Japanese study, the 5-year survival rate for total gastrectomy was 19.8%, for proximal gastrectomy 23.1% and for distal gastrectomy 50.3%; the 5-year survival rate for distal gastrectomy excising less than four-fifths of the stomach was 52.0%, and for resections excising more than four-fifths of the stomach it was 45.8%. It is true that many of the types of gastrectomy described in the Japanese studies were chosen because of the site and extent of the lesion, so these groups are not strictly comparable. The argument in favour of total gastrectomy to remove a possible site of recurrence would be sensible if the postoperative mortality and morbidity rates were the same for all procedures.

The necessity for the lymphadenectomy in curative operations for gastric cancer is supported by the increased survival rate obtained by R2 resections compared with R1 resections and R0 resections. Further support is gained from the report of 59 patients with apparently benign gastric ulcers removed surgically and subsequently proved by histological examination to be carcinomas. All these patients initially had a non-radical gastrectomy. Twenty-four then had revisional radical operations, and the 5-year survival rate in this group was 56%. Thirty-five patients had no further resection and a 23% 5-year survival rate. These results support the concept of wide surgical resection and lymphadenectomy as the treatment of choice for gastric cancer and suggests that extent of surgical resection can influence the natural history of the disease.

A limiting factor to extensive resections is postoperative mortality. Longmire,[72] in a review of the literature, reported an overall operative mortality of 21% for total gastrectomy and believed that this was unacceptably high. Pichlmayr and Meyer's[70] reported mortality was 9.3%, and the Japanese mortality after total gastrectomy of 6.2% was similar to that of other, less radical gastrectomies.[69] However, Gilbertson[73] noted a large increase in mortality with R3 resections contributing to a reduction in the 5-year survival rate from 28 to 17%, but the operative mortality in Japan was similar for all types of lymphadenectomy.[69] The low mortality rates reported are from large series from a small number of surgeons. Thus, when a surgeon is not undertaking many gastric operations, his or her postoperative mortality for total gastrectomy is likely to be too high; for such surgeons a subtotal gastrectomy (R2) is the operation of choice.

(a)

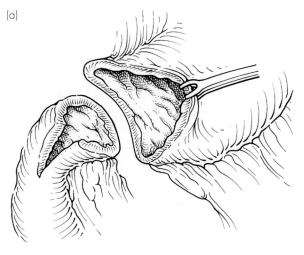

Figure 37.17

Reconstruction after a partial gastrectomy. (a) Billroth II; (b) Billroth I; (c) Roux-en-Y.

(b)

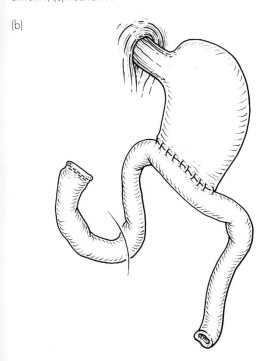

(c)

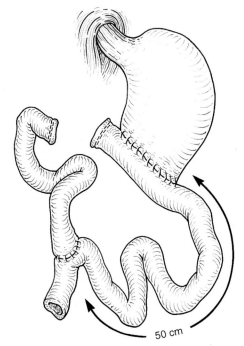

50 cm

Principles of reconstruction

All the features that have been so closely examined in relation to reconstructive procedures for benign disease must be considered in restoring gastrointestinal continuity to the patient with cancer. The reconstructive procedure may produce more severe symptoms than does the cancer itself.

Recurrent disease may produce further gastrointestinal complications. This most frequently occurs locally at the site of the previous resection, either in the gastric remnant or in residual nodes.[74-76] To prevent recurrent disease precipitating intestinal obstruction, it is best to construct a wide stoma at a distance from the site of likely recurrence. This is best achieved by a Billroth II anastomosis (Figure 37.17a). If a Billroth I (Figure 37.17b) reconstruction is performed, a wide stoma can be achieved by anastomosing the proximal stomach to the duodenum, which has been opened on its inner border (Figure 25-5A).

The incidence of postgastrectomy problems, such as vomiting, diarrhoea, dumping and haematological and nutritional effects, is similar in the classical Billroth I anastomosis and in this modified technique.[77] Bile reflux can occur after a reconstructive procedure for a partial gastrectomy; its relation to postoperative symptoms is not clear. It may be associated with symptoms, but these usually occur when the bile reflux is into the oesophagus.[78,79] Thus, there is an argument in favour of reconstructing partial as well as total gastrectomies by a Roux-en-Y technique to provide effective bile diversion (Figure 37.17c).

The reconstructive procedure following a total gastrectomy is also important. Total gastrectomy is often associated with adverse long-term nutritional effects. The sequelae of this operative procedure are best evaluated after total gastrectomy for the Zollinger–Ellison syndrome, for massive bleeding from the stomach or for polyposis. Many patients lost weight after total gastrectomy, although this can be corrected by dietary supplementation.[80-82] Megaloblastic and iron deficiency anaemia may also develop in these patients.[83]

Malabsorption of fat and protein is common in patients after total gastrectomy, and the absorption of glucose usually shows a pattern of early hyperglycaemia and late hypoglycaemia.[84] The most significant malnutrition occurs in patients who have severe postgastrectomy syndromes,[85] which indicates the importance of the reconstructive procedure. The construction of gastric pouches and the use of jejunal segments to ensure duodenal passage of food have been used as reconstructive procedures in an attempt to reduce these problems,[86] but there is no evidence that they reduce the metabolic consequences.

The most commonly employed reconstructions are the Roux-en-Y, the Henley jejunal interposition and the omega loop (Figure 37.18). The incidence of many postgastrectomy syndromes, such as distension, dumping and diarrhoea, is similar for all three methods, occurring in about 20% of all patients.[87] In addition, bile reflux is commonly associated with significant morbidity.[79] Bile reflux was investigated using a [99mTc]HIDA scan (Figure 37.19). A scan with isotopic activity in the oesophageal area correlated well with the presence of endoscopic and microscopic oesophagitis. Eight of ten patients with oesophageal reflux were evaluated as Visick grade 3 or 4, in comparison with only two patients in Visick grade 3 among 17 patients with no reflux. Reflux was related to the length of the diverting limb. It occurred in Roux-en-Y reconstructions with limbs of 35 cm or less and in five of six omega loop reconstructions. This study was unable to evaluate the Henley interposition loop,[88] but it has been reported to be a satisfactory method of diverting bile if the length of the interposition loop is 25 cm or more.[89] A 50 cm Roux-en-Y reconstruction appears to be the operation of choice because it is simpler to perform than the Henley reconstruction. It has fewer anastomoses and ensures a more certain blood supply at the region of the oesophagojejunostomy. Lygidakis[86] described a further development of the Roux-en-Y method of reconstruction and reported improved quality of life with minimal postgastrectomy symptoms.

Surgical procedure (resection)

The incision for laparotomy depends on the site of the primary lesion. For lesions of the cardia for which proximal, partial or total gastrectomy may be envisioned, the patient may be placed on the right side for an abdominothoracic approach. For the more common lesions of the antrum and body of the stomach, adequate exposure is obtained through the abdomen. At laparotomy the possibility of cure is assessed first. Curative resection should be considered impossible only in the presence of peritoneal seedlings, distant metastases, extension to unresectable adjacent structures, or massive involvement of preaortic lymph nodes. Macroscopic surgical evaluation of lymph nodes adjacent to a gastric tumour is not accurate, and treatment should not be limited because of the presence of palpable nodes.

The definitive radical surgical resection must be the equivalent of the R2 resection reported in the Japanese literature. This is a resection that includes the removal of all the N2 tiers of nodes. The precise N1 and N2 nodes vary according to the site of the primary lesion (see Table 37.6 and Figure 37.7). The two most appropriate operations for gastric cancer are a radical subtotal distal gastrectomy and a total gastrectomy. For the common carcinoma of the lower one-third of the stomach, a subtotal distal gastrectomy will remove the N1 and N2 lymph nodes, although it is necessary to undertake extra dissection to clear the right cardiac, common hepatic and coeliac axis nodes. For lesions of the middle third of the stomach, it may be appropriate to undertake a total gastrectomy, in which case the N1 and N2 nodes should be removed *en bloc* with the primary lesion. For lesions of the upper third, the most appropriate resection is a total gastrectomy. In all resections, at least 5 cm clearance of the primary lesion should be achieved, and frozen section should be used to confirm microscopic clearance at the resection lines. As involvement of preaortic nodes is associated with a poor prognosis and indicates N4 node involvement, the initial step in an operation should be to have a preaortic (infratolic) node examined by frozen section. If this proves to be involved, curative surgery is not possible and suitable

(a)

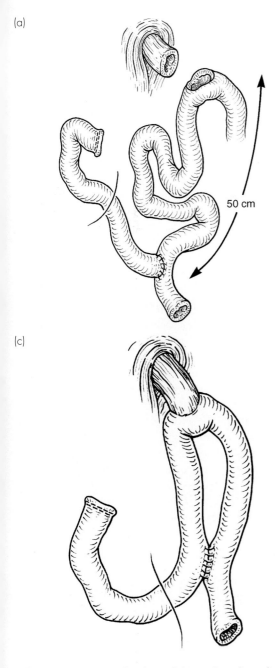

50 cm

(c)

(b)

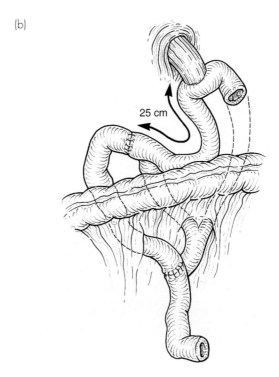

25 cm

Figure 37.18

Reconstruction after a total gastrectomy. (a) Roux-en-Y; (b) Henley jejunal interposition; (c) Omega loop.

to the oesophageal hiatus, followed by the separation of the anterior leaf of the hepatic duodenal ligament, downward to the origin of the right gastric vessels. These vessels are divided and ligated, with removal of the appropriate lymph nodes.

The duodenum is divided, and the distal stomach with the attached omentum is reflected out of the left costal margin of the incision. A portion of duodenal cuff is excised for frozen section examination. Thereafter, the lymph nodes of the hepatoduodenal ligament and those behind the pancreas are dissected *en bloc* from right to left through the foramen of Winslow, and the dissection is continued to the nodes along the common hepatic artery. The left gastric artery is isolated, divided and ligated, with removal of appropriate nodes. The lymph nodes along the splenic artery are dissected toward the splenic hilus. If the presence of pancreatic nodal metastases demands it, resection of the pancreas and spleen can be performed for complete clearance. The attachments of the right cardia to the oesophageal hiatus are separated, both the vagus nerves are divided, and the lymph nodes of the right cardia are removed, completing the mobilization of the stomach and the lymphadenectomy. Now a partial or total gastrectomy is performed. In a total gastrectomy, the spleen is mobilized by dividing the lienorenal ligament; the splenic artery and vein and then the oesophagus are divided, and the stomach is removed.

Method of reconstruction

After a partial gastrectomy, gastrointestinal continuity is restored either by a modification of the Billroth I anastomosis or by a Billroth II anastomosis.

palliative surgery is undertaken. If this node is free of tumour the patient is suitable for curative surgery.

This procedure of gastrectomy and lymph node dissection was described by Nakajima and Kajitani[90] (Figure 37.20). The first step is a detachment of the greater omentum from the transverse colon from left to right. The anterior leaf of the mesocolon is also removed with the omentum. At the inferior margin of the pancreas the right gastroepiploic vessel is ligated, with the dissection of lymph nodes along the superior mesenteric vein. The pancreatic capsule – the serous floor of the omental bursa – is removed upward to the common hepatic artery. The gastroduodenal artery is then dissected downward to the right gastroepiploic artery. It is divided and ligated.

The next step includes the detachment of the lesser omentum from the undersurface of the left lobe of the liver upward

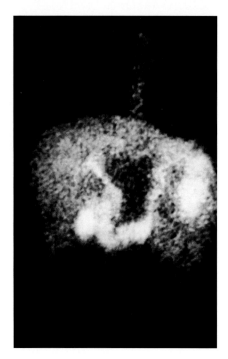

Figure 37.19
[^{99m}Tc]HIDA scan demonstrating bile reflux after a total gastrectomy.

In the modified Billroth I gastrectomy, the whole of the divided end of the stomach is anastomosed end to end to the duodenum. To facilitate this and to obtain a gastroduodenal stoma of 6–8 cm, the incision across the duodenum is extended along the inferomedial border (see Figure 37.17b). The gastroduodenal anastomosis is usually performed in two

layers. For a Billroth II (see Figure 37.17a) reconstruction the duodenal stump is closed in two layers, as is the gastrojejunal anastomosis. For a Roux-en-Y reconstruction the duodenal stump is closed as in a Billroth II gastrectomy; the jejunum is divided 7–10 cm distal to the duodenal flexure, the distal end of the jejunum is closed, and the stomach is anastomosed end to side to this portion of jejunum. The proximal end of jejunum is then anastomosed to the small intestine, 50 cm distal to the gastrojejunal anastomosis (see Figure 37.17c).

After a total gastrectomy the best reconstruction is a Roux-en-Y (see Figure 37.18a). This can be achieved either by hand-sewn anastomosis or by the use of the circular stapling device. In a Henley reconstruction, a 25 cm or longer portion of small intestine is dissected, starting 10 cm from the duodenojejunal flexure. This is anastomosed in an isoperistaltic manner to the oesophagus and duodenum. Small intestinal continuity is re-established by an end-to-end anastomosis (see Figure 37.18b).

Postoperative complications

In addition to the general complications that may be associated with any surgical procedure (e.g. wound sepsis, pneumonia, etc.) there are specific complications of gastric resection, such as reactionary haemorrhage and, later, dehiscence.

Reactionary haemorrhage is not common if a two-layer suture technique or the circular staple gun is used because both methods produce an inner haemostatic layer. However, the principle of the stapling machines is that there are staggered rows of staples that are not totally haemostatic, and great care must be taken to ensure that there is no bleeding. In the event of reactionary haemorrhage, early reoperation is necessary to control the bleeding vessel.

Anastomotic dehiscence is an unusual complication of

(a)
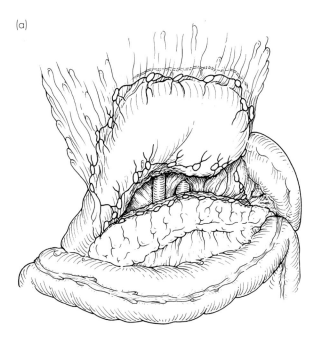

(b)
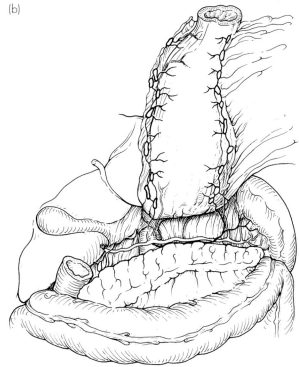

Figure 37.20
(a) and (b) R2 nodal dissection in a gastrectomy.

gastroduodenal or gastrojejunal anastomoses, but it is an important cause of morbidity and mortality following oeso-phagojejunal anastomosis. This complication can be reduced to a minimum by the use of meticulous suture technique.

After total gastrectomy the patient should be maintained on intravenous fluids or nutrition until the integrity of the oesophageal anastomosis has been established, on postopera-tive day 7–10, with a water-soluble contrast examination. If there is a small leak, parenteral nutrition should be continued until the leak has closed. An anastomotic leak following a total or partial gastrectomy may present as an enterocutaneous fistula, and parenteral nutrition is essential until this closes. Fortunately, it is rare for there to be complete dehiscence; if it does occur, it is often associated with sepsis. The only hope for survival is to isolate the ends of intestine as cutaneous fistu-las; for the oesophagus, this necessitates bringing the cervical oesophagus to the surface as an oesophagostomy. Long-term parenteral nutrition is needed until the patient is well enough to undergo a second reconstructive procedure.

Palliative surgical treatment

The ideal form of palliative treatment must be determined indi-vidually for each patient after evaluating the symptoms to be palliated and the quality of life afforded by the procedure. The symptoms most commonly requiring palliation are obstruction, haemorrhage and pain, and the procedures available are bypass, intubation, exclusion and resection. Pyloric obstruction may be effectively corrected by resection or gastroenterostomy, although the results of bypass are so disappointing as to make it hardly worth considering. Obstruction at the cardia is relieved by resection, if feasible; if not, endoscopic intubation is preferred to operative intubation. Haemorrhage, if acute, must be treated by resection. In chronic blood loss, however, radiotherapy may be considered.[91]

Pain is a frequent symptom. It may be intermittent, like peptic ulcer pain, or constant and related to extragastric spread of the neoplasm, either locally or distantly. Resection of the carcinoma, is effective for ulcer-type pain, but pain related to extragastric extension or metastatic disease is seldom relieved by resection. Symptomatic relief can often be achieved only by analgesics, although occasionally radiotherapy or chemo-therapy may help. The best palliation for symptomatic relief follows resection, and the surgeon should always attempt this even if macroscopic disease is left in situ.

Follow-up care

The object of follow-up care in cancer patients is to detect recurrent disease at a sufficiently early stage, to allow further treatment and to give moral support to the patient and the family. In addition, postgastrectomy syndromes should be sought; it should never be assumed that the recurrence of symptoms is related to recurrent disease.

Most patients with gastric cancer will die of recurrent disease within 5 years of resection. Conventional methods of follow-up care include symptomatic assessment and physical examination. Symptomatic evaluation is important if recurrence

is to be detected at an early stage, and the development of any symptoms in the absence of physical signs should be an indi-cation for upper gastrointestinal investigation. Such investiga-tion should be by endoscopy because radiological assessment of the gastric remnant is inaccurate. Physical examination will only detect gross recurrent disease, and the chance of curative surgical treatment in this group is remote. However, palliative treatment should always be considered with reference to the patient's symptoms.

In asymptomatic patients followed up by regular endo-scopy, 11% have been demonstrated to develop remnant recur-rence;[92] however, none of these were suitable for further curative surgery. In a study of 503 patients with early gastric cancer,[93] five developed recurrence in the gastric remnant. Even in this group the recurrence proved to be advanced and a palliative resection was only possible in three cases. Neither of these studies support endoscopic surveillance as a necessary follow-up procedure: remnant recurrence is usually associated with untreatable extragastric disease.

Nutritional indices must be monitored in the follow-up care of all gastrectomy patients. Vitamin B_{12} supplements are neces-sary after total gastrectomy. Among the long-term survivors with partial gastrectomy, a considerable proportion will have iron deficiency anaemia and require iron supplements.

Reasons for failure

Recurrent disease following radical resection is caused by the progressive development of micrometastases. The sites of recurrence are both local and distant. The local recurrences may be in the gastric bed, gastric stump or residual local lymph nodes. Distant metastases may occur at many sites but they occur most commonly in the liver or peritoneal cavity, and, more rarely, in the lungs and bones. In a post-mortem study of 92 patients who had previously had curative subtotal gastrectomy, McNeer et al.[76] found some form of local recur-rence in 80.5%, and at distal sites alone in 15.2%. Gunderson and Sosin[74] analysed the patients in Minnesota who had reoperations. There was evidence of recurrent cancer in 80.4%, and the only site of recurrence was local in 53.7% of the group.

Perhaps the most important group to study for sites of failure are those patients who underwent surgery for 'early' lesions: in this group it is unlikely site of recurrence does not reflect surgical inability to clear disease. Ichiyoshi and his col-leagues[93] reported 17 of 503 patients with 'early' cancer who died from recurrent disease. There was a recurrence mortality of 2.2% at 9 years for mucosal cancer and 8.4% at 8 years for submucosal cancer. The cancer recurred as a result of haematogenous spread (liver, lung, bone) in nine cases, lym-phatic spread in three cases, and in the gastric remnant in five cases. The high incidence of recurrent disease caused by micrometastases after surgical intervention, and the possibility that a more extensive operation might reduce this, has already been explored. Radical resection (R2) may reduce the inci-dence of local recurrence, but extended radical resection (R3) is associated with a high postoperative mortality, and long-term survival is not increased. The inability of an operation to eradicate all disease and prevent the development of recurrence highlights the limitations of surgical treatment as a single modality in the management of gastric cancer. It is clear that adjuvant therapies must be evaluated in an attempt to improve control of this disease.

Non-surgical management

Many non-surgical therapies have been evaluated in patients with gastric cancer, both in the treatment of advanced disease and as an adjuvant to curative resection.

Phase II studies have been valuable in identifying active agents in stomach cancer, so that well-conducted controlled randomized studies could be set up to test those agents. In 1974, Comis and Carter[94] stated that only three drugs had been adequately tested in stomach cancer – 5-fluorouracil (5-FU), Mitomycin C (MMC), and 1,3-bis (2-chloroethyl)-1-nitrosurea (BCNU) – although at that stage only 33 patients had been evaluated with BCNU. Since then, doxorubicin, cis-platinum and etoposide in the West, and chromomycin A3 and carbazilquinone in Japan, can be added. These latter two drugs have generated very little interest in the West despite response rates of 39 and 25%, respectively. The single agents so far evaluated have been summarized by Earl et al.[95] and Ogawa.[96] Only a handful have been properly evaluated, and yet many have now been assessed in randomized single agent and combination studies.

The question of randomization raises the issue of control groups and what they should be. In the USA, the standard comparison has been with 5-FU, despite the fact that in 1974 Moertel et al.[97] pointed out that it had minimal therapeutic value, and more recently Schien et al.[98] stated that the treatment of advanced disease with single agents, including 5-FU, is 'an established exercise in futility'. Both Fielding et al.[99] in the UK and Douglas[100] in the USA have shown concurrently that no-treatment controls have a better survival than historical controls in adjuvant studies.

In addition to lack of adequate evaluation for response prior to trials, and the lack of no-treatment or placebo controls, other general criticisms of the majority of published randomized trials are as follow:

- The numbers are too small in each arm (to have a 95% chance of showing a 20% difference requires over 100 patients in each arm).

- Response rate is used as an end-point, rather than survival. The response rate is notoriously difficult to assess in gastric cancer and has rarely related to significant benefit in survival.

- There has been poor stratification for the 'known' prognostic factors. In advanced disease the most important appears to be initial performance status.[97] Lavin et al.[101] in a multivariate analysis of data collected prospectively for a large randomized study in 322 patients, confirmed the prognostic value of performance status and added blood chemistries, measurable disease status and differential counts as independent prognostic variables in advanced disease.

In adjuvant studies the most important prognostic factor is the stage of disease, to which may be added length of history and histological type (Lauren classification). In most adjuvant studies in the West, comparisons have been made within conventional stage groups. This approach may lead to unrecognized inequalities within stage groups that could have a greater effect on prognosis than any benefit of treatment.

Advanced disease

Radiotherapy There are no 'pure' randomized trials of radiotherapeutic regimens. Those in which radiotherapy is one of the treatment arms will be discussed in a later section concerning combined modality treatment.

Chemotherapy The response rates for the major studies of combinations of chemotherapeutic agents are summarized below.

Kovach et al.[102] at the Mayo Clinic compared 5-FU (13.5 mg/kg per day × 5 every 5 weeks i.v.) to BCNU (50 mg/m² per day × 5 every 8 weeks i.v.) and BCNU (40 mg/m² per day × 5 every 8 weeks i.v.). There were only 28, 23 and 34 patients in each group. Their conclusion (that 5-FU alone and 5-FU and BCNU were superior in response rate and survival to BCNU alone) is undermined by the poorer performance status of the BCNU group.

Moertel et al.[103] compared 1-(2-chloroethyl)-3-(4-methylcyclohex)-1-nitrosourea (MeCCNU) (200 mg/m² every 7 weeks orally) to MeCCNU (276 mg/m² every 7 weeks orally) plus 5-FU (300 mg/m² day × 5 every 7 weeks i.v.), with or without an induction course of cyclophosphamide (1200 mg/m² single dose i.v.). This study suggests that addition of cyclophosphamide increases toxicity and reduces survival and response rate. Although the numbers are rather small in each group, the groups were well stratified and it is hard to criticize the finding that the 5-FU – MeCCNU combination had a better survival at the 5% level. Taken in conjunction with the study by Kovach et al.[102] it looked at this stage as though 5-FU and nitrosurea combinations might have been a significant advance. Kingston et al.[104] reported the results of a double-blind controlled trial of 5-FU (20 mg/kg i.v. weekly) and MeCCNU (125 mg/m² every 6–10 weeks orally) versus placebo. The groups were stratified for age and length of history but not for performance status, but they were found to be equivalent in this respect. This is an important study as a placebo control was used and there were nearly 100 patients in each arm. Contrary to the previous study, no survival advantage was found. This result, however, has failed to be conclusive for two reasons. The inclusion of palliative procedures in unequal proportions in the two arms and the inability of 59% of patients to take both the drugs have biased the result against the treatment arm.

In 1979[105] the Eastern Co-operative Oncology Group (ECOG) reported on two further studies which included 5-FU and MeCCNU. In the first, 139 patients were evaluable from 191 entered into a study of 5-FU (325 mg/m² per day on days 1–5 and 375 mg/m² per day on days 36–40 every 10 weeks i.v.) plus MeCCNU (150 mg/m² orally every 10 weeks) versus 5-FU (325 mg/m² days 1–5 every 5 weeks) plus MMC (3.75 mg/m² per day × 5 every 5 weeks) versus doxorubicin

(60 mg/m² on days 1, 22, 43 every 4 weeks i.v. to a total dose of 550 mg/m². Those patients with a cardiac history were not randomized to doxorubicin, so only 115 patients were properly stratified and randomized to the three groups and eligible for survival analysis. There were no differences between the groups in this respect but the numbers are too small in each group to consider the results definitive. It is an interesting comment on response rate data that the reported response rate for 5-FU and MeCCNU in this study was 24%, compared with the same group's reported response for this regimen in 1976 of 41%.

The second study[106] randomly compared 5-FU alone (450 mg/m² per day on days 1–5 i.v. every 5 weeks) with 5-FU (325 mg/m² per day on days 1–5 i.v. and 375 mg/m² per day on days 36–40 i.v. every 10 weeks) plus MeCCNU (150 mg/m² orally 9–10 weeks) and additionally randomized to concomitant testolactone or no testolactone (50 mg orally × 3 per day until death or intolerance). When disease progression occurred patients were all reassigned to secondary treatment with doxorubicin alone. A total of 179 were randomized after stratification for performance status, degree of differentation and resection of primary. The combined treatment was not superior to 5-FU alone, and there was no benefit from the addition of testolactone.

The same year, the South West Oncology Group (SWOG)[107] presented their results of a comparison of 5-FU (1000 mg/m² per day on days 1–4 i.v. every 4 weeks) plus either MeCCNU (150–175 mg/m² orally every 8 weeks). The groups were stratified for measurable disease but not for performance status, and it is not clear whether the groups were well matched. A total of 167 patients were analysed but no difference in survival was found. The study was unusual in having very low response rates for these two combinations: 14% for 5-FU and MMC and only 9% for 5-FU and MeCCNU.

The SWOG study[107] and the ECOG study[105] already referred to are two of the three main studies reporting 5-FU and MMC combinations; response rates of 14 and 31%, respectively, are quoted, but survival is identical and in neither study is it different from that of doxorubicin.

Rake et al.[108] reported one of the few studies of advanced disease to use a no-treatment control arm. They assessed 5-FU (10 mg/kg × 5 every 6 weeks) in combination with MMC (100 µg/kg × 5 every 6 weeks) after an induction course of vincristine, methotrexate, cyclophosphamide and 5-FU. Only 76 patients were studied, and these were split between 37 inoperable patients and 39 with a palliative primary resection with no stratification. Survival was identical between treatment and controls in these two subgroups. This study has since been repeated in an adjuvant setting.

The ECOG study[105] also showed that doxorubicin had activity in stomach cancer and was as good as 5-FU in combination with MeCCNU or MMC. The Gastrointestinal Tumour Study Group (GITSG)[109] compared doxorubicin (60 mg/m² days 1, 22, 43 every 4 weeks to a total dose of 550 mg/m²) with FMC (5-FU 300 mg/m² per day × 5, MMC 1 mg/m² per day × 5 and cytosine arabinoside (ARA-C) 50 mg/m² per day × 5 every 5 weeks) and FAMe (5-FU 350 mg/m² per day on days 1–5,

36–40 i.v., doxorubicin 40 mg/m² on days 1, 36 i.v. and MeCCNU 150 mg/m² orally on day 1 every 10 weeks). Of 134 patients stratified (for measurable disease, performance status and resection of primary) and randomized, 110 patients were evaluated. Response rates were 24% for doxorubicin, 17% for FMC and an encouraging 47% for FAMe, which also had an improved survival over doxorubicin ($P < 0.03$) and FMC ($P < 0.04$) after correction for prognostic factors with a Cox multivariant analysis.

FMC (5-FU 10 mg/kg, MMC 0.8 mg/kg and ARA-C 0.8 mg/kg i.v. × 2 per week for 2 weeks then weekly indefinitely) has been compared with 5-FU alone (13.5 mg/kg per day, then alternate days to toxicity, then 15 mg/kg i.v. weekly after recovery from toxicity).[110] No stratification was used but the groups were very well matched. No difference was found between the two groups in response rate or survival, but the small numbers used once more make the result inconclusive.

FAMe has since been reported in two further studies from the GITSG[111,112] and one from the ECOG.[113] The first study[111] compared 5-FU and MeCCNU (FMe) with FAMe (using a slightly lower dose of 5-FU and MeCCNU than the first arm), FIMe (with the same dose of 5-FU and MeCCNU as FAMe but substituting IRCF 159 razoxane for doxorubicin) and FAM (5-FU 275 mg/m² i.v. on days 1–5 every 5 weeks + doxorubicin 30 mg/m² on days 1–5 every 5 weeks + MMC 10 mg/m² every 10 weeks). Patients were stratified for measurable disease, prior chemotherapy, resection of the primary and performance status, but there was a final imbalance in the distribution of good performance status patients in favour of the FAMe and FMe patient groups. An unbalanced randomization was used to produce higher numbers in the previously unstudied groups; 205 were randomized and 181 were evaluated. Despite the small numbers, a significantly improved survival ($P < 0.01$) was claimed for FAM that purports to take account of the imbalance of prognostic factors in the groups. On this occasion, FAMe was not better than FM3, and the FIMe was rather worse. The toxicity of the FMe (higher dose) regimen was greater than the other combinations.

The next study from the GITSG[112] produced the opposite result. FAMe was compared with FAM and FA. This was a similar well-constructed study with well-matched groups (although there were slight imbalances to the disadvantage of the FA group). It was a large study with 232 patients equally divided, and on this occasion there was a just statistically significant survival advantage for FAMe over FA ($P < 0.03$) but not FAM, and FAM was no better than FA.

The ECOG study[113] is only available in abstract form so far. A total of 196 patients were evaluated from 241 randomized to FMe, FAMe, FAM or doxorubicin + MMC (AM). Although the regimens are similar, none of the doses exactly correspond to the previous GITSG studies. FAM and FAMe are very similar in response rate and survival, and both appear to be better than FMe in these two respects and better than AM in survival but not response rate. The final results are awaited. On the basis of the combination of the best response rate (40%), the best survival and the best toxicity, this group has chosen FAM for further adjuvant studies. Prior to these latter studies, an interesting co-operative study between Japan and the USA had been reported.[114] 5-FU plus doxorubicin was used as a common arm between the two centres and compared with tegafur (Ftorafur) + doxorubicin + BCNU in the USA and with tegafur + doxorubicin + MMC in Japan. The definitive report is still awaited, but no differences in survival were found either between the centres or the study groups.

In a study from the Mayo clinic,[115] with approximately 100 patients in each arm and 98% of those randomized evaluable, FAM (the standard Georgetown regimen) was compared with FA (5-FU 400 mg/m^2 per day on days 1–4, doxorubicin 40 mg/m^2 every 4 weeks) and 5-FU alone (500 mg/m^2 per day days 1–5 every 4 weeks). No difference in response rate or survival was found. FAM was the most toxic, and neither FAM nor FA could be recommended as standard treatment.

Cis-platinum used in combination with other agents has been reported[116] to produce high response rates. Cis-platinum (40 mg/m^2 i.v. on days 2 and 8), etoposide (120 mg/m^2 on days 4, 5 and 6) and doxorubicin (20 mg/m^2 on days 1 and 7) have been used in 56 patients with a reported response rate of 73%.

This latest study is encouraging: the response rates documented are higher than reported previously and may be sufficient to result in long-term benefit.

Radiotherapy and chemotherapy In 1969, Moertel and co-workers[117] reported the results of a prospective double-blind controlled study of 48 patients with locally unresectable gastric cancer. All received 3500–4000 rads in 150–200 rad (1.5–2 Gy) fractions, followed by either 5-FU (25 patients) to a total dose of 45 mg/kg over 3 days, or placebo (23 patients). There was a statistically significant survival advantage in favour of the 5-FU group ($P < 0.01$), the mean survival being more than double that in controls (13 versus 5.9 months). After 5 years of complete follow-up, there was a 12% survival in the patients receiving chemotherapy (3/25), whereas none of the radiotherapy-only group survived more than 15 months.[34] This study needs to be repeated with better stratification and larger numbers.

The study by Falkson et al.[118] compared 5-FU (12.5 mg/kg per day × 5 i.v. every 5 weeks) and radiotherapy (2000 rad (20 Gy) over 12 days then 1200 rad (12 Gy) with second and fifth courses) and radiotherapy with a four-drug combination (5-FU, vincristine, BCNU and dacarbazine (DTICO)). Unfortunately, the study was not stratified. The authors concluded that a larger group of patients, which would permit adequate stratification, might show an advantage for the four-drug combination. There is, however, little evidence in phase II studies for the usefulness of these particular drugs, and there are now better combinations to evaluate.

The GITSG[119] study of 5-FU plus MeCCNU with or without radiotherapy (5000 rad (50 Gy) in 8 weeks) in locally advanced disease has produced interesting data. Overall, radiotherapy plus chemotherapy (5-FU + MeCCNU) is not statistically different from chemotherapy alone, but the pattern of survival is statistically different when tested by a non-proportional hazard model. At 1 year, the results in the radiotherapy arm are inferior to those of chemotherapy alone, but the survival curve

for radiotherapy plateaus, whereas that for the chemotherapy arm continues to fall, so that at 5 years there is a superior survival for the radiotherapy plus chemotherapy arm. It is suggested that the combination of radiotherapy and chemotherapy, when treating locally advanced disease, is possibly effective but toxic. Further studies are needed to test different delivery schedules to try to reduce this toxicity.

Adjuvant therapy

Radiotherapy The rationale for adjuvant radiotherapy in gastric cancer has been defined by Gunderson and Sosin.[74] When evaluating the sites of failure at second-look operations after a potentially curative resection, 54% of 86 patients had local failure only, and 88% had a local or regional component of failure.

The only randomized study so far reported used intraoperative radiotherapy (IORT).[120] This was undertaken over a period of 20 years and involved 26 institutions in Japan. Following resection and before anastomosis, the patient is given 2800–4000 rad (28–40 Gy) as a single dose using a special pentagonal sterile treatment cone, while vital organs are shielded as much as possible. The anastomosis is then completed. This treatment has been used on an alternate patient basis as a form of randomization. A total of 110 patients had potentially curative surgery only, and 84 patients had IORT. No serious postoperative complications were reported, and no intestinal disturbances were found. While no statistical analysis has been given and the numbers remain small, the increased survival in the higher risk groups, particularly for those with local invasion but no distant spread, is encouraging.

Further work on IORT is currently being undertaken by Sindelar and co-workers at the National Cancer Institute. Patients with serosal or lymph node involvement who have had a 'curative' resection being randomized to external beam radiotherapy (EBRT), 4500 cGy in a single fraction, plus the hypoxic cell sensitizer misonidazole 3.5 mg/m^2. The lack of a control group weakens the value of this study. The low dose of radiation, compared with that of Abe and Takahashi,[120] was used because results of preliminary studies showed portal fibrosis and complete loss of kidney function at or above these levels. Abe and Takahashi[120] reported no such complications. IORT is an expensive form of therapy and would be difficult to institute widely, even if of considerable proven benefit.

In 1981, the British Stomach Cancer Group[122] instituted a randomized controlled study comparing surgery only to surgery plus postoperative adjuvant external radiotherapy (4500 cGy in 25 fractions over 5 weeks) or chemotherapy (MMC, doxorubicin and 5-FU); 436 patients were randomly allocated to one of the three treatment groups. Within a 12-month minimum follow-up, 334 patients died, 292 from recurrent cancer. The median survival for all patients treated was 15 months. Neither form of adjuvant therapy provides a survival benefit.

Chemotherapy When most currently reported adjuvant studies were established in the 1970s, there was a general optimism that drugs that were only partially effective in advanced disease might still be effective in the adjuvant setting. This is now widely recognized as false, and, in fact, the results of adjuvant studies have been even more disappointing than studies of tumour responsiveness. To date, no Western study of adjuvant therapy has shown a survival advantage for treatment over controls, whereas Japanese studies with impressive numbers have shown statistically significant but small benefits in specific situations.

Single agents In 1968, Longmire et al.[123] reported an adjuvant study of thio-tepa (triethylenethiophosphoramide). At 3 years the lymph node-negative groups showed a survival advantage, but at 10 years no difference persisted.[124] This early lesson has frequently repeated itself and must not be forgotten when evaluating interim reports. The fact that the only stratification was for type of surgery detracts somewhat from the conclusions. However, the groups were matched for age, extent of disease, type of surgery and concomitant diseases. It is very likely, therefore, that thio-tepa in these doses is not beneficial in the adjuvant setting.

Serlin et al.[125] reported the results of the Veterans Administration Surgical Oncology Group (VASOG) study of 5-FUDR (5-fluoro-2-deoxyuridine) versus an untreated control. There were no differences in survival, operative mortality or complications between the two groups. The groups were only stratified for type of surgery, and it is not clear whether the groups were well matched in other respects, but with nearly 200 patients in each group, stratification becomes less important and the result is probably valid.

The study by Fujimoto et al.[126] compared an oral regimen of 5-FU + Futraful (FT207) given continuously on a daily basis for 24–36 months to toxicity, with no-treatment controls. A total of 249 patients were randomized but, when reported, 32 patients were excluded from the treatment arm but none from the control arm because it was 'too soon for evaluation'. No stratification was used and it is not clear whether the groups are comparable, apart from age and stage. Despite these deficiencies, the results are impressive. There was an overall survival benefit of approximately 20% throughout the 5-year-period ($P < 0.001$). This was true for the serosa-positive groups but not for the serosa-negative group. The deficiencies in this study detract from the impact of these results, but there are good grounds for repeating this approach with a tighter protocol.

Imanaga and Nakazato[127] reported the results of a large study of 2636 patients given MMC under four different treatment protocols. In 714 stage I–IV patients given a low dose (0.08 mg/kg) twice weekly for 5 weeks (protocol 1) a 13.5% overall 5-year survival advantage over no-treatment controls was reported ($P < 0.05$). (This was 36.6% in serosa-negative patients.) Protocols 2 and 3 with high-dose short-term treatments showed no benefit. Protocol 4 repeated the study of protocol 1 but had an additional FMC arm. At 3 years no differences were apparent. No stratification was used, and insufficient data were given to assess the comparability of these groups. It would be difficult to repeat this study in the West with such large numbers, but it is interesting to note that

it would appear that this institution has not been able to repeat its own results and, perhaps wisely, still feels the need for no-treatment controls.

Two agents

1. 5-FU + MeCCNU There have been three major adjuvant studies of this combination against no-treatment controls. The GITSG study[128] and the ECOG study[129] used identical regimens, and both were stratified for depth of invasion, lymph node status and tumour site, but the GITSG stratified for histology and type of gastrectomy as well. The GITSG had 142 evaluable patients of 165 randomized, and treatment had to start within 6 weeks of surgery. The two groups were extremely well matched for the stratification characteristics, as well as for sex, race, age and performance status. At the time of reporting, the median follow-up was 4 years, and at that point there was a statistically significant survival advantage in favour of treatment, demonstrated by a covariate analysis to allow for what small group differences there were ($P = 0.06$). This slender advantage may be confirmed on continued follow-up, but if it follows the pattern of other studies reported before the 5-year figures were available, it may equally well disappear.

The ECOG study would appear to be an almost identical study to that of the GITSG, but the 2-year survival figures after a median follow-up in excess of 4 years is identical in both groups.

The third major study was conducted by the VASOG.[130] The regimen was slightly different, using a potentially higher dose of both drugs given on a 7-week cycle (rather than 10-week) but also started within 7 weeks of surgery. Although 321 patients entered the trial, of which a commendable 312 were evaluable, they were only stratified for extent of disease and not for other factors. Retrospectively, analysis shows the groups to be as well matched for prognostic factors as those in the GITSG study. Only the first stratification group, with 156 patients, is comparable with the GITSG study, which used very strict criteria to try to ensure that only 'curative' resections were included. A potential weakness of the VASOG study is that their 'curative' group included patients with suspected but not histologically proven residual disease. They found no differences in survival on log rank analysis in any of the groups ($P = 0.88$ for the curative group). Overall, it would appear that there is, as yet, no justification for the use of adjuvant 5-FU and MeCCNU.

2. FT207 Futraful) + MMC The first Japanese co-operative study[131] evaluated FT207 (60 g over 3 months) combined with either high-dose short-term or lower dose long-term MMC against these two MMC regimens alone. A total of 1673 patients were studied. A survival advantage for the combination is claimed.

A second Japanese co-operative study[132,133] evaluated MMC + FT207. High-dose short-term MMC was given to group A, a 1-year course of FT207 was given to group B, and the two were combined in group C. Over 3000 patients were evaluated and a statistically significant advantage is claimed at 3 years for FT207 over MMC and for the combined treatment over the other two. Only the authors' abstracts are available in English, and therefore a detailed assessment of both studies is not possible. The 5-year figures should be available shortly, and it is to be hoped that full details will be published in the West.

3. 5-FU + MMC The British Stomach Cancer Group[134] reported a study of 411 evaluable patients of 455 randomized to receive either long-term (up to 2 years) MMC + 5-FU with or without an induction course (5-FU, methotrexate, vincristine and cyclophosphamide) or placebo. (The surgery to first treatment interval was rather long at up to 3 months.) Stratification was for age, sex, length of history and stage, and the groups proved to be well matched. Overall, there were no differences in survival. An early advantage seen in those receiving treatment started within 1 month of surgery was not sustained at 2 years, but suggested further adjuvant studies should have as short a surgery-to-treatment time as possible. This study reported 16 drug-related deaths which would have abolished any beneficial effect of the treatment. Of these, 11 were due to the haemolytic uraemic syndrome, which would appear to be a serious dose-limiting effect of MMC. This study supports the importance of untreated controls in all future adjuvant trials.

Multiple agents Nakajima et al.[135] reported a trial comparing FMC, MMC alone, and no-treatment controls. Only 126 patients were evaluable but, despite these small numbers, a statistically significant superior survival was found for FMC over no-treatment controls but not over MMC alone.

Radiotherapy and chemotherapy In the largest series to date, Dent et al.[136] reported a randomized study of 142 surgically treated patients stratified according to TNM stage into division 1 (T1–3, N1–2, MO) or 2 (T4 or M1). Division 1 was randomized, without further stratification, to receive either no further treatment or radiotherapy (2000 rad (20 Gy) in eight fractions over 10 days), followed by 5-FU (500 mg daily × 4 preradiation then 12.5 mg/kg daily for 5 days every 4 weeks for six courses). Division 2 (T4 or M1) was randomized to receive either no treatment, the same radiotherapy and 5-FU, or into a third group who received thiotepa 45 mg i.v. for 3 days, repeated monthly for 6 months. At 2 years minimum follow-up, when 86% had died, no difference in survival was found between treated and control patients in either division. Only division 1 is truly an adjuvant study. A total of 66 patients were randomized to the two groups, and 58 were evaluable. They ranged from T1 to T3 N2, and, whereas the two groups are well matched, the numbers within each TNM stage became too small for these data to be considered reliable.

Moertel et al.[137] have reported a study of 62 patients with resected tumours that involved the regional nodes or were locally invasive. A non-stratified unbalanced randomization was used to allocate either no further treatment or 3750 rad (37.5 Gy) radiotherapy plus 5-FU (15 mg/kg per day for 3 days). Patients were asked for consent after randomization: 10 of 39 refused treatment.

The 5-year survival rate for the groups as randomized was 23% for the treatment and 4% for the control arm; a significant result at *P* < 0.024. When, however, the ten patients who refused the treatment as randomized were analysed separately, the 5-year survival proved to be 20% for those who received the randomized treatment and a surprising 30% for the treatment refusers. There was now no significant difference between the three groups. This raises interesting questions about the nature of survival in active and passive patients, as well as giving a timely reminder of the continuing need for no-treatment controls and the problems arising from interference with randomized procedures.

There is, therefore, contradictory evidence about the value of 5-FU and radiotherapy in the adjuvant setting. Although Moertel's success may have been due to the larger treatment field and the higher radiotherapy dose than that used by Dent et al.,[136] the latter used a higher and longer dose of 5-FU. Radiotherapy and 5-FU cannot be recommended for routine use in the adjuvant setting, but further studies are warranted.

Summary

Surgery remains the only conclusively beneficial therapy for gastric cancer. On the basis of the evidence reviewed here, no patient with gastric cancer should receive radiotherapy or chemotherapy outside of controlled trials. The lack of placebo or no-treatment controls has reduced the value of many years of expensive and otherwise well-conducted research; many patients have suffered toxic treatment without benefit to themselves or posterity.

Future trials need to have sufficient numbers to: (1) have a chance of showing a true positive effect – far too many studies were bound to fail on this count alone; and (2) limit stratification requirements. As trial numbers increase, the group differences even out; this would mean that a study would be likely to withstand retrospective criticism based on newly discovered prognostic factors not originally stratified for.

There are suggestions from these data that real improvements in patient treatment may be possible with currently available drugs. Dramatic changes in the management of gastric cancer, however, are not likely to be achieved until new, more effective agents are found.

Overall results and prognosis

Over 100 years ago, Theodore Billroth operated on Theresa Hellor for a gastric adenocarcinoma.[138] At the laparotomy a few hazelnut-sized mesenteric lymph nodes were found and resected with the stomach. Microscopically, these nodes were involved with a medullary type of cancer. A few months later, Mrs Hellor died of recurrent disease. This story is familiar to the modern surgeon and is still typical of the presentation and course of gastric cancer in the Western world.

However, there have been advances since Billroth's initial operation. His achievement was that his patients survive the operation, a rare event 100 years ago for surgery of such magnitude. Perhaps the most significant advance in the twentieth century has been to make partial gastrectomy a safer operation. In 1896 the operative mortality for gastrectomy was 54.4%,[139] compared with 4% in modern times. This reduction in postoperative mortality has been due mainly to improvements in surgical techniques, anaesthesia and supportive care.

The overall results of treatment are dependent on certain features:

- Laparotomy rates
- Operative mortality
- Prognostic factors.

Laparotomy rate

Generally, there has been an increase in the number of patients undergoing laparotomy (Table 37.8). In hospital-based areas, this can be as high as 90%. However, in population-based studies the rate is usually lower, but even these demonstrate a trend towards increased laparotomy rate, which has been followed by an increase in the resection rate, particularly in the proportion undergoing curative resection. Throughout the period of the West Midlands Cancer Registry study there was an increase in both laparotomy and resection rates: in 1957–1961 54 and 28%, respectively; in 1977–1981 58 and 33%, respectively (Figure 37.21). The fact that more patients have undergone laparotomy, with the corresponding improved assessment of the spread of disease, may account for the increased resection rate for both curative and palliative intent in the last decade.

Although it is proposed that the lower laparotomy rate is simply related to the stage of the disease, such that many are considered to have disease too advanced to be considered for treatment, the data do not support this. There are other factors which determine whether a patient is offered the opportunity of surgical treatment. Age has a marked influence on treatment, resection and laparotomy rates. In all patients offered laparotomy, the resection rates are comparable. However, of 1959 in the age group 0–49 years, 5141 in the age group

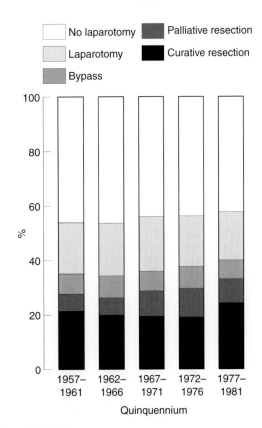

Figure 37.21

Distribution by treatment and quinquennium.

50–59 years, 9853 in the age group 60–69 years, 9995 in the age group 70–79 years, and 4619 above the age of 80 years, the percentages offered no treatment were 17.7, 21.5, 31.5, 51.6 and 80.1%, respectively (Figure 37.22).

Table 37.8 Rates and results of an international comparison of the surgical treatment of gastric cancer in Europe, the USA and Japan

AUTHORS	YEAR	OPERATION RATE (%)	RESECTION RATE (%)	CURATIVE RESECTION RATE (%)	OVERALL 5-YEAR SURVIVAL RATE (%)
Europe					
Brookes et al.	1950–1959	63.5	42.5	26.5	4.9
Desmond	1944–1970	—	54.0	18.4	8.0
Svennevig and Nysted	1959–1968	71.3	45.0	32.3	10.0
Inberg et al.	1946–1955	53.9	21.1	17.1	3.7
	1956–1965	62.0	32.1	25.2	6.5
	1966–1972	69.3	45.1	23.6	10.8
USA					
Dupont et al.	1948–1973	76.0	48.0	22.5	7.5
Cady et al.	1940–1949	80.0	—	37.0	7.0
	1957–1966	94.0	58.0	44.0	11.0
Hoerr	1950–1972	96.0	54.6	46.4	15.1
Adashek et al.	1956–1965	71.0	39.0	24.0	8.0
	1966–1975	76.0	51.0	31.0	10.0
Scott et al.	1960–1983	90.0	71.0	42.0	15.0
Japan					
Mine et al.	1955–1963	93.2	63.2	52.3	14.4
Muto et al.	1941–1961	98.7	79.4	—	19.0
Kajitani and Takagi	1946–1970	97.7	—	67.0	33.3
Kajitani and Miwa	1963–1966	94.3	63.4	44.7	16.4

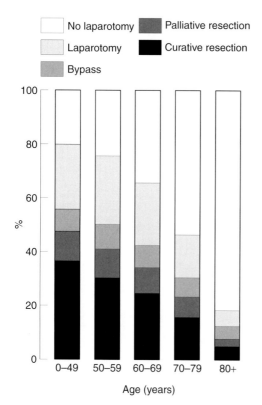

Figure 37.22
Distribution by type of treatment and age.

Table 37.9 Distribution (%) by treatment within site

TREATMENT	CARDIA	BODY	PYLORIC ANTRUM	OTHER SINGLE SITES	UNSPECIFIED OR MULTIPLE
Curative resection					
Total	7.4	10.1	1.7	7.3	2.4
Partial	25.4	14.0	33.6	24.2	5.3
Palliative resection					
Total	2.5	3.0	0.6	2.6	1.1
Partial	8.6	5.2	13.1	10.5	3.0
Other treatments					
Bypass	1.7	4.2	18.5	4.6	4.8
Laparotomy + intubation	13.6	3.8	0.1	0.9	1.2
Laparotomy + adjuvant therapy	1.0	1.8	0.6	1.6	1.2
Laparotomy only	9.8	20.4	8.2	16.3	18.6
No laparotomy					
Intubation	4.9	1.2	0.6	0.4	0.6
Chemotherapy or radiotherapy	0.8	1.2	0.5	0.7	1.1
No treatment	24.3	35.1	22.5	30.9	60.7
Total	100.0	100.0	100.0	100.0	100.0
Based on	2826	3340	6687	4393	14321

The site of the primary lesion has an effect on both laparotomy and resection rates. Resection rates are highest for pyloric and antral lesions. For both cardia and pyloric tumours, the combined rates for intubation and bypass are highest, indicating attempts to overcome the obstructive complications of these tumours. Lesions in the body are associated with lowest resection rates and highest rates of non-treatment, indicating the limited treatment for these tumours. The lower laparotomy rate of 37.6% for tumours involving multiple unspecified sites not only reflects the extent of tumours involving multiple sites, but also accounts for the limited information available about these sites (Table 37.9).

Operative mortality

The number of patients dying in the postoperative period is of particular concern. Postoperative mortality, as assessed by 1-month mortality, varies with the aim of therapy (Table 37.10). It is lowest for those undergoing resection but increases significantly in patients undergoing bypass procedures or having laparotomy alone, and, of particular interest, the 1-month mortality is highest in the group offered no treatment. In a population-based study reported by Allum et al.,[140] resection was undertaken in 9247 patients: for cure in 6588 and as palliation in 2659. The operative mortality (as defined as death within 30 days of operation) for total gastrectomy was 28.8% and for partial gastrectomy 13%. The operative mortality rate for palliative resections was 36.6% for total gastrectomy and 23.0% for partial gastrectomy. The 30-day mortality rate for those undergoing laparotomy was 35.8%, contrasting with a rate of 49% for those having no treatment.

In an attempt to establish which factors influence the outcome of surgery, the number of curative resections performed annually by each surgeon has been calculated and this has been related to subsequent mortality. The median number of resections was 4.6 per year, i.e. 50% of all resections were done by surgeons doing less than five procedures a year. For partial gastrectomy, the operative mortality was not influenced by the number of procedures performed. However, for total gastrectomy, the operative mortality declined with increasing experience. For surgeons performing an average of more than nine resections per year, the operative mortality was 21.6%, compared with 30.8% for those performing six or less. This population-based study highlights the importance of surgical

Table 37.10 One-month mortality (%) by treatment and decade

TREATMENT	1962–1971	1972–1981
Curative resection		
Total gastrectomy	28.6	26.6
Partial gastrectomy	11.4	14.4
Palliative resection		
Total gastrectomy	35.5	38.6
Partial gastrectomy	22.6	23.7
Other treatments		
By-pass	24.2	30.4
Laparotomy + intubation	42.0	41.3
Laparotomy + adjuvant therapy	18.4	16.5
Laparotomy only	35.3	39.9
No laparotomy		
Intubation	38.6	33.1
Chemotherapy or radiotherapy	27.5	33.1
No treatment	48.8	50.5
Total	35.4	36.7

experience, and the results reported from other International Centres with a particular expertise in gastrectomy demonstrate that lower operative mortality can be achieved by specialists. Pilchmayr and Mayer,[70] in the Federal Republic of Germany, reported an operative mortality rate for total gastrectomy of 8%; the overall Japanese figure is 3%.[69] Furthermore, recent series from individual surgeons with a specific interest in this disease clearly demonstrate acceptably low operative mortality for radical resection. In a personal series[141,142] of radical resections from the UK, surgeons' operative mortality rates of 5% and zero have been reported. These studies all highlight the facts that an improvement can be made in the results of treatment of this condition if acceptable operative mortality can be achieved and that there is a need for the development of specialist gastric surgeons.

Prognosis and factors affecting prognosis

The prognosis of gastric carcinoma is poor. Many factors influence prognosis, perhaps the most important being the extent of disease and the depth of penetration of the primary lesion. The majority of patients have advanced disease at presentation: 10% are unfit for any operation, resection is only possible in 50% and radical surgery in 25%.[143] The overall 5-year survival is low. Gilbertson[73] in the USA reported a 5-year survival of 8.8% and Brookes et al.[14] 4.9%. More recent studies show there has been little alteration in the UK. The overall age-adjusted 5-year survival in the West Midlands over the last 25 years remains low, at 5%.[140] However, this study shows that there has been a significant increase in survival time for those treated by curative resection between 1972 and 1981 when compared to the previous decade. In Japan, there has been an improvement in the overall results. The Japanese Research Society's results of treatment of 24982 patients from 103 centres between 1963 and 1966 reported a 5-year survival of 16.4%, which is significantly better than any other international figure. Identifiable factors that influence prognosis have evolved from all these data.

Clinical The sex and age of the patient and the preoperative length of history are clinical features that relate to prognosis in malignant disease. Waterhouse[144] reported over 40000 patients with malignant disease and demonstrated a corrected 5-year survival of all cancers in males of 18.5% and in females of 34.5%. This difference was also present in those having radical treatment: the 5-year survival was 42.9 and 55.1% in males and females, respectively. However, these findings were not confirmed in gastric cancer, the 5-year survival for males and females being 4.9 and 4.2%, respectively.[7] Prognosis of cancers for all sites decreases with increasing age;[144] however, when corrected this apparent difference is less marked. The role of age has been evaluated for its overall effect on survival and 1-month mortality (Figure 37.23). This demonstrates that, with increasing age, there is an increased operative mortality following any resection. The overall survival of older patients is closely related to treatment, and the proportion undergoing curative resection decreases significantly with age. When patients are studied by stage and age, it is quite clear that in

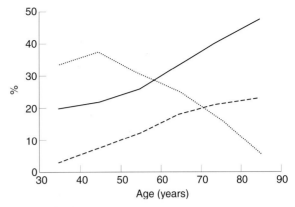

Figure 37.23

Effect of age on 1-month mortality rates. —, All cases; ------, curative resection; — — —, proportion curative resection.

most stages of disease it is the stage that is important and not the age. Age alone does not have an influence on survival (Figure 37.24).

An interesting correlation between length of history prior to diagnosis and survival has been established for gastric cancers.[14,48] Brookes et al.[14] reported an 11.1% 5-year survival in 433 patients with a history of less than 3 months, increasing to 28.1% in 96 patients with a history of more than 3 years. This finding also pertained to early gastric cancers: 13 of 14 patients with a history of more than 12 months survived 5 years, whereas the crude 5-year survival in 56 with a history of less than 12 months was 48%.[50] In a more recent study[7] the 5-year survival rates for 15858 patients with a history of less than 6 months was 4.2%, whereas in 4970 patients with a history of more than 6 months the survival rate was 9.2%. This is also maintained in those patients who have had a curative resection: the 5-year survival of 3440 patients with a history of less than 6 months was 16.9%, and in 1685 with a history of more than 6 months it was 25.2%. The effect of duration of symptoms appeared to be maintained within each stage of disease, particularly in stages I, II and III (i.e. those resected for cure) (Figure 37.25).

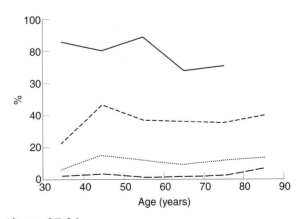

Figure 37.24

Five-year, age-adjusted survival by age and stage excluding deaths within 1 month. —, stage I; ------, stage II; ......, stage III; — — —, stage IVa.

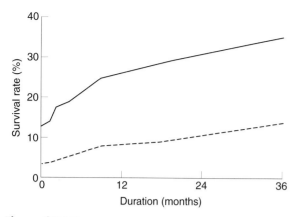

Figure 37.25

One- (—) and 5-year (----) age-adjusted survival rates by duration of symptoms.

Surgical Certain factors determined at laparotomy and the extent of surgical excision affect prognosis. The most important factor is complete surgical excision (curative or radical surgery). A radical resection is one which excises the primary growth and appropriate lymph nodes and, when completed, leaves no evidence of macroscopic residual disease. Palliative resections are often undertaken to relieve symptoms but tumour clearance is incomplete, either in the gastric bed or because of distant metastases.

The 5-year survival for all cases of gastric cancer is about 5%. Long-term survival in inoperable cases is unusual; Thomson et al.[145] reported only two 5-year survivors out of 348 patients and the 5-year survival was only 0.2–0.7%.[7,14,72] Palliative surgery was done in 8.4–54.7% of cases and the 5-year survival was 1.4–2.4%. In the recent series, in 478 patients undergoing a palliative total gastrectomy there was not a single 5-year survivor. However, of 2181 patients undergoing a palliative partial gastrectomy 2.6% survived 5 years.

After curative resection, widely differing 5-year survivals are reported and the variation in figures reflects the type of series – whether it is a population-based, a personal or hospital series. Kajitani and Takagi[72] reported a 5-year survival of 49% for 3145 cases undergoing curative surgery between 1946 and 1960 in the Cancer Institute Hospital in Tokyo. This had improved from 39.3% in 1946–1950 to 59% in 1966–1970. This hospital series has to be compared with a population-based study reported by Kajitani in which the 5-year survival for 10 771 cases having curative surgery between 1963 and 1966 was 33.4%. Similarly, in European and American studies these differences are apparent. At the University Hospital of Los Angeles the 5-year survival of patients undergoing curative resection at two hospitals between 1950 and 1970 was 32%,[147] compared with English figures of 18.9–25% in population-based studies. It is of note that the differences in results of treatment between America, Europe and Japan are only apparent in patients undergoing curative surgery and not in the inoperable or paliative cases, probably reflecting the stage of disease at surgical resection. In addition to surgical excision being considered curative and palliative, there is much debate on the amount of stomach that should be excised and the

extent of lymphadenectomy. Without doubt the most significant influence on prognosis is whether the resection is curative or palliative.

Pathological The pathological features of a tumour are important prognostic factors, particularly the depth of penetration of the primary and the involvement of lymph nodes. Although the morphology of gastric neoplasms has been studied in detail, most of the descriptive methods have been of little value as prognostic indicators, except for the classification of Lauren.[39] His description of the two main histological types, diffuse and intestinal, has related well to epidemiological findings and has demonstrated that the intestinal type is associated with improved prognosis.[148] In recent years interest has focused on early gastric cancer. The incidence of this lesion has increased in Japan as a result of their mass screening programme.[149] However, this lesion is rare in the UK (less than 1%) and there is no evidence that it is increasing.[50,140] Early gastric cancers are defined as lesions confined to the mucosa and submucosa of the gastric wall independent of lymph node metastases, which occur in 8.4% of these lesions. The rate of metastasis is 3% for mucosal and 15.2% for submucosal lesions. The 5-year survival rate for early cancers in Japan exceeds 90%, whereas European studies reported a survival of 70–75%.[50,51,72,140] All other gastric cancers are considered advanced, and the 5-year survival in Japan was 41.8% compared with 17.4% in the West Midlands.

Lymph node status has always been reported as an important factor. Hawley et al.[150] studied lymph node status in 205 patients and reported a 5-year survival of 40% in patients with no nodal involvement and 11% in patients with nodal involvement. Cantrell[151] investigated the influence of the number of involved nodes and reported a 5-year survival of 46% for no nodal involvement, 35% if less than half the nodes examined were involved and 8% if the majority were involved. The Japanese have extended this work and classified nodes into four groups. Group I (N1) nodes were strictly perigastric, including right and left cardiac, lesser and greater curvature and supra/intrapyloric nodes. Group II (N2) nodes were more distant than N1 and included nodes located along the left gastric, hepatic and splenic arteries and around the splenic artery and splenic hilus. Group III (N3) nodes were more distant than N2 and included nodes in the hepatoduodenal ligament on the posterior aspect of the pancreas at the root of the mesentery and the superior mesenteric artery and at the diaphragm and perioesophageal nodes in the lower thorax. Group IV (N4) nodes included all nodes located more distant than N3, including lymph nodes around the middle colic artery and the abdominal para-aortic nodes. These groups were applicable when the tumour occupied the major part of the stomach and they were modified for more localized lesions. If the major part of the tumour was localized to the upper third of the stomach, supra- and infrapyloric nodes were replaced with N2 nodes.

For tumours in the middle third of the stomach, the left cardiac nodes were placed in group II and the diaphragmatic and paraoesophageal nodes in group IV. With tumours located in the lower third, the right gastric nodes were placed in group II, the left cardiac nodes in group III, the splenic hilar nodes along the splenic artery in group III and the diaphragmatic and paraoesophageal nodes in group IV.[72] This very elaborate identification of lymph node groups was done in 5706 resected cases; in 1260 insufficient data was available for classification. There was no node involvement in 1592 cases and the 5-year survival was 79.8%; 1004 were in group I; 1119 in group II; 206 in group III and 71 in group IV. The corrected 5-year survival rates were 38.5, 22.8, 11.1 and 8.5%, respectively.

Adeshek et al.[147] reported similar trends in nodes classified as primary and secondary, with respective 5-year survivals of 34 and 18% compared with 44% in the node–negative group. In the Japanese study,[72] an equally detailed assessment was made of depth of penetration of the primary lesion in 5706 resected cases. Examined microscopically, the depth of penetration was defined as M if limited to the mucosa, SM to the submucosa, PM to the muscularis propria, SS to the serosa, S1 with extension and confinement to the serosa, S2 when exposed on the surface of the serosa and S3 when crossing the serosa and extending up into neighbouring organs. The number of cases were: 362 M; 433 SM; 658 PM; 796 SS; 752 S1; 1515 S2; and 565 S3. The 5-year survival rates were, respectively, 100, 90.3, 70.2, 48.9, 39.6, 22.1 and 7.35%. In most of these groups the 5-year survival was best when no nodes were involved, and decreased with involvement of each group of nodes. A point of particular interest was the effect of the combination of depth of penetration and nodal involvement on survival. The 5-year corrected survival of 273 serosa-negative, node-negative patients was 88.1%; that of 200 serosa-positive, node-negative patients was 48.3%; that of 149 serosa-negative, node-positive was 71.1%; and that of 317 serosa-positive, node-positive was 33.2%.

Clinicopathological staging The identification of various prognostic factors has allowed a clinicopathological staging system to be evolved. This takes account of the important features, namely:

- Curative or palliative surgery
- Depth of penetration of the primary lesion
- Presence or absence of distant metastases.

This staging system (see Table 36.5) results in the identification of groups of patients with highly significant survival differences (Figure 37.26); this system should form the basis for comparative studies, and any other prognostic factor should be shown to have an effect independent of those already taken into account before being accommodated in such a system.

Early detection

A number of criteria must be met by a screening programme to ensure that subjects will derive benefit from being screened. The disease must be an important cause of morbidity and mortality in the population to be screened; there must be a suitable screening test which is acceptable to the population; and the treatment must be demonstrated to influence the natural history of the disease. The features of an ideal screening test are that it must be:

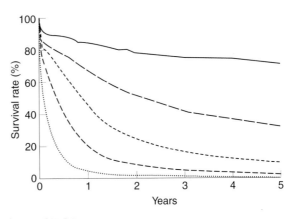

Figure 37.26
Annual age-adjusted survival by stage of disease. —, stage I; ———, stage II; ------, stage III; — — —, stage IVa; ...., stage IVb.

- Simple
- Acceptable
- Accurate
- Cheap
- Repeatable
- Sensitive (the ability of a test to be positive in the presence of disease)
- Specific (the ability of a test to be negative in the absence of disease).

Screening reduces the delay in diagnosis and can only be considered valuable if it can be demonstrated that the treatment of early lesions is more effective than that of conventionally diagnosed lesions. This assumes that there is treatment that is capable of influencing the natural history of the disease. The evaluation of results by analysis of 5-year survival rates ceases to be meaningful in studies of screening because survival may be improved by reducing the 'lead-in' time.

There is, at present, no evidence of an effective adjuvant to surgery (e.g chemotherapy or radiotherapy). Thus, surgery remains the mainstay of therapy. Surgery effectively relieves symptoms and there is evidence that it prolongs survival. The Japanese have demonstrated that extensive lymphadenectomy increases survival.[72] Additionally, Desmond et al.[71] reported on 59 patients with apparently benign ulcers which were removed surgically and proved on subsequent histological examination to be malignant. Twenty-four of the patients had further surgery and the 5-year survival in this group was 56%, compared with 23% in the remainder. More recently, the long-term results of surgical treatment of early gastric cancer supports the premise that surgery can influence the natural history of this early disease. The survival of over 90% is maintained in this group of patients to beyond 15 years.

Screening for gastric carcinoma in Japan

The Japanese now have extensive experience of screening for gastric carcinoma. In Japan, the incidence rate of gastric cancer is approximately 120 per 100 000 population. The Japanese initiated screening programmes for gastric cancer in 1960. Approximately five million people were screened annually (however, there are 37 million over the age of 40). There has been a decline in mortality for gastric carcinoma and the tendency is for this decline to be greatest in the areas where the rate of screening is highest. The screened populations have lower death rates from gastric carcinoma than the non-screened populations. In 1969–1972,[152] in a population in which 17.7% were screened, the death rate per 100 000 was 97.5. This fell to 73 in the years 1973–1977, compared with a low-screened population in which only 7.7% were screened and the mortality rate in the first period was 84.9 per 100 000 and was 84.3 in the latter period. This demonstrates that the mortality rate is down by 24.5% in the area of high screening.

The screening test was a double-contrast barium meal, performed in mobile vehicles. The sensitivity of the test can be 100% if ten films are taken for each subject.[153] This method yields a gastric carcinoma in 0.1–0.2 subjects screened, or a carcinoma for every 500–1000 examinations.[154]

The advantage of screening is that carcinomas detected are at an early stage: the proportion of early gastric cancer diagnosed was 40–45% in the screened population, compared with 25% for a group of patients with gastric carcinoma presenting to an outpatient clinic.[155] In common with mammographic screening for breast cancer, there is a potential risk of irradiation-induced leukaemia in programmes of screening for gastric cancer with a barium meal. However, there has been no increase in the incidence of leukaemia reported from Japanese Cancer Registries since the onset of the gastric mass screening survey. Japanese programmes have shown that, in common with other screening programmes, the education level of the subjects has a direct effect on the likelihood of their accepting screening. Subjects are also more likely to accept screening if it is offered at the work place and if there is a positive family history of the disease.

Frequency of rescreening

In any cancer screening programme there must clearly be a commitment to repeating the screening of the population. The early data suggested that screening should be repeated at yearly intervals. However, more recently it appears that the optimal rescreening period is every 3 years.[156]

Population to be screened

Although in large Japanese surveys an asymptomatic population has been investigated, the value of this approach is limited by its cost-effectiveness. The detection rate is 1 in 1000 and only 14% of the population at risk are screened.[157] In populations with a lower incidence of gastric cancer, these limitations would be further compounded. Such problems can be minimized by selecting high-risk populations who would find conventional forms of upper gastrointestinal investigation acceptable.

High-risk groups

There are international variations in the incidence of gastric cancer. Each country must determine the significance of this

health problem and whether its significance is such that they need to embark on screening programmes or encourage early diagnosis. The latter can be established by the identification of high-risk groups (Table 37.11).

Table 37.11 Risk factors for gastric cancer

Epidemiological
Genetic
Geographic
Occupational

Predisposing lesions
Pernicious anaemia
Postoperative stomach

Precancerous lesions
Autoimmune gastritis
Environmental gastritis
Dysplasia
Gastric polyps

Symptomatic patients
40 years or more with dyspepsia

The relationship of each of these groups to gastric cancer has been discussed earlier. The significance is such that continued surveillance of these groups is necessary in an early diagnosis programme. However, screening directed only to specific groups is not the answer to early detection because a majority of patients with gastric cancer do not have a predisposing condition and precancerous lesions can only be established at endoscopy on the basis of examination of biopsies. Of 2030 patients reported in three series, only 28 (less than 2%) had pernicious anaemia, and of the 1026 patients reported by Ellis et al., only 4.5% had had a previous operation for a benign condition.[27,48,49]

All patients with gastric cancer will ultimately develop symptoms and yet the diagnosis is commonly made when the disease is advanced. The difficulty for the physician is to differentiate between the symptoms of benign and malignant upper gastrointestinal disorders. It is important to identify the 'symptomatic at-risk' patients in whom a precise diagnosis can be established before instituting therapy. This can be done by studying the features of patients with gastric cancer and the differences between early and advanced disease (see earlier text on clinical features).

Early diagnosis

Investigation of dyspeptic patients has been undertaken by Barnes and colleagues.[159] They detected one early gastric cancer in 50 patients and found a cause for symptoms in the majority of others. A larger programme has been undertaken in Italy. In this study the population was canvassed through the media: 9276 patients came forward voluntarily or were referred by their general practitioners to diagnostic centres. A total of 819 (8.8%) gastric cancers were detected and, additionally, 364 were found to have polyps and 1361 had peptic ulcers.[160] More recently an early diagnosis programme in the UK has offered early diagnosis to patients over the age of 40 presenting to their family doctor for the first time with dyspepsia. Patients with high-risk conditions, such as chronic atrophic gastritis, intestinal metaplasia, dysplasia or polyps, have been entered into a follow-up programme of annual endoscopy. This approach has demonstrated that 1 in 50 patients have gastric cancer. A total of 57 gastric cancers have been detected and 27% of these are early.[59]

Methods of screening (Table 37.12)

The aim of any screening method must be to increase the number of patients suitable for treatment. A successful screening procedure should either establish the diagnosis or select patients for further investigation. It should be simple, cost-effective, easy to perform, of minimal inconvenience to those screened and have no long-term risks. In addition, it should have an acceptable false-positive and false-negative rate.

Table 37.12   Methods of diagnosis

Conventional
  Direct radiology
  Endoscopy
Screening methods
  Indirect radiology
  Gastric juice factors
    Fetal sialoglycoprotein
    Lactic dehydrogenase
  Serum tests
    Tetracycline test
  Urine testing
    Diagnex Blue test
Other possible tests
  Gastric juice
    pH
    α-Acid glycoprotein
    Carcinoembryonic antigen
  Serological
    α-fetoprotein
    Carcinoembryonic antigen
    Pepsinogen I

Conventional methods of investigation

The conventional methods of investigation of the upper gastrointestinal tract are double-contrast radiology and fibreoptic endoscopy. The latter allows direct visualization and biopsy of the lesion and a minimum of six biopsies should be taken.[53] Using radiology and endoscopy in combination, the accuracy of diagnosis is 98%.[54]

These two investigations cannot realistically be considered for mass screening of asymptomatic populations. Fibreoptic endoscopy is an invasive procedure that requires extensive facilities. It is time consuming to perform and unlikely to be acceptable to an asymptomatic population. Many of these criticisms can be levelled at radiological screening studies and, additionally, there is the hazard to the individual of radiation exposure. However, it must be stressed that these remain the definitive investigations for establishing the diagnosis in patients selected by other methods.

Screening tests

To date, a number of screening programmes that select patients for definite investigation have been undertaken.

Indirect radiology   Because of the limitations of conventional radiology as a screening procedure, the Japanese introduced indirect radiology for mass screening. Radiography is undertaken in a mobile unit by technicians. Six double-contrast radiographs are taken to provide accurate visualization of the areas of the stomach in which carcinomas most frequently occur.[52] Each investigation takes about 3–4 minutes and 60–70 persons can be examined in 1 day. Those with abnormal radiology are called up for detailed radiology and endoscopy. Screening has detected 0.92–1.45 cases of gastric cancer per 1000 screened patients. The detection rate decreased during the period of the study and this has been attributed to (1) an increased proportion of repeatedly-examined patients, and (2) a decrease in the incidence of gastric cancer. During 1975, in addition to 2804 gastric cancers, 8326 gastric polyps, 41 725 gastric ulcers, 24 430 duodenal ulcer and 5226 gastroduodenal ulcers were detected. In the Osaka mass screening programme, 33 221 patients were examined and 7670 recommended for further examination, at which 123 (3.7% of total screened) gastric carcinomas were detected, 31 being 'early' gastric cancers. The false-positive rate was 22.8% (the number of patients referred for further examination who did not have carcinomas, but including those who had other pathology). A further 25 cases were diagnosed within a year of a normal screening, a false-negative rate of 16.9%.

Radiology provides valuable information about gastroduodenal disease and, as well as identifying gastric carcinomas, detects patients who could be considered at risk of developing a carcinoma (i.e. those with polyps). However, it is not reliable in detecting other premalignant lesions and is inaccurate in assessing the postoperative stomach. Repeated radiological examination is necessary for follow-up, which, of course, increases the radiation exposure. As yet, no long-term side-effects have been demonstrated in Japan: there has been no increase in leukaemia in the screened populations.

Markers in gastric juice   The collection of gastric juice requires intubation to obtain the specimen. This may be undertaken by family doctors or nurses and specimens can be stored for further examination.

Fetal sialoglycoprotein antigen (FSA)[161] is present in gastric juice and has been used for screening in Finland. Samples were collected from 39 706 persons, aged 40–70 years and living in rural areas; 3508 (8.8%) were FSA-positive and these patients were endoscoped. Thirty-five (0.9%) gastric carcinomas were found; 1462 (3.7%) patients had other pathology. At follow-up, 27 FSA-positive patients were found to have gastric carcinomas during the first year, and a further seven during the next 2 years.

Ten carcinomas developed in 36 187 FSA-negative patients during the first year. The number of patients requiring further examination, when no carcinoma was found, was 3743, a false-positive rate of 8.7%. In a further study of patients with established diagnosis, FSA was positive, as shown in Table 37.6. This method of screening not only identifies gastric carcinomas but also selects those patients who may be at risk in the future.

Lactic dehydrogenase (LDH) and β-glucoronidase may be elevated in the gastric juice of patients with cancer, polyps, gastritis or metaplasia. In a screening programme,[162] 289 of 1534 patients had an elevated LDH level and seven had gastric carcinomas (of which three were 'early'). The false-positive rate was 18.3%. Rogers et al.[163] have demonstrated that LDH and β-glucuronidase were both elevated in gastric carcinoma.

Serum tests The ear-puncture tetracycline test has been used in China for mass screening; this test is based on the affinity of tetracycline for malignant tissue.[164] This test was positive in 74.4% of 446 cases of gastric cancer. In a mass survey of 57 164 persons, 22 cases of gastric cancer were found and 17 were positive in the test. The test was used in this screening programme as part of an integrated panel of tests. It was found to be positive in 1.1–3.4% of the general population and, as such, has high false-positive and false-negative rates, a factor which limits its usefulness.

Urine tests In Italy, acidity was tested in 26 712 asymptomatic persons by a calorific test in urine: the Diagnex Blue test.[165] Impaired acid secretion was detected in 5624 persons, who then underwent blind abrasive cytology with a retractable nylon brush; 709 individuals had abnormal cytology, and definitive endoscopy diagnosed gastric cancer in 11 (including eight early gastric cancers), severe atrophic gastritis in 144, gastric ulcers in 11 and gastric polyps in six.

Other tests There are a number of other investigations that may prove useful as screening tests. These have been evaluated in scientific studies but none has been tested in screening programmes.

Gastric juice Hypochlorhydria may occur in gastric cancer.[166] However, it is more often a reflection of the size of the carcinoma and therefore measurement of acid level would prove an unreliable method of detecting early lesions.[167] α-Acid glycoprotein, an acute phase protein, was present in the gastric juice of 94% of patients with gastric cancer and, in addition, present in 4–40% of patients with other gastric pathology, but was not present in those with normal stomachs.[168] Carcinoembryonic antigen may be elevated in the gastric juice of patients with cancer and atrophic gastritis.[169]

Serological tests Carcinoembryonic antigen and α-fetoprotein may be elevated in patients with gastric cancer but this elevation is usually associated with advanced disease.[170,171] This, together with the non-specificity of the tests, make them inappropriate investigations for mass screening programmes.

Serum pepsinogen levels may be low in patients with pernicious anaemia and atrophic gastritis.[172] Stemmerman et al.[173] predicted the presence of gastric cancer or intestinal metaplasia. Hallisey and Fielding[174] demonstrated that a low pepsinogen I (<30 mg/ml) or a raised gastrin (>70 pg/ml) identify 60% of cancers and 61% of the high-risk groups.

GASTRIC LYMPHOMA

The stomach is the most common site for extranodal lymphoma but this remains an uncommon neoplasm. The diagnosis requires fulfilment of the criteria established by Dawson et al.[175] (Table 37.13).

Table 37.13 Criteria for diagnosis of gastric lymphoma

1. Absence of palpable superficial nodes
2. No mediastinal disease on chest radiograph
3. No leukaemia on blood film or bone marrow
4. No tumour in liver or spleen
5. Only regional gastric nodes involved
6. Predominantly gastric lesion

Epidemiology

Gastric lymphoma represents 1.5–3.0% of all gastric malignancies and 40% of all gastrointestinal lymphomas. Adults dying of nodal lymphoma have gastric involvement in 29–50% of cases. There is evidence that the incidence has increased from 1.5 to 3.0 per million population per annum over a 20-year period. The mean age at presentation is 62.8 years for females and 58.8 years for males. There are a higher proportion under 35 years of age than for carcinoma (5.1 versus 0.4%). The incidence for males is higher than for females at all ages (M:F = 1.75:1).

Aetiology

The aetiology remains unknown. Gastric lymphomas are a submucosal disease. The development of nodal lymphomas may be related to systemic factors, such as herbicides, or occupation or social class but there is no proven link between these factors and gastric disease. Interestingly, *Helicobacter pylori* infection has been associated with an increased risk for gastric lymphoma, particularly for low-grade B-cell lymphomas originating from mucosa-associated lymphoid tissue (MALT).[176]

Pathology

Gastric lymphoma is primarily a non-Hodgkin's B-cell lymphoma (Hodgkin's 3.1% and T-cell lymphoma 1%). The classifications commonly reported are the Kiel, the Rappaport and the Working Formulation (Table 37.14) that is becoming standard for nodal lymphoma in the USA. Although useful in nodal lymphoma, none have so far been proved to have prognostic value in gastric disease. Immunohistochemistry now largely differentiates anaplastic carcinoma from lymphoma. Macroscopically the lesions may be polypoid, fungating or diffusely infiltrating. Microscopically, the tumours arise in lymphoid tissue in the lamina propria and extend submucosally.

MALT lymphomas

One of the most conspicuous histopathological features of *H. pylori* gastritis is the presence of lymphoid follicles in the gastric mucosa. Size and distribution of lymphoid follicles

Table 37.14 Histological classifications of lymphomas

CLASSIFICATION	%[a]
Keil	
High grade	46
Immunoblastic	15
Lymphoblastic	9
Centroblastic	9
Histiocytic	2
Unclassified	11
Low Grade	51
Immunocytic	23
Lymphocytic	11
Centroblastic–centrocytic	14
Centrocytic	3
Rappaport	
Diffuse, histiocytic	57
Diffuse, well-differentiated lymphocytic	18
Diffuse, mixed	12
Diffuse, poorly-differentiated lymphocytic	5
Nodular, mixed	1
Nodular, histiocytic	0
Nodular, poorly differentiated lymphocytic	0
Lymphoblastic	1
Unclassified	5
New Working Formulation (NCI)	
I Low grade	
A ML, diffuse, small lymphocytic	4
B ML, follicular, small cleaved cell	0
ML, follicular, mixed cell	0
C ML, follicular, large cell	0
II Intermediate grade	
D ML, diffuse, polymorphic plasmacytoid	0
E ML, follicular and diffuse small cleaved cell	1
F ML, diffuse mixed	32
III High grade	
G ML, diffuse, large cell, immunoblastic	63
H ML, diffuse, lymphoblastic	0
I ML, Burkitt's type	0

[a]Percentages taken from single published series.

shows great variability in different subjects and in different regions of the stomach of each subject, but if a sufficient sample is obtained, all infected stomachs will reveal the presence of lymphoid follicles. When the consistent nature of this response to *H. pylori* was established, it became possible to consolidate a number of previously separate observations into a unifying theory. The normal gastric mucosa does not normally harbour mucosa-associated lymphoid tissue (MALT), yet primary gastric MALT lymphomas (low-grade B cell lymphomas arising in MALT) are not infrequent. Since *H. pylori* gastritis is the only condition known to be consistently associated with the development of gastric MALT, it became apparent that *H. pylori* could represent, if not the cause, at the very least the necessary precursor for the development of primary gastric MALT lymphomas.[177] These low-grade, indolent, often patchy gastric lymphomas have been shown to be identical to the entity previously known as 'pseudolymphoma,' a term whose use is now discouraged.

Diagnosis

The presentation of PGL does not differ from carcinoma (Table 37.15). The mean duration of symptoms is 3.2 months. A palpable mass is present in 21%. This is important because the presence of a mass does not rule out a resection with macroscopic clearance of disease. Eighteen percent of patients are admitted as emergencies, usually with bleeding or perforation.

MALT lymphoma can be diagnosed histologically in the presence of a diffuse lymphocytic infiltrate consisting of centrocyte-like cells and forming lymphoepithelial lesions. Centrocyte-like cells have been described as 'irregular cells with cleaved nuclei that may bear close resemblance to small lymphocytes and that have a clearing of cytoplasma which may result in a monocytoid appearance'.[177] The cells are CD-20 positive and CD-45 RO, CD-5 and CD-10 negative.

Table 37.15 Presenting symptoms for gastric lymphomas

SYMPTOM	%
Pain (including dyspepsia)	70
Weight loss	15
Vomiting	14
Bleeding and anaemia	9
Anorexia	7
Dysphagia	5
Flatulence	3
Malaise and lassitude	3
Bowel change	2
Mass	1
Not known	5

Investigations

The diagnosis is not made before the laparotomy in two-thirds of cases. The definitive diagnostic test is biopsy, therefore endoscopy is the first line investigation.

Endoscopy

This is diagnostic in 44–95% of cases but the biopsy can be misleading. Lymphoma is a submucosal disease and biopsy is difficult. If an abnormality is seen and the biopsy is negative, investigation must be rigorously pursued with repeat multiple deep biopsies. If symptoms, especially weight loss, persist and biopsies remain negative, lymphoma should be borne in mind and laparotomy considered.

Barium meal

This suggests the diagnosis in up to 71% of cases. Features indicative of lymphoma are:

● Diffuse mucosal hypertrophy with irregular thickened folds.

● Multiple ulcerations.

● Single ulcers and diffuse mucosal thickening.

● Mass lesions or mucosal irregularity extending across the pylorus. Lesions greater than 15 cm are usually lymphoma, less than 5 cm usually carcinoma.

Ultrasonography and CT

These provide useful staging information but are not primarily diagnostic.

Staging

Staging requires clinical, surgical and endoscopic findings, a full blood count, blood film, liver function tests, bone marrow and liver biopsy, chest radiograph, CT and/or lymphangiography. Even with the Muschoff modification, the Ann Arbor staging system, which is standard for nodal lymphoma, is inappropriate for gastric lesions. The modified TNM staging system is easier to apply and prognostic.

Treatment

Primary therapy

Surgery At present the only proven treatment of benefit is surgical resection. If fit enough, all patients should have an exploratory laparotomy and surgical resection where possible.

Primary chemotherapy This has been associated with perforation and bleeding but improved survival has not been proven.

Primary radiotherapy This has shown some benefit but suggestions that it is as good as surgery are unsubstantiated. No patient should be offered primary chemotherapy or radiotherapy unless surgical resection is not possible.

Antibiotic therapy In 1991 Wotherspoon et al.[178] demonstrated that virtually all primary gastric MALT lymphomas were associated with active H. pylori infection and showed for the first time that some of these lymphomas could be treated by curing the infection.[179] Many subsequent clinical investigations have confirmed the validity of this therapeutic approach, although it is clear that not all such lymphomas respond to antibiotic treatment of H. pylori.[180] Rigorously controlled clinical studies are necessary before treatment of H. pylori infection can be recommended as the sole therapy for primary gastric MALT lymphomas.

Adjuvant therapy

Adjuvant chemotherapy Current evidence suggests that chemotherapy regimens which are effective in nodal disease are less effective in extranodal disease of gastric lymphomas. However, evidence for the effectiveness as adjuvant treatment is accumulating, e.g. recent data from the Birmingham Cancer Registry give a 100% 5-year survival for those patients with involved local nodes who had a curative resection and adjuvant therapy, while those not given adjuvant chemotherapy had a 29% 5-year survival. This difference is statistically significant.

Radiotherapy This has universally given an improvement in survival but no series has ever proved the benefit statistically.

Prognosis

The overall age-adjusted 5-year survival is 32%,[181] which compares very favourably with carcinoma at 8.5%. Neither age, sex nor histology affects the prognosis. For resected cases the 5-year survival is 41% when the nodes are involved, 58% when the disease is confined to the stomach wall and 80–92% if the serosa is not involved.

GASTRIC CARCINOID

This is an exceptionally rare malignant neoplasm of the stomach. McDonald[182] reviewed 418 116 surgical specimens and 16 401 autopsies: 356 gastrointestinal carcinoids were found, an incidence of 0.8%. They can have their primary location in the stomach. Of 31 716 neoplasms of the stomach, only 13 (0.1%) were carcinoids.[7]

Classification and histology

Orbendorfer[183] introduced the term 'carcinoid' to describe a group of gastrointestinal tumours that grow more slowly and have a more benign course than adenocarcinomas. Mason[184] established that the tumour arises from enterochromaffin cells at the base of the crypts of Lieberkuhn. These tumours were shown to contain 5-hydroxytryptamine (5-HT, serotonin), and there is an excessive amount of the serotonin metabolite 5-hydroxyindoleacetic acid (5-HIAA) in the urine of patients with carcinoid syndrome. Pearse[185] and Pearse et al.[186] described a group of neuroendocrine cells with similar ultrastructure and cytochemical features – the APUD (amine, precursor, uptake and decarboxylation) system; they suggested that they have a common embryological origin from neuroectoderm.[185,186] Carcinoids demonstrate five generally accepted histological growth patterns: insular, trabecular, glandular, differentiated and mixed. The pattern is of prognostic significance, with mixed insular plus glandular having the best prognosis, followed by insular, trebecular, mixed insular plus trebecular in descending order. The rare glandular and undifferentiated patterns occur in 6% of cases and have the worst prognosis (median survival 0.5 months).[187] The tumours are classically composed of small polypoid or round cells with basophilic nuclei which are round and central. The cytoplasm usually contains granules and in some carcinoids psammoma bodies are found.

Carcinoid tumours are classically stained by silver stains, which may be argyrophil and/or argentaffin. It is probable that the 5-HT reduces the silver salts so that the cells with small amounts will be argyrophil and those with large amounts argentaffin.

General pathology

The most common site of gastrointestinal carcinoids is the appendix, followed by the ileum and rectum. Only 2–3% of carcinoids are found in the stomach. Twenty-three per cent of patients with gastric carcinoid have metastatic disease. Gastric carcinoids tend to be trabecular in histological structure and are usually negative to argentaffin and diazo reactions. They are frequently associated with the carcinoid syndrome; the 5HT content of the tumours is low but the urinary 5-HIAA is high and they may frequently secrete 5-hydroxytryptophan. Metastases commonly occur to bone (osteoblastic) and skin.

They are frequently associated with other endocrine secretions.[188]

Malignant carcinoid syndrome

Clinical development

All patients with this syndrome arising from the gastrointestinal tract have metastatic disease. The symptoms are due to humoral secretions, and systemic symptoms do not usually occur until hepatic metastases are present. This is probably because the liver metabolizes the secretions and, until it can be bypassed, the syndrome does not develop. There are rare exceptions to this and the syndrome has developed in patients with nodal peritoneal or retroperitoneal disease. The main features of the disease are flushing, diarrhoea, wheezing and cardiac lesions.

Flushing Four different types of flushing have been described[189]:

1. A diffuse erythematous flush affecting not only the normal flushing area but also the skin of the back, abdomen and palms. It usually lasts 2–5 minutes.

2. A violaceous flush associated with dilated facial veins, telangectasia, watery eyes and conjunctival secretion. This flush may be permanent.

3. A bright-red patchy flush (geographical) associated with gastric carcinomas and excess histamine release.

4. A type much commoner in bronchial carcinoids associated with flushes lasting for hours, facial skin swelling, lacrimation, swelling of the salivary glands, high blood tension, exacerbation of diarrhoea and palpitations – this is the most severe type. It can be precipitated by factors such as eating, hot drinks, exercise, alcohol, excitement, sexual intercourse, defecation and postural change.

It was thought that 5-HT was the main mediator, but there is no correlation of flushing with urinary 5-HIAA excretion. 5-HT may be responsible for the cyanotic type of flush. Bradykinin may be important. It is probable that alcohol stimulates the release of adrenaline, resulting in the release of kallikrein from the tumour. Alcohol-induced flushing can be blocked by α-blocking drugs such as phentolamine. Adrenaline isoproterenol and calcium can also stimulate the flush and cause gastrin release. Doses of pentagastrin stimulate flushing in carcinoid patients.

Diarrhoea and abdominal pain This is nearly as common as flushing. The diarrhoea may not be associated with flushing, suggesting that the mediators are different. Watery stools accompanied by colicky abdominal pain and urgency of defecation are common. 5-HT stimulates the small bowel and pharmacological agents often block the diarrhoea without affecting flushing. Abdominal pain is the initial symptom in many patients. Differentiation needs to be made between abdominal pain related to mechanical obstruction due to tumour and that which is the result of the syndrome. An attempt can be made to differentiate between the two on the basis of symptoms and on the detection of metastatic disease.

Pulmonary manifestations Asthma-like episodes are frequently associated with flushing attacks; this is often the result of hyperventilation rather than bronchospasm, which itself is rare. Definite wheezing can be relieved by isoproterenol.

Heart disease Fibrosis involves the right side of the heart more than the left. The smooth plaques involve pulmonary and tricuspid valves. The most common lesions are those of pulmonary valve stenosis and tricuspid incompetence. The clinical features of tricuspid incompetence predominate and this may be a potentiator during a flush when cardiac output increases. The cause of the lesions is probably 5-HT, although the mechanism is unknown. These patients tend to have a very high urinary 5-HIAA.

Gastric carcinoids and pernicious anaemia

In pernicious anaemia, the absence of hydrochloric acid in the stomach may lead to hyperplasia of the gastrin-producing G endocrine cells. There is a strong association between gastric carcinoids and pernicious anaemia. The carcinoid tumours may be multiple and arise in association with G endocrine cells, or enterochromic-like cell hyperplasia. The tumours may contain gastrin and can metastasize.

Diagnosis

The diagnosis of a non-functioning carcinoid tumour will not commonly be made on clinical grounds alone and may only be made at laparotomy. It is usually detected when investigating the patient for obstructive symptoms. In metastatic disease, the patient can develop a carcinoid syndrome. If it is suspected, a flush provocation can be tried – with a measure of spirits being rapidly swallowed. If this is not successful, noradrenaline, or adrenaline can be used. Careful assessment of the liver by CT is the most appropriate way of detecting disease. Hepatic angiography can be of value, particularly in patients being considered for surgery.

The quantitative measurement of urinary 5-HIAA is important. A screening test will pick up levels of either 30 mg in 24 hours and, if positive, a 24-hour urinary 5-HIAA should be measured. Chlorpromazine can interfere with the assay. Reserpine, bananas, avocados, pineapples and walnuts may elevate urinary 5-HIAA. If the urinary 5-HIAA is not elevated and a carcinoid syndrome is suspected, chromatography of the urine for 5-HT should be carried out.

Treatment

Localized gastric carcinoid

Conservative local removal is all that is necessary for tumours less than 1 cm in diameter. More extensive resection is necessary for those of 2 cm or above.

Carcinoids of regional spread

Radical resection is advised in patients with metastases confined to regional nodes or regional invasion. Gastric carcinoids are slow growing and long-term survival will occur. In 17 patients with gastrointestinal carcinoids with both regional and peritoneal metastases, and where all visible disease was removed, there was a 71% 5-year survival. If the disease is not resectable, attempt at debulking can lead to apparent seeding and worsen the matting that occurs between the loops of bowel. Areas of small bowel obstruction will need to be bypassed, regardless of resectability.

Advanced carcinoid disease

Surgery The first therapeutic option to be considered should be surgery; relief of intestinal obstruction may help the common gastrointestinal symptoms. Resection of nodal masses or metastatic disease can relieve the syndrome in many cases without liver metastases.

Liver metastases If the metastatic disease is confined to one lobe and the patient has severe symptoms from either local disease or the syndrome, it is worth resecting or shelling out the secondaries. Patients with cardiac disease and resectable tumours should also be considered for this treatment to try and prevent progressive cardiac damage. Even apparently small lesions, if confined to one side, can be the cause of some of the syndrome.

Anaesthesia for the carcinoid syndrome needs to be carefully considered and severe hypertension and flushing may occur during surgery, even in patients with non-metastatic carcinoid.

Hepatic artery occlusion Because liver secondaries are usually multiple in both lobes, other approaches are necessary. The oxygen supply to secondaries is arterial (90% of oxygenation) compared with only 50% to the normal liver. Hepatic artery ligation has a mortality of 10–22%. Causes of death include hepatic necrosis, hepatorenal syndrome, liver abscess, carcinoid crisis, gall bladder necrosis, cardiovascular collapse and septicaemia. High fevers occur; transaminases are grossly elevated but there are only small rises in bilirubin and alkaline phosphatase. Objective tumour regression can be demonstrated when urinary 5-HIAA falls rapidly. However, the median response is short (5–14 months). Collaterals can develop rapidly after ligation of the hepatic artery. Specific embolization of a hepatic artery has many theoretical advantages because it is directed at the specific secondary lesion, and is repeatable if the tumour revascularizes. In four of six patients treated by gelfoam embolization there was good symptomatic improvement and an 80% fall of urinary 5-HIAA.[190]

Cardiac disease This is managed along conventional lines for heart failure. Surgery can be considered for those with severe valve disease. Strickman and colleagues[191] (1982) reported on 13 valve replacements; six patients were alive from 4 months to 8 years and seven had died from 1 month to 6 years after surgery.

Pharmacological therapy Before considering interfering with the blood supply to the liver, there is a series of trials showing symptomatic relief with pharmacological blocking agents. These have been well summarized by Harris[188] (Figure 37.27 and Table 37.16).

Table 37.16 Agents that can produce symptomatic relief of carcinoid syndrome

Adrenergic blocking agents
  Clonidine
  Phenoxybenzamine
  Phentolamine
  Propanolol

Inhibition of 5-HT synthesis
  α-Methyldopa
  5-Flurotryptophan
  Parachlorophenylalanine

Peripheral serotonin antagonists
  Cyproheptadine
  Methysergide

Oestrogen-receptor antagonist
  Tamoxifen

Histamine H₁ antagonist
  Cyproheptadine

Histamine H₂ antagonist
  Cimetidine

Unknown mechanisms
  Corticosteroids (? kallikrein release)
  Chlorpromazine (? kinin antagonist)
  Somatostatin (release inhibitor)
  Fenfluramine (5-HT depletion)
  Interferon

Chemotherapy This should only be considered for patients with major symptoms from a carcinoid syndrome or from metastases not responsive to pharmacological therapy and not suitable for surgery. Few drugs have been assessed in more than five patients: doxorubicin (60 mg/m^2) has been assessed in the largest number of patients and could be recommended as first line treatment. Other agents that have been used in small numbers include BCNU, chlorambucil, hydroxyurea nitrogen and MMC. The median duration of response from various series is 3–7 months, and the objective response rate varies from 18% for most single agents to up to 55% for combination chemotherapy.[188]

Prognosis

The median survival from the onset of flushing is 38 months. The 5-HIAA level is of prognostic value. The median survival was 29 months if levels were 10–49 mg/24 hours, 21 months if the levels were 50–149 mg/24 hours and 13 months if greater than 150 mg/24 hours.[192] The 5-year survival of those with non-functioning tumours was better, at 54%.[187]

LEIOMYOSARCOMAS

Differentiation between benign and malignant smooth muscle tumours is difficult. Malignant smooth muscle tumours are characterized by walls and pallisades of cells and they are usually without a capsule.[193] Evans[193] described the criteria for malignancy as:

- Increased cell size.
- Increased irregularity of cell size and shape.

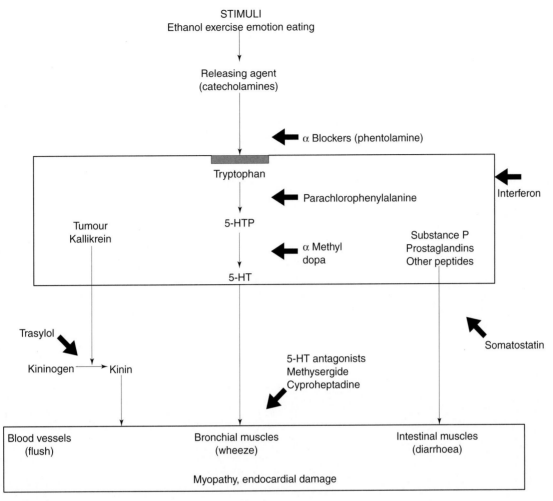

Figure 37.27

Sites of action of pharmacological blocking agents in carcinoid syndrome.

- Lack of complete cell differentiation.
- Presence of short, plump cells with oval nuclei.
- Presence of hypochromic and multiple nuclei with variable reactions.
- Presence of mitotic figures, some of which are atypical.

Leiomyosarcomas are uncommon: of 31 716 malignant tumours of the stomach reported over a 25-year period, only 99 were classified as leiomyosarcomas.[7] The male:female sex ratio is 1:1. These tumours occur most commonly between the ages of 40 and 80 years with the highest incidence in the 60–79-year age group. The age distribution is, however, somewhat younger than in carcinoma. In men, 40% with leiomyosarcomas are under 60 years of age, compared with 27% for carcinomas. The difference is less striking in women: 30% compared with 16%.

Leiomyosarcomas represent 95% of gastric sarcomas, and 10% are multiple. Half are found in the body of the stomach, 25% in the fundus, 9–16% in the pyloric antrum and 8–16% in the cardiac region. Macroscopically, these tumours are submucosal lesions but they can occasionally have central ulceration. Microscopically, the criteria described by Evans still pertain.

These have now been further extended: Shiu et al.[194] used ten histological features to describe the grading malignancy of a leiomyosarcoma. One of the ten criteria was the number of mitoses: 1–9 per ten high-power fields equals low-grade tumour (5-year survival 81%); more than ten per high-power field equals high-grade tumour (5-year survival 32%).

These smooth muscle tumours usually arise from the muscularis propria. When small, they retain an intermural position, but once they enlarge they bulge on to the mucosal or serosal cells, or both (dumb-bell tumours). Submucosal tumours often show ulceration of the apices – the cut surface has a whorled appearance and cystic spaces are often present. Histologically, they typically show the appearances of recognizable smooth muscle cells with nuclei in abundance; cytoplasm is arranged in walls of insulating bundles and nuclei often lie in parallel rows. A variant in the stomach is the epithelioid small muscle tumour which is composed of polygonal round cells with a clear perinuclear zone.

The tumours grow locally and can extend into adjacent and retroperitoneal structures. Metastases to lymph nodes have been described, local nodes being involved in up to 11%. Distant sites of metastatic disease, such as liver, lung and peritoneum, can also be found.

Clinical presentation

Melaena and haematemesis are the most common form of presentation, occurring in just over half the patients. The second most common symptom is pain. Neither the position in the gastric wall nor the location in the stomach is diagnostic. The diagnosis is made by a combination of endoscopy and radiology. At endoscopy, a submucosal lesion may be apparent. In addition, there is often an area of central ulceration. Biopsies are often unhelpful as it is a submucosal lesion. Barium examination is helpful in identifying the extent of a submucosal lesion and may be supplemented by CT.

Treatment

Surgical excision is the most appropriate treatment: partial or total gastrectomy with local node excision is recommended. Interestingly, the results from local excision do appear to be similar to those of gastrectomy. Of 16 patients treated by local excision, 46.1 survived 5 years. Sixty-two patients underwent a definitive gastrectomy and survival at 5 years in this group was 47.5%.[7] Resection was possible in nearly 80% of all cases. Radiotherapy and chemotherapy have little to offer in the management of this neoplasm.

REFERENCES

1. Ming EC. The adenoma–carcinoma sequence in the stomach and colon. II. Malignant potential of gastric polyps; *Gastrointest Radiol* 1976; **1**: 121.
2. Skandalakis JE & Gray SW. Smooth muscle tumours of the alimentary tract. In Ariel IM (ed.) *Progress in Clinical Cancer*. New York: Grune & Stratton, 1965: 692.
3. *United Nations Demographic Year Book.* 1986.
4. Muir C, Waterhouse J, Mack T, Powell J & Whelan S (eds). Cancer incidence in the continents, vol. V. *IARC Sci Publ* 1987; **88**.
5. Haenszel W. Variation of incidence and mortality from stomach cancer with particular reference to the United States. *J Natl Cancer Inst* 1958; **21**: 213.
6. Hirayama T. Changing patterns in the incidence of gastric cancer. In Fielding JWL, Newman CN, Ford CHJ & Jones BG (eds) *Gastric Cancer*, Advances in the Biosciences, Vol. 32. Oxford: Pergamon Press, 1981: 1.
7. Fielding JWL, Powell J, Allum WH, Waterhouse JAH & McConkey C. *Carcinoma of the Stomach.* Clinical Cancer Monograph vol. III. Basingstoke: MacMillan, 1989.
8. Haenszel W & Kurihara M. Studies of Japanese migrants. 1. Mortality from cancer and other diseases among Japanese in the United States; *J Natl Cancer Inst* 1968; **40**: 43.
9. Dublin LI & Marks HH. The inheritance of longevity – a study based on life insurance records. *Proc Assoc Life Insur Dir Am* 1941; **28**: 89.
10. Videbaek A & Mosbech J. The aetiology of gastric carcinoma elucidated by a study of 302 pedigrees. *Acta Med Scand* 1954; **149**: 137.
11. Aird I, Bentall HH & Roberts JAF. A relationship between cancer of the stomach and ABO blood groups. *BMJ* 1953; **1**: 799.
12. Stukonis M & Doll R. Gastric cancer in man and physical activity at work. *Int J Cancer* 1969; **4**: 248.
13. Craven JL, Baum M & West RR. Variations in gastric cancer mortality in South Wales. *Clin Oncol* 1979; **5**: 341.
14. Brookes VS, Waterhouse JAH & Powell DJ. Carcinoma of the stomach: 10-year survey of results and of factors affecting prognosis. *BMJ*, 1965; **1**: 1577.
15. Hammond EC & Horn D. The relationship between human smoking habits and death rates. *JAMA* 1954; **155**: 1316.
16. Hill MJ, Hawksworth G & Tattersall G. Bacteria, nitrosamines, and cancer of the stomach. *Br J Cancer* 1973; **28**: 562.
17. Haenszel W, Kurihara N, Locke W et al. Stomach cancer in Japan. *J Natl Cancer Inst* 1976; 56: 265.
18. Hill MJ. In vivo bacterial *N* nitrosation and its possible role in human cancer. In Miller EC et al (eds) *Naturally Occurring Carcinogens–Mutagens and Modulators of Carcinogenesis*. Tokyo: Japan Scientific Society Press, 1979: 229.
19. Gatehouse D, Dimock F, Burdon DW, Alexander-Williams J & Keighley MRB. Prediction of wound sepsis following gastric operations. *Br J Surg* 1978; **65**: 551.
20. Correa P, Haenszel W, Cuello C et al. A model for gastric cancer epidemiology. *Lancet* 1975; **ii**: 58.
21. Keighley MRB, Youngs D, Poxon V et al. Intra-gastric *N*-nitrosation is unlikely to be responsible for gastric carcinoma developing after operation for duodenal ulcer. *Gut* 1984; **25**: 238.
22. Meyrick-Thomas J, Misiewicz J, Schaub N et al. Effect of treatment for one year with ranitidine and of truncal vagotomy and pyloroplasty on intra-gastric pH, total and nitrate-reducing bacteria and nitrate and *N*-nitroso compounds in patients with peptic ulcers. *Gut* 1985; (in press).
23. Hill MJ. Aetiology of gastric cancer. *Clinical Oncol* 1984; **3**: 237.
24. Stocks P & Davies RI. Epidemiological evidence for chemical and spectrographical analysis that soil is concerned in the causation of cancer. *Br J Cancer* 1960; **14**: 8.
25. Tromp SW & Diehl JC. A statistical study of possible relationship between carcinoma of the stomach and soil. *Br J Cancer* 1955; **3**: 349.
26. Stalsberg H & Taksdal S. Stomach cancer following gastric surgery for benign surgical conditions. *Lancet* 1971; **ii**: 1175.
27. Ellis DJ, Kingston RD, Brookes VS & Waterhouse JAH. Gastric carcinoma and previous peptic ulceration. *Br J Surg* 1979; **66**: 117.
28. Freisen G, Dockerty M & Remine MD. Superficial carcinoma of the stomach. *Surgery* 1962; **51**: 300.
29. Crespi IM & Munoz N. Gastric precancer states. In Fielding JWL, Newman CN, Ford CHJ & Jones BG (eds) *Gastric Cancer*, Advances in the Biosciences, vol. 32. Oxford: Pergamon Press, 1981: 64.
30. Correa P. The epidemiology and pathogenesis of chronic gastritis; three aetiologic entities. *Front Gastrointest Res* 1980; **6**: 98.
31. Strickland RG & Mackay IR. A re-appraisal of the nature and significance of chronic atrophic gastritis. *Am J Dig Dis* 1973; **18**: 426.
32. Stemmerman G, Haenszel W & Locke F. Epidemiological pathology of gastric ulcer and gastric carcinoma among Japanese in Hawaii. *J Natl Cancer Inst* 1977; **58**: 13.
33. Stadelmann O, Elster K, Stolte M et al. The peptic gastric ulcer. Histographic and functional investigations. *Scand J Gastroenterol* 1971; **6**: 613.
34. Correa P, Cuello C, Duque E et al. Gastric cancer in Colombia. III. The natural history of precursor lesions. *J Natl Cancer Inst* 1976; **57**: 1027.
35. Imai T, Kubo T & Watarnabe H. Chronic gastritis in Japanese with reference to high incidence of gastric carcinoma. *J Natl Cancer Inst* 1971; **47**: 179.
36. Jass JR. Role of intestinal metaplasia in the histogenesis of gastric carcinoma. *J Clin Pathol* 1980; **33**: 801.
37. Filipe MF, Potet F, Bogomoletz WV et al. Incomplete sulphamucin secreting intestinal metaplasia for gastric cancer. Preliminary data from a prospective study from three centres. *Gut* 1985; **26**: 1319.
38. Farinati F and the Interdisciplinary Group on Gastric Epithelial Dysplasia (IGGED). Gastric epithelial dysplasia: a prospective multicentre follow-up study. *Gut* 1988; **29**: A1453.
39. Lauren P. The two main histological types of gastric carcinoma: diffuse and so-called intestinal type carcinoma. *Acta Pathol Microbiol Scand* 1965; **64**: 31.
40. Morson BC, Sobin LH, Grundimann E et al. Precancerous conditions and epithelial dysplasia in the stomach. *J Clin Pathol* 1980; **33**: 711.
41. Sogo J, Kobayashi K, Saito J, Fujimaki M & Muto T. The role of lymphadenectomy in curative surgery for gastric cancer. *World J Surg* 1979; **3**: 701.
42. Oota. *Histological Typing of Gastric and Oesophageal Tumours.* Geneva: WHO, 1977.
43. Ming SS. Gastric carcinoma: a pathological classification. *Cancer* 1977; **39**: 2475.
44. Mulligan RM & Rember RR. Histogenesis and biologic behaviour of gastric cancer. *Arch Pathol* 1954; **58**: 1.
45. Carnett JB & Howell JC. A case of coarctation of the aorta and gastric carcinoma with a discussion of metastases. *Surg Clin North Am* 1932; **12**: 1351.
46. Coller FA, Kay EB & McIntyre RS. Regional lymphatic metastasis of carcinoma of the stomach. *Arch Surg* 1941; **43**: 748.
47. Zinniger M & Collins W. Extension of carcinoma of the stomach into the duodenum and oesophagus. *Ann Surg* 1949; **130**: 557.
48. Swynnerton BF & Truelove SC. Carcinoma of the stomach. *BMJ* 1952; **1**: 287.

49. Lundh G, Burn JI, Kalig G et al. A co-operative international study of gastric cancer. *Ann R Coll Surg Engl* 1974; **54**: 219.

50. Fielding JWL, Ellis DJ, Jones BG et al. Natural history of 'early' gastric cancer: results of a 10-year regional survey. *BMJ* 1980; **281**: 965.

51. Green P, O'Toole K, Weinberg L & Goldfarb J. Early gastric cancer. *Gastroenterology* 1981; **81**: 247.

52. Hisamichi S, Nuzaki K, Kitagana M et al. Evaluation of mass screening programme for stomach cancer. *Tohuku J Exp Med* 1976; **118** (Suppl.): 69.

53. Dekker W & Tytgat GN. Diagnostic accuracy of fibre-endoscopy in the detection of upper intestinal malignancy. A follow-up analysis. *Gastroenterology* 1977; **73**: 710.

54. Nagao F & Takahishi MD. Diagnosis of advanced gastric cancer. *World J Surg* 1979; **3**: 693.

55. Tsuda Y. A study in the diagnosis of gastric lesions choosing the fibro-gastroscope combined with a new staining process. *Jpn J Gastroenterol Endosc* 1972; **14**: 261.

56. Tatsuta M, Okuda S, Tamura H & Taniguchi H. Endoscopic diagnosis of early gastric cancer by endoscopic Congo-red methylene blue test. *Cancer* 1982; **50**: 2956.

57. Hallisey MT & Fielding JWL. In-vivo staining for gastric cancer. *Lancet* 1988; **1**: 115.

58. Dodley CP, Weiner JM & Larson AW. Endoscopy or radiography: the patient's choice. *Am J Med* 1986; **80**: 203.

59. Hallisey MT, Allum WH, Jewkes AJ, Ellis DJ & Fielding JWL. Screening paper. Early detection of gastric cancer. *BMJ* 1990; **301**: 513.

60. Heyder M & Lux G. Malignant lesions of the upper gastrointestinal tract. *Scand J Gastroenterol* 1986; **21**(suppl. 123): 47.

61. Dehn T, Reznek RH, Nockler IB & White FE. The preoperative assessment of advanced gastric cancer by computer tomography. *Br J Surg* 1974; **71**: 413.

62. Efsen F & Fischerman K. Angiography in gastric tumours. *Acta Radiol Diagn* 1974; **15**: 193.

63. Cederqvist C & Nielsen J. Value of liver function tests in predicting resectability in patients with gastric cancer. *Acta Chir Scand* 1973; **139**: 656.

64. Allum W, Mcdonald F, Anderson P & Fielding JWL. Localisation of gastrointestinal cancer with 131-iodine labelled monoclonal antibody to CEA. *Br J Cancer*.

65. Cushieri A. Laparoscopy in general surgery and gastroenterology. *Br J Hosp Med* 1980; **24**: 252.

66. Gross E, Bancewicz J & Ingram G. Assessment of gastric cancer by laparoscopy. *BMJ* 1984; **288**: 1577.

67. Fabricus P, Hawker P & Dykes P. Reduction of anastomotic leakage after total gastrectomy by pre-operative bleeding. Presented at the *World Congress of Gastroenterology*, 1982, Stockholm.

68. Hockey M, Fielding JWL, Kelly KA et al. Resection line involvement in stomach cancer. *BMJ* 1984; **289**: 601.

69. Kajitani T & Miwa K. Treatment results of stomach cancer in Japan 1963–1966. *WHO-CC Monogr* 1979; **2**: 1963.

70. Pichlmayr R & Meyer MJ. Patterns of recurrence in relation to therapeutic strategy. In Fielding JWL, Newman CN, Ford CHJ & Jones BG (eds) *Gastric Cancer*, Advances in the Biosciences, vol. 32. Oxford: Pergamon Press, 1981: 171.

71. Desmond A, Nicholls J & Brown C. Further surgical management of gastric ulcer with unsuspected malignant change. *Ann R Coll Surg Engl* 1975; **57**: 101.

72. Longmire WP. Gastric carcinoma: is radical gastrectomy worthwhile? *Ann R Coll Surg Engl* 1980; **62**: 25.

73. Gilbertson VA. Results of treatment of stomach cancer. *Cancer* 1969; **23**: 1305.

74. Gunderson L & Sosin H. Adenocarcinoma of the stomach: areas of failure in a re-operative series (second or symptomatic looks). Clinicopathological correlation and implications for adjuvant therapy. *Int J Radiat Oncol Biol Phys* 1982; **8**: 1.

75. Gunderson L. Radiation therapy: results and future possibilities. *Clin Gastroenterol* 1976; **5**: 743.

76. McNeer G, Vandenberg H, Down FY & Boden A. A critical evaluation of subtotal gastrectomy for cure of cancer of the stomach. *Ann Surg* 1951; **134**: 2.

77. Brookes VS, Meynell MJ, Bold AM & Kingston RD. A review of symptoms, haematology and clinical chemistry following a partial gastrectomy. *Br J Surg* 1974; **61**: 9.

78. Alexander-Williams J. Duodenogastric reflux after gastric operations. *Br J Surg* 1981; **68**: 685.

79. Donovan IA, Fielding JWL, Bradby H, Sorgi M & Harding LK. Bile diversion after total gastrectomy. *Br J Surg* 1982; **69**: 389.

80. Adams JF. The clinical and metabolic consequences of total gastrectomy. I. Morbidity, weight and nutrition. *Scand J Gastroenterol* 1967; **2**: 137.

81. Bradley EF, Isaacs J, Hersh T, Davidson ED & Millikan W. Nutritional consequences of total gastrectomy. *Ann Surg* 1975; **182**: 415.

82. Seifert RR & Way LW. Total gastrectomy. *Am J Surg* 1978; **135**: 348.

83. Adams JF. The clinical and metabolic consequences of total gastrectomy. II. Anaemia, metabolism of iron, vitamin B_{12} and folic acid. *Scand J Gastroenterol* 1968; **3**: 145.

84. Goebell H. Pathophysiological consequences of total gastrectomy in gastric cancer. Herfath C & Schlag P (eds) Berlin: Springer, 1979.

85. Alexander-Williams J. Post-gastrectomy problems. *BMJ* 1967; **4**: 403.

86. Lygidakis NJ. Total gastrectomy for gastric carcinoma: a retrospective study of different procedures and assessment of a new technique of gastric reconstruction. *Br J Surg* 1981; **68**: 649.

87. Huguier M, Lancret JM, Bernard PF, Baschet C & Le Henand F. Functional results of different reconstructive procedures after total gastrectomy. *Br J Surg* 1976; **63**: 704.

88. Henley FA. Gastrectomy with replacement. A preliminary communication. *Br J Surg* 1952; **41**: 118.

89. Tonelli F, Corazziari E & Spireli F. Evaluation of alkaline reflux after total gastrectomy in Henley and Roux-en-Y reconstructive procedures. *World J Surg* 1978; **2**: 233.

90. Nakajima T & Kajitani T. Surgical treatment of gastric cancer with special reference to lymph node dissection. In Friedman M, Ogawa M & Kisner D (eds) *Diagnosis and Treatment of Upper Gastrointestinal Tumours*. Amsterdam: Excerpta Medica 1981: 207.

91. Remine WH. Pre-operative assessment and palliative surgery. In Fielding JWL, Newman CN, Ford CHJ & Jones BG (eds) *Gastric Cancer*, Advances in the Biosciences, vol. 32. Oxford: Pergamon Press, 1981: 123.

92. Allum WH, Hockey MS & Fielding JWL. Gastric remnant recurrence: detection and implications for the management of gastric cancer. *Clin Oncol* 1984; **10**: 333.

93. Ichiyoshi Y, Toda T, Minamisono Y et al. Recurrence in early gastric cancer. *Surgery* 1990; **107**: 489.

94. Comis RL & Carter SK. A review of chemotherapy in gastric cancer. *Cancer* 1974; **34**: 1576.

95. Earl HM, Coombes RC & Schien PS. Cytotoxic chemotherapy for cancer of the stomach. *Clin Oncol* 1984; **3**: 351.

96. Ogawa M. A recent overview of chemotherapy for advanced stomach cancer in Japan. In Schabel FM (ed.) *Application of Cancer Chemotherapy* 1978: 149.

97. Moertel CG, Schutt AJ, Halin RG et al. Effects of patient selection on results of phase II chemotherapy trials in gastrointestinal cancer. *Cancer Chemother Rep* 1974; **58**: 257.

98. Schien PS, Coffey R & Smith FP. Chemotherapy and combined modality treatment of gastric cancer. In Fielding JWL, Newman CE, Ford CHJ & Jones BG (eds) *Gastric Cancer, Advances in the Biosciences*, vol. 32. Oxford: Pergamon Press, 1981: 139.

99. Fielding JWL, Fagg SL, Jones BG et al. An interim report of a prospective randomised controlled study of adjuvant chemotherapy in operable gastric cancer. *World J Surg* 1983; **7**: 390.

100. Douglas HO Jr. Adjuvant chemotherapy after curative resection for gastric cancer: demonstration of necessity for randomised concurrent controls. *Proc Am J Soc Clin Oncol* 1980; C21 (abstract).

101. Lavin PT, Brukner HW & Plaxe SC. Studies in prognostic factors relating to chemotherapy for advanced gastric cancer – for the Gastrointestinal Tumour Study Group. *Cancer* 1982; **50**: 2106.

102. Kovach JS, Moertel GG, Schutt AJ et al. A controlled study of combined 1,3-bis (2-chloroethyl C)-1-nitrosurea and 5-fluorouracil therapy for advanced gastric and pancreatic cancer. *Cancer* 1974; **33**: 563.

103. Moertel CG, Mittelman JA, Bakemeir RF et al. Sequential and combination chemotherapy of advanced gastric cancer. *Cancer* 1976; **38**: 678.

104. Kingston RD, Ellis DJ, Powell J et al. The West Midlands Gastric Carcinoma Trial: planning and results. *Clin Oncol* 1978; **4**: 55.

105. Moertel CG & Lavin PT. Phase II–III chemotherapy studies in advanced gastric cancer. *Cancer Treat Rep* 1979; **63**: 1863.

106. Moertel CG, Engstrom P, Lavin PT, Gelber RD & Carbone PP. Chemotherapy of gastric and pancreatic carcinoma. A controlled evaluation of combinations of 5-fluorouracil with nitrosurea and 'lactones'. *Surgery* 1979; **85**: 509.

107. Buroker JT, Kim PN & Groppe ME. 5-FU infusion with mitomycin C versus 5-FU infusion with methyl CCNU in the treatment of advanced upper gastrointestinal cancer. A South West Oncology Group Study. *Cancer* 1979; **44**: 1215.

108. Rake MO, Mallinson CN, Cocking JB et al. Chemotherapy in advanced gastric cancer; a controlled, prospective, randomised multicentre study. *Gut* 1979; **20**: 797.

109. Gastrointestinal Tumour Study Group. Phase II–III chemotherapy studies in advanced gastric cancer. *Cancer Treat Rep* 1979; **63**: 1871.

110. Cocconi G, De Lisi V & Di Blasio B. Randomised comparison of 5-FU alone or combined with Mitomycin C and cytarabine (MFC) in the treatment of advanced gastric cancer. *Cancer Treat Rep* 1982; **66**: 1263.

111. Gastrointestinal Tumour Study Group. A comparative clinical assessment of combination chemotherapy in the management of advanced gastric carcinomas. *Cancer* 1982; **49**: 1362.

112. Gastrointestinal Tumour Study Group. Randomised study of combination chemotherapy in unresectable gastric cancer. *Cancer* 1984; **53**: 13.

113. Douglas HO, Lavin PT, Goudsmit A & Klaasen DJ. Phase II–III evaluation of combinations of methyl CCNU, Mitomycin C, Adriamycin and 5-FU in advanced measurable gastric cancer. *Proc Am Soc Clin Oncol* 1983; C473.

114. Friedman MA, Kimura K, Sakurai Y et al. Chemotherapy of advanced gastric cancer – a Northern California Oncology Group study (NCOG) and Japanese Gastric Chemotherapy Group trial. *Proc Am Soc Clin Oncol* 1979; **21**: 418 (abstract).

115. Cullinan S, Moertel C, Fleming T, Enerson L, Krook J & Schutt A. A randomised comparison of 5-FU alone (F), 5-FU + Adriamycin and Mitomycin C (FAM) in gastric and pancreatic cancer. *Proc Am Soc Clin Oncol* 1984; C536.

116. Preusser P, Wilke H, Achterrath W et al. Advanced gastric cancer: a Phase II study with etoposide (E), Adriamycin (A) and split course cis platinum (P) = EAP. *Proc Am Soc Clin Oncol* 1987; **6**: 75 (abstract).

117. Moertel CG, Childs DS Jr, Reitimeier RJ et al. Combined 5-fluorouracil and super voltage radiation therapy of locally unresectable gastrointestinal cancer. *Lancet* 1969; **ii**: 865.

118. Falkson G, Van Eden EB & Sandison AG. A controlled clinical trial of fluorouracil plus imidazole carboxamide dimethyl triazeno plus vincristine plus bis-chloroethyl nitrosurea plus radiotherapy in stomach cancer. *Med Pediatr Oncol* 1976; **2**: 111.

119. Gastrointestinal Tumour Study Group. A comparison of combination modality therapy for locally advanced gastric cancer. *Cancer* 1982; **49**: 1771.

120. Abe M & Takahashi M. Intraoperative radiotherapy: the Japanese experience. *Int J Radiat Oncol Biol Phys* 1981; **7**: 863.

121. Sindelar WF, Kinsella T, Tepper J et al. Experimental clinical studies with intra-operative radiotherapy. *Surg Gynecol Obstet*, 1983; **157**: 205.

122. Allum WH, Hallissey MT, Ward LC & Hockey MS. A controlled, prospective, randomised trial of adjuvant chemotherapy or radiotherapy in resectable gastric cancer; interim report. *Br J Cancer* 1989; **60**: 739.

123. Longmire WP, Kuzma JW & Dixon JW. The use of triethylene thiophosphoramide as an adjuvant to the surgical treatment of gastric carcinoma. *Ann Surg* 1968; **167**: 293.

124. Dixon WJ, Longmire WP & Holden W. Use of triethlene thiophosphamide as an adjuvant to the surgical treatment of gastric and colorectal carcinoma – 10-year follow-up. *Am Surg* 1971; **173**: 26.

125. Serlin O, Wolkoff TS, Amadeo JM & Keohn RJ. Use of 5-fluorodeoxyuridine (FUDR) as an adjuvant to the surgical management of carcinoma of the stomach. *Cancer* 1969; **24**: 223.

126. Fujimoto S, Akao T, Itoh B et al. Protracted oral chemotherapy with fluorinated pyrimidines as an adjuvant to surgical treatment for stomach cancer. *Ann Surg* 1977; **185**: 462.

127. Imanaga H & Nakazato H. Results of surgery for gastric cancer and effect of adjuvant Mitomycin C on cancer for recurrence. *World J Surg* 1977; **1**: 213.

128. Gastrointestinal Tumour Study Group. Controlled trial of adjuvant chemotherapy following curative resection for gastric cancer. *Cancer* 1982; **49**: 1116.

129. Engstrom P & Lavin P for the Eastern Corporative Oncology Group. Post-operative adjuvant therapy of gastric cancer patients. *Proc Am Soc Clin Oncol* 1983; C446.

130. Higgins GA, Amadeo J, Smith DE, Humphrey EW & Keehn RJ. Efficacy of prolonged intermittent therapy with combined 5-FU and methyl-CCNU following resection for gastric carcinoma. *Cancer* 1983; **52**: 1102.

131. Kondo T, Inokuchi K & Hattori T. Multi-hospital randomised study on the adjuvant chemotherapy with Mitomycin C and Futrafal for gastric cancer versus estimation of 5-year survival rate. *Gan To Kagaku Ryoho* 1982; **9**: 2016.

132. Abe O, Inokuchi K, Hattori T et al. Randomised study on the long-term adjuvant chemotherapy with Ftorafur and Mitomycin C for stomach cancer: Second Report. *Gan To Kagaku Ryoho* 1983; **10**: 2408.

133. Kasai Y, Inokuchi K, Hattori T et al. Effect of post-operative long-term chemotherapy of stomach cancer using Mitomycin C and Futrafal – the secondary study. *Gan To Kagaku Ryoho* 1982; **9**: 1449.

134. Allum WH, Hallissey MT & Kelly KA for the British Stomach Cancer Group. Adjuvant chemotherapy in operable gastric cancer. *Lancet* 1989; **i**: 571.

135. Nakajima T, Fukami A, Takagi K & Kajtani T. Adjuvant chemotherapy with Mitomycin C and with a multi-drug combination of Mitomycin C, 5-fluorouracil and cytosine arabinoside after curative resection of gastric cancer. *Jpn J Clin Oncol* 1980; **10**: 187.

136. Dent DM, Werner ID, Novis B, Cheverton P & Brice P. Prospective randomised trial of combined oncological therapy for gastric carcinoma. *Cancer* 1979; **44**: 385.

137. Moertel CG, Childs DS, O'Follow JR et al. Combined 5-fluorouracil and radiation therapy as a surgical adjuvant for poor prognosis gastric carcinoma. *J Clin Oncol* 1984; **2**: 1249.

138. Billroth T. Offenes Schreiben an Herrn Dr L. Wittelshofer. *Wien Med Wochenschr* 1881; **31**: 161.

139. Haberkant H. Ueber die bis-erzielten unmittelbaren und weiteren Erfolge der verschiendenen Operationen am Magen. *Arch Klin Chir* 1896; **51**: 484.

140. Allum WH, Powell DJ, McConkey & Fielding JWL. Gastric cancer – a 25-year review. *Br J Surg* 1989; **76**: 535.

141. Doggory RT & Cuschieri A. Paper $R_{2/3}$ gastrectomy for gastric carcinoma: an audited experience of a consecutive series. *Br J Surg* 1985; **72**: 146.

142. Irbin TT & Bridger JE. Gastric cancer – an audit of 122 consecutive cases and the results of R_1 gastrectomy. *Br J Surg* 1988; **75**: 106.

143. Burn IA & Welbourn RB. Cancer of the stomach. In Smith R (ed.) *Gastric Surgery: Surgical Forum*. London: Butterworth, 1975: 121.

144. Waterhouse JAH. *Cancer Handbook of Epidemiology and Prognosis*. Edinburgh: Churchill Livingstone, 1974.

145. Thomson JW, MacGregor AB & MacLoed DA. Some aspects of cancer of the stomach. *J R Coll Surg Edinb* 1971; **16**: 287.

146. Kajitani T & Takagi K. Cancer of the stomach at the Cancer Institute Hospital Tokyo. *Gann Monogr Cancer Res* 1979; **22**: 77.

147. Adashek K, Sangel J & Longmire WP. Cancer of the stomach. Review of 10-year intervals. *Ann Surg* 1979; **189**: 6.

148. Inberg MV, Heinonen R, Rantakokko V & Viikari SJ. Surgical treatment of gastric carcinoma. *Arch Surg* 1975; **110**: 703.

149. Miwa K. Cancer of the stomach in Japan. *Gann Monogr Cancer Res* 1979; **22**: 61.

150. Hawley PR, Westerholm P & Morson BC. Pathology and prognosis of carcinoma of the stomach. *Br J Surg* 1970; **57**: 877.

151. Cantrell EG. The importance of lymph nodes in the assessment of gastric carcinoma at operation. *Br J Surg* 1971; **58**: 384.

152. Hirayama T. Gastric cancer: epidemiology and screening. In Bouchier IA, Allan RN, Hodgson HJ & Keighley MRB (eds) *Textbook of Gastroenterology*. London: Baillière Tindall, 1984: 219.

153. Ishikawa H. Detectability of early gastric cancer with indirect fluro-radiotherapy. *Gann Monogr Cancer Res* 1971; **11**: 27.

154. Kaneko E, Makamura T, Umeda L, Fujino N & Niwa H. Outcome of gastric carcinoma detected by gastric mass survey in Japan. *Gut* 1977; **18**: 626.

155. Kaibara N, Kawaguchi H, Nishioi H et al. Significance of mass survey for gastric cancer from a stand point of surgery. *Am J Surg* 1981; **140**: 543.

156. Kohrogi N. A study on the efficiency of gastric cancer screening with special reference to the appropriate frequency of screening. *Fukuoka Igaku Zasshi* 1987; **78**: 67.

157. Hirayama T. Methods and results (cost-effectiveness) of gastric cancer screening. In Fielding JWL, Newman CE, Ford CHJ & Jones BG (eds) *Gastric Cancer*, Advances in the Biosciences, vol. 32. Oxford: Pergamon Press, 1981: 77.

158. Takagi K. Stages of gastric cancer and reconstruction after surgery. In Fielding JWL, Newman CE, Ford CHJ & Jones BG (eds) *Gastric Cancer*, Advances in the Biosciences, vol. 32. Oxford: Pergamon Press, 1981: 191.

159. Barnes RJ, Gear MWL, Nicol A & Drew AB. Study of dyspepsia in a general practice as assessed by endoscopy and radiology. *BMJ* 1974; **4**: 214.
160. Aste H, Amadori D & Maltoni G. Early gastric cancer detection in four areas at different gastric cancer death rate. *Acta Endosc* 1981; **11**: 123.
161. Hakkinen I. Application of serum and gastric juice tumour markers to early diagnosis and screening of gastric cancer. In Fielding JWL, Newman CE, Ford CHJ & Jones BG (eds) *Gastric Cancer*, Advances in the Biosciences, vol. 32. Oxford: Pergamon Press, 1981: 85.
162. Figus AI. Gastroenterological welfare centre and early gastric cancer in Hungary. In Grundmann E, Grunze H & Witte S (eds) *Early Gastric Cancer: Current Status of Diagnosis*. Berlin: Springer, 1974: 185.
163. Rogers K, Roberts GM & Williams GT. Gastric juice enzymes – an aid in the diagnosis of gastric cancer? *Lancet* 1981; **i**: 1124.
164. Coordinating Group for Detection of Gastric Cancer, the People's Republic of China. Gastric cancer mass screening by ear-puncture tetracycline test. In Thatcher N (ed.) *Digestive Cancer: Advances in Medical Oncology, Research and Education*, vol. IX. Oxford: Pergamon Press, 1979: 221.
165. Crespi M. Mass Screening: Europe 2. In Cotton P (ed.) *Early Gastric Cancer*. Welwyn Garden City: SmithKline & French, 1982; 80.
166. Wangensteen OH. *Cancer of the Oesophagus and Stomach*. New York: American Cancer Society, 1951.
167. Misaki F & Kawai K. Acid secretion in different stages of gastric carcinoma. *Gut* 1981; **22**: 877A.
168. Rapp W, Heim M, Mikulicz-Radecki JGV & Ludwig R. Alpha-acid glycoprotein in gastric cancer juice. *Klin Wochenschr* 1975; **53**: 139.
169. Bunn PA, Cohen MI, Widerlite L, Nugent JL, Matthews MJ & Minna ID. Simultaneous gastric and plasma immunoreactive plasma carcinoembryonic antigen in 108 patients undergoing gastroscopy. *Gastroenterology* 1979; **76**: 734.
170. Booth SN, King PG, Leonard JC & Dykes PW. Serum carcinoembryonic antigen in clinical disorders. *Gut* 1973; **14**: 794.
171. Holyoke ED, Chu TM, Douglas HO & Goldrosen MH. The role of immunological methods in the diagnosis of cancer of the stomach. In Thatcher N (ed.) *Digestive Cancer: Advances in Medical Oncology, Research and Education*, vol. ix. Oxford: Pergamon Press, 1979: 227.
172. Bock OAA, Arapakis G, Witts LJ & Richard WCD. The serum pepsinogen level with special reference to the histology of the gastric mucosa. *Gut* 1963; **4**: 106.
173. Stemmermann GN, Samloff IM, Nomura A & Walsh JH. Serum pepsinogen I and gastrin in relation to extent and location of intestinal metaplasia in the surgically resected stomach. *Dig Dis Sci* 1980; **25**: 680.
174. Hallissey M & Fielding J. Pepsinogen I and gastrin: a screening test for gastric cancer. *Gut* 1989; **30**: A711.
175. Dawson IMP, Cornes JS & Morrson BC. Primary malignant lymphoid tumours of the gastrointestinal tract. *Br J Surg* 1960; **40**: 80.
176. Parsonnet J, Hansen S, Rodriguez L et al. *Helicobacter pylori* infection and gastric lymphoma. *N Engl J Med* 1994; **330**: 1310.
177. Isaacson PG. Gastrointestinal lymphoma. *Hum Pathol* 1994; **25(10)**: 1020–9.
178. Wotherspoon AC, Ortiz HC, Falzon MR, Isaacson PG. *Helicobacter pylori* associated gastritis and primary B-cell gastric lymphoma. *Lancet* 1991; **338**: 1175.
179. Wotherspoon AC, Doglioni C, Diss TC et al. Regression of primary low-grade B-cell gastric lymphoma of mucosa associated lymphoid tissue type after eradication of *H. pylori*. *Lancet* 1993; **342**: 575.
180. Bayerdörffer E, Neubauer A, Rudolph B et al. Regression of primary gastric lymphoma of mucosa-associated lymphoid tissue type after cure of Helicobacter pylori infection. MALT Lymphoma Study Group. *Lancet* 1995; **345**: 1591.
181. Hockey MS, Powell J, Crocker J & Fielding J. Primary gastric lymphoma. *Br J Surg* 1987; **74**: 483.
182. McDonald RA. A study of 356 carcinoids of the gastrointestinal tract. *Am J Surg* 1956; **21**: 876.
183. Orbendorfer SL. Karzenoide Tumoren des Dunndarns. *Z Pathol* 1907; 1426.
184. Masson P. Carcinoids and nerve hyperplasia of the appendicular mucosa. *Am J Pathol* 1928; **4**: 1981.
185. Pearse AGE. The cytochemistry and structure of polypeptide hormone-producing cells of the APUD series and the embryological physiological and pathological implications of the concept. *J Histochem Cytochem* 1969; **17**: 303.
186. Pearse AGE, Polak JM & Bloom SR. The newer gut hormones: cellular sources, physiology, pathology, and clinical aspects. *Gastroenterology* 1977; **72**: 746.
187. Goodwin JD. Carcinoid Tumours – analysis of 2837 cases. *Cancer* 1975; **36**: 560.
188. Harris AL. Carcinoid tumour. In Fielding JWL & Priestman TJ (eds) *Gastrointestinal Oncology*. Tunbridge Wells: Castle House, 1986: 256.
189. Grahame-Smith DJ. *The Carcinoid Syndrome*. London: William Hilum, 1972.
190. Melia WN, Nunnerley HB, Johnson PJ et al. Use of arterial re-vascularisation and cytotoxic drugs in 30 patients with carcinoid syndrome. *Br J Surg* 1982; **46**: 231.
191. Strickman et al. 1982.
192. Davies Z, Moertel CG & Magilrath DC. The malignant carcinoid syndrome. *Surg Gynecol Obstet* 1973; **137**: 637.
193. Evans RW. *Histological Appearances of Tumours*. Edinburgh: Livingstone, 1956.
194. Shiu MH, Farr GH, Papachristou DN & Hajdu SI. Myosarcomas of the stomach. Natural history, prognostic factors and management. *Cancer* 1982; **49**: 177.

38

UPPER GASTROINTESTINAL TRACT BLEEDING

PW Dykes
RP Walt

Bleeding from the gastrointestinal tract reflects pathology of four major anatomical areas: the upper gastrointestinal tract, the small and large intestine, and the liver. This review deals with only the first two of these.

Its clinical presentation is extraordinarily variable, ranging from the extremes of death due to rapid exsanguination to an apparently obscure iron deficiency anaemia. Between these extremes lie many syndromes, all requiring intelligent awareness and all fraught with danger to life and prolonged health.

The problem is essentially one of management, with mortality as its ultimate index, and although contributory and fascinating to various degrees, all other facets of the question are secondary to this.

Historical

The twentieth century has seen an enormous output of publication on gastrointestinal bleeding from the first clinical reports, and has spanned the introduction of ambulance services and blood transfusion, diagnostic radiology and endoscopy, the evolution of surgical thinking, pharmacological studies, and more recently an explosion of effort in therapeutic endoscopy.

Early mortality rates were high by modern standards, but definitions were imprecise, diagnosis inaccurate, and many patients never even reached hospital. In 1927 the late Ernest Bulmer, reporting from the General Hospital, Birmingham, UK in the *Lancet*,[1] observed an increase in mortality for bleeding ulcers from nil in 1902 to 16% in 1925. He commented that: 'it seemed to be a reasonable supposition that cases of such severity as in the old days would have been allowed to die comfortably at home are at the present time entrusted to a fast motor ambulance with a good prospect of arriving at hospital before a fatal issue has occurred.' It is indeed difficult to believe that the true mortality from gastrointestinal bleeding early this century could have been less than 20–30%, particularly as: 'at the present time, the treatment is morphine, a period of starvation with rectal salines, and later a graduated diet with alkalis.'[1] It is possible to follow mortality through the century, with an initial improvement in the 1930s coincident with the introduction of blood transfusion, and a slower and more variable improvement thereafter (Figure 38.1). Overall mortality, regardless of diagnosis, is often now reported as 10%, with 4–5% for bleeding peptic ulceration in units committed to a careful management policy.[2–4] The slowness of the improvement has none the less been frustrating and its variability is intriguing. The variations between reports provide most of the clues to improved management. Apart from changing proportions of community and hospital management, there have also been significant demographic changes, of which age is the most obvious and important.

Seventy years ago the condition was a problem of young people, with as few as 10% over the age of 60.[5,6] Since then, the mean age has risen with that of the community, and today more than 60% are older than 60 years[3,4] (Figure 38.1). Sixty is indeed the vital age point for gastrointestinal bleeding, as mortality in younger persons is rare in well-run units, and usually avoidable. From 60 onwards, the risk steadily increases, and

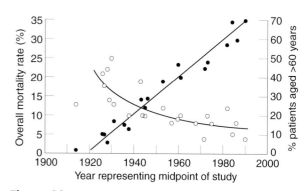

Figure 38.1

Changing mortality (O) and age distribution (●) of gastrointestinal bleeding through the twentieth century.

with it the need for clinical vigilance. The development of designated geriatric wards with direct admission of emergencies complicates the situation further, and it is important that these patients receive at least as much care as those younger and more robust.

In most hospitals, surgery remains the definitive therapy, with the key problems being supportive therapy, the skill of the surgeon, and the timing and nature of the operation. Many pharmacological therapies have been tried, involving predominantly suppression of gastric acidity and of tissue and luminal fibrinolysis, but so far with disappointing results. More recently the development of therapeutic endoscopy has opened an exciting new dimension to the problem, with the possibility arising that the endoscopist might supplant the surgeon as the major mediator of treatment.

Definitions

It is important to be precise as to usage of clinical terms, and in this chapter we offer the following definitions:

- **Haematemesis** The vomiting of fresh or altered blood in observable amounts.
- **Melaena** The passage of visible altered blood in or associated with the faeces.
- **Rectal bleeding** The passage of bright-red blood per rectum.
- **Continued bleeding** Bleeding which apparently continues from the initial haemorrhage.
- **Rebleeding** Bleeding which recurs after initial cessation and clinical stability.
- **Further bleeding** Either continuous or rebleeding.

CLINICAL DISORDERS

Bleeding from the oesophagus

The importance of the oesophagus as a source of upper alimentary bleeding has often been underestimated. Oesophageal sources have been reported as accounting for between 11 and 37% of reported series of patients, of which the minority are due to oesophageal varices.[7] The widespread use of endoscopy in diagnosis has greatly improved the accuracy of reporting, in particular of Mallory–Weiss tears. The oesophagus is also a common source of chronic blood loss, particularly in the elderly where oesophagitis may produce few local symptoms yet cause severe iron deficiency anaemia.

Hiatal hernia

The radiological demonstration of a hiatal hernia is now recognized to be a common and usually irrelevant finding in the diagnosis of upper gastrointestinal bleeding. Hiatal hernia may cause alimentary bleeding from oesophagitis, but the resulting erythema and erosions in the gastric mucosa are more likely to cause chronic than acute bleeding and such patients more commonly present with iron deficiency anaemia. Ulceration occurs more often in association with paraoesophageal than with sliding hernias,[8] and it has been estimated that a fifth of

patients with a large paraoesophageal hernia suffer a major haemorrhage. Trauma at the hiatal level, usually due to a tight hiatus, causes a chronic gastric ulcer (riding ulcer) to develop astride the hiatus, which may be the source of massive bleeding.

Barrett's oesophagus

This disorder, described by Barrett[9] in 1950, is characterized by columnar epithelium lining the lower oesophagus and was found to be present in 196 of 1196 patients with peptic oesophagitis examined endoscopically by Savary and Miller.[10] The squamocolumnar junction lies at a variable distance above the cardia and the squamous mucosa is often the site of severe oesophagitis, which may cause stricture formation in the mid-oesophagus and bleeding. Bleeding from this source is usually mild, but overt upper alimentary bleeding may on occasion be massive and then is usually due to chronic ulceration (Barrett's ulcer) of the columnar epithelial-lined oesophagus. These ulcers closely resemble the chronic type of gastric ulcer, in that they are deep and solitary with a white base and a sharply defined edge. Rarely, penetration of the descending aorta, which lies in close proximity to the posterior aspect of the lower oesophagus, causes torrential and usually fatal bleeding. Adenocarcinoma is a recognized complication of Barrett's oesophagus,[11] representing yet another but much less frequent cause of bleeding.

Reflux oesophagitis

Reflux oesophagitis frequently occurs in association with duodenal or gastric ulceration but is a relatively uncommon source of acute bleeding. Bleeding from an already inflamed oesophageal mucosa may be precipitated by irritant tablets such as non-steroidal anti-inflammatory drugs (NSAIDs) which sometimes remain in the oesophageal lumen for long periods because of defective oesophageal clearance. Oesophagitis first develops on the crests of mucosal folds above the cardia and, when these are obliterated by distension with air at endoscopy, linear longitudinal areas of reddening are seen in the lower oesophagus. When oesophagitis is sufficiently severe as to cause acute bleeding, erosions are superimposed upon a background of erythema, and appear as multiple small bleeding points often interspersed with areas of adherent fibrinous exudate. Areas of deeper ulceration, sometimes in association with stricture formation, may be the source of localized haemorrhage.

Mallory–Weiss tear

In this disorder one or occasionally more longitudinal mucosal tears are sustained at the cardia at or just below the squamocolumnar mucosal junction. In this region the submucosa contains a plexus of thin-walled vessels which constitute the source of bleeding. A small sliding hiatal hernia can be found in the majority of patients who develop a Mallory–Weiss lesion, and tearing occurs when the cardia is in the thorax, at which time any violent diaphragmatic contraction with increased intra-abdominal pressure will subject the region of the cardia to a very high gradient of pressure across its wall.[12] This mechanism closely resembles that of spontaneous perforation of the oesophagus. Mallory–Weiss tears account for between 5 and 15% of all acute upper alimentary bleeding episodes necessitating admission of the patient to hospital,[7] and it seems likely that many more tears cause bleeding which is too trivial to warrant admission. After 2–3 days the tear is converted into a linear ulcer with a greyish base and most are undetectable after 7–10 days. Graham and Schwartz[13] found additional upper alimentary pathology in 32 of 93 patients with Mallory–Weiss tears, and in 14 this appeared to be the source of the bleeding. Endoscopy is, therefore, important not only in deciding whether a tear is present but also in determining whether this or some other lesion is the actual cause of bleeding. Bleeding from Mallory–Weiss tears is usually mild and blood transfusion is required only in a minority of patients unless a second source of haemorrhage is present.

Neoplasms of the oesophagus

Squamous carcinoma and gastric adenocarcinoma account for a very small proportion of hospital admissions for acute upper alimentary bleeding. Angioma of the oesophagus is rare, but presents to the endoscopist as a bluish nodule which can cause profuse blood loss.

Corrosives and drugs

Corrosive poisons taken accidentally or with suicidal intent cause necrosis of the wall of the upper alimentary tract. In recent years irritant tablets lodging in the oesophagus and sometimes remaining there for long periods have been recognized as causing mucosal ulceration and bleeding. Potassium, doxycycline and NSAIDs are the most commonly incriminated.[14] The degree of mucosal damage will depend not only upon the irritant nature of the contents of the tablet but also upon the duration of exposure, which is prolonged if oesophageal motility is impaired.

Peptic ulceration

Ulceration of the gastric or duodenal mucosa is the most common cause of haematemesis or melaena. It is a frequent cause of admission to acute hospitals and bleeding seriously interferes with the life and activity of the patient with peptic ulcer. Haemorrhage was at one time believed to be a rare complication of an unusual condition, largely because it was accepted as the only satisfactory clinical evidence of the very existence of ulceration. Autopsy statistics obtained in the early part of the twentieth century show that bleeding ulceration was the cause of death in about 0.4% of hospital autopsies, whereas peptic ulceration was present in 6%.[15] A careful longitudinal study of 1435 ulcer patients by Emery and Monroe[16] in 1935 showed that 27% bled during a 4-year period of observation. In 1944, Stolte[17] showed that, with careful attention to a detailed history, it is likely that the incidence of bleeding episodes is probably higher still. Set against a similar rate for perforation of 13%,[18] it seems that haemorrhage occurs with about twice the frequency. The longer the duration of ulcer disease, the greater the chance that the patient will have bled. In examining the histories of 333 ulcer patients, Stolte found the annual incidence of haemorrhage to be 8.4, 5.4, 5 and 5.9% for each of the first 4 years after commencement of symptoms. Jordan and Kiefer[19] have also found a slightly greater tendency to haemorrhage in the first year, and it appears that the incidence then remains constant at about 5% per annum for up to 10 years, when there may be some reduction. Within this overall incidence, however, some patients remain in remission for more than 20 years[16] where there may be a further group with a special and repeated tendency to bleed. Jordan and Kiefer showed that the rate of further haemorrhage was greater in patients who had already bled, especially if it had occurred two or more times. Further studies on duodenal ulcer patients indicated a rate of recurrent haemorrhage of 11% in those presenting with indigestion, but 75% where the initial presentation was haemorrhage without pain.

The mean age of patients with gastrointestinal bleeding continues to rise, and reflects the increasing age of the community (Figure 38.1). Furthermore, the risk of bleeding also continues to rise with age, particularly in females (Figure 38.2). Although these data relate to population rather than ulcer incidence, it is probable that bleeding from ulcers is more common later in life. Stolte[17] calculated annual frequency rates for each decade at 4.2% (under 20 years), 2.8% (20–30 years), 5.8% (30–40 years), 7.2% (40–50 years), 9.2% (50–60 years), 15.4% (60–70 years) and 24% (80+ years). Further analysis in this study suggested that this increasing incidence was because an ulcer which began later in life is more prone to bleeding than a long-standing ulcer present before the age of 30. We further analysed this problem and showed it to apply to both gastric and duodenal ulcers for both sexes, but not to mucosal erosions (Figure 38.3). Apart from a substantial number of bleeding duodenal ulcers in younger men, the rates for haemorrhage in both types of ulcer were at least five times higher over the age of 50. The considerable incidence of bleeding duodenal ulcers in younger men is striking and suggests a subpopulation separate from all other ulcer groups. This could result from alcohol, smoking or stress, but no other convincing sex difference or incidence has been described.

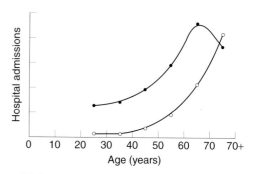

Figure 38.2

Hospital admissions for gastrointestinal bleeding for males (●) and females (O) related for each decade to total community population figures. (NB. There are no absolute numbers on y axis, as admissions came from a wider area than the local population.)

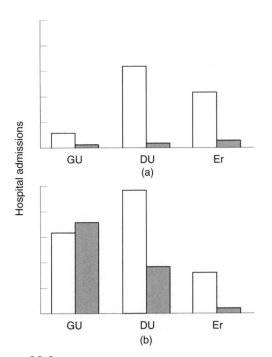

Figure 38.3
Hospital admissions following haemorrhage from each of the three major diagnoses related to the community population. (a) 0–50 years; (b) 50+ years. □, Males; ■, females; GU, gastric ulcer; DU, duodenal ulcer; Er, erosions. (See note under Figure 38.2.)

There also appears to be an increased incidence (approximately 30%) of bleeding in autumn and early winter,[20] but curiously these rates fall again in February and March when human morale and physical well-being in the northern hemisphere must be low.

Studies on the pathology of a bleeding ulcer confirm that two-thirds can be classed as chronic,[21] although the distinction is impossible to define accurately. The causation of bleeding is likely to be very different because diffuse slow bleeding is more common in an oedematous inflamed lesion, whereas profuse haemorrhage is more frequently associated with a ruptured major artery in the base of a penetrating ulcer. Acute ulcers which bleed are usually flat and may involve small arteries or veins before they have had time to undergo thrombotic obliteration, but much haemorrhagic oozing may occur if the area is particularly vascular and acutely inflamed. Even whilst healing, vessels may rupture, and then commonly project, nipple-like, from the centre. These changes are proliferative, causing endarteritis obliterans in arteries and thrombosis in veins. Haemorrhage occurs despite these protective mechanisms and a breach in the vessel wall can often be demonstrated. Usually only part of the vessel wall is involved, and a circular aneurysm may then develop prior to rupture. In cases of repeated haematemesis, several obliterated arterial orifices have been observed, often in different loops of the same vessel.[15] The most common sites for bleeding ulcers are the lesser curvature or posterior wall of the stomach and the posterior wall of the duodenum.

Erosive disease

The term 'erosive disease' includes small haemorrhagic lesions, usually multiple, occurring in the gastric and duodenal mucosa. The lesions sometime become ulcerated and are variously known as acute erosions, acute ulcers or haemorrhagic gastro-duodenitis. The erosions are shallow, usually less than 5 mm in diameter and oval or circular. Their edges are sharply defined, raised and congested and their base greyish-yellow. They are commonly multiple and may involve any part of the gastric or duodenal mucosa. They have, however, a tendency to be present in chains or clusters, most commonly in the antrum.[22] The intervening mucosa is often congested and oedematous, and coated by large amounts of mucus. There may be well-defined petechial haemorrhage, larger zones of confluent mucosal or submucosal bleeding, or free bleeding from the surface of the erosion. Microscopically, the predominant lesion is patchy inflammation with focal cell necrosis in an otherwise normal mucosa.

Since Dupuytren recorded acute gastric ulceration in burned patients in 1832, many apparent precipitating factors have been proposed[23] (Table 38.1). Burns, head injury, cerebrovascular accidents, infections, respiratory failure and many metabolic derangements have all been proposed as precipitating factors, together with drug and alcohol ingestion. Curling's ulceration in burned patients is a particularly interesting example, and Sevitt[24] has suggested two main groups. In the largest (14% of burned patients), usually where the burns are more extensive, acute multiple superficial ulcers develop within 48 hours in the fundic portion of the stomach. In the second group (9% of burned patients), bleeding occurs later, erosions are deeper, larger, and sited in the duodenum. It is the first group which are generally called stress ulcers, whilst the second may represent reactivation in patients with latent peptic ulcer disease. Ulcers associated with intracranial lesions (Cushing's ulcer) are larger and deeper[25] and have been shown to have normal gastric mucosal permeability, thus distinguishing them from the multiple shallow erosions.[26]

Table 38.1 Causes of gastric erosion

Burns
Drugs
   Aspirin
   Non-steroidal anti-inflammatory drugs
   Corticosteroids
   Alcohol
Head injuries
Hepatic failure
Intracranial surgery
Intracranial vascular accidents
Overwhelming infection
Pancreatitis
Renal failure
Respiratory failure
Shock

Drugs as gastric irritants

Although 40 years have elapsed since the first reports of an association between aspirin ingestion and gastric haemorrhage, the precise relationship between anti-inflammatory drug therapy and clinically significant intestinal bleeding remains unclear. Nearly all reports document a higher aspirin consumption among bleeding patients than control.[27-29] The selection of controls is the issue which determines the validity of these investigations, but the difficulties inherent in this exercise and the weaknesses of many existing studies have been extensively exposed.[30,31] The study of Levy[32] avoided many of the pitfalls and was based on the prehospital drug intake of patients admitted to 24 hospitals in the Boston area serving a population of 2.8 million. The methods for determining drug-taking habits were strict and uniform and investigators confined their analyses to subjects who were taking aspirin regularly. The results show a higher proportion of heavy aspirin users (defined as at least 4 days per week for more than 12 weeks) amongst those admitted with acute bleeding than in a large control group. The differences were most marked for those bleeding from gastritis or gastric ulcers. In contrast, light aspirin intake was not associated with increased bleeding in any of the diagnostic subgroups. The crucial findings were twofold. Firstly, even in the heavy intake group the excess risk of haemorrhage attributed to aspirin consumption was only 15 per 100 000 users each year. Secondly, the increased incidence of hospital admission for uncomplicated gastric ulcer was 10 per 100 000 each year in the same group. There was no evidence that light intake of aspirin was at all related to these complications, or that duodenal ulceration was related to any level of aspirin intake. A further and very useful study has been performed in Nottingham. A comparison was made between the recent drug intake of patients admitted with haematemesis and melaena with that of a random control population from two general practices. Account was taken of all analgesic and anti-inflammatory drugs, although the analysis applied particularly to aspirin and paracetamol. It was evident that the intake of both aspirin and paracetamol was associated with the haematemesis patients, but that more patients had taken aspirin than paracetamol. It was concluded that ill patients will take analgesics, but that aspirin was associated with a small and significant increase in the incidence of upper gastrointestinal haemorrhage.

More recent case control and retrospective studies from Nottingham,[33] Tayside[34] and Tennesee[35] have more clearly defined the problem. The relative risk of bleeding from peptic ulcer (*both* duodenal and gastric) ranges between 2 and 10 in patients receiving non-steroidals or aspirin. These increased risks are substantial because there is a large usage of anti-inflammatory drugs (22 million prescriptions annually in England and Wales alone). It is not yet clear whether individual drugs carry greater risks. One study has shown that the problem is at least as great, if not greater, in patients who are in the first week of using a NSAID.[35] The group at greatest risk are the elderly, who form the majority of users of the drugs and also run the highest chance of succumbing to gastrointestinal bleeding. The suggestion, under investigation, that patients should all receive concurrent prostaglandin replacement therapy in order to prevent complications of NSAID-related ulcers has been aired.[36] The problem is complicated by variable

assessments of risk and the present assumption that prevention of endoscopic ulcers in prospective studies would decrease complications. Present evidence does not support the use of prophylactic therapy for NSAID users, where advice must be to stop the NSAID if at all possible. It seems reasonable to use treatment to prevent known ulcer recurrences, although even this has not so far been shown to alter the frequency of complications.

Vascular anomalies of the stomach and duodenum

Hereditary haemorrhagic telangiectasia

Gastrointestinal bleeding may occur in 13% of patients with the Rendu–Osler–Weber syndrome (hereditary haemorrhagic telangiectasia).[37] There is nearly always a family history of the condition and bleeding may occur from lesions in any part of the gastrointestinal tract.[38] The history is usually one of repeated gastrointestinal blood loss requiring transfusion and sometimes presenting as haematemesis. The frequency and severity of bleeding tends to increase with age.

An important epidemiological study has been published in Denmark where a well-confined area of population in one large and a number of smaller islands represents 9% of the total population of the country.[39] The authors identified 139 cases of haemorrhagic telangiectasia and, of these, 35 had gastrointestinal bleeding and 28 showed gastrointestinal telangiectasia. Extensive endoscopic examination showed that the main areas affected were the stomach and duodenum, with positive findings in 89 and 61%, respectively. Five patients showed oesophageal lesions and five colorectal lesions. The mean age at which gastrointestinal bleeding presented was 55 years, as distinct from 11 years for the onset of epistaxis. A typical endoscopic finding was multiple nodular angiomas, sometimes with stellate projections; occasionally the lesion was surrounded by an anaemic halo. The condition was also shown to occur to a significantly increased degree in patients with blood group O. Bleeding did not seem to be dangerous.

Angiodysplasia

Angiodysplasia of the gastrointestinal tract has attracted much attention and similar lesions are described in the stomach, duodenum and colon. Angiodysplasia has been described as 'a sharply delineated red mucosal lesions with a flat or slightly raised surface; histological examination reveals dilated thin walled mucosal blood vessels'.[40] The microanatomy of the gastric lesions is similar to that in the colon and comprises dilated tortuous submucosal veins surrounded by a tangle of dilated tiny vessels. The lesions are more common in the stomach than the duodenum, but can occur right through the small intestine. The causes are unknown, but the presence of dilated tortuous submucosal veins arouses attention and a theory of submucosal venous obstruction is popular. This would account for the greater prevalence of the lesion in the larger right colon and also in the stomach, where there is vigorous churning and peristaltic activity. A relationship has been described with aortic stenosis and renal failure,[41] and indeed replacement of the aortic valve has induced disappearance of the lesion. The lesion commonly occurs in the sixth or seventh decade; the endoscopic appearance is of a bright spot 3–10 mm in diameter, often with a frond-like margin and little or no protrusion.[42] Others show a telangiectatic appearance, and half are apparently covered by normal mucosa.

Dieulafoy's erosion

A complicated vascular anomaly is that of Dieulafoy's erosion, which has been reviewed.[43,44] The lesion is most commonly sited on the posterior wall of the stomach and is associated with a localized vascular abnormality that can be demonstrated by angiography. Endoscopically the condition is diagnosed by the fortunate endoscopist who sees a spurt of arterial blood jetting from the posterior wall of the stomach.

Blue rubber bleb naevi

Cavernous haemangiomas of the skin may be associated with haemangiomas of the gut, and are sometimes the source of gastrointestinal bleeding. The inheritance is by autosomal dominant gene. The skin lesions are either intracutaneous or subcutaneous and may be seen on the lip. The mouth should always be inspected for such anomalies in patients with gastrointestinal bleeding. The intestinal lesions are often submucous, bleed easily and are more common in the small bowel than in the colon.[45]

Bleeding from the ampulla of Vater

Haematobilia is a rare but important cause of gastrointestinal bleeding and can be torrential. Bleeding from the liver occurs usually following injury, either as a result of blunt trauma[46] or from liver biopsy.[47] Bleeding from biopsies can be several days after the procedure and can be aggravated by coagulation defects which commonly occur in patients with liver disease. Vascular abnormalities, particularly hepatic artery aneurysm or vascular tumours, are responsible for probably a third of cases. Apart from overt blood loss, clinical features include biliary colic and intermittent jaundice. The gall bladder is often distended with blood and may, therefore, be palpable. Diagnosis is established by arteriography or duodenoscopy, when blood may be seen issuing from the papilla.

Bleeding down the pancreatic duct may arise following rupture of a splenic artery aneurysm, but more frequently this is a complication of acute or chronic alcoholic pancreatitis.[48] Patients present with recurrent abdominal pain complicated by haematemesis or melaena.

Arterioenteric fistulas

The most common site of arterial fistula into the intestinal tract is from the aorta to the third part of the duodenum.[49] Aortoduodenal fistulas are usually a complication of abdominal aortic aneurysm and are reported most frequently following a previously successful aneurysectomy.[50] Spontaneous rupture of an aneurysm into the duodenum is uncommon. Other less common sites of fistulas include the aorta or iliac artery into the ileum, sigmoid colon or rectum[51] (Table 38.2). Also

Table 38.2   Site of aortoenteric fistulas[51]

SITE	INCIDENCE (%)
Stomach	5
Duodenum: total	81
1st part	1
2nd part	4
3rd part	57
4th part	5
5th part	14
Small bowel: total	8
Jejunum	5
Ileum	2
Unspecified	1
Large bowel: total	6
Caecum	1
Ascending colon	1
Sigmoid colon	3
Rectum	1

included as a cause of arteriointestinal fistulas are gunshot wounds and ingested foreign bodies. The symptoms are those of central abdominal pain radiating to the back and haematemesis. Quite astonishingly, such fistulas are not usually immediately fatal, but include a clinical syndrome sufficiently prolonged to allow useful diagnosis and therapy. Clinical examination will often reveal a previous long midline incision or a pulsatile epigastric mass with a bruit. If the diagnosis is considered, endoscopy should never be carried out in the endoscopy suite but in or adjacent to an operating theatre with a vascular surgeon at hand.

Other rare causes

Other unusual disorders which can cause bleeding from the gut include pseudoxanthoma elasticum,[52] the Ehlers–Danlos syndrome and the Peutz–Jeghers syndrome.[53] These disorders are extraordinarily uncommon and more frequently present with chronic blood loss than with haematemesis and melaena. They should, however, always be looked for in the undiagnosed patient.

Disordered haemostasis

Platelet deficiency

Gastrointestinal bleeding secondary to haematological disorders is either secondary to liver disease or involves deficiency of thrombocytes or clotting factors. There is no significant risk of bleeding from platelet disorders when the platelet count is above $100 \times 10^9/l$. The risk of haemorrhage is moderate between 30 and $100 \times 10^9/l$, but there is a very high risk of spontaneous bleeding with platelet counts below $30 \times 10^9/l$. Low platelet counts themselves have a wide variety of causes and arise from bone marrow defects as in leukaemia and myelofibrosis, from decreased platelet survival due to the effect of drugs or hypersplenism, or from increased platelet consumption as in disseminated intravascular coagulation. Thrombocytopenic patients are more liable to bleed if the platelet count has recently fallen or if infection coexists. Conversely, patients in a steady state of chronic thrombocytopenia will often tolerate very low platelet counts surprisingly well. Treatment by means of a platelet concentrate should be restricted to patients in whom gastrointestinal bleeding is a major clinical problem. The unnecessary use of such concentrates renders the patient refractory to future transfusions by the induction of platelet antibodies. Transfusion should not be given to a stable patient with platelet counts around or above $30 \times 10^9/l$. Overt bleeding or fresh purpura are much more definite indices for urgent transfusion. Once a concentrate is given, usually prepared from six blood donation packs, then successful arrest of bleeding is often achieved without a demonstrable rise in the platelet count.

It must also be remembered that defective platelet function can occur in a wide range of clinical conditions. These include the effect of aspirin, renal failure, myelomatosis and myeloproliferative disorders. Dangerously low levels of platelets can occur in patients being treated with cytotoxic drugs, adding to the problems of patients with leukaemia.

Deficiencies of clotting factors

Gastrointestinal bleeding in patients with haemophilia (factor VIII deficiency) is usually caused by a coexisting peptic ulcer.[54] Although aspirin ingestion is potentially an important cause of bleeding, most haemophiliacs are careful to avoid it. Thus haematemesis should be investigated and treated in a manner similar to that required for the patient with normal haemostasis. The full support of a haemophilia centre is required, however, and the plasma factor VIII level should be raised from the 1% level of the severely affected patient to above 60%, and maintained above 30% until the bleeding has stopped. Screening of the patient's blood for hepatitis antigen and human immunodeficiency virus (HIV) should be urgently performed to determine the risk to attending staff.

Patients with von Willebrand's disease have the combination of a coagulation defect (factor VIII), an endothelial cell defect and a platelet function defect. These patients bleed more readily from the mucous membranes than do haemophiliacs and gastrointestinal bleeding can be particularly troublesome. When these patients undergo an abdominal operation, the surgeon should pay meticulous attention to local haemostasis.

Anticoagulation

Therapeutic anticoagulation with warfarin is not uncommon in patients admitted to hospital with all manner of conditions, including gastrointestinal bleeding. Provided the anticoagulation has been well controlled, there is no evidence for an increased risk of haemorrhage. Spontaneous bleeding from an otherwise normal mucosa will not occur unless the prothrombin time is beyond five times the control value, when bleeding can be torrential. Correction of an abnormal prothrombin time can be done with intravenous vitamin K_1, which does, however, take 2 hours to have an effect, and the prothrombin time is then likely to overcorrect at 24 hours. This can be a significant problem in patients with a cardiac valve prosthesis.

Temporary correction of a prolonged prothrombin time may be achieved using fresh frozen plasma or a prothrombin complex concentrate, although the latter has become less favoured with the rise of the problem of infection with HIV.

Liver disease causing a bleeding diathesis

A coagulation abnormality can be demonstrated in almost all patients with liver failure, and upper alimentary tract bleeding has been shown to be the cause of death in up to 20% of patients with fulminant hepatic failure.[55] The liver has a complex role in the synthesis of both precursor and inhibitory proteins of the coagulation and fibrinolytic pathways and, by means of its reticuloendothelial cells, also clears activated products of both pathways from the plasma. The plasma level of many coagulation factors, particularly those which are vitamin K dependent (II, VII, IX and X), is reduced as a result of impaired liver synthesis. Cirrhotic patients have also been described to have an exaggerated fibrinolytic response, and antifibrinolytic therapy has, therefore, been recommended for patients bleeding following portocaval anastomosis.[56] In addition, thrombocytopenia is frequently seen, despite an active marrow production of platelets. This reduction is usually caused by pooling and destruction of platelets in the spleen enlarged from portal hypertension. This situation can be complicated by consumption of platelets in disseminated intravascular coagulation associated with acute hepatic failure. The coagulation defects in liver disease are so complex that skilled haematological advice should always be sought in this extremely difficult situation. Bleeding due to portal hypertension is covered in detail in Chapter 39.

ASSESSMENT

Clinical

Despite highly developed methods of interventional investigation, it is important to assess the patient carefully at the bedside to avoid missing clues which may lead to important and even unusual diagnoses.

A history of preceding dyspepsia with nocturnal chest pains and sour regurgitation into the mouth suggests reflux oesophagitis as a cause of bleeding. However, the severity of dyspeptic symptoms does not correlate closely with the intensity of the oesophagitis, and about a third of those admitted to hospital with acute bleeding from reflux oesophagitis will admit to no antecedent dyspepsia. Bleeding from an already inflamed oesophageal mucosa may be precipitated by irritant tablets which sometimes remain in the oesophageal lumen for long periods because of defective oesophageal clearance. A Mallory–Weiss tear is suggested by the sequence of vomiting following by haematemesis, but more than 50% of patients give no history of retching or vomiting. In a few instances violent diaphragmatic contractions, as occur in epileptic convulsions, status asthmaticus and paroxysms of coughing, precede bleeding from a Mallory–Weiss tear but, in many, haematemesis is the first symptom.

The diagnosis of peptic ulceration from the history is even more indefinite, and indeed the incidence of haemorrhage from symptomless ulcers is quite high. Between $1:6$ and $1:2$ patients have been described as bleeding from symptomless ulcers[57,58] and it has been pointed out that this bleeding from a symptomless lesion occurs three times as often from a gastric ulcer as it does from a duodenal ulcer.[59]

Patients with erosions of the upper gastrointestinal tract, without preceding symptoms, are commonly to be found in intensive care units. Fortunately, with the improving standard of intensive care, the incidence of these erosions with complicating haemorrhage is declining.[60]

Clinical examination is extremely important, with a careful search for evidence of the less common diagnoses. Spider naevi, Dupuytren's contracture or splenomegaly indicate the possibility of portal hypertension. Bruising and joint swelling must be looked for, indicating coagulation disorders, taken in conjunction with a careful family and past history. The skin should be looked at carefully for evidence of angiomas, which can be of many types. These include telangiectases on the nose, the lips and in the mouth, but often more widely spread as in hereditary haemorrhagic telangiectasia, and cavernous haemangiomas of the skin and particularly the lip from the so-called blue rubber bleb naevi. Extremely rarely, fortunate physicians will come across and diagnose pseudoxanthoma elasticum and the Ehler–Danlos syndrome from the characteristic appearances of the skin and hyperextensibility of the joints.

Probably more important than anything in today's patient is obtaining a careful history to elicit the ingestion of irritating drugs such as aspirin and other NSAIDs and, of course, alcohol. In an attempt to extract the maximum from the clinical features several attempts have been made to computerize the clinical findings and eliminate, as far as possible, factors arising from human error. Unfortunately this accuracy is no more impressive than can be obtained by a careful clinician at the bedside, and even in the best hands the computer-aided diagnostic predictions are never terribly satisfactory[61] (Table 38.3).

Table 38.3 Accuracy of computer-aided prediction in 307 cases of upper gastrointestinal bleeding (from Airedale, UK and Marburg, West Germany)[61]

DIAGNOSIS	CORRECTLY PREDICTED (%)
Varices	93
Mallory–Weiss	78
Hiatal hernia	67
Neoplasm	57
Normal endoscopy	55
Peptic ulcer	55
Erosions	50
Overall	59

Blood urea nitrogen:creatinine ratio

It has been shown that the blood urea nitrogen rises in patients with gastrointestinal bleeding, and this finding is largely confined to those with bleeding from the upper gastrointestinal tract as distinct from the colon.[62] More recently this technique has been applied to the diagnosis in children, in whom the

localization of the bleeding point is often even more difficult than in adults.[63] The separation of the two groups is convincing but not close enough to 100% to be very helpful in terms of diagnosis.

Endoscopy

Emergency endoscopy requires more technical skill and clinical judgment than routine examinations and carries greater risks. These procedures should not be delegated to inexperienced staff: a hospital should have its own rota of experienced endoscopists available to carry out these procedures at the appropriate time.

Although emergency endoscopy is sometimes carried out out-of-hours in annexes to an operating theatre, this is usually because of difficulty in providing skilled endoscopy staff. It has been our experience that these examinations are better performed in the endoscopy unit with endoscopy staff, often supported by a ward nurse. It cannot be stressed too strongly that this procedure is much more difficult than routine endoscopy and both staff and environment should be of the highest possible standard.

It is logical to perform the endoscopy as soon as possible and most of the studies where the value of the procedure has been assessed have been done with the endoscopy carried out within 12 hours of the patient's arrival at hospital, often within an hour or two. This ideal situation is not often transferred into practice, and it is a fair compromise for these patients to be placed on the first endoscopy list after hospital admission, except for the occasional patient operated on during the course of an evening. Clearly, resuscitation takes precedence, but there is no need to delay the examination until blood transfusion is complete. These patients are more anxious than patients on routine lists, and will need at least as much sedation. Indeed, the incidence of alcoholism in these emergency patients is much higher than usual and such patients are often resistant to sedation.

A forward-viewing instrument should always be used to examine the oesophagus, stomach and duodenum, and a substantial channel for suction and irrigation is essential. Endoscopists should take care to advance the instrument with caution, particularly in the oesophagus, as vital information on the presence of fresh bleeding might be lost if the instrument abrades the lower end of the oesophagus. The oesophagus should be carefully examined for the presence of fresh blood, oesophageal varices and erosive oesophagitis; the gastro-oesophageal junction for Mallory–Weiss tears. The stomach often contains a substantial amount of blood and may need to be carefully washed. A lot of information can be obtained without washing, simply by rotating the patient backwards and forwards and placing the endoscope carefully in the uppermost part of the stomach. Experienced endoscopists are not put off by substantial amounts of clot or even fresh blood, and a spurting vessel, as in a Dieulafoy erosion, is of vital importance to a surgeon performing an emergency laparotomy. The maximum obtainable information should be balanced against the time of the procedure, which should never exceed 10–15 minutes. In both the stomach and the duodenum the examination may be able to localize the site of adherent blood clot, which probably represents the site of bleeding, and once again an experienced endoscopist can gently wash away the clot, exposing the presence of an ulcer and its contained bleeding vessel. Provided this is done gently there is no reason to fear further haemorrhage as spurting arterial lesions would prob-ably rebleed in any case, and will encourage urgent surgical intervention and a reduction in the ultimate risk. Highly skilled endoscopists claim a diagnostic accuracy of 80–95% – these procedures should not be carried out by anyone else.

Finally, in the undiagnosed patient severe haemorrhage which necessitates emergency laparotomy can be investigated by endoscopy carried out in the anteroom to the operating theatre. In this situation the patient is rendered even more safe by the presence of a cuffed endotracheal tube, with tight control on the circulatory system through intravenous transfusion.

Imaging

Contrast radiology

Contrast radiology has been extensively applied for diagnostic purposes but is today seldom used, having been supplanted by endoscopy, which is considerably more accurate and applicable in virtually all patients. None the less, in the appropriate hospital with an enthusiastic radiologist, contrast radiology remains a valuable tool which should not be ignored.[64] The technique involves the use of double contrast (barium and air) which, in the best hands, has the most remarkable degree of precision. If the patient has a nasogastric tube it is convenient to administer both barium and air through this and the radiologist normally introduces 100 ml of barium solution followed by 300–400 ml of air. Rotating the patient several times will produce adequate coating of the mucosa with the best possible chance of demonstrating a lesion. When the duodenal cap is filled with barium, 20 mg of hyoscine or 0.25 mg of glucagon is injected intravenously to render the duodenal cap hypotonic. The technique can be adapted to examination of the oesophagus by withdrawing the nasogastric tube into the gullet and it is occasionally possible to demonstrate lesions as small as a mucosal tear.

Arteriography

Arteriography can be of value in the diagnosis of acute gastrointestinal bleeding, but the bleeding rate has to be considerable and success has only been found in units where radiologists are committed and highly specialized in this area. Application of the technique in other units has usually been found disappointing and the rewards are not worth the delay and the increased hazard to the patient. None the less, in the best hands it is an extremely valuable technique and capable of application to patients when actively bleeding and even when severely ill. It has been widely developed in certain specialized areas and has been extensively reviewed.[64] More recently, digital subtraction angiography has been applied to this area,[65] a technique which has been found more useful for bleeding from the upper than the lower gastrointestinal tract.

Scintigraphy

Radiolabelled colloids have been applied to undiagnosed patients with gastrointestinal bleeding, but more commonly in those bleeding from the lower gut.[64] ^{99m}Tc-sulphur colloid has been the most popular agent, but the same isotope has recently been applied to red blood cells.[66] This relatively noninvasive technique deserves wider use in hospitals with nuclear medicine facilities.

PROGNOSIS

Causes of death

Much can be learnt from examining the causes of death because management must address the most obvious complications. It has been argued that surgery itself could be a major contributory factor as so many deaths are postoperative. Clearly a zero rate for surgery implies zero surgical complications. Many publications describe the deaths in their series, and several have set out to devise risk factors, either for rebleeding or mortality.

Of those series in which there are a substantial number of reasonably documented cases and the cause of death is identifiable, these fall into fairly well defined groups (Table 38.4). Persistent and sometimes unrecognized bleeding was described in 1966 from Canada,[67] where Devitt and his colleagues described 50 consecutive deaths from bleeding peptic ulceration over a 9-year period. They found the natural history of fatal bleeding ulcer to be that of multiple self-limited haemorrhages, with the median number before death as five. This paper must be of largely historical interest because five rebleeds would never today be allowed before action was taken to close the bleeding point. The authors examined errors in management and pointed to delayed surgery, inadequate transfusion, avoidable technical surgical complications, and inexperience of the attending physician. In 1976 an Edinburgh group[68] attributed most of their 21 deaths to surgical complications, and surprisingly concluded: 'how difficult it would be to

Table 38.4   Factors attributed to deaths in upper gastrointestinal bleeding

ORIGIN OF STUDY (YEAR)	FURTHER HAEMORRHAGE	SURGERY	COINCIDENT DISEASE	TOTAL DEATHS/ CASES REPORTED
Ottawa[67] (1966)	44	13	35	50/?
Edinburgh[68] (1976)	5	13	3	21/?
Birmingham[69] (1976)	3	8	4	10/147
Birmingham[2] (1984)	3	4	3	10/142
Newport[70] (1986)[a]	15	13	31	50/330
Bath[3] (1990)	3	8	12	15/217
Birmingham[4] (1990)	—	2	13	13/342

[a]Includes non-ulcer cases.

reduce the mortality of upper gastrointestinal bleeding.' Allan and Dykes[69] also emphasized the number of deaths which related to surgery and its complications; in their series, 8 of the 10 deaths followed an operation. Although the postoperative deaths occurred in patients who had previously been in reasonable health, most suffered from cardiovascular or respiratory disease. In several, leakage had occurred from an anastomotic site and the importance of avoiding unnecessary gastric resection was stressed. This factor still applies, and surgery should be well planned and not involve larger procedures than are necessary. A valuable retrospective audit of results in a district general hospital, published in 1986,[70] revealed a peptic ulcer mortality of 11% with a low operation rate (16%). The authors blamed surgical delay for a higher operative mortality, and it would seem logical that this played a role in the overall and rather high mortality rate. Fully 14 deaths were ascribed to continued bleeding in patients who did not have an operation, although the paper does not allow separation of peptic ulcer deaths. This report probably reflects a wider pattern of management and results than is generally believed, but one which should be alterable by regular audit of clinical results, and attention to detail of management.

In more recent studies where mortality for peptic ulcer bleeding has been reduced to approximately 4%, exsanguination appears less and less. Two studies from Birmingham, covering nearly 500 consecutive peptic ulcer patients admitted between 1980 and 1988,[2,4] show that, with careful adherence to an early emergency surgery protocol, exsanguination has virtually been eliminated as a cause of death. There was a significant number of patients who were purposely not resuscitated: those suffering from advanced malignancy and elderly patients with other fatal illness. Apart from this, mortality was invariably associated with other coincident disease: cardiovascular, renal, respiratory or cerebrovascular. Only one patient died from septic complications. A similar study from Bath[3] reported 15 deaths in 217 patients, and again nearly all of these had serious concomitant pathology. More than 80% of deaths were in patients over the age of 70. Thus, exsanguination and leakage from surgical anastomosis seem to have subsided as factors responsible for death, and in the 1990s we are left with deaths occurring in perhaps 4% of bleeding ulcer patients; all of these have severe coincident disease, and most of them are elderly.

Predictive risk factors

Several groups have carried out a more careful statistical evaluation of factors associated with rebleeding and mortality, and calculated indices such as relative risk and predictive factors. Additionally, formulae have been calculated to indicate high- and low-risk groups, and to indicate which patients should go immediately to surgery.

The relative risk of rebleeding indicates how much more commonly any feature was present in rebleeding patients than in those who settled.[71] Such indices are calculated in slightly different ways in different series and comparison is difficult. None the less comparable data are available for peptic ulcer patients from three groups[71-73] (Table 38.5). Age, shock and

Table 38.5 Relative risk of rebleeding associated with clinical factors

| | RELATIVE RISK | | |
INDICES	1988[71]	1986[72]	1987[73]
Age	1.4	1.5	1.7
Concurrent disease	3.8	1.6	—
Shock	5.6	2.5	2.0
Hb (low)	1.7	4.3	2.0
Endoscopic stigmata	—	1.9	6.1
Continued bleeding	2.0	—	—
Gastric ulcer	—	—	1.7
Medication	—	—	1.7

anaemia on admission appear regularly as associated with an increased risk of rebleeding, and in two of the three studies coincident disease and endoscopic stigmata also showed increased hazards. Clason and colleagues[72] applied the technique of stepwise logistic regression to examine independence of these factors, and only age, shock and endoscopic stigmata emerged as having independent significance.

Interesting data are included in the Organisation Mondiale de Gastroenterologie (OMGE) report[71] on the remaining risk of rebleeding each day of the hospital admission. This has been plotted graphically (Figure 38.4) and it is apparent that the risk falls exponentially with time until it reaches the residual risk, 10 days after admission. For the low-risk group, the residual risk appears to have been reached 3–4 days after admission. These data are helpful in deciding when the patient is ready to go home.

Risk factor calculations carried out for mortality have generally been assessed as the level of significance with which death is associated with any given factor (Table 38.6). Once again, age, shock, anaemia and concurrent disease appear regularly in the analyses, together now with rebleeding. Again applying the technique of stepwise logistic regression, Clason et al.[72] identified age, shock and rebleeding as independent predictors of hazard to life. The data from Newport in Wales[70] was unfortunately analysed including all diagnoses but is still in broad agreement with the other two studies.

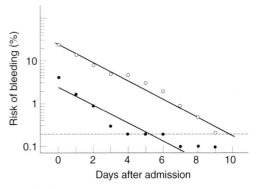

Figure 38.4

Remaining risk (%) of rebleeding during hospital stay each day after admission for all patients (O) and for the low-risk group (●). The residual risk for non-bleeding ulcer patients is indicated by the dotted line.[71]

Table 38.6 Mortality and risk factors: level of statistical significance associated with clinical factors as predictors of mortality

INDICES	SIGNIFICANCE		
	1986[70]	1986[72]	1990[3]
Age	0.001	0.0001[a]	0.005
Coincident disease	0.01	0.0001	0.005
Shock	—	0.0001[a]	0.001
Hb (low)	0.01	0.0001	0.001
Endoscopic stigmata	—	0.0001	—
Rebleeding	0.05	0.0001[a]	0.001

[a]Shown to be an independent variable by stepwise logistic regression analysis.

Applying stepwise logistic regression, Brearley et al.[73] derived a formula including age, history of previous ulcer surgery, anaemia, gastric ulcer, major stigmata and concurrent illness; all of these had an independent influence. Inclusion of major stigmata resulted in a high false-positive rate, and a formula was therefore devised separating this variable. Application of the formula to 70 further patients correctly predicted rebleeding in 84% of the high-risk group. Rebleeding in the low-risk group was never severe. A similar attempt to produce a formula useful to clinicians using computer anlysis was undertaken by the OMGE.[71] Of 592 patients placed in the highest risk category, 60% rebled and 32% died. By contrast, amongst 870 patients placed in the lowest risk category, 4% rebled and only two patients (0.2%) died. An extension of this study to data from Sikkim and China[74] showed that simplification of this formula did not seriously impair its predictive value, whilst apparently being applicable in any hospital throughout the world and without requiring computer back-up.

Whether or not a formula is helpful to the clinician in indicating a high-risk group or the need for emergency surgery is not entirely clear and is indeed a matter for personal preference. Patients who are over 60 years of age (see Table 38.5), are anaemic or at endoscopy have major stigmata of recent haemorrhage, are none the less at increased risk of rebleeding, and these, together with patients suffering significant concurrent disease, those shocked on admission or those who rebleed, are all at increased hazard to life. Such, at least, are the patients who should be cared for in a unit for 'bleeding patients'.

Long-term prognosis

What happens subsequently to patients discharged after a bleeding episode? Several authors have followed the fortunes of patients admitted with acute haemorrhage from peptic ulceration. Chinn and colleagues[75] studied 310 patients admitted between 1936 and 1948, and followed them until mid-1951. The only substantial and well-defined group within this study comprised 173 patients admitted for bleeding duodenal ulcer without previous hospitalization. Of these, 31% rebled within 5 years and 48% within 10 years. Corresponding figures for mortality related to this bleeding were 3 and 7%, respectively. This was a relatively young group by today's experience, with only

24% over the age of 60. Harvey and Langman[76] using life tables, found only 24% of such patients to have had a relevant complication 10 years later, whilst, from Australia, Duggan[77] gave a figure of 49%. Patients admitted for a second time for bleeding duodenal ulcers have a greater subsequent tendency to further complication (at 5 years: 64% from Chinn et al.,[75] 35% from Harvey and Langman[76]). Age did not appear to influence the rate of later complications in any study. Mortality is also similar for the index and all subsequent admissions.

Data on gastric ulceration are more sparse, the only group of any size coming from Nottingham.[78] A careful study of 152 patients showed a better prognosis than for duodenal ulcer, and fewer than 20% suffered further haemorrhage, perforation or ulcer-related death within 10 years.

The risk of ulcer complications recedes with time, and in the Nottingham studies there were no further ulcer incidents for either gastric or duodenal ulcer patients after 6–7 years. Division of bleeding patients into two age spans showed no difference in risk of recurrence between young and older patients. Another curious association emerged from these studies. Although 10-year mortality figures in gastric ulcer patients are as expected from anticipated life tables, deaths from duodenal ulcer patients for males were 17 (eight expected) and for females six (one expected).[77] The excess of deaths from duodenal ulcer follow-up were attributable to diseases of the circulatory system. This association received some support from two large autopsy studies showing a highly significant relationship between duodenal ulceration, coronary artery disease and aortic aneurysm. This association might be due to different levels of smoking. These studies span the introduction of adequate medical therapy for peptic ulceration and a continuing rise in the age of the patient groups. Further studies should be done in units with low mortality figures, careful follow-up and a substantial proportion of older patients.

SUPPORTIVE MANAGEMENT

Where

It is odd that these acutely ill patients are admitted under the care of physicians, when definitive therapy is in the hands of surgeons. This division of responsibility is one of the most dangerous aspects of gastrointestinal bleeding, and introduces a potentially lethal recipe for delay, requiring decision on action from two, often separate teams. It is for this reason that designation of 'bleeding' beds in a combined medical–surgical gastrointestinal unit has been proposed for the average patient.[69,79–81] A few, such as those severely shocked, those bleeding from oesophageal varices, or those at high risk of rebleeding, should be in intensive care. There are also many patients in whom bleeding has been so minimal that they can correctly be cared for in a general ward. These include particularly the young, patients with Mallory–Weiss tears and those with superficial erosions. The average patient, however, requires high dependency observation, sometimes available adjacent to an intensive care unit, but better still in a designated gastrointestinal unit. This concept, proposed by Tanner and Desmond[79] in 1950, was extended later in Australia by

Hunt et al.[80] and later used in Birmingham.[2] Both possibilities are helpful, but we believe the gastrointestinal unit to be superior, involving both regular and joint supervision by an experienced medicosurgical team and close access to endoscopic facilities.

Perhaps the most important advantage of these patients being in a designated gastrointestinal ward area is the development of expertise by the nursing staff in the early detection of rebleeding and circulatory problems and in providing additional support for an overall plan of management. Resident medical staff change too rapidly for satisfactory continuity to be established and it has been our experience that skilled and dedicated nursing staff cover this transition extremely well. We have been extremely well served by our own nursing staff in this context and others have made similar tributes.[79,80]

How

The crucial principle of management is the maintenance of a stable cardiovascular system, and most danger comes from inadequate and tardy correction of oligaemic shock, failure to quickly recognize and treat rebleeding, or the precipitation of cardiac failure by overzealous transfusion. Blood volume measurements have been used but are generally unnecessary and will delay obviously-required replacement therapy. Continuous monitoring of central venous pressure is a more rapid and flexible method of controlling circulatory problems and there is now widespread skill in its use in intensive care units where it is almost routine. It is none the less a substantially invasive procedure requiring continual experience in its safe use and interpretation, and it is neither generally necessary nor wise to use it outside intensive care units.

It is sufficient on admission to the emergency department for an immediate assessment to be made of the circulatory system through simple clinical criteria such as skin warmth and moisture, pulse, blood pressure and its postural relationship, haemoglobin and red cell indices. Where volume replacement is necessary an intravenous infusion line should be established quickly, with initial infusion of crystalloid and colloid as required. It is seldom necessary to infuse blood before adequate cross-matching, but the clinical object is to restore rapidly the circulation to normal. There is, of course, a danger of overtransfusion, particularly with the increasing number of older patients with cardiovascular pathology. It has also been shown that transfusion itself impairs coagulation,[82] but the evidence that this has clinical importance is meagre. The restoration and maintenance of circulatory normality is the first and urgent aim of treatment. This is usually accomplished initially by infusion of saline, often with 2 or more units of colloid (e.g. Haemaccel) before blood is available. Whilst a normal haemoglobin concentration is desirable, a normal circulation is much more important. The major hazard here is rapid overtransfusion, putting unnecessary stress on a pathological heart; a careful watch on neck veins and lung bases is usually sufficient without recourse to central venous pressure measurements. The increasing age and degree of illness of these patients demands close observation, with particular reference to chest infection, cardiac arrhythmias, diabetes, renal function and cerebrovascular complications. Appropriate treatment must be rapidly instituted to avoid additional hazard, underlining the importance of the principles of high dependency.

It is our experience that the desirable duration of this dependency is not difficult to judge but should be as long as the hazard of serious rebleeding remains. In this context, the recent data from the International Study of Clinical Criteria[71] are important, indicating the substantial difference in rebleeding rates between those at high and low risk (Figure 38.5). Clearly those at low risk need not be admitted to high dependency at all, and may in fact be rapidly discharged from hospital. The high-risk patient should be closely observed for several days and may then be transferred to a general ward before discharge.

Further haemorrhage

The most important event of all at this time is continued or recurrent haemorrhage, as permanent cessation of bleeding would eliminate the need for intervention and minimize the circulatory problems. In this ideal state, mortality would probably be negligible. Thus the aim of clinical management is to detect any further bleeding at the earliest possible moment. Failure to maintain satisfactory circulation despite apparently adequate transfusion generally indicates further bleeding, and the most important indices are pulse, blood pressure, central venous pressure and urine flow. All these should rapidly return to normal but their continued observation is vital.

Rebleeding can be rapid and clinically obvious or slowly continuous and concealed. Volume replacement should be equally rapid as long as bleeding continues, and care must be taken not to let bleeding go on too long. Rapid rebleeding is evident by the vomiting of fresh or altered blood, a sudden drop in blood pressure or an increase in pulse rate. Slow rebleeding often does not declare itself for some time, usually by a slowly increasing pulse rate, postural hypotension, the appearance of melaena, or even simply by a drop in haemoglobin concentration. Whatever the signs are, rebleeding indicates the presence of danger and is the major late indication for surgical intervention. It is extremely important neither to miss its onset nor to misjudge its extent. A transfusion requirement of 12 units or more in a young patient, and 8 units or more in someone over 60 implies the necessity for surgical intervention.

CONTROL OF HAEMORRHAGE

Pharmacological therapy

The desire for a simple 'medical' therapy which can be started as soon as bleeding is diagnosed is understandable. Unfortunately, no treatment has fulfilled this role although many units routinely prescribe drugs. The principle has been to improve clotting or limit the degradation of clot which has formed. The major therapies have therefore been gastric antisecretory agents, which theoretically aid haemostasis by inactivating peptic digestion of clot. Antifibrinolytic agents have also been used with some success. However, the body of data available does not allow one to recommend the routine use of any pharmacological agent. It is reasonable to start oral therapy for peptic ulcer healing as soon as a diagnosis is made but clinicians should be clear that such treatment is not aimed particularly at bleeding.

Ansecretory therapy

H$_2$-receptor antagonists Conflicting results abound but the consensus is that little important (or measurable) benefit is associated with the use of intravenous antisecretory agents.[83] An argument for increasing doses which render patients achlorhydric is prevalent[84] but initial results are not encouraging. There now seems little justification for routine use of H$_2$-receptor antagonists in upper gastrointestinal bleeding.

Proton pump inhibitors Omeprazole is the only drug which has been widely studied from this group and only one trial in gastrointestinal bleeding of adequate size has been reported. The result suggested that an early diminution of stigmata of bleeding occured but rebleeding and mortality were not significantly altered.[85]

Somatostatin Evidence of benefit with this drug is also conflicting and conclusive recommendations cannot be made[86] but routine use can not presently be condoned.

Antifibrinolytic therapy

Tranexamic acid has been tested in reasonable numbers of patients. Few individual studies are large enough to give conclusive answers but a combined analysis has identified a poss-ible important benefit.[87] The difficulties of meta-analysis include publication bias, whereby 'positive' studies are favoured. This aside, there is reason to believe that systemic antifibrinolytic therapy could reduce rebleeding, operation and mortality rates. However, on present evidence routine use cannot be justified.

Endoscopic intervention

Emergency endoscopy offers the ability to make a diagnosis and should therefore influence management. This has never been satisfactorily proven in clinical trial, yet the logic seems sound and more benefit seems to come from early rather than delayed endoscopy.[88] The other, and perhaps more important, advantage of early endoscopy lies in the ability to apply haemostatic devices to bleeding lesions. The use of sclerotherapy for oesophageal varices is discussed elsewhere and few now dispute the value of the technique. The main techniques used in peptic ulcer bleeding are laser photocoagulation, heater probe coagulation, electrocoagulation with mono-, bi- and multipolar electrodes, balloon tamponade and injection sclerotherapy. Microwave coagulation may be available in the future. Most emphasis has been placed on laser photocoagulation but expense and technical difficulties may mean that it will be superseded.

With all techniques a learning curve probably applies, so results from centres where the procedures are established and practised by experienced operators may not be reproducible in other places planning to provide the new service. The results of trials must also be viewed in context and cannot necessarily be translated to ordinary practice. In all trials some patients who may require treatment are excluded and assumptions have to be made about their potential responses.

All the techniques discussed below have been associated with perforation or increasing ulcer size in a small number of cases. Generally the techniques appear safe but long-term effects on vasculature or ulceration are not yet clear.

Laser photocoagulation

Laser light causes vaporization and heat-induced coagulation when applied to tissue. Two laser types have been used. The argon laser is avidly absorbed by haemoglobin and has limited tissue penetration. The neodymium yttrium–aluminium–garnet (NdYAG) laser has greater tissue penetration. A number of

Table 38.7 Results of trials of laser treatment of upper gastrointestinal bleeding

AUTHORS	N[a]	RANDOMIZED		REBLEEDING		SURGERY		DEATH		SIGNIFICANCE
		LAS.	CON.	LAS.	CON.	LAS.	CON.	LAS.	CON.	
Laurence et al.[89] (argon)	60	60	—	5(8)	—	13(22)	—	5(8)	—	No control
Vallon et al.[90] (argon)	178	68	68	20(29)	23(34)	17(25)	19(28)	5(7)	10(15)	NS[b]
Swain et al.[91] 1981 (argon)	155	36	40	11(31)	17(43)	8(22)	14(35)	0	7(18)	P<0.02 for death[c]
Krejs et al.[92] (NdYAG)	174	85	89	19(22)	18(20)	14(16)	15(17)	1(1)	1(1)	NS
Rutgeerts et al.[93] (NdYAG)	†	52	58	5(10)	12(21)	3(6)	9(16)	8(15)	8(14)	NS
Swain et al.[91] (NdYAG)[91]	164	70	68	7(10)	27(40)	7(10)	24(35)	1(1)	8(12)	P<0.01 for rebleed, <0.05 for death
Macleod et al.[95] (NdYAG)	45	21	24	6(29)	8(33)	5(24)	8(33)	1(5)	2(8)	NS[d]

Values in parentheses are percentages.
Las., laser treatment; Con., controls; NS, not significant.
[a]Where possible total number given rather than only those randomized.
† Total number unclear; arterial spurters excluded, 16% technical failures.
[b]P<0.05 if patients with spurting only are considered and two are excluded from laser group because of failure to apply the beam accurately.
[c]P<0.05 for rebleeding if analysis confined to non-bleeding visible vessels or a combination of bleeding and non-bleeding visible vessels.
[d]P<0.01 for rebleeding and operation in arterial spurters which received laser treatment (33% did not for technical reasons).

controlled trials have been performed, although some are too small to be confident of the results (Table 38.7). Some vessels in ulcers are inaccessible at endoscopy. If such patients are included in studies of laser application it is difficult to demonstrate a benefit. However, where the ulcers have been treatable a reduction in emergency surgery or mortality has been shown for ulcers with visible vessels[91] and with arterial bleeding[90,91] using argon lasers. Similar results have been achieved with NdYAG lasers but in most studies approximately 20% of patients could not be treated for technical reasons. Overall results with laser photocoagulation are not very impressive and the capital expense and technical difficulties should be considered. Where ulcer bleeding is brisk and the vessels are accessible the role of laser appears greatest. Injection of adrenaline around the ulcer base may also improve the effect of the laser.

Heater probe coagulation

The major problem with all methods which cause coagulation by heat at the end of a probe is that subsequent movement of the probe can dislodge the coagulum because it tends to stick to the probe. 'Non-stick' coatings and water jets have been developed in an attempt to eliminate this problem. Published experience is limited with the Teflon-covered heater probe, although uncontrolled studies have demonstrated that the device can produce haemostasis. Access in duodenal ulcer bleeding is reputedly difficult. One small controlled trial[96] is insufficient to recommend the widespread use of this technique. Compared with NdYAG laser treatment the heater probe was less (but not significantly) effective.[97] Comparison of the heater probe with pure alcohol injection and controls has shown a significant reduction in surgical intervention.[98]

Electrocoagulation

Two general methods exist: bipolar and monopolar. The latter requires a ground plate and the electric current flows through the patient to it. Bipolar probes have two electrodes or more, separated by 1–2 mm, between which current flows across tissue in contact. Indeed many electrodes are commonly arranged around the probe (multipolar). A water pump is also necessary to limit the tendency for the probe to stick. The

results of controlled trials (Table 38.8), although encouraging, are no better than those using other haemostatic methods. Where direct comparisons have been made electrocoagulation is no more nor less effective than laser photocoagulation.[105,106]

Injection sclerotherapy

The recent and potentially most practical endoscopic intervention involves injection of sclerosant (polidocanol, alcohol) and/or adrenaline in and around the ulcer base. Most endoscopists already inject oesophageal varices and are therefore familiar with the equipment which is generally available. Repeated injection is required in a substantial proportion of cases for optimum results. Controlled experience is limited but encouraging (Table 38.9). Uncontrolled data are unhelpful. Injection therapy has been shown to give similar results to laser photocoagulation, yet poorer initial haemostasis than the heater probe.[98,106] There is some evidence that laser photocoagulation is aided by injection of adrenaline beforehand.

Overall position regarding endoscopic intervention

Trials of endoscopic therapy have been subjected to a comprehensive meta-analysis.[111] Thirty randomized controlled trials were identified, and analysis demonstrated that such therapy significantly reduced rates of further bleeding (odds ratio, 0.38: confidence interval, 0.32–0.45), surgery (odds ratio, 0.36; 95% confidence interval 0.28–0.45), and mortality (odds ratio 0.55; 95% confidence interval, 0.40–0.76). Further examination of subgroups indicated that this improvement applied only to those patients with the high-risk endoscopic features of active bleeding or non-bleeding visible vessels, and not to those with adherent clots or flat pigmented spots. No convincing differences were demonstrable between the separate techniques. It therefore seems that endoscopic intervention is beneficial for high-risk lesions, and that clinicians should choose their method based on experience, predictability and cost.

Other methods

Ingenious balloons and clips have been reported but none are in common use. Controlled data with these techniques are still

Table 38.8 Controlled trials of bipolar electrocoagulation for upper gastrointestinal bleeding

AUTHORS	N[a]	RANDOMIZED ELE.	RANDOMIZED CON.	REBLEEDING ELE.	REBLEEDING CON.	SURGERY ELE.	SURGERY CON.	DEATH ELE.	DEATH CON.	SIGNIFICANCE
Goudie et al.[99]	54	21	25	7(33)	5(20)	2(10)	2(8)	0	0	NS
Kernohan et al.[100]	45	21	24	9(43)	7(29)	3(14)	5(21)	0	1(4)	NS
Laine[101]	44	21	23	—	—	3(14)	13(57)	3(14)	0	P<0.03 for surgery[b]
O'Brien[102]	204	101	103	17(17)	34(33)	7(7)	10(10)	13(13)	14(14)	P<0.002 for rebleeding
Brearley et al.[103]	45	21	21	6(29)	8(38)	5(24)	4(19)	0	0	NS
Laine[104]	60	31	29	6(19)	12(41)	3(10)	8(28)	1(3)	0	NS

Values in parentheses are percentages.
Ele., electrocoagulation; Con., controls; NS, not significant.
[a]Where possible total number given rather than only those randomized.
[b]Half the patients had Mallory–Weiss tears or vascular malformations; no significant difference between surgery rates in peptic ulcer bleeds.

Table 38.9 Controlled trials of injection sclerotherapy for upper gastrointestinal bleeding

AUTHORS	N	RANDOMIZED		REBLEEDING		SURGERY		DEATH		SIGNIFICANCE
		INJ.	CON.	INJ.	CON.	INJ.	CON.	INJ.	CON.	
Panes et al.[107] (poli +)	113	55	58	3(6)	25(43)	3(6)	20(34)	2(4)	4(7)	P<0.02 for rebleed or surgery
Balanzo[108] (poli +)	72	36	36	7(19)	7(19)	7(19)	12(33)	1(3)	1(3)	NS
Chung et al.[109] (adrenaline)	68	34	34	—	—	5(15)	14(41)	3(9)	2(6)	P<0.02 for surgery
Rutgeerts[a] (poli +)		40	20	3(8)	12(60)	3(8)	11(55)	2(5)	2(10)	P<0.05 for rebleeding
(adrenaline)		40	—	7(18)	—	6(15)	—	4(10)	—	NS

Values in parentheses are percentages.
Inj., injection sclerotherapy; Con., controls; poli +, polidocanol plus adrenaline; NS, not significant.
[a]Trial also compared laser photocoagulation and control group not strictly comparable. Polidocanol plus adrenaline injection was most effective but not significantly more so than laser plus adrenaline injection.

awaited. Microwave energy produces coagulation and has also been used but widespread application is unlikely.

Surgical intervention

Although the steady improvement in therapeutic endoscopy gives encouragement for the future, its practical application now to the overall problem is minimal. There are hospitals where these techniques are under study and form the first line of definitive therapy but, for most, surgery provides the only way in which uncontrolled or repeated bleeding can be stopped.

It is self-evident that continued arterial bleeding requires a surgical ligature, and this situation can be clinically obvious even though the presence of the bleeding lesion can only be inferred from the bedside. Erosion of a major vessel in the base of an ulcer or bleeding from Dieulafoy's erosion will induce such torrential bleeding as to produce the almost immediate vomiting of large amounts of fresh blood, rapidly followed by circulatory collapse. Alternatively the endoscopist may be fortunate enough to observe arterial spurting despite the difficulties associated with large amounts of retained blood clot in the stomach. Improving endoscopic skill renders this situation more common than might be expected, but in general a skilled nurse is usually just as accurate and certainly much quicker in reaching a diagnosis.

Much more difficult is the decision of if and when to operate on the patient who is bleeding slowly or repeatedly, in whom circulatory stability is maintained either by vasoconstriction or by adequate transfusion. It is not, therefore, surprising to find widely varying operation rates; reported values range from 20 to 64% and the indications when specified are equally variable.

It is important to distinguish between emergency and early elective surgery, a separation first proposed by Schiller and colleagues in 1970.[112] Although the immediate aftermath of an acute gastrointestinal bleed is not the most appropriate time to consider major definitive surgery, it is none the less inevitable that a long recurrent history of ulcer relapse and healing, despite adequate medical therapy, does influence the decision to operate and the choice of the most appropriate procedure. This was becoming increasingly so with many patients having multiple courses of H2-receptor antagonists, but the recent introduction of the proton pump inhibitor omeprazole has again altered the balance against early elective surgery. Even in the most skilled and dedicated units there is a definable mortality, higher in the elderly and in those with severe coincident disease. The aim of surgery is to save life by reliably stopping bleeding, not to embark on complex operations just because the abdomen is open. It is now better surgical policy to render the patient safe and to embark on prolonged effective medical therapy for the peptic ulcer.

As already indicated it is important to site these seriously ill patients appropriately. Those with bleeding varices, severe forms of shock or at major risk of rebleeding are often best nursed in intensive care units, as are the most seriously ill in the immediate postoperative period. Apart from those clearly at low risk, all remaining patients must be under more careful observation than is possible in a general ward. For reasons previously outlined, this should be in an area of high dependency, preferably in a designated gastrointestinal ward.

Infections, both in the wound and systemically, e.g. pneumonia and septicaemia, are serious potential disasters and must be treated energetically. Gatehouse et al.[113] showed that patients have abnormally high bacterial counts in the gastric lumen after a gastrointestinal bleed. They further showed a relationship between these counts and the liability to postoperative sepsis. It is likely that this is mediated partly by inhibition of gastric acidity and protein lysis, and partly by the substantial amount of blood clot often present in the stomach. Gastric acidity can also be affected by H2-receptor antagonist therapy and the potential for infection is therefore substantially increased. The place of prophylactic antibiotics in major abdominal surgery is well established, and the same policy must equally be applied to these seriously ill patients. A cephalosporin given as a single dose immediately before surgery, followed by two postoperative doses at 12-hourly intervals, is our current policy.

The use of anticoagulants in conditions of major haemorrhage might well appear to be dangerous, but we were impressed by the high incidence of thromboembolic deaths previously reported.[69] Heparin given subcutaneously in low dosage has, in other situations, been shown to be effective in decreasing the incidence of fatal postoperative thromboembolism.[114] We have, therefore, been using low-dose heparin routinely postoperatively in these patients since 1979, with a marked absence of fatal pulmonary embolism and postoperative bleeding complications. We have not used heparin in non-surgical patients, although it has been shown that any bleeding episode is followed by a hypercoagulable state.[82] Anticoagulation, either complete or partial, requires clinical evaluation.

Surgery in undiagnosed bleeding

Rarely, patients will present in the emergency department with massive continuing undiagnosed bleeding, taxing all efforts at resuscitation and rendering endoscopy impracticable. Such patients must be taken immediately to the operating theatre, and induction of anaesthesia is sometimes followed by reduction or even cessation of the bleeding. Once the airway is protected, endoscopy is safe and should always be performed. Finding the causative lesion can be difficult in patients where the ulcer may be shallow and impalpable, and any disadvantage from the short delay in commencing the operation is well counterbalanced by the valuable diagnostic information often produced. Clearly, if the bleeding stops and gastroscopy reveals an intact mucosa, the patient should be reawakened without laparotomy. Gastroscopy has also been used intraoperatively, and occasionally there may well be value in this.

Duodenal ulceration

Truncal vagotomy and pyloroplasty For the majority of surgeons truncal vagotomy and pyloroplasty combined with under-running of the bleeding vessel remains the operation of choice,[115] and has indeed been the operation performed in more than half of our own patients over the last 5 years. If the patient is not actively bleeding at the time of surgery it is advisable to start with the vagotomy, whereas in the presence of bleeding it is better to control blood loss first by under-running the ulcer.

About 3 cm of each vagal trunk should be excised and the lower 5 cm of oesophagus carefully cleared of all vagal fibres. Care must be taken not to perforate the oesophagus. If a bleeding vessel is present it should be tied off separately with figure-of-eight stitches proximal and distal to the bleeding point. The mucosa may then be approximated with a few deep sutures. Smaller ulcers without a vessel should be sutured with the deep sutures alone. The common bile duct is usually at a safe distance but great care should be taken to avoid damaging it, especially if there is duodenal deformity, when the anatomy may be gravely distorted. The preferred suture material may be any one of the synthetic absorbable materials. After under-running the ulcer, the gastroduodenotomy is closed transversely as a Heineke–Mikulicz pyloroplasty. With severe duodenal scarring due to anterior and posterior duodenal ulceration the pyloroduodenal incision may be closed as a Finney pyloroplasty to prevent gastric outlet obstruction.

Truncal vagotomy and antrectomy Herrington and Davidson[116] advocate truncal vagotomy with antrectomy and Billroth I reconstruction, as well as under-running of the bleeding ulcer for the good-risk patient, provided the inflammatory process in the duodenum allows resection and a safe gastroduodenal anastomosis. They report a satisfactory overall mortality for the procedure of 5.5% and an incidence of early rebleeding of less than 1% in a total of 250 emergency and semiemergency operations. They advise truncal vagotomy and pyloroplasty for the high-risk patient, but unfortunately there have been no controlled clinical trials to compare the results of these procedures with under-running alone in high- and low-risk patients.

Billroth II gastrectomy For a large duodenal ulcer a Billroth II gastrectomy may still be required to control bleeding, especially when rebleeding follows a more conservative operation. Suture line leakage and duodenal stump complications are major sources of morbidity and mortality, limiting the desirability of this operation. Great care must be taken to suture firmly and without tension and provide temporary drainage when necessary.

Proximal gastric vagotomy Proximal gastric vagotomy has become the preferred definitive surgical treatment of duodenal ulceration. Protagonists of this procedure have also recommended its use for selected patients with bleeding duodenal ulceration, under-running the ulcer via a duodenotomy. Proximal gastric vagotomy was used in this way by Johnston et al.[117] in a series of 26 patients, with no deaths; more recently from Charleston, West Virginia, Hoake et al.[118] have described a further 22 parietal cell vagotomies carried out for acute haemorrhage. Five of these patients were in shock, and the group as a whole appeared to be a fairly average case mix. There were no deaths, and long-term follow-up indicated an excellent functional result. Proximal gastric vagotomy is not yet widely accepted for this purpose as it is a more lengthy procedure than vagotomy and drainage and can only be done by an appropriately skilled surgeon. It is associated with a high rate of ulcer recurrence, but it must again be emphasized that saving life is more important than definitive therapy.

Under-running alone In 1963 Foster et al.[119] commented: 'the advisability of lesser procedures in seriously ill patients with peptic ulcer haemorrhage is obvious.' They suggested the use of vagotomy and pyloroplasty with suture ligation of the bleeding point, and reported the successful treatment of seven such patients. In Birmingham an analysis of the specific causes of death led us to a similar belief that the operation itself produced most of the fatal complications. A high incidence of anastomotic leakage induced a recommendation that, whenever practicable, gastrectomy should be replaced by more conservative procedures. Since that time, mortality has fallen further and operations now appear safer.[4] Pharmacological treatment of the ulcer has, however, also continued to improve and there is less need for the surgeon to feel the ulcer diathesis must be cured while the vagus nerve is at hand. Improvements in surgical technique are balanced by an increase in the proportion of patients decrepit with the diseases of age, and the same concerns therefore still apply to limiting the extent of surgical interference.

We have therefore often adopted the policy of simply under-running the ulcer to stop bleeding effectively. Treatment of the ulcer diathesis is then left to a pharmacological approach, with definitive surgery being a consideration for the future. Naturally this approach began for patients at particularly high risk, but there are other complications of surgical treatment apart from infection, thrombosis and death. It is unfortunate to have an initially satisfactory outcome but be left with problems of dumping, diarrhoea and ulcer recurrence. We therefore believe that this more conservative policy requires proper assessment, and a European study has started to examine the question.

The operation can usually be done through a duodenotomy, leaving the pylorus intact, but if exposure is inadequate the sphincter itself must be transected. Reconstruction is done in the line of incision, provided the duodenum is not grossly deformed, in which case there could be a risk of postoperative gastric outlet obstruction.[120] If there is a stricture limited to the duodenum the duodenotomy should be closed as a duodenoplasty, thus avoiding pyloroplasty. Location of a duodenal ulcer may occasionally be difficult, in which case a Perspex proctoscope or vaginal speculum can be very useful.

Gastric ulceration

It has been standard practice to perform gastrectomy, usually Billroth I, and this if often associated with a low risk of rebleeding and a high probability for long-term cure. It does, however, carry a high mortality rate, even in the best hands,[121] and again these patients are frequently aged.[122] Location high on the lesser curvature and posterior erosions into the pancreas and splenic artery can also present additional serious problems. Finally, there can be no assurance that any gastric ulcer is necessarily benign, thus adding to the complexity of the surgical decision.

Gastrectomy is now less used as the operation of choice and appears to be giving way to truncal vagotomy and pyloroplasty with ulcer excision or biopsy, and arterial ligation or under-running.[116] A lower mortality rate has been reported to follow this procedure (7%) but with a high rate of rebleeding (7%), and also of recurrent ulceration (15%). Proximal gastric vagotomy is even more difficult in gastric ulcer patients, particularly when the ulcer is sited high on the lesser curvature. It has not been used extensively in this situation and is not recommended.

Under-running and biopsy or excision of the ulcer without any attempt at an ulcer curative procedure have in the past been reserved for the very high-risk patient, but recently this conservative approach has been more seriously examined. Early results from Rogers et al.[122] are impressive, with an operative mortality of 10% for under-running alone, compared with 26% for partial gastrectomy, and an extremely high 45% for vagotomy and under-running. Only one of the 20 patients treated by under-running alone rebled, but this study was not controlled and the patients were collected over 8 years, suggesting an element of selection bias. At the General Hospital in Birmingham our choice has been for this conservative surgical option in a third of gastric ulcer patients.

A gastric ulcer should always be excised rather than biopsied, in order to decrease the rebleeding rate and to avoid missing a cancer due to having insufficient material for histological examination. Transgastric excision of a high gastric

ulcer is the preferred procedure as attempts to excise the ulcer by wedge excision from the lesser curvature endangers the nerves of Latarget and may thus lead to antral stasis and recurrent ulceration.[123] All patients should be placed on a long-term follow-up programme after non-resectional gastric surgery.

Our own low surgical mortality might be explained by many factors other than the choice of the correct procedure. Such factors include a high diagnostic rate, establishment of the optimal timing of surgery, improvement in collaboration between physicians, surgeons and nurses, and insistence on an adequate level of experience of surgeon and anaesthetist. The question of which is the best operation remains unanswered and should be addressed by clinical trial only within a framework established by these favourable contributory factors.

Surgical treatment of other bleeding lesions

Mallory–Weiss tears Mallory–Weiss tears rarely induce dangerous bleeding and seldom require surgery. They usually heal spontaneously but vasopressin can be useful when bleeding is persistent. If an operation is required, exposure through a high longitudinal gastrotomy is satisfactory for oversewing the tear; a Perspex proctoscope may be helpful in determining the extent of the lesions. One absolute indication for operation is in patients with a full-thickness oesophageal tear with perforation into the mediastinum (Boerhaave syndrome). These patients are gravely ill, often presenting shocked, with severe retrosternal and abdominal pain, surgical emphysema in the neck, radiological evidence of air in the mediastinum and neck and sometimes under the diaphragm. Treatment is directed to dealing with the perforation.

Stress bleeding As a result of the high standard of intensive care therapy, stress ulceration is becoming a rare condition. As the mortality of patients operated on for haemorrhage exceeds 30%,[124] attempts at reducing mortality are best directed at prevention. Antacid and H₂-receptor antagonist therapy have been shown to be beneficial for the prevention of these ulcers,[125] and tranexamic acid has been proposed as effective treatment.[126] Increasing use of endoscopic injection with adrenaline and sclerosing agents for bleeding ulcers should be extended to this problem by those with the appropriate experience. If bleeding persists and operation becomes mandatory, the stomach should be opened and attempts made to under-run individual bleeding points because the haemorrhage may be coming from deeper erosions involving small arteries. This should always be combined with vagotomy and pyloroplasty. For the rare patient with recurrent bleeding or multifocal bleeding, total gastrectomy may be necessary. In such situations mortality is high and may exceed 50%.[127]

Dieulafoy vascular malformations (exulceratio simplex) This is a rare cause of upper gastrointestinal bleeding which can easily be overlooked at endoscopy and at operation as a cause of massive, often recurrent haematemesis. Bleeding is caused by an unusually large (1–3 mm) artery that runs in the submucosa in close contact with the mucous membrane. Massive bleeding can occur if erosion of the mucous membrane and arterial wall are present. The mucosal defect is usually 2–5 mm, and in more than 80% of patients the site of bleeding is found within 6 cm of the gastro-oesophageal junction, usually along the lesser curve. It can occur at any age (mean age 52 years) and is twice as frequent in men as in women.[128] A high mortality is associated with delayed diagnosis. The endoscopic appearances of the Dieulafoy lesion are variable. Sometimes no abnormality is seen and sometimes it is only after repeated endoscopies that one suddenly sees active bleeding from a pin-point mucosal lesion. Sometimes there is a small erosive defect with a tiny visible vessel or adherent clot. If endoscopic treatment fails, wedge resection without vagotomy is recommended.

Cushing and Curling ulcers Management depends on the endoscopic findings. Discrete deep ulcers are likely to involve larger vessels and are usually treated in the same way as peptic ulcers. Diffuse shallow ulceration is best managed in a fashion similar to that outlined for stress ulceration.

Stomal and recurrent (postoperative) ulceration Occasionally bleeding may occur from a stomal ulcer. This can usually be managed with H$_2$-receptor antagonists as bleeding from stomal ulcers is rarely catastrophic. Indications for operation are more conservative than those outlined for peptic ulcers. As reoperation after previous gastrectomy may be technically extremely demanding, especially under emergency conditions, only experienced surgeons should operate on these patients. The type of operation will depend upon the site of ulceration, the fitness of the patient and the nature of the original operation. Thus vagotomy, revagotomy, gastric resection or ulcer excision and reconstruction are all possible solutions to this difficult problem.

Tumours Bleeding from a mesenchymal tumour, of which leiomyoma is the most common, is a relatively rare cause of massive upper gastrointestinal bleeding. It is usually a well-circumscribed submucosal tumour, with ulceration of the overlying mucosa causing the bleeding. The same criteria for the timing of surgical intervention are used as for peptic ulcers; local resection is sufficient. Tumours near the oesophagogastric junction can be treated by incising the overlying mucosa and enucleating the tumour.

Gastric lymphomas may present with bleeding and should, if possible, be managed by radical excision. Depending on the histological type, adjuvant chemotherapy and radiotherapy may be advisable.

The prognosis of patients with bleeding gastric adenocarcinoma is generally poor.[70] Most tumours are advanced and in only a few patients is radical excision justified. Bleeding duodenal or pancreatic cancers are almost never salvageable by surgery. It is important that an ulcer with the appearance of cancer but negative histology and cytology be treated as a peptic ulcer. If it is clinically indicated, surgery should not be withheld from these patients.

Aortoenteric haemorrhage This serious cause of both minor and major upper gastrointestinal bleeding has an increasing incidence. The crucial issue for successful management is to suspect the diagnosis in any patient with a history of previous aortic surgery who presents with an upper gastrointestinal bleed. The patient should be endoscoped in the operating theatre, preferably under general anaesthesia. If the diagnosis of aortoenteric fistula is confirmed, or if in such a patient bleeding from another source in the oesophagus, stomach or duodenum is excluded, laparotomy should proceed immediately with a team including an experienced vascular surgeon. The traditional approach is to oversew the aorta, remove the graft and perform an axillobifemoral bypass.

Haematobilia Operation is best avoided and selective arterial catheterization with embolization is the treatment of choice.

Timing of surgery

There has been extensive debate as to whether it is safer to support the circulation and postpone surgery or to operate early on the increasing numbers of patients with life-threatening haemorrhage who are aged and suffer from severe coincident disease. There is often clinical reluctance to take such apparently poor-risk patients to theatre, with all the inherent circulatory and respiratory complications. There are very few patients indeed who are admitted with gastrointestinal bleeding but who are also suffering from such advanced malignant or other terminal disease that it is kinder not to resuscitate and not to operate. This tiny group, however, must not be confused with the very substantial number of elderly patients suffering from coincident disease, such as bronchitis, cardiac failure, coronary ischaemia or peripheral vascular disease, where the haemorrhage poses yet another threat to life. There is no question that in these patients it is vital to offer the best possible medical management, and the question here is whether to operate early or to resuscitate, monitor carefully and operate later only if required.

Some evidence was presented from Nottingham in 1979[129] comparing the clinical results at two separate hospitals applying different policies. One hospital had a consistently higher operation rate (46%) and an earlier time for surgery, whereas the other tended to operate later and less often (21%). Three hundred and two patients were studied and there was no apparent difference in risk factors in the two groups of patients. As the operative mortality was similar in the two hospitals (22%), the total mortality was much higher in the hospital with an aggressive policy (18%) than where the policy was more conservative (11%). Applying the principle deduced from this study, the authors reduced the overall operation rate from 34 to 21% in a subsequent 3-year period.[130] The surgical mortality increased slightly but the overall mortality for peptic ulcer bleeding remained constant at 11%. It was concluded that surgery should not be pressed in such ill patients unless it was almost inevitable.

Advocates for a more aggressive policy are not difficult to find, and in 1950 Tanner and Desmond[79] reviewed the results of surgery in bleeding peptic ulcer disease involving 622 admissions with chronic peptic ulceration over a 10-year period. Early in this study operation was avoided wherever possible, but in the latter period patients were treated with early surgery whenever certain minimal criteria were breached.

The rate of surgical intervention increased from 5 to 60%, but despite a marked increase in the average age of the patients, the overall mortality fell from 10 to 7%. The study was uncontrolled and the authors correctly attributed part of the success to a dedicated team of medical and nursing staff. Indeed, results can always be improved when the group responsible is welded into an efficient watchful unit. Adoption of a similar policy in Montreal led on to a study of 211 peptic ulcer patients managed to a fairly aggressive protocol. Surgery was indicated for all patients with gastric ulcers, for older patients with duodenal ulceration, and wherever the initial transfusion was 5 or more units of whole blood. Overall mortality reduced from 7.3 to 2.4% in a historical period of comparison. The policy of tight management and early surgery was further developed by Hunt et al.[80] in Melbourne, who described the results achieved by their unit over a 6-year period from 1972 to 1978. Good results were obtained, with a mortality for peptic ulcer bleeding of 6%, achieved through an operation rate of 43% (surgical mortality 10%). Curiously, when the study period was broken into three 2-year periods, mortality in the last of these was significantly lower, at 1.5%, although the operation rate and case mix remained the same. Any suggestion that a permanent change had been effected was unfortunately refuted by a subsequent report,[131] when the mortality had returned to 7.4% with an operation rate of 27% (surgical mortality 19%).

The only prospective randomized study carried out on this question was published from this unit in Birmingham in 1984,[2] in which patients with proven peptic ulcers were stratified by age (above and below 60 years) and randomized to receive either early or delayed surgical intervention according to defined criteria. Endoscopy was carried out within 12 hours of admission and patients were managed in a designated unit. In younger patients mortality was negligible, no advantage was found from early operation, and the operation rate of 50% in the early group was regarded as excessive. The study was therefore stopped earlier in the younger group. In the older group, however, mortality in the gastric ulcer patients receiving early surgery was significantly lower and in all ulcer patients mortality was 4% for early surgery against 15% for delayed. It was deduced that minimal mortality was associated with urgent and skilled surgical intervention when certain criteria were satisfied.

This policy was adopted for the succeeding 5-year period (1984–1988), except that stigmata of recent haemorrhage were no longer considered an indication for surgery. The results of this audit, together with the results reported recently from Bath, UK, using almost identical criteria, are listed in Table 38.10. In both of these studies even advanced inoperable malignant disease was included and, at least in the Birmingham series, supportive treatment was withdrawn in several patients. Mortality was low in both, totalling 25 of the 559 (4.5%) patients available for study. There is a remarkable similarity in the mortality rate at different ages, which for the over 60s was 6% in both and in the over 80s 10% in Bath and 9% in Birmingham (Figure 38.5). Both studies give excellent results, reflecting the continued success of integrated bleeding units with clearly defined protocols of management.

Table 38.10 Results currently achieved applying a clear aggressive surgical policy

	BATH[3]	BIRMINGHAM[4]
Type of ulcer		
Gastric	109	124
Duodenal	108	218
Total	217	342
Surgery		
Vagotomy + pyloroplasty	26	33
Resection	13	27
Minimal	7	9
Total	46(21%)	69(20%)
Deaths		
Surgical	7(15%)	3(4%)
Non-surgical	5	11
Total	12(6%)	13(4%)

Mortality for bleeding peptic ulceration should not exceed 5% and the results from Bath and Birmingham indicate that this is possible using a very clearly defined and aggressive surgical policy. If the criteria are applied vigorously, the surgeon and the anaesthetist are skilled and experienced, and the patient is managed with care, preferably in an area designated for this problem, then these results should be obtainable in any hospital. The present evidence indicates that it is a fallacy to postpone or avoid surgery in older people with severe coincident disease.

RECOMMENDATIONS

A low level of mortality for bleeding peptic ulceration will probably remain unavoidable in older patients. Present evidence suggests that this should be negligible below the age of 60, and in the region of 6% for those above this age. The risk rises further with age, but should still not exceed 10% for those older than 80. This mortality will still include many patients severely ill from other causes, and otherwise healthy old people bleeding from their ulcers should normally survive. There will be others with, for example, disseminated malignant disease in whom it may be judged more humane to withdraw resuscitation.

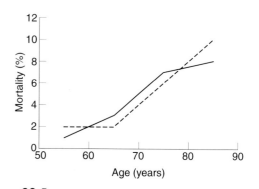

Figure 38.5

Relationship between mortality and age in recent published series: Bath, UK[3] (------); Birmingham, UK[4] (——).

We believe avoidable deaths follow mismanagement in three major areas:

1. Failure to take quick action to stop bleeding.

2. Inadequate resuscitation on admission or following further haemorrhage.

3. The absence or lack of adherence to a clear protocol of management.

Management should be based on a number of important principles. Firstly, there must be efficient and competent assessment and diagnosis. Resuscitation must be quick and management alert to further bleeding. The majority of patients should be in a high-dependency area with gastroenterological input, a few in an intensive care unit, and those with a number of minor bleeds (e.g. Mallory–Weiss) may be cared for in general medical wards. It is essential to establish a firm protocol of management geared to the particular skills available. Finally, results must be subjected to regular audit, with feedback into the agreed protocol.

Intervention to stop or prevent haemorrhage has traditionally been surgical and currently remains so in the majority of European hospitals. Steady improvement in techniques, skill and therapeutic endoscopy indicates that this is likely to change, and we look forward to a potential decline in reliance on surgery, with all of its complications. The same principles of speedy resuscitation, watchful management and alertness for intervention will, however, remain and form the essential basis of a protocol. Drug therapy, although important in the medium term to heal lesions, does not form an essential part in the acute episode. We have steadily refined our own protocol and offer it as the best we know for any hospital dependent upon surgery as its interventional weapon.

Protocol for the management of acute upper gastrointestinal bleeding: the General Hospital, Birmingham, 1991

1. All patients to be admitted under the care of the physician on duty on the day they enter hospital.

2. All admissions to be promptly notified to the resident medical officer (RMO). The RMO then informs the resident surgical officer (RSO) and the on-call endoscopist, who together form the 'bleeding team' – they are jointly responsible for the management decisions.

3. Patients to be gastroscoped as soon as possible, normally by the endoscopist on call. This is usually done by addition to the next standard list. Out of hours it is done in the endoscopy suite with the help of two nurses, one trained in endoscopy.

4. Responsibility for the care of these patients during the whole of their stay in hospital will remain with the same medical and surgical firms on duty on admission day, unless other individual arrangements are made.

5. Patients with minor bleeds are usually admitted to general medical wards, but the following patients are admitted to reserved 'bleeding beds' in the gastrointestinal ward.

   (a) All patients who have had a substantial gastrointestinal bleed.
   (b) Patients over 60 years of age.
   (c) Patients known to have cirrhosis/varices.

   Severely ill patients including patients injected for bleeding varices should be in the intensive care unit.

6. *Indications for Surgery*
   (a) Immediate surgery (all ages).
      (i) Exsanguinating haemorrhage: if the patient's condition cannot be stabilized during initial resuscitation because of continued blood loss.
      (ii) Spurting vessel at endoscopy which cannot be controlled by local injection.
   (b) Patients older than 60 years.
      (i) Four units of blood/plasma expander required on admission to secure haemodynamic stability.
      (ii) One rebleed in hospital.
      (iii) Persistent bleeding requiring transfusion of 8 units in 48 hours.
   (c) Patients younger than 60 years.
      (i) Eight units of blood/plasma expander required on admission to ensure haemodynamic stability.
      (ii) Two rebleeds in hospital.
      (iii) Persistent bleeding requiring transfusion of 12 units in 48 hours.

7. Operations on bleeding patients to be performed by a surgeon of specialist registrar status or above, with a correspondingly experienced anaesthetist. The surgeon on call to be consulted about any difficult cases.

This protocol represents a collective series of guidelines developed from the experience of ourselves and others. Of these guidelines, only the timing of surgery has been subject to a prospective randomized clinical trial.[2] It has none the less been further applied by ourselves and others, always with similarly satisfactory results.[3,4,132] Although this protocol has been developed in relationship to surgery as the definitive therapy for the control of haemorrhage, we believe the principles apply equally to the rapidly developing endoscopic therapy. Major deviations from this protocol should also be assessed by randomized prospective clinical trials. At this time, however, we believe the protocol to be applicable in any district general hospital, where it can produce acceptably low levels of mortality and morbidity.

REFERENCES

1. Bulmer E. The mortality from haematemesis. *Lancet* 1927; **ii**: 720.
2. Morris DL, Hawker PC, Brearley S, Simms M, Dykes PW & Keighley MRB. Optimal timing of operation for bleeding peptic ulcer: prospective randomized trial. *BMJ* 1984; **228**: 1277.
3. Holman RAE, Davis M, Gough KR, Gartell P, Britton DC & Smith RB. Value of a centralised approach in the management of haematemesis and melaena: experience in a district general hospital. *Gut* 1990; **31**: 504.
4. Wheatley KE, Snyman JH, Brearley S, Keighley MRB & Dykes PW. Mortality in patients with bleeding peptic ulcer when those aged 60 or over are operated on early. *BMJ* 1990; **301**: 272.
5. Burger F & Hartfall SJ. Haematemesis in peptic ulcer. *Guy's Hosp Rep* 1934; **84**: 197.

6. Cullinan ER & Price RK. Haematemesis following peptic ulceration. *St Bart's Hosp Rev* 1932; **65**: 185.

7. Atkinson M. Bleeding from the oesophagus. In Dykes PW & Keighley MRB (eds) *Gastrointestinal Haemorrhage*. Bristol: Wright, 1981: 23.

8. Windsor CWO & Collins JL. Anaemia and hiatus hernia: experience of 450 patients. *Thorax* 1967; **22**: 73.

9. Barrett NR. Chronic peptic ulcer of oesophagus 'oesophagitis'. *Br J Surg* 1950; **38**: 175.

10. Savary M & Miller G. The esophagus. In Gassman AG (ed.) *Handbook and Atlas of Endoscopy*. Switzerland: Solothurn, 1978.

11. McDonald GB, Brand DL & Thorning DR. Multiple adenomatous neoplasms arising in columnar lined (Barrett's) oesophagus. *Gastroenterology* 1977; **72**: 1317.

12. Atkinson M, Bottrill MB, Edwards AT et al. Mucosal tears at the oesophago-gastric junction (Mallory–Weiss syndrome). *Gut* 1961; **2**: 1.

13. Graham DY & Schwartz JT. The spectrum of the Mallory–Weiss tear. *Medicine (Baltimore)* 1977; **57**: 307.

14. Collins FJ, Mathews HR, Baker SE et al. Drug induced oesophageal injury. *BMJ* 1979; **1**: 1673.

15. Hurst AF & Stewart MJ. Etiology. In Hurst AF & Stewart MJ (eds) *Gastric and Duodenal Ulcer*. London: Oxford University Press, 1929: 29.

16. Emery ES & Monroe RT. Peptic ulcer. *Arch Intern Med* 1935; **55**: 271.

17. Stolte JB. The frequency of manifest bleeding in peptic ulcer with regard to the duration of the disease and to the age of the diseased. *Acta Med Scand* 1944; **116**: 584.

18. DeBakey M. Acute perforated gastroduodenal ulceration. *Surgery* 1940; **8**: 852.

19. Jordan SM & Kiefer ED. Complications of peptic ulcer: their prognostic significance. *JAMA* 1934; **103**: 2004.

20. Johnston SJ, Jones PF, Kyle J & Needham CD. Epidemiology and course of gastrointestinal haemorrhage in north-east Scotland. *BMJ* 1973; **3**: 655.

21. Heuer GJ. The surgical aspects of haemorrhage from peptic ulcer. *N Engl Med J* 1946; **235**: 777.

22. Green PHR, Fevere DI, Barrett PJ et al. Chronic erosive (verrucous) gastritis. *Endoscopy* 1977; **9**: 74.

23. Bennett JR & Dykes PW. Ulcerative disease of the stomach and duodenum. In Dykes PW & Keighley MRB (eds) *Gastrointestinal Haemorrhage*. Bristol: Wright, 1981: 23.

24. Sevitt S. Duodenal and gastric ulceration after burning. *Br J Surg* 1967; **54**: 32.

25. Cushing H. Peptic ulcers and the interbrain. *Surg Gynecol Obstet* 1932; **55**: 1.

26. Skillman JJ & Silen W. Stress ulcers. *Lancet* 1972; **ii**: 1303.

27. Muir A & Cossar IA. Aspirin and ulcer. *BMJ* 1955; **2**: 7.

28. Alvares AS & Summerskill WHJ. Gastrointestinal haemorrhage and salicylates. *Lancet* 1958; **ii**: 920.

29. Lange HF. Salicylates and gastric haemorrhage. *Gastroenterology* 1957; **33**: 778.

30. Cooke AR. Drugs and peptic ulceration. In Sleisenger MH & Fordtran JA (eds) *Gastrointestinal Disease*. Philadelphia: WB Saunders, 1973: 642.

31. Langman MJS. Aspirin is not a major cause of acute gastrointestinal bleeding. In Ingelfinger FJ, Ebert RV, Finland RV et al (eds) *Controversy in Internal Medicine*. Philadelphia: WB Saunders, 1974: 493.

32. Levy M. Aspirin use in patients with major gastrointestinal bleeding and peptic ulcer disease. *N Engl J Med* 1974; **290**: 1158.

33. Somerville K, Faulkner G & Langman MJS. Non-steroidal anti-inflammatory drugs and bleeding peptic ulcer. *Lancet* 1986; **i**: 462.

34. Beardon PHG, Brown SV & McDevitt DF. Gastrointestinal events in patients prescribed non-steroidal anti-inflammatory drugs: a controlled study using record linkage in Tayside. *Q J Med* 1989; **71**: 497.

35. Griffin MR, Piper JM, Daugherty JR, Snowden MR & Ray WA. Non-steroidal anti-inflammatory drug use and increased risk for peptic ulcer disease in elderly persons. *Ann Intern Med* 1991; **114**: 257.

36. Hawkey CJ. Non-steroidal anti-inflammatory drugs and peptic ulcers: facts and figures multiply but do they add up? *BMJ* 1990; **300**: 278.

37. Russell Smith C, Bartholomew LC & Cain JC. Hereditary haemorrhagic telangiectasia and gastrointestinal haemorrhage. *Gastroenterology* 1963; **44**: 1.

38. Jacobson G & Krause V. Hereditary haemorrhagic telangiectasia localised to the gastrointestinal tract. *Scand J Gastroenterol* 1970; **5**: 283.

39. Vase P & Grove O. Gastrointestinal lesions in hereditary haemorrhagic telangiectasia. *Gastroenterology* 1986; **91**: 1079.

40. Gilmore PR. Angioplasia of the upper gastrointestinal tract. *J Clin Gastroenterol* 1988; **10**: 386.

41. Tai D-I, Chou F-F, Lee T-Y & Lin C-C. Vascular ectasia of the duodenum detected by duodenoscopy. *Am J Gastroenterol* 1987; **82**: 1071.

42. Moreto M, Figa M, Ojembarrena E & Zeballa M. Vascular malformations of the stomach and duodenum: an endoscopic classification. *Endoscopy* 1986; **18**: 227.

43. Bakka A & Rosseland AR. Massive gastric bleeding from exulceratio simplex (Dieulafoy). *Acta Chir Scand* 1986; **152**: 285.

44. Boron B & Mobarhan S. Endoscopic treatment of Dieulafoy haemorrhage. *J Clin Gastroenterol* 1987; **9**: 518.

45. Berlyne GM & Berlyne N. Anaemia due to 'blue-rubber-bleb' naevus disease. *Lancet* 1960; **ii**: 1275.

46. Berenson MM & Freston JW. Intrahepatic artery aneurysm associated with haemobilia. *Gastroenterology* 1974; **66**: 254.

47. Harlaflis NN & Akin JT. Haemobilia from ruptured hepatic artery aneurysm. *Am J Surg* 1977; **133**: 229.

48. Wu TK, Zaman SN, Gullick HD et al. Spontaneous haemorrhage due to pseudocysts of the pancreas. *Am J Surg* 1977; **134**: 408.

49. Garrett HE, Beall AC, Jordan GL et al. Surgical considerations of massive haemorrhage caused by aorto-duodenal fistula. *Am J Surg* 1963; **105**: 6.

50. Cordell AR, Wright RH & Johnston FR. Gastrointestinal haemorrhage after abdominal aortic operation. *Surgery* 1960; **48**: 997.

51. Reckless JPD, McColl I & Taylor GW. Aorto-enteric fistulae: an uncommon complication of abdominal aortic aneurysms. *Br J Surg* 1972; **59**: 458.

52. Kundrotas L, Novak J, Kremzier J, Meenaghan M & Hassett J. Gastric bleeding in pseudoxanthoma elasticum. *Am J Gastroenterol* 1988; **83**: 868.

53. Callender ST. Chronic blood loss. In Dykes PW & Keighley MRB (eds) *Gastrointestinal Haemorrhage*. Bristol: Wright, 1981: 112.

54. Carron DB, Boon TH & Walker FC. Peptic ulcer in the haemophiliac and its relation to gastrointestinal bleeding. *Lancet* 1965; **ii**: 1036.

55. Gazzard BG, Portmann B, Murray-Lyon IM et al. Causes of death in fulminant hepatic failure and relationship to quantitative histological assessment of parenchymal damage. *Q J Med* 1975; **44**: 615.

56. Fletcher AP, Biederman O, Moore D et al. Abnormal plasminogen–plasmin system activity (fibrinolysis) in patients with hepatic cirrhosis: its cause and consequences. *J Clin Invest* 1964; **43**: 681.

57. Forrest JAH & Finlayson NDC. The investigation of acute upper gastrointestinal haemorrhage. *Br J Hosp Med* 1974; **12**: 160.

58. Chandler GN & Watkinson G. The early diagnosis of the cause of haematemesis. *Q J Med* 1959; **28**: 371.

59. Kalk H. Einiges uber die gross Blutung du des Geschwurskrankheit du Magens und Zwolffingerdarmes. *Dtsch Med Wochenschr* 1936; **62**: 1202.

60. Matthews JB, Tortella BJ & Silen W. Gastroduodenal haemorrhage and perforation in the post-operative period. *Surg Gynecol Obstet* 1988; **167**: 389.

61. de Dombal FT, Morgan AG, Staniland JR & Ohmann C. Clinical features – computer analysis. In Dykes PW & Keighley MRB (eds) *Gastrointestinal Haemorrhage*. Bristol: Wright, 1981: 155.

62. Snook JA, Holdstock GE & Banforth J. Value of a simple biochemical ratio in distinguishing upper and lower sites of gastrointestinal haemorrhage. *Lancet* 1986; **i**: 1064.

63. Felber S, Rosenthal P & Henton D. The BUN/creatinine ratio in localizing gastrointestinal bleeding in paediatric patients. *J Pediatr Gastroenterol Nutr* 1988; **7**: 685.

64. Gordon R, Herlinger H & Baum S. Arteriography and scintiscanning. In Dykes PW & Keighley MRB (eds) *Gastrointestinal Haemorrhage*. Bristol: Wright, 1981: 209.

65. Rees CR, Palmaz JC, Alvarado R, Tyrrell R, Ciarvino V & Register T. DSA in acute gastrointestinal haemorrhage – clinical and in vitro studies. *Radiology* 1988; **169**: 499.

66. Annual Scientific Meeting: Gastroenterological Society of Australia. 'GI bleeding' workshop. *Aust N Z J Med* 1986; **16**: (Suppl. 3): 591.

67. Devitt JE, Brown FN & Beattie WG. Fatal bleeding ulcer. *Ann Surg* 1966; **164**: 840.

68. Logan RFA & Finlayson NDC. Death in acute upper gastrointestinal bleeding. Can endoscopy reduce mortality? *Lancet* 1976; **i**: 1173.

69. Allan RN & Dykes PW. A study of the factors influencing mortality rates from gastrointestinal haemorrhage. *Q J Med* 1976; **54**: 533.

70. Madden MV & Griffith GH. Management of upper gastrointestinal bleeding in a district general hospital. *J R Coll Physicians Lond* 1986; **20**: 212.

71. Morgan AG & Clamp SE. OMGE international upper gastrointestinal bleeding survey, 1978–1986. *Scand J Gastroenterol Suppl* 1988; **144**: 51.

72. Clason AE, Macleod DAD & Elton RA. Clinical factors in the prediction of further haemorrhage or mortality in acute upper gastrointestinal haemorrhage. *Br J Surg* 1986; **73**: 985.

73. Brearley S, Hawker PC, Morris DL, Dykes PW & Keighley MRB. Selection of patients for surgery following peptic ulcer haemorrhage. *Br J Surg* 1987; **74**: 893.

74. Clamp SE, Morgan AG, Kotwol MR et al. Use of a multi-centre survey to provide clinical guidelines for upper gastrointestinal bleeding in developing countries. *Scand J Gastroenterol Suppl* 1988; **144**: 63.

75. Chinn AB, Littell AS, Badger GF & Beams AJ. Acute haemorrhage from peptic ulcer. A follow-up study of 310 patients. *N Engl J Med* 1956; **255**: 973.

76. Harvey RF & Langman MJS. The late results of medical and surgical treatment for bleeding duodenal ulcer. *Q J Med* 1970; **156**: 539.

77. Duggan JM. Ten year follow up of gastrointestinal haemorrhage patients. *Aust N Z J Med* 1986; **16**: 33.

78. Smart HL & Langman MJS. Late outcome of bleeding gastric ulcers. *Gut* 1986; **27**: 926.

79. Tanner NC & Desmond AM. The surgical treatment of haematemesis and melaena. *Postgrad Med J* 1950; **26**: 253.

80. Hunt PS, Hanskey J & Korman MG. Mortality in patients with haematemesis and melaena: a prospective trial. *BMJ* 1979; **1**: 1238.

81. Sanderson JD, Taylor RFH, Pugh S & Vicary FR. Specialized gastrointestinal units for the management of upper gastrointestinal haemorrhage. *Postgrad Med J* 1990; **66**: 654.

82. Blair SD, Javrin SB, McCollum CN & Greenhalgh RM. Effect of early blood transfusion on gastrointestinal haemorhage. *Br J Surg* 1986; **73**: 783.

83. Collins R & Langman MJS. Treatment with histamine H₂ antagonists in acute upper gastrointestinal haemorrhage. Implications of randomised trials. *N Engl J Med* 1985; **313**: 660.

84. Merki HS, Witzel L, Kaufman D et al. Continuous intravenous infusions of famotidine maintain high intragastric pH in duodenal ulcer. *Gut* 1988; **29**: 453.

85. Daneshmend TK, Hawkey CJ, Langman MJS, Logan RFA, Long RG & Walt RP. Omeprazole versus placebo for acute upper gastrointestinal bleeding: randomised double-blind controlled trial. *BMJ* 1992; **304**: 143.

86. Christiansen J, Ottenjann R & Von Arx F. Placebo-controlled trial with the somatostatin analogue SMS 201–995 in peptic ulcer bleeding. *Gastroenterology* 1989; **97**: 568.

87. Henry DA & O'Connell DL. Effects of fibrinolytic inhibitors on mortality from upper gastrointestinal haemorrhage. *BMJ* 1989; **298**: 1142.

88. Forrest JAH, Finlayson NDC & Shearman DJC. Endoscopy in gastrointestinal bleeding. *Lancet* 1974; **ii**: 394.

89. Laurence BH, Vallon AG, Cotton PB et al. Endoscopic laser photocoagulation for bleeding peptic ulcers. *Lancet* 1980; **i**: 124.

90. Vallon AG, Cotton PB, Laurence BH, Miro JRA & Oses JCS. Randomised trial of endoscopic argon laser photocoagulation in bleeding peptic ulcer. *Gut* 1981; **22**: 228.

91. Swain CP, Bown SG, Storey DW, Kirkham JS, Northfield TC & Salmon PR. Controlled trial of argon laser photoccoagulation in bleeding peptic ulcer. *Lancet* 1981; **ii**: 1313.

92. Krejs GJ, Little KH, Westergaard H, Hamilton JK, Spady DK & Polter DE. Laser photocoagulation for the treatment of acute peptic ulcer bleeding. *N Engl J Med* 1987; **316**: 1618.

93. Rutgeerts P, Vantrappen G, Broeckaert L et al. Controlled trial of YAG laser treatment of upper digestive haemorrhage. *Gastroenterology* 1982; **83**: 410.

94. Swain CP, Kirkham JS, Salmon PR, Bown SG & Northfield TC. Controlled trial of Nd YAG laser photocoagulation in bleeding peptic ulcers. *Lancet* 1986; **i**: 1113.

95. Macleod IA, Mills PR, Mackenzie JF, Joffe SN, Russell RI & Carter DC. Neodymium yttrium aluminium garnet laser photocoagulation for major haemorrhage from peptic ulcer and single vessels: a single blind controlled study. *BMJ* 1983; **286**: 345.

96. Fullarton GM, Birnie GG, Macdonald A & Murray WR. Controlled trial of heater probe treatment in bleeding peptic ulcers. *Br J Surg* 1989; **76**: 541.

97. Matthewson K, Swain CP, Bland M, Kirkham JS, Bown SG & Northfield TC. Randomised comparison of Nd YAG laser, heater probe and no endoscopic therapy for bleeding peptic ulcer. *Gastroenterology* 1990; **98**: 1239.

98. Lin HJ, Lee FY, Kang WM, Tsai YT, Lee SD & Lee CH. Heat probe thermocoagulation and pure alcohol injection in massive peptic ulcer haemorrhage: a prospective, randomised controlled trial. *Gut* 1990; **31**: 753.

99. Goudie BM, Mitchell KG, Birnie GG & Mackay C. Controlled trial of endoscopic bipolar electrocoagulation in the treatment of bleeding peptic ulcers. *Gut* 1984; **25**: A1185.

100. Kernohan RM, Anderson JR, McKelvey STD & Kennedy TL. A controlled trial of bipolar electrocoagulation in patients with upper gastrointestinal bleeding. *Br J Surg* 1984; **71**: 889.

101. Laine L. Multipolar electrocoagulation in the treatment of ulcers with non-bleeding visible vessels: a prospective controlled trial. *Gut* 1987; **28**: A1342.

102. O'Brien JD, Day SJ & Burnham WR. Controlled trial of small bipolar probe in bleeding peptic ulcers. *Lancet* 1985; **i**: 464.

103. Brearley S, Hawker PC, Dykes PW & Keighley MRB. Perendoscopic bipolar diathermy coagulation of visible vessels uing a 3.2 mm probe: a randomised trial. *Endoscopy* 1987; **19**: 160.

104. Laine L. Multipolar electrocoagulation in the treatment of active upper gastrointestinal tract haemorrhage: a prospective controlled trial. *N Engl J Med* 1987; **26**: 1613.

105. Goff JS. Bipolar electrocoagulation versus Nd-YAG laser photocoagulation for upper gastrointestinal bleeding lesions. *Dig Dis Sci* 1986; **31**: 906.

106. Rutgeerts P, Vantrappen G, Van Hootgem PH et al. Neodymium YAG laser photocoagulation versus multipolar electrocoagulation for the treatment of severely bleeding ulcers: a randomized comparison. *Gastrointest Endosc* 1987; **33**: 199.

107. Panes J, Viver M, Forne E, Garcia EO, Marco C & Garau J. Controlled trial of endoscopic sclerosis in bleeding peptic ulcers. *Lancet* 1987; **ii**: 1292.

108. Balanzo J, Salnz S, Such J et al. Endoscopic hemostasis by local injection of epinephrine and volidocanol in bleeding ulcer. A prospective randomised trial. *Endoscopy* 1988; **20**: 289.

109. Chung SCS, Leung JWC, Steele RJC, Crofts TJ & Li AJC. Endoscopic adrenaline injection for actively bleeding ulcers: a randomised trial. *BMJ* 1988; **296**: 1631.

110. Rutgeerts P, Vantrappen G, Broeckaert L, Coremans G, Janssans J & Hiele M. Companion of endoscopic polidocanol injection and YAG Laser therapy for bleeding peptic ulcers. *Lancet* 1989; **i**: 1164.

111. Cook DJ, Guyatt GH, Salena BJ & Laine LA. Endoscopic therapy for acute momvariceal upper gastrointestinal hemorrhage: a meta-analysis. Gastroenterology 1992; **102**: 139.

112. Schiller KFR, Truelove SC & Williams DG. Haematemesis and melaena with special reference to factors influencing the outcome. *BMJ* 1970; **2**: 7.

113. Gatehouse D, Dimock F, Burdon DW et al. Prediction of wound sepsis following gastric operations. *Br J Surg* 1978; **65**: 551.

114. Kakkar VV, Corrigan TP, Fossard DP et al. Prevention of fatal pulmonary embolism by low doses of heparin. An international multicentre trial. *Lancet* 1975; **ii**: 7924.

115. Stringer MD & Cameron AEP. Surgeons' attitudes to the operative management of duodenal ulcer perforation and haemorrhage. *Ann R Coll Surg Engl* 1988; **70**: 220.

116. Herrington JL & Davidson JR III. Bleeding gastroduodenal ulcers: choice of operations. *World J Surg* 1987; **11**: 304.

117. Johnston D, Lyndon PJ, Smith RB & Humphrey CS. Highly selective vagotomy without a drainage procedure in the treatment of haemorrhage, perforation and pyloric stenosis due to peptic ulcer. *Br J Surg* 1973; **60**: 790.

118. Hoak BA, Tiley E, Kusminsky R & Boland JP. Parietal cell vagotomy for bleeding duodenal ulcers. *Am Surg* 1988; **54**: 249.

119. Foster JH, Hickok DF & Dunphy JE. Factors influencing mortality following emergency operation for massive upper gastrointestinal hemorrhage. *Surg Gynecol Obstet* 1963; **117**: 257.

120. Johnston D. Division and repair of the sphincteric mechanism at the gastric outlet in emergency operations for bleeding peptic ulcer. *Ann Surg* 1977; **186**: 723.

121. Ovaska JT & Havia T. Surgical treatment of high gastric ulcer. *Ann Chir Gynaecol* 1988; **77**: 6.

122. Rogers PN, Murray WR, Shaw R & Brar S. Surgical management of bleeding gastric ulceration. *Br J Surg* 1988; **75**: 16.

123. Johnston D. Duodenal and gastric ulcer. In Schwartz BI & Ellis H (eds) *Maingot's Abdominal Operations*. New York: Appleton-Century-Crofts, 1985: 767.

124. Cheung LY. Treatment of established stress ulcer disease. *World J Surg* 1981; **5**: 235.

125. Shuman RB, Schuster DP & Zuckerman GR. Prophylactic therapy for stress ulcer bleeding: a reappraisal. *Ann Intern Med* 1987; **106**: 562.

126. Biggs JC, Hugh TB & Dodds AJ. Tranexamic acid and upper gastrointestinal haemorrhage – a double blind trial. *Gut* 1976; **17**: 729.

127. Hubert JP, Kiernan PD, Welch JB, ReMine WH & Bears OH. The surgical management of bleeding stress ulcers. *Ann Surg* 1980; **191**: 672.

128. Veldhuyzen van Zantan SJO, Bartelsman JFMW, Schipper MEI & Tytgat GNJ. Recurrent massive haematemsis from Dieulafoy vascular malformations – a review of 101 cases. *Gut* 1986; **27**: 213.

129. Dronfield MW, Atkinson M & Langman MJS. Effect of different operation policies on mortality from bleeding peptic ulcer. *Lancet* 1979; **i**: 1126.

130. Vellacott KD, Dronfield MW, Atkinson M & Langman MJS. Comparison of surgical and medical management of bleeding peptic ulcers. *BMJ* 1982; **284**: 548.

131. Hunt PS. Bleeding gastroduodenal ulcers: selection of patients for surgery. *World J Surg* 1987; **11**: 289.

132. Clements D, Aslan S, Foster D, Stamatakis J, Wilkins WE & Morris JS. Acute upper gastrointestinal haemorrhage in a district general hospital: audit of an agreed management policy. *J R Coll Physicians Lond* 1991; **25**: 27.

39

THE STOMACH IN PORTAL HYPERTENSION

AG Johnson

The underlying causes of portal hypertension are discussed in the oesophageal section (Table 39.1 and see p. 264). Here we are concerned with the features of portal hypertension that show in the stomach; these are gastric varices and portal hypertensive gastropathy, although clinicians must always remember that straightforward chronic peptic gastric ulcers can also occur in patients with portal hypertension.

Table 39.1 Classification of causes of portal hypertension

A	Presinusoidal	
	I Extrahepatic obstruction	
	(a) Intrinsic thrombosis	– neonatal sepsis
		– pyelophlebitis
		– increased coagulability
	(b) Extrinsic compression	– pancreatic tumour
		– pancreatitis
		– enlarged lymph nodes
	II Intraphepatic	– schistosomiasis
		– congenital hepatic fibrosis
		– sarcoidosis
		– reticuloendothelial disease
		– early stages of primary biliary cirrhosis
B	Intrahepatic	– mainly cirrhosis, e.g. alcohol, viral, haemochromatosis, chemical poisons, idiopathic
C	Postsinusoidal	– obstruction of hepatic veins or inferior vena cava (Budd–Chiari syndrome)
D	Increased portal flow	– AV fistula
		– increased hepatic flow

GASTRIC VARICES

Gastric varices occur mainly in the upper half of the stomach and may or may not be associated with oesophageal varices. They only give symptoms if they impinge on the mucosa and then bleed. The mere presence of varices does not appear to affect gastric function. They are a far less frequent site of bleeding than oesophageal varices (5 versus 77%; see p. 266)

and are covered by a glandular rather than a squamous mucosa.

Classification

We have proposed a classification based on approach to treatment as well as anatomy:[1]

Type I High, usually lesser curve varices which are an inferior extension of oesophageal varices across the squamo-columnar junction. They are treated by sclerotherapy.

Type II Gastric varices in the fundus associated with oesophageal varices. They can coexist with type I varices but do not respond well to sclerotherapy with standard agents. If they bleed they should be treated by undersewing, shunt or devascularization.

Type III Gastric varices in the fundus and body, in the absence of oesophageal varices, which are usually the result of segmented portal hypertension due to splenic vein thrombosis. The blood bypasses the block via the gastric vessels to reach the portal vein (see Figure 17.1). Splenectomy is usually curative, with under-running if there is active bleeding.

Does sclerotherapy of oesophageal varices cause or enlarge gastric varices?

In our experience, the appearance of type II varices is independent of the injection of oesophageal varices. They disappear in some and appear in others. Type I varices appeared in 20 of 208 patients, from 1 week to 3 years after starting a sclerotherapy programme. Whether this is cause and effect or merely the progression of the portal hypertension is difficult to determine, but the relationship of the injections to the lowest perforating vein may be important (see p. 271): if the oesophageal vein is thrombosed just above the perforator then the flow may be diverted retrogradely down the lesser curve. By contrast, retrograde thrombosis from the oesophagus of type I gastric varices has been well documented.

Diagnosis

The endoscopic diagnosis of gastric varices is more difficult than that of oesophageal varices, particularly when the fundus is full of blood clot. The diagnosis may have to be made by exclusion if the oesophagus, body and antrum of the stomach and duodenum are all seen not to be the site of bleeding. Gastropathy (see below) gives diffuse oozing and the crater of a gastric ulcer is usually identifiable. Blood spurting from an apparently intact mucosa is characteristic of gastric variceal bleeding, even if the underlying vein cannot be seen.

When they are not bleeding, gastric varices can also be difficult to identify when the rugal folds are prominent. Varices often run across the direction of the rugae and do not flatten during moderate distension of the stomach with air, when the bluish colour becomes more obvious (see Figure 17.2). In a study on observer variation[2] there was good agreement between observers on the presence or absence of gastric varices, but other authors have found poor correlation, especially if grading is taken into account. Angiography may be used both to identify the presence of gastric varices and to distinguish type III varices, which need a different surgical approach.

Management of bleeding gastric varices

There is no indication to treat gastric varices that have not bled, but about 60% will bleed eventually on long-term follow-up if further serious oesophageal bleeding is prevented.

Tamponade

A Linton balloon or the gastric balloon of a Sengstaken–Blakemore tube, distended with 400 ml of air and put on traction, can be used to compress bleeding varices, particularly if they are around the cardia. However, it is very difficult to exert any effective pressure against the distensible gastric fundus.

Drugs

Drugs such as metoclopramide, which are effective in stopping the bleeding from oesophageal varices by constricting the lower oesophageal sphincter, will not be effective for gastric varices. It is not known whether somatostatin is effective for gastric varices. The first line treatment for temporary control of gastric varices is vasopressin plus glyceryl trinitrate.

Sclerotherapy

A prospective randomised trial has shown that 50% glucose water controls bleeding as well as tetradecyl sulphate (92% v 80%) and has a significantly lower rate of rebleeding (30% v 70%) and gastric ulcers (30% v 92%). The mortality was the same and it now needs to be compared with cyanoacrylate.[3]

Emergency surgery

If bleeding is not quickly controlled, operation is indicated before further blood loss puts the patient's hepatic and renal function at risk. A devascularization or portacaval shunt may be performed but in both cases the bleeding varix must be undersewn to control the immediate haemorrhage.

Prevention of rebleeding

There is little evidence that beta blockers taken continuously reduce rebleeding of gastric varices as opposed to gastropathy or oesophageal varices.

Surgery as an elective procedure after the bleeding is controlled is the surest method. Either devascularization or a shunt is required for type II varices, depending on the state of the liver, a shunt being contraindicated in the elderly or in those of Child's grade C. A preoperation doppler ultrascans or venogram is advisable to confirm the state of the portal and splenic veins.

End-to-side or side-to-side portacaval shunts are the simplest procedures to perform technically. They are extremely effective at preventing rebleeding but are complicated by a significant incidence of hepatic encephalopathy. Selective shunts have a lower encephalopathy but a higher rebleeding rate.

CONGESTIVE GASTROPATHY

For many years changes in the gastric mucosa were observed in patients with cirrhosis and portal hypertension, but because most of the patients had alcohol-related disease it was assumed that there was an 'inflammatory gastritis' due to alcohol. When similar changes were also seen in patients with non-alcoholic portal hypertension and biopsies showed dilatation of vessels and congestion rather than inflammatory gastritis, the condition was renamed *congestive gastropathy*[4] or, more recently, *vasculopathy*.[5]

Incidence

In early endoscopic observations it was noted that nearly half the bleeding episodes of cirrhotic patients admitted to a liver unit were not from varices but from 'gastritis'.[6] In the Sheffield patients who were being followed up after sclerotherapy for their first bleed from oesophageal varices 35% of the subsequent bleeds were from gastropathy (Table 39.2). The steady diffuse oozing from the gastric mucosa may be just as life threatening as intermittent brisk bleeding from varices.

Diagnosis

The diagnosis can only be made by endoscopy and biopsy. The appearances are classified as mild or severe.

Table 39.2 Source of gastrointestinal bleeding on first presentation and subsequent episodes (over 4 years)

SITE	PRESENTING BLEEDS	SUBSEQUENT BLEEDS
Oesophageal varices	88(77.2)	64(31.5)
Gastric varices	6(5.3)	11(5.4)
Gastropathy	9(7.9)	71(35.0)
Peptic ulcer	4(3.5)	3(1.5)
Postinjection slough	—	16(7.9)
Rectal varices	3(2.6)	2(1.0)
Others	4(3.5)	36(17.7)
Total	114(100)	203(100)

Values in parentheses are percentages.

Mild changes

- Fine pink speckling.
- Superficial reddening.
- A reticular or mosaic pattern with red patches bordered by pale lines (snake skin).

This last appearance is characteristic of portal hypertension, whereas the other two are less specific and only biopsy can distinguish between inflammatory gastritis and congestive gastropathy. Mosaic (snake skin) pattern (Figure 39.1) was found in 94% of 100 patients with cirrhosis and portal hypertension but in only 0.3% of 300 controls; however, observer variation in identifying this pattern is quite marked. These 'mild' changes do not, however, give rise to bleeding.

Severe changes

- Discrete cherry-red spots
- Confluent superficial vascular dilatation (often with diffuse oozing from the surface).

These changes are associated with a high risk of serious haemorrhage. The lesions are usually in the body and fundus but sometimes the whole stomach may be affected.

Association of gastropathy with other lesions

Gastropathy may coexist with oesophageal and/or gastric varices or may be independent of both. It also occurs in noncirrhotic portal hypertension but is very rare after a successful portal – systemic shunt operation. There is no evidence that oesophageal variceal sclerotherapy makes it worse, but any development is more likely to be due to the progression of the portal hypertension. It represents portal hypertension affecting the submucosal and intramucosal vessels.

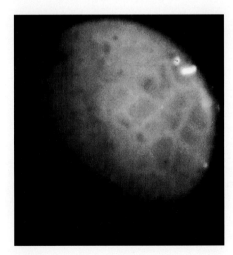

Figure 39.1
Endoscopic view of severe congestive gastropathy showing discrete cherry-red spots on a background of mosaic (snake skin) pattern.

It must not be forgotten that peptic gastric ulcers and mucosal erosion from non-steroidal anti-inflammatory drugs can occur in patients with portal hypertension as in others.

Treatment

As it is not an inflammatory or acid-related gastritis, antacids, H_2-receptor blockers and similar drugs are ineffective. When there is acute bleeding, neither sclerotherapy nor balloon tamponade is appropriate because of the large area involved.

Beta blockers

There is good evidence that beta blockers can not only control bleeding[7] but also improve the appearances and prevent haemorrhage.[8]

Surgery

If drugs should fail, shunt surgery can be life saving; for acute bleeding most surgeons would favour an end-to-side portacaval shunt. Devascularization operations do not necessarily stop bleeding or cure the gastropathy.

IN CONCLUSION

Gastric varices are a rare but important site of haemorrhage in patients with portal hypertension. The diagnosis may be difficult but urgent effective treatment is essential and occasionally this must be major surgery. To procrastinate by attempting repeatedly to inject large spurting fundal varices is to court disaster. Diffuse gastropathy, on the other hand, nearly always responds to beta blockers, which should be taken to prevent further trouble in the long term. It is important that this condition is appreciated and diagnosed by endoscopy as it is becoming increasingly common because more patients survive their first oesophageal bleed and have a fairly good prognosis. More research on the pathophysiology of gastropathy and new drug treatments is urgently needed.

REFERENCES

1. Hosking SW & Johnson AG. Gastric varices: a proposed classification leading to management. *Br J Surg* 1988; **75**: 195.
2. Calès P, Zabatto B, Meskens C et al. Gastroesophageal endoscopic features in cirrhosis. Observer variability, interassociations, and relationship to hepatic dysfunction. *Gastroenterology* 1990; **98**: 156.
3. Chang KY, Wu CS & Chen PC. Prospective, randomised trial of hypertonic glucose water and sodium tetradecyl sulphate for gastric variceal bleeding in patients with advanced liver cirrhosis. *Endoscopy* 1996; **28**: 481.
4. McCormack TT, Sims I, Eyre-Brook IA et al. Gastric lesions in portal hypertension: inflammatory gastritis or congestive gastropathy? *Gut* 1985; **26**: 1226.
5. Sarfeh IJ & Tarnawski A. Gastric mucosal vasculopathy in portal hypertension. *Gastroenterology* 1987; **93**: 1129.
6. Waldram R, Davis M, Minnerly H et al. Emergency endoscopy of the gastrointestinal haemorrhage in 50 patients with portal hypertension. *BMJ* 1984; **4**: 194.
7. Hosking SW, Kennedy HJ, Seddon I et al. The role of propranolol in congestive gastropathy of portal hypertension. *Hepatology* 1987; **7**: 437.
8. Lebrec D, Poynard T, Bernnan J et al. A randomised controlled study of propranolol for prevention of recurrent gastrointestinal bleeding in patients with cirrhosis: a final report. *Hepatology* 1984; **4**:355.

40

SURGERY FOR OBESITY

RA Forse
LD MacLean

INTRODUCTION

The evidence is now overwhelming that obesity, defined as excessive storage of energy in the form of fat, has adverse effects on health and longevity. This conclusion of the National Institutes of Health Consensus Panel on the Health Implications of Obesity in the USA is supported by data which associate obesity with hypertension, hypercholesterolaemia, non-insulin dependent diabetes mellitus and an excess mortality from cancers of the colorectum, prostate, endometrium, gall bladder, cervix, ovary and breast.[1] About 34 million adult Americans are overweight, that is with a body mass index (weight (kg)/height (m^2)) greater than 28 which approximates a level of 20% above normal weight. Put another way, 26% of Americans aged 20–75 years are overweight,[2] and there is an estimate that six million Americans suffer from life-threatening morbid obesity.[3]

Depending on the criteria used, studies on the prevalence of obesity in children indicate that between 5 and 25% of children in North America from preschool age through to adolescence are overweight. Finally, 80% of obese children become obese adults. In addition, if an obese child has not reduced to a healthy body weight by the end of adolescence, the odds against his or her doing so as an adult are 28:1.[4] Patients with their onset of obesity in infancy have a lower tolerance for fasting than those who become obese later in life.[5] Similar risks and incidence of obesity are reported from other regions of the world, and these studies conclude that obesity and its related disease lower life expectancy.[6]

Conclusions from the Framingham study are that overweight, non-smoking men and women have mortality rates that are 3.9 times higher than those of non-smokers who have a desirable weight (100–109%). This study did not indicate that there is a 'safe' level of overweight, or that weight gain in middle age is healthy or that desirable weights increase with age.[7] Most data on the risks of obesity relate to life expectancy, but of equal importance is the absence of illness or a healthy existence, including good psychosocial adjustment, in patients who were never obese or who lost and maintained weight to a normal level. Obesity that increases weight over twice normal

(morbid obesity) accelerates the incidence and severity of the known risks of obesity – diabetes mellitus, hypertension, asthma, sleep apnoea, hyperlipidaemia, and coronary heart disease – and adds several risks encountered especially in this group of very obese individuals (Table 40.1). The present recommendations are that these patients be referred to as clinically severe or significant obesity rather then using the pejorative term morbid.

Data on risks of mortality in clinically significant obesity are not readily available because these individuals are usually not accepted for life insurance and therefore do not enter actuarial assessments. One study of this group of patients widely reported in the surgical literature is that of Drenick et al.[8] They followed 200 men for a mean of 7.6 years, most of whom were at least twice normal weight. The mortality rate over that period was judged to be 12 times that expected in normal weight men of the same age (25–34 years) in the general population. In fact, 50 of the 200 patients died during the follow-up period. Cardiovascular disease was the most common cause

Table 40.1 Special risks associated with morbid obesity

Cardiorespiratory
  Hypervolaemia
  Increased left ventricular filling pressure
  Hypoventilation syndrome
  Cor pulmonale
  Sleep apnoea syndrome
Osteoarthritis of weight-bearing joints
Gout
Psychosocial incapacity
Operation risks
  Anaesthesia and operation risk increase
  Impaired pulmonary function
  Increased risk of wound
    infection; wound dehiscence; late hernia formation
Abnormalities of liver function
Venous stasis of lower extremities
  Stasis ulcers
  Thromboembolism

of death in the obese patients, almost 30% higher than for American men as a whole. Accidental deaths were also higher in the obese. In one study of middle age women, body weight and mortality from all causes were directly related. The study indicated that lean women did not have excess mortality and that the lowest mortality was observed in women 15% the current average American women's weight.[9]

The economics of the care of patients with obesity is not insignificant as it should include the cost of the associated morbidity. A conservative estimate was set at 39.3 billion dollars for 1986 or 5.5% of the cost of illness.[10]

As emphasized by Van Itallie,[11] it is quite clear that conventional, non-operative treatments (a low-calorie, balanced diet, anorectic drugs, behavioural therapy and exercise) have little or nothing to offer the patient with clinically significant obesity. This is the case even though with severe fasting large amounts of weight can be lost often with dramatic and impressive health and social benefits. These same patients almost invariably regain the weight after concluding the period of severe fasting.

Currently there is a growing experience with drugs to control obesity. There are several classes of drugs that are being used, which can be categorized as follows. The centrally active catecholaminergic agents, the centrally active serotoninergic agents, drugs affecting absorption and combined adrenergic and serotonergic agents. Currently there are limitations set on the type and the duration that patients can be exposed to these drugs. The other problems are that the average weight loss with the agents is only 30–40 pounds (13–18 kg), although there has been a great deal of experience with the clinically significantly obese, and that there is a high rate of weight regain when the patients come off the medications.[12,13] In addition, there is concern about pulmonary hypertension, a complication that is rare but could be more of an issue in clinically significantly obese patients who have a history of having a higher incidence of pulmonary hypertension. Much more work will have to be done with these agents before their role in the overall therapy of the clinically significantly obese patient is known.

It follows and one can conclude that surgery for clinically significant obesity is based on the dual premise that this degree of obesity is not amenable to non-surgical treatments and is hazardous to the health of the individual. Most but not all students of the problem agree.[5,14,15] The question that remains is: Can surgery improve the prognosis of these very obese patients? In order to compare results and to determine the relative efficacy of treatments, readily available and inexpensive acceptable criteria must be used to quantitate the degree of obesity in individual patients and in populations of obese patients.

HOW TO QUANTITATE OBESITY

Apart from the technique of densitometry, which is a measurement used in research, five measures are in common use to assess the degree of obesity and thereby the degree of risk. All have demonstrated epidemiological support related to morbidity and mortality for both men and women in all age groups.[16]

1. Height and weight tables are most widely used but have the disadvantage of lacking a measure for body frame;

2. Skin-fold measurements are not suitably reliable and do not document the distribution of obesity.

3. The ratio of the waist circumference to hip circumference (WHR) is strongly associated with risk factors and can be measured more reliably than skin-fold thickness.[17,18] The specific WHR values recommended by Bjorntorp[17] are 1.0 for men and 0.8 for women. There is increasing health risk with increased WHR values but at this time no scale of measurement showing increased probability of health problems with increasing WHR ratios is available. The other problem is the ability to determine accurately the waist in the patient with clinically significant obesity.

4. Circumferences other than waist and hip, e.g. arm or leg circumferences, have been measured, but few population studies are available relating these measures independently to morbidity or mortality.

5. The body mass index (BMI) (weight (kg)/height (m²) is highly correlated with body fat,[19] is easily measured and is a valid measure of weight in relation to health.

Many studies now show that a BMI greater than 27 is associated with an increased occurrence of hypertension, hyperlipidaemia, diabetes, cancers of the endometrium, breast and colon and coronary heart disease.[16] The mortality rate increases as BMI increases from normal levels of 20–25 to 40, which is morbid obesity (Figure 40.1). A BMI of 20–25 has the lowest risk. A BMI <20 and between 25 and 30 has a low risk; from 30 to 40 moderate risk and >40 high risk. A BMI of 25–30 is termed by Garrow[15] as grade I obesity, 30–40 is grade II obesity, and >40 is grade III obesity (morbid obesity).

In the UK, the proportion of men aged 16–64 years in grade I, II and III is 34%, 6% and 0.1%. The corresponding figures for women are 24%, 8% and 0.3%. Reports from other European countries, Australia, Canada and the USA indicate a similar prevalence of obesity. The more severe grades of obesity are more commonly encountered in women. Few data are available for the group of patients being considered for surgery

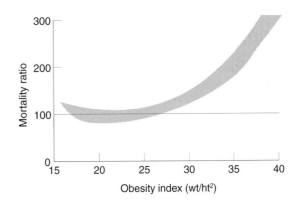

Figure 40.1

Relation of obesity index (wt/ht²) to mortality ratio. Average mortality = 100. (Data of Seltzer.[20] Reproduced with permission from Garrow.[15])

(morbid or superobesity) because of their inability to obtain life insurance. We define morbid obesity or medically significant obesity as a BMI of 40–50. Patients with a body mass index greater than 50 are classed as superobese.

The WHR should be added to the BMI as a more sensitive indicator of health risk and thereby could be a useful measure to subdivide obese people into high and possibly lower risk groups. These measures are useful to assess patients after surgery to document the degree of obesity and incumbent risks that persist after this radical form of therapy. It is now well established that the distribution of adipose tissue is of prognostic importance. Excess body fat in the lower trunk or abdominal area – the android distribution – is associated with increased risk particularly for stroke, myocardial infarction and diabetes in both men[20,21] and women.[20,22] Furthermore, this phenotype has a strong genetic basis. The site of fat distribution is largely determined by genotype.[23]

There is evidence that an accurate assessment of the distribution of body fat is a computed tomography (CT) scan with a single abdominal cut at the lumbar 4 level. This will provide a measure of the subcutaneous versus the central fat distribution, a relationship that appears to have a significant bearing on obesity-related morbidity. The problem with this assessment is the cost and the fact that many CT scan tables will not accommodate morbidly obese patients.

There is evidence that patients who were obese and who subsequently reduced to normal weight and maintained that weight thereafter enjoyed normal life expectancy.[24]

AETIOLOGY

Obesity is an excess of storage of energy as adipose tissue and always results from an imbalance of food intake and caloric expenditure. Most people, whether lean or obese, remain at the same weight for long periods which indicates that there is no change in their stored energy. Therefore, the energy content of the food ingested is in balance with their energy expenditure and this is referred to as their set point. This is accomplished by most of us without an awareness of controlling caloric intake or physical activity.

Since high energy content of stored fat is the identifying feature of obesity and since food intake is controllable, it is often mistakenly assumed that obesity is a disorder of food intake, pure and simple.[25] Although it is true that obese people have eaten more than they require, the eating behaviour of the great majority of obese people is not systematically different from that of the great majority of normal weight people. It is also true that obese people do not have a more efficient system for absorption of foodstuffs.[26]

Metabolic rate

Evidence is now accumulating that the metabolic rate at rest may be lower in individuals predisposed to obesity and that this trait may be inherited. One convincing investigation by Ravussin et al.[27] studied the energy expenditure among Southwestern American Indians (the Pima), a population

prone to obesity. The metabolic rate at rest was measured with a ventilated-hood indirect calorimeter,[28] and energy expenditure was calculated from the rates of oxygen consumption and carbon dioxide production. Energy expenditure correlated in a prospective fashion with the rate of change in body weight over a 2-year follow-up period. The risk of gaining more than 7.5 kg in body weight was increased fourfold in persons with a low 24-hour energy expenditure as compared with persons with a high 24-hour expenditure. This low energy expenditure, which led to abnormal weight gain, had a strong familial bias.

This agrees with the observation by Fontaine et al.[29] who showed in monozygotic and dizygotic twins that the metabolic rate at rest was determined by genetic background. Monozygotic twins, regardless of environment after birth, develop obesity at a similar rate. If one monozygotic twin becomes obese, the other is very likely to do so also even though they have been separated and are in different environments. Monozygotic twins who have been given a larger caloric intake than normal over a three-month period may gain weight or remain stable, but each twin behaves the same in terms of weight change.

Bouchard[30] measured resting metabolic rate (RMR), the thermic effect of food intake (TFM) and the energy cost of submaximal energy expenditure (TEE) to see if an inherited predisposition to obesity was related to expenditure and if this was genetically determined. These variables were measured in parent–child pairs, dizygotic and monozygotic twins. Genotype accounted for a highly significant fraction (equal to or greater than 40%) of the individual differences in RMR, TFM and TEE.

A Danish study examined the weight of adopted, as compared with full biological siblings and with half-siblings, raised in different environments. If the adoptees were obese, the full siblings living elsewhere were very likely to be obese also, as measured by an elevated body mass index. There was a similar but weaker relation between adoptees and their half-siblings.[31] No correlation existed between the degree of obesity of adoptees and non-biological siblings.

Energy expenditure at rest and over a period of 24 hours are both known to vary considerably from person to person and is directly related to body size. However, even after adjustment for differences in body size and composition, age and sex, the variability in energy expenditure is larger than can be accounted for by methodological errors or by day-to-day individual variations.[28,32] This implies that subjects with similar physical characteristics can require more or less energy to maintain their body weights, and can, therefore, be more or less 'energy efficient'. It follows that more 'energy efficient' individuals would have a predisposition to obesity.

After weight gain, the new adjusted metabolic rate in the affected patients was similar in the study by Ravussin et al.[27] to that measured in the subjects who were of normal weight. Weight gain is a compensatory mechanism that results in increased energy expenditure, perhaps because of a requirement for a larger body cell mass to carry the increased load inherent in the gain in weight.

Genetic influences

There is still further evidence linking obesity to decreased energy expenditure and in turn to a genetic predisposition. Roberts et al.[33] documented in a prospective study the contributions of low energy expenditure and high energy intake to excessive weight gain in infants born to overweight mothers. They used a new doubly labelled water technique to determine energy expenditure and metabolizable energy intake.[34] Of the babies of obese mothers 50% became obese by one year. At three months, when the infants of overweight and lean mothers were indistinguishable in regard to body mass index and skinfold thickness, there had already occurred a marked decrease in the total energy expenditure of the infants who later became overweight. In fact, the energy expenditure at three months of age was 21% lower in the infants who later became obese.

There is probably genomic control of thermogenesis, and certain populations such as the Pima Indians of southwestern USA in whom a high incidence of obesity exists, required a genetic make-up that preserved calories in order to survive times of famine known to have existed in their environment from 1880 to the 1930s.[25] Hirsch and Leibel[25] speculate that the genetic make-up of the survivors is now a detriment to survival in an environment which provides food in abundance. It is also likely that genetic predisposition to obesity is not likely to respond to usual treatments aimed at dietary regulation and behaviour modification.

A more recent breakthrough has been the discovery of an obese gene and its protein product leptin. The gene is expressed in adipose tissue where the leptin is released in response to the metabolic state of the adipocyte.[35] There are leptin receptors in the brain including the hypothalamus, which are active and help to control the appetite centre.[36] Low levels of circulating leptin and/or a decreased response of the leptin receptor to leptin results in obesity in animals. The exact role and relationship of this gene and its product to human obesity is still under investigation. At present it appears that in humans in a similar fashion, leptin is produced by the adipocyte and regulates the appetite centre. Human obesity, however, is still thought to be multifactorial and as such would not be expected to be regulated by a single gene or gene product.

HISTORY OF SURGERY FOR OBESITY

The surgical treatment of obesity is a relatively recent development and has encountered resistance within the profession for many reasons. Obesity is considered by many to be no more than an unfettered drive for pleasure derived from eating rather than a metabolic defect characterized by an economical use of foodstuffs. Many believe that even morbid obesity can be reversed by a sensible change in life style, even though 5-year treatment successes based on this are practically non-existent. Obesity is thought to exist because of an abundance of food and a sedentary life style, even though the evidence is strong that obesity is frequently genetically determined.

Kremen et al.[37] kindled the interest of many surgeons in the possibility that there could be a surgical role in the treatment of dangerous obesity. He and his colleagues in 1954 asked the innocent question; 'If large sections of the small intestine must be resected, should one make every effort to preserve the ileocaecal valve?' On the basis of a study on animals they concluded that the ileocaecal valve did prevent weight loss, especially when large portions of the ileum were out of circuit. They performed a jejunoileal bypass on a single patient, a 34-year-old white female whose maximum weight had been 385 lb (175 kg). About 90 cm of jejunum was anastomosed to 45 cm of ileum and the distal end of the bypassed small intestine was anastomosed to the transverse colon.

In 1971 the patient's bypass was revised by shortening the functioning jejunum to 40 cm and the ileum to 15 cm. Her weight then decreased from 240 lb (109 kg) to 171 lb and levelled off at 190 lb (86 kg). She was pleased with the weight loss and increased mobility, but required intermittent supplements of magnesium, calcium and potassium. She died in 1981 of myocardial infarct at 61 years of age having experienced angina pectoris for at least 1 year before her death. She maintained a low serum cholesterol from the time of her original operation (60–120 mg%).[38]

This experience had been preceded by resection of a large segment of small intestine in an obese patient by Henrikson in 1952,[38] but the surgery had the disadvantage of not being reversible.

There followed a series of operations, the first of which was a jejunocolic bypass designed to lower weight rapidly to a normal level and then restore normal intestinal continuity. This was done with the expectation that patients would be able to maintain the new decreased weight after re-operation. This procedure proved risky because of severe malnutrition and metabolic imbalances and was quickly abandoned.[39]

Between 1962 and 1975 there were trials of several types of jejunoileal bypass. These operations had various lengths of jejunum and ileum in circuit which ranged from 40 to over 100 cm, with either an end-to-side or an end-to-end anastomosis. If the operation was performed end-to-end, the bypassed segment was drained usually into the colon and even into the stomach to prevent backwash enteritis[40–43] (Figures 40.2–40.4).

The intestinal bypass is still used to treat hypercholesterolaemia that is unresponsive to pharmacological treatment. The POSCH study is still ongoing and continues to show excellent results for this condition.[44]

The rationale for inducing weight loss has now enlarged to include not only decreased absorption but also restriction of intake (Table 40.2).

INDICATIONS FOR SURGERY

Strict criteria should be followed in the selection of patients for this radical form of therapy. These concepts were reviewed and accepted by the National Institutes of Health (NIH) consensus conference. The factors to be considered include weight, age, medical problems that may improve with weight loss, genetic background, dietary, emotional, social and behavioural problems that may help predict success or failure.

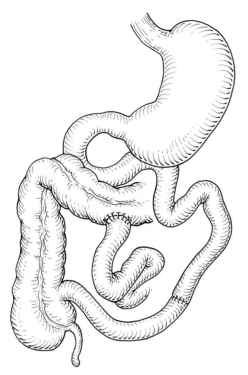

Figure 40.2
Jejunoileal bypass with end-to-end anastomosis. The bypassed segment has been drained into the transverse colon. The intestine in circuit from the ligament of Treitz to the colon was usually 50–75 cm long.

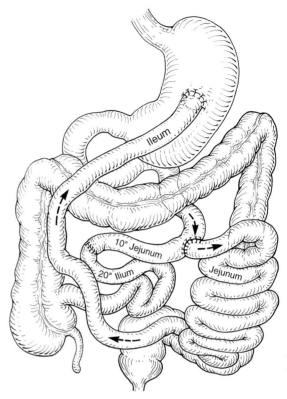

Figure 40.4
The operation of Gourlay. After end-to-end jejunoileal bypass has been performed, the bypassed segment is drained into the stomach to avoid bypass enteritis believed to be due to contamination and stenosis in the bypass segment when it is drained into the colon as in Figure 40.2. (Reproduced with the permission from Cleater and Goulay.[43])

We suggest surgical treatment in patients who have a BMI > 40 kg/m² for at least 5 years. Patients who have a number of weight-related co-morbidities, and who are continuing to gain weight, yet who are not quite at a BMI of 40 kg/m² can also be considered for surgery. We have operated on patients with few exceptions between 21 and 50 years of age. The younger age group may represent patients with early onset obesity with a poor prognosis for non-operative treatments, but we have reasoned that patients should be old enough to take responsibility for their decisions on this therapy. In occasional cases after considerable scrutiny young patients can be operated on but there is a need for careful supervision. In most patients over 50, the damage has frequently been done, but there are exceptions

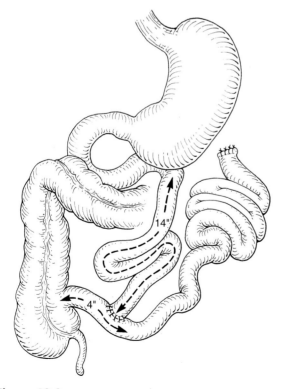

Figure 40.3
Jejunoileal bypass with end-to-side anastomosis: 35 to 10 cm of ileum.

Table 40.2 Procedures used for treating obesity

PRINCIPLE	PROCEDURE
Reduction of absorption	Jejunoileal bypass
	Biliointestinal bypass
	Biliopancreatic bypass
Reduction of intake	Dental occlusion
	Intragastric prosthesis
	Gastroplasty
Reduction of intake and absorption	Gastric bypass

with patients who have severe disability due to degeneration of weight-bearing joints or sleep apnoea. In these instances we would consider this therapy in older patients.

For many years we arranged for all of our patients to be interviewed by interested psychiatrists. They very rarely excluded a patient even though we did encounter emotional problems which required dismantling the operation at a later date (less than 1% of patients). We do not currently request psychiatric consultation before surgery. Stunkard et al.[45] have summarized the psychological aspects of the surgical treatment of obesity. They state: 'There is no substantial difference between the obese and non-obese on psychological testing.' In general, emotional state and self-confidence improve after surgically induced weight loss, and there is resolution of depression. Some patients with psychiatric problems can be surgically treated for their obesity. They must be treated in conjunction with the pyschiatric team, and these patients may have their pyschiatric problem improve with the weight loss and increased patient confidence. These patients are very much an exception rather than the rule.

All patients should have tried non-operative treatment of severe obesity. The most effective methods are peer-pressure groups such as Weightwatchers or TOPS (Take Off Pounds Sensibly).

Many patients are referred for surgery because they have some complications of obesity. The most common are hypertension, diabetes mellitus, sleep apnoea, very rarely the pickwickian syndrome, degenerative bone of joint disease in weight-bearing extremities and in women, amenorrhoea or menorrhagia, stress incontinence and cholecystitis. Successful weight loss is especially gratifying in these groups.

The patient should be free of any endocrine or metabolic disorder which could be corrected by measures other than caloric restriction.

A history of alcoholism, drug addiction, frank psychosis and liver disease are absolute contraindications for the surgery. If the patient is able to deal with the alcohol and drug addiction and go through rehabilitation then the surgeon can reassess the patient after a period of observation.

Emphasis must be placed on postoperative care and follow-up, and be agreed to by the patient before operation. Group sessions with patients who have been operated on and their experiences should be available to preoperative patients. The nature of their food intake should be freely discussed. Some insight into their eating behaviour is important for the patient, as with either operation the success will be related to changes in the patient's eating habit. This is especially important for patients undergoing gastroplasty after which a near-liquid diet is taken by some patients.

The names, addresses and phone number of relatives or friends who are willing to contact the patient must be obtained before operation. The patients must agree to return to a follow-up clinic monthly for the first year, every three months for the second year, and at least every 6 months thereafter. The patients must realize it is important to have blood samples taken and to be endoscoped at follow-up visits. The operation must be explained by the operating surgeon. A video tape can be used effectively to show the procedure and the status of patients after the operation.

We do not routinely obtain pulmonary function or exercise tolerance tests. These are performed in the patient with a history of pulmonary or cardiac problems, or with an abnormal electrocardiogram. Grace[46] has listed criteria for selecting patients who may lose more weight or have fewer complications after surgery for obesity. These include the following.

1. Less obese – the operations are usually easier and return to normal weight is much more frequent in the morbidly obese as compared to the superobese.

2. Young patients who are married with an active job and no history of admissions for psychiatric problems – coping skills are superior;

3. No previous operation for obesity. This is an especially difficult problem if the operation appears to be technically sound and the patient has not lost significant weight;

4. Social support, fewer negative life events, co-operative in follow-up, mature attitude, adequate intelligence and very low alcohol intake are all very favourable signs.

Many of the indicators of success become obvious only after prolonged follow-up. The science of selection is poorly developed at this time, but the guidelines above should be helpful to those initiating a programme.

MALABSORPTION TECHNIQUES

Jejunoileal bypass

The various types of jejunoileal bypass produced varying amounts of weight loss that was roughly inversely related to the length of intestine remaining in circuit. With lengths longer than 100 cm, weight loss usually proved to be unsatisfactory. With lengths shorter than 45 cm, the incidence of protein malnutrition rose sharply. Baddeley[47] in a randomized trial compared the end-to-end with the end-to-side anastomosis using the same lengths in both: 35 cm of jejunum and 10 cm of ileum. He reported that there was no statistical difference in weight loss or morbidity between the two groups.

Although some[48] reported that weight loss after jejunoileal bypass was due primarily to decreased intake rather than caloric loss through malabsorption, the complications related to loss of essential nutrients or minerals in the stool led to an intolerable rate of complications.

The late complications are summarized in Table 40.3. Liver failure was especially alarming and had been the main complication leading to death in the abandoned jejunocolic bypass operation. Patients with liver failure present with weakness, lethargy, anorexia, nausea, vomiting and can progress rapidly into encephalopathy with abnormal liver function.

In a study from our own institution[49] we measured body composition in 44 morbidly obese patients who underwent jejunoileal bypass. These body composition measurements which accurately quantitate the fat, protein and extracellular components of body composition were performed before the operation and at regular intervals after surgery. In 33 of these

Table 40.3 Late complications of jejunoileal bypass

	NO. OF PATIENTS
Renal stones	22 (12.8)
Arthritis	17 (9.9)
Severe persistent diarrhoea	13 (7.6)
Malnutrition and dehydration	11 (6.4)
Hernia (incisional)	10 (5.8)
Cholecystitis and cholelithiasis	8 (4.6)
Hypomagnesaemia	3 (1.7)
Acidosis (symptomatic)	2 (1.2)
Intussusception (reoperated upon)	2 (1.2)
Pancreatitis	2 (1.2)
Hypoglycaemia	2 (1.2)
Hepatic dysfunction	2 (1.2)
Hepatic failure and death	2 (1.2)
Dermatitis	2 (1.2)
Duodenal ulcer with haemorrhage	1 (0.6)
Gastric ulcer	1 (0.6)
Erythema nodosum	1 (0.6)
Persistent vomiting	1 (0.6)
Perforated sigmoid diverticulitis	1 (0.6)
Carcinoma of sigmoid colon	1 (0.6)
Encephalopathy	1 (0.6)
Death	3 (1.7)

Values in parentheses are percentages.
From Linner[38] with permission.

patients at 1 year, body weights had decreased by 24.4±2.1% whereas the body cell mass (the energy producing, oxygen utilizing cells of the body) had decreased by only 21±7.1%. The body composition before and after intestinal bypass (7 months to 3 years) showed weight loss that is principally due to a loss of fat in the group which did well nutritionally, and weight loss due to not only a loss of fat but also of body cell mass in those who became malnourished and did not do well clinically. In the latter patients, body weights at one year had decreased by 27.0±3.0% and the body cell mass had decreased by an alarming 22.0±6.1%. The latter patients had developed protein malnutrition with accompanying liver failure in many. In their acute phase of kwashiorkor, all were treated successfully with intravenous amino acids, but all ultimately required restoration of normal intestinal continuity. There were no deaths. It was not possible to determine before surgery which patients would develop a malnourished state.

Jejunoileal bypass was abandoned for several reasons: the high rate of late complications, including malnutrition, but also failure to maintain a satisfactory weight loss. There were several patient deaths from the liver failure secondary to hepatic cirrhosis resulting from the jejunoileal bypass. Late weight gain after 5–10 years was common.[49] Especially significant was the importance of long and thorough follow-up to establish the limitations of these operations.

Biliary intestinal bypass

Eriksson[50] reported a modification of the jejunoileal bypass in which the bypassed segment after the end-to-side procedure was not closed but anastomosed to the gall bladder. The postulated advantage of this operation was the preservation of

normal enterohepatic circulation of bile salts from the distal ileum. In the jejunoileal bypass as usually performed, the bile salts are converted into bile acids in the jejunum because of bacterial overgrowth with irritation of the colon and diarrhoea.

In a similar operation by Hallberg and Holmgren,[51] an end-to-side jejunoileal bypass was constructed 15–20 cm proximal to the caecum with 40–45 cm of jejunum in circuit (Figure 40.5). The proximal end of the defunctioned jejunum was anastomosed to the gall bladder. If the gall bladder contained stones, they were removed.

Biliopancreatic bypass

Scopinaro et al.[52] developed an operation for obesity based on the idea that one could induce selective absorption of foodstuffs and retain normal bile salt absorption. The operation (Figure 40.6) consists of a gastrectomy with a Roux-en-Y gastroenterostomy. The gastrectomy was performed to prevent stomal ulcers and to limit intake. Others have substituted either a parietal cell vagotomy[53] or truncal vagotomy instead of a gastrectomy.[54] Because of diarrhoea, the latter is not currently recommended.[54] The length of bowel from the gastroenterostomy to the ileocaecal valve, as well as the length of the common channel, have been varied by Scopinaro and colleagues. There is theoretically a selective malabsorption of fat and starch and the enterohepatic circulation of bile salts is maintained. The flow of bile and pancreatic juice through the excluded segment

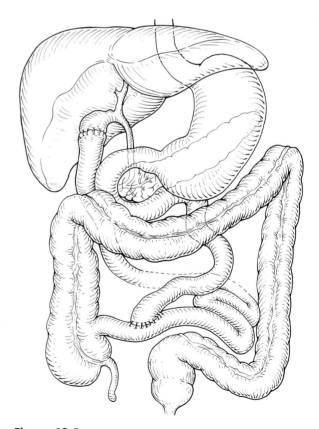

Figure 40.5
Biliointestinal bypass designed to maintain normal enterohepatic bile salt circulation and thereby cause less diarrhoea due to conversion of bile salts into bile acids.

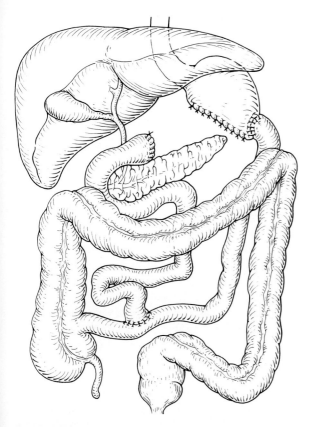

Figure 40.6
Biliopancreatic bypass of Scopinaro. There is a two-thirds
gastric resection with duodenal closure and construction of a
long Roux-en-Y limb which diverts the pancreaticobiliary flow to
the terminal ileum. Currently, the alimentary limb of jejunoileum
is 200 cm in length, the Roux limb is anastomosed to the
terminal ileum 50 cm proximal to the ileocaecal valve.[54]

of small intestine might be expected to reduce bacterial overgrowth.[54] Diarrhoea is reported to be less severe than with conventional jejunoileal bypass, with only two or three fatty-type
stools per day and seldom any liquid movements. There is a
large amount of foul flatus because of starch digestion in the
colon.

Late follow-up of metabolic complications in these operations is limited in the literature. In one study of 41 patients
with biliopancreatic bypass seen 1–5 years after operation,
metabolic bone disease was present in 30 patients (73%).[55] The
defect was characterized by defective mineralization, decreased
bone formation and increased resorption. Nine patients were
also hypocalcaemic. This is similar to bone disease due to
calcium loss and vitamin D deficiency seen after jejunoileal
bypass. A total of 380 biliopancreatic bypass operations were
done by Scopinaro et al. at the University of Genoa between
May 1976 and April 1984. The results reported in 1987[56,57]
showed that 21% had protein malnutrition with follow-up of at
least 1 year.

The first operations of Scopinaro divided the small intestine
at midpoint so that the alimentary tract and the biliopancreatic
tract were of equal length. The common tract after end-to-side
ileoileostomy was made 50 cm in length to provide absorption

of proteins and bile salts and to reduce to a minimum fat and
starch absorption. A partial gastrectomy was initially added to
prevent stomal ulcer. Gallstone formation was common and
cholecystectomy was soon also performed. If there is a channel
in the ileum which drains the jejunum and mixes with the
ingested food, the procedure is called a 'partial biliopancreatic
bypass'. If this mixing in the ileum is not permitted by anastomosing each loop separately into the colon, this is referred to
as a 'total biliopancreatic bypass'. The latter has a high incidence of protein malnutrition and is not currently recommended for clinical application.

Weight loss was not adequate or late weight gain occurred
with partial biliopancreatic bypass, which prompted Scopinaro
et al. to use a 'short loop' partial biliopancreatic bypass. In this
modification the loop of ileum draining the stomach was made
200 cm in length. This caused an increase in stomal ulcers which
led to a further modification: more extensive gastrectomy.

Their current operation for super obesity is a very small
stomach (200 ml capacity) partial biliopancreatic bypass, with
200 cm of ileum in continuity with the stomach and an end-to-
side enteroenterostomy of the biliopancreatic tract 50 cm proximal to the ileocaecal valve.

For the morbidly obese they advise a larger gastric volume
of 300–400 ml. This operation leads to less protein malnutrition
(Figure 40.6).

Complications following these operations include a significant incidence of microcytic, hypochromic anaemia, low calcium absorption, protein malnutrition, metabolic bone disease,
reduced cell-mediated immunity and a high incidence of
stomal ulcers. Favourable results have been reported in
patients afflicted with the pickwickian syndrome, somnolence,
hypertension, abnormal liver function, hypercholesterolaemia,
diabetes mellitus and hyperuricaemia.

Weight losses expressed as residual percentage over ideal
weight show satisfactory results in the majority of patients at 2
and 5 years, but the metabolic price to pay for this has not as
yet been clearly documented.

Many surgeons will try to duplicate these results using gastric bypass instead of gastrectomy to avoid the irreversible
nature of the Scopinaro operation. These operations appear to
depend substantially on malabsorption for their effectiveness.
Whether the undesirable features of malabsorption will domi-
nate the longterm results awaits further studies and confirmation of the work of Scopinaro and his colleagues.

REDUCTION OF ORAL INTAKE

Another approach to the surgery of the obese patient is based
on the concept of reducing the nutritional intake. This was an
obvious extension of the diet. The points in the enteric system
where the intake could practically be physically limited
included the mouth and the stomach.

Dental occlusion

Garrow[58] is the main advocate of jaw wiring. A milk diet is
instituted for at least two months before the procedure. His
patients are all admitted to a clinical research centre before the

operation and all have the opportunity to speak with other patients who have the same treatment. They invoke several conditions: the patients should never remove the wires for any reason; the patients must return to the hospital at monthly intervals for medical supervision; and the patient must agree to wear a waist cord indefinitely after the wires are removed.

The results of this programme on 35 patients showed that nine patients dropped out before significant weight loss, 12 completed the wiring schedule but then dropped out; 14 continued with the waist cord and at 3 years had lost 33% of pre-operative weight or 62% of their excess weight.

In our clinic we performed jaw wiring on 72 patients. This study was based on the hypothesis that if one returned patients to normal weight they would remain at this weight even after the wires were removed. This idea followed an experience with patients who had an effective result after gastroplasty and continued to have an excellent result even though it was proved by endoscopy that the operation had failed technically. A disruption of the staple line or massive enlargement of the stoma were the principal causes of failure of the operation in these patients. Our experience (L.D. MacLean and B. Rhode, unpublished data) with 72 patients was much less successful than that described by Garrow and Webster.[59] We followed the patients from 2 to 5 years and found that even though some patients lost weight down to a normal weight, all patients regained most of the weight lost after the wires were removed. In many patients the wires were reapplied and again a significant weight loss resulted, but failure again followed removal of the fixation. An abdominal belt was not used in this study, but we do not believe that this will be a suitable long-term treatment for patients with clinically significant obesity.

This was also the experience of Drenick and Hargis[60] who documented an important weight loss with tooth wiring, but in long-term follow-up after removal of the jaw fixation, weight gain occurred which frequently exceeded the weight before treatment. Most workers now agree that jaw wiring at this time is only useful in preparation of very obese patients for surgery.

Intragastric bubble

The intragastric balloon was introduced for use in humans in Europe in 1982 and the Garren bubble was approved for use in the USA in 1985. They are filled with 200 ml of air and are free-floating and designed to produce satiety with less intake by the patients. Over 20 000 of these devices were implanted[61] without any evidence of significant, long-term weight loss. At least one death and significant morbidity have been reported.[61] A substantial percentage of balloons deflate spontaneously before the end of the 4-month recommended period of use, and migration into the small intestine can occur with subsequent bowel obstruction. No long-term studies of benefits have as yet been reported. T.V. Taylor (personal communication) uses a silicone rather than a latex balloon which may be more durable. This silicone balloon has a volume of 550 ml as apposed to the 200 ml of the Garren bubble. Significant weight loss has been reported but only in the short term. No long-term efficacy has been shown.

Gastroplasty

These operations were designed to divide the stomach into a smaller proximal pouch and a larger distal. There are three main components of the operation, the pouch size, the staple line and the outlet connecting the two pouches. The horizontal stapling of the stomach with a reinforced greater curvature channel, or reinforced gastrogastrostomy, are unsatisfactory procedures.[38]

Vertical stapling without support was introduced by Tretbar et al.[62] Eckhout and Prinzing,[63] O'Leary[64] and Laws and Piantadosi[65] (Figure 40.7) developed similar procedures but added external support to control the size of the orifice and thereby limit eating. Mason developed the gastroplasty which has gained widest acceptance (Figure 40.8). He emphasized that the vertical staple lines must be parallel and close together (the TA-90B instrument now makes this easier). The vertical line must be at the Angle of His and not to the left in the gastric fundus. The orifice size must be 5.0 cm in external circumference and be measured and supported with a band of Marlex 5 mm wide and 50 mm long. The pouch must be less than 30 ml when measured at surgery using a 70 cm height of water pressure.

Similar requirements for the vertical ring gastroplasty (VRG) have been summarized by Willbanks.[66] The pouch must be less than 50 ml and pouches of 15–20 ml are common. The orifice must be less than 12 mm in diameter (36F). Willbanks advises a stoma of 9.5–10 mm (30–32F). There must be some method to prevent stoma enlargement. He uses a silastic tubing 4.3 cm in length through which a monofilament suture is threaded which permits fixation at the appropriate site on the stomach. The staple line must be reinforced with a non-absorbable suture (2/0 polypropylene). Willbanks believes a vertical pouch is less likely to dilate than a horizontal pouch because the gastric wall is thicker on the lesser curve of the stomach.

The results of vertical banded gastroplasty (VBG) are much more variable than other bariatric procedures (Table 40.4). Sugerman and colleagues[67] found only 33% of patients achieved good or excellent results at three years, whereas Dietel et al.[68] had 83% in these categories after two years. We

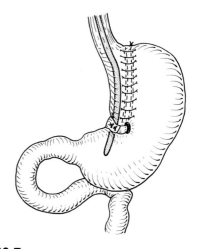

Figure 40.7
Vertical ring gastroplasty.

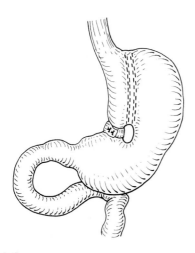

Figure 40.8
Vertical banded gastroplasty.

found a 60% good or excellent result after 3 years but with a 30% reoperation rate. We did notice that 47 patients after vertical banded gastroplasty who maintained an orifice less than 11 mm in diameter, as measured at endoscopy, and in whom the staple lines remained intact achieved an excellent result in 57% of cases and a good result in 32% or, combined, an 89% success rate after 4 years.[69] If the operation remains as Mason designed it, the results can be very gratifying but this was the case in only 47 of 201 patients in our experience.

COMBINED GASTRIC RESTRICTION AND MALABSORPTION

Mason, who found the jejunoileal bypass an unsatisfactory treatment for obese patients, reasoned that limiting intake might be a more physiological approach. He had observed that patients with extensive gastrectomy for other reasons such as duodenal ulcer frequently lost weight and that many of these patients had difficulty maintaining a normal weight. He also knew that, if the gastric pouch was small enough, stomal ulcer was very infrequent even in patients with duodenal ulcer. He reasoned that if the distal stomach is not resected, the antrum is not isolated and it remains in continuity with most of the acid-producing stomach. Acid peptic ulceration has not been a significant problem after gastric bypass.

Mason and Ito[73] first reported their operation, a gastric bypass with division of the stomach and loop gastroenterostomy in 1969 (Figure 40.9). Several modifications have been introduced since that time (Figures 40.10 and 40.11): gastric bypass with or without division of the stomach, and using

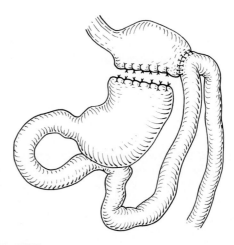

Figure 40.9
Loop, large pouch gastric bypass first advocated by Mason and Ito.[73]

Table 40.4 Weight loss after gastric operations for obesity

AUTHORS(S)	n	FOLLOW-UP (YEARS)	TYPE OF OPERATION	AVERAGE WT LOSS (%)	EXCESS WT LOST (%)	AVERAGE RESULTS IN PERCENTAGE OF EXCESS WEIGHT 0–25% (%)	26–50% (%)	51–75% (%)	76–100% (%)	>100% (%)
Linner[38]	223	4	Roux (GB)	38	86	55	28	10	5	1
Linner[38]	47	4	Loop (GB)	24	55	25	27	30	10	8
Linner[38]	187	4	Horizontal (GB)	20	40	20	37	25	11	7
Thompson et al.[80]	63	3	Loop (GB)	—	—	51	36	10	2	1
Sugerman et al.[67]	18	3	Roux (GB)	—	—	33	55	6	0	6
Sugerman et al.[67]	15	3	VBG	—	—	0	33	33	14	20
Deitel et al.[68]	87	2	VBG	—	—	83		12		5
MacLean et al.[69]	196	3	VBG	34	63	28	32	18	8	3
MacLean et al.[69a]	47	4	VBG	—	—	57	32	11	0	0
Willbanks[70]	305	2	VBG	36	61	—	—	—	—	—
Flickinger et al.[71]	99	4	Roux (GB)	35	61	—	—	—	—	—
Mason et al.[73]	58	5	VBG	29	60	—	—	—	—	—
Yale[72b]	225	5	Roux (GB)	31 ± 12	60 ± 23	—	—	—	—	—
Yale[72c]	89	3	VBG	25 ± 11	50 ± 22	—	—	—	—	—

GB, gastric bypass; VBG, vertical banded gastroplasty.
[a] Selected – technically satisfactory over 4 years, i.e. staple line intact and orifice <11 mm diameter, morbid obesity only.
[b] Twenty-six percent of patients failed to lose 25% of original weight at 5 years.
[c] Forty-five percent of patients failed to lose 25% of original weight at 3 years.

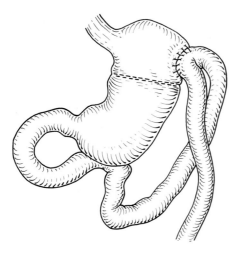

Figure 40.10
Loop gastric bypass with staple partition of the stomach.[74]

Roux-en-Y or loop anastomosis.[74-76] The anastomosis to jejunum can be made after a horizontal or vertical stapling of the stomach. The orifice size is made 1 cm in diameter and pouch size as small as possible, but certainly less than 30 ml.

Our own experience with gastric bypass with a silicone ring about the anastomosis to prevent enlargement was not good. The ring, even though not sutured to the stomach or intestine, eroded into the area of the anastomosis and caused stenosis

which frequently necessitated reoperation.[77] It had been previously noted that external support of a small stoma, as in horizontal gastroplasty, provided by suturing through the gastric wall will fail because of internal migration of the material used. External support of a stoma not adjacent to an anastomosis, as in vertical-banded gastroplasty, is much more likely to function without migration.

Complications of gastric surgery

Early and late complications after gastric operations are summarized in Tables 40.5 and 40.6. Early complications, including mortality, probably do not vary between the vertical banded gastroplasty and the gastric bypass.

The most threatening early complication is a leak with peritonitis which has a high fatality rate if not diagnosed and treated promptly. To help avoid this complication, intraoperative testing for leaks is important and should be done with a methylene blue solution passed through a nasogastric tube. Early leaks within the first 24 hours are especially treacherous. The patients have an elevated pulse rate (over 120 beats/minute), and become increasingly dyspenic and can be misdiagnosed as having a pulmonary embolus. Fever is usually present with abdominal tenderness. Water-soluble contrast material can be given by mouth to document the leak but not always positive. In patients with the above signs and leucocytosis with left shoulder tip pain occurring in the first 48

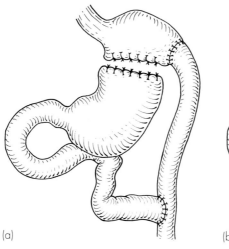 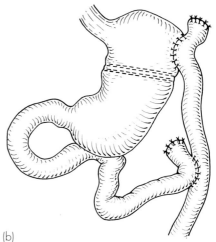

(a)   (b)

Figure 40.11
(a) and (b) Roux-en-Y gastric bypass with transection of the stomach.[75]

Table 40.5 Early complications after gastric surgery for obesity

AUTHOR(S)	N	PULMONARY EMBOLUS	PNEUMONIA ATELECTASIS	WOUND INFECTION	WOUND DEHISCENCE	SPLENECTOMY	GASTRIC LEAK	MORTALITY
Thompson et al.[78]	150	—	6.7%	4.7%	0	2.6%	1.4%	1.4%
Pories et al.[79]	102	—	—	7 (7%)	—	—	—	0
Benotti et al.[80]	289	1	27 (9%)	21 (7%)	5 (2%)	—	10 (4%)	1%
Hornberger[81]	31	6%	—	15%	3%	—	0	6%
Vaughan et al.[82]	210	—	—	32 (15.2%)	1 (0.5%)	—	—	1%
Linner[18]	285	0	7 (2.5%)	6 (2.1%)	0	1 (0.3%)	2 (0.7%)	0.7%

Table 40.6 Late complications after gastric surgery for obesity

AUTHORS	TYPE OF SURGERY	n	STAPLE LINE DISRUPTION (%)	STOMAL ULCER (%)	VENTRAL HERNIA (%)	CHOLELITHIASIS (%)	REVISION RATE (%)
Thompson et al.[78]	GB	150	6	0	18	24	10.8
MacLean et al.[69]	VBG	201	48	0	—	—	36

GB, gastric bypass; VBG, vertical banded gastroplasty.

hours, there is strong evidence that a leak has occurred and the patient should be returned to the operating room for repair and drainage of the area without radiological confirmation. Leaks occurring later, after 5 days, can be managed by percutaneously placed drainage tubes using radiographic control.

Splenic injury requiring splenectomy rarely occurs. We have done over 600 operations on the stomach for control of obesity and only one splenectomy was necessary due to late bleeding from a splenic haematoma.

The most important late complication in our hands has been staple line disruption, which is not always readily seen on endoscopy or with upper gastrointestinal series. Many of our patients who had a less than satisfactory weight loss proved on careful examination to have this complication. Repair of the disruption can produce a dramatically improved result.

Our own results with vertical banded gastroplasty are shown in Table 40.7.[69] Evaluation was made on an annual basis and the results listed as good, satisfactory and unsatisfactory. A good result indicates a patient who has lost at least 25% of preoperative weight and is within 30% of normal, a satisfactory result indicates a loss of at least 25% and an unsatisfactory result a loss of less than 25% of preoperative weight.[69]

The Reinhold classification is also used with results represented as excellent, good, fair, poor or failure. The mean percentage weight loss varies between 31.0±0.7% and 33.8±0.9%

over the 5 years of follow-up. The percentage excess weight loss varies over a 5-year period between 60±2 and 65±2% but despite these favourable indicators, there were 40% of patients who failed to lose weight or stabilized their weights at greater than 50% above ideal. This was principally due to a significant incidence of disruption of the vertical staple line (48%), and 36% of the total number of patients required a re-operation to repair the staple line.

This experience has prompted us to utilize an operation not dependent on staples (Figure 40.12) in which the Mueller stapler is used and division is made between two double rows of vertical staples. The divided, stapled tissue is oversewn with 3/0 polyethylene suture to prevent staple line disruption. Follow-up is not long enough to give a final result for this operation, but staple line disruption has been markedly diminished but surprisingly not eliminated.

LATE RESULTS OF GASTRIC BYPASS

The Reinhold classification[77] describes how closely a patient's weight approaches ideal (Table 40.8) and is a good way to compare the value of different operations. It is preferable to giving results as a mean weight loss or mean percentage excess weight loss, which can appear quite good and mask the fact that significant numbers of patients have a fair or poor

Table 40.7 Clinical results at 1 to 5 years after vertical banded gastroplasty

RESULTS	1 YEAR (n = 201)	2 YEARS (n = 200)	3 YEARS (n = 196)	4 YEARS (n = 139)	5 YEARS (n = 57)
Good	61(30)	64(32)	60(31)	37(27)	21(37)
Satisfactory	98(49)	84(42)	95(48)	73(53)	23(40)
Unsatisfactory	32(16)	22(11)	20(10)	24(17)	12(21)
Excellent (<25% excess wt.)	53(26)	60(30)	54(28)	30(22)	16(28)
Good (26–50% excess wt.)	62(31)	53(27)	64(33)	50(36)	15(26)
Fair (51–75% excess wt.)	42(21)	44(22)	36(18)	37(27)	19(33)
Poor (76–100% excess wt.)	20(10)	7(4)	16(8)	13(9)	5(9)
Failure (>100% excess wt.)	14(7)	6(3)	5(3)	4(3)	1(2)
Mean % wt. loss	31.0 ± 0.7	33.8 ± 0.9	33.0 ± 0.9	31.4 ± 1.1	32.1 ± 1.8
% excess wt.	46 ± 2	40 ± 2	43 ± 2	45 ± 2	46 ± 3
% excess wt. loss	61 ± 2	65 ± 2	63 ± 2	60 ± 2	60 ± 3
Lost to follow-up	9(4.5)	29(14.5)	20(10)	5(4)	1(2)
Deaths	1	1	1	0	0
Disruption of staple line	27	28	25	15	10
Reoperations	7	21	32	11	11

Values in parentheses are percentages.
From MacLean[68] et al. with permission.

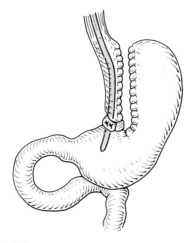

Figure 40.12
Vertical banded gastroplasty with division between the staple lines. This operation is not dependent on staples.

result or even be a frank failure of surgery for obesity. This classification displays results on an individual basis. It permits one to determine how many failures exist as well as the excellent results.

Results currently in the literature with long follow-up are summarized in Table 40.4.

The results of gastric bypass in Table 40.4 are designated GB with either a 'Roux' or 'Loop' anastomosis. The number of patients and minimal follow-up, as well as average percentage weight lost and average percentage excess weight lost, are listed. This should be compared with the Reinhold classification which shows how many patients achieved an excellent or good result (had 50% or less excess weight over ideal) and how many had a fair, poor or failed result in which they did not lose excess weight to within 50% of ideal. A reasonable goal should be to return all patients to a state where they do not exceed 50% excess weight. Very few reports permit one to evaluate the results of an operation because the data on weight loss are not individualized. When this is done as by Linner,[38] Thompson et al.[78] and Sugerman et al.[67] the superiority of gastric bypass over other operations is clearly illustrated. Linner[38] found 55% of patients with gastric bypass Roux-en-Y had an excellent result and were within 25% of ideal weight at 4 years after surgery. Only 7% were in the poor or failed category. Thompson et al.[78] with a follow-up at 3 years had 87% in the excellent or good category and only 3% were poor or failed results.

Table 40.8 Reinhold classification of results after surgery for obesity

RESULT	APPROXIMATION TO NORMAL WEIGHT[a]
Excellent	0–25% excess weight
Good	26–50% excess weight
Fair	51–75% excess weight
Poor	76–100% excess weight
Failure	100% excess weight

[a]Ideal weight based on Metropolitan life insurance tables, 1983.[112]

Sugerman and colleagues[67] using a GB Roux achieved an 88% good or excellent result in 18 patients followed for 3 years and a 6% failure rate. Although others have documented a mean percentage weight loss of 31–35% and a mean excess weight loss of 60% or greater, one cannot be certain how many patients achieved a good or excellent result and how many failed, because there is a large standard error of the mean when a range of weights is given at final assessment.[79]

Limb length

The standard gastric bypass operation uses a limb length of 45 cm. There is evidence that by adding more limb length there is increased weight loss, but there are increased co-morbidities. The extreme of the limb length, the biliopancreatic bypass uses only a common length of 50 cm, with a greater weight loss, but complications of malabsorption particularly vitamin and mineral deficiencies. Protein malnutrition can occur, whereas this complication is not seen in the gastric bypass. Limb lengths of up to 100 cm have been shown to increase weight loss but not add co-morbidities.[83] At this time there are modifications of the gastric bypass with limb lengths between 45 and 100 cm.

The other problem with the surgery is the staple line and incidence of staple line dehiscence of up to 35%. There are differences in staplers with the Mueller staple line apparently more susceptible to breakdown as opposed to the TA 90 (Autosuture Co., US Surgical Corp, Norwalk, CT). However, the single application of thc TA 90B is still associated with a high incidence of staple line fistulas. There are now two schools of thought developing to deal with this complication. The first is to add staple applications one on top of the other, and in some cases there are three applications used, with reported staple line dehiscence of 2%. The other option is to divide the staple line with oversewing of the staple lines. In these series the staple line dehiscence is also decreased to less than 5%.

Success

There continues to be controversy about the definition of success with this operation. Although obtaining a weight close to the ideal weight is a good objective, considerable benefit can be obtained outside the mere change in body weight. Most of the objective of the surgery for the patient is weight reduction but the focus should be on improving health. In terms of improved health, the reduction in co-morbidities is important. In a review of this subject Kral[84] pooled published data from 1000 patients. In this he defined cure as off all medications and improved as a reduction of medications. He found that the degree of consistent weight loss from the surgery had a major impact on these co-morbidities: hypertension (60–65% cured and 90% improved); diabetes (90–95% cured and 100% improved); dyslipidaemia (70% cured and 85% improved); asthma (greater than 95% cured and 100% improved); heart failure (60% cured and 90% improved) and sleep apnoea (100% cured and 100% improved). Additional problems such as degenerative arthritis, reflux oesophagitis, stress incontinence, irregular menses and psychosocial problems are also improved but the published data are not as conclusive. Based on these data it is very apparent that the effect of bariatric surgery on the overall health of these patients is very profound.

Morbid obesity versus superobesity

Results of gastroplasty for superobesity (BMI >50) are not as good as for patients with morbid obesity (BMI 40–50) (Table 40.9).[69,85] Only 8% of superobese patients go back to a weight within 25% of normal (an excellent result), as compared to 39% of morbidly obese patients. Other data, including our own, have shown that superobese patients with a gastric bypass, also do not have the same weight loss as compared to the morbidly obese. In view of these results we do not recommend the use gastroplasty for the superobese. In addition, the gastric bypass for the superobese patients should also be adjusted. Brolin et al.[83] demonstrated that an afferent limb length of 100 cm improved the weight loss but did not increase the postoperative complications. Currently, both of the authors are using a longer limb gastric bypass for the superobese patients, including the afferent limb (MacLean) and the efferent limb (Forse).

Table 40.9   Final results in patients with morbid obesity or superobesity

	MORBID OBESITY	SUPEROBESITY
n	140(70)	59(30)
Follow-up (months)	46.6 ± 1.0	50.4 ± 1.2
Results		
Good	62(44)	7(12)
Satisfactory	52(37)	46(78)
Unsatisfactory	26(19)	6(10)
Excellent (<25% excess wt.)	54(39)	5(8)
Good (26–50% excess wt.)	52(37)	19(32)
Fair (51–75% excess wt.)	30(21)	17(29)
Poor (76–100% excess wt.)	3(2)	14(24)
Failure (>100% excess wt.)	1(1)	4(7)
Lost	1	0
Death	1	0

Values in parentheses are percentages.
From MacLean et al.[69] with permission.

Gastric pouch

The data from both gastroplasty and gastric bypass have indicated that the gastric pouch should be no greater than 50 ml in volume. The problem that has developed in both operations has been the staple line as outlined previously. The other issue was the position of the gastric pouch in the stomach. If kept close to the lesser curve, pouch enlargement appeared to be less than in those created in the fundus where distention resulted in a very large pouch over time.

Laparoscopic surgery

There is currently a growing experience with laparoscopic bariatric surgery in morbid obesity. The advantages of this surgery include the smaller incisions, decreased incisional hernias, reduced wound pain, reduced handling of tissues, decreased narcotic use, earlier return of intestinal function, and a reduced metabolic response to surgery reflecting the decreased surgical stress. These advantages are a great asset to the patient with clinically significant obesity undergoing abdominal surgery. Presently morbid obesity is listed as a relative contraindication to laparoscopic surgery. In 1992 Unger et al.[86] reported the successful use of laparoscopic cholecystectomy in morbid obese patients with cholelithiais and this has been confirmed more recently by Deitel.[87] These surgeons concluded that morbid obesity was an indication rather than a contraindication for laparoscopic surgery due to the reduction in surgical morbidity and improved recovery.

The adaptation of this surgical approach to bariatric surgery is well underway. The first operation was a restrictive operation, designed as a gastric banding operation. The initial series was reported by Catona in 1993.[88] There were 40 patients who had a gastric banding with weight loss over 6 months similar to those who had a formal gastroplasty. The operations used five ports in the upper abdomen in a fashion similar to a hiatal hernia repair. The authors used 36 silastic and four Vycril bands all permanently placed, with the greatest problem being the tightness of the band for a stoma of 12–13 mm. In three patients the operation had to be revised due to stenosis. In this study the patient's weight went from 118±8 kg preoperatively to 107±14 kg at 6 months. The next step was to use an adjustable band rather than a fixed band, and this approach is currently being studied. The initial reports were encouraging but the experience was limited.[89] Both traditional gastroplasties and gastric bypass operations have been performed laparoscopically but with difficulty and with no long-term data. There are currently a number of centres using new equipment to facilitate the development of the laparoscopic approach. One would expect that the studies will show some advantage for this surgery over open surgery and based on previous experience, the gastric bypass will yield better results than the gastroplasty.

WOUND INFECTION

Morbidly obese patients with a large abdominal pannus and abundant subcutaneous fat have a higher risk for wound infections than normal weight individuals.[90] In addition, many of these patients have metabolic problems, particularly diabetes mellitus which may also increase this risk. Review of the literature indicates that the wound infection rate in severely obese patients ranges from 1.3 to 21%.[90–92] Treatment of wound infections can be difficult, often requiring prolonged hospitalization and long programmes of home care to obtain secondary healing. Several prophylactic measures have been utilized. There is continued interest in using drains for large wounds with deep subcutaneous spaces. However, in a recent randomized trial, it has been shown that there is no advantage in using a closed drainage system in these wounds.[93]

The approach of most surgeons to the abdominal wound in the morbidly obese is to avoid suture closure of the subcutaneous tissue. The wound is irrigated with saline and the skin closed with sutures or staples.

Another approach to the prophylaxis against wound infections has been the use of antibiotics, even though with their use, the rate of wound infections has still been reported to be high. In a recent study the wound infection rate was 16% compared to the wound infection rate of 2.8% for clean contaminated surgery in normal weight controls.[94] To investigate the possible failure of prophylactic antibiotics, we studied a number of regimens for administering them to these patients. The study investigated the administration of 1 g of cefazolin subcutaneously, intramuscularly or intravenously, preoperatively. The serum and subcutaneous tissue levels of the antibiotic were measured at the initiation of surgery and at the time the wound was closed. These measurements indicated that all three routes of administration failed to produce adequate tissue levels of the antibiotic during and at the end of the surgery. The tissue levels were well below the therapeutic levels for Gram-negative organisms.

A fourth group of morbidly obese patients was given 2 g of cefazolin intravenously at the beginning of the operation. Concentration of the antibiotic in the subcutaneous tissue at the time of wound closure in this group reached therapeutic levels for Gram-negative organisms. Subsequent to this, the regimen for antibiotic prophylaxis was changed to 2 g intravenously at the time of induction of anaesthesia. Using this regimen, the wound infection rate dropped from 16.5% to 5.6% over the same period in the subsequent year.

This study suggests that the pharmacodynamics of other drugs which depend on specific limits or concentrations to be effective should be studied in obese patients, an example being prophylactic heparin.

REMEDIAL SURGERY

Failure to lose adequate weight or late weight gain after successful reductions is common after surgery for obesity, especially in reports with long-term (3–6 years) and complete follow-up. In our own follow-up we have been impressed that failures to lose weight or late weight gain after surgery are frequently due to the technical failure of the operation rather than failure of the patient. When the original operation is reconstructed, impressive weight loss again occurs in most of these 'patient failures'. In a recent review of 201 patients with vertical banded gastroplasty, followed for a minimum of 3 years to over 5 years staple line disruption occurred in 105 or 52%.[69] About 36% were reoperated upon and the staple line restapled or restapled and divided. The improvement in results over the subsequent 2 years is shown in Table 40.10. There were four reperforations in the 10 patients in whom no division between the staple lines was made, but only one of 44 when there was division between the staple lines. A good result is classed as a patient who is within 30% of ideal weight. A satisfactory result is a loss of at least 25% of preoperative weight and an unsatisfactory result, failure to lose at least 25% of preoperative weight. There was an increase in good results after reoperation but the follow-up period is not long enough to be absolutely certain of this result. This treatment of staple line disruption may not ultimately prove satisfactory.

Table 40.10 Late results of reoperation for staple line disruption after vertical banded gastroplasty

	NO DIVISION	WITH DIVISION	TOTAL
n	10	44	54
Follow-up (months)	35.7 ± 1.4	17.5 ± 1.4	—
Too early (<6 months)	0	9	9
Results			
Before reoperation[a]			
Good	0	6(17)	6(13)
Satisfactory	5(50)	18(52)	23(51)
Unsatisfactory	5(50)	11(31)	16(36)
After reoperation[a]			
Good	2(20)	15(43)	17(38)
Satisfactory	6(60)	16(46)	22(49)
Unsatisfactory	2(20)	4(11)	6(13)

Values in parentheses are percentages.
[a] χ^2 Outcome before versus after, $P = 0.007$.
Adapted from MacLean et al.[69] with permission.

Remedial operations for intestinal bypass have been restoration of normal intestinal continuity with or without vertical banded gastroplasty or gastric bypass. In patients with severe diarrhoea and protein malnutrition who have end-to-end jejunoileal bypass with the bypassed segment implanted into the colon, there is another option. Based on the idea that some of the difficulty is due to overgrowth of bacteria in the bypassed segment it might be transferred from the colon to the stomach as suggested by Cleator and Gourlay.[43] No controlled trial to support this concept exists.

If vertical banded or vertical ring gastroplasty fails because of stenosis of the outlet or erosion of the banding material into the lumen which can cause pain and bleeding, we favour removal of the material and conversion to gastric bypass. The end of the gastric pouch is anastomosed side-to-side or end-to-side to a Roux-en-Y loop of jejunum brought up in the retrocolic and retrogastric positions (Figure 40.13). We tend to try and remove the failed outlet and its material and then use the open end of the pouch to anastomose end-to-side to the jejunal limb. If the gastric pouch exceeds 50 ml or if there is a hole in the staple line, this should be restapled. We favour the TA90B with oversewing using 3/0 polyethylene sutures. This approach to the failed gastroplasty has also been successful with other surgeons.[95]

If there is failure of a gastric bypass with an obvious cause, this should be repaired. Stomal ulcer in our experience has always coexisted with a perforation in the staple line, so that the Roux loop is exposed to the entire stomach' acid production rather than a small pouch. Closure of the staple line with the TA90B and oversewing is effective treatment.

Correction of late weight gain after gastric bypass with a large anastomosis or enlarged pouch but intact staple line is less amenable to treatment. Schwartz et al.[96] found in these settings a high incidence of major complications and subsequently negligible weight loss. Lengthening the Roux limb or conversion to a Scopinaro-type operation is being used by

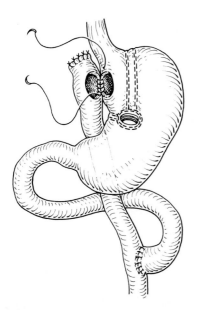

Figure 40.13
Roux-en-Y gastric bypass using a small vertical gastric pouch as for gastroplasty. The vertical staple lines must be oversewn or divided. The end of the pouch must also be oversutured and divided or used for the anastomosis.

some surgeons in this setting, but no long-term results are as yet reported.

Our own policy is to convert failed jejunoileal bypasses into either gastric bypass Roux-en-Y, or vertical banded gastroplasty with reanastomosis of the intestine. Failed horizontal gastroplasty is best converted into gastric bypass Roux-en-Y on the lesser curvature using a small vertical pouch. The lateral pouch must be drained by the previously constructed gastrogastrostomy. Failed vertical banded gastroplasty is best converted to gastric bypass Roux-en-Y as it eliminates further difficulty with outlet obstruction if the reoperation is being done for staple line disruption. We are presently following failed gastric bypass Roux-en-Y without obvious cause or for possibly enlarged stoma or pouch size, awaiting the studies of others on lengthening the Roux limb or performing biliointestinal or biliopancreatic bypass.

Despite the controversies that exist with revisional surgery, we have looked at the safety and long-term results. In 63 patients undergoing revisional surgery between 1981 and 1994 there was no mortality and serious complications occurred in 16%.[97] The follow-up was 68% and showed that these patients had an original BMI of 50 ± 10 kg/m^2, at revisional surgery a BMI of 39 ± 9 kg/m^2 and at the follow-up a BMI of 34 ± 10 kg/m^2. Those patients whose original BMI was greater than 50 kg/m^2 making them superobese had a greater weight loss than those with BMI <50 kg/m^2. These data re-emphasize the need to use more aggressive surgery initially for the superobese patient. All of these data support our confidence in using revisional surgery.

ANAESTHESIA FOR OBESE PATIENTS

Severely obese individuals require increased oxygen consumption ($\dot{V}o_2$) and produce increased amounts of carbon dioxide ($\dot{V}co_2$) because increased cardiac output and alveolar ventilation are necessary to maintain the fat, but especially the body cell mass supporting it. This leads to increased alveolar ventilation at rest. This further adds to the work of breathing because of decreased chest wall compliance due to the weight of fat. Functional residual capacity decreases so that alveolar closure occurs over the range of normal tidal volumes. As a result, alveolar perfusion continues, resulting in blood flow to non-ventilated or intermittently ventilated lung units. Resting arterial oxygenation predicted for age is reduced in both the sitting and supine positions and is especially aggravated in the reverse Trendelenburg position.

The pulmonary investigation of a patient who is a candidate for surgery for obesity should emphasize primarily a good clinical history to determine the degree of dyspnoea and the presence of asthma or bronchitis. A chest radiograph and arterial blood gases are routinely obtained. There is a need for pulmonary function tests only when the initial evaluation is clearly abnormal. If patients are asthmatic, function tests with and without bronchodilators should be available to optimize pulmonary function during and after surgery.

Two, well-recognized clinical syndromes which impair pulmonary function are the obstructive sleep apnoea syndrome, and the obesity hypoventilation syndrome or pickwickian syndrome. The former should be suspected when the patient has a history of loud snoring, frequent nocturnal awakening and daytime somnolence and is due to repeated attacks of upper airway obstruction. This increases with increasing body weight but may occur without obesity, and loss of weight does not guarantee amelioration of the problem. The syndrome is confirmed by sleep polysomnography which documents cessation of airflow with persistent respiratory efforts which are relieved by arousal. Weight loss induced by gastric restrictive procedures has been very effective.[3]

The pickwickian syndrome is a much more serious and fortunately very rare condition first described by Burwell et al.[98] who were recalling the sleepy obese boy Tom in *Pickwick Papers*. Their first patient was a 52-year-old markedly obese man who fell asleep in a poker game holding a hand containing two aces and three kings. After finishing the hand his 'friends' aroused him and took him to the hospital assuming he was ill. In this syndrome there is an attenuated response to hypercapnia and to hypoxia. There is decreased forced vital capacity, expiratory reserve volume, functional residual capacity and maximum minute volume of ventilation, usually without obstruction to airflow. The impairment is restrictive rather than obstructive.

As a result of hypoxaemia, these patients become polycythaemic which may cause pulmonary artery vasoconstriction and pulmonary hypertension, right heart strain and ultimately right heart failure or cor pulmonale.

Even without pulmonary insufficiency, anaesthetic management of the morbidly obese can be demanding, and endotracheal intubation difficult. An oral airway is inserted following muscle relaxation with vercuronium and sodium thiopental induction. An anaesthesiologist and an assistant are usually required to oxygenate an obese patient adequately before intubation. The patients are operated on in the reverse Trendelenburg position (15–20°) using a four-point fixation table-mounted retractor. Excellent relaxation is required to make this retraction most effective. Most patients are extubated in the operating room and returned to their room after a period of observation in the recovery room.

Epidural analgesia is more effective than routine pain medication and can be used with safety, even though prophylactic heparin 5000 iu given every 12 hours is used routinely starting preoperatively and continuing until the patient is fully mobile.

Prolonged ventilation in an intensive care unit may be required for patients with sleep apnoea syndrome or the obesity hypoventilation syndrome.

Surgically induced weight loss is capable of improving arterial oxygenation, minimizing carbon dioxide retention, expanding lung volumes, correcting polycythaemia and eliminating apnoea. The respiratory insufficiency of obesity should be considered a major indication for surgery.

In patients without overt pulmonary failure, pulmonary function is still a major consideration. We followed functional residual capacity in obese patients after surgery and found a 30% decrease immediately after surgery.[99] This worsened over the first 24 hours if the patient was left in bed rather than moving to a chair. The decrease in functional residual capacity persists longer in obese patients than in normal subjects. By the fifth postoperative day, functional residual capacity had returned to 80% of preoperative values in the obese but was completely normal in controls. Early ambulation, even on the day of surgery, is possible with epidural analgesia and produces a 10–15% improvement in functional residual capacity in the obese.

CARDIAC FUNCTION IN THE MORBIDLY OBESE

Morbidly obese patients may have significant cardiac dysfunction. The evidence for this has been accumulating over the years with the initial studies having been done by pathologists, who identified ventricular hypertrophy.[100] The hearts of these patients did not have fat infiltration nor did they have accelerated atherosclerotic muscular disease, but a thickened left ventricular wall.[101] There have been a number of echocardiography studies that have revealed that the ventricular hypertrophy of the morbidly obese patient is present without significant changes in chamber size.[102] Further investigations have shown that ventricular dysfunction is associated with ventricular hypertrophy.[103] These studies have shown that the filling pressures of the heart are increased. A study by Agarwal et al.[104] investigated the ventricular function of the heart during surgery. It was found that there were abnormal elevations of the filling pressures with a decrease in the ventricular function in morbidly obese patients compared with normal weight individuals.

We have conducted a study on 30 morbidly obese patients using echocardiography, a radionucleotide angiography scan and right heart catheterization.[105] In these studies we found evidence of hypertrophy of the ventricle in 32% of the patients

and a calculated ventricular mass of 430 g (normal value 300 g). Associated with this there was evidence of a non-compliant ventricle when the heart of the morbidly obese patient was stressed either by exercise or fluid challenges. When the ventricle was challenged, the stroke volume remained fixed and increased cardiac output was dependent on an increase in heart rate.

Cardiac output was not increased to the degree expected by the increased filling pressures which resulted from exercise or a fluid load. Although most physicians caring for these patients recognize that cardiac reserve is limited, this is most clearly seen in those more morbidly obese patients who have immediate postoperative complications, such as sepsis.

There is optimism that weight loss will improve cardiac function (Table 40.11).[106] There are reports that show that the incidence of hypertension is significantly decreased after weight loss.[107] Improvement in left ventricular function with weight loss has been documented.[108] It is disturbing that a corresponding decrease in left ventricular hypertrophy has not been demonstrated after weight loss in morbidly obese patients as it has been in the mildly obese.[109] Confirmation of these findings, using invasive as well as non-invasive techniques, should make it possible to be more reliant on the non-invasive techniques in the thorough evaluation of the morbidly obese patient. It is reasonable to expect a greater refinement of risk related to cardiac function and more progressive management of obesity.

Table 40.11 Cardiovascular benefits of weight loss

Total body oxygen requirements decrease
Arteriovenous oxygen difference decreases
Cardiac output decreases
Systemic arterial pressure decreases
Total blood volume decreases
Stroke volume at rest decreases
Left ventricular stroke work at rest decreases

NUTRITION AFTER OPERATIONS FOR OBESITY

Malnutrition occurs commonly in patients who have had significant weight loss after operations for morbid obesity. The malnutrition that develops after jejunoileal bypass is kwashiorkor in type, as it is associated with hepatic dysfunction and is similar to that which occurs with protein deprivation without carbohydrate restriction. These patients usually have a reduction in the plasma concentration of essential amino acids, an elevation of plasma glycine and a favourable therapeutic response either to intravenous amino acids or to restoration of intestinal continuity.

In contrast, operations designed to limit intake result in a decreased intake of both calories and protein and this state of malnutrition more closely mimics marasmus, in which liver failure is rare but vitamin deficiencies are common. Patients with malnutrition after intake limiting procedures exhibit weakness, easy fatiguability, a failure to return to former occupation, repeated infections, immunological incompetence,

Wernicke–Korsakoff syndrome and vitamin B_{12} and folic acid deficiencies.

The malnutrition that develops after all operations is characterized by an abnormal contraction of the body cell mass with an expansion of the extracellular mass. Body composition can be determined by isotope dilution techniques. The totally exchangeable sodium (Na_e) can be determined from the equilibrated plasma sodium-22 specific activity at 24 hours; total body water can be calculated from the equilibrated plasma tritium concentration at 24 hours and total exchangeable potassium (K_e) can be calculated from total body water, Na_e and the ratio in whole blood of the sodium plus potassium content divided by its water content.[110]

Lean body mass, body fat and body cell mass can be calculated from equations readily available. The total exchangeable sodium to total exchangeable potassium ratio (Na_e/K_e) is a sensitive index of nutritional state. In the normally nourished, this ratio approximates unity with an upper 95% confidence limit of 1.22. Malnutrition is defined as a loss of body cell mass accompanied by an expansion of extracellular mass and thus an increase in the Na_e/K_e ratio. Malnutrition is defined as a Na_e/K_e ratio greater than 1.22.[104]

Figures 40.14 and 40.15 show results, after intestinal bypass and gastric bypass, of the two types of nutritional deficiencies both characterized by a contraction of body cell mass in patients undergoing surgery for obesity.

Our own results on nutritional consequences of vertical banded gastroplasty showed that no patient developed malnutrition when studied one year after surgery despite regaining normal weight.[105] Unfortunately, many of these patients failed at a later date probably because of the small size of the orifice which permitted them to regain normal weight which ultimately led to breakdown of the vertical staple line.

Gastric restrictive operations which returned patients to within 25% of normal weight are associated with many good nutritional consequences. These include amelioration of diabetes mellitus and correction of liver function abnormalities.

Steatosis with abnormalities of liver function occurs commonly in obesity. In 45 of 60 patients who underwent vertical

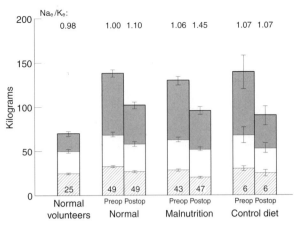

Figure 40.15

The body composition (■, fat; □ extracellular mass; ▨, body cell mass) before and after gastroplasty and gastric bypass in 47 patients with and 49 patients without malnutrition. The body composition in six patients who remained on a control diet of 750 kcal (178 kJ) daily by gastrostomy is also illustrated. The body composition of 25 normal volunteers is included.

banded gastroplasty, one or more liver function tests were abnormally elevated before surgery. At 1 year after surgery, liver function tests were normal in all but six of the 60 patients.[105] The weight loss was good in one of these liver failures, satisfactory in three and unsatisfactory in two. In contrast, liver dysfunction is common after intestinal bypass and is especially severe in patients who develop malnutrition. Correction of the contracted body cell mass by intravenous amino acids or by surgical restoration of normal intestinal continuity promptly reverses even severe liver failure.[111]

CONCLUSIONS

Surgery for morbid and superobesity or clinically significant obesity is still developmental. Long-term follow-up is essential and minimally must be 3–5 years to establish the value of a given operation. Gastric bypass has given the optimal long-term results at this time, with weight loss, a reduction in weight related co-morbidities and a low risk for complications. The most important benefits have been socioeconomic rehabilitation, amelioration of diabetes mellitus, improvement in liver function, lowering of blood uric acid levels, improvement in hypertension, fall in blood triglyceride levels, greater mobility and decrease in symptoms in weight-bearing joints.

It is possible that the surgically induced weight loss will be associated with improvement in major areas of weight-related dysfunction such as cardiac function. The Swedish obesity study comparing surgery to diet is still underway, but there are initial data indicating that there is a reduction in morbidity and mortality with bariatric surgery.

As we wait for the biology of obesity to be understood and our ability to determine the patient at risk with their obesity to improve, surgery is the proven treatment for this degree of obesity. Selection of patients on the basis of propensity to obesity and ways to determine the relative risks of different types of obesity hold promise for the future. The effect of surgically

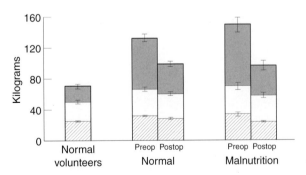

Figure 40.14

The body composition (■, fat; □, extracellular mass; ▨, body cell mass) before and after jejunoileal bypass in 11 patients with and 33 patients without malnutrition. The body composition of 25 normal weight volunteers is included for comparison.

induced weight loss on morbidity and long-term life expectancy has not been clearly defined.

REFERENCES

1. National Institutes of Health Consensus Development Panel on the Health Implications of Obesity. Health implications of obesity. *Ann Intern Med* 1985; **103**: 1073.
2. Van Itallie TB. Health implications of overweight and obesity in the United States. *Ann Intern Med* 1985; **103**: 983.
3. Sugarman HJ. Pulmonary function in morbid obesity. *Gastroenterol Clin North Am* 1987; **16**: 225.
4. Brownell KD. Obesity: understanding and treating a serious, prevalent, and refractory disorder. *J Consult Clin Psychol* 1982; **50**: 820.
5. Drenick EJ & Johnson D. Weight reduction by fasting and semistarvation in morbid obesity: long-term follow-up. *Int J Obes* 1978; **2**: 123.
6. Kluthe R & Schubert A. Obesity in Europe. *Ann Intern Med* 1985; **103**: 1037.
7. Garrison RJ & Castelli WP. Weight and thirty-year mortality in men in the Framingham study. *Ann Intern Med* 1985; **103**: 1006.
8. Drenick EJ, Bale GS, Seltzer F & Johnson DG. Excessive mortality and causes of death in morbidly obese men. *JAMA* 1980; **243**: 443.
9. Manson JE, Willett WC, Stampfer MJ et al. Body weight and mortality among women. *N Engl J Med* 1995; **333**: 677–685.
10. Colditz GA. Economic costs of obesity. *Am J Clin Nutr* 1992; **55** (Suppl.): 503S–507S.
11. Van Itallie TB. 'Morbid' obesity: a hazardous disorder that resists conservative treatment. *Am J Clin Nutr* 1980; **33**: 358.
12. Bray GA. Use and abuse of appetite-suppressant drugs in the treatment of obesity. *Ann Intern Med* 1993; **119**: 707–713.
13. Bray GA, Ryan DH, Gordon D, Heidingsfelder S, Cerise F & Wilson K. A double-blind randomized placebo-controlled trial of silbutramine. *Obes Res* 1996; **4**: 263–270.
14. Currey H, Malcolm R, Riddle E & Schachte M. Behavioral treatment of obesity. Limitations and results with the chronically obese. *JAMA* 1977; **237**: 2829.
15. Garrow JS. *Obesity and Related Diseases*. Edinburgh and London: Churchill Livingstone, 1988.
16. *Canadian Guidelines for Health Weights*. Ottawa: Health and Welfare Canada, 1988.
17. Bjorntorp P. Obesity and the risk of cardiovascular disease. *Ann Clin Res* 1985; **17**: 3.
18. Bray GA. Definition, measurement, and classification of the syndromes of obesity. In Bray G (ed.) *Obesity KROC Foundation Symposium on Comparative Methods of Weight Control*. London: John Libbey, 1980.
19. Norgan NG & Ferro-Luzzi A. Principal components as indicators of body fatness and subcutaneous fat patterning. *Hum Nutr Clin Nutr* 1985; **39**: 45.
20. Seltzer CC. Some re-evaluations of the build and blood pressure study, 1959 as related to ponderal index, somatotype and mortality. *N Engl J Med* 1966; **274**: 254.
21. Larsson B. Regional obesity as a health hazard in men – prospective studies. *Acta Med Scand Suppl* 1988; **723**: 45.
22. Lapidus L & Bengtsson C. Regional obesity as a health hazard in women – a prospective study. *Acta Med Scand Suppl* 1988; **723**: 53.
23. Bouchard C. Genetic factors in the regulation of adipose tissue distribution. *Acta Med Scand Suppl* 1988; **723**: 135.
24. Dublin LI. Relation of obesity to longevity. *N Engl J Med* 1953; **248**: 971.
25. Hirsch J & Leibel RL. New light on obesity. *N Engl J Med* 1988; **318**: 509.
26. Garrow JS & Wright D. Burning off unwanted energy. *Lancet* 1980; **i**: 377.
27. Ravussin E, Lillioja S, Knowler WC et al. Reduced rate of energy expenditure as a risk factor for body-weight gain. *N Engl J Med* 1988; **318**: 467.
28. Bogardus C, Lillioja S, Ravussin E et al. Familial dependence of the resting metabolic rate. *N Engl J Med* 1986; **315**: 96.
29. Fontaine E, Savard R, Tremblay A, Despres JP, Poehlman E & Bouchard C. Resting metabolic rate in monozygotic and dizygotic twins. *Acta Genet Med Gemellol (Roma)* 1985; **34**: 41.
30. Bouchard C. Genetic factors in obesity. *Med Clin North Am* 1989; **73**: 67.
31. Sorensen TIA, Price RA, Stunkard AJ & Schulsinger F. Genetics of obesity in adult adoptees and their biological siblings. *BMJ* 1989; **298**: 87.
32. Ravussin E, Lillioja S, Anderson TE, Christin L & Bogardus C. Determinants of 24-hour energy expenditure in man: methods and results using a respiratory chamber. *J Clin Invest* 1986; **78**: 1568.
33. Roberts SB, Savage J, Coward WA, Chew B & Lucas A. Energy expenditure and intake in infants born to lean and overweight mothers. *N Engl J Med* 1988; **318**: 461.
34. Jones PJH, Winthrop AL, Schoeller DA et al. Validation of doubly labeled water for assessing energy expenditure in infants. *Pediatr Res* 1987; **21**: 242.
35. Zhang Y, Proenca R, Maffei M, Barone M, Leopold L & Freidman JM. Positional cloning of the mouse obese gene and its human homoloque. *Nature* 1994; **372**: 425–431.
36. Tartaglia LA, Dembski M, Weng X et al. Identification and expression cloning of a leptin receptor, OB-R. *Cell* 1995; **83**: 1263–1271.
37. Kremen AJ, Linner JH & Nelson CH. An experimental evaluation of the nutritional importance of proximal and distal small intestine. *Ann Surg* 1954; **140**: 439.
38. Linner JH. *Surgery for Morbid Obesity*. New York: Springer-Verlag, 1984.
39. Payne JH, De Wind L, Schwab CE & Kern WH. Surgical treatment of morbid obesity – sixteen years of experience. *Arch Surg* 1973; **106**: 423.
40. Scott HW Jr, Dean R, Shull HJ et al. New considerations in use of jejunoileal bypass in patients with morbid obesity. *Ann Surg* 1973; **177**: 723.
41. Buchwald H, Varco RL, Moore RB & Schwartz MZ. Intestinal bypass procedures. Partial ileal bypass for hyperlipidemia and jejunoileal bypass for obesity. *Curr Probl Surg* 1975; **12 (4)**: 1.
42. Salmon PA. The results of small intestine bypass operations for the treatment of obesity. *Surg Gynecol Obstet* 1971; **132**: 965.
43. Cleator IGM & Gourlay RH. Ileogastrostomy for morbid obesity. *Can J Surg* 1988; **31**: 114.
44. Buchwald H, Campos CT, Boen JR, Nguyen PA & Williams SE. Disease-free intervals after partial ileal bypass in patients with coronary heart disease and hypercholesterolemia: report from the Program on the Surgical Control of the Hyperlipidemia (POSCH) *J. Am. Coll Cardiol* 1995; **26**: 351–357.
45. Stunkard AJ, Stinnett JL & Smoller JW. Psychological and social aspects of the surgical treatment of obesity. *Am J Psychiatry* 1986; **143**: 417.
46. Grace DM. Patient selection for obesity surgery. *Gastroenterol Clin North Am* 1987; **16**: 399.
47. Baddeley RM. The management of gross refractory obesity by jejuno-ileal bypass. *Br J Surg* 1979; **66**: 525.
48. Bray GA, Barry RE, Benfield JR, Castelnuovo-Tedesco P & Rodin J. Intestinal bypass surgery for obesity decreases food intake and taste preferences. *Am J Clin Nutr* 1976; **29**: 779.
49. MacLean LD, Rochon G, Munro M, Watson KEL & Shizgal HM. Intestinal bypass for morbid obesity: a consecutive personal series. *Can J Surg* 1980; **23**: 54.
50. Eriksson F. Biliointestinal bypass. *Int J Obes* 1981; **5**: 437.
51. Hallberg D & Holmgren U. Bilio-intestinal shunt. A method and a pilot study for treatment of obesity. *Acta Chir Scand* 1979; **145**: 405.
52. Scopinaro N, Gianetta E, Civalleri D, Bonalumi U & Bachi V. Bilio-pancreatic bypass for obesity: II. Initial experience in man. *Br J Surg* 1979; **66**: 618.
53. Biron S, Plamondon H, Bourque RA, Marceau P, Potvin M & Piche P. Clinical experience with biliopancreatic bypass and gastrectomy or selective vagotomy for morbid obesity. *Can J Surg* 1986; **29**: 408.
54. Holian DK. Biliopancreatic bypass for morbid obesity. *Contemp Surg* 1982; **21**: 55.
55. Compston JE, Vedi S, Gianetta E, Watson G, Civalleri D & Scopinaro N. Bone histomorphometry and vitamin D status after biliopancreatic bypass for obesity. *Gastroenterology* 1984; **87**: 350.
56. Gianetti E, Friedman D, Adami GF et al. Etiological factors of protein malnutrition after biliopancreatic diversion. *Gast Clin NA* 1987; **16**: 503.
57. Gianetta E, Adami GF, Friedman D et al. Protein malnutrition after biliopancreatic division (BPD). *Int J Obes* 1987; **11**: 206.
58. Garrow JS. Dental splinting in the treatment of hyperphagic obesity. *Proc Nutr Soc* 1974; **33**: 29A.
59. Garrow JS & Webster JD. Long-term results of treatment of severe obesity with jaw wiring and waist cord. *Proc Nutr Soc* 1986; **45**: 119A.
60. Drenick E & Hargis H. Wiring for weight reduction. *Obes Bariatr Med* 1978; **7**: 210.
61. Lerman RH & Cave DR. Medical and surgical management of obesity. *Adv Intern Med* 1989; **34**: 127.

62. Tretbar LL, Taylor TL & Sifers EC. Weight reduction. Gastric plication for morbid obesity. *J Kans Med Soc* 1976; **77**: 488.

63. Eckhout GV & Prinzing JF. Surgery for morbid obesity: comparison of gastric bypass with vertically stapled gastroplasty. *Colo Med* 1981; **78**: 117.

64. O'Leary JP. Partition of the lesser curvature of the stomach in morbid obesity. *Surg Gynecol Obstet* 1982; **154**: 85.

65. Laws HL & Piantadosi S. Superior gastric reduction procedure for morbid obesity. A prospective, randomized trial. *Ann Surg* 1981; **193**: 334.

66. Willbanks OL. Gastric restrictive procedures: gastroplasty. *Gastroenterol Clin North Am* 1987; **16**: 273.

67. Sugerman HJ, Starkey JV & Birkenhauer R. A randomized prospective trial of gastric bypass versus vertical banded gastroplasty for morbid obesity and their effects on sweets versus non-sweets eaters. *Ann Surg* 1987; **205**: 613.

68. Deitel M, Jones BA, Petrov I, Wlodarczyk SR and Basi S. Vertical banded gastroplasty: results in 233 patients. *Can J Surg* 1986; **29**: 322.

69. MacLean LD, Rhode BM & Forse RA. Late results of vertical banded gastroplasty for morbid and super obesity. *Surgery* 1990; **107**: 20–27.

70. Willbanks OL. Long-term results of silicone elastomer ring vertical gastroplasty for the treatment of morbid obesity. *Surgery* 1987; **101**: 606.

71. Flickinger EG, Sinar DR & Swanson M. Gastric bypass. *Gastroenterol Clin North Am* 1987; **16**: 283.

72. Yale CE. Gastric surgery for morbid obesity: Complications and long-term weight control. (In press).

73. Mason EE & Ito C. Gastric bypass. *Ann Surg* 1969; **170**: 329.

74. Alden JF. Gastric and jejunoileal bypass. A comparison in the treatment of morbid obesity. *Arch Surg* 1977; **112**: 799.

75. Griffen WO Jr. Gastric bypass for morbid obesity. *Surg Clin North Am* 1979; **59**: 1103.

76. Griffen WO Jr, Young VL & Stevenson CC. A prospective comparison of gastric and jejunoileal bypass procedures for morbid obesity. *Ann Surg* 1977; **186**: 500.

77. Reinhold RB. Critical analysis of long-term weight loss following gastric bypass. *Surg Gynecol Obstet* 1982; **155**: 385.

78. Thompson WR, Amaral JF, Caldwell MD, Martin HF & Randall HT. Complications and weight loss in 150 consecutive gastric exclusion patients – critical review. *Am J Surg* 1983; **146**: 602.

79. Pories WJ, Flickinger EG, Meelheim D, van Rij AM & Thomas FT. The effectiveness of gastric bypass over gastric partition in morbid obesity. Consequence of distal gastric and duodenal exclusion. *Ann Surg* 1982; **196**: 389.

80. Benotti PN, Hollingshead J, Mascioli EA, Bothe A Jr, Bistrian BR & Blackburn GL. Gastric restrictive operation for morbid obesity. *Am J Surg* 1989; **157**: 150.

81. Hornberger HR. Gastric bypass. *Am J Surg* 1976; **131**: 415.

82. Vaughan RW & Wise L. Choice of abdominal operative incision in the obese patient: a study using blood gas measurements. *Ann Surg* 1975; **181**: 829.

83. Brolin RE, Kenler HA, Gorman JH & Cody RP. Long-limb gastric bypass in the superobese. A prospective randomized study. *Ann Surg* 1992; **215**: 387–95.

84. Kral JG. Surgical treatment of obesity. In Wadden TA & Van Itallic (eds) *Treatment of the Seriously Obese Patient*. New York: The Guillford Press, 1992.

85. Mason EE, Doherty C, Maher JW, Scott DH, Rodriguez EM & Blommers TJ. Super obesity and gastric reduction procedures. *Gastroenterol Clin North Am* 1987; **16**: 495.

86. Unger SW, Unger HM, Edelman DS, Scott JS & Rosenbaum G. Obesity: an indication rather than a contraindication to laparoscopic surgery. *Obes Surg* 1992; **2**: 29–31.

87. Deitel M, Smith L & Harmantas A. Laparoscopic cholecystectomy after vertical banded gastroplasty. *Obes Surg* 1994; **4**: 13–15.

88. Catona A, Gossenberg M, LaManna A & Mussini G. Laparoscopic gastric banding: preliminary series *Obes Surg* 1993; **3**: 207–209.

89. Belachew M, Legrand M, Vincent V et al. Laparoscopic Adjustable Silicone Gastric Banding (LASGB) in the Treatment of Morbid Obesity. Presentation at the 7th ICO Satellite Symposium on the Surgical Treatment of Obesity, 1995.

90. Pories WJ, van Rij AM, Burlingham BT, Fulghum RS & Meelheim D. Prophylactic cefazolin in gastric bypass surgery. *Surgery* 1981; **90**: 426.

91. Joffe SN. A review: surgery for morbid obesity. *J Surg Res* 1982; **33**: 74.

92. Mason EE. *Surgery for Morbid Obesity – Major Problems in Clinical Surgery*. Philadelphia: WB Saunders, 1987.

93. Shaffer D, Benotti PN, Bothe A Jr, Jenkins RL & Blackburn GL. A prospective, randomized trial of abdominal wound drainage in gastric bypass surgery. *Ann Surg* 1987; **206**: 134.

94. Forse RA, Karam B, MacLean LD & Christou NV. Antibiotic prophylaxis for surgery in morbidly obese patients. *Surgery* 1989; **106**: 750–757.

95. Sugerman HJ, Kellum JM, DeMaria EJ & Reines HD. Conversion of failed or complicated vertical banded gastroplasty to gastric bypass in morbid obesity. *Am J Surg* 1996; **171**: 263–269.

96. Schwartz RW, Strodel WE, Simpson WS & Griffen WO Jr. Gastric bypass revision: lessons learned from 920 cases. *Surgery* 1988; **104**: 806.

97. Benotti PN & Forse RA. Safety and long-term efficacy of revisional surgery in severe obesity. *Am J Surg* 1996; **172**: 232–235.

98. Burwell CS, Robin ED, Whaley RD & Bickelmann AG. Extreme obesity associated with alveolar hypoventilation – a pickwickian syndrome. *Am J Med* 1956; **21**: 811.

99. Tin LK, Martin TJ, Ramsey J et al. The functional residual capacity in morbidly obese patients after gastroplasty. *Int J Obes* 1988; **12**: 608.

100. Smith HL & Willius FA. Adiposity of the heart. A clinical and pathologic study of one hundred and thirty-six obese patients. *Intern Med* 1933; **52**: 911.

101. Amad KH, Brennan JC & Alexander JK. The cardiac pathology of chronic exogenous obesity. *Circulation* 1965; **32**: 740.

102. Alpert MA, Terry BE & Kelly DL. Effect of weight loss on cardiac chamber size, wall thickness and left ventricular function in morbid obesity. *Am J Cardiol* 1985; **55**: 783.

103. de Divitiis O, Fazio S, Petitto M, Maddalena G, Contaldo F & Mancini M. Obesity and cardiac function. *Circulation* 1981; **64**: 477.

104. Agarwal N, Shibutani K, San Filippo JA & Del Guercio LRM. Hemodynamic and respiratory changes in surgery of the morbidly obese. *Surgery* 1982; **92**: 226.

105. Meterissian S, Din AA, Lisbona R, MacLean LD & Forse RA. Assessment of cardiac function in the morbidly obese. *Surgery* 1990; **108**: 809–820.

106. Mason EE, Printen KJ, Barron P, Lewis JW, Kealey GP & Blommers TJ. Risk reduction in gastric operations for obesity. *Ann Surg* 1979; **190**: 158.

107. Brolin RE. Results of obesity surgery. *Gastroenterol Clin North Am* 1987; **16**: 317.

108. Archibald HE, Stallings VA, Pencharz PB et al. Changes in intraventricular septal thickness, left ventricular volume in obese adolescents on a high protein weight reducing diet. *Int J Obes* 1989; **13**: 265.

109. Messerli FH. Cardiovascular effects of obesity and hypertension. *Lancet* 1982; **i**: 1165.

110. Shizgal HM, Forse RA, Spanier AH & MacLean LD. Protein malnutrition following intestinal bypass for morbid obesity. *Surgery* 1979; **86**: 60.

111. MacLean LD, Rhode B & Shizgal HM. Nutrition after vertical banded gastroplasty. *Ann Surg* 1987; **206**: 555.

112. 1983 Metropolitan height and weight tables. *Stat Bull Metrop Insur Co* 1983; **64**: 2.

41

MISCELLANEOUS CONDITIONS OF THE STOMACH

CP Armstrong

GASTRIC DIVERTICULA

Incidence

Gastric diverticula are relatively rare when compared with other sites of diverticula in the gastrointestinal tract. In order of frequency, diverticula are found in the colon, duodenum, jejunum, oesophagus and stomach.[1] Palmer,[2] in the most complete review to date on the subject, collected 412 cases of gastric diverticula. Fifty-nine of these cases were found in 1 371 000 general hospital admissions; an incidence of 0.0043%. A total of 165 cases were diagnosed during 380 099 routine barium examinations; an incidence of 0.043%. In contrast Meeroff et al.[3] found 30 cases from 7500 radiological examinations; an incidence of 0.4%, which is ten times higher than that of Palmer. Gastric diverticula have been reported in 0.03–0.3% of routine endoscopies.[4,5] The true incidence of gastric diverticula is unknown because reported series often reflect enthusiasm for identifying these elusive anomalies. In asymptomatic individuals the incidence, based on autopsy studies, is approximately 0.02%. In patients with gastrointestinal complaints the incidence is probably around 0.1–0.5%.

Classification

Gastric diverticula have been classified by Rivers et al.[6,7] as:

1. True acquired: include all coats of the gastric wall, and are almost always located in the juxtacardiac region of the stomach. These diverticula will be discussed at length in this chapter.
2. Acquired: are caused by organic disease and are related to either (a) pulsion, caused by raised intragastric pressure; or (b) traction, caused by traction from extragastric structures, e.g. healing inflammatory processes such as pancreatitis and cholecystitis.
3. False: contain only some of the gastric layers.

Pathology

Gastric diverticula have an equal sex incidence and are found

at all ages. Most have been reported in patients aged between 20 and 60 years and this age incidence may reflect the ages at which radiological and endoscopic examination is most commonly performed. Several cases have been reported in infants.[8] Gastric diverticula are almost exclusively single and in Palmer's[2] extensive review only six of 412 patients had two diverticula. The diverticula are usually 1–5 cm in length, although rare cases of up to 11 cm have been reported. Their size varies from that of a pea to a lemon. The ostium of the diverticulum is usually 2–4 cm in diameter and the width of the neck has been related to symptoms. Diverticula with narrow necks are the most symptomatic and these diverticula may be commonly missed on routine radiology or endoscopy. Over three-quarters of true gastric diverticula are found in a strikingly constant site.[9,10] This area is high on the posterior wall of the fundus, 2 cm below the gastro-oesophageal junction and 3 cm from the lesser curve.

The position of gastric diverticula in Palmer's series of 412 patients is shown in Figure 40.1. The pyloric and antral areas account for approximately 15% of gastric diverticula. Rarely are diverticula found on the curvatures of the stomach.

Partial diverticula A variant from the ordinary type of diverticulum is described in the prepyloric area and has been termed a

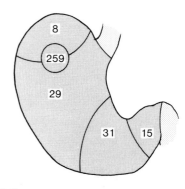

Figure 41.1
Position of gastric diverticula (posterior view of stomach). (Adapted with permission from Palmer.[2])

'partial' or 'intramural' diverticulum.[11-13] In these diverticula mucosa projects into, but not through, the muscular wall of the stomach, resulting in a normal external appearance. These diverticula are usually clinically insignificant but may cause diagnostic confusion.

Pathogenesis

Most authors consider juxtacardiac gastric diverticula to be of congenital origin. Various workers[7,14-17] have subscribed to the concept of the presence of a 'locus minoris resistentiae' in the gastric wall, through which diverticula form. The underlying anatomical basis for this weakness relates to division of the longitudinal muscle fibres in the region of the cardia, creating a weak point in which the wall is formed mostly of circular and oblique fibres. Large penetrating branches of the left gastric artery further weaken the area, and another reason for weakness may be the deficiency in peritoneal covering of the posterior wall of the stomach for 2–3 cm below the cardia.

Kurgan and Hoffmann[18] advanced an elegant hypothesis as to the aetiology of juxtacardiac diverticula. Their theory is based on the posterior vagal trunk, its attachments to the coeliac plexus, and the presence in 91% of individuals of a fundal branch, the criminal nerve of Grassi.[19] This nerve enters the stomach at a constant position at the back of the fundus, a site which coincides with that of juxtacardiac gastric diverticula. During embryological development the stomach rotates, producing tension on the posterior vagal trunk which is fixed at the coeliac plexus. Tension is transmitted down Grassi's nerve to its site of insertion, leading to the formation of a true traction diverticulum (Figure 41.2). Grassi's nerve has a variable site of origin from the posterior vagus nerve and only a distal origin will give enough 'pull' to produce a diverticulum. Most other vagal nerve fibres enter the lesser curvature of the stomach and are not stretched during rotation. This hypothesis is an attractive explanation for both the site and frequency of juxtacardiac gastric diverticula. Final proof of this hypothesis requires the demonstration of a Grassi nerve emerging from the apex of a diverticulum.

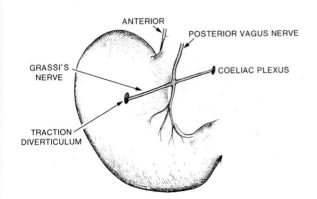

Figure 41.2

Aetiology of gastric diverticulum; the importance of the vagal nerve. (Reproduced with permission from Kurgan and Hoffman.[18]) Courtesy of Longmans Group Ltd.

Clinical features

The clinical importance of gastric diverticula has been a contentious issue for years as it appears that most are completely asymptomatic. Palmer[20] followed 50 patients with gastric diverticula for many years. Eleven remained asymptomatic, 30 developed symptoms from other gastrointestinal diseases, and in only nine patients were symptoms attributable to the diverticulum. Diverticulectomy was performed in six of the nine symptomatic cases with excellent results.

The most common symptoms attributable to gastric diverticula are those of postprandial epigastric fullness and uneasiness, nausea, vomiting, heartburn, epigastric pain and flatulent dyspepsia. This discomfort is usually intermittent and may be related to distension of the diverticular sac with food and gastric secretions. Anaise and colleagues[21] have described a patient with the above symptoms and endoscopic visualization of the diverticulum was associated with typical pain after gentle probing of the diverticular sac with biopsy forceps. Endoscopic pressure elsewhere on the gastric wall produced no discomfort. This case suggests that pain from a gastric diverticulum may relate to pressure or stretching of the diverticular wall. Furthermore it may be that reproduction of symptoms by gentle endoscopic pressure is a valid criterion for attributing them to the diverticulum. The non-specific symptoms of clinically relevant gastric diverticulum are frequency attributed to more common upper gastrointestinal pathology such as reflux oesophagitis, peptic ulceration, gastritis, oesophagogastric neoplasia, cholelithiasis and pancreatic disease.

A variety of complications from gastric diverticula have been described:

- *Haemorrhage.* Several cases of massive bleeding from a gastric diverticulum have been reported.[22-24] Gibbons and Harvey[25] demonstrated that bleeding originated from a benign peptic ulcer within the diverticulum. It seems likely that the mucosal lining of a gastric diverticulum is particularly predisposed to ulceration and haemorrhage.[23,25]
- *Acute diverticulitis* is more common in diverticula with a narrow neck and is associated with symptoms similar to those of an acutely penetrating gastric ulcer.
- *Perforation* is usually associated with acute diverticulitis or peptic ulceration and produces symptoms and signs indistinguishable from those of a perforated gastric ulcer. Ward et al.[26] have reported a case of massive haemoperitoneum due to bleeding from a perforated gastric diverticulum.
- *Torsion* of a diverticulum resulting in gangrene has been described.[27]
- *Dysphagia* has been related to juxtacardiac diverticula invaginating into the oesophagus, giving a pseudotumour appearance at endoscopy.[28]

Rarely diverticula may contain enteroliths or foreign bodies. A gastric diverticulum has even been described in an inguinal hernia sac.[29] There is no obvious tendency toward carcinogenesis in gastric diverticula but occasionally incidental tumours may be found inside. Pyloroantral diverticula commonly contain heterotopic pancreatic tissue.[2]

Diagnosis

As most gastric diverticula are asymptomatic the finding of these sacs is largely incidental. The condition is most frequently diagnosed by barium radiology. Akerlund[30] in 1923 was the first to describe the radiological findings. Gastric diverticula are shown as sac-like smooth outpouchings with an even contour and narrow neck. In the erect position the diverticulum will often show a fluid level capped with air. The contour may change with position and its size may increase on expiration. However, even the expert radiologist will on occasion have difficulty in filling the diverticular sac and may experience further problems in the interpretation of radiological images. Radiologically the juxtacardiac diverticulum fills by a small neck and varying angles of projection are sometimes necessary to demonstrate the pouch in profile because of its posterior location. It is best seen in the upright position, in the right anterior oblique projection (Figure 41.3). During screening it is sometimes possible to fill and empty a diverticulum by a change of position.[24] Juxtacardiac diverticula may be misdiagnosed as a large penetrating gastric ulcer, although the juxtacardiac location of most diverticula is a rare site for benign peptic ulceration. Identification of diverticula may be aided by the following criteria:

● Location.

● Demonstration of a connecting neck.

● Recognition of the mucosal surface in the neck and body.

● Muscular contraction with change in size and shape.

'Partial' gastric diverticula have several radiological characteristics, namely a site close to the pylorus, a pit of barium 1–2 mm deep contained entirely within the gastric wall, a well defined edge and a surrounding mound 1–2 cm in diameter.[11-13]

The widespread use of gastroscopy occasionally demonstrates an incidental gastric diverticulum. The juxtacardiac area is a relative 'blind spot' to the endoscopist and requires skilled examination with retroversion of the gastroscope (Figure 41.4). Endoscopy has rarely demonstrated a diverticular source for major gastrointestinal haemorrhage.[25] A large gastric diverticulum may be diagnosed by computed tomography (CT) with the stomach containing contrast medium. Coeliac angiography may be of benefit in patients with active haemorrhage from a gastric diverticulum.[22]

Treatment

As most diverticula are asymptomatic it would seem prudent to leave them alone unless they can be reasonably shown to be the cause of symptoms. When finding a gastric diverticulum in a patient with non-specific dyspepsia, it may be extremely difficult to causally relate the diverticulum to symptoms. Medical management has been advocated for symptomatic cases, although the results of such treatment are almost invariably disappointing. Postural drainage may be used in those patients unfit for surgery where pouch retention has been demonstrated.

The mainstay of treatment for symptomatic gastric diverticula lies with surgical resection. Operation has been advised under the following conditions.[31]

● Severe symptoms unresponsive to medical treatment.

● Complications such as haemorrhage or diverticulitis.

● Uncertain diagnosis, especially when malignancy is suspected.

(a)

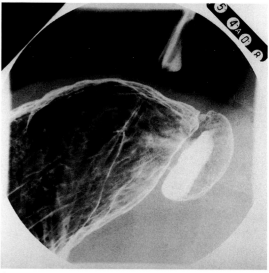

(b)

Figure 41.3
Barium meal ((a) AP view, (b) Lateral view) demonstrating a juxtacardiac gastric diverticulum. (Courtesy of Dr J. Virjee.)

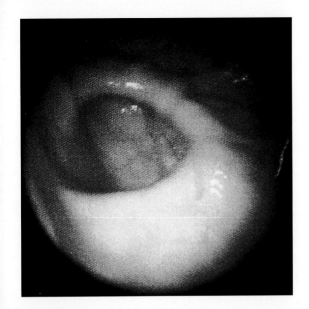

Figure 41.4
Endoscopic appearance of a juxtacardiac gastric diverticulum.

- When symptoms are undoubtedly from the diverticulum and other causes of upper abdominal dyspepsia have been excluded.
- Diverticula with a narrow neck and a wide sac.

Surgical excision may be difficult as most diverticula are in a relatively inaccessible area and there are frequent examples of these diverticula being missed at operation.[2,21] Difficulty in finding a juxtacardiac diverticulum may be eased by endoscopic localization of the sac immediately before or during surgery.[21] Hejboer and Nieuwenhuizen[32] have suggested cross-clamping the antrum and filling the stomach via a nasogastric tube to highlight the diverticular sac. Juxtacardiac diverticula are best exposed by dividing the gastrosplenic ligament and short gastric vessels. The stomach is then rotated to expose the posteriorly placed diverticula sac. Local excision with primary closure of the gastric defect is the treatment of choice. In Palmer's collected series[2] simple diverticulectomy was performed in 86 patients, invagination in 12 and partial gastrectomy in 16 with satisfactory results for each surgical procedure.

Diverticula in the pyloroantral region, when symptomatic, are best treated by partial gastrectomy with a Billroth I anastamosis.

GASTRIC DUPLICATION

The widespread use of the term duplication derives from the work of Ladd, Gross and Holcomb.[33–35] The use of the term duplication simplifies the nomenclature of these conditions which had previously been synonymously termed enteric cysts, enterogenous cysts, gastrogenous cysts, gastric enterocystoma and reduplication. Gastric duplication is defined as a mass lesion which develops in the stomach, that is distinct from it, and that contains all layers of the gastric wall.[36,37]

Incidence

Duplications of the alimentary tract can occur at any site from the mouth to the anus. Duplications have been regarded as relative rarities although they are now being reported with increasing frequency. Recent studies have shown that duplications occur in order of frequency in the ileum, oesophagus, colon, jejunum and stomach. Gross[38] had two cases of gastric duplication in a total of 68 intra-abdominal duplications. Bower and colleagues[39] from Pittsburgh, described 64 intra-abdominal duplications, of which six were of the stomach. Kremer et al.[40] saw nine cases of gastric duplications in 5 years and Abrami and Dennison[41] reported five cases. Bartels[42] in 1967 presented 55 cases of gastric duplication and Tabrisky et al.[43] reviewed 65 cases. Holcomb and colleagues[44] from Philadelphia reported their experience with 101 intestinal duplications in 96 children over a period of 38 years. The location and type of these duplications are shown in Table 41.1. These studies have shown that gastric duplications account for approximately 5–10% of all gastrointestinal duplications. The largest series of gastric duplications has been reported by Wieczorek and associates[45] who found 109 cases from an extensive analysis of the literature.

Table 41.1 Location of intestinal duplications

LOCATION	CYSTIC	TUBULAR	TOTAL
Oesophagus	21	—	21
Thoracoabdominal	—	3	3
Gastroduodenal	10	—	10
Jejunal	10	2	12
Ileal	25	10	35
Colonic	8	12	20
Total	74	27	101

After Holcomb et al.[44] with permission.

Pathology

In 1959 Rowling[46] summarized three essential criteria for making the diagnosis of gastric duplication:

1. The wall of the cyst is contiguous with the stomach wall.

2. The cyst is surrounded by smooth muscle which is continuous with the muscle of the stomach.

3. The wall of the cyst is lined by alimentary epithelium.

Gastric duplications usually have a common blood supply with the stomach from the gastroepiploic vessels. The lining mucosal epithelium secretes typical gastric juice containing acid and pepsin and the duplication is under the same hormonal and nervous influences as the stomach itself. Two-thirds of gastric duplications occur in females and one-third in males. This is contrary to other alimentary duplications in which most (70%) occur in males. The majority of cases are diagnosed in the first 3 months of life, although a significant number (25%) are found in teenagers and young adults. Rarely gastric duplications present with symptoms in late adult life.[47]

The most common location is along the greater curvature,

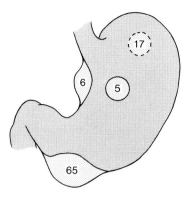

Figure 41.5
Position of gastric duplications. (Reproduced with permission from Wieczorek et al.[45])

Table 41.2 Location of heterotopic gastric and pancreatic tissue

DUPLICATIONS	NUMBER	HETEROTOPIC TISSUE	
		GASTRIC	PANCREATIC
Oesophagus	21	7	—
Thoracoabdominal	3	1	—
Gastroduodenal	10	—	3
Jejunal	12	1	1
Ileal	35	11	—
Colonic	20	1	1
Total	101	21	5

From Holcomb et al.[44] with permission.

with most being found in the antrum. Several cases of complete gastric duplication extending from the oesophagus to the pylorus have been reported. In the series of Wieczorek et al.[45] seven of 109 cases were complete duplications and it is of note that no duplication was reported solely at the cardia or oesophagogastric junction. The relative position of gastric duplications is shown in Figure 41.5. Gastric duplications may be tubular or cystic. The tubular type usually communicates with the stomach whereas the cystic type rarely does. In the review by Wieczorek and colleagues[45] 69 cases (82%) were cystic and did not communicate, whereas 14 (18%) were tubular and did communicate. Bartels[42] has also reported communication between the gastric duplication and either the umbilicus or a Meckel's diverticulum. If the duplication communicates with the true gastric lumen then the fluid it secretes will pass into the gut. However, since most are closed and cystic, high pressure rapidly develops within the duplication, leading to mucosal inflammation and eventual necrosis. The final pathological process is that of mucosal destruction and perforation. The volume of gastric duplications varies from 15 ml to over 1000 ml.[48] In infants the duplication may be three to four times the size of the normal stomach. Generally gastric duplications are filled with a viscid and mucoid material that is sometimes clear and at other times dark and contains blood.

The mucosal lining of gastric duplications is usually gastric although duodenal, colonic, ileal and jejunal linings also occur.[43] Heterotopic pancreatic tissue is found in approximately 10% of gastric duplications[40,42] and Bartels[42] reported that five of his 55 cases contained heterotopic pancreatic tissue. Gastric mucosa may also be present in duplications at other gastrointestinal sites. Favara et al.[49] described 38 intestinal duplications, of which two were in the stomach. Ten of these 38 duplications contained heterotopic gastric mucosa. Holcomb and colleagues[44] have summarized their experience with heterotopic gastric and pancreatic tissue in intestinal duplications as shown in Table 41.2. There are several cases of abdominal cysts lined with gastric mucosa and having a smooth muscle wall. However, these cysts do not satisfy Rowling's[46] criteria for gastric duplication as they do not share a common muscular wall with the stomach. Wieczorek and associates[45] describe 12 such cysts lined with gastric mucosa and two also had pancreatic

tissue in the submucosa. Seven of these 12 cysts had ulcerated linings.

Occasionally gastric duplications communicate with the pancreatic ductal system and Hoffman and colleagues[50] described six cases with this abnormality. In four patients the duplications were contiguous with the stomach and in two the duplications were separate. All four patients with contiguous gastric duplications had recurrent episodes of pancreatitis, whereas the non-contiguous duplications did not have hyperamylasaemia. The four patients with contiguous duplications had an accessory lobe of pancreatic tissue originating from the main pancreas. This accessory lobe contained a duct that communicated with both the gastric duplication and the main pancreatic duct. Torma[51] has further commented on the association between gastric duplication and malunion of the pancreatic anlage. He describes a stringy portion of pancreatic duct tissue from the ventral bud that is pulled anterior and cephalad to the developing gastric duplication.

Pathogenesis

Duplications arise from disturbances in the embryonic development of the gastrointestinal tract. Several theories have been proposed for the formation of intestinal duplications at varying sites.[52] These theories are the diverticular theory of Lewis and Thyng,[53] the split notochord or neuroenteric theory of Saunders,[54] Bentley and Smith[55] and McLetchie et al.[56] and the suggestion by Mellish and Koop[57] that environmental factors such as trauma or hypoxia in early fetal development are responsible. The most plausible explanation is the aberrant recanalization theory of Bremer.[58,59] In the 6-week embryo the intestinal tract is increasing in length more rapidly than the embryo as a whole. This rapid growth in length is preceded by an increase of its epithelial cells to such an extent that in some regions the lumen of the gut tube becomes reduced or even occluded. This is known as the solid stage of the intestinal tract. Normally the cells of the epithelial mass secrete a fluid that gathers into vacuoles. The vacuoles tend to coalesce with one another, forming the intestinal lumen. In rare cases the chains of fused vacuoles may retain their form and cause intestinal duplications. If the vacuoles only coalesce with one another the resultant cyst does not communicate with the main lumen. If the vacuoles coalesce with one another to form a cyst and then one opens into the main lumen, there will be a communication between the duplication and the lumen of the bowel. Bremer[58] postulated that with growth the two lumina move apart and that the wall of the bowel grows in between them so that ultimately two complete walls form. There are, however, some difficulties with Bremer's theory and it seems that no one explanation is tenable for every alimentary duplication. The association of pancreatic abnormalities with gastric duplications is better explained by the neuroenteric theory of McLetchie.[56]

Clinical features

The symptoms of a gastric duplication will depend on its size, position, communication with the gastrointestinal tract and the coexistence of other abnormalities. Most duplications are found in infants and young children, although 25–30% are found after 12 years of age. Wieczorek and colleagues[45] tabulated the symptoms in their review of gastric duplications (Table 41.3). Gastric outlet obstruction manifested by vomiting was noted in over one-third of Wieczorek's series and was particularly common in infants. Many duplications attain a large size before detection and in the report of Tabrisky et al.[43] two-thirds of patients presented with a palpable, often tender, epigastric mass. Anaemia or bleeding episodes are seen in one-third of gastric duplications and are particularly noticeable in the older patient. Occasionally gastric duplications are associated with pneumonia or pleural effusion. One case[60] involved a gastric duplication that extended into the thorax through the oesophageal hiatus. The duplication communicated with the main pancreatic duct and the right pleural cavity, resulting in chronic pancreatitis and a chronic pleural effusion.

Table 41.3 Symptoms associated with 109 gastric duplications

SYMPTOM	NUMBER
Mass	65
Vomiting	61
Abdominal pain	35
Weight loss; failure to thrive	32
Anaemia	26
Malaena	17
Haematemesis	12
Abdominal distension	12
Fever	8
Asymptomatic	3

Other rare symptoms included diarrhoea, dehydration, constipation, dyspnoea, cyanosis, pneumonia and pleural effusion.
From Wieczorek et al.[45] with permission.

Several potentially serious complications have been reported with gastric duplications.

Perforation may occur either into adjacent structures, with fistulation, or directly into the peritoneal cavity. Several of these perforations have been fatal and Bower et al.[39] describe

a perforated gastric duplication that was found at autopsy and was the cause of death. In the series of 109 cases reported by Wieczorek et al.[45] 13 perforations were described. Perforation is due to either necrosis of the duplication resulting from high pressure or as a result of peptic ulceration in the duplication.

Bleeding may occur into a non-communicating duplication, resulting in anaemia. Bleeding into the gut may be the result of a communicating duplication or of erosions or ulceration in the adjacent stomach. The bleeding of gastric duplications is usually a result of gastric juice acting on the duplication mucosa to produce gastritis and peptic ulceration. Occasionally intractable peptic ulceration is found in association with a gastric duplication and this has been related to either hypersecretion of gastrin[61] or the duplication acting as an antral pouch.[62] One large ulcer in a gastric duplication penetrated the aorta and caused exsanguinating haemorrhage.[63]

Pyloric stenosis occurs as a result of duplications in the pyloric region. This situation is often misinterpreted as congenital hypertrophic pyloric stenosis.

Pancreatitis may develop as a result of communication with the pancreatic duct.[44,50,64] It has been postulated that pancreatitis develops as a result of blood or gastric juice causing obstruction and inflammation in the pancreatic duct.

Carcinoma is a rare complication of duplications. Orr and Edwards[65] reported eight cases of carcinoma developing in intestinal duplications. One case[66] was in a 64-year-old woman who developed a well-differentiated adenocarcinoma with nodal involvement in a gastric duplication. Another carcinoma developed in an ileal duplication lined with gastric mucosa.[67]

Coexisting anomalies are frequently found and have been reported in 33–50% of all cases of gastric duplication. The coexisting anomalies in the report of Wieczorek and associates[45] are shown in Table 41.4. Further intestinal duplications are commonly seen in association with gastric duplications. In the review of Tabrisky and colleagues[43] 12 of 65 patients with gastric duplications had a second intestinal duplication and these were present in the oesophagus in four, stomach in three, duodenum in three, ileum in one and colon in one.

Table 41.4 Gastric duplications[109]: coexisting anomalies

ANOMALY	NUMBER
Oesophageal duplication	9
Vertebral anomalies	8
Aberrant pancreas	7
Duodenal duplication	4
Malrotation of gut	3
Pulmonary sequestration	3
Splenic abnormality	2
Urinary tract abnormality	2
Turner's syndrome	2
Patent ductus arteriosus	2
Ventricular septal defect	2
Meckel's diverticulum	2

From Wieczorek et al.[45] with permission.

Diagnosis

The most important investigations in the diagnosis of gastric duplications are radiological. A plain abdominal radiograph may show an abdominal mass, a distended stomach from gastric outlet obstruction or rarely calcification in the wall of the duplication.[68] A chest radiograph can demonstrate associated thoracic abnormalities such as oesophageal duplication, pulmonary sequestration and vertebral abnormalities. Barium radiology usually illustrates an extrinsic filling defect along the greater curvature or signs of gastric outlet obstruction (Figure 41.6a). Only 15–18% of gastric duplications communicate with the gastric lumen,[43,45] and thus barium rarely demonstrates the lining of the duplication.

Gastroscopy may be helpful in the diagnosis of a gastric duplication by showing an extrinsic mass indenting the greater curvature, a peptic ulcer, gastritis and rarely communication with the duplication.

Ultrasonography has recently been used in the diagnosis of intestinal duplication. Lamont and colleagues[69] reported excellent results with this technique and showed that duplications have a highly echogenic inner rim, due to the mucosal lining, with active contractility in the muscular wall. Extensive ulceration of the mucosa by gastric juice may destroy the inner lining so that the duplication may resemble an abscess, a haematoma or a pseudocyst of the pancreas.

CT has also been used, particularly when associated oesophageal duplications are suspected.[44] A gastric duplication will show as a smooth, well-marginated, circumscribed mass of homogeneous material. The mass is contiguous with the stomach, with a low attenuation of 15–30 Hounsfield units. The outer rim enhances with contrast material, whereas the central core remains dark. Magnetic resonance imaging may also be used to visualize associated vertebral anomalies and thus help to identify individuals at risk for neurological injury associated with surgical resection.[63] Technetium-99m scanning is useful in the detection of gastric mucosa in the same way as in the detection of a Meckel's diverticulum (Figure 41.6b). Promising results have been reported with technetium scanning in patients with intestinal duplications containing gastric mucosa.[70,71]

Endoscopic retrograde cholangiopancreatography (ERCP) is used in those rare patients who have pancreatitis resulting from communication with a gastric duplication. Hoffman and colleagues[50] used this technique to identify an anomalous pancreatic duct communicating with a gastric duplication in a patient with recurrent pancreatitis. They also remarked on the ease of making a misdiagnosis of a pancreatic pseudocyst.

Treatment

The treatment for the vast majority of gastric duplication patients is surgical. According to Torma[51] the reasons for operation are gastric outlet obstruction, gastrointestinal bleeding, perforation, fistulation, suspected malignancy and to confirm the diagnosis. The surgical procedure should not be more radical than necessary to eliminate the patient's complaints and prevent further recurrence.[44] Ravitch[52] emphasizes that surgical preference should be for an operation that removes all of the duplication lining. The operative technique consists of dissecting the duplication from the common muscle wall or excising the duplication with a margin of normal stomach and primary

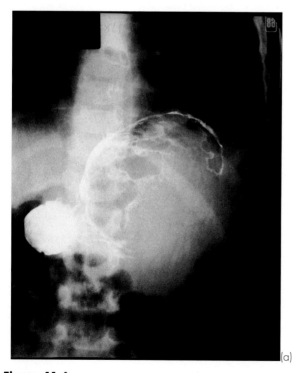

(a)

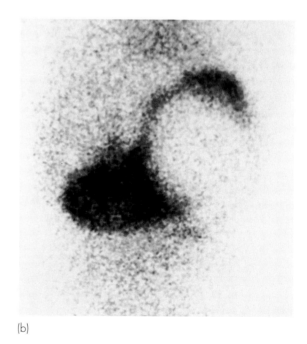

(b)

Figure 41.6
(a) Barium meal in a child demonstrating a large filling defect along the greater curvature of the stomach. (Courtesy of Dr J. Virjee.)
(b) Technetium-99m scan demonstrating a filling defect along the greater curvature of the stomach. (Courtesy of Dr J. Virjee.)

closure. Some cases may require partial excision of the duplication with mucosal stripping from the common wall. Surgery may be facilitated by needle aspiration of the duplication before dissection. After removal of the duplication small gastric perforations should be ruled out by distending the stomach with air via a nasogastric tube. Simple marsupialization is usually unsuccessful and in the series of Wieczorek et al.[45] four of eight marsupializations had disappointing results leading to eventual total excision of the duplication. In some infants, however, large duplications are best managed by wide gastrogastrostomy to prevent a small stomach syndrome. In rare cases the duplication cannot be excised and in these cases internal drainage is needed – either by gastrogastrostomy or by using a Roux loop of intestine. In infants with gastric outlet obstruction Torma[51] has emphasized the importance of testing the patency of the true pylorus as there may be intrinsic fibrous obliteration as well as extrinsic compression of the lumen. In patients with pancreatitis associated with gastric duplication, excision of both the duplication and the anomalous pancreas has resulted in relief of symptoms.[50]

RUPTURE OF THE STOMACH

Stomach rupture may occur spontaneously or as a result of external trauma. External trauma may be penetrating, nonpenetrating or iatrogenic.

Incidence

Traumatic rupture

Blunt Blunt trauma to the abdomen uncommonly results in rupture of the stomach. This is because the stomach is relatively protected in its anatomical location, has a thick wall, is usually empty and is highly mobile and distensible. Yajko and associates[72] reviewed the incidence of gastric rupture following severe blunt abdominal trauma, as shown in Table 41.5. The relative rarity of traumatic gastric rupture was further highlighted by Luccioni and Mammucari[78] who found only four cases of gastric rupture in a series of 6000 patients with less severe blunt abdominal trauma. Further reports[79–82] have shown that, although traumatic gastric rupture is relatively uncommon, it occurs sufficiently frequently to be clinically important.

Penetrating Penetrating injuries of the abdomen and chest are most frequently caused by gunshot and stab wounds. Nance

Table 41.5 Blunt abdominal trauma and gastric rupture in five reported series

REPORT	NUMBER OF CASES	GASTROINTESTINAL TRACT INJURY	STOMACH RUPTURE
Allen and Curry[73]	297	32 (11)	3 (1.0)
Fitzgerald et al.[74]	200	30 (15)	3 (1.5)
Rodkey[75]	177	29 (16)	3 (1.7)
Morton et al.[76]	120	13 (11)	2 (1.7)
Clarke[77]	107	19 (18)	1 (0.9)
Total	901	123 (13.7)	12 (1.3)

Values in parentheses are percentages.

and colleagues[83] from New Orleans reported their experience with penetrating wounds of the abdomen in 2212 patients (Table 41.6). This study showed that the stomach was the fourth most commonly injured intra-abdominal organ following penetrating trauma by either gunshot or stab.

Table 41.6 Penetrating abdominal wounds and the incidence of visceral injuries

VISCUS	WOUND	
	GUNSHOT (n=1032)	STAB (n=1180)
Small bowel	348	74
Colon	296	48
Liver	296	95
Stomach	184	47
Pancreas	82	8
Duodenum	60	10
Gall bladder	32	4

From Nance et al.[83] with permission.

Iatrogenic The increasing use of invasive investigations and non-operative treatments has resulted in an expanding number of iatrogenic injuries to the stomach. The most common of these injuries is gastric perforation following gastroscopy. The American Society for Gastrointestinal Endoscopy published the results of its survey in 1976.[84] They reviewed 211 410 gastroscopies and found 70 incidences of perforation, an incidence of 0.03%. Previous studies have found nine stomach perforations in 49 000 gastroscopies[85] (incidence 0.018%) and 75 gastric perforations in 267 175 gastroscopies[86] (incidence 0.028%). Schiller et al.[87] reported on 23 500 gastroscopies performed by 63 endoscopists and found 26 perforations, an incidence of 0.11%.

Spontaneous rupture

Spontaneous rupture of the stomach without any trauma to the abdominal wall or with a pre-existing pathological condition in the stomach is rare. Albo and colleagues[88] collected 43 cases in an extensive review in 1963. Evans[89] in 1968 reported 49 cases and Harling[90] in 1984 was able to find 70 cases in a collective review of all published reports. Similar gastro-oesophageal pathologies, such as spontaneous rupture of the oesophagus (Boerhaave syndrome) and mucosal lacerations (Mallory–Weiss tears), should not be confused with spontaneous gastric rupture.

Pathology

Traumatic rupture

Blunt Blunt traumatic rupture of the stomach usually occurs as a result of abdominal trauma shortly after eating a large meal. In the series of Yajko and colleagues[72] of 35 cases the average age was 31 years with a strong male preponderance. In adults rupture most frequently occurs near the lesser curvature, whereas in children most ruptures are located close to the greater curvature. Traumatic rupture of the stomach is followed by massive contamination of the upper abdomen which leads to rapid clinical deterioration.[91] Siemens and Fulton[91] have emphasized that blunt traumatic rupture of the stomach is often associated with injuries to other intra-abdominal viscera, including most commonly the spleen, liver, pancreas, colon, duodenum and mesentery. Complete stomach transection can rarely occur, with shearing of the stomach from its points of fixation at the oesophagus and stomach, following a direct, localized high velocity blow.[92]

Penetrating The stomach is the fourth most commonly injured intra-abdominal organ injured following gunshot or stab wounds.[82] Most penetrating wounds occur in young men and these injuries are often complicated by the prior ingestion of alcohol and drugs. Stab wounds to the stomach usually cause little damage to the stomach other than the entry and exit wounds. These gastric wounds can often be complicated by haemorrhage, particularly if a major artery or vein is transected. Associated wounds in surrounding structures are common and usually follow the direction of the stab. Stab wounds of the abdomen are most common in the upper anterior quadrants of the abdomen and are multiple in 20% of cases. The left side is more frequently involved, presumably related to the predominance of right-handed assailants.[93] Penetrating wounds to the lower chest inflict intra-abdominal injury in 15% of cases as a result of the ascent of the diaphragm and intra-abdominal contents during expiration. Stab wounds to the back are also associated with a 14% incidence of visceral injury. The parietal peritoneum is penetrated in 70% of cases of anterior and lateral abdominal stab wounds, although visceral injury is present in only one-third to one-half of these patients.[93]

Gunshot wounds are associated with more severe disruption of the stomach wall and frequently there is widespread intra-abdominal injury. Gunshots in the proximity of the abdomen enter the peritoneum in 80% of cases and cause visceral injury in 96–98% of these patients.[93] Low-velocity bullets tend to produce small wounds, whereas high-velocity projectiles cause gross disruption to the surrounding tissue as they impart large quantities of energy. Contamination by external material is frequent in gunshot wounds.

Spontaneous rupture

Spontaneous rupture of the stomach is more frequent in females and occurs at a mean age of 43 years.[88] In the reports of Harling[90] and Saul et al.[94] women accounted for 72 and 67%, respectively, of all cases of spontaneous rupture. Most spontaneous ruptures in adult stomachs occur on the proximal lesser curvature and this was the site in 73% of Albo and associates' series,[88] 60% in the report of Baglio and Futtal[95] and 63% in the review of Saul et al.[94] In most cases the rupture is single and in only three cases have multiple perforations been observed.[88] The size of the tear ranges from 1 cm to over 10 cm in length[95,96] and pathological examination of the stomach usually shows extreme thinning of the gastric wall around the site of rupture. In most cases there is no inflammatory response, although oedema and haemorrhage are present. The most marked histological abnormality is that of tearing and diastases

of isolated muscle bundles in a thin translucent wall. A recent case report[97] confirmed these pathological findings and further highlighted the extreme thinning of the stomach wall and the lack of inflammatory changes. Harling[90] has suggested that rupture begins as a mucosal tear followed by dissection in the deeper layers of the stomach and a longer tear in the serosa.

Pathogenesis

Traumatic rupture

Blunt The stomach is relatively protected against the forces of blunt trauma. Siemens and Fulton[91] suggested that blunt trauma resulted in gastric rupture as a result of (1) rapid deceleration injuries such as a fall or pressure from the steering wheel in motor accidents, (2) direct trauma to the abdomen, and (3) cardiopulmonary resuscitation. In their series 59% of patients had a full stomach before traumatic gastric rupture and most had multiple other injuries. Siemens and Fulton[91] postulated that inertia and rapid deceleration cause the full stomach to move forward while the lesser curvature remains fixed. The resultant shearing force leads, in most cases, to tearing along the anterior wall or lesser curvature, whereas the freely mobile and more distensible greater curvature can better tolerate rapid changes in tension. Yajko and colleagues[72] related blunt traumatic rupture to a rapid rise in intra-abdominal and intraluminal pressure. By Laplace's law, the transmural pressure P is related to intramural tension T and the radius of curvature R by the formula $P = k$ T/R. In the intestine, rupture occurs at the position of greatest radius. In the stomach, however, rupture is related to increasing intramural tension rather than increased intraluminal pressure.

Penetrating The protected location and pliability of the stomach renders this organ far more susceptible to penetrating injuries than to blunt trauma. Penetrating trauma often results in unrecognized, potentially lethal injuries to associated vascular structures.[93] Overall gunshot wounds are five times as lethal as stab wounds.[93]

Iatrogenic Iatrogenic injury and rupture of the stomach is most commonly related to endoscopic procedures such as gastroscopy, ERCP and laparoscopy. During gastroscopy air is introduced into the stomach under high pressure and this can rarely result in pneumoperitoneum.[98] or gastric perforation. The use of drainage tubes for thoracentesis, abdominal paracentesis and peritoneal dialysis has also caused gastric perforations. The widespread use of percutaneous endoscopic gastrostomy (PEG) has also resulted in gastric perforations. External cardiac massage and inadvertent oxygen insufflation during cardiopulmonary resuscitation are further causes of iatrogenic gastric rupture.[97]

Spontaneous rupture

The exact mechanism of spontaneous gastric rupture is unknown, although there appear to be two prerequisites for its pathogenesis, namely gastric distension and raised intra-abdominal pressure. Gastric distension alone is generally insufficient to cause gastric rupture. Revilloid[99] in 1885 demonstrated that over 4 litres of fluid were needed to rupture the stomachs of fresh cadavers. This reflects the stomach's extreme distensibility and shows that tremendous expansion must occur before rupture. Over half the reported cases of spontaneous gastric rupture are associated with the recent ingestion of a large meal. Albo and coworkers[88] found that 27 of 43 instances of gastric rupture were related to overeating and overdrinking. When the stomach is overdistended the angle between the stomach and the oesophagus is increased and the oesophagus is angulated against the fixed fibres of the right crus of the diaphragm. This rapidly leads to occlusion of the gastro-oesophageal junction, which then acts as a one-way valve, with aerophagia and gastric secretion adding to further distension.[88,97,100] Once acute gastric distension has developed, factors that increase intra-abdominal pressure like coughing, vomiting, exertion and grand mal seizures can precipitate rupture. Experimentally tears can be produced by the introduction of gas, fluid and an acid–bicarbonate mixture into cadaver stomachs.[88]

Distension causes the stomach to assume a spherical shape. The lesser curvature, with fewer folds and less elasticity, has a reduced capacity to distend than the rest of the stomach, which results in acute stretching of the gastric wall in this site. It is postulated that marked stretching of the relatively fixed mucosa along the lesser curvature results in ischaemic necrosis, and Glassman[101] thought that rupture was due to paralysis of the gastric wall with areas of softening and infarction. Infarction of the stomach wall does not usually occur with arterial insufficiency, as demonstrated by the Somervell operation performed in over 400 patients with duodenal ulceration.[88] Intragastric pressure must increase above gastric venous pressure to cause ischaemia and infarction. In dogs, gastric infarction only occurs when gastric veins, and not the arteries alone, are ligated.[90]

Spontaneous rupture of the stomach can occur in acute gastric dilatation and Saul et al.[94] reported 12 cases of rupture complicating acute gastric dilatation in patients with anorexia nervosa. One of these patients had over 8 litres of fluid in the stomach and peritoneum. Other aetiologies for spontanous gastric rupture include oxygen insufflation,[102] massive gastric haemorrhage[103] and ingestion of sodium bicarbonate.[104] Cramer and Heimbach[102] have reported a case of spontaneous rupture of the stomach as result of gastrointestinal barotrauma in a scuba diver. The probable mechanism in this case was the swallowing of water and the filling of the stomach with air when the diver became trapped at a depth of 27 metres. When he rose to the surface the pressure in his stomach increased, according to Boyle's law, more than twofold, resulting in stomach rupture.

When sodium bicarbonate is added to acidic gastric juice large quantities of carbon dioxide are released. Fordtran and colleagues[105] demonstrated that even if hydrochloric acid and bicarbonate react instantaneously, the resulting gas development is slow, mainly because the carbon dioxide dissolves in the fluid and is only slowly released to the gas phase. The most important exogenous features determining the rate of gas release were the volume of solution, the quantity of reactants, the air volume over the reaction mixture, the partial pressure of carbon dioxide in the solution before the bicarbonate was added, and the rate of mixing. Owing to the uncertainty in these factors, Fordtran and colleagues[105] speculated that the amount of gas released after ingestion of sodium bicarbonate would be difficult to predict. At the recommended dose of bicarbonate (1.8 g) 20 ml of gas as produced within 3 minutes, but 8.4 g of bicarbonate would give 470 ml of carbon dioxide in the same time. In the case of Brismar et al.[104] over 30 g of bicarbonate was ingested, resulting in enormous gas production and a ruptured stomach.

Clinical features

Traumatic rupture

Blunt The clinical features of blunt traumatic stomach rupture are often masked by coexisting serious injuries to the head, chest and extremities. The external signs of trauma to the abdomen may be minimal, despite the presence of marked intra-abdominal injuries. Examination may show abdominal bruising and associated chest injuries, such as fractured ribs and a pneumothorax. Clinically patients with ruptured stomachs are usually shocked and this may be further compounded by intra-abdominal bleeding from injuries to the liver and spleen. The abdomen is distended and painful due to the large amounts of intraperitoneal air and gastric contents. The patient is usually cyanosed and dyspnoeic owing to respiratory embarrassment caused by the abdominal distension and there may be cervical surgical emphysema due to mediastinal tracking of air. Passing a nasogastric tube will invariably reveal a bloody aspirate indicative of gastric injury.

Penetrating These injuries to the stomach are usually obvious with an external abdominal wound. However, care should be taken with lower thoracic and posterior trunk wounds which can also enter the peritoneum and damage the stomach.[93]

Iatrogenic These injuries to the stomach are manifest by their preceding history, although pain and other signs do not always occur immediately. Several days may elapse before stomach rupture presents to the surgeon and this is particularly related to day-case procedures such as endoscopy, laparoscopy and liver biopsy.

Spontaneous rupture

Spontaneous rupture of the stomach is usually preceded by a history of ingestion of a large meal followed by vomiting and sudden development of upper abdominal pain. Rapid clinical deterioration follows as a result of the massive release of air and gastric contents into the peritoneum and mediastinum. The cardinal early symptoms are those of dyspnoea, distension and abdominal tenderness. Vomiting is often absent, although it may be bloody in nature, and this may be related to the occluded gastro-oesophageal junction. Some patients develop surgical emphysema in the neck and this sign was present in seven of 43 (16%) patients in the report of Albo and colleagues.[88] Millar and associates[100] suggested a tetralogy of symptoms indicating spontaneous gastric rupture:

- Abdominal distension
- Signs of peritonitis
- Shock
- Air in the subcutaneous tissues of the neck.

A distinctive feature of spontaneous rupture is the rapid and often irreversible deterioration in the patient's clinical condition. The outpouring of serum, blood and gastric contents from the rupture site and bacterial contamination of the peritoneum combine to produce severe shock. Air and fluid escaping into the peritoneal cavity through the large gastric hole cause abdominal distension, splinting of the diaphragm and respiratory embarrassment. Frequently the diagnosis of spontaneous rupture of the stomach is made late, and in the report of Albo et al.[88] 25 of 43 patients with this condition had no operation and in many the diagnosis was first made at autopsy.

Diagnosis

Traumatic rupture

Blunt The diagnosis of blunt traumatic rupture of the stomach is often made late owing to the presence of concomitant injuries. Radiology of the chest and abdomen must be performed in all patients following major blunt trauma. Chest radiographs may demonstrate fractured ribs, haemo- or pneumothorax, mediastinal emphysema, raised or ruptured hemidiaphragm and gas under the diaphragm. Abdominal radiographs often show free abdominal fluid and gas, with the lateral decubitus film being of particular value. When the diagnosis of gastric rupture is uncertain the instillation of radiographic contrast via a nasogastric tube can be beneficial. Paracentesis may be helpful and Vassy et al.[81] report three cases of blunt traumatic gastric rupture in which paracentesis obtained fluid distinguishable from blood and suggestive of gastric contents. Peritoneal lavage is frequently used in the diagnosis of clinically significant blunt abdominal trauma. Fischer and associates[106] reported their experience in 2586 patients undergoing peritoneal lavage. The diagnostic accuracy in that large series was 98.5%, with 0.2% false positives and 1.2% false negatives. In the patient with gastric trauma peritoneal lavage may show free air, bloody fluid or gastric contents which are acidic on pH testing. Diagnostic laparoscopy can be very helpful, although care should be taken not to miss posterior perforations. CT is also useful, especially when combined with the instillation of contrast material into the stomach. Federle and coworkers[107] reported the use of CT scanning in 200 patients after blunt abdominal trauma with no false positives or negatives.

Penetrating Penetrating wounds of the abdomen and lower chest must always be considered to have entered the abdominal cavity. Chest radiographs will often show a haemo- or pneumothorax, with free gas under the diaphragm on an erect film. Abdominal radiographs demonstrate free gas and fluid and projectiles may also be visualized following gunshot injuries.

Spontaneous rupture

Spontaneous rupture of the stomach is rarely diagnosed before operation or death and in the report of Albo and colleagues[88] only one of 43 cases had a correct preoperative diagnosis. Radiology is the most helpful investigation and chest films may demonstrate mediastinal gas, lung collapse, pnemothorax and gas under the diaphragm. Abdominal radiology invariably shows large amounts of intraperitoneal fluid or gas. The use of contrast material (Gastrografin) can help differentiate a spontaneous rupture of the stomach from the more common oesophageal rupture (Boerhaave syndrome).

Treatment

Traumatic rupture

Blunt Blunt trauma to the abdomen requires rapid assessment of the extent of all coexisting injuries. Prompt resuscitation is mandatory and this must initially comprise the maintenance of adequate cardiorespiratory function through the use of oxygen, intravenous fluids, chest intubation and ventilation if required. Patients with suspected intra-abdominal trauma should have a nasogastric tube and urinary catheter passed and an intravenous line inserted and an early decision should be made as to whether laparotomy is needed. Laparotomy should be performed through a midline incision, with the perioperative use of broad-spectrum antibiotics. In the case of stomach injuries careful inspection of the anterior and posterior walls is needed. The lesser sac must always be opened and coexisting injuries to the spleen, liver, pancreas, duodenum, diaphragm and bowel excluded by meticulous examination. The site of stomach rupture is exposed, devitalized tissue removed, and the defect closed in two layers. Careful peritoneal toilet is an absolute requirement and may be aided by the use of large volumes of saline or antibiotic solution. Pieces of food are often present in the peritoneal cavity and must all be removed to prevent later infection. The healing capacity of the stomach is impressive and only one suture line leak has been reported.[91] Postoperative intra-abdominal sepsis is common, although its incidence can be markedly reduced by meticulous operative technique, careful peritoneal toilet and the use of the newer broad-spectrum antibiotics. In the series of Yajko et al.[72] the mortality following blunt traumatic rupture of the stomach was 46%, and this was reduced to 33% in 1977 at the time of the report of the Siemens and Fulton.[91] Mortality following this injury can be related to coexisting injuries, late diagnosis and intra-abdominal sepsis.

Penetrating Two reports[82,83] have shown that not all penetrating stab wounds of the abdomen require laparotomy and these same authors have demonstrated the efficacy of a selective policy for exploratory laparotomy. If the patient's condition is stable and there are no signs of significant intra-abdominal injury a policy of close observation can be followed. If there is doubt as to whether the stab wound enters the peritoneum, either exploration of the wound under local anaesthetic or the use of radiological contrast may be helpful. Briggs et al.[93] reported the results of exploration under local anaesthetic in a collected series of 753 patients with stab wounds to the anterior abdomen. In 28% an initial physical examination indicated the need for laparotomy. The remaining 541 patients (72%) were without suspicious physical findings and underwent local wound exploration. Of these cases 293 patients had positive findings and underwent laparotomy, with 46% having visceral injuries. The 248 patients with negative findings were all managed conservatively without further problems. In this report[93] local exploration prevented 248 of 541 (46%) patients from undergoing an unnecessary laparotomy.

At laparotomy the stab wound should be carefully followed because multiple intra-abdominal organs can be involved. Penetrating wounds of the stomach are usually anterior and in these cases the posterior wall must also be examined to exclude unsuspected through-and-through injuries. Penetrating stab wounds high on the greater curvature, around the cardia or through the posterior wall of the stomach alone can easily be missed and in these difficult cases the use of nasogastric instillation of air or can be helpful.

All gunshot wounds of the abdomen require exploratory laparotomy as there is invariably significant intra-abdominal trauma. Gunshot wounds of the stomach can result in loss of gastric tissue, which may necessitate gastric reconstruction or gastrectomy.

Nance and colleagues[83] reported 17 deaths from 1180 stab wounds of the abdomen (including 47 stomach injuries), a mortality rate of 1.4%. In contrast, gunshot wounds were associated with 129 deaths in 1032 patients (184 stomach wounds), a mortality rate of 12.5%.

Iatrogenic Iatrogenic perforations of the stomach require prompt recognition, laparotomy and closure of the defect. Unfortunately the diagnosis is often made late and this has resulted in several fatalities.[84]

Spontaneous rupture

Spontaneous rupture of the stomach is a serious clinical problem which has an extremely high mortality. The two main reasons for the lethality of this condition are:

1. The diagnosis is often made very late and stomach rupture may not be recognized until autopsy.
2. There is a rapid and often irreversible clinical deterioration.

In the series of Albo et al.[88] only six of 43 patients survived, no patient survived without surgery and the mortality of 18 operated cases was 65%. Demetriades et al.[108] in 1982 reported that 75% of patients died following spontaneous gastric rupture. Evans[89] reviewed 49 cases in 1968 and found 11 survivors; all the survivors were numbered among the 22 patients who were operated on. Early death following spontaneous rupture of the stomach is frequent and has been related to acute cardiorespiratory failure. Millar and colleagues[100] postulated that air might enter the venous system through the torn gastric veins along the lesser curvature of the stomach. This theory appears unlikely as it is doubtful whether air could pass through the liver into the systemic circulation.

Patients with suspected spontaneous rupture of the stomach require rigorous early resuscitative measures, and it is imperative to make the diagnosis of intra-abdominal perforation at an early stage in view of the rapidity of clinical deterioration. At operation there is invariably gross peritoneal contamination related to the preceding gastric distension. The stomach must be carefully inspected and the defect exposed. The edges of the defect should be freshened and tissue sent for histology to exclude primary gastric pathology. The whole stomach is decompressed through the defect and the mucosa carefully inspected, with mucosal tears being under-run to prevent bleeding. The stomach is closed in two layers and nasogastric suction is maintained for several days to prevent gastric dilatation. Meticulous peritoneal toilet is mandatory and may be aided by saline or antibiotic lavage. Distal gastric obstruction in the pylorus or duodenum may require pyloroplasty or gastrojejunostomy. Advances in perioperative care will continue to improve the results of treatment for spontaneous rupture of the stomach. Despite these advances Matikainen[109] has recently reported the fatal outcome of an 18-year-old girl who was operated on within 2 hours of spontaneous gastric perforation.

GASTRIC VOLVULUS

Gastric volvulus has been described either as an acquired torsion of the stomach[110] or as an abnormal rotation of the stomach of more than 180° which causes partial or complete closed loop obstruction.[111]

Incidence

Gastric volvulus is a relatively uncommon clinical entity. The initial description of this condition was given by Berti[112] in 1866 after performing an autopsy on a 60-year-old woman who had died quickly of a high closed loop intestinal obstruction. At post mortem the patient was found to have an acute gastric volvulus with obstruction of the lower oesophagus and duodenum. Collective reviews of more than 250 cases by Buchanan,[113] Dalgaard,[114] Gurnsey and Connolly[115] and Wastell and Ellis[116] have brought this condition into clinical focus. Cole and Dickinson[117] reported on 250 cases of gastric volvulus, of which 44 occurred in infants or children under 12 years of age. The number of case reports increases yearly as the condition becomes better recognized and Llaneza and Salt[110] have suggested that gastric volvulus is more common than previously thought. Carter and colleagues[118] have recently reported on 25 cases of acute gastric volvulus and the total number of reported cases is now approximately 400.

Classification

The initial classification of gastric volvulus was introduced by Von Haberer[119] in 1912 and has since been modified by Singleton[120] in 1940 and later by Wastell and Ellis[116] in 1971. The characteristics on which this classification is made include type, extent, direction, aetiology and severity.

1. *Type* (based on axis of rotation) (Figure 41.7).
   (a) Organoaxial (Figure 41.8). Rotation of the stomach occurs upward around the long (cardiopyloric) axis, an

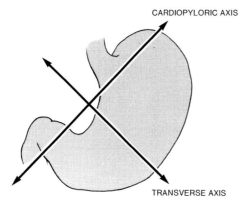

Figure 41.7
Axis of gastric rotation; organoaxial and mesenteroaxial.

imaginary line drawn from the gastric cardia to the pylorus. This type of gastric volvulus is the upside-down stomach seen with the large paraoesophageal hiatus hernia.

(b) Mesenteroaxial (Figure 41.9). Rotation of the stomach occurs around the long axis of the gastric mesenteries, a line approximately perpendicular to the cardiopyloric line. The twist usually occurs right to left, although occasionally it is left to right.

(c) Combined or unclassified type. A combination of the organoaxial and mesenteroaxial types.

2. *Extent*

(a) Total: entire stomach rotates except for the part attached to the diaphragm.

(b) Partial: rotation is limited to one segment of the stomach, usually the pyloric portion.

3. *Direction*

(a) Anterior: rotating part passes anteriorly.

(b) Posterior: rotating part passes posteriorly.

4. *Aetiology*

(a) Secondary: results from disease in the stomach or adjoining organs.

(b) Idiopathic: no specific cause-and-effect relationship established.

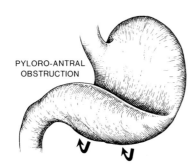

Figure 41.8
Organoaxial gastric volvulus.

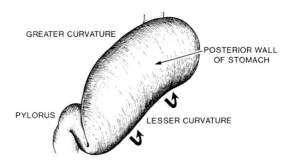

Figure 41.9
Mesenteroaxial gastric volvulus.

5. *Severity*

(a) Acute: acute symptoms, emergency surgery is necessary.

(b) Chronic: symptoms are chronic or may be asymptomatic.

Table 41.7 summarizes the relative frequency of the different types of gastric volvulus from the report of Wastell and Ellis.[116]

Table 41.7   Gastric volvulus: relative frequency of different types in a series of 206 patients

	NUMBER	PERCENTAGE
1. *Type*		
Mesenteroaxial	60	29
Organoaxial	122	59
Combined	5	2
Not classified	19	10
2. *Extent*	*Total*	*Partial*
Mesenteroaxial	57	3
Organoaxial	111	11
Mixed	5	0
Total	173(93)	14(7)
3. *Direction*	*Anterior*	*Posterior*
Mesenteroaxial	37	10
Organoaxial	85	8
Total	122(87)	18(13)
4. *Aetiology*	*Primary*	*Secondary*
Mesenteroaxial	22	38
Organoaxial	32	90
Total	54(30)	128(70)
5. *Severity*	*Acute*	*Chronic*
Mesenteroaxial	36	24
Organoaxial	73	49
Total	109(60)	73(40)

Values in parentheses are percentages.
From Wastell and Ellis[116] with permission.

Pathology

Gastric volvulus has an equal sex incidence and has been most frequently reported in adults in the fifth decade of life, with 10% of cases being seen in children.[117] The degree of rotation varies, although partial volvulus usually involves a rotation of less than 180°, whereas acute or total volvulus is usually 180–360°.[118]

Most cases of acute or total gastric volvulus are organoaxial and these accounted for 16 of the 25 cases (64%) in the report of Carter et al.[118] The greater curvature usually rotates upwards in front of the lesser curvature so that the posterior wall of the stomach lies anterior (Figure 41.8). Often acute organoaxial volvulus is associated with an abnormality such as eventration of the diaphragm, paraoesophageal hiatus hernia or displacement of neighbouring viscera such as the spleen or colon. Organoaxial volvulus initially results in pyloric obstruction, followed by obstruction at the cardia and the development of a closed loop obstruction. In the series of Carter and associates[118] almost all cases of acute organoaxial volvulus were associated with hiatus hernia or diaphragmatic defects.

Mesenteroaxial volvulus is more frequently idiopathic and partial in extent.[118] In these cases the rotation is usually limited to the mobile pyloric end where obstruction occurs. The anterior gastric wall is folded back upon itself and separates the cardia from the pylorus (Figure 41.9). Mesenteroaxial volvulus causes obstruction in the mid-portion of the stomach. Because the twist is often partial, spontaneous detorsion with recurrent acute episodes is more common.

Several complications have been reported in association with gastric volvulus, namely gastric outlet obstruction, strangulation, haemorrhage from the stomach, perforation, pulmonary complications, splenic rupture, pancreatic necrosis, omental avulsion and shock.[118,121–123] Strangulation from acute gastric volvulus leading to gangrene is reported to be uncommon because of the stomach's good blood supply. Unlike most viscera with a mesentery the stomach has an abundant blood supply and is quite resistant to infarction unless unrelieved torsion occurs.[124,125] In the series of acute gastric volvulus reported by Carter and colleagues[118] 28% of cases were associated with acute gastric necrosis and all but one case was organoaxial in nature. In the same series[118] diaphragmatic defects, such as traumatic hernia, eventration and congenital hernia, were particularly prone to cause strangulation following gastric volvulus. Splenic rupture has been reported[118] due to disruption of splenic vessels in the twisting process and occasionally severe gastric haemorrhage can develop.[126]

Pathogenesis

The stomach is a very mobile intra-abdominal organ and intermittent episodes of rotation without symptoms probably occur more often than is appreciated.[114,116] Relaxation of the ligamentous supports of the stomach is a major factor permitting volvulus to occur. The stomach is held firmly in place proximally at the cardia and distally at the retroperitoneal fixation of the duodenum. Between these points the gastrophrenic, gastrosplenic, gastrocolic and gastrohepatic ligaments tether it in place. The highest ligamentous support is the gastrophrenic ligament and the lowest consists of the peritoneum covering the second part of the duodenum.[127] Gastric fixation is usually limited by the length and mobility of the lesser curvature as well as that of the

gastrohepatic omentum. When the ligaments are congenitally absent or become lax, volvulus can occur. From cadaver studies, Dalgaard[114] showed that the stomach cannot be rotated 180° unless the gastrosplenic or gastrocolic ligament, or both, is severed. Thus for volvulus to occur in vivo, abnormal relaxation of the ligamentous attachments of the stomach must be present, allowing torsion of 180° along or perpendicular to the cardiopyloric axis to occur. Occasionally one or more ligaments may be congenitally absent, which predisposes the patient to gastric volvulus. When the ligaments are relaxed the weight of a large fluid-filled stomach may cause approximation of the pylorus and cardia, setting the stage for volvulus to occur. It is easy to twist a large atonic stomach and a fluid-filled one may be twisted more easily than an empty one. However, a stomach with intact ligaments will at once glide back into its normal location.[128]

Adhesions, either congenital or acquired, may form an axis for rotation of the stomach. Extrinsic pressure from adjoining masses or organs, or intrinsic lesions of the stomach, such as an ulcer or neoplasm, that may obstruct or distend the stomach, may initiate gastric volvulus.[111,118] Intractable vomiting, rapid increases in intra-abdominal pressure, trauma and acute gastric dilatation are also precipitating factors.

A second pathophysiological process in the formation of gastric volvulus is the presence of an abnormal extension of the abdominal cavity, which permits the stomach to enter and twist. Such extensions are caused by: (1) a paraoesophageal hiatus hernia in which the gastric volvulus is usually organoaxial;[118] (2) eventration of the left part of the diaphragm, which may be related to left phrenic nerve paralysis or be the consequence of pneumonectomy[129] or lobectomy,[130] in which the volvulus is usually mesenteroaxial; (3) a large incisional hernia; and (4) traumatic injury to the diaphragm.[118,131] In the series of Tanner[132] eventration of the diaphragm was present in 21 of 27 cases of chronic gastric volvulus. It has been suggested[133] that in the presence of a raised left hemidiaphragm the increased subphrenic space becomes filled with the greater curvature of the stomach, which in turn draws up the transverse colon and leads to volvulus of the stomach. Aerocolia (distension of the large bowel with gas) of the transverse colon has been considered an important aetiological factor.[132,134] However, although large bowel distension can cause displacement of the stomach, volvulus is unlikely to occur if the ligaments supporting the stomach are normal. Rare associations with gastric volvulus include a long redundant mesocolon,[135] pneumatosis cystoides intestinalis,[136] congenital obstructive bands and abnormal abdominal adhesions such as choledochoduodenal bands.[111]

Recently Yin and Nowak[137] described the familial occurrence of intrathoracic gastric volvulus. They described chronic volvulus in a mother and daughter and suggested that a genetic factor might be involved in the pathogenesis of this disorder. It is also of interest that ligamentous laxity in the Ehlers–Danlos syndrome is associated with recurrent gastric volvulus.[138]

Clinical features

The clinical features of gastric volvulus are primarily determined by the severity (acute or chronic) and type of volvulus.

Acute gastric volvulus

This is a surgical emergency and presents with a striking clinical picture. The onset is generally abrupt, with severe upper abdominal or lower thoracic pain that may radiate to the back, neck or interscapular region. Early vomiting (usually non-bilious) is replaced by unproductive retching, and copious emesis of stomach contents is unusual when the cardia is completely obstructed. The organoaxial type tends to cause obstruction at the cardia and pylorus, resulting in a closed loop obstruction, rapid gastric distension and acute symptoms. In the mesenteroaxial type, the pylorus and cardio-oesophageal junction approximate, resulting in occlusion of only one orifice and a less acute clinical presentation.

The clinical features of acute gastric volvulus with strangulation are either abdominal, thoracic or both.[118] The abdominal manifestations include sudden excruiating upper abdominal pain with tenderness and early vomiting, followed by unproductive retching. Gastrointestinal bleeding from ischaemic necrosis and hypovolaemic shock from blood and fluid loss may also occur. The thoracic manifestations include severe lower chest or substernal pain with radiation to the neck or shoulder, dyspnoea, and cyanosis resulting from a mediastinal shift produced by massive distension from herniated viscera or a pleural effusion.[118]

Examination in patients with acute gastric volvulus reveals progressive distension and tympany of the upper abdomen but the lower abdomen remains soft and lax. Occasionally a succussion splash may be detected, and auscultation of the chest may reveal bowel sounds.[124] If the stomach is intrathoracic, abdominal findings may be minimal.[118]

Borchardt[139] in 1904 described a clinical triad which is of great value in the diagnosis of an acute gastric volvulus:

1. Severe epigastric pain and distension.
2. Vomiting followed by violent retching with an inability to vomit.
3. Difficulty or inability to pass a nasogastric tube.

This triad can be closely related to the pathological changes of acute gastric volvulus, namely an initial block at the pylorus, obstruction at the cardia and the development of closed loop obstruction with distension of the stomach by gas and fluid. This triad is present in most cases of acute gastric volvulus in adults, although the classic triad can be difficult to recognize in infants and children.[140]

Carter and colleagues[118] have suggested that there are at least three additional clinical features that facilitate early diagnosis of acute gastric volvulus:

1. Minimal abdominal findings when the stomach is in the thorax.
2. A gas-filled viscus in the lower chest or abdomen, shown by the chest radiograph, especially when associated with a paraoesophageal hiatus hernia.
3. Obstruction at the site of volvulus shown by emergency upper gastrointestinal series.

Acute gastric volvulus results in rapid clinical deterioration as vascular occlusion and infarction of the stomach occur. Shock, perforation and death are the final result if surgery is not performed promptly. The diagnosis is rarely made before surgery because most physicians are unfamiliar with this condition.[124] The differential diagnosis includes myocardial infarction, perforated peptic ulcer, pancreatitis and ruptured aortic aneurysm. The most frequent misdiagnosis is that of acute myocardial infarction and this diagnostic difficulty can be further compounded by acute gastric volvulus producing electrocardiographic changes that mimic those of myocardial infarction.[141]

Chronic gastric volvulus

This is usually of the organoaxial type and has an entirely different clinical picture from acute volvulus which may remain undiagnosed for years. The symptoms of this condition are variable and include pyrosis, epigastric pain, belching, bloating, nausea, vomiting, early satiety and fullness, and the patient may even notice a mass. These symptoms frequently come on after a heavy meal and last for a variable period of time, after which they are completely relieved. The patient may find that discomfort is relieved by self-induced vomiting or a change in position.[124] Symptomatic gastro-oesophageal reflux disease is not common, although oesophagoscopy will often identify oesophagitis.[142] Since chronic gastric volvulus is often found in elderly patients with a paraoesophageal hiatus hernia, the diagnosis can be missed if symptoms are attributed to the hernia.[110] It is therefore important to consider chronic gastric volvulus in any elderly patient who has a diaphragmatic hernia and complains of vomiting.[123] The main differential diagnoses of chronic gastric volvulus include reflux oesophagitis with hiatus hernia, oesophageal neoplasia, peptic ulceration, gastritis, gastric cancer, cholelithiasis and pancreatic neoplasm.

Investigations

The definitive diagnosis of gastric volvulus is based on radiographic assessment.[110] The classic appearance of gastric volvulus on a chest radiograph with the patient erect includes two abnormal air–fluid levels: one beneath the left hemidiaphragm and the other in the retrocardiac mediastinum.[143] The one in the retrocardiac mediastinum represents the dilated, herniated distal stomach with partial or complete obstruction of its outlet. The one beneath the diaphragm represents an air–fluid level in the normally-positioned fundus which may be partially obstructed at the inlet to the twisted and herniated segment. Symptoms suggesting gastric outlet obstruction usually occur when the rotation increases so that both the inlet and outlet of the rotated stomach become obstructed, and radiologically the retrocardiac air–fluid level is then replaced by a homogenous soft tissue mass, the fluid-filled antrum.

These findings can be confirmed by barium examination of the upper gastrointestinal tract. The upper gastrointestinal series in mesenteroaxial volvulus shows the oesophagogastric junction to be below the diaphragmatic level. The distal part of the stomach appears to be cephalad, and a 'beak' appears where the oesophagogastric junction is normally located. A stomach with organoaxial volvulus may appear inverted or upside-down, with the cardia and pylorus positioned at the same level and pointing downward. Askew[111] has emphasized that the radiological appearances of gastric volvulus must be carefully distinguished from those of a cascade (cup and spill) stomach, in which there is loculation and dilatation of the fundus, the contrast medium first filling the fundus and then spilling over into the body and antrum. A gastric volvulus has two fluid levels, whereas a cascade stomach has only one level.

The pertinent radiological criteria in the diagnosis of an *acute* gastric volvulus (Figure 41.10) have been summarized by DeLorimier and Penn[144] as:

- A localized massive distension of the upper abdomen.
- Visualization of the outlines of a 'hair-pin' loop with the incisura directed towards the right upper quadrant or posteriorly.
- Fixation of the loop regardless of the position of the patient.
- Delimitation of barium at the tapered end of the oesophagus.
- Possible evidence of hiatal or diaphragmatic herniation.
- Deviation in splenic position.

- Segmental distension of loops of small intestine and colon, indicating an associated ileus.

Clearfield and Stahlgren[128] have summarized the radiological signs of *chronic* volvulus (Figure 41.11):

- A double fluid level.
- The stomach is inverted, with the greater curvature above the level of the lesser curvature.
- The cardia and pylorus may be at the same level.
- The pylorus and duodenum point downwards.
- Greater than normal gastric mobility.
- The mucosal folds may show evidence of torsion or twisting.
- The abdominal portion of the oesophagus may be longer than normal.
- There may be a demonstrable hourglass stomach or a diaphragmatic defect.

Endoscopy is useful in the diagnosis of patients with chronic gastric volvulus as it also allows a close inspection of the upper gastrointestinal tract.[133] In patients with a gastric volvulus gastroscopy often demonstrates a large hiatus hernia and the endoscopist may get 'lost' in the stomach as the normal landmarks are reversed. Such a situation encountered by an experienced endoscopist is virtually diagnostic of a chronic intrathoracic gastric volvulus. When the diagnosis is recognized, careful manoeuvring will often reveal the anatomy of the volvulus and allow endoscopic derotation to be performed.[133,145]

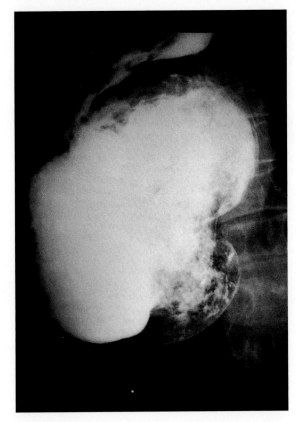

Figure 41.10
Barium meal showing acute gastric volvulus with gastric dilatation and pyloric obstruction. (Courtesy of Dr J. Virjee.)

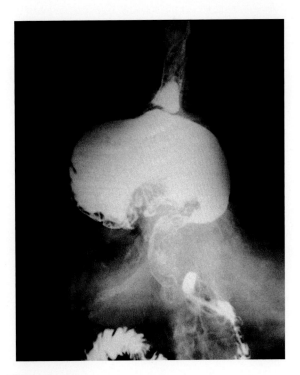

Figure 41.11
Barium meal showing chronic intrathoracic gastric volvulus. (Courtesy of Dr J. Virjee.)

Treatment

Acute

Acute gastric volvulus may be treated without surgery if a nasogastric tube can be successfully passed and the stomach emptied. This is much more likely in the mesenteroaxial type in which the cardia is open. In the more common organoaxial variety, in which the cardia is obstructed, a nasogastric tube cannot usually be passed, and an immediate operation is mandatory. Askew[111] has suggested that with gentle persistence it is possible to pass a nasogastric tube into the stomach but extreme care should be exercised as oesophageal perforation can result.[128] A radiographic nasogastric tube can be passed under fluoroscopic guidance if necessary.[110] Endoscopic correction of acute gastric volvulus has been described,[121] although this is not considered to be the most acceptable mode of therapy.

Acute gastric volvulus requires emergency laparotomy after initial resuscitation with intravenous fluids and parenteral antibiotics. The operative objectives include gastric decompression, reduction of the torsion and correction of any causative abnormalities such as diaphragmatic hernia or eventration.[110] The abdomen is opened through a long upper midline incision. Marked distension is usually first noted in the upper abdomen, with the transverse colon lying high under the diaphragm. Inexperienced surgeons may have difficulty both in recognizing the anatomical landmarks and in appreciating the pathological process. It is usually impossible to reduce the volvulus while gastric distension is present and therefore the stomach is emptied with a needle or via a gastrostomy. Several litres of bloody fluid and gas are usually removed, and this allows easy reduction of the volvulus. Care must be taken during deflation and detorting of the stomach to avoid accidental splenic injury.[124] After reduction of the volvulus, areas of stomach necrosis must be carefully identified and these may necessitate local excision or gastric resection, depending on the extent of the ischaemic injury. In the report of Carter et al.[118] 28% of cases of acute gastric volvulus were associated with gastric necrosis and two cases of gangrene of the transverse colon requiring colectomy were seen. Diaphragmatic defects such as paraoesophageal hiatus hernia, traumatic and congenital hernia and eventration must be repaired if possible. The simplest method of fixation of the stomach to prevent rerotation is an anterior gastropexy, suturing the stomach along the length of the gastrocolic omentum to the anterior abdominal wall. In the poor-risk patient a temporary gastrostomy may be all that is required. More extensive fixation procedures are not indicated in acute volvulus. In situations with coexisting gastric pathology, such as a peptic ulcer, partial gastrectomy may be necessary. After the volvulus is corrected a nasogastric tube is passed into the stomach and this should be maintained for several days postoperatively.

The reported high mortality of 30–50% associated with acute gastric volvulus reflects delay in recognition and treatment of this condition. Delay also increases the risk of strangulation, which is the chief cause of the high death rate. Many of the reported deaths from acute volvulus occurred before 1950 and this fact undoubtedly accounts for the high reported mortality. A recent report by Carter et al.[118] demonstrated an 8.5% mortality from acute gastric volvulus and this is a closer reflection of the true figure in the present era. Early recognition and treatment of acute gastric volvulus remains the main determinant of outcome and in the same series[118] one case was found at autopsy after the patient had been treated as having pneumonia on the medical service.

Chronic

In contrast to the acute variety, chronic gastric volvulus does not require surgical intervention unless symptoms such as persistent vomiting, epigastric pain and haematemesis become unbearable. Concomitant disease must be excluded and treated. In some patients conservative measures such as the use of a bland diet of frequent small feedings and repeated passage of a nasogastric tube may afford symptomatic relief.

Chronic gastric volvulus may on occasion be corrected by endoscopic manipulation, as described by Patel.[133] With air insufflation at a minimum, the endoscope is put in a loop form and the endoscope rotated 180° in an anticlockwise or clockwise direction. This results in a sudden 'jar', indicating derotation of the stomach, and immediate endoscopic examination will usually reveal the stomach to be in a normal position. In patients unsuitable for surgery endoscopic derotation can be repeatedly performed[133] and good long-term results have been published.[145,146] Recurrent volvulus after endoscopic derotation is usually an indication for surgery; however, dual percutaneous endoscopic gastrostomy in the antrum and body of the stomach was used successfully in one patient with chronic intermittent gastric volvulus.[147]

Surgery is the mainstay of treatment in medically suitable patients with severe symptoms from a radiologically proven chronic gastric volvulus. At operation associated diaphragmatic abnormalities are repaired, adhesions and other significant intra-abdominal pathologies corrected and some form of gastropexy performed. Most surgeons performed a gastropexy after repairing the diaphragm, although Askew[111] has found no case of recurrence following repair of the diaphragmatic abnormality and simple reduction of the volvulus without additional fixation. In children simple reduction of the volvulus with or without gastric fixation by means of a gastrostomy gives excellent results irrespective of associated diaphragmatic abnormalities.[117] Laparoscopic repairs of chronic gastric volvulus is well described. The stomach is reduced and sutured to the diaphragm and oesophageal hiatus.

Simple anterior gastropexy by suturing the stomach to the liver, ligamentum teres or the posterior rectus sheath is associated with a high recurrence rate.[132] Posterior gastroenterostomy has been suggested for the simple chronic volvulus as an easy method of providing fixation and adequate drainage of the stomach,[134] and Farkas and Celestin[148] have reported excellent long-term results with retrocolic gastrojejunostomy in nine patients with chronic gastric volvulus. They emphasize the importance of making the anastamosis very close the duodenojejunal junction.

Stremple[149] devised a new operation for the anatomical correction of chronic intermittent gastric volvulus. He recommends suturing part of the greater curvature of the stomach to the colon mesentery, thus forming a new gastrocolic ligament. The rest of the greater curvature is fixed to the posterior parietal peritoneum to prevent gastric rotation when eventration of the diaphragm is present. Tanner[132] and Schreiber et al.[150] have described a colonic displacement operation. In this procedure the transverse colon is separated from the stomach by dividing the gastrocolic omentum from the duodenum to the gastric fundus. After division of adhesions, and provided there is a reasonable length of mesocolon, the whole mobilized transverse colon and greater omentum can be positioned in the left subdiaphragmatic space. An anterior gastropexy is then added. Twelve of 15 of Tanner's[132] cases were asymptomatic at follow-up 5–12 years after surgery. Singh and Garg[151] have further suggested adding a gastrojejunal hitch to Tanner's procedure. In this operation the posterior wall of the stomach is sutured to the jejunal wall close to the duodenojejunal junction. No stoma is made and this hitch provides a continuous pull and fixation to the posterior wall of the stomach and thereby prevents rotation.

GASTRIC BEZOARS

Bezoars are defined as concretions of various foreign or intrinsic substances found in the stomach and intestine of both man and animals.[152,153] The name bezoar derives from either the Arabian word badzahr or the Persian padzahr, both of which mean protecting against poison or an antidote. Bezoars have long been surrounded by mystique and have been greatly prized as a remedy of multiple ailments.

Incidence

The bezoar is the most common foreign body that lodges and stays in the stomach.[154] Although bezoars are encountered infrequently they are not rare. In 1938 DeBakey and Oschner published two classical articles on the subject of bezoars and reviewed 311 cases collected from the literature.[152,153] More recently Zarling and Thompson[155] reported 52 bezoars found over a 5-year period, Diettrich and Gau[156] found 38 postgastrectomy bezoars over 8 years and Cain et al.[157] were able to review 99 postgastrectomy bezoars.

Ahn and colleagues[158] reviewed 3247 gastroscopies performed in one institution over 7 years and found 14 bezoars, an incidence of 0.4%. Diettrich and Gau[156] have suggested that the prevalence of bezoars in the postgastrectomy state is more common than is usually appreciated, although the increasing number of endoscopies performed over the last two decades have revealed that bezoars are still uncommon.

Classification (DeBakey and Oschner[152,153])

1. Trichobezoar: composed of hair.
2. Phytobezoar: composed of vegetable matter. These have been subdivided into diospyrobezoar (persimmon associated) and ordinary phytobezoar (no persimmon aetiology).
3. Trichophytobezoar: composed of hair and vegetable matter.
4. Concretions and miscellaneous intragastric bodies; lactobezoars (from milk products in infancy).

Pathology

In the review of DeBakey and Oschner[152,153] 55% of 311 bezoars were trichobezoars, 41% were phytobezoars (30% persimmon, 11% others) and 4% concretions. Since then there has been a marked change and phytobezoars are now much more commonly seen than trichobezoars.

Trichobezoars

Trichobezoars consist of hair casts, which may attain enormous size, eventually filling and assuming the shape of the stomach. Trichobezoars most frequently occur in nervous children and mentally disturbed adults. Most cases are seen in young women, and in one report[152,153] 90% were found in women under 30 years of age. Trichobezoars consist of a glairy, mucoid coat which contains decaying foodstuff enmeshed amongst enormous amounts of hair. They are always black in colour (even in blondes) and this is thought to be secondary to chemical changes in the hair fibres. Trichobezoars have an extremely fetid odour which is related to the presence of undigested fat and a heavy bacterial colonization. The largest trichobezoars have weighed 3 kg wet weight and when fully developed they can assume a perfect cast of the stomach. Occasionally trichobezoars extend through the pylorus and into the small bowel, producing the so-called Rapunzel syndrome.[159] It is of interest that only occasionally do these patients have overt psychiatric illness, although it is generally assumed that most cases are related to a personality disorder.[152,153]

Phytobezoars

The most commonly seen bezoar is now the phytobezoar and these are most frequently related to persimmon ingestion (diospyrobezoars) or postgastric surgery. Phytobezoars are composed of organic plant matter and may occur when vegetables or fruit fibres are ingested in great quantities. Numerous causative agents for phytobezoars have been reported, ranging from oranges to grapes and celery fibres to leeks.[152,153,160] In the series of DeBakey and Oschner[152,153] 77% of phytobezoars occurred in men with most occurring in the sixth decade. Phytobezoars vary in weight from 1 to 200 g, in length from 5 to 10 cm and in diameter from 3 to 6 cm. They are usually a greenish-red colour and shrink remarkably on drying. One reported phytobezoar shrank from a weight of 460 g and physical dimensions of 14 × 9 cm to 60 g and 4 × 2 cm over a 2-week period.[152,153] Most phytobezoars are single, although in 17% of cases more than one bezoar is present.[152,153] Their surface is either smooth or pitted and sectioning reveals an amorphous composition with no evidence of lamination. They are almost entirely composed of organic matter and if burnt very little ash remains. Phytobezoars can also be found in the oesophagus and intestine and in one report[152,153] 78% were in the stomach, 17% were in the small bowel and 5% were in both the stomach and intestine. Phytobezoars cause symptoms by either acting as a ball valve and giving obstructive problems or by causing local irritation, with gastritis or peptic ulceration.

Diospyrobezoars or persimmon phytobezoars account for a large proportion of all bezoars in certain areas of the world. The persimmon berry derives from a tree of the ebony family, *Diospyros virginiana*, which is found in south-eastern USA and Japan. The persimmon is a true berry which measures 2–4 cm in diameter and has an orange colour. When unripe the berries are hard and sour but on ripening they become soft and sweet.

Postgastrectomy phytobezoars are now relatively common, whereas none were described in DeBakey and Oschner's review, presumably on account of the large amount of ulcer surgery performed since 1940. Diettrich and Gau[156] reported 33 patients with 37 phytobezoars and one concretion. Twenty-nine of their patients (88%) had undergone various gastric procedures and the other four had varying gastro-oesophageal pathology (Table 41.8). Vagotomy and antrectomy was the most commonly performed operation although no comparison of the various gastric procedures was possible. Cain and colleagues[157] also reported on postgastrectomy phytobezoars. They described 99 cases, of whom 65 were men, with the most common age being in the fifth decade. Sixty of the 99 cases were associated with oranges, with only four bezoars in the stomach and 95 in the intestine. This distribution does, however, suggest that most of these bezoars were strictly food boluses.

Table 41.8 Gastric surgical procedures performed before formation of phytobezoar in 33 patients

PROCEDURE	NUMBER	INTERVAL BETWEEN SURGERY AND BEZOAR (YEARS)
Vagotomy and antrectomy	15 (45.5)	10.0
Billroth I	5 (15.1)	10.7
Billroth II	7 (21.1)	12.0
Unknown	3 (9.1)	5.0
Vagotomy and pyloroplasty	8 (24.2)	3.6
Vagotomy and gastroenterostomy	3 (9.1)	10.0
Wedge resection	3 (9.1)	5.3
None	4 (12.1)	—

Values in parentheses are percentages.
From Diettrich and Gau[156] with permission.

Concretions

These are relatively unusual forms of bezoar and account for less than 5% of reported cases.[161] They can be related to ingestion of medications that in bulk will adhere, such as barium for radiological examinations, magnesium and calcium carbonate, paraffin, aluminium, hydroxide gel, cholestyramine and sucralfate.[162] Classically gastric concretions have been described in furniture polishers who drank large quantities of polish containing shellac and alcohol. These resinous contents agglutinate into a solid mass which grows by laminar accretion to enormous size. A polystyrene bezoar has also been reported in a

patient following styrofoam cup ingestion.[163] Fungal or yeast bezoars have been described in the postgastrectomy patient.[164] Most reported cases are from Scandinavia and the bezoars are observed following vagotomy and Billroth I gastrectomy.[165] *Candida albicans* and *Torulopsis glabrata*, both human saprophytes, are the most common organisms found in yeast bezoars. Lactobezoars occur in low birth weight neonates fed a highly concentrated milk formula within the first week of life. Because of poor neonatal gastric motility, relative dehydration and the concentrated milk formula, milk products like casein congeal to form a lactobezoar.[162]

Pathogenesis

Trichobezoars develop primarily from the habitual ingestion of hair (trichophagia). It is unclear why the hair tends to accumulate in the stomach instead of passing down into the gut. DeBakey and Oschner[152,153] suggested that the amount of fat in the diet is important in the movement of hair through the bowel. Large quantities of fat in the diet cause gastric stasis of hair, whereas low quantities of fat are associated with hair transit through the intestine. It has also been postulated that hair strands, too slippery to be propulsed, are initially retained by the mucosal folds of the stomach and gradually become enmeshed in the bezoar matrix.[159]

Phytobezoars The pathogenesis of phytobezoars is related to either aberrant gastric motility or consumption of non-digestible vegetable fibres.[154,166] Vegetable fibres may accumulate in the stomach on account of improper mastication by edentulous subjects or as a result of excessive ingestion of causative agents such as persimmons or oranges. The formation of non-persimmon phytobezoars is primarily mechanical and occurs by entanglement of insoluble and indigestible vegetable fibres.

The formation of persimmon phytobezoars (diospyrobezoars) has been much researched and appears related to the presence of tannins.[167] Most fruits and vegetables contain tannin in the form of soluble polymers, which are acted on by gastric acid to release insoluble tannin monomers such as catechin and leucoanthrocyanidin. Unripe persimmons and the skin of ripe fruit have a very high concentration of catechin and leucoanthrocyanidin (six times that of an apple). When unripe persimmons are added to 0.1 mmol/l hydrochloric acid or gastric juice they turn brown and form a solid mass. Biochemically leucoanthrocyanidin is acted on by an enzyme leucodelphinidin-3-glucosidase in the presence of acid to form red-brown polymers or phlobathenes, which form a rigid insoluble mass by hydrogen bonding to proteins and cell walls. Thus persimmon phytobezoars consist of tannins, cellulose, hemicellulose, proteins and glycoproteins. Other fruits and vegetables contain far less tannins and so the formation of insoluble masses in the presence of acid is unusual.

Endogenous factors that are important in the genesis of gastric bezoars are connected to the ability of the stomach to break the ingested material chemically and to mobilize the fragments down to the intestine. These factors include impaired gastric motility, changes in the quantity or quality of gastric acid secretion, changes in mucus production and mechanical or functional pyloric dysfunction.[168] Aberrant gastric motility and phytobezoar formation is associated with the postgastrectomy stomach, diabetes,[158] myotonic muscular dystrophy and cimetidine therapy.[169] Postgastrectomy bezoars are now the most common type of bezoar and the gastric procedure most frequently associated with their formation is vagotomy and antrectomy.[170] Billroth I anastamoses tend to produce gastric bezoars and Billroth II anastamoses are associated with small bowel bezoars.[170] Postgastrectomy bezoars may be caused by decreased gastric motility and reduced acid–pepsin secretion, leading to impaired chyme breakdown.[156] The normally poor digestion of cellulose deteriorates further in the postgastrectomy patient and this substance forms an excellent nucleus for bezoar formation.[171] The loss of the grinding and sieving mechanism of the antropyloric pump may impair the ability of the stomach to reduce the size of ingested particles.[169,172] Delayed gastric emptying has been described in patients with postgastrectomy bezoars and it has been suggested that this is the fundamental mechanism for their formation.[173]

Calabuig and associates[169] recently studied gastric emptying of a solid meal in ten patients who developed a bezoar after previous gastric surgery. Patients were studied 1 year after the bezoars had been removed and the results were compared with gastric emptying data of similarly operated patients without bezoars. No differences were found in gastric emptying between patients with and without bezoar formation, although the vagotomy and antrectomy subgroup did have significant gastric hold-up. Calabuig and coworkers concluded that factors other than the gastric digestive phase were the main contributors to bezoar formation. These same workers suggested that other alterations in motility during the postoperative period might be involved and postulated that disruption of phase II of the interdigestive migrating motor complex in the stomach following vagotomy and the abolishment of phase III activity following antrectomy might be important factors. As a result of these changes Calabuig et al thought that large undigested particles might remain in the stomach as a result of reduced gastric emptying during the digestive period. These particles could aggregate and form bezoars. This study raises many questions and further investigation of gastric motility is needed to ascertain the causes of postgastrectomy bezoar formation.

Recently, delayed gastric emptying and bezoar formation has been recognized as a major problem following Roux-en-Y biliary diversion for alkaline reflux gastritis. Vogel and Woodward[174] documented gastroparesis and objective evidence of delayed gastric emptying in 10–50% of patients undergoing Roux-en-Y diversion. This delayed emptying is for solids only as studies of liquid emptying have been normal. Vogel and Woodward[174] reported on 37 cases with post-Roux-en-Y gastric retention who required further surgical therapy, and 25 of these patients (68%) had bezoars, with symptoms of nausea, vomiting and abdominal pain. The reasons for gastric stasis after Roux-en-Y diversion are complex, but may include the antrectomy, the vagotomy and the Roux-en-Y loop of jejunum where the migrating motor complex is disrupted.

Diabetes mellitus has also been related to phytobezoar

formation.[158,175,176] Zarling and Thompson[155] found that bezoar formation could be related to systemic disease in 17 patients without prior gastric surgery or persimmon ingestion. They described gastric phytobezoars in 12 diabetics, two patients with chronic renal failure, two taking psychotropic drugs and one with scleroderma. Ahn and associates[158] further examined the relationship of diabetes to bezoar formation in 14 patients, of whom seven were diabetics who all showed signs of autonomic neuropathy. Further studies have described gastric motility disorders in 20–30% of diabetic patients despite the absence of clinical manifestations.[177] Ahn and coworkers[158] concluded that bezoars are commonly associated with diabetes as a result of autonomic neuropathy and decreased gastric motility.

Clinical features

Trichobezoars

In spite of their enormous size trichobezoars can be asymptomatic for years. The first symptoms are usually vague and consist of anorexia, dyspepsia, malaise, weakness, headaches and a feeling of heaviness in the epigastrium. These symptoms run an insidious course and are followed by nausea, vomiting and abdominal pain, ranging from a dull ache to severe colic, with patients eventually developing weight loss and complications. Complications occur as a result of interference with the normal physiological activity of the gut, leading to obstructive symptoms and weight loss, and traumatic irritation to the stomach, leading to gastritis, ulceration and perforation. Haematemsis and melaena are not infrequent late complications of trichobezoar and were seen in 6% of cases in one report.[152,153]

Up to 10% of trichobezoars are associated with gastric ulcers, which have the same pathophysiological characteristics as the normal gastric ulcer, with 80% occurring on the lesser curvature. Gastric ulcers can bleed torrentially or perforate, which is potentially extremely dangerous because of the marked bacterial contamination of trichobezoar. Rarely small pieces of hair can break off the main trichobezoar mass and pass down the intestine to give obstruction. Trichobezoars are rarely associated with chronic megaloblastic anaemia secondary to vitamin B_{12} deficiency, steatorrhoea, pancreatitis, obstructive jaundice, intussusception and appendicitis.[159] Examination of a patient with a trichobezoar almost always demonstrates a large epigastric mass which may demonstrate crepitus on palpation.[178] These patients frequently have severe halitosis and there may be scanty hair in the frontal and temporal regions of the scalp.

Phytobezoars

The clinical features of phytobezoars are often non-specific and it may be easy, particularly in the postgastrectomy patient, to attribute the symptoms to more common conditions.[156] The symptoms of persimmon phytobezoars (diospyrobezoars) begin soon after ingestion of persimmons and are potentiated by drinking copious amounts of water.[166] After ingestion many patients develop severe abdominal distress, and haematemesis or melaena may be accompanying symptoms. This acute attack is generally followed by recurrent attacks of a milder character interspersed between varying intervals of almost complete relief. Non-persimmon phytobezoars have no acute attack, although the later symptoms are generally similar to those associated with persimmons. The symptoms of a phytobezoar are determined by its size, location and degree of disturbance in gastric pathology. The patient may complain of a dragging feeling, fullness, a mass or heaviness in the epigastrium. Cramp-like epigastric pain is frequent and later nausea and vomiting may occur. The vomitus in these patients is characteristically small in amount as the bezoar acts as a ball valve, preventing ejection of large amounts from the stomach.

Postgastrectomy phytobezoars usually present in a similar way. Diettrich and Gau[156] documented the clinical features in their 33 patients as: vague epigastric distress (83%), weight loss of 1–17 kg (31%), fullness or bloating (28%), nausea and vomiting (22%), upper gastrointestinal bleeding (16%), dysphagia (12%) and foul eructations (8%). In their report the average duration of symptoms was 9 weeks.

The most serious complication of a phytobezoar is the development of gastrointestinal haemorrhage as a result of gastritis or peptic ulceration. this is more commonly seen with persimmon bezoars and in a recent report 12 of 17 gastric diospyrobezoars were associated with bleeding from a gastric ulcer.[166] Perforation may occur, although this is generally less serious than with a trichobezoar on account of the relatively sterile gastric contents. Obstruction can develop at the pylorus due to a ball-valve effect or the bezoar extending through the pylorus. The whole bezoar may pass into the intestine or small bits can break off the main mass, leading to small bowel obstruction. Weight loss minimicking gastric neoplasm can occur and protein-losing gastropathies have been reported with massive bezoars.[179] The association of bezoars with weight loss has been the stimulus to the use of intragastric balloons in the treatment of obesity.[180,181] However, careful perusal of the literature on bezoars reveals that weight loss is relatively unusual and occurs at a late stage in association with other symptoms, such as bleeding. These factors may account for the poor results associated with intragastric balloons. Rarely gastric carcinoma may accompany the presence of a phytobezoar and one has been reported in association with a linitis plastica carcinoma with reduced gastric motility.[156]

Examination of patients with phytobezoars may reveal a large epigastric mass with well-defined edges, uniform firmness and no crepitus. In the report of DeBakey and Oschner[152,153] 57% of patients with a phytobezoar had a palpable mass.

Investigations

Most bezoars are associated with mild iron deficiency anaemia and in late cases hypoproteinaemia will occur. Plain abdominal radiology may demonstrate an epigastric mass invading the gastric air bubble[171] and the mass usually shows irregular mottling due to small pockets of air trapped within the bezoar. Barium radiology demonstrates a large filling defect within the lumen of the stomach which, unlike a large gastric neoplasm,

is freely mobile. A delayed film at approximately 6 hours will frequently show contrast material caught up in the interstices of the bezoar. This appearance is more frequent and more pronounced with trichobezoars as there is less permeation of barium contrast into the phytobezoar bulk. Difficulty in the radiological diagnosis of bezoars is frequently encountered in the postgastrectomy patient (Figure 41.12)[182] and in the report of Diettrich and Gau[156] only 24% of barium studies were positive for a bezoar. Ultrasonography of the epigastrium is reported as being helpful in the diagnosis of bezoars, with the finding of an echogenic solid mass which casts a complete sonic shadow in the left upper quadrant of the abdomen.[183,184] The 'clean' acoustic shadow obtained might relate to multiple tiny interfaces in the densely packed bezoar.

Endoscopy is now the investigation of choice because treatment can be instituted at the same time. Phytobezoars are seen as large, firm three-dimensional masses of a greenish-yellow material (Figure 41.13), whereas trichobezoars are invariably black and tarry with hair often visualized. Gastroscopy allows a complete examination for associated gastric pathology, such as gastritis, peptic ulceration and carcinoma, and is particularly helpful in the postgastrectomy patient where radiology is frequently misleading. Diettrich and Gau[156] reported their endoscopic findings in 33 patients when the bezoars were all clearly visualized and the upper gastrointestinal tract carefully examined. In their report the size of the bezoar was assessed as

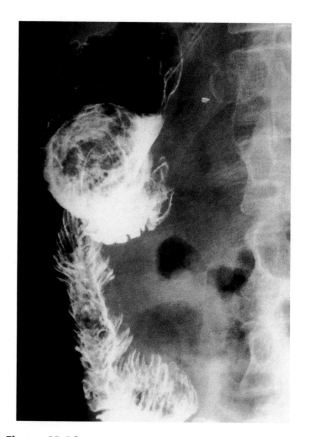

Figure 41.12
Barium meal showing previous gastric surgery (antrectomy with Roux-en-Y anastomosis) with phytobezoar in the gastric remnant. (Courtesy of Dr J. Virjee.)

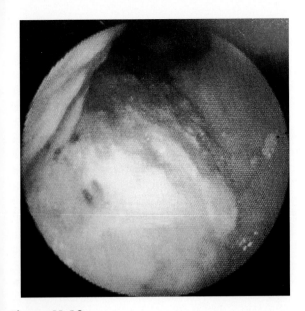

Figure 41.13
Endoscopic appearance of a gastric phytobezoar.

medium in 47%, large in 34% and excessively large in 19%. The stoma from previous gastric surgery was closely examined in all cases and was normal in 66%, stenosed in 8% and ulcerated in 26%. Associated gastric pathology, highlighting the effectiveness of gastroscopy, was identified in a high proportion: gastritis in 26%, peptic ulceration in 10% paraoesophageal hiatus hernia in 3%, oesophageal stricture in 3% and gastric carcinoma in 3%. In the rare case where endoscopy is not immediately diagnostic the finding on biopsy of hair or vegetable fibres is pathognomonic for bezoars.

Treatment

The treatment of gastric bezoars has undergone marked changes since the report of DeBakey and Oschner.[151,153] The currently accepted treatments for patients with gastric bezoars include observation, dissolution, fragmentation and surgery. Gastric bezoars have been known to resolve spontaneously and Kadian et al.[185] observed that four of six patients passed their bezoars without intervention, although complete resolution took as long as 10 months.

Enzymatic dissolution of gastric phytobezoars has given varying results, perhaps because of their different chemical composition. Proteolytic enzymes, to dissolve the proteins trapped in the bezoar matrix, have been most frequently used and the agents employed include papain, Adolph's meat tenderizer, pancrelipase and pancreatin. Papain is given to patients as two 10 000-unit tablets chewed with each meal and Adolph's meat tenderizer as 10–15 ml in water before each meal. Klamer and Max[154] tested the effect of different dissolution therapies on fragments of bezoar obtained at gastroscopy and found that dissolution was most effective when either papain or pancrelipase was used. They suggested that a single reagent might not act predictably on all phytobezoars on account of their heterogeneous make-up and advised that

testing various solutions on an endoscopic biopsy of the bezoar on which they are expected to work might improve the chances of successful dissolution therapy. The overall success rate for proteolytic therapy is 67–77%.[162] Cellulase, which breaks down cellulose, has also been successfully used to dissolve phytobezoars[167] and appears to act more quickly than proteolytic agents.[186] Holloway and associates[167] confirmed the effectiveness of cellulase in vitro and successfully cleared ten bezoars with a treatment protocol using 0.5 g/dl cellulase in 1 litre over 24 hours. The overall success rate for cellulase is 83–100%.[167] Other agents that have been employed with a varying degree of success in the dissolution of phytobezoars include acetylcysteine (success rate 50%), sodium bicarbonate, zinc chloride and vitamin C.[154,156,162,186] Enzymatic dissolution of bezoars is undoubtedly an effective therapeutic option, although the process may be prolonged and complications have been reported.[186]

Endoscopic manipulation is now undoubtedly the most useful and effective therapy for gastric phytobezoars.[156] This method has several advantages over other treatments as it is highly effective and has a short duration of therapy that is not dependent on patient compliance with diet or medication. Diettrich and Gau[156] described their technique of endoscopic fragmentation of bezoars with biopsy forceps. In all their 33 patients the stomach was successfully cleared with a treatment time of 15–35 minutes. Phytobezoars may also be removed by using a Water Pik.[160,187] A long plastic tube 2 mm in diameter is inserted through a gastroscope which is visualizing the bezoar. The plastic tube is attached to the Water Pik and under direct vision a jet of water is directed at the bezoar. After the bezoar is fragmented the stomach is lavaged and broken particles of bezoar removed. Rider and colleagues[160] found this to be a highly effective method of treating gastric phytobezoars and reported disintegration of the bezoar after only a few minutes. Chen[188] has also reported success in using an endoscopic drill for fragmenting particularly hard bezoars and concretions, and neodymium-YAG laser therapy has been effectively employed in a few cases.[189]

Occasionally surgery will be needed to remove large symptomatic bezoars, and this is necessary in all cases with trichobezoars.[159] The bezoar is removed in one piece by simple gastrostomy performed under antibiotic cover. Care should be exercised to avoid missing further bezoars in the intestine and, if found, they are removed by enterotomy or milked into the large intestine.

Treatment of bezoars must include careful follow-up as a proportion of bezoars will recur. This is particularly important in patients with gastric motility problems; in the report of Diettrich and Gau[156] 13.6% of bezoars recurred. The patient is counselled as to proper diet and preparation of food, and gastric motility stimulants, such as metoclopramide, domperidone and cisapride may be helpful in the postgastrectomy or diabetic patient. For those patients with recurrent phytobezoars that are all demonstrated to be chemically similar, long-term maintenance on a specific solvent regime is indicated.[154] Patients with trichobezoars always require psychological evaluation to prevent recurrence.[159]

GASTRIC FOREIGN BODIES

The most frequently encountered foreign bodies in the gastrointestinal tract are either accidentally or deliberately swallowed.[161] Although most swallowed foreign bodies are completely harmless, some objects are still associated with a significant morbidity and mortality. In the USA over 1500 people per year die from foreign bodies in the upper gastrointestinal tract.[190,191] Approximately 90% of all ingested foreign bodies pass into the gastrointestinal tract, with 10% entering the tracheobronchial tree.[192] Over 80% of all foreign bodies are swallowed by children, with the highest incidence in the 1–3-year age range. Adults with dentures are prone to swallowing foreign bodies on account of their reduced oral tactile sensation.[161] Ingested foreign bodies are also commonly associated with smugglers, professional entertainers, prisoners and psychiatric patients. These latter two groups of patients often have recurrent episodes of foreign body ingestion and this may occur on a regular basis over a period of years. In the case described by Chalk and Foucar,[193] of a manic depressive patient, 2533 foreign bodies were removed at laparotomy.

Certain factors influence the fate of ingested foreign bodies, namely their size, shape and the presence of pre-existing intestinal disease. There are several sites of possible lodgement in the gastrointestinal tract. In the oesophagus a foreign body may lodge at the cricopharyngeus, at the aortic arch or at the gastro-oesophageal junction. Approximately 10% of patients with oesophageal foreign bodies have pre-existing oesophageal disease.[194] Once foreign bodies have entered the stomach, 95% will pass and only 5% will remain in the gastric lumen. The duodenal curve is a further site of lodgement and this is particularly so with long objects. Once in the small bowel the foreign body may obstruct at the ileocaecal valve, although most objects will pass into the colon. Occasionally a foreign body will impact in a Mechel's diverticulum or in the appendix and cause local inflammation.[195]

Children most commonly swallow small objects such as pins, coins, small toys, buttons, nails, screws and small batteries. Once these foreign bodies have entered the stomach almost all will pass spontaneously without incident.[196] Alkaline disc batteries are often swallowed by children. There have been reports of perforation within the gastrointestinal system associated with leakage of the alkaline battery contents, and late oesophageal strictures can occur. These problems are invariably preceded by breakage of the battery case, which can be seen on plain radiographs.[197]

Adults swallow a variety of objects and in a recent report from Hong Kong[194] fish and chicken bones were the most common causative agents. The number of foreign bodies may be extremely large and Devaneson et al.[190] recently described a case of 648 metallic objects that formed an intertwining mass in the stomach. Smooth foreign bodies, such as coins, buttons, marbles and small keys, usually pass without difficulty. Large pointed objects are the most troublesome. Of these, open safety pins, razor blades, hair pins and table cutlery are the most frequently associated with problems. In the adult it has been stated that objects thicker than 2 cm and longer than 5 cm tend to lodge in the stomach.[191]

Although over 90% of ingested foreign bodies pass through the intestine without complications, there are numerous reports of life-threatening complications. Foreign bodies may cause obstruction, particularly in the lower oesophagus and in the small bowel. Perforation can occur with sharp objects and this may occur throughout the gastrointestinal tract (Figure 41.14). Lodgement of a foreign body, particularly when sharp, can lead to local erosion and perforation. Perforation may result in the formation of a local abscess or widespread peritonitis. Perforation is a rare complication of foreign body ingestion and in a series of 800 cases this complication was seen in only 1% of patients.[198] The same authors found that the stomach and duodenum were the sites of perforation in approximately half of a collected series of 71 perforated cases; the remaining perforations were equally divided among the small intestine, the caecum and the colon. Gastrointestinal bleeding has been reported and is related to sharp trauma to the mucosa or the development of local ulceration. Rarely an aortoduodenal fistula may develop with local erosion.[161] Migration through the intestinal wall occasionally occurs and foreign bodies have been found in the liver[199] and the right kidney[200] with tracts extending from the stomach and duodenum, respectively. Rarely foreign metallic bodies can spontaneously disintegrate in the intestine over a period of time.[201]

Foreign bodies in the stomach are usually asymptomatic and

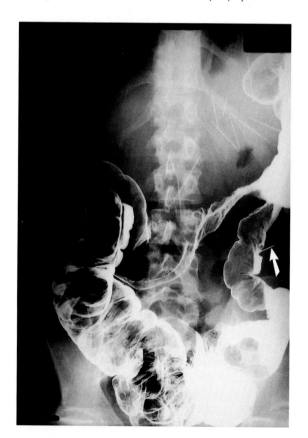

Figure 41.14
Barium enema demonstrating perforation of descending colon by a needle (arrowed). Note multiple needles in the stomach. (Courtesy of Dr J. Virjee.)

will progress down the gastrointestinal tract without discomfort. Some patients may complain of vague cramps, vomiting, heaviness in the epigastrium, anorexia and malnutrition. With pre-existing pyloric obstruction foreign bodies may cause complete gastric outlet obstruction. Perforation is indicated by peritonitis or local tenderness with distension and pyrexia. Many of the cases of the multiple foreign bodies in the stomach of mental patients have produced no symptoms. Teimourian et al.[201] reported foreign body ingestion in 101 psychotic patients. They found that one-third of patients died as a direct result of an ingested metallic body, regardless of whether the patient was subjected to operative or non-operative management. They related these results to the basic inability of most of these patients to communicate early symptoms. Moreover the basic difficulty of interpreting physical signs of perforation in obviously psychotic individuals often resulted in late operative intervention.

The diagnosis can usually be made from the clinical history and radiological examination. Difficulty may be encountered with oesophageal and gastric foreign bodies which are comparatively radiolucent, such as chicken bones and plastic material of various shapes and sizes. In the report of Nandi and Ong[194] positive plain radiographs were obtained in only 14% of oesophageal foreign bodies. Endoscopy may be needed to find the foreign body in a proportion of cases.

The treatment of foreign bodies depends on their size and shape and the point of lodgement. All foreign bodies in the oesophagus should be removed to prevent perforation. This is usually performed endoscopically using a variety of instruments to grasp the object. Sharp objects such as razors can be pulled into an overture to prevent trauma on withdrawal. Open safety pins are pulled blunt end first to conform to the old axiom 'advancing points puncture, trailing do not'. In some pediatric patients the Foley catheter technique is useful for smooth objects such as coins. Most foreign bodies in the stomach will pass and they should be observed radiologically, as long as the patient is asymptomatic, to monitor forward progress. Smooth foreign bodies, except alkaline disc batteries, can be watched for several weeks, whereas large foreign bodies or sharp objects require endoscopic intervention. Advances in endoscopy have made it possible to remove almost any object from the stomach. Foreign bodies can be removed, even when impacted in the wall of the bowel, and the patient managed conservatively to good effect. Occasionally magnets may be used for removal of metallic foreign bodies.[161]

Surgery for foreign bodies is now rare and is generally for complications such as perforation and haemorrhage. Objects that fail to progress through the bowel or that are sharp (e.g. open safety pins) require enterotomy and removal. Immediately before laparotomy a radiograph should be taken to confirm the position of the foreign body; fluoroscopic screening may be needed at surgery, both to find the object and to ensure complete removal of multiple objects.

REFERENCES

1. Feldman D. *Clinical Roentgenology of the Digestive Tract*, 4th edn. Baltimore, MD: Williams & Wilkins, 1957.

2. Palmer ED. Collective review: gastric diverticula. *Int Abstr Surg* 1951; **92**: 417–428.

3. Meeroff M, Gollan JR & Meeroff JC. Gastric diverticulum. *Am J Gastroenterol* 1967; **47**: 189–203.

4. Raffin SB. Diverticula, rupture and volvulus. In Sleisenger MH & Fortran JS (eds) *Gastrointestinal Disease: Pathophysiology, Diagnosis and Management*, 4th Edn. London: WB Saunders, 1989: 735–736.

5. Localio SA & Stahl WM. Diverticula of the stomach. *Curr Prob Surg* 1968; **Jan**: 6–14.

6. Rivers AB, Stevens G & Kirklin BR. Diverticula of the stomach. *Surg Gynecol Obstet* 1935; **60**: 106–113.

7. Herrera AF. Diverticula of the stomach. In Bockus HL (ed.) *Gastroenterology*, 3rd edn. Philadelphia: WB Saunders, 1974: 1093–1098.

8. Burke T. Gastric diverticula in childhood: a report of two cases and a review of the literature. *J Singapore Pediatr Soc* 1965; **7**: 101–105.

9. Rotterdam H & Enterline HT. *Pathology of the Stomach and Duodenum*. New York: Springer, 1989: 27–28.

10. Neblett WM & O'Neill JA Jr. Gastric diverticulum. In Scott HW & Sawyers JL (eds) *Surgery of the Stomach, Duodenum and Small Intestine*. Boston: Blackwell, 1987: 361–363.

11. Dickinson RJ & Freeman AH. Partial gastric diverticula: radiological and endoscopic features in six patients. *Gut* 1986; **27**: 954–957.

12. Cockrell CH, Cho SR, Messmer JM, Shaw CI & Liu CI. Intramural gastric diverticula: a report of three cases. *Br J Radiol* 1984; **57**: 285–288.

13. Treichel J, Gerstenberg E, Palme G & Klemm T. Diagnosis of partial gastric diverticula. *Radiology* 1976; **119**: 13–18.

14. Bigg RL & Judd ES. Gastric diverticula. *Am J Surg* 1963; **105**: 239–243.

15. Buckstein J. *The Digestive Tract in Roentgenology*, 2nd edn, vol. I, Philadelphia: Lippincott, 1953: 298.

16. Condon RE. In Nyhus LM & Wastell C. *Surgery of the Stomach and Duodenum*, 4th edn. Boston: Little Brown, 1986: 583–584.

17. Gray SW & Skandalakis JE. *Embryology for Surgeons*. Philadelphia: WB Saunders, 1972: 113–115.

18. Kurgan A & Hoffman J. Aetiology of gastric diverticula – an hypothesis. *Med Hypotheses* 1981; **7**: 1471–1476.

19. Grassi G. Highly selective vagotomy with intra-operative acid testing of completeness of vagal section. *Surg Gynecol Obstet* 1975; **140**: 259–264.

20. Palmer ED. Gastric diverticulosis. *Am Fam Physician* 1973; **7**: 114–117.

21. Anaise D, Brand DL, Smith NL & Soroff HS. Pitfalls in the diagnosis and treatment of a symptomatic gastric diverticulum. *Gastrointest Endosc* 1984; **30**: 28–30.

22. Graham DY & Kimbrough RC. Congenital gastric diverticulum as a cause of massive haemorrhage. *Am J Dig Dis* 1974; **19**: 174–178.

23. Cosman B, Kollum J & Kingsbury H. Gastric diverticula and massive gastro-intestinal haemorrhage. *Am J Surg* 1957; **94**: 144–148.

24. Eras P & Bernbaum SL. Gastric diverticula: congenital and acquired. *Am J Gastroenterol* 1972; **57**: 120–132.

25. Gibbons CP & Harvey L. An ulcerated gastric diverticulum – a rare cause of haematemesis and malaena. *Postgrad Med J* 1984; **60**: 693–695.

26. Ward WW, Oca CF & Carty CB. Massive haemoperitoneum due to gastric diverticula. *JAMA* 1966; **196**: 798–801.

27. Sinclair N. Congenital diverticulum of the stomach in an infant. *Br J Surg* 1929; **17**: 182–183.

28. Dragomiresco L, Freschin D, Pawn C & Bandila TR. Deux cas de diverticule gastrique invaginé dans l'ésophage. *J Chir (Paris)* 1963; **86**: 192–194.

29. Hartley JB. Diverticulum of stomach found to enter left inguinal hernial sac. *Br J Radiol* 1945; **18**: 231–232.

30. Akerlund D. Gastric diverticulum. *Acta Radiol* 1923; **2**: 476–485.

31. Ellis H. Diverticula, volvulus and ileus. In Schwarts SI & Ellis H (eds) *Maingot's Abdominal Operations*, 8th edn. Norwalk, CT: Appleton-Century-Crofts, 1985: 643–646.

32. Hejboer LP & Nieuwenhuizen LN. Gastric diverticula. *Neth J Surg* 1980; **32**: 16–18.

33. Ladd WE. Duplications of the alimentary tract. *South Med. J.* 1937; **30**: 363–371.

34. Gross RE, Holcomb GW Jr & Farber S. Duplications of the alimentary tract. *Paediatrics* 1952; **9**: 449–468.

35. Ladd WE & Gross RE. Surgical treatment of duplications of the alimentary tract: enterogenous cysts, enteric cysts or ileum duplex. *Surg Gynecol Obstet* 1940; **70**: 295–302.

36. Gray SW & Skandalakis JE. *Embryology for Surgeons*. Philadelphia: WB Saunders, 1972.

37. Sleisenger MH & Fortran JS. *Gastrointestinal Disease: Pathophysiology,*

Diagnosis and Management, 4th edn. Philadelphia: WB Saunders, 1989: 667.

38. Gross RE. *The Surgery of Infancy and Childhood.* Philadelphia, WB Saunders, 1953.

39. Bower RJ, Sieber WK & Kiesewetter WB. Alimentary tract duplications in children. *Ann Surg* 1978; **188**: 669–674.

40. Kremer RM, Lepoff BB & Izant RJ Jr. *Duplication of the stomach. J Pediatr Surg* 1970; **5**: 360–364.

41. Abrami G & Dennison WM. Duplications of the stomach. *Surgery* 1961; **49**: 794–801.

42. Bartels RJ. Duplication of the stomach: case report and review of the literature. *Am Surg* 1967; **33**: 747–752.

43. Tabrisky J, Szalay GC & Meade WS. Duplication of the stomach. *Am J Gastroenterol* 1973; **59**: 327–339.

44. Holcomb GW, Ali Gheissari, O'Neill JA, Shorter NA & Bishop HC. Surgical mangement of alimentary tract duplications. *Ann Surg* 1989; **209**: 167–174.

45. Wieczorek RL, Seidman I & Ranson JH. Congenital duplication of the stomach. Case report and review of the English literature. *Am J Gastroenterol* 1984; **79**: 597–602.

46. Rowling JT. Some observations on gastric cysts. *Br J Surg* 1959; **46**: 441–445.

47. Rotterdam H & Enterline HT. *Pathology of the Stomach and Duodenum.* New York: Springer, 1989: 26–27.

48. Clement KW & Escamilla HA. Duplication of the stomach. *J Nat Med Assoc* 1974; **66**: 292–304.

49. Favara BE, Franciosi RA & Akers DR. Enteric duplications. *Am J Dis Child* 1971; **122**: 501–505.

50. Hoffman M, Sugerman HJ & Herman D. Gastric duplication cyst communicating with aberrant pancreatic duct: a rare cause of recurrent acute pancreatitis. *Surgery* 1987; **101**: 369–372.

51. Torma MJ. Of double stomachs. *Arch Surg* 1974; **109**: 555–557.

52. Ravitch MM. Duplications of the gastrointestinal tract. In KJ Welch, JG Randolph, MM Ravitch, JA O'Neill & MI Rower (eds) *Paediatric Surgery,* 4th edn. Chicago: Year Book, 1986: 911–920.

53. Lewis FT & Thyng FW. Regular occurence of intestinal diverticula in embryos of pig, rabbit and man. *Am J Anat* 1908; **7**: 505–519.

54. Saunders RL. Combined anterior and posterior spina bifida in a living neonatal human female. *Anat Rec* 1953; **87**: 255–278.

55. Bentley JFR & Smith JR. Development posterior enteric remnants and spinal malformations. *Arch Dis Child* 1960; **35**: 76–86.

56. McLetchie NGB, Purves JK & Saunders RL. The genesis of gastric and certain intestinal diverticula and enterogenous cysts. *Surg Gynecol Obstet* 1954; **99**: 135–141.

57. Mellish RWL & Koop CE. Clinical manifestations of duplication of the bowel. *Pediatrics* 1961; **27**: 397–407.

58. Bremer JL. Diverticula and duplications of the intestinal tract. *Arch Pathol* 1944; **38**: 132–140.

59. Bockus HL. *Gastroenterology* 3rd edn. Philadelphia: WB Saunders, 1974: 1103–1114.

60. Fitzgibbons RJ Jr, Nugent FW & Ellis FH. Unusual thoraco-abdominal duplication associated with pancreaticopleural fistulae. *Gastroenterology* 1980; **79**: 344–347.

61. Condon RE. In Nyhus LM & Wastell C (eds) *Surgery of the Stomach and Duodenum,* 4th ed. Boston: Little Brown, 1986: 584–585.

62. Garnjobst W. Antral duplication with intractable duodenal ulcer. *Gastroenterology* 1965; **49**: 419–421.

63. Noblett WW & O'Neill JA Jr. In Scott HW Jr & Sawyers JL (eds) *Surgery of the Stomach, Duodenum and Small Intestine.* Boston: Blackwell, 1987: 363–366.

64. Traverso LW, Damus PS & Longmire WL. Pancreatitis of unusual origin. *Surg Gynecol Obstet* 1975; **141**: 383–386.

65. Orr MM & Edwards AJ. Neoplastic change in duplications of the alimentary tract. *Br J Surg* 1975; **62**: 269–274.

66. Mayo HW, McKee EE & Anderson RM. Carcinoma arising in reduplication of stomach (gastrogenous cyst): a case report. *Ann Surg* 1955; **141**: 550–555.

67. Micolonghi T & Meissner GF. Gastric type carcinoma arising in duplication of the small intestine. *Ann Surg* 1958; **147**: 124–127.

68. Onojola MF, Hood IC & Stevenson GW. Calcified gastric duplication. *Gastrointest Radiol* 1980; **5**: 232–238.

69. Lamont AC, Starinsky R & Cremin BJ. Ultrasonic diagnosis of duplication cysts in children. *Br J Radiol* 1984; **57**: 463–467.

70. Curran JP, Behbahani M & Kim BH. Ectopic gastric duplication cyst in an infant. *Clin Pediatr* 1984; **23**: 50–55.

71. Teele RL, Henschke CL & Tapper D. The radiographic and ultrasonographic evaluation of enteric duplication cysts. *Pediatr Radiol* 1980; **10**: 9–14.

72. Yajko R, Seydett F & Trimble C. Rupture of the stomach from blunt abdominal trauma. *J Trauma* 1975; **15**: 177–183.

73. Allen RB & Curry GJ. Abdominal trauma: a study of 297 consecutive cases. *Am J Surg* 1957; **93**: 398–402.

74. Fitzgerald JB, Crawford ES & DeBakey ME. Surgical considerations of non-penetrating abdominal injuries: an analysis of 200 cases. *Am J Surg* 1960; **100**: 22–30.

75. Rodkey GR. The management of abdominal injuries. *Surg Clin North Am* 1966; **46**: 627–639.

76. Morton JH, Hinshaw HR & Morton JJ. Blunt trauma to the abdomen. *Ann Surg* 1957; **145**: 699–704.

77. Clarke R. Closed abdominal injuries. *Lancet* 1954; **ii**: 877–879.

78. Luccioni L & Mammucari R. Temaditraumichiusi dell'addone; considerazioni anatomo-cliniche e terapeutiche chirurgiche su alcune osservazioni di lesioni gastriche da scoppio. *Ann Ital Chir* 1969; **45**: 226–236.

79. Asch JR, Coran AG & Johnson PW. Gastric perforation secondary to blunt trauma in children. *J Trauma* 1975; **15**: 196–197.

80. Bussey HJ, McGhee RN & Tyson KRT. Isolated gastric rupture due to blunt trauma. *J Trauma* 1975; **15**: 193–195.

81. Vassy LE, Klecker RL, Koch E & Morse TS. Traumatic gastric perforation in children from blunt trauma. *J Trauma* 1975; **15**: 190–192.

82. Andersen CB & Ballinger WF. Abdominal injuries. In Zuidema GD, Rutherford PB & Ballinger WB (eds) *The Management of Trauma,* 4th edn. Philadephia: WB Saunders, 1985: 449–504.

83. Nance FC, Wennar MH, Johnson LW, Ingram JC & Cohn I Jr. Surgical judgement in the management of penetrating wounds of the abdomen: experience with 2212 patients. *Ann Surg* 1974; **179**: 639–645.

84. Mandelstam P, Sugawa C & Silvis CE. Complications associated with oesophagogastroduodenoscopy and with oesophageal dilation. *Gastrointest Endosc* 1976; **23**: 16–19.

85. Jones F, Doll R & Fletcher C. The risks of gastroscopy. *Lancet* 1951; **i**: 226–230.

86. Palmer ED & Wirst C. Survey of gastroscopic and oesophagoscopic accidents. *JAMA* 1957; **164**: 2012–2015.

87. Schiller KF, Cotton PB & Albert RK. The hazards of digestive fibre-endoscopy: a survey of British experience. *Gut* 1972; **13**: 1027.

88. Albo R, De Lorimier AA & Silen W. Spontaneous rupture of the stomach in the adult. *Surgery* 1963; **53**: 797–805.

89. Evans DS. Acute dilatation and spontaneous rupture of the stomach. *Br J Surg* 1968; **55**: 940–942.

90. Harling H. Spontaneous rupture of the stomach. *Acta Chir Scand* 1984; **150**: 101–103.

91. Siemens RA & Fulton RL. Gastric rupture as a result of blunt trauma. *Am Surg* 1977; **43**: 229–233.

92. Rooney JA & Pesek IG. Transection of the stomach due to blunt abdominal trauma. *J Trauma* 1968; **8**: 487–492.

93. Briggs SE, Hendricks D & Flint LM Jr. Penetrating abdominal trauma: resuscitation, diagnostic evaluation and definite management. *Adv Surg* 1987; **20**: 1–46.

94. Saul SH, Decker A & Watson CG. Acute gastric dilatation with infarction and perforation. *Gut* 1981; **22**: 978–983.

95. Baglio CM & Fattal GA. Spontaneous rupture of the stomach in the adult. *Am J Dig Dis* 1962; **7**: 75–83.

96. Le Duox MS, Sillers MJ & Atkins CP. Spontaneous rupture of the stomach in the adult. *South Med J* 1991; **84**: 399–401.

97. Chandrasekhara KL, Iyer SK, Sutton AL & Starek AE. Spontaneous rupture of the stomach. *Am J Med* 1986; **81**: 1062–1064.

98. Madura M, Craig R & Shields T. Unusual causes of spontaneous pneumoperitoneum. *Surg Gynecol Obstet* 1982; **154**: 417–420.

99. Revilliod E. Rupture l'estomac. *Rev Med Suisse Romande* 1985; **5**: 5.

100. Millar TM, Bruce J & Paterson JRS. Spontaneous rupture of the stomach. *Br J Surg* 1957; **44**: 513–516.

101. Glassman O. Subcutaneous rupture of the stomach; traumatic and spontaneous. *Ann Surg* 1929; **89**: 247–263.

102. Cramer FS & Heimbach RD. Stomach rupture as a result of gastrointestinal barotrauma in a scuba diver. *J Trauma* 1982; **22**: 238–240.

103. Bolt DE & Hennessy WB. Rupture of the stomach complicating gastric haemorrhage. *Lancet* 1955; **ii**: 485–486.

104. Brismer B, Strandberg A & Wilklund B. Stomach rupture following ingestion of sodium bicarbonate. *Acta Chir Scand* 1986; (Suppl. **530**): 97–99.

105. Fordtran JS, Morawski SG, Santa Ana CA & Rector FC. Gas production after reaction of sodium bicarbonate and hydrochloric acid. *Gastroenterology* 1984; **87**: 1014–1021.

106. Fischer RP, Beverlin BC, Engrav LH, Benjamin CI & Perry JF Jr. diagnostic peritoneal lavage. Fourteen years and 2586 patients later. *Am J Surg* 1979; **136**: 701–705.

107. Federle MP, Crass RA, Jeffrey RB & Trunkey DD. Computed tomography in blunt abdominal trauma. *Arch Surg* 1982; **117**: 645–650.

108. Demetriades D, Van Der Veen BW & Hatzitheophilous C. Spontaneous rupture of the stomach in an adult. *S Afr Med J* 1982; **61**: 23–26.

109. Matikainen M. Rupture of the stomach: a rare complication of resuscitation. Case report. *Acta Chir Scand* 1978; **144**: 61–62.

110. Llaneza PP & Salt WB. Gastric volvulus: more common than previously thought? *Postgrad Med J* 1986; **80**: 279–288.

111. Askew AR. Treatment of acute and chronic gastric volvulus. *Ann R Coll Surg Engl* 1978; **60**: 326–328.

112. Berti A. Sigolare attortiglamento dell'esofago col duodeno sequito da rapida morte. *Gazz Med Ital Prov Ver* 1866; **9**: 139.

113. Buchanan J. Volvulus of the stomach. *Br J Surg* 1930; **18**: 99–112.

114. Dalgaard JB. Volvulus of the stomach. *Acta Clin Scand* 1952; **103**: 131–153.

115. Gurnsey JM & Connolly JE. Acute, complete gastric volvulus: collective review and report of 2 cases. *Arch Surg* 1963; **86**: 423–429.

116. Wastell C & Ellis H. Volvulus of the stomach: a review with a report of 8 cases. *Br J Surg* 1971; **58**: 557–562.

117. Cole BC & Dickinson SJ. Acute volvulus of the stomach in infants and children. *Surgery* 1971; **70**: 707–717.

118. Carter R, Brewer LA & Linshaw DB. Acute gastric volvulus: a study of 25 cases. *Am J Surg* 1980; **140**: 99–106.

119. Von Haberer H. Volvulus des Magens bei Carcinoma. *Dtsch Z Chir* 1912; **115**: 497–504.

120. Singleton AC. Chronic gastric volvulus. *Radiology* 1940; **34**: 53–61.

121. Haddad JK, Doherty C & Clark RE. Acute gastric volvulus: endoscopic derotation. *West J Med* 1977; **127**: 341–346.

122. Giblin TR & Martin JD. Volvulus of the stomach. *Am Surg* 1960; **26**: 759–762.

123. Chessick KC & Hoye SJ. Paraoesophageal hernia and gastric volvulus. *J Fla Med Assoc* 1973; **62**: 30–34.

124. Smith RJ. Volvulus of the stomach. *J Natl Med Assoc* 1983; **75**: 393–397.

125. Ziprkowski MN & Teele RL. Gastric volvulus in childhood. *AJR* 1979; **132**: 921–925.

126. Metcalfe-Gibson C. A case of haemorrhage from volvulus of the gastric fundus. *Br J Surg* 1975; **62**: 224–225.

127. Camblos JF. Acute volvulus of the stomach. *Am Surg* 1969; **35**: 505–509.

128. Clearfield HR & Stahlgren. Acute dilatation, volvulus and torsion of the stomach. In JE Berk (ed.) *Bockus Gastroenterology*, 4th edn. Philadelphia: WB Saunders, 1984: 1373–1380.

129. Carlisle BB & Hayes CW. Gastric volvulus: an unusual complication after pneumonectomy. *Am J Surg* 1967; **113**: 579–582.

130. Creedon PJ & Burman JF. Volvulus of the stomach: report of a case with complications. *Am J Surg* 1965; **110**: 964–966.

131. Pillay SB, Angorn IB & Baker LW. Gastric volvulus unassociated with hiatal hernia. *S Afr Med J* 1977; **52**: 880–885.

132. Tanner NC. Chronic and recurrent volvulus of the stomach with late results of 'colonic displacement'. *Am J Surg* 1968; **115**: 505–515.

133. Patel NM. Chronic gastric volvulus: report of a case and review of literature. *Am J Gastroenterol* 1985; **80**: 170–173.

134. Thorpe JAC. Chronic gastric volvulus: aetiology and treatment. *Br J Clin Pract* 1981; **35**: 161–162.

135. Jones WM & Jones CD. Volvulus of the transverse colon associated with organoaxial volvulus of the stomach. *Am J Surg* 1972; **124**: 404–406.

136. Elidan J, Gimmon Z & Schwartz A. Pneumoperitonuem induced by pneumatosis cystoides intestinalis associated with volvulus of the stomach. *Am J Gastroenterol* 1980; **74**: 189–195.

137. Yin RL & Nowak TV. Familial occurrence of intrathoracic gastric volvulus. *Dig Dis Sci* 1988; **33**: 1483–1487.

138. Linnemann MP & Johnson VW. Ehlers–Danlos syndrome presenting with torsion of the stomach. *Proc R Soc Med* 1975; **68**: 330–333.

139. Borchardt M. Zur Pathologie und Therapie des Magenvolvulus. *Arch Klin Chir* 1904; **74**: 243–260.

140. Campbell JB. Neonatal gastric volvulus. *AJR* 1979; **132**: 723–725.

141. Farr C, Graver K & Curry RW. Electrocardiographic changes with gastric volvulus. *N Engl J Med* 1984; **310**: 1747–1748.

142. Pearson FG, Cooper JD & Ives R. Massive hiatal hernia with incarceration: a report of 53 cases. *Ann Thorac Surg* 1983; **35**: 45–51.

143. Menuck L. Plain film findings of gastric volvulus herniating into the chest. *AJR* 1976; **126**: 1169–1174.

144. DeLorimier AA & Penn L. Acute volvulus of the stomach emphasizing management hazards. *AJR* 1957; **77**: 627–633.

145. Bhasin DK, Nagi B, Kochhar R, Singh K & Mehta SK. Endoscopic correction of organo-axial volvulus. *Endoscopy* 1988; **20**: 283.

146. Bhasin DK, Nagi B, Kochhar R, Sihgn K, Gupta NM & Mehta SK. Endoscopic management of chronic organo-axial volvulus of the stomach. *Am J Gastroenterol* 1990; **85**: 1486–1489.

147. Eckhauser ML & Ferron JP. The use of dual percutaneous endoscopic gastrostomy in the management of chronic intermittent gastric volvulus. *Gastrointest Endosc* 1985; **31**: 340–342.

148. Farkas AG & Celestin LR. Gastrojejunostomy: a simple method of treatment of gastric volvulus. *Ann R Coll Surg Engl* 1986; **68**: 107–109.

149. Stremple JF. A new operation for the anatomic correction of chronic intermittent gastric volvulus. *Am J Surg* 1973; **125**: 360–363.

150. Schreiber H, Flickinger EG & Eichelbergen MR. Colonic displacement: proposed treatment for gastric remnant volvulus due to eventration of the diaphragm. *Am J Surg* 1980; **139**: 719–722.

151. Singh J & Garg P. Gastrojejunal hitch in gastric volvulus. *Am J Gastroenterol* 1989; **84**: 693–694.

152. DeBakey M & Oschner A. Part I: Bezoars and concretions. *Surgery* 1938; **4**: 934–963.

153. DeBakey M & Oschner A. Part II: Bezoars and concretions. *Surgery* 1938; **5**: 132–160.

154. Klamer TW & Max MH. Recurrent gastric bezoars. A new approach to treatment and prevention. *Am J Surg* 1983; **145**: 417–419.

155. Zarling J & Thompson LE. Non persimmon gastric phytobezoar: a benign recurrent condition. *Arch Intern Med* 1984; **144**: 959–961.

156. Diettrich NA & Gau FC. Post gastrectomy phytobezoars – endoscopic diagnosis and treatment. *Arch Surg* 1985; **120**: 432–435.

157. Cain GD, Moore P & Pattersen M. Bezoars – a complication of the post gastrectomy state. *Dig Dis Sci* 1968; **13**: 801–809.

158. Ahn YH, Maturu P, Steinheber FU & Goldman JM. Association of diabetes mellitus with gastric bezoar formation. *Arch Intern Med* 1987; **147**: 527–528.

159. Wolfsen PJ, Fabius RJ & Leibowitz AN. The Rapunzel syndrome: an unusual trichobezoar. *Am J Gastroenterol* 1987; **82**: 365–367.

160. Rider JA, Foresti-Lorente RF, Garrido J & Puletti EJ. Gastric bezoars: treatment and prevention. *Am J Gastroenterol* 1984; **79**: 357–359.

161. DeBakey M & Jordan GL. Foreign bodies in the oesophagus, stomach and duodenum. In Schwartz SL & Ellis H (eds) *Maingot's Abdominal Operations*, 8th edn. Norwalk, CT: Appleton-Century-Crofts, 1985: 667–683.

162. Andrus CH & Ponsky JL. Bezoars: classification, pathophysiology and treatment. *Am J Gastroenterol* 1988; **83**: 476–478.

163. Finley CR, Hellmuth EW & Schubert TT. Polystyrene bezoar in a patient with polystyrenomania. *Am J Gastroenterol* 1988; **83**: 74–76.

164. Borg I, Heijkenskyold F & Nihlen B. Massive growth of yeasts in resected stomachs. *Gut* 1966; **7**: 244–247.

165. Perttala Y, Peltokallio P, Leiviska T & Sipponen J. Yeast bezoar formation following gastric surgery. *AJR* 1975; **125**: 365–368.

166. Dolan P & Thompson B. Management of persimmon bezoars (diospyrobezoars). *South Med J* 1979; **72**: 1527–1529.

167. Holloway WD, Lee SP & Nicholson GI. the composition and dissolution of phytobezoars. *Arch Pathol Lab Med* 1980; **104**: 159–161.

168. Meeroff JC, Squires PA & Grasman K. Gastric lupinoma: a new variety of phytobezoar. *Am J Gastroenterol* 1989; **84**: 650–652.

169. Calabuig R, Navarro S, Carrio I, Artigas V & Puig LaCalle J. Gastric emptying and bezoars. *Am J Surg* 1989; **157**: 287–290.

170. Jay BS & Burrell M. Iatrogenic problems following gastric surgery. *Gastrointest Radiol* 1977; **2**: 239–257.

171. Szemes G & Amberg J. Gastric bezoars after partial gastrectomy. *Radiology* 1968; **90**: 765–768.

172. Stanten A & Peters H. Enzymatic dissolution of phytobezoars. *Am J Surg* 1975; **130**: 259–261.

173. Brady PG. Gastric phytobezoars consequent to delayed gastric emptying. *Gastrointest Endosc* 1978; **24**: 159–161.

174. Vogel SB & Woodward ER. The surgical treatment of chronic gastrectomy following Roux-Y diversion for alkaline reflux gastritis. *Ann Surg* 1989; **209**: 756–763.

175. Brady PG & Richardson R. Gastric bezoar formation secondary to gastroparesis diabeticorum. *Arch Intern Med* 1977; **137**: 1729.

176. Silver BJ, Rhodes JB & Schimke RN. Bezoars: a complication of diabetic gastroparesis. *J Kansas Med Soc* 1983; **84**: 249–250.

177. Goyal RK & Spiro HM. Gastrointestinal manifestations of diabetes mellitus. *Med Clin North Am* 1971; **55**: 1031–1044.

178. Das Gupta H, Chandra S & Gupta M. Trichobezoar – clinical diagnosis. *J Postgrad Med* 1979; **25**: 181–183.

179. Hossenbocus A & Colin-Jones D. Trichobezoar, gastric polysis, protein losing gastroenteropathy and steatorrhoea. *Gut* 1973; **14**: 730–732.

180. McFarland RJ, Grundy A, Gazet J-C & Pilkington TRE. The intragastric balloon: a novel idea proved ineffective. *Br J Surg* 1987; **74**: 137–139.

181. Kral JG. Gastric balloons: a plea for sanity in the midst of balloonacy. *Gastroenterology* 1988; **95**: 213–215.

182. Bowden TA, Hooks VH & Mansberger AR. The stomach after surgery. *Ann Surg* 1983; **197**: 637–644.

183. Ratcliffe JF. The ultrasonic appearance of a trichobezoar. *Br J Radiol* 1982; **55**: 166–167.

184. McCracken S, Jongeward R, Silver TM & Jafri SZ. Gastric trichobezoar: sonographic findings. *Radiology* 1986; **161**: 123–124.

185. Kadian RS, Rose JF & Mann MS. Gastric bezoars – spontaneous resolution. *Am J Gastroenterol* 1978; **70**: 79–82.

186. Zarling EJ & Moeller DD. Bezoar therapy. Complications of using Adolph's meat tenderizer and alternative from literature review. *Arch Intern Med* 1981; **191**: 1669–1670.

187. Madsen R, Skibba RM & Galvan A. Gastric bezoars: a technique of endoscopic removal. *Dig Dis Sci* 1978; **23**: 717–719.

188. Chen GH. Removal of bezoars from stomach using an endoscopic drill. *Gastrointest Endosc* 1985; **31**: 355.

189. Naveau S, Poynard T & Zourabichvili O. Gastric phytobezoar destruction by ND:YAG laser therapy. *Gastrointest Endosc* 1986; **32**: 430–431.

190. Devaneson J Pisani P & Sharman P. Metallic foreign bodies in the stomach. *Arch Surg* 1977; **112**: 664–665.

191. Webb WA, McDaniel L & Jones L. Foreign bodies of the upper gastrointestinal tract. Current management. *South Med J* 1984; **77**: 1083–1086.

192. Schwartz GF & Polsky HS. Ingested foreign bodies of the gastrointestinal tract. *Am Surg* 1976; **42**: 236–238.

193. Chalk GF & Foucar HO. Foreign bodies in the stomach. *Arch Surg* 1928; **16**: 494–499.

194. Nandi P & Ong GB. Foreign body in the oesophagus: review of 2394 cases. *Br J Surg* 1978; **65**: 5–9.

195. Willis GA & Ho WC. Perforation of a Meckel's diverticulum by an alkaline hearing aid battery. *Can Med Assoc J* 1982; **126**: 497–498.

196. Groff DB III. Foreign bodies and bezoars. In KJ Welch, JG Randolp, MM Ravitch, JA O'Neill & M. Rower (eds) *Paediatric Surgery*, 4th edn. Chicago: Year Book 1986: 907–911.

197. Kuling K, Rumack CM & Rumack BH. Disc battery ingestion. *JAMA* 1983; **249**: 2502–2504.

198. Henderson FF & Gaston EA. Ingested foreign body in the gastrointestinal tract. *Arch Surg* 1938; **36**: 66–69.

199. Abel RM, Fischer JE & Hendren WH. Penetration of the alimentary tract by a foreign body with migration to the liver. *Arch Surg* 1971; **102**: 227–228.

200. Baird JM & Spence HM. Ingested foreign bodies migrating to the kidney from the gastrointestinal tract. *J Urol* 1968; **99**: 675–680.

201. Dixon JM, Armstrong CP & Davies GC. Corrosion of swallowed foreign body. *J R Soc Med* 1982; **75**: 567–568.

202. Teimourian B, Cigtay AS & Smyth NPD. Management of ingested foreign bodies in the psychotic patient. *Arch Surg* 1964; **88**: 915–920.

PART

THREE

Small Intestine

edited by RCN Williamson

42

ANATOMY OF THE SMALL INTESTINE

RCN Williamson

INTRODUCTION

Segments

The small intestine is the most prominent occupant of the infra-colic compartment of the abdominal cavity. It is a continuous tube, divided into three segments for descriptive purposes. The *duodenum* is the proximal fixed portion extending from the pylorus to the duodenojejunal flexure. The word duodenum derives from the Latin word *duodeni* (12 apiece) and reflects the fact that this segment is the length of 12 fingers' breadth, i.e. 10 inches or 25 cm. The succeeding segment is termed *jejunum* after the Latin word for empty (fasting). Since food passes rapidly through it, the jejunum is usually empty at autopsy (or operation). The third and longest segment of small bowel is the *ileum* (Latin *ilia* = intestines; Greek *eileos* = colic). When present, Meckel's diverticulum arises from the terminal ileum.

Watersheds

The commencement of the duodenum is clearly marked by the pylorus. External inspection during laparotomy usually reveals an indentation roughly at this point, and the pylorus is crossed anteriorly by the vein of Mayo*. Palpation confirms the muscular ring of the pyloric sphincter. From the luminal aspect the pylorus can be identified during gastroscopy as the distal orifice of the stomach; it is usually partly closed and can be seen to contract. The termination of the duodenum is also clearly marked. At this point the small bowel passes forward to leave its retroperitoneal site and acquire a complete mesentery. A peritoneal fold known as the ligament of Treitz† is attached to the antimesenteric border of the bowel as it passes from its fixed to its free part and marks the approximate position of the duodenojejunal junction. The junction between jejunum and ileum is imperceptible. By convention, the proximal 40% of mesenteric small bowel is termed the jejunum and the distal

60% the ileum. Although a typical loop of jejunum has a thicker wall and a wider lumen than a typical loop of ileum, accurate measurements would therefore be necessary before ascribing an individual segment of mid-small bowel to one or other category. The termination of the ileum, however, is precisely delineated by the ileocaecal junction.

Length

Measurements of small bowel length in vivo are notoriously inaccurate. They are always lower than figures obtained after death, either in situ or following removal of the bowel from the body, because of the loss of muscle tone and the telescopic effect of the mesenteric attachment. Estimates of small bowel length in living adults range from about 3.0 to 3.5 m. Two cadaveric studies have shown great variability in length (between 3.0 and 8.6 m) with an average of around 6 m.[1,2] The small bowel is longer in men than women and in tall subjects than short.[3] Its length is independent of age or body weight but may be affected by diet. Because of these inconsistencies, it is better to measure the length of the intestinal remnant than the length of the resected segment after surgical shortening of the gut.

Development

The embryology of the small bowel is considered in detail in Chapter 62. Apart from the proximal 8–10 cm it develops from the primitive midgut, i.e. that part of the fetal intestine that is displaced into the physiological hernia by the growing liver between the 6th and 10th weeks of intrauterine life. The midgut extends from the major duodenal papilla almost to the splenic flexure of the colon. Its apex is marked by the attachment of the vitelline duct, the proximal portion of which may persist into postnatal life as Meckel's diverticulum. The first and upper second parts of the duodenum develop from the foregut. Thus nearly all the small intestine is supplied by the superior mesenteric artery, the artery of the midgut, but the proximal duodenum receives blood from the coeliac axis (foregut artery) via the gastroduodenal artery.

---

* The brothers Mayo, Charles Horace (1865–1939) and William James (1861–1939), described the prepyloric vein in 1900.

† Wenzel Treitz (1819–1872) was Professor of Pathology at Prague and described the suspensory ligament of the duodenum in 1853.

GROSS ANATOMY

The duodenum

Some 20–25 cm in length, the duodenum extends from pylorus to ligament of Treitz as a C-shaped loop, partly encircling the head of pancreas. It shares a common blood supply with the head of pancreas, to which it is closely applied and firmly adherent. Except at its origin, the duodenum has no mesentery and is only covered with peritoneum on its anterior aspect. It is the widest portion of the small bowel with a diameter of 4–5 cm. The duodenum is subdivided into four portions of unequal length, which run in different directions.

The first or superior part

This is about 5 cm long and passes to the right from the pylorus to the neck of the gall bladder. It lies in the transpyloric plane at the level of the lower border of the first lumbar vertebra. Its proximal 1–2 cm are invested with peritoneum and form part of the anterior wall of the lesser sac; thereafter the duodenum is retroperitoneal. Its upper border is attached to the right-hand end of the lesser omentum. Its lower border is attached to the greater omentum before becoming applied to the head of pancreas. The relations of the first part of the duodenum are as follows: in front, gall bladder and quadrate lobe (segment IV) of liver; above, epiploic foramen of Winslow[*]; behind, gastroduodenal artery, bile duct and portal vein; below, head and neck of pancreas. The duodenal bulb or cap is a radiological term applied to that part of the viscus shown on a barium meal examination immediately beyond the pyloric constriction.

The second or descending part

Opposite the neck of the gall bladder, the duodenum curves sharply downwards and descends for 7–10 cm before turning to the left at the level of the third lumbar vertebra to enter its horizontal portion. About 8–10 cm distal to the pylorus, the posteromedial aspect of the descending duodenum is marked by the *major duodenal papilla*, which juts into the lumen as a tiny nipple. On the summit of the papilla open the terminal portions of the bile duct and pancreatic duct, which usually unite to form a short common channel, some 5 mm long. Immediately behind its duodenal orifice this common channel shows a variable degree of dilatation, called the hepatopancreatic ampulla, better known as the ampulla of Vater.[*] In fact, others had already described the ampulla; this and other anatomical misattributions in this region are clarified by Stern.[4] The terminal bile duct and pancreatic duct each have their own sphincter of circular muscle fibres, and the common channel is surrounded by a similar thickening of muscle (the sphincter of Oddi[‡]) as it passes through the duodenal wall.

Although the major papilla usually lies just below the midpoint of the descending duodenum, its position is somewhat variable. It can enter the second part of the duodenum at any level, or even enter the third part. Likewise, the anatomy of the terminal bile and pancreatic ducts shows various different patterns. Often there is no ampulla and sometimes the two ducts open independently at the apex of the papilla. Rarely there is a long common channel (>15 mm), in which case the pancreatobiliary ductal union takes place outside the duodenal wall; this anomaly may be associated with choledochal cyst.

At duodenoscopy the position of the major papilla is marked by a small hood or fold of mucosa. At operation the papilla can usually be palpated through the duodenal wall. After incising the papilla superiorly, the firm whiteish mucosa of the terminal bile duct can be differentiated from the exuberant, pink duodenal mucosa. The orifice of the major pancreatic duct (of Wirsung[*]) occupies a relatively constant position on the lower lip of the bile duct at 5 o'clock and will normally accept a 4 Fr catheter. When present, the *minor duodenal papilla* lies about 2 cm proximal to the major papilla and again on the posteromedial wall. It is generally very tiny and marks the termination of the accessory (minor) pancreatic duct (of Santorini[†]). Occasionally the accessory papilla is ectopic.

The descending duodenum is crossed anteriorly by the transverse colon, to which it is loosely attached by areolar tissue. Above and below the transverse colon its anterior surface is covered with peritoneum. Incision of the peritoneum along its lateral border (Kocher's manoeuvre[‡]) is required to recreate a duodenal mesentery and mobilize the organ. Above the colon the duodenum is related anteriorly to the right lobe of the liver (segment V), which bears a faint duodenal impression; below the colon and mesocolon, loops of jejunum overlie it. Posteriorly the descending duodenum is closely related to the hilum of the right kidney, with the renal vein and inferior vena cava to the left of this organ. Medially it is related to the head of pancreas and laterally to the right colic (hepatic) flexure.

The third or horizontal part

This passes from right to left at the level of the lower border of the third lumbar vertebra and is 8–10 cm long. It crosses the right ureter, right psoas major muscle, right gonadal vessels, inferior vena cava and aorta. It is itself crossed by the superior mesenteric vein, superior mesenteric artery and root of the mesentery in that order; elsewhere it is covered with peritoneum. In thin patients with an acute angle of origin of the superior mesenteric artery, the third part of the duodenum may be trapped and partly obstructed between that vessel and the

---

* Jacob Benignus Winslow (1669–1760) was a Dane who described the aditus to the lesser sac in 1732 and became Professor of Anatomy, Physic and Surgery at the University of Paris 11 years later at the age of 74 years.
† Abraham Vater (1684–1751) was Professor of Anatomy and Botany at Wittenberg in Germany and described the ampulla in 1720.
‡ Ruggero Oddi (1845–1906) was a physiologist at Perugia and later a surgeon and anatomist at Rome. He described the sphincter in 1887.

* Johann Georg Wirsung (1600–1643) was a Bavarian who became Professor of Anatomy at Padua. He described the major pancreatic duct the year before he was murdered.
† Giovanni Domenico Santorini (1681–1737) described the accessory pancreatic duct in 1724 when Professor of Anatomy and Medicine in his native city of Venice. According to Stern,[4] several others had previously described this duct.
‡ Emil Theodor Kocher (1841–1917) was Professor of Clinical Surgery at Berne and the first surgeon to win a Nobel Prize (in 1909).

aorta (see Chapter 61). Its upper surface is attached to the head of pancreas and to the uncinate process behind the superior mesenteric vessels. Its lower surface is related to the jejunum in the infracolic compartment.

The fourth or ascending part

This commences in front of the aorta and runs upwards for 2–3 cm before turning downwards and forwards at the duodenojejunal flexure. In front lie the transverse colon and mesocolon. Its right border is attached to the root of the mesentery, from which the peritoneum sweeps across its anterior surface. Behind, from right to left, lie the aorta, left sympathetic trunk, left psoas muscle, left renal and gonadal vessels and the inferior mesenteric vein. The left kidney and ureter are left-sided relations.

Duodenojejunal flexure

At this point the duodenum regains a mesentery to continue as the freely mobile jejunum. The duodenojejunal flexure lies at the level of the upper border of the second lumbar vertebra just to the left of the midline. It is related above to the body of the pancreas. The ligament of Treitz is attached to the bowel at this point. It contains both striated muscle fibres (connected with the diaphragm) and a band of fibrous tissue and smooth muscle. Both portions blend with connective tissue overlying the aorta. Thus the ligament anchors the fourth part of the duodenum and the first few centimetres of jejunum.

The peritoneal attachments in this region create a number of potential *fossae*, in which a knuckle of bowel may very occasionally become trapped. Just to the left of the duodenojejunal flexure the inferior mesenteric vein arches upwards and to the right, raising a fold of peritoneum which forms the anterior wall of the paraduodenal fossa. A retroduodenal fossa may sometimes extend behind the flexure itself, and folds of peritoneum can give rise to superior and inferior duodenal fossae between the lateral edge of the bowel and the posterior abdominal wall. The mouths of all four fossae face inwards towards each other.[5]

The jejunum and ileum

Together these segments comprise the mesenteric small bowel and extend as a series of loops some 3 m in total length from the duodenojejunal flexure to the ileocaecal junction. Thanks to its mesentery, which suspends it from the posterior abdominal wall, the jejunoileum is the most mobile organ in the abdomen, if not the entire body. Its coils are distributed throughout the infracolic compartment and occupy the pelvis, particularly in the erect position. There is a gradual decrease in calibre and mural thickness between the proximal jejunum and the terminal ileum, consistent with the fact that most nutrients are absorbed from the upper small bowel. As already stated, however, the precise boundary between jejunum and ileum 40% of the way along the bowel cannot readily be identified.

The jejunum has a diameter of about 4 cm and the ileum slightly less (3.5 cm). The jejunum is thicker and more vascular and has a redder colouration. Feeling the jejunal wall between finger and thumb gives the sensation of a double layer, as opposed to a single layer for the thinner ileum. The valvular folds (valvulae conniventes) of mucous membrane are much more prominent in the jejunum, whereas the aggregated lymphoid follicles in the bowel wall are larger and more numerous in the ileum. The jejunum generally occupies the left lumbar and umbilical regions of the abdomen. The ileum lies in the hypogastric region and the pelvis. Its final loop is relatively fixed low in the right iliac fossa before ascending to open into the medial wall of the large intestine (caecum).

The terminal ileum joins the caecum at its junction with the ascending colon about 2 cm above and slightly anterior to the entry of the vermiform appendix. The surface projection of the *ileocaecal junction* is marked by the junction of the intertubercular plane (L5) and the right lateral plane, a vertical line joining the mid-clavicular and mid-inguinal points. McBurney's point*, which is defined as the junction of the outer and middle thirds of a line running between umbilicus and right anterior superior iliac spine, is thus a better marker of the ileocaecal junction than of the base of the appendix, which lies just below and medial to this point.

The junction between small and large intestines is marked by the *ileocaecal valve*. The two semilunar lips of this valve run in an approximately horizontal direction and project into the caecal lumen. They fuse at either end and continue as a frenulum or narrow ridge of mucosa. At the medial end of the valve the frenulum is continuous with the lower border of the terminal ileum. Apposition of the lips of the ileocaecal 'valve' during distension of the caecum will tend to lessen the reflux of faeces into the ileum, but this antireflux action often appears to be incompetent when studied radiologically. The major purpose of the valve may be to serve as a brake on ileal emptying. The sphincter is thought to relax in response to food entering the stomach, the so-called gastroileal reflex.

Like the duodenojejunal flexure, the ileocaecal junction can be the site of certain peritoneal *fossae*, which tend to be deeper in children than adults. The superior ileocaecal fossa lies between the vascular fold of the caecum (containing the anterior caecal artery) in front and the terminal ileum with its mesentery behind. The inferior ileocaecal fossa lies between the ileocaecal fold in front and the 'bloodless' fold of Treves† (sometimes a misnomer) and mesoappendix behind. Thirdly, the retrocaecal fossa lies between the caecum and posterior parietal peritoneum, sometimes extending upwards behind the lower ascending colon. It is bounded by two folds of peritoneum passing from the posterior abdominal wall to the caecum, and it often contains the appendix.

---

* Charles McBurney (1845–1913) described the point of maximal tenderness in acute appendicitis in 1889, when Surgeon-in-Chief to the Roosevelt Hospital, New York.
† Sir Frederick Treves (1853–1923) described the ileocaecal fold in 1885. He was surgeon to the London Hospital. He operated on King Edward VII for appendix abscess in June 1902, thus delaying the Coronation for 6 weeks.

Meckel's diverticulum

This embyological remnant of the vitellointestinal duct occurs in about 3% of the population. Meckel's diverticulum*, the diverticulum ilei, arises from the terminal ileum at a point 1 m or less from the ileocaecal junction. Its size is variable but it averages 5 cm in length and 3–4 cm in diameter. Although attached to the antimesenteric border of the bowel, it is supplied by a small artery and vein which run across the ileum from the mesentery. The diverticulum usually terminates freely within the peritoneal cavity, but sometimes it is anchored by a fibrous band passing from its tip to the adjacent bowel or abdominal wall; this band can lead to volvulus of one or more loops of intestine.

The lining of Meckel's diverticulum is identical to that of the terminal ileum from which it springs. However, small foci of heterotopic mucosa may be found in about a quarter of these diverticula. The most common type of 'foreign' mucosa is gastric, generally containing oxyntic cells but sometimes resembling pyloric mucosa. Peptic ulceration may occur in such cases (see Chapter 57). It usually presents as brisk rectal bleeding in a child or young adult. Since the ectopic tissue takes up the isotope technetium, just like orthotopic oxyntic mucosa in the stomach, such patients are likely to have a positive Meckel scan. Exocrine pancreatic tissue and colonic mucosa have also been described in Meckel's diverticulum.

The mesentery

The root (base) of the mesentery of the small bowel is approximately 15 cm long. It extends obliquely downwards and to the right from the body of the second lumbar vertebra (to the left of the midline) to the front of the right sacroiliac joint. It crosses the third part of the duodenum, the aorta, inferior vena cava, right ureter and psoas major. From this relatively narrow base the mesentery fans out over a radius of about 20 cm to gain attachment to the entire length of small intestine distal to the duodenojejunal flexure. Thus the jejunum and ileum are suspended from the posterior abdominal wall.

The mesentery consists of a double layer of peritoneum, the two layers being continuous with one another over the surface of the bowel. It contains a variable quantity of fat together with the arterial, venous, lymphatic and autonomic nerve supply to the small intestine. In addition, the mesentery is the site of numerous lymph nodes that drain the bowel. Its voluminous attachment imparts a great deal of mobility to the loops of the gut.

VASCULAR AND NERVOUS SUPPLY

Arteries

Consistent with its embryonic origin (see above), the proximal duodenum receives its blood mainly from the coeliac axis. The gastroduodenal artery is given off from the hepatic artery at a genu as the parent vessel bends sharply upwards to enter the

---

* Johann Friedrich Meckel (the younger, 1781–1833) succeeded his father as Professor of Anatomy and Surgery at Halle in 1808 and described the diverticulum ilei the following year.

---

free edge of the lesser omentum. The *gastroduodenal artery* runs down behind the pylorus closely applied to the neck of pancreas. When it reaches the lower border of the duodenum it gives off its right gastroepiploic branch, which passes along the greater curve of the stomach, and then continues as the superior pancreaticoduodenal artery. This vessel soon divides into an anterior and posterior branch, which run around the concavity of the duodenal loop in the anterior and posterior groove between the duodenum and the head of pancreas. They anastomose end-on to the anterior and posterior branches of the inferior pancreaticoduodenal artery, the first branch of the superior mesenteric artery.

Thus the entire duodenum is supplied by the *pancreaticoduodenal arcades* through branches that communicate freely with one another. Should the coeliac axis be compressed by the median arcuate ligament, these arcade vessels can become dilated and allow the superior mesenteric artery to supply the liver. Ligature of either the superior or the inferior pancreatoduodenal artery will not ordinarily embarrass the duodenum. Ligature of both renders it partly ischaemic, though it will usually survive on vessels running in the wall of the bowel from each end. There is overlap in the blood supply to the watershed territory (descending duodenum) between foregut and midgut. However, about 97% of the small intestine (distal duodenum, jejunoileum) is supplied by the superior mesenteric artery, together with the right half of the large intestine, the head of pancreas and sometimes the liver.

The *superior mesenteric artery* arises from the front of the abdominal aorta at the level of the superior border of the neck of pancreas and the first lumbar vertebra. Its origin is usually about 5 mm below that of the coeliac axis (T12), but the distance between the two vessels is variable.[6] Sometimes the superior mesenteric artery has a low take-off from the aorta (L2) and rarely there is a common coeliacomesenteric trunk, in which case the left gastric artery may arise independently at a higher level. Either the right hepatic or an accessory hepatic or the entire hepatic supply come from the superior mesenteric artery in about 25% of persons. Much less common is a large vessel running between the origins of the coeliac and superior mesenteric arteries, the ramus anastomoticus of Bühler. Occasional variants include origin of the dorsal and transverse pancreatic arteries, the right gastroepiploic, gastroduodenal, splenic and even the cystic artery from the main superior mesenteric trunk.[7]

The superior mesenteric artery passes steeply downwards behind the neck of pancreas and splenic vein to gain the left-hand side of the superior mesenteric vein. Together they pass over the left renal vein, uncinate process of the pancreas and third (horizontal) part of the duodenum to enter the mesentery. Occasionally in very thin subjects or those with an exaggerated lordosis the superior mesenteric artery can partly obstruct the duodenum at this point (see Chapter 61).

Normally the first branch of the superior mesenteric artery is the inferior pancreaticoduodenal artery, which arises from its right side just above the uncinate process. Subsequently the three colic branches (middle colic, right colic and ileocolic) are given off in that order, again from the right side of the parent vessel. As the superior mesenteric artery courses downwards and slightly to the right along the base of the mesentery, it gives origin to a succession of *jejunal* and *ileal* branches, 12–20 in number, from its left side. The highest of these supplies the fourth part of the duodenum and duodenojejunal flexure. The superior mesenteric artery ends at the terminal ileum 50–60 cm proximal to the ileocaecal junction, i.e. at the site of Meckel's diverticulum (when present).

Each jejunal and ileal artery runs between the layers of the mesentery towards the bowel wall. After 5–10 cm the artery divides into branches which anastomose with branches from the neighbouring vessel to form a series of *arcades*. Short branches from the primary arcades arborize to form secondary and tertiary arcades, and ultimately blood reaches the mesenteric border of the gut through a series of straight arteries, the *vasa recta*. A few of these vasa recta may arise from the primary arcade and short-circuit the subsequent arcades. The greater absorptive function of the jejunum predicates a better blood supply than that of the ileum, and the arterial patterns differ. The jejunal arteries are longer and wider and the arcades are better developed. The stem arteries and the ultimate vasa recta for the ileum become progressively shorter. The blood supply of the upper jejunum is particularly variable. There may be one large stem artery forming up to four arcades or several smaller arteries that intercommunicate. Often the first two or three jejunal arteries arise from the anterior or posterior pancreaticoduodenal arcades[7] rather than from the main superior mesenteric trunk.

Once the vasa recta reach the edge of the bowel, they break up into several branches which pierce the outer coat and form an extensive vascular plexus within the submucosa. Some vessels pass around to the antimesenteric border of the bowel beneath the serosa before entering the muscularis. Tiny vessels arising from the submucosal plexus supply the mucosa, and each villus has a central core containing its feeding arteriole.

The small intestine, especially the duodenum and proximal jejunum, has a rich blood supply. It differs from the large intestine in the extent of arcade formation and the large number of primary stem arteries. Although the vasa recta cannot be considered as end-arteries, the extent of anastomosis between the terminal intestinal branches is limited and interruption of 2–3 vasa recta may embarrass a short segment of bowel.

Veins

The small intestine drains into the portal system which carries blood to the liver and thence, after filtration, via the hepatic veins and inferior vena cava to the heart. The venous drainage of the jejunum and ileum mirrors the arterial disposition, but that of the duodenum is somewhat different. There is no gastroduodenal vein. Instead, blood from the duodenal loop and head of pancreas enters a variable number of short pancreaticoduodenal veins which, together with the right gastroepiploic vein, pass directly into the terminal 2 cm of the superior mesenteric vein or the portal vein itself.

Thus the *superior mesenteric vein* drains virtually the entire small intestine (plus the right colon). Commencing opposite the terminal ileum, it runs at first obliquely upwards to the left and then vertically upwards in the base of the mesentery. *En route* it receives colic branches from the right and jejunoileal branches from the left. It lies to the right and slightly in front of the superior mesenteric artery. As it traverses the third part of the duodenum and uncinate process of the pancreas, the vein begins to diverge from the artery. In this region it is joined by one or more pancreatic and pancreaticoduodenal veins and lastly by the right gastroepiploic vein, before uniting with the splenic vein to continue as the portal vein. The T-junction of superior mesenteric and splenic veins lies behind the neck of pancreas, and at this point the superior mesenteric artery is placed more deeply and to the left as it arises from the aorta.

The portal venous system contains no valves. Thus portal hypertension is transmitted directly to the veins of the small intestine, which become enlarged and congested. For most of the body arterial anatomy tends to be more constant than venous anatomy. In the case of the small intestine, particularly the main branches of the superior mesenteric vessels, the reverse probably holds true. However, there are some common variants affecting the disposition of the great veins. The inferior mesenteric vein usually joins the splenic vein just short of its junction with the superior mesenteric vein, but the three vessels may unite at the same point. The coronary (left gastric) vein may also enter this junction rather than draining into the portal (or splenic) vein. Similarly the right gastric and superior pancreaticoduodenal vein(s) can enter either the portal or the superior mesenteric vein.

Lymphatics

Each villus throughout the small intestine contains a central lacteal. The lacteal runs down the villus and communicates at its base with tiny lymph vessels draining the adjacent crypts to form an extensive submucosal lymphatic plexus. From this plexus small vessels pass through the muscularis to form a second network of lymphatics in the subserosal layer. The main lacteals leaving the small intestine and passing through the mesentery can usually be seen quite easily in a thin subject. Their fat content gives them a milky-white appearance. The course followed by lymph vessels from individual segments of the small intestine is determined by the arterial supply, which has already been described in detail.

Over a hundred lymph nodes lying between the leaves of the mesentery act as staging posts for the lymph during its upward passage from the bowel. The larger nodes lie in the root of mesentery, and these drain through quite sizeable lymphatic channels to the *superior mesenteric nodes* surrounding the origin of the superior mesenteric artery. Duodenal and pancreatic lymph drains to nodes lying in the anterior and posterior pancreaticoduodenal grooves and thence to the *coeliac nodes* surrounding the origin of the coeliac axis. The short intestinal lymph trunk conveys afferent lymph from the coeliac and superior mesenteric nodes to the cisterna chyli, a sac-like dilatation at the level of the T12 and the origin of the thoracic duct.

The small intestine contains a large amount of lymphoid

tissue within its wall, partly in the form of solitary follicles in the mucosa but mostly as aggregated lymphoid follicles or Peyer's patches*. This lymphoid tissue is a rich source of IgA. Peyer's patches are especially numerous in the terminal ileum. Their structure is described below.

Nerves

The small intestine receives sympathetic innervation from the splanchic nerves and parasympathetic innervation from the vagus nerves. The *sympathetic* supply originates in cells in the lateral columns of the lower 6–7 thoracic segments of the spinal cord. The preganglionic fibres leave the cord through white rami communicantes to the two ganglionated sympathetic trunks. They pass straight through these trunks without synapsing and travel in the thoracic splanchnic nerves (greater, lesser and least) to the coeliac plexus and on to the preaortic and superior mesenteric plexus. Here they relay with ganglia in each plexus. Postganglionic fibres are then distributed along the superior mesenteric artery (and branches of the coeliac artery) to the entire small bowel.

The *parasympathetic* supply derives from the right (posterior) vagus nerve and coeliac plexus. Preganglionic efferent fibres pass through the coeliac and superior mesenteric plexuses without relaying and are then distributed to the gut along the feeding arteries. They finally synapse with cells in the autonomic plexus on and within the bowel wall, so that the postganglionic fibres are very short.

These autonomic efferent nerves ramify in the *myenteric* (*Auerbach's*) *plexus*†, which lies between the longitudinal and circular muscle layers of the bowel and supplies each layer. Branches pass onwards to the *submucous* (*Meissner's*) *plexus*‡ and thence to the mucosa. The function of the autonomic innervation of the small intestine can be summarized (and simplified) as follows: the sympathetic inhibits peristalsis but causes contraction of the muscularis mucosae (and intestinal sphincters), while the parasympathetic is excitatory to the muscle coat and secretory glands. Both components probably convey afferent impulses from the intestine.

MICROSCOPIC ANATOMY

Intestinal wall

In common with the rest of the alimentary canal, the small intestine has four layers or coats.

1. The outermost coat is the *serosa* or visceral peritoneum. It comprises a single layer of mesothelial cells resting on a layer of loose areolar connective tissue. It completely invests the jejunoileum except for a strip along the mesenteric border. It only covers the anterior surface of the duodenum.

2. Beneath the serosa lies the *muscularis* (externa), which is disposed in two layers, a thin outer longitudinal layer and a thicker inner circular layer. These two layers of smooth muscle are connected by transitional fascicles. Between the two lie the non-myelinated nerve fibres and parasympathetic ganglion cells of the myenteric plexus of Auerbach. Once thought to be a syncytium, the smooth muscle fibres have been shown by electron microscopy to be discrete spindle-shaped cells about 250 μm long.[8]

3. The *submucosa* is sandwiched between the muscular and mucosal coats. It contains a mixture of areolar and dense fibroelastic connective tissue interspersed with blood vessels, lymphatics and the submucous autonomic plexus of Meissner. The intestinal submucosa is a tough layer which helps to retain sutures inserted through the bowel wall. Within the duodenum (only) the submucosa contains compound tubuloalveolar glands called *Brunner's glands*.* The ducts of these glands pierce the muscularis mucosa to enter the crypt. Brunner's glands secrete an alkaline mucinous material. They are more plentiful in proximal than distal duodenum.

4. The innermost layer of the bowel wall is the *mucosa*. This is the thickest and most complex layer, and it is described in detail below.

Mucosa

Circular folds

The luminal surface of the small intestine is distinguished by the presence of innumerable folds of mucosa, each of which passes transversely around much or all of the circumference of the bowel. These circular folds differ from the gastric rugae in that they are not effaced by distension of the viscus. They are also termed plicae circulares, valvulae conniventes or valves of Kerckring†. Folds are absent from the proximal 3–5 cm of duodenum and rudimentary in the terminal ileum, but they are particularly prominent in the distal duodenum and upper jejunum, diminishing in size thereafter. Besides increasing the absorptive surface area, they may delay intestinal transit to some extent and thus improve digestion.

Villi and crypts

The velvety appearance of the small bowel lining is due to the presence of myriads of tiny mucosal projections called villi. They are closely packed together with a density of up to 40 villi/mm.[2] Villi diminish progressively in height between the duodenum and upper jejunum (c. 1 mm long) and the lower ileum (0.5 mm). Moreover, villous morphology changes between these sites, with a decreasing aboral gradient in breadth as well as height. Like the circular folds, villi greatly increase the epithelial surface available for the absorption of nutrients.

---

*Johann Conrad Peyer (1653–1712) was Professor of Logic, Rhetoric and Medicine in Schaffhausen, Switzerland. His patches (described in 1677) had already been described by the Danish polymath, Niels Stensen.

†Leopold Auerbach (1828–1897) described the myenteric plexus in 1862, 10 years before he became Professor of Neuropathology in Breslau.

‡Georg Meissner (1829–1905), a peripatetic German professor, described the submucous nerve plexus in 1853.

---

*Johann Brunner (1653–1727) described the duodenal glands in 1687 when Professor of Anatomy at Heidelberg

†Theodor Kerckring (1640–1693), German anatomist in Amsterdam, first described these circular folds.

In between the villi are the simple tubular intestinal glands or crypts (of Lieberkühn*). The crypts extend deeply into the mucosa, almost to the muscularis mucosae. Each villus and crypt is lined by a single layer of epithelial cells resting on a basement membrane. The villus has a central core of connective tissue containing capillaries, nerves and a central lacteal surrounded by a small bundle of smooth muscle fibres derived from the muscularis mucosae. Likewise the crypt epithelium is supported by mesenchyme containing tiny blood and lymphatic vessels.

Mucosal layers

The deepest layer is the muscularis mucosae, which consists of a mixture of longitudinal and circular non-striated fibres and extends into the circular folds. The most superficial layer is the intestinal epithelium, essentially a single layer of tall columnar cells. In between lies the lamina propria, which is composed of loose fibrous connective tissue containing vessels, nerves, lymphocytes, macrophages, eosinophils and mast cells as well as fibroblasts.

Lymphatic follicles

Lymphoid tissue is plentiful within the enteric mucosa, especially in children. Individual lymphocytes can be seen in the epithelium and lamina propria. In addition, collections of lymphocytes form lymphatic follicles, which are distributed throughout the small bowel but particularly in the ileum. Follicles are either solitary or aggregated in the form of elliptical Peyer's patches visible to the naked eye. Each follicle contains a fibrous network stuffed with lymphocytes and a rich supply of capillaries. The overlying epithelium loses its villous pattern and contains membrane (M) cells specialized for antigen transport.[9] This tissue seems likely to be responsible for the immunological surveillance of ingested antigens.

Regional differences

One segment of small intestine closely resembles another in terms of structural anatomy, but subtle differences can be recognized. The duodenum is characterized by the presence of Brunner's glands in the submucosa. The ileum has abundant lymphoid tissue. Mural and especially mucosal thickness is greater in proximal than distal intestine; villi and crypts are longer and mucosal folds are more prominent. These differences reflect the much greater concentration of nutrients to which jejunum rather than ileum is exposed. They are not immutable. Ileum experimentally transposed to a jejunal environment grows to resemble the adjacent gut (see Chapter 46).[10]

Epithelial cells

Cell types

Besides the wandering lymphocyte, there are four types of cell within the small bowel epithelium. *Columnar cells* predominate.

They form a regular palisade with basal nuclei and granular cytoplasm. Their absorptive function is reflected in the presence of a brush border of microvilli, each about 1 μm long and ranged in parallel disposition along the luminal border of the cell. *Mucous* (goblet) cells are less plentiful than in the colon. Microvilli are rudimentary, but the cytoplasm is distended with mucin, making these cells easily recognizable in histological sections. Their mucinous secretion acts as a lubricant. *Enteroendocrine cells* are scattered through the crypts and to a lesser extent can be found within the villous epithelium. When stained with silver salts these cells can be seen to contain black cytoplasmic granules. These granules contain several different biologically active polypeptides, such as secretin, cholecystokinin, enteroglucagon, neurotensin, somatostatin, bombesin and vasoactive intestinal polypeptide. The secretory product(s) of the endocrine cells varies with the anatomical site of that segment of bowel. Lastly, *Paneth* cells* are confined to the basal region of the small bowel crypt. They too have prominent cytoplasmic granules which stain with phosphotungstic acid and may contain digestive enzymes.

Cytokinetics

The small bowel epithelium is in a constant state of flux. It is replaced every 2 days in rodents and every 3–6 days in humans.[10] The reason for this apparently wasteful turnover, which exceeds that of any other healthy tissue, remains obscure. Cells replicate at the crypt base, migrate up the crypt and on to the villus and are lost by extrusion into the lumen of the bowel at the villus tip. As they migrate they differentiate, and columnar cells develop the enzyme complement enabling them to function as mature absorptive cells. Thus the lower two-thirds of the crypt represents the proliferative compartment and the villus the functional compartment. Under normal circumstances mitotic figures are confined to the crypt. At the base of each crypt is a population of slowly-cycling stem cells, which give rise to each new generation of cells. Mucous cells and endocrine cells appear to undergo the same process of replication (from undifferentiated precursors) and migration.[11] Paneth cells do not migrate but differentiate within the crypt base, where they ultimately degenerate and undergo phagocytosis.

The villus with its associated 'feeding' crypts may be regarded as the basic functional unit of the small bowel epithelium. In steady-state conditions in the adult, loss of cells by extrusion is precisely balanced by the birth of new cells. Minor circadian fluctuations may be governed by dietary habits. This dynamic equilibrium requires delicate homeostatic control. Data suggest that cell division in the crypt is regulated by the number of cells present in the functional compartment (the villus), suggesting a feedback mechanism possibly dependent on the secretion of a chalone (local inhibitor).[10] Beyond this intrinsic regulation, however, intestinal cytokinetics can be profoundly affected by a variety of extrinsic factors, chief of which are alterations in nutrient intake and surgical shortening of the gut.[12] Thus the small bowel is exquisitely sensitive to the effects

---

† Johann Lieberkühn (1711–1756), anatomist in Berlin, described the crypts in 1745, 57 years after Marcello Malpighi and 30 years after Johann Brunner.

* Josef Paneth (1857–1890), Viennese physiologist, described these cells at the crypt base 2 years before his untimely death.

of starvation, showing disproportionate loss of mucosal mass (hypoplasia), whereas hyperphagia stimulates growth. The adaptive response to surgical operations and the mechanisms that control it are discussed in Chapter 46, but, in brief, resection causes compensatory hyperplasia (in the portions that remain) and bypass causes hypoplastic changes similar to those seen in starvation. Both refeeding and restoration of continuity restore the normal integrity of the mucosa.

REFERENCES

1. Bryant J. Observations upon the growth and length of the human intestine. *Am J Med Sci* 1924; **167**: 499–520.
2. Underhill BML. Intestinal length in man. *BMJ* 1955; **2**: 1243–1246.
3. Jit I & Grewal SS. Lengths of the small and large intestines in North Indian subjects. *J Anat India* 1975; **24**: 89–100.
4. Stern CD. A historical perspective on the discovery of the accessory duct of the pancreas, the ampulla 'of Vater' and *pancreas divisum. Gut* 1986; **27**: 203–212.
5. Last RJ. *Anatomy: Regional and Applied.* Edinburgh: Churchill Livingstone, 1984.
6. Michels NA. The variant blood supply of the small and large intestine: its import in regional resections. *J Int Coll Surg* 1963; **39**: 127–138.
7. Netter F. Blood supply of small and large intestine. In Oppenheimer E (ed.) *CIBA Collection of Medical Illustrations,* vol. 3, Digestive System, part 2, Lower Digestive Tract. New York: Ciba, 1962: 64–74.
8. Ishitani MB & Jones RS. Functional anatomy and applied physiology of the small intestine. In Scott HW Jr & Sawyers JL (eds) *Surgery of the Stomach, Duodenum and Small Intestine.* Oxford: Blackwell, 1987: 61–77.
9. Owen RL & Jones AL. Epithelial cell specialization within human Peyer's patches. An ultrastructural study of intestinal lymphoid follicles. *Gastroenterology* 1974; **66**: 189–203.
10. Williamson RCN. Intestinal adaptation. *N Engl J Med* 1978; **298**: 1393–1402, 1444–1450.
11. Cheng H & Leblond CP. Origin, differentiation and renewal of the four main epithelial cell types in the mouse small intestine V. Unitarian theory of the origin of the four epithelial cell types. *Am J Anat* 1974; **141**: 537–562.
12. Williamson RCN. Intestinal adaptation: factors that influence morphology. *Scand J Gastroenterol* 1982; **17** (suppl. 74): 21–29.

43

PHYSIOLOGY OF THE SMALL INTESTINE

WR Fleming

The small intestine has crucial responsibilities in the survival of its host. The major function is the absorption of nutrients, such as carbohydrates, protein and fat, together with vitamins, minerals and trace elements. It modifies some dietary constituents by enzymatic action to render them absorbable and mixes and propels the contents onwards, allowing maximum exposure of the digested nutrients to the absorptive surfaces. In addition, the small intestine plays a key role in water and electrolyte balance by both secretory and absorptive processes. It must absorb 6–7 litres of endogenous secretions per day produced by various intestinal organs and glands, and allow the efficient recycling of bile acids, digestive enzymes and electrolytes. The gut has a vital excretory function as well, acting as a conduit for unabsorbable substances such as dietary fibre and allowing the elimination of breakdown products of bilirubin, sex hormones and some drugs. Finally, the small bowel acts as a gastrointestinal endocrine organ and plays a part in the immune protection of the body.

DIGESTION AND ABSORPTION

General features

The small intestine digests and absorbs food by a complex series of intraluminal and mucosal processes, involving salivary, gastric, biliary, pancreatic and intestinal movements and secretions. It is fast: a complete meal may be fully digested and absorbed within 3 hours. It is also extremely efficient: the absorptive efficiency of both fat and protein exceeds 95%.[1] In health, the digestion and absorption of carbohydrates, proteins, fats, fluid and electrolytes, iron and folate is completed in the jejunum, leaving a large residual functional capacity.[2] The ileum can adapt and subsume the prime functions of the jejunum after removal of the proximal small bowel, however the reverse is not the case. Certain functions of the ileum remain exclusively ileal, such as the absorption of vitamin B_{12} and bile salts, where the specialized transport mechanisms are confined to this segment. Excision of more than 150 cm of ileum will invariably result in malabsorption of fat (from depletion of the bile salt

pool) and vitamin B_{12}. The duodenum, jejunum and ileum differ in their absorption of water, electrolytes and nutrients (Table 43.1).

Table 43.1 Absorption in the small intestine[3]

	DUODENUM	JEJUNUM	ILEUM
Water	+	+++	++
Sodium	+	+++	++
Potassium	+	+++	+
Chloride	+	++	+++
Fats	++	+++	+
Proteins	++	+++	+
Carbohydrates	++	+++	+
Bile salts	0	0	+++
Fat-soluble vitamins[a]	+	+++	+
Water-soluble vitamins			
Vitamin B_{12}	0	0	+++
Folic acid	+	+++	++
Ascorbic acid	?	+	+++
Minerals			
Iron	+++	++	0
Calcium	++	+++	+
Magnesium	+	++	++

[a]Vitamin K (endogenously produced fraction) absorbed in the colon.

Intestinal microflora

The gastrointestinal tract is sterile at birth but quickly becomes colonized via the oral route, so that by 3–4 weeks after birth the normal adult enteric microflora is established. The healthy proximal small intestine contains only a transient microbial population, comprising mostly oral aerobes and anaerobes, reflecting the regulatory conditions of gastric acidity and gastric and small bowel peristalsis.[4–6] The distal ileum has a different and constant microflora that contains higher bacterial counts and organisms resembling those found in the large bowel. Backwash through the ileocaecal valve contaminates the distal ileum with faecal aerobes and anaerobes,[7] allowing the distal ileum to act as a transitional zone between the relatively sterile proximal gut and the bacterially rich colon.

The functions of the intestinal microflora are incompletely understood. It appears to play an important protective role against bacterial overgrowth and infection by prevention of colonization by pathogenic bacteria and the production of some toxic substances and antibiotic-like molecules. Enteric micro-organisms are also involved in intraluminal digestion, but the major site for this is in the colon with its vastly greater population of bacteria. Disease states such as intestinal obstruction, inflammatory bowel diseases and blind loops and pouches dramatically change the intestinal microflora. Bacterial overgrowth due to stasis and diminished or absent gastric acidity results in malabsorption, diarrhoea and steatorrhoea.

Carbohydrate absorption

In the Western diet, carbohydrates supply half the calories ingested by man. They are ingested as polysaccharides, such as starch (60%), and disaccharides such as sucrose (30%) and lactose (10%).[8] Starch is the major dietary form of carbohydrate, consisting of large polysaccharides of two types (amylopectin and amylose), depending on the linking pattern of their glucose molecules. Digestion of carbohydrate involves hydrolysis of starch by salivary and pancreatic amylase, followed by surface digestion of oligosaccharides at the brush border. Absorption of the resulting monosaccharides takes place by carrier-mediated cellular transport and some paracellular absorption, predominantly in the proximal small intestine and probably within the first 70 cm.[2,9]

Starch digestion begins in the mouth by the hydrolytic action of salivary amylase, resulting in the formation of maltose, maltotriose and α-limited dextrins. This process continues in the stomach until the bolus is macerated and broken into smaller particles. Pancreatic enzymes continue the hydrolysis, generating further di- and trisaccharides, but they cannot complete digestion to monosaccharides. Salivary and pancreatic α-amylases act on the interior 1,4 links of starch but cannot break outermost 1,4 linkages or 1,6 glucose links, leaving partially digested oligosaccharides. Other polysaccharides, such as cellulose, cannot be digested at all and so pass down the gut to contribute to dietary fibre. The action of amylase is rapid because of the large quantities of the enzyme secreted by the pancreas, and amylase-induced digestion of starches is usually completed within the duodenum.[8]

The final stage of carbohydrate digestion is mediated by the oligosaccharidases present on the brush border of the enterocyte. Man is born with a full complement of these enzymes, but they are only present in the mature columnar epithelial cells of the intestinal villus. There is a tendency for DNA synthesis, protein synthesis and then the appearance of oligosaccharidase activity to occur sequentially in the enterocyte as crypt cells migrate and mature into villus columnar cells. Although oligosaccharidases are present in highest concentration in the jejunum, they persist at physiologically important levels throughout most of the ileum but are absent in the colon. Oligosaccharides produced as the result of starch hydrolysis, as well as those ingested, such as sucrose and lactose, are hydrolysed by several specific oligosaccharidases, as shown in Table 43.2. The most important of these are lactase, sucrase and α-dextrinase (isomaltase). The monosaccharides produced by this final hydrolysis at the brush border (glucose, galactose and fructose) are therefore available for absorption in a locally high concentration at the site of their production.

Table 43.2 Oligosaccharide enzymes on the brush border of the enterocyte

ENZYME	OLIGOSACCHARIDE SUBSTRATE	PRODUCT
Lactase	Lactose	Glucose, galactose
α-Dextrinase (isomaltase)	α-Dextrins	Glucose
Sucrase	Sucrose, maltose, maltotriose and some α-dextrins	Glucose, fructose
Glucoamylase	Malto-oligosaccharides	Glucose
Trehalase	Trehalose	Glucose

Hydrolysis of oligosaccharides to form monosaccharides must occur at the same rate as monosaccharide absorption to prevent excessive osmotic movement of water into the lumen of the gut. Whenever monosaccharide transport capacity is exceeded, the excessive luminal monosaccharide products retard the hydrolysis of their parent oligosaccharide by limiting enzyme activity, thus bringing balance back into the system.[8] Oligosaccharidase activity is also inhibited by pancreatic and bacterial proteases, bile salts and a prolonged period of fasting.[10]

Absorption of monosaccharides into the cell occurs rapidly by saturable active transport mechanisms and passive facilitated diffusion, supplemented by absorption by the paracellular junctions of the jejunum which have some permeability to monosaccharides. Glucose and galactose are actively and competitively transported into the enterocyte against a concentration gradient by a highly specific sodium-mediated transport mechanism (see below), requiring energy, oxygen and the active cotransport of sodium at the basolateral membrane. Fructose, the other major monosaccharide, is absorbed by a process of energy-independent facilitated diffusion. The carbohydrates are not metabolized to any extent within the cell but are transported out of the enterocyte into the interstitial space by a sodium-independent carrier mechanism present in the basolateral membrane.[1]

Protein absorption

Protein is needed in the diet to provide essential amino acids that cannot be created by endogenous means and are required for the maintenance of effective protein synthesis. Although most is digested and absorbed in the proximal jejunum,[9] protein digestion starts in the stomach, where the physical actions of mixing and churning by gastric peristalsis, the acidic environment and the enzymatic action of pepsin begin the process of hydrolysis of protein into polypeptides. Once the chyme reaches the duodenum, the acid is neutralized and pepsin is inactivated, allowing the next phase of protein digestion to begin.

The exocrine pancreas secretes proteases as proenzymes that are activated by duodenal mucosal enteropeptidase (enterokinase). This process converts trypsinogen (the inactive proenzyme) into the active form, trypsin. Activated trypsin takes over subsequent activation of trypsinogen and other pancreatic endo- and exopeptidases, which convert the peptides to oligopeptides, dipetides and basic and neutral amino acids. The endopeptidases (trypsin, chymotrypsin and elastase) produce oligopeptides that are then digested by the exopeptidases (carboxypeptidases A and B).

At the surface of the enterocyte, further hydrolysis of the peptide products of luminal digestion by aminopeptidases occurs, although not all oligopeptides are converted to amino acids. Some dipeptides and tripeptides, especially those containing glycine and proline, may be absorbed intact, undergoing intracellular hydrolysis. Free amino acids represent only one-third of the product of intraluminal digestion of protein, the remainder being oligopeptides, which are either digested by brush-border enzymes or absorbed intact.[3] There are specific hydrolysis–transport proteins for dipeptides, which simultaneously hydrolyse the dipeptides and transport the amino acids so formed; absorption of some of these dipeptides is more rapid than absorption of their constituent amino acids.

Amino acid absorption occurs by a rapid, active, energy-dependent, carrier-mediated, saturable transport mechanism. There are at least four of these systems, depending on the structure of the amino acid, with separate mechanisms for neutral, dibasic and dicarboxylic acids, imino acids and glycine. Amino acids pass through the enterocyte rapidly with only a small proportion being used for intracellular protein synthesis, the remainder passing out through the basolateral membrane, probably by a carrier mechanism. In healthy adults over 70% of protein digestion and absorption is completed in the jejunum.

Fat absorption

Dietary fat consists primarily of the triglycerides of long chain fatty acids (palmitic, stearic, oleic and linoleic) and is an important source of calories as it generates more than double the number of calories per gram of either carbohydrate or protein. Triglyceride molecules are insoluble in water and so must be hydrolysed and the resulting products solubilized by the formation of mixed micelles with bile acids. Micellar solubilization is very effective, and by mid-jejunum nearly all the dietary fats (and fat-soluble vitamins) in the lumen of the gut will have been absorbed.

Hydrolysis of triglycerides

Most fat enters the small intestine in its original form because gastric lipase activity is minimal and little digestion takes place in the stomach. When a fatty meal enters the small intestine, cholecystokinin and secretin are released, these being the principal humoral stimulants of pancreatic enzyme and bicarbonate secretion, respectively (see below). Similar to the process in

protein digestion, pancreatic lipases are released as proenzymes that must be activated. Duodenal enteropeptidase (enterokinase) activates trypsin, which acts on prophospholipase, procarboxyl ester hydrolase, chymotrypsinogen, proelastase and the procarboxypeptidases to form the active enzymes. In addition, trypsin acts on procolipase to form the active cofactor, colipase.

Triglycerides are emulsified by bile salts and hydrolysed by the actions of pancreatic lipase and colipase to form fatty acids and a monoglyceride. The colipase binds triglyceride in the presence of bile salts and aids the anchoring of lipase at the oil–water interface.[11] This process is dependent on an alkaline pH and optimal bile salt concentration.[12] The dissolution of the lipolytic products by bile salts is essential for their successful absorption in the aqueous contents of the intestinal lumen.

Human bile is composed of bile salts, phospholipids, cholesterol, proteins, bilirubin and other substances (Figure 43.1). Bile salts are a source of endogenous lipid and detergent. They are soluble amphiphiles, having a hydrophobic side, a hydrophilic side and a hydrophilic tail.[13] Many other endogenous substances may be secreted in bile in small amounts and undergo enterohepatic recycling (see below).[14] Bacterial reduction products of bilirubin, fat-soluble vitamins (especially the biologically active forms of vitamin D), water-soluble vitamins (especially vitamin B_{12}), folic acid, pyridoxine and many oestrogenic steroids can appear in bile. Several exogenous substances are also secreted in bile, such as common drugs like indomethacin, antibiotics and chlorpromazine.

The mixture of free fatty acids, monoglycerides, phospholipids and cholesterol is rendered water soluble by entering into molecular aggregation with bile salts to form mixed micelles. Fatty acids within the micelles are neutralized by pancreatic bicarbonate. Formation of micelles depends on the concentration of bile salt, the particular bile salt structure, state of conjugation, pH, temperature and counter ion concentration.

At the surface of the enterocyte the micellar structure allows the rapid absorption of free fatty acids, monoglycerides and phospholipids by a process of diffusion across the unstirred water layer and cell membrane, leaving the bile salts within the lumen for subsequent recycling via the terminal ileum. Once the free fatty acids have entered the cell, resyn-

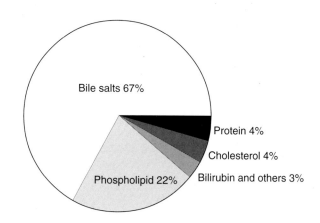

Figure 42.1

Composition of bile.

thesis into triglycerides occurs rapidly. Fatty acids are bound to special proteins (fatty acid binding protein)[15,16] and transported from the cytoplasm to the smooth endoplasmic reticulum to begin the process of re-esterification. Here they are activated to form fatty acid coenzyme A derivatives, which subsequently esterify to reform the triglyceride molecule. In the endoplasmic reticulum, triglyceride combines with phospholipids, cholesterol and cholesterol esters to form chylomicrons. The chylomicron has an oily central core of triglycerides, cholesterol esters and trace lipids covered by a stabilizing layer of phopholipids and apoproteins. The Golgi apparatus subsequently packages the chylomicrons into secretory vesicles which migrate through the cytoplasm to the basolateral membrane of the cell. The vesicles discharge their contents by exocytosis, and the chylomicrons enter the central lacteal of the villus. From there they travel via larger lymphatic channels to the thoracic duct and eventually into the bloodstream via the subclavian vein (Figure 43.2).

Medium and short chain fatty acids

The absorption of medium and short chain fatty acids differs from that of the far more common long chain triglycerides found in the diet (Table 43.3). Medium and short chain fatty acids are water soluble and do not require micellar solubilization for

Table 43.3 Differences in digestion and absorption of fatty acids

	LONG CHAIN	SHORT AND MEDIUM CHAIN
Size	Large; >C12	Small; <C5 and C5–C11
Water solubility	Poor	Excellent
Intraluminal hydrolysis		
Required	Yes	No
Efficiency	Incomplete	Complete and rapid
Paracellular absorption	Minimal	Major role
Intracellular processes		
Re-esterification	Yes	No
Lipolytic product	Triglyceride	Fatty acid
Transport	Chylomicron and lymphatics	Direct to portal blood

absorption. They are sufficiently small to pass paracellularly as well as transcellularly and are not incorporated into chylomicrons. Thus medium and short chain fatty acids can be absorbed directly into the enterocyte without hydrolysis or micelle formation, and they pass unchanged directly into the portal circulation. This fact has important therapeutic implications in the management of patients with defects in digestion and absorption of fats.

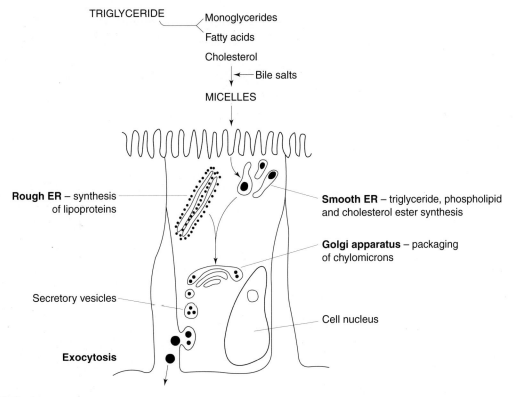

Figure 42.2
Absorption of triglycerides and cholesterol. Triglycerides are hydrolysed by pancreatic lipase and colipase to fatty acids and monoglycerides, then rendered soluble by aggregation with bile salts into micelles. Once in the enterocyte, re-esterification of lipolytic products into triglyceride occurs in smooth endoplasmic reticulum (ER). Lipoproteins are synthesized within rough ER. Chylomicrons are formed from triglyceride, combined with phospholipid, lipoproteins and cholesterol. Packaged into secretory vesicles in the Golgi apparatus, chylomicrons are discharged from the basolateral membrane of the cell by exocytosis, entering the central lacteal.

Cholesterol

Cholesterol in the small intestine originates from dietary and biliary sources and is poorly absorbed from the gut. It follows a similar pathway to long chain fatty acids, but is solubilized poorly by mixed micelles and does not bind to intracellular fatty acid binding proteins. It is slowly released from the enterocyte in the hydrophobic centre of chylomicrons.

Bile salt reabsorption

Bile salts are left behind in the lumen of the small intestine after absorption of the lipolytic products of fat digestion, maintaining a relatively high concentration throughout the small bowel. Although there is some passive reabsorption in the jejunum, the predominant site of bile salt reabsorption is the terminal ileum. Enterocytes actively transport bile salts in a highly efficient manner, with approximately 95% of bile salts entering the ileum being reabsorbed. Once transported across the cell, bile salts are returned to the liver via the portal circulation, efficiently extracted for recycling and resecreted into canalicular bile.

The total pool contains 2–4 g of bile salts, and as the enterohepatic circulation turns over six times a day some 20–25 g of bile salts traverse the small intestine daily. The combination of passive reabsorption in the jejunum and active reabsorption in the ileum means that only 5% of the total pool per cycle, or 30% per day, enters the colon through the ileocaecal valve. In the colon bile salts are metabolized, and about 50% are reabsorbed by passive diffusion. In the steady state, faecal excretion of some 600–800 mg per day is adequately balanced by the equivalent production of new bile salts in the liver.[17]

Ileal resections of less than 100 cm will cause bile salt depletion, but the losses can usually be adequately compensated by increased hepatic production. The increased load of bile salts in the colon will produce a secretory diarrhoea. Once ileal resection exceeds 100 cm or extensive ileal disease is present, such as in ileal Crohn's disease, bile salt deficiency occurs and triglyceride and fat-soluble vitamin malabsorption follow.[18]

Vitamin absorption

Fat soluble vitamins

The fat-soluble vitamins A, D, E and K are absorbed in the proximal intestine largely by passive processes similar to those responsible for dietary fat absorption. As with triglyceride, they have limited solubility in water and must be solubilized with bile salts in mixed micelles for diffusion through the cell membrane. They are incorporated into chylomicrons in the enterocyte and transported from the cell by lymphatics.

Vitamin A is a lipid-soluble micronutrient necessary for the support of growth and differentiation of epithelial tissues, and the preservation of vision. The major dietary source is β-carotene from plant sources, but it is also ingested as fatty acid esters of retinyl from animal sources.[16] It possesses virtually no aqueous solubility, so bile salts are needed for active conversion of β-carotene to retinol and for micellar solubilization.[19]

Hydrolysis to retinol occurs at the cell surface by pancreatic and mucosal enzymes, followed by solubilization in mixed micelles and absorption. Once inside the cell, the retinol is esterified with palmitic acid to form retinyl esters, which are transported via lymphatics in chylomicrons.[13] Vitamin A and its other active forms undergo enterohepatic circulation once synthesis is completed.[14]

Vitamin D is derived from exogenous and endogenous sources and is intimately involved in calcium and phosphate metabolism. Endogenous production, from exposure of the cholesterol-derived precursor provitamin D_3 to sunlight, appears to be the most important source. Dietary vitamin D is absorbed unchanged and incorporated into chylomicrons for processing by the liver and kidney to produce the active form.[20]

The antioxidant Vitamin E, the most active compound being α-tocopherol, is found in leafy vegetables and is absorbed in the proximal intestine with micellar solubilization.

Vitamin K has both exogenous sources (dietary) and endogenous sources (production in the colon by bacteria). Both require bile salt solubilization in micelles for absorption, but the predominant site is in the small bowel. Bile salt deficiency or lack of dietary vitamin K can result in abnormalities in the clotting process because of diminished hepatic production of prothrombin.

Water-soluble vitamins

The water-soluble vitamins are absorbed by passive diffusion or by several active transport mechanisms, involving sodium-dependent membrane-bound carriers.

Vitamin C absorption appears similar to that of the monosaccharides, involving an energy-dependent sodium-coupled process at the mucosal membrane, with energy supplied by the basolateral membrane Na^+, K^+-ATPase.[21] In contrast to the monosaccharides, however, ascorbic acid is mostly absorbed in the ileum.

Vitamin B_{12} (cobalamin) is present in the diet in a variety of coenzyme forms bound to dietary protein. Its absorption is a complex process that begins with the release of cobalamin from dietary protein by gastric pepsin, followed by its attachment to carrier proteins, known as R proteins, which are present in salivary secretions, gastric juices and bile.[22,23] The R protein, which has a very high affinity for cobalamin, enters the duodenum in the cobalamin–R protein complex, which is degraded by pancreatic proteases. The released cobalamin is subsequently bound to intrinsic factor, a mucopolypeptide produced by the gastric parietal cell. Cobalamin is also present in bile bound to R proteins, so that endogenous and dietary cobalamin are absorbed together in the distal ileum.

The intrinsic factor–cobalamin complex then binds to specific brush-border receptor sites in the terminal ileum, mostly in the distal 100 cm.[24] The intact complex is absorbed in an energy-dependent process that requires calcium and a neutral pH. Once inside the cell, the cobalamin is released from intrinsic factor and transferred to another carrier, transcobalamin, exiting via the basolateral membrane.

Folate occurs in the diet in various conjugates with gluta-mate molecules, which must be hydrolysed by a specific brush-border enzyme to the monoglutamate form for absorp-tion.[3,22] The enzyme is found throughout the small intestine but is most active in the jejunum. The monoglutamate is then absorbed by a carrier-mediated, specific active transport mech-anism and metabolized intracellularly to reduced monoglu-tamic methyl folate for transport to the liver by the mesenteric circulation. Folate deficiency is particularly common in Crohn's disease, with malabsorption of folate being demonstrated in some 28% of patients.[25] Sulphasalazine therapy has also been associated with folate deficiency because of its ability competi-tively to inhibit folate transport and metabolism.[26]

Thiamine and riboflavin are large polar molecules that require carrier systems for their absorption from the proximal small intestine,[1] and similar active sodium-dependent systems exist for nicotinic acid, biotin, inositol and choline.[27]

Mineral absorption

The small intestine absorbs calcium, phosphorus and iron, as well as other important minerals and trace elements such as magnesium, copper and zinc.

Calcium

Calcium is a vital body mineral involved in neurotransmitter release and nerve impulse propagation, contraction of muscle, blood clotting, exocrine and endocrine secretory processes and cell proliferation.[28] Control of calcium homeostasis occurs at three sites: bone, the primary reservoir of the cation; kidney, the organ that regulates excretion; and the intestine, the pre-dominant site of exogenous calcium absorption. Calcium is a small cation and should be freely permeable across the paracellular junctions of the proximal small bowel, provided it is in solution. Although the efficiency of calcium transport is greatest in the duodenum and decreases along the bowel, the slower transit time through the ileum results in the greatest contribution to absorption.[28]

Calcium is first bound to a specific calcium-binding protein, whose synthesis within mucosal goblet cells is controlled by the active form of vitamin D_3 (1,25-dihydroxycholecalciferol). The calcium–protein complex is absorbed into the enterocyte, where the binding protein is removed and the calcium exported via a Ca^{2+}-ATPase in the basolateral membrane. Absorption is normally inefficient (about 33%) but can be increased in calcium deficiency by the actions of vitamin D and parathyroid hormone. Together, these agents increase absorp-tion by increasing brush-border permeability to calcium, increasing calcium-binding protein and stimulating activity of the basolateral membrane Ca^{2+}-ATPase.

Phosphorus

Inorganic phosphate has roles in bone metabolism and acid–base balance, while organic phosphate has roles in the energetic machinery of the cell (e.g. ATP) and transmission of genetic information (nucleic acids); it is an important con-stituent of cellular membranes (phospholipids) and it plays a crucial role in hormone-controlled functions (cyclic AMP, etc.).[29] Phosphorus is absorbed as phosphate throughout the small intestine via sodium-dependent active absorption, but mainly in the jejunum.

Iron

Iron absorption occurs primarily in the duodenum and upper jejunum, with only small amounts absorbed from elsewhere in the gastrointestinal tract. Iron can be absorbed from haem, from haemoglobin and myoglobin, and by binding of inorganic iron by a saturable active transport mechanism in the brush border. Because iron has limited solubility at small intestinal pH, luminal conditions are important:[3,30] gastric acid, ascorbic acid and certain amino acids dissolve iron and increase absorp-tion, whereas phosphates, citrate and fibre decrease absorp-tion. Iron that enters the enterocyte is stored as ferritin unless the body is iron deficient, when it is released by an active transport mechanism into the plasma with transferrin. If the need for iron is low and the stores in the cell are not mobilized before the enterocyte is shed, the absorbed iron is lost in the faeces.

Trace elements

The importance of trace elements in humans became obvious with the introduction of total parenteral nutrition, which uncovered a number of previously unrecognized syndromes indicating dietary deficiency.

Zinc is necessary for nucleic acid and protein synthesis and is a key constituent of many enzymes. It is absorbed most rapidly in the duodenum and upper jejunum, by an active energy-dependent process,[13] but the gut is also the main excre-tory route for zinc. Up to 25% of endogenous zinc lost in the faeces is contributed by pancreatic secretions,[31] although the contribution of intestinal secretion and enterocyte desquama-tion to faecal zinc levels remains undefined.

Copper is absorbed in the stomach and duodenum and excreted in the bile. Although absorption increases as dietary intake increases, the excretion of copper in bile also increases to maintain steady body levels.[23]

ABSORPTION OF WATER AND ELECTROLYTES

General features

Digestion and absorption from the lumen of the bowel requires water for maintenance of liquid enteric contents, which in turn allows the efficient interaction of digestive enzymes and food particles and the diffusion of nutrients to the surface of the epithelial cells where absorption takes place.[32] The total quantity of fluid that the gut must absorb each day is 8–9 litres, made up of 1.5–2 litres of ingested dietary fluid and 6–7 litres of endogenously produced secre-tions from the intestine and its attached organs and glands (Table 43.4). All but 1500 ml is absorbed in the small intestine and the colon accounts for most of what is left, leaving about 100 ml to be excreted in the faeces each day.

Table 43.4 Small intestinal daily fluid load

SOURCE	VOLUME (ML/DAY)
Oral intake	1500–2000
Saliva	1500
Gastric juice	2500
Bile	500
Pancreatic juice	1500
Intestine	1000

The small intestine has a prodigious reserve capacity for absorption and secretion because of its huge 250 m² surface area. Valvulae conniventes increase the surface area threefold, the intestinal villi a further tenfold and the millions of microvilli a further 20-fold, thus amplifying the intestinal surface area by 600 times over a flat surface.[33,34] The motility of the gut adds a further physiological amplification by altering the flow of chyme and adjusting its contact time with the mucosal absorptive surface.

Water movement, whether absorptive or secretory, is intimately coupled to the movements of electrolytes, which are moved by active transport processes; Na⁺ is the principal ion driving absorption of water. Although 20–30 g of sodium is secreted in the intestinal juices and up to 10 g is ingested each day, less than 0.5% is lost in the faeces per day.[33] A number of general features about these efficient active mechanisms are apparent:[35]

- The ultimate driving force for all active monovalent ion transport in the small bowel is the Na⁺–K⁺ exchange pump, powered by Na⁺,K⁺-ATPase, located in the basolateral membranes of the enterocytes.

- Na⁺ is absorbed actively throughout the small intestine; other transport processes that move solutes against their electrochemical gradients (e.g. those for Cl⁻, HCO₃⁻, H⁺ and bile salts) and those for neutral solutes (e.g. amino acids and sugars) are coupled directly or indirectly to the transport of Na⁺.

Passive movements

The permeability of the intestinal mucosa to water and electrolytes is greatest in the duodenum and jejunum, gradually diminishing down the length of the gut as pore size decreases.[36] The junctional complexes between enterocytes are leaky, allowing a large bidirectional flow from lumen to blood and vice versa. Not only does the permeability of the gut decrease as one moves distally, but there are also local variations so it appears that the villus cells are the predominant site of absorption and the crypt cells the main site of secretion.

Water movement, and the passage of small water-soluble molecules, across the gastrointestinal epithelium occurs passively via the paracellular path, depending on the osmotic gradient across the epithelium. To promote water absorption from luminal fluid, an osmotic gradient must be set up, and this is achieved predominantly in vivo by the active transport of solutes such as glucose or amino acids across the enterocyte.[13]

Water movement in response to the generated osmotic gradient results in the non-electrogenic transport of sodium and chloride by solvent drag. Up to 80% of the glucose-stimulated sodium absorption in the human jejunum may be by this mechanism.[37] The remainder of sodium absorption takes place by a number of active processes detailed below.

Active electrolyte transport processes

Basal sodium pump

The sodium pump, powered by Na⁺,K⁺-ATPase, in the basolateral membrane of the enterocyte extrudes sodium into the intercellular space and keeps a low sodium concentration and a negative electrical charge within the cell. This process creates an electrical and chemical gradient for reabsorption of sodium into the cell. The active absorption of positively-charged sodium into the intercellular space allows negatively-charged chloride to follow passively down the electrical gradient. In the duodenum and upper jejunum the paracellular paths are very leaky, so net inward movement of sodium is low. In the ileum, however, permeability of the epithelium is less, which allows net flow of sodium and water from the lumen to the intestinal epithelium.

Sodium–glucose cotransport

The absorption of glucose is achieved by a Na⁺–glucose cotransport carrier at the brush border of the enterocyte.[37] Because the entry of sodium raises the cell's electrical charge, net absorption is dependent on the extrusion of sodium from the basolateral membrane. The absorbed glucose is removed by a sodium-independent carrier, while the sodium is pushed out by the sodium pump. The positive charge of the Na⁺ attracts an anion (principally Cl⁻) for absorption by the paracellular pathway, and water follows passively to maintain osmolarity in the intercellular space. Thus, intestinal glucose transport also drives water and electrolyte absorption.

Electroneutral sodium chloride absorption

This process forms the major mechanism of sodium absorption in the ileum where the epithelium is less permeable. It comprises a Na⁺–H⁺ exchange and a Cl⁻–HCO₃⁻ exchange working together so that Na⁺ and Cl⁻ are absorbed into the cell, while H⁺ and HCO₃⁻ are secreted into the lumen of the gut.[38,39] The hydrogen and bicarbonate ions are converted to water and carbon dioxide in the bowel lumen, with the water contributing to the chyme and the carbon dioxide being reabsorbed and excreted in the expired air without the need for another transport mechanism. This process results in net absorption of sodium chloride and water.

INTESTINAL SECRETION

General features

In addition to the absorption promoted by various luminal solutes, the epithelium of the small bowel actively secretes fluid and electrolytes in response to a variety of gastrointestinal hormones. The mechanisms of secretion usually involve the chloride ion, with a contribution from active bicarbonate secretion, especially in the ileum.

Chloride secretion

The enterocyte takes up chloride from the plasma via a basolateral membrane-coupled Na$^+$–K$^+$–Cl$^-$ transport mechanism. The sodium pump provides the driving energy, recycling Na$^+$, while K$^+$ channels allow potassium to passively re-enter the plasma. As chloride ions accumulate in the cell an electrochemical gradient is established, and chloride is thus actively secreted via apical membrane Cl$^-$ channels into the intestinal lumen. Na$^+$,K$^+$ and water follow passively down the paracellular path.[40]

Bicarbonate secretion

Bicarbonate is the predominant ion in both bile and pancreatic secretions, serving to neutralize gastric acid and provide optimal conditions for enzyme function and nutrient absorption from the gut lumen. The neutralization of acid has an important cytoprotective role in preventing duodenal ulceration,[41-43] in conjunction with the secretion of neutral mucus by Brunner's glands. Bicarbonate is produced by intracellular carbonic anhydrase (found in greatest concentration in the apical cells of the villi and absent in the crypts)[41] and actively secreted in exchange for absorbed chloride ions. This process is particularly important in the ileum as a means of conserving chloride.

Regulation of duodenal bicarbonate secretion is on several levels:[41]

- Luminal acid, which acts via local mucosal prostaglandins and can be inhibited by agents that decrease prostaglandin synthesis, such as aspirin.[44]
- Neural control, via the vagal stimulation triggered by feeding.
- Humoral factors, such as cholecystokinin (CCK), pancreatic polypeptide (PP), neurotensin, glucagon, gastric inhibitory peptide (GIP) and vasoactive intestinal polypeptide (VIP), which all stimulate bicarbonate secretion.

Gastric acid inhibitors, such as H$_2$ antagonists and H$^+$,K$^+$-ATPase blockers, do not influence duodenal bicarbonate secretion.

INTESTINAL MOTILITY

General features

Investigation of small intestinal function is technically difficult, so relatively little is known about the normal transit of chyme along the bowel. The gastrointestinal tract can be regarded as a series of coupled propelling and receiving segments, providing alternation of resistance and active propulsion.[45] The effect of this combination is to provide a net distal flow while allowing adequate mixing of luminal contents. The interaction of intestinal smooth muscle movements, motion of the mucosal surface and even of the villi allows maximum exposure of the nutrients and fluid for absorption. Chyme does not progress as a bolus, but spreads out to cover the whole of the small intestine, with liquids moving faster than solids. The input of a meal into the gut is variable, depending on the gastric emptying rate, and a variety of controls operate to moderate the flow of chyme after a meal. Motility patterns differ between the fed and fasting state, with the latter governed by the migrating motor complex.

Fasting state motility

The migrating motor complex (MMC) consists of a number of phases of muscular activity, characterized by bursts of action potentials that sweep along the gut. At any one point in the intestine this cycle of activity and inactivity lasts about 90 minutes. In man the MMC begins in the stomach and progresses through the whole gut, although the associated rhythmic muscle contractions or 'activity fronts' rarely traverse the terminal ileum.[46] Periodic changes occur in lower oesophageal sphincter and gastric antral activity and in contraction of the gall bladder in association with the MMC. It appears that control of the MMC rests mainly with an external neurogenic mechanism, as this fasting motor pattern is promptly abolished by feeding.

Abnormalities in the MMC are found in a number of clinical disorders characterized by gut motility disturbances, in particular diabetic enteropathy,[47] and in patients with cirrhosis.[48]

Postprandial motility

For about 3–4 hours after a meal the MMC is completely disrupted and replaced by a series of irregular contractions in characteristic patterns.

Segmentation

Segmentation contractions are unpropagated tonic contractions of intestinal circular smooth muscle. They divide the lumen of the gut into a series of segments that promotes mixing of chyme with gastrointestinal enzymes and secretions. Because of the slightly faster rate of contractions in the duodenum compared with the ileum, there is a slow net distal movement of the contents.

Discrete propulsive contractions

These are bursts of contractions lasting 30–60 seconds, mostly found in the proximal jejunum, propagated down the intestine over short distances. They allow slow flow of chyme while maximizing absorption.

Peristalsis

This is a contraction ring of circular smooth muscle that may develop anywhere in the gut, but mainly the ileum, and move distally over a variable distance at speeds of 60–120 cm per minute. They rush fluid through the bowel, distributing it over the luminal surface, and move the intestinal contents distally. They are particularly associated with complete intestinal obstruction and are grossly exaggerated in the presence of enterotoxins.[49]

Mucosal movements

Contraction of the muscularis mucosae causes shifts in the valvulae conniventes over the surface of the intestinal smooth muscle, further mixing the luminal contents.

The villi also exhibit motility independent of the contractions of the outer muscle coat, consisting of piston-like retractions and pendular movements, particularly in the proximal gut.[50] These movements increase markedly after a meal, especially one containing long chain fatty acids or amino acids, but their control is unclear. Possible functions include a villous pump, to empty the contents of the central lacteal into larger lymph vessels, and promoting intestinal mucosal blood flow or nutrient absorption.

Control of intestinal motility

Motor patterns in the small bowel are controlled on a number of levels by a complex interaction of local, hormonal and neurological factors.

Local mechanisms

Rhythmic contractions are governed by slow waves which act as pacemaking potentials, setting the frequency, velocity and direction of peristaltic movements. An intestinal pacemaker in the proximal duodenum initiates this sequence of slow waves that migrate distally. Although the electrical potential is present, contraction of the smooth muscle occurs with only 30–40% of the slow wave cycles by a superimposed spike discharge. This whole process is modulated by the extrinsic and intrinsic nervous systems, although the vagus controls the force and likelihood of contraction rather than the rhythm.

Gut neural controls

There are a number of regional reflexes, mediated by the vagus, that influence small intestinal activity:

- Intestinal distension produces gastric relaxation and induces peristaltic contraction above the point of distension, with inhibition of contraction below it.
- Composition of the gastric chyme delivered to the intestine moderates the level of antral contractility, with fat, acid and the products of protein digestion inhibiting it.
- Food in the ileal region interacts with local receptors that slow gastric emptying and intestinal transit and suppress food intake[45] – the 'ileal brake'.

Hormonal controls

Hormones can act locally as neurotransmitters or humorally via the bloodstream, but this area is still under intense investigation. Motilin, a 23 amino acid peptide found predominantly in duodenal muscle, has been implicated as the main hormone governing the responsiveness of the gut to intrinsic neural activity. In the stomach, gastrin and motilin increase antral motility, while secretin, neurotensin and CCK inhibit it. In the intestine, motilin and substance P stimulate motility, whereas neurotensin and somatostatin inhibit motility.

Cerebral factors

Cerebral controls act via neural mechanisms such as the autonomic nervous system, spinal reflexes and the central nervous system, and via humoral mechanisms such as centrally released peptides and non-gastrointestinal hormones acting as neurotransmitters.[46]

GASTROINTESTINAL HORMONES

General features

Since 1970, over 35 additional peptides have been discovered within the gut and central nervous systems.[51] During their isolation and investigation a number of matters have become clear: (1) identical or closely related peptides occur both in gut endocrine cells and in neurones, either in gut or elsewhere, including the central nervous system; (2) particular peptides may function not only as local gut hormones or paracrine regulators but also as central or peripheral neurotransmitters.[52] Gut endocrine peptides are confined either to mucosa (e.g. gastrin, secretin, CCK, motilin, neurotensin and enteroglucagon) or within pancreatic islets (e.g. insulin, glucagon, somatostatin and PP). Most neuropeptides, such as VIP, substance P and somatostatin (SS), are present within intrinsic nerve plexuses and nerve fibres. With the exception of secretin, glucagon, glucose-dependent insulinotropic polypeptide (GIP) and peptide YY, all of the gut regulatory peptides are found in brain tissue. In general, the distribution of gut hormones reflects their functions and sites of action (Table 43.5). A number of these hormones have been discussed elsewhere (see Chapter 20) in relation to gastric physiology, but will be briefly detailed here.

Small bowel hormones

Gastrin

Gastrin is mainly found in the gastric antrum and is the most potent known stimulus to gastric acid secretion. It exists in several forms, depending on the number of amino acid residues, including Big gastrin (consisting of 34 amino acids) mainly in the duodenum and upper jejunum in small amounts, and the more common and abundant Little gastrin (consisting of 17 amino acids) found in the gastric antrum. Besides its actions on acid secretion, gastrin stimulates pepsin secretion, gal bladder contraction, hepatic bile flow and gastric blood flow. It has effects on intestinal motility, inhibiting pyloric and ileocaecal sphincter function and stimulating small bowel tone and motility, and has tropic effects on gastric and small intestinal mucosa and on the pancreas.[53]

Cholecystokinin

Existing in a number of forms depending on the number of amino acid residues, CCK has an identical terminal amino acid sequence to gastrin, suggesting a common evolutionary history. It is found in three main forms: CCK-39, CCK-33 and CCK-8 with the last being the active form. It is principally found in the duodenal mucosa but also to a lesser extent in the jejunum and ileum. It has major roles in stimulating gall bladder contraction (as its name would imply) and promoting

Table 43.5 Gastrointestinal hormones

HORMONE	AMINO ACIDS	PRINCIPAL DISTRIBUTION	MAJOR ACTIONS
Gastrin			
Big gastrin	34	Duodenum, upper jejunum	↑ Acid and pepsin secretion, gall bladder contraction and ↑ bile flow, ↑ gastrointestinal tone and motility,
Little gastrin	17	Gastric antrum	tropic effects on stomach, pancreas
Cholecystokinin			
CCK-39	39	Duodenum, jejunum	Gall bladder contraction,
CCK-33	33		↑ pancreatic enzyme secretion
CCK-8	8		
Secretin	27	Duodenum, upper jejunum	↓ Gastric secretion, ↑ pancreatic bicarbonate secretion
Glucose-dependent insulinotropic peptide	42	Duodenum, jejunum	↑ Insulin release after a meal
Motilin	23	Duodenum, jejunum	↑ Gut motility
Vasoactive intestinal peptide	28	All gut nerves	Mesenteric vasodilatation, ↑ electrolyte and water secretion
Substance P	11	All gut	↑ Gut motility, gall bladder contraction and ↑ bile flow, ↑ pancreatic juice
Somatostatin			
SS-28	28	All gut mucosa, pancreas	↓ Saliva, acid, pepsin, intrinsic factor, ↓ pancreatic enzymes and bicarbonate, ↓ gall bladder contraction and bile flow,
SS-14	14	Nerves	↓ gastrointestinal hormones, ↓ secretion of fluid and electrolytes
Neurotensin	13	Ileum	Mesenteric vasodilatation, ↓ gut motility
Peptide YY	36	Ileum, colon	'Ileal brake'
Enteroglucagon			
Glicentin	69	Ileum	Gut motility, intestinal growth and differentiation

pancreatic enzyme secretion. In addition, CCK has secondary roles in stimulating pancreatic bicarbonate and insulin secretion, bile flow and Brunner's gland mucus secretion.

Secretin

Secretin has been extensively studied and has a wide variety of actions on many areas of the gastrointestinal tract.[54] It is a 27 amino acid polypeptide principally found in the duodenum, but also in lesser amounts in the upper jejunum. Its main actions involve inhibition of gastric acid secretion and the production of bicarbonate-rich pancreatic juice.

Glucose-dependent insulinotropic peptide

This 42 amino acid polypeptide found in the upper small intestine was formerly known as gastric inhibitory peptide, having been thought to inhibit gastric acid secretion. It appears that this effect only occurs in pharmacological doses, and it has little effect on the stomach in physiological amounts. Its most important function is in potentiating insulin release after a meal, hence the name change to reflect its physiological role.

Motilin

This has been discussed earlier in relation to its effects on gastrointestinal motility. Motilin is a 23 amino acid residue molecule found principally in the duodenum, but also the gastric antrum and jejunum. It is the main hormonal mediator of gut motility, stimulating the production of migrating motor complexes when injected intravenously during the fasting state.[46] It is not the only mediator, however; a wide range of other hormones is implicated, including CCK, SS, neurotensin and PP.

Vasoactive intestinal peptide

This is a 28 amino acid polypeptide found throughout the gut but in greatest amount in the colon, with the least quantity in the stomach. It functions as a neuropeptide, being found in the intestinal nerve plexuses and nerve fibres. Primary physiological functions include mesenteric vasodilatation and the stimulation of intestinal fluid and electrolyte secretion by the promotion of active chloride secretion. Pharmacological doses inhibit acid and pepsin secretion but these do not appear to be important roles physiologically.

Substance P

Substance P acts as a non-cholinergic excitatory neurotransmitter, regulating gut motility. It is found throughout the gut but principally in the duodenum, with the least amounts in the stomach. It increases intestinal smooth muscle contraction and gall bladder contraction, stimulates bile flow and pancreatic juice output.

Somatostatin

Existing in two forms with either 14 (SS-14) or 28 (SS-28) amino acid residues, somatostatin is a naturally occurring, virtually universal inhibitory substance.[55] It was originally described as an inhibitor of growth hormone release, being found in the hypothalamus, but has now been found widely distributed, acting as a neuropeptide and endocrine peptide in various parts of the body and exerting a negative effect on many physiological functions. In the gut SS-14, found in nerve cells, acts as a neuropeptide, whereas the larger form, SS-28, is found in the gastrointestinal mucosa and pancreatic δ cells acting as a gut endocrine peptide. SS is found throughout the gut, but is in highest concentration in the jejunum, ileum and gastric antrum.

SS functions as an inhibitory peptide, decreasing all secretions from saliva and gastric acid to pepsin and intrinsic factor. It inhibits pancreatic enzyme and bicarbonate secretion, decreases bile flow and inhibits the secretion of gastrointestinal hormones, such as gastrin, secretin, CCK, GIP, VIP, insulin and motilin. SS diminishes gut and gall bladder motility, inhibits secretion of intestinal fluid and electrolytes, and decreases nutrient absorption and splanchnic blood flow.

Other hormones

Neurotensin, a 13 amino acid polypeptide, is mainly found in the ileum, with lesser amounts in the jejunum. It acts both as a neuropeptide and endocrine peptide, inhibiting small bowel motility but also increasing mesenteric vasodilatation.

Peptide YY, a 36 amino acid molecule, is mostly found in the colon, with less in the ileum. It has been implicated as a mediator of the 'ileal brake.'

Enteroglucagon is found in a number of forms, but the largest is glicentin, a polypeptide of 69 amino acid residues. It is different from pancreatic glucagon, found in pancreatic A cells, which is involved in carbohydrate metabolism. The functions of glicentin, found in the mucosa of the distal small intestine, are unclear but may involve gut motility or intestinal growth and differentiation.

OTHER FUNCTIONS OF THE SMALL INTESTINE

Lipoprotein production

The small intestine is an active site of lipoprotein assembly and secretion, producing half of the daily output of apolipoprotein A-I, a major component of high density lipoproteins.[16] Production takes place in the rough endoplasmic reticulum and export is via exocytosis in high density, low density and very low density lipoproteins, as well as chylomicrons. Synthesis occurs throughout the gut but principally in the proximal jejunum. Although there are other sites for lipoprotein production, such as the liver, the small bowel plays a major role in the metabolism of plasma lipoproteins.

Immunological functions

As a major area of exposure to exogenous toxins and microbiological agents the small intestine has a well-developed immune defence system to protect the body from ingestion of bacteria and other micro-organisms. The bowel contains plasma cells and lymphocytes and is the major site of production of IgA, which is secreted into the gut lumen as a dimer, combined with a locally produced protein from the enterocyte, the secretory component. The intraepithelial lymphocytes comprise both helper and suppressor T cells, whereas the lamina propria population is mainly B cells producing immunoglobulins.

Once in the gut lumen, the combined dimeric IgA–secretory component molecule inhibits the adherence of coated micro-organisms to the surface of the enterocyte, preventing entry, but it may also activate the complement pathway in immune defence when aggregated on the surface of bacteria.[23]

Epithelial repair

The gut not only has immunological defences but has a sophisticated repair mechanism when damage is sustained, either by direct trauma or in ulcerating diseases such as peptic ulceration and Crohn's disease. The duodenum has a particularly well-developed defence to cope with the hostile conditions, which can be considered on a number of levels.[41] Pre-epithelial protection is provided in two ways: (1) a viscoelastic mucous gel of variable thickness, secreted by Brunner's glands, which increases in thickness to protect areas of re-epithelializing mucosa; and (2) bicarbonate secretion into this mucous gel by the duodenal mucosa, so that the pH at the cell surface is near neutral, despite a pH of around 2 in the lumen bulk solution.[42] At the epithelium itself, phopholipids acts as surfactants to prevent water-soluble agents in the lumen from damaging cells and the enterocytes have selective permeability to hydrogen ions. Subepithelial protection is provided by rapid blood flow to maximize oxygen delivery to the mucosa and allow rapid removal of neutrients, water and metabolic end-products.

Small superficial defects in the mucosa are repaired by very rapid restitution, involving cell migration across an intact basal membrane. With larger defects an ulcer-associated cell line (UACL) is stimulated into action, forming a 'gastrointestinal repair kit'. Previously known as pyloric metaplasia, the UACL typically arises where there is enteric ulceration, notably in the ulcerated gut of Crohn's disease. This cell lineage produces neutral mucin, is non-proliferative and secretes abundant epidermal growth factor (EGF).[56] EGF is a significant mitogen, secreted directly into the small intestine by Brunner's glands and via salivary and biliary secretion. It is also found in a wide variety of external secretions, in blood and amniotic fluid.[57] EGF receptors are found on the basolateral membranes of enterocytes,[58] strongly suggesting its role in mucosal repair and maintenance.

By studying ileal resection specimens from patients with Crohn's disease, Roberts and Stoddart[59] confirmed the development of mucus-secreting glands, resembling Brunner's glands, within mucosa adjacent to ulceration. The UACL is formed by extrusion from the base of the intestinal crypt, forming a new gland in the lamina propria that secretes EGF. Enterocytes are thus stimulated to migrate from the proliferative zone in the base of the crypts, differentiate and move towards villi tips.

Brunner's glands can thus be regarded as a 'permanent first-aid post' in a hostile area, while the UACL develops in response to damage wherever it occurs.

REFERENCES

1. Hofmann AF. Digestion and absorption. In West JB (ed.) *Best and Taylor's Physiological Basis of Medical Practice*, 12th edn. Baltimore, MD: Williams & Wilkins, 1990: 693–706.
2. Borgstrom B, Dahlqvist G, Lundh G & Sjovall J. Studies of intestinal digestion and absorption in the human. *J Clin Invest* 1957; **36**: 1521–1536.

3. Wilson JAP & Owyang C. Physiology of digestion and absorption. In Nelson RL & Nyhus LM (eds) *Surgery of the Small Intestine.* Norwalk, CT: Appleton & Lange, 1987: 21–28.

4. Cushieri A. The small intestine and vermiform appendix. In Cushieri A, Giles GR & Mossa AR (eds) *Essential Surgical Practice*, 2nd edn. London: Wright, 1988: 1136–1163.

5. Frederiksen W, Bruusgaard A & Thaysen EH. Assessment of the relationship between gastric secretory capacity and jejunal bacteriology. *Scand J Gastroenterol* 1973; **8**: 353.

6. Geray JDA & Shiner M. Influence of gastric pH on gastric and jejunal flora. *Gut* 1967; **8**: 574.

7. Adinolfi MF, Cerise EJ & Nichols RL. Microbiology of the small intestine. In Nelson RL & Nyhus LM (eds) *Surgery of the Small Intestine.* Norwalk, CT: Appleton & Lange, 1987: 39–46.

8. Gray GM. Carbohydrate digestion and absorption: role of the small intestine. *N Engl J Med* 1975; **292**: 1225–1230.

9. Johannson C. Studies of gastrointestinal interactions: VII Characteristics of the absorption pattern of sugar, fat and protein from composite meals in man. A quantitative study. *Scand J Gastroenterol* 1975; **10**: 33–42.

10. Alpers DH & Seetharam B. Physiology of diseases involving intestinal brush-border proteins. *N Engl J Med* 1977; **296**: 1047–1050.

11. Borgstrom B. On the interactions between pancreatic lipase and colipase and the substrate, and the importance of bile salts. *J Lipid Res* 1975; **16**: 411–417.

12. Hofmann AF. Clinical implications of physiochemical studies on bile salts. *Gastroenterology* 1965; **48**: 484–494.

13. Chadwick VS & Camilleri M. Pathophysiology of small intestinal function and the effect of Crohn's disease. In Allan RN, Keighley MRB, Alexander-Williams J & Hawkins CF (eds) *Inflammatory Bowel Diseases*, 2nd Edn. London: Churchill Livingstone, 1990: 37–54.

14. Borgstrom B & Patton JS. Luminal events in gastrointestinal lipid digestion. In Schultz SG (ed) *Handbook of Physiology*, sect. 6, The Gastrointestinal System, vol. IV, Intestinal Absorption and Secretion. Washington, DC: American Physiological Society, 1991: 475–504.

15. Ockner RK & Manning JA. Fatty acid binding protein in small intestine. Identification, isolation and evidence for its role in cellular fatty acid transport. *J Clin Invest* 1974; **54**: 326–338.

16. Davidson NO, Magun AM & Glickman RM. Enterocyte lipid absorption and secretion. In Schultz SG (ed.) *Handbook of Physiology*, sect. 6, The Gastrointestinal System, vol. IV, Intestinal Absorption and Secretion. Washington, DC: American Physiological Society, 1991: 505–526.

17. Lack L & Weiner IM. Intestinal bile acid transport: structure–activity relationships and other properties. *Am J Physiol* 1966; **210**: 1142–1152.

18. Hofmann AF. The syndrome of ileal disease and the broken enterohepatic circulation: cholerteic enteropathy. *Gastroenterology* 1967; **52**: 752–757.

19. Hollander D & Ruble PE Jr β-carotene intestinal absorption: bile, fatty acid, pH and flow rate effects on transport. *Am J Physiol* 1978; **235**: E686–691.

20. DeLuca HF. Function of the fat-soluble vitamins. *Am J Clin Nutr* 1975; **28**: 339–345.

21. Mellors AJ, Nahrwold DL & Rose RC. Ascorbic acid flux across the mucosal border of guinea pig and human ileum. *Am J Physiol* 1977; **233**: 274–279.

22. Lindenbaum J. Aspects of vitamin B_{12} and folate metabolism in malabsorption syndromes. *Am J Med* 1979; **67**: 1037–1048.

23. Ishitani MB & Jones RS. Part II: Functional anatomy and applied physiology of the small intestine. In Scott HW Jr & Sawyers JL (eds) *Surgery of the Stomach, Duodenum and Small Intestine.* London: Blackwell, 1987: 61–77.

24. Katz M & Cooper BA. Solubilised receptor for vitamin B_{12} intrinsic factor complex from human intestine. *Br J Haematol* 1974; **25**: 569–579.

25. Hoffbrand AV, Stewart JS, Booth CC & Mollin DL. Folate deficiency in Crohn's disease: incidence, pathogenesis and treatment. *BMJ* 1968; **2**: 71–75.

26. Selhub J, Dhar GJ & Rosenberg IH. Inhibition of folate enzymes by sulfasalazine. *J Clin Invest* 1978; **61**: 221–224.

27. Rose RC. Water-soluble vitamin absorption in intestine. *Annu Rev Physiol* 1980; **42**: 157–171.

28. Nemere I & Norman AW. Transport of calcium. In Schultz SG (ed.) *Handbook of Physiology*, sect. 6, The Gastrointestinal System, vol. IV, Intestinal Absorption and Secretion. Washington, DC: American Physiological Society, 1991: 337–360.

29. Danisi G & Murer H. Inorganic phosphate absorption in small intestine. In Schultz SG (ed.) *Handbook of Physiology*, sect. 6, The Gastrointestinal System, vol. IV, Intestinal Absorption and Secretion. Washington, DC: American Physiological Society, 1991: 323–336.

30. Finch CA & Huebers HA. Iron absorption. In Schultz SG (ed.) *Handbook of Physiology*, sect. 6, The Gastrointestinal System. vol. IV, Intestinal Absorption and Secretion. Washington, DC: American Physiological Society, 1991: 361–369.

31. Stake PE, Miller WJ, Blackmon DM, Gentry RP & Neathery MW. Role of pancreas in endogenous zinc excretion in the bovine. *J Nutr* 1974; **104**: 1279–1284.

32. Dharmsathaphorn K. Intestinal water and electrolyte secretion and absorption. In West JB (ed.) *Best and Taylor's Physiological Basis of Medical Practice*, 12th edn. Baltimore, MD: Williams & Wilkins, 1990: 707–721.

33. Guyton AC. *Textbook of Medical Physiology*, 8th edn. Philadelphia: WB Saunders, 1991.

34. Madara JL. Functional morphology of epithelium of the small intestine. In Schultz SG (ed.) *Handbook of Physiology*, sect. 6, The Gastrointestinal System, vol. IV, Intestinal Absorption and Secretion. Washington, DC: American Physiological Society, 1991: 83–120.

35. Sullivan SK & Field M. Ion transport across mammalian small intestine. In Schultz SG (ed.) *Handbook of Physiology*, sect. 6, The Gastrointestinal System, vol. IV, Intestinal Absorption and Secretion. Washington, DC: American Physiological Society, 1991: 287–301.

36. Fordtran JS, Rector FC, Ewton MF, Soter N & Kinney J. Permeability characteristics of the human small intestine. *J Clin Invest* 1965; **44**: 1935–1944.

37. Fordtran JS. Stimulation of active and passive sodium absorption by sugars in the human jejunum. *J Clin Invest* 1975; **55**: 728–737.

38. Turnberg LA, Fordtran JS, Carter NW & Rector FC Jr Mechanism of bicarbonate absorption and its relationship to sodium transport in the human jejunum. *J Clin Invest* 1970; **49**: 548–556.

39. Turnberg LA, Bieberdorf FA, Morowski SG & Fordtran JS. Interrelationships of chloride, bicarbonate, sodium and hydrogen transport into the human ileum. *J Clin Invest* 1970; **49**: 557–567.

40. Davis G, Santa Ana C, Morowski SG & Fordtran JS. Active chloride secretion in the normal human jejunum. *J Clin Invest* 1980; **66**: 1326–1333.

41. Safsten B. Duodenal bicarbonate secretion and mucosal protection. *Acta Physiol Scand Suppl* 1993; **613**: 1–43.

42. Quigley EMM & Turnberg LA. pH of the microclimate lining human gastric and duodenal mucosa in vivo. Studies in control subjects and duodenal ulcer patients. *Gastroenterology* 1987; **92**: 1876–1884.

43. Isenberg JI, Selling JA, Hogan DL & Koss MA. Impaired proximal duodenal mucosal bicarbonate secretion in patients with duodenal ulcer. *N Engl J Med* 1987; **316**: 374–379.

44. Selling JA, Hogan DL, Aly A, Koss MA & Isenberg JI. Indomethacin inhibits duodenal mucosal bicarbonate secretion and endogenous prostaglandin E_2 output in human subjects. *Ann Intern Med* 1987; **106**: 368–371.

45. Malagelada JR & Azpiroz F. Determinants of gastric emptying and transit in the small intestine. In Schultz SG (ed.) *Handbook of Physiology*, sect. 6, The Gastrointestinal System, vol. I, part 2, Motility and Circulation. Washington, DC: American Physiological Society, 1991: 909–937.

46. Borody TJ & Phillips SF. Motility of the small intestine. In Nelson RL & Nyhus LM (eds) *Surgery of the Small Intestine.* Norwalk, CT: Appleton & Lange, 1987: 29–38.

47. Christensen J. Gastrointestinal motility. In West JB (ed.) *Best and Taylor's Physiological Basis of Medical Practice*, 12th edn. Baltimore, MD: Williams & Wilkins, 1990.

48. Chesta J, Defilippi C & Defil C. Abnormalities in proximal small bowel motility in patients with cirrhosis. *Hepatology* 1993; **17**: 828–832.

49. Mathias JR, Carlson GM, DiMarino AJ, Bertiger G, Morton HE & Cohen S. Intestinal myoelectric activity in response to live *Vibrio cholerae* and cholera enterotoxin. *J Clin Invest* 1976; **58**: 91–96.

50. Wormack WA, Kvietys PR & Granger DN. Villous motility. In Schultz SG (ed.) *Handbook of Physiology*, sect. 6, The Gastrointestinal System, vol. I, part 2, Motility and Circulation. Washington, DC: American Physiological Society, 1991: 975–986.

51. Go VLW & Koch TR. Distribution of gut peptides. In Schultz SG (ed.) *Handbook of Physiology*, sect. 6, The Gastrointestinal System, vol. II, Neural and Endocrine Biology. Washington, DC: American Physiological Society, 1991: 111–122.

52. Dockray GJ. Comparative neuroendocrinology of gut peptides. In Schultz SG. (ed.) *Handbook of Physiology*, sect. 6, The Gastrointestinal System, vol. II, Neural and Endocrine Biology. Washington, DC: American Physiological Society, 1991: 133–170.

53. Dockray GJ & Gregory RA. Gastrin. In Schultz SG (ed.) *Handbook of Physiology*, sect. 6, The Gastrointestinal System, vol. II, Neural and Endocrine Biology. Washington, DC: American Physiological Society, 1991: 311–336.

54. Chey WY & Chang TM. Secretin. In Schultz SG (ed.) *Handbook of Physiology*, sect. 6, The Gastrointestinal System, vol. II, Neural and Endocrine Biology. Washington, DC: American Physiological Society, 1991: 359–402.

55. Yamada T & Chiba T. Somatostatin. In Schultz SG (ed.) *Handbook of Physiology*, sect. 6, The Gastrointestinal System, vol. II, Neural and Endocrine Biology. Washington, DC: American Physiological Society, 1991: 431–453.

56. Wright NA, Pike C & Elia G. Induction of a novel epidermal growth factor-secreting cell lineage by mucosal ulceration in human gastrointestinal stem cells. *Nature* 1990; **343**: 82–85.

57. Marti U, Burwen SJ & Jones AL. Biological effects of epidermal growth factor, with emphasis on the gastrointestinal tract and liver: an update. *Hepatology* 1989; **9**: 126–138.

58. Mynott CL, Pinches SA, Gamer A & Shirazi-Beechey SP. Location and characteristics of epidermal growth factor binding to enterocyte plasma membranes. *Biochem Soc Trans* 1991; **19**: 307S.

59. Roberts ISD & Stoddart RW. Ulcer-associated cell lineage ('pyloric metaplasia') in Crohn's disease: a lectin histochemical study. *J Pathol* 1993; **171**: 13–19.

44

INVESTIGATION AND DIAGNOSIS OF SMALL INTESTINAL DISEASE

RE Barry

The small intestine is a large organ which performs many functions, the most obvious of which is digestion and absorption. It is also an important barrier between the internal and external environment and provides an important protective role in excluding pathogenic organisms and harmful macromolecules. For this reason the small intestine acts as an immunological organ of considerable importance.

The small intestine functions in concert with other organs in the digestive tract and is subject to similar neurohumoral control mechanisms. It can also influence the various functions of the rest of the gastrointestinal tract through its actions as a hormone-producing organ. It produces a large variety of biologically active peptides and amines, some of which are known to have an important role in normal physiology (e.g. gastrin, cholecystokinin). Others are known to be important in the pathogenesis of certain disease states (e.g. vasoactive intestinal peptide), whereas others are known to produce biological effects in experimental systems but have no recognized role as yet in normal physiology or disease states.

In addition to its digestive, absorptive, immunological and hormonal roles, the small intestine has a large secretory capacity which is independent of its absorptive function.

Diseases of the small intestine can occur primarily as a failure of any of these functions; but equally, primary disease of the small intestine can result in secondary effects on digestion, absorption, secretion, host defence mechanisms and humoral control.

CLINICAL FEATURES

Small bowel disease usually presents with a pattern of symptoms that is not unique to the small intestine. For example, malabsorption or steatorrhoea is frequently a manifestation of gastric, pancreatic or hepatic disorder rather than small intestinal disease, and the manifestations of inflammatory disease of the small intestine can be almost identical to those of colonic inflammation. Diagnosis is none the less usually straightforward, provided the clinican is careful to take a full history with appropriate attention to detail and examines the abdomen skilfully.

Abdominal examination always includes rectal examination and the testing of the stool for occult blood, the presence of which indicates a breach in mucosal integrity. Examination of the stool for the presence of blood, pus, parasites and undigested food has obvious diagnostic importance. Eosinophils and Charcot–Leyden crystals suggest eosinophilic enteritis. Culture of fresh stool may be diagnostic for *Shigella, Salmonella, Yersinia, Campylobacter* and, if appropriate, *Clostridium difficile* and *Escherichia coli.*

Most inflammatory and neoplastic diseases of the small intestine are likely to be diagnosed clinically with the additional information provided by simple radiology, but simple haematological investigations can provide isolated diagnostic clues:

Diseases causing malabsorption may be suggested by:

- Mixed deficiencies e.g. low serum ferritin, low red cell folate levels, low serum vitamin B_{12}
- Macrocytosis
- Low serum calcium
- Raised alkaline phosphatase
- Prolonged prothrombin time.

Inflammatory disease may be suggested by:

- Anaemia
- Raised viscosity and ESR
- Thrombocythaemia
- Low plasma proteins
- Raised acute phase proteins, e.g. C-reactive protein
- (Care is required with Crohn's disease, in which inflammatory indices are often misleading.)

Protein-losing enteropathy may be suggested by:

- Lymphopenia (especially in intestinal lymphangiectasia)
- Low albumin and low IgG.

Secretory diarrhoea may be suggested by:

- Hypokalaemia.

Abnormal haematological findings should never be ignored in the diagnosis of small intestinal disease.

Although long-standing and extensive small intestinal disease, e.g. coeliac disease, may be quite asymptomatic, the pattern of presentation of overt small intestinal disease is remarkably uniform. Patients commonly present with frequent passage of loose stools which may or may not be accompanied by weight loss, abdominal pain and symptoms and signs of inflammation. Unlike the very frequent, watery, small-volume stool characteristic of colonic disease and accompanied by urgency, incontinence and tenesmus, the stool in small intestinal disease is characteristically less frequent, semiformed, bulky and pale.

The loose stool of small bowel disease may be caused by steatorrhoea (too much fat in the faeces) or diarrhoea (too much water in the faeces). The diagnostic principles for each will be considered separately.

MALABSORPTION AND STEATORRHOEA

Malabsorption is a common consequence of small intestinal disease. It may present as an acute syndrome, with steatorrhoea, diarrhoea and weight loss, or more commonly have an insidious onset presenting with one or other consequential deficiency states, such as a mixed deficiency anaemia.

In the investigation and diagnosis of small intestinal disease, when the patient's symptoms suggest a malabsorptive syndrome, it is usually important (1) to establish whether malabsorption is present and (2) to investigate which disease process is causing the malabsorption.

Physiological considerations

The three major components of food are carbohydrate, protein and fats.

Carbohydrates

Carbohydrates are ingested mainly as starch (amylose and amylopectin) or dissacharides (lactose, sucrose). Starch is digested within the small intestinal lumen by pancreatic amylase. The product of the luminal digestion of amylose (a straight-chain polysaccharide) is glucose, which is then absorbed through the small intestinal mucosal cell by an active transport process which is sodium- and energy-dependent. Pancreatic amylase has a stereospecificity as a consequence of which the products of luminal digestion of amylopectin are, in addition to glucose, branched chain oligosaccharides. These oligosaccharides are then adsorbed on to the brush border of the small intestinal cells, where further digestion by the brush-border oligosaccharidase enzymes complete the digestion to glucose, which is then absorbed by the active transport mechanism. The products of carbohydrate digestion and absorption are transported via the portal circulation.

There is no luminal phase for the digestion of disaccharides such as sucrose and lactose. Digestion to the constituent monosaccharides takes place on the brush border of the intestinal epithelial cell where the lactase and sucrase enzymes are situated.

Protein

The pancreas again plays a key role in the digestion of protein. Pancreatic proteases digest proteins within the small intestinal lumen. The products of luminal digestion are free amino acids and oligopeptides. There are, however, several different transport systems within the intestinal brush border for the different groups of amino acids. As with carbohydrate digestion, oligopeptides are adsorbed on to the brush border, where brush-border peptidases can complete the digestion to free amino acids, which are then absorbed. However, unlike the situation in carbohydrate absorption, some dipeptdes and tripeptides can be absorbed intact without further digestion. The absorbed products of protein digestion are also transported via the portal circulation.

Fat

Fat is triglyceride: three long chain fatty acids linked by a glycerol molecule. In quantitative terms the pancreas is again the key organ for the luminal digestion of fat under normal circumstances. Pancreatic lipases digest the triglyceride to two free fatty acids and a β-monoglyceride. Each of these products of digestion is poorly soluble in the water phase but is amphipathic. Bile salt molecules are detergent. Provided bile salts are present in the small intestinal lumen in sufficient concentration ('critical micellar concentration'), bile salt micelles will form and the products of fat digestion will be incorporated into mixed micelles. Being 'solubilized' in micelles, the fatty acids and monoglycerides are transported to the intestinal cells where absorption takes place.

Once inside the epithelial cells, the fatty acids and monoglycerides are re-esterified to form triglyceride again, which is then coated with β-lipoprotein to form chylomicrons. These particles are then extruded through the intestinal epithelial cell and delivered into the lacteals, not the portal circulation; they reach the systemic circulation via the thoracic duct.

It can be seen from the above that the digestion and absorption of carbohydrate and protein require a functioning pancreas, an enterocyte (small intestinal mucosal cell) and an intact portal circulation. For the digestion and absorption of fat, however, additional steps are required: a functioning liver and biliary tract to produce an appropriate luminal concentration of bile acids; a mucosal ability to re-esterify the products of fat digestion and to synthesize and transport β-lipoproteins; and a lymphatic delivery system which is unimpeded. Since there are more opportunities for fat absorption to become disordered, and since those sites at which disease influences the absorption of carbohydrate and protein would also influence the absorption of fat, it is preferable to *investigate only fat absorption when establishing the presence or absence of malabsorption.* Steatorrhoea is, therefore, the hallmark of malabsorption. Tests of carbohydrate or protein absorption do not produce additional useful information.

Diagnosis of steatorrhoea
Faecal fat estimation

Steatorrhoea is the presence of excess fat in the stool. The normal fat content of the stool is less than 15 mmol per day, approximately half of which is endogenous. To detect the presence of small intestinal disease producing malabsorption, it is often necessary to stress the intestinal absorptive capacity by increasing the ingested fat load to 100 g per day and to collect the faecal output and measure the fat content over a minimum of 3 days during the period of fat loading. Because such a formal fat balance is tedious, time consuming and unpopular with laboratory staff, many surrogate tests have been developed to estimate fat absorption. The fat balance remains the most sensitive and gives an indication of absorption integrated over a 3-day period, which contrasts with the isolated 'snapshot' provided by most surrogate fat absorption tests. In the presence of intestinal disease, fat absorption varies at different times (e.g. in the fasting versus the non-fasting state). Such 'sampling' errors are avoided by the 3-day collection of a formal fat balance.

Triolein breath test

After an overnight fast, an oral dose of 5 μCi glyceryl-[14C]triolein is administered with a standard test meal. Each of the three oleic acid molecules is labelled with the 14C istotope. After digestion and absorption of the triglyceride, the oleic acid is metabolized to carbon dioxide and water. The labelled carbon dioxide is excreted in the breath, trapped in hyamine hydroxide and assayed by liquid scintillation counting.[1] The output of [14C]carbon dioxide is expressed as percentage dose excreted per hour. Peak excretion is greater than 3.5%/h in normals.

Other lipids and other isotopes have been used.

Surrogate markers for fat absorption such as serum turbidity after a standard oral fat load cannot be recommended.

Investigating the cause of malabsorption and steatorrhoea

Almost all diseases that affect the small intestine can cause malabsorption, and since the number of such diseases is large a logical sequence of investigation is imperative. Having established the presence of malabsorption, the gross anatomy of the small intestine is *first* investigated by barium follow-through examination (see Chapter 45). This examination permits the diagnosis of a variety of diseases causing intestinal malabsorption. Examples are listed in Table 44.1.

In the case of strictures, fistulas and diverticulosis, the malabsorption arises as a consequence of a large bowel flora,

which is related to the anatomical lesion and causes dehydroxylation and deconjugation of the luminal bile acids. As a result the concentration of effective bile acids falls below the critical micellar concentration required for solubilization of the products of fat digestion. Although in other cases the mechanisms causing the malabsorption are less well understood, the diagnosis of the intestinal disease is obtained by this single first investigation.

If the barium follow-through fails to demonstrate a gross anatomical lesion to account for the malabsorption, the microscopic anatomy of the small intestinal mucosa should *next* be examined on a peroral jejunal biopsy. Confusion can be caused by non-specific mucosal architectural changes which occur in the proximal duodenum and by the small size of endoscopic biopsies. It is therefore preferable to obtain jejunal biopsies with a Watson capsule screened to a position just distal to the ligament of Treitz. In experienced hands it rarely takes more than a few minutes to obtain a suitable biopsy. Careful orientation of the biopsy before fixation will permit the histological diagnosis of a variety of small intestinal mucosal diseases that cause malabsorption. Examples are shown in Table 44.2.

Table 44.2 Mucosal diseases of the small intestine that can be diagnosed by peroral jejunal biopsy

Coeliac disease
Dermatitis herpetiformis
A-β-lipoproteinaemia
Intestinal lymphangiectasia
Amyloidosis
Whipple's disease
Giardiasis
Common variable immune deficiency
Intestinal lymphoma and its variants (e.g. α-chain disease)
Tropical sprue

If the gross intestinal anatomy assessed on barium follow-through and the microscopic mucosal anatomy assessed on jejunal biopsy are both normal, then *the likely cause of the malapsorption is pancreatic or biliary disease*. Assessment of pancreatic anatomy and function is now indicated, but other intestinal causes of malabsorption such as small intestinal bacterial colonization syndromes or hypolactasia may also be investigated.

BACTERIAL COLONIZATION OF THE SMALL INTESTINE

The proximal small intestine rarely contains more than 10^3 (predominantly aerobic) organisms per millilitre. The density of the flora increases in the distal ileum, where the organisms are predominantly obligate anaerobes.

The mechanisms that preserve the relative sterility of the upper small intestine are inadequately understood. Important roles may be played by the low gastric pH, normal intestinal motility and normal immunoglobulin synthesis and secretion by the immune system of the small intestinal mucosa. In conditions

Table 44.1 Diseases causing intestinal malabsorption that can be diagnosed by barium follow-through examination

Small intestinal strictures
Intestinal carcinoma and lymphoma
Jejunal diverticulosis
Crohn's disease
Enteric fistulas
Systemic sclerosis
Radiation enteritis

that impair intestinal motility, such as partial obstruction by stricture, jejunal diverticulosis or systemic sclerosis, the small intestine becomes colonized by a predominantly anaerobic bacterial flora, which can cause steatorrhoea by dehydroxylation and deconjugation of the luminal bile salts. The severe malabsorption of coloenteric fistula is caused not by 'short-circuit' of the intestine, but by anaerobic colonization of the small intestine.

Specific deficiency of vitamin B_{12} can result from the ability of this anaerobic flora to split the intrinsic factor–vitamin B_{12} complex, thus rendering the vitamin non-absorbable. As with terminal ileal disease, the Schilling test in intestinal colonization remains positive despite the addition of intrinsic factor to the orally administered labelled vitamin B_{12}.

Small intestinal bacterial colonization commonly occurs secondarily to a structural abnormality of the intestine, and this can be diagnosed radiologically. However, colonization can also occur in the absence of an identifiable gross anatomical abnormality – for example in achlorhydria, pseudo-obstruction, various immune deficiency states and old age. A number of simple tests can be used to diagnose colonization.

Investigation of small intestinal colonization

Small intestinal bacterial colonization results in an excess of indicans in the patient's urine, and this compound can be directly assayed. However, specific non-invasive tests for the detection of colonization have been developed. The most widely used are the glucose–hydrogen breath test[2] and the [¹⁴C]glycocholate breath test.[3]

Glucose–hydrogen breath test

Mammalian cells do not produce hydrogen. The small amounts of hydrogen (approximately 5–10 ppm) found in exhaled air are the product of bacterial metabolism absorbed from the colon. Several robust and inexpensive gas chromatographs specifically designed to measure the concentration of hydrogen in expired air are now marketed.

Glucose taken by mouth in health is absorbed completely in the small intestine and does not reach the colonic flora. In normal subjects there is therefore no rise above basal levels of hydrogen in the breath following an oral glucose load. In the presence of proximal small intestinal colonization, ingestion of a standard oral glucose load results in a large rise above basal levels of hydrogen in the breath. This characteristic rise is used as a marker of small intestinal colonization.

Not all organisms are capable of producing free hydrogen. As a consequence, the test has a false-negative rate of approximately 30%. Care is required in interpreting the test in the presence of poor oral hygiene and biliary tract disease. The false-positive rate is approximately 10%.

[¹⁴C]Glycocholate breath test

Natural and orally administered bile acids, such as the glycine conjugate of cholic acid, are absorbed by the specific transport mechanisms for bile acids in the terminal ileum. In the presence of small intestinal bacterial colonization the bacterial flora deconjugate the bile acid, releasing the glycine, which is absorbed and metabolized so that the carbon moiety of the glycine eventually appears in expired air as carbon dioxide. Using peroral synthetic glycocholate in which the glycine is labelled with ¹⁴C, administered with a test meal, the exhaled [¹⁴C]-carbon dioxide is trapped in hyamine, and the ¹⁴C is assayed by liquid scintillation counting to quantitate the deconjugation of the bile acid. There is no appreciable production of [¹⁴C]-carbon dioxide in normals. In the presence of small intestinal colonization the output of labelled CO_2 is proportional to the degree of colonization. Sensitivity and specificity are similar to the glucose–hydrogen breath test.[4]

The investigations described above detect the presence of intestinal colonization. To show that the colonization is causing symptoms requires a trial of antibiotic treatment using an antibiotic such as metronidazole that is effective against obligate anaerobes. Symptoms usually respond within 12 hours of starting treatment with an effective antibiotic.

Other hydrogen breath tests

Lactose–hydrogen test Lactase deficiency can be diagnosed using an isotonic lactose solution instead of glucose. Under physiological conditions lactose is digested by brush-border lactase, and the monosaccharide products glucose and galactose are absorbed. In alactasia and hypolactasia, orally administered lactose is unabsorbed and reaches the colon, where it is metabolized by the normal colonic flora with a resultant rise in exhaled hydrogen (which is not seen in normals). The test cannot be interpreted in the presence of small intestinal colonization.

Lactulose–hydrogen test This test is used to measure small intestinal transit time. Lactulose is not absorbed in the small intestine. The time from ingestion of an isotonic lactulose solution to the beginning of the rise in breath hydrogen output above basal indicates the time taken for the lactulose to traverse the small intestine to reach the normal colonic flora.

SMALL INTESTINAL DIARRHOEA

In addition to the daily oral fluid intake of approximately 2 litres, there is a further daily fluid load of about 8 litres entering the small intestine from the exocrine secretions of the salivary glands, stomach, pancreas, biliary tract and the small intestine itself. At least 80% of this fluid is reabsorbed in the small intestine, so that only approximately 1–2 litres fluid per day enters the colon and less than 200 ml appears in the stool. Small intestinal diseases that increase the net fluid output of the intestine soon result in diarrhoea despite the absorptive capacity of the colon.

The permeability of the jejunum is ten times greater than that of the ileum. Much of the large flux of fluids in the upper small intestine is osmotically determined and dependent on luminal concentration of electrolytes and unabsorbed products of digestion. Because of the osmotic drag of unabsorbed food products, the output of a high jejunostomy can exceed by severalfold the normal oral fluid intake. The sodium-coupled absorption of glucose (e.g. from glucose–electrolyte mixtures) stimulates water absorption and reduces this loss.

In addition to this osmotically determined fluid flux, the small intestinal mucosa can actively secrete electrolytes and water. The secretory and absorptive mechanisms are independent of each other. Except for rare congenital abnormalities such a congenital chloridorrhoea, the diarrhoeas caused by excessive intestinal secretion are mediated by the activation of various cyclic nucleotides in the small intestinal mucosa (cAMP, cGMP). This process occurs when biologically active molecules such as hormones or enterotoxins bind with an appropriate receptor on the surface of the intestinal epithelial cell.

Small intestinal diarrhoea may, therefore, be predominantly osmotic or predominantly secretory. Examples of the relevant diseases are listed in Table 44.3.

Table 44.3   Causes of osmotic and secretory diarrhoea

Osmotic diarrhoea
- Malabsorption (especially carbohydrates)
- Disaccharidase deficiencies
- Ingestions of osmotic laxatives

Secretory diarrhoea
- Excessive hormone production
    Vasoactive intestinal peptide
    Gastrin
    Calcitonin
    Glucagon
    Thyroxine
- Infection by enterotoxin-producing organisms
    Vibrio cholerae
    Enteropathogenic *E. coli*
    Staphylococcus aureus
    Clostridium perfringens
    Clostridium difficile
    Shigella
    Yersinia enterocolitica
    Various salmonellae
- Other biologically active molecules
    Serotonin
    Prostaglandins

When the cause of small intestinal diarrhoea is not immediately obvious, it becomes useful to *establish whether the diarrhoea is secretory or osmotic*. Two simple tests usually suffice:

1. Measurement of the daily stool volume on a normal diet, then measurement of the stool volume during a 48–72 h fast, while replacing fluids and electrolytes intravenously. Osmotic diarrhoea is food related and output falls considerably during fasting, whereas secretory diarrhoea is largely uninfluenced by fasting.

2. Centrifugation of the liquid stool to obtain supernatant stool water and measurement of the osmolality and electrolyte content of the stool water. The osmolality *calculated* from the electrolyte content (approximately 2 × total concentration of major cations) approximates to the *measured* osmolality in secretory diarrhoeas and is approximately isotonic

with plasma. In osmotic diarrhoeas there is a marked gap between the observed and calculated values caused by unabsorbed solutes or surreptitious abuse of osmotic laxatives.

When these simple investigations indicate a secretory diarrhoea, assay of the serum levels of appropriate hormones (especially vasoactive intestinal peptide) is indicated as the next step towards the diagnosis of an endocrine tumour if a careful search for toxigenic organisms proves negative.

Bile salt diarrhoea

Bile salts and free fatty acids cause a secretory diarrhoea by similar mechanisms acting on the colon. Although outside the scope of this chapter, such colonic secretion occurs as a consequence of failure of the small intestine to reabsorb luminal bile salts, which consequently enter the colon. This failure is commonly caused by disease or resection of the terminal ileum where the specific transport mechanisms for bile salt absorption are to be found.

Since the specific transport mechanism for vitamin B_{12} absorption also resides in the terminal ileum, the Schilling test incorporating intrinsic factor with the orally administered labelled vitamin B_{12} can be used as a test for the integrity of the terminal ileum. The [^{14}C]-glycocholate breath test[3] is a more specific indicator of bile salt malabsorption.

A therapeutic trial of a bile salt-binding resin such as cholestyramine is a useful simple diagnostic tool for bile salt-induced diarrhoea, providing the ileal disease or resection is limited. When more than 100 cm of terminal ileum is affected, bile salt loss into the colon exceeds the capacity of the liver to replace them and bile salt deficiency and consequential malabsorption of fat will ensure.[5] In these circumstances, because fatty acids can cause a similar colonic diarrhoea, a trial of cholestyramine plus a low-fat diet is required for diagnosis.

INFLAMMATORY DISEASE OF THE SMALL INTESTINE

By far the most common inflammatory conditions of the small intestine are enteric infections and Crohn's disease. Other causes include bacterial overgrowth, Whipple's disease, radiation enteritis, eosinophilic enteritis and concomitant involvement of the small intestine in systemic disease such as connective tissue diseases and Henoch–Schönlein vasculitis.

Diarrhoea due to enteric infections is extremely common but usually self-limiting and infrequently presents to hospital practice. In childhood a causative organism can be identified in 80% of patients; it is generally viral in origin, rotavirus being the most common virus. In adults the infective agent is usually bacterial. Until recently, only a minority of causative organisms has been identified. Diagnostic success rates are increasing (over 60% in one survey in north-west London), due partly to the increased recognition of *Campylobacter* species and *Clostridium difficile* and partly to increased sophistication of routine laboratories.

Organisms such as *Salmonella typhi* and other salmonellae,

Campylobacter, Shigella and *Yersinia enterocolitica*, are invasive; pus and blood are detectable in the stool. Enterotoxin-producing organisms cause a secretory diarrhoea and a stool devoid of pus or occult blood. Stool microscopy and culture remain the basis for the diagnosis of enteric infections.

The presence of non-infective intestinal inflammatory lesions is often suggested by the usual inflammatory indicators: fever, leucocytosis, raised viscosity/ESR and elevated acute phase protein levels. Several acute phase protiens have been used to detect inflammation, none of which has any clear advantage over the commonly used C-reactive protein. Most inflammatory conditions can usually be located by barium follow-through examination or enteroclysis. Definitive diagnosis may require biopsy of the affected mucosa.

Radioisotope scanning

The localization of obscure intestinal inflammation can be achieved by ^{111}In-labelled leucocyte scanning.[6] Autologous leucocytes are labelled with ^{111}In before intravenous reinfusion. The labelled leucocytes tend to localize at sites of inflammation which can then be located by scanning with a gamma camera. This test gives an indication of the extent and localization of the inflammatory process, e.g. non-steroidal drug-induced terminal ileal inflammation, Crohn's disease, etc. Counting the ^{111}In excreted in the faeces gives a reasonable correlation with the severity of the inflammatory process. Similar techniques using ^{67}Ga-citrate which localizes to tumours and inflammatory lesions, and ^{99m}Tc-sucralfate (inflammatory lesions) have also been employed.

Enteric protein loss

Excessive protein loss into the gastrointestinal tract is a non-specific feature of many small intestinal diseases including inflammatory lesions. Unlike the situation with urinary protein loss, the loss of protein into the gastrointestinal tract occurs independently of protein size, charge or other characteristics. Consequently, in intestinal protein loss those proteins with low fractional catabolic rates such as albumin and IgG tend to have lower serum levels than those of higher fractional catabolic rates.

Various isotopically labelled proteins and non-protein molecules have been used to measure enteric protein loss. ^{51}Cr-albumin has been widely used because ^{51}Cr is not excreted into the gastrointestinal tract unless it is attached to protein. However, ^{51}Cr-chloride is more widely available and, when given intravenously, it labels many proteins directly; the amount of ^{51}Cr excreted into the gut reflects a similar clearance regardless of the proteins to which it is attached. Counting the ^{51}Cr in blood and a pooled faecal collection over several days will allow the protein clearance (fraction of intravascular compartment cleared into the gut per day) to be calculated.[7] In health, clearance is less than 2%.

α_1-Antitrypsin clearance is a useful alternative. It utilizes the main serum α_1-globulin, which can be easily assayed in the stool. Using this endogenous protein avoids the use of radioisotopes.[8]

Detection of inflammation by isotope scanning or demonstration of protein-losing enteropathy gives no indication of the causative disease process, which must then be determined on clinical grounds or on intestinal biopsy.

VASCULAR DISORDERS

Vascular disorders usually present as

- Occult bleeding, e.g. in angiodysplasia, telangiectasia, haemangioma
- Chronic ischaemia, e.g. 'mesenteric angina' due to atheroma
- Vasculitis, e.g. Behçet's disease, Henoch–Schönlein purpura, systemic lupus erythematosus.

The investigation of vascular disorders of the small intestine remains unsatisfactory (see also Chapters 45 and 54). The diagnosis often rests ultimately on clinical criteria. Angiography will commonly demonstrate severe atheroma in the mesenteric vessels of a patient with a history suggestive of small intestinal ischaemia, but equally severe changes can be found in totally asymptomatic patients. Measurement of superior mesenteric blood flow by Doppler ultrasonography is under extensive study but is not yet interpretable as a diagnostic tool.

Enteric vasculitis usually occurs as part of the manifestation of systemic disease. Its presence may be indicated by serological evidence of complement consumption, the presence of occult faecal blood and radiological evidence of mucosal oedema or ulceration. Protein-losing enteropathy is often present.

Enteric bleeding may be demonstrated directly by extravasation of contrast into the lumen during selective mesenteric angiography if the bleeding is sufficiently brisk. The approximate site of acute bleeding can also be estimated by scanning the abdomen with a gamma camera following the intravenous injection of ^{99m}Tc-colloid.

To identify slow or intermittently bleeding lesions requires a label that circulates continuously over a prolonged time. Autologous red cells labelled in vitro with ^{99m}Tc and reinfused intravenously allow monitoring by gamma camera over at least 24 hours. In one study 47% of patients yielded a positive result at 6 hours, a figure that would not have been achieved using technetium-colloid.[9] This test has been modified in various ways. The labelling of the red cells is now often performed in vivo by intravenous injection of stannous chloride and sodium pyrophosphate. These agents combine in vivo to form stannous pyrophosphate, which complexes with the patient's red cells. After 30 minutes an intravenous injection of ^{99m}Tc is given, which binds with the complex on the red cells. Free ^{99m}Tc is secreted by gastric mucosa in the stomach or Meckel's diverticulum, which may complicate the interpretation of the scans.

The radioisotope scanning techniques have totally replaced the previously used fluorescein string test and its modifications for the localization of chronic gastrointestinal bleeding.

Reinfusion of autologous red cells labelled in vitro with ^{51}Cr will allow the faecal blood loss to be quantitated over many days because the isotope has a long half-life (27.8 days) and is not reabsorbed from the intestinal tract.[10]

REFERENCES

1. Mylvaganum K, Hudson PR, Ross A & Williams CP. ^{14}C-Triolein breath test. A routine test in the gastroenterology clinic? *Gut* 1986; **27**: 1347–1352.
2. Metz G, Gassull MA, Drasar BS et al. Breath hydrogen test for small intestinal bacterial colonisation. *Lancet* 1976; **i**: 668–669.
3. Fromm H & Hoffman AF. Breath test for altered bile acid metabolism. *Lancet* 1971; **ii**: 621–625.
4. Caspary WF. Breath tests. *Clin Gastroenterol* 1978; **7**: 351–374.
5. Hoffman A. The enterohepatic circulation of bile acids. In Sleisenger M & Fordtran JS (eds) *Gastrointestinal Disease*. Philadelphia: WB Saunders, 1978: 418–492.
6. Peters AM, Saverymuttu SH, Reavy HJ et al. Imaging of inflammation with indium-111 troplolonate labelled leycocytes. *J Nucl Med* 1983; **24**: 39–44.
7. Van Tongeren JHM & Reichert WJ. Demonstration of protein-losing gastro-enteropathy: the quantitative estimation of gastrointestinal protein loss using ^{51}Cr-labelled plasma proteins. *Clin Chim Acta* 1966; **14**: 42–48.
8. Florent C, L'Hirondel C, Desmazures C et al. Intestinal clearance of alpha-1-antitrypsin. A sensitive method for the detection of protein-losing enteropathy. *Gastroenterology* 1981; **81**: 777–780.
9. Markisz JA, Front D, Royal HD et al. An evaluation of ^{99m}Tc-labelled red blood cell scientigraphy for the detection and localisation of gastrointestinal bleeding sites. *Gastroenterology* 1982; **83**: 394–398.
10. Cameron AD. Gastrointestinal blood loss measured by radioactive chrominum. *Gut* 1960; **1**: 177–182.

45

RADIOLOGICAL INVESTIGATION OF THE SMALL INTESTINE

DJ Nolan

Radiological imaging plays an important role in the diagnosis and assessment of disorders of the small intestine. Plain radiographs continue to be the investigation of choice in patients who present with acute symptoms, while barium contrast studies are used to show the lumen of the intestine in patients who develop symptoms less acutely. Ultrasonography and computed tomography (CT) are playing an increasing role in the evaluation of the acute abdomen and in the management of some chronic disorders. Angiography is an essential investigation in patients with suspected recurrent or obscure intestinal bleeding. Radionuclide imagine has a limited role in the small intestine, but it can be helpful in finding the approximate location of obscure bleeding, for detecting Meckel's diverticulum and in the evaluation of inflammatory bowel disease.

PLAIN RADIOGRAPHS

The plain radiographic views that are taken will depend on the presenting clinical features. The supine abdominal radiograph and the upright chest are the basic views.[1] The lower edge of the supine abdominal view should show the symphysis pubis and hernial orifices, and at the upper end the diaphragm should be included.[2,3] The supine abdominal radiograph is likely to be the most useful single view. Additional views of the abdomen need only be taken if clinically indicated or if features are detected on the supine film radiography that require further evaluation.[1,4,5] If plain radiographs are unhelpful or inconclusive, contrast studies, ultrasonography or CT may be necessary to obtain further diagnostic information.

Plain radiographic abnormalities

Mechanical intestinal obstruction

Intestinal obstruction can be diagnosed on plain abdominal radiographs in 60–70% of cases.[6,7] The supine abdominal radiograph is the most reliable view.[4,8] The characteristic features of obstruction on the supine view are gas-distended loops of jejunum and ileum arranged in transverse layers across the centre of the abdomen, the 'ladder-rung' pattern (Figure 45.1).

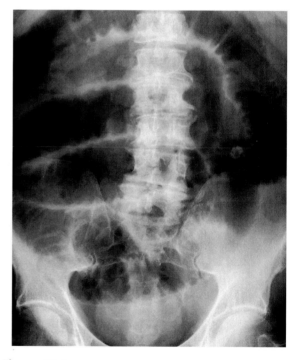

Figure 45.1
Plain radiograph – small intestinal obstruction. The characteristic features of gas-filled dilated loops of small intestine are seen.

Stretched-out valvulae conniventes are seen in the dilated jejunal loops in the upper left and central parts of the abdomen. Ileal loops are lower, further to the right and contain fewer valvulae. Fluid is more likely to collect in loops of intestine located in the flanks and in the ileum. In the mainly fluid-filled loops, small collections of gas may be seen outlining the central portion of the valvulae conniventes. If loops of fluid-filled intestine lie close together, it may be difficult or even impossible to distinguish individual loops. There is little gas or faecal material seen in the colon in cases of small intestinal obstruction. However, a moderate-to-normal amount of colonic gas may be present when obstruction is incomplete. When there is

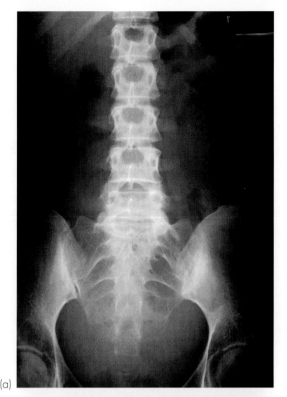

(a)

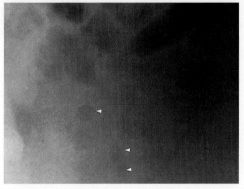

(b)

Figure 45.2
Plain abdominal radiograph – fluid-filled intestinal obstruction.
(a) The fluid-filled loops are opaque and cannot be identified.
Some small collections of gas are noted above the fluid in
jejunal loops located in the left upper quadrant. (b) A close-up
view of the small gas collections in the fluid-filled loops
(arrowheads).

high small intestinal obstruction, the jejunal loops may be
decompressed due to repeated vomiting.

In the upright view the characteristic air-filled levels in
obstruction are seen as hoop-shaped small intestinal loops
forming an inverted U over horizontal fluid levels. The loops
are arranged one above the other, upwards and to the left.[3] A
fluid level is seen in a limb of each loop. Fluid levels at a different height in the same intestinal loop have previously been
considered confirmatory evidence of mechanical obstruction.
In a recent study, however, differential air–fluid levels were not
found to be a sensitive method of determining the presence of
mechanical obstruction.[9] Long immobile fluid levels, on the
other hand, are likely to indicate paralytic ileus.

Fluid levels on the upright view are not reliable evidence of
obstruction as they may be seen in a number of non-obstructive
disorders, including gastroenteritis, hypercalcaemia, uraemia
and jejunal diverticulosis and after the use of saline cathartics.
Between three and five short fluid levels can be a normal finding, particularly if they are located in the right lower quadrant.
In patients with marked obstruction of the distal small intestine,
the obstructed loops may be filled with fluid. The fluid-filled
loops may be opaque or may be seen as oval or round soft tissue masses and can be difficult to identify (Figure 45.2). If fluid-
filled obstruction is suspected on the supine view, an upright
view can confirm the diagnosis by showing the characteristic
'string of beads' sign (Figure 45.3). These are small collections
of gas trapped between the valvulae above the fluid, and this
finding confirms the diagnosis of intestinal obstruction, even in
the absence of gas-distended intestinal loops.

Closed-loop obstruction

'Closed-loop' obstruction has a characteristic radiological
appearance due to the fairly constant anatomical arrangement
produced by the incarcerated or twisted loop.[10] The diagnosis
should be suspected when the strangulated loop is filled with
air and sometimes distended out of proportion to the remaining small intestine (Figure 45.4). The incarcerated loop may
show the 'coffee bean' sign on an upright or decubitus view.
This appearance is produced by the gas in the closed loop

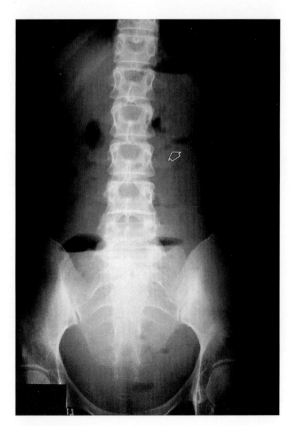

Figure 45.3
Plain abdominal radiograph – fluid-filled intestinal obstruction.
An upright abdominal radiograph shows the characteristic
'string of beads' appearance (arrow).

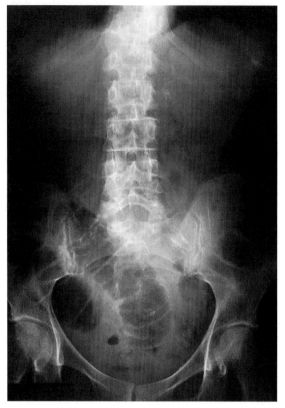

Figure 45.4
Plain abdominal radiograph – closed-loop obstruction. The dilated gas-filled closed loop is seen arising out of the pelvis on the right side. The more proximal small intestine has decompressed as a result of vomiting. Gas is noted in the sigmoid colon.

forcing the opposed, oedematous intestinal wall together to form the centrally placed shadow.[10] Gas and faecal material are more likely to remain in the caecum and ascending colon in closed-loop obstruction than in other types of obstruction because of the paralysing effect of strangulation. The closed loop may be filled with fluid, making it difficult to see, but it may be identified as a round or oval soft tissue mass in the mid-abdomen or pelvis. Distended gas-filled loops, characteristic of obstruction, may be seen proximal to the closed loop.

Other types of obstruction

In volvulus, intestinal loops may be seen as radiating strips converging at the centre of the torsion, positioned anywhere in the abdomen, with a tendency to go upwards and to the right.[3] However, it is usually not possible to distinguish volvulus from closed-loop or simple obstruction.

Gallstone ileus, which is intestinal obstruction caused by an impacted gallstone, characteristically shows evidence of mechanical obstruction with visualization of the obstructing calculus. Air in the biliary tree is identified radiographically in about one-third of patients.[11]

In paralytic ileus, the extent of intestinal distension may vary considerably, from local dilatation of a short segment of intestine to general distension of all the intestine.[1] When there is localized inflammation, such as cholecystitis or pancreatitis, the ileus may develop in an adjacent loop of small intestine, termed a 'sentinel loop'. When paralytic ileus involves the small and large intestine it may be difficult to differentiate it from obstruction, and contrast studies may be necessary to establish the correct diagnosis.[12]

Mesenteric vascular disease

Intestinal infarction has a high mortality rate and can be difficult to diagnose.[13] Embolism, thrombosis or trauma to the superior mesenteric artery are the most frequent causes of mesenteric infarction. The condition is irreversible and occurs mainly in the small intestine, ascending colon and transverse colon. Identification of the characteristic plain radiographic signs is most important as the clinical diagnosis is often uncertain. In the early stages dilatation of the small intestine, ascending colon and transverse colon are characteristic. Specific radiological signs may be seen in 60% of patients.[14] These include oedematous thickened valvulae conniventes, thickening of the intestinal wall, intramural air (Figure 45.5) and air within the intrahepatic portal venous system. Intramural gas is diagnostic of intestinal necrosis and, like gas in the portal veins, it indicates a poor prognosis.

Mesenteric venous thrombosis may be seen as a rigid thickened segment of intestine, outlined by intraluminal gas, not changing in decubitus or upright radiographs.[16]

BARIUM STUDIES

The two principal barium techniques used for investigating the small intestine are the barium follow-through and enteroclysis

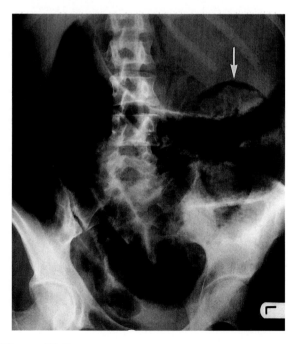

Figure 45.5
Plain abdominal radiograph – intestinal infarction. Gas in the intestinal wall is shown as crescentic shadowing (arrow) and as widespread, small, slightly irregular shadows. (Reproduced with permission from Nolan.[15])

(small bowel enema). The follow-through is still the method of choice in most centres, although enteroclysis is being more widely adopted.

Barium that refluxes through the ileocaecal valve during barium enema examination can provide useful diagnostic information about the terminal ileum. Miller[17] described a method of refluxing a large volume of barium in a retrograde manner through the ileocaecal valve to outline all the small intestine, and called it the complete reflux examination. This technique is now rarely used. Long intestinal tubes[18] used to decompress obstructed small intestine can be used as a means of introducing barium to the site of obstruction for diagnostic purposes.[19]

Good visualization of the ileocaecal area can be obtained by performing a 'peroral pneumocolon' examination.[20] This technique is a modification of the barium follow-through. Air is introduced into the colon per rectum when the head of the barium column has reached the ascending colon. This air is refluxed into the caecum and terminal ileum, providing good double-contrast views of the terminal ileum and caecum. The peroral pneumocolon examination can give useful further information about the ileocaecal area when conventional methods have not shown the area adequately.

Barium follow-through

The follow-through examination of the small intestine normally follows a barium examination of the oesophagus, stomach and duodenum, although it may be performed as a dedicated examination of the jejunum and ileum. The patient ingests a large volume of barium suspension. Radiographs of the abdomen are taken at half-hourly intervals until barium reaches the terminal ileum. Spot views are taken of the terminal ileum and any segments that are suspected to be abnormal.

Enteroclysis

Excellent visualization of the jujunum and ileum is achieved when barium suspension is introduced directly into the small intestine through a tube. The dilute single-contrast technique described by Sellink[21] is used in some departments,[22] others prefer the double-contrast method, using barium and an aqueous suspension of methylcellulose.[19] A double-contrast method using barium suspension and air is not widely used except in Japan and some centres in Europe.

During enteroclysis the jejunum and ileum are distended with dilute barium suspension, thereby making it easier to identify any morphological abnormalities that might be present. A high degree of diagnostic accuracy is possible when enteroclysis is used. A review of our own material[23] showed a sensitivity of 93.1% and a specificity of 96.9% for demonstrating disorders that accounted for the patient's presenting symptoms. It is easier for the radiologist to become more skilled at performing and interpreting enteroclysis than the time-consuming repeated fluoroscopy that is necessary during the barium follow-through.[24] The reasons why enteroclysis is not more widely adopted are because the patient may suffer discomfort during intubation, because of the potentially high patient radiation dose and because it is considered to be time consuming. Most patients only experience minor discomfort when a 10 Fr tube[25] by the nasogastric route is used for gastroduodenal intubation.[26] By using a low fluoroscopy current and rare earth screens, we calculated that the mean effective patient dose was 1.5 mSv during enteroclysis.[27] This dose compares favourably with a dose of 0.9 mSv for barium meals and 2.8 mSv for barium enemas using the same equipment.[28] Routine CT of the abdomen gives a much higher radiation dose of about 7.0–8.0 mSv.[29] The procedure takes only slightly longer than a barium enema examination and considerably less than a barium follow-through examination.

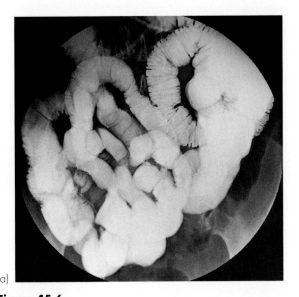

(a)

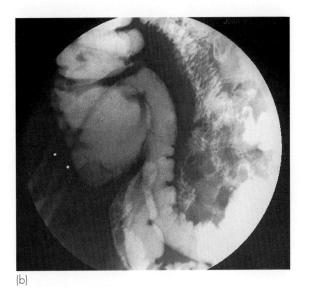

(b)

Figure 45.6

Enteroclysis – normal examination. (a) Jejunal and ileal loops are distended with dilute barium suspension. (b) A spot view of the terminal ileum.

In the author's opinion enteroclysis is the examination of choice for suspected disorders causing morphological changes of the small intestine, such as Crohn's disease, neoplasms, chronic radiation enteritis, ischaemia, Meckel's diverticulum or obstruction.[30] Barium is contraindicated in perforation of the small intestine, although if a small leak is suspected the ability of barium suspension to demonstrate the site outweighs the theoretical consideration of toxicity due to leakage of barium.[31]

The enteroclysis technique recommended here is similar to that described by Sellink.[22,32] The 10 Fr radiopaque tube is introduced via the nasogastric route and passed to the duodenum, so that the tip is positioned at or just distal to the duodenojejunal junction (ligament of Treitz). Dilute barium is infused, using a pump, at about 75 ml per minute. A total volume of 1000–1200 ml is infused. The head of the barium column normally reaches the terminal ileum in 10–20 minutes. Radiographs of the jejunum and ileum, outlined with barium, are obtained (Figure 45.6a). Spot compression views of the terminal ileum (Figure 45.6b), pelvic loops of ileum and any other segments of interest are taken. When the double-contrast technique is performed, 200 ml of moderate density barium suspension is injected, followed by 1000–2000 ml of a 0.5% aqueous suspension of methylcellulose. This technique give excellent mucosal detail of normal intestine, but abnormal segments are not always well shown.

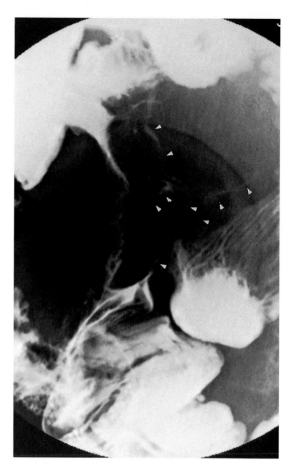

Figure 45.8
Enteroclysis – Crohn's disease. There is marked narrowing and distortion of the terminal ileum and multiple communicating sinus tracks (arrowheads) are outlined by the barium suspension.

Diagnosis of disorders on barium examination

Crohn's disease

Crohn's disease is well shown by enteroclysis.[33] The most frequently seen signs include ulceration, thickening and distortion of the valvulae conniventes, strictures, dilatation proximal to the strictures, thickening of the intestinal wall and a right iliac fossa mass displacing adjacent intestine. Characteristic ulceration includes discrete ulcers, fissure ulcers (Figure 45.7), longitudinal ulcers and cobblestoning. Fissure ulceration may progress to sinuses (Figure 45.8) and fistulae. The disease process may be discontinuous, characteristically seen as asymmetry or skip lesions. The changes of Crohn's disease may be localized to the terminal ileum or the ileum proximal to an ileocolic anastomosis site (Figure 45.9), or it may be more extensive, sometimes involving almost all the intestine (Figure 45.10).

Neoplasms

Primary malignant neoplasms are uncommon in the small intestine.[34] Adenocarcinoma, lymphomas and carcinoid tumours

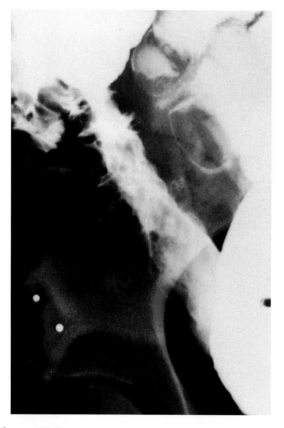

Figure 45.7
Enteroclysis – Crohn's disease. The mucosal pattern of the terminal ileum has been completely effaced, there is slight narrowing and irregularity of the lumen and multiple fissure ulcers are seen projecting into the thickened ileal wall.

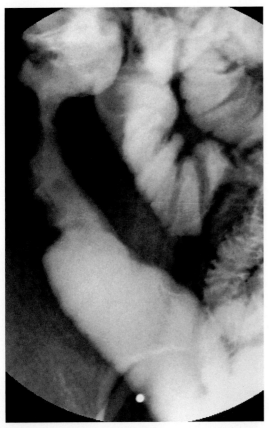

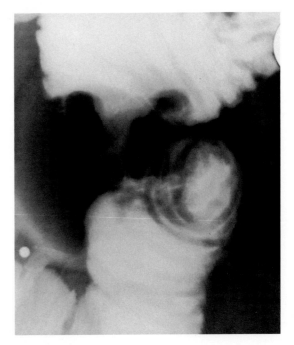

Figure 45.11
Enteroclysis – carcinoma. A spot compression view of a proximal jejunal segment shows a short tight stricture with mucosal destruction and shouldering of the margins, characteristic of carcinoma. There is slight dilatation of the intestine proximal to the stricture.

Figure 45.9
Enteroclysis – recurrent Crohn's disease. A short segment of recurrent Crohn's disease is seen in the ileum just proximal to an ileocolic anastomosis in a patient who had a previous right hemicolectomy for Crohn's disease.

are the types most frequently encountered. Leiomyosarcomas are less frequently seen. The characteristic location and appearances of these different neoplasms make it possible to

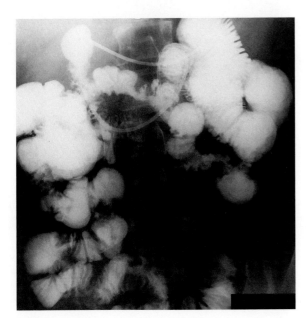

Figure 45.10
Enteroclysis – Crohn's disease. Extensive changes of Crohn's disease are seen in the small intestine with multiple segments of narrowing and asymmetry. Short segments of slight dilatation are also seen proximal to some of the strictures.

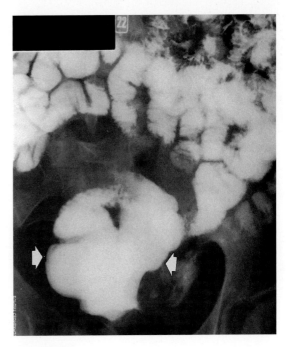

Figure 45.12
Enteroclysis – lymphoma. (a) A large mass with a central irregular cavity (arrows) is seen displacing adjacent loops of intestine. (Reproduced with permission from Gourtsoyannis and Nolan.[37])

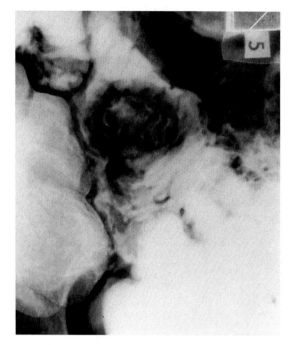

Figure 45.13
Enteroclysis – carcinoid tumour. A round intraluminal filling defect is shown in the terminal ileum of a patient who presented with the carcinoid syndrome.

reach the correct diagnosis with a certain degree of confidence.[35]

Adenocarcinomas are mostly located in the duodenum and proximal jejunum.[36] The radiological appearances are similar to those of carcinoma of the colon; they are shown on barium studies as strictures with mucosal destruction and shouldering of the margins (Figure 45.11), irregular polypoid masses or ulcerating lesions. In lymphoma the lesions are mostly located in the ileum and are multiple in about 40% of cases.[37] The radiological signs include strictures with mucosal destruction, broad-based ulceration, cavitation (Figure 45.12), thickening of the valvulae, polypoid intraluminal filling defects, an eccentric mass and the characteristic, but rarely

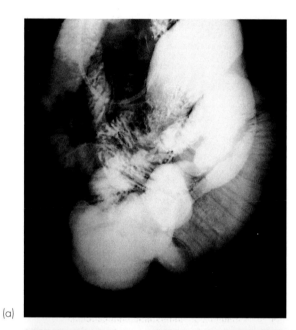

(a)

(b)

Figure 45.15
Enteroclysis – chronic radiation enteritis causing obstruction. (a) There is considerable dilatation of the proximal small intestine. (b) A spot view of the area of obstruction shows adherent loops of intestine with marked mural thickening (arrows).

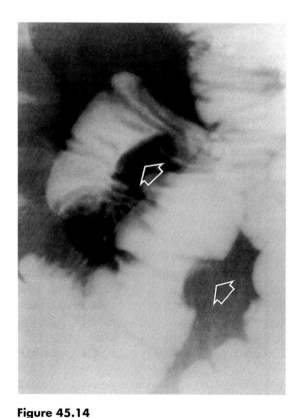

Figure 45.14
Enteroclysis – carcinoid tumour. A spot view of a segment of distal ileum shows two intramural filling defects (arrows) in a patient with multiple primary ileal carcinoids. (Reproduced with permission from Jeffree and Nolan.[39])

seen, 'aneurysmal dilatation.' Carcinoid tumours are mostly seen as single or multiple intraluminal (Figure 45.13). or intramural (Figure 45.14) filling defects located in the distal ileum.[38,39] Sometimes carcinoids present as ileal strictures. In cases with extensive mesenteric fibrosis, adjacent loops of intestine are compressed by a mainly eccentric mass and it may not be possible to identify the primary tumour. Leiomyosarcomas may be seen as a solitary small or large cavitating mass, often with a fairly large extraluminal component. Metastases, particularly malignant melanoma, may also present as cavitating masses in the small intestine.

Radiation enteritis

Patients with chronic radiation enteritis may develop symptoms at any time from the end of radiotherapy treatment up to 25 years later. This disorder should be considered in any patient with a history of previous radiotherapy who develops intestinal symptoms. Many patients with chronic radiation enteritis develop intestinal obstruction (Figure 45.15). Characteristic appearances of chronic radiation enteritis, shown on enteroclysis, include thickening of the valvulae conniventes (Figure 45.16), stenosis (Figure 45.17), adhesions, mural thickening, mucosal tacking and effacement of the mucosal pattern.[40] Sinuses and fistulae, are occasionally seen.

Ischaemia

Intestinal ischaemia causes separation of intestinal loops, with oedema and marked thickening of the valvulae conniventes.[41] The intestine usually returns to normal, although occasionally strictures may develop. Blunt abdominal trauma can cause localized ischaemia and result in stricture formation[42] (Figure 45.18).

Meckel's diverticulum

Meckel's diverticulum can be difficult to detect preoperatively. Radionuclide imaging is more accurate for detecting Meckel's diverticulum in children than in adults.[44] Enteroclysis is superior

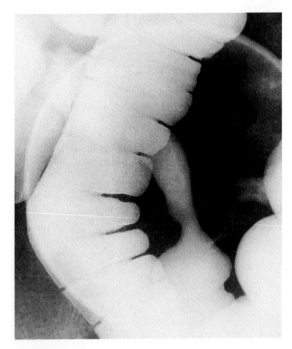

Figure 45.17
Enteroclysis – radiation stricture. A spot compression view of a segment of distal ileum shows a short tight stricture causing partial obstruction. (Reproduced with permission from Mendelson and Nolan.[40])

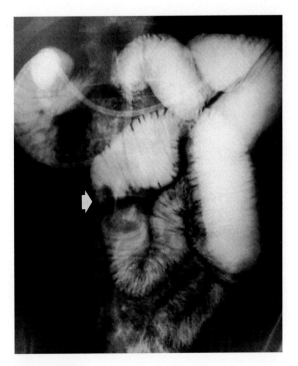

Figure 45.18
Enteroclysis – ischaemic intestinal stricture. A short tight stricture in the mid-jejunum (arrow) is shown causing some degree of obstruction with dilatation of the intestine proximal to the narrowing. The ischaemic stricture developed shortly after the patient sustained blunt abdominal trauma. (Reproduced with permission from Nolan.[43])

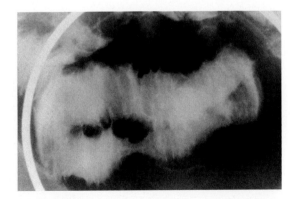

Figure 45.16
Enteroclysis – chronic radiation enteritis. A spot compression view of a pelvic loop of ileum showing thickening of the valvulae conniventes and mucosal tacking. The segment of apparent narrowing was not constant. (Reproduced with permission from Mendelson and Nolan.[40])

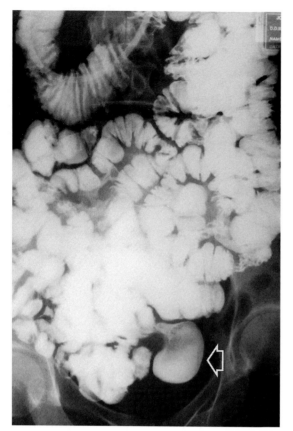

Figure 45.19
Enteroclysis – Meckel's diverticulum. A Meckel's diverticulum is seen as a sac-like structure (arrow) arising from the antimesenteric border of the ileum. (Reproduced with permission from Nolan and Cadman.[32])

to the barium follow-through for demonstrating Meckel's diverticulum.[45,46] Meckel's diverticulum is seen as a blind-ending sac arising from the antemesenteric border of the ileum[47] (Figure

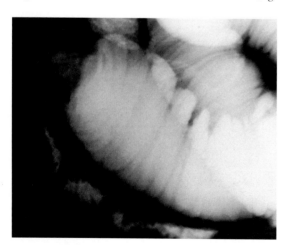

Figure 45.20
Enteroclysis – intestinal obstruction. There is marked obstruction of a pelvic loop of ileum. This spot view shows the abrupt transition between dilated intestine and collapsed intestine that identifies the site of obstruction. The obstruction was caused by infiltration from recurrent sigmoid carcinoma.

45.19). A characteristic triradiate fold or a triangular plateau may be present at the neck of the diverticulum.[45]

Intestinal obstruction

Barium studies can play an important role in the diagnosis and assessment of suspected or known small intestinal obstruction. Barium suspension is safe in partial or complete obstruction and does not become impacted in the small intestine.[48] Barium is superior to water-soluble contrast medium because of its greater density; it has fewer side-effects and produces less crampy abdominal pain and vomiting.[49,50] Enteroclysis is a particularly useful technique for investigating suspected intestinal obstruction.[51] The site of obstruction is recognized by showing the zone of acute transition in calibre between the distended

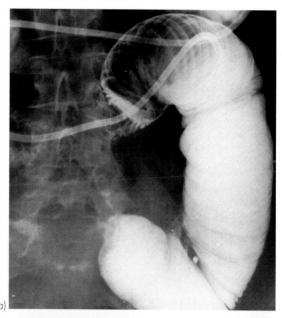

(a)

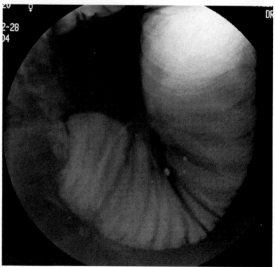

(b)

Figure 45.21
Enteroclysis – intestinal obstruction. (a) and (b) Obstruction in the proximal jejunum is shown as an abrupt termination in the barium column. The obstruction was due to adhesions that developed following an abdominal operation.

loops proximal to the obstruction site and the collapsed loops distally (Figure 45.20). Occasionally the obstructing lesion causes an abrupt halt in the passage of barium (Figure 45.21).

Closed-loop obstruction may be diagnosed on enteroclysis.[52] The diagnosis is made when the barium suspension is seen outlining the closed loop, with the related segments of narrowing at the neck of the loop (Figure 45.22). Intestinal obstruction can be difficult to diagnose clinically and on plain abdominal radiographs in the early postoperative period. Enteroclysis can be most useful in the postoperative period following abdominal surgery to distinguish obstruction from paralytic ileus.

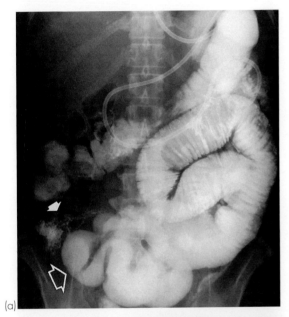

(a)

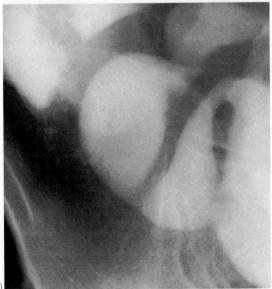

(b)

Figure 45.22

Enteroclysis – closed-loop obstruction. (a) There is marked intestinal obstruction with dilatation of the small intestine. A closed loop can be identified in the distal ileum (open arrow). Collapsed loops of ileum are seen distal to the site of obstruction (closed arrow). (b) A spot view of the closed loop. An adhesive band was found at laparotomy.

Obstruction can be confirmed, the site of obstruction is clearly seen (see Figure 45.21) and the cause is frequently identified.[53]

ARTERIOGRAPHY

Diagnostic arteriography plays an important role in the diagnosis and localization of lesions causing acute, chronic or obscure bleeding from the small intestine. 'Obscure intestinal bleeding' is a term used to denote that the cause is unknown, after routine investigation of the upper gastrointestinal tract and colon have failed to identify the cause.[54] The rate of bleeding must be at least 0.5 ml/min for successful visualization at arteriography.[55]

High-quality arteriography should always be performed before laparotomy is considered in patients who present with obscure bleeding. It may be necessary to perform superselective studies to accurately identify and locate a lesion in the small intestine.

When a small lesion is detected in the intestine at angiography, it may be necessary to perform intraoperative arteriography to confirm its precise location during laparotomy. At the end of the arteriographic examination the superselective catheter is left in the branch vessel supplying the lesion. The abnormality can then be located at operation by performing angiography in the operating theatre. The other alternative is to inject methylene blue into the indwelling superselective catheter. This manoeuvre results in a bluish discoloration of the short segment of intestine supplied by that arterial branch.[56]

A variety of intestinal abnormalities may cause obscure bleeding into the small intestine. These conditions include arteriovenous malformations (Figure 45.23), haemangiomas, neoplasms, Meckel's diverticulum, solitary ulcers of the small intestine, localized ischaemic ulceration and jejunal diverticula.[54] Arteriovenous malformations and haemangiomas are seen as an abnormal small vascular blush. Neoplasms normally show characteristic angiographic appearances. Leiomyomas show a well-defined homogeneous blush with rapid arterial filling and early venous drainage (Figure 45.24).[57,58] Carcinoids have a stellate arterial configuration with kinking and irregularity of the mesenteric artery branches and poor tumour accumulation of contrast medium with non-filling veins.[38,59] In adenocarcinomas, characteristic hypervascularity is seen with occlusion of arteries and encasement of jejunal artery branches by the neoplasm.[60]

Meckel's diverticulum may be diagnosed in a number of ways by arteriography. Active bleeding into the diverticulum may be seen. A localized area of hypervascularity, representing richly vascular gastric tissue, may be identified. The characteristic remnant of the right vitelline artery, the end-artery of the superior mesenteric artery that supplies the diverticulum, may be demonstrated.[61]

COMPUTED TOMOGRAPHY

There is an increasing role for the use of CT in the evaluation of acute and chronic disorders of the small intestine. CT can be invaluable for diagnosing intestinal infarction[62,63] and for diagnosing intestinal obstruction and establishing the site and cause

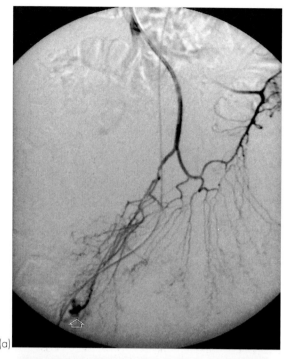

(a)

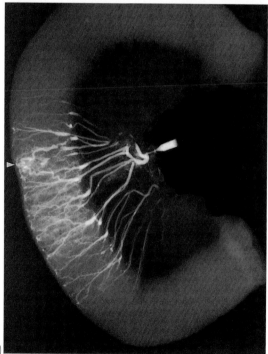

(b)

Figure 45.23

Angiography – arteriovenous malformation. (a) Contrast medium injected through a catheter selectively positioned in the last jejunal branch artery demonstrates an arteriovenous malformation (arrow) in the wall of the intestine. The catheter was then introduced more selectively into the branch feeding the malformation before the patient was transferred to the operating theatre. Fluorescein was then injected via the catheter to identify the short segment of intestine before it was resected. (b) The specimen was injected with barium and the presence of the arteriovenous malformation (arrowhead) was confirmed. (Courtesy of Dr J.E. Jackson.)

of obstruction.[64–66] CT plays a useful role in the management of problems in patients with Crohn's disease.[67] It is used to assess small intestinal neoplasms and it can provide important information about the extraluminal component of intestinal disorders, the relationship of adjacent organs and tissues and ancillary intra-abdominal findings.[68]

When the small intestine is examined in patients who do not present acutely, opacification of the intestinal lumen with contrast medium is necessary for CT evaluation. A dilute barium suspension or dilute iodinated water-soluble contrast medium is used. Barium suspension is more palatable and is preferred for routine CT.

Abnormalities on CT

Mesenteric vascular disease

CT is now frequently being used in the evaluation of abdominal pain, and it can play an important role in the early diagnosis and management of intestinal infarction.[62] Characteristic findings on CT include intramural gas, portal mesenteric

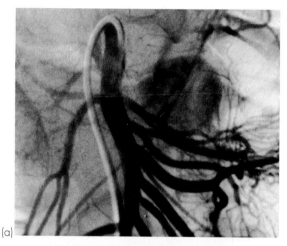

(a)

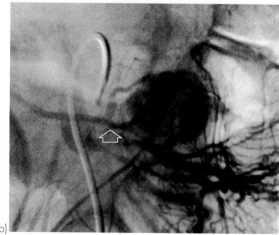

(b)

Figure 45.24

Angiography – leiomyoma. Selective superior mesenteric angiography shows (a) a well-defined homogeneous vascular neoplasm supplied by the first jejunal branch, and (b) early draining veins in the late arterial phase (arrow). (Reproduced with permission from Forbes et al.[58])

venous gas, focal thickening of the intestinal wall, focal or diffuse fluid-filled dilated intestine and clot in the superior mesenteric artery.[62] In patients with suspected intestinal infarction in whom CT findings are normal or non-specific, plain radiographs should be taken as they may identify findings that will suggest the diagnosis.[63]

Intestinal obstruction

CT is now proving to be the examination of choice in patients with suspected small intestinal obstruction.[64] It is particularly sensitive at diagnosing complete obstruction (Figure 45.25) and determining the location and cause. This technique is useful in patients with small intestinal dilatation in whom it can aid both the diagnosis of obstruction and differentiate it from other conditions likely to cause intestinal dilation.[65] The ability to diag-

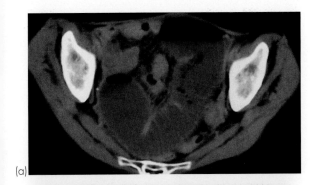

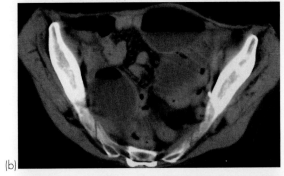

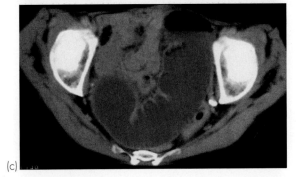

Figure 45.25

Computed tomography – intestinal obstruction. (a) Dilated, mainly fluid-filled loops of small intestine are seen. The stretched valvulae conniventes can be identified. Note the small collections of air in the fluid. (b) and (c) Two sections through the pelvis show a dilated fluid-filled loop terminating abruptly. The obstruction was due to adhesions. (Courtesy of Dr C.H. Woodham.)

nose small intestinal obstruction and differentiate it from paralytic ileus is based on the detection of a definite transition zone between dilated loops of small intestine proximal to the site of obstruction and collapsed loops of small intestine or colon distal to the site of obstruction.[66] The larger the discrepancy at the transition zone and the greater the degree of collapse of the distal loops, the more convincing and reliable are the CT findings. Enteroclysis is, however, more reliable in patients with partial, incomplete or intermittent obstruction.[66]

In patients with adhesions, the exact point of obstruction is sometimes visualized at CT as a beak-like narrowing.[69-72] If a neoplasm, abscess, inflammation or hernia is not shown during a careful CT examination, the findings indicate adhesions as the cause of obstruction.[66]

Closed-loop obstruction

The CT signs are characteristic in closed-loop strangulated small intestinal obstruction.[73-75] Sequential cross-sections through an elongated U- or C-shaped closed loop reveal a characteristic fixed radial distribution of several dilated intestinal loops with stretched and prominent mesenteric vessels converging towards the point of torsion.[66] The incarcerated loop is entirely or almost entirely filled with fluid; the proximal intestinal loops normally contain large amounts of air. Ischaemic changes in the wall of the closed loop are indicative of strangulation. The wall of the closed loop of intestine is slightly and circumferentially thickened; it may show increased attenuation and there may be concentric rings of slightly different density – the 'target' or 'halo' sign. In advanced cases pneumatosis intestinalis may develop.[66] The most reliable CT findings of strangulation are air in the intestinal wall and haemorrhagic mesenteric changes selectively involving the incarcerated loops.

Crohn's disease

In Crohn's disease CT is useful for evaluating suspected complications.[67,76,77] The scans can show mural, serosal and mesenteric abnormalities such as thickening of the intestinal wall (Figure 45.26), an inflammatory mass (Figure 45.27), mesenteric abscess and mesenteric lymphadenopathy.[67] CT demonstrates the presence, and precise location and size of abscess cavities and allows the progressional resolution of the abscess to be monitored.[76] Unsuspected sinuses and fistulas and associated abscess cavities can be demonstrated, together with their location in relation to the retroperitoneum, intraperitoneal spaces and abdominal wall.[67] A fluid collection in the mesentery or retroperitoneum adjacent to intestine strongly suggests an abscess, especially if it is bordered by a thick contrast-enhancing rim. If air bubbles or gas–fluid levels are present within the fluid, the appearances are virtually pathognomonic of an abscess.[78]

Lymphoma

CT can demonstrate the size and extent of the neoplasm (Figure 45.28) and mesenteric infiltration in patients with lymphoma. Characteristic appearances on both ultrasonography

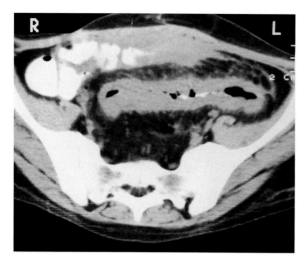

Figure 45.26
Computed tomography – Crohn's disease. Asymmetrical thickening of a segment of ileum characteristic of Crohn's disease is seen. Air and contrast medium can be identified in the lumen. (Courtesy of Dr L. Engelholm.)

and CT may be seen; lymphomatous tissue is shown as a lobulated confluent mass infiltrating the mesenteric leaves and encasing the superior mesenteric artery and vein, producing a characteristic 'sandwich-like' appearance.[79]

ULTRASONOGRAPHY

Ultrasonography has a limited role in the diagnosis and management of disorders of the small intestine. It is rarely used as the initial diagnostic procedure in suspected intestinal disorders, but because it is widely used for investigating the abdomen small intestinal abnormalities are encountered frequently.[80,81] The ultrasonographer should, therefore, recognize normal and abnormal intestinal patterns so that appropriate investigations can be recommended.[82]

Obstruction of the small intestine may be diagnosed on

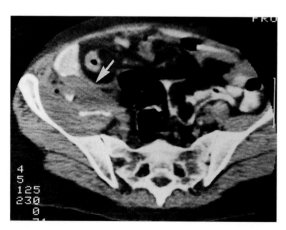

Figure 45.27
Computed tomography – Crohn's disease. An inflammatory mass is shown encasing the terminal ileum (arrow), which is outlined with contrast medium. The thickened wall of a more proximal ileal loop can also be identified. (Courtesy of Dr L. Engelholm.)

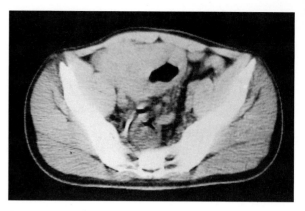

Figure 45.28
Computed tomography – lymphoma. CT shows a thick-walled pelvic mass with a central cavity adjacent to the anterior abdominal wall (same case as Figure 45.12).

ultrasonography; the valvulae conniventes are recognized when they project into the fluid-filled intestine.[83,84] Ultrasonography can be used to demonstrate thickening of the intestinal wall in Crohn's disease, for detecting complications (Figure 45.29) and for assessing response to treatment.[85-87] It is possible to identify primary intestinal neoplasms (Figure 45.30) using a dedicated ultrasonographic technique.[88]

RADIONUCLIDE SCANNING

Radionuclide scintigraphy has a role in screening patients with suspected intestinal bleeding, detecting Meckel's deverticulum and in assessing inflammatory bowel disease. In patients who present with intestinal bleeding the general anatomical location of the bleeding may be identified using

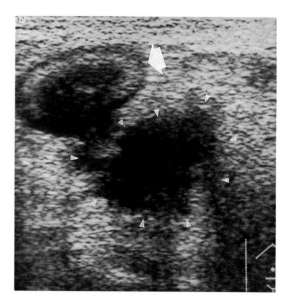

Figure 45.29
Ultrasonography – Crohn's disease. Characteristic thickening of the ileal wall (arrow) is seen on a transverse scan of the lower abdomen. An abscess cavity (arrowheads) is shown communicating with the abnormal ileum. (Courtesy of Dr D.R.M. Lindsell.)

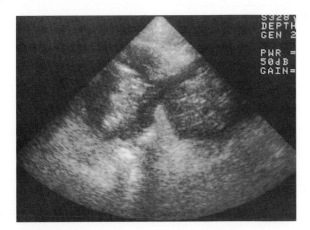

Figure 45.30
Ultrasonography – lymphoma. An intestinal related mass containing two large cavities is shown in a patient with lymphoma. (Courtesy of Dr D.R.M. Lindsell.)

radionuclide scintigraphy; further investigations, such as angiography, can then be performed to define the bleeding site more precisely.[55]

Two radionuclide imaging tests are currently recommended for detecting bleeding. One involves the use of ^{99m}Tc-sulphur colloid and the other red cells labelled with ^{99m}Tc by a modified in vivo technique.[55] ^{99m}Tc is given as an intravenous injection.[89] A small amount of radionuclide extravasates at the bleeding site, and this increases with each circulation. The site of bleeding can be identified in 5–10 minutes. This technique is remarkably sensitive, detecting bleeding rates as low as 0.1 ml/min.[55] The limitation of this method is that the patient has to be actively bleeding at the time of the examination for the test to be positive.

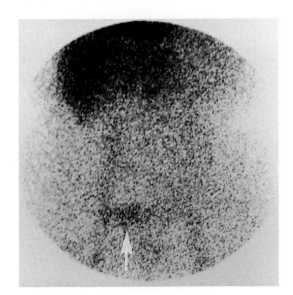

Figure 45.31
Radionuclide scan – Meckel's diverticulum. An area of increased uptake of radionuclide (arrow) is seen in the right lower quadrant, identifying the site of ectopic gastric mucosa in a Meckel's diverticulum. (Courtesy of Dr B.J. Shepstone and reproduced with permission from Nolan.[15])

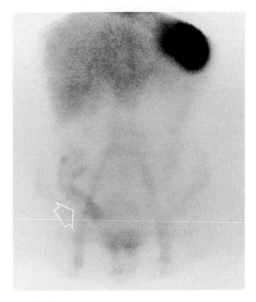

Figure 45.32
Radionuclide scan – Crohn's disease. A high uptake of radionuclide (arrow) is shown in a segment of ileal Crohn's disease. (Courtesy of Dr B.J. Shepstone.)

When the ^{99m}Tc-labelled red cell technique is used, the red cells remain in the circulation and imaging can be repeated for up to 24 hours.[90] Two quoted disadvantages of this technique are the high background activity and the fact that radioactivity may move along the intestine if the bleeding stops, so that a later scan may show the activity at another site.[55] Nevertheless, the ^{99m}Tc-labelled red cell technique is more accurate than technetium alone, with a sensitivity of 93% and a specificity of 95%.[91]

Radionuclide imaging using ^{99m}Tc-pertechnetate can be a useful technique for detecting Meckel's diverticulum[92] (Figure 45.31). However, there is a high false-negative rate in adults,[43,44] and its greatest diagnostic yield is in the paediatric age group.[93,94]

Radionuclide scanning using ^{111}In-labelled leucocytes can be used to image inflammatory bowel disease (Figure 45.32). The labelled leucocytes migrate to the actively inflamed segment of intestine, making it possible to estimate the extent of disease. The technique is particularly useful for detecting recurrent Crohn's disease following previous resections and for assessing activity in patients with known disease.[95] Octreotide scintigraphy may help in localising carcinoid tumours, both primary and metastatic (see Chapter 59).

REFERENCES

1. Field S. The plain abdominal radiograph – the acute abdomen. In Grainger RG & Allison DJ (eds) *Diagnostic Radiology – An Anglo-American Textbook of Imaging*, 3rd edn. Edinburgh: Churchill Livingstone, 1997: 885–907.
2. Miller RE. The technical approach to the acute abdomen. *Semin Roentgenol* 1973; **8**: 267–269.
3. Frimman-Dahl J. *Rontgen Examinations in Acute Abdominal Diseases*, 3rd edn. Springfield, IL: CC Thomas, 1974.
4. Field S, Guy PJ, Upsdell SM & Scourfield AE. The erect abdominal radiograph in the acute abdomen: should its routine use be abandoned? *BMJ* 1985; **290**: 1934–1936.

5. Mirvis SE, Young JWR, Keramati B, McCrea ES & Tarr R. Plain film evaluation of patients with abdominal pain: are three radiographs necessary? *AJR* 1986; **147**: 501–503.

6. Lo AM, Evans WE & Carey LC. Review of small bowel obstruction at Milwaukee County General Hospital. *Am J Surg* 1966; **111**: 884–887.

7. Gough IR. Strangulating adhesive small bowel obstruction with normal radiographs. *Br J Surg* 1978; **65**: 431–434.

8. Hodges PC & Miller RE. Intestinal obstruction. *AJR* 1955; **74**: 1015–1025.

9. Harlow CL, Stears RLG, Zeligman BE & Archer PG. Diagnosis of bowel obstruction on plain abdominal radiographs: significance of air–fluid levels at different heights in the same loop of bowel. *AJR* 1993; **161**: 291–295.

10. Mellins HZ & Rigler LG. The roentgen findings in strangulating obstructions of the small intestine. *AJR* 1954; **71**: 404–415.

11. Day EA & Marks C. Gallstone ileus. Review of the literature and presentation of thirty-four new cases. *Am J Surg* 1975; **129**: 552–558.

12. Vest B & Margulis AR. The roentgen diagnosis of postoperative ileus-obstruction. *Surg Gynecol Obstet* 1962; **115**: 421–427.

13. Hessen I. Roentgen examination in cases of occlusion of the mesenteric vessels. *Acta Radiol* 1955; **44**: 293–305.

14. Scott JR, Miller WT, Urso M & Stadalnik RC. Acute mesenteric infarction. *AJR* 1971; **113**: 269–279.

15. Nolan DJ. Radiology of the small intestine. In Nelson RL & Nyhus LM (eds) *Surgery of the Small Intestine*. Norwalk, CT: Appleton & Lange, 1987: 59–83.

16. Nelson SW & Eggleston W. Findings on plain roentgenograms of the abdomen associated with mesenteric vascular occlusion with a possible new sign of mesenteric venous thrombosis. *AJR* 1960; **83**: 886–894.

17. Miller RE. Complete reflux small bowel examination. *Radiology* 1965; **84**: 457–463.

18. Miller TG & Abbott WO. Intestinal intubation: a practical technique. *Am J Med Sci* 1934; **187**: 595–599.

19. Herlinger H. A modified technique for the double-contrast small bowel enema. *Gastrointest Radiol* 1978; **3**: 201–207.

20. Kellett MJ, Zboralske FF & Margulis AR. Peroral pneumocolon examination of the ileocaecal region. *Gastrointest Radiol* 1977; **1**: 361–365.

21. Sellink JL. *Examination of the Small Intestine by Duodenal Intubation*. Leiden: Stenfert Kroese, 1971.

22. Nolan DJ. The small intestine. In Whitehouse GW & Worthington BS (eds) *Techniques in Diagnostic Imaging*, 3rd edn. Oxford: Blackwell, 1996: 34–49.

23. Dixon PM, Roulston ME & Nolan DJ. The small bowel enema: a ten year reivew. *Clin Radiol* 1993; **47**: 46–48.

24. Thoeni RF. Radiography of the small bowel and enteroclysis: a perspective. *Invest Radiol* 1987; **22**: 930–936.

25. Traill ZT & Nolan DJ. Intubation times using a new enteroclysis tube. *Clin Radiol* 1995; **50**: 339–340.

26. Maglinte DDT, Lappas JC, Chernish SM & Sellink JL. Intubation routes for enteroclysis. *Radiology* 1986; **158**: 553–534.

27. Hart D, Haggett PJ, Boardman P, Nolan DJ & Wall BF. Patient radiation doses from enteroclysis. *Br J Radiol* 1994; **67**: 997–1000.

28. Hart D & Wall LBF. Estimation of effective dose from dose–area product measurements for barium meals and barium enemas. *Br J Radiol* 1994; **67**: 485–489.

29. Shrimpton PC, Jones DG, Hillier MC et al. *Survey of CT Practice in the UK*, part II, Dosimetric Aspects. NRPB-R249. London: HMSO, 1991.

30. Nolan DJ & Traill ZC. Review: the current role of the barium examination of the small intestine. *Clin Radiol.*

31. Freeark RJ, Love L & Baker RJ. An active diagnostic approach to blunt abdominal trauma. *Surg Clin North Am* 1968; **48**: 97–109.

32. Nolan DJ & Cadman P. The small bowel enema made easy. *Clin Radiol* 1987; **38**: 295–301.

33. Nolan DJ & Gourtsoyiannis NC. Crohn's disease of the small intestine: a review of the radiological appearances in 100 consecutive patients examined by a barium infusion technique. *Clin Radiol* 1980; **30**: 597–603.

34. Viamonte M & Viamonte M. Primary squamous cell carcinoma of the small bowel. *Dis Colon Rectum* 1992; **35**: 806–809.

35. Gourtsoyiannis NC & Nolan DJ. *Imaging of Small Intestinal Tumours*. Amsterdam: Elsevier Science, 1997.

36. Papadopoulos VD & Nolan DJ. Carcinoma of the small intestine. *Clin Radiol* 1985; **36**: 409–413.

37. Gourtsoyiannis NC & Nolan DJ. Lymphoma of the small intestine; radiological features. *Clin Radiol* 1988; **39**: 639–645.

38. Jeffree MA, Barter DJ, Hemingway AP & Nolan DJ. Primary carcinoid tumours of the ileum: the radiological appearances. *Clin Radiol* 1984; **35**: 451–455.

39. Jeffree MA & Nolan DJ. Multiple ileal carcinoid tumours. Case report. *Br J Radiol* 1987; **60**: 402–403.

40. Mendelson RM & Nolan DJ. The radiological features of radiation enteritis. *Clin Radiol* 1985; **36**: 141–148.

41. Marshak RH, Lindner AE & Maklansky D. Ischaemia of the small intestine. *Am J Gastroenterol* 1976; **66**: 390–400.

42. Marks CG, Nolan DJ, Piris J & Webster CU. Small bowel strictures after blunt abdominal trauma. *Br J Surg* 1979; **66**: 663–664.

43. Nolan DJ. *Radiological Atlas of Gastrointestinal Disease*. Chichester, New York: Wiley, 1983.

44. Schwartz MJ & Lewis JH. Meckel's diverticulum: pitfalls in scintigraphic detection in the adult. *Am J Gastroenterol* 1984; **79**: 611–618.

45. Maglinte DDT, Elmore MF, Isenberg M & Dolan PA. Meckel's diverticulum: radiologic demonstration by enteroclysis. *AJR* 1980; **134**: 925–932.

46. Dixon PM & Nolan DJ. The diagnosis of Meckel's diverticulum: a continuing challenge. *Clin Radiol* 1987; **38**: 615–619.

47. Meyers MA. Clinical involvement of mesenteric and antimesenteric borders of small bowel loops. II. Radiologic interpretation of pathologic alterations. *Gastrointest Radiol* 1976; **1**: 49–58.

48. Miller RE & Brahme F. Large amounts of orally administered barium for obstruction of the small intestine. *Surg Gynecol Obstet* 1969; **129**: 1185–1188.

49. Donato H, Mayo HW & Barr LH. The effect of peroral barium in partial obstruction of the small bowel. *Surgery* 1954; **35**: 719–723.

50. Nelson SW, Christoforidis AJ & Roenigk WJ. Barium suspensions vs water-soluble iodine compounds in the study of obstruction of the small bowel. An experimental study of physiologic characteristics and radiographic value. *Radiology* 1963; **80**: 252–254.

51. Nolan DJ & Marks CG. The barium infusion in small intestinal obstruction. *Clin Radiol* 1981; **32**: 651–655.

52. Price J & Nolan DJ. Closed loop obstruction: diagnosis by enteroclysis. *Gastrointest Radiol* 1989; **14**: 251–254.

53. Dehn TCB & Nolan DJ. Enteroclysis in the diagnosis of intestinal obstruction in the early postoperative period. *Gastrointest Radiol* 1989; **14**: 15–21.

54. Thompson JN, Hemingway AP, McPherson GAD et al. Obscure gastrointestinal haemorrhage of small bowel origin. *BMJ* 1980; **23**: 1663.

55. Baum S. Angiography and the gastrointestinal bleeder. *Radiology* 1982; **143**: 569–572.

56. Athanasoulis CA, Moncure AC, Greenfield AJ et al. Intraoperative localization of small bowel bleeding sites with combined use of angiographic methods and methylene blue injection. *Surgery* 1980; **87**: 77–84.

57. Boijsen E & Reuter SR. Mesenteric angiography in the evaluation of inflammatory and neoplastic disease of the intestine. *Radiology* 1966; **87**: 1028–1036.

58. Forbes ESC, Nolan DJ, Fletcher EWL & Lee E. Small bowel melaena: two cases diagnosed by angiography. *Radiology* 1978; **65**: 168–170.

59. Reuter SR & Boijsen E. Angiographic findings in two ileal carcinoid tumours. *Radiology* 1966; **87**: 836–840.

60. Ekberg O & Ekholm S. Radiology in primary small bowel adenocarcinoma. *Gastrointest Radiol* 1980; **5**: 49–53.

61. Okazaki M, Higashihara H, Saida Y et al. Angiographic findings of Meckel's diverticulum: the characteristic appearances of the vitelline artery. *Abdom Imaging* 1993; **18**: 15–19.

62. Federle MP, Chun G, Jeffery RB & Rayor R. Computed tomographic findings in bowel infarction. *AJR* 1984; **142**: 91–95.

63. Smerud MJ, Johnson CD & Stephens DH. Diagnosis of bowel infarction: a comparison of plain films and CT scans in 23 cases. *AJR* 1990; **154**: 99–103.

64. Frager D, Medwid SW, Baer JW et al. CT of small bowel obstruction: value in establishing the diagnosis and determining the degree and cause. *AJR* 1994; **162**: 37–41.

65. Gazelle GS, Goldberg MA, Wittenberg J et al. Efficacy of CT in distinguishing small-bowel obstruction from other causes of small-bowel dilation. *AJR* 1994; **162**: 43–47.

66. Balthazar EJ. CT of small bowel obstruction. *AJR* 1994; **162**: 255–261.

67. Goldberg HI, Gore RM, Margulis AR, Moss AA & Baker EL. Computed tomography in the evaluation of Crohn's disease. *AJR* 1983; **140**: 277–282.

68. Hulnick DH. Small intestine. In Megibow AJ & Balthazar EJ (eds)

Computed Tomography of the Gastrointestinal Tract. St Louis: CV Mosby, 1986: 217–278.

69. Megibow AJ, Balthazar EJ, Cho KC, Medwid SW, Birnbaum BA & Noz ME. Bowel obstruction: evaluation with CT. *Radiology* 1991; **180**: 313–318.

70. Fukuya T, Hawes DR, Lu CC, Chang PJ & Barloon TJ. CT diagnosis of small bowel obstruction: efficacy in 60 patients. *AJR* 1992; **158**: 765–769.

71. Ha HK, Park CH, Kim SK et al. CT analysis of intestinal obstruction due to adhesions: early detection of strangulation. *J Comput Assist Tomogr* 1993; **17**: 386-389.

72. Maglinte DDT, Gage SN, Harmon BH et al. Obstruction of the small intestine: accuracy and role of CT in diagnosis. *Radiology* 1993; **188**: 61.

73. Balthazar EJ, Baumann JS & Megibow AJ. CT diagnosis of closed loop obstruction. *J Comput Assist Tomogr* 1985; **9**: 953–955.

74. Jaramillo D & Raval B. CT diagnosis of primary small bowel volvulus. *AJR* 1986; **147**: 941–942.

75. Balthazar EJ, Birnbaum BA, Megibow AJ, Gordon RB, Whelan CA & Hulnick DH. Closed-loop and strangulating intestinal obstruction: CT signs. *Radiology* 1992; **185**: 769–775.

76. Berliner L, Redmond P, Purrow E et al. Computed tomography in Crohn's disease. *Am J Gastroenterol* 1982; **77**: 548–553.

77. Frick MP, Feinberg SB, Stenlund RR & Gedgaudas E. Evaluation of abdominal fistulas with computed tomography. *Comput Radiol* 1982; **6**: 17–25.

78. Knochel JQ, Kochler PR, Lee TG & Welch DM. Diagnosis of abdominal abscesses with computed tomography, ultrasound, and in leukocyte scans. *Radiology* 1980; **137**: 425–432.

79. Mueller PR, Ferrucci JT, Harbin WP, Kirkpatrick RH, Simeone JF & Wittenberg J. Appearances of lymphomatous involvement of the mesentery by ultrasonography and computed body tomography. *Radiology* 1980; **134**: 467–473.

80. Dubbins PA & Kurtz AB. Normal and abnormal bowel. In Goldberg BB (ed.) *Abdominal Ultrasound.* New York: Wiley, 1984: 287–305.

81. Somers S & Stevenson GW. The small bowel: anatomy and nontube examinations. In Freeny PC & Stevenson GW (eds) *Margulis and Burhenne's Alimentary Tract Radiology.* St Louis: CV Mosby, 1994: 512–532.

82. Vecchioli A, De Franco A, Maresca G & Gore RM. Cross-sectional imaging of the small intestine. In Gore RM, Levine MS & Laufer I (eds) *Textbook of Gastrointestinal Radiology.* Philadelphia: WB Saunders, 1994: 789–801.

83. Scheible W & Goldberger LE. Diagnosis of small bowel obstruction: the contribution of diagnostic ultrasound. *AJR* 1979; 133: 685–688.

84. Fleischer AC, Dowling AD, Weingstein L & Jones AE. Sonographic patterns of distended fluid filled bowel. *Radiology* 1979; 133: 681–685.

85. Holt S & Samuel E. Grey scale ultrasound in Crohn's disease. *Gut* 1979; **20**: 590–595.

86. Sonnenberg A, Erckenbrecht J, Peter P & Niederau C. Detection of Crohn's disease by ultrasound. *Gastroenterology* 1982; **83**: 430–434.

87. Dubbins PA. Ultrasound demonstration of bowel wall thickness in inflammatory bowel disease. *Clin Radiol* 1984; **35**: 227–231.

88. Bin W, Jianguo L & Baowei D. The sonographic appearances of small bowel tumours. *Clin Radiol* 1992; **46**: 30–31.

89. Alavi A & Ring EJ. Localization of gastrointestinal bleeding: superiority of ^{99m}Tc sulphur colloid compared to angiography. *AJR* 1981; **137**: 741–748.

90. McKusick KA, Froelich J, Callahan RJ, Winzelberg GG & Strauss HW. ^{99m}Tc red blood cells for detection of gastrointestinal bleeding: experience with 80 patients. *AJR* 1981; **137**: 1113–1118.

91. Bunker SR, Lull RJ, Tanasescu DU et al. Scintigraphy of gastrointestinal haemorrhage: superiority of ^{99m}Tc red blood cells over ^{99m}Tc sulphur colloid. *AJR* 1984; **143**: 543–548.

92. Conway JJ. Radionuclide diagnosis of Meckel's diverticulum. *Gastrointest Radiol* 1980; **5**: 209–213.

93. Sfakianakis GN & Conway JJ. Detection of ectopic gastric mucosa in Meckel's diverticulum and in other aberrations by scintigraphy: 1. Pathophysiology and 10-year clinical experience. *J Nucl Med* 1981; **22**: 647–654.

94. Cooney DR, Duszynski DO, Camboa E, Karp MP & Jewett TCJR. The abdominal technetium scan (a decade experience). *J Pediatr Surg* 1982; **17**: 611–619.

95. Saverymuttu SH, Peters AM, Hodgson HJ, Chadwick VS & Lavender JP. ^{111}Indium leukocyte scanning in small-bowel Crohn's disease. *Gastrointest Radiol* 1983; **8**: 157–161.

46

ADAPTATION AND FAILURE OF THE SMALL BOWEL

E Weser
RCN Williamson

SHORT BOWEL SYNDROME

CAUSES

There are numerous causes for surgical resection of small intestine leading to short bowel syndrome or 'failure of the small bowel' (Table 46.1). Most commonly, bowel infarction (including volvulus/strangulation) and abdominal trauma account for acute surgical intervention with resection of varying lengths of small intestine. Patients with jejunoileal bypass for the treatment of morbid obesity and those with granulomatous enteritis (Crohn's disease) and multiple resections comprise most of the remaining group. Some patients with extensive radiation enteropathy even without resection of small intestine may functionally exhibit small bowel failure. Proper management for this condition, whatever its original cause, depends on a thorough understanding of the altered physiology of the shortened small intestine.

MALABSORPTION
The effects of small bowel resection

Small bowel resection results in a reduction of absorbing mucosal surface area and usually of transit time through the remaining intestine. The decreased contact time between luminal nutrients and mucosal surface in a shortened small bowel therefore contributes both to maldigestion and malabsorption of nutrients. Nevertheless, the small intestine has a large functional reserve capacity, allowing 40–50% of small bowel to be removed without noticeable impairment of nutrient absorption and overall nutrition. As indicated below, the anatomical location of excised intestine is an important consideration in determining the degree of malabsorption and metabolic sequelae of the resection. Although the minimum length of small intestine required to support adequate nutrition by oral or

Table 46.1 Causes for failure of the small bowel

1. Alterations of blood flow to small intestine
   (a) Superior mesenteric artery thrombosis (or embolus)
   (b) Superior mesenteric vein thrombosis
   (c) Strangulated hernia
   (d) Volvulus

2. Primary surgical resection or bypass of small intestine
   (a) Abdominal trauma
   (b) Jejunoileal bypass for morbid obesity
   (c) Unintended gastroileal amastomosis for peptic ulcer

3. Primary small bowel disease
   (a) Regional enteritis requiring one or more resections of small bowel
   (b) Small bowel cancer or intra-abdominal neoplasms involving small bowel (and colon)
   (c) Radiation enteropathy

enteral feeding alone is not known, there are occasional reports of extended survival after near-total excision of small bowel.[1,2] Removal of mid-small bowel or jejunum is generally tolerated better than resection of duodenum or terminal ileum. Often the loss of the ileocaecal junction is an additional detriment imposed on the patient with ileal resection (for reasons given below). The important factors influencing nutrient absorption and metabolic status after small bowel resection are listed in Table 46.2.

Under normal circumstances, digestion and absorption of nutrients consisting of fat, carbohydrate, protein, minerals and water-soluble vitamins (excluding vitamin B_{12}) are accomplished in the duodenum and jejunum (see also Chapter 43). The ileum receives relatively little demand for nutrient absorption and represents a large functional reserve capacity. With large resections of proximal small bowel, there will be reduced production of cholecystokinin and secretin and thus reduced stimulation of pancreaticobiliary secretions. Removal

Table 46.2 Important factors affecting nutrient absorption and metabolic status after small bowel resection

1. Length of removed intestine
2. Anatomical location of removed intestine
3. Exclusion or inclusion of ileocaecal valve
4. Functional status of remaining small and large bowel
5. Functional status of liver, gall bladder, pancreas and stomach
6. Adaptive changes in remaining small and large bowel, pancreas and stomach

of ileum generally results in greater metabolic sequelae than the loss of comparable lengths of jejunum, because the ileum is the selective site for active reabsorption of conjugated bile salts, of vitamin B_{12} complexed with intrinsic factor and probably of hydroxy-vitamin D metabolites found in bile. After loss of ileum, some adaptive increase in absorption by diffusion of bile salts and vitamin B_{12} occurs in the remnant jejunum.[3-5] Also, active bile salt transport may undergo induction in the remaining jejunum and ileum,[3,4] and there is a limited increase in hepatic bile salt synthesis.[6] The excessive loss of bile salts that follows decreased ileal reabsorption may result in a diminished pool of circulating bile salts and lowered bile salt concentrations in the lumen of the small intestine. This process results in impaired formation of bile salt micelles in the lumen and consequent reduction in the absorption of fatty acids, monoglycerides and fat-soluble vitamins (A, D, E, K). Increased amounts of fat, fatty acids and conjugated bile salts enter the colon, where bacterial metabolism produces hydroxy fatty acids and deconjugated bile salts. These products alter water and electrolyte absorption from the colon[7,8] and produce a secretory diarrhoea as well as steatorrhoea.

Removal of limited amounts of ileum (usually less than 100 cm of distal ileum) may result in marked diarrhoea with only modest, if any, steatorrhoea, primarily because of the increase in bile salts entering the colon. Usually, an increase in hepatic synthesis of bile salts maintains adequacy of their small bowel concentrations, so that steatorrhoea is not a problem. Increased lithogenicity of hepatic bile may also occur when small bowel resection interrupts the ileohepatic recirculation of bile salts. Insufficient absorption of vitamin B_{12} can lead to a depletion of body stores over several years, and in the presence of vitamin B_{12} deficiency intestinal mucosal morphology and transport function may be impaired.[9]

Associated with steatorrhoea, malabsorption of fat-soluble vitamins may produce clinical signs of their deficiency. Particularly important in this regard are vitamins K and D. Reduced serum concentrations of 25-hydroxy vitamin D have been noted after intestinal resection and represent both decreased vitamin D absorption and insufficient intake.[10] An enterohepatic circulation of hydroxy vitamin D metabolites may be an important factor in reduced serum concentrations, since it is known that intravenous injection of 25-hydroxy vitamin D is followed by its appearance into the intestinal lumen in both experimental animals and humans.[11,12]

Resection of the ileocaecal valve and colon

Diarrhoea may be additionally increased by removal of the ileocaecal valve together with distal ileal resection (and often also segmental colectomy). Several mechanisms contribute to this result. The degree of bacterial seeding in existing shortened small intestine may increase,[13,14] thereby enhancing bacterial deconjugation of bile salts in the bowel lumen. Thus there is further reduction in the active reabsorption of conjugated bile salts and an increase of both conjugated and deconjugated bile salts entering the colon. This further reduction of bile salt reabsorption would also increase fat malabsorption. Bacterial overgrowth in the shortened small intestine may also metabolise intraluminal vitamin B_{12} sufficiently to reduce availability for absorption and thus increase the probability of vitamin B_{12} deficiency. The existence of the ileocaecal valve may also lengthen small bowel transit time[15] and permit small bowel nutrients to have longer contact time with mucosa, resulting in better absorption.

The colon is not only a storage organ for small bowel effluent, but it is also important for absorption and maintenance of water and electrolyte balance, particularly sodium. The absence of varying amounts of colon, as commonly accompanies resection of the ileocaecal junction, may worsen diarrhoea, dehydration, hypovolaemia and electrolyte depletion. Intestinal transit time has been correlated with increasing lengths of preserved colon as has the faecal electrolyte content.[16] Therefore, it is important to stress the role of the large bowel in maintaining water and electrolyte balances.[17]

The colon is also an important site for the absorption of soluble dietary oxalate.[18] Under normal circumstances, most dietary oxalate combines with intraluminal calcium and forms insoluble calcium oxalate, which remains unabsorbed. When steatorrhoea exists, calcium in the lumen of the intestine binds with unabsorbed fats and fatty acids, decreasing the availability of calcium for oxalate binding. Therefore, patients with steatorrhoea or ileectomy and intact colons may have greater absorption of dietary oxalate and subsequent excretion into the urine. Oxalate stones can develop in the urinary tract (see below).

Additional effects

The duodenal mucosa is the site of maximal rates of absorption for iron, calcium and magnesium. Nevertheless, appreciable absorption of these ions takes place along the entire length of the small bowel because of longer mucosal contact time and exposure to a greater mucosal surface area. Resection of upper or lower small intestine may therefore cause decreased absorption of these ions, resulting in clinical evidence of deficiency. Reduced serum concentrations of 25-hydroxy vitamin D in patients with short bowel[10] may be associated with further decreases in calcium absorption. Steatorrhoea may also cause excessive binding of luminal magnesium, as well as calcium, with unabsorbed fatty acids and thereby reduce absorption. In short bowel patients, decreased absorption of these ions and metabolic bone disease have been reported.[19] Intraluminal zinc and other trace metals may also be sequestered by unabsorbed fatty acids, resulting in deficiencies with clinical manifestations.[19,20]

With the exception of vitamin B$_{12}$, deficiencies of water-soluble vitamins seem to be less frequent than those of fat-soluble vitamins after small bowel resection. Dietary folate (pteroylpolyglutamate) is absorbed in the proximal intestine after deconjugation by the mucosa to pteroylmonoglutamates. Except in patients with minimal residual small intestine, sufficient compensatory deconjugation and transport of folate must occur, perhaps involving a significant enterohepatic recirculation.[21]

Some patients with extensive small bowel resection develop gastric hypersecretion in the months after operation.[2,22] There is some correlation between the length of bowel removed and the degree of hypersecretion,[22] which appears to diminish with time. Serum gastrin concentrations may increase after small bowel resection,[23] presumably because of reduced catabolism by small bowel tissue and tropic changes in gastric mucosa resulting in an increased parietal cell mass.[24] A reduction of enteric hormones (removed with small bowel tissue) that normally inhibit the tropic effects of gastrin (such as secretion, cholecystokinin and others) may also play a role in enhancing gastric secretion. The increased volume of gastric juice contributes to an increase in intraluminal fluid in the residual small bowel, thereby diluting pancreatic enzymes and bile acids as well as stimulating peristalsis. Pancreatic digestive function is also impaired by the low pH of luminal fluid and together with inhibited bile salt micelle formation may cause diarrhoea, steatorrhoea, peptic ulceration and breakdown of surgical anastomoses. This situation is not unlike a patient with Zollinger–Ellison syndrome further complicated by a shortened gastrointestinal tract. With reduced pancreatic stimulation from less cholecystokinin and secretion production as well as malnutrition, some patients may ultimately develop reduced pancreatic exocrine secretion and even pancreatic atrophy.

Removal of small bowel tissue may also be accompanied by a total reduction in mucosal disaccharidases and thus impair the hydrolysis and absorption of disaccharides. Lactase deficiency is most commonly seen, and ingested lactose may add an osmotic diarrhoea to the patient's already impaired absorptive state.

The functional state of the remaining small and large bowel after resection is extremely important in determining the patient's long-term outcome and complications. Although intestinal adaptation is discussed later in this chapter, it is important to emphasize that the condition of the remaining intestine, liver and pancreas influences the ability of the patient to digest and absorb oral nutrients. Patients with residual disease in the gastrointestinal tract, such as granulomatous enterocolitis, radiation enteritis, ischaemic enteropathy or other primary enteropathies as well as liver and pancreatic insufficiency have a worse prognosis as regards maintaining adequate nutrition.

CLINICAL MANIFESTATIONS

The extent and site of the small bowel resection largely determine the severity of clinical manifestations. Radiological examination of the small bowel may help to determine the relative length and dilatation of the residual intestine (Figure 46.1).

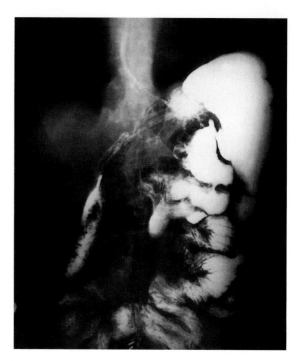

Figure 46.1
Radiological examination of patient with extensive small bowel resection and partial colectomy showing gastroduodenal jejunal segment emptying into remaining left colon.

Troublesome diarrhoea and steatorrhoea may be found in patients with resections limited to the ileum and ileocaecal junction (less than 30% of total small bowel), mainly due to the interruption of the enterohepatic circulation of bile acids and the entry of cathartic bile acids into the large bowel.

Obviously, patients with extensive small bowel resections will experience an important reduction in overall nutrient absorption and develop severe weight loss, weakness and fatigue associated with frequent stools. The malabsorption of vitamin D, calcium and protein may eventually cause metabolic bone disease (osteomalacia and osteoporosis) manifested by spontaneous fractures and bone pain. If hypocalcaemia and hypomagnesaemia develop, patients may present with tetany or carpopedal spasm. With excessive losses of dietary and endogenous sources of vitamin K in the stools, coagulation defects may occur and lead to ecchymoses, purpura or generalized bleeding phenomena. Hypoalbuminaemia and vitamin B complex deficiencies are common and may respectively produce oedema and peripheral neuropathies. Likewise, anaemia occurs in many patients and may represent combined deficiencies of folic acid, vitamin B$_{12}$ and iron.

As noted previously, gastric hypersecretion may occur in the weeks or months following extensive resection of the small bowel and contribute to the clinical picture. Not only are patients at risk of peptic ulcer disease, but steatorrhoea and diarrhoea may be worsened. Gastric hypersecretion appears, however, to be a relatively transient event and it improves with time.[22]

Related to the loss of ileum, patients may develop sufficient depletion of the bile acid pool to produce lithogenic bile, resulting in a threefold increase in the incidence of gall-stones.[25,26] Some patients may also absorb greater quantities of dietary oxalate depending on the degree of steatorrhoea, calcium-fatty acid binding and the existence of sufficient colon to absorb the soluble oxalate. Chronic hyperoxaluria may cause calcium oxalate kidney stones.[18,27] Patients with an ileostomy are less likely to develop oxalate stones even if they have steatorrhoea.[28]

Other clinical manifestations can occur because of intestinal bacteria. Malabsorption of fat and vitamin B_{12} may be further impaired because of bacterial overgrowth in the remaining small bowel. Intraluminal proliferation of bacteria may occur more readily in the absence of the ileocaecal valve. Additionally, bacterial metabolism of unabsorbed nutrients in the colon may be the mechanism by which some patients develop a D-lactic acidosis associated with neurological abnormalities.[29]

LABORATORY ABNORMALITIES

The laboratory findings in many patients with insufficient small bowel may usually be anticipated from the degree of malabsorption and the extent of fluid and electrolyte losses. Commonly, hypokalaemia and a depleted sodium and water condition are found. Faecal losses of calcium and magnesium are often associated with low serum concentrations of the cation. These patients have varying degrees of faecal fat excretion, depending on the amount of ingested fat in the diet, and may have low serum prothrombin (increased prothrombin times) and carotene levels. Unless adequately replaced, both vitamin B_{12} and iron deficiency anaemias may exist. Because absorption of protein is likely to be impaired, hypoalbuminaemia is also common. A variety of sugar absorption tests is abnormal including D-xylose and lactose absorption.

TREATMENT

Treatment of short bowel syndrome logically follows an understanding of the aforementioned pathophysiology. Patients with underlying small bowel disease, such as Crohn's disease and with multiple small bowel resections should obviously have residual inflammation in the remaining intestine treated with optimal medical therapy, i.e. sulphasalazine, aminosalicylates, steroids and/or antibiotics or azathioprine. The main approach to treatment can be divided into nutritional or dietary measures and the use of specific drugs.

Diet therapy

In the period immediately following resection, patients will benefit from *total parenteral nutrition*. If the resection was extensive, rapid transition to full oral nutrition may not be possible. Intestinal adaptation usually requires weeks or months (indeed if ever the case) before absorption of orally ingested nutrients is adequate to furnish the patient's energy requirements. In patients with less extensive resections or those with a relatively long remaining jejunal segment, tolerance of enteral feedings may develop more rapidly.

Usually *enteral feeding* may be started within the first week after operation. It is important to continue parenteral nutrition until it is apparent that the patient can tolerate and sustain adequate calorie intake via the enteral route. Implementation of enteral nutrition is accomplished by using defined formula diets. These products (1) have low-to-absent concentrations of long-chain triglycerides; (2) have calories provided by a mixture of essential amino acids and carbohydrates (usually glucose); (3) possess balanced electrolytes as well as other nutrients such as medium-chain triglycerides.[30] These enteral diets are thought to be more readily absorbed in a shortened intestine, since minimal digestion is required before absorption. Because of their low or absent fat content, these preparations are usually unpalatable and are given via a fine-bore nasogastric tube. They are also hyperosmolar solutions and may themselves cause vomiting or diarrhoea; thus they are usually given at first diluted one in three or four. It is best to administer these solutions by a slow, continuous drip over 24 hours and increase their strength in stepwise doses.

Some success has been achieved with the additional use of colonic infusions of fluids and electrolytes in patients who have all or part of their colon bypassed.[31] This procedure may help maintain positive fluid and electrolyte balance, plasma volume and normal renal function.

When the patient is able to progress to a more conventional food intake, it may prove useful at first to limit the daily fat intake to 40 g or less. Fat absorption is likely to remain appreciably reduced in patients with short bowel, and unabsorbed fat may obligate important faecal losses of fluid and electrolytes (particularly calcium and magnesium). However, recent studies have shown that a more liberal intake of dietary fat is not accompanied by such severe losses and will permit the patient to benefit from a greater caloric intake.[32] These patients should receive replacement or supplemental calcium plus fat-soluble vitamin D therapy to correct or prevent hypocalcaemia and metabolic bone disease. Magnesium deficiency may require parenteral injections of magnesium sulphate or citrate, since use of oral magnesium therapy usually worsens diarrhoea and is unsuccessful.

With continuous steatorrhoea, deficiency of the fat-soluble vitamin K may develop and result in hypoprothrombinaemia, which may be corrected by periodic injections of vitamin K. Although vitamin A deficiency seems to occur less often, patients should be evaluated for impairment of retinal dark adaptation and be treated accordingly. Usually improved fat absorption occurs with intestinal adaptation over a period of time, and patients begin to tolerate increased amounts of dietary fat.

In most patients with small bowel resection, absorption of water-soluble vitamins remains relatively well preserved and deficiencies are less common. In patients with extensive resections involving both the ileum and jejunum, large doses of liquid oral multivitamin preparations are usually successful in preventing or treating deficiencies of water-soluble vitamins. As previously mentioned, absorption of vitamin B_{12} is an active process in the ileum. In patients with ileal resections, usually greater than 2 metres, periodic injections of vitamin B_{12} are required to prevent eventual deficiency of this vitamin. Some patients also require iron and calcium therapy when the duodenum is either bypassed or included in the small bowel resection, even though the extent of the enterectomy is relatively limited. Since the rates of absorption of these minerals are most rapid from the duodenum, its absence may be just enough to cause inadequate absorption (even though absorption does occur along the entire length of remaining bowel).

Patients with extensive small bowel resection lose much intestinal lactase (and other disaccharidases) so as to impair hydrolysis of dietary disaccharides. Additionally, rapid transit through a shortened intestine may deliver increased quantities of sugars to the colon, where bacterial fermentation can worsen diarrhoea and add to the patient's symptoms. Therefore, it is frequently necessary to limit milk (lactose) products unless exogenous lactase is given (as mentioned below). Without milk products, the need for calcium supplementation cannot be overemphasized. In some patients, restriction of dietary sucrose and use of increased dietary starch results in decreased jejunostomy and ileostomy fluid outputs, suggesting that starch carbohydrate is better tolerated.[32]

As discussed earlier, some patients with short bowel and an intact colon may have hyperoxaluria and subsequently develop calcium oxalate kidney stones. Patients on a stable dietary intake should have several measurements of 24 hour urinary oxalate excretion performed and, if elevated, be placed on a low oxalate intake (Table 46.3). Calcium supplementation will also decrease dietary oxalate absorption and reduce oxalate excretion in the urine. It is necessary, however, to avoid excessive urinary calcium excretion. A large daily fluid intake to assure greater urine volumes may also help prevent kidney stones but may worsen diarrhoea. Whatever diet seems optimally to help the patient, food intake should be divided into multiple small feeds. Fewer, larger-volume meals are likely to exceed the absorptive capability of the remaining small bowel and worsen the osmotic diarrhoea.

Table 46.3 Foods with high concentrations of oxalate

Fruits	Oranges, strawberries, plums, concord grapes, raspberries, gooseberries, red currants, cranberries, blackberries, figs
Vegetables	Spinach, beets, beet greens, green onions, parsley, okra, sweet potatoes, yams, sweet and green peppers, carrots, celery, wax beans, artichokes, rhubarb, chard, endive
Other	Tea, cocoa, chocolate, cola beverages

Drug treatment

The primary aim of drug therapy is to reduce debilitating diarrhoea and allow the patient to assume as near-normal activities as possible. Codeine, diphenoxylate, loperamide and possibly anticholinergic drugs should be given in effective doses sufficient to increase transit time and reduce the frequency of bowel movements. Liquid preparations rather than tablets seem to be absorbed more rapidly and completely. Although not commonly used, parenteral administration of anticholinergics

may be more effective in some patients.[33] Bacterial colonization of residual small bowel is common in these patients and may contribute to their diarrhoea. Therefore, 7–14-day courses of antibiotics, such as ampicillin, tetracycline or low doses of neomycin may be helpful in altering the bacterial flora and in improving absorption for many weeks following their use. Bacterial culture of intestinal contents may be helpful in selecting the initial choice of antibiotic. In circumstances in which gastric hypersecretion is evident, treatment with H_2 antagonists has proved effective in controlling gastric secretory volumes and acid production.[34,35] These agents are preferable to antacids and/or anticholinergic drugs. Additional use of pancreatic supplements high in lipase activity given with meals, in adequate doses, may be helpful in reducing steatorrhoea. Patients with a short bowel may have relative (or absolute) pancreatic insufficiency owing to dilution or inactivation of pancreatic enzymes by gastric acid as well as impaired stimulation of pancreatic secretion and enzyme mixing with ingested food. Recently, the use of lactase enzymes added either to whole milk or taken together with the ingestion of lactose-containing foods has proved useful in individuals with lactase deficit, and it should be tried in short-bowel patients.

For those patients with ileal resections limited to less than 100 cm and a related bile acid-induced diarrhoea, treatment with cholestyramine 8–12 g daily may dramatically improve their symptoms.[36] Cholestyramine will bind with unabsorbed bile acids and prevent their secretory stimulus in the colon. Diarrhoea in patients with more extensive resections is additionally caused by the secretory effects of unabsorbed hydroxy fatty acids and the osmotic influences of unabsorbed nutrients, so that cholestyramine is usually not helpful. In fact, cholestyramine in these instances may further deplete the bile acid pool and worsen steatorrhoea and diarrhoea. If cholestyramine is used, it may also bind dietary oxalate and reduce its absorption, resulting in a decrease in urinary oxalate excretion.

Studies with a parenterally administered somatostatin analogue (octreotide) offer promise as an agent to reduce intestinal secretions and diarrhoea, but these efforts must still be regarded as experimental.[37,38]

Home parenteral nutrition

For patients with intractable short bowel syndrome, long-term parenteral nutrition is necessary to support life. Growing sophistication with this modality of treatment has made it possible to provide all nutrient requirements via silastic catheters placed in the superior vena cava while patients live at home and, in many cases, pursue routine work and leisure activities. Sometimes, continuing intestinal adaptation allows parenteral nutrition to be discontinued after a period of months, though patients may remain unstable and require intermittent support for episodes of electrolyte imbalance or nutritional failure. Other patients with short bowel syndrome remain dependent on intravenous alimentation indefinitely, and this is especially so if there is less than one metre of jejunoileum in association with loss of the ileocaecal valve and/or part of the large intestine.

Home parenteral nutrition is a complex and time-consuming treatment for the patient and requires a period of approximately three weeks in hospital for training in the technique.[39] The patients look after their own central line and are only admitted to hospital when complications arise, notably episodes of sepsis or venous thrombosis related to the catheter and acute metabolic derangements.[40] The only non-surgical alternative that permits patients with total gut failure to survive is to keep the patients in hospital or readmit them for intermittent therapy, but this is less cost-effective and may be impossible with a scattered population.[41,42] The limitations of intestinal transplantation are such that home parenteral nutrition can be justified in selected patients (despite its cost) as the only practicable means of preventing death from a combination of dehydration and malnutrition.[43] Although results vary quite widely between centres,[39] a 5-year survival of up to 75% can be achieved.[44]

Surgical techniques

In patients who respond poorly to dietary and drug therapies, a variety of surgical operations short of intestinal transplantation have been tried in an attempt to increase transit time and/or improve intestinal absorption. Thompson and colleagues[45–47] have described the following surgical options.

1. Tapering enteroplasty. The intestinal circumference is reduced by imbrication (turning-in) or actual excision of the redundant bowel along the antimesenteric border. This technique may be appropriate in patients (especially children) in whom gross intestinal dilatation leads to bacterial overgrowth and malabsorption, and improved function can be anticipated at least in the short term.[46]

2. Intestinal lengthening. A dilated loop of small bowel is divided in two longitudinally (between the mesenteric and antimesenteric borders), and the two new segments of intestine are anastomosed end-to-end.[47] Elongation by at least 20 cm can be achieved in suitable cases.

3. Creation of an artificial intestinal valve by intussusception of a segment of small bowel.

4. Segmental reversal of the small bowel. Promising medium-term results have recently been reported in a small series of patients who received antiperistaltic interposition of a short segment of bowel (8–15 cm in length).[48] The reversed segment acts as a brake, prolonging transit time and thus contact between luminal nutrients and the residual small bowel mucosa. There is a risk of episodic intestinal obstruction, however.

Other available techniques include colonic interposition, stricturoplasty to deal with stenotic areas, creation of a recirculating bowel loop and intestinal pacing. The experience is generally greatest in the paediatric population. Although individual patients have clearly received benefit, the improvement may be short-lived and there are several potential complications that could even exacerbate the original short bowel syndrome. Therefore at the present time these operations must still be regarded as experimental.

Small bowel transplantation

The definitive cure of short bowel syndrome ought to be the transplantation of a 'new' and complete small intestine. Unfortunately the combined effects of ischaemic injury during organ harvesting plus early rejection of the transplant can damage the mucosal barrier sufficiently to cause septicaemia, which threatens the survival of the recipient as well as the graft.[49] In addition, the substantial lymphoid component in the transplanted bowel and its mesenteric lymph nodes can lead to graft versus-host-disease (GVHD). These several problems meant that the early clinical attempts at small bowel transplantation were uniformly fatal, patients dying from systemic sepsis within days or weeks of the operation.

The advent of new immunosuppressive agents (notably cyclosporin and FK506) has greatly improved the prospect of preventing rejection of the graft, allowing repopulation of the transplanted organ by host lymphocytes. A small number of long-term survivors has now been reported, and a two-year survival rate (for patient and graft) of approximately 50% can be achieved.[50] For reasons that are still unclear, a concomitant liver graft may improve the chances of success.[46,49] Many problems remain to be solved before intestinal transplantation becomes a routine technique, notably opportunistic infection and the control of GVHD, but the pace of progress in this field is very rapid at the present time.

POSTOPERATIVE ADAPTATION OF THE SMALL BOWEL

COMPENSATORY HYPERPLASIA

Like the kidney and the liver, the small bowel possesses both a considerable functional reserve and a remarkable capacity to grow in response to loss of part of its mass. As already stated (p. 722), up to half the small intestine can be resected (or bypassed) without much impairment in nutritional status or any marked increase in stool frequency. Even a remnant of 20–30% may suffice to support independent life (i.e. without the need for parenteral nutrition), provided that the residual bowel is healthy and that appropriate dietary adjustments are made.

The phenomenon of intestinal adaptation is of considerable relevance to modern surgical practice. Many patients now survive massive intestinal loss, either suddenly as a consequence of extensive infarction or cumulatively from repeated resections, as in Crohn's disease (see Chapter 51). Moreover, well over 100 000 patients are estimated to have undergone subtotal jejunoileal bypass for obesity before this operation fell into relative disrepute.[51] An understanding of the phenomenon of adaptation and its mechanisms of control is thus of importance if the functional legacy of losing large amounts of tissue is to be minimized.

The small bowel responds to tissue loss not by elongation (except to a minor degree) but by increased mucosal mass leading to a thickening of its wall.[52] This compensatory hypertrophy was first observed in experimental animals by Senn in 1888.[53] Subsequently Flint recognized that postresectional adaptation involved both villi and crypts and, to a lesser extent, the muscularis propria.[54] He observed that there was epithelial hyperplasia with an increase in the size of the villi but not in their number. That the small bowel mucosa can undergo hyperplasia is remarkable considering that it is already the most rapidly renewing tissue in the body, with a turnover time of only a few days.[52]

Intestinal adaptation is a two-way process, occurring in response to a reduced as well as an increased demand on the gut. This dual response is most clearly seen in intestinal bypass, where the hyperplastic loops of bowel that remain in continuity with the nutrient stream stand in sharp contrast to the atrophic defunctioned loops (Figure 46.2). Surgical operations are not the only factors that produce adaptive change; food intake also has a profound effect on the bowel. Thus, hyperphagia (over-eating) leads to mucosal hyperplasia, whereas starvation causes hypoplasia.[55] Parenteral nutrition maintains the mass of the body organs but does nothing to reverse the disuse atrophy that occurs with fasting. The integrity of the small bowel lumen is maintained by the absorption of nutrients from chyme, and it is exquisitely sensitive to the withdrawal of this supply.[56] Knowledge of this fact should encourage surgeons to reintroduce enteral feeding as soon as possible after an operation. Dowling has identified two main categories of intestinal adaptation:[57] type 1 or physiological, which occurs in response to surgical operations and dietary manipulation (Table 46.4) and type 2 or pathological, which occurs in response to a disease process (e.g. coeliac disease, bacterial infection, irradiation) and is strictly a repair process that follows trauma. This section is chiefly concerned with postoperative adaptation but will also consider the response to alterations in food intake.

Table 46.4 Intestinal adaptation to surgical or dietary factors

	HYPERPLASIA	HYPOPLASIA
Surgical operations		
Small bowel resection	+ (espc. downstream)	–
Small bowel bypass	+ (functioning loops)	+ (defunctioned loops)
Ileojejunal transposition	+ (transposed ileum)	± (transposed jejunum)
Pancreatobiliary diversion	+ (downstream)	? (upstream)
Dietary manipulation		
Fasting	–	+
Refeeding	+	–
Hyperphagia	+	–
Parenteral nutrition	–	+

STRUCTURAL AND FUNCTIONAL CHANGES

Postresectional hyperplasia is manifested by increased villous height and crypt depth and a greater number of epithelial cells per unit length of villus and crypt.[58] Ileal villi also change their shape to resemble jejunal villi. An increased rate of crypt cell proliferation can be shown by an enhanced uptake of tritiated thymidine or bromodeoxyuridine and by measuring crypt cell production rate in microdissected whole crypts (following administration of a metaphase-arresting drug such as vincristine).

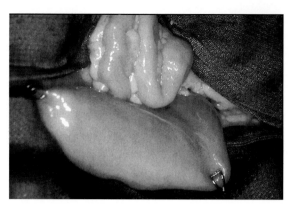

Figure 46.2
Laparotomy findings in a middle-aged woman who was undergoing reversal of a jejunoileal bypass operation carried out five years previously for morbid obesity. The dilated and hyperplastic segment of jejunum that remains in continuity with the nutrient stream contrasts sharply with the atrophic segments of the long defunctioned ('blind') loop.

Thus the adaptive response is truly one of hyperplasia. The phenomenon has mostly been studied in laboratory animals, but available data in man are generally in accord.

The enterocytes that are produced as a result of more rapid proliferation at the crypt base are often considered functionally immature. They spend a shorter time in the differentiation zone of the crypt and therefore possess fewer transport sites as they emerge onto the villus. This immaturity is cancelled out by the increase in overall cell number, so that enzyme activity per unit length of bowel is enhanced in hyperplastic segments of bowel. As a result there is a net enhancement of glucose, water and electrolyte absorption after enteric resection. This simple concept may not hold true for all aspects of enterocyte function, since some enzymes develop more rapidly in hyperplastic mucosa.[59]

Adaptive hyperplasia is greater after a proximal small bowel resection than after an equivalent distal small bowel resection.[58] This fact may reflect the greater mucosal mass that is normally present in the jejunum than the ileum, i.e. the proximal bowel is already closer to its maximum potential. The adaptive response is greatest in bowel close to the anastomosis, and it tapers off distally. It also occurs proximal to the site of anastomosis, though to a lesser extent. Thus the stomach and duodenum share in the compensatory response to jejunal resection, and there is some ileal adaptation to colectomy. Gastric hypersecretion after small bowel resection and bypass and diminishing ileostomy effluent with time after colectomy may be clinical consequences of this upstream adaptation. Lastly, the magnitude of the adaptive hyperplasia is roughly proportional to the length of bowel resected.

The downstream response to enteric bypass is broadly similar to that of enteric resection. By contrast, there is a sharp reduction in crypt cell production rate within the bypassed loop of bowel, and this reduction is reflected by lower mucosal mass and reduced contents of protein and DNA.[58] Bypassed jejunum shows a greater degree of defunction hypoplasia than bypassed ileum (at least in rats). The hypoplasia is accompanied by reduced segmental absorption of glucose and amino acids and by lower mucosal enzyme levels. All these changes are rapidly reversed by restoration of the bypassed segment of bowel to normal intestinal continuity. If jejunoileal transposition is carried out experimentally, the transposed ileum undergoes a similar hyperplastic response to that of jejunal resection, whereas the fate of the transposed jejunum is less clear-cut.[60]

After six days of total starvation in rats the weight of the small bowel diminishes by one half, whereas body weight falls only by one third. Crypt cell production rate declines, especially in the jejunum, and the villi and crypts decrease in size.[55] Refeeding promptly reverses the atrophy of starvation. Hyperphagia can be induced experimentally by various means, including hyperthyroidism, diabetes and lactation. All these conditions are associated with increased mucosal mass and proliferative indices. The use of total parenteral nutrition (TPN) in laboratory animals leads to a small bowel (especially jejunum) that is both hypoplastic and hypofunctional. Apart from the small bowel, gastric fundus, pancreas and colon, all other organs maintain their weight. The atrophic effect of TPN on the gut can be prevented by giving elemental diets or by infusions of cholecystokinin (CCK) or secretin. Importantly, the hyperplastic response to bowel resection fails to develop in animals that are fed by TPN.[61]

MECHANISMS OF CONTROL

Many of the features of compensatory intestinal hyperplasia can be explained by the theory of luminal nutrition, which states that the integrity of the mucosa is maintained by the presence of nutrient substances within the lumen of the small intestine.[62] It suggests that the enterocytes have first call on the energy sources that they absorb on behalf of the other organs in the body. Any procedure that renders the distal bowel subject to a greater nutrient load will produce hyperplasia of the mucosa within that segment. Thus after jejunal resection the ileum becomes exposed to a richer chyme than before, and it undergoes adaptive growth as a direct consequence. This concept explains the adaptive response of ileal segments transposed to a jejunal environment, although the metamorphosis is not total because the ectopic ileum retains its specific transport functions (e.g. for vitamin B_{12}).[60] The theory of luminal nutrition is also supported by the profound hypoplasia that is seen either in fasting animals or in bowel defunctioned by a surgical bypass. It accounts for the hyperplasia of experimental hyperplagia, which is abolished by pair feeding of experimental and control animals.

There can be no doubt that the nutrient load is a major determinant of the structural, functional and kinetic status of the small bowel, and luminal bulk also plays a part in maintaining the mucosal mass of the colon (which atrophies with parenteral or elemental alimentation). Part of the effect is probably indirect and results from the digestive fluids and enzymes that are secreted in response to food in the gut. Pancreatobiliary secretions are relatively easy to isolate, and their effect has been

studied experimentally in some detail.[62] The evidence indicates that bile and pancreatic juice have an important role in maintaining the normal aboral (i.e. proximodistal) gradient in mucosal mass. Distal diversion of the pancreatobiliary effluent causes ileal hyperplasia with or without jejunal resection. Increased pancreatic and biliary secretion may be the key intermediary in the ability of CCK/secretin infusion to prevent the hypoplasia of TPN, though these hormones could theoretically have a direct tropic effect on the bowel.

Luminal factors do not adequately explain all aspects of intestinal adaptation, for example adaptive changes seen in bowel proximal to the site of anastomosis (even if the food intake remains normal) or in segments excluded from the nutrient stream as a Thiry-Vella fistula, which can still respond to a small bowel resection or the onset of lactation. More direct evidence for a circulating (systemic) factor comes from parabiotic experiments, when enterectomy in one animal causes a proliferative response in its partner.[52]

Several different gastrointestinal peptides have been considered for the role of enterotropic hormone.[62] The tropic effect of gastrin seems to be restricted to the stomach and duodenum. The related hormone CCK probably does not have a direct effect on the jejunoileal mucosa (though it is tropic to the pancreas), but influences adaptive events by stimulating the flow of bile and pancreatic juice. Epidermal growth factor can prevent the hypoplasia of TPN in rats and can enhance cell turnover throughout the gut. Other peptides such as motilin, bombesin and vasoactive intestinal polypeptide (VIP) may have modest effects on the bowel mucosa, but enteroglucagon emerges as the strongest candidate for the title of enterotropin. There is a good relationship between circulating levels of enteroglucagon (but not gastrin) and cell proliferation rates in a wide variety of experimental models of adaptation.[63] The ileal site of enteroglucagon secretion fits with the fact that the ileal response to jejunal resection is greater than the jejunal response to ileal resection. Marked intestinal dilatation and villous hyperplasia were noted in one patient with a renal tumour that secreted enteroglucagon, and these feaatures disappeared after resection of the tumour.[64] Somatostatin probably exerts an antitropic effect on the small bowel, in part by preventing enteroglucagon release.

Luminal nutrients and endogenous secretions may stimulate adaptive change by triggering the release of peptides that act either systemically or locally in a paracrine fashion. Alternatively, they could directly stimulate intracellular growth regulators such as polyamines. The proliferative activity of the bowel mucosa depends not only on the presence or absence of food in the lumen of the gut but also on the nature of that food and the timing of its ingestion. Complex mechanisms are clearly involved in permitting the gastrointestinal tract to respond so precisely to its inconstant environment.

CLINICAL IMPLICATIONS OF INTESTINAL ADAPTATION

Most of the features of the compensatory response of the gut have been explored in laboratory animals, but limited clinical data broadly support a similar set of events in humans. The relative frequency of reversal operations for jejunoileal bypass has provided an excellent opportunity to compare the structural and functional adaptation of the short functioning segments with the hypoplasia of the long blind loop.[62] Sometimes excessive hyperplasia thwarted the primary objective of the operation and led to a failure to maintain the initial loss of weight.[65] Following massive small bowel resection, there is a variable period in which the patient passes frequent watery motions and then displays a gradual ability to change from parenteral to enteral nutrition as stool consistency improves. Eventually a plateau is reached beyond which there is no further improvement. The time scale of this clinical adaptation depends on the extent and site of the resected bowel, the functional state of the remaining bowel and the individual's own ability to adapt.

There are various guidelines to surgical practice when major interventions on the small intestine are contemplated, though these clearly have to be modified to suit the exact clinical circumstances. These guidelines can be summarized as follows.[62]

1. Resect as little as possible. The adaptive reserve of the jejunoileum is not unlimited, and long-term survival may be impossible without parenteral support when much less than one metre remains in continuity (though children may eventually tolerate extensive resections better than adults).

2. Resect (or bypass) jejunum in preference to ileum, since the ileum has specific transport functions (for vitamin B_{12} and bile salts) as well as a greater capacity to adapt. Thus vitamin B_{12} deficiency, bile salt catharsis and gallstones may complicate an extensive ileal resection.

3. Institute enteral nutrition as soon as possible after the operation. The crucial impact of food on mucosal growth means that the adaptive response is largely ineffective in its absence.

4. Control gastric hypersecretion after massive enterectomy and bacterial contamination of the small bowel after excision of the ileocaecal valve.

5. Remember that full adaptation in humans may take weeks or even months to develop, especially if the patient's general health is compromised, so that an expectant and optimistic attitude may well be appropriate.

REFERENCES

1. Anderson C. Long term survival with six inches of small intestine. *BMJ* 1965; **1**: 419.
2. Winawar SJ, Broitman SA, Wolochow DA et al. Successful management of massive small bowel resection based on assessment of absorption defects and nutritional needs. *N Engl J Med* 1966; **274**: 72.
3. Tilson DM, Boyer JL & Wright KH. Jejunal absorption of bile salts after resection of the ileum. *Surgery* 1975; **77**: 231.
4. Heubi JE, Balistreri WF, Partin JC, et al. Enterohepatic circulation of bile acids in infants and children with ileal resection. *J Lab Clin Med* 1980; **95**: 231.
5. Mackinnon AM, Short MD, Elias E et al. Adaptive changes in vitamin B_{12} absorption in celiac disease and after proximal small bowel resection in man. *Am J Dig Dis* 1975; **20**: 835.
6. Ho KJ & Bondi JL. Cholesterol metabolism in patients with resection of ileum and proximal colon. *Am J Clin Nutr* 1977; **30**: 151.
7. Ammon HV & Phillips SF. Inhibition of colonic water and electrolyte absorption by fatty acids in man. *Gastroenterology* 1973; **65**: 774.
8. Mekhjian HS, Phillips SF & Hofman AF. Colonic secretion of water and electrolytes induced by bile acids: perfusion studies in man. *J Clin Invest* 1971; **50**: 1569.
9. Arvanitakis C. Functional and morphologic abnormalities of the small intestinal mucosa in pernicious anemia. *Acta HepatoGastroenterol* 1978; **25**: 313.
10. Compston JE & Creamer B. Plasma levels and intestinal absorption of 25-hydroxy vitamin D in patients with small bowel resection. *Gut* 1977; **18**: 171.
11. Kumar R, Nagubandi S, Mattox VR et al. Enterohepatic physiology of 1,25-dihydroxy vitamin D_3. *J Clin Invest* 1980; **65**: 277.
12. Arnaud SB, Coldsmith RS, Lambert PW et al. 25-Hydroxy vitamin D_3. Evidence of an enterohepatic circulation in man. *Proc Soc Exp Biol Med* 1975; **149**: 570.
13. Isaacs PET & Kim YS. The contaminated small bowel syndrome. *Am J Med* 1979; **67**: 1049.
14. Simon GL & Gorbach SL. Intestinal microflora. *Med Clin North Am* 1982; **66**: 563.
15. Gazet JC & Kopp J. Surgical significance of ileo-cecal junction. *Surgery* 1964; **56**: 565.
16. Cummins JH, James WPT & Wiggins HS. Role of the colon in ileal-resection diarrhea. *Lancet* 1973; **i**: 344.
17. Mitchel JE, Breuer RI, Zuckerman L et al. The colon influences ileal resection diarrhea. *Dig Dis Sci* 1980; **25**: 33.
18. Earnest DL. *Advances in Internal Medicine*. Chicago: Year Book Medical Publishers, 1978.
19. Ladeioged KK, Nicolaidou P & Jarnum S. Calcium, phosphorus, magnesium, zinc and nitrogen balance in patients with severe short bowel syndrome. *Am J Clin Nutr* 1980; **33**: 2137.
20. Catalanotto FA. The trace metal zinc and taste. *Am J Clin Nutr* 1978; **31**: 1098.
21. Steinberg SE, Campbell CL & Hellman RS. Kinetics of the normal folate enterohepatic cycle. *J Clin Invest* 1979; **64**: 83.
22. Buxton B. Samll bowel resection and gastric hypersecretion. *Gut* 1974; **15**: 229.
23. Straus E, Gerson CD & Yalow R. Hypersecretion of gastrin associated with the short bowel syndrome. *Gastroenterology* 1974; **66**: 175.
24. Seelig LL, Winborn WB & Weser E. Effects of small bowel resection on the gastric mucosa in the rat. *Gastroenterology* 1977; **72**: 421.
25. Heaton KW & Read AE. Gallstones in patients with disorders of the terminal ileum and disturbed bile salt metabolism. *BMJ* 1969; **3**: 494.
26. Hill GL, Mair WSJ & Goligher JC. Gallstones after ileostomy and ileal resection. *Gut* 1975; **16**: 932.
27. Dharmsathaphorn K, Freeman DH, Binder HJ et al. Increased risk of nephrolithiasis in patients with steatorrhea. *Dig Dis Sci* 1982; **27**: 401.
28. Dobbins JW & Binder HJ. Importance of the colon in enteric hyperoxaluria. *N Engl J Med* 1977; **296**: 298.
29. Stolberg L, Rolfe R, Gitlin N et al. D-Lactic acidosis due to abnormal gut flora. *N Engl J Med* 1982; **306**: 1344.
30. Young EA, Heuler N, Russell P et al. Comparative nutritional analysis of chemically defined diets. *Gastroenterology* 1975; **69**: 1338.
31. Rodgers JB, Bernard HR & Balint JA. Colonic infusion in the management of the short bowel syndrome. *Gastroenterology* 1976; **70**: 186.
32. Woolf GM & Jeejeebhoy KN. Diet for the patient with short bowel: high fat or high carbohydrate? *Gastroenterology* 1982; **82**: 1260.
33. Greenberger NJ. State of the art: The management of the patient with short bowel syndrome. *Am J Gastroenterol* 1978; **70**: 528.
34. Cortot A, Fleming R & Malagelada JR. Improved nutrient absorption after cimetidine in short bowel syndrome with gastric hypersecretion. *N Engl J Med* 1979; **300**: 79.
35. Murphy JP, King DR & Dubois A. Treatment of gastric hypersecretion with cimetidine in the short bowel syndrome. *N Engl J Med* 1979; **300**: 80.
36. Hofmann AF & Poley JR. Role of bile acid malabsorption in pathogenesis of diarrhea and steatorrhea in patients with ileal resection. I. Response to cholestyramine or replacement of dietary long chain triglyceride by medium chain triglyceride. *Gastroenterology* 1972; **69**: 918.
37. Dharmsathaphorn K, Gorelick FS, Sherwin RS et al. Somatostatin decreases diarrhea in patients with the short-bowel syndrome. *J Clin Gastroenterol* 1982; **4**: 521.
38. Nightingale JMD, Walker ER, Burnham WR et al. Octreotide (a somatostatin analogue) improves the quality of life in some patients with a short intestine. *Aliment Pharmacol Therap* 1989; **3**: 367.

39. O'Hanrahan T & Irving MH. The role of home parenteral nutrition in the management of intestinal failure: report of 400 cases. *Clin Nutr* 1992; **11**: 331–336.

40. Johnston DA, Richards J & Pennington CR. Auditing the effect of experience and change on home parenteral nutrition related complications. *Clin Nutr* 1994; **13**: 341–344.

41. Detsky AS, McLaughlin JR, Abrams AB et al. A cost–utility analysis of the home parenteral nutrition program at Toronto General Hospital: 1970–1982. *J Parenter Enteral Nutr* 1986; **10**: 49–57.

42. Richards DM & Irving MH. Cost–utility analysis of home parenteral nutrition. *Br J Surg* 1996; **83**: 1226–1229.

43. Irving MH. Ethical problems associated with the treatment of intestinal failure. *Aust NZ J Surg* 1986; **56**: 425–427.

44. Messing B, Lémann M, Landais P et al. Prognosis of patients with nonmalignant chronic intestinal failure receiving long-term home parenteral nutrition. *Gastroenterology* 1995; **108**: 1005–1010.

45. Thompson JS. Surgical considerations in the short bowel syndrome. *Surg Gynecol Obstet* 1993; **176**: 89–101.

46. Thompson JS, Langnas AN, Pinch LW, Kaufman S, Quigley EMM & Vanderhoof JA. Surgical approach to short bowel syndrome. Experience in a population of 160 patients. *Ann Surg* 1995; **222**: 600–607.

47. Thompson JS, Pinch LW, Murray N et al. Experience with intestinal lengthening for the short bowel syndrome. *J Pediatr Surg* 1991; **26**: 721–724.

48. Panis Y, Messing B, Rivet P et al. Segmental reversal of the small bowel as an alternative to intestinal transplantation in patients with short bowel syndrome. *Ann Surg* 1997; **225**: 401–407.

49. Wood RFM. Small bowel transplantation. *Br J Surg* 1992; **79**: 193–194.

50. Todo S, Reyes J, Furukawa H et al. Outcome analysis of 71 clinical intestinal transplantations. *Ann Surg* 1995; **222**: 170–282.

51. Mason EE. Development of gastric bypass and gastroplasty. In Maxwell JD, Gazet J-C & Pilkington TR (eds) *Surgical Management of Obesity*. London: Academic Press, 1980: 29–39.

52. Williamson RCN. Intestinal adaptation. Structural, functional and cytokinetic changes. *N Engl J Med* 1978; **298**: 1393–1402.

53. Senn N. An experimental contribution to intestinal surgery with special reference to the treatment of intestinal obstruction. II. Enterectomy. *Ann Surg* 1888; **7**: 99–115.

54. Flint JM. The effect of extensive resections of the small intestine. *Bull Johns Hopkins Hosp* 1912; **23**: 127–144.

55. Bristol JB & Williamson RCN. Nutrition, operations and intestinal adaptation. *J Parenter Enteral Nutr* 1988; **12**: 299–309.

56. Williamson RCN. Disuse atrophy of the intestinal tract. *Clin Nutr* 1984; **3**: 169–170.

57. Dowling RH. Small bowel adaptation and its regulation. *Scand J Gastroenterol* 1982; **17** (Suppl 174): 53–74.

58. Bristol JB & Williamson RCN. Postoperative adaptation of the small intestine. *World J Surg* 1985; **9**: 825–832.

59. Chaves M, Smith MW & Williamson RCN. Increased activity of digestive enzymes in ileal enterocytes adapting to proximal small bowel resection. *Gut* 1987; **28**: 981–987.

60. Grönqvist B, Engström B & Grimelius L. Morphological studies of the rat small intestine after jejuno-ileal transposition. *Acta Chir Scand* 1975; **141**: 208–217.

61. Feldman EJ, Dowling RH, McNaughton J et al. Effect of oral versus intravenous nutrition on intestinal adaptation after small bowel resection in the dog. *Gastroenterology* 1976; **70**: 712–719.

62. Bristol JB & Williamson RCN. Mechanisms of intestinal adaptation. *Pediatr Surg Int* 1988; **4**: 233–241.

63. Sagor GR, Ghatei MA, Al-Mukhtar MYT, Wright NA & Bloom SR Evidence for a humoral mechanism after small intestinal resection. Exclusion of gastrin but not enteroglucagon. *Gastroenterology* 1983; **84**: 902–906.

64. Gleeson MH, Bloom SR, Polak J, Henry K & Dowling RH. Endocrine tumour in kidney affecting small bowel structure, motility and absorptive function. *Gut* 1971; **12**: 773–782

65. Miskowiak J & Andersen B. Intestinal adaptation after jejunoileal bypass for morbid obesity: a possible explanation for inadequate weight loss. *Br J Surg* 1983; **70**: 27–30.

47

INJURIES TO THE SMALL INTESTINE

DB McConnell
DD Trunkey

The incidence of injury to the small bowel in penetrating trauma is high. It occurs in 60% of patients with gunshot wounds and 18% of patients with stab wounds to the abdomen.[1,2] By contrast, small bowel injury in patients with blunt abdominal trauma is less frequent but still occurs in 12% of patients.[3] Interestingly, small bowel injury is much less frequent in children than it is in adults who have blunt trauma to the torso.

Although small bowel leads the list in terms of being the most frequently injured organ in penetrating trauma, other organs are often injured at the same time. Only 25% of patients will have a single organ injury with gunshot wounds. Colon, liver, stomach and kidney follow small bowel as the organs most often injured in penetrating abdominal trauma.[1] In blunt trauma, however, small bowel injury trails splenic injury, liver injury and renal injury in frequency. Small bowel injury is about one-third as frequent as splenic injury and one-half as frequent as liver or kidney injury.

It is useful for the trauma surgeon to conceptualize the torso of the trauma patient as a cylinder divided into zones. We have divided the torso into three primary zones, going from cephalad to caudad.[4] Zone I comprises the upper torso from clavicles to nipples. Zone II consists of the area between the nipples and umbilicus. Zone III comprises the remaining lower torso, including the pelvis (Figure 47.1). Blunt or penetrating trauma to zones II or III may produce small bowel injury regardless of whether the injury is centrally or laterally located.

This chapter reviews some of the common mechanisms of injury resulting in duodenal, small bowel and mesenteric injury, plus diagnostic methods in current use and technical aspects of small bowel repair. Current methods of evaluating small bowel viability are also discussed.

DIAGNOSTIC METHODS

Patients greatly benefit from the early diagnosis and treatment of serious injuries, and injuries to the small bowel and duodenum are no exception. Let us examine the diagnostic methods

in current use in the trauma patient. The enormous value of the history of injury which can be obtained from the patient, the ambulance or air transport crew or other members of the family should not be overlooked. Information of particular value with regard to abdominal trauma includes whether or not a seat-belt was worn, use of an air-bag in the vehicle, time of last meal, use of alcohol or drugs, condition and kind of vehicle, steering column injury, difficulty with extraction, presence or absence of

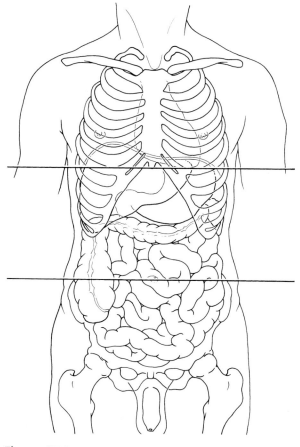

Figure 47.1
Sagittal zones of the torso.

ejection from the vehicle at time of injury, time of transport and estimated speed of vehicle. The patient's past medical history is relevant and should be obtained from the patient, if possible, or family members if necessary. In penetrating injuries valuable facts in assessment include calibre of weapon, distance from the assailant (particularly relevant with shotgun injuries), knife length and an estimate of the amount of blood loss at the scene. Although the patient may contribute some of this information, the investigating police or ambulance personnel will be a valid source of information as well.

The purpose of the initial physical examination and subsequent serial examinations is to detect all important injuries, to determine the need for further diagnostic studies and to evaluate the necessity and timing of operation. A positive physical examination is very reliable; however, many patients with injuries requiring operation have either an equivocal examination or a negative examination. Patients with multiple injuries may have pain in so many locations that the abdominal examination is misleading. Patients with head injury and those with paraplegia need diagnostic studies beyond physical examination. Many injured patients present with high levels of blood alcohol or other chemical substances that may alter mental status and lead to a false-negative physical examination. Although patients with small bowel or duodenal injury may demonstrate enough peritoneal irritation to indicate laparotomy on physical examination, patients with multiple injuries may need diagnostic peritoneal lavage or contrast-enhanced computed tomography (CT) to aid in the decision for laparotomy. Both of these diagnostic aids have been extensively evaluated in the past few years, yet complete agreement about the indications for laparotomy has not yet been reached, particularly as they pertain to small bowel injury.

Diagnostic peritoneal lavage

Diagnostic peritoneal lavage (DPL) is useful in blunt abdominal trauma and in certain patients with penetrating abdominal trauma.

Indications[5]

● Multiply injured patient with equivocal abdominal examination.

● Multiply injured patient with head injury, evidence of intoxication, presence of paraplegia.

● Multiply injured patient with anticipated lengthy radiological diagnostic procedures requiring general anaesthesia for other injuries.

● Patients with unexplained hypotension or blood loss.

Although it is usually stated that the haemodynamically unstable patient does not need a DPL because the need for laparotomy is obvious, exceptions are easily found. For instance, a patient with a pelvic fracture may be haemodynamically unstable from retroperitoneal bleeding or intraperitoneal bleeding. In this example, a supraumbilical DPL may be of value. DPL has been particularly useful in our experience in the multiply injured patient who is unconscious and needs to

be rushed to the operating room for care of extra-abdominal injuries. The DPL can be performed quickly, usually, in less than 5 minutes, and will help to prioritize decision-making. In a few instances, craniotomy has been done at the same time as laparotomy because of simultaneous acute epidural haematoma and splenic rupture, the diagnosis of which was suggested by an intraoperative DPL.

Findings that indicate the need for laparotomy[5]

1. < 5 ml gross blood

2. Obvious intestinal content

3. Lavage fluid observed to exit via chest tube or indwelling urinary catheter

4. Laboratory analysis of lavage fluid:
   (a) > 100 000 red blood cells/mm^3
   (b) > 500 white blood cells/mm^3.

The DPL has excellent sensitivity for intraperitoneal bleeding; however, it is known to have a 2% false-negative rate.[6,7] Typically the injuries missed by DPL are pancreatic, retroperitoneal duodenal, bladder or small bowel injuries. The first three are missed because of the retroperitoneal location. Small bowel injuries may be missed because of their paucity of bleeding. It should be emphasized that the DPL only evaluates intraperitoneal injuries. It will probably not detect an injury to the diaphragm unless this is associated with bleeding. Furthermore, patients with previous abdominal surgery may have some quadrants of the abdomen walled off by adhesions, limiting distribution of the lavage fluid and creating and false-negative examination.

Technical aspects

Ideally, patients selected for DPL should not have previous lower abdominal incisions. Both the stomach and bladder should be decompressed with appropriate tubes. A standard surgical skin preparation is employed. Using 1% lignocaine with adrenaline, the midline is anaesthetized; the incision is centred about one-third of the distance from the unbilicus to the symphysis pubis. We prefer to open the peritoneum directly rather than puncturing it blindly. A peritoneal dialysis catheter is advanced into the pelvis. A syringe is then directly connected to the dialysis catheter and aspirated. If no blood is withdrawn, 10 ml/kg of Ringer-Lactate solution warmed to 37°C is infused into the peritoneal cavity. After a few minutes to allow distribution throughout the peritoneal cavity, the collection bottle is placed on the floor and the periotneal fluid is collected. This fluid is analysed for red cells, white cells, and gestrointestinal content. In most patients, inspection of the aspirate is sufficient for clinical decision making. Equipment needed for a DPL is minimal and is available in kit form from many suppliers.

Contrast-enhanced computed tomography

At the Oregon Health Sciences University we use a GE Hi Speed/i Helical CT Scanner, version 3.5. The typical abdominal CT scan takes 15–20 minutes to complete, not counting transportation time. CT scanning is of cnormous value in patients with abdominal trauma; however, *its use should apply to only haemodynamically stable patients.* If the study is deemed important, even the uncooperative patient can be successfully studied by intubating, providing mechanical ventilation and maintaining a state of paralysis with non-depolarizing paralysing agents. CT is particularly applicable to patients with blunt abdominal trauma. Federle et al.[8] found it useful in splenic injuries, hepatic injuries, pancreatic injuries, duodenal trauma and renal trauma. Intraperitoneal structures can be evaluated as well as retroperitoneal structures. Rib fractures, spinal fractures and pelvic fractures are readily identified via bone windows in the course of performing abdominal and pelvic CT. With regard to duodenal injury, CT may demonstrate small amounts of retroperitoneal gas and extravasated intestinal contrast, thus making the need for laparotomy obvious. Similarly, small bowel injury may be detected by either extravasation of contrast or identification of localized bowel oedema.[9]

Most trauma centres now consider DPL and CT to be complementary studies, not competitive. Goldstein and associates[10] recommend CT over DPL, finding it to be more sensitive and specific; they also noted that no important injuries were missed by CT. Fischer et al.[3] point out that blunt abdominal trauma resulted in small bowel injury in 26% of adults and 7% of children, emphasizing the need for early diagnosis and management. Unlike Goldstein, Fischer concluded that CT was insufficiently sensitive for the reliable detection of gastrointestinal disruption, apparently recommending exploratory laparotomy as a diagnostic tool in questionable cases. We continue to recommend well-performed CT in appropriately selected patients. Interpretation by a senior radiologist is an instrumental part of the successful use of this technique in the trauma patient. Although we currently prefer double-contrast CT in awake, stable patients, we are willing to do a DPL, if it can be done quickly, or an exploratory laparotomy in the unstable patient with multiple injuries. Thus in certain patients laparotomy becomes the ultimate diagnostic tool for evaluating serious intra-abdominal injury.

Caution should be applied to interpretation of CT in patients who have had a preceding DPL. The DPL will introduce air into the peritoneal cavity, which negates the most reliable CT sign of gastrointestinal disruption. Similarly, residual lavage fluid can be misinterpreted as blood, misleading the radiologist in interpretation of the CT scan.

BLUNT TRAUMA TO THE DUODENUM

The anatomy of the duodenum, particularly its retroperitoneal position and integral relationship with the spine, figures heavily in understanding blunt duodenal trauma.[11] Similarly, the intimate relationship between the head of the pancreas and the first, second and third parts of the duodenum provides an opportunity for complex combined duodenal and pancreatic injury. Thus we see a spectrum of injuries ranging from submucosal haematoma to complete duodenal wall disruption with pancreatic and bile duct injury. Centred over the right lateral border of L1 and L2, the duodenum becomes relatively

fixed in a retroperitoneal position, subsequently emerging anterior to the body of L2 to again become intraperitoneal as the jejunum. Although the duodenum and pancreas are located deep in the upper abdomen, blows to the anterior abdomen can compress the duodenum and pancreas against the spine, producing serious injury. In children the rib-cage provides even less protection to upper abdominal structures than it does in adults.

Intramural haematoma

Blunt duodenal trauma can produce a shear injury, which results in an intramural haematoma of the duodenum. Although this clinical entity can occur at any age, the highest proportion of patients is among the paediatric age group. Patients present with progressive signs and symptoms of an upper abdominal bowel obstruction, i.e. bilious vomiting. A right upper quadrant mass may be palpated in 40%, but contrast-enhanced CT usually demonstrates the duodenal injury. Other clinical findings include a large gastric air–fluid level, little gas in the small bowel and an absent right psoas shadow on an abdominal radiograph. Contrast-enhanced CT has superseded Gastrografin studies of the upper gastrointestinal tract because CT provides the advantage of visualizing and locating other intraperitoneal and retroperitoneal pathology. Experienced paediatric surgeons are divided over routine non-operative versus operative therapy for intramural duodenal hematoma. Fullen and associates[12] described successful non-operative management in 11 patients with this condition. If early laparotomy is not dictated by associated injuries, one has the option of supportive care, hoping for spontaneous reabsorption of the haematoma. Some surgeons indicate a 75% success rate with non-operative management. Supportive care will consist of nasogastric suction, nutritional support and periodic physical examination. If there is no improvement after 2 weeks, laparotomy should be performed. Walt[13] has recommended that operation should be chosen if obstruction persists beyond 10 days, if pain seems to be increasing or if there is evidence of bleeding into the lumen of the bowel or into the peritoneal cavity. In adult patients we prefer early evacuation of the haematoma, exploration for other injuries and feeding jejunostomy.

Should operation be chosen for duodenal haematoma, the operative procedure consists of a generous Kocher manoeuvre to evaluate the duodenum for perforation. The duodenal wall is then incised directly over the haematoma, taking care to not enter the duodenal lumen. After evacuating the haematoma and assuring hemostasis, the duodenal wall is repaired with interrupted silk sutures. We prefer to leave a closed suction drain near the repair. A gastrojejunostomy is rarely needed if the injury is a proven duodenal wall haematoma. Gastrojejunostomy is reserved for patients whose duodenal obstruction persists postoperatively or whose injury is more extensive.

Disruption of the integrity of the duodenal wall

There are many options for management when a full-thickness duodenal wall injury is present (Figure 47.2). The optimal

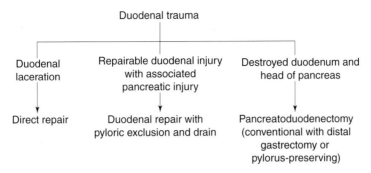

Figure 47.2
Duodenal trauma decision tree.

method of repair depends on location of injury, associated injury to adjacent structures and, in some cases, severity of local peritonitis. Clearly, early diagnosis of duodenal injury is advantageous and leads to the lowest possible morbidity and mortality.

At operation, full-thickness duodenal injury should be suspected if bile staining is noted near the duodenum. The adjacent retroperitoneum may take on a glistening appearance. Retroperitoneal crepitus indicating gas extravasation is another certain sign of disruption of the integrity of the duodenal wall.

Successful repair of duodenal wall laceration requires meticulous attention to technical aspects of the closure. The closure must reapproximate the injured wall in such a way that leakage as well as obstruction of the lumen is avoided. We prefer a two-layer closure, with a mucosal closure of running, absorbable monofilament suture protected by an outer layer of interrupted 3/0 or 4/0 silk Lembert sutures. If possible the wound is closed transversely. To ensure no tension on the suture line, a generous Kocher manoeuvre is carried out. In general the duodenal blood supply is so rich that viability of the injured wall is seldom an issue.

Simple laceration of the duodenal wall accounts for the majority of duodenal injuries. On rare occasions, however, a larger portion of the duodenal wall is non-viable, necessitating more extensive debridement. In these few instances other more intricate methods of repair are advocated. Options available include resection with end-to-end anastomosis, Roux-en-Y duodenojejunostomy, serosal patch with jejunum and jejunal patch.[14]

Resection of the injured portion of duodenum with end-to-end anastamosis is most applicable to injury in the proximal first part and the distal third and fourth parts of the duodenum, where the medial wall of the duodenum is not firmly adherent to the pancreas. The Roux-en-Y duodenojejunostomy is both extremely useful and the preferred method of repair of large defects of the second and third parts of the duodenum. Advantages of the Roux loop are related to its ability to provide closure of large, odd-shaped defects and the loop brings with it its own blood supply. In instances where complete transection has occurred at the level of the ampulla and end-to-end anastomosis would appear to be difficult because of tension, closure of the distal end and Roux-en-Y anastomosis to the proximal end provides an acceptable solution. By contrast, transection

injuries in the proximal duodenum may best be handled by closure of the distal duodenal stump, antrectomy and gastrojejunostomy.

Confusion exists over indications for duodenal diverticulization as described by Berne et al.,[15] or duodenal exclusion as described by Vaughan et al.[16] This kind of procedure is needed when the duodenal repair is possible, but there is such concern about postoperative fistula that it is best to divert the gastrointestinal stream away from the injured duodenum.

Duodenal diverticulization or duodenal exclusion

The indications are:

- Duodenal repair or postoperative oedema that may compromise the lumen;
- Concern that duodenal fistula is a strong possibilty;
- Combined duodenal and pancreatic injury.

The essential components of the Berne operation consist of closure of the duodenal injury, antrectomy with gastrojejunostomy (end of stomach to side of jejunum), tube duodenostomy and complementary drainage. By diverting the gastroenteric stream away from the duodenum, the duodenum is said to be 'diverticulized'. In Berne's original publication in 1968, this procedure was reported done in 16 patients, with three deaths. In 1974, the series was updated with an additional 34 patients. Overall, the combined mortality rate was 16%. Complications reported with this operation included seven duodenal fistulas (14%), five pancreatic fistulas (10%) and 11 patients (22%) with minor sepsis not requiring drainage of an abscess. It is notable that all the pancreatic fistulas and four of seven duodenal fistulas closed spontaneously. The feared complication of lateral duodenal fistula with its notoriously high mortality rate is aborted by the Berne 'diverticulization'. Any fistula that occurs has been converted to an end fistula with much less dire consequences. In essence, the diverticulization procedure is said to be a middle-of-the-road therapeutic concept between simple duodenal closure or patch repair on the one hand and pancreatoduodenectomy on the other. In their 1974 publication Berne and his associates[3] also recommended drainage of the common duct if the pancreatic injury lies near its intrapancreatic portion, but advised cholecystostomy if the common duct was small. We do not believe these manoeuvres are necessary.

In 1977 Vaughan et al.[16] introduced the pyloric exclusion operation as a means of producing duodenal diverticulization. This procedure was carried out in 75 patients out of a larger group of 175 patients with duodenal and pancreatic trauma. This technically easier procedure achieved temporary diverticularization of the duodenum and eliminated the antrectomy. Devised by Jordan, this operation consists of repair of the duodenal wound by measures judged most appropriate. As a last stage of the operation, a site is chosen for gastrojejunostomy near the pylorus. Once the gastrotomy is made, the pylorus is visualized, then oversewn with absorbable suture. The gastrojejunostomy is completed without adding a vagotomy. The mortality rate in patients in Vaughan et al.'s series for those needing pyloric exclusion was 19%; however, the incidence of duodenal fistula was only 5%. It is noteworthy that only one patient died as a result of formation of a duodenal fistula in this series. Certainly this represents an advance because the complication of a lateral duodenal fistula has previously been associated with high mortality and considerable morbidity rates. Apparently, by using absorbable sutures, the pyloric closure reopens remotely enough from the time of injury and operation to provide temporary diversion of the gastroenteric stream when needed. Commenting on diverticulization procedures, Walt[13] stated that these procedures are not often necessary, but when there is an associated pancreatic injury, the exclusion procedure has been very effective. Walt also advocates liberal use of postoperative drains as well as a lateral duodenostomy, which is kept on gentle suction for 14 days as a controlled fistula. The procedure described by Vaughan has generally replaced the earlier procedure described by Berne. The pylorus tends to reopen in 3–4 weeks. In the 10% of patients who develop a pancreatic fistula, most will spontaneously cease. Recent availability of somatostatin has facilitated the care of pancreatic fistulas and shortened their course.

Duodenal resection procedures are reserved for the few patients who have such extensive duodenal and pancreatic injury that these structures are essentially unrepairable or nonvital. Depending on the extent and specific site of injury, two operations may be applicable in this setting. The first is the standard pancreatoduodenectomy. In this procedure the reconstruction consists of an end-to-end pancreatojejunostomy with the end of pancreas invaginated deeply into the jejunum. An end-to-side choledochojejunostomy is then constructed several centimetres from the first anastomosis. Finally an end-to-side gastrojejunostomy is constructed in the antecolic position. If the injury lends itself to preservation of the pylorus, a pylorus-preserving pancreatoduodenectomy can be done, resulting in less physiological disturbance than the standard pancreatoduodenectomy. The reconstruction in this instance consists of an end-to-end pancreatojejunostomy, choledochojejunostomy and end-to-side duodenojejunostomy. In both methods of reconstruction, the pancreas is invaginated for several centimetres into the end of the jejunum. A stent may be left in the pancreatic duct to divert pancreatic secretions until healing has occurred.

Resection of the pancreas and duodenum for injury is carried out in the presence of a normal-sized (i.e. small) common bile duct, which can make the choledochojejunostomy technically difficult. A useful technique is to use a modified Carrel patch technique, which is illustrated in Figures 47.3.

BLUNT TRAUMA TO THE SMALL BOWEL

An important mechanism of small bowel injury is that which occurs in patients wearing a lap seat-belt.[17-19] Small bowel may be trapped between the patient's spine and the seat-belt. This can result in loss of integrity of the bowel wall by direct contusion, laceration or a blow-out effect of a closed loop. A high index of suspicion should lead to early diagnosis and management of patients with this injury. Typically, patients may have an associated lumbar spine fracture when trunk flexion is severe. In Appleby and Nagy's series,[17] 19% had associated lumbar spine injury. Although the mechanism of injury should alert the physician to the possibility of injury diagnosis of small bowel injury is sometimes unfortunately delayed. Delay occurs because many of these patients have multiple injuries which make typical peritoneal signs difficult to elicit. Characteristically, patients may have seat-belt markings on their abdominal wall skin (Figures 47.4, 47.5 and 47.6). In some, necrotic subcutaneous fat will need sharp debridement. We have recently cared for a child with a severe seat belt injury, including abdominal wall injury, small

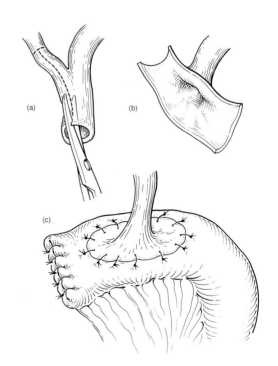

Figure 47.3
Following trauma to the common duct it may be necessary to reimplant the duct into a Roux-en-Y loop of jejunum. Since the common duct is often small, in these instances it may be necessary to do a 'patch'. In (a) the cystic duct is transected and the gall bladder removed. An incision in the common and cystic duct is made as shown by the dotted line. The patch shown in (b) is then sewn into the Roux-en-Y (c).

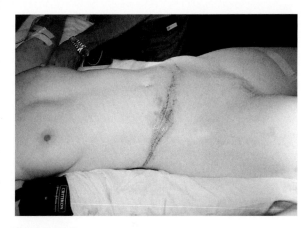

Figure 47.4
A typical seat belt injury.

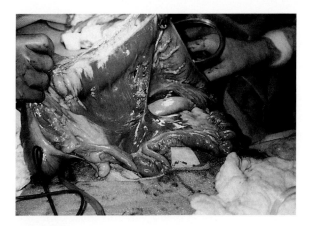

Figure 47.6
The operative picture shows the extensive bleeding into the mesentery (Figure 47.5).

bowel and colon injury, and spine injury which unfortunately included paraplegia.

STAB WOUND TO THE ABDOMEN

The management of stab wounds to the lower torso has changed from a policy of mandatory laparotomy to one of selective management[2,20–22] (Figure 47.7). Under the mandatory operation rule, many patients had a non-therapeutic operation. The role of physical examination in patients with abdominal stab wounds is recognized as the diagnostic method that results in the fewest unnecessary laparotomies, yet definitive treatment is often delayed. Patients with peritoneal irritation, absent bowel sounds or evidence of shock clearly need immediate laparotomy. Stable patients with none of these findings may undergo local wound exploration. If the wound appears to be simply a tangential slash, it can be properly cared for and the patient discharged. In patients with possible peritoneal penetration, hospitalization is needed for serial physical examinations, haematocrit and white cell counts and amylase estimations. If blood is found in the nasogastric aspirate, stools or

urine, laparotomy should be considered. Similarly patients who require greater volumes of crystalloid solutions than expected should be re-evaluated for possible laparotomy. Some centres recommend a DPL to aid in their decision for operation. It should be noted that the number of RBC/mm^3 for a positive DPL is much lower in penetrating wounds because intestinal injuries often do not bleed very much. Others advocate contrast-enhanced CT, which allows detection of retroperitoneal injury as well as intraperitoneal injury. CT has been particularly useful when the stab wound is located between the anterior axillary line and the paraspinous muscles.

At exploration for an abdominal stab wound, the objective is usually to identify and control all bleeding sites and repair all holes in the intestine. Although it is often stated that an even number of holes should be detected, this is not always the case. With regard to small bowel stab wounds, we prefer a two-layer closure, converting longitudinal wounds into transverse closure only if the wounds are large. Before carrying out a repair, the surgeon should debride any devitalized tissue. If

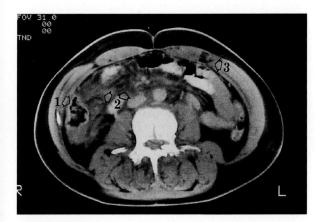

Figure 47.5
CT scan performed on the patient in Figure 47.4, showing air within the right colon wall (1) and extensive bleeding into the mesentery (2). Note also the disruption of the left rectus muscle (3).

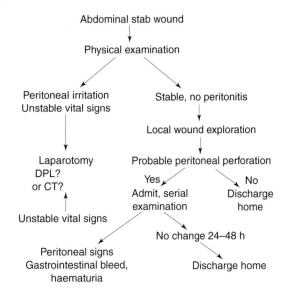

Figure 47.7
Management of the abdominal stab wound.

several intestinal holes are found in close proximity it may be wise to carry out a segmental resection and reanastomosis, including all of the injuries in the resected specimen. To avoid overlooking a rent, the entire intestine should be inspected methodically from the oesophageal hiatus to the rectosigmoid junction. It may be necessary to take down the ligament of Treitz or to completely mobilize the duodenum for adequate inspection of the entire bowel.

GUNSHOT WOUND TO THE ABDOMEN

Experience over several wars has revealed a steadily declining mortality rate with gunshot wounds of the abdomen; the current figure is 12% when optimally treated.[23] Small bowel leads the list of organs most frequently injured by a gunshot wound of the abdomen. About 25% of patients have a single organ injury, 33% have two organs injured, 20% have three organs injured and 10% have four organs injured.[1] Morbidity and mortality rates steadily increase as the number of injured organs increases.

In contrast to stab wounds, we take the categorical position that all patients with gunshot wounds to the abdomen should have a laparotomy (Figure 47.8). Only patients who can be shown to have tangential wounding with no entry into the peritoneal cavity are candidates for a non-operative approach.[24] Moore et al.[25] have cautioned us that occasionally patients with tangential wounds will have visceral injury due to high missile velocity and/or blast effect. Thus, these patients should be observed for an additional time even though they at first appear not to have any intraperitoneal injury. About half the patients with gunshot wounds in zone 2 will have entry of the missile into the abdomen with serious injury. An argument can be made for routine laparotomy in this group of patients even though their abdominal examination is initially benign. Small bowel injury was present in 20% of patients with gunshot wounds to the lower chest in Moore's series in 37% of patients with abdominal gunshot wounds.

At operation, management objectives for patients with abdominal gunshot wounds are similar to those for patients with stab wounds: repair if possible, resect if necessary. Resuscitation, which begins in the emergency department, continues in the operating room. In unstable patients the initial priority is control of haemorrhage. Repair of injury to the small bowel is deferred until haemorrhage is under control and other

life-threatening problems are dealt with. All holes must be identified, debrided and closed. If there is injury to adjacent mesentery resulting in a haematoma, the surgeon may wish to carry out simple evacuation of the haematoma and ligation of bleeding vessels.

Patients may have a haematoma located more proximally in the mesentery. Here it may be useful to gain proximal arterial and venous control before opening the haematoma to carry out ligation or arterial repair, as necessary.[26] Once the bleeding is controlled, the bowel must be carefully evaluated for adequacy of its arterial supply and venous drainage. To facilitate proximal control, the right colon can be mobilized. This allows proximal visualization and control of the superior mesenteric artery and vein as they emerge from the pancreas to cross over the duodenum. After evacuating the haematoma, small bleeding vessels may be ligated as needed. If the main trunk of the superior mesenteric artery has been injured, it may be segmentally repaired by using reversed saphenous vein or patched by using saphenous vein as needed. Proximal mesenteric venous injury may rapidly lead to intestinal infarction unless venous repair is done. This disastrous event may not be set in play until venous ligation is done. Venous collateral circulation is not reliable. If the distal mesenteric circulation is injured close to the bowel, the patient is best served by segmental bowel resection and end-to-end anastomosis. Although survival will occur with as little as 50 cm of small bowel, as much length as possible should be saved because quality of life is poor with a short gut syndrome. After completion of the vessel ligation or repair, the mesentery is reapproximated to avoid later entrapment of a small bowel loop. After debridement of devitalized tissue, the bowel is repaired using two-layer closure technique. In patients who undergo a segmental resection, a standard two-layer end-to-end anastomosis is most frequently used to restore continuity. A side-to-side anastomosis is seldom necessary.

Feliciano et al.[1] point out that there is a higher mortality rate from gunshot wounds to the abdomen when vascular structures are injured. Patients without vascular injuries have a 97% survival. The overall survival in their series was 88.3%.

ASSESSMENT OF SMALL BOWEL VIABILITY

Resection of a large segment of small bowel is not often necessary in the trauma patient. Conventional methods, i.e. visual

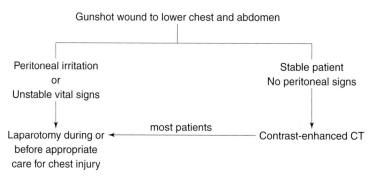

Figure 47.8
Management of gunshot wounds to the lower chest and abdomen.

inspection, palpation of arterial pulses, colour and peristalsis and bleeding from the cut ends of the bowel can be used to choose the points of resection. In the patient in whom a major portion of small bowel is threatened because of arterial or venous injury, it may be useful for the surgeon to have more sensitive means of assessing intestinal viability in the operating room. Furthermore, traditional means of assessing viability, such as bowel colour, presence of peristalsis and bleeding from the cut edge, are now regarded as unreliable predictors of viability.[27]

Several techniques for assessing viability have been described, including methods of evaluating blood flow and methods of detecting electrical activity of the bowel wall.[28-30] At the present time, assessment of bowel electrical activity is not yet perfected but appears promising.

Doppler ultrasonography was shown to be a useful clinical method for assessing intestinal viability by O'Donnell, Wright and Hobson[31-32] in 1975. In their study of bowel subjected to differing durations of ischaemia, the Doppler probe detected pulsatile flow and predicted viability when visual means could not distinguish between viable and non-viable bowel. These authors concluded that when intestinal blood flow could be detected in the serosa and mesentery–bowel junction, ultimate viability of the intestine was assured.

A second study by Cooperman and associates[33] determined that viability was predicted by the presence of a Doppler signal in the bowel wall. As the probe was moved further away from the point of the last signal, progressive degrees of necrosis were observed. The starting point for progressive necrosis was 1 cm from the last Doppler signal. Lynch and associates[34] compared Doppler ultrasonography with laser Doppler velocimetry and perfusion fluorometry in experimental ischaemic bowel segments. Although they found the laser Doppler index and perfusion fluorometry to be more sensitive than the simple hand-held Doppler in predicting non-viability, they concluded that standard Doppler compared favourably with these more refined studies. Because of low cost and ready availability, the standard Doppler will remain a useful adjunct in the operating room. Tollefson et al.[35] studied transserosal photoplethysmographic pulse oximetry and compared it with Doppler ultrasonography and a fluorescein test. In this animal study histological examination was used for control. No significant differences could be found among these three methods of assessing intestinal viability. The authors concluded that pulse oximetry was readily available in most operating rooms, operator independent and easy to interpret. It is the preferred alternative for objective intraoperative assessment of intestinal viability. Alos and associates[36] studied experimental jejunoileal anastomoses in dogs and similarly concluded that photoplethysmography was the preferred method of assessing intestinal viability in the presence of ischaemia. This method of assessment was found to be superior to Doppler ultrasonography in this study.

Carter and associates[37] evaluated qualitative fluorescence, quantitative fluorescence and clinical evaluation in predicting intestinal viability and expressed the results in terms of sensitivity and specificity. They found all three methods to have 100% specificity, but only quantitative fluorescence had 100% sensitivity. Clinical judgement and qualitative fluorescence had 33% and 11% sensitivity, respectively. These authors found that visual inspection led to misinterpretation, because a hyperfluorescent pattern often progressed to necrosis.

Qualitative fluorescence is a second inexpensive and readily available technique for evaluating intestinal viability in the operating room. In adults and children, 7.5 mg/kg injected intravenously should result in even distribution of fluorescein in the mesentery and intestinal wall in 1–2 minutes. When the operating room is darkened and ultraviolet illumination is provided by a Wood's lamp, an even distribution of bright-yellow fluorescense should normally be present. Non-viable intestine should remain dark. Bowel of questionable viability may have patchy areas of bright-yellow and darkened bowel wall. It has been our experience that the combination of the fluorescein and Doppler tests together with clinical judgement has allowed accurate prediction of intestinal viability with a very high confidence level. In fact, we use the Doppler to evaluate only areas thought to be questionable with the fluorescein test. In a review paper Horgan and Gorey[38] concluded that fluorescein tests and Doppler studies via ultrasonography or laser velocimetry were the most practical assessment tools in operating rooms today. There is not 100% correlation between perfusion and viability and Carters' and colleagues'[36] data contradict our clinical impression. Thus at the present time, when intestinal viability is uncertain even after the fluorescein test and the Doppler examination, and the segment to be resected is not trival, we re-explore the patient 18–24 hours later. We find this 'second look' operation to be an extremely valuable manoeuvre if bowel viability is marginal during the first laparotomy.[26]

REFERENCES

1. Feliciano DV, Burch JM, Jordan GL Jr et al. Abdominal gunshot wounds: an urban trauma center's experience with 300 consecutive patients. *Ann Surg* 1988; **208**: 362–370.
2. Steyn M. The management of abdominal stab wounds: the optimal algorithm. *S Afr J Surg* 1985; **23**: 18–22.
3. Fischer DP, Miller-Crotchett P & Reed L. Gastrointestinal disruption: the hazard of non-operative management in adults with blunt abdominal injury. *J Trauma* 1988; **28**: 1445–1449.
4. Trunkey DD. Torso trauma. *Curr Probl Surg* 1987; **24**: 164.
5. Committee on Trauma, American College of Surgeons. *Advanced Trauma Life Support Program for Physicians*. Chicago: American College of Surgeons, 1993.
6. Danne PD. Early management of abdominal trauma: the role of diagnostic peritoneal lavage. *Aust NZ J Surg* 1988; **58**: 879–887.
7. Thal ER, May RA & Beesinger D. Peritoneal lavage: its unreliability in gunshot wounds of the lower chest and abdomen. *Arch Surg* 1980; **115**: 430–433.
8. Federle MD, Crass R, Jeffrey B & Trunkey D. Computed tomography in blunt abdominal trauma. *Arch Surg* 1982; **117**: 645–650.
9. Donahue JH, Federle MP, Trunkey DD et al. Computed tomography in the diagnosis of blunt intestinal and mesenteric injuries. *J Trauma* 1987; **27**: 11–17.
10. Goldstein AS, Salvatore JA & Shafton GW. The diagnostic superiority of computéd tomography. *J Trauma* 1985; **25**: 938–943.
11. Snyder WH, Weigelt JA & Beitz DS. The surgical management of duodenal trauma – precepts based on a review of 247 cases. *Arch Surg* 1980; **115**: 422.
12. Fullen WD, Selle JG & Altemier WA. Intramural duodenal hematoma. *Ann Surg* 1974; **179**: 549–555.

13. Walt AJ. Chapter 40, Complications of gastrointestinal trauma. In Lazar JG (ed.) *Complications in Surgery and Trauma.* Philodelphia: Lippencott, 1984: chap. 40.

14. Jordan GL Jr. Injury to the pancreas and duodenum. In Matton KL, Moore EE & Feliciano DV (eds) *Trauma.* Norwalk, CT: Appleton & Lange, 1988: chap. 33.

15. Berne CJ, Donovan AJ, Yellin AE et al. Duodenal 'diverticularization' for duodenal and pancreatic injury. *Am J Surg* 1974; **127**: 503–507.

16. Vaughan GD III, Frazier OH & Jordan GL Jr. The use of pyloric exclusion in the management of severe duodenal injuries. *Am J Surg* 1977; **134**: 785–790.

17. Appleby JP & Nagy AG. Abdominal injuries associated with the use of seat belts. *Am J Surg* 1989; **157**: 457–458.

18. Denis R, Allad M, Allas H et al. Changing trends in abdominal injury in seat belt wearers. *J Trauma* 1983; **23**: 1007.

19. Williams JS & Kirkpatrick JR. The nature of seat belt injuries. *J Trauma* 1971; **11**: 207.

20. Coppa GF. Management of penetrating wounds of the back and flank. *Surg Gynecol Obstet* 1984; **159**: 514–518.

21. Nance FC, Wennar MH, Johnson LW, ingram JC & Cohn I Jr. Surgical judgment in the mangement of penetrating wounds of the abdomen: experience with 2212 patients. *Ann Surg* 1974; **179**: 639–646.

22. Zubowski R, Nallathambi M, Ivatuny R & Stahl W. Selective conservatism in abdominal stab wounds: the efficacy of serial physical examination. *J Trauma* 1988; **28**: 1665–1668.

23. Adams DB. Abdominal gunshot wounds in warfare: a historical review. *Milit Med* 1983; **148**: 15–20.

24. Lowe JR, Saletta JD, Read DR, Radhakrisman J & Moss GS. Should laparotomy be mandatory or selective in GSW of the abdomen? *J Trauma* 1977; **17**: 903–907.

25. Moore EE, Van Duzer-Moore & Thompson JS Mandatory laparotomy for gunshot wounds penetrating the abdomen. *Am J Surg* 1980; **140**: 847–851.

26. Christensen N. Small bowel and mesentery. In Blaisdell FW & Trunkey DD (eds) *Trauma Management*, vol. 1, New York: Thieme-Stratton, 1982: 149–163.

27. Boley S. Symposium on small and large bowel problems: determination of intestinal viability. *Contemp Surg* 1988; **33**: 100–101.

28. Brolin RE, Semmlow JL, Mackenzie JW et al. Quantitative myoeletric determination of bowel viability. *J Surg Res* 1986; **41**: 557–562.

29. Brolin RD, Semmlow JL, Koch RA et al. Myoelectric assessment of bowel viability. *Surgery* 1987; **102**: 32–38.

30. Orland PJ, Cazi GA & Brolin RE. Determination of small bowel viability using quantitative myoelectric and color analysis. *J Surg Res* 1993; **55**: 581–587.

31. O'Donnell JA & Hobson RW II. Operative confirmation of doppler ultrasound in evaluation of intestinal ischemia. *Surgery* 1980; **87**: 109–112.

32. Wright CB & Hobson RW II. Prediction of intestinal viability using doppler ultrasound technics. *Am J Surg* 1975; **129**: 642–645.

33. Cooperman M, Pace, WG, Carey LC et al. Determination of viability of ischemic intestine by doppler ultrasound. *Surgery* 1978; **83**: 705–710.

34. Lynch TG, Hobson RW, Keer JC et al. Doppler ultrasound, laser doppler and perfusion fluorometry in bowel ischemia. *Arch Surg* 1988; **123**: 483–486.

35. Tollefson DF, Wright DJ & Reddy DJ. Intraoperative determination of intestinal viability by pulse oximetry. *Ann Vasc Surg* 1995; **9**: 357–360.

36. Alos R, Garcia-Gonera E, Calvete J & Uribe W. The use of photoplethysmography and Doppler ultrasound to predict anastomotic viability after segmental intestinal ischaemia in dogs. *Eur J Surg* 1993; **159**: 35–41.

37. Carter MS, Fontini GA & Boley SJ. Qualitative and quantitative fluorescence in determining intestinal viability. *Am J Surg* 1984; **147**: 117–123.

38. Horgan PG & Gorey TF. Operative assessment of intestinal viability. *Surg Clin North Am* 1992; **72**: 153–155.

48

EXTERNAL FISTULAS OF THE SMALL BOWEL

P Frileux
Y Parc

'Modern times' in the management of enterocutaneous fistulas began in the early 1960s. Edmunds et al.[1] produced their classical study on 157 patients, reporting a high mortality rate and advocating early surgical repair. Trémolières et al.[2] proposed a concept of conservative management based on specialized local care and high calorie enteral intake, aiming at obtaining either spontaneous closure or suitable conditions for elective surgical closure.

In the following decade, MacFadyen et al.[3] reported the results obtained with parenteral hyperalimentation: a 6.5% mortality rate and a 70% rate of spontaneous closure. Although these results probably reflect some selection in the patient population, total parenteral nutrition (TPN) has since proved to be a mode of nutrition that is particularly well adapted to this condition and has become the mainstay of treatment in the English-speaking world. Lévy et al.[4] tested their method of continuous enteral nutrition (CEN) in patients with fistulas assuming that the slow transit obtained with continuous infusion of nutrients in a viscous solution could represent an appropriate mode of artificial nutrition, despite the exclusion of a segment of small bowel. Together with this policy of enteral nutrition, Lévy and co-workers[5,6] developed various procedures of fistula obturation and chyme reinfusion.

Enterocutaneous fistulas represent an emergency in two respects: local care and nutrition. Any fistula patient is at risk of surgical complications (evisceration, abdominal abscess, ileus, haemorrhage) and eventual organ failure. The cornerstones of successful treatment are the assiduous presence of both physician and surgeon at the patient's bedside, cohesion among the medical staff, precision and cautiousness in fistula assessment, and attention to detail in local care and general monitoring.

Current management of enterocutaneous fistulas does not include any early surgical attempt to repair the fistula. The basis of the treatment is a long period of medical support allowing for restoration of general condition and nutritional state, and resolution of the intense inflammatory peritoneal reaction. During this period, spontaneous closure of the fistula is sought and may be obtained in the presence of favourable anatomical conditions. Otherwise, closure of the fistula is realized by elective surgical repair in a well-prepared patient (Figure 48.1).

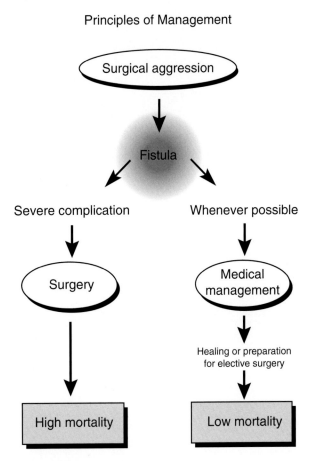

Figure 48.1
Principles of management of enterocutaneous fistulas.

Unfortunately, the presence of severe surgical complications may necessitate resorting to emergency operation. The principle of surgical management in such conditions is to exteriorize the bowel as a temporary stoma, leaving re-establishment of continuity for a subsequent stage. Emergency operation is associated with a high mortality rate.

Although they illustrate the failure of surgery (and of the surgeon), patients with fistulas should not be overlooked. They need strong and friendly psychological support from medical and nursing staff to face the long period of medical treatment and the possible re-operations required by their condition.

GENERAL CONSIDERATIONS

Definitions

A fistula is an abnormal communication between two epithelialized surfaces. An external fistula connects a hollow viscus (or several) to the skin; those arising from the small bowel are usually named 'enterocutaneous'.

Classification according to the type of intestinal orifice

Site Jejunal fistulas represent one-third of the total.[5] They are characterized by a high output (1500–7000 ml/24 h) and poor prognosis, and they are easily identified by the aspect of the effluent: clear, yellow or light green, with little solid debris and a pH above 7. Transit time from mouth to fistula is less than 30 minutes. Ileal fistulas have a lower output (50–3000 ml/24 h) and are indicated by the faeculent nature of the fluid, which is brown and contains solid debris. Both jejunal and ileal fistulas are injurious to the skin; in the setting of a combined fistula this fact allows recognition of the existence of an enteric component.

Number Single fistulas are those with one intestinal opening only, regardless of the number of external orifices on the skin. Multiple fistulas have several openings in the small bowel. Combined fistulas are those involving another hollow viscus in addition to the small bowel, such as colon, urinary bladder or vagina.

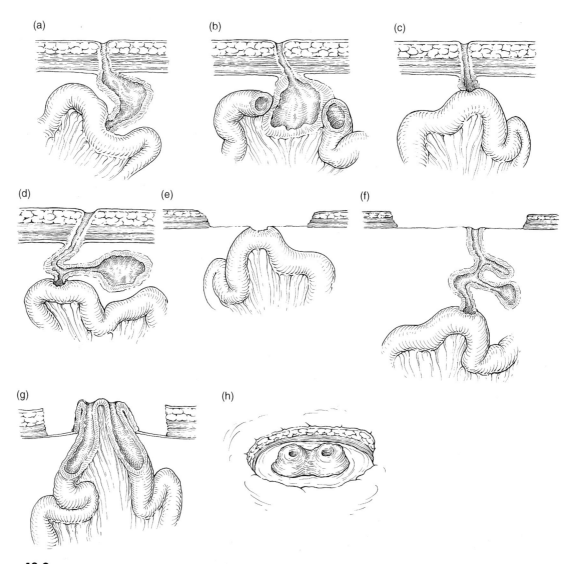

Figure 48.2

Definitions. (a) Lateral fistula; (b) end fistula; (c) direct fistula; (d) indirect fistula; (e) exposed fistula, direct type; (f) exposed fistula, indirect type; (g,h) exposed fistula with eversion of the intestine on to the granulation tissue (g, in section, h, external aspect);

Circumferential extent Lateral fistulas derive from a side opening in the bowel, which otherwise retains continuity, and are thus liable to close spontaneously. End fistulas result from a complete disruption of the bowel ends (Figure 48.2a,b); they are uncommon.[5]

Classification according to the fistula track and the external orifice

Track Direct fistulas are those in which the intestinal opening is visible from the outside. Indirect fistulas are those with a long, sinuous or multiple track with possible interposed pockets of pus forming intermediary cavities (Figure 48.2).

External opening Most enterocutaneous fistulas open into a surgical incision or a drainage site, and no major dehiscence of the abdominal wall is associated. Exposed fistulas[6] (Figure 48.2e–i) are those that open into a large dehiscence of the abdominal wall (greater than 20 cm²). Exposed fistulas have two distinct mechanisms of formation (Figure 48.3): bowel-to-wall fistulas (80% of the total) arise secondary to a leak from the small intestine and lead to an abscess draining spontaneously through the dehisced incision. Wall-to-bowel fistulas (20% of the total) arise secondary to external trauma inflicted on a superficial bowel loop exposed in an evisceration; they are always of direct type, whereas bowel-to-wall fistulas may be either direct or indirect (Figure 48.2).

Distinction between fistula and peritonitis associated with exteriorization of digestive fluid

In theory, these two conditions are fundamentally different. A fistula is an established communication with a track that is well walled off from the peritoneal cavity; it commonly requires conservative treatment. A leak with peritonitis and general effusion of digestive fluid, some of which escapes through the incision, requires urgent operation. However, the distinction may be subtle; these two situations may represent two different stages of evolution in the same patient, and the difference may be minimal between a fistula associated with multiple abscesses and a multiloculated peritonitis.

Aetiopathology

Spontaneous fistulas

Although it was not uncommon in the past to observe spontaneous enterocutaneous fistulas as a result of grossly advanced disease, they have become very rare outside the context of Crohn's disease.

Congenital fistulas occurring in adults result from persistent patency of the vitellointestinal duct; the opening of the track may be triggered by an episode of intestinal obstruction.

Traumatic fistulas follow injuries that have been unrecognized or underestimated. They are uncommon, although some

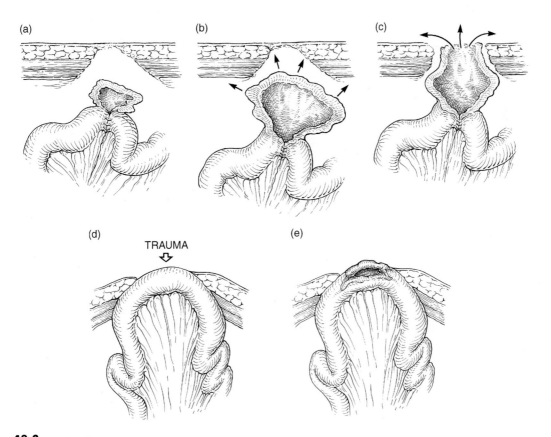

Figure 48.3

Exposed fistulas. Mechanisms of formation. a,b,c: bowel-to-wall; d,e: wall-to-bowel. (a) Anastomotic leak; (b) expanding sepsis; (c) abdominal wall dehiscence, spontaneous drainage of the purulent material and fistula; (d) superficial loop of intestine exposed in an evisceration (e.g. following laparostomy); (e) trauma – fistula.

bizarre enterocutaneous fistulas involving either the duodenum or the colon have been reported. Foreign bodies may lead to ileal perforation with abscess and fistula formation.

Fistulas related to specific diseases

Crohn's disease accounts for a substantial proportion of fistulas in Scandinavian, US and UK series (see also Chapter 51).[7,8] Two types are now clearly distinguished:[9] *type 1* represents the fistulas arising from a segment of bowel grossly involved by Crohn's disease and occurring either spontaneously or after a minor procedure (e.g. appendicectomy). They are rarely amenable to closure by medical treatment, although occasional cases of cure by 6-mercaptopurine have been reported. Radical cure can be obtained by a relatively simple surgical procedure with little or no risk. *Type 2* fistulas occur after resectional surgery for Crohn's disease and arise from a leak at the suture line. They represent a high-risk group because the general condition of the patient is poor, deep-seated abscesses are frequent, and satisfactory intestinal absorption may be impaired by the previous resection. However, type 2 fistulas may heal with conservative treatment since the leaking segment is free of major involvement by Crohn's disease. Conservative treatment is therefore the treatment of choice for a type 2 fistula. Should it not close, elective surgical repair becomes necessary; the procedure is frequently complex and associated with a high mortality and morbidity rate. In the Manchester series reporting 71 cases of Crohn's fistula, mortality rate was zero for type 1 fistula (0/49) and 18% for type 2 fistula (4/22).[10] In the Hospital Saint-Antoine (HSA) series including 21 type 2 Crohn's fistulas among a total of 335 postoperative high-output fistulas, six patients died (28%), six healed spontaneously (28%) and nine underwent surgical repair of the fistula (44%).[5]

Postirradiation fistulas represent the most difficult and can be the most distressing situation in fistula care (see also Chapter 52). They are either *spontaneous* following formation of an abscess due to a sealed perforation of the intestine or to an obstruction, or *postoperative* after re-operation for incisional hernia, intestinal obstruction or local recurrence. Spontaneous healing is possible provided the bowel bearing the fistulous orifice is not grossly involved by radiation disease. But the intestinal fistula is frequently combined with urinary or rectosigmoid damage, and often a complex repair is required. The series from Hôpital Saint-Antoine (HSA) included 38 postoperative fistulas associated with radiation-damaged bowel;[5] the mortality rate was 31%, the spontaneous closure rate 26% and the surgical closure rate 43%.

Fistulas associated with tuberculosis or actinomycosis are the basis of anecdotal case reports and develop either spontaneously or postoperatively.

Factors underlying common postoperative fistulas

There are two factors in the aetiopathology of common postoperative fistulas which form the bulk, if not the total, of many published series:[1,5,8] patient-related factors and operation-related factors.

Patient-related factors

Patient-related factors are diseases such as obesity, cirrhosis, diabetes, arteriosclerosis, respiratory insufficiency or steroid treatment. In these circumstances the healing capacity is decreased and there is an appreciable risk of sepsis after major abdominal procedures, thus explaining why these patients are prone to develop a fistula in their postoperative course. These chronic diseases also complicate the management and prognosis of the patient.

Acute surgical emergencies are not uncommonly followed by fistula formation. Thus in acute intestinal obstruction, hypoxia and inflammation of the bowel wall and intraluminal bacterial overgrowth create a 'high-risk' situation. However, if care is taken to evacuate bowel contents, perform peritoneal lavage and resect any bowel of questionable viability, an anastomosis may be carried out with reasonable safety. Trocar enterotomy for evacuation of bowel contents is the origin of several fistulas in our series, and this dangerous procedure should be abandoned. Acute peritonitis is associated with maximal impairment of the healing capacity of the bowel wall. It has been our recommendation for many years[11] to perform temporary enterostomy instead of primary suture under such conditions. In the HSA series, 40% of the operations responsible for fistula formation had been performed in an emergency setting. Anastomosis in an infected field was responsible for 12.5% of the fistulas.

Another patient-related factor is represented by situations leading to repeated laparotomies. Difficulty in dissection, bleeding and bowel loop injuries are frequent in reoperative surgery, putting the patient at risk of fistula development. In the HSA series, 72% of the fistulas followed reoperative surgery.

Operation-related factors

There are three anatomic mechanisms of fistula formation: anastomotic leakage, accounting for approximately 50% of cases; surgical trauma (35%); and bowel necrosis (15%). Within each category, inappropriate surgical procedures are often involved in the genesis of the fistula.

In fistulas due to anastomotic leakage the main error is intestinal suture in a grossly infected field, not only in the context of primary peritonitis (see above) but also in the context of early reoperation for a septic complication. It is true that temporary enterostomy – the procedure we advocate in such conditions – can pose difficulties of management, but the development of TPN, inhibitors of digestive secretion, modern appliances and chyme reinfusion[11] has solved virtually all these problems.

In fistulas due to surgical trauma there is a great variety of causative procedures.

1. Dissection of bowel loops in reoperative surgery may provoke lesions which, if unrecognized or overlooked, will lead to fistula.
2. Drains (tubes or corrugated drains) placed in contact with bowel loops are dangerous and ineffective, regardless of the material from which they are manufactured. With the

exception of capillary drainage (Mikulicz/packing) for severe peritonitis,[12] there is no place for tubes and drains in the infracolic compartment of the peritoneal cavity.

3. Bowel plication by suture of bowel loops or mesentery (Noble procedure, Childs–Phillips procedure), once recommended in the management of recurrent intestinal obstruction, was responsible for five fistulas in the HSA series, all five cases being extremely severe (multiple fistulas exposed in a wide evisceration).

4. Open abdomen (laparostomy) combined with scheduled relaparotomy is a technique proposed in the treatment of diffuse severe peritonitis and necrotizing pancreatitis. Although it may save lives, it is responsible for 10% of fistulas of the exposed 'wall-to-bowel' type, arising from the loops situated at the surface of the evisceration.[12] These exposed fistulas have a 30% mortality rate and are particularly difficult to handle in terms of local care. This technique should be restricted to extreme situations and practised only in specialist institutions where maximal experience may minimize the incidence of fistula formation.[12]

5. Abdominal wall closure using aggressive techniques – through and through retention suture, non-absorbable mesh in a septic field – are responsible for an appreciable number of exposed fistulas of the small bowel. The absorbable meshes now available (Vicryl®) are well tolerated in a contaminated abdomen and should be preferred. External binding by adhesive band provides a further protection against evisceration in the early postoperative period.

Fistulas in relation to bowel necrosis may occur in the context of a postoperative ileus, in which limited damage to a bowel loop at operation eventually becomes a transmural necrosis. Bowel necrosis leading to fistula may also follow operations in which a segment of intestine of dubious viability has been left in place – for example, with intestinal infarction, obstruction or involvement of the small bowel with a malignant tumour.

CHARACTERISTICS OF ENTEROCUTANEOUS FISTULAS

Circumstances of fistula formation and initial assessment

Time

Enterocutaneous fistulas usually occur between the third and 15th postoperative day. The earlier the onset of the fistula, the worse the prognosis, except when the fistula follows a limited reoperation, such as drainage of abscess. Late fistulas, appearing more than three months after operation, are usually 'benign'.

Diagnosis

Diagnosis of an external fistula poses few problems: there is spontaneous evacuation of gas and digestive fluid irritating the skin. The presence of fever, abdominal signs and discharge of pus in the preceding days is common; these signs usually subside as the fistula appears. In rare instances of low output fistulas combined with profuse suppuration, dye-markers or radiological studies may be necessary to make the diagnosis.

Clinical history

Immediate past clinical history should be established with the aim of finding one or several factors for fistula formation, whether patient-related or operation-related (see above). If no factor is found, the diagnosis of the primary disease should be critically reconsidered in the light of the postoperative complication represented by the fistula.

Assessment

Anatomical assessment is both clinical and radiological.

Clinical assessment The body surface should be inspected with sufficient light and sufficient time with the help of an atraumatic sucker and after removal of all dressings. All wounds and orifices are examined, allowing one to see the intestinal orifice in case of a direct fistula. Probing wounds and tracks with metal instruments or stiff tubes is prohibited. Coloured markers (methylene blue in high fistulas and carmine red in ileal fistulas) may give a rough indication of the level of the fistula and the speed of intestinal transit, and may indicate other external orifices communicating with the main track; dye tests may also help clarify the problem of combined fistulas.

Radiological assessment This is the cornerstone of investigation and the main guide to further management. Fistulography (Figure 48.4) is possible in indirect fistula only; a Foley catheter is inserted through the external orifice(s), the balloon is inflated and water-soluble contrast medium is injected. This examination requires the presence of both surgeon and radiologist. Progression of the contrast medium is followed under fluoroscopy, and films are taken at various angles. The aim of fistulography is to give a detailed assessment of the fistula track and to identify the organs involved. Gastrointestinal contrast studies allow precise evaluation of the bowel proximal to the fistula, show whether there is passage of medium distal to the point of leakage, and give complementary information in case of a combined fistula. Barium meal and follow-through is the basic examination. Colonic contrast studies are required if colonic or rectal involvement is suspected and also in the search for an obstruction at this level. Intravenous urography is performed if a communication with the urinary tract is indicated by clinical or radiological signs. Endoscopic retrograde catheterization of the papilla and pancreatography is occasionally required in enterocutaneous fistulas occurring after operations for acute necrotizing pancreatitis.

Endoscopic assessment has not been widely used in the past in the investigation and management of enterocutaneous fistulas, but its role is growing. Fibrescopes of various calibres may be introduced by a natural orifice (mouth or anus), a stoma or a fistula orifice and can explore both the bowel adjacent to the fistula and the track. Endoscopic injection of fibrin

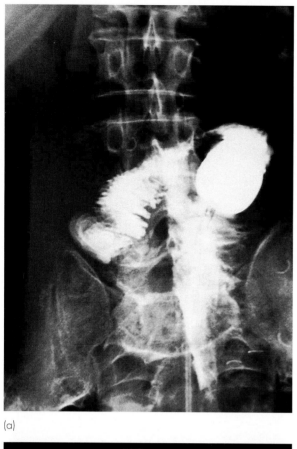

(a)

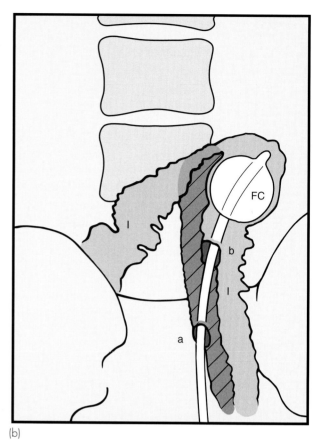

(b)

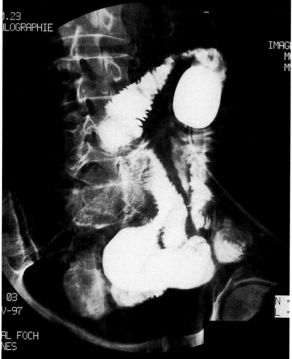

(c)

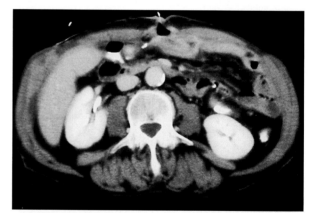

(d)

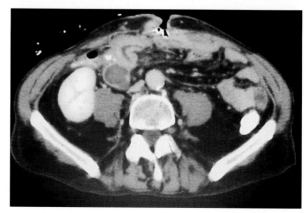

(e)

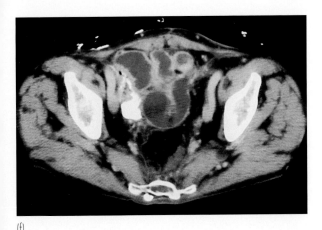
(f)

Figure 48.4
Imaging in a 73-year-old patient operated for obstructive radiation enteritis (dissection of adhesions plus short ileal resection). Recurrence of obstruction plus ileal fistula. (a) and (b). *Fistulography and diagram.* A Foley catheter (**FC**) is inserted through the external opening (**a**). It passes straight into a bowel loop (**I**). Contrast media shows a long intermediary cavity (hatched surface) communicating with the bowel (**b**) and situated below the midline scar. (c). *Fistulography.* Oblique view of the same opacification. (d) *CT Scan.* The sub-parietal cavity is clearly visible, filled with air. (e) *CT Scan.* Section showing the external opening. A thickened loop of intestine is visible on the right side, beneath the abdominal wall. (f) *CT Scan.* Section of the lower abdomen showing dilated loops of bowel, proximal to the fistula.

sealant from the lumen of the gut into the track has been reported as a successful means of management.[13]

Imaging by CT scan, ultrasound or MRI may help assess both abscess formation and the extent of the underlying disease. Demonstration of local recurrence or distant metastases clearly influences the choice of therapy in cancer patients.

Condition of the digestive tract

The total remaining length of small intestine, its nature and condition and the possible presence of an obstruction distal to the fistula will guide both nutritional management and local care. In cases of short bowel (i.e. remaining length of bowel less than 150 cm), nutritional problems predominate. Not only must fistula closure be obtained, but bowel adaptation must also be achieved before the patient is weaned off TPN. Enteral nutrition by means of CEN associated with obturation or chyme reinfusion should be undertaken as soon as possible provided it does not interfere with spontaneous healing, as it encourages intestinal adaptation to resection[14] (see Chapter 46).

Impact of the fistula

Amount of fistula effluent

'High-output' fistulas are those with daily volumes greater than 500 ml.[5,7] Measurement of the volume of fistula discharge should be carried out in a patient receiving nil by mouth, either by simple collection of the fluid or by subtraction between total output and volume of irrigation.

Preservation of spontaneous intestinal transit distal to the fistula is a favourable sign, indicating a partial fistula, whereas absence of distal transit is a symptom of distal obstruction or of an end fistula. Thus bowel actions should be measured and recorded.

Metabolic problems are common in high-output fistulas. In addition to loss of water, the fistula causes a large deficit in sodium, chloride, bicarbonate and potassium, leading to dehydration, hyponatraemia, metabolic acidosis and hypokalaemia. Water and electrolyte replacement is based on plasma and urine estimations. It should also be guided by the electrolyte composition of the fistula fluid as it may differ from physiological values in the presence of transit modification, plasma exudation and peritoneal inflammation.

Malnutrition affects virtually all patients with a high-output enterocutaneous fistula, being the cumulative consequence of primary disease, operation, sepsis and loss of chyme.[15] It is an important prognostic index and one of the elements leading to failure of early operative attempts at fistula repair. Malnutrition is reflected by weight loss, fall in indices such as serum albumin and impairment of delayed hypersensitivity skin tests. Although interesting in theory, sophisticated methods such as anthropometric measurements and total body composition analysis have little place in the routine monitoring of patients with fistula. In severe malnourished patients bedridden for a long time, complications such as pressure sores, deep vein thrombosis and muscle contractures are frequent; their prevention is difficult and tedious, and it requires a dedicated team of physiotherapists.

Factors predisposing to persistence of the fistula

Apart from general factors, such as malnutrition, some local characteristics of the fistula may impede spontaneous healing.

Intestinal obstruction distal to the fistula due to either tumour or inflammation will clearly require surgical correction. In addition to resection of the fistulated bowel, resection or bypass of the obstructed area will be necessary.

Direct contact between intestinal mucosa and body surface, which is frequent in the case of an exposed fistula (Figure 48.2f,h), precludes any possibility of closure. However, if the mucosa lies below the surface of the granulating tissue and if it is not everted, healing remains possible with the help of an obturating device (Figure 48.2e).

Deleterious action of the enzyme-rich fistula fluid, associated with purulent discharge from an undrained cavity, may attack the superficial part of the fistula track at the level of the skin and subcutaneous layer. This process leads to further cavitation instead of healing by granulation. Either irrigation of the track or decrease of enzyme concentration and fluid volume by TPN or an elemental diet may avoid this adverse effect.

Intra-abdominal abscesses prevent fistula closure in two ways: (1) they maintain the state of malnutrition, catabolism and ileus; and (2) when close to the fistula track, they impede the local healing process. When elective drainage can be efficiently carried out, fistula closure may occur. Failure of healing when an abscess is present and inaccessible to drainage has been stressed by many authors.[1,7] In the HSA series, of the patients presenting with a deep-seated abscess, only 13% healed spontaneously.

Total discontinuity of the bowel ends, a rare condition outside exposed fistulas with everted mucosa, does not allow spontaneous closure. The same applies to involvement of the fistulated bowel by a specific disease (carcinoma, Crohn's disease, severe radiation enteritis). The configuration of the fistula track also affects the chance of healing. A long, fine and straight track is favourable: the presence of multiple tracks and of intermediary cavities is unfavourable. If the fistula opens at the far end of a 'canopy' formed by a flap of abdominal wall (Figure 48.5), this is also an adverse factor.

Combined fistulas with the participation of another hollow viscus are unable to close spontaneously, regardless of the organ involved (colon, rectum, vagina, urinary tract).

Acute complications of enterocutaneous fistulas

Many prognostic scores have been described. This section details the current prognostic elements used at HSA[6] in the field of gastrointestinal intensive care (Table 48.1).

Multiple fistulas and combined fistulas These represent 35% of the cases in the HSA series. Their severity stems from the fact that they often follow extensive operations undertaken for serious diseases. Likewise, they require complex surgical procedures at the time of elective repair.

Intra-abdominal abscesses A moderate discharge from the external orifice or the wound is of little importance and warrants neither culture nor treatment. Deep-seated abscesses represent a major complication of external fistulas.[16,17] Whereas before the 1970s the prognostic determinants were electrolyte imbalance, nutritional problems and difficulty with local care,[1,18] the problem of sepsis now predominates for many reasons:[7] increased malnutrition, system or organ failure, poor healing and the necessity for

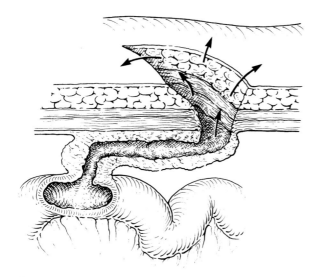

Figure 48.5
'Canopy' fistula.

Table 48.1 Complicating factors of enterocutaneous fistulas that affect prognosis: the experience of Hôpital St. Antoine[5] (335 cases)

Factor	Patients		Mortality rate when factor present	Mortality rate when factor absent
	n	%		
Multiple fistulas	116	35	48	26
Intra-abdominal abscesses	150	45	51	20
Septicaemia	130	39	55	20
Ileus	63	19	62	27
ARDS	104	31	69	18
Acute bleeding	60	18	62	28
Renal hepatic failure	120	36	66	16
Thromboembolic complications	39	12	64	30

ARDS, adult respiratory distress syndrome.

an urgent surgical procedure (elective drainage at the least, radical surgery at the most). In the HSA series 150 intra-abdominal abscesses were documented at operation, autopsy or by spontaneous evacuation (Table 48.1), and of these 85 (56%) required urgent operation because of evidence of major sepsis. Fifteen patients (10%) underwent elective drainage, 52 (35%) underwent radical operation with complete peritoneal dissection and creation of temporary enterostomies, whereas 18 (11%) were considered too ill to sustain such a procedure; they received a simple supportive therapy and died shortly after admission. In the other 65 patients (44%) the collection drained spontaneously or could be left in situ until time of elective operation.

Intra-abdominal sepsis is suspected in the presence of general signs of infection, abundant discharge of pus, a palpable mass or remote organ failure. Persisting malnutrition and absence of wound healing also indicate the presence of sepsis.[4,16] Although plain radiography studies may show air–fluid levels and abscess cavities, diagnosis of an intra-abdominal collection generally requires further imaging. Ultrasound scanning requires a dedicated and highly skilled operator as it is often a difficult and tedious enterprise, most frequently performed at the bedside with many dressings to undo. However, ultrasonography can be highly productive. It shows collections, allows percutaneous puncture and drainage and gives some information on the condition of the bowel.

CT scanning accurately demonstrates collections situated in the upper abdomen and retroperitoneum, but it is less reliable for the exploration of the infracolic compartment. In patients with complex dressings and/or organ failure, ultrasonography at the bedside is far more practical and represents the routine method of exploration.

Septicaemia Septicaemia originates from either intra-abdominal collections or an intravenous catheter. Abdominal collections are more frequent in the early period of management, and they provide a strong indication for emergency operation. In the HSA series, 58 of 130 patients (45%) with documented septicaemia required an emergency laparotomy.

The micro-organisms encountered in patients with fistulas are primarily enterococci, anaerobes and Gram-negative rods. After multiple laparotomies, recurrent septic events and repeated antibiotic therapy, patients are prone to nosocomial infections including *Staphylococcus* sp, fungi and *Acinetobacter* sp. In the most severe cases septicaemia may be complicated by endocarditis or metastatic abscess formation.

Ileus Ileus may be due to either peritoneal inflammation or adhesions surrounding a septic focus or the fistula site. Among the 63 HSA patients presenting with persisting ileus, 11 died at an early stage (18%); 17 (27%) resumed a normal transit within 15 days and could be managed conservatively, and 35 (55%) were reoperated for persistence of the obstruction or associated sepsis. Ultrasound or CT scanning may help to distinguish between inflammatory and mechanical obstruction, but the distinction is usually made on clinical grounds. Time may resolve the issue.

Adult respiratory distress syndrome (ARDS) ARDS requiring prolonged mechanical ventilation may be due to an intra-abdominal septic complication ('shock lung syndrome'), in which case early operation is required. Alternatively it may be due to other causes such as pre-existing respiratory insufficiency, aspiration pneumonia, pleural effusion, fluid overload, abdominal meteorism, functional incompetence of the abdominal wall or parenteral overload of glucose. Detailed analysis of the respiratory symptoms, a search for other signs of abdominal sepsis and evaluation of the patient's progress allows identification of the aetiology and the appropriate therapy. Among 104 patients with ARDS in the HSA series, one-third died early, one-third were reoperated as an emergency and one-third were managed conservatively and could be weaned from the ventilator.

Bleeding Acute bleeding may originate from either the upper gastrointestinal tract or the fistula track.

Acute 'stress' ulcers have become infrequent with the advent of prophylactic drugs, such as H_2-blockers, sucralfate and omeprazole. They can still occur at an early stage of management in unstable patients. Bleeding should if possible be managed conservatively or by endoscopic means, but acute ulcer is frequently a sign of severe sepsis. If a deep-seated abscess is found, it is a strong indication for urgent operation; intra-abdominal sepsis and fistula should be dealt with, and acute ulcer should be managed conservatively. The most complex situation is presented by acute bleeding from a chronic cavitating ulcer plus intra-abdominal sepsis; urgent operation should deal with both sepsis, fistula and bleeding ulcer.

Bleeding from the fistula track may arise from the granulation tissue, particularly in jejunal fistulas and in cases of poor drainage. Irrigation of the track, sometimes requiring massive volumes of fluid (10–20 litres/24 h), represents an effective treatment. Bleeding may also result from erosion of a major blood vessel; it then demands immediate operation (or embolization if interventional radiological facilities are readily available). Among 60 patients with acute bleeding in the HSA series, 36 underwent urgent operation and 24 were successfully managed conservatively.

Renal and/or hepatic failure This is indicated by levels of serum creatinine > 250 μmol/l, serum bilirubin > 60 μmol/l and transaminases greater than three times normal.[5] It is often a warning sign of severe sepsis. In the absence of chronic renal or hepatic disease and lack of improvement despite appropriate resuscitation, failure of these organs is a strong indication for surgical exploration; although the likelihood of cure is small, urgent operation provides the only choice. In profound renal failure haemodialysis may be required before operation. Among the 120 HSA patients presenting with hepatic/renal failure, 34 died early (28%), 46 were operated on (38%) and 40 were managed conservatively (34%).

Thromboembolic complications Deep vein thrombosis and pulmonary embolism are major threats in fistula patients who display all the risk factors for venous thrombosis. All available means are to be used: low-molecular-weight heparin, elastic stockings, active and passive mobilization, elevation of the legs.

INITIAL MANAGEMENT

Initial therapeutic indications

On presentation of the patient the programme includes four stages.

1. Scrutinize the operative reports and patient records to detect surgical pitfalls, overlooked chronic diseases and potential complications.

2. Assess the patient's general condition and begin resuscitation.

3. Examine the patient after removal of all dressings.

4. Reassure the patient and his family. Patients referred with a fistula are extremely anxious, and the first contact with the doctor in charge is of great importance.

In rare cases, emergency operation is immediately selected, e.g. for fulminating sepsis, massive bleeding and free evisceration. Most often a detailed evaluation is carried out over 3–5 days.[19] When severe general signs of sepsis are associated with a documented intra-abdominal abscess, percutaneous drainage or elective surgical drainage may be attempted to drain a single and accessible abscess cavity; otherwise a radical procedure is required. Radical emergency operation includes complete abdominal exploration and transformation of fistulas into enterostomies.

Emergency 'salvage' surgery

When indicated, salvage operation should be carried out without delay. Delayed salvage operations performed after a so-called 'period of preparation' of 3–4 weeks have uniformly poor results.[6,16,17] Thanks to the progress of intensive care, these patients can sustain the aggression of a full laparotomy after only a short preparation. However, preoperative and immediate postoperative intensive care are critical, as mobilization of septic material during dissection leads to bacteraemia and severe septic signs: fall in blood pressure, hypoxaemia, hepatic or renal failure and coagulation abnormalities. Broad-spectrum antibiotic cover is necessary, as is replacement of blood loss and repeated monitoring of coagulation parameters.

The technique of elective and percutaneous drainage is purposefully omitted as it has been widely described in the literature and has no special features in fistula patients.

Technique of radical emergency surgery

The technique of 'salvage' operation is similar to that described for the treatment of diffuse postoperative peritonitis.[20] It includes the following steps.

1. Complete exposure of the abdominal cavity, which presents even more difficulties in fistula patients than in postoperative peritonitis. The dissection is long, tedious and bloody. When dissection of the upper abdomen appears difficult and hazardous, provided that imaging has shown no lesion in this sector, exploration may be restricted to the infracolic compartment. Dissection begins from free spaces, when available, and progresses from flanks to midline and from the depths to the surface; it involves both digital and sharp dissection.

2. Meticulous peritoneal toilet and gentle debridement of fibrinous material.

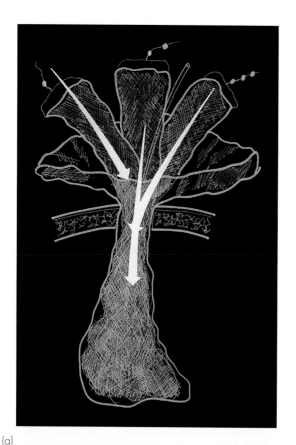

(a)

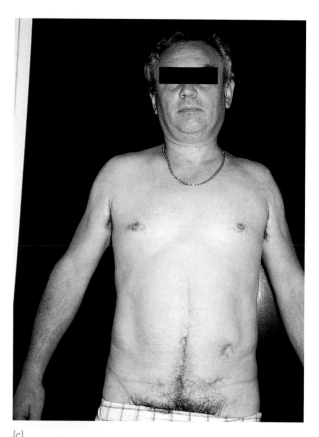

(c)

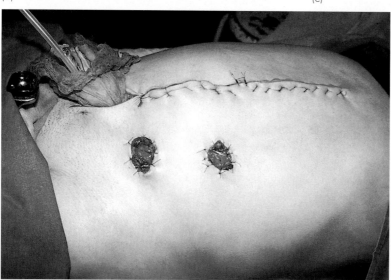

(b)

Figure 48.6

The Mikulicz packing. (a) Components: gauze bag filled with long gauze swabs (arrows). (b) A view of a Mikulicz packing just after abdominal wall closure. Two end stomas are visible. (c) Same patient after restoration of continuity (six months later).

3. Creation of enterostomies at the site of the fistula: loop stoma if the orifice is small, resection plus end stomas otherwise. Anastomoses are avoided.

4. Active drainage is achieved by sump tubes and corrugated drains in the upper abdomen. Mikulicz packing (Figure 48.6a,b)[20] provides capillary aspiration in the pouch of Douglas and in abscess cavities (Figure 48.11).

5. Tension-free closure of the abdominal wall. It may be feas-ible with conventional fascial and skin closure. When the fascial plane is necrotic but the skin is accessible to tension-free closure, a Vicryl® mesh may be inserted, taking care to place the mesh deep in the flanks; the skin only is then closed. When closure without tension is impossible, the technique favoured at the HSA is to create lateral myocutaneous advancement flaps and to close the skin in the midline (Figure 48.7);[12] an absorbable mesh is used as a supplementary protection (Figure 48.7). Advancement flaps should be made before creation of the stomas.

Salvage operations transform the problem of fistula management into one of temporary enterostomies.

CONSERVATIVE MANAGEMENT

Metabolic and nutritional therapy

Enterocutaneous fistulas represent an emergency as regards fluid and electrolyte balance and nutrition.

Water and electrolyte requirements

A water and electrolyte regimen should include the following two elements.

1. An invariable part representing the basal requirements, which is approximately estimated for an adult weighing 70 kg by the following formula: 2500 ml water or 5% glucose, 100 mEq sodium, 125 mEq chloride, 20 mEq potassium, plus calcium, magnesium, vitamins and trace elements.

2. A variable part aiming at compensating the fluid and electrolyte loss through the fistula. This part of the regimen is based on daily measurement of the fistula effluent and on repeated analysis of the electrolyte and protein content of the fistula fluid, together with routine clinical and biological

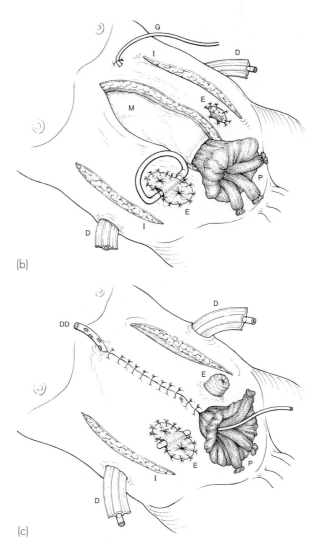

Figure 48.7
Schematics of 'salvage' surgery. (a) Tracing of the relaxation incisions. (b) Intraoperative view, immediately before skin closure showing Vicryl® mesh (M) Mikulicz packing (P), relaxation incisions (I), temporary enterostomies (E), drains from upper abdomen and paracolic gutters (D) and a feeding gastrostomy (G). (c) Immediate postoperative view. A drain (DD) is placed between mesh and skin layer.

monitoring. A basic compensatory regimen can be proposed for the initial period of management: to each litre of extra fluid (5% glucose) is added 8 g NaCl, 2 g KCl plus calcium and magnesium as appropriate. In the case of jejunal fistulas, this compensatory fluid may be mixed 1:4 with isotonic bicarbonate solution.

The initial route of infusion for water and electrolytes is by means of an intracaval catheter. As inflammation subsides and intestinal transit resumes, the enteral route may be utilized and may eventually become the exclusive route of administration.

Energy and protein requirements

Formerly overlooked, the nutritional failure induced by enterocutaneous fistulas is now fully appreciated and receives appropriate treatment. Fistula patients fall into the category of depleted and stressed patients. Their requirements in terms of intravenous nutrition, as measured by neutron activation analysis,[21] are equal to 45–50 kcal/kg body weight/day with 350 mg/kg/day of nitrogen. Due to the particular avidity of depleted patients for protein,[22] energy intake need not greatly exceed energy expenditure to allow laying down of protein. In such patients there is a marked preference for fat as the energy source. Excess glucose may result in increased energy expenditure, a rise in respiratory quotient and excessive lipogenesis. Therefore, energy should be provided in a 50:50 glucose–fat ratio.[21] Amino acid solutions used in TPN should contain essential amino acids at a level of about 40%.[21]

Conclusions drawn from studies undertaken in patients receiving intravenous nutrition cannot be extended to patients receiving enteral support. Prospective studies have shown that the energy intake required to maintain weight in depleted but non-stressed surgical patients on continuous enteral nutrition (CEN) equals 35 kcal/kg/day.[4] The energy requirement on CEN in depleted and stressed patients reaches 65 kcal/kg/day.[4] The nitrogen intake required to maintain balance on CEN varies between 19 and 22 g per day.[4]

The energy and protein levels required to ensure a weight gain of 3% over 15 days have been established in prospective studies of different types of patients on CEN. Depending on the presence of a fistula and/or severe sepsis, calorie intake ranged between 55–90 kcal/kg/day and nitrogen between 28 and 32 g per day.[4] These levels represent net intake and should be increased when part of the feed is lost through a fistula.

Tolerance of high loads of energy and glucose is satisfactory when provided enterally in contrast to TPN, even in patients with critical respiratory status.[4]

Practicalities of TPN

Short-term TPN may be considered in patients with a low output fistula or patients likely to be transferred shortly to exclusive enteral support. It is defined as a period of TPN less than 14 days in duration. Short-term TPN may be achieved through a peripheral vein, by a soft plastic needle, using solutions of osmolarity < 600 mosmol/l to avoid venous inflammation and thrombosis.

Long-term TPN (>15 days) is carried out with a catheter positioned in the superior vena cava. Silicone and polyurethane catheters are now available and can be inserted percutaneously. The nutrition line should be restricted to nutritional use and not be 'broken' for other purposes. Currently TPN bags providing all the nutrients for a 24 h period are available, thus allowing for maximum safety. Preferably all aspects of the TPN line and catheter maintenance should be managed by a specialized team. Protein, glucose and fat should be infused simultaneously, a regular infusion speed being achieved by an infusion pump.

The TPN regimen begins with a moderate intake (20 kcal/kg/day) and is progressively increased until the plateau of 45–50 kcal/kg/day is attained. Protein (including glutamine) represents 15% of the energy intake (2–2.5 g/kg/day), carbohydrate 45% (5–6 g/kg/day) and fat 35% (1.5–2 g/kg/day). The nitrogen:calorie ratio ranges between 1:130 and 1:150. Vitamins and trace elements are provided in generous quantities.

TPN bags are supplied either from the manufacturer or from the hospital pharmacy department. At the beginning of treatment, when a patient's requirements vary from day to day, it is best to give the basic water/electrolyte requirement into the TPN bag and to provide the extra fluid by peripheral venous access. When requirements become stable, the extra fluid may be included in the 'big bag'.

Complications of TPN become more infrequent as the materials and experience improve. Septic complications represent the main threat in those patients with intra-abdominal sepsis and intestinal and/or purulent discharge. Metabolic, mechanical and thrombotic complications can occur at any time of the fistula management, even in a stablized patient. The possibility of serious complications should lead the clinician to seek an alternative to TPN when suitable conditions are present.

Continuous enteral nutrition (CEN)

CEN represents a rational, continuous and automatic enteral infusion system currently using large-capacity refrigerated infusion pumps or sterile containers to allow for minimal manipulation. CEN may be undertaken as soon as intestinal transit has resumed, in the absence of contraindications, such as ultrashort bowel, neurological disorders or the risk of aspiration. Enteral autonomy is attained in an average of 10 days. The problem of loss of feed through the fistula is resolved by various techniques.

In ileal fistulas, absorption in the bowel proximal to the fistula is usually sufficient, due to the high intake, the viscosity of the diet and the continuous infusion. Fluid and electrolytes may be simultaneously infused by another route (peripheral vein, distal bowel, colon) to maintain a low osmolarity of the diet.

In jejunal fistulas, the high output is not a major obstacle to enteral support: obturation or chyme reinfusion have been shown to be efficient and feasible.[5]

Diets used in fistula patients have precise specifications. Carbohydrate is provided in the form of oligosaccharides/ polyglycosides (Caloreen®, Maltrinex®, Sopharga Laboratories F 92086 Puteaux, France) and accounts for 50–65% of energy intake. Fat (20–25% of energy intake) is in the form of medium-chain triglycerides supplemented with linoleic acid and fat-soluble vitamins (Liprocil®, Liprogram® iii). Protein (15% of energy intake) is in the form of protein hydrolysates (Alburone®, Proteofon® iii) or small peptides (Reabilan®). Osmolarity is in the range of 250–350 mosmol/l. Mean nitrogen : calorie ratio is 1 : 190. A viscous additive such as tapioca solution[4] or Indian corn starch (Amidon Visco®, Gallia Laboratories F 92203 Levallois, France) can produce a viscosity of 10 viscosity units, i.e. eight times the viscosity of glycerine at 37°C. Elemental and semi-elemental diets (Vivonex®, Flexical®, Steraldiet®, Precitene®) are only used in a minority of patients and are restricted to the early stage of management, as the theoretical advantage of quick absorption is offset by their high osmolarity.[14] Vitamins and trace elements (egg yolk) are included in the diet.

Infusion is made by nasogastric tube or a gastrostomy catheter made of soft silicone elastomer (Vygon Inc.) with a large bore (12–14Fr). When sterile, ready-to-use and complete diets are used, infusion may be achieved by a small portable pump. In fistula patients, as already mentioned, it is preferable to constitute a special diet from basic nutrients. All the components required for a 24 hour period are mixed in a large capacity can (4–5 litres), which is an integral part of a refrigerated nutrition pump (Nutripompe®).

CEN is started as intestinal transit has resumed, after a test infusion of coloured dialysate, and it begins at a volume of 1000–1500 ml/24 h. The volume infused and the calorie concentration is progressively increased until the desired amount is reached. This quantity varies between 60 and 100 kcal/kg/day according to the severity of sepsis and the fistula output; the mean calorie concentration is 1 kcal/ml.

Provided the diet is prepared with strict asepsis and is kept at 4°C, complications are infrequent. Major complications such as aspiration pneumonia are exceptional and are due to failure to respect the contraindications. Minor complications such as pharyngitis, transient diarrhoea, nausea and meteorism are often due to technical mistakes and should not lead to interruption of CEN.

In the HSA series,[5] 85% of the patients were managed exclusively by CEN, either from the beginning of the management or after an initial period of nutrition by TPN (mean duration 17 days).

Duration of artificial nutrition

Artificial nutrition, either enteral or parenteral, should cover the whole period of conservative management. When closure of the fistula is obtained without reoperation, it is advisable to maintain artificial nutritional support for several days after closure before resuming oral intake. Weaning to oral intake should also progress gradually.

Which mode of nutrition is best?

Advocates of TPN claim that it not only provides appropriate nutritional support but is also an efficient means to obtain fistula closure by the reduction of the volume of effluent and enzyme concentration induced by bowel rest.[3] However, the impact of TPN on closure rate remains controversial. In Reber's experience,[23] the rate of spontaneous closure was 26% in the period 1968–1971, when 24% of patients received TPN, and only 30% in the period 1971–1977, when 71% of patients received TPN. Soeters et al.[24] noted a progression from 10% to 22% over approximately the same period of time. Although a spontaneous closure rate of 70% may be attained in selected patient populations,[3,25] the mean figures reported in large series are in the range 20–40%.[8,10,23,24,26–28]

Advocates of enteral nutrition claim that CEN is the 'physiological' method of nutrition, with favourable effects on intestinal adaptation, gut barrier efficiency and bacterial translocation.[29] Some authors use elemental diets with the aim of limiting the fistula output[30–32] and thereby obtain a spontaneous closure rate similar to that obtained by TPN. Lévy and co-workers favour polymeric/semi-elemental solutions mixed with a viscous additive so as to attain high energy levels. This approach requires CEN to be associated with special techniques: irrigation of the fistula track at least and obturation/reinfusion at the most. Provided these procedures are applied, a 38% spontaneous closure rate is obtained in high-output fistulas,[5] including a 23% spontaneous closure rate in exposed fistulas.

In conclusion, it appears that both methods are currently worthwhile, although enteral support is likely to enjoy increasing development in forthcoming years for two main reasons. First technology will provide improved materials for fistula obturation and chyme reinfusion, together with new high-viscosity/low-osmolarity diets; and second, further studies seem likely to demonstrate favourable effects of enteral nutrition in stressed ICU patients.

Somatostatin

The advent of somatostatin and its analogues to existing therapeutic means has been promising. Some preliminary studies report a prompt spontaneous closure of fistulas under TPN combined with somatostatin.[33] However, these results have subsequently been challenged,[34] and several specialized centres have embarked on an international multicentre randomized trial. Unfortunately, fistulas of the small intestine represent such an heterogeneous group that the number of patients meeting the inclusion criteria was insufficient.

Somatostatin decreases fistula output by 30–60% and may accelerate closure of some cases of fistula, provided there is no anatomical obstacle. The effect of somatostatin is maximal in high (proximal) fistulas and in the early period of fistula formation. Although it may represent a useful adjunct, somatostatin treatment does not represent a radical transformation in fistula management.

Local care

The aim of local care is to achieve (1) drainage of the fistula track including any interposed pockets, (2) leak-proof collection of the fistula fluid and (3) an efficient support of the abdominal wall. Wounds are left open for inspection, either

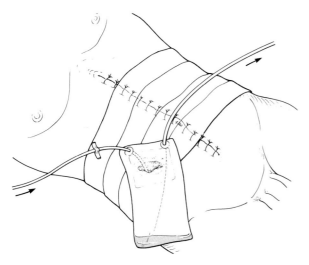

Figure 48.8
Closed system of irrigation and collection of fistula fluid.

completely open (the sheets being stented by a cradle) or under closed transparent appliances.

Irrigation of the fistula track is not compulsory and is in fact seldom used in the Anglo-Saxon scientific community; it is popular in France and Continental Europe after the work of Trémolières.[2] Irrigation is necessary if the nutritional support is CEN, as it dilutes and neutralizes the corrosive effect of the enzyme-rich digestive fluid; it is also helpful in cases of gross suppuration. The irrigation fluid commonly used is a 0.45% solution of lactic acid buffered at pH 4.5 and coloured blue, infused at a rate depending on the fistula output (1500–2500 ml/24 h). In the early postoperative period dialysate may be preferred. Irrigation is achieved by a fine-bore silicone elastomer soft tube (8–12 Fr). The tip of the irrigation tube should be positioned as close as possible to the intestinal opening to irrigate the whole track and to let the irrigation fluid flow in the same direction as the fistula fluid, i.e. from intestine to skin.

Collection of the fluid

Collection of the fluid may be achieved by (1) closed systems or (2) open systems.

(a)

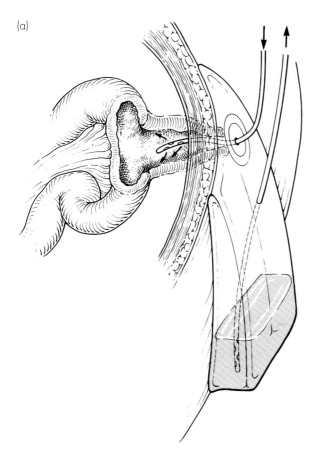

(b)

(c)

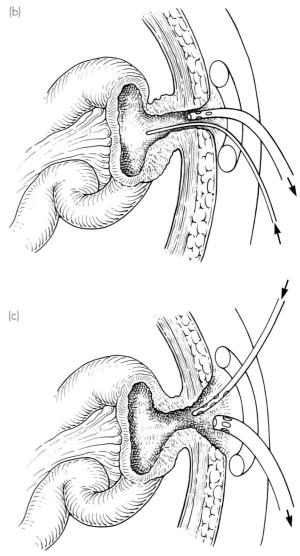

Figure 48.9
Various system of irrigation/fluid collection: (a) closed system (simple fistula); (b) open system for a fistula with limited dehiscence; (c) open system for an exposed fistula.

Closed systems These represent the simplest method; a sealed appliance collects the fluid by gravity, and permanent suction is applied to the appliance (Figure 48.8). The seal may be separate from the appliance. A ring of home-made karaya paste is the cheapest available material. Stomahesive® wafers may be cut to the size and shape of the orifice, massaged with warm hands and applied to the skin. Many other barrier sheets are currently available (e.g. Comfeel®, Holliesive®), and in this case any ordinary appliance is appropriate. Appliance and seal may be provided as a ready-to-use unit and are now available under many trade names, the Draina-S® (Biotrol Laboratories) being currently the most efficient in terms of adhesion.

Open systems These are required in fistulas with parietal dehiscence or with an irregular surface around the fistulous orifice that impedes the placement of an appliance. The basic system is made of a karaya dam circumscribing the wound and ensuring a leakproof enclosure for irrigation and aspiration (Figures.48.9a,b). The karaya roll forming the dam is homemade; equal parts of karaya powder and glycerine are mixed, and 5–20% water is added until the desired consistency is obtained. Aspiration is provided by atraumatic large-bore (>30 F) Dacron®, woven carbon or silicone tubes with an air aspiration channel; the vacuum does not exceed –50 cm H_2O. A capillary silicone tube has been developed to provide a self-limitation of the vacuum (Figure 48.10). The tip of the aspiration tube is positioned at the dependent end of the surface circumscribed by the karaya dam by means of copper wire attached to the surrounding skin or to the roll of karaya. An isobaric cupula (Figure 48.11) placed on a non-vulcanized silicone foam base is useful in exposed fistulas as the base sticks to granulation tissue and does not melt in contact with

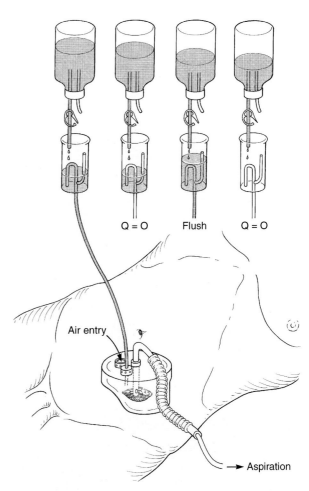

Figure 48.11
Isobaric cupula and intermittent irrigation system.

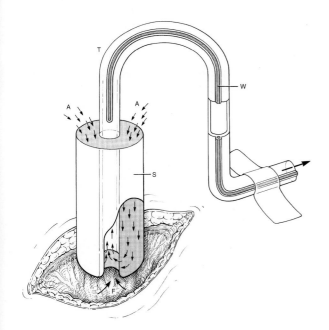

Figure 48.10
Capillary aspiration unit with vacuum self-limiting system. S, soft silicone foam surrounding the tube; W, wire; T, tube; A, air penetrating by the permeable part of the silicone surface; F, aspiration of the fluid.

digestive fluid. It includes a system of discontinuous irrigation (flushing) which eliminates all debris and ensures the permeability of the suction line.

Practicalities of local care Local care begins by removal of all dressings and topical agents. The skin is cleaned with saline and dried with a hair-dryer while the fistula fluid is aspirated by an atraumatic sucker held by an assistant. Barrier powder (Stomahesive® or Karaya) may be applied to the skin in the presence of erosions. The appropriate system is selected according to the shape and size of the fistula orifice and parietal dehiscence. In the presence of multiple fistula tracks, each track should be fitted with a separate collection system. The co-operation of the patient is an absolute requirement and is obtained only through the establishment of a close patient–staff relationship. Frequent bedside visits of the consultant for an informal chat are required, and occasionally supportive drug treatment may be useful.

Special systems: obturation and chyme reinfusion

In the case of a high-output fistula, it may be valuable to limit the discharge or to recycle the chyme in the distal intestine.

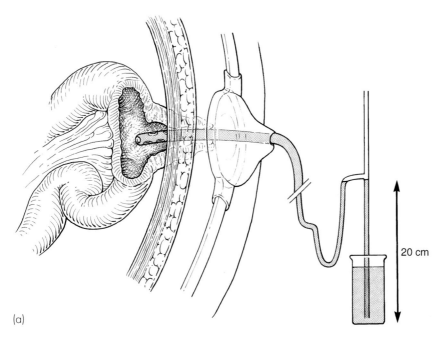

(a)

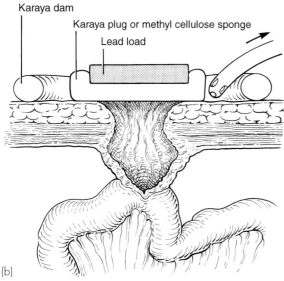

Karaya dam

Karaya plug or methyl cellulose sponge

Lead load

(b)

Figure 48.12

Obturation. (a) System of output limitation: obturation with evacuation of fistula fluid over a pressure of 20 cm H_2O – *'Belt and nipple'* system appropriate for fistulas with little or no parietal dehiscence; (b) System of total obturation. Occasional overflow is collected by suction inside a perimeter circumscribed by a karaya dam lead load system, which is convenient for exposed fistulas.

20 cm

Obturators are used in cases of lateral fistulas. Direct fistulas, provided they are not everted, may be 'plugged' by a cellulose sponge or a karaya paste disc applied with a pressure of 10 g/cm² by means of a lead load. At the initial stage of obturation the pressure of the fluid beneath the obturation device is maintained at a low level, and the overflow is collected (Figure 48.12a). At a later stage total obturation is achieved (Figure 48.12a). This system not only limits the output but also favours spontaneous healing. Exposed fistulas without a surrounding surface which allows counterpressure or plugging may, nevertheless, be obturated by means of a twin-disc device (Figure 48.13a–e). Although efficient, this device prevents spontaneous healing.

Chyme recycling applies to exposed fistulas everted on to the granulation tissue. The chyme collected at the proximal orifice is reinfused into the distal small bowel.[11]

In the HSA fistula series, obturation was used in 64 patients (29% of the conservative management group) and chyme reinfusion in 28 patients (12%).

ELECTIVE REPAIR SURGERY

Principles and indications

The principles of the surgical repair of a fistula are now well established. The surgical procedure should be radical, any lesser operation invariably resulting in recurrence.[15,17,23] Any attempt at suture in a septic field is doomed to failure.[11,16,24,35] Any attempt at surgical repair at an early phase of the fistula course puts the patient at major risk of further fistulisation and death from sepsis.[1,17,18,28] As postoperative fistulas appear after a phase of diffuse intra-abdominal sepsis, time is necessary for the obliterative peritonitis to relapse, usually two months at the least. Therefore, in agreement with other authors,[10,17,36,37] we recommend that repair surgery should be performed at least eight weeks after the onset of the fistula, i.e. ten weeks on average after the causative operation. The timing of the repair operation also should take into consideration the possibility of spontaneous healing. If anatomical conditions are favourable, an effective period of conservative treatment should be carried out for a minimum period of six weeks before reaching the decision to operate. If anatomical conditions preclude closure, repair surgery should be performed directly when two months have passed since the phase of intra-abdominal sepsis and/or fistula onset. Fistulas occurring at a late period after operation (e.g. a traumatic fistula complicating a long-standing evisceration) may be operated on without delay, provided that there is no associated intra-abdominal sepsis.

Preparation of the patient

Operations for fistula repair often represent a lengthy, taxing and haemorrhagic enterprise; intraoperative bacteraemia and septic shock are not uncommon after mobilization of septic material. Coagulation abnormalities are frequently associated

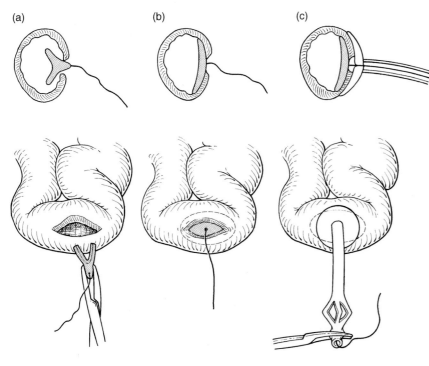

(a) (b) (c)

Figure 48.13
Twin disc obturation. (a,b,c)
Positioning in the bowel; (d,e)
open/closed positions.

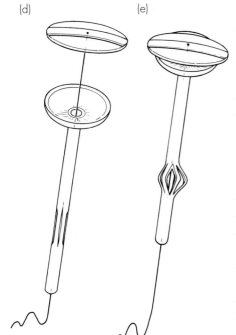

(d) (e)

anastomose the ends. But the situation may be complex due to the presence of a residual lesion (inflammation, cancer) or to combination with another fistula. However complex the problems may be, they should all be resolved in one operation. If necessary, a defunctioning stoma may be created provided that it can be closed by an elective approach; no further extensive laparotomy should be required as a second stage.

Technique

There is no remaining abdominal cavity. The bowel loops are tightly adherent to the deep aspect of the abdominal wall and to the intra-abdominal components.

Approach is usually by a long midline incision, except in particular cases of exposed fistula with a large transverse evisceration. A relatively free section is sought for the beginning of the dissection, either a scar-free portion of the midline or the upper part of it. Skin is incised slowly and cautiously, blood being constantly sucked as bowel may be close to the dermal layer. If a free portion of the deep aspect of the midline is found, dissection between the bowel and the scar is undertaken from this point. The opening of the deep layer of the midline incision progresses as the loops are freed from its deep aspect (Figure 48.14a,b).

If the loops are encrusted in the abdominal wall, sharp dissection should continue in the wall itself until an easier site of dissection is reached more laterally (Figure 48.14c). Once the incision is completed, both edges of the wound are held upwards and dissection proceeds (a) between the intestine and the parietal peritonum, going far laterally, (b) within the loops of intestine, beginning from the easier parts and progressing from depth to surface, from flanks to midline and from mesentery to intestine, and (c) at the fistula site and in the pelvis, this always being the most difficult part.

with haemorrhagic dissection of inflamed tissue, sepsis and impaired liver function. Preparation for operation includes checking laboratory data, bacterial sampling of any discharge and systemic antibiotic cover. Intraoperative monitoring of central venous pressure is routinely performed; blood losses are replaced by blood and fresh frozen plasma (avoiding haemodilution) and blood/plasma substitutes to maintain coagulation factors at a normal level.

Strategy

The basic principle of repair surgery is simple: dissect out the whole bowel, resect the portion of fistulous bowel and

(a)

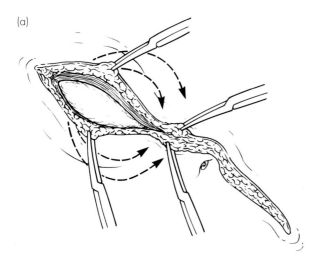

Figure 48.14

Repair surgery. (a) Incision and progression of the dissection from the upper midline downwards. Dissection goes laterally first and then back to the midline. Wound edges are held by strong forceps. (b) Dissection of the loops from the deep aspect of the midline; in 'easy' cases finger dissection can almost reach the midline and prepare for safe scissors section; (c) Dissection of the loops from the deep aspect of the midline; in 'difficult' cases where the loops are encrusted in the abdominal wall sharp dissection in the depths of the wall is required until free space is reached.

(b)

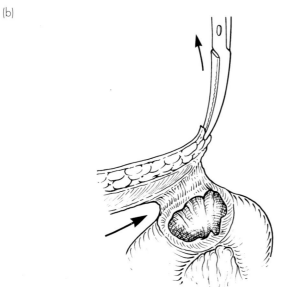
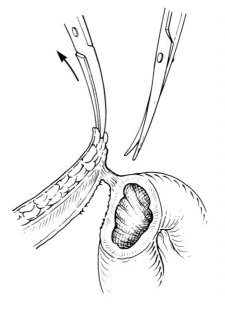

(c)

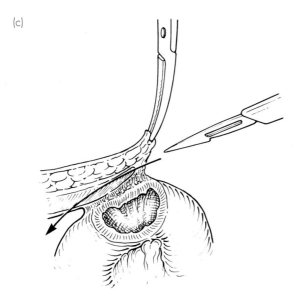

technique alone may suffice, or at least it can prepare for a safe sharp dissection.

Resection of the fistulous bowel is carried out: either a single resection in cases of a single or multiple adjacent lesions, or two or more segmental resections in cases of multiple and distant fistulas. When multiple lesions are present, some may be limited in size and be accessible to suture after resection of the edges. Anastomoses are performed end-to-end, using running 4/0 or 5/0 absorbable sutures and taking care to use the finest possible needles. A fibrin adhesive (Tissucol®, Biocol®) may be laid on the suture line.

Peritoneal toilet and haemostasis of the dissected surfaces comprise the next stage; haemostasis requires time and patience. Drains may be used in the upper abdomen provided they are in a dependent position and far from the intestinal loops; drains should be avoided in the lower abdomen.

Closure of the abdominal wall may be carried out in a conventional fashion if the fascial layer is preserved and is amenable to closure without tension. Even in this favourable case it is advisable to interpose an absorbable mesh (Vicryl®) between the loops of intestine and the abdominal wall (Figure

Separation of intestinal loops is initiated by finger dissection, pressing the adhesions between thumb and index: this

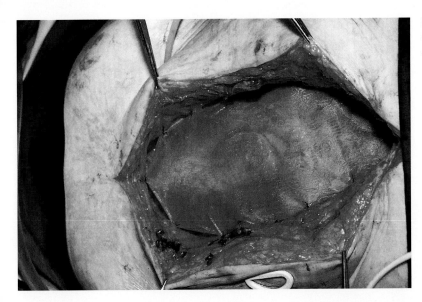

Figure 48.15
Closure of the abdominal wall in simple cases; positioning of the Vicryl® mesh.

48.15). Frequently the fascia is absent, necrotic or retracted, and only the skin can be closed without tension; then an absorbable mesh should be placed and positioned as far laterally as possible and in the pelvis to 'wrap' the small bowel and provide an efficient protection. Soft silicone tubes (18–20 F) may be placed between the mesh and the skin to collect any exudate that may accumulate in this space, and they are connected to a closed appliance. The skin is closed using interrupted mattress sutures. Abdominal binding is performed with adhesive bands positioned far laterally.

The most difficult situation is represented by large losses of the parietal wall; lateral relaxation incisions are then required[12]

Exposed fistulas represent a particular problem for dissection. The incision should circumscribe the area of granulation tissue bearing the fistula and this area is dissected last, proceeding from depth to surface and separating each individual loop of bowel from the fistulous area. At first sight all the loops attached to the granulating tissue seem to be involved in the fistula process but, in reality, many are intact and may be separated from the other loops, sometimes by leaving bits of granulating tissue or skin on the surface of the bowel, which is of no consequence.

Postoperative care

Antibiotic cover is maintained for a minimum of three days. TPN is maintained until transit has resumed, when enteral support may be substituted. It is not uncommon in the early postoperative period to observe substantial exudation through the drains or the incision.

Complications

Although the early postoperative course may be difficult, abnormal signs generally subside after 4–6 days. A complication should be suspected if symptoms of sepsis are either delayed in their onset, prolonged and surprisingly severe, or associated with physical signs (pain, swelling, tenderness).

The main complication is recurrence of a fistula. Persistent peritoneal bleeding may occur and be life threatening.

Results of fistula repair operations show a low mortality

Table 48.2   Overall mortality rate and spontaneous closure rate

Authors	Year	No. of patients	No. of small bowel fistulas	Mortality rate (small bowel fistulas) (%)	Spontaneous closure rate (small bowel fistulas) %
McFadyen et al.[3]	1973	62	26	6	69
Reber et al.[23]	1978	186	120	22	20
Coutsofides and Fazio[17]	1979	174	174	22	17
Soeters et al.[24]	1979	128	52	21	38
Hill and Bambach[28]	1981	50	50	20	42
Sitges-Serra et al.[25]	1982	87	87	21	71
Allardyce[27]	1983	52	NS	38	43
MacIntyre et al.[8]	1984	114	114	5.3	24
Sansoni and Irving[10]	1985	51	51	23	16
Lévy et al.[5]	1989	335	335	34	26

NS, not stated.

rate, ranging between zero[26,28] and 15%.[17,23] The refistulisation rate varies between 5 and 15%.[17,23,26,28] In the HSA series,[5] 147 patients underwent surgical repair of the fistula: 120 after conservative management and 27 after salvage surgery (see Figure 48.17); 22 patients died (15%). Complications occurred in 43% of the patients, either medical complications (16%) or surgical complications (27%), including refistulisation, bleeding and wound infection.

RESULTS, OVERALL PROGNOSIS AND FUTURE TRENDS

Mortality rate

Table 48.2 shows the overall mortality rate and the rate of spontaneous closure reported in recent series. The incidence of death remains high in major referral centres collecting complicated cases of patients admitted after failure of previous

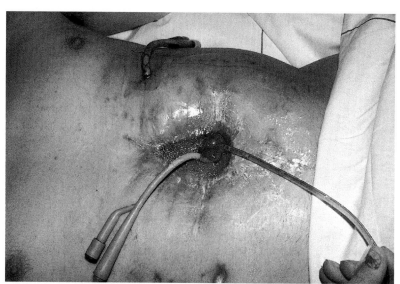

(a)

Figure 48.16
Closure of the abdominal wall using relaxation incisions.
(a) Preoperative view, exposed-fistula; (b) intraoperative view showing parietal defect, Vicryl® mesh and lateral counterincisions; (c) postoperative view showing expansion of the rectus muscle within the relaxation incisions and sliding of the flaps towards the midline; (d) and (e) post operative result.

(b)

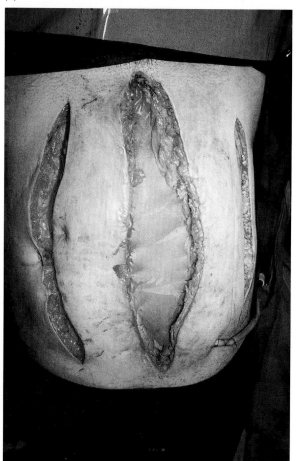

(c)

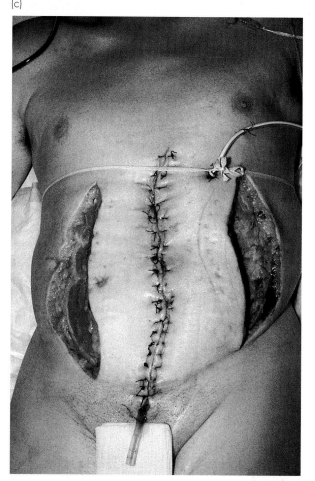

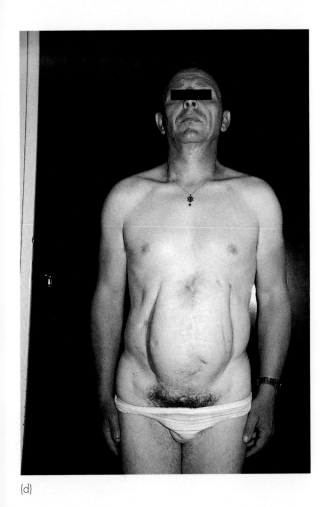

(d)

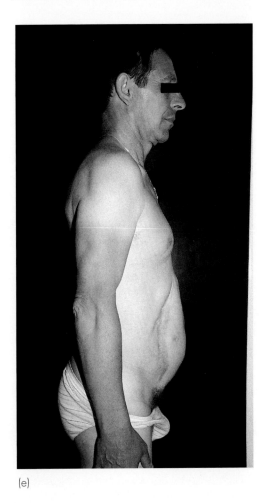

(e)

therapy;[5,10,24] even in the most recent years the mortality rate has scarcely fallen below 20%.[5,10,38] Lack of improvement in mortality rate with the passage of time has been emphasized by previous workers,[23,24] and it is probably related to the increased severity of cases referred since simple fistulas are now managed in the original institutions.

Prognostic factors

Four types of prognostic factors have been identified:

1. Age
2. Chronic intercurrent disease
3. Characteristics of the fistula
4. Acute complications

The main factors are summarized in Figure 48.18.

Age The mortality rate remains low until the age of 50 years and then increases until the age of 70 years, remaining stable

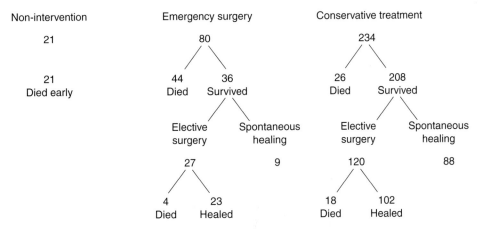

Figure 48.17
Flow diagram showing the therapeutic pathways of patients in the HSA series.[5]

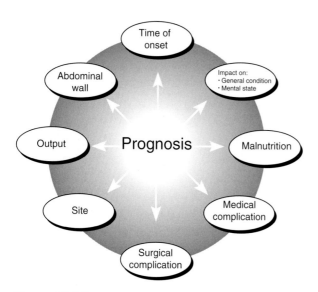

Figure 48.18
Diagram of the main prognostic factors.

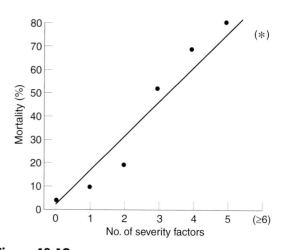

Figure 48.19
Correlation between the number of cumulative complicating factors of prognosis (Table 48.1) and mortality rate in the HSA series of 335 cases.[5]

thereafter.[5] Age also affects the complication rate and the incidence of late sequelae.

Chronic diseases Digestive diseases such as radiation enteritis or Crohn's disease complicate the management of a fistula but do not result in an increased mortality rate. General conditions, such as atherosclerosis, diabetes or chronic respiratory insufficiency adversely affect the prognosis.[5]

Characteristics of the fistula Exposed fistulas and high-output (>1500 ml/24h) fistulas have a significantly poorer prognosis.[5] The site of the fistula (jejunal vs ileal) and the time of occurrence (<15 days vs >15 days after operation) have an apparent, though not significant, impact on mortality rate.

Acute complications All complications have significant impact on survival (Table 48.1). The cumulative number of complicating factors has a close linear correlation with mortality rate (Figure 48.19). In the absence of such complications, the risk of death is close to zero.[5]

Another way to illustrate the prognostic factors is to relate the mortality rate to the therapeutic pathways (Figure 48.17). All authors have reported a higher mortality rate in patients requiring operation; this fact only means that surgical cases are more severe. Those patients requiring emergency operation have serious complications, but although the mortality rate in this situation exceeds 50%, emergency operation is the only chance for the patient and should therefore be attempted. Patients requiring repair surgery have intractable fistulas, and it is useless to prolong conservative treatment.

Recently, prognostic indexes have been proposed for patients on intensive care, providing each patient at a given time with a severity score that affects their chance of survival. Altomare et al.[38] have proposed a severity index for fistula patients that combines the Apache II score and the serum albumin concentration.

Future trends

In the section on aetiopathology it was stressed that questionable surgical procedures are responsible for an appreciable proportion of postoperative fistulas, e.g. 45% in the HSA series (152/335).[5] About 72% of postoperative fistulas follow reoperative surgery.[5] These figures suggest that future trends in fistula management should be orientated toward fistula prevention.

Once the fistula is present, the management can be conducted in simple cases in the original institution. Otherwise the patient should be promptly referred to a specialized unit, which provides the best chance of survival and spontaneous closure. In the management of a fistula patient, constant attention to all

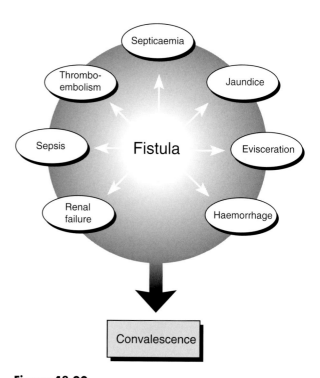

Figure 48.20
The multiple obstacles between fistula and home.

details is required, both in local and general care. Assiduous presence of the senior medical staff at the patient's bedside and strong psychological support from the whole staff will help the patient to overcome this distressing situation. In the most severe cases with repeated incidents (Figure 48.20), the medical and nursing staff need to persevere. Such perseverance will not uncommonly be rewarded by an unexpectedly favourable outcome. Rehabilitation of such patients, who are often young, and have a benign primary disease and are referred in a critical condition, is one of the most satisfactory enterprises in the whole of surgical practice.

REFERENCES

1. Edmunds LH, Williams GM & Welch CE. External fistulas arising from the gastrointestinal tract. *Ann Surg* 1960; **152**: 445.
2. Trémolières J, Bonfils S & Gros J. L'irrigation par l'acide lactique: traitement des fistules cutanées digestives avec sécretion trypsique et autodigestion pariétale. *Arch Fr Mal App Dig* 1961; **50**: 636.
3. MacFadyen BV, Dudrick SJ & Ruberg JL. Management of gastrointestinal fistulas with parenteral hyperalimentation. *Surgery* 1973; **74**: 100.
4. Lévy E, Huguet C, Parc R et al. Continuous high-energy low-flow-rate enteral support: a panoramic view of 1000 cases. *Life Support Syst* 1985; **3**: 247.
5. Lévy E, Frileux P, Cugnenc PH, Honiger J, Ollivier JM, Parc R. High-output external fistulae of the small bowel; management with continuous enteral nutrition. *Br J Surg* 1989; **76**: 676.
6. Lévy E, Cugnenc PH, Parc R, Bloch P, Huguet C, Frileux P. Fistules jejuno-iléales s'ouvrant dans une éviscération: expérience de 120 cas. *Gastroentérol Clin Biol* 1981; **5**: 497.
7. Alexander-Williams J & Irving M. *Intestinal Fistulas.* Bristol: John Wright, 1982.
8. MacIntyre PB, Ritchie JK, Hawley PR, Bartram CI & Lennard-Jones JE. Management of enterocutaneous fistulas: a review of 132 cases. *Br J Surg* 1984; **71**: 293.
9. Irving M. Assessment and management of external fistulas in Crohn's disease. *Br J Surg* 1983; **70**: 233.
10. Sansoni B & Irving M. Small bowel fistulas. *World J Surg* 1985; **9**: 897.
11. Lévy E, Parc R & Loygue J. Stomies terminales, jéjunales ou iléales temporaires de sauvetage avec réinstillation autoregulee. *Nouv Presse Med* 1977; **6**: 461.
12. Lévy E, Palmer D, Frileux P et al. Septic necrosis of the midline wound in postoperative peritonitis: successful management by debridement, myocutaneous advancement and primary skin closure. *Ann Surg*, 1988; **207**: 470.
13. Waclawiczeck HW. Progress in fibrin sealing. Berlin: Springer, 1989.
14. Lévy E, Frileux P, Sandrucci S et al. Continuous enteral nutrition in the early adaptive stage of the short bowel syndrome. *Br J Surg* 1988; **75**: 549.
15. Blackett RL & Hill GL. Postoperative small bowel fistulas: a study of a consecutive series of patients treated with intravenous hyperalimentation. *Br J Surg* 1978; **65**: 775.
16. Aguirre A & Fischer J. The role of surgery and hyperalimentation in therapy of gastrointestinal–cutaneous fistulae. *Ann Surg* 1974; **180**: 393.
17. Coutsofides T & Fazio VW. Small intestine cutaneous fistulas. *Surg Gynecol Obstet* 1979; **149**: 333.
18. Chapman R, Foran R & Dunphy JE. Management of intestinal fistulas. *Ann J Surg* 1964; **108**: 157.
19. Sheldon GF, Gardiner BN, Way LW et al. Management of gastrointestinal fistulas. *Surg Gynecol Obstet* 1971; **133**: 385–389.
20. Parc R, Lévy E & Loygue J. Principes d'une intervention pour péritonite. *Ann Chir* 1985; **39**: 541.
21. Hill GL & Church J. Energy and protein requirements of general surgical patients requiring intravenous nutrition. *Br J Surg* 1984; **71**: 1.
22. Elwyn DH. Nutritional requirements in adult surgical patients. *Crit Care Med*, 1980; **8**: 9–20.
23. Reber HA, Roberts C, Way LW & Dunphy JE. Management of external gastrointestinal fistulas. *Ann Surg* 1978; **188**: 460.
24. Soeters PB, Ebeid AM & Fischer JE. Review of 404 patients with gastrointestinal fistulas: impact of parenteral nutrition. *Ann Surg* 1979; **190**: 189.
25. Sitges-Serra A, Jaruieta E & Sitges-Creus A. Management of enterocutaneous fistulas: the roles of parenteral nutrition and surgery. *Br J Surg* 1982; **69**: 147.
26. Hollender LF, Meyer C, Avet D & Meyer B. Postoperative fistulas of the small intestine. Therapeutic principles. *World J Surg* 1983; **7**: 474.
27. Allardyce DB. Management of small bowel fistulas. *Am J Surg* 1983; **145**: 593.
28. Hill GL & Bambach CP. A technique for the operative closure of persistent external small bowel fistulas. *Aust NZ J Surg* 1981; **51**: 477.
29. Saadia R, Schein M, MacFarlane C & Boffard KD. Gut barrier function and the surgeon. *Br J Surg* 1990; **77**: 487.
30. Wolfe BM, Keltner RM & Willmann VL. Intestinal output in regular, elemental and intravenous alimentation. *Am J Surg* 1972; **124**: 803.
31. Deitel M. Elemental diet and enterocutaneous fistula. *World J Surg* 1983; **7**: 451.
32. Holmes JT. Nutritional support of fistulas. *Br J Surg* 1977; **64**: 695.
33. Di Costanzo J, Cano N & Martin JO. Somatostatin in gastro-intestinal fistulas treated by total parenteral nutrition. *Lancet* 1982; **ii**: 338.
34. Kingsnorth AN, Moss JG & Small WP. Failure of somatostatin to accelerate close of enterocutaneous fistulas in patients receiving total parenteral nutrition. *Lancet* 1986; **i**: 1271.
35. Goligher JC. Resection with exteriorisation in the management of faecal fistulas originating in the small intestine. *Br J Surg* 1971; **58**: 163.
36. Fazio VW, Coutsofides T & Steiger E. Factors influencing the outcome of treatment of small bowel cutaneous fistula. *World J Surg* 1983; **7**: 481.
37. Hill GL. Operative strategy in the treatment of enterocutaneous fistulas. *World J Surg* 1983; **7**: 495.
38. Altomare DF, Serio G, Pannarale OC et al. Prediction of mortality by logistic regression analysis in patients with postoperative enterocutaneous fistulae. *Br J Surg* 1990; **77**: 450.

49

INTERNAL FISTULAS OF THE SMALL INTESTINE

EP Levy
P Frileux
Y Parc

DUODENOGASTRIC FISTULAS

The 'double pylorus' connecting the distal antrum to the duodenum through an accessory channel is usually a complication of peptic ulceration. It is more a curiosity than an actual complication, and it does not deserve specific therapy. Since its initial description by Christien in 1971, about 60 cases have been described in the literature.[1]

Aetiology

Acquired fistulas

The main source of acquired duodenogastric fistulas is the development of a peptic ulcer in the distal gastric antrum, on either curvature, leading to adhesions between the ulcer and the base of the duodenal bulb. Depending on the ulcer location, the connection to the duodenum lies either at the superior or the inferior aspect of the bulb (Figure 49.1). The fistula tract becomes epithelialized soon after formation.[1]

It has been assumed in the past that a possible mechanism of fistula formation was the junction of two opposing ulcers, one gastric and one duodenal. In fact, an initial duodenal ulcer is exceptional.[1] In an early report by Gould and associates,[2] gastroduodenal fistula was reported as joining *either* the posterior wall of the stomach to the third part of the duodenum *or* the body of the stomach to the duodenal bulb, but all these variants seem to be rare.

The other cause of acquired gastroduodenal fistula is carcinoma of the stomach developing within the distal antrum and involving the duodenal wall. Two cases have been described to date;[3,4] in each the endoscopic appearance was of a double channel with partition of the tumour at the level of the pylorus.

Congenital fistulas

Congenital double pylorus is related either to a duplication of the digestive tract or to a diverticulum.[5] This condition differs from acquired fistulas by the fact that each lumen is lined by a mucosal and muscular coat. Two cases of actual congenital double pylorus have been described in the literature,[5] whereas many so-called 'congenital gastroduodenal fistulas' are in reality secondary to gastric ulcers.

(a)

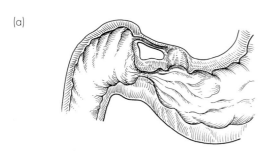

(b)

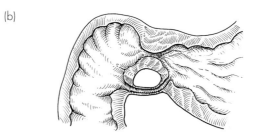

Figure 49.1
The two possible locations of duodenogastric fistulas (schematics from upper GI series). (a) Duodenogastric fistula which has developed at the site of lesser curve. (b) Duodenogastric fistula at site of greater curve.

Symptoms

In the setting of gastroduodenal fistulas secondary to peptic ulcer disease, the clinical presentation includes a long history of epigastric pain and overt or occult gastrointestinal haemorrhage. Peptic ulcer disease has generally been established for more than two years. No specific symptom can be related to the fistula. In the case of a malignant fistula, epigastric pain may be relieved at the time of fistula formation. The two patients with congenital double pylorus had a history of epigastric pain.[5]

Diagnosis

The double channel pylorus complicating gastric ulcer is a radiological finding in most instances. The appearance is characteristic, but one must appreciate the existence of this condition for correct interpretation of the contrast series. The long and narrow connection between antrum and duodenum is clearly outlined with barium and separated from the normal pylorus by a radiolucent band[1] (Figure 49.1). At endoscopy, both the pylorus and the fistula may be visualized and cannulated with a polyethylene catheter.[1] However, the mucosal oedema, hypertrophic folds and blood clot may suggest the presence of a tumour and lead to an unnecessary gastric resection.[1] The double pylorus may also be discovered during the healing period at follow-up endoscopy.

Malignant fistulas are demonstrated either radiologically or endoscopically. They need to be distinguished from mere protrusion of a gastric carcinoma into the pyloric channel, mimicking the double pylorus.

Treatment

The incidence of double-channel pylorus in relation to peptic ulcer has decreased with the advent of efficient medical therapy for this disease. Once established, this complication responds well to antisecretory drugs. It either disappears or persists in the form of an epithelialized track. The fistula may remains as the only patent channel, the native pylorus being obstructed by the inflammatory process. Operation, which should be restricted to patients with intractable pain, recurrent haemorrhage or suspicion of malignancy, usually consists of partial gastrectomy.

Treatment of malignant gastroduodenal fistulas consists of Whipple's operation with an extensive gastrectomy when no distant or local spread precludes curative intent. Otherwise simple gastroenterostomy is indicated.

Treatment of the exceptional congenital double pylorus has been operative in the two cases reported: Billroth I gastrectomy in one, division of the septum in the other. It is uncertain whether operation was really justified.

Conclusion

Gastroduodenal fistula complicating peptic ulcer disease is rare. It should be recognized on upper gastrointestinal series and should not be mistaken for a malignant lesion. It should be treated as any gastric ulcer. Other types of double channel pylorus are exceptional.

GASTROJEJUNOCOLIC FISTULAS

Gastrojejunocolic fistulas are extremely rare nowadays and were only sporadically reported in the older literature. Probably less than 100 cases have been described since the beginning of the century.

Aetiology

The most common cause of gastrojejunocolic fistula is recurrent peptic ulcer or anastomotic ulcer following gastric resection with gastrojejunal anastomosis (Billroth II procedure).[6] The surgical procedure explains the involvement of the small bowel (Figure 49.2). In non-operated patients, a communication between stomach, large bowel and jejunum is distinctly uncommon, but it may be produced by malignant tumours of the stomach, transverse colon or splenic flexure.[6,7] Although most of these tumours are adenocarcinomas, it is important to note that gastric (or, rarely, colonic) lymphoma can lead to this kind of fistula, especially in patients undergoing chemotherapy.[8,9]

There are anecdotal cases of benign peptic ulcer reaching the colonic lumen through the transverse mesocolon or via a confined perforation, and secondarily involving a jejunal loop;[6] most authors have emphasized the role of steroidal or non-steroidal anti-inflammatory agents[10] in the genesis of primary gastrocolic or gastrojejunocolic fistulas. The ulcerogenic properties of these drugs plus the decreased local inflammatory phenomenon could explain such extensive fistulas.[7] Fistula related to tuberculosis, syphilis and mycosis are of historical interest.[10] One case related to regional enteritis (Crohn's disease) has been reported.[11]

Incidence

At the beginning of gastric surgery for ulcer disease, gastrojejunocolic fistula was reported to complicate 10–15% of cases of marginal ulceration following gastrojejunostomy.[11] The incidence has decreased since the practice of vagotomy and higher

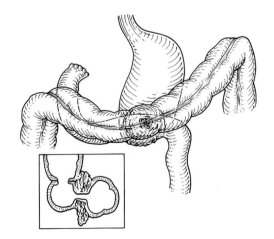

Figure 49.2

Gastrojejunocolic fistula. The transverse colon has become adherent to the mass of a recurrent (marginal) ulcer at the site of previous gastrojejunostomy following Billroth II (Polya) partial gastrectomy for duodenal ulcer disease. A fistula between upper and lower gastrointestinal tract has ensued.

gastrectomy and since the discovery of H$_2$ blockers and proton pump inhibitors. Gastroscopy allows a close watch to be kept on patients operated on for peptic ulcer disease and permits early treatment in cases of marginal ulceration. Palliative gastroenterostomies performed without vagotomy for gastric or pancreatic cancer led to anastomotic ulcer in 10% of cases, but antisecretory drugs commonly allow healing.

Symptoms

Abdominal pain, severe diarrhoea and weight loss are the most common clinical findings.[11] Malnutrition is also a common presenting sign. Faecal vomiting is considered to be a classic symptom of the disease, but it is found in less than 50% of cases.[7,10,11] Upper gastrointestinal bleeding occurs in one-third of patients.[7,10] Rarely, a free perforation may occur, leading to diffuse or localized peritonitis.[6]

The contamination of the upper gastrointestinal tract with faecal organisms seems to be important in the sometimes devastating clinical syndrome that is manifested by weight loss, anaemia and severe diarrhoea[12] (Figure 49.3). The transit of faecal material through the small bowel causes gross disturbances in absorptive and digestive function. Passage of chyme from the upper digestive tract into the colon has little importance in the genesis of clinical symptoms. Moreover, upper endoscopic examinations frequently show faecal material flowing from the colon, giving evidence of the higher intraluminal pressure in the colon than in the stomach or jejunum.[6]

Diagnosis

Laboratory findings usually reflect dehydration, malnutrition and sepsis. They are more important for the preoperative assessment of the patient's condition than for diagnosis. Barium enema leads to diagnosis in 95% of cases.[7,11] An upper gastrointestinal series, which has only a 25% yield in demonstrating the fistula, gives useful information about the stomach and the jejunum. Gastroscopy demonstrates the fistula by

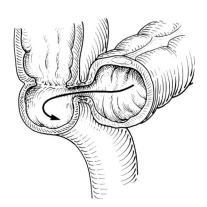

Figure 49.3
Diagram to show lateral view of gastrojejunocolic fistula. The fistula develops between adherent transverse colon and the site of previous gastrojejunostomy as a result of a stomal ulcer. The arrow shows the route by which faeces contaminate the upper small bowel to cause a severe enteritis leading to weight loss, diarrhoea and malnutrition.

showing faecal material in the gastric lumen. It also shows the marginal ulcer and allows biopsy of the ulcer to exclude the possibility of malignancy. Passing through the fistula from the stomach to the colon with the fibroscope is not helpful and possibly dangerous. Tests using dyes (e.g. indigo carmine) in an enema which are collected by a nasogastric tube are seldom needed to prove the communication between stomach and colon. Colonoscopy is rarely performed and should be restricted to patients in whom a specific disease of the colon is suspected, e.g. Crohn's disease, or cancer.

Treatment

The goals of treatment of gastrojejunocolic fistula are twofold:

1. To interrupt the vicious circle of faecal contamination of the upper digestive tract, and lead the patient to a better nutritional state;
2. To cure the fistula and prevent recurrence of the underlying ulcer disease (which is the most frequent cause of fistula).

Different techniques have been described for attaining these goals. Staged procedures were at first the preferred techniques, ranging from simple colostomy to three-stage procedures consisting of colostomy followed by resection of the fistula and closure of the colostomy. Lahey in 1938 proposed a two-stage procedure whereby ileosigmoid bypass was followed by fistula resection, thus avoiding both the need for a third stage and the period of colostomy. All procedures had in common the diversion of the faecal stream away from the upper gastrointestinal tract as a first stage. Since the 1940s progress in nutrition and antibiotic therapy has allowed surgeons to consider the cure of the fistula in one stage. The first step in management is medical therapy comprising antibiotics, antisecretory drugs and nutritional support. Correction of metabolic abnormalities, enema or whole gut irrigations to clean the colon, bowel rest, total parenteral nutrition, and H$_2$ blockers or omeprazole should then prepare the patient for a safe surgical procedure. These measures frequently allow spontaneous closure of the fistula tract. Except in a high-risk patient with poor life expectancy, it is necessary to achieve complete treatment by surgical resection to suppress the remaining part of the fistula and cure the ulcer disease.[7,10] Controlling the ulcer diathesis is important. Localio et al.[13] reviewed 115 cases between 1943 and 1953 and found a recurrence rate of 50% among those treated with cure of the fistula only, as compared to 4% among those treated with correction of the ulcer diathesis as well.

The surgical procedure combines en bloc resection of the gastrojejunal anastomosis with colectomy, followed by a new gastrojejunostomy, or a Roux-en-Y limb and vagotomy (if not previously performed). Colonic anastomosis may be undertaken at the same time. In emergency procedures related to free perforation, the gastric defect may be oversewn, but the involved large bowel has to be resected and exteriorized.[6]

In rare cases when the general condition of the patient remains poor despite medical treatment, then staged operation is advised. Rather than performing a right colostomy that will impede performance of fistula resection, it is preferable to raise a lateral ileostomy. This stoma allows complete exclusion of the colon, irrigation of the distal bowel and later elective cure of the fistula under good conditions. The ileostomy can either be taken down at this second operation or left for a third stage.

In each patient long-term treatment with H_2-receptor antagonists must be considered, and a close surveillance of the new gastrojejunostomy must be planned. If no risk factor is found for a gastrojejunocolic fistula, Zollinger–Ellison syndrome has to be excluded by measuring serum gastrin levels. Surreptitious salicylate abuse has been described[10] to explain recurrences after correct management of gastrojejunocolic fistula.

Results

As early as 1960, Barber et al.[14] reported a mortality rate as low as 2–6% among 76 patients after a one-stage procedure. Marshall[15] emphasized the decrease in the mortality rate of this condition from 25% in 1927–1936 to 4% in 1937–1946 and zero in 1947–1955. These satisfactory results have been obtained in selected patients, who were found fit enough to sustain a one-stage major operation. However, the progress of medical treatment now makes it possible to improve the condition of most patients to a point where such operation is feasible.

Conclusion

Gastrojejunocolic fistulas may disappear from the list of postoperative complications of ulcer disease, thanks to a careful follow-up of patients, avoidance of injurious drugs and powerful antisecretory agents that are able to cure most of the recurrent anastomotic ulcers. In the case of an established gastrojejunocolic fistula, progress in medical care facilitates a one-stage surgical procedure.

DUODENOCOLIC FISTULAS (excluding Crohn's disease)

Communication between the duodenal and colonic lumens is a rare entity. The main cause is colonic carcinoma at the hepatic flexure, but non-malignant cases have also been reported. Symptoms arise from the contamination of the upper digestive tract by faecal material, as with gastrojejunocolic fistula. Parenteral nutritional support allows sufficient improvement in general condition to achieve radical cure in one operation.

Incidence

Several reports have estimated the incidence of malignant duodenocolic fistula at 1–2 per 1000 cases of right colonic carcinoma.[16,17] Up to 1989 only 60 patients with duodenocolic fistulas secondary to colon cancer were reported in the literature. Benign causes were thought to be rare, but more and more cases have been reported in the past few years; in an exhaustive survey of the world literature in 1986, 62 such cases were collected.[18]

Aetiology

Malignant duodenocolic fistulas are usually the final stage of duodenal wall involvement arising from a right colonic cancer

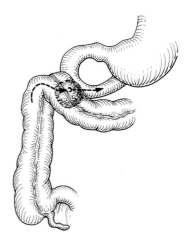

Figure 49.4
Malignant duodenocolic fistula. A large primary carcinoma arising from the hepatic flexure of the colon has become adherent to the third part of the duodenum, and a fistula has developed at this site. The arrow shows the direction by which faeces can enter the duodenum to contaminate the small bowel.

(Figure 49.4). The primary malignant condition is an adenocarcinoma but, exceptionally, a lymphosarcoma has been reported. In other rare cases the malignant process is situated in the duodenal wall, pancreas or gall bladder.[19]

Benign duodenocolic fistulas are related to duodenal ulcer, duodenal diverticulum, inflammatory diseases (ulcerative colitis) and infectious diseases (tuberculosis, typhoid, amoebiasis).[18] They may also follow operations on the duodenum, biliary tract or colon[18] (Table 49.1).

Table 49.1   Causes of benign duodenocolic fistulas in the literature.

CAUSES	NO. OF CASES
Duodenal ulcer	14
Duodenal diverticulum	9
Tuberculosis	8
Regional ileitis	7
Congenital anomalies	4
Iatrogenic (postoperative)	4
Appendicitis	3
Ulcerative colitis	3
Trauma	2
Typoid	1
Amoebiasis	1
Unknown	6
Total	62

After Lopez and Hreno.[18]

Symptoms

The presenting signs and symptoms are the same as for gastrojejunocolic fistula but they are worsened by the underlying malignant disease. The mechanism of the disorder is a two-way bypass. First, gastric, pancreatic and biliary secretions pass into the colonic lumen and cause diarrhoea related to the presence of acid and unconjugated bile salts. Secondly, there is a faecal contamination of the duodenum, leading to bacterial overgrowth in the small intestine, causing enteritis and impairing absorptive function (Figure 49.4). These two facts explain the clinical features of diarrhoea, weight loss, malnutrition and anaemia in about 80% of cases.[19] Pain is usual, but may be related to the malignant tumour with or without fistula. Faecal vomiting or belching is pathognomonic but only present in 17% of cases. A palpable mass is found in 40–65% of cases.[20]

Diagnosis

Barium enema is the investigation of choice to document a duodenocolic fistula. It shows sudden filling of the duodenal lumen from the transverse colon and, if present, the colonic tumour. Upper gastrointestinal studies may demonstrate air or contrast material in the biliary tree when the fistula is secondary to cholelithiasis, or a normal colonic mucosal outline when it is due to primary duodenal disease. Gastroduodenoscopy may demonstrate the fistula, showing faecal material in the stomach itself or the fistulous tract. Colonoscopy allows identification and biopsy of the primary colonic disease. Laboratory findings reflect both dehydration and an inflammatory process.

In the case of malignant disease, assessment must include hepatic ultrasonography, computed tomography (CT), chest radiography and serum tumour markers. The stage of malignant disease at the time of diagnosis is an important prognostic factor and will influence the choice of surgical procedure.

Treatment

The therapeutic approach aims at (1) correction of the metabolic disorders induced by the fistula and (2) resection or exclusion of the fistula. Total parenteral nutrition, antisecretory drugs, whole gut irrigations and enemas will improve the general status in the first instance.

Treatment of malignant fistulas

The surgical procedure should be tailored to the extent of disease, but even if there are distant metastases resection provides the best palliation. Two possibilities may be considered with a view to cure.

1. Right colectomy with pancreatoduodenectomy is mandatory when the extent of the malignant disease makes duodenal wall closure impossible. In resectable cases it probably represents the procedure of choice in terms of early postoperative mortality and long-term results.[16,20,21] The causes of unresectability are the involvement of the retroperitoneal space or the superior mesenteric vessels. Thirteen cases have been reported to date,[21] with a 46% 2.5-year survival and one local recurrence. There was no postoperative death.

2. Right colectomy with duodenal wall resection is advocated when the involvement of duodenal wall is small or when distant metastasis rules out curative resection. The main

difficulty remains the closure of the duodenal defect. If it is small, primary closure by means of transverse suture is possible, perhaps with gastroenterostomy to protect the suture line.[16] Several procedures have been described to achieve closure of major duodenal defects, including a serosal jejunal patch and lateral duodenoenterostomy with an omega loop; although frequently proposed, a Roux-en-Y loop has not given a successful outcome in this condition.[16] Although this procedure is the most commonly performed (about 60% of cases), the risk of anastomotic leakage is high due to adverse local conditions and poor nutritional status. It is associated with a 28% early postoperative mortality rate, mainly attributed to difficulty with the duodenal closure.[21] Several cases of prolonged survival have been reported, suggesting that use of a Roux loop could be an efficient treatment in some patients and that the fistula may be related to an inflammatory process rather than extensive cancer.[16] However, long-term results of limited resection of the duodenum are impaired by the high rate of local recurrence. In a review of the literature including 16 cases of right hemicolectomy and duodenal excision, Le Treut et al.[16] reported six survivors with no evidence of disease and nine deaths, including seven documented local recurrences.

None of the various diverting procedures is really satisfactory, although many are described. The choice of procedure should be based on the anatomical condition, bearing in mind that the aim is to isolate the upper digestive tract from faecal soiling, and to permit the discharge of the fistulous tract. Such procedures combine gastrojejunostomy with ileotransversostomy, or the duodenocolic mass is bypassed by a distal ileostomy.[16] Such techniques should be reserved for patients in whom a right colectomy is not feasible.

Treatment of benign duodenocolic fistulas

Surgical correction of a benign duodenocolic fistula may be almost as challenging when major inflammatory changes are present. As Starzl and associates have suggested,[22] corrective surgery is performed either for direct closure of the fistula or to enhance the possibility of closure. The standard technique of fistula closure entails colonic resection and closure of the duodenal defect. Closure of a major defect may require serosal patching, duodenojejunostomy or partial duodenal exclusion with vagotomy and gastroenterostomy.[18] Pancreatoduodenectomy has not been used among cases reported to date. Among 61 patients collected from the literature, there were only two deaths and the long-term results were mostly satisfactory.[18]

Operative difficulties

The right upper quadrant is difficult to dissect in both benign and malignant fistulas. It is best first to expose the retroperitoneal region and identify the right kidney, the right renal vessels, the ureter and the inferior vena cava. The porta hepatis and the mesenteric vessels represent the other points of possible invasion and should be checked before division of the fistula. At this point, it may be possible to carry out an *en bloc* resection (in case of malignancy) or a division of fistula followed by excision of the duodenal margin and duodenal closure (in case of benign fistula).

INTERNAL FISTULAS IN CROHN'S DISEASE

Internal fistulas represent a common complication of Crohn's disease, affecting 15–30% of the patients in surgical series.[23-25] Their pathophysiology remains unclear; it was originally thought that they were the consequence of transmural extension of the inflammatory process with deep fissures leading to subacute perforation, abscess and fistula.[26] Steinberg et al.[27] and Farmer et al.[24] also pointed out the frequent association of an internal fistula with an abscess. However, more recent studies suggest that fistula formation without abscess may be more frequent, only 10–30% of the patients having an abscess at operation.[28,29]

Development of an internal fistula is usually heralded by severe yet non-specific clinical symptoms: fever, weight loss, diarrhoea, obstruction and sepsis. Internal fistulas have few specific symptoms, except the enterovesical type yet they represent an expression of severe Crohn's disease. Approximately 25% of patients with internal fistulas have multiple internal communications, and another 10% present with simultaneous enterocutaneous fistulas.[29] Most of these patients (approximately 60%) have evidence of Crohn's disease affecting both ileum and colon, whereas 25% have ileitis and 15% have colitis only.[28,29]

The fistula usually connects a segment of bowel affected by specific lesions of Crohn's with a viscus free from disease. The segment of bowel generating the fistula should be resected. The viscus connected to this segment is frequently inflamed and shows mucosal lesions but, in most cases, these changes are localized and allow a conservative approach. Nevertheless, the surgical treatment of these patients is difficult and is associated with a high morbidity rate for many reasons. The patient is often septic and malnourished;[23,26] in 30% of cases fistula formation represents a recurrence of Crohn's disease[30] and difficulties of dissection are common. A temporary defunctioning stoma may be required. Extensive intestinal Crohn's lesions are not uncommon and may lead to wide resection.

Therefore, surgical indications need careful thought. Immediate operation is required in the presence of peritonitis, abscess and intractable obstruction or sepsis. With disabling symptoms such as diarrhoea, weight loss, abdominal pain or features such as pneumaturia and urinary infection, medical treatment should be attempted first. Eventually 75–95% of the patients will require surgical therapy,[29,31] but some will escape operation and an appreciable proportion will benefit from a delay of one to six years before operation, being reasonably comfortable during this time.[29] Thus the fistula *per se* is not necessarily an indication for operation unless medical treatment fails (see Chapter 50). The principles of the surgical treatment of Crohn's disease are considered in Chapter 51.

Duodenoenteric fistula

This is a rare entity, and a review of the literature[32,33] could enumerate only 40 cases. Its incidence in large surgical series of Crohn's disease ranges between 1 and 3%[32] of the total number of patients and represents 5–10% of all internal fistulas complicating Crohn's disease. It affects mainly male patients (mean sex ratio 2.8 : 1). Two types are recognized: fistulas following ileocaecal resection and primary fistulas. Fistulas after ileocaecal resection connect the second part of the duodenum with the site of the ileocolostomy and result from either sepsis following resection or recurrence of Crohn's disease at the site of anastomosis. Primary fistulas affect various parts of the duodenum and are due to ileal and/or colonic lesions; multiple fistulas are common. In both instances the origin of the fistula is on the ileal or colonic side; the duodenum represents the 'receiving viscus' and is seldom affected by specific Crohn's lesions.

Symptoms include abdominal pain, diarrhoea, intestinal obstruction, weight loss, fever and abdominal mass. Faeculent vomiting is rare. The fistula is shown by radiography and/or endoscopy. Preoperative work-up includes CT or ultrasound scanning, upper and lower endoscopy, and contrast radiographs of stomach, colon and small bowel. This imaging allows an evaluation of duodenal and enteric lesions. It is important to demonstrate the extent of duodenal lesions and to look for duodenal stenosis, as this will affect the choice of the procedure on the duodenum.

Operation is not an emergency requirement as the communication between duodenum and colon/ileum is of small calibre and does not produce diarrhoea. The indication for operation stems from complications and intractability, though most patients will require operation eventually.

In all patients operation includes the resection of the ileum and/or colon responsible for the fistula formation plus the repair of the duodenal defect. In cases of duodenocolic fistula, it is unusual to find a limited extension of the colonic disease allowing for a segmental resection, and a formal right hemicolectomy or an ileocolic resection (including the previous anastomosis) is required. Resection is followed by an ileocolostomy. This anastomosis should be located in the left part of the transverse colon to avoid contact with the duodenum; extensive colonic lesions may require even wider resections. As for the duodenal repair, debridement and primary closure is usually feasible, but a large defect may require a duodenojejunostomy or a Roux loop. The extent of the duodenal disease is best evaluated by preoperative duodenoscopy showing the mucosal side. This investigation plus the operative findings allows an appropriate choice of duodenal procedure to be made. Protection of the duodenal suture line by an omental patch, temporary decompression by a nasogastric tube, and placement of a jejunal feeding catheter, are strongly advised. Whether protective means, such as serosal patch, fibrin sealant or somatostatin should be used in these patients is still a matter for debate.

After surgical treatment for duodenoenteric fistula, the mortality rate is approximately 10% and the morbidity rate is 20%;[32] the main complications are sepsis and fistula from the duodenal suture line. Recurrence of Crohn's disease is common but affects the ileum and colon only. Recurrent duodenal disease is rare, and recurrent duodenoenteric fisula is exceptional.

Prevention of duodenoenteric fistulas lies in proper positioning of the ileocolostomy following the ileocaecal resection; either the anastomosis is placed low in the ascending colon or an omentoplasty separates the anastomosis from the duodenum.

In summary, duodenoenteric fistula is a rare complication of Crohn's disease and the expression of severe and multiple lesions. The extent of the disease warrants surgical treatment in most cases. Operation for a duodenoenteric fistula is a complex procedure, the main risk being leakage from the duodenal repair.

Enteroenteric fistulas (ileum to jejunum, ileum to ileum)

These represent 20% of all internal Crohn's fistulas. They are characterized by the absence of specific symptoms and, therefore, do not constitute by themselves an indication for operation.

At operation, an enteroenteric fistula may present as an inflammatory mass of diseased bowel in which only examination of the resected specimen reveals a communication between the two diseased segments. Another form, equally frequent, is a fistula originating from a segment of diseased bowel but opening into normal intestine. In this case, the fistula can and should be identified when adhesions between the inflamed and healthy intestine are divided but, as the orifice is small, this requires careful inspection and probing of any suspect area. It should be borne in mind that 25–40% of internal fistulas are not diagnosed preoperatively but only at operation or on pathological examination.[28,29] It is necessary, therefore, to check routinely any segment of bowel tightly adherent to inflammatory tissue. Alexander-Williams[34] has proposed insufflation of the bowel after dissection to detect any stenosis and fistula.

Are there any clinical features that may be attributed to enteroenteral fistulas? Patients with this condition usually present with abdominal pain, weight loss and diarrhoea; an abdominal mass can be palpated in 20% of cases. About 10% of patients have an enterocutaneous fistula in addition to the internal communication.[28] It has been suggested that fistula formation could decompress an obstructed segment and therefore provide relief after an acute episode of abdominal pain, but the fistulous tracts are invariably small and seldom permit passage of appreciable amounts of intestinal content. Similarly, it is difficult to imagine that passage of intestinal contents through such fine channels can cause diarrhoea by means of a short circuit. Therefore, an internal enteroenteric fistula is only a feature of severe Crohn's lesions and carries no specific deleterious effect. Preoperative diagnosis of internal enteroenteric fistula is made in 50–75% of patients, mainly on radiological studies, by the demonstration of a fine tract connecting two (or more) loops of intestine.

Indications for treatment

Although enteroenteric fistulas were once considered in many institutions as a formal indication for operation, attitudes have changed. Nowadays most surgeons prefer to operate for the same criteria as in any Crohn's patient: intestinal obstruction, abscess formation, haemorrhage and failure to control symptoms with medical therapy. Abscesses complicate the course of internal fistulas in Crohn's disease in approximately 15% of cases, and they should be routinely sought by ultrasonography and/or CT scanning. In the absence of abscess or other clinical criteria warranting operation, there is no specific risk in maintaining the patient on medical treatment.

In one series, among 33 patients with an internal fistula diagnosed before operation, 10 underwent immediate operation, 15 came to delayed operation after a mean period of one year (range 1 month–6 years) and eight had no operation. Among 11 enteroenteric fistulas, one was managed non-operatively. Although the rate of abscess was increased in the 'delayed surgery' group (53% v 18%), no difference in mortality and morbidity rates could be found. The type of operation performed was independent of its timing.[29]

The clinical experience from the Johns Hopkins Hospital is similar: among 48 patients with an ileoileal or ileocolic fistula, 24 were operated upon immediately, 10 within one year, eight after a mean of 3.5 years and six had no operation.[28]

In both series, all non-operated patients were on active medical treatment: steroids, sulphasalazine or azathioprine. They remained relatively asymptomatic during the course of follow-up but the majority were on maintenance therapy.[28,29] Azathioprine has been advocated in the treatment of Crohn's fistulas but has proven of little benefit in enteroenteric fistula: only one of seven patients achieved closure in a recent report from the Mount Sinai Hospital.[35] Therefore, in enteroenteric fistulas, azathioprine is indicated for the same reasons as in ordinary Crohn's ileitis.

Approximately two-thirds of the patients with enteroenteric fistula have severe lesions of Crohn's disease and require surgical treatment either immediately or after a short period of preparation. The remaining third, however, show a good response to medical therapy and may escape operation for years, or even completely. The risk of operation after a prolonged period of maintenance therapy is not increased provided undue delay is avoided in the presence of intractable symptoms.

Technique and results of operation in enteroenteric fistulas

In the past many patients underwent diversion of the faecal stream as a first stage,[26] but the routine approach is now to perform a resection of the diseased bowel followed by immediate anastomosis. In the St Mark's series, among 42 resections other than coloproctectomy, 38 had an immediate anastomosis and four a staged operation.[29] However, in the presence of severe sepsis, free perforation and/or malnutrition, exteriorization of bowel ends after resection remains the safest procedure. When the fistula connects two inflamed segments of intestine, double resection is required; this situation is found in 60% of cases.[28,29] When the fistula opens in healthy small bowel, the secondary orifice may simply be closed after limited excision of the edges. As the secondary fistula orifice is usually situated on the mesenteric border, closure may seem difficult. In fact, clearing the edges is easy and does not interfere with the blood supply. When the fistula connects a diseased loop with a normal loop, but both orifices lie within a short distance, a single resection including the diseased bowel and the secondary orifice may be the best choice.

As in any operation dealing with Crohn's ileitis, it is mandatory to explore the whole intestine and to treat all tight stenoses[34] and any other important lesion that might be encountered. Patients with a large abscess in conjunction with a fistula are better managed by drainage alone, as this may suffice to provide long-term relief with no great risk of a serious cutaneous fistula. If a formal laparotomy is required for drainage, exteriorization of the bowel ends is the safest choice.

The postoperative mortality rate of fistula surgery is low, ranging from zero to 2%;[28,29] the main threat is pulmonary embolism. Other complications include intra-abdominal sepsis (10%), faecal fistula (10%) and intestinal obstruction (5%). Postoperative faecal fistulas, or type II Crohn's enterocutaneous fistulas, usually heal with conservative therapy.[36] Prevention of anastomotic leakage by somatostatin analogues or fibrin sealants requires further evaluation.

Ileosigmoid fistulas

Communication between the ileum and sigmoid colon in Crohn's disease is the commonest type of Crohn's internal fistula (30–50%). It is the indication for operation in 5–10% of patients.[28,29,37] The usual pattern of Crohn's disease is ileocaecal involvement, with the occasional case of extensive colitis in association with ileitis. Ileosigmoid fistulization is the result of ileal lesions extending into the sigmoid mesentery and the sigmoid wall, with or without abscess formation (Figure 49.5). Abscess is found at operation in 20% of patients.[28,29,34] Colonic lesions are merely the consequence of fistula formation and take the form of pericolic inflammation and localized mucosal changes: oedema, friability, pseudopolyps. The principle of

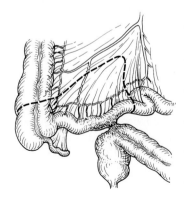

Figure 49.5
Ileosigmoid fistula in Crohn's disease. The primary site of disease is the terminal ileum, and this is to be resected by means of ileocaecal excision. The sigmoid colon is often healthy except immediately around the fistula, and the colon is to be managed by simple closure, wedge excision or formal resection according to the extent of involvement.

surgical treatment is now clarified: ileocaecal resection plus a limited procedure on the sigmoid, either simple closure or wedge resection.

Many Crohn's patients presenting with ileosigmoid fistula have already undergone laparotomy, and evaluation of the length of remaining bowel is required to determine the best treatment. Half of these patients have multiple fistulas:[37] enterocutaneous fistulas, enterovesical communication or multiple enteroenteric tracts. A search for such associated conditions will be part of the preoperative work-up.

There is no specific symptom of ileosigmoid fistula. The communication is of small calibre and does not produce diarrhoea, *per se*. Yet it bears witness to severe Crohn's disease and generally requires operation. In the St Mark's series,[29] where conservative treatment was firmly attempted in all cases, only 3 out of 46 patients with ileosigmoid fistula escaped operation. In the Johns Hopkins series one patient among 17 with ileosigmoid fistula 'was not operated on soon enough and spontaneously closed his fistula'.[38] Medical treatment, including azathioprine, is ineffective at closing an ileosigmoid communication,[35] but it is clear for any experienced clinician that the aim of medical therapy is to relieve the symptoms related to active Crohn's disease and that conservative treatment must be continued if effective, even if the ileosigmoid fistula persists.

The indications for operation are therefore failure of medical treatment to control symptoms, intestinal obstruction, abscess or free perforation. The preparation for operation includes adequate nutrition, prograde bowel preparation and antibiotics. Exploration of the whole peritoneal cavity is carried out to obtain an accurate evaluation of the extent of the disease and exclude other internal fistulas.

Operation for ileosigmoid fistula requiring ileocaecal resection plus either simple closure or formal resection of the sigmoid[39] (Figure 49.5) has been a matter of debate. Supporters of the double resection[29,39] argue that severe pericolic inflammation and true Crohn's mucosal lesions in the sigmoid – even if localized – are strong enough elements to warrant sigmoid resection. Supporters of simple closure/wedge resection[37,38,40,41] claim that sigmoid mucosal changes are a mere extension of the ileal lesions and that a simple closure of the sigmoid defect, after limited excision, is a safe manoeuvre in terms of both immediate and long-term results. This attitude is strongly supported by a report from the Chicago University Hospital showing no leak, no death and no sigmoid recurrence after simple closure of the colonic defect among 48 ileosigmoid fistulas.[37] In comparison, double resection was followed by a 10% incidence of faecal fistula in the St Mark's series.[29]

However, there is a small proportion of patients with extensive colitis who require a wider excision. In this regard, Greenstein[42] has suggested adaptation of the procedure on the sigmoid according to the extent of colonic inflammation as evaluated at endoscopy. In cases in which colonic lesions are absent or minimal, simple closure may suffice, but should the colonic involvement be extensive or take the form of multiple fistulas or stricture, then formal resection is required. Such an eclectic approach has been adopted at our institution.

When endoscopy has been normal or shown limited disease, which is the case in 90% of patients, the procedure is simple. Adhesions are divided at first by blunt dissection and then by sharp dissection at the site of the fistula track. Inspection and probing of the track indicates whether it opens blindly or into the sigmoid itself. An actual communication with the lumen of the sigmoid is signalled by the site of attachment (antimesenteric or lateral walls of the colon) and by the characteristic aspect of the track showing granulation tissue or colonic mucosa. Suspicious areas may be probed gently for confirmation of a suspected fistula. Once the fistula has been diagnosed, the first step is to excise the fistula track plus the edges of the orifice in the sigmoid. This procedure allows inspection of the surrounding mucosa; if mucosal changes are minimal or absent, then the defect may be simply closed. If mucosal lesions or stricture is found, then a wedge resection or a short segmental resection is performed. When the fistula track involves an appreciable segment of colon or shows considerable inflammation or multiple tracks, it may be necessary to perform a formal resection, although even in this situation Block and Schraut[37] has performed a simple closure of the defect combined with a loop colostomy.

Should no endoscopic examination have been performed before operation, palpation of the colon above and below the site of attachment allows evaluation of the extent of the disease. This evaluation, combined with inspection of the mucosa after fistula excision, may provide sufficient information to make a safe choice of procedure.

Although most patients are operated on without performing a stoma there are two situations in which an enterostomy is required.

1. In the 10% of cases showing extensive colonic Crohn's disease; either an anterior resection or a suture line within inflammatory tissue may be necessary. Rectosigmoid lesions may remain distal to the site of fistula closure. In all such instances, it is best to perform a defunctioning stoma.[42,43]

2. In the presence of peritonitis, large abscess or severe malnutrition,[23,37] it is safest to exteriorize both ends of intestine after ileocaecal resection instead of performing an anastomosis.

In addition to these two clear cases for a stoma, some surgeons prefer to perform a loop colostomy proximal to the sigmoid suture line whenever local inflammation is marked.

Ileovesical fistulas

Ileovesical fistulas in Crohn's disease arise secondary to an ileal inflammatory process with either abscess formation or progressive extension toward the urinary bladder.[31] The site of urinary communication is the dome of the bladder. Fistulas originating in a Meckel's diverticulum,[43] or an opening in the right ureter,[44] have also been described. Ileovesical fistula is more frequent in males because of the protective effect of the uterus in women.

The incidence of enterovesical fistula in series of patients with Crohn's disease ranges from 2–6%.[30] Among all enterovesical fistulas, the ileovesical type represents the commonest form, ranging from 60 to 80%.[30,31] Crohn's disease accounts for 6% of all enterovesical fistulas.[45] The pattern of Crohn's disease in a patient with ileovesical fistula is dominated by ileitis and ileocolitis.[30,31] Although usually benign, the inflammatory lesions at the site of the fistula may have undergone malignant degeneration after a longstanding course of Crohn's disease; Greenstein et al.[31] report three such cases among a series of 38 patients.

The occurrence of an ileovesical fistula signals an exacerbation of the disease and is frequently associated with an increase of both digestive and septic symptoms. At presentation, 40% of the patients suffer from severe malnutrition, and 30% have a documented pelvic abscess.[30,46] The clinical presentation is usually suggestive, urinary symptoms being predominant in two-thirds of patients. Dysuria and frequency (95% of patients), pneumaturia (80%) and faecaluria (65%) are associated with urinary tract infection (90%) showing multiple bacterial strains. In one-third of patients septic or intestinal signs predominate.

Preoperative diagnosis of ileovesical fistula can be made by either demonstration of the communication or signs of bullous oedema on the bladder dome at cystoscopic examination. Plain abdominal radiology or CT scanning may demonstrate the presence of air in the bladder. Small bowel series provide an accurate evaluation of the ileal and caecal lesions but seldom show the communication with the bladder. Intravenous pyelography rarely shows passage of contrast medium to the ileum, but it may show mucosal irregularity and a mass effect at the dome of the bladder. It may also demonstrate hydronephrosis when the termination of the right ureter is involved in the inflammatory process, and this finding indicates a difficult surgical dissection. Radiological and endoscopic examinations of the colon are required to look for an ileosigmoid fistula, which is associated in 40% of cases.[47] Contrast enema may demonstrate the fistula, whereas endoscopy rarely shows the communication but is useful to evaluate the extent of sigmoid disease.

CT scan and ultrasonography are required in searching for an intra-abdominal abscess; such a complication will frequently lead to a multiple-stage procedure. Cystoscopic examination is the most efficient examination in terms of diagnosis, showing an obvious defect or at least revealing indirect signs at the dome of the bladder: localized 'bullous' oedema, pseudopolyps, erythema. Cystoscopy provides positive findings in 60–80% of cases.

In summary, preoperative evaluation leads to a precise diagnosis in 70% of cases and strong suspicion in 20% (mainly on the clinical history), whereas the fistula is an intraoperative finding in 10%. Lack of preoperative diagnosis of an ileovesical fistula does not represent a major problem as the treatment is simple and requires no more preparation than the placement of a urinary catheter, which is routine practice in major procedures for Crohn's disease.

Associated fistulas are a frequent feature, and up to 65% of patients have another fistula, mainly ileosigmoid but also ileocutaneous, ileovaginal or enteroenteric. Intraoperative exploration of the whole length of bowel is therefore required, together with gentle probing of any suspicious adhesion or granulating track.

Medical treatment comprises bowel rest, total parenteral nutrition, steroids and/or azathioprine, plus symptomatic treatment of urinary infection. In the absence of abscess, medical treatment may provide long-term relief in terms of intestinal and urinary symptoms. If not, medical treatment may be prolonged without the risk of severe renal complication. It may even allow closure of the fistula, as in four of 16 cases with azathioprine in the St Mark's series,[29] and in one of 38 untreated patients reported by Schraut and Block.[46] Occasional urinary infections may be treated as required. Eventually, 75–100% of the patients came to operation, not merely for the presence of an ileovesical fistula but also for associated conditions, such as intestinal obstruction, abscess, tender abdominal mass, or just intractability. About 80% of the patients requiring operation are operated upon early after presentation owing to the severity of symptoms or previous failure of medical treatment.

The operative principles are simple: resect the diseased ileocaecal segment and close the vesical orifice. Ileocaecal resection may be difficult in the presence of a mass involving the bladder, sigmoid and retroperitoneum. In these cases, careful and patient dissection should aim at achieving a resection despite adverse conditions, as bypass operations seldom provide long-term relief. Closure of the bladder defect should be managed as simply as possible by 'pinching off' the fistula or carrying out a limited resection of the inflammatory tissue. Absorbable sutures are used; thick through-and-through stitches should be avoided as they can provoke haematuria in the postoperative period.[30] Many techniques have been suggested, including omentoplasty,[30] suture with peritoneal patch[46] and no suture at all.[30] Formal cystectomy is avoided. Although pelvic drainage is advocated by some authors,[30] it is restricted to drainage of adjacent abscess cavities by others.[46] A Foley catheter is left in place for 7–10 days and removed after a control cystogram.

In favourable cases this operation can be conducted in one stage, but there are certain situations in which a stoma should be performed. Approximately 25% of patients undergo a two-stage operation;[30,31,46] options include an ileostomy as the first stage followed by a definitive procedure, an ileocaecal resection with exteriorization or an ileocaecal resection plus a sigmoid procedure plus colostomy. Two-stage procedures are required in the presence of major purulent contamination or peritonitis, the presence of a large abscess, extensive colonic disease, multiple fistulas or malnutrition.[23] Associated ileosigmoid fistulas should be treated according to the standard principles set out above.[29,30,46,47]

The immediate results of operation are satisfactory, with a mortality rate ranging from 0 to 5% and an equally low incidence of complications, such as fistula, intra-abdominal sepsis and wound abscess. Urinary fistulas following operation usually settle with vesical drainage alone.

The mean postoperative hospital stay is two weeks. It might be anticipated that a patient with an ileovesical and frequently another associated fistula would be prone to early recurrence due to the aggressive form of the disease.[25,48] However, follow-up of patients in reported series fails to indicate either a higher or an earlier incidence of clinically recurrent Crohn's disease. In the Cleveland Clinic series, 61 patients were followed for a mean of 106 months; 11 (17%) were re-operated for recurrent Crohn's disease, and a further group of seven patients (11%) were on permanent medication.[30] In the Mount Sinai series, 50% of patients were re-operated for recurrence.[31] These relatively high figures were not found in the series from the Johns Hopkins Hospital, in which 10 of 11 patients remained well after a mean follow-up of four years.[44] In the report by Schraut et al.[47] describing the outcome of 22 patients with ileocolovesical fistula, the rate of recurrence was 45%. Rarely does the recurrence take the form of an enterovesical fistula, except when the Crohn's disease or the fistula itself was undiagnosed at the time of the first operation.

In summary, enterovesical fistula in Crohn's disease represents a severe form of the disease, and operation is required in about 90% of cases. In the absence of abscess or hydronephrosis, medical treatment may be attempted and can provide lasting relief, if not cure, with little risk for renal function.[49] Operation consists of ileocaecal resection, closure of the bladder defect and treatment of associated fistulas. Immediate and long-term results after operation are satisfactory; recurrence is no more frequent than after operation for non-fistulous Crohn's disease.

COLOENTERIC FISTULAS IN DIVERTICULAR DISEASE

Ileocolic fistulas in diverticular disease are either primary or postoperative. They may occur spontaneously after a long period of inflammation; presence of a palpable mass is common. Treatment of such forms poses few problems. They may also occur after colonic resection for diverticulosis, usually after operations performed for either acute or chronic complications of the disease.

Primary ileosigmoid fistulas

These represent 7–20% of all internal fistulas in diverticular disease and approximately 1% of all surgically treated cases of diverticulosis.[50,51] Diverticulosis, cancer and Crohn's disease are the three main causes of coloenteric fistula[50] (Figure 49.6). Diverticular coloenteric fistulas may be associated with colovesical fistulas in up to 50% of cases,[50] but they are much less often associated with colovaginal fistulas. They are accompanied by an inflammatory pseudotumour in 80% of cases.[52]

In these patients the disease has been symptomatic for a minimum duration of one year before fistula formation. There are few specific symptoms, and the actual diagnosis of coloenteric fistula is often made only at operation. Diarrhoea is a common feature; it may be due to the direct passage of intestinal contents from ileum to sigmoid (20% of cases) or to bacterial enteritis related to regurgitation of clonic contents into the small bowel.[50,52] Fever, abdominal pain, weight loss and palpation of a tender pelvic mass are usually present. Barium enema is the best means of diagnosis, demonstrating the abnormal communication in 11/12 cases in Abacarian and Udezue's series[50] and often showing evidence of diverticulosis.

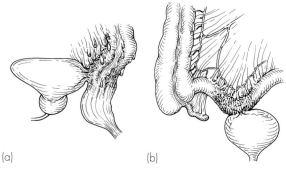

(a) (b)

Figure 49.6
Two common types of vesicointestinal fistula. (a) Colovesical
fistula secondary to diverticulitis affecting the sigmoid colon to
produce a local inflammatory mass ('diverticuloma').
(b) Enterovesical fistula complicating Crohn's disease of the
terminal ileum.

At operation, the ileal loops are tightly adherent to the
inflammatory sigmoid mass (or abscess). The fistula is clearly
visible after division of the adhesions. The ileal side of the
problem is solved by a short small bowel resection followed
by immediate anastomosis. The procedure on the sigmoid is
similar to that performed in the presence of an inflammatory
pseudotumour, i.e. resection with primary anastomosis. The
colorectal anastomosis should be created at the level of the
peritoneal reflection to avoid contact with areas of peritoneal
inflammation and remaining parts of the abscess wall. The
results of primary resection and anastomosis may be summarized as follows: mortality rate 2–5%, morbidity rate around
20% mainly due to anastomotic leakage and wound infection.[50-52]

There is no place for medical treatment in patients whose
symptoms are numerous, severe, longstanding and not relieved
by drug therapy. There is little place for operations such as
colostomy or Hartmann's procedure.

Postoperative coloenteric fistula

This is one of the numerous complications that may follow
resection for diverticular disease. The fistula usually occurs
when the primary operation has been carried out in the context of an acute or chronic complication of the disease, i.e.
obstruction, abscess, pseudotumour or re-operation for a
previous complication. The following two cases illustrate this
condition.

Case 1 Diverticular disease was associated with an abscess in
the pouch of Douglas, which was drained per vaginam. One
year later, resection was carried out with primary anastomosis,
but the postoperative course was complicated by a colocutaneous fistula which was treated by transverse colostomy. A
complex fistula then ensued: ileocolonic, colocutaneous and
colovaginal. The problem was resolved by re-operation including ileal resection and a Hartmann's procedure, with colostomy
closure four months later.

Case 2 An acute onset of diverticular disease presented as
intestinal obstruction. Sigmoid resection was performed as an

emergency, but a subsequent anastomotic leak was treated by
Hartmann's operation. The patient developed an ileocolic fistula associated with an ileocutaneous fistula. After a six week
period of conservative treatment, re-operation entailed small
bowel resection and colorectal anastomosis.

These two cases show that each patient must be managed
on an individual basis and may require either emergency operation or conservative management according to the severity of
sepsis at the time of referral. Ultrasonography and CT scanning
help to determine the presence of an intra-abdominal abscess
or other complication.

AORTOENTERIC FISTULAS

Erosion of the aorta into the adjacent gastrointestinal tract is a
rare cause of digestive haemorrhage. Aortoenteric fistulas may
occur either primarily, originating from aneurysmal degeneration of the aorta, or secondarily following placement of a prosthetic graft (Figure 49.7). To remain within the scope of
gastrointestinal surgery, fistulas secondary to vascular reconstruction are excluded from this study and attention is focused
on the spontaneous forms of the disease.

Bleeding into the gastrointestinal tract from the aorta
inevitably proceeds to exsanguination unless the disease is
treated surgically. But immediate massive bleeding is not the
rule; repetitive episodes of haemorrhage over a 24–28 h period
usually precede the actual rupture of the aneurysm. This delay
makes it possible to attempt surgical repair of the fistula before
the patient collapses, provided that early diagnosis is made.

Pathogenesis and incidence

The incidence of primary aortoenteric fistulas in autopsy series
ranges between 0.04 and 0.07%. No more than 150 cases have
been published to date;[53] 80% of the patients are male, and the
average age is 60 years. Atherosclerosis accounts for the majority of cases, whereas rare diseases may be involved in younger
patients such as mycotic aneurysms, tuberculous degeneration
of the aortic wall adjacent to intestinal lesions and false
aneurysm following vascular trauma.[54-56] Infection is associated
with aortoenteric fistulas in 50% of cases. It may be:

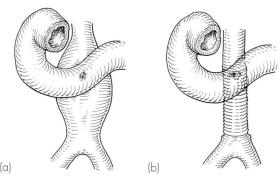

(a) (b)

Figure 49.7
The two common types of aortoenteric fistula. (a) A primary
fistula between an aortic aneurysm and the third part of the
duodenum. (b) A fistula that has arisen secondarily between an
aortic graft and the duodenum after previous aneurysm surgery.

1. A true mycotic lesion due to primary bacterial colonization of an aorta affected by atherosclerosis, leading to aneurysm and fistula formation;

2. an atherosclerotic aneurysm colonized by bacterial seeding with secondary fistulation;

3. an atherosclerotic aneurysm free from bacterial colonization, primarily fistulating into the duodenum and secondarily contaminated by the digestive flora.

Contamination by intestinal bacteria may not occur when the fistula is at duodenal level, but it is common at a more distal location in the intestine. A primary mode of infection may be suspected in the presence of organisms such as *Streptococcus* D, *Staphylococcus*, *Klebsiella* and *Salmonella*, whereas nothing may be concluded when enteric pathogens are found.

Aortoenteric fistulas in the absence of aneurysm are rare, less than 10 cases having been described.[57] The exact process initiating the fistula is unknown.

Anatomical characteristics

Aortic lesions

The fistula is situated on the anterior aspect of the aorta, anywhere between the origin of the renal arteries and the aortic bifurcation. The diameter of the aneurysm is variable, ranging from a few millimetres to over 10 cm. Most of these aneurysms are of fusiform type, yet saccular aneurysms are encountered in an unusually high incidence of 20%.[58,59]

Intestinal lesions

About 80% of aortoenteric fistulas are situated at the level of the third and fourth parts of the duodenum. The jejunum is involved in 10% of cases, the ileum in 20% and the colon (mostly sigmoid) in 70%.[53] The size of the intestinal orifice is 10 mm on average, rarely exceeding 30 mm. When infection is present, it is localized and rarely spreads to the retroperitoneal space.

Clinical presentation

Aortoenteric fistula invariably presents with some form of gastrointestinal bleeding. A transient, self-limiting 'herald-bleed' before gross intestinal blood loss is noted in 75% of the patients, with repeat episodes of bleeding over a 1–7 day period.[60] The limited size of the fistula probably allows the formation of a plug formed by clot and inflammatory debris until progressive enlargement of the fistula eventually leads to exsanguination. Chronic anaemia with guaiac-positive stools may rarely be the presenting picture and this, of course, is highly misleading. Septic signs – fever, positive blood culture, high white cell count – are a strong argument in favour of the diagnosis and are present in approximately 30% of cases.[53]

There are several possible diagnostic procedures. Plain abdominal radiology and ultrasonography may demonstrate the presence of the aneurysm, if not already clinically diagnosed. CT scan is the main diagnostic procedure; it should be carried out with intravenous injection of contrast medium and without opacification of the gastrointestinal tract. It confirms the presence of the aneurysm and may demonstrate the abnormal communication.[61,62] Indirect signs include a close proximity or even an apparent continuity between duodenum and aorta; the direct sign is the passage of contrast medium from the aorta to the duodenal lumen (Figure 49.7). The CT scan may also show local signs of infection: gas or fluid collection around the aorta, enlarged lymph nodes and remote septic foci.

Magnetic resonance imaging is not usually available in the emergency situation. Barium swallow may identify a filling defect or an irregularity in the duodenum as an indirect sign of the aneurysm.[63]

Upper gastrointestinal endoscopy is also an effective means of diagnosis. Passage of the endoscope into the third and fourth part of the duodenum or beyond the duodenojejunal flexure by a skilled endoscopist permits direct visualization of the intestinal side of the fistula.[64] It appears as a posterior ulcer situated on a pulsatile mass; bleeding is exceptionally seen. Any biopsy or brisk lavage should be avoided. Passage of the endoscope beyond the second part of the duodenum may prove difficult in the emergency setting, and then only indirect signs are available. The oesophagus, stomach and duodenum are normal. Bright red blood is seen coming from the distal duodenum. Endoscopy may be misleading when a gastric or duodenal ulcer is found. As such lesions are associated with aortic aneurysms in 25% of cases,[66] unless they are actively bleeding at endoscopy, they should not be taken as an argument against the diagnosis of aortoenteric fistula.

Aortography is rarely able to show the fistula by extravasation of contrast medium.[67] Furthermore, this diagnostic procedure is less effective than ultrasound scan. However, it may be useful in showing associated iliac, femoral and visceral arterial lesions.

Practical management

The case of massive haemorrhage leading to immediate laparotomy poses few difficulties of diagnosis and management. Operation in extreme emergency is mandatory, but the outcome is likely to be fatal.

In the patient presenting with episodes of moderate haemorrhage, advantage should be drawn from this herald bleeding to permit early operation. The following programme of management is currently the most effective.

1. Gastrointestinal bleeding plus an aortic aneurysm means immediate suspicion of the diagnosis. This suspicion is to be borne in mind unless an evident cause of active bleeding is documented.

2. Upper gastrointestinal endoscopy is carried out with the aim of exploring the whole length of the duodenum. Direct signs lead to operation.

3. In the absence of direct visualization of the fistula, CT scan is undertaken at once with the following precautions: the time of transportation of the patient to the radiological facility should be short, and during the transport the patient should

remain under close supervision. CT scan usually provides strong evidence in favour of the diagnosis.

4. Aortography is restricted to patients presenting with simultaneous lesions in the iliac and femoral arteries.

5. Both CT scan and aortography seldom show direct passage of contrast into the duodenum. However, suspicion based on indirect signs plus the absence of another site of active bleeding is sufficient to warrant immediate laparotomy. Rare cases of aortoenteric fistulas without aneurysm pose a difficult problem of diagnosis, and all reported cases have been recognized at laparotomy only.[58]

Treatment

Laparotomy must be carried out by a surgeon trained in vascular surgery, even if the diagnosis remains unconfirmed. The diagnosis is not unveiled immediately at abdominal exploration; exploration of the whole retroperitoneal space with mobilization of the third and fourth portions of the duodenum is required to obtain a clear view of the fistula. Failure to carry out this manoeuvre could lead to misguided and irrelevant operations. A recent survey of the literature reveals that in 10% of cases the correct diagnosis was made either at autopsy or at a second operation after a negative first exploration.[57,68] Before dismantling the fistula, the aorta should be controlled, either at the infrarenal level (if feasible) or in the coeliac region. Control of the aorta at the lower thoracic or coeliac level is expeditious and allows the infrarenal aorta to be exposed in a more leisurely and precise manner, following which the clamp is replaced in the infrarenal position, and the fistula is entered.

A search for other sources of bleeding should only be considered if full mobilization of duodenum, jejunum and ileum fails to demonstrate any fistula. Once the fistula has been identified, samples are taken of the surrounding tissues, of blood clots and from the margins of resected tissue for bacteriological study.

The first procedure is repair of the intestinal defect; in most instances this can be done by simple suture after minimal resection of the fistula margin.[57] In the presence of a large opening, other methods may be required; closure of the duodenum followed by duodenojejunostomy seems to be preferred to other techniques.[57,69] Protection of the suture line by a gastrostomy or a gastroenterostomy is unnecessary; placement of fibrin sealant (authors' technique, unpublished data) or the use of a serosal patch may represent a useful adjunct. Once the digestive tract has been closed, necrotic tissue is excised and the duodenum is separated from the rest of the operative field. A clean set of instruments is now used.

The vascular procedure includes resection of the anterior wall of the aneurysm and a thromboendarterectomy, leaving in place the posterior and lateral wall of the aorta. Although some cases have been treated by resection without revascularization or anterior patching, the routine procedure is to revascularize the lower limbs either with a prosthetic graft or by means of axillofemoral bypass. Bypass procedures should be restricted to cases with major contamination.[70,71] Recently, results of fresh aortic transplants used in a septic milieu have been shown to

have a remarkable tolerance.[57] Such grafts may become increasingly available with the development of transplant surgery. They may be conserved for 15 days and thus be available in an emergency.

Separation of the graft from the duodenum is a key point. Omentoplasty is the basic technique when feasible. Otherwise, a pediculated fragment of transverse mesocolon, or even a bowel loop, should be interposed. Drainage is achieved by means of fine-bore suction drains.

Systemic antibiotic therapy is provided pre- and peroperatively, and it is maintained for several days after operation. In the postoperative period a contrast study of the upper gastrointestinal tract should be obtained. CT scan is also useful to monitor the local evolution and to detect residual collections. Percutaneous needle aspirations under CT guidance may identify a microbial pathogen. In the long-term follow-up, clinical and CT scan assessments are required.

Results

The overall mortality rate obtained from the literature is approximately 50%. Causes of death may be exsanguination, leakage from the duodenal suture line, infection of the graft or other complications of atherosclerosis.

Initial infection has an important impact on mortality rate, survival rate being 35% in the presence of infection and 65% in its absence.[57] The technique of revascularization also plays an important role. In the group of patients initially free from infection, in situ revascularization is followed by a 72% survival rate versus 33% after axillofemoral bypass.[53] In the group of infected patients, axillofemoral bypass has no advantage over in situ revascularization.[57] In this latter group, replacement of the aorta by a fresh aortic homograft may be the solution of choice in the near future.

There are several possible explanations for the more favourable results following in situ revascularization.

1. In aortoenteric fistulas, infection remains localized and does not diffuse extensively in the retroperitoneal space in the way that secondary paraprosthetic fistulas often do.

2. After in situ revascularization there is no risk of rupture of the aortic stump.

3. In situ revascularization carries a lower risk of sigmoid ischaemia.

4. Monitoring of local complications is easier after placement of an in situ prosthesis.

Conclusion

Aortoenteric fistulas are currently associated with a high mortality rate (50%). Early recognition at the stage of the 'herald bleed' and immediate treatment by a team of well-trained vascular surgeons is likely to improve these figures.

ACKNOWLEDGEMENTS

The authors are grateful to Anne Berger, Jean-Marc Chevallier, Guy-Noel Francoval and Jean-Patrick Sales for their helpful contributions in the preparation of the manuscript.

REFERENCES

1. Ghahrremani GG, Gore RM & Fields WR. Acquired double pylorus due to gastroduodenal fistula complicating peptic ulceration. *Arch Surg* 1980; **115**: 194–198.
2. Gould LV. Spontaneous gastroduodenal fistula. *Br J Radiol* 1961; **34**: 619–621.
3. Fine M, Kavin H & Grant T. Double pylorus as a complication of carcinoma of the stomach. *Gastrointest Endosc* 1987; **33**: 39–41.
4. Friehling JS & Rosenthal LE. Gastric carcinoma presenting as a double-channel pylorus on upper gastrointestinal series. *Dig Dis Sci* 1985; **30**: 269–273.
5. Sufian S, Oinski S & Matsuomoto T. Congenital double pylorus. A case report and review of the literature. *Gastroenterology* 1977; **73**: 154–157.
6. Schein M. Free perforation of benign gastrojejunocolic and gastrocolic fistula. *Dis Colon Rectum* 1987; **30**: 705–706.
7. Valette H & Salas J. Les fistules gastro-coliques. Une complication rare de l'ulcère gastrique. *J Chir (Paris)* 1990; **127**: 299–300.
8. Cessot F, Sautereau D, Gainant A, Devalois B, Le Sidaner A, & Pillegand B. Fistule jéjuno-colique revelant un lymphome colique pléiomorphe. *Gastroentérol Clin Biol* 1990; **14**: 511–512.
9. Laufer I, Jopffe N & Stolberg H. Unusual causes of gastrocolic fistula. *Gastrointest Radiol* 1977; **2**: 21–25.
10. Soybel DI, Kestenberg A, Brunt EM & Becker JM. Gastrocolic fistula as a complication of benign gastric ulcer: a report of four cases and update of the literature. *Br J Surg* 1989; **76**: 1298–1300.
11. Cody JH, DiVicenti FC, Cowick DR & Mahanes JR. Gastrocolic and gastrojejunocolic fistulae: report of twelve cases and review of the literature. *Ann Surg* 1975; **181**: 376–380.
12. Kiskaddon RM, Templeton FE & Fenshaw RJF. Gastrocolic fistula: a new concept of pathologic physiology; mechanism of production of the syndrome. *Cleve Clin Q* 1947; **14**: 94–97.
13. Localio SA, Stone P & Hinton JW. Gastrojejunocolic fistula. *Surg Gynecol Obstet* 1953; **96**: 455–461.
14. Barber KW, Waugh JK & Priestley JT. Operation in one-stage for gastrojejunocolic fistula. *Surg Clin North Am* 1962; **42**: 1443–1445.
15. Marshall SF & Knud-Hansen J. Gastrojejunocolic and gastrocolic fistulas. *Ann Surg* 1957; **145**: 770–778.
16. Le Treut YP, Echimane A, Maurin B, Maillet B & Bricot R. La chirurgie d'exérèse des fistules duodéno-coliques malignes. *J Chir (Paris)* 1984; **121**: 411–418.
17. Roberts PL, Coller JA, Corriveau S & Nielsen-Whitcomb FF. Malignant duodenocolic fistula diagnosed by endoscopy. *Surg Endosc* 1989; **3**: 112–114.
18. Lopez MJ & Hreno A. Iatrogenic duodenocolic fistula. *Can J Surg* 1986; **29**: 439–442.
19. Bastiaens MT, Wittens CHA, Van Deursen CTB, Lens J, & Lustermans FAT. A patient with a duodenocolic fistula. *Neth J Surg* 1989; **41**: 74–76.
20. Guisto F, Arzillo G, Lodo N, Falchero F & Gramegna A. Malignant duodenocolic fistula. A case report. *Ital J Surg Sci* 1986; **16**: 47–49.
21. Barton DJ, Walsh TN, Keane T & Duignan JP. Malignant duodenocolic fistula. *Dis Colon Rectum* 1987; **30**: 636–637.
22. Starzl TE, Dorr TW & Meyer WJ Jr. Benign duodenocolic fistula. *Arch Surg* 1959; **78**: 611–619.
23. Pettit SH & Irving MH. The operative management of fistulous Crohn's disease. *Surg Gynecol Obstet* 1988; **167**: 223–228.
24. Farmer RG, Hawk WA & Turnbull RB Jr. Indication for surgery in Crohn's disease: analysis of 500 cases. *Gastroenterology* 1976; **71**: 245–250.
25. Whelan G, Farmer RG, Fazio VW & Goormastic M. Recurrence after surgery in Crohn's disease. Relationship to location of disease (clinical pattern) and surgical indication. *Gastroenterology* 1985; **88**: 1826–1833.
26. Greenstein AJ, Kark AE & Dreiling DA. Crohn's disease of the colon. I – Fistula in Crohn's disease of the colon, classification, presenting features and management in 63 patients. *Am J Gastroenterol* 1974; **62**: 419–429.
27. Steinberg DM, Cooke WT & Alexander-Williams J. Abscess and fistulae in Crohn's disease. *Gut* 1973; **14**: 865–869.
28. Broe PJ, Bayless TM & Cameron JL. Crohn's disease: are enteroenteral fistulas an indication for surgery? *Surgery* 1982; **91**: 249–253.
29. Glass RE, Ritchie JK, Lennard-Jones JE, Hawley PR & Todd IP. Internal fistulas in Crohn's disease. *Dis Colon Rectum* 1985; **28**: 557–561.
30. McNamara MJ, Fazio VW, Lavery IC, Weakley FL & Farmer RG. Surgical treatment of enterovesical fistulas in Crohn's disease. *Dis Colon Rectum* 1990; **33**: 271–276.
31. Greenstein AJ, Sachar DB, Tzakis A, Sher L, Heimann T & Aufses AH. Course of enterovesical fistulas in Crohn's disease. *Am J Surg* 1984; **147**: 788–792.
32. Lee KKW & Schraut WH. Diagnosis and treatment of duodenoenteric fistulas complicating Crohn's disease. *Arch Surg* 1989; **124**: 712–715.
33. Wilk PJ, Fazio VW & Turnbull RB. The dilemma of Crohn's disease: ileoduodenal fistula complicating Crohn's disease. *Dis Colon Rectum* 1977; **20**: 387–392.
34. Alexander-Williams J. The technique of intestinal stricturoplasty. *Int J Colorect Dis* 1986; **1**: 54–57.
35. Korelitz BI & Present DH. Favourable effect of 6-mercaptopirine on fistulae of Crohn's disease. *Dig Dis Sci* 1985; **30**: 58–64.
36. Irving MH. Assessment and management of external fistulas in Crohn's disease. *Br J Surg* 1983; **70**: 223–236.
37. Block GE & Schraut WH. The operative treatment of Crohn's enteritis complicated by ileosigmoid fistula. *Ann Surg* 1982; **196**: 356–360.
38. Cameron JL. Discussion, in The operative treatment of Crohn's enteritis complicated by ileosigmoid fistula. *Ann Surg* 1982; **196**: 356–360.
39. Fazio VW, Wilk P, Turnbull RB & Jagelman DG. The dilemma of Crohn's disease: ileosigmoidal fistula complicating Crohn's disease. *Dis Colon Rectum* 1977; **20**: 381–386.
40. Heimann T, Greenstein AJ & Aufses AH. Surgical management of ileosigmoid fistula in Crohn's disease. *Am J Gastroenterol* 1979; **72**: 21–24.
41. Garlock JH. *Garlock's Surgery of the Alimentary Tract.* New York: Appleton Century Crofts, 1967; 270–276.
42. Greenstein AJ. The surgery of Crohn's disease. *Surg Clin North Am* 1987; **67**: 573–596.
43. Petros JG & Argy O. Enterovesical fistula from Meckel's diverticulum in a patient with Crohn's ileitis. *Dig Dis Sci* 1990; **35**: 133–136.
44. Talamini MA, Broe PJ & Cameron JL. Urinary fistulas in Crohn's disease. *Surg Gynecol Obstet* 1982; **154**: 553–556.
45. Marti MC & Simmen U. Les fistules enétro-vésicales. *J Chir (Paris)* 1980; **117**: 469–474.
46. Schraut WH & Block GE. Enterovesical fistula complicating Crophn's ileocolitis. *Am J Gastroenterol* 1984; **79**: 186–190.
47. Schraut WH, Chapman C & Abraham VS. Operative treatment of Crohn's ileocolitis complicated by ileosigmoid and ileovesical fistulae. *Ann Surg* 1988; **207**: 48–51.
48. Greenstein AJ, Lachman P, Sachar DB et al. Perforating and non-perforating indications for repeated operations in Crohn's disease: evidence for two clinical forms. *Gut* 1988; **29**: 588–592.
49. Margolin ML & Korelitz BI. The management of enterovesical fistulas in Crohn's disease. *Gastroenterology* 1986; **90**: 1534 (abstract).
50. Abcarian H & Udezue N. Coloenteric fistulas. *Dis Colon Rectum* 1978; **21**: 281–286.
51. Woods RJ, Lavery IC, Fazio VW, Jagelman DG & Weakley FL. Internal fistulas in diverticular disease. *Dis Colon Rectum* 1988; **31**: 591–596.
52. Parc R & Chevallier JM. Indications chirurgicales dans la diverticulose colique. *Rev Prat* 1988; **38**: 25–33.
53. Steffes BC & O'Leary JP. Primary aorta-duodenal fistula: a case report and a review of the literature. *Ann Surg* 1980; **46**: 121–129.
54. Bergqvist D. Arterio enteric fistula. *Acta Chir Scand* 1987; **153**: 81–86.
55. Sweeney MS & Gadacz TR. Primary aorto duodenal fistula: manifestation, diagnosis and treatment. *Surgery* 1984; **96**: 492–495.
56. Simeliere TH, Chevallier JM, Enon B et al. Fistule aorto duodénale primaire d'origine tuberculeuse. *J Chir (Paris)* 1987; **124**: 464–466.
57. Bacourt F, Gompel H., Bergemer AM. Fistules aorto digestives primaires. In: Kieffer E (ed.) *Les Anéuysmes de l'Aorte sous-rénale*, Paris; AERCV, 1990; 405–411.
58. Gad A. Aorta duodenal fistula revisited. *Scand J Gastroenterol* 1989; **24**: 97–100.
59. Vetto JT, Steven CC, Smythe TB et al. Iliac arterial-enteric fistulas occurring after pelvic irradiation. *Surgery* 1987; **101**: 643–645.
60. Kleinmann LH, Toanne JB & Bernhard VM. A diagnostic and therapeutic approach to aorto-enteric fistulas. Clinical experience with 20 patients. *Surgery* 1979; **86**: 868–874.
61. Ibrahim MI, Raccuia JS, Micale J & Zafar A. Primary aorto duodenal fistula. Diagnosis by computed tomography. *Arch Surg* 1989; **124**: 870–871.
62. Kukora JS, Rushton FW & Cranston PE. New computed tomographic signs of aorto enteric fistula. *Arch Surg* 1984; **119**: 1073–1075.
63. Bacourt F. Fistules aorto digestives. *Nouv Presse Med* 1984; **23**: 1447–1451.
64. Konigsrainer A, Pointner R, Reissingl H & Weimann S. Endoscopic aspects of aorto intestina fistula. *Surg Endosc* 1987; **1**: 37–40.
65. Benhamou G & Duron JJ. Aorto digestive fistulae. *Int Surg* 1982; **67**: 307–310.

66. Jones AW, Kirk RS & Bloor K. The association between aneurysm of the abdominal aorta and peptic ulceration. *Gut* 1970; **11**: 679–684.

67. Dendooven D, Deroose J, Hamerline G et al. A case of a primary aorto duodenal fistula detected by arteriography. *J Belge Radiol* 1987; **67**: 417–420.

68. Elliott JP, Smith RF & Szilagyl DE. Aorto-enteric and para prosthetic enteric fistulas. *Arch Surg* 1974; **108**: 479–490.

69. Bacourt F. Fistules aorto digestives prothetiques. In: Barral X (ed.) Paris: Masson, 1988; 96–105.

70. Fastrez J, Mabaix M, Rettmann R & Lega A. Les fistules aorto-duodénales primitives, a propos de deux cas. *Acta Chir Belg* 1985; **85**: 61–66.

71. Daugherty M, Shearer G & Ernst CB. Primary aorto duodenal fistula: extra anatomic vascular reconstruction is not required for successful management. *Surgery* 1979; **86**: 399–408.

72. Yeager RA, Monet GL, Taylor LM et al. Improving survival and limb salvage in patients with aortic graft infection. *Am J Surg* 1990; **159**: 466–469.

50

MEDICAL ASPECTS OF CROHN'S DISEASE

KL Collings
PB Miner

INTRODUCTION

Crohn's disease is an inflammatory condition of the small intestine and colon related to aggressive activity of the gastrointestinal immune system manifest by symptoms of diarrhoea, abdominal pain, intestinal obstruction, gastrointestinal bleeding and malnutrition. The potential involvement of any area of the gastrointestinal tract demonstrates the diversity of the disease and emphasizes the variety of possible disease presentations. Although symptoms may present at any age, Crohn's disease is most common in the young, often delaying full body growth and development. Numerous advances in treatment of symptoms, inflammation and nutrition have improved the health of patients with Crohn's disease, but surgical intervention continues to play a major role in management. This chapter discusses the medical aspects of Crohn's disease.

INCIDENCE

Extensive epidemiologic research in inflammatory bowel disease (IBD) has been conducted over the past 50 years. Numerous problems surround the interpretation of these data as the advancements in diagnosis and the emergence of more refined definitions of these diseases have changed during the period of data collection in these studies. A prime example involves the endoscopic definition of colonic disease. With the development and utilization of fibreoptic colonoscopy in the 1960s and 1970s, Crohn's colitis emerged as a distinct diagnostic entity reshuffling the distribution of colonic disease between ulcerative colitis and colonic Crohn's disease. A second example is the recognition of indeterminant colitis, a hybrid disease which begins with the appearance of ulcerative colitis and gradually transforms into a disease resembling Crohn's colitis. The increasing incidence of indeterminant colitis may reflect a better understanding of the natural history of IBD, but an alternative hypothesis is that there is an iatrogenic component to the change in the appearance of the colon related to chemical sensitivity of the colon to mesalamine.[1]

Published studies in the United States report incidence rates of Crohn's disease between 1.2 and 8.8 per 100,000 population.[2-10] Since the natural history of this disease is measured in decades, prevalence figures more accurately reflect the population at risk for medical problems than do annual incidence figures. In North America, the prevalence of Crohn's disease has been reported to be 44–106 per 100,000.[4-6,11] Internationally the figures vary widely with prevalence rates as high as 2000 per 100,000 Jews in Newport, Wales, reflecting the geographic and ethnic differences in distribution of the disease.[12]

Several risk factors have emerged from large epidemiologic studies. There is a female preponderance of patients with Crohn's disease in about half the studies.[13] The disease often presents at a young age with a bimodal distribution peaking in the early twenties and again emerging in the mid-sixties.[14] Ethnicity is a complex problem. The risk of presenting with Crohn's disease is higher in the Jewish than non-Jewish population in the United States, Sweden, southeast Wales and South Africa whereas the incidence for Jews in Israel is similar to that found in the non-Jewish population in Westernized countries.[15-19] These data have been used to emphasize the role of the environment in influencing the presentation of a disease with genetic linkage. Familial aggregation has been recognized from early demographic studies.[20] The current emphasis on human genome studies should clarify the genetic issues in Crohn's disease, but it is immediately apparent that the risk of a second individual appearing in a proband's family is between 1 and 8%.[21-29]

THEORIES REGARDING PATHOGENESIS

Genetic

The epidemiologic studies have always stimulated an interest in the genetic influences on the presentation of inflammatory bowel disease. A number of studies from the premolecular biology era convincingly demonstrated a genetic predisposition for the development of IBD, but studies in identical twins just as firmly established that genetic predisposition was insufficient by itself for presentation of the disease.[20,30-33] Other confounding observations include the familial predisposition to inflammatory bowel disease, but a variation in the phenotypic expression of the disease. The lack of fidelity to phenotypic expression suggests a genetic susceptibility to intestinal inflammation with other non-genetic factors influencing expression of the disease. Extensive genetic description using histocompatability antigens (HLAs) support genetic patterns of the disease, but the number of HLA comparisons and relatively low odds ratios of most comparisons make this a tedious and difficult endeavour.[13] The best data should come from the mapping of the human genome. It is now clear that genes on chromosome 16 are linked to Crohn's disease.[34] Currently, thousands of candidate genes on chromosome 16 are being actively explored. The final gene, or more likely, the constellation of genes implicated in Crohn's disease may soon be delineated. Despite these advances, it is clear from animal models as well as the epidemiologic data in mean, that genetic predisposition may be necessary, but is not alone sufficient for the expression of the disease.[35-38]

Infectious

Infections have always been a focus for investigation into inflammatory bowel disease because ulcerative colitis and Crohn's disease have symptoms and clinical findings similar to recognized infectious diseases. The reported response of patients with Crohn's disease to antibiotics provides the strongest corroborative evidence for a role of bacteria in inflammatory bowel disease.[39] Moss et al.[39] presented intriguing data from an open-labelled, uncontrolled study of antibiotics in Crohn's disease showed unexpected clinical improvement. Subsequent studies have confirmed a role for metronidazole, ciprofloxacin, and erythromycin (and the related macrolide, clarithromycin) in improving patients with Crohn's disease.[40-43] Unfortunately, non-antibiotic effects of these drugs can confuse the expected role of antibiotics as primary anti-infective agents. For example, both ciprofloxacin and metronidazole have effects on the immune system that may be as important as their effects on bacterial proliferation.[44]

Three roles for infectious pathogens are possible in IBD:

1. activating the immune system with a specific primary pathogen;
2. inducing relapse through a specific organism;
3. sensitizing the mucosal immune system through bacterial antigens, bacterial metabolic products or alteration of the luminal microenvironment.

Specific primary pathogen

Several infectious agents have been suggested to cause Crohn's disease including Chlamydia, *Pseudomonas maltophilia*, RNA retrovirus, *Mycobacterium kansassi*, *Mycobacterium paratuberculosis* and *Paramyxovirus* (measles) virus.[45,50] Investigations have long been based on animal models of human pathology

studies. Animal studies using human tissue to cause granuloma formation created great interest in the 1970s.[51,52] The enthusiasm for each of these agents was justified by the early studies, however, in each instance attempted validation in independent laboratories failed to find an infectious aetiology. High quality investigators vigorously debate each specific organism identified in Crohn's disease, reporting either the presence or absence of a specific infectious association. The careful observer finds it difficult to dismiss or accept the concept of a specific infectious agent as important in Crohn's disease. A unifying concept for these apparently disparate data promulgates activation of the genetically primed gastrointestinal immune system by a specific infection so that downregulation of the overactive and injurious immune process is difficult. This model supports diffuse infectious organisms which may activate the genetically primed patient to allow expression of the disease. Following epidemics of routine enteric infections, persistent intestinal inflammation occurs in a small percentage of patients. Since no infection is detectable at the time of diagnosis of inflammatory bowel disease, it is assumed that the infection activates a primed immune system and is the initiating environmental event that established the inflammatory bowel disease. With the sophistication of the techniques applied to the exploration of an infectious aetiology for Crohn's disease and the failure to discover a specific bacterium, fungus or virus, it seems unlikely that a specific infection will be determined to cause Crohn's disease.

Inducing relapse

There is clear evidence for the exacerbation of inflammatory bowel disease by intercurrent infections. The respiratory linkage is most interesting because activation of inflammatory bowel disease through a non-enteric infection suggests upregulation of the immune system is sufficient to tip the balance of controlled inflammation in the intestine toward active inflammation. Respiratory infections that are linked to activation of disease include influenza A or B virus, respiratory syncytial virus, parainfluenza virus and *Mycoplasma pneumoniae*.[53] The suggestion that enteric infections induce relapse requires very little justification as inflammation in the intestinal tract following an enteric infection is expected.[54] Exacerbations of inflammatory bowel disease are associated with *Clostridium difficile*, *Campylobacter*, *Cytomegalovirus*, *Salmonella sp.*, *Aeromonas sp.*, *Eschersichia coli* and *Mycobacterium avium*.[53,55] Although the evidence supports these infections in activating inflammation in patients with established disease, there is little support for their role in the pathogenesis of Crohn's disease.

Luminal microenvironment

The effect of luminal bacteria, their bacterial products and their effect on food constituents forms the best support for a role of bacteria in the pathogenesis of inflammatory bowel disease. The support begins with the experimental genetic models of inflammatory bowel disease in which activation of mucosal inflammation does not occur if the animals are raised in a germ-free environment.[36,56] The mechanism of the permissive effect of intestinal flora on the development of inflammation is unclear. Other observations that support the importance of the microenvironment are the clinical improvement seen after defined low antigen diets, bowel rest, bowel diversion and luminal antibiotics. Considerable investigative effort is focused on this aspect of disease activation and changes in the luminal microenvironment that may perpetuate remission of the disease.

Allergic

Inflammatory bowel disease is not an allergic disorder, but mast cells and eosinophils play a critical role in the pathogenesis and expression of the disease. Early studies of the histopathology of inflammatory bowel disease describe numerous eosinophils in the mucosa of the intestinal tract.[57–61] Since the principal role of eosinophils was felt to be allergic, considerable effort was expended to prove that there was an allergic component to the disease. These efforts failed to define an allergic component to the disease. Renewed interest in the role of the eosinophil in inflammatory bowel disease occurred with the observation of tissue toxicity which accompanied the hypereosinophilia of the Tryptophan–Eosinophilia–Myalgia syndrome and the recognition that eosinophils have an immunoregulatory function independent of immunoglobulin E (IgE)-mediated activation.[62–64] Paralleling the changes in the understanding of eosinophil function was the recognition of the role of the mast cell in the neuroimmune system and the regulatory role the mast cell plays at the interface of the body and the environment. There is insufficient information to detail the role of the mast cell and eosinophil in inflammatory bowel disease at this juncture. Although this role does not appear to be mediated through an allergic pathway, allergic stimulation may activate a relapse in the disease through non-specific induction of eosinophil function.[65]

Autoimmune

The autoimmune hypothesis is immediately attractive in diseases of unknown origin in which immunosuppression improves some of the symptoms. Several colon specific antigens have been identified (e.g. anticolon lipopolysccharide, colitis colon-bound antibody, antiepithelial cell-associated components). However, the significance of these antigens is unknown as their presence and location in the intestinal tract does not correlate with the expression of the disease by location or extent. Furthermore, these antigens have been isolated in diseases in which there is no colonic inflammation.[66] Cells with cytotoxicity for colonic epithelial cells have been isolated from the peripheral blood of patients with inflammatory bowel disease. These cells are present in the mucosa of such patients, raising the possibility that they play a role in mucosal cell injury. Although it is possible the identification of specific colonic mucosal antibodies represents the tip of the iceberg with regard to autoantibodies, it is difficult to explain the pathophysiology of the transmural inflammation seen in Crohn's disease with antibodies to the surface mucosa. This remains a possible, though unlikely aetiology for Crohn's disease.

Increased intestinal permeability

Hollander et al.[67] proposed the hypothesis that the genetic susceptibility to Crohn's disease was related to an inherent increase in intestinal permeability. There has been considerable debate over this observation and the potential importance of these changes. More extensive research is needed in this area, but this important hypothesis could explain how the immune system may be activated in Crohn's disease as well as integrate the information related to relapses of inflammatory bowel disease. Intestinal permeability could also be used to explain the self-perpetuating inflammation characteristic of inflammatory bowel disease.

Thromboembolic

The thromboembolic hypothesis regarding the aetiology of inflammatory bowel disease has always drifted around the periphery of ideas about intestinal inflammation. The changes that can be seen in patients with clearly demonstrable ischaemia have features similar to the histologic changes of microvascular thrombosis found in resected small intestinal and colonic specimens from patients with inflammatory bowel disease. A surge of momentum for this hypothesis was prompted by the publication of the value of heparin in management of ulcerative colitis.[68,69] This interesting and important observation is probably related to the immunological suppression accompanying heparin rather than the action of the drug in preventing thrombus formation.

FACTORS RELATED TO DISEASE ACTIVITY

Diet

Since the immune system provides an effective defensive barrier protecting the host from the environment, it is reasonable to assume there is a relationship between the luminal contents of the gastrointestinal tract and the overactive immune mucosal system in patients with inflammatory bowel disease. Unfortunately, there are few data to support or contest the notion that diet is related to disease activity. The supposition that diet may profoundly influence symptoms could be explained by numerous complex pathophysiological events. Simple sugars in the diet may lead to symptoms from either their osmotic effect passing through an intestine with compromised absorptive capacity, or from decreased disaccharidase itself. Bacterial degradation into gas causes abdominal pain, bloating and flatulence in the presence of bacterial overgrowth of the small bowel or when simple sugars enter the colon. Fats are difficult to digest and absorb due to the loss of bile salts from an impaired terminal ileum and loss of mucosal surface from active inflammation. Fat malabsorption and maldigestion cause diarrhoea and the unpleasant symptom of steatorrhoea while the discomfort of excessive intestinal contractions aggravate the symptoms. Several specific foods seem to cause symptoms in most patients with Crohn's disease, but the reasons are obscure. A few of the frequently mentioned foods to be avoided are beef, wheat, alcohol, citrus juices, onions, fibrous fruits and vegetables. Consistent with the hypothesis that luminal factors are important in Crohn's disease, the observation that elemental diets and well-defined oral feeding can decrease the symptoms of inflammatory bowel disease and actually improve growth in children with Crohn's disease support a role for diet, or at least dietary manipulation, as a factor that influences disease activity.[70-72]

Smoking

The relationship between smoking and activity of ulcerative colitis was described by Harries et al. in 1982.[73] Since then, smoking status has been well established as a relative protective factor in ulcerative colitis and an exacerbating factor in Crohn's disease.[74] The reasons for this divergence are unclear. Nicotine patches have been tried in ulcerative colitis with limited success suggesting a more complex interaction with cigarette smoke and the gastrointestinal immune system. Patients with Crohn's disease should not smoke.

Non-steroidal Anti-inflammatory drugs (NSAIDs)

Strong evidence supports a detrimental role of NSAIDs in inflammatory bowel disease.[75-77] There are many possible reasons including the suppression of protective prostaglandin synthesis, decreased oxidative phosphorylation in the enterocyte, altered fatty acid synthesis and increased intestinal permeability. Until the exact mechanism of disease activation is identified, every effort should be made to avoid NSAID use in inflammatory bowel disease.

Stress

Debates regarding the pathogenesis of inflammatory bowel disease in the 1950s included vigorous support for the psychiatric aetiology of intestinal inflammation. As it became apparent that IBD was not a psychiatric disease, the pendulum of opinion swung to the other extreme with the denial that stress could influence clinical presentation or course. A newly appreciated area of immunological research involves the relationship between the enteric nervous system and the gastrointestinal immune system focusing on the juxtapositioning of the gastrointestinal mast cell and the nerve endings in the enteric nervous system.[78-81] Studies evaluating mast cell degranulation in response to a Pavlovian stimulus support the suspected link between central nervous system events and intestinal immune response.[82] The precise role played by stress in IBD is unknown, but it can at least activate the symptoms of IBD, while current evidence suggests that active inflammation may also be induced by stress.

PATHOPHYSIOLOGY OF SYMPTOMS

The predominant symptoms of Crohn's disease are diarrhoea, abdominal pain and weight loss. The distribution of symptoms and the relative importance of symptoms in an individual patient may vary widely making management a difficult task.

Discussion of the pathophysiology of each of the symptoms is useful in the medical decision making process.

Diarrhoea

The diarrhoea of Crohn's disease has numerous dimensions, many of which can be acting at the same time. The principal stimulus for diarrhoea is the mucosal immune response accompanied by the secretion of numerous cytokines. These inflammatory products stimulate myoelectric activity in the small bowel and colon in conjunction with changes in intestinal fluid secretion. Accompanying these changes is the stimulation for relaxation of the internal anal sphincter caused by the release of histamine. These cytokine-related changes in intestinal and colonic physiology are responsible for the diarrhoea whereas the symptom of tenesmus is associated with internal anal sphincter relaxation in conjunction with rectal contractility. The interrelationship between mast cells and eosinophils and their role in the inflammatory process presents an opportunity to deal with the diarrhoea not only through the control of cytokine release but with the addition of antihistamines to the medical management regimen. The diurnal variation in eosinophil function provides an important clinical clue to the origin of the diarrhoea. Since eosinophils have the greatest sensitivity and activation between 11 p.m. and 2 a.m., a patient awakened from sleep with diarrhoea in this time period likely has an eosinophilic component to the symptoms and should benefit by the addition of antihistamine therapy to the medical regimen.

There are numerous other factors which influence diarrhoea to a variable extent in each patient. The decreased small intestinal absorptive surface from disease or surgical extirpation presents the colon with excessive fluids and nutrients to handle. If the colon is involved by disease or removed by operation, inadequate surface for the absorption of the normal amount of ileal effluent will result in large volume diarrhoea. Independent of surface area of the small intestine, disaccharidase deficiency contributes to osmotic load of poorly digested sugars entering the colon with the additional subsequent burden of gas from colonic bacterial metabolism of these simple sugars. Dietary restriction is often helpful. With ileal inflammation, compromise of the active absorption of bile acids leads to an increase in the concentration of bile acids in the colon. Cholerrhetic enteropathy results due to stimulation of colonic contractility, colonic fluid secretion and relaxation of the internal anal sphincter. The hallmark of cholerrhetic enteropathy is faecal incontinence due to the magnitude of changes stimulated by bile in the colon. The only study of faecal incontinence in patients with Crohn's disease without fistulizing perineal disease demonstrated that the probable cause of incontinence was ileal malabsorption of bile acids.[83] It has been recently recognized that cholerrhetic enteropathy is due to bile acid-induced mast cell degranulation.[84] The excessive numbers of mast cells seen in the colon and small bowel of patients with Crohn's disease amplifies the sensitivity to small amounts of bile acids.

Changes in anorectal physiology are more important in

ulcerative colitis than in Crohn's disease because the rectum is often spared in the inflammatory process in Crohn's disease. When the rectum is inflamed, the problem of increased internal anal sphincter relaxation is compounded by decreased rectal compliance with a concomitant increase in rectal contractility. These changes lead to the symptom of tenesmus and increased stool frequency.

Nutrient malabsorption also influences the symptom of diarrhoea. Carbohydrate malabsorption contributes to fluid accumulation and the osmotic load in the colon and the formation of gas from bacterial degredation of carbohydrates. In patients with rapid rectal filling, the sensory discrimination between fluid and gas is difficult. Since the patient recognizes that he/she cannot distinguish between gas and liquid, there is no safety in passing flatus outside the security of a toilet. Symptomatic management to control the intestinal production of gas can have an important effect on quality of life by decreasing the number of trips to the toilet. Fat malabsorption occurs for numerous reasons and contributes not only to nutritional failure but symptoms as well. Fat malabsorption due to loss of mucosal surface may occur when the primary fat absorptive surface of the proximal intestine is involved with disease or removed by resection or when there is a loss of bile acids into the colon from disease or resection of the terminal ileum. When the concentration of bile acids is too low to form micelles, impaired fat absorption occurs. Bacterial overgrowth in the small intestine compromises nutritional status and may result from a number of immunological or structural abnormalities. Most often it occurs in the intestine proximal to a small intestinal stricture. Bacterial overgrowth deconjugates bile salts, thus decreasing the efficiency of micelle formation and increasing the loss into the colon through less effective ileal absorption. Bacteria in the small intestine also break down pancreatic enzymes and further compromise normal fat digestion. As fats are broken down into short chain fatty acids, peristalsis and colonic fluid secretion are stimulated causing an increase in the number of stools. Less frequently, diarrhoea may occur as a consequence of entero-enteric or enterocolic fistulas with either bacterial overgrowth in the small intestine or by intestinal chyme passing from the absorptive surface of the small intestine into the colon.

Pain

The most common explanation for pain in patients with Crohn's disease is partial obstruction of the intestinal lumen, which can occur at any level. The pain is generally related to eating. A common reason for hospitalization is partial or transient complete bowel obstruction related to dietary indiscretion. Intravenous fluids and limited oral intake usually manage these symptoms easily, though surgical consultation should occur early in the hospital course. Luminal distension related to impaired motility or the gas produced by bacterial overgrowth also contribute to the pain of partial obstruction. A second reason for pain is visceral hyperalgesia, a problem of increased sensitivity to distension of the lumen. Recent investigation has provided the link between inflammation and this increased sensitivity.[85,86] Although many aspects are unexplained, elevated histamine and serotonin are involved in the visceral pain pathway and both are products of the intestinal inflammation found in Crohn's disease.

Pain in patients with Crohn's disease may also arise from gallstones, which are common concomitants partly owing to the abnormalities of bile acid metabolism. The diagnosis is often difficult because of the complex pathophysiology of Crohn's disease and the numerous sources of pain in these patients. Abscesses and fistulas represent another category of pathologic problems that cause pain. The most difficult problem is pain due to an abscess or fistula in the perineum. The pain is caused by the physical presence of the abnormality and the secondary effects of skin and tissue injury surrounding the leakage of purulent fluid or intestinal contents onto the perineal skin. Skilled surgical consultation is essential to provide drainage of the abscesses and management of the fistula tracts while preserving the muscular integrity of the anal sphincter complex.

Two causes of pain indirectly related to the gastrointestinal tract can also give rise to management problems. Ureteric obstruction, which can be very painful, results either from direct extension of the inflammatory process in the intestine, or more often from nephrolithiasis. Calcium oxalate stones form because of oxalate absorption from the colon. Generally they occur in patients who have intact pancreatic function but impaired small intestinal absorption of fat. The pancreatic enzymes breakdown triglycerides into fatty acids, which cannot be absorbed. Subsequently the fatty acids compete with oxalate for calcium binding allowing free oxalate to enter the colon and be absorbed. Oxalate is excreted in the urine and precipitates with calcium. Often Crohn's patients are chronically dehydrated from inadequate oral intake of fluid and the fluid losses from diarrhoea further complicate the renal handling of oxalate. The second non-intestinal source of pain is arthritis. Pain management is challenging as the NSAIDs commonly used to manage arthritis carry the risk of exacerbating the disease.

Nutritional failure

Weight loss in adults and failure to thrive in children are two serious medical problems. It is clear that the malabsorption due to the intestinal disease plays an important role in nutritional failure. Fat, protein and carbohydrate malabsorption and the specific deficits of mineral and vitamin absorption, particularly vitamin B_{12}, are obvious problems faced by Crohn's patients. Other related nutritional problems are often overlooked. Anorexia is common due to the physiological consequence of active cytokine release from the inflamed tissue, as well as psychological anorexia due to the fear of pain from obstructive symptoms that can follow eating. Nausea occurs in response to inflammatory products and as a result of the altered peristalsis accompanying small bowel obstruction. Gastric pain or associated nausea may reflect involvement of the stomach by Crohn's disease or the medications (e.g. metronidazole, azulfidine, prednisone) given for disease management. Finally, active inflammation leads to a catabolic state complicating the nutritional needs and the ability to maintain good nutrition. Many of the problems listed above have nutritional consequences. Bacterial overgrowth, obstruction and decreased mucosal surface all contribute to the nutritional problems and need to be carefully addressed.

Perineal symptoms

Perineal symptoms deserve special attention. The most common problem is chemical dermatitis related to the problem of frequent diarrhoeal stools which leach the protective fatty acids from the skin and enhance the perineal injury by making hygiene and dry skin difficult to achieve. In patients using immunosuppressive agents or antibiotics, infective dermatitis (usually candidiasis) can be overlooked by the physician, but is very uncomfortable for the patient. Fistulas and abscesses are usually not overlooked because of the associated symptoms. Sphincter disruption may follow infection, obstetric trauma or surgical intervention and should be sought by physical examination or rectal ultrasonography. Quality surgical consultation is essential since preserving function in the pelvic floor is a priority for long-term management both medically and psychologically.

Extraintestinal manifestations of Crohn's disease (Table 50.1)

The numerous extraintestinal manifestations of Crohn's disease include ophthalmological, rheumatological, haematological and dermatological problems recognized and managed with variable degrees of success and they usually are of greater interest to the gastroenterologist than the surgeon. Hepatobiliary problems often require surgical intervention. Gallstones commonly require cholecystectomy. More seriously sclerosing cholangitis can progress to the point of liver failure, with the need to perform liver transplantation.

Table 50.1 Common extraintestinal manifestations of inflammatory bowel disease

BODY SYSTEM	CONDITION
Hepatobiliary	Hepatic steatosis (fatty change) Cholelithiasis Primary sclerosing cholangitis
Rheumatological	Peripheral ('enteropathic') arthritis Ankylosing spondylitis Sacroilitis
Dermatological	Erythema nodosum Pyoderma gangrenosum 'Metatastic' Crohn's disease of the skin Perianal skin tags Aphthous stomatitis Changes of nutritional deficiency
Ocular	Uveitis/iritis Episcleritis
Genitourinary	Nephrolithiasis Obstructive uropathy secondary to inflammation Enterovesical/enteroureteral/enterovaginal fistulas

EVALUATION

History

The definition of the disease includes the symptoms and course of illness in each patient. A positive family history is an extremely useful clue in patients with IBD. Most of the attention is directed at the principal symptoms of diarrhoea and abdominal pain. Other important symptoms occur less frequently such as bleeding, nutritional failure, extraintestinal manifestations of disease and fistulous complications.

Physical examination

General appearance is important as it often reflects nutritional problems which are related to the distribution and severity of the disease. Height and weight reflect the severity of nutritional deficiency. An adult of short stature who is found to have Crohn's disease suggests the disease has been present since early adolescence. The general examination seeks to discover extraintestinal manifestations of inflammatory bowel disease such as eye, joint or skin pathology. The abdominal examination may suggest partial obstruction, an inflammatory mass, focal areas of tenderness or enterocutaneous fistula. Perineal examination reveals fistulas or abscesses, chemical dermatitis from diarrhoea, or 'elephant ears' associated with perineal disease. Rectal examination may document a stricture, palpable rectal ulcers, perirectal abscesses or bleeding into the gastrointestinal tract.

Nuances of the pathophysiology of inflammatory bowel disease arise from the component of disease severity. *Bowel frequency* is related to the amount of colonic mucosal involvement and the degree of inflammation. Rectal sensitivity to luminal distention is the principal factor that determines the number of bowel movements. Reactive contractility of the inflamed distal colon with coordinated internal anal sphincter relaxation causes the symptom of tenesmus and the passage of small volume stools. Rectal sensitivity has a good, but imperfect, relationship to obvious mucosal inflammation. The changes in anorectal physiology may be present in patients with Crohn's disease involving only the terminal ileum. In these patients, the increased colonic concentration of bile acids leads to increased myoelectric activity of the normal appearing colon, fluid secretion from the colonic mucosa and internal anal sphincter relaxation. Nocturnal diarrhoea occurs in severe disease and suggests a prominent role for eosinophils, since the diurnal variation of eosinophil activation parallels the nocturnal pattern of diarrhoea in these patients. *Bloody diarrhoea* is proportional to the degree of mucosal injury making this symptom a central element in estimating disease severity. *Fever* accompanies cytokine release from colonic inflammation or related systemic infection, a complication that increases morbidity and mortality rates in patients with ulcerative colitis. *Tachycardia* is an important, multifaceted physical finding in the severity index reflecting (1) the state of dehydration from anorexia, fever and diarrhoea and (2) vascular dilation in response to fever and cytokine release. *Anaemia* reflects acute and chronic blood loss as well as suppression of haematopoiesis associated with chronic illness. Vitamin B_{12} malabsorption due to ileal disease is also an important factor in anaemia and needs to be assessed by specific measurement of circulating vitamin B_{12} as well as the capacity to absorb vitamin B_{12}. This information is obtained through a Shilling's test with intrinsic factor. *Erythrocyte sedimentation rate* (ESR) greater than 30 mm/h indicates the systemic response to inflammation. In the absence of systemic manifestations of disease, the ESR is directly related to the severity of intestinal inflammation. If systemic features are present, it reflects the summation of the immunological response to the disease. *Hypoalbuminaemia* is highly predictive of serious disease. Although the intestinal loss of albumin occurs in relation to the severity of colonic inflammation, an equally important issue is the suppression of albumin synthesis reflected by falling prealbumin in response to the stress of severe disease.[87] In this capacity, serum albumin is a 'negative acute phase reactant' and an excellent monitor of severity of illness.

Imaging Studies

A variety of imaging studies are available for making the diagnosis and for determining the extent and severity of Crohn's disease and its extraintestinal complications. Plain abdominal radiographs provide important information in the acute presentation of symptoms as they can demonstrate intestinal obstruction or evidence of perforation. They may also reveal renal and biliary calculi axial arthropathy, compressed vertebral bodies or osteoporosis. To some extent, barium contrast studies of the proximal gastrointestinal tract and colon have been supplanted by videoendoscopy which provides a better differential diagnosis and the opportunity to obtain biopsies. Contrast examinations do have an important role in cases where endoscopy is precluded by strictures or external compression of the bowel. Enteroclysis with intubation and controlled delivery of a methylcellulose and barium mixture or the newer technique using *Enterovue* provides a translucent image of the small intestine which allows examination of fine detail. It enhances the visualization of the distal small intestine and provides an excellent estimate of the extent of disease. Fistulograms provide useful information regarding the surgical approach that may be required. A fistula exiting the intestinal tract proximal to a stricture is unlikely to respond to medical management. Computerized axial tomography and magnetic resonance imaging have improved management significantly by providing detailed information about thickened bowel loops, abscesses and fistula tracts. This information is especially useful in directing surgical intervention. Ultrasonography has several useful roles in evaluating patients with Crohn's disease. Examination of the right lower quadrant may provide the earliest evidence of thickened terminal ileum. Pain in the right upper quadrant may be explored for the presence of gallstones. Recent descriptions of ultrasonographic findings which reflect disease within the liver parenchyma such as sclerosing cholangitis help clinical assessment. Ultrasonic examination of the ureters for obstruction from nephrolithiasis or an inflammatory intra-abdominal mass provides a painless and effective tool for leading the clinician toward an otherwise difficult diagnosis. Endoscopic

ultrasonography is in it's infancy, but has the potential of defining pelvic floor problems with high resolution images. Dual energy X-ray absorptiometry (DEXA) scanning for bone density has become an important tool for the assessment of osteoporosis – a problem of profound significance to patients of all ages with Crohn's disease. Susceptibility to osteoporosis arises from malabsorption of Vitamin D and calcium, increased urinary excretion of calcium and magnesium due to the effect of interleukin-1 on the kidney, and the untoward effects of treatment with glucocorticoids.

Endoscopy allows the visualization of the gastrointestinal mucosa in newly diagnosed patients, those in remission or patients with relapse and complications. The diagnosis of isolated Crohn's colitis could not be made until fibreoptic endoscopy improved the visual definition of ulcerative colitis and Crohn's colitis in the late 1960s and early 1970s. Improved instruments allow safer and better imaging of the mucosa which can be complemented by mucosal biopsies to differentiate varying types of mucosal inflammation and estimate dysplasia for cancer surveillance. In addition to the routine upper endoscopic examinations and colonoscopy, ileoscopy has become far easier with the smaller endoscope diameters and the greater flexibility of the tip of the scope. Hepatobiliary disease can be explored by endoscopic retrograde cholangiography which also allows dilatation of a dominant stricture.

Biopsies through the endoscope provide mucosal specimens for histological evaluation. The purpose of the biopsy is to exclude other causes of intestinal inflammation and to assess the criteria consistent with a diagnosis of Crohn's disease.

MANAGEMENT

Medical management of Crohn's disease can be separated into three separate medical considerations; symptoms, nutrition, and mucosal inflammation, the fourth component of management is surgical intervention.

Symptoms

The principal symptoms of Crohn's disease are abdominal pain and diarrhoea with secondary symptoms of bleeding, fever, fatigue, perineal pain and arthralgia. Most of these symptoms are managed by addressing the intestinal inflammation, but adjunctive symptomatic therapy can also be useful. Abdominal pain occurs for several reasons including sensitivity to normal stimuli due to inflammation, distension related to obstruction or bacterial overgrowth, and painful peristalsis secondary to partial intestinal obstruction. Visceral hyperalgesia is an area of intense research interest. Currently, it is believed that the hypersensitivity in patients with Crohn's disease is related to their intestinal inflammation. The close interrelationship of the enteric nervous system and mucosal and submucosal mast cells has led to the hypothesis that antihistamine and antiserotonin medications may be helpful in allaying the pain. This hypothesis is being tested in a randomized and double blind fashion. Our positive experience with open-labelled antihistamines makes us optimistic that this will be a useful strategy. Clonidine has been used in a number of different abdominal pain problems and it is useful in Crohn's patients through modulation of abdominal pain and a positive effect on reducing intestinal secretion. Bacterial overgrowth is often overlooked because of the difficulty of making the diagnosis since symptoms parallel the symptoms of Crohn's disease. Confirming bacterial overgrowth with a lactulose breath test is useful, but an empiric trial of antibiotics may provide convincing clinical evidence sufficient to continue to manage this component of the symptoms. Suppressing peristalsis should be done with caution since antiperistaltic drugs may exacerbate the disease. Cautious use of loperamide, Lomotil or anticholinergics may improve pain due to increased intestinal contractility.

Diarrhoea is the second prominent symptom of Crohn's disease and it generally improves with medical management of intestinal inflammation. Dietary management focused on decreasing the simple sugars that enter the colon decreases the formation of intestinal gas and reduces the colonic stimulant effect of short-chain fatty acids produced as a consequence of bacterial metabolism. Antihistamines and anticholinergics improve diarrhoea as well as abdominal cramping. In Crohn's disease, functional compromise of the terminal ileum leads to bile acid malabsorption with subsequent cholerrhetic enteropathy. This can be managed with colestipol or cholestyramine. Nocturnal symptoms may be particularly disabling due to the symptoms themselves and the sleep deprivation they cause. Eosinophils are an active part of the intestinal inflammatory response in Crohn's disease and the predilection for eosinophil degranulation between 11 p.m. and 2 a.m. aggravates the nocturnal symptoms which often improve with antihistamine therapy.

Pain management is a serious problem since NSAIDs should be avoided and narcotics can cause addiction. Analgesics such as Acetaminophen, Tramadol HCl and Darvocet™ (propoxyphene napsylate and acetaminophen) are often effective in dealing with both somatic and intestinal pain. Tricyclic antidepressants interfere with pain perception pathways and may help to decrease the diarrhoea, modulate pain and improve sleep patterns. Managing arthralgia is difficult. Omega-3 fatty acids are currently being explored to shift the leukotriene pathway away from the leukotrienes associated with arthritis and arthralgia.[88,89] The use of the omega-3 fatty acids in maintaining remission in Crohn's disease following surgical resection makes this a logical therapeutic step, though unproven for the management of joint symptoms. Perineal pain is complex as the origin is often obscure. Abscesses and fistulas are obvious problems and require attention to the underlying inflammatory bowel disease. Perineal dermatitis, chemical and infectious, is a common problem associated with diarrhoea and immunosuppression or antibiotic treatment. Chemical dermatitis arises when the diarrhoea causes a wet perineum which leaches the protective fatty acids from the skin and leaves it susceptible the chemical contents of the diarrhoea. Protective lotions such as Balneol ™ (a perianal cleansing lotion containing mineral oil, lanolino oil and methyl paraben) improve the integrity of the skin and reduce the pain. The thickened weeping dermatitis seen with infection should be recognized and treated aggressively with topical or systemic medications. In women, treatment of infectious perineal dermatitis must also include treatment of vaginitis and consideration of a rectovaginal fistula as the aetiology for persistent perineal infectious dermatitis.

Diet

Nutritional issues are difficult in patients with Crohn's disease due to the symptoms caused by many foods. Patients who experience nausea or pain from dietary elements decrease their oral intake and are at risk of malnutrition. Few valid guidelines are available for patients. A diet low in simple sugars and fat is recommended because these two elements seem to aggravate the symptoms of Crohn's disease. Patients with either inflammatory or fibrotic strictures need to avoid the foods known to cause obstruction: oranges, grapefruits, nuts of all kinds including legumes, peanuts, shredded coconut and fibrous vegetables. Most Crohn's patients do not tolerate beef (the reason is unknown) or milk (lactose intolerance is partly responsible). The apparent response of the inflammation of Crohn's disease to an elemental diet is unknown, but thought to be related to a change in the luminal contents which may, in turn, be related to the inflammatory process. Total parenteral nutrition (TPN) has special application in the patient being considered for surgery, as improved nutrition improves postoperative recovery and may decrease the intestinal inflammation.

Inflammation

The greatest focus of management revolves around decreasing the intestinal inflammation that causes strictures, mucosal inflammation, mucosal ulcers and the systemic consequences of inflammation. Most of the management directed toward mucosal inflammation has been derived from the treatment of ulcerative colitis or has become accepted on the basis of empirical treatment. Properly controlled trials are difficult to conduct and the complexity of Crohn's disease always opens these trials to scholarly criticism.

Glucocorticoids

These have been the mainstay of the acute treatment of Crohn's disease. There is often a rapid symptomatic response to parenteral or oral steroids. However, the difficulty of long-term management and the problem of drug toxicity has led to the search for drugs that will permit patients to be weaned off steroids. Further concern has been expressed regarding the possibility that steroids early in the course of Crohn's disease might make long-term management more difficult. This is supported by the observation that 20% of patients will require chronic steroids once they have been initiated.[90,91] The important message is to try to treat the presenting disease without steroids. If steroids are needed, the life-time dose should be kept as low as possible, and steroid-sparing drugs should be used to get patients off steroids as soon as possible. When necessary, parenteral steroids can be used in doses up to 60 mg of methylprednisolone or 40–80 mg of oral prednisone. Once the disease is stable, a tapering regimen (approximately 1 mg decrease in dose per day) is a relatively standard approach to decreasing the steroids. Little objective information is available regarding the use of glucocorticoids but rapidly tapering steroid doses and alternate-day regimens are reportedly useful in decreasing the complications of steroid use. It is important to recognize that many patients who require hospitalization have symptoms due to transient bowel obstruction from food. Common food items that cause these symptoms include oranges, grapefruit, carrots, popcorn, nuts, peanuts and shredded coconut. Careful dietary inquire is needed before treating with steroids as most of these patients will do well with a clear liquid diet and intravenous hydration. Newly developed steroids have the potential of a topically active glucocorticoid with little systemic toxicity. Budesonide is a potent steroid with efficient first-pass clearance by metabolism in the liver. Theoretically, since most of the venous blood flow from the gastrointestinal tract goes through the portal circulation, the low glucocorticoid activity of the metabolic products decrease the systemic toxicity of the steroids allowing local effects to induce disease remission. A recent study demonstrated twice as many responders to budesonide than conventional steroids with no side effects in patients with Crohn's disease involving the terminal ileum.[92] These drugs are not yet proven as some early studies indicate the effective dose for therapy is accompanied by a systemic effect significant enough to suppress adrenal function.

5-Aminosalicylic acid (5-ASA) or mesalamine

Azulfidine (sulphasalazine) consists of 5-aminosalicylic acid and sulphapyridine. Azad-Kahn et al. demonstrated that the 5-ASA component was as effective as Azulfidine when given as an enema in patients with left-sided ulcerative colitis.[93] This observation led to the development of numerous 5-ASA compounds including olsalazine, balsalazide, Asacol, Pentasa and Rowasa enemas and suppositories (Table 50.2). Each of these

drugs has a distribution pattern that may allow it to be used in management of patients with ulcerative colitis or Crohn's disease. The major mechanism of action of 5-ASA is unclear and the 5-ASA drugs are only mildly effective in the management of Crohn's disease. The low toxicity in all patients and effectiveness of these drugs in ulcerative colitis provides sufficient support for most gastroenterologists to use the mesalamine derivatives in managing patients with Crohn's disease.

6-Mercaptopurine (6-MP)

Largely due to the scholarly and advocacy efforts of Dan Present[94-95], 6-MP has become part of the standard panel of drugs to be used in the management of Crohn's disease. It has the benefit of steroid sparing in these patients and has proven to be a relatively safe drug for long-term management of Crohn's disease. The major side-effects of bone marrow suppression, hepatitis and pancreatitis are uncommon and usually can be caught early enough to prevent any long-term complications. The principal disadvantage is the 60–90-day period necessary for a beneficial effect to emerge. Studies are currently underway to investigate high-dose, short-term treatment to determine whether this waiting period can be shortened. Doses of 6-MP of 50–125 mg may be used to suppress the immune system while monitoring white blood cell count, liver tests and amylase/lipase levels for drug toxicity.[94-98] Response rates in all categories of Crohn's disease are at least as effective as the response with glucocorticoids with a long-term reduction in side-effects.

Antibiotics

Antibiotic treatment of Crohn's disease has been pursued with a particular fascination since the disease has been linked to infectious colitis by the nature of the pathological findings.

Table 50.2   Options for mesalamine treatment

OPTION	UNIT DOSE	DELIVERED TO	DAILY DOSE	PROBLEMS
Direct contact				
Rowasa suppository	500 mg	Distal 20 cm	1.0–1.5 g	Expulsion due to rectal
Rowasa enema	4 g	Distal 50 cm	4 g	sensitivity
Bacterial azoreductase-dependent release				
Azulfidine	500 mg	Colon	3–6 g (Acute)	Headache, nausea, vomiting,
			2–4 g (Maint)	other effects of sulphapyridine
				Only 192 mg 5-ASA per tablet
Osalazine	250 mg	Colon	1–3 g	Diarrhoea limits dose
			6.75 g (Acute)	
Balsalazide	750 mg	Colon	3 g (Maint)	
Luminal pH dependent release				
Asacol	400 mg	Ileum/colon	2.4–4.8 g (Acute)	Capsules may pass through colon
			0.8–4.8 g (Maint)	without releasing 5-ASA
Sustained release				
Pentasa	250 mg	Entire gastrointestinal tract	2–4 g (Acute) 1.5–4 g (Maint)	Release is time dependent and influenced by delayed transit due to strictures or accelerated transit due to bacterial toxins

5-ASA, 5-aminosalicylic acid.

Moss et al.[39] brought the topic into focus with the presentation of 50 patients with Crohn's disease treated with various antibiotics with success in improving not only the symptoms but the radiographic features of the disease. Metronidazole has been used as an antibiotic for the treatment of fistula and also viewed as a possible treatment for the disease itself. The success of metronidazole may be attributed to several possible pharmacological effects. The first possibility is that the disease is related to a specific infection that is treated by the metronidazole. This is highly unlikely as no specific infection has been isolated despite aggressive techniques for identification. The second issue is an alteration in the luminal flora. This is an attractive hypothesis as the luminal factors which influence the disease are becoming an important topic of research. The third issue is related to the non-antibiotic effects of metronidazole. It improves wound healing in germ-free animal and has a distinct effect on the immune system possibly modulated by its effect on selectins and integrins. The improvement in activity of disease is modest as is the improvement in fistula healing. Recent information supports a role for metronidazole in maintenance of remission. Metronidazole has a positive, though small, effect on the course of Crohn's disease. Ciprofloxacin is another antibiotic with an effect on Crohn's disease that may be modulated, not by its antibiotic effect, but by its effect on the immune system. It is particularly interesting that the combination of ciprofloxacin and metronidazole can be as effective as prednisone in the management of acute Crohn's disease.[99] New quinilones are also being studied that influence the role of interleukin-2 (IL-2), an interferon in the immune process. Clarithromycin may be useful,[100] which is in line with an earlier study of erythromycin in the treatment of Crohn's disease.[39] At the present time, the exact role of antibiotics in Crohn's disease is still being explored with the weight of opinion focused on the change in luminal composition as the principal factor that improves the intestinal inflammation due to the exuberant activity of the immune system.

Methotrexate

Methotrexate has been used in a variety of immunologically mediated diseases. It has molecular homology with interleukin-1 (IL-1) and acts as an (IL-1) receptor antagonist (IL-1ra). Since there is an imbalance of IL-1 and IL-1ra in Crohn's disease, it would be expected that methotrexate would correct this ratio. Patients with Crohn's disease respond in about 75% of cases, but there is a high relapse rate in the 6–12 months after the initiation of therapy.[101] The role of methotrexate in IBD is minimal; but it does have a more rapid onset of action than 6-MP.

Cyclosporin

Cyclosporin changed the face of organ transplantation. Its use in inflammatory bowel disease was based on the ability to suppress the immune system. In a small study in patients with ulcerative colitis, cyclosporin was very effective in improving patients who were at high risk of surgery.[102] In a 3-month study of patients with active chronic Crohn's disease it was less effective with 59% improving with oral cyclosporin compared to 32% on placebo.[103] Intravenous therapy is more effective and it is difficult to manage patients by long-term cyclosporin therapy. It is interesting to speculate on the long-term benefit of cyclosporin when the disease appears to remain active in both ulcerative colitis and Crohn's colitis after organ transplantation and long-term cyclosporin therapy.

Anti tumour necrosis factor

Tumour necrosis factor (TNF) is present in high quantities in the stool of patients with IBD and there is an increase in the number of cells producing TNF in patients with IBD. This observation and the recognition that TNF is pivotal in the amplification of immunological and inflammatory processes, led to the development of anti-TNF compounds to treat Crohn's disease. Although relatively few patients have been treated with the chimeric monoclonal antibiody cA2 for TNF, it is effective in short-term management of moderate-to-severe

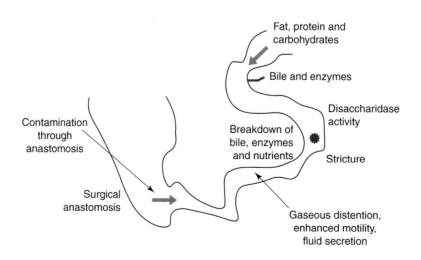

Figure 50.1

Pathogenesis of bacterial overgrowth and consequences. Strictures from Crohn's disease lead to proximal stasis of small bowel contents. Patent anastomosis after ileal resection allows colonic contents to reflux into the small bowel.

treatment-resistant Crohn's disease,[104] long-term prevention of relapse and fistula improvement.[105] The long-term value of anti-TNF therapy needs to be evaluated more carefully, but there is great hope that this will be a major improvement in the management of Crohn's disease.

Other cytokines

Development of new cytokine therapies with IL-11 and IL-10 holds promise. IL-10 acts to suppress inflammation and in a pilot study it improved the Crohn's Disease Activity Index in 46 patients receiving IL-10 compared with controls.[106] In a more extensive study of IL-10, remission was reported in 29% of patients at a dose of 5 µg/kg/day.[107] Recombinant human interleukin-11 (rhIL-11) may be useful in the treatment of Crohn's disease, but the data are insufficient to confirm its efficacy at this point.[108]

Surgical management

Although surgical management of Crohn's disease is not the topic of this chapter, it is our opinion that surgical management of Crohn's disease is often necessary and preferable to long-term medical management of several of the problems associated with Crohn's disease.

REFERENCES

1. Sturgeon JB, Bhatia PS, Hermens DJ & Miner PB. Exacerbation of chronic ulcerative colitis with mesalamine. *Gastroenterology* 1993; **104**:A785.
2. Calkins BM, Lilienfeld AM, Garland CF & Mendeloff AI. Trends in incidence rates of ulcerative colitis and Crohn's disease. *Dig Dis Sci* 1984; **29**:913.
3. Garland CF, Lilienfeld AM, Mendeloff AI, Markowitz JA, Terrell KB & Garland FC. Incidence rates of ulcerative colitis and Crohn's disease in fifteen areas of the United States. *Gastroenterology* 1981; **81**:1115.
4. Gollop JH, Phillips SF, Melton III, LJ & Sinsmeister AR. Epidemiologic aspects of Crohn's disease: a population-based study in Olmsted County, Minnesota, 1943–82. *Gut* 1988; **29**:49.
5. Sedlack RE, Nobrega FR, Kurland LT & Sauer WG. Inflammatory colon disease in Rochester, Minnesota, 1935–1964. *Gastroenterology* 1972; **62**:935.
6. Gelpi A. Inflammatory bowel disease among college students. *West J Med* 1978; **129**:369.
7. Stowe SP, Redmond SR, Stormont JM et al. An epidemiologic study of inflammatory bowel disease in Rochester, New York: Hospital incidence. *Gastroenterology* 1990; **98**:104.
8. Nunes GC & Ahlquist RE. Increasing incidence of Crohn's disease. *Am J Surg* 1983; **145**:578.
9. Haitt RA & Kaufman L. Epidemiology of inflammatory bowel disease in a defined northern California population. *West J Med* 1988; **149**:541.
10. Kurata JH, Kantor-Fish S, Frankl H, Godby P & Vandheim CM. Crohn's disease among ethnic groups in a large health maintenance organization. *Gastroenterology* 1992; **102**:1940.
11. Pinchbeck BR, Kirdeikis J & Thomsom ABR. Inflammatory bowel disease in northern Alberta. *J Clin Gastroenterol* 1988; **10**:505.
12. Mayberry JF, Judd D, Smart H, Rhodes J, Calcraft B & Morris JS. Crohn's disease in Jewish people – an epidemiologic study in southeast Wales. *Digestion* 1986; **35**:237.
13. Calkins BM & Mendeloff AI. The epidemiology of idopathic inflammatory bowel disease. In Kirsner JB & Shorter RG (eds) *Inflammatory Bowel Disease*, 4th edn. Baltimore; Williams & Wilkins, 1995.
14. Evans JF & Acheson ED. An epidemiological study of ulcerative colitis and regional enteritis in the Oxford area. *Gut* 1965; **6**:311.
15. Krawiec J, Odes HS, Lasry Y, Krugliak P & Weitzman S. Aspects of the epidemiology of Crohn's disease in the Jewish population in Beer Sheva, Israel. *Isr J Med Sci* 1984; **20**:16.
16. Fireman Z, Grossman A, Lilos P, Eshchar Y, Theodor E & Gilat T. Epidemiology of Crohn's disease in the Jewish population of central Israel, 1970–1980. *Am J Gastroenterol* 1989; **84**:255.
17. Odes HS, Fraser D & Krawiec J. Ulcerative colitis in the Jewish population of southern Israel 1961–1958: Epidemiological and clinical study. *Gut* 1987; **28**:854.
18. Odes HS, Fraser D & Drawiec J. Incidence of idiopathic ulcerative colitis in Jewish population subgroups in the Beer Sheva region of Israel. *Am J Gastroenterol* 1987; **82**:854.
19. Niv Y & Abukasis G. Prevalence of ulcerative colitis in the Israeli kibbutz population. *J Clin Gastroenterol* 1991; **13**:98.
20. Calkins BM & Mendeloff AI. Epidemiology of inflammatory bowel disease. *Epidemiol Rev* 1986; **8**:60.
21. Almy TP & Sherlock P. Genetic aspects of ulcerative colitis and regional enteritis. *Gastroenterology* 1966; **51**:757.
22. Sategna-Guidetti C, Bianco L. Bracco E & Marucco E. Familial incidence of Crohn's disease in Italy. *Dig Dis Sci* 1986; **31**:557.
23. Monsen U, Brostrom O, Nordenvail B, Sorstad J & Hellers G. Prevalence of inflammatory bowel disease among relatives of patients with ulcerative colitis. *Scand J Gastroenterol* 1987; **22**:214.
24. Lashner BA, Evans AA, Kirsner JB & Hanauer SB. Prevalence and incidence of inflammatory bowel disease in family members. *Gastroenterology* 1986; **91**:1396.
25. Kirsner JB & Spencer JA. Family occurrence of ulcerative colitis, regional enteritis and ileocolitis. *Ann Intern Med* 1963; **59**:133.
26. Binder V, Weeke E, Olsen JH, Anthonisen P & Riis P. A genetic study of ulcerative colitis. *Gastroenterology* 1966; **1**:49.
27. Leukonia RM & McConnell RB. Familial inflammatory bowel disease-hereditary or environment? *Gut* 1976; **17**:235.
28. Fielding JF. The relative risk of inflammatory bowel disease among parents and siblings of Crohn's disease patients. *J Clin Gastroenterol* 1986; **8**:655.
29. McConnell RB. Genetic aspects of idiopathic inflammatory bowel disease. In Kirsner JB & Shorter RG (eds) *Inflammatory Bowel Disease*. Philadelphia, Lea & Febiger, 1988.
30. Mendeloff AI & Calkins BM. The epidemiology of idiopathic inflammatory bowel disease. In Kirsner JB & Shorter RG (eds) *Inflammatory Bowel Disease*, 3rd edn. Philadelphia, Lea & Febiger, 1988.
31. Tattersall RB & Pyke DA. Diabetes in identical twins. *Lancet* 1972; **ii**:1120.
32. Tysk C, Lindberg E, Jarnerot G & Floderus-Myrhed B. Ulcerative colitis and Crohn's disease in an unselected population of monozygotic and dizygotic twins. A study of heritability and the influence of smoking. *Gut* 1988; **29**:990.
33. Zlotogora J & Rachmilewitz D: Letter: Are individuals born as twins at higher risk of developing Crohn's disease? *Gut* 1989; **30**:141.
34. Mirza MM, Lee J, Teare D et al. Evidence of linkage of the inflammatory bowel disease susceptibility locus on chromosome 16 (IBDI) to ulcerative colitis. *J Med Genet* 1998; **35**:218.
35. Noam I, Ford D, Bowman SJ et al. Analysis of the contribution of HLA genes to genetic predisposition in inflammatory bowel disease. *Am J Hum Genet* 1996; **59**:226.
36. Podolsky DK. Lessons from genetic models of inflammatory bowel disease. *Acta Gastroenterol Belg* 1997; **60**:163.
37. Alsenberg J & Janowitz HD. Cluster of inflammatory bowel disease in three close college friends? *J Clin Gastroenterol* 1993; **17**:18.
38. Koutroubakis I, Manoussos ON, Meuwissen SG & Pena AS. Environmental risk factors in inflammatory bowel disease. *Hepatogastroenterology* 1996; **43**:381.
39. Moss AA, Carbone JV & Kressel HY. Radiologic and clinical assessment of broad spectrum antibiotic therapy in Crohn's disease. *Am J Roentgenol* 1978; **131**:787.
40. Rutgeerts P, Hiele M, Geboes K et al. Controlled trial of metronidazole treatment for prevention of Crohn's recurrence after ileal resection. *Gastroenterology* 1995; **108**:1617.
41. Ursing B, Alm T, Barany F et al. A comparative study of metronidazole and sulfasalazine for active Crohn's disease: the cooperative Crohn's disease study in Sweden (results). *Gastroenterology* 1982; **83**:550.
42. Bernstein LH, Frank MS, Brandt LJ & Boley SJ. Healing of perineal Crohn's disease with metronidazole. *Gastroenterology* 1980; **79**:357.
43. Prantera C, Zannoni F, Scribano ML et al. An antibiotic regimen for the treatment of active Crohn's disease: A randomized, controlled clinical trial of metronidazole plus ciprofloxacin. *Am J Gastroenterol* 1996; **91**:328.

44. Tawfik AF, Shoeb HA, Bishop SJ, al-Shammary FJ & Shibl AM. Influence of new quinolones on normal immune capabilities. *J Chemother* 1990; **2**:300.

45. Munro J, Mayberry JF, Matthews N & Rhodes J. Chlamydia and Crohn's disease. *Lancet* 1979; **ii**:45.

46. Parent K & Mitchel P. Cell wall defective variants of pseudomonas like (Group Va) bacteria in Crohn's disease. *Gastroenterology* 1978; **75**:368.

47. Whorwell PJ, Phillips CA, Beeken WL, Little PK & Roessner KD. Isolation of reovirus-like agents from patients with Crohn's disease. *Lancet* 1977; **i**:1169.

48. Burnham WR, Lennard-Jones JE, Stanford JL & Bird RG. Mycobacteria as a possible cause of inflammatory bowel disease. *Lancet* 1978; **ii**:693.

49. Chlodini RJ, Van Kruiningen HJ, Thayer WR, Merkal RS & Coutu JA. Possible role of mycobacteria in inflammatory bowel disease. I. An unclassified mycobacterium species isolated from patients with Crohn's disease. *Dig Dis Sci* 1984; **29**:1073.

50. Wakefield AJ, Pittilo RM, Sim R et al. Evidence of pesistent measles virus infection in Crohn's disease. *J Med Virol* 1993; **39**:345.

51. Taub RN, Sachar D, Siltzbach LE & Janowitz H. Transmission of ileitis and sarcoid granulomas to mice. *Trans Assoc Am Phys* 1975; **87**:219.

52. Cave DR, Mitchell DN & Brooke BN. Experimental animal studies of the etiology and pathogenesis of Crohn's disease. *Gastroenterology* 1975; **69**:618–624.

53. Kangro HO, Chong SK, Hardiman A, Heath RB & Walker-Smith JA. A prospective study of viral and mycoplasma infections in chronic inflammatory bowel disease. *Gastroenterology* 1990; **98**:549.

54. Weber P, Koch M, Heizmann WR, Scheurlen M, Jenss H & Hartmann F. Microbic superinfection in relapse of inflammatory bowel disease. *J Clin Gastroenterol* 1992; **14**:302.

55. Greenfield C, Aguilar Ramiriz JR, Pounder RE et al. *Clostridium difficile* and inflammatory bowel disease. *Gut* 1983; **24**:713.

56. Powrie F & Leach MW. Genetic and spontanious models of inflammatory bowel disease in rodents: evidence for abnormalities in mucosal immune regulation. *Ther Immunol* 1995; **2**:115.

57. O'Donoghue DP & Kumar P. Rectal IgE cells in inflammatory bowel disease. *Gut* 1979; **20**:149.

58. Willoughby CP, Piris J & Truelove SC. Tissue eosinophils in ulcerative colitis. *Scand J Gastroenterol* 1979; **14**:395.

59. Heatley RV & James PD. Eosinophils in the rectal mucosa. A simple method of predicting the outcome of ulcerative procitis? *Gut* 1978; **20**:787.

60. Naylor AR & Pollet JE. Eosinophilic colitis. *Dis Colon Rectum* 1985; **28**:615.

61. Lewin K, Riddell RH & Weinstein WM. *Gastrointestinal Pathology and its Clinical Implications.* New York: Igaku-Shoin, 1992.

62. De Schryver-Kecskemeti KJ, Bennert KW, Cooper GS & Yang P. Gastrointestinal involvement in L-tryptophan (L-Trp) associated eosinophilia–myalgia syndrome (EMS). *Dig Dis Sci* 1992; **37**:697.

63. De Schryver-Kecskemeti KJ, Gramlich TL, Crofford LJ et al. Mast cell and eosinophil infiltrates in gastrointestinal mucosa of Lewis rats treated with L-tryptophan implicated in human eosinophilia–myalgia syndrome. *Mod Pathol* 1991; **4**:354.

64. Crofford LJ, Rader JI, Dalakas MC et al. L-Tryptophan implicated in human eosinophilia-myalgia syndrome causes fasclitis and perimyositis in the Lewis rat. *J Clin Invest* 1990; **86**:1757.

65. Miner PB. Newer aspects of the eosinophil in IBD: Insights in Gastroenterology. *Clin Persp Gastroenterol* 1999; **1**.

66. Elson CO. The immunology of inflammatory bowel disease. In Kirsner JB & Shorter RG (eds) *Inflammatory Bowel Disease,* 3rd edn. Philadelphia: Lea & Febiger, 1988.

67. Hollander D, Vandheim CM, Brettholz E, Petersen GM, Delahunty T & Rotter JI. Increased intestinal permeability in patients with Crohn's disease and their relatives. *Ann Intern Med* 1986; **105**:883.

68. Gaffney PR, O'Leary JJ, Doyle CT et al. Response to heparin in patients with ulcerative colitis. *Lancet* 1991; **337**:238.

69. Evans RC, Wong VS, Morris AI & Rhodes JM. Treatment of corticosteroid-resistant ulcerative colitis with heparin – a report of 16 cases. *Aliment Pharmacol Ther* 1997; **11**:1037.

70. Fleming CR. Nutrition in patients with Crohn's disease: another piece of the puzzle. *J Parent Ent Nutr* 1995; **19**:93.

71. Greenberg GR. Nutritional support in inflammatory bowel disease: current status and future directions. *Scand J Gastroenterol* 1992; **192**:117.

72. Teahon K, Pearson M, Smith T & Bjarnason I. Alterations in nutritional status and disease activity during treatment of Crohn's disease with elemental diet. *Scand J Gastroenterol* 1995; **30**:54.

73. Harries AD, Baird A & Rhodes J. Non-smoking: a feature of ulcerative colitis. *Br Med J* 1982; **284**:706.

74. Sutherland LR, Ramcharan S, Bryant H & Fick G. Effect of cigarette smoking on recurrence of Crohn's disease. *Gastroenterology* 1990; **98**:1123.

75. Kaufmann HF & Taubin HL. Nonsteroidal anti-inflammatory drugs activate quiescent inflammatory bowel disease. *Ann Intern Med* 1987; **107**:513.

76. Evans JM, McMahon AD, Murray FE, McDevitt DG & MacDonald TM. Non-steroidal anti-inflammatory drugs are associated with emergency admission to hospital for colitis due to inflammatory bowel disease. *Gut* 1997; **40**:619.

77. Bielecki JW & Filippini L. Side effects of non-steroidal antirheumatic agents in the lower intestinal tract. *Schweiz Med Wochenschr* 1993; **123**:1419.

78. Drossman DA. Psychosocial considerations in gastroenterology. In Sleisenger MG, Fordtran JS, Cello JP, Feldman M (eds) *Gastrointestinal Disease: Pathophysiology, Diagnosis, Management.* Philadelphia: WB Saunders, 1993.

79. Mayer EA & Raybould HE. Role of visceral afferent mechanisms in functional bowel disorders. *Gastroenterology* 1990; **99**:1688.

80. Shanahan F & Anton P. Neuroendocrine modulation of the immune system: possible implications for inflammatory bowel disease. *Dig Dis Sci* 1988; **33**:41S.

81. Bellinger DL, Lorton D, Romano TD, Olschowka JA, Telten SY & Felten DL. Neuropeptide innervation of lymphoid organs. *Ann NY Acad Sci* 1990; **594**:17.

82. Gauci M, Husband AJ, Saxarra H & King MG. Pavlovian conditioning of nasal tryptase release in human subjects with allergic rhinitis. *Physiol Behav* 1994; **55**:823.

83. Buchman P, Dolb E & Alexander-Williams J. Pathogenesis of urgency in defaecation in Crohn's disease. *Digestion* 1981; **22**:310.

84. Gelbmann CM, Schteingart CD, Thompson SM, Hofmann AF & Barrett KE. Mast cells and histamine contribute to bile acid-stimulated secretion in the mouse colon. *J Clin Invest* 1995; **95**:2831.

85. Junien JL & Riviere P. Review article: the hypersensitive gut— peripheral kappa agonists as a new pharmacological approach. *Aliment Pharmacol Ther* 1995; **9**:117.

86. Mayer EA & Gebhart GF. Basic and clinical aspects of visceral hyperalgesia. *Gastroenterology* 1994; **107**:271.

87. Buckell NA, Lennare-Jones JE, Hernandez MA, Kohn J, Riches PG & Wedsworth J. Measurement of serum proteins during attacks of ulcerative colitis as a guide to patient management. *Gut* 1979; **20**:22.

88. Ikehata A, Hiwatashi N, Kinouchi Y et al. Effect of intravenously infused eicosapentaenoic acid on the leukotriene generation in patients with active Crohn's disease. *Am J Clin Nutr* 1992; **56**:938.

89. Heller A, Koch T, Schmeck J & van Ackern K. Lipid mediators in inflammatory disorders. *Drugs* 1998; **55**:487.

90. Munkolm P, Langholz E, Davidsen M & Binder V. Frequency of glucocorticoid resistance and dependency in Crohn's disease. *Gut* 1994; **35**:360.

91. Reinisch W, Gasche C, Wyatt J et al. Steroid dependency in Crohn's disease. *Lancet* 1995; **345**:859.

92. Bar-Meir S, Chowers Y, Lavy A et al. and the Israeli Budesonlde Study Group. Budesonide versus prednisone in the treatment of active Crohn's disease. *Gastroenterology* 1998; **115**:835.

93. Azad Khan AK, Piris J & Truelove SL. An experiment to determine the active therapeutic moiety of sulphasalazine. *Lancet* 1977; **ii**:892.

94. Present DH, Meltzer SJ, Krumholz MP & Wolke A. 6-Mercaptopurine in the management of inflammatory bowel disease: short- and long-term toxicity. *Ann Intern Med* 1989; **111**:641.

95. Present DH, Korelitz BI, Wisch N, Glass JL, Sachar DB & Pasternack BS. Treatment of Crohn's disease with 6-Mercaptopurine. *N Engl J Med* 1980; **302**:981.

96. Singleton JW, Law DH, Kelley ML Fr, Merkhjian HS & Sturdevant RA. National Cooperative Crohn's Disease Study: adverse reactions to study drugs. *Gastroenterology* 1979; **77**:887.

97. Markowitz J, Daum F, Cohen SA et al. Immunology of inflammatory bowel disease: Summary of the proceedings of the Subcommittee on Immunosuppressive Use in IBD. *J Pediatr Gastroenterol Nutr* 1991; **12**:411.

98. Colonna T & Korelitz BI. The role of leukopenia in the 6-mercatopurine-induced remission of refractory Crohn's disease. *Am J Gastroenterol* 1994; **89**:362.

99. Greenbloom SL, Steinheart AH & Greenberg GR. Combination ciprofloxacin and metronidazole for active Crohn's disease. *Can J Gastroenterol* 1998; **12**:53.

100. Graham D, Al-Assi M & Robinson M. Prolonged remission in Crohn's disease following therapy for *Mycobacterium paratuberculosis* infection. *Gastroenterology* 1995; **108**:826.

101. Kozarek RA, Patterson DJ, Gelfand MD, Botoman VA, Ball TJ & Wilske KR. Methotrexate induces clinical and histologic remission in patients with refractory inflammatory bowel disease. *Ann Intern Med* 1989; **110**:353.

102. Lichtiger S, Present DH, Kornbluth A et al. Cyclosporine in severe ulcerative colitis refractory to steroid therapy. *N Engl J Med* 1994; **330**:1841.

103. Brynskov J, Freund L, Rasmussen SN et al. A placebo-controlled, double-blind, randomized trial of cyclosporine therapy in active chronic Crohn's disease. *N Engl J Med* 1989; **321**:845.

104. Targan SR, Hanauer SB, vanDeventer SJH et al. for the Crohn's Disease cA2 Study Group. A Short-term study of chimeric monoclonal antibody cA2 to tumor necrosis factor α for Chron's disease. *N Engl J Med* 1997; **337**:1029.

105. D'Haens GR, vanDeventer SJH, Van Hogezand R et al. Anti-TNF α monoclonal antibody (cA2) produces endoscopic healing in patients with treatment resistant, active Crohn's disease. *Gastroenterology* 1998; **114**:A-1108.

106. vanDeventer SJH, Elson CO, Fedorak RN for the Crohn's disease study group. Multiple doses of intravenous interleukin-10 in steroid-refractory Crohn's disease. *Gastroenterology* 1997; **113**:383.

107. Fedorak RN, Gangl A, Elson Co et al. and the IL10 IBD cooperative study group: safety, tolerance and efficacy of multiple doses of subcutaneous Interleukin-10 in mild to moderate active Crohn's disease. *Gastroenterology* 1998; **114**:A-1108.

108. Bank S, Sninsky C, Robinson M et al. Safety and activity evaluation of rhIL-11 in subjects with active Crohn's disease. *Gastroenterology* 1997; **112**:A927.

51

CROHN'S ENTERITIS: SURGICAL TREATMENT

BG Wolff

SURGICAL PRINCIPLES

Crohn's disease may involve nearly the entire gastrointestinal tract in many patients, and electron microscopic abnormalities have been documented throughout the intestine in patients with Crohn's disease. Therefore, the concept of complete excision of the disease is impractical. Efforts are concentrated towards treatment of the areas most responsible for syndromes such as intractability, stricture, bleeding, perforation or obstruction.

For young patients with Crohn's disease the cumulative risk of undergoing operation in their lifetime is nearly 90%, and the cumulative risk of recurrent disease at 20 years is 70%, but a nihilistic approach to the surgical treatment of Crohn's disease on the theory that recrudescence or recurrence is inevitable is not justified. Most series do show a high recurrence rate after operative treatment.[1-4] Many of the data are derived from retrospective studies in tertiary care centres and therefore suffer a referral bias. The crude surgical intervention rate (41%) in one population-controlled study[5] was lower than in other previous studies, possibly reflecting a treatment bias toward earlier operation in those other reviews. Furthermore, over a 40-year period in Olmsted County, Minnesota, over half the patients with Crohn's disease were managed quite satisfactorily nonoperatively in spite of a high risk of periodic recrudescence.[5]

Despite the surgeon's inability completely to resect or cure Crohn's disease surgically, operation should not be delayed because of fears of recurrence. This approach is unrealistic because: (1) resection is conservative at the present time and usually constitutes only the involved bowel, which will never be normal; (2) as many as 50% of patients will never have a symptomatic recurrence; (3) those that do have a recurrence may gain several years of improved quality of life and be off medication.

The latter point is supported by data from a recent prospective randomized trial of drug prophylaxis (5-aminosalicylic

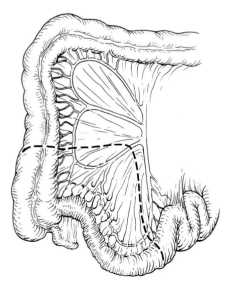
(a)

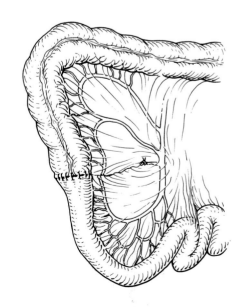
(b)

Figure 51.1
Right hemicolectomy for Crohn's disease.

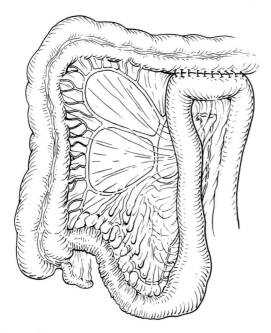

Figure 51.2
Bypass without exclusion.

acid) after surgical resections in patients grossly free of disease at the time of operation.[6] After predicting a postoperative recurrence rate based on the literature of approximately 12% a year, the authors of this study found that the annual recurrence rate was nearly twice this figure in a prospective study in which patients had yearly, complete gastrointestinal examinations. Of 163 patients entered into the trial, 31% in the treatment group have developed symptomatic recurrence, and 14% in the control group have developed symptomatic recurrence. This does not include those with asymptomatic recurrence. Therefore, when investigated prospectively, many more patients

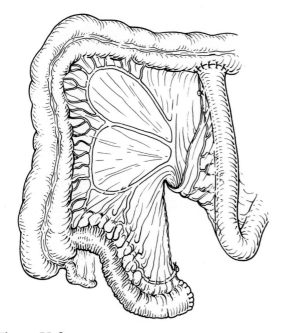

Figure 51.3
Bypass with exclusion.

($P = 0.031$) than previously believed will have recurrence that may or may not become symptomatic at a later time.

In the past, small intestinal Crohn's disease was treated by two main operative approaches, either excision or bypass of the lesions, with or without exclusion. Examples of excision and bypass are shown in Figures 51.1–51.3. Bypass has been almost completely eliminated in the operative treatment of Crohn's disease, since the bypassed segment continues to cause symptoms requiring treatment and may even harbour malignancy (Figures 51.4 and 51.5).[7] The risk of carcinoma in a small bowel affected with Crohn's disease is substantially greater than the risk in healthy bowel.[8]

More recently, the management of small bowel strictures in Crohn's disease has undergone change. Strictureplasty has been popularized by Lee[9] and Alexander-Williams in the UK.[10] This technique, adapted from surgery for tubercular strictures in India, allows the surgeon to preserve small bowel and avoid excessively large resections or multiple resections in patients whose primary disorder is stricture and resultant partial obstruction from Crohn's disease.

The principal controversy in the operative treatment of Crohn's disease has concerned the length of disease-free margins, and whether disease-free margins reduce the rate of recrudescence or recurrence following resection. In an update of their original series, Krause and colleagues[11] reported long-term follow-up (>14 years) of their patients who had radical resections at the first operation (10 cm of normal bowel excised on either side of the involved bowel) with a recurrence rate of 31%, with fewer reoperations, and a better quality of life compared with those who underwent non-radical resections (recurrence rate 83%). This position has been supported by others.[12,13] In the Mayo Clinic experience, 89% of those with microscopically involved margins recurred within seven years, and the institutional 10-year recurrence rate was 55%. In a Norwegian study,[13] 60% of those with microscopic signs of disease at the anastomosis were found to have developed recurrence, as opposed to 14% when the margins of resection were free of disease. On the other hand, Pennington et al.[14] found that there was no difference in those who had microscopically normal margins and those who had microscopically involved margins; this study has been supported by work

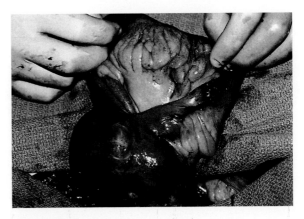

Figure 51.4
Active Crohn's disease in bypassed small bowel segment.

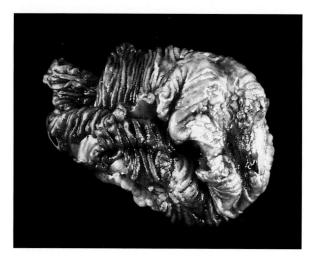

Figure 51.5
Active Crohn's disease in bypassed small bowel segment.

from Sweden[15] and France.[16] Moreover, this controversy seems to revolve around the pathological description of microscopic Crohn's disease, and this issue is not likely to be settled in a retrospective study. In the prospective study described above, there was no difference in recurrence rates between patients who had a 5 cm or greater margin compared to those with less than 5 cm margins (Figure 51.6). Most surgeons performing a resection on the small bowel affected with Crohn's disease would attempt to obtain a disease-free margin of 2–5 cm on both sides of the area of involvement. Although frozen section margins are used in some centres, disease-free margins are generally established by gross inspection of the mucosa. Certainly in a patient with multiple skip areas, obtaining microscopic borders free of disease is counterproductive: and may lead to short bowel syndrome. Patients with this problem do not have enough remaining intestine to digest and absorb food properly. Therefore, judgement must be exercised in performing resections. Although resections are conservative in a patient with an isolated area of active Crohn's disease, complete removal should be obtained. If margins are positive, the risk of intestinal anastomosis is not inherently greater than in normal uninvolved bowel.[12,17]

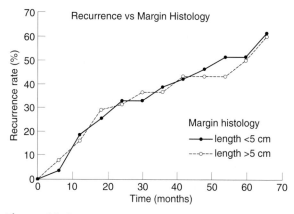

Figure 51.6
Recurrence versus margin histology.

INDICATIONS FOR OPERATION

The commonest sites of primary involvement with Crohn's disease are terminal ileum and caecum. Ileocolitis seems to confer the highest recurrence rate after operation, but this is still a matter of debate.[18] The commonest emergency indications for operation are perforation, fistula formation and abscess or, more rarely, bleeding. Obstruction is usually partial; rarely does Crohn's disease of the small intestine present as complete obstruction. Nevertheless, nasogastric suction and intravenous nutrition can be instituted in these patients, and the distended small bowel will usually decompress with resumption of bowel action. Failure of such a resolution with resumption of oral feeding generally leads to operation. Perforation of the terminal ileum is uncommon, but it mimics appendicitis and the diagnosis is often confused.

Severe systemic symptoms in small bowel disease that is intractable to medical therapy (Chapter 50), including weight loss and growth failure in children, lead to elective surgery. Extraintestinal manifestations of inflammatory bowel disease contribute to the decision to operate, and most of these complications, with the exception of ankylosing spondylitis and hepatic complications, will resolve with the excision of intestine grossly involved with Crohn's disease.

PREPARATION

Patients undergoing emergency operation for Crohn's disease are given prompt fluid, electrolyte resuscitation and triple agent antibiotic coverage e.g. metronidazole, gentamicin and ampicillin; other broad-spectrum antibiotics can be used. If time allows, the preoperative marking site for a stoma should be made, since this is a very likely outcome of such operations. Patients with peritonitis should have a nasogastric tube inserted preoperatively, and this should remain in place for several days postoperatively. Those patients undergoing elective operation may benefit from total parenteral nutrition depending on their nutritional status preoperatively. Even though elemental diets have not been effective as primary treatment for exacerbations of Crohn's disease, there is evidence that such preparation will produce a better outcome in the severely debilitated patient. Anaemia should also be corrected by transfusion, although the effect of intraoperative transfusion on recurrence rate is unknown.[18] Patients who have been receiving corticosteroids should receive additional steroid preparation in the perioperative period, usually 100 mg hydrocortisone intravenously every 8 hours, to provide support during operative stress.

Bowel preparation consists of either a cathartic/enema preparation or an oral lavage solution of 4 l of a balanced electrolyte solution, such as Golytely™, which can be given on the day before operation. Clear liquid is the diet of choice before operation. Some surgeons prefer to perform an on-table bowel preparation, and some even provide only intravenous antibiotics with no preoperative bowel preparation, but it has been shown definitively that the reduction of the amount of stool in the bowel reduces the infection rate postoperatively. Oral antibiotics consisting of neomycin and erythromycin base can be given the day before operation in a dose of 1 g of each every 4 h. Alternatively, after the lavage preparation, 2 g each of metronidazole and neomycin can be given, with the dosage repeated 4 hours later. This regime has been shown to be as effective as the cathartic/enema preparation.[19] Intravenous antibiotics in addition to oral antibiotics have not proven to be more effective than oral antibiotics alone.

PROCEDURE

Resection

A vertical midline abdominal incision is made to the left of the umbilicus, which leaves the right lower quadrant unscarred and available for use as the site of an ileostomy, should one be required. The abdominal contents are carefully inspected and some assessment is made of the extent of disease. Generally, small bowel Crohn's disease will affect the terminal ileum and it is usually necessary to resect the terminal ileum, caecum, appendix and perhaps a portion of the ascending colon (Figures 51.7–51.10). An end-to-end anastomosis can then be made with an absorbable suture material, such as PDS™, or a side-to-side anastomosis can be constructed using linear staplers such as the GIA™. After resection, it is customary to measure the remaining amount of small bowel, so that some assessment will be available for use when considering future operations. The overriding concern in resection of the small bowel is to preserve as much normal functioning small bowel as possible.

Skip areas may be found more proximally, and subtle strictures can be recognized by performing an enterotomy and passing a Baker® tube through the lumen of the intestine. The size of the strictures can be gauged by measuring the size of the balloon when inflated, and the strictures are detected as an impediment as the catheter is drawn back through the bowel. Such strictures may not be apparent by simply examining the bowel externally with palpation or by inspection. In performing resections for small bowel Crohn's disease, it is not necessary to perform a lymphadenectomy or to excise all of the thickened mesentery, as this has no bearing on recurrence rate and may compromise blood supply to the anastomosis (Figures 51.11 and 51.12).

Strictureplasty

If multiple strictures are found throughout the small intestine with or without an area that must be resected, the option of strictureplasty becomes apparent. Strictureplasties have been performed successfully in very active areas of disease, as well as in areas of burned-out fibrotic disease. After identifying areas of stricture, the strictureplasty is performed by making a

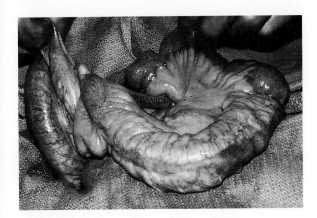

Figure 51.7

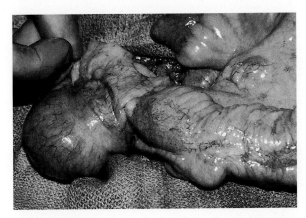

Figure 51.8

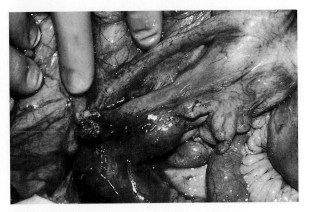

Figure 51.9

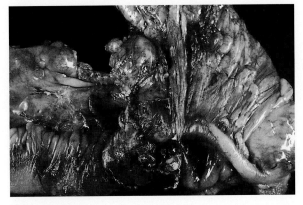

Figure 51.10

Ileocolic Crohn's disease with fistula into tip of appendix.

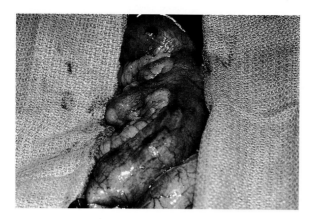

Figure 51.11
Terminal ileal Crohn's disease with involvement of Meckel's diverticulum.

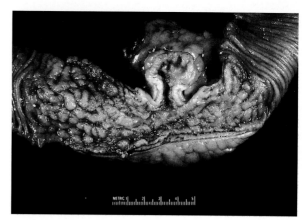

Figure 51.12
Terminal ileal Crohn's with involvement of Meckel's diverticulum.

longitudinal incision over the area of stricture and then closing this incision in a transverse direction (Figures 51.13–51.18). Either a single or two-layer technique can be performed with a durable monofilament absorbable or non-absorbable suture. It is our policy to place a Weck™ clip at the base of the stricture-plasty for future identification. Strictured areas up to 20 cm long have been treated in such a manner by performing a Finney type anastomosis, but this is uncommon. Areas of severe involvement of that length should be considered more appropriate for resection.

Experience with strictureplasties is growing, and to date the results have been good. In one series,[20] 24 patients were operated on and 86 strictures were treated with strictureplasty. Obstruction was relieved in all patients and there was no fistula formation. One recurrent stricture appeared during a mean follow-up of 40 months. A series of 145 patients from the Cleveland Clinic have undergone 700 strictureplasties. Similar results were obtained as to complications and low morbidity.[21] A comparison of results from different studies is shown in Table 51.1.[22a,b]

Ileoproctostomy

Ileoproctostomy (ileorectostomy) is an option that may be performed in patients with minimal or no rectal disease. Nevertheless, experience with this procedure has not been good.[23–26] In one study of ileocolic anastomosis,[27] there was aphthous ulcer recurrence proximal to the anastomosis in 72% of the patients followed colonoscopically within one year of operation. Nevertheless, approximately one-third of patients undergoing ileoproctostomy will have long-term benefit without the need for medication.

Other continence-preserving procedures

Rarely, ileal pouch–anal anastomosis has been done in patients with Crohn's colitis as a planned procedure. There are too few patients available for a knowledgeable assessment. However, in our own series,[28] two patients had ileal pouch–anal anastomosis for Crohn's colitis as a planned procedure. One patient did well and the other did not. Of the remaining 14 patients who had a diagnosis made of Crohn's disease after ileal

Table 51.1 Results with strictureplasty

REFERENCE[1]	DATE	NO. PATIENTS	TOTAL OPERATIONS	NO. OF STRICTUREPLASTIES	CONCOMITANT RESECTION (%)	PERIOPERATIVE COMPLICATIONS (%)	RECURRENT SYMPTOMS (%)	AVERAGE FOLLOW-UP
Silvermen et al. Toronto	1989	14	16	36	93	21	26	16 months
Pritchard et al. Lahey	1990	13	16	52	31	15	69	2 years
Fazio et al. Cleveland	1989	50	54	225	60	16	22	8.3 months
Dehn et al. Oxford	1989	24	30	86	62	1	46	40 months
Alexander-Williams Birmingham	1987	57		146		14	40	6 months
Kendall et al. St Mark's	1986	5	5	26	80	2	100	6 months
Mayo	1991	35	36	71	66	14	20	2 years

[1] From Ref. 22a,b.

pouch–anal anastomosis, five have abdominal stomas and 11 still have an ileoanal anastomosis. Of these 11, eight have good pouch function and three have fair pouch function. There is some evidence that patients who have had anorectal pathology before ileal–pouch anastomosis have a much worse prognosis than those who have not had anorectal problems preoperatively in the event that a later diagnosis of Crohn's disease is established.[29]

In one report[30] a series of seven patients underwent proctocolectomy for Crohn's disease and were followed-up for a mean disease-free interval of 7.7 years. At this point, three patients underwent revision of their ileostomy to a Kock continent ileostomy. Postoperative complication and revision rates (28%) were comparable to continent ileostomy results for individuals with other pathology, and all patients were fully continent to gas and ileal effluent. Nevertheless, in an earlier series of 52 patients with Crohn's disease,[31] there was considerable morbidity and even mortality in constructing continent ileostomies.

Ileosigmoid fistula

A common occurrence with small bowel Crohn's disease is the presence of an ileosigmoid fistula. There has been some debate as to whether the sigmoid segment should be resected as opposed to performing a separation of the fistula and simple excision with closure of the fistulous site (Figures 51.19–51.21). It is generally believed that the ileum form as a fistula into the sigmoid colon and, in most cases, that the sigmoid colon does not have *de facto* involvement with Crohn's disease. This question could easily be settled with preoperative colonoscopy or intraoperative colonoscopy. If the sigmoid colon is not involved, excision of the fistulous site in the colon and simple closure is the procedure of choice.[32,33] In our own series, there was no difference in short-term complications of recurrence rate among two groups of patients who underwent either simple detachment of the fistula and oversewing of the sigmoid ($n = 26$) or combined sigmoid and ileal resection ($n = 27$). Nevertheless, if isolated Crohn's colitis appears in conjunction with an ileosigmoid fistula, a joint resection should be undertaken. Ileosigmoid and other internal fistulas in Crohn's disease are considered in detail in Chapter 49.

Ureteric obstruction

Rarely, with small intestinal Crohn's disease and abscess formation or formation of a psoas abscess, obstruction of the ureters may result in hydronephrosis. At one time, it was believed that ureterolysis should be undertaken to relieve ureteric obstruction, but there is evidence that this procedure is unnecessary[34] and that if the offending segment of bowel is resected and the

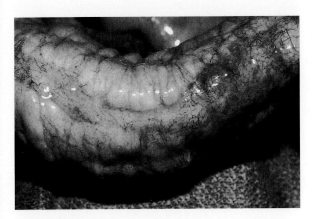

Figure 51.13
'Fat wrapping' in Crohn's disease.

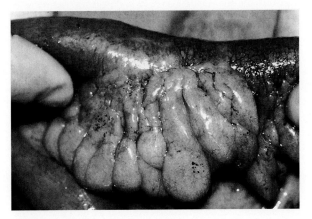

Figure 51.14
Crohn's disease stricture of small bowel.

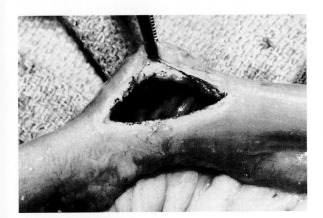

Figure 51.15
Transverse incision through stricture.

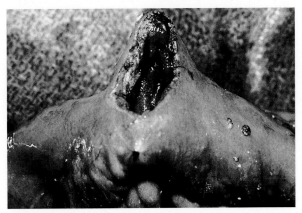

Figure 51.16
Vertical opposition for closure.

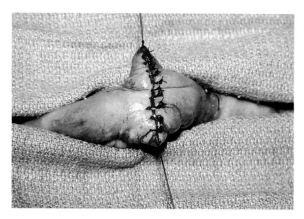

Figure 51.17
Vertical closure.

abscess adequately drained, the retroperitoneal obstruction will be relieved in time with no further manoeuvres. Complications from ureterolysis can be serious and include nephrectomy as well as ureteral fistulas and pyelonephritis.

STOMAL COMPLICATIONS

Brooke ileostomy is a frequent component of operations for Crohn's disease and is thus a frequent site of recurrence, the most distressing consequence being paraileostomy fistula (see also Chapter 56). Unfortunately, it is frequently necessary to resite the stoma in the opposite lower quadrant of the abdomen or at another abdominal site.[35] Ileostomy has also been used as a diversionary procedure for Crohn's colitis and particularly for anorectal Crohn's disease. In several series, reanastomosis of the ileum and distal colon or rectum was possible in less than one-third of patients.[36-38]

More controversy stems from the question of resection of active proximal disease in a setting of small bowel disease in conjunction with anorectal disease. In a long-term follow-up of patients with anorectal Crohn's disease,[39] resection of active proximal Crohn's disease seemed to correlate with improved anorectal disease in many cases; however, *lasting* benefit occurred fortuitously in patients who had all proximal disease removed and who did not have recurrence or recrudescence

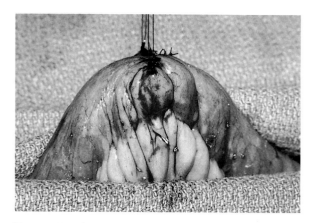

Figure 51.18
Clip placed at base of mesentery to mark site.

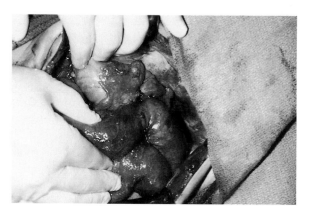

Figure 51.19
Ileosigmoid fistula with cystoenteric component.

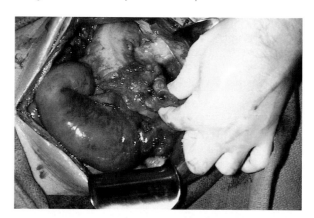

Figure 51.20
Ileosigmoid fistula – separated sigmoid colon site.

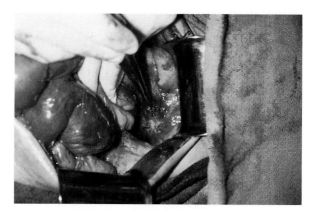

Figure 51.21
Bladder extension of cystoenteric fistula.

proximally. If recurrence became evident in the proximal bowel, in almost all cases anorectal Crohn's became active as well.

Challenging the bowel with intestinal contents often temporary ileostomy and defunctioned colonic Crohn's disease has been undertaken to predict the long-term course after reestablishment of bowel continuity. The authors found no correlation with the results of reestablishment of continuity when patients with an ileostomy were challenged with their own ileostomy contents inserted into the defunctioned colon.[40]

CROHN'S DISEASE IN CHILDHOOD

Crohn's disease in children is uncommon and carries an estimated prevalence of one case per 10 000 of the paediatric population. The most common indication for operation in the paediatric age group is failure to thrive. Unlike the adult group, initial site of disease seems to affect outcome with the best results being found in disease confined to the small bowel or to the ileocaecal region.[41] Children with proctocolectomy and ileostomy fared better than those who had staged colonic resections or diverting ileostomy. In 90% of the children, an acceleration in growth activity was observed during the first year after operation.

The same question of proximal resection in children with active perianal or anorectal disease has been studied. Most children eventually require proctocolectomy because of severe anorectal disease, despite manipulation with faecal diversion and resection of proximal active intra-abdominal disease.[42]

PREGNANCY AND CROHN'S DISEASE

The combination of pregnancy with Crohn's disease is one that is particularly difficult for patients and clinicians. In one series of 50 patients,[43] 78 pregnancies were reviewed and the results suggested that the outcome of pregnancy was not adversely affected by Crohn's disease. However, patients who had active disease at conception or had an exacerbation during the pregnancy had poor outcomes independent of the use of medication or the need for operation. Neither pregnancy nor the medications that were taken affected the course of the disease. The risk of spontaneous abortions and of complicated live births in pregnant women with Crohn's disease was similar to that seen in the general population.

GASTRODUODENAL CROHN'S DISEASE

STOMACH

Gastric Crohn's disease is very uncommon and is almost always managed medically. If perforations, bleeding or fistulas occur, local excision of the grossly involved tissue is undertaken and anastomosis at the site of excision is performed.[44] An instance of isolated Crohn's disease of the stomach has been

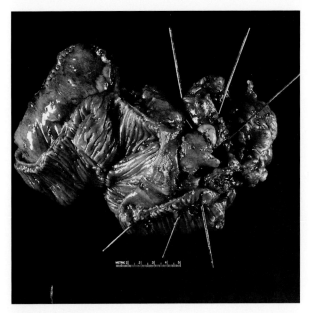

Figure 51.23
Small bowel fistulae, from the duodenum in Crohn's disease.

reported,[45] and this was treated successfully with total gastrectomy. In this situation, it is almost impossible to differentiate preoperatively Crohn's disease from gastric lymphoma or other malignancy.

Duodenum

Gastroduodenal involvement with Crohn's disease occurs in up to 4% of cases (see also Chapter 50). Duodenal Crohn's disease is generally associated with ileal Crohn's disease (Figures 51.22 and 51.23). Duodenal Crohn's disease may also mimic lymphoma and most commonly causes duodenal obstruction, but duodenal perforation may occur with fistula formation into the pancreas or into the transverse colon or small bowel. When operation is required, gastrojejunostomy rather than duodenal resection is the procedure of choice, although duodenal strictureplasty has been done in selected patients. A truncal vagotomy has been carried out in conjunction with gastrojejunostomy,[46] but since the incidence of marginal ulcer is low (less than 5%), these ulcers can usually be managed more satisfactorily with medical therapy, such as the new generation of H_2-receptor blockers.

REFERENCES

1. Whelan G, Farmer RG, Fazio VW & Goormastic M. Recurrence after surgery in Crohn's disease: relationship to location of disease (clinical pattern) and surgical indication. *Gastroenterology* 1985; **88**: 1826.
2. Farmer RG, Whelan G & Fazio VW. Long-term follow-up of patients with Crohn's disease: relationship between the clinical pattern and prognosis. *Gastroenterology* 1985; **88**: 1818.
3. Shivananda S, Hordijk ML, Pena AS & Mayberry JF. Crohn's disease: risk of recurrence and reoperation in a defined population. *Gut* 1989; **30**: 990.
4. Ekelund GW & Lindhagen T. Controversies in the surgical management of Crohn's disease. *Perspect Colon Rectal Surg* 1989; **2**: 1.
5. Agrez MV, Valente RM, Pierce W, Melton III LJ, van Heerden JA & Beart Jr RW. Surgical history of Crohn's disease in a well-defined population. *Mayo Clin Proc* 1982; **57**: 747.

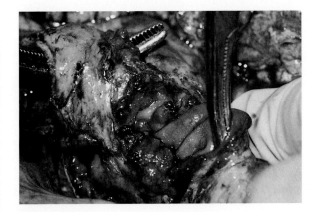

Figure 51.22
Duodenal fistulas of Crohn's disease

6. McLeod RS, Wolff BG & Steinhart AH et al. Prophylactic mesalamine treatment decreases postoperative recurrence of Crohn's disease. *Gastroenterology* 1995; **109**: 404.

7. Homan WP & Dineen P. Comparison of the results of resection, bypass, and bypass with exclusion for ileocecal Crohn's disease. *Ann Surg* 1978; **187**: 530.

8. Traube J, Simpson S, Riddell RH, Levin B & Kirsner JB. Crohn's disease and adenocarcinoma of the bowel. *Dig Dis Sci* 1980; **12**: 939.

9. Lee ECG. Limited surgery in the management of strictures in Crohn's disease. *Inflam Bowel Dis* 1985; **35**: 265.

10. Alexander-Williams JA & Fornaro M. Strictureplasty in Crohn's disease. *Chirug* 1982; **53**: 799.

11. Krause U, Ejerblad S & Bergman L. Crohn's disease: a long-term study of the clinical course in 186 patients. *Scand J Gastroenterol* 1985; **20**: 516.

12. Wolff BG, Beart Jr, RW, Frydenberg HB, Weiland LH, Agrez MV & Ilstrup DM. The importance of disease-free margins in resections for Crohn's disease. *Dis Col Rectum* 1983; **26**: 239.

13. Karesen R, Serch-Hanssen A, Thoresen BO & Hertzberg J. Crohn's disease: long-term results of surgical treatment. *Scand J Gastroenterol* 1981; **16**: 57.

14. Pennington L, Hamilton PSR, Bayless TM & Cameron JL. Surgical management of Crohn's disease: influence of disease at margin of resection. *Ann Surg* 1981; **192**: 311.

15. Heuman R, Boeryd B, Bolin T & Sjodahl R. The influence of disease at the margin of resection on the outcome of Crohn's disease. *Br J Surg* 1983; **70**: 519.

16. Adloff M, Arnaud JP & Ollier JC. Does the histologic appearance at the margin of resection affect the postoperative recurrence rate in Crohn's disease? *Am Surg* 1987; **53**: 543.

17. Post S, Betzler M, von Ditfurth B, Schurmann G, Kuppers P & Herfarth C. Risks of intestinal anastomoses in Crohn's disease. *Ann Surg* 1991; **213**: 37.

18. Williams JG, Wong WD, Rothenberger DA & Goldberg SM. Recurrence of Crohn's disease after resection. *Br J Surg* 1991; **78**: 10.

19. Wolff BG, Beart Jr, RW, Dozois RR et al. A new bowel preparation for elective colon and rectal surgery: a prospective, randomized clinical trial. *Arch Surg* 1988; **123**: 895.

20. Dehn TCB, Kettlewell MGW, Mortensen NJ et al. Ten-year experience of strictureplasty for obstructive Crohn's disease. *Br J Surg* 1989; **76**: 339.

21. Fazio VW & Galandiuk S. Strictureplasty: newer conservative surgery in Crohn's disease. *Pract Gastroenterol* 1990; **14**: 23.

22a. Spencer MP, Wolff BG: Strictureplasty: An intestine-conserving surgical option for obstructive Crohn's disease. *Probl Gen Surg, Surgical Treatment of Inflammatory Bowel Disease.* 1993; **10** : 180.

22b. Spencer MP, Nelson H. Wolff, BG, Dozois RR: Strictureplasty for obstructive Crohn's disease: *The Mayo Experience. Mayo Clinic Proceedings* 1994; **69**: 33.

23. Goligher JC. The long-term results of excisional surgery for primary and recurrent Crohn's disease of the large intestine. *Dis Colon Rectum* 1985; **28**: 51.

24. Hulten L. Surgical options in the treatment of ulcerative colitis and Crohn's colitis. *Schweiz Med Wochenschr* 1988; **118**: 745.

25. Buchmann P, Weterman IT, Keighley MB, Pena SA, Allan RN & Alexander-Williams J. The prognosis of ileorectal anastomosis in Crohn's disease. *Br J Surg* 1981; **68**: 7.

26. Farnell MB, van Heerden JA, Beart Jr RW & Weiland LH. Rectal preservation in nonspecific inflammatory disease of the colon. *Ann Surg* 1980; **192**: 249.

27. Rutgeerts P, Geboes K, van Trappen G et al. Natural history of recurrent Crohn's disease at the ileocolonic anastomosis after curative surgery. *Gut* 1984; **25**: 665.

28. Johnson GP & Wolff BG. Complications and functional outcome in patients with ileal pouch-anal anastomosis in Crohn's disease. Presented at the American Society of Colon and Rectal Surgeons Meeting, St Louis, Missouri, April 1990.

29. Hyman NH, Fazio VW, Tuxen WB & Lavery IC. Consequences of ileal pouch-anal anastomosis for Crohn's colitis. *Dis Colon Rectum* 1991; **34**: 653.

30. Bloom RJ, Larsen CP, Watt R, Oberhelman, Jr HA. A reappraisal of the Kock continent ileostomy in patients with Crohn's disease. *Surg Gynecol Obstet* 1986; **162**: 105.

31. Myrbold HE & Kock NG. Continent ileostomy in patients with Crohn's disease. *Gastroenterology* 1981; **80**: 1237.

32. Block GE & Schraut WH. The operative treatment of Crohn's enteritis complicated by ileosgimoid fistula. *Ann Surg* 1983; **196**: 356.

33. Young-Fadok TM, Wolff BG & Meagher A et al. Surgical management of ileosigmoid fistulas in Crohn's disease. *Dis Colon Rectum* 1997; **40**: 558.

34. Siminovitch JMP & Fazio VW. Ureteral obstruction secondary to Crohn's disease: a need for ureterolysis? *Am J Surg* 1980; **139**: 95.

35. Greenstein AJ, Dicker A, Meyers S & Aufses Jr AH. Periileostomy fistulae in Crohn's disease. *Ann Surg* 1983; **197**: 179.

36. McIlrath DC. Diverting ileostomy or colostomy in the management of Crohn's disease of the colon. *Arch Surg* 1971; **103**: 308.

37. Oberhelman HA. The effect of intestinal diversion by ileostomy in Crohn's disease of the colon. In Weterman It, Pena S & Booh CC (eds) *The Management of Crohn's Disease.* Amsterdam, Oxford: Excerpta Medica, 1976: 216.

38. Aufses AH & Kreel I. Ileostomy for granulomatous ileal colitis. *Ann Surg* 1971; **173**: 91.

39. Wolff BG, Culp CE, Beart Jr RW, Ilstrup DM & Ready RL. Anorectal Crohn's disease: a long-term perspective. *Dis Colon Rectum* 1985; **28**: 709.

40. Fasoli R, Kettlewell MGW, Mortensen N & Jewell DP. Response to faecal challenge in defunctioned colonic Crohn's disease: prediction of long-term course. *Br J Surg* 1990; **77**: 616.

41. Davies G, Evans CM, Shand WS & Walker-Smith JA. Surgery for Crohn's disease in childhood: influence of site of disease and operative procedure on outcome. *Br J Surg* 1990; **77**: 891.

42. Orkin BA & Telander RL. The effect of intra-abdominal resection or fecal diversion on perianal disease in pediatric Crohn's disease. *J Pediatr Surg* 1985; **20**: 343.

43. Woolfson K, Cohen Z & McLeod RS. Crohn's disease and pregnancy. *Dis Colon Rectum* 1990; **33**: 869.

44. Lee KKW & Schraut WH. Diagnosis and treatment of duodenoenteric fistulas complicating Crohn's disease. *Arch Surg* 1989; **124**: 712.

45. Cary ER, Tremaine WJ, Banks PM & Nagorney DM. Isolated Crohn's disease of the stomach. *Mayo Clin Proc* 1989; **64**: 776.

46. Murray JJ, Schoetz Jr DJ, Nugent FW, Coller JA & Veidenheimer MC. Surgical management of Crohn's disease involving the duodenum. *Am J Surg* 1984; **147**: 58.

52

RADIATION ENTERITIS AND OTHER INFLAMMATORY CONDITIONS

J Spencer

RADIATION ENTEROPATHY

The discovery by Roentgen in 1895 of a 'new kind of ray' introduced therapeutic as well as diagnostic possibilities. Within 2 years the acute gastrointestinal effects of abdominopelvic radiotherapy had been reported, under the name of 'deep tissue traumatism'.[1] Before the end of World War I, Futh and Ebeler[2] had already reported patients with radiation-induced strictures and fistulas. Today, about a half of all patients with malignant disease undergo some form of radiotherapy, and many of these can reasonably hope for cure. Unfortunately, radiation-induced damage to the gut may lead to disability and death long after the original disease has been controlled.

Incidence

The incidence of radiation enteropathy is difficult to assess. If all gastrointestinal symptoms are considered, then it may be as high as 50–75%.[3] In most patients such symptoms will be transient. Early series describe the incidence of those going on to operation as 2–17%.[4,5] The incidence of 'surgical disease' appears to be increasing. In a London Hospital series the overall incidence of all bowel complications rose over a 20-year period from 4.9 to 7.5%.[6] At Hammersmith Hospital in London, of nearly 80 patients presenting with 'surgical' complications between 1958 and 1988, well over half presented in the third decade.[7] This apparent rise in incidence partly reflects changes in radiotherapy practice, and partly the chronic nature of the induced bowel disease, with surgical referral sometimes being made very late in the history of the disease. Intracavitary radiation has been shown to be particularly damaging, and combined internal and external therapy even more so. In the London Hospital series,[6] patients treated for cervical cancer were more at risk than those with endometrial malignancy, but this difference reflected a later presentation of disease, which more often necessitated combined radiation.

Less severe enteropathy, not needing surgical intervention, is much more common than is often realized. After the common acute symptoms of adbominopelvic radiation such as nausea and diarrhoea have settled, patients may be asymptomatic. Studies of 17 such asymptomatic patients attending a follow-up radiotherapy clinic revealed that 16 had evidence of malabsorption on ^{14}C breath testing.[8] Similarly, in a series of patients who had undergone radiotherapy for bladder tumours, eight of 14 had abnormal Schilling tests, indicating deficient ileal function.[9]

Gut tolerance to radiotherapy

Radiation therapy relies on a damaging effect that differentiates between malignant and normal tissue. This differentiation is of course incomplete, so it is not possible to avoid damage to adjacent organs when destroying a tumour. How much damage occurs depends on a number of factors, one of which is the tolerance of the particular tissue.

Doses of radiation producing damage in up to 5% or 50% within 5 years are termed $TD_{5/5}$ and $TD_{50/5}$, respectively. The ranges for different parts of the gut are shown in Table 52.1. It will be noted that these doses are very close to the therapeutic doses required to control common tumours. For example, average doses used in the treatment of cervical or endometrial cancer are between 4000 and 8000 cGy. The higher the dose used, the greater the risk of damage.

Table 52.1 Tolerance of normal gut tissue to radiotherapy

TISSUE	$TD_{5/5}$ (cGy)	$TD_{50/5}$ (cGy)
Oesophagus	6000	7500
Stomach	4500	5000
Small bowel	4500	6500
Colon	4500	6500
Rectum	5500	8000

$TD_{5/5}$ and $TD_{50/5}$ are explained in the text.

Pathophysiology

Ionizing radiation affects the gut in two principal ways. There is a direct effect, and then an indirect effect due to progressive obliterative vasculitis. The direct or acute effects of radiation consist mainly of the depletion of actively proliferating cells in what was previously a stable cell-renewal system. Within hours of a therapeutic dose of radiation histological changes can be detected. In the small bowel mucosa cell, mitoses are reduced and villi are shortened, reducing absorptive area. Over the next 2–4 weeks a cellular infiltrate, principally of leucocytes, is seen, with the formation of crypt abscesses. Within 6 months complete histological recovery may occur. During this acute phase malabsorption may be demonstrated for bile salts, fat, carbohydrates, protein and vitamin B_{12}.

The late sequelae of radiation enteritis are macroscopically apparent as thickened gut with areas of telangiectasia. Mucosal ulceration may occur, and indeed it can progress to extend through the gut wall. This process may lead to perforation, fistulas or local abscesses, while resolution may result in fibrous strictures. In such strictures there is always an element of inflammatory oedema, the state of which may determine clinical patency. Microscopic features of late damage include obliterative enteritis, submucosal fibrosis and oedema, lymphatic ectasia and abnormal, stellate fibroblasts. Studies of the microvasculature of resected gut have demonstrated reduced and abnormal vessels in irradiated bowel, with some avascular areas corresponding to areas of infarction.[10]

Predisposing factors

In many patients no predisposing factors can be identified, but such factors do exist. The following are among the most important.

Excessive radiotherapy This was clearly very important in the early days of therapy, and may still be important when treating large or recurrent tumours.

Combined chemotherapy It can be shown that chemotherapeutic agents enhance the effects of radiotherapy. Unfortunately this fact applies to normal as well as malignant tissue. This effect has been demonstrated with many drugs, including actinomycin D, 5-fluorouracil, methotrexate and doxorubicin (Adriamycin).[11,12]

Physical build Thin patients, women and the elderly all carry more small intestine in the pelvis.[13] This distribution increases the risks to the gut of pelvic radiotherapy.

Previous abdominopelvic surgery There is good evidence to suggest that previous operations predispose to radiation enteropathy. In one study[14] patients who had suffered radiation damage to the gut were compared with a well-matched group who had not. Previous operations had occurred significantly more often in those with damaged gut. The mechanism usually assumed is that postoperative adhesions reduce the mobility of gut, thus exposing the same segments of intestine to excessive radiation. Such fixity was confirmed by Green,[15] who found in a radiological study that gut was more likely to be relatively or completely immobile after previous operations. However, the mobility of gut filled with heavy contrast medium may not reflect its motility in everyday life.

Vascular occlusion As radiation produces its effects by causing a vasculitis, it might be expected that predisposing vascular disease would exaggerate this process. A significant association between the presence of hypertension, diabetes or cardiovascular disease at the time of radiotherapy and subsequent injury was found by DeCosse et al.[16]

Prevention

Radiation damage is more likely to occur if a large volume of small bowel is irradiated. Fixation in the pelvis due to previous adhesions adds to the risk, likewise the physical build (see above). It has been shown that treatment in the prone position, with a head-down tilt, and with a full bladder, reduces the volume of gut irradiated. Such manoeuvres appear to reduce the incidence of acute radiation enteritis.[17] Modifying the fractionation of treatment may also benefit the bowel.[18]

Various mechanical devices have been used to reduce risk, such as the insertion of a polyglycolic acid mesh sling to hold the small bowel out of the pelvis during therapy.[19,20] Filling the pelvis with omentum may also have a similar protective effect. No such methods have been evaluated by controlled trials, and they are not widely used.

There is some evidence that the use of elemental diets during abdominal radiotherapy reduces bowel damage. This phenomenon may be the result of a reduction in bowel volume, an indirect effect related to the reduction of pancreatic enzymes or bile salts, or the result of the demonstrable improvement in nitrogen balance, or any combination of these or other factors. Such diets are unpalatable and expensive and are not used routinely. Total parenteral nutrition is useful in the management of established radiation bowel disease, and may have a preventive role during therapy. This possibility has not been studied carefully.

Non-steroidal anti-inflammatory drugs (NSAIDs) might theoretically help to alleviate or prevent gut damage, as circulating prostaglandins rise during therapy.[21] However, results of their use have not been encouraging. Similarly, steroids have not been definitely shown to be clinically effective in prophylaxis. In experimental dog studies the *Ascaris lumbricoides* body wall protease inhibitor protected jejunal loops during radiotherapy.[22] No clinical studies of the use of this inhibitor have been reported.

Natural history

Acute effects

Most patients experience gut symptoms during a course of abdominal radiotherapy. These symptoms consist of diarrhoea, nausea, vomiting or pain. Within a few weeks the symptoms have settled, usually never to return. Absence of symptoms during this acute phase is no guarantee of long-term freedom, but there is some evidence that the worst acute reactions are associated with an increased risk of later complications.[23]

Subclinical effects

Chronic damage may develop without the occurrence of symptoms. In one study 17 patients were studied in a radiotherapy clinic, none of whom had any complaints. However, 12 had an altered bowel habit, and 16 had evidence of malabsorption.[8] In another study of patients undergoing radiotherapy for bladder cancer, malabsorption of B_{12} indicated ileal damage, such as that illustrated in Figure 52.1.[9] One surgical implication is that subsequent removal of small bowel may have a much greater than expected effect on absorption. What is more, damaged bowel may perforate after unrelated operations, even when it appears macroscopically normal and the patient is previously asymptomatic.[24]

Late effects

The latent period between a course of radiation therapy and the development of bowel damage is usually between 6 months and 2 years. It can, however, be more protracted, even as long as 30 years. The diagnosis of radiation enteritis must always be considered whenever previous radiotherapy has been given. It is often overlooked or misdiagnosed as recurrent malignancy.

Malabsorption is common, but may be subclinical. The most common clinical problem is proctosigmoiditis; in one series nearly three-quarters of the patients presented in this way.[25] The degree of disability varies: in some cases mild symptoms may persist for years without progression; in others, bowel disturbance might be severe, and haemorrhage demands transfusion. When bleeding occurs, spontaneous remission is very unlikely and most patients eventually need surgical treatment.[26]

Radiation enteritis is a progressive disease. If the disease is severe enough to necessitate surgical treatment, on subsequent follow-up most patients will have further problems. These may consist of complications directly related to surgical operations, persistence of original symptoms, new radiation-related disease,

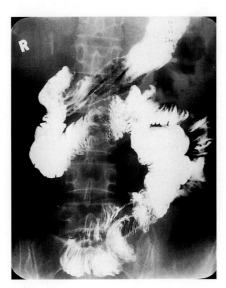

Figure 52.1
Radiograph of a patient who had undergone radiotherapy for cervical carcinoma. The small bowel mucosa shows oedema, and there is dilatation above ileal strictures.

or any combination of these events.[27] If a diversion colostomy is performed in rectal disease, rectal bleeding may persist. Bypass of small bowel or ileocaecal disease may be followed by progression of disease in the excluded bowel, with fistula formation. The vasculitis induced by radiation may continue to progress, causing new lesions after successful initial treatment.

Investigation

In any patient who has previously undergone abdominal radiotherapy, gut symptoms should raise suspicions of radiation damage. The major differential diagnosis, in the early years after radiation, is residual or recurrent malignancy.

Acute disease involving the rectum may mimic ulcerative colitis very closely. Sigmoidoscopy is important, but it must be performed with extreme care. Computed tomography (CT), done for example to search for recurrent tumours, may show oedema of the bowel wall.[28]

In chronic disease malabsorption may be an important feature. The haemoglobin, red cell indices, transferrin, folate, calcium, albumin and prothrombin time are important clues to the nutritional status. Faecal fats will indicate the degree of steatorrhoea. Use of the $[1\text{-}^{14}C]$cholylglycine breath test may indicate bile salt malabsorption[8] and a Schilling test assesses B_{12} absorption. Other assessments may be made of bacterial overgrowth when obstructive lesions are present.

The small bowel enema is most helpful in assessing enteric damage, and a double-contrast barium enema is essential for colonic disease. In the small bowel, differentiation from other inflammatory bowel disease is not always possible, and the extent of disease cannot be reliably noted. However, characteristic features are thickened valvulae conniventes, stenosis, mural thickening, adhesions, effacement of mucosal pattern, ulceration and evidence of sinuses and fistulas. These features have been reviewed by Mendelson and Nolan.[29]

Visceral arteriography is not commonly performed, but it may show arterial stenosis at injury sites, the lesions themselves being avascular.[30] This fact is of interest in view of the obliterative arteritis known to be the key pathological feature.

Technetium-99m leucocyte scans have demonstrated gut involvement, with changes similar to those seen in other inflammatory bowel disease,[31] and may indicate involvement beyond what is macroscopically noticeable. However, no investigation denotes accurately the extent of disease, which cannot be assessed thoroughly even at laparotomy. It must also always be borne in mind that both small and large bowel will be affected in most patients, although the more severe lesions may seem well localized.

Complications

The major complications of radiation enteropathy are perforation, haemorrhage, fistula and stricture. Figure 52.2[32] illustrates the latent period seen in a series of patients between radiotherapy and the presentation of various complications. It can be seen that perforation and haemorrhage tend to occur relatively early in the disease, being manifestations of acute inflammation. Fistulas and particularly strictures, which occur later, are

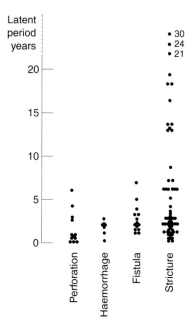

Figure 52.2
Time of presentation of various radiation-induced lesions. Data from the Hammersmith series.[39]

the result of a progressive obliterative endarteritis. There is a tendency for complications to occur earlier in the large bowel than in the small bowel.

Perforation

Perforation of either the large bowel (usually the sigmoid colon) or the small bowel (usually the ileum) may occur early after, or even during, therapy. In the first 6 months, perforation usually occurs as an apparently isolated lesion, presumably the result of direct trauma to a specific area of gut wall. Another group of patients present later, in whom the perforation is in dilated diseased gut proximal to a radiation-induced stricture. Another situation arises in patients who have never had symptoms of radiation enteritis, but who develop apparently spontaneous fistulas from the small bowel after operations performed for other pathology.[24] The possibility of the latter type of lesion emphasizes the potential fragility of irradiated gut. Even adhesiolysis may jeopardize the blood supply in such bowel.[34]

Perforation may lead to a generalized peritonitis, or be locally contained by adhesions, giving rise to an abscess. Such abscesses may later rupture to produce a fistula.

Haemorrhage

Bleeding usually occurs in the first few months or years after therapy, but once it occurs it can become a chronic problem. The bleeding is almost always from the rectum and sigmoid colon, arising from a proctosigmoiditis, often with ulceration. As there is an underlying gut ischaemia, healing does not readily occur. The persistent bloody discharge, sometimes with intermittent brisker bleeding, gives rise to intolerable symptoms with anaemia and secondary debility. Surgical diversion of the bowel contents reduces but does not eliminate symptoms, and more radical surgery is often required.

Bleeding from the small bowel is not common; occult blood will not uncommonly be present, but brisk episodes of haemorrhage occur much more rarely.

Fistulas

Fistulas represent a severe form of radiation disease. Synchronous lesions (including other fistulas) are common[35] and the prognosis of people presenting with fistulas is poor.[26]

Conservative treatment results in the healing of over 60% of other gastrointestinal fistulas, but it is rarely successful in radiation disease. Most fistulas involve the ileum or rectosigmoid, and the bladder and vagina are commonly involved. They are very often associated with more distal stricture formation.

The site of fistula formation indicates the high dose of radiation received during therapy for gynaecological or bladder malignancy. It is particularly difficult in such patients to exclude recurrent malignancy. Malnutrition may be a considerable problem in patients with fistulas. Synchronous urinary tract problems, such as ascending infection secondary to fistulation, often occur. When fistulas are multiple there may also be sinuses into localized peritoneal abscesses, with associated sepsis and malaise.

Strictures

Strictures may occur very early in the disease, but the tendency to fibrosis and luminal obstruction persists. Thus strictures may form very late, in some cases as long as 30 years after therapy. In late presentations it is crucial that the previous radiation therapy is not forgotten; to misdiagnose radiation enteritis is to court surgical disaster.

Partially obstructing strictures may give rise to bacterial overgrowth and malabsorption syndromes. Symptoms of recurrent subacute obstruction may occur. Strictures are often multiple, and stasis in segmented small bowel may occasionally give rise to enterolith formation (Figure 52.3, see colour plate also). Dilated, diseased and fistulated bowel above a stricture commonly perforates or fistulates, as described earlier.

As with other lesions, small bowel strictures occur most often in the ileum. The rectosigmoid may also become strictured, complicating the treatment of small bowel disease.

All enteric strictures have elements of spasm and oedema as well as fibrosis, which probably explains the intermittent nature of the initial symptoms. With time, however, fibrous stenosis leads to clinical obstruction.

Malignancy

Ionizing radiation is carcinogenic; recognition of this fact led to the abandoning of radiotherapy for benign disease many years ago. Theoretically, therefore, bowel damaged by radiation might be at an increased risk of malignancy.

Some 20 cases of squamous oesophageal cancer have been attributed to radiation.[36] The writer performed a splenectomy on a 20-year-old female with Hodgkin's lymphoma, who subsequently received mediastinal radiotherapy. Ten years later she presented with a squamous oesophageal carcinoma, which was treated successfully by oesophagectomy.[37]

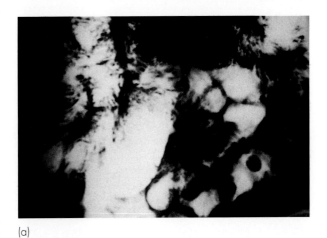

(a)

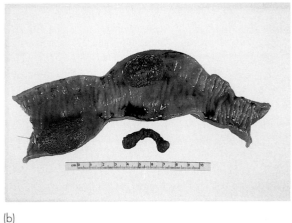

(b)

Figure 52.3

(a) Radiograph indicating the presence of enteroliths in ileum affected by radiation. (b) In the opened resection specimen the causative strictures are clearly seen.

The colorectum is clearly at risk of radiation-induced cancer, but this risk appears to be small. Some series would suggest that there is no increased risk. Ingelmann-Sundberg[38] studied 3392 patients with cervical cancer and found no excess incidence of colorectal cancer. A larger study of 7127 women (of whom 5997 received radiotherapy) revealed a relative risk of developing second primary cancers of 1.4, the excess incidence occurring after 15 years.[39]

The Committee on the Biological Effects of Ionizing Radiation (BEIR)[40] estimated the radiation-induced colonic cancer risk at between 0.1 and 1.7 additional cases per year for each million persons exposed to 1 cGy at the colon. Based on this estimate assuming (rather conservatively) a radiation dose of 30 Gy for women irradiated for gynaecological tumours, Sandler and Sandler[41] concluded that the 'second cancer' risk lay between 1.4 and 8.3 times that in the normal population. Their calculations assumed treatment between the ages of 40 and 50 years and a 20–30-year follow-up.

Radiation-induced bowel cancer is thus uncommon, but it does occur. Mucin abnormalities of a type found in association with malignancy have been observed in irradiated colon.[42] It appears that the risk is principally in the rectum rather than the colon, which makes screening by sigmoidoscopy at least a theoretical option. Screening should certainly be borne in mind when 10 years have elapsed since therapy, particularly in patients who develop bowel symptoms. However, induction of small bowel tumours by previous radiotherapy does not seem to be a problem.

Conservative treatment

Radiation-induced bowel damage should always be treated conservatively if at all possible. Operations should be reserved for complications or genuine failure of medical treatment. In each patient an individual treatment plan must be made, and co-operation between physician and surgeon may be of great importance in formulating this plan.

Medical management is determined by the pathological and clinical features outlined above. In *acute radiation enteritis* the aim is to tide patients over what is in most cases a transient problem. Treatment is largely symptomatic, with antiemetic and antidiarrhoeal agents as appropriate. There may also be a case for using NSAIDs, which help to alleviate both nausea and diarrhoea.[43] Elemental diets have been used during therapy, but routine use could not be seriously entertained. Such diets should be considered if the acute phase becomes intense.[44]

In *chronic radiation enteritis* symptoms and signs are more diverse and depend on the site and nature of the underlying pathology. It is a mistake to oversimplify in this disease, which is almost always more extensive than is apparent and usually affects both small and large bowel. Some problems, such as malabsorption, may need prolonged treatment. Others, such as pain, may be more variable. *Any* sudden changes need careful assessment; perforation in particular can occur suddenly and lead to localized or generalized sepsis.

There are three main aspects to be considered in conservative management; they are best described in turn, although together they comprise overall treatment.

Management of metabolic sequelae

Ileal involvement leads to malabsorption of both bile salts and vitamin B_{12}. The former can give rise to fat malabsorption if severe, but smaller losses of bile salts into the colon can produce a cholereic diarrhoea.

If steatorrhoea occurs, then vitamin D and calcium deficiency may result. Osteomalacia and even tetany have been described in radiation enteritis on this basis.[45] Vitamin K deficiency may lead to bruising, and vitamin E deficiency has been known to cause a peripheral neuropathy. Increased colonic oxalate absorption may lead to hyperoxaluria, but adequate fluids should compensate for this. Vitamin A deficiency sufficiently severe to cause night blindness has been seen. One such patient seen by the author was an amateur astronomer, who noticed a visual deficiency which was later attributed to a low Vitamin A.

Steatorrhoea will normally respond to a low-fat diet, supplemented with medium-chain triglycerides. Cholereic diarrhoea can be treated with cholestyramine, although compliance is often a problem.

Vitamin B$_{12}$ malabsorption may result directly from ileal malabsorption, or indirectly as the result of bacterial overgrowth. A Schilling test, before and after antibiotics, helps to distinguish these causes and indicates appropriate treatment. If B$_{12}$ is deficient a megaloblastic anaemia may result, and even subacute combined degeneration of the cord has been seen in radiation enteritis.[46] Vitamin B$_{12}$ stores can easily be replenished and maintained by injection.

Management of functional problems

Intermittent subacute small bowel obstruction is always treated conservatively in the first instance. Intravenous fluids and nasogastric aspiration may be sufficient. In the long term most patients with obstruction come to laparotomy, and this fact has been used as an argument for early operation. It is of great importance that out-of-hours operations by inexperienced surgeons are avoided at all costs. Adequate preparation is essential, and no operation for this disease should be undertaken lightly. Conservative treatment should not be unnecessarily prolonged, however, particularly as about two-thirds of patients will eventually need a laparotomy.[47] 'Pseudo-obstruction' may sometimes occur, presumably a motility disorder due to a radiation myopathy.[48]

If strictures do not warrant resection, then clearly the avoidance of high-residue foods may be important. The metabolic effects of stricture formation have been discussed above. In extreme cases of 'short bowel syndrome' fluid and electrolyte problems may also occur, compounded by large bowel abnormalities or previous resections. Oral or even long-term intravenous therapy may be required.

Management of inflammation

Experience of the treatment of other inflammatory bowel disease has led inevitably to the trial of anti-inflammatory drugs in radiation enterocolitis. An early report of the use of sulphasalazine and prednisone was very encouraging,[49] as have been several subsequent studies. For example Morgenstern et al.[34] reported improvement in both diarrhoea and malabsorption. No controlled studies have confirmed efficacy in this complicated and variable disease.

Surgical management

General principles

It has already been emphasized that surgical treatment is never undertaken lightly in this disease. Indications must be strong, preparation and timing considered very seriously, and risks balanced against possible gains. Persistent tumour should, as far as possible, be excluded.

It is important that the patient understands potential risks and can co-operate in care. In rectosigmoid disease, patients who can cope well with an existing stoma should be encouraged as far as possible to live with it, rather than proceed to further operation. However, in each case all these factors must be judged carefully. Even in the presence of obstruction, unplanned emergency operations by inexperienced staff should be avoided if at all possible.

As most lesions result from pelvic radiotherapy, radiation damage affects principally (and often solely) the ileum. The exact extent, however, cannot be accurately determined. If radiotherapy has been for non-pelvic disease, other parts of the bowel may be affected. For example duodenal disease has followed radiation for hypernephroma, and occasionally the small bowel can be diffusely affected.

If operative treatment is indicated, preoperative care must be taken to optimize fluid and electrolyte balance, nutrition and haemoglobin level. At operation, the basic underlying lesion must be remembered as dictating action. That is to say, obliterative endarteritis must be assumed to exist in all visible lesions and to extend well beyond these, as this will affect healing. It has been shown for example that skin flaps raised in a pig and sutured back into position remain viable for 6 weeks after irradiation, but from then on their viability falls off rapidly;[50] small vessel loss is the reason for this phenomenon. Clinical experience early after radiotherapy generally supports this; later after therapy the vascular changes, although invisible, are well established. Collateral blood supply is sometimes dependent on adhesions.

Based on these observations, if extensive adhesions are found at laparotomy, it is best to avoid complete adhesiolysis, which may promote subsequent fistula formation. Tissues must be handled gently, and unnecessary clamping or use of tissue forceps on the bowel should be avoided.

Resection

Because of the difficulty in assessing the extent of the disease, wide resection is often recommended. Such advice begs the question: 'How wide is wide?' The suggestion that at least 50 cm of gut should be removed[51] cannot be universally applicable, given the patchy distribution of partially invisible disease. It is extremely likely that anastomosing two diseased ends together will lead to leakage, with fistula or sepsis and death. Resection and primary anastomosis carries a reported high risk of 31–45% leakage, and 2–9% death.[16,33,52,53]

Fortunately, these risks can largely be averted by application of a simple principle. If for one 'end' at least of the anastomosis, gut is derived from outside the radiation field, then the risk of anastomotic problems is minimal. As the disease is mainly ileal, this principle can be achieved by a resection that removes ileum together with ascending colon; an ileotransverse anastomosis is then performed, utilizing the hepatic flexure. In the case of pelvic radiotherapy, this flexure is well protected from irradiation. Such an anastomosis will heal safely, even if the ileal component has some measure of disease. Although we are not concerned here with large bowel disease, it is of interest to note that the same principle can be applied to rectosigmoid disease, in which the splenic flexure can be brought down to be anastomosed with the rectum with a high likelihood of success. Good results have been reported in two series using this technique[32,54], which is illustrated in

Figure 52.4. Such a method may be less applicable if there has been any previous small bowel resection, or if the disease is diffuse.

In the rare situation of proximal jejunal disease, or the (unfortunately) more common situation of diffuse small bowel enteritis, then localized resections may be unavoidable. Great care must be taken with anastomosis in such cases. The writer has used stapling techniques with success in these circumstances, closing the ends of the bowel and performing a side-to-side enteroenterostomy. There are no data to show whether this technique is advantageous; it certainly works in a difficult situation, and in a limited series fistulation has been avoided.

Bypass

Bypass or exclusion procedures should be avoided if at all possible. A study by Swan et al.[55] in 1976 compared retrospectively the results of bypass operations and those of resection with primary anastomosis. Better results were found with bypass, and these authors confirmed the good results by utilizing bypass in their own patients. Unfortunately, the initial good results of bypass are not maintained, as disease often progresses in the excluded gut, giving rise to perforation, fistula or bleeding. Thus Smith et al.[56] found that 22% of 54 patients developed fistula or necrosis of bypassed bowel. In the author's experience, in seven of 22 patients problems arose in the excluded gut. What is more, exclusion has not improved the results of primary anastomosis. Bypass should therefore be a last-resort procedure, used only in the presence of extensive or irresectable disease.

Stomas

Radiation bowel disease adds to the risks of stoma surgery. Colostomies raised in the vicinity of radiated bowel often need refashioning because of retraction, stenosis or gangrene. Similar risks are incurred if an ileostomy is prepared during the manage-

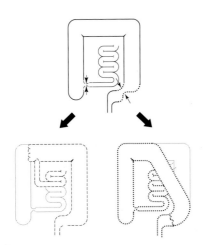

Figure 52.4
Diagram illustrating preferred anastomosis in radiation enteritis. The principle involves the use of unirradiated bowel for one 'end' of the anastomosis. The hepatic and splenic flexures of the colon can be used for ileal and rectosigmoid resections respectively (see text).

ment of colorectal radiation disease, as the ileum is commonly affected. This fact can seriously complicate the management of combined small bowel and large bowel disease.

Adhesions

It should perhaps be stressed once again that complete adhesiolysis may be disadvantageous at laparotomy for this disease. Sufficient dissection must be carried out to ensure that important pathology is not overlooked, such as a stricture buried under adhesions. Where to draw the line may be difficult because adhesiolysis is believed to precipitate necrosis and subsequent perforation.

Incisions

It is often advised that laparotomy incisions should as far as possible avoid heavily irradiated skin to minimize problems with healing. In practice this does not seem to be a serious problem, probably because modern therapy spreads the radiation load between several areas of skin. In the author's experience, even after fast-neutron therapy, which has caused many problems due to late necrosis of tissues, laparotomy wounds in the radiation field have healed satisfactorily[57].

Fistulas

As mentioned earlier, fistulas from irradiated small bowel do not heal on conservative treatment. As they are most often distal rather than proximal, fluid losses and electrolyte problems, although important, can usually be managed without great difficulty.

Because of failure to heal, enterocutaneous fistulas are best resected.[58] Similarly, ileovaginal fistulas, which cause considerable distress, are treated by resection. However, they are often accompanied by severe rectosigmoid disease, and complex fistulas may involve both large and small intestine. In such cases the diseased small bowel should be resected using the principles outlined earlier, and a diverting colostomy performed as the first stage of treating the rectal disease.

Summary

Radiation enteritis is a common sequel of abdominal and pelvic radiotherapy. It is often asymptomatic, and usually mild and transient.

In its more severe form it is a dangerous and progressive disease. Conservative treatment should be employed as far as possible, with surgical treatment being used as a last resort. Operations, when necessary, must be carefully planned and executed. Emergency procedures should be avoided, or when necessary carried out by experienced staff. Where possible, resections should be planned to avoid anastomosis between two involved segments of intestine.

ACUTE INFECTIONS
Staphylococcal enteritis

Staphylococcus aureus was once considered to be responsible for most cases of antibiotic-associated colitis. Early data on this association are now considered unreliable, and it is no longer believed that the organism has any important role in this condition.[59]

Staph. aureus is an important cause of diarrhoea associated with food poisoning, being (along with *Clostridium perfringens* and *Bacillus cereus*) an organism that can form enterotoxins in contaminated food. These bacteria give rise to acute diarrhoea which is usually short-lived, rarely lasting more than 48 hours.[60]

The symptom complex is that of 'gastroenteritis', namely anorexia, malaise, nausea, vomiting, abdominal cramps and sudden-onset diarrhoea. The episode usually occurs in a group context, several patients having consumed the same contaminated food.

The only clinical problem is to guard against dehydration, but the self-limiting disease rarely needs intensive investigation or therapy, and surgical complications do not occur.

Coliforms

Acute diarrhoea may be caused by enteropathic foms of *Escherichia coli*. It was recognized relatively recently that *E. coli* is one of the common causes of 'traveller's diarrhoea', this discovery following on the development of appropriate methods of toxin detection.[61] Enterotoxic *E. coli* (ETEC) produce both heat-labile and heat-stable toxins, both of which greatly increase fluid secretion from enterocytes without damaging the mucosa. A third group of cytopathic toxins is also recognized.

Other forms of *E. coli* are enteroinvasive (EIEC) or enteropathogenic (EPEC). The former produce mucosal damage, mainly in the colon, and give rise to acute bloody diarrhoea. The second cause diarrhoea, usually in children, by inducing secretion of fluid by a means still not fully defined.

Clinically, *E. coli* produces watery diarrhoea lasting from 1 to 5 days, often accompanied by nausea, vomiting and colicky pain. A mild fever and headache may be present. Spontaneous recovery occurs, although in the case of traveller's diarrhoea infection with more than one agent is always possible and may alter the clinical course appreciably. Occasionally protracted diarrhoea may follow the acute illness, associated with bacterial colonization of the upper small bowel. Stool investigations aid in diagnosis, but the more sophisticated studies used for the detection of coliform toxins are not usually necessary in so self-limiting a disease.

Treatment is supportive, early use of oral rehydration therapy is wise and antidiarrhoeal agents may be helpful. Antibiotics should seldom be used. Surgical complications do not occur.

Salmonella

Enteric fever is caused by the organism *Salmonella typhi* and is endemic in most tropical countries. Spread is by the orofaecal (or faeco-oral) route, and after ingestion the organism colonizes the ileum, involving the Peyer's patches in particular. There is an early bacteraemia which exposes most organs to salmonella, but the gut infection predominates.

The fever may be accompanied by headaches, joint pains, weakness, cough, rash and abdominal pain. Leucopenia is characteristic. Clinical manifestations of salmonella infection are protean and include a pyrexia (PUO), meningitis, abdominal signs suggesting appendicitis, acute gastrintestinal haemorrhage, bowel perforation, orchitis, arthropathy or osteomyelitis.

Most typically, fever and diarrhoea with green 'pea-soup' stools are accompanied by abdominal pain. Perforation is very common, occurring in up to 20% of cases, and is a common cause of death. It tends to occur in the third week of the disease, but may occur during the early septicaemic phase.

Acute salmonella cholecystitis may occur or, after the acute illness has settled, the gall bladder may remain chronically infected, giving rise to the carrier state with constant excretion of organisms in the stools.

Diagnosis is initially clinical, and treatment in most cases must not await laboratory confirmation. Leucopenia is a useful supportive early finding. Stool culture is the essential confirmatory step.

Treatment is supportive, with adequate and appropriate fluids, and with the use of antibiotics, especially chloramphenicol. When perforation occurs, meteorism may be a striking feature. A case has been argued for the conservative management of perforation, but this policy was based on data obtained in a rural epidemic in Africa when large numbers of patients were treated with inadequate facilities. It was shown that conservative treatment, including the use of intraperitoneal fluid infusions, could improve survival.[62] Given the improved facilities available in most parts of the world today, it is generally agreed that perforation should be treated by operation. Even then the mortality rate is high – up to 15%. Simple suture of perforations is recommended. A striking feature at laparotomy is the absence of any sealing of perforations by omentum.

Because of the underlying pathology, perforations are almost always in the terminal ileum; they are often multiple.

Campylobacter

It is only in the last 20 years that infection with *Campylobacter* species has been recognized as an important cause of acute diarrhoea in both children and adults. *C. fetus* (subsp. *jejuni* and *intestinalis*) is a Gram-negative microaerophilic spiral organism with a polar flagellum. Infections are more prevalent in the summer. The organisms may be acquired from chicken that has been badly prepared, from dogs with diarrhoea, from unpasteurized milk or from water. Epidemics may arise from these sources. Small and large bowel are involved, with marked ileitis being seen at laparotomy. Sigmoidoscopy may reveal appearances mimicking ulcerative colitis.

Campylobacter gastroenteritis usually presents as a self-limiting mild episode of diarrhoea lasting 2–10 (usually 3–5) days. A mild fever with malaise, myalgia and headache may precede the diarrhoea, and colicky abdominal pain may be a feature. Vomiting is uncommon. Rarely, haemorrhage occurs from the ileum, which may be severe. Extraintestinal features occasionally occur: septicaemia with meningitis, pneumonia or endocarditis and reactive arthropathy. Endocarditis in this condition carries a high mortality note, which has been attributed to inappropriate antibiotic therapy.[63]

Therapy in most cases is supportive. Antibiotic treatment, usually with erythromycin, is rapidly effective but is not routinely necessary or advisable. Central nervous system infections should be treated with chloramphenicol. Except in rare instances of prolonged haemorrhage there is no need for surgical treatment. Appendicectomy is often performed because of a mistaken diagnosis, and is uneventful.

Cholera

This infectious disease is caused by colonization of the small bowel by *Vibrio cholerae*. Classically it takes the form of severe watery diarrhoea. It is endemic in the tropics. Serious epidemics occur, with high mortality rates.

The cholera vibrio is a small Gram-negative organism with terminal flagellae. Usually ingested in infected water, organisms enter the small bowel, penetrate its mucous lining and adhere to the brush border of the mucosa. Vibrios produce an enterotoxin which stimulates active secretion of chloride and bicarbonate ions and inhibits sodium chloride absorption; this process results in a severe diarrhoea, with volumes that may exceed 1 litre per hour. The enterotoxin consists of several subunits, one of which binds irreversibly to adenylate cyclase in the basolateral membrane of the enterocyte in a manner that leaves it in a continuously active state. In addition, protein kinases cause conformational changes in proteins associated with the chloride channel (second-messenger secretion coupling). The net result is a massive secretion of sodium, chloride and water.[64] Hypovolaemic shock may ensue with metabolic acidosis, often proceeding to renal failure in the absence of treatment. The diarrhoea is usually painless. Death (if it occurs) is due to metabolic disturbance; 'surgical' complications are not a feature of this disease.

Treatment consists of replacing lost fluid intravenously, oral rehydration therapy and antibiotics. Tetracycline is the antibiotic of choice. The widespread introduction of oral rehydration therapy has had a profound effect in reducing the mortality rate in cholera epidemics. It is based on the recognition that sodium and glucose absorption are linked. Simple and cheaply produced preparations can be made available in epidemic situations, although in the very sick intravenous rehydration is also necessary.

Improvements in sanitation and hygiene to prevent cholera are crucial; health education is vital in this context. Vaccination is effective in most but not all individuals.

Viruses

Viruses are important causes of acute gastroenteritis throughout the world. In healthy adults the effects are inconvenient rather than serious. In developing countries where children may be malnourished, the results are very different, with a mortality rate of 1–4% representing the deaths of up to 18 million children a year.[65]

Acute epidemic non-bacterial gastroenteritis (winter vomiting disease) is a self-limiting disease associated with fever, myalgia, colic, vomiting and diarrhoea. It usually lasts only a few days. Spread is usually from contaminated food, water or shellfish, or by faeco-oral contact. The Norwalk virus is the agent most frequently involved. There are many strains, some antigenically closely related and others quite distinct. In an oyster-related epidemic in New South Wales, virus was detected in stools in 39% of cases, but Norwalk antibodies rose in 75%.[66]

Rotavirus infections are often hospital-acquired; the stability of these viruses contributes to environmental contamination. Although resulting in mild illness, hospital stay may be prolonged and lactose intolerance has occurred. The problem is greatest in children's wards and neonatal units. The viruses recognized as causing gastroenteritis most commonly are listed in Table 52.2.

Table 52.2 Viruses that commonly cause gastroenteritis

VIRUS	EPIDEMIOLOGY
Small round structured (Norwalk)	World-wide; community outbreaks
Small round featureless	Water or shellfish contamination
Rotavirus	World-wide; winter disease of infants and children; about 50% of UK 'diarrhoea and vomiting'
Fastidious adenovirus	Probably world-wide; less common than rotavirus
Astrovirus	Mild disease in children
Calcivirus	Mild disease in children and elderly; winter vomiting
Coronavirus-like	Possible association with neonatal necrotizing enterocolitis

HIV infection

Infection with the human immunodeficiency virus (HIV) predisposes to diarrhoea, which is usually due to secondary infection in the immunocompromised patient. *Salmonella* and *Campylobacter* are likely to cause a more severe illness than in otherwise healthy individuals. *Cryptosporidium* species cause opportunist infections, which were exceedingly rare before the acquired immune deficiency syndrome (AIDS) era. About 50% of patients with AIDS develop diarrhoea due to a *cryptosporidium*, usually *C. parvum*.[67] Very mild inflammatory changes are present, and no toxins have been identified. The diarrhoea appears to be largely secretory in type.

Cytomegalovirus (CMV) and herpes simplex virus cause diarrhoea in AIDS but mostly affect the colon rather than the small bowel. CMV occasionally causes small bowel ulceration and haemorrhage, and even perforation has been attributed to this virus in a leukaemic patient. *Mycobacterium avium-intracellulare* infects the small bowel, and its finding on jejunal biopsy helps in the diagnosis of AIDS. Its pathogenicity remains unclear.

Whether HIV itself produces a functional defect in the small bowel is debated; indeed enterocyte invasion by HIV is uncertain, and the frequent association with other pathogens makes assessment more difficult.

MANAGEMENT OF GASTROENTERITIS

The syndrome of anorexia, nausea, vomiting, abdominal pain and diarrhoea, usually occurring in a group context, is commonly known as gastroenteritis. A variety of viruses, bacteria or protozoa may be implicated. These disorders are usually brief and self-limiting.

In most social circumstances the general diagnosis is clear, and search for a specific cause or organism is not appropriate. If an outbreak occurs in hospital or a similar context then a 'point' source may be defined with benefit, and identifying a specific organism may limit further spread. The presence of a high fever or rectal bleeding is an indication to pursue a more precise diagnosis.

If abdominal pain is a marked feature, then signs such as tenderness or guarding may suggest a localized lesion such as appendicitis. If plain abdominal radiographs are taken, it is important to recognize that multiple fluid levels are often seen in acute gastroenteritis. The association of this appearance with diarrhoea excludes both ileus and obstruction. Just occasionally more localized 'radiological ileus' may indicate an inflammatory lesion, such as a retroileal appendicitis. A chronic obstruction of the small bowel may occasionally present with diarrhoea if there is bacterial overgrowth proximal to a distal stricture. Similar appearances can occur in invasive parasitic infections, especially hyperinfestation with *Strongyloides*.

Acute gastroenteritis is self-limiting, so clinical management is merely supportive. Early use of oral rehydration therapy may be beneficial, and antidiarrhoeals such as loperamide or codeine phosphate may be employed.

CHRONIC INFECTIONS

Tuberculosis

Any part of the gut may be affected by tuberculosis, though ileocaecal infection (Figure 52.5) is most common. In developed countries *Mycobacterium bovis* is not now commonly seen because of the strict control of infection in cattle and the routine use of pasteurized milk. It is still, however, a fairly common cause of disease in the gut, and in many countries such as the UK and the USA there has been a great increase in this disease over recent decades, predominantly in immigrant populations.[68,69]

Intestinal tuberculosis may present as a chronic inflammatory illness with no obvious localization until investigations are performed. Alternatively the presentation may be of localized or abdominal disease from the outset.

Tuberculous *peritonitis* may result in ascites or, in its hypertrophic form, produce matting together of omentum and bowel.

Intestinal infection may be ulcerative. This form is most often associated with pulmonary infection. The ileum shows multiple mucosal ulcers, which tend to lie transversely across the bowel wall, contrasting with the longitudinal ulcers seen in typhoid. The wall tends to be thickened, so perforation is uncommon. On healing, cicatricial scarring may result in intestinal obstruction.

More commonly ileocaecal infection is *hyperplastic*, with caseation. Acute-on-chronic obstructive symptoms may be the first evidence of such disease, although a palpable mass may be present on examination.

Tuberculosis has emerged as an important disease in HIV-infected patients, in whom it is more likely to present as an extrapulmonary disease. Such patients will frequently have a negative Mantoux test.[70]

Diagnosis In European countries the major diagnostic problem relates to the differentiation from Crohn's disease. General indices of inflammatory disease are usually present. Plain abdominal radiographs may give evidence of free fluid, intestinal fluid levels or abscesses. In ascites, ultrasonographic examination is very useful and aids satisfactory aspiration of fluid for microscopy and culture. Some have emphasized the value of laparoscopy in ascites: it permits visualization and biopsy of tubercles in addition to aspiration of fluid.[71] The collection of multiple stool specimens for culture is important. Small bowel capsule biopsy may occasionally be helpful, but is unlikely to be so in distal disease. CT-guided aspiration of visceral lesions or of a mesenteric mass can provide a diagnosis without recourse to laparoscopy or laparotomy.[72]

Clinical features that can help in the differentiation from Crohn's disease are listed in Table 52.3. The major reason why this differentiation is so important is included in the list, namely the potential danger of steroid therapy in tuberculosis.

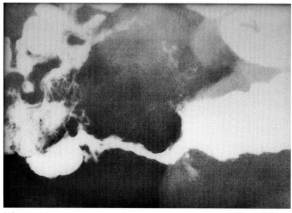

(a)

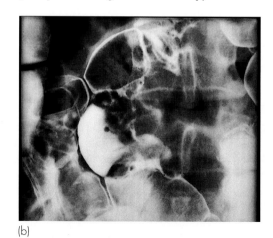

(b)

Figure 52.5

(a) Dilated ileum proximal to a stricture in ileocaecal tuberculosis. (b) A large ileal tuberculous ulcer.

Table 52.3 Clinical differentiation between ileocaecal Crohn's disease and tuberculosis

CROHN'S	TUBERCULOSIS
No	Phlyctenular conjunctivitis
Uveitis	No
Clubbing	Unlikely
Ascending cholangitis	No
Sclerosing cholangitis	No
Bluish perianal skin	No
No	Lupus vulgaris (*M. bovis* only)
Spondylitis, sacroilitis	No
Distal arthropathy	Larger joints involved
Ascites rare	Ascites common
Aphthous ulcers	No
Steroids often helpful	Steroids may be dangerous

Treatment General and chemotherapeutic medical treatment is indicated in most patients. If diagnosis can be confirmed without laparotomy, antituberculous therapy may be completely successful. Occasionally, healing of disease may lead to subsequent small bowel stenosis.[73] Sometimes a diagnostic laparotomy is necessary. Occasionally acute signs suggest appendicitis, and if at laparotomy characteristic tuberculosis is seen, biopsies should be taken (of tubercles, omentum or nodes) and resection avoided.

Laparoscopy may be a useful alternative to laparotomy in cases with ascites. In the absence of ascites, it may be dangerous unless an open-insertion technique is used to avoid perforation of adherent bowel.[71]

Obstruction is a clear indication for surgical intervention if medical treatment fails. It was once believed that chemotherapy increased fibrosis, thus causing obstruction and perforation.[74] More recent reports suggest that most patients respond well to treatment, and operation may be reserved for the few failures.[74] In acute obstruction resection and anastomosis should be performed – usually a right hemicolectomy. Chronic obstruction, which may present with diarrhoea due to bacterial overgrowth, is treated similarly. Bypass operations are best avoided as long-term sequelae can arise in the excluded segment. As in Crohn's disease, some have advocated stricture-plasty for ileal strictures; this may be appropriate for fibrous strictures seen after prolonged medical therapy, and good results have been reported.[75] The one situation in which bypass may be necessary is duodenal tuberculosis, for which a gastroenterostomy may be necessary to relieve vomiting.

Both haemorrhage and perforation may necessitate urgent surgical treatment in this disease, but both are rare. Local resection or hemicolectomy are indicated depending on the circumstances. After such acute interventions, appropriate chemotherapy is essential.

Yersinia

Two species of *Yersinia*, *Y. enterolitica* and *Y. pseudotuberculosis*, cause gastrointestinal disease in man; the former is more common. *Y. pseudotuberculosis* is more likely to cause the pseudoappendicitis syndrome, which is surgically most

important. Both organisms cause disease after oral ingestion of contaminated food, milk or water. Several different strains are recognized; they differ in geographical distribution and possibly in virulence. Epidemiologically, these are typically infections of colder-temperate climates, with a particularly high incidence in Canada and Scandinavia. There is evidence of an increasing incidence over recent decades.[76]

Acute yersinial enterocolitis occurs after a 4–10-day incubation period. The ileum and colon are invaded and focal ulcerations occur. This process is associated with diarrhoea and fever, and occasionally other features develop such as arthritis, liver involvement or even central nervous system changes. In immunosuppressed patients a particularly severe invasive disease may occur which has a high mortality rate. Sufferers from AIDS may be susceptible to such infections. Usually, however, the disease is self-limiting, and recovery is complete. Although the organism can be shown to be sensitive to antibiotics, for example the newer cephalosporins, use of these agents does not alter the course of the common form of the disease. It is best therefore to reserve antibiotics for rare, complicated forms of the disease.

During acute episodes there is typically a leucocytosis, and barium studies may show mucosal oedema with 'cobblestoning' of the ileum. Unlike Crohn's disease, strictures and fistulas do not occur. Sigmoidoscopy may reveal an inflamed friable mucosa, or ulceration (often aphthous in appearance) may be seen.

Pseudoappendicitis/mesenteric adenitis are more locally invasive forms of the disease, characteristically due to *Y. pseudotuberculosis*. This condition frequently presents as a differential diagnosis of appendicitis; indeed, it may be diagnosed at laparotomy. Under these circumstances the appendix may be removed safely, but mesenteric nodes should be taken and sent for both culture and histology. Culture of free fluid found at laparotomy may be adequate for diagnosis.

Severe ileal ulceration with haemorrhage occurs very rarely, usually in children under 5 years of age. Perforation may also occur in such cases.

Diagnosis is made by culture from peritoneal fluid or mesenteric node. If fever lasting several days and diarrhoea are prominent features in a patient presenting with possible appendicitis, then yersiniosis should be considered in the differential diagnosis. If the diagnosis is suggested at *diagnostic laparoscopy*, then nodes or free fluid can be obtained. Laparoscopic appendicectomy may still be entertained at this stage, or at open laparotomy.

Treatment is supportive. There is no evidence that the routine use of antibiotics has any effect on the clinical course of the disease. They are best reserved for use in severe sepsis, or in 'at-risk' immunosuppressed subjects.[77]

Actinomycosis

Actinomyces israelii is an anaerobic Gram-positive bacterium with branching filamentous hyphae. It is widely distributed in nature, and the pathogenic forms occur as commensals in the normal mouth. It is not known what predisposes to tissue invasion.

Characteristic actinomycotic lesions consist of firm nodular granulomas giving rise to indurated tissue masses with indefinite borders. Such infection is locally progressive, organisms spreading along and through tissue planes. The lesions are chronic and give rise to minimal systemic disturbance.

Four clinical forms of infection are recognized: cervicofacial, thoracic, hepatic and ileocaecal. This last form is the one that involves the small bowel, although the principal organ involved is the caecum. Clinical presentation is either of subacute right iliac fossa inflammation, mistaken as appendicitis, or as a more chronic caecal mass, often resected as a supposed carcinoma. Differential diagnosis is always problematic as more serious lesions cannot be excluded radiologically. When sinuses occur, the discharge of pus containing characteristic 'sulphur granules' is virtually diagnostic, and culture gives confirmation. Most often ileocaecal disease is diagnosed at or after laparotomy. Treatment is with benzylpenicillin, given in large doses over a period of 6 weeks.

Fungal infections

Fungal involvement of the small intestine is a rare event, and is almost invariably associated with immunosuppressed states. *Candida* and *Aspergillus* species are almost always responsible. In a 10-year review from a regional cancer centre in Manchester, 14 cases were seen in patients being treated for malignancy.[78] Lesions found at autopsy included ulcers of varying configurations, sloughed mucous membranes, polypoid masses and segmental lesions.

Candida tends to be localized to the mucosa, but *Aspergillus* more often invades transmurally. Both small and large bowel may be involved. From a clinical viewpoint variable patterns may be seen on endoscopy, most often resembling a pseudomembranous colitis. Very often such infections are not diagnosed in life.

Occasionally invasive aspergillosis causes small bowel obstruction, which has led to surgical resection during therapy for leukaemia in childhood.[79] The penetrative nature of *Aspergillus* has also been known to cause bowel infarction[80] or even appendicitis.[81]

Treatment with amphotericin B and flucocytosine may be helpful, though the former is a toxic drug and side-effects are common. Imidazole antifungal drugs are not effective against *Aspergillus*.

INFESTATIONS

Schistosomiasis

Four schistosomes are topical parasites of man. Of these *Schistosoma haematobium* and *S. mansoni* are the most important, *S. japonicum* being limited to China and Japan and some other Far Eastern countries, and *S. intercalatum* being an African species of very limited distribution. Schistomosomes are trematodes, which actively penetrate the skin of man and have fresh-water snails as their intermediate host. Human disease therefore occurs in relation to rivers and lakes in the tropics, and it is estimated that 200 million people are infested,[82] *S. haematobium* affects the urinary tract in man and does not cause digestive disease. *S. mansoni* (and the other species) principally affect the large bowel. Eggs from the parasites are passed in the faeces and hatch to form miracidial larvae, which enter a snail. Within the snail multiplication takes place, with the eventual release into the water of cercaria which penetrate human skin. Adult trematodes eventually inhabit the mesenteric veins. In heavy intestations eggs are trapped in the mucosa and submucosa of the colon; pseudotubercles produced may coalesce to form pseudopapillomas.

Direct foregut involvement does not usually occur, but eggs carried to the liver become lodged in the portal tracts. Eventual fibrosis may give rise to portal hypertension with hepatosplenomegaly. Variceal haemorrhage occurs as in other forms of portal hypertension. Because the small bowel is much less affected than the colon, malabsorption is rare. Protein-losing enteropathy has been described in Egypt in patients who have developed polyposis.[83] This condition is extremely rare in other countries.

Ascariasis

It has been estimated that 26% of the world's population are infested with *Ascaris lumbricoides*. Adult worms inhabit the small bowel lumen. They are stout nematodes 200–400 × 3–6 mm (female) or 150–300 × 2–4 mm (male) in size. A female lays about 200 000 eggs a day, which are passed in the faeces. The larval stages occur in soil, and the second-stage larvae may eventually be ingested. From the duodenum they pass through the liver to the lungs, then via the trachea to enter the upper gut. This migration is accompanied by respiratory symptoms of varying severity – death due to pneumonitis is common in children in the tropics – but gut involvement gives rise to nausea, vomiting, colic and, in heavy infestation, intestinal obstruction.[84] Worms may be seen on a barium study of the small bowel.

Ascaris may migrate up the bile ducts or pancreatic duct, causing cholangitis, liver abscess or pancreatitis. The propensity of this nematode to travel up any convenient tube is illustrated in Figure 52.6 (see colour plate also). Occasionally worms will develop in the peritoneal cavity or pass out

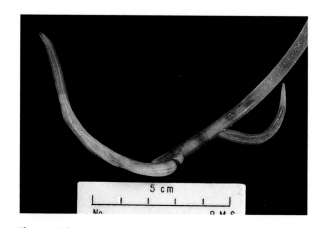

Figure 52.6
Ascaris lumbricodies found on withdrawal of a gastroduodenal tube inserted at vagotomy.

through orifices such as the nose. Roundworms are not limited to the tropics, and although the incidence is related to overall standards of hygiene, ascaris complications can appear sporadically in surprising contexts.

Treatment, after diagnosis by examination of the faeces, is with anthelmintics such as piperazine adipate. If laparotomy is needed for obstruction, an attempt is made to 'milk' the worm bolus into the caecum. This manoeuvre usually fails and an enterotomy is needed. There is a pronounced tendency for ascaris to migrate through suture lines, so adequate clearance should be achieved, followed by drug therapy.

The presence of ascaris should be taken seriously in preoperative situations. If ova are present in faeces, it is imperative to eliminate the parasites by appropriate therapy before any planned operation on the gut. If this is not done, the worm is prone to penetrate surgical suture lines and cause leakage and peritonitis.

Hookworms

Hookworm infestations occur in the tropics but extend into temperate zones. Both organisms involved, *Necator americanus* and *Ancylostoma duodenale*, live principally in the duodenum, though in heavy infestation they may be found as far down as the caecum. Soil larvae enter via the skin, or may sometimes be ingested. Eosinophilia is a feature of early infestation but is not typical of the chronic phase.

The only clinically important feature of infection is anaemia, which is due to blood loss and may not occur if iron intake and general nutrition are adequate. In severe infestations, however, profound anaemia may occur. It is not now believed that hookworms produce malabsorption.

In the tropics tetrachloroethylene is widely used for treatment because it is cheap and effective. It is, however, hepatotoxic, and treatment with mebendazole or thiabendazole, or with bephenium or pyrantel, is to be preferred. The side-effects of these agents are limited to occasional nausea or vomiting.

Tapeworms

Adult cestodes inhabit the small intestine. The common species affecting man are the fish tapeworm *Diphyllobothrium latum*, the beef tapeworm *Taenia saginata* and the pork tapeworm *Taenia solium*. *Hymenolepsis nana* is a smaller worm which is very common in children in some parts of the world, notably in Eastern Europe. *Echinococcus* species are of great importance as a cause of disease in man, but it is the larval form that causes such disease and the human small bowel is not inhabited by adult worms.

Fish tapeworms may produce macrocytic anaemia by competitive take-up of vitamin B_{12}, although this phenomenon is rare outside Northern Europe. *Taenia* species may cause epigastric and central abdominal pain, nausea and weight loss. Localized inflammation of the ileal mucosa may occur; very rarely intestinal obstruction, perforation or appendicitis are reported.

The presence of tapeworms is diagnosed by the presence of gravid proglottids in the faeces. Treatment with anthelmintics should be accompanied by B_{12} therapy where appropriate.

Anisakis (herringworm)

Anisakis is a parasite of fish-eating mammals, and infests man when insufficiently cooked fish is eaten. Although described mainly in Holland and Japan, cases are seen with increasing frequency in the West with the proliferation of Japanese restaurants. Larvae are found in abscesses in the wall of the stomach and intestine. Pain, nausea and colic may occur, and laparotomy for obstruction reveals an inflammatory mass. It has been suggested[85] that a history of recent ingestion of raw fish is sufficient to permit non-operative treatment in this brief self-limiting disease, but clearly a laparotomy may be safer when clinical doubt is present. A fluorescent antibody test for anisakiasis is available.

Eustrongyloides

Eustrongyloides is a parasite of fish-eating birds, and like *Anisakis* infects man when fish is eaten in an insufficiently cooked state. Although rare, its importance relates to the fact that it may perforate the small intestine, causing acute peritonitis. A bright-pink worm is found wriggling in the peritoneal cavity at laparotomy.[86]

Angiostrongylus

Angiostrongylus costaricensis lives in adult form in rodents and in larval form in slugs. Ingestion by man of small slugs or their mucous secretions may give rise to intestinal infestation with larvae. These penetrate the intestinal wall, usually about 20–30 days after infestation, in the ileocaecal area. The resulting illness, usually in children, is mistaken for appendicitis or intestinal obstruction, but if untreated may last for several weeks and then regress. There is no satisfactory drug therapy.[87]

Strongyloides

Strongyloides stercoralis is widespread in the tropics, but occurs sporadically in Europe and North America. The parasite may live freely in the soil, in several forms. One larval form may penetrate human skin. Penetration is followed by a complex migration, with ultimate infection of the small intestine by female adult parasites, 2.0–2.2 mm in length. Most frequently the ileal crypts are infested. The female lays eggs there, and larvae burrow into the mucosa causing a superficial ileitis, with excess mucus production.

The main significance of strongyloidiasis is that it may occur in a severe invasive form known as hyperinfestation. In this condition autoinfestation becomes more widespread, and parasites are found in the submucosa (Figure 52.7, see colour plate also), which becomes oedematous and atrophic. The gut becomes congested and inelastic. The clinical picture may be of a paralytic ileus (Figure 52.8) or of small bowel obstruction, or of a haemorrhagic ulcerative enterocolitis or necrotizing jejunitis. Septicaemic death is common. Severe illness with abdominal signs may lead to laparotomy, which in this condition is almost universally fatal.[88] Disseminated strongyloidiasis is usually related to immunodeficiency states. It has

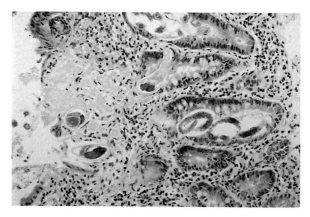

Figure 52.7
Strongyloides stercoralis in duodenal mucosa. The patient presented with an acute abdomen with multiple fluid levels on radiography. Hyperinfestation was treated successfully, but the patient was subsequently found to have a malignant lymphoma.

been associated with immunosuppressive therapy, with malignant lymphoma and more recently with AIDS.

The relevance of this parasite is threefold. First, the presence of *Strongyloides* in the faeces should never be ignored; treatment should always be instituted because symptomless infection may later become lethal. Secondly, parasitic infection should be excluded (though this is never completely possible) by examination of faeces before immunosuppressive treatment is instituted. Thirdly, if the diagnosis is suspected attempts should be made to confirm it. Apart from examination of the faeces, duodenal aspiration by intubation, or better still by duodenoscopy with mucosal biopsy, is likely to be diagnostic.

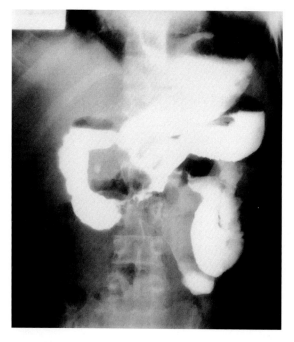

Figure 52.8
Barium follow-through showing oedematous ulcerated small bowel in a patient heavily infested with strongyloides.

Chemotherapy with thiabendazole is usually effective in simple infestation, and it may be life saving in hyperinfestation states. Complete eradication may be difficult, however. Repeated short courses of therapy, including newer agents such as albendazole or ivermectin, may be necessary.[89]

Oesophagostomum

Nematodes of the superfamily Strongyloidea occasionally give rise to serious surgical complications. Worms of the genus *Oesophagostomum* are most frequently responsible. These are common parasites of ruminants, monkeys and apes, and humans appear to be accidental hosts. The worm in its histotropic phase is confined to the bowel wall. Occasionally it fails to enter the lumen but migrates into surrounding tissues. The most common result is a tumour-like inflammatory mass or abscess, most often in the ileocaecal region.

This disease was recognized as early as 1902,[90] and it has been described in many parts of the world, as reviewed by Anthony and McAdam.[91] It is a disease of the tropics, but occurs in both indigenous and 'expatriate' populations. Thirty-four cases were described from Uganda,[91] usually presenting with a 4–6 cm mass, often containing an abscess. A worm 'track' is usually found on sectioning the mass, often containing the parasite. Lesions may be multiple.

The clinical diagnosis may be difficult: differential diagnosis at operation including malignancy, tuberculosis or an amoeboma. Cases have been seen in Europe in patients returning from the tropics, emphasizing the need to be aware of such apparently exotic diseases.

Pentastomes

Pentastomes are not strictly helminths but belong to a phylum that lies somewhere between annelids and arthropods. *Armillifer armillatus* is a parasite of snakes in the tropics. Ingestion of eggs by humans leads to liberation of the parasite, which bores through the small intestine and encysts in the mesentery or the liver. Severe pathology is rare, but a calcified nodule may present on X-ray examination or at laparotomy. This nodule is easily mistaken for a metastasis if malignant disease is present. The author has seen two such cases in West London in patients who each had a gastric carcinoma and a white liver nodule at laparotomy (Figure 52.9, see colour plate also). Infestation is very common in some tropical countries; for example, the incidence is 45% in Malaysian aborigines. Sporadic cases are seen in Europe, particularly in patients from the former Yugoslavia.[92]

Giardia

Giardia lamblia is a flagellated protozoan which is endemic in many countries. The incidence of infection in the UK has been reported as between 5 and 16%, and in the USA 4%. Infection occurs by the ingestion of mature cysts, which 'excystate' in the stomach. The trophozoites inhabit the upper two-thirds of the small bowel. Spread is by contamination of water and food with cysts. Person-to-person infection can occur during anal sexual intercourse.

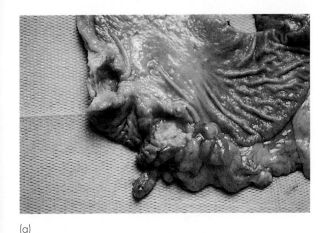

(a)

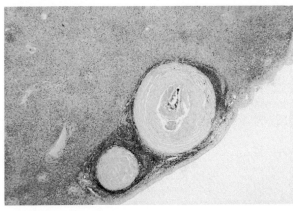

(b)

Figure 52.9

(a) Carcinoma of the antrum; an ulcerated lesion is seen in the prepyloric area. (b) Histological section of a white liver nodule from the same patient. It was not a metastasis, but an encysted larva of *Armillifer armillatus*.

Most infections are asymptomatic. Acute diarrhoea may occur, with explosive foul-smelling watery stools, belching, distension and cramps. Chronic malabsorption also occurs, with steatorrhoea. It is suggested that *Giardia* infection may also predispose to biliary tract infections and pancreatitis, and a mild reactive hepatitis may occur.[93]

Chemotherapy with tinidazole, mepacrine or furazolidone is usually effective. From a surgical viewpoint the major importance of giardiasis relates to the differential diagnosis of acute and chronic diarrhoea. No direct surgical complications result from the infestation itself.

Amoebae

Entamoeba histolytica infestation is contracted by the faeco-oral route via the ingestion of contaminated food or water or by homosexual activity, especially oroanal sexual contact. The incidence in Western temperate countries has risen considerably in recent years in association with widespread homosexual activity.

Infection affects mainly the large bowel, and especially the caecum and rectosigmoid. The small bowel is rarely involved, although in severe caecal disease lesions may 'overflow' into the terminal ileum. It has been postulated that invasion of intestinal mucosa by amoebae may be facilitated by gut bacteria, and that the relative sterility of the small bowel may protect it from invasion. Haematogenous spread may lead to liver abscess as a presenting feature. In acute 'typhlitic' involvement of the caecum, a considerable inflammatory mass may be formed. The mass occasionally results in distal small bowel obstruction, but this is rare. Very mild inflammatory changes are present and no toxins have been identified. The diarrhoea appears to be largely secretory in type.

Diagnosis is usually made by examination of the stools, but this has been shown to be somewhat suspect. Antigen detection enzyme-linked immunosorbent assay for galactose inhibitable adherence protein antigen in serum and faeces may offer a more reliable means of diagnosis.[94]

EOSINOPHILIC GASTROENTERITIS

This is an uncommon disorder which usually involves the gastric antrum and the upper jejunum. It has three main forms, distinguished by the layer of the gut involved. Thus *mucosal* involvement presents as protein-losing enteropathy and malabsorption and is associated with allergic disorders. *Muscle* involvement produces thickening and obstruction, and occasionally fistula or haemorrhage. *Serosal* involvement produces pain, peritonitis and sometimes ascites.[95] In all forms there are areas of thickening with dense eosinophil infiltrates. The disease occurs mainly in young adults but can be seen at any age. It is twice as common in males as in females. The aetiology is unknown.

The disease may occur as a brief episode, or in some cases be prolonged over several years. Ileocolitis is a less common form and mimics Crohn's disease. The more common proximal disease is difficult to diagnose if the antrum is not involved, as the jejunum is not readily accessible to endoscopy. In ascitic forms the fluid may contain up to 99% eosinophils, but a high count may occur in other conditions. Only about 20% of cases show an eosinophilia in peripheral blood.

Eosinophilic gastroenteritis has been seen in epidemic form, and found to be associated with the dog hookworm *Ancylostoma caninum*.[96] Some cases presented as surgical emergencies, mimicking appendicitis.[97] It is not known whether the epidemic form, seen in North Queensland, Australia, is a separate form or an indicator that unidentified parasites may play a role more commonly in the aetiology of eosinophilic gastroenteritis.

If a diagnosis can be made without laparotomy, steroids should be employed. In the absence of complications operation is not helpful. The disease tends to be self-limiting with a good prognosis.

ENTERIC ULCERATION

Ulceration of the small bowel can occur in a large variety of clinical conditions, as illustrated in Table 52.4, many of which are

Table 52.4 Ulceration of the small bowel.

Congenital	Drug-induced	Endometriosis
Intestinal atresia	Enteric-coated potassium	Coeliac disease
Ectopic gastric mucosa	Corticosteroids	Jejunal diverticulosis
Intestinal reduplication	Indomethacin	Post-irradiation
Meconium ileus	Phenylbutazone	
Meckel's diverticulum	Immunosuppression	*Hormonal*
		Zollinger-Ellison syndrome
	Traumatic	Phaeochromocytoma
Acquired	External	
Bacterial	Bands	*Neoplastic*
Tuberculosis	Volvulus	Benign
Typhoid	Hernia	Leiomyoma
Cholera	Luminal	Adenoma
Shigella dysentery	Foreign bodies	Malignant
Syphilis	Bolus impaction	Adenocarcinoma
Viral	Gallstone ileus	Lymphoma
Cytomegalovirus	Intubation	Carcinoid
Other enteropathic viruses		Leiomyosarcoma
Fungal	*Vascular*	Malignant histiocytosis
Histoplasmosis	Embolic	Secondary tumour
Aspergillosis	Thrombotic	
Protozoal	Intussusception	*Metabolic*
Amoebiasis	Polyarteritis nodosa	Uraemia
Parasitic	Thromboangitis obliterans	Anastomotic
Ancyclostomiasis		
Ascariasis	*Inflammatory*	*Idiopathic*
	Crohn's disease	

Modified from Thomas and Williamson.[117]

discussed earlier (see also Chapter 54). The diversity emphasizes the need for care in diagnosis in small bowel ulceration.

Peptic ulcer (postbulbar)

Peptic ulcer occurring in the distal duodenum or uppermost jejunum of an unoperated patient is always associated with the Zollinger–Ellison syndrome (see Chapter 36). Other associated features are usually present, such as diarrhoea and a history of aggressive complicated peptic ulcer disease. Other endocrine disorders, notably hyperparathyroidism, may be associated. Diagnosis is confirmed by an elevated fasting plasma gastrin.

Complications of such ulcers are common, and patients often present with haemorrhage or perforation. In the absence of such complications, management consists of establishing the diagnosis, attempting to localize the underlying gastrinoma (or gastrinomas), and addressing the gastric hypersecretion of acid which is the major cause of morbidity. The advent of proton pump inhibitors such as omeprazole and lansoprazole has transformed the treatment of this condition, as adequate control of acid is now always possible, and more time is available for assessment and decision-making. The widespread use of other acid-reducing agents (H_2 antagonists) in the community has also altered the clinical pattern, fewer patients presenting with acute severe complications. Details of management are discussed further in Chapter 34.

Peptic ulcer (stomal)

The operation of gastrojejunostomy, with or without gastric resection, exposes the upper jejunum to gastric secretions to an abnormal degree. Peptic ulcer may result, and always lies on the jejunal side of the stoma immediately adjacent to the suture line (see Chapter 35).

The incidence of such ulcers was high when inadequate gastrectomy was performed early in the twentieth century, and it lessened when higher resections were performed routinely. When vagotomy took over from gastrectomy in the management of duodenal ulcer, stomal ulcers were seen when gastrojejunostomy was associated with an incomplete vagotomy.

The main importance of stomal ulcers relates to the high incidence of complications, which are twofold. *Haemorrhage* is a common feature and tends to occur in brisk and repeated episodes associated with high morbidity and mortality rates. The second problem relates to the anatomical proximity of the transverse colon and is the formation of *gastrocolic fistula*. Such fistulas present with diarrhoea, which is due to the colonization of small bowel with colonic flora. The metabolic effects of this contamination in a malnourished postgastrectomy patient can be very profound.

Both complications are very dangerous, which implies that stomal ulcers must be treated with profound respect. Diagnosis is usually made easily by endoscopy. Because of the risks, until recently all stomal ulcers were considered an indication for surgical treatment, usually by excision and vagotomy (or completion of an inadequate vagotomy). With the advent of omeprazole some stomal ulcers are now treated conservatively with success; such treatment should be considered permanent, however. Late cessation of treatment in an ageing patient can lead to a lethal recurrence.

Haemorrhage from a stomal ulcer may be treated endoscopically (by injection, heat probe or laser), but the general principles of surgery for bleeding peptic ulcer should be applied, and operation should be considered early on in the elderly. Gastrocolic fistula almost always requires surgical treatment. Before the mechanisms involved in producing the diarrhoea were understood, this involved a staged operation in a sick patient. Prior control of the diarrhoea with antibiotics plus careful control of fluid balance and nutrition has been a considerable advance. It permits a single operation, which usually involves closure of a colonic defect and an appropriate gastric resection, often with a vagotomy.

Meckel's ulcer

Peptic ulcers can form within a Meckel's diverticulum and are often complicated by haemorrhage or perforation. The ulcer occurs most frequently near the neck of the diverticulum. Such ulcers are discussed in Chapter 57 under the heading of small bowel diverticula.

Potassium-induced ulcer

During the 1960s enteric coated potassium was implicated in the aetiology of some cases of non-specific ulceration of the small bowel[98,99] (see also Chapter 54). Administration of such agents was found to produce similar lesions in dogs.[100] A typical such agent has an outer sugar coat of cyclopenthiazide, and an inner slow-release wax core of potassium. It is thought that sudden release of high local concentrations of potassium in the small bowel are responsible for the pathology, although the pathological changes are the same as those found in non-specific ulcers, as described later. The clinical presentation is also identical.

Non-steroidal anti-inflammatory drugs

It has long been known that NSAIDs, which are in very wide use, especially in the elderly, produce ulceration of the stomach and duodenum with a high incidence of complications. It has been recognized more recently that such drugs also cause ulceration of the jejunum and ileum. This fact has been recognized in particular by the use of jejunoscopy. Patients on therapy for rheumatoid arthritis may have demonstrable intestinal blood loss, and in such patients almost a half can be shown to have ulceration in the small bowel.[101]

Ulcerative jejunoileitis

Ulcerative jejunitis is characterized by chronic multiple and apparently benign ulcers. Occasionally the ileum is also affected.[102] It occurs mainly in patients between 40 and 60 years of age. The clinical picture is usually of fever, anorexia, weight loss, abdominal pain and diarrhoea. Anaemia is usually present, with steatorrhoea and sometimes a protein-losing enteropathy. Pathologically, ulceration is present in a flat mucosa as found in coeliac disease. It has been reported that a few patients have demonstrated the *HLA-DR3* genotype which is also present in coeliac disease.[103]

Complications such as haemorrhage and perforation are common, and strictures may occur. Surgical treatment is

therefore often precipitated, and satisfactory local treatment by an appropriate resection improves the prognosis, which in general is very poor.

Patients with coeliac disease tend to suffer ulcerative jejunitis and lymphoma at a similar stage in life, and progression from one to the other may be seen. It has been suggested that ulcerative jejunitis itself is part of the spectrum of malignant lymphoma[104] (see Chapter 60).

Non-specific ulcer

Ulceration of the small bowel may occur in a large variety of clinical conditions, as listed in Table 52.4.[105] Rarely, ulcers occur that do not fit into any of the pathological groupings listed, and they are known as 'non-specific' or 'idiopathic' ulcers. First described by Baillie[106] in 1795, 'simple' ulcers of the small bowel were reviewed by Combes[107] in 1897. The lesion was described by Grasman[108] in 1925 as 'sharp-bordered, solitary ulceration with no surrounding inflammation, of unknown cause, indefinite pathogenesis, and an acute or chronic course'. The aetiology of such ulcers remains obscure, although they have a typical histological picture. There is a zone of granulation tissue which is well circumscribed; local hyperplasia of the muscularis mucosae and foci of pyloric metaplasia are present in the adjacent mucosa. A typical ulcer occurring in an elderly woman who presented with ileal obstruction is seen in Figure 52.10 (see colour plate also).

When enteric coated potassium was first implicated in enteric ulceration,[98] it was soon realized that it was not the cause of all similar ulcers. In a review of 395 patients from around the world with solitary ulcers, less than half were taking enteric coated potassium.[109] In a review of similar patients from the Mayo Clinic only 10% were receiving such medication.[110]

Such ulcers present with either obstruction or haemorrhage, or more rarely with perforation.[111] Bleeding may be acute, or chronic, in the latter case giving rise to anaemia. There appears to be a tendency towards obstruction as the presenting feature in recent years, whereas earlier reports emphasized perforation. Anaemia was a rare feature in early reports of this condition.[112,113] Later studies suggest that patients with bleeding tend to be younger than those with obstruction.[114]

Treatment is by local excision and is curative.[105,115] Simple closure of perforation has been advocated, but this has the disadvantages of not providing adequate histology and of risking recurrence.[116,105]

Anastomotic ulcer

Gastrointestinal blood loss in a patient who has undergone a previous enteroenteroanastomosis is occasionally found to originate from a non-specific ulcer at the site of this anastomosis. The reason for such ulcers is not clear, as histological examination reveals focal ulceration and chronic inflammation but no crypt abscesses or granulomas. Clinical presentation may be acute with melaena, or with anaemia secondary to chronic blood loss. Localization has occasionally been made using labelled red cells. Excision of the anastomosis is always curative.[117]

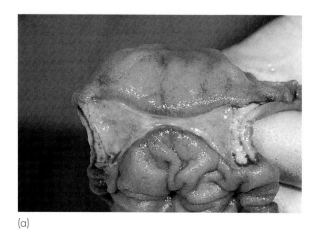

(a)

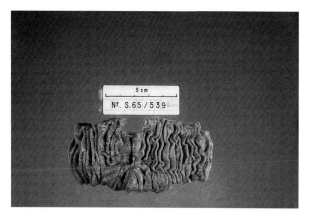

(b)

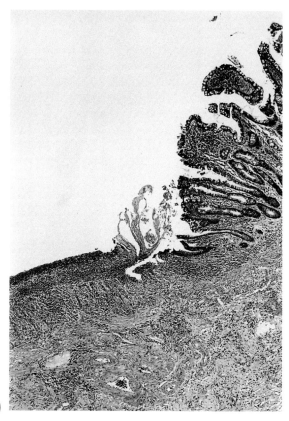

(c)

Figure 52.10
Non-specific ileal ulcers. (a) From a patient who presented with haemorrhage, and (b) From another who presented with ileal obstruction. (c) The histological appearances of the ulcer illustrated in (b). There is complete loss of the mucosa and an ulcer base of granulation tissue.

Graft-versus-host disease

This occurs principally after bone marrow transplantation, when immunocompetent cells present in the transplant recognize foreign histocompatibility antigens present in the host. It has been very rarely reported after blood transfusion or after solid organ transplantation. Gut and liver involvement may occur in 10% of HLA-identical marrow recipients, but in 60% of cases of HLA-non-identical family member recipients.

Where the gut is involved, stomach, small and large bowel may be affected. The ileocaecal region is most involved. Watery diarrhoea, anorexia, vomiting and cramps are present, and there may be haemorrhage. Radiological studies show mucosal oedema and rapid transit.

Management consists of bowel rest, parenteral nutrition and electrolyte replacement, together with appropriate immunosuppression, usually with cyclosporin and methylprednisolone. Intercurrent infections must be treated promptly. Acute disease (occurring within 100 days of transplant) has a high mortality rate, approaching 50% for moderate-to-severe disease. The chronic form of graft-versus-host disease occurs later and typically affects more organs, although the small bowel is usually less affected.[118]

REFERENCES

1. Walsh D. Deep tissue traumatism from Roentgen ray exposure. *Br Med J* 1897; **2**: 272

2. Futh H & Ebeler F. Roentgen und radium Therapie des Uterus Karzinoms. *Zentralbl Gynakol* 1915; **39**: 217.

3. Maas JM. Intestinal changes secondary to irradiation of pelvic malignancies. *Am J Obstet Gynecol* 1948; **56**: 249.

4. Aldridge AH. Intestinal injuries resulting from irradiation treatment of uterine carcinoma. *Am J Obstet Gynecol* 1942; **44**: 833.

5. Requarth W & Roberts S. Intestinal injuries following irradiation of pelvic viscera for malignancy. *Arch Surg* 1956; **73**: 682.

6. Allen-Mersh TG, Wilson EJ, Hope-Stone HF & Mann CV. Has the incidence of radiation-induced bowel damage changed in the last 20 years? *J R Soc Med* 1986; **79**: 387.

7. Galland RB & Spencer J. Natural history and surgical management of radiation enteritis. *Br J Surg* 1987; **74**: 742.

8. Newman A, Datssaris J, Blendis LM, Charlesworth M & Walter LH. Small-intestinal injury in women who have had pelvic radiotherapy. *Lancet* 1973; **ii**: 1471.

9. McBrien MP. Vitamin B_{12} malabsorption after cobalt teletherapy for carcinoma of the bladder. *BMJ* 1973; **1**: 648.

10. Carr ND, Pullen BR, Hasleton PS & Schofield PF. Microvascular studies in human radiation bowel disease. *Gut* 1984; **25**: 448.

11. Donaldson SS, Jundt S, Ricour C, Sarrizin D, Lemerle J & Schweisguth O. Radiation enteritis in childhood. A retrospective review, clinicopathological correlation and dietary management. *Cancer* 1975; **35**: 1167.

12. Shehata WM & Meyer RL. The enhancement effect of irradiation by methotrexate: report of three complications. *Cancer* 1980; **46**: 1349.

13. Green N, Iba G & Smith WR. Measures to minimise small intestine injury in the irradiated pelvis. *Cancer* 1975; **35**: 1633.

14. Loiudice T, Baxter D & Balint J. Effects of abdominal surgery on the development of radiation enteropathy. *Gastroenterology* 1977; **73**: 1093.

15. Green N. The avoidance of small intestine injury in gynecologic cancer. *Int J Radiat Oncol Biol Phys* 1983; **9**: 1385.

16. De Cosse JJ, Rhodes RS, Wentz WB, Reagan JW, Dworken HJ & Holden WD. The natural history and management of radiation induced injury of the gastrointestinal tract. *Ann Surg* 1969; **170**: 369.

17. Gallagher MJ. A prospective study of treatment techniques to minimise the volume of pelvic small bowel with reduction of acute and late effects associated with radiation. *Int J Radiat Oncol Biol Phys* 1986; **12**: 1565.

18. Fowler JF. Non-standard fractionation in radiotherapy. *Int J Radiat Oncol Biol Phys* 1982; **8**: 50.

19. Devereux DF, Chandler JJ, Einsentat T & Zinkin L. Efficacy of an absorbable mesh in keeping the small bowel out of the human pelvis following surgery. *Dis Colon Rectum* 1988; **29**: 283.

20. Soper JT, Clance-Pearson DL & Creasman WT. Absorbable synthetic mesh (910-polyglactin) intestinal sling to reduce radiation small bowel injury in patients with pelvic malignancies. *Gynecol Oncol* 1988; **29**: 283.

21. Tanner NS, Stamford IF & Bennett A. Plasma prostaglandins in mucositis due to radiotherapy and chemotherapy for head and neck cancer. *Br J Cancer* 1981; **43**: 767.

22. Rachootin S, Shepiro S & Yamakawa T. Potent antiproteases derived from *Ascaris lumbricoides*: efficacy in amelioration of post-radiation enteropathy. *Gastroenterology* 1972; **62**: 797.

23. Buchler DA, Kline JC, Peckham BM, Boone MLM & Carr WF. Radiation reactions in cervical cancer therapy. *Am J Obstet Gynecol* 1971; **111**: 745.

24. Galland RB & Spencer J. Spontaneous postoperative perforation of previously asymptomatic irradiated bowel. *Br J Surg* 1985; **72**: 285.

25. Bosch A & Frias Z. Complications after radiation therapy for cervical carcinoma. *Acta Radiol (Ther)(Stockh)* 1977; **16**: 53.

26. Gilinsky NH, Burns DG, Barbezat GO, Levin W, Myers HS & Marks IN. The natural history of radiation-induced proctosigmoiditis: an analysis of 88 patients. *Q J Med* 1983; **205**: 40.

27. Galland RB & Spencer J. The natural history of established radiation enteritis. *Lancet* 1985; **i**: 1275.

28. Soloman A, Papo J & Stern D. Computed tomographic investigation of serosal and intramural gastrointestinal pathology. *Gastrointest Radiol* 1987; **12**: 25.

29. Mendelson RM & Nolan DJ. The radiological features of radiation enteritis. *Clin Radiol* 1985; **36**: 141.

30. Dencker H, Holidahl KH & Lunderquist AE. Mesenteric angiography in patients with radiation injury of the bowel after pelvis irradiation. *AJR* 1972; **114**: 476.

31. Levi S, Hodgson HJ, Calam J & Lavender JP. Detecting radiation enterocolitis with Tc-99m HMPAO-labelled leucocytes. Unpublished data.

32. Galland RB & Spencer J. Surgical management of radiation enteritis. *Surgery* 1986; **99**: 133.

33. Galland RB & Spencer J. Surgical aspects of radiation injury to the intestine. *Br J Surg* 1979; **66**: 135.

34. Morgenstern L, Thompson R & Friedman NB. The modern enigma of radiation enteropathy: sequelae and solutions. *Am J Surg* 1977; **134**: 166.

35. Cooke SAR & DeMoor NG. The surgical treatment of the radiation-damaged rectum. *Br J Surg* 1981; **68**: 488.

36. Sherrill DJ, Grishkin BA & Gellal FS. Radiation associated malignancies of the oesophagus. *Cancer* 1984; **54**: 726.

37. Jones DA, Steger A & Goolden AWG. Carcinoma of the oesophagus after radiotherapy for Hodgkin's disease. *Br J Radiol* 1985; **58**: 1131.

38. Ingleman-Sundberg A. Rectal injuries following radiation treatment of the cervix uteri. *Acta Radiol Suppl (Stockh)* 1947; **64**: 3.

39. Kleinerman RA, Curtin RE, Boice JD et al. Second cancers following radiotherapy for cervical cancer. *J Natl Cancer Inst* 1982; **69**: 1027.

40. Committee on the Biological Effects of Ionizing Radiation. *The Effects on Populations of Exposures to Low Levels of Ionising Radiation 1980*. Washington, DC: National Academy Press, 1980: 367.

41. Sandler RS & Sandler DP. Radiation-induced cancers of the colon and rectum. Assessing the risk. *Gastroenterology* 1983; **84**: 51.

42. Dawson PM, Galland RB & Rees HC. Mucin abnormalities in the radiation damaged colon. *Dig Surg* 1987; **4**: 19.

43. Stryker JA, Demers LM & Mortel R. Prophylactic ibuprofen administration during pelvic irradiation. *Int J Radiat Oncol Biol Phys* 1979; **5**: 2049.

44. McArdle A, Reid EC & Laplante MP. Prophylaxis against radiation injury. *Arch Surg* 1986; **121**: 879.

45. Wellwood JM & Jackson BT. The intestinal complications of radiotherapy. *Br J Surg* 1973; **60**: 814.

46. Duncan W & Leonard J. The malabsorption syndrome following radiotherapy. *Q J Med* 1965; **34**: 319.

47. Helmkamp BF & Kimmel J. Conservative management of small bowel obstruction. *Am J Obstet Gynecol* 1985; **152**: 677.

48. Conklin JL & Anuras S. Radiation-induced recurrent intestinal pseudo-obstruction. *Am J Gastroenterol* 1981; **75**: 440.

49. Goldstein F, Khoury J & Thornton JJ. Treatment of chronic radiation enteritis and colitis with salicazosulfapyridine and systemic corticosteroids. *Am J Gastroenterol* 1976; **65**: 201.

50. Patterson TJS, Berry J & Wiernick G. The effect of X-irradiation on the survival of skin flaps in the pig. *Br J Plast Surg* 1972; **25**: 17.

51. Schofield PF, Carr ND & Holden D. Pathogenesis and treatment of radiation bowel disease: discussion paper. *J R Soc Med* 1986; **79**: 30.

52. Deitel M & Vasic V. Major intestinal complications of radiotherapy. *Am J Gastroenterol* 1979; **72**: 65.

53. Russell JC & Welsh JP. Operative management of radiation injuries to the intestinal tract. *Am J Surg* 1979; **137**: 433.

54. Marks G & Mohiudden M. The surgical management of the radiation-injured intestine. *Surg Clin North Am* 1983; **63**: 81.

55. Swan RW, Fowler WC & Boronow RC. Surgical management of radiation injury to the small intestine. *Surg Gynecol Obstet* 1976; **142**: 325.

56. Smith ST, Seski JC, Copeland LJ, Gershenson DM, Edwards CL & Herson J. Surgical management of irradiation-induced small bowel damage. *Obstet Gynecol* 1985; **65**: 563.

57. Catterall M, Kingsley D, Lawrence G, Grainger J & Spencer J. The effect of fast neutrons on inoperable carcinoma of the stomach. *Gut* 1975; **16**: 150.

58. Durdey P & Williams NS. Radiation fistulae – general principles of management. In Galland RB & Spencer J (eds) *Radiation Enteritis*. London: Edward Arnold, 1990: 215.

59. Keusch GT & Present DH. Summary of workshop on clindamycin colitis. *J Infect Dis* 1976; **133**: 578.

60. Bishop FR. Spectrum of infectious agents in acute diarrhoeas. In Chadwick VS & Phillips S (eds) *Gastroenterology 2: Small Intestine*. London: Butterworth, 1982: 319.

61. Gorbach SL, Kean BH & Evans DG. Traveller's diarrhoea and toxigenic *Escherichia coli*. *N Engl J Med* 1975; **292**: 933.

62. Huckstep RL. Recent advances in the surgery of typhoid fever. *Ann R Coll Surg Eng* 1960; **26**: 207.

63. Schmidt W, Chmel H, Karundki Z & Sen P. The clinical spectrum of *Campylobacter fetus* infections: report of five cases and review of the literature. *Q J Med* 1980; **73**: 431.

64. Rao MC. Molecular mechanisms of bacterial endotoxins. In Farthing MJG & Keusch GT (eds) *Enteric Infection*. London: Chapman & Hall, 1987: 87.

65. Rohde JE & Northrup RS. Taking science where the diarrhoea is. In Elliott K & Knight J (eds) *Acute Diarrhoea* (CIBA Foundation Symposium 42). Amsterdam: Elsevier, 1976: 339.

66. Murphy AM, Grohmann GS, Christopher PJ et al. An Australia-wide outbreak of gastroenteritis from oysters caused by Norwalk virus. *Med J Aust* 1979; **2**: 329.

67. Connolly GM, Dryden MS, Shanson DE et al. Cryptosporidial diarrhoea in AIDS and its treatment. *Gut* 1988; **29**: 593.

68. Addison NV. Abdominal tuberculosis – a disease revived. *Ann R Coll Surg Engl* 1983; **65**: 105.

69. Probert CSF, Jayanthi V, Wicks AC, Carr-Locke DL, Garner P & Mayberry JF. Epidemiological study of abdominal tuberculosis among Indian migrants and the indigenous population of Leicester, 1972–1989. *Gut* 1992; **33**: 1085.

70. Braun MM, Byers RH, Heyward RL et al. Acquired immunodeficiency syndrome (AIDS) and extrapulmonary tuberculosis in the United States. *Arch Intern Med* 1990; **150**: 1913.

71. Mimica M. Usefulness and limitations of laparoscopy in the diagnosis of tuberculous peritonitis. *Endoscopy* 1992; **24**: 588.

72. Finker M, Perchick A & Burnstein DE. Fine needle aspiration biopsy of tuberculous lymphadenitis in patients with and without the acquired immune deficiency syndrome. *Acta Cytol* 1991; **35**: 325.

73. Kapoor VK & Sharma LK. Abdominal tuberculosis. *Br J Surg* 1988; **75**: 2.

74. Gilinsky NH, Marks IN, Kotter RE & Price SK. Abdominal tuberculosis: a 10-year review. *S Afr Med J* 1983; **64**: 849.

75. Katariya RN, Sood S, Rao PG & Rao PL. Stricture-plasty for tubercular strictures of the gastrointestinal tract. *Br J Surg* 1977; **64**: 496.

76. Bottone EJ. *Yersinia enterocolitica*: a panoramic view of a charismatic microorganism. *CRC Crit Rev Microbiol* 1977; **5**: 211.

77. Hoogkamp-Karstanje JA. Antibiotics in *Yersinia enterocolitica* infections. *J Antimicrob Chemother* 1987; **20**: 123.

78. Prescott RJ, Harris M & Banerjee SS. Fungal infections of the small and large intestines. *J Clin Pathol* 1992; **45**: 806.

79. Martierre WF, Mong AT & Pulito AR. Locally invasive aspergillosis of the bowel. *J Pediatr Surg* 1992; **27**: 1611.

80. Cohen R & Heffner JE. Bowel infarction as the initial manifestation of disseminated aspergillosis. *Chest* 1992; **101**: 877.

81. Rogers S, Potter MN & Slade RR. Aspergillus appendicitis in acute myeloid leukaemia. *Clin Lab Haematol* 1990; **12**: 471.

82. Webbe G. Schistosomiasis: some advances. *B M J* 1981; **283**: 1104.

83. Lehman JS, Farid Z, Bassily S, Haxton J, Abdel Wahab MF & Kent DC. Intestinal protein loss in schistosomal polyposis of the colon. *Gastroenterology* 1970; **59**: 433.

84. Ihekwaba FN. Intestinal ascariasis and the acute abdomen in the tropics. *J R Coll Surg Edinb* 1980; **25**: 452.

85. Verhamme MAM & Ramboer CHR. Anisakiasis caused by herring in vinegar: a little known medical problem. *Gut* 1988; **29**: 843.

86. Wittner M, Turner JW, Jacquette G, Ash LR, Salgo MP & Tanowitz HB. Eustrongyloidiasis – a parasitic infection acquired by eating sushi. *N Engl J Med* 1989; **320**: 1124.

87. Marsden PD. Other nematodes. *Clin Gastroenterol* 1978; **7**: 219.

88. Ali-Khan Z & Seemayer TA. Fatal bowel infarction and sepsis: an unusual complication of systemic strongyloidiasis. *Trans R Soc Trop Med Hyg* 1975; **69**: 473.

89. Grove DI. Strongyloidiasis: a conundrum for gastroenterologists. *Gut* 1994; 35: 437.

90. Brumpt E. *Précis de Parasitologie*, 6th edn vol. 1. Paris: Masson, 1902: 879.

91. Anthony PP & McAdam IWJ. Helminthic pseudotumours of the bowel: thirty-four cases of helminthoma. *Gut* 1972; **13**: 8.

92. Muller R. Pentastomes. In *Worms and Disease*. London: Heinemann, 1975: 129.

93. Farthing MJG. Giardiasis In Bouchier IAD, Allan RN, Hodgson HJF & Keighley MRB, (eds) *Gastroenterology, Clinical Science and Practice*, 2nd edn. London: WB Saunders, 1993: 1363.

94. Ravdin JI. Diagnosis of invasive amoebiasis – time to end the morphology era. *Gut* 1994; **35**: 1018.

95. Marshak RH, Lindner A, Maklansky D & Gelb A. Eosinophilic gastroenteritis. *JAMA* 1981; **245**: 1677.

96. Croese J. Human eosinophilic gastroenteritis caused by dog hookworm, *Ancylostoma caninum*. *Lancet* 1990; **336**: 571.

97. Croese J, Prociv P, Magguire EJ & Crawford AP. Eosinophilic enteritis presenting as surgical emergencies: a report of six cases. *Med J Aust* 1990; **153**: 415.

98. Morgenstern L, Freilich M & Panish JF. The circumferential small-bowel ulcer: clinical aspects in 17 patients. *JAMA* 1965; **191**: 637.

99. Campbell JR & Knapp RW. Small bowel ulceration associated with thiazide and potassium therapy: review of 13 cases. *Ann Surg* 1966; **163**: 291.

100. Boley SJ, Schultz L, Krieger H, Schwartz S, Elguezebal A & Allen AC. Experimental evaluation of thiazides and potassium as a cause of small bowel ulcer. *JAMA* 1965; **192**: 763.

101. Morris AJ, Wasson L, Park RHR & McKenzie JS. Small bowel enteroscopy with water insufflation – the first 80 cases. *Gut* 1991; **32**: A1226.

102. Bayless TM, Kapelowitz RF, Shelley WM, Ballinger WR & Hendrik TR. Intestinal ulceration, a complication of coeliac disease. *New Engl J Med* 1967; **776**: 996.

103. Swinson CMM, Storm G, Coles FC & Booth CC. Coeliac disease and malignancy. *Lancet* 1983; **i**: 111.

104. Isaacson PG, O'Connor NRJ, Spencer JO et al. Malignant histiocytosis of the intestine: a T-cell lymphoma. *Lancet* 1985; **ii**: 616.

105. Thomas WEG, Williamson RCN. Enteric ulceration and its complications *World J Surg* 1985; **9**: 876.

106. Baillie M. *The Morbid Anatomy of Some of the Most Important Parts of the Human Body* 1st American edn. Albany, Barbar and Southwick, 1795. Cited by Guest JL. *Int Abst Surg* 1963; **117**: 409.

107. Combes C. Des ulceres simples de l'intestin. Thèse de doct, Faculté de Médecine et de Pharmacie de Toulouse, 1897. Cited by Grasman M, *Arch Klin Chir* 1925; 136: 449.

108. Grasman M. Zur Frage des Ulcus Simplex des Dunndarmes. *Arch Klin Chir* 1925; **136**: 449.

109. Lawrason FD, Alpert E, Moht FL & McMahon FG. Ulcerative obstructive lesions of the small intestine. *JAMA* 1965; **191**: 641.

110. Baydstun JS, Gaffey TA & Bartholomew LG. Clinico pathologic study of non-specific ulcers of the small intestine. *Dig Dis Sci* 1981; **26**: 911.

111. Watson MR. Primary non-specific ulceration of the small intestine. *Arch Surg* 1963; **87**: 600.

112. Billig DM & Jordan GL. Non-specific ulcers of the small intestine. *Am J Surg* 1965; **110**: 745.

113. Morlock CG, Goehrs HR & Dockerty MB. Primary non-specific ulcers of the small intestine. clinicopathological study of 18 cases with follow-up of 14 previously reported cases. *Gastroenterology* 1956; **31**: 667.

114. Grosfeld JL, Schiller M, Weinberger M & Clatworthy HW. Primary non-specific ileal ulcers in children. *Am J Dis Child* 1970; **120**: 447.

115. Thomas WEG & Williamson RCN. Nonspecific small bowel ulceration. *Postgrad Med J* 1985; **61**: 587.

116. Guest JL. Nonspecific ulceration of the intestine. *Int Abst Surg* 1963; **117**: 409.

117. Bosmans L, Storms P & Gruwez JA. Chronic anaemia secondary to side-to-side distal small bowel anastomosis. *Acta Chir Belg* 1993; **93**: 25.

118. Glucksberg H, Storb R, Fefer A et al. Clinical manifestations of graft-versus-host disease in human recipients of marrow from HLA-matched sibling donors. *Transplantation* 1974; **18**: 295.

53

SMALL BOWEL OBSTRUCTION

H Ellis

INTRODUCTION

Excellent accounts of the early history of intestinal obstruction are given by Cope[1] and Wangensteen.[2] Nearly every form of fatal acute abdominal disease, from the earliest times until the beginning of the sixteenth century, was regarded as being due to obstruction of the bowels, termed ileus or iliac passion. Many of these cases were examples of peritonitis, terminating in paralytic ileus. During the seventeenth and eighteenth centuries, the more frequent performance of post-mortem examinations led to the recognition of peritonitis and later to knowledge of the various causes of peritonitis.

However, from early days, one form of intestinal obstruction to be diagnosed with accuracy was that consequent on obstruction or strangulation of the intestine in an external hernia, most often inguinal. The gravity of the acute symptoms that accompanied the sudden onset of pain and swelling in an external hernia was fully realized by the earliest surgical practitioners. Treatment comprised violent attempts at reducing the hernia, with the patient in the head-down position, supplemented by the use of cold water, hot applications, purgation and bleeding. Where this failed, in a small minority of cases the crisis may have been resolved by gangrene of the gut, abscess formation and the development of a faecal fistula, but most patients must surely have perished. Attempts at surgical division of the obstructing neck of the hernia were reported from the earliest times, and the procedure was certainly advocated by Pierre Franco in the sixteenth century.

Although colostomies were carried out for occasional examples of large bowel obstruction due to imperforate anus or rectal cancers in the pre-anaesthetic days, the management of small bowel obstruction, for practical purposes, awaited the introduction of anaesthesia and of antiseptic surgery towards the end of the nineteenth century.

Obstruction of the small intestine is a grave and life-threatening complication. If recognized and treated with speed and efficiency in its earliest stages, the immediate and long-term results are extremely gratifying in the great majority of patients. Regretfully, there is often delay which, although sometimes due to the patient, may all too frequently be attributed to the surgeon. As a result of this, distended or strangulated intestine become seriously or irreparably damaged or may even rupture, so that the situation changes to one of extreme danger when even the most skilful surgery may fail to prevent serious complications or even death. Whether the operation is carried out by the most skilful surgeon or one less experienced is infinitely less important than whether it is carried out at an early or at a late stage of the progressive changes which accompany intestinal obstruction. Much of the success of treating this condition depends on early diagnosis, skilful and prompt management and an appreciation of the importance of treating the biochemical and pathological effects of the obstruction just as much as the cause of the obstruction itself.

Obstruction of the small intestine is divided into two major groups, mechanical and neurogenic.

Mechanical obstruction implies that the intestinal contents are prevented from their passage along the bowel by obstruction of the gut lumen. Mechanical obstruction, in turn, is subdivided into two major categories, simple and strangulated.

In *simple obstruction*, the problem is purely one of obstruction to the passage of intestinal contents. However, as progressive distension of the gut occurs, the blood supply of its wall may become compromised and necrosis may follow. In *strangulated obstruction*, however, there is also an immediate occlusion to the blood supply of the involved segment of the intestine which, if unrelieved, must inevitably lead to gangrene.

In *neurogenic* or *adynamic obstruction* (or ileus) the intestinal contents do not traverse the bowel because of intestinal paralysis. The two common examples of this are postoperative ileus and mesenteric infarction.

Classification of the enormous variety of causes of mechanical small bowel obstruction is considered under the three headings that apply to any obstructed tube within the body:[3]

1. Causes in the lumen, e.g. gallstone ileus, food bolus obstruction;

2. Causes in the wall, e.g. congenital atresias, inflammatory strictures, small bowel neoplasms;

3. Causes outside the wall, e.g. strangulated hernia, obstruction due to adhesions or bands, volvulus and intussusception.

Mechanical obstruction may also be classified according to its site (high or low in the small intestine) and its speed of onset, which determines whether the obstruction is acute, chronic or acute superimposed on a chronic obstruction.

Aetiology

An interesting and quite remarkable change has taken place in the aetiology of acute small bowel obstruction within the lifetime of today's surgeons. Up to World War II, strangulated external hernias accounted for a high percentage of the total cases of intestinal obstruction, whereas obstruction due to adhesions was relatively uncommon (as was large bowel obstruction due to cancer). Thus, Vick[4] carried out an important review in 1932 of 6892 patients with acute intestinal obstruction admitted to 21 hospitals in the UK between 1925 and 1930. Of these, 49% were due to strangulated external hernias whereas adhesions were responsible for only 7% (tumours accounted for 13% of the total). Since then, strangulated hernias have fallen in incidence, no doubt due to the fact that elective operations are performed more frequently even in relatively old and feeble subjects. However, in keeping with the enormous increase in the frequency of abdominal operations, postoperative adhesions have become far more common as a cause of intestinal obstruction. Waldron and Hampton[5] reported in 1961 that 40% of their 493 cases of intestinal obstruction were due to adhesions, compared with only 12% of strangulated hernias. The same authors reviewed five large series of cases published between 1905 and 1931 and found 7.5% were due to adhesions compared with 58.2% resulting from strangulated hernias. They compared this percentage with an analysis of another five large series of cases carried out between 1940 and 1953, in which the incidence of adhesions had risen to 38.2% whereas that of strangulated hernias had fallen to 24.1%. McEntee et al.[6] have reviewed 228 patients admitted to four district hospitals in the North of England (draining an estimated population of 591 000) over a 12-month period. Strangulated hernias accounted for 25% of the total,

whereas adhesions amounted to 32%. In our own series[7] at Westminster Hospital, of 279 patients admitted between 1962 and 1983, 31% had obstruction due to adhesions and 23% had strangulated hernias. These cases included both large and small bowel obstruction, the latter accounting for 36% of the admissions. This pattern reflects our particular interest in neoplastic disease, since 84 of the patients had malignant obstruction of the large intestine. In most published series in the Western World, between 70 and 80% of all cases of intestinal obstruction involve the small intestine.

Geographical distribution

There are wide and interesting differences between the common causes of small bowel obstruction through the world. These differences depend on a wide variety of factors, including dietary habits, genetic differences, anatomical variations, differences in life expectancy and, as will be discussed, to a very considerable extent on the provision of surgical facilities in a particular community. Thus, in many undeveloped parts of the world, strangulated external hernia remains the most common cause of small bowel obstruction, just as pertained 50 or 60 years ago in the Western World. In contrast, intestinal obstruction due to adhesions in these same communities is at a much lower level than in the Western World, and this correlates very well with the comparatively low incidence of sophisticated abdominal surgery with its resultant intra-abdominal adhesions. Those cases of adhesive obstruction that are found in these areas very often result from pelvic inflammatory disease. Some noteworthy figures for the causes of obstruction reported from parts of India, East, Central and West Africa, and from the West Indies are presented in Table 53.1.[8-14]

It is interesting that Ti and Yong[15] found that the sophisticated local Chinese population in Malaysia has adhesions as the most common cause of small bowel obstruction whereas the less sophisticated Malay and Indian patients presented

Table 53.1 Causes of obstruction in India, Africa and the West Indies

STUDY (LOCALE)	NO. OF CASES	TYPE OF OBSTRUCTION (%)					VOLVULUS	
		ADHESION	HERNIA	INTUSUSS-CEPTION	MALIGNANCY	TUBERCU-LOSIS	LARGE BOWEL	SMALL BOWEL
Gill and Eggleston[8] (Punjab)	147	15	27	12	–	3	9	16
McAdam[9] (Kampala, Uganda)	794	4	75	4	1	–	13	0.4
White[10] (Bulawayo, Zimbabwe)	172	17	36	7	–	–	11	8
Chiedozi[11] (Benin City, Nigeria)	316	10.8	65	11.4	0.3	–	–	8
Cole[12] (Ibadan, Nigeria)	436	10	35	27	1	0.7	0.7	3
Badoe[13] (Accra, Ghana)	782	10	77.6	4	0.6	–	4	1
Brooks and Butler[14] (Jamaica)	250	23	25	19	5	–	6	0.4

Modified from Ellis.[3]

most frequently with strangulated hernias. It could be that the medical sophistication of a community can be judged by the extent to which postoperative adhesion obstruction outweighs the incidence of strangulated external hernia.

In India, tuberculosis of the ileocaecal region is relatively common. There was a 3% incidence noted in the series from the Punjab,[8] although in the Western World it is practically non-existent except among the immigrant population. By contrast, Crohn's disease is uncommon in developing communities. Tandon and Prakash[16] reviewed 212 patients with chronic or subacute small bowel obstruction in Delhi. Of these, 159 were diagnosed as tuberculosis, whereas the authors could identify only 10 examples of Crohn's disease of the terminal ileum.

There is a surprisingly high incidence of intussusception in West Nigeria[12] where it occurs in both children and young adults, and a similarly high incidence of idiopathic intussusception in the adult black population of Natal.[17]

There is a remarkable variation in the incidence of volvulus of both the large and small intestine throughout the world, its incidence being particularly high in Third World countries. Although rare in most communities in the West, it is common in Finland.[18] In Zimbabwe, White[10] reported that nearly 20% of 112 obstructions were caused by sigmoid volvulus, but volvulus of the small intestine was also remarkably common in that country (11.6%). In the Punjab, volvulus of both small and large intestine is common.[8] In Iran, Saidi[19] noted that of 286 obstructions, 13.6% had volvulus of the sigmoid, 5.7% volvulus of the caecum and 22.7% volvulus of the small intestine.

En passant, it should be noted that the low incidence of carcinoma in less developed countries becomes obvious and may merely reflect the lower life expectancy in these communities. Dietary and genetic factors may also play a part.

PATHOPHYSIOLOGY OF SMALL BOWEL OBSTRUCTION

It has already been noted that obstruction of the small bowel lumen may be produced by causes in the lumen, causes in the gut wall and extrinsic causes. It is in the third group, together with instances of mesenteric infarction, that strangulation of the bowel may supervene. However, even in the absence of strangulation, ischaemia progressing to necrosis and eventually to perforation of the dead bowel can occur in simple obstruction. This complication may be due to pressure necrosis at the site where a tight band passes across a loop of bowel, or a stercoral ulceration of the gut wall may occur as a result of pressure necrosis produced by a foreign body or impacted bowel contents within the gut lumen. Gross distension of the intestine may impair the blood supply to the wall to such a degree that patchy necrosis occurs and can progress to perforation.

In simple obstruction, there are important and progressive changes that take place in the bacteriological content of the bowel above the obstruction, in the amount of gas contained therein, in the circulation of the distended bowel wall and in the fluid and electrolyte fluxes that take place across it. When the picture is complicated by strangulation, these changes are compounded by the progressive vascular alterations in the affected intestine, eventually leading to peritonitis associated with death or even perforation of the gut wall.

Microbiology of bowel obstruction

The normal upper small intestine contains only transient flora. More distally, the small bowel contents yields a scanty growth of faecal organisms. However, in the presence of obstruction, rapid colonization of organisms, predominantly faecal in type, occurs above the point of obstruction. The longer the period of occlusion, the higher up the bowel contamination extends, whereas the small bowel below the obstruction remains either sterile or contains only a few transient colonies. Normally, bacteria traverse the small intestine so quickly that appreciable growth does not occur. In the presence of the stasis produced by obstruction, proliferation by geometrical progression results in rapid colonization of the gut lumen.

Sykes and his colleagues[20] performed needle aspiration of the intestine in patients with small bowel obstruction or acute large bowel obstruction and in a control group of patients undergoing surgery for gallstones. They were able to demonstrate an increase in organisms above the obstruction with a considerable increase in the anaerobic bacteria, especially *Bacteroides*. This growth was particularly evident in patients with large bowel obstruction. Jejunal specimens were obtained by intubation during the early period of postoperative recovery after operation for the relief of small bowel obstruction. The bacterial flora returned to normal by the fourth or fifth postoperative day, the greatest reduction in organisms occurring on the second and third days.

Distension

The distended bowel above an obstruction contains both gas and fluid. Although gas may be seen radiologically in the small intestine in normal children, it is absent after the age of about seven years. Originally it was thought that the gas accumulating above an obstruction originated from putrefaction of the bowel contents. However, in the classical study by Wangensteen and Rea,[21] cervical oesophagostomies in dogs, which had obstruction of the terminal ileum, virtually prevented abdominal distension apart from the 20 cm of intestine immediately above the obstruction. Provided that they were maintained on intravenous fluids, these animals could live for an average of 35 days. However, dogs without an oesophagostomy rapidly became distended and did not survive for more than five days. This experiment showed that the distension, at least in this experimental model, was mainly due to swallowed air. It is well known that serial radiographs taken of patients undergoing intravenous pyelography show progressive dilatation of the bowel with air, especially in nervous patients, and can be prevented by gastric aspiration. Excessive air swallowing is likely to occur in patients suffering from any acute abdominal pain. Faecal organisms can ferment cellulose, so part of the gaseous distension of the colon may be due to such fermentation, but there is little doubt that the bulk of the gas distending the small bowel in obstruction results from aerophagy.

Fluid loss

There are two factors that account for the fluid accumulation above the level of the obstruction: (1) loss of absorptive surface and (2) alteration in the fluid and electrolyte flux across the bowel wall proximal to the obstruction.

In the healthy subject, approximately 7 litres of gastrointestinal secretions pour into the alimentary tract each 24 hours. Almost all of this fluid is absorbed in the colon. In the presence of an obstruction of the small intestine, the colonic absorptive surface is lost and this large amount of fluid accumulates above the obstruction. This loss of water and electrolytes into the bowel is compounded by a decreased absorption across the gut mucosa and an increased secretion into the bowel lumen from the bloodstream. The experiments by Shields[22] in the dog using isotopes of water, sodium and potassium, demonstrated that within 12 hours of obstruction there is a decrease in absorption of water from the gut into the bloodstream which is accompanied, after 36 hours, by an increase in water shift from the blood into the gut lumen, with a net accumulation of water in the intestine. The potassium in the bowel lumen is also increased by a similar mechanism. The diminution of movement of sodium from the lumen of the gut into the blood is not so great, but the movement in the opposite direction is increased fourfold within 48 hours.

Circulatory changes

Although simple mechanical obstruction can be defined as a compromise of the lumen of the bowel without compromise of its blood supply, progressive distension, even in the absence of strangulation, can impair the intramural circulation of the bowel. As the bowel becomes increasingly distended, although the intraluminal pressure may only rise moderately, there may be considerable tension in the bowel wall itself, and this is evident when the distended gut is examined at operation. This tension produces increased resistance in the capillaries, which eventually leads to complete stagnation of the bowel wall circulation in the advanced case. Obliteration of the blood supply probably results from a combination of progressive thinning of the wall of the bowel, narrowing of the lumen of its vessels and the increased pressure within the bowel lumen. The least blood supply is at the antimesenteric border of the intestine, and it is here that the bowel eventually tends to perforate from ischaemic necrosis.

PATHOLOGY OF STRANGULATED OBSTRUCTION

Strangulated intestinal obstruction presents a considerably more complex pathological problem than simple gut occlusion.[23] In addition to the physiological disturbances that accompany simple obstruction, there are the additional factors of blood loss into the infarcted bowel, death of tissue within the strangulated segment of intestine, passage of toxins across the damaged bowel wall into the peritoneal cavity and, in advanced cases, the toxaemia produced by frank perforation of the gangrenous segment.

As progressive increase of pressure occurs within the obstructed bowel loop, this first exceeds the venous pressure in the gut wall with consequent venous engorgement of these vessels, followed by capillary rupture and haemorrhagic infiltration. This process occurs first in the submucosa, then the mucosa and then throughout all layers of the gut wall. Thrombosis in the intramural and mesenteric veins hastens this ischaemic process. Necrosis appears first on the mucosal surface of the gut[24] because of the relative vulnerability of the gut epithelium to anoxia. It is quite common when examining a resected specimen of ischaemic gut to note a fairly healthy external appearance accompanied by a marked degree of mucosal damage. Eventually ischaemic changes take place throughout the thickness of the gut wall, leading finally to perforation of the totally necrotic segment.

During the evolution of these changes in strangulation, there is increasing exudate of fluid across the damaged bowel wall into the peritoneal cavity. This changes from an initial clear serous fluid into a haemorrhagic, and finally a stinking black exudation. This loss of protein-rich and blood containing fluid is a contributing factor to the hypovolaemic shock in these patients.

Initially, the exudate is sterile, but within a few hours it teems with both aerobic and anaerobic organisms. It is not surprising that this exudate can be shown experimentally to be highly toxic. Much of this toxicity is probably the effect of the endotoxins produced by Gram-negative faecal organisms.

Postischaemic stenosis

If a segment of strangulated bowel is encountered at operation, the involved segment is resected if considered non-viable. If the circulation improves and the bowel recovers its normal appearance, it is replaced into the abdominal cavity, usually with total recovery. Very occasionally, however, although the strangulated gut may appear viable, it may undergo slow progressive stenosis over a matter of weeks, months or even years. Obviously infarction of the muscle wall has taken place in such cases with subsequent fibrous replacement of the damaged tissues. Early cases were described in which reduction by taxis had been carried out for strangulated hernias. Obre[24] in 1851 gave the first example of this phenomenon following operation; this was a woman of 34 years operated on for a strangulated inguinal hernia, at which time ischaemic small intestine was found in the sac and reduced. Seven months later she developed obstructive symptoms, and she eventually died 10 months after her initial hernia reduction. At autopsy, there was a stricture of the intestine at the site of the originally obstructed small intestine.

Barry[25] gives an historical review of this condition. It is a little surprising that such lesions following gut infarction are unusual. Presumably in clinical practice there is an 'all or none' situation in which either the gut undergoes total necrosis or virtual complete recovery.

Similar strictures of the small intestine have been reported after mesenteric infarction and after crush injury to the abdomen, presumably as a result of a tear of the mesentery insufficient to produce complete necrosis but enough to produce partial infarction of the bowel. Lien and colleagues[26] have reviewed four examples of this phenomenon.

DIAGNOSIS

Clinical features

The patient with acute abdominal pain remains one of the main purely clinical problems that confront the medical practitioner today. In no other common situation is reliance on the clinical features, immediate decision and accurate diagnosis of such great importance.[3] A delay of even a few hours in initiating the correct line of treatment may make all the difference between a smooth or a stormy course or, indeed, even place the patient in mortal danger. Nowhere else in this more true than when the emergency is due to a small bowel obstruction.

Not only is this an important diagnostic problem but it is also often an extremely difficult one. It may be difficult to obtain an accurate history from a patient who is rolling around with agonizing abdominal pain, nor is it a simple matter to examine an exquisitely tender abdomen. To compound the problem, laboratory and radiological investigations, although often helpful, may at other times yield little more information than the clinical findings and can even be frankly misleading. A patient with a gangrenous loop of small intestine may have entirely normal abdominal radiographs, a white count within normal limits and nothing on the battery of biochemical investigations to suggest a potentially lethal situation within the abdomen.

Diagnosis depends on the classical triad of a carefully taken history, a meticulously performed physical examination and special investigations, but it must be stressed that the first two are by far the most important. It is a very good general clinical rule (and nowhere more apposite than in the acute abdominal emergency), that if the special investigations fit in with the diagnosis made as a result of clinical findings, then these provide most helpful confirmatory evidence. However, if there is disagreement between the laboratory findings and the diagnosis based on a careful clinical assessment, then it is a wise surgeon who sides with the latter rather than the former.

Accurate diagnosis of intestinal obstruction comprises four steps.

1. Is the patient suffering from intestinal obstruction or not?
2. If so, can its level in the bowel be located?
3. Can we attempt to differentiate between a simple and strangulated obstruction? (As will be shown later, this is often little more than an inspired guess.)
4. Can we diagnose the exact cause of the obstruction?

The classical quartet of clinical features of intestinal obstruction is colicky abdominal pain, vomiting, absolute constipation and abdominal distension. It might be thought that the diagnosis of obstruction would therefore be a relatively simple matter. However, in practice, one or more of these features might not be present. The pain may have been disguised by opiates given before the surgeon has seen the patient; vomiting is delayed in a low intestinal obstruction; if the obstruction is incomplete, flatus may still pass; moreover, a loaded large bowel below the obstruction can still provide one or two faecal actions before constipation becomes total; finally, distension may not be an obvious feature in a very high small bowel obstruction.

Symptoms

The surgeon must use a fine economy in taking a history from the patient with acute abdominal pain. Care must be taken not to exhaust and exasperate a sick patient who is in considerable pain with a lot of irrelevant questions.

Pain is by far the commonest symptom in acute intestinal obstruction. The onset may be either insidious or relatively abrupt in simple occlusion, but with a strangulation obstruction the onset is more often sudden and severe. The pain occurs in colicky spasms which last for 2–3 minutes, rising to a peak and then falling or even stopping completely before the next spasm occurs. During the pain, the patient is anxious and restless. He or she may draw up the knees or roll over onto one side in a curled-up position in an effort to find some comfort. The whole attitude is in contrast to the patient with peritonitis, who tries to keep entirely still and finds the slightest movement agonizing.

Synchronous with the spasms of pain, noisy borborygmi may be heard. *Vomiting* classically occurs at an early stage in a high small intestinal obstruction but is delayed or even absent when the obstruction is in the distal small intestine or, particularly, in the large bowel. Initially the vomit comprises recently ingested food and clear gastric juice, but within hours it becomes bile-stained and then becomes dark brown with a characteristic and unforgettable stench – so-called faeculent vomiting. This smell results from the profuse bacterial growth in the stagnant intestinal contents above the obstruction (as described above). Copious fluid loss results in dehydration; which soon becomes clinically obvious as extreme thirst, dry tongue and skin, and scanty urine.

Distension depends on the site of the obstruction and the length of time that the bowel has been occluded. If the obstruction is in the proximal jejunum, the stomach becomes distended with gas and secretions so that there may be a swelling in the epigastric region, but the rest of the abdomen remains unremarkable. A low small bowel obstruction is accompanied by a distension of the central part of the abdomen, but gross distension often means a colonic obstruction. Indeed, the most remarkable distension of the abdomen is usually seen in sigmoid volvulus.

Constipation is commonly absolute, by which is meant that neither flatus nor faeces have been passed. However, as has already been noted, there may be exceptions to the rule. A partial obstruction may allow gas to pass in a Richter's hernia, where only part of the bowel wall is implicated, and there may be normal bowel function. There may be a natural or enema-produced evacuation of faecal contents that are lying distal to the obstruction.

It was once the practice to administer an enema or even to give two diagnostic enemas in order to determine whether the patient was capable of passing flatus or faeces. It was assumed that if no flatus had passed even after the administration of a second enema then complete intestinal obstruction was present. This test is unreliable and exhausting to the patient and should be relegated to the shelves of surgical history.

Other points in the history include details of any previous abdominal operations, since a scar on the abdomen in a patient with intestinal obstruction strongly suggests a diagnosis of intra-abdominal adhesions or a band. A history of change in bowel habit, together perhaps with the presence of blood and mucus in the faeces, suggests a large bowel obstruction due to a carcinoma. The history may reveal such rare information as: the recent ingestion of potassium chloride tablets, suggesting the possibility of a small bowel stricture; pain down the inner side of the thigh in a thin elderly woman, which suggests the possibility of a strangulated obturator hernia; or previous episodes of biliary pain, which raises the question of a gallstone ileus.

Examination

The clinical examination also requires its own particular skill. It is a mistake to rush ahead and palpate the abdomen at once. Time should be spent in careful observation of the patient as a whole and of the abdomen in particular. In the early stages of obstruction, the temperature, pulse, respiration and blood pressure are usually within normal limits but as the obstruction progresses, the patient becomes anxious and pale, the pulse rate rises and there may be a drop in temperature and blood pressure. Shock tends to be more marked in a case of strangulated obstruction. As the condition progresses, there are obvious signs of dehydration.

Careful inspection of the abdomen may reveal localized or general distension and also visible peristalsis. This sign is not itself pathognomonic of obstruction and may be seen in a normal individual who has a particularly thin abdominal wall or a ventral hernia. However, visible peristalsis associated with severe colicky pain is certainly strongly suggestive of a bowel obstruction. A previous laparotomy scar should be carefully searched for as this may have been almost forgotten by the patient but is a vital clue. (The author operated on a patient of 95 whose adhesive obstruction resulted from her ovarian cystectomy 50 years previously.) Next, scrutinize and carefully palpate the hernial orifices. Perhaps the most common sign to be missed is the small strangulated inguinal, umbilical or, more especially, femoral hernia particularly in an obese woman. It may seem unbelievable that a patient with intestinal obstruction does not know that he or she has an irreducible hernia but this is frequently the case. Some years ago a distinguished anaesthetist was admitted who, when seized with acute abdominal pain, realized that this was due to an intestinal obstruction but was quite unaware that he had a strangulated inguinal hernia. A cardinal rule that must never be omitted in any patient with acute abdominal pain is to inspect and palpate the hernial orifices.

Next the abdomen is palpated with the greatest delicacy. An abdomen that will relax completely under gentle palpation and allow the posterior abdominal wall to be massaged rarely, if ever, harbours an acute surgical pathology. Tenderness, release tenderness and muscle guarding are all features of intestinal obstruction and tend to be more marked in the strangulated case, although this is by no means an invariable rule. A mass may be detected on palpation and this may be due to a tumour, Crohn's disease, an inflammatory mass or an intussusception.

Particular skill is required in palpation of the abdomen in children. Utmost gentleness is essential. The child is best held in the mother's arms and the examiner's warmed hand is then insinuated beneath the blankets and under the cover of soothing words. If all else fails, the patient must be examined again after sedation.

Auscultation nearly always reveals increased bowel sounds in mechanical obstruction. Indeed, they may be so loud that borborygmi may be heard without the aid of any instrument. Loud, splashing, rushing or tinkling sounds may be heard with the stethoscope, and these exaggerated noises may correspond to the spasms of colicky pain. By contrast, the silent abdomen suggests ileus or infarction of the intestine. If large amounts of free fluid are present, transmitted heart and breath sounds may be detected on auscultation.

A rectal examination should never be omitted. Typically in intestinal obstruction the rectum is ballooned. This is an undoubted clinical phenomenon, and yet I have not come across any satisfactory explanation of · its aetiology. Occasionally a low lying obstructive tumour may be found or an impacted mass of faeces. A pelvic swelling may be palpable through the rectal mucosa, and blood or slime on the examining finger again suggests a large bowel pathology. Rarely the tip of an intussusception may be felt.

Special investigations

A full blood count, serum electrolytes and blood urea estimation should be performed. A raised white cell count is suggestive of strangulation but, as is discussed later, this is not at all a reliable feature. A raised haemoglobin level indicates haemoconcentration and is a guide to subsequent fluid replacement. Severe electrolyte depletion due to loss of gastrointestinal fluid in vomit and gut sequestration will be indicated by diminution in the serum sodium, potassium, chloride and bicarbonate and an elevation of the blood urea.

If the diagnosis of the patient's acute abdominal pain is in any doubt, it is valuable to do a serum amylase estimation, since acute pancreatitis always enters into the differential diagnosis of such a case.

Radiological investigations

The radiological investigations of a patient with acute small bowel obstruction are important, but it is essential to remember that at least 5% of patients with this condition have entirely normal abdominal radiographs. A strangulated loop of small intestine, completely filled with fluid, is radiolucent. A normal radiograph must *never* be considered to exclude a sound clinical diagnosis of intestinal obstruction.[27]

Plain radiographs of the abdomen are taken in the erect and lying positions. With the patient supine, the radiographs show the amount and distribution of gas in the gut (Figure 53.1). Distended loops of small intestine lie transversely in a stepladder manner across the centre of the abdomen (Figure 53.2). The small bowel folds traverse the complete width of the gut shadow and are spaced at regular intervals. The gas shadows of the large intestine are located peripherally and show haustral folds that do not completely traverse the width of the intestine. The distended caecum is smooth-walled and usually easily identified in the right iliac fossa. In complete obstruction, gas is absent within the rectum. With the patient erect, the association of gas and fluid gives rise to a series of fluid levels. If perforation has occurred, there will be free gas beneath the diaphragm (Figure 53.3).

A number of specific forms of intestinal obstruction may give typical appearances on plain radiographs. Although it should be evident on clinical examination, a strangulated groin hernia may demonstrate a bubble of gas in the strangulated bowel in the groin region. Gallstone ileus may show air in the biliary system, as a result of the fistula between the gall bladder and duodenum, and the gallstone itself may be visualized. Volvulus of the colon usually reveals a tremendously distended large bowel loop.

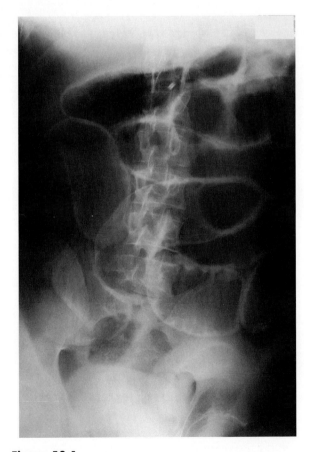

Figure 53.1
Supine radiograph of the abdomen showing gross small bowel distension. The patient had had an abdominal operation a few months previously. Obstruction at any time after laparotomy makes adhesions a likely cause, as was found in this case.

In doubtful cases or in partial small bowel obstruction, follow-through radiographs after ingestion of an aqueous contrast medium such as gastrografin may be extremely helpful. However, this material rapidly loses density in transit owing to dilution with gut contents. In practice, it is quite safe to use barium sulphate, which maintains its opacity, and there is very little danger of its impaction above the small bowel obstruction because the considerable fluid accumulation above the occlusion rapidly dilutes the medium. Another useful technique, particularly if the patient has a nasogastric tube already in place, is to inject the barium suspension through the nasogastric tube.[28]

If the diagnosis lies between obstruction of the large or small bowel, an emergency water-soluble contrast enema can be extremely valuable. It will confirm the diagnosis of mechanical large bowel obstruction and, most importantly, eliminate the diagnosis of colonic pseudo-obstruction, where there will be free flow of the contrast to the caecum.[29,30]

Location of the obstruction in the small bowel

Having diagnosed a small bowel obstruction, it may be possible to make a reasonable guess as to its level. An obstruction high in the small bowel, in the upper jejunal area, is suggested by rapid onset of copious and frequent vomiting with early development of dehydration owing to this fluid loss. Abdominal distension may be absent at least in the early stages, although later the upper abdomen becomes distended.

By contrast, an obstruction low down in the small intestine is likely to be associated with later and less profuse vomiting and with more marked abdominal distension, which involves the central abdomen.

These clinical clues may be reinforced by examination of the distended loops seen on the plain abdominal radiographs and confirmed, in doubtful or subacute cases, by a limited barium meal and follow-through examination, as described above (Figure 53.3).

DIFFERENTIATION BETWEEN A SIMPLE AND STRANGULATED OBSTRUCTION

Textbook descriptions and many surgical articles imply that the differential diagnosis between a strangulated and simple obstruction is a fairly straightforward affair. Different authorities stress different clinical or laboratory features. Those suggesting that the obstruction is associated with a strangulated loop of bowel include:

1. A sudden onset of the abdominal pain, which tends to be continuous rather than the classical colicky attacks;

2. The early appearance of shock;

3. The presence of fever and progressive elevation of the pulse;

4. Abdominal palpation which reveals marked tenderness, the presence of a positive release tenderness test with abdominal guarding and a tender abdominal mass;

5. An early elevation of the white blood count.

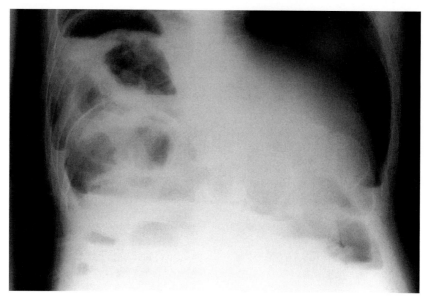

Figure 53.2
Plain abdominal radiograph (supine) showing low small bowel obstruction secondary to a strangulated hernia. Besides adhesions, strangulated hernia is the other common cause of obstruction of the small intestine.

In point of fact, analysis of any series of cases of small bowel obstruction or, better still, a critical study of one's own experience, soon demonstrates that attempts at the differential

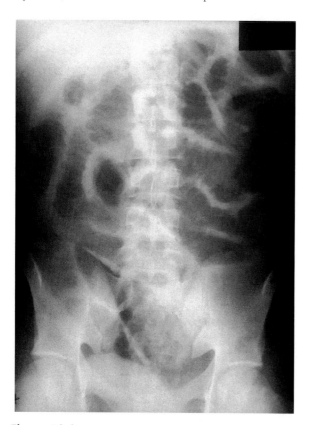

Figure 53.3
Erect abdominal radiograph showing gas under each cupola of the diaphragm in a patient with a neglected adhesion obstruction of the small bowel that had proceeded to strangulation and perforation of the bowel.

diagnosis between these two forms of obstruction are often little more than an academic exercise. Any experienced surgical registrar will soon recall examples that he has operated on of patients with obstruction who seemed relatively fit, who lacked any of the features listed above and yet who, at laparotomy, were found to have a strangulated, even gangrenous, loop of small bowel within the abdominal cavity.

Cooke[31] in a survey among senior surgical registrars in the UK found that nearly all of them felt unable to distinguish with any degree of certainty between a simple and a strangulated obstruction. Silen and colleagues[32] found that only 15% of 112 cases of strangulated obstruction were correctly diagnosed at initial hospital admission, and in more than a third of the cases the presence of intestinal obstruction was not even suspected at this stage. Simple obstruction of the small bowel was the initial diagnosis in the remaining 48% of cases, and 18% of the abdominal radiographs in this series were interpreted as being normal.

Careful studies comparing the clinical and laboratory features of simple and strangulated obstructions have been carried out by Becker[33] and by Zollinger and Kinsey,[34] which show that none of the features listed above are of any real help in differentiating between simple and strangulated obstructions. Their comparative figures are presented in Table 53.2.

It is true that in the extreme example of bowel infarction – mesenteric vascular occlusion – the physical signs and laboratory data suggest a rapid and progressive abdominal catastrophy. Thus, in a compilation of symptoms and signs based on some 1500 patients with this condition, Jackson[35] found pain, vomiting and an elevated white blood count to be present in almost every case. It was not uncommon for the white count to be $20 \times 10^9/l$ in the early hours of the disease, and it could reach up to $40 \times 10^9/l$ when gangrene of the bowel was

Table 53.2 Clinical features of simple and strangulated obstructions

	SIMPLE CASES (%)	STRANGULATED CASES (%)
Becker (1952)[35] *New Orleans*	(*n*=324)	(*n*=88)
Temperature >37.7°C	16	23
P >100	15	23
Abdominal or pelvic tenderness	73	82
Mass	5	10
Leucocytosis	44	50
All these signs absent	12	7
Zollinger and Kinsey (1964)[34] *Columbus, Ohio*	(*n* = 387)	(*n* = 45)
Temperature >37.2°C	38	45
P >100	38	52
Mass	22	32
Constant pain	18	20
White blood cells > 15,000	27	38

Modified from Ellis.[3]

established. Two-thirds of the patients were in shock, and about 70% showed abdominal tenderness.

In this context, Wilson and Imrie[36] performed serum amylase estimations on 63 patients with mesenteric infarction on admission to hospital. Fifteen of these patients had levels that reached greater than twice normal, and five patients had amylase levels that were in the diagnostic range of acute pancreatitis (above 1200 units/l), leading to inappropriate non-operative treatment in four cases. The magnitude of the hyperamylasaemia appeared to be related to the extent of the bowel infarction, the highest levels occurring when this involved the small bowel and colon. This increase was not due to associated acute pancreatitis, as no evidence of pancreatitis was found in those patients coming to autopsy. They postulate transudation of amylase across the dead bowel wall into the peritoneal cavity and its subsequent absorption into the bloodstream as the probable explanation of this phenomenon.

Perhaps in the future more use will be made of the computer and multivariate analysis of data in predicting whether or not gut is strangulated. Pain and colleagues[37] fed into a computer with multivariate analysis the details of 120 patients with simple small bowel obstruction that settled with conservative treatment, 38 patients with viable strangulation of the small bowel and 39 with non-viable strangulated small bowel obstruction found at operation. The thresholds used were; age of the patient; duration of symptoms; absence or presence of pain and whether this was colicky or continuous; increased, normal, decreased or absent bowel sounds; temperature; heart rate and white cell count. The computer was then able to identify correctly 85% of patients with simple obstruction, 61% with viable strangulation and 74% with non-viable strangulation. More importantly, it allocated correctly 82% of patients with viable strangulation and 90% of those with non-viable strangulation to categories in which strangulation was present or would occur. This performance contrasted

with the diagnostic accuracy of the surgeon, since only 66% of patients with viable strangulation and 46% of patients with non-viable strangulation had been correctly diagnosed by the surgeon as requiring immediate operation. Although the authors do not advocate that the decision to operate or not should be made by the computer, they suggest that the computer may assist in those patients whom the surgeon initially decides to treat conservatively. This assistance may reduce the number of patients who are subsequently found to have strangulation after a period of non-operative treatment.

Computer or no computer, the fact of the matter remains that there is no reliable technique currently available that can differentiate with certainty between a strangulated or non-strangulated obstruction.

ACCURATE DETERMINATION OF THE CAUSE OF THE OBSTRUCTION

The last step in the diagnostic cascade is an attempt to diagnose the exact aetiology of the small bowel obstruction. In many cases this may be obvious, such as the presence of a strangulated external hernia, the presence of a mass highly suggestive of an intussusception in a young child or the presence of a scar on the abdominal wall, which always means obstruction due to adhesions or a band until proved otherwise. A previous history of peritoneal or pelvic infection is also suggestive of adhesive obstruction.

The age of the patient gives a useful clue as to the likely causes of intestinal obstruction. Table 53.3 lists the common causes of obstruction at the various age groups.

Some special forms of obstruction and their specific diagnoses are considered later in this chapter.

Differential diagnosis

Nothing can be so easy, nor can present with such difficulty, as the diagnosis of a patient with an 'acute' abdomen. The novice

Table 53.3 Common causes of small bowel obstruction according to age group

AGE GROUP	CAUSES OF OBSTRUCTION
Neonatal	Congenital atresia Volvulus neonatorum Meconium ileus
Infancy	Strangulated inguinal hernia Intussusception Complications of Meckel's diverticulum
Young adults	Adhesions and bands Strangulated inguinal hernia
Middle age	Adhesions and bands Strangulated inguinal hernia Strangulated femoral hernia (females)
Elderly	Adhesions and bands Strangulated inguinal hernia Strangulated femoral hernia (females) Strangulated umbilical hernia Internal herniations (e.g. obturator)

may be amused at the long list of differential diagnoses given in the textbooks yet, with more experience, he or she has the chagrin of crossing off one by one the mistakes made in this long and sometimes surprising list of possibilities.

Intra-abdominal causes

It may be difficult to differentiate between an acute small bowel and a large bowel mechanical obstruction. As the lines of treatment are very similar, this error is not usually of serious consequence. The other causes of acute abdominal colicky pain include biliary and ureteric colic, usually due to calculous disease, and acute appendicitis. Indeed, a retroileal acutely inflamed appendix, particularly in an elderly subject, may well present with fairly centrally placed abdominal pain and marked abdominal distension closely mimicking a low small bowel obstruction. Acute pancreatitis and ruptured aortic aneurysm both present with abdominal distension, severe pain and collapse. Both are usually accompanied by severe lumbar pain, and detection of a pulsating mass in the case of the ruptured aneurysm is an important diagnostic aid. The differential diagnosis from a patient with advanced peritonitis may be extremely difficult; indeed, as has already been discussed, the patient with advanced strangulated obstruction will have an associated peritonitis from transudation of toxins and bacteria across the damaged bowel wall (or even through the perforated necrotic intestine).

Extra-abdominal causes

Upper abdominal pain, tenderness and guarding may be associated with acute pulmonary or pleural infection and may be experienced in an acute myocardial infarction.

Neurological conditions include herpes zoster affecting the lower thoracic segments, epidemic myalgia (Bornholm disease) and acute lead poisoning.

Medical conditions include abdominal pain and vomiting which may accompany diabetic keto-acidosis. It is essential to test the urine for sugar as a routine in all patients with acute abdominal pain and to perform a blood sugar estimation if there is any doubt. Sickle-cell anaemia may produce abdominal pain and tenderness during an acute haemolytic episode, although the nature of this pain is not understood.

Special diagnostic difficulties[38]

If one asks any group of surgeons to list the real difficulties in diagnosis of patients presenting with the features of intestinal obstruction, they will probably include four categories: the very young patient, the elderly, the postoperative case and the malingerer.

In children, the history is often hard to obtain, examination is difficult and the infant's condition can deteriorate with surprising and alarming speed. The history in the elderly patient can also present problems; moreover, perhaps because of the higher pain threshold in these subjects, the whole clinical picture tends to be obscured. During the postoperative period, there is also the background discomfort of the operation itself, the heavy sedation which has often been given and the natural

reluctance of the surgeon to re-open the abdomen. However, the patient whose adynamic ileus quietly slips into an acute mechanical obstruction due to adhesions presents a serious problem both in diagnosis and management, which is often resolved only by the most careful and often repeated examinations.

Finally, there is the malingerer who all too often haunts the casualty departments and who has an extraordinary facility for imitating most of the acute abdominal emergencies to perfection. Such patients are usually mentally abnormal or drug addicts. Always be on guard. There was the famous case in Scandinavia of a sailor who presented with all the features of a perforated peptic ulcer, the scars of two previous operations for the same condition, and a magnificent ship in full sail tattoed on his chest. The surgeon recognized this description as that of a well known case of the 'Munchausen syndrome' and sent him home. Unfortunately, there were two sailors in Sweden who possessed two scars on the abdomen and a ship in full sail tattooed on the chest; sad to say, this was the one with the genuine perforation.

PRINCIPLES OF TREATMENT

This section considers general principles of treatment. Specific operative details for particular types and causes of obstruction of the small intestine are considered later in this chapter.

With only a few exceptions, once the diagnosis of organic obstruction of the small intestine is diagnosed, urgent surgical intervention is required as soon as the necessary preoperative steps have been taken. This general rule, sometimes summed up with the aphorism 'do not let the sun rise or set on an intestinal obstruction' is because of the difficulty, indeed the impossibility, of the surgeon being able to differentiate with any confidence at all between a simple and a strangulated obstruction. As a consequence, delay may result in what was a viable loop of strangulated intestine being converted into a gangrenous or even perforated segment of bowel with all its associated problems and its increased risk of complications and death.

The principal exceptions to this excellent general rule of early surgical intervention are:

1. Obstruction occurring early in the postoperative period after laparotomy;

2. Recurrent obstruction due to adhesions;

3. Where the small bowel obstruction appears to be incomplete, as demonstrated by passage of flatus per rectum;

4. Patients with adynamic ileus and pseudo-obstruction of the small bowel are treated conservatively, as is discussed in later sections.

Where the obstruction is caused by adhesions in the immediate postoperative period, or where we are dealing with a known case of recurrent episodes of obstruction due to adhesions, then certainly a trial of conservative treatment with nasogastric suction and intravenous fluid and electrolyte replacement can be attempted; it must be abandoned at once at any sign of deterioration in the patient's condition. It is mandatory that such a patient, (1) be constantly re-examined with meticulous care, (2) be maintained on repeated observations of his vital signs and (3) be subjected to repeated radiological assessment by means of plain abdominal radiographs Wolfson and colleagues[39] give an interesting account of 127 episodes of obstruction of the small intestine due to adhesions in 112 patients. Of these, 113 episodes were treated conservatively and two-thirds of these responded to non-operative management. These authors advocate the use of an aspirating tube passed beyond the duodenum, but Bizer and colleagues[40] found no difference in successful results between patients managed with long tubes compared to those who had the conventional nasogastric tube passed. These authors describe 22 patients who developed obstruction during the early postoperative period (within 30 days of operation); 21 were treated conservatively, and in nine cases the obstruction was relieved. This rate was not significantly different from the 278 patients with late adhesive obstruction. In 21 patients with obstruction secondary to Crohn's disease, 20 were relieved by conservative management. Brolin[41] was successful in treating 91 of 175 cases of partial small bowel obstruction by drip and suction.

Preoperative measures

Preparation for operation comprises the initiation of gastric suction, administration of intravenous fluid and electrolytes and commencement of suitable antibiotic therapy. Once the decision has been taken that operation is indicated, an adequate dose of opiate is given, which mitigates the unpleasantness of having a large-bore nasogastric tube passed. It is essential that the stomach be emptied of its foul contents before induction of anaesthesia.

Operation must not be delayed for the many hours that it would take to restore normality to a grossly dehydrated patient. One or two litres can be replaced in the hour or so necessary to make preparation for operation, and this should take the form of normal saline or Hartmann's solution. Fluid replacement is then continued during and after the operation and is monitored by the patient's general condition, urine output, the results of haematocrit or haemoglobin estimation and the serum electrolytes. A grossly dehydrated adult patient may have a total deficiency of 6–8 litres of what is, in effect, normal saline. In the seriously ill patient, a central venous pressure line can be valuable as a guide in monitoring fluid replacement. A blood transfusion may be necessary in the presence of shock or obvious anaemia.

Before performing the laparotomy in a case of small bowel obstruction, the surgeon cannot tell what will be found; there may be a non-viable or perforated segment of bowel or a situation in which intestinal resection will be necessary. Under all these conditions, the risk of intraperitoneal and wound infection is high. This risk can be reduced by commencement of a suitable broad-spectrum antibiotic cover preoperatively. My own current practice is to use a third generation cephalosporin (Cefuroxime) and metronidazole; these provide a broad spectrum that deals with both the aerobic and anaerobic bowel organisms.

OPERATIVE TREATMENT

General principles

In the treatment of acute small bowel obstruction, the following operations may be indicated:

1. Exploration and repair of a strangulated external hernia;
2. Exploratory laparotomy for obstruction of uncertain origin;
3. Resection of the small intestine, either to remove the obstructing lesion (e.g. a stricture or tumour of the small bowel) or because a strangulated segment of intestine has undergone irreversible ischaemic change;
4. A short-circuiting operation, e.g. enteroanastomosis or an ileocolic anastomosis, to bypass an unresectable obstruction;
5. Division of an obstructing band or adhesions;
6. Enterotomy to remove an obstructing food bolus or gallstones;
7. Planned operations for specific obstructive lesions, e.g. reduction of an intussusception in a child or a stricturoplasty in a short-segment Crohn's obstruction.

General principles of treatment of strangulated external hernis

The detailed operative management of strangulated external hernias is outside the remit of this volume, but there are certain general principles to be stated here.

Although conservative attempts at reduction are fully justified in dealing with an irreducible inguinal hernia in a child, for practical purposes a strangulated hernia in an adult patient requires immediate operative reduction and repair. In early cases, it is perfectly reasonable to apply gentle pressure to the hernia with the patient lying in the head-down position under suitable sedation. Even if the hernia reduces, it is still wise to repair it, either at once or at the next convenient operating list. Indeed, it is not unusual for the hernia to reduce spontaneously once the patient has been anaesthetized and given a muscle relaxant. Under these circumstances the surgeon should certainly go ahead and repair the hernia. Violent attempts at manipulative reduction should never be performed.

Ideally, a general anaesthetic with muscle relaxant should be used, since this undoubtedly gives the best operative conditions for the surgeon. However, if the patient is in poor general condition a local anaesthetic can be employed supplemented by intravenous diazepam.

At operation, the sac is opened and bowel viability is determined (as discussed below). Viable intestine is returned to the abdominal cavity after releasing the obstructing neck of the hernia. If the bowel is obviously dead, it is resected with end-to-end anastomosis. It is perfectly sound practice simply to invert and oversew a localized zone of necrosis that may be seen at the site of the constriction ring when the rest of the obstructed loop appears perfectly viable. A series of interrupted serosal sutures of catgut or Dexon should be used (Figure 53.4).

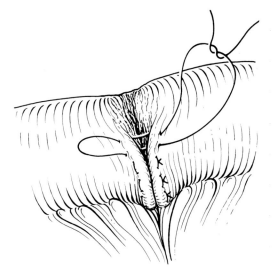

Figure 53.4
Oversewing a localized zone of necrosis by means of a series of interrupted serosal sutures.

In the great majority of cases, the resection can be safely performed through the opened sac, and the anastomosis is returned to the abdomen through the widened hernial orifice. In some cases, it may be necessary to perform a laparotomy if adequate exposure cannot be obtained.

From time to time, and this is especially so in emerging communities, a patient will be seen with gangrenous strangulated bowel within the hernial sac, perhaps complicated by necrosis and sloughing of the overlying tissues and even with established clostridial infection. Under such circumstances the necrotic bowel and gangrenous tissues are simply cut away with the production of a faecal fistula at the hernial orifice – the only safe way of dealing with this critical situation. The fistula can be closed electively as soon as the patient's general condition allows. The author has never had to perform this procedure, but has seen patients in Third World hospitals whose lives have undoubtedly been saved by this technique.

Exploratory laparotomy

If the abdomen is explored for small bowel obstruction of uncertain origin, the primary object is to save life by the simplest procedure consistent with ultimate recovery. The three essential steps at operation are:

1. To discover and deal with the obstructing pathology;
2. To decompress the dilated loops of bowel proximal to the obstruction;
3. To determine the state of viability of the liberated segment of gut.

Specific attention is concentrated, from this last point of view, to the bowel at the exact site of obstruction, as it is here that necrosis is likely to commence.

When the obstruction (and indeed the diagnosis) is of uncertain origin, the abdomen should be explored through a right paramedian paraumbilical incision or through a central midline incision. Recently I have carried the midline incision straight through the umbilicus without (as is usually practised) deviating around it. This manoeuvre gives a satisfactory scar, with no increased risk of herniation. In passing, it should be mentioned that closure of the incision in such cases should be by the mass closure technique using unabsorbable suture material such as nylon. Such a closure will almost eliminate the risk of wound dehiscence.[42] The incision should be small in the first instance, about 10 cm in length, but it should be enlarged without hesitation if the operative findings make further access necessary.

Extreme care should be exercised in opening the peritoneum since, in so many patients, the obstruction is due to adhesions from previous surgery, and loops of bowel may be closely adherent to the parietal wall immediately deep to the incision. Even in the intact abdominal cavity, grossly distended loops of gut pressing against the abdominal wall are at special risk of damage.

Exploration should be carried out on definite set lines. When the peritoneum is opened, the caecum should first be palpated. If it is distended, then the obstruction must be in the colon and the large bowel is further explored. However, if the caecum is collapsed, then obstruction of the small bowel is confirmed, and this should be sought by tracing collapsed gut through the fingers until the junction with the distended bowel is met. Here the definitive pathology will be seen and can be dealt with in most cases. When the cause is irremovable or it is deemed inadvisable not to remove it at once, it may be bypassed by a short-circuit operation. Rarely, in grave cases, the dilated intestine above the intestine may be drained by an enterostomy.

Decompression of the distended intestine

In many cases, once the cause of the occlusion has been demonstrated, it is desirable to decompress the grossly dilated loops of proximal bowel before carrying out any further procedure. Indeed, in some cases the mass of dilated loops makes it difficult for the surgeon to expose the site of the obstruction before decompression is performed. Moreover, distended gut is difficult to handle and may even rupture during manipulation. Certainly, closure of the abdominal incision if the bowel has not been decompressed is a tiresome task both for the surgeon and the anaesthetist.

A wide-bore needle or trocar attached to the suction pump may be used to puncture a distended loop of intestine but, unfortunately, the lumen usually rapidly blocks with faecal material and it is difficult to decompress adjacent distended loops. Savage[43] has devised a useful long trocar and cannula which is inserted through a purse-string suture and enables the cannula to be threaded a considerable distance proximally along the distended bowel. Intermittent suction is applied and the cannula, if blocked, can be cleared by re-introducing the trocar along its length (Figure 53.5).

Although very useful, this does have the disadvantage of opening the bowel with the very real risk of wound contamination. A most useful technique was described by Jones and

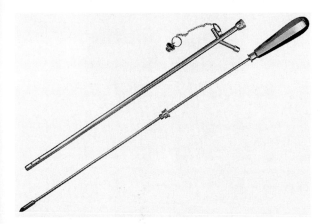

Figure 53.5
The Savage decompressor. This has been dismantled to demonstrate the trocar above and the introducer below.

Matheson[44] in which the small bowel is emptied in a retrograde manner back into the stomach, from which the contents are aspirated via a nasogastric tube. The great advantage of this method is that there is no danger of spillage of infected bowel contents and no risk of the puncture wound leaking either at the time of operation or thereafter. These authors state:

> We are now satisfied that the small bowel content can regularly be emptied back into the stomach by simple retrograde stripping, whence it is removed by aspiration through a wide-bore tube, therefore avoiding enterotomy. There is a common impression that the duodenal loop and pylorus offer undue opposition to this manoeuvre but this is not correct. In a low ileal obstruction, we gently empty the jejunum first, starting at about the jejuno-ileal junction and milking the contents proximally between the straight index and middle fingers. Some firm pressure is needed on the proximal jejunum but it always empties safely and easily into duodenum and stomach; reflux of fluid does not occur back into the jejunum. The ileal content is then brought up into the empty jejunum afterwards and emptied through the duodenum.

Having used this technique on many occasions the author can vouch for its efficiency in the great majority of cases (Figure 53.6).

Determination of viability of the intestine

Having relieved the obstruction, the surgeon's next duty is to determine the viability of the affected bowel. In cases of obstruction of the small intestine, this problem occurs under the following circumstances.[3]

1. When a segment of bowel has been strangulated (internal or external hernia, a band, intussusception, etc.), and a decision must be made concerning the viability of the whole affected loop;

2. In similar circumstances where the surgeon is confident of the viability of the affected loop but is concerned about the constriction line at the actual level of the obstruction;

3. In cases of mesenteric infarction when there is the problem of deciding the extent of non-viable intestine.

Ver Steeg and Broders[45] give a useful analysis of the aetiology of 88 consecutive cases of intestinal gangrene, with adhesions, strangulated hernia and mesenteric vascular occlusions as the principal causes (Table 53.4).

Table 53.4   Aetiology of intestinal ischaemia

Strangulated obstructions (*n*=57)		
	Adhesions	33
	External hernias	15
	Volvulus	4
	Internal hernias	3
	Blunt trauma	1
	Intussusception	1
Mesenteric vascular occlusions (*n*=31)		
	Arterial	11
	Non-occlusive	9
	Venous	4
	Ruptured aortic aneurysms	4
	Postoperative aortic surgery	2
	Moniliasis	1

From Ver Steeg and Broders.[45]

Most surgeons rely heavily on clinical judgement in the assessment of bowel viability after release of a strangulated obstruction. Certainly, with increasing experience, they are unlikely to err either on the side of pessimism, with early resort to bowel resection, or on the side of excessive optimism, with its risk of perforation or at least a stricture of a non-viable segment.

An excellent sign of perfectly viable intestine is rapid return of normal healthy reddish-pink colour to the cyanosed loop of bowel. This sign is reinforced if a good pulsation is seen and/or felt in the supplying mesentery. A glistening serosa is also reassuring. It is still important to carry out a careful inspection of the constriction ring, which may remain thinned and discoloured even though the rest of the intestine has returned to normal. Under these circumstances resection may not be necessary, as the constriction line can often be treated by oversewing (see Figure 53.4).

At a further stage, haemorrhages will have occurred in the affected segment of bowel wall and the adjacent mesentery. The thickened oedematous mesentery may make it difficult to feel for pulsation. However, the bowel returns to normal colour on release of the constriction, its consistency is normal and peristalsis may be visible. This is the stage which can give considerable anxiety to the surgeon. I recommend that the affected segment be wrapped in a pack soaked in warm normal saline and inspected again after 5–10 minutes. This time can be spent usefully in decompressing the intestine above the obstruction and this manoeuvre, itself, is often associated with improvement in the appearance of the bowel. If at a still further stage the bowel fails to return to its normal

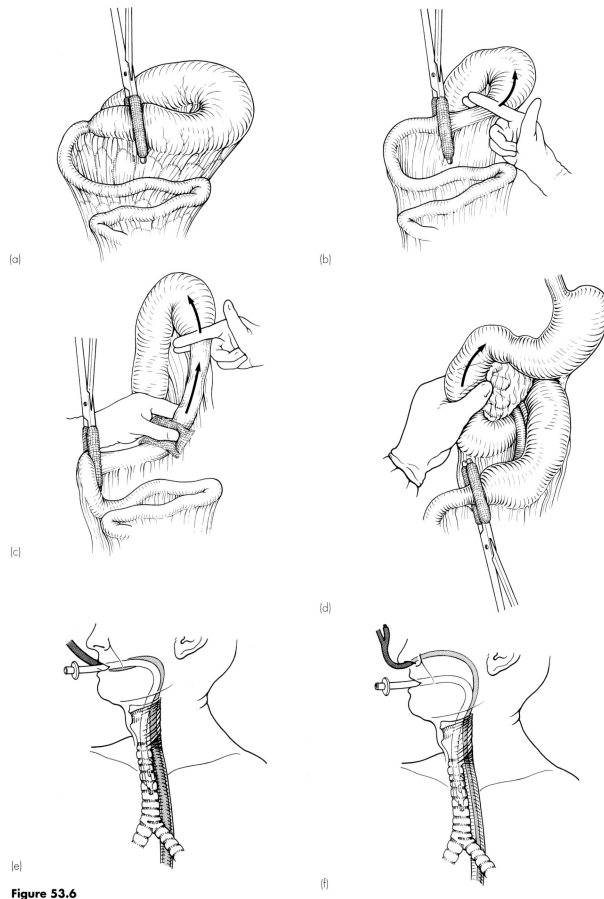

(a)

(b)

(c)

(d)

(e)

(f)

Figure 53.6

Retrograde decompression of the distended small intestine.

colour, feels thin and papery and shows no peristaltic activity then it should be considered non-viable.

Of course there is the final stage about which there is no doubt at all. The bowel is black or even greenish in colour, the serosa matt, the bowel consistency feels thin and lifeless, exactly like the gut encountered in the autopsy room, and there is a malodorous darkly blood-stained peritoneal exudate. There may even be frank perforation of the gangrenous segment. Under these circumstances irreversible necrosis has undoubtedly occurred.

Many experimental and clinical studies have been expended on attempts to improve the blood supply of jeopardized intestine or to determine whether or not gut of borderline viability can be conserved with safety. The administration of 100% oxygen to the patient is often advocated, and certainly there is no harm in trying this. Others have advised injection of novocaine into the supplying mesentery or into the intestinal wall and the use of papaverine intravenously. It is unlikely that any of these techniques are of clinical value.

A wide variety of dye injections have been used as tests of bowel viability. These include intravenous fluorescein with observation of the bowel by means of ultraviolet light, and the use of methylene blue, indigo carmine and trypan blue. Operative angiography and electromyographic studies of the affected bowel wall segment are hardly applicable to the clinical situation.

There have been many reports of the use of Doppler ultrasound to determine the viability of ischaemic intestine and several groups have reported favourable results. Thus Cooperman and colleagues[46,47] report their use of the Doppler proble in 23 patients with 25 segments of questionably viable intestine. Ten segments judged to be non-viable on clinical lines had satisfactory arterial flow detected on the Doppler probe and were preserved; all had a benign clinical course. Two were judged clinically viable and showed no flow on the probe and were resected. Nine cases had non-viable intestine both on clinical and on probe assessment, and all were resected.

Technique of resection of infarcted small intestine

Since resection of ischaemic small gut is so often indicated in the management of strangulated obstruction or of mesenteric vascular occlusion, the technique of this procedure needs to be considered in some detail.

The operative steps comprise division of the mesenteric vessels, resection of the ischaemic bowel back to tissues of undoubted viability and restoration of continuity. Mesenteric division is carried out as conservatively as possible to avoid damage to main mesenteric trunks and risk of jeopardizing the blood supply to healthy intestine.

In a thin subject, visualization of the vascular arcades is easy enough in the translucent mesentery (Figure 53.7). Under these circumstances, the leaves of peritoneum are divided using scissors and the area of mesentery to be resected is thus outlined (Figure 53.8). By picking up individual vessels and

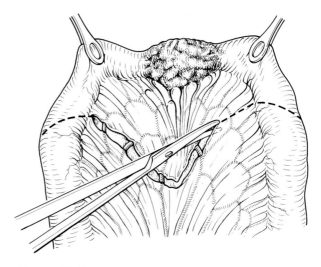

Figure 53.7
Resection of the small intestine. Preliminary inspection of the mesentery. Note the proposed line of incision of the bowel which slopes downward from the mesenteric to the antimesenteric border in order to preserve the blood supplies of the latter.

tying them with linen thread before their division, it is possible to produce a neat and bloodless section of the mesentery (Figure 53.9). However, if the patient is obese and the mesentery fatty, or if the mesentery is (as so often occurs in this circumstance) oedematous or even haemorrhagic, serial division of the mesentery is carried out between a succession of closely placed artery forceps applied close to the bowel wall (Figure 53.9).

Only small bites of mesentery should be taken; this avoids large pedicles from which it is easy for the mesenteric vessels to escape during ligation. This event will result in either unpleasant bleeding or the development of a large mesenteric haematoma. The mesentery is divided up to the edge of the bowel wall on either side of the obviously ischaemic segment.

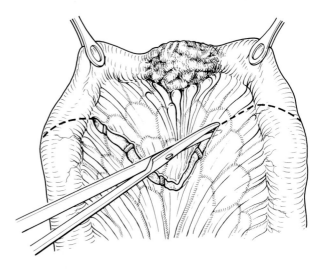

Figure 53.8
Resection of small intestine. Division of the mesenteric peritoneum.

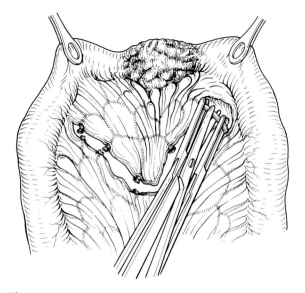

Figure 53.9

Resection of small intestine. The mesenteric vessels are best ligated individually and then divided (as shown on the left-hand side). If the mesentery is fatty, it is divided seriatim between artery forceps (right-hand side).

The exact site of resection is decided upon when the surgeon is certain that there is an adequate blood supply to the proposed anastomosis. Good vascularization is shown by the healthy colour of the bowel, a normal appearance of its serosa and the presence of obvious pulsating arteries at the proposed site of division.

A non-crushing intestinal clamp is placed proximal to the proposed site of gut division and a crushing clamp is placed at the line at which section is to take place. A pair of clamps is placed similarly at the distal end of the proposed division. The intestine is then carefully packed off by large moist swabs to prevent contamination from bowel contents, and the intestine is divided close against the two crushing clamps (Figure 53.10).

The two well-vascularized divided ends of intestine, projecting from their soft clamps, are apposed in preparation for anastomosis. The bowel lumen (particularly of the distal end) can, if necessary, be enlarged by judiciously incising the antimesenteric border (Figure 53.11). A simple two-layer anastomosis is now performed using 2/0 chromic catgut sutures or a similar synthetic alternative such as Vicryl. The first layer comprises the serosal (Lembert) stitch which commences at the antimesenteric border. The all-coats through-and-through suture line is then commenced, and the sutures are inserted close together at intervals of about 2–3 mm; they should be placed tightly so that haemostasis is ensured (Figures 53.12 and 53.13). Having reached the extremity of the posterior internal layer, the corner is turned by means of a loop-on-mucosa suture, performed by passing the needle from within the lumen of the bowel outward and then passing from within to without the bowel lumen on the opposite side. This manoeuvre may be repeated once or twice more and will result in a neat turn of the corner, so that the second layer of the continuous all-coats suture can be brought back along the length of the intestine by means of a simple over-and-over stitch. This stitch is tied to the end with which it was commenced (Figure 53.14).

The non-crushing clamps are now removed, and the serosal suture is completed to cover the anterior aspect of the anastomosis (Figure 53.15). The anastomotic line is then re-assessed for a satisfactory blood supply, and its lumen is checked between the index finger and the thumb to ensure patency (Figure 53.16).

The divided edges of the mesentery should now be united by means of a continuous catgut suture, carefully avoiding the mesenteric blood vessels (Figure 53.17). In a very fatty or oedematous mesentery, where it is impossible to identify individual vessels, a safe technique is to pick up the opposing points of mesentery with artery forceps and to tie these together with thread or catgut ligatures. This obviates the risk of pricking the mesenteric vessels with consequent haematoma. Finally, the anastomotic line, where possible, is wrapped in omentum.

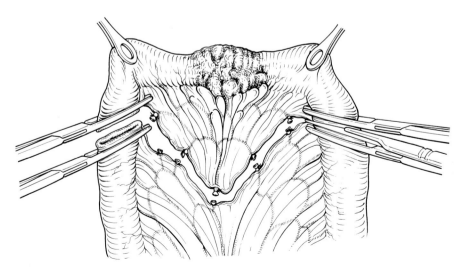

Figure 53.10

The intestine is resected between clamps.

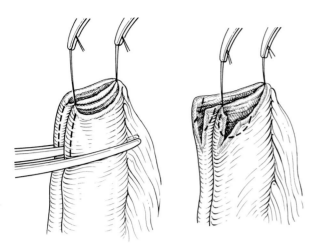

Figure 53.11
The open ends of the small bowel are apposed for anastomosis. The bowel lumen can be enlarged by judiciously slitting the antimesenteric border as shown on the right-hand side.

Small bowel anastomosis is seldom a difficult surgical procedure. This simple end-to-end technique can almost always be employed, and it is rarely necessary for an end-to-side or side-to-side anastomosis to be indicated in the adult.

Mortality and prognosis factors

Although small bowel obstruction remains a dangerous surgical emergency, over the decades there has been a steady overall decline in mortality rate. The published mortality figures for large series of cases (mostly lumping together small and large bowel obstructions, both simple and strangulated) demonstrate that the mortality in the 1890s was in the region of 40%, and came down to approximately 25% of all cases in the period preceding World War II until, in modern times, the published figures show a mortality in the range of 5–10%.

Table 53.5 provides a spectrum of published figures over the last century. Very accurate figures are available from the

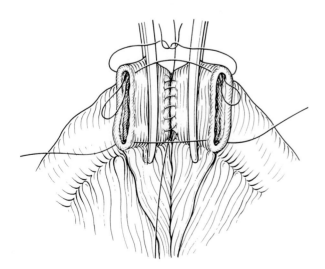

Figure 53.12
The posterior serosal continuous suture is inserted.

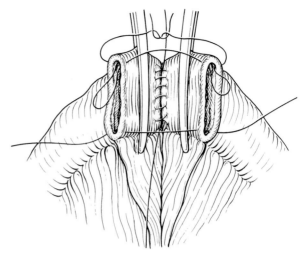

Figure 53.13
The posterior all coats layer. The stages of the loop on the mucosa suture are shown.

statistics of the Registrar General for England and Wales for the mortality rate for intestinal obstruction. These are published under two headings: (1) intestinal obstruction without mention of hernia; and (2) hernias of the abdominal cavity with obstruction. The death rate per million for intestinal obstruction without mention of hernia fell from 50 in 1940 to 30 in 1950 and has continued to decline, although rather less sharply, since then. In 1980 there were 17 deaths per million in males and 26 per million in females. In 1955 a total of 2603 patients died from intestinal obstruction, of which 1253 were due to strangulated hernias. By 1984, the total had fallen to 1531, of which 339 were strangulated hernias.

Table 53.5 Spectrum of mortality for intestinal obstruction (small and large bowel) over 100 years

SOURCE	YEAR	COUNTRY	NO. OF CASES	MORTALITY (%)
Gibson[48]	1900	Collected papers from 1888	1000	43
Souttar[49]	1925	UK	3064	26
Vick[4]	1932	UK	6892	26
Smith[50]	1955	USA	1252	14.5
Becker[51]	1955	USA	1007	18.7
Barling[52]	1956	Australia	355	20
Waldron and Hampton[5]	1961	USA	493	14
Kaltiala et al.[18]	1972	Finland	558	8
Stewardson et al.[53]	1978	USA	238[a]	5.5
Nelson and Ellis[7]	1984	UK	279	7.9
McEntee[6]	1987	UK	228	11.4
Mucha[54]	1987	USA	289[a]	10.4

[a]Small intestine only.

It is interesting to contrast this relatively modest decline in death rate with the figures published from the same source for acute appendicitis. Today this amounts to about four deaths per million, compared with 60 per million in 1940.

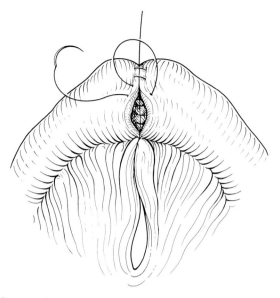

Figure 53.14
The anterior all coats layer is inserted.

The improvement in prognosis of intestinal obstruction is no doubt due to a combination of factors. These include: (1) improved anaesthesia, with consequent reduction in the very real hazards of aspiration of regurgitated stomach contents; (2) improved technique of abdominal muscle relaxation, which makes operations on patients with gross abdominal distension safer and, perhaps more important, helps in closing the laparotomy incisions efficiently; (3) better knowledge of fluid and electrolyte replacement, efficient blood transfusion services and the introduction of broad-spectrum antibiotics. It is also hoped that decades of teaching have instructed surgeons in the importance of early intervention, especially when there is any question at all that a strangulation has occurred.

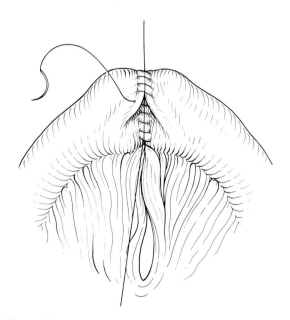

Figure 53.15
The anterior serosal layer.

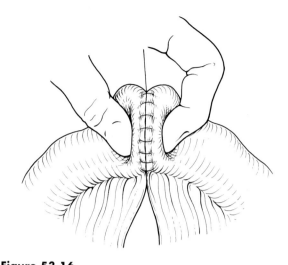

Figure 53.16
The completed anastomosis is inspected, haemostasis is ensured and the lumen of the anastomosis checked betwen the finger and the thumb.

The major factors influencing the survival rate of intestinal obstruction may be summed up as follows.

1. Extremes of age – the mortality rate is especially high in infancy and in the elderly. Mucha,[54] for example, noted that of 30 deaths that occurred in a series of 289 patients undergoing 314 operations for small bowel obstruction, 15 were in their eighth or ninth decade.

2. Correlating with their age, the general condition of the patient is of extreme importance. This includes the complicating elements of preoperative chest infection, cardiac failure and gross electrolyte depletion and dehydration.

3. The most important local factor, which has an intense bearing on the patient's general condition, is the presence of strangulation of the bowel with gangrene or, worse still, perforation of the affected segment of gut.

4. The underlying pathology producing the obstruction is obviously of crucial importance, and this is particularly so

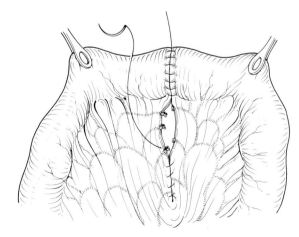

Figure 53.17
Finally, the divided mesentary is reconstituted.

when the obstruction is due to the presence of intra-abdominal neoplastic disease (usually secondary deposits or lymphoma). Thus in the series presented by Mucha[54] the mortality rate for patients with strangulated hernia was 4.3% and for adhesions 4.6%. However, the mortality rate among patients whose obstruction was due to neoplastic disease rose to 21.3%.

The effect of strangulation on mortality rates is striking. Table 53.6 presents a selection of mortality figures for patients with simple obstruction compared with those complicated by strangulation.

ADYNAMIC ILEUS

Besides the various mechanical lesions that may occlude the small bowel from within the lumen on the wall and from outside the wall, a functional obstruction may result from loss of propulsive activity in all or part of the intestine. This important, potentially dangerous and rather poorly understood situation of functional obstruction has been termed *paralytic ileus*, but in many cases it probably results from a reflex inhibition of the gut rather than paralysis and is better termed *neurogenic* or *adynamic ileus*.

It is important to note that a wide range of aetiologies may produce this clinical syndrome. These include:

1. Postoperative adynamic ileus;
2. Ileus resulting from peritonitis;
3. The retroperitoneal syndrome;
4. Spinal injuries;
5. Metabolic disturbances;
6. Drug-induced.

Clinical features

The classical picture of adynamic ileus is the same whatever the underlying aetiology. There is abdominal distension, absolute constipation (the patient passes neither flatus nor faeces) and there is effortless vomiting. If the patient has a nasogastric tube in place, copious aspirates are obtained. The patient is anxious and complains of abdominal discomfort, but this is compatible with the abdominal distension or the amount of pain (in the postoperative case) that might be expected from the abdominal wound. The pulse shows progressive elevation during the evolution of the syndrome, but the temperature is normal unless there is an associated peritonitis or the complicating factor of a postoperative pulmonary collapse.

On examination of the abdomen, there is distension and generalized tenderness; very typically, the abdomen is silent on prolonged auscultation. A plain radiograph of the abdomen demonstrates gas distributed throughout the small and large intestine, whereas the erect film demonstrates multiple fluid levels.

Postoperative adynamic ileus

Postoperative ileus is by far and away the most common of the aetiologies listed above. Indeed, some degree of adynamic ileus is almost inevitable no matter how minor the intra-abdominal procedure. Its exact mechanism is still not completely understood. An important factor is probable stress-induced sympathetic hyperactivity, but in many cases the syndrome is probably multifactorial. Other factors are the associated peritoneal irritation caused by pus or blood, electrolyte imbalance, especially potassium depletion, the effects of analgesic and other postoperative drugs and, in prolonged and serious cases, the complicating factor that a mechanical element may be induced by the matting together of loops of small intestine by postoperative fibrinous adhesions. When a bowel anastomosis is present, oedema at the stoma may produce a temporary mechanical obstruction, which again may complicate the clinical situation.

There is good evidence that postoperative adynamic ileus, in the uncomplicated case, is principally the result of a reflex mediated via the sympathetic nervous system. In the classical experiments of Bayliss and Starling in 1899,[56] the intestine of dogs submitted to laparotomy was found to be collapsed and motionless. Inhibition of intestinal peristalsis was produced by stimulation of the splanchnic nerves, and splanchnicectomy abolished the intestinal inhibition induced by laparotomy. Neely and Catchpole[57] and Nadrowski[58] give excellent summaries of the large mass of experimental and clinical studies that reinforce these early experiments and that demonstrate the protective effect of either splanchnic division, spinal cord destruction or spinal anaesthesia on the evolution of postoperative adynamic ileus. Adrenergic nerve blockade and chemical sympathectomy with 6-hydroxydopamine also suppress the appearance of postoperative experimental ileus, whereas adrenalectomy does not alter the course of the ileus. All these findings are consistent with the hypothesis that postoperative

Table 53.6 Mortality simple and strangulated obstruction

SOURCE	YEAR	COUNTRY	NO. OF CASES	MORTALITY (%)	
				SIMPLE	STRANGULATED
Becker[51]	1955	USA	1007	14	30.5
Savage[43]	1960	UK	179	12	21
Waldron and Hampton[5]	1961	USA	493	11.3	28.8
Leffall et al.[55]	1965	USA	1700	3	30.7
Kaltiala et al.[18]	1972	Finland	558	5	30

ileus is related to intestinal sympathetic neuronal hyperactivity. It is noteworthy that Petri[59] demonstrated increased levels of both adrenaline and noradrenaline in the plasma of patients with adynamic ileus, and Smith and colleagues[60] showed an increase in noradrenaline level in the plasma of dogs undergoing abdominal exploration.

Nadrowski[58] suggests two types of sympathetic reflex pathways. Low-threshold spinal reflexes, originating from stimuli of lesser peritoneal irritation, pass via somatic afferents to the spinal cord and can be abolished by spinal anaesthesia. However, high-threshold reflexes, which are only initiated by severe peritoneal irritation, have their cell station in the prevertebral ganglia, bypass the CNS and are not therefore blocked by spinal anaesthesia. Both types of reflex are blocked by guanethidine, an adrenergic neurone-blocking agent, because they both rely on transmission through efferent adrenergic neurones.

Rennie and colleagues[61] have demonstrated two possible humoral inhibitory mechanisms that may occur in the colon and may contribute to postoperative adynamic ileus. Dopamine (a precursor of adrenaline and noradrenaline) was shown to inhibit isolated colonic smooth muscle strips by a direct effect in longitudinal muscle and by a nerve-mediated mechanism in circular muscle. Motilin is one of several gastrointestinal peptides that have been shown to stimulate colonic activity (others include gastrin and cholecystokinin). These investigators demonstrated that plasma motilin levels were suppressed during operation but returned to normal level postoperatively, and this correlated with the return of normal gut motility. The duration of suppression of the plasma motilin level was found to be related to the severity of the operation.

Pathophysiology

Classically it was considered that after abdominal exploration the whole of the gut became paralysed. However, a series of interesting clinical investigations by Wells and co-workers in Liverpool[62] and Rothnie and co-workers[63] at St Bartholomew's Hospital challenged this simplistic concept. Their investigations included prolonged auscultation of the abdomen using a microphone, pressure studies via a fine nasogastric tube introduced into the upper jejunum, serial plain radiograph studies of the abdomen in the postoperative period and radiological investigations of contrast material introduced into the stomach or the jejunum at the time of operation. These studies demonstrated that gastric stasis occurs after any operation but more especially when the abdominal cavity has been opened. Under these circumstances, gastric stasis lasts from 18 hours to four days. By contrast, small intestinal peristalsis returns within a few hours of operation in the absence of any complicating factors. Thus, contrast material placed into the duodenum spreads rapidly throughout the small intestine and reaches the caecum within 24 hours. However, the colon shows stasis that persists for one or two days after laparotomy. In the normal subject, swallowed air rapidly transits through the alimentary canal and is passed per rectum within about half an hour. However, the situation is very different

in the postoperative patient. In such cases, air swallowing is often marked, especially among those who are apprehensive, retching or in pain. The atonic stomach becomes distended with swallowed air, and a good deal of this passes through the pyloric sphincter. It is then rapidly transmitted by the normal small bowel peristalsis and enters the colon, which is atonic, so that the usual cause of postoperative distension is gas dilating the inert large intestine.

The absence of bowel sounds in the early postoperative period appears to be due to an empty small intestine. When fluid and air are injected into the duodenum through a nasogastric tube, bowel sounds are heard at once. It appears that the return of bowel sounds indicates the restoration of normal gastric and colonic motility and not (as was previously thought) the return of function to the small intestine. This phenomenon is soon followed by the passage of flatus and the relief of the patient's symptoms.

Further clinical and experimental studies, using more sophisticated techniques, have confirmed these simple clinical observations. Ross and colleagues[64] placed radiotelemeter capsules in the jejunum and recorded the postoperative return of motility to the small intestine. Small bowel peristalsis was recorded within one hour in those operations that did not involve laparotomy (for example, haemorrhoidectomy or hernia repair), after approximately four hours after surgery to the upper gastrointestinal tract that did not involve vagotomy (for example gastrectomy and gastrojejunostomy) and in about 10 hours after vagotomy with drainage. Studies of postoperative motility of the large intestine in man using radiotelemetering capsules, radio-opaque markers that could be identified on radiographs of the abdomen and faeces, and serial abdominal radiographs have confirmed that colonic activity returns in about 16 hours after an operation that does not involve the abdomen but is delayed for approximately 48 hours if the abdominal cavity is entered.[65] This study was noteworthy in showing that return of colonic activity did not appear to be related to the length of time that the operation took to perform nor did it demonstrate any influence of the amount of post-operative analgesia on the duration of colonic inactivity.

The extensive laboratory studies by Graber and colleagues[66] are of particular note. They used strain-gauge force transducers and bipolar electrodes placed on the gastric antrum, the midsmall bowel, the right colon and the sigmoid colon in stumptailed monkeys. Animals were subjected to either extensive right-sided abdominal dissection and mobilization or the same procedure on the left side or a midline incision with gentle digital manipulation of the intestines. The first two procedures involved much more intestinal handling and dissection and took some five to six times longer than the minimal laparotomy procedure. The mean time required for return of normal contraction frequencies was 3.4 hours for the antrum, 6.5 hours for the small bowel, 45 hours for the right colon and 55 hours for the sigmoid colon. A most interesting finding was that the duration and pattern of postoperative ileus in these experiments were independent of the extent, site and duration of the operative procedure.

Peritonitis

General peritonitis is invariably accompanied by adynamic ileus. One would imagine that this was due to the fact that there would be a toxic effect of purulent peritoneal fluid on the intestine itself. However, it is well known that a segment of small intestine, obtained from an animal with experimentally produced peritonitis, will continue to undergo rhythmic contraction when placed in a saline bath. In clinical practice, peristalsis may be observed in early cases of peritonitis, but in advanced instances the soggy, distended, inflamed gut, covered by adherent plaques of slough, seems totally atonic.

The exact mechanism of adynamic ileus in advanced peritonitis is probably multifactorial, a compound of sympathetic stimulation, metabolic disturbances, gaseous distension and the effects (in postoperative cases) of surgical handling. In addition, in many cases there are the exacerbating mechanical factors of kinking and twisting of the bowel from fibrinous adhesions and, where an anastomosis has been performed, of the oedematous swelling of the sutured bowel.

The retroperitoneal syndrome

Anything that results in disturbance of the retroperitoneal tissues may result in adynamic ileus and is believed to be the result of reflex stimulation of the sympathetic splanchnic outflow. Thus, ileus commonly follows any extensive retroperitoneal surgery (bilateral lumbar sympathectomy, nephrectomy and resection of an abdominal aortic aneurysm). It may occur in retroperitoneal haemorrhage and is particularly likely to be seen in patients who have developed a ruptured aortic aneurysm, with extensive retroperitoneal extravasation of blood, followed by extensive surgery for operative repair.

During World War II it became well recognized that a gunshot wound producing retroperitoneal haemorrhage would frequently result in an ileus that closely simulated the features of intraperitoneal injury and yet, at laparotomy, the peritoneal cavity would be found to be entirely intact, the gut grossly dilated and the damage to lie in the retroperitoneal plane. Blackburn and Rob[67] popularized the term 'retroperitoneal syndrome' for this phenomenon.

The silent distended abdomen associated with acute pancreatitis is another variant of this phenomenon, and a similar state of affairs may often be seen in a patient with severe ureteric colic.

It is noteworthy that this syndrome can be reproduced in experimental animals. Lindquist[68] produced prolonged ileus in rats by injecting blood, turpentine or pus into the retroperitoneal space. Woods et al.[69] produced ileus in monkeys by retroperitoneal dissection accompanied by cross-clamping of the right renal pedicle. They were able to demonstrate decreased myoelectric activity in the antrum, small bowel and right colon for 24 hours after this procedure, and in the sigmoid colon the depressed activity persisted for 72 hours.

Spinal injuries

It is well known that spinal trauma, spinal fractures and transection of the cord may result in functional intestinal obstruction.

In an extensive and important review of this subject, Watkin[70] uses the term 'spinal ileus' to denote this syndrome.

In clinical practice, it is important to distinguish these cases of adynamic ileus after spinal injury from the acute gastric dilatation that may follow the application of a plaster cast to the trunk or hip – the so-called 'cast syndrome'.[71] Here, the third part of the duodenum is 'nipped' between the superior mesenteric pedicle anteriorly and the lumbar vertebrae posteriorly by the acute lordosis. The syndrome may also occur in the absence of a plaster cast in patients placed on lower limb or skull traction and nursed in an immobile supine position. Obviously this is a very different state of affairs from 'spinal ileus' but one that can be differentiated by plain and contrast radiography of the abdomen. The radiographs demonstrate gastric dilatation, dilatation of the second and third portions of the duodenum and a sharp cut-off at the level of the superior mesenteric vessels.

Metabolic disturbances

Adynamic ileus may complicate the severe metabolic disturbances of diabetic coma and uraemia. It has been reported in cases of severe myxoedema, and here the features may lead to inappropriate surgical intervention.[72]

Severe changes in the internal environment due to acute anaemia, serum hypo-osmolarity and depletion of serum chloride, sodium, potassium and magnesium may all induce adynamic ileus. Potassium depletion below 2.5 mequiv/l in particular has a well-known association with ileus. The potassium ion accelerates the production or release of acetylcholine and plays a part in nerve impulse transmission. It is important, therefore, to replace potassium in patients with severe postoperative ileus in which loss of potassium in the gastric aspirate aggravates the obligatory urinary loss of potassium in the postoperative catabolic phase.

Hypomagnesaemia may also produce adynamic ileus, and magnesium administration is advisable in patients with prolonged ileus.

Drug-induced adynamic ileus

There is a wide variety of drugs affecting smooth muscle that are well known to produce constipation and have been reported to induce a picture of adynamic ileus; there have been examples of unnecessary laparotomies in this situation. Table 53.7, summarizes the drug groups most commonly implicated. All the opiate or narcotic types of analgesic have this effect, and it is well known that drug addicts may present with features that suggest an acute abdomen as a result of heroin, methadone and other addictive opiates.[73]

Antihistamines are particularly likely to produce an ileus in patients with Parkinson's disease. Clonidine, a potent antihypertensive agent, also has a direct effect on intestinal smooth muscle, and cases of pseudo-obstruction have been reported due to this drug. Autonomic ganglion-blocking drugs may cause adynamic ileus, as may the tricyclic antidepressants, as a result of their powerful anticholinergic action. Milner and Hills[74] give an account of three examples of adynamic ileus complicating

Table 53.7 Drugs which may induce adynamic ileus

Analgesics	Morphia
	Heroin
	Methadone
Antihistamines (especially in Parkinson's disease)	
Antihypertensives	Clonidine
Autonomic ganglion blocking drugs	Probanthine (propantheline bromide)
	Hexamethonium bromide
Tricyclic antidepressants	Imipramine
	Amitriptyline
	Nortriptyline

nortriptyline therapy, including one patient actually submitted to laparotomy, at which time gross dilatation of the large bowel down to the rectum was discovered. These authors quote five other reported examples of ileus complicating amitriptyline therapy.

Pathological changes in adynamic ileus

At post-mortem examination of a patient who has succumbed with advanced adynamic ileus, the stomach and the whole of the intestine will be found to be thin-walled and distended. The bowel is cyanosed and contains large amounts of gas together with faecal fluid. The peritoneal cavity may contain purulent fluid, and the loops of small bowel will be tethered to each other by fibrinous adhesions.

The pathological effects of the ileus are as follows:

1. There is severe water, electrolyte and protein depletion. Congestion and increased permeability of the bowel wall allows transudation of plasma into the gut lumen and into the peritoneal cavity. This compounds the fluid loss in vomit, gastric aspiration or merely sequestration into the distended bowel lumen. There may eventually be oligaemic shock, with resultant circulatory failure and oliguria due to tubular necrosis.

2. The gross distension of the intestine impairs its blood supply and allows toxic absorption to occur from the gut lumen in a manner similar to that observed in gross mechanical intestinal obstruction.

3. The gross abdominal distension impairs both respiratory and cardiac function. Pressure on the vena cava and iliac veins predisposes to massive venous thrombosis with a high risk of consequent pulmonary embolism – a not infrequent terminal affair in such cases.

Differential diagnosis

It is vitally important, and also sometimes extremely difficult, to differentiate in the postoperative period between adynamic ileus and postoperative mechanical intestinal obstruction. The latter might be the result of fibrinous bands or adhesions between loops of small intestine or tethering of a bowel loop to the abdominal incision. There may be strangulation of a loop of small bowel through a partial dehiscence of the

laparotomy wound or of the pelvic floor after major rectal or gynaecological surgery.

This accurate diagnosis is of great importance, because as a general rule adynamic ileus is treated conservatively and is aggravated by an unnecessary secondary exploratory operation, whereas mechanical obstruction in these circumstances usually requires urgent surgical relief. To compound the difficulty, in so many cases what is first an adynamic ileus passes insidiously into a true mechanical intestinal obstruction.

Careful consideration of the following five criteria will suggest a mechanical rather than an adynamic postoperative obstruction.[75]

1. Persistence of the clinical picture of ileus for four or more days following operation. Although a time limit cannot be laid down, certainly each day following the fourth makes it more likely that the obstruction has become mechanical rather than being a persistence of the adynamic state.

2. The patient has passed flatus or even had his bowels open but then ceases all such passage. Obviously there is no reason why an adynamic ileus, once overcome, should return; the situation now suggests the onset of mechanical obstruction.

3. The presence of noisy peristaltic rushes on abdominal auscultation in the absence of the passage of flatus. It is important to notice that in gross ileus splashing sounds may occasionally be heard in the fluid-filled distended loops of intestine and that, moreover, there may be transmitted breath and heart sounds in such circumstances.

4. The presence of colicky abdominal pain.

5. Radiographs of the abdomen demonstrate a local loop of distended small intestine in the absence of gas shadows in the large bowel.

Radiology

There is no doubt that the single most useful special investigation in adynamic ileus is plain radiography of the abdomen in the erect and supine position, repeated if necessary within a few hours. A comprehensive review of this subject is given by Gammill and Nice,[76] who compared the abdominal radiographs of 300 normal subjects (including some who had received a purgative or castor oil combined with an enema) with cases of mechanical intestinal obstruction and with adynamic ileus. They recorded that more than two air-fluid levels in dilated small intestine was always pathological, being associated with either mechanical or adynamic ileus. If the small intestine was dilated in the absence of colonic gas, this was found to be strongly suggestive of small bowel obstruction. Distended small bowel, together with gas in the undistended colon, suggested either partial or resolving small intestinal obstruction or adynamic ileus. In such circumstances, a further radiograph 2–4 hours later was useful. An unchanged pattern was likely to be due to adynamic obstruction. Dilatation of the small intestine with associated gas in distended colon suggested either an adynamic ileus or a large bowel obstruction, and an emergency barium enema would demonstrate the presence of a mechanical block in the large bowel. In spite of previous suggestions, these authors were unable to confirm that the presence of two air–fluid levels in the same loop at different heights with relation to the vertical axis was not of any use in distinguishing between dynamic and adynamic ileus. It is noteworthy that these authorities conclude that occasionally the plain radiographs give completely confusing findings and under such circumstances the only safe rule is reliance on clinical judgement.

In difficult cases, the use of the water-soluble contrast medium gastrografin may be helpful, if administered either orally or through the nasogastric tube. Passage of the contrast into the large bowel over the next few hours suggests adynamic ileus, whereas failure of the medium to enter the colon would suggest mechanical obstruction.

In spite of all available aids, the differential diagnosis between mechanical and adynamic postoperative obstruction is often difficult and requires the highest degree of clinical judgement. It is aided by the most meticulous and often repeated examination of the patient. Noisy bowel sounds and cramping pains may represent mechanical obstruction, but they also occur quite frequently just as the adynamic ileus is about to relieve itself and flatus to be passed. Under such circumstances, a short period of further delay, together with the study of additional radiographs of the abdomen, may resolve the differential diagnosis one way or the other.

Management of adynamic ileus

Prophylaxis

Nowadays, with modern well-established principles of pre- and postoperative care combined with meticulous surgery, it is unusual to see a case of persistent adynamic ileus following straightforward abdominal surgery. Those examples that are encountered usually follow operations complicated by severe peritonitis, extensive retroperitoneal dissection or where there has been an anastomotic leak.

Whenever possible, the surgeon should ensure that the patient is in normal fluid and electrolyte balance before operation and that this is maintained postoperatively, especially in those patients in whom there is excessive fluid loss (e.g. from the gastric aspirate or a gastrointestinal fistula). It goes without saying that at laparotomy a sound technique is essential to reduce the possibility of leakage of intestinal contents into the peritoneal cavity.

Postoperative anxiety is relieved by reassurance and the judicious use of regular doses of opiates. Chlorpromazine is particularly useful in the anxious patient. Aerophagy should be discouraged, and the early use of gastric suction is instituted if vomiting or excessive belching occurs. There is no evidence, in any controlled trial, that the routine use of nasogastric aspiration is a prophylaxis against adynamic ileus. In my own practice, for example, a nasogastric tube is not routinely employed after elective biliary, gastric or large bowel surgery.

The established case

The vast majority of cases of adynamic ileus respond to the following simple but carefully conducted regime.

Firstly, fluid and electrolyte balance are maintained by means of an intravenous drip. The amounts given are estimated by combination of sound clinical assessment, scrupulously kept fluid balance charts and repeated serum electrolyte estimations. Particular care is taken to maintain a normal serum potassium level. Many surgeons commence intravenous alimentation via a caval line. It is unlikely, however, that this is required in the vast majority of cases where the period of ileus is likely to last only a number of days. Therefore, unless there is some other good indication for this therapy – particularly a high intestinal fistula – simple replacement of fluid and electrolytes alone will suffice.

Secondly a nasogastric tube is passed and put onto free drainage together with hourly aspirations; both modalities are carefully measured and recorded. By this means, swallowed air is removed and further gaseous distension prevented, nausea is improved and the concomitant gastric dilatation and retention are relieved. Once the tube is in place, there is no need to restrict the patient from small hourly drinks of clear fluids – 30–60 ml per hour. These are comforting and help keep the mouth clean.

Intestinal intubation by means of a Miller–Abbott or other nasogastric tube appears attractive in theory but is difficult to achieve in practice because of the failure to pass the tube onwards from the stomach to the lower alimentary tract in the great majority of patients. Most surgeons in the UK have abandoned its use in cases of adynamic ileus. I certainly have not used this technique once in the past 27 years in my own unit, and I do not believe that I have harmed my patients. However, they have certainly been saved a great deal of unnecessary discomfort.

Thirdly, pethidine (meperidine), morphine or omnopon are prescribed at regular four-hourly intervals, together with chlorpromazine, the dose being adjusted to the size and age of the patient.

Finally, strict and repeated clinical observations, together with radiographs of the abdomen, are carried out in order to monitor the progress of the ileus and to detect whether or not a mechanical obstruction may be supervening.

Under this regime, after several anxious days, bowel sounds are detected, griping 'wind' pains may be experienced by the patient, then flatus is passed and the crisis is over. Often a glance is enough to tell that all is well – the patient is sitting up in bed and asking for food!

Naturally, with such a common phenomenon, all sorts of means have been tried in order to stir the paralysed bowel into activity. These include the use of enemas, purgatives, prostigmine, pitressin, vitamin B and electrical pacemaking via a tube in the stomach together with an electrode on the abdominal wall or by electrodes applied externally. Pantothenic acid and metoclopramide have both had their advocates. In a situation in which the vast majority of patients get better under the conservative treatment outlined above, it is very difficult to assess the value of these techniques since they are usually reported by enthusiasts in entirely uncontrolled and anecdotal trials.

Pharmacological treatment

Based on the theory of reflex sympathetic inhibition of the bowel as the aetiology of adynamic ileus, it is attractive to use the concept of sympathetic blockade and/or parasympathetic stimulation in cases of recalcitrant ileus.

Guanethidine, an α- and β-adrenergic blocking agent, prevents sympathetic neuronal inhibition of the intestine and inhibition exacerbated by abnormally high levels of circulating catecholamine. Bethanechol, which structurally resembles acetylcholine, initiates gastrointestinal muscle contraction by direct stimulant action on acetylcholine receptors. The use of these two drugs in combination has been advocated by Neely and Catchpole.[77] More recently, cisapride has been introduced as an agent that selectively enhances acetylcholine release from the postganglionic cholinergic nerve endings in the myenteric plexus. Verlinden et al.[78] report a controlled trial in patients with postoperative ileus lasting from 48 to 72 hours who were given one or two intravenous doses of cisapride and compared with a control group. The first occurrence of flatus was taken to mark the cessation of ileus. There was no significant difference in remission of ileus between the groups in the first hour after injection. However, patients not responding to treatment in the first hour were given a repeat dose and observed for the following three hours. In this group, there was a significant remission of ileus in those receiving cisapride, which was particularly marked in those who had undergone intraperitoneal surgery.

There is no reason to doubt that as knowledge of the fundamental pharmacological disturbances of ileus improve, specific means of overcoming this syndrome should prove effective.

PSEUDO-OBSTRUCTION OF THE SMALL INTESTINE

Pseudo-obstruction of the small intestine is an extremely uncommon syndrome – even rarer than pseudo-obstruction of the colon, with which it may occasionally co-exist. It can be defined as a condition in which there are all the features of acute, or more often subacute or chronic, mechanical obstruction of the small bowel but with no obvious cause to be found at laparotomy on macroscopic examination of the dilated small bowel.

The subject has been well reviewed by Richards and Williams[79] and by Ishitani and Jones.[80] The condition may be subdivided into a primary group, with either an abnormality of the small bowel smooth muscle or a degeneration of the myenteric and submucosal plexuses of nerves, and a secondary group where intestinal dysfunction occurs as part of some recognized underlying defect.

Schuffler and colleagues[81] describe four infants who had chronic intestinal pseudo-obstruction caused by visceral myopathy. All had abdominal distension and emaciation and all died within 10–18 months of birth. Three, in addition, had signs of urological obstruction. The pathological features of visceral myopathy were identified in sample sites from the oesophagus, stomach, small and large intestine, ureter and bladder of all four infants.

The secondary group includes patients with diabetes mellitus, collagen disease, such as progressive systemic sclerosis (scleroderma) and systemic lupus, amyloid disease, neurological diseases such as Parkinson's disease, Chagas' disease, electrolyte disturbances (hypokalaemia and hypomagnesaemia), as well as pharmacologically induced disorders due to drugs already listed in the section on adynamic ileus.

Clinical features

It can be very difficult to differentiate between partial mechanical obstruction of the small intestine and chronic pseudo-obstruction. There are recurrent attacks of colicky abdominal pain, distension, nausea and vomiting together with constipation, although there may be episodes of diarrhoea associated with the attacks. The episodes may be intermittent, with periods of complete relief, but eventually the attacks may become frequent and even unrelenting. Symptoms usually commence in childhood or adolescence. Clinical examination reveals abdominal distension with noisy bowel sounds. In chronic cases, weight loss may be profound. In the secondary group of patients, there may be clinical features associated with the various syndromes listed above.

Plain abdominal radiographs show gaseous dilatation of the small intestine, but this may be associated with increased large bowel gas. A barium meal and follow-through or small bowel enema demonstrates a prolonged transit time of barium to the large bowel and excludes a mechanical obstruction. Prolonged bowel transit time may be demonstrated by special techniques such as the use of ingested technetium-99-labelled pellets. Oesophageal manometry can be useful in confirming chronic intestinal pseudo-obstruction. Although most patients do not complain of dysphagia, some 80% have abnormal oesophageal motility.

Definitive diagnosis may be made by a full-thickness biopsy of the intestine, which may be able to identify the smooth muscle degeneration or, with the help of special silver stains, nerve degeneration of the myenteric plexus. However, operation should be avoided whenever possible in these patients if the diagnosis can be established by any other means.

Management

Episodes of obstruction are dealt with conservatively by nasogastric aspiration and intravenous fluid replacement. Between attacks, the patient should be maintained on a low-bulk highly nutritious diet with vitamin supplements. Total parenteral nutrition may be necessary in occasional severe cases. Naturally a wide variety of drugs has been used in this condition with little effect, although cisapride may prove useful. Occasionally the surgeon will be forced into the situation of performing a laparotomy in such a patient where mechanical obstruction cannot be excluded. Here, the bare minimum should be performed if no mechanical obstructive lesion is found, and the surgeon should be content to merely carry out a full-thickness bowel biopsy.

SPECIAL TYPES OF SMALL BOWEL OBSTRUCTION

Many of the specific forms of small bowel obstruction detailed in the general section above are dealt with elsewhere, for example the neonatal obstructions (Chapter 62), small bowel tumours (Chapter 60), Meckel's diverticulum and potassium-induced ulcers of the small bowel (Chapter 54).

In this chapter the following special types of small bowel obstruction are detailed:

1. Bolus obstruction due to ingested food and other substances;
2. Gallstone ileus;
3. Adult intussusception;
4. Adhesions and bands.

Bolus obstruction

Obstruction due to food and other ingested materials

An extraordinary variety of foreign substances may be ingested into the alimentary tract. Fortunately the great majority pass spontaneously with few if any symptoms. Occasionally, impaction occurs, and this may produce perforation, ulceration or obstruction anywhere along the gut. This section concentrates on the last of these complications as it pertains to the small intestine.

Swallowed foreign bodies are particularly likely to be found in children, prisoners, mental defectives, psychiatric patients and circus performers. A modern variant is the ingestion of balloons filled with drugs in an attempt to smuggle these through customs or into prison. Rupture of the container can produce a fatal overdose, and in other cases impaction of the balloon causes intestinal obstruction. Trent and Kim[82] described two patients who had ingested packets of cocaine and who required urgent operation, one because of toxic manifestations of the ingested cocaine and the other because of small bowel obstruction. Another unusual problem presented by drug containers is noted by Muhletaler et al.[83] who report two cases of partial intestinal obstruction due to swallowing the desiccant packing in bottles of medicinal tablets. They warn that this may be swallowed inadvertently by people with poor eyesight instead of their tablets.

In the great majority of cases, if a swallowed object can pass from the oesophagus into the stomach it is likely to traverse the alimentary tract without causing further harm. For this reason, intestinal obstruction due to food is rare. Ward-McQuaid[84] collected 178 examples with no fewer than 45 different obstructing agents. Stephens[85] raised this number to 63 varieties of foodstuffs. Heading the list of obstructing agents was the persimmon. The skin of this fruit contains a cement-like substance termed shiboul which is precipitated by gastric juice and agglutinates the fibres and seeds of the fruit. Most obstructing food materials are, indeed, those rich in fibre or desiccated fruits that swell when they take up fluid or substances that are resistant to the gut enzymes. Two further

factors may predispose to obstruction. The first is inefficient mastication, either because the patient lacks teeth or because he has bolted the food. The second is that the patient may have had a previous partial gastrectomy or gastric short-circuit. In such cases, the stoma allows the food bolus to pass readily into the upper small gut. It is noteworthy that Norberg,[86] in a review of 26 patients undergoing 28 examples of intestinal obstruction due to swallowed food, found that every one had undergone a previous partial gastrectomy. The obstructing agents were oranges in 25 cases, one example each of apple and of grapefruit and the remaining one being of some unidentified fruit.

McClurken and Carp[87] report a patient who developed complete obstruction of the small bowel after the ingestion of two bowls of bran cereal. The obstructing mass had formed a toothpaste-like plug which required an enterotomy for its removal. Perhaps more examples may be expected of this phenomenon in today's diet-conscious society.

Diagnosis

Most patients never seek medical advice and settle down after an attack of 'green apple colic'. The features of the fully developed case are those of a typical intestinal obstruction, but the diagnosis can be suspected if the following triad co-exists:

1. The patient is edentulous;
2. The patient has undergone a previous partial gastrectomy;
3. The patient admits to the ingestion of a large amount of fruit material.

Treatment

If the surgeon is fairly certain of the diagnosis, a period of conservative treatment with nasogastric aspiration and intravenous fluid replacement is indicated. In most patients who present with the full-blown syndrome of small bowel obstruction, the diagnosis is not made until laparotomy. The site of impaction is usually the lower small bowel; the impacted loop is oedematous, inflamed and distended by what is obviously an intraluminal mass. The mass can usually be broken up with the fingers and coaxed into the caecum, which then allows normal evacuation subsequently to take place. If this manoeuvre is impossible, it may be necessary to open the bowel to remove the occluded material or even to carry out a localized resection. I have had to perform this on one occasion when a mass of compacted mushrooms in the terminal ileum perforated the distended segment of ileum.

Intestinal parasites

Obstruction of the small bowel due to masses of roundworms (*Ascaris lumbricoides*) is not unusual in Africa and in the Far East. Occasional cases will be seen in Western countries in travellers returning from overseas. Obstruction is especially likely to take place in children.[88,89] Impaction may occur anywhere throughout the small bowel but is particularly likely to take place in the terminal ileum. Obstruction may be precipitated in patients who have recently been given a vermifuge, which produces a solid mass of dead worms in the gut.

Diagnosis is made on the basis of a history of previous passage of worms or vomiting of worms, the presence of worms or their eggs in the stools and a palpable putty-like mass in one or other iliac fossae. Small bowel volvulus may complicate intestinal ascariasis; Wiersma and Hadley[90] give an account of 29 patients undergoing this complication.

Treatment

Mild and subacute cases are treated conservatively. Purgatives and anthelmintics are avoided until the obstructive episode has settled since the dead worms may impact, thus converting a partial into a complete occlusion. If the symptoms do not subside or if the diagnosis is in doubt, laparotomy is performed. If possible the mass of worms should be milked through the ileocaecal valve into the colon. If this is not possible or if the gut is obviously not viable, then resection is probably safer than enterotomy.[91] The installation of intraluminal vermifuge at the time of operation will minimize postoperative worm migration through the suture line or anastomosis.[92]

Gallstone ileus

Obstruction of the bowel by impaction of a gallstone within its lumen is an unusual phenomenon. According to the review by Raiford,[91] the condition was first noted at autopsy by Bartholin in 1654. Courvoisier[92] gave a detailed account of 131 cases in 1890. A full account of the pathology of this condition in 127 collected cases was given two years later by Naunyn,[93] who noted that large gallstones could ulcerate into the duodenum and become impacted at a lower level in the bowel.

Gallstone ileus accounts for 1–2% of all cases of intestinal obstruction. Thus, in a collected series of nearly 20 000 cases of intestinal obstruction, McLaughlin and Raines[94] found that 1.9% were due to gallstone obstruction. It is noteworthy that the phenomenon appears to be extremely rare in Japan where only 112 cases were recorded from the beginning of the century to 1978.[95]

The great majority of patients are elderly women – about 80% female with an average age of 75 years.

Pathology

It is well known that small gallstones may traverse the common bile duct and be passed per rectum, where they can be recovered from the stools. In some patients such stones might form the nucleus of an enterolith, which may enlarge sufficiently to obstruct the gut lumen.[96] To obstruct the lumen of the small intestine the gallstone must be at least 2.5 cm in diameter and it can only enter the alimentary canal by a process of ulceration. In most cases entry takes place via a fistula into the duodenum, but in others ulceration occurs into the small or large intestine or, rarely, into the stomach. Moreover, a large stone impacted at the lower end of the common bile duct may ulcerate its way through the ampulla into the duodenum. Courvoisier[92] noted the situation of the fistula in 36 post-mortems on cases of gallstone ileus. In 25 the fistula was located into the duodenum, there was one example each into the small intestine and the colon and two examples where the fistula occurred into both duodenum and colon. In

the remaining seven patients the stone had apparently passed through the ampulla. Impaction may occur anywhere along the alimentary canal from the duodenum to the colon but the site of election is in the lower ileum.

Even if a cholecystoenteric fistula forms, in many cases the causative gallstone may still be able to pass spontaneously per rectum and this probably happens in the majority of cases. The causative gallstone may still be able to pass spontaneously per rectum and this probably happens in the majority of cases. It is important to note that recurrent episodes of gallstone ileus and the presence of multiple stones within the gut are not at all uncommon. In some instances recurrence of the obstruction occurs within days or weeks of the first episode, suggesting that more than one stone is already present in the alimentary canal. Multiplicity is especially likely if the obstructing stone is found to be barrel-shaped with one end concave. When recurrences take place months or years later, they may well represent passage of further stones from the gall bladder through the fistula.

Clinical features

The typical patient is an old lady with acute small bowel obstruction in whom the actual cause is not suspected preoperatively. There is often a history of previous attacks of biliary colic, for example in 60% of a collected series of 154 patients.[97] In many cases, the obstruction is first partial and may remain so as a relatively mild or intermittent attack for some hours or even days. This sequence is probably due to the stone being pushed along the alimentary canal before it eventually impacts. Although the clinical diagnosis may be elusive, it should be remembered when an elderly female presents with the clinical features of intestinal obstruction and gives a previous history suggestive of biliary disease, especially if there is no other obvious cause.

Radiology

The presence of air in the biliary tree on plain radiographs of the abdomen in a patient with features of intestinal obstruction is all but diagnostic of gallstone ileus (Figure 53.18). The biliary air reflects the fact that there is a fistula into the alimentary tract. There are other causes of gas in the bile passages on radiological examination: the recent passage of a stone through the common duct; a previous sphincterotomy; a previous choledochoenterostomy or an emphysematous cholecystitis.

The stone itself may be visualized as a radio-opaque object and this may be seen to have changed in position from a previous radiograph. Thus Haffner and co-workers[98] found air within the biliary tree in 15 of 20 patients with gallstone ileus and visualized the stone itself in 10 of them.

Treatment

The usual preoperative care is instituted: nasogastric suction, intravenous fluid and electrolyte replacement and broad-spectrum antibiotic cover commencing with the premedication. At laparotomy the diagnosis becomes obvious when a hard mass is palpated at the junction of dilated and collapsed intestine, usually in the lower ileum. In most cases, the calculus is

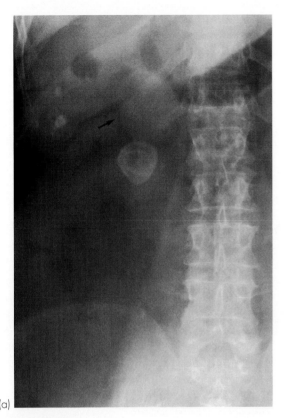

(a)

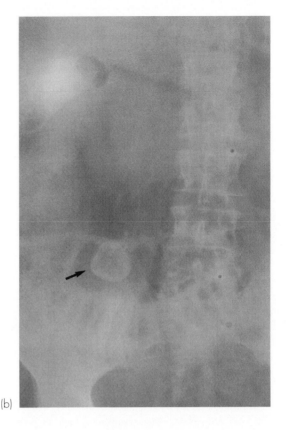

(b)

Figure 53.18

Plain abdominal radiograph (supine) in a 73-year-old woman with gallstone ileus. A large radiopaque calculus can be seen in the right lumbar region of the abdomen, and there is gas in the biliary tree (a). The patient had had six days of intermittent abdominal pain and vomiting, and she was dehydrated on admission to hospital with evidence of pre-renal uraemia. She was treated conservatively at first, but a repeat radiograph three days later showed that the calculus had moved to the right iliac fossa and lay within a dilated loop of bowel (b). Laparotomy was now performed. (Photograph supplied by Professor RCN Williamson).

found to be lying quite loosely within the bowel lumen. Non-crushing clamps are applied above and below the stone, the whole area is carefully isolated with wet packs and the stone is removed through a longitudinal enterotomy, which is then sutured transversely with two layers of continuous catgut (Figure 53.19, see colour plate also).

Occasionally, the stone may be found firmly impacted with threatened gangrene or even perforation. In such instances, resection of the affected portion of intestine is carried out with end-to-end anastomosis. If the proximal bowel is grossly distended, retrograde stripping is performed and the contents are aspirated through the nasogastric tube.

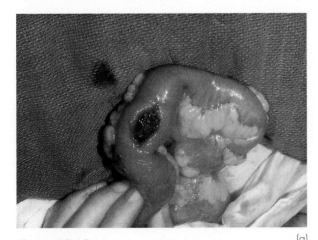

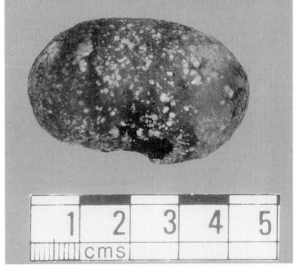

(a)

(b)

Figure 53.19

Gallstone ileus. A calculus has been exposed through an enterotomy in the ileum (a), and it is then removed (b). See legend to Figure 53.18 for the patient's clinical details.

A systematic search must be made throughout the small and large intestine for the presence of other stones. This procedure is especially important if the calculus that has been removed is found to be facetted, has a concave surface or has obviously fragmented. The gall bladder is then palpated. If a large stone is felt, it should be removed by incising into the gall bladder. The incision is closed with a continuous catgut suture. It is not necessary to insert a cholecystotomy tube into the gall bladder since it is already decompressed by the fistula. If no stones are left in the gall bladder and if the duct system is patent, the fistula will usually close spontaneously. Provided that the bowel is carefully examined for a second stone and that any remaining large stone within the gall bladder is removed by cholecystotomy, it is unlikely that additional stones will fistulate from the gall bladder into the bowel lumen and most fistulas will shrink down and close once the stone has passed. It is not advisable to perform a routine cholecystectomy, since these are often elderly sick patients and the operative steps outlined above suffice.

In the postoperative period it is certainly worthwhile performing ultrasonography to demonstrate whether or not there are residual gallstones. If one or more large stones have been overlooked or if the patient subsequently develops recurrent attacks of biliary colic, then an elective cholecystectomy can be recommended, but in most cases this will not be necessary.

Andersson and Zederfeldt[99] report that of their 44 patients with gallstone ileus, five were subjected to cholecystectomy and closure of the fistula at the time of operation for the gallstone obstruction. Three of these patients died, two of them because of peritonitis secondary to failure of healing of the duodenal closure. However, of the 31 surviving patients, only eight subsequently had symptoms of biliary disease and only four of these required operation for their symptoms.

Adult intussusception

In spite of a good deal of overlap, there are aetiological, pathological and clinical differences that divide cases of intussusception into those occurring in children (peak incidence under two years of age) and those occurring in adults. Childhood intussusception is dealt with in Chapter 62. It is common, and in the great majority of patients there is no obvious aetiological factor. In adults intussusception is rather unusual, but nearly all patients have an obvious cause, usually a tumour, which is likely to be benign in the small bowel and malignant in cases of colonic intussusception.

Occasionally, a non-tumorous lesion is found at the apex of an intussusception. Among these, an inverted Meckel's diverticulum is probably the commonest. Other causes include a granuloma of the appendix stump, the excluded small bowel segment following jejunoileal bypass for morbid obesity, mucocele of the appendix and the swollen bowel associated with typhoid or with bacillary or amoebic dysentery.

Among the benign tumours, a submucous lipoma is frequently reported and this is most often found in the caecum and ascending colon. Although the benign pedunculated tumour of the small intestine associated with the Peutz–Jeghers

syndrome is an unusual lesion, it has a strong association with intussusception. Intussusception is a common finding in patients with metastatic melanoma who have gastrointestinal obstructive symptoms. The metastasis may be solitary, and under such circumstances resection should be performed.[100]

Although in the Western world adult intussusception usually has an underlying cause, this is not so in some African communities where there is a high incidence of idiopathic adult intussusception. In a review of 436 cases of intestinal obstruction in Ibadan, Nigeria, Cole[12] recorded 76 examples of idiopathic caecocolic intussusception out of a total of 119 examples of intussusception.

Clinical features

The adult patient with intussusception may present with the typical features of acute intestinal obstruction, but quite often there are repeated incidents of subacute obstruction; during these attacks an obvious mass may be found in the abdomen or even be noted by the patient. Rarely, the intussuscepting tumour of the colon may prolapse through the anal verge or be seen at sigmoidoscopy. The presence of typical pigment spots on the face, lips and buccal mucosa would suggest the diagnosis of Peutz–Jeghers syndrome.

Radiological examination

Plain radiographs of the abdomen may demonstrate dilated loops of small bowel with fluid levels. A chronic small bowel intussusception can be shown by a barium small bowel meal, whereas an intussuscepting large bowel growth may be visualized on a barium enema examination. The barium enema may produce at least a temporary reduction of the intussusception. One of three typical pictures may be seen (Figure 53.20): the so-called 'pitch fork sign', a crescentic defect or, most typical of all, a coiled spring appearance around the apex of the intussusception.

Treatment

The treatment of adult intussusception is invariably surgical. The diagnosis at operation is not difficult to make, but the exact underlying aetiology may be obscure until the specimen has been reduced and dissected. Because of the high risk of underlying malignancy in large bowel intussusception, it is advisable to proceed at once to resection without any attempt

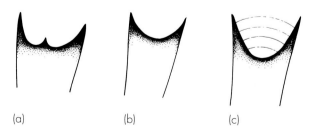

(a)   (b)   (c)

Figure 53.20
Diagrams of the typical barium enema appearances of the 'head' of an intussusception in the adult. (a) 'pitch fork'; (b) 'crescent'; (c) 'coiled spring'.

to reduce the intussusception. However, with intussusception of the small bowel, a cautious attempt at reduction should be made. If the lesion is found to be necrotic, then immediate resection is carried out. If there is no obvious cause, nothing further than reduction need be performed. A benign tumour should be locally removed through an enterotomy, but if there is any question of malignancy an adequate resection should be performed. In cases of Peutz–Jeghers syndrome, in which further episodes of intussusception can be anticipated, it is important to preserve as much bowel as possible, so that a simple enterotomy with removal of the intussuscepting polyp is all that is necessary provided that the bowel is viable.

Adhesion obstruction

Aetiology of postoperative adhesions

The process of adhesion formation has been carefully studied in humans and in laboratory animals. There is first hyperaemia and oedema of the damaged or inflamed serosa, then rapid deposition of fibrin. Involved surfaces become adherent to each other by means of an inflammatory exudate of fibrin and polymorphs. This fibrinous anlage may absorb within a few days, as observed by Jackson[106] in dogs in whom a plastic observation window was inserted into the abdominal wall. In other cases, organization may occur, with ingrowth of blood vessels and fibroblasts and the development of established fibrous adhesions.

It soon became obvious that the important factor to determine was what decides whether fibrinous adhesions absorb completely and without trace or become organized into persistent (and potentially dangerous) fibrous strands. By armchair reasoning rather than experimental observations, and based on the analogy of the healing of cutaneous wounds, surgeons and pathologists assumed that it was the mesothelium that determined whether the fibrinous exudate became absorbed or organized. If this layer was intact, they argued, then the fibrin would disappear. If destroyed, then persistent fibrous adhesions must inevitably develop. It was this theory that led surgeons to believe that peritoneal denudation must be avoided at all costs, i.e. that peritoneal defects must be oversewn, patched or covered by grafts and that raw areas must be eliminated. The surgeon visualizes that a large peritoneal defect following an abdominoperineal excision of the rectum, for example, can only heal by massive fibrosis, in much the same way that a similar mangled area of skin would heal by extensive scar tissue. However, when put to the test, it has been found both clinically and in the laboratory that extensive areas of denuded serosa heal without adhesion formation. In my own studies,[107] large defects produced by excision of the parietal peritoneum in the rat healed within days to produce a glistening smooth serosa without adhesions. However, when the peritoneal defect was repaired by sutures or peritoneal graft, adhesion formation was almost invariable. Injection studies and even naked-eye examination of these adhesions revealed tiny blood vessels running along the adhesive strand into the sutured or grafted tissue. This observation suggested that it was not the peritoneal defect itself that produced adhesions but rather the presence of devascularized tissue that must inevitably result from either the suturing of the defect or the application of a free graft to the area. Similar adhesion production could be obtained by any other method that resulted in the formation of ischaemic tissue within the abdominal cavity, for example by crushing the parietal peritoneum. This ischaemic concept was reinforced by demonstrating that division of the mesentery of the small intestine would result in dense adhesions forming to the ischaemic segment of bowel. Vascular injection studies confirmed that these adhesions carried vessels into the damaged gut wall and could often maintain the viability of the intestine.

Ischaemic tissues are not unique in stimulating an inflammatory vascular response and adhesion formation. Many of the substances that may contaminate the peritoneal cavity at the time of laparotomy may be responsible for the formation of granulomas and the development of fibrous intra-abdominal strands. These include fragments of gauze, lint, cotton wool, clumps of antibiotic powder, powerful antiseptics, and above all, the various dusting powders that have been introduced for use with surgical gloves.[108,109]

The most detailed account of the extent of this problem is that by Myllarniemi,[110] of 309 cases of postoperative adhesions, biopsy showed foreign body reactions in 61% and the incidence was particularly high after major or repeated operations. In half the cases, the foreign material was talc, in a quarter it was lint or thread, and the remaining examples showed starch, extruded gut contents, suture materials or a mixture of materials, usually talc associated with thread.

Peritoneal fibrinolysis

Studies on the fibrinolytic activity of the peritoneum have cast important light on the exact mechanism of adhesion formation and may provide an important clue to prophylaxis. Buckman et al.[111,112] and Raftery[113] have shown that the peritoneum has a high plasminogen activity measured by the areas of lysis produced on fibrin plates by standard biopsy specimens of the tissues under investigation. Plasminogen activator converts plasminogen into plasmin, which in turn lyses fibrin. This plasminogen activity is lost in peritoneum rendered ischaemic by grafting, diathermy coagulation or tight suturing. Thus, the intact peritoneum can lyse the fibrinous coagulum. When this activity is reduced, as in the presence of trauma, ischaemia or infection, fibrin organization occurs and fibrous adhesions result.

In our laboratory, Lennox (unpublished observations) has demonstrated that the peritoneal mesothelium possesses a high plasminogen activator activity, but the underlying tissues also contain plasminogen activator properties, probably from the endothelial cells of the submesothelial blood vessels. This activity is less than that of the mesothelial cells but is still present. If the mesothelial layer has an activity of 100%, the submesothelial tissues have an activity of 58%. When an area of peritoneum is excised, the underlying tissues may well lie in contact with a fully peritonealized organ with its full complement of plasminogen activator activity. Between them, the two surfaces are able to lyse the fibrinous adhesions. When two denuded areas are in apposition, the level of plasminogen activator may be insufficient to lyse the fibrin and persistent adhesions result. To study this matter further, we conducted a series of experiments in rats.[114] Of 15 animals with parietal peritoneal defects, none developed adhesions. When the caecum was denuded in another 15 animals, three developed adhesions. When both caecum and adjacent parietal peritoneum were denuded in 15 further rats, 12 developed adhesions ($P < 0.01$).

Prevention of adhesions

During this century there has been a great deal of work on attempts to prevent adhesions. The problem has been approached from a number of aspects, which can be classified as follows:[115]

1. The prevention of the deposition of fibrin in the postoperative peritoneal exudate by use of anticoagulants, e.g. heparin, dicoumarol, sodium citrate and dextran.

2. The removal of fibrin which has already been deposited. This has included lavage with saline, the use of enzymes such as pepsin and trypsin, and both local and systemic fibrinolytic agents including streptokinase, actase, streptodornase and urokinase.

3. The mechanical separation of loops of intestine from each other. This has included distending the abdominal cavity with oxygen, the use of olive oil, liquid paraffin, etc. and the use of every variety of membrane and of silicones to cover traumatized peritoneum.

4. The inhibition of fibroblastic proliferation in order to prevent fibroplasia within the deposits of fibrin. This has included the use of antihistamines, steroids and cytotoxic drugs.

Reviewing many hundreds of papers in this field, the overall picture is of enthusiastic reports on experimental studies, progressing in some cases to actual clinical use, then further reports showing either no effect at all or an actual increase in adhesion formation compared with controls. Eventually each particular fashion has been abandoned.

Based on the studies quoted above on the fibrinolytic action of normal peritoneum, removal of the fibrin exudate would be the most attractive concept for adhesion prevention. We were able to show that a highly purified preparation of streptokinase[116] undoubtedly inhibited adhesion formation in the rabbit, but it was necessary to give the streptokinase intraperitoneally on two or three consecutive days immediately after operation.

Menzies and Ellis[117] have demonstrated that recombinant tissue plasminogen activator, applied as a topical preparation, can prevent the re-formation of divided adhesions in the rabbit. There was no evidence in this study of excessive haemorrhage or delayed wound healing, and a clinical trial is now justified in the use of this material when patients are submitted to laparotomy for recurrent adhesion obstruction.

Treatment of obstruction due to adhesions

It is a good general rule that an acute small bowel mechanical obstruction is a mandatory indication for urgent operation.

There are two instances, however, when there may be qualifications to this rule.

First, it is not uncommon to see a patient in the early days after a major operation complicated by severe ileus, who complains of abdominal pains and whose previously silent abdomen now reveals bowel sounds. In some circumstances, there may be a period of doubt as to whether these signs represent a recovering ileus, soon to be rewarded by the passage of flatus, or the development of mechanical adhesive obstruction. Obviously it is wise to continue conservative treatment for a little longer. Fresh radiographs of the abdomen are taken which may be very helpful; gas extended through the large bowel suggests a recovering ileus, whereas loops of distended small intestine with fluid levels suggest mechanical obstruction. If the patient has already passed flatus or has had a bowel action and then becomes distended with colicky pain, the diagnosis must be one of adhesive obstruction and operation will be indicated.

The second indication, fortunately seen less often nowadays, is in a patient who has suffered repeated previous episodes of intestinal obstruction with several previous operations for division of adhesions. Under these circumstances one is encouraged by the fact that matted loops of intestine, stuck one to the other, are unlikely to be strangulated. Here a trial period of nasogastric aspiration and intravenous fluid replacement is certainly justified in the hope that the obstruction is incomplete and that spontaneous remission will occur. Often, indeed, there may be a history of previous admissions in which such a period of conservative treatment has proved successful. The most careful observation must be carried out, however, and any deterioration in the patient's condition indicates that immediate operative intervention is advisable.

When operation is indicated in the early postoperative period, the second laparotomy is carried out through the recent abdominal wound. A loop of bowel may be found adherent to the wound itself (not uncommonly to a small defect in the peritoneum where early dehiscence is taking place). More often it will be found that the site of the obstruction is in association with the operative area itself. For example, a loop of small intestine will be found adherent to the pelvic floor after an abdominoperineal excision of the rectum, or herniation develops through a mesenteric defect which has been imperfectly closed. Having freed the obstruction, the surgeon decompresses the bowel by retrograde milking of the intestine back into the stomach, and any anatomical defect such as a hole in the mesentery is then repaired.

When laparotomy is being performed for adhesive obstruction late after previous abdominal surgery, again it is usually possible to perform this through the old incision. If the previous wound is re-opened, once again great care must be taken in case a loop of bowel is adherent to the undersurface of the scar. It is a useful manoeuvre to extend the incision a little higher or lower beyond the reaches of the original scar, so that intact peritoneal cavity can hopefully be entered at the extremity of the wound.

The operation for late intestinal obstruction due to adhesions can be one of the simplest or one of the most testing in

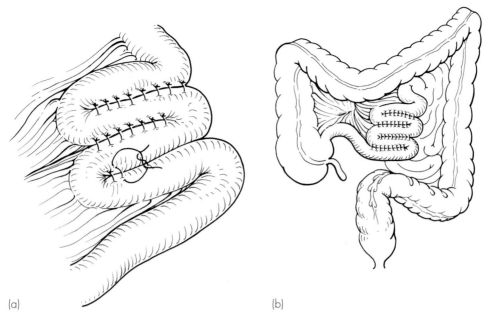

(a)   (b)

Figure 53.21
Plication of the intestine in diagrammatic form. (a) The operation in progress; (b) the procedure completed.

surgery. At one end of the spectrum, there may be a solitary adhesive band that requires simple division. At the other, the surgeon finds a matted mass of intestines that requires the greatest care and patience to free by sharp dissection. In some cases it may be wise to resect or bypass an inextricably fused clump of obstructed bowel.

Having divided the obstructing adhesions, is there any way to prevent further episodes of obstruction? A number of plication procedures have been advocated which are designed to avoid further acute kinking of the matted bowel. This technique was first reported by Wichmann[118] and popularized by Noble,[119] after whom the operation is often named. Plication is a major procedure that requires extensive division of the adhesions and then meticulous suture of loop after loop of intestine into place (Figure 53.21). More recently, transmesenteric plication of loops of small intestine in a serpentine pattern has been put forward as a simpler and safer procedure.[120] This procedure is depicted in Figure 53.22. I have no personal experience of

these operations, and I am not convinced from my reading of the results of others that the incidence of recurrent intestinal obstruction in their patients is any lower than in those subjected to simple division of the obstructing bands. Only a prospective multicentre trial would provide an answer.

I employ the Baker tube[121] (Figure 53.23) introduced through a jejunostomy and threaded through the whole length of the small intestine. The Foley-type balloon at its end assists its being threaded through the bowel. Its intrinsice stiffness prevents kinking while adhesions develop. Munro and Jones[122] give an excellent account of operative intubation in the treatment of complicated small bowel obstruction. Again, there are only anecdotal reports of the value of this tube. Where there is

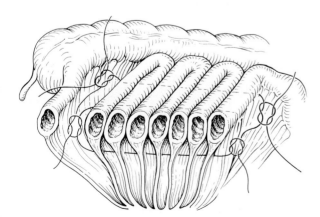

Figure 53.22
Two diagrammatic views of transmesenteric plication.

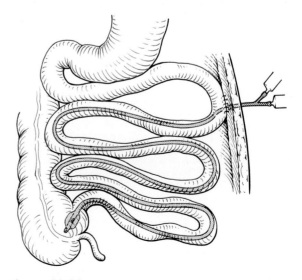

Figure 53.23
Intestinal intubation via a jejunostomy (based on Munro and Jones[122]).

a single band or a few adhesions, simple division alone is all that is indicated. When multiple severe adhesions are present, we still need more information regarding the wisest procedure to adopt: plication, intubation or simple lysis.

The experimental studies using topical plasminogen activator are most encouraging, and we are now ready for a clinical trial in which, following division of the adhesions, the plasminogen activator is applied in a suitable topical vehicle. At present we are simply using vaseline for this purpose, but much further work needs to be done in this fascinating and important field.

REFERENCES

1. Cope Z. *A History of the Acute Abdomen.* London: Oxford University Press, 1965.
2. Wangensteen OH. Historical aspects of the management of acute intestinal obstruction. *Surgery* 1969; **65:** 363.
3. Ellis H. *Intestinal Obstruction.* New York, Appleton Century Crofts, 1982.
4. Vick RH. Statistics of acute intestinal obstruction. *BMJ* 1932; **2:** 546.
5. Waldron GW & Hampton JM. Intestinal obstruction: a half century comparative analysis. *Ann Surg* 1961; **153:** 839.
6. McEntee G, Pender D, Mulvin D et al. Current spectrum of intestinal obstruction. *Br J Surg* 1987; **74:** 975.
7. Nelson IW & Ellis H. The spectrum of intestinal obstruction to-day. *Br J Clin Pract* 1984; **38:** 249.
8. Gill SS & Eggleston FC. Acute intestinal obstruction. *Arch Surg* 1965; **91:** 589.
9. McAdam IWJ. A three year review of intestinal obstruction: Mulago Hospital, Kampala, Uganda. *East Afr Med J* 1961; **38:** 536.
10. White A. Intestinal obstruction in the Rhodesian African: a review of 112 cases. *East Afr Med J* 1961; **38:** 525.
11. Chiedozi LC, Abo IO & Piserchia NE. Mechanical bowel obstruction. Review of 316 cases in Benin city. *Am J Surg* 1980; **139:** 389.
12. Cole GJ. A review of 436 cases of intestinal obstruction in Ibadan. *Gut* 1965; **6:** 151.
13. Badoe EA. Patterns of acute intestinal obstruction in Ghana. *West Afr Med J* 1968; **17:** 194.
14. Brooks VEH & Butler A. Acute intestinal obstruction in Jamaica. *Surg Gynecol Obstet* 1966; **122:** 261.
15. Ti TK & Yong NK. The pattern of intestinal obstruction in Malaysia. *Br J Surg* 1976; **63:** 963.
16. Tandon HD & Prakash A. Pathology of intestinal tuberculosis and its distinction from Crohn's disease. *Gut* 1972; **13:** 260.
17. Kark AE & Rundle WJ. The pattern of intussusception in Africans in Natal. *Br J Surg* 1960; **48:** 296.
18. Kaltiala EH, Lenkkeri H & Larmi TK. Mechanical intestinal obstruction. An analysis of 577 cases. *Ann Chir Gynaecol Fenn* 1972; **61:** 87.
19. Saidi F. The high incidence of intestinal volvulus in Iran. *Gut* 1969; **10:** 838.
20. Sykes PA, Boulter KH & Schofield PF. The microflora of the obstructed bowel. *Br J Surg* 1976; **63:** 721.
21. Wangensteen OH & Rea CE. The distension factor in simple intestinal obstruction; experimental study with exclusion of swallowed air by cervical esophagostomy. *Surgery* 1939; **5:** 327.
22. Shields R. The absorption and secretion of fluid and electrolytes by the obstructed bowel. *Br J Surg* 1965; **52:** 774.
23. Laufman H & Nora PF. Physiological problems underlying strangulation obstruction. *Surg Clin North Am* 1962; **42:** 219.
24. Obre H. Distension of intestine following strangulation eleven months previously. *Trans Pathol Soc Lond* 1851; **3:** 95.
25. Barry HC. Fibrous stricture of the small intestine following strangulated hernia. *Br J Surg* 1942; **30:** 64.
26. Lien GS, Mori M & Enjoji M. Delayed post traumatic ischemic stricture of the small intestine. A clinicopathologic study of four cases. *Acta Pathol Jpn* 1987; **37:** 1367.
27. Kingsnorth AN. Fluid-filled intestinal obstruction. *Br J Surg* 1976; **63:** 289.
28. Maglinte DDT, Peterson LA, Vahey TN, Miller RE & Chenish SM. Enteroclysis in partial small bowel obstruction. *Am J Surg* 1984; **147:** 325.
29. Koruth NM, Koruth A & Matheson NA. The place of contrast enema in the management of large bowel obstruction. *J R Coll Surg Edinb* 1985; **30:** 258.
30. Stewart J, Finan PJ, Courtney DF & Brennan TG. Does a water soluble contrast enema assist in the management of acute large bowel obstruction: a prospective study of 117 cases. *Br J Surg* 1984; **71:** 799.
31. Cooke RV. Discussion on small bowel obstruction. *Proc R Soc Med* 1958; **51:** 503.
32. Silen W, Hein MF & Goldman L. Strangulation obstruction of the small intestine. *Arch Surg* 1962; **85:** 121.
33. Becker WF. Acute adhesive ileus: a study of 412 cases with particular reference to the abuse of tube decompression in treatment. *Surg Gynecol Obstet* 1952; **95:** 472.
34. Zollinger RM & Kinsey DL. Diagnosis and management of intestinal obstruction. *Am Surg* 1964; **30:** 1.
35. Jackson BB. *Occlusion of the Superior Mesenteric Artery.* Springfield Illinois: CC Thomas, 1963.
36. Wilson C & Imrie CW. Amylase and gut infarction. *Br J Surg* 1986; **73:** 219.
37. Pain JA, Collier DS & Hanka R. Small bowel obstruction: computer-assisted prediction of strangulation at presentation. *Br J Surg* 1987; **74:** 981.
38. Ellis H. Diagnosis of the acute abdomen. *BMJ* 1968; **1:** 491.
39. Wolfson PJ, Bauer JJ, Galernt IM, Kreel I & Aufses AH. Use of the long tube in the management of patients with small-intestinal obstruction due to adhesions. *Arch Surg* 1985; **120:** 1001.
40. Bizer LS, Liebling RW, Delaney HM & Gliedman ML. Small bowel obstruction. The role of nonoperative treatment in simple intestinal obstruction and predictive cirteria for strangulation obstruction. *Surgery* 1981; **89:** 407.
41. Brolin RE. Partial small bowel obstruction. *Surgery* 1984; **95:** 145.
42. Ellis H, Bucknall TE & Cox PJ. Abdominal incisions and their closure. *Curr Probl Surg* 1985; **22:** 1–51.
43. Savage PT. The management of acute intestinal obstruction. A critical review of 179 personal cases. *Br J Surg* 1960; **47:** 643.
44. Jones PF & Matheson NA. Operative decompression of intestinal obstruction. *Lancet* 1969; **i:** 1197.
45. Ver Steeg KR & Broders CW. Gangrene of the bowel. *Surg Clin North Am* 1979; **59:** 869.
46. Cooperman M, Martin EW & Carey LC. Evaluation of ischemic intestine by Doppler ultrasound. *Am J Surg* 1980; **139:** 73.
47. Cooperman M, Martin EW & Carey LC. Determination of intestinal viability by Doppler ultrasonography in venous infarction. *Ann Surg* 1980; **191:** 57.
48. Gibson CL. A study of 1000 operations for acute intestinal obstruction. *Ann Surg* 1900; **32:** 486.
49. Souttar HS. Acute intestinal obstruction. *BMJ* 1925; **2:** 1000.
50. Smith CA, Perry JF & Onehiro EG. Mechanical intestinal obstructions. A study of 1252 cases. *Surg Gynecol Obstet* 1955; **100:** 651.
51. Becker WF. Intestinal obstruction. An analysis of 1007 cases. *South Med J* 1955; **48:** 41.
52. Barling EV. Intestinal obstruction. *Aust NZ J Surg* 1956; **285:** 25.
53. Stewardson RH, Bombeck T & Nyhus LM. Critical operative management of small bowel obstruction. *Ann Surg* 1978; **187:** 189.
54. Mucha P. Small intestinal obstruction. *Surg Clin North Am* 1987; **67:** 597.
55. Leffall LD, Quander J & Symphax B. Strangulation intestinal obstruction: a clinical appraisal. *Arch Surg* 1965; **91:** 592.
56. Bayliss WM & Starling EH. The movements and innervation of the small intestine. *J Physiol* 1899; **24:** 99.
57. Neely J & Catchpole B. Ileus; the restoration of alimentary motility by pharmacological means. *Br J Surg* 1971; **58:** 21.
58. Nadrowski L. Paralytic ileus: recent advances in pathophysiology and treatment. *Curr Surg* 1983; **40:** 260.
59. Petri G. Invited commentary on the use of chlorpromazine in the treatment of adynamic ileus. *World J Surg* 1977; **1:** 659.
60. Smith J Kelly KA & Weinshilboum RM. Pathophysiology of postoperative ileus. *Arch Surg* 1977; **112:** 203.
61. Rennie JA, Christofides, ND, Mitchenere P et al. Neural and humoral factors in postoperative ileus. *Br J Surg* 1980; **67:** 694.
62. Wells C, Tinkler I, Rawlinson K, Jones H & Saunders J. Postoperative gastrointestinal motility. *Lancet* 1964; **i:** 4.
63. Rothnie NG, Harper RAK & Catchpole BN. Early postoperative gastrointestinal motility. *Lancet* 1963; **ii:** 64.

64. Ross B, Watson BW & Kay AW. Studies on the effect of vagotomy on small intestinal motility using the radio-telemetering capsule. *Gut* 1963; **4**: 77.

65. Wilson JP. Postoperative motility of the large intestine in man. *Gut* 1975; **16**: 689.

66. Graber JN, Schulte WJ, Condon RE & Cowles VE. Relationship of duration of postoperative ileus to extent and site of operative dissection. *Surgery* 1982; **92**: 87.

67. Blackburn G & Rob CG. The abdominal wound in the field. *Br J Surg* 1945; **33**: 46.

68. Lindquist B. Propulsive gastrointestinal motility related to retroperitoneal irritation. An experimental study in the rat. *Acta Chir Scand* 1968; Suppl. **384**: 44.

69. Woods JH, Erickson LW, Condon RE & Schulte WJ. Postoperative ileus: a colonic problem. *Surgery* 1978; **84**: 527.

70. Watkin DFL. Spinal ileus. *Br J Surg* 1970; **57**: 142.

71. Schwartz DR & Wilks HW. Acetabular development after reduction of congenital dislocation of the hip: a follow up study of fifty hips. *J Bone Joint Surg* (Am) 1964; **46**: 1549.

72. Boruchow IB, Miller LD & Fitts WT. Paralytic ileus in myxedema. *Arch Surg* 1966; **92**: 960.

73. Spira IA, Rubenstein R, Wolf D & Wolff WI. Fecal impaction following methadone ingestion simulating intestinal obstruction. *Ann Surg* 1975; **181**: 15.

74. Milner G & Hills NF. Adynamic ileus and nortriptyline. *BMJ* 1966; **1**: 841.

75. Ellis H. In Schwartz S & Ellis H (eds) *Maingot's Abdominal Operations*, 8th edn, vol. 2. New York, Appleton Century Crofts, 1985: 1179.

76. Gammill SL & Nice CM. Air fluid levels: their occurrence in normal patients and their role in the analysis of ileus. *Surgery* 1972; **71**: 771.

77. Neely J & Catchpole B. Ileus, the restoration of alimentary motility by pharmacological means. *Br J Surg* 1971; **58**: 21.

78. Verlinden M, Michiels G, Boghaert A, Coster M & Dehertoy P. Treatment of postoperative gastrointestinal atony. *Br J Surg* 1987; **74**: 614.

79. Richards WO & Williams LF. Obstruction of the large and small intestine. *Surg Clin North Am* 1988; **68**: 355.

80. Ishitani MB & Jones RS. Intestinal obstruction in Adults. In Scott HW, Sawyers JL (eds) *Surgery of the Stomach Duodenum and Small Intestine*. Boston: Blackwell Scientific, 1987: 893.

81. Schuffler MD, Pagon RA, Schwartz R & Bill AH. Visceral myopathy of the gastrointestinal tract in infants. *Gastroenterology* 1988; **94**: 892.

82. Trent MS & Kim U. Cocaine packet ingestion. Surgical or medical management? *Arch Surg* 1987; **122**: 1179.

83. Muhletaler CA, Gerlock AJ, Shull HJ & Adkins RB. The pill bottle desiccant; a cause of partial gastrointestinal obstruction. *JAMA* 1980; **243**: 1921.

84. Ward-McQuaid N. Intestinal obstruction due to food. *BMJ* 1950; **2**: 1106.

85. Stephens FO. Intestinal colic caused by food. *Gut* 1966; **7**: 581.

86. Norberg PB. Intestinal obstruction due to food. *Surg Gynecol Obstet* 1961; **113**: 149.

87. McClurken JB & Carp NZ. Bran-inducted small-intestinal obstruction in a patient with no history of abdominal operation. *Arch Surg* 1988; **123**: 98.

88. Ihekwaba FN. Intestinal ascariasis and the acute abdomen in the tropics. *J R Coll Surg Edinb* 1980; **25**: 452.

89. Louw JH. Abdominal complications of *Ascaris lumbricoides* infestation in children. *Br J Surg* 1966; **53**: 510.

90. Wiersma R & Hadley GP. Small bowel volvulus complicating intestinal ascariasis in children. *Br J Surg* 1988; **75**: 86.

91. Raiford TS. Intestinal obstruction due to gallstones (gallstone ileus). *Ann Surg* 1961; **153**: 830.

92. Courvoisier LG. *Beitrage zu Pathologie und Chirurgie der Gallenwage*. Leipzig: FCW Vogel, 1890.

93. Naunyn B. *A Treatise on Cholelithiathis*. London: New Sydenham Society, 1892.

94. McLaughlin CW & Raines M. Obstruction of the alimentary tract from gallstones. *Am J Surg* 1951; **81**: 424.

95. Kasahara Y, Amemura H & Shiraha S. *Am J Surg* 1980; **140**: 437.

96. Newman JH. A case of gall-stone ileus in the absence of a biliary enteric fistula. *Br J Surg* 1972; **59**: 573.

97. Kirkland KC & Croce EJ. Gallstone intestinal obstruction. A review of the literature and presentation of 12 cases including 3 recurrences. *JAMA* 1961; **176**: 494.

98. Haffner JFW, Semb LS & Aakus T. Gallstone ileus. A report of 22 cases. *Acta Chir Scand* 1969; **135**: 707.

99. Andersson A & Zederfeldt B. Gallstone ileus. *Acta Chir Scand* 1969; **135**: 713.

100. Klausner JM, Skornick Y, Lelcuk S, Baratz M & Merhav A. Acute complications of metastatic melanoma to the gastrointestinal tract. *Br J Surg* 1982; **69**: 195.

101. Playforth RH, Holloway JB & Griffen WO. Mechanical small bowel obstruction. A plea for earlier intervention. *Ann Surg* 1970; **171**: 783.

102. Stewardson RH, Bombeck T & Nyhus LM. Critical operative management of small bowel obstruction. *Ann Surg* 1987; **187**: 189.

103. Perry JF, Smith GA & Yonehiro EG. Intestinal obstruction due to adhesions; a review of 388 cases. *Ann Surg* 1955; **142**: 810.

104. Raf LE. Causes of abdominal adhesions in cases of intestinal obstruction. *Acta Chir Scand* 1969; **135**: 75.

105. Weibel MA & Majno G. Peritoneal adhesions and their relation to abdominal surgery. *Am J Surg* 1973; **126**: 345.

106. Jackson BB. Observations on intraperitoneal adhesions – an experimental study. *Surgery* 1958; **44**: 507.

107. Ellis H. The aetiology of postoperative adhesions. *Br J Surg* 1962; **50**: 10.

108. Cade D & Ellis H. The peritoneal reaction to starch and its modification by prednisone. *Exp Surg Res* 1976; **8**: 471.

109. Jagelman DG & Ellis H. Starch and intraperitoneal adhesion formation. *Br J Surg* 1973; **60**: 111.

110. Myllarniemi H. Foreign material in adhesion formation after abdominal surgery. *Acta Chir Scand* (Suppl) 1967; 377.

111. Buckman RF, Woods M, Sargent L & Gervin AS. A unifying pathogenetic mechanism in the etiology of intraperitoneal adhesions. *J Surg Res* 1976; **20**: 1.

112. Buckman RF, Buckman PD, Hufnagel HV & Gervin AS. A physiologic basis for the adhesion-free healing of deperitonealized surfaces. *J Surg Res* 1976; **21**: 67.

113. Raftery AT. Effect of peritoneal trauma on peritoneal fibrinolytic activity and intraperitoneal adhesion formation. An experimental study in the rat. *Eur Surg Res* 1981; **13**: 397.

114. Lamont P & Ellis H. 1989 (in press).

115. Ellis H. The cause and prevention of post-operative adhesions. *Surg Gynecol Obstet* 1971; **133**: 497.

116. James DCO, Ellis H & Hugh TB. The effect of streptokinase on experimental intraperitoneal adhesion formation. *J Pathol Bacteriol* 1965; **90**: 279.

117. Menzies D & Ellis H. Intra-abdominal adhesions and their prevention by topical tissue plasminogen activator. *J R Soc Med* 1989 (in press).

118. Wichmann SE. Uber die peritonisierung von wundflachen am dunndarm. *Langenbeck Arch Klin Chir* 1934; **179**: 589.

119. Noble TB. Plication of small intestine as prophylaxis against adhesions. *Am J Surg* 1937; **35**: 41.

120. Childs WA & Phillips RB. Experience with intestinal plication and a proposed modification. *Ann Surg* 1960; **152**: 258.

121. Baker JW. A historical overview of surgical decompression in advanced intestinal obstruction. *Surg Gynecol Obstet* 1984; **158**: 593.

122. Munro A & Jones PF. Operative intubation in the treatment of complicated small bowel obstruction. *Br J Surg* 1978; **65**: 123.

54

HAEMORRHAGE AND PERFORATION OF THE SMALL BOWEL

WEG Thomas

The small bowel may well be referred to as the 'Cinderella' of the gastrointestinal tract, as it is all too often neglected with regard to differential diagnosis in cases of hemorrhage and perforation. This is because it is the part of the bowel most remote from both the mouth and the anus, and is consequently relatively inaccessible and difficult to investigate. Endoscopy, the current mainstay of upper and lower gastrointestinal investigation, is technically complex when it comes to examination of the small bowel and is seldom possible except at laparotomy. Barium follow-through studies, although easy to perform, have a very low 'pick-up' rate, and although enteroclysis (small bowel enema) has now superseded the standard follow-through study (see Chapter 45), it will still fail to identify many cases of small bowel pathology. Coupled to the relative rarity of many of the conditions that present with small bowel bleeding or perforation, this difficulty in investigation often results in delay in diagnosis. The unfortunate patient has to undergo an extensive and unnecessary series of investigations with a disproportionate amount of time and resources being expended. Furthermore, laparotomy may not always provide an easy option for diagnosis, as many of the lesions that will be described are impalpable. It is therefore highly desirable that a preoperative diagnosis should be obtained whenever possible.

Diagnosis should be achieved by judicious use of available investigative procedures. Any temptation to employ the 'blunderbus' approach of throwing every possible investigation at the suffering patient should be resisted. The actual choice or sequence of investigations will depend on an accurate history and a meticulous examination of the patient. These age-old clinical principles are never so important as when chasing an obscure cause of gastrointestinal haemorrhage and, if forgotten, will often result in unnecessary suffering for the patient and inefficient resource management.

SMALL BOWEL HAEMORRHAGE

Causes

The differential diagnosis of enteric haemorrhage is vast (Table 54.1) and includes any form of ulceration, tumour or vascular anomaly. The clinical picture is therefore variable, often with a fluctuating pattern of hemorrhage. Bleeding may be (1) occult throughout (presenting as iron deficiency anemia and positive faecal occult blood), (2) initially occult and then subsequently overt, or (3) sudden and dramatic from the outset. The pattern of bleeding depends upon the nature of the underlying pathological process; for example, overt bleeding may be encountered in certain cases of small bowel ulceration, Meckel's diverticulum or vascular malformation, while occult haemorrhage is usually seen in cases of drug-induced ulceration, small bowel tumours or inflammatory bowel diseases such as Crohn's disease.

Small bowel ulceration

Ulceration of the small bowel distal to the duodenum is rare.[1] Most of the cases of enteric ulceration listed in Table 54.1 are uncommon causes of small bowel haemorrhage. Some of them may even cause anemia of a non-specific nature, owing to systemic disease, which can confuse the clinical picture. It is therefore important to exclude ischaemic, traumatic, nutritional and hormonal causes of ulceration, as well as to look for evidence of infective, inflammatory or drug-induced lesions. Congenital conditions may present in neonates as intestinal atresia or meconium ileus, in which case the obstructive element will usually be the predominant clinical problem. However, congenital conditions that present in adult life, such as intestinal reduplication or Meckel's diverticulum, will often present with ulceration, haemorrhage or perforation.

Associated disease processes will often provide valuable clues to the aetiology of enteric ulceration. In a patient with severe cardiac or vascular disease, the ulceration may be ischaemic in origin,[2] whereas if ulceration is associated with malabsorption it is important to exclude coeliac disease and intestinal lymphoma.[3,4] Geographical associations also need to be taken into account when considering the differential diagnosis of enteric ulceration – typhoid and tuberculous enteritis are common in tropical climates.

Certain cases of small bowel ulceration do not fit into any

Table 54.1   Causes of small bowel ulceration and haemorrhage

Congenital	Phenylbutazone	Coeliac disease
Intestinal atresia	Immunosuppression	Jejunal diverticulosis
Ectopic gastric mucosa		Chronic pancreatitis
Intestinal reduplication	*Traumatic*	Postirradiation
Meconium ileus	External	
Meckel's diverticulum	Bands	*Hormonal*
	Volvulus	Zollinger–Ellison syndrome
	Hernia	Phaeochromocytoma
Acquired	Luminal	
Infective	Foreign bodies	*Neoplastic*
Bacterial	Bolus impaction	Benign
Tuberculosis	Gallstone ileus	Leiomyoma
Typhoid	Intubation	Adenoma
Cholera		Malignant
Shigella dysentery	*Vascular*	Adenocarcinoma
Syphilis	Embolic	Lymphoma
Viral	Thrombotic	Carcinoid
Cytomegalovirus	Intussusception	Leiomyosarcoma
Other enteropathic viruses	Polyarteritis nodosa	Malignant histiocytosis
Fungal	Thromboangiitis obliterans	Secondary tumour
Histoplasmosis		
Aspergillosis	*Anomalies*	*Metabolic*
Protozoal	Telangiectasia	Uraemia
Amoebiasis	Arteriovenous malformations	
Parasitic	Angiodysplasia	*Haematological*
Ancylostomiasis	Phlebectasia	Thrombocytopaenia purpura
Ascariasis	Haemangioma	Thrombocythaemia
	Aortoenteric fistula	Haemophilia
Drug-induced		Von Willebrand's disease
Enteric coated potassium	*Inflammatory*	Poorly controlled anticoagulation
Corticosteroids	Crohn's disease	
Indomethacin	Endometriosis	*Idiopathic*

clear pathological grouping and are called 'non-specific' or 'idiopathic'.[5,6] *Non-specific ulcers* were first described by Baillie in 1795[7] and have a classical appearance (Figure 54.1). They tend to be sharp-bordered solitary ulcers with little or no surrounding inflammation. Their aetiology remains unknown, but during the 1960s enteric coated potassium was implicated in certain cases[8,9] and its administration to dogs has been shown to produce similar lesions.[10] However, other reviews have shown that 10% or less of patients with these lesions were

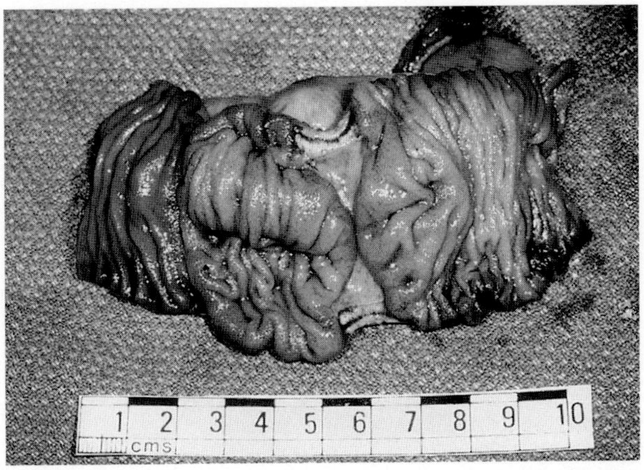

Figure 54.1
Non-specific small bowel ulceration that presented with chronic blood loss. (By kind permission of *World J Surgery*.)

receiving such medication.[1,5] Similar lesions can be caused by non-steroidal anti-inflammatory agents.[11] In time it is likely that other agents will be implicated, and the truly idiopathic ulcer will become less frequently seen.

There appears to be a changing pattern in the clinical presentation of non-specific small bowel ulceration. Early reports described a high incidence of perforation,[12,13] whereas more recent studies document a higher incidence of intestinal obstruction[1] or gastrointestinal haemorrhage.[5] Such bleeding may be acute or chronic, although anaemia was a rare feature in early reports. Later studies suggest that bleeding tends to occur in younger patients, whereas older patients may present with obstruction due to cicatrization.[1,14] All reports tend to stress the delay in diagnosis, apart from in those patients who present with perforation or acute intestinal obstruction.

Small bowel diverticula

Both the congenital Meckel's diverticulum and the acquired jejunoileal diverticula can present with gastrointestinal haemorrhage (see also Chapter 57). Up to 25% of patients with a symptomatic *Meckel's diverticulum* (Figure 54.2) present with bleeding,[15] which occurs as a result of peptic ulceration of the ileal mucosa associated with acid secretion from ectopic gastric mucosa (Figure 54.3); this figure rises to 50% in children under the age of 2 years. The pattern of bleeding ranges from occult blood loss[16] to the passage of large amounts of bright-red blood per rectum.[15] The bleeding in certain cases may be so

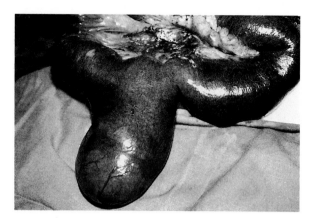

Figure 54.2
Asymptomatic Meckel's diverticulum.

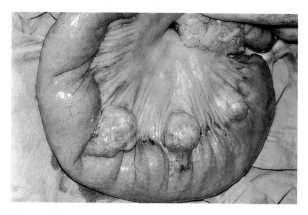

Figure 54.4
Multiple jejunoileal diverticula that presented with intestinal haemorrhage. Intraoperative enteroscopy was used to identify the bleeding diverticulum.

severe that the patient can rapidly exsanguinate, and cases of intestinal obstruction secondary to intraluminal thrombus have also been reported.[17] Early diagnosis is therefore essential.[18]

Jejunoileal diverticula (Figure 54.4) are unusual causes of gastrointestinal blood loss but must be remembered in any case of chronic or recurrent blood loss in an elderly patient. As with Meckel's diverticulum, the bleeding can be either acute and severe[19] or chronic and occult.[20] Most patients present with melaena, which is uncommon with Meckel's diverticulum, and a few cases have been reported presenting with haematemesis. In patients with acute haemorrhage, almost 25% have evidence of previous chronic blood loss,[20,21] thus presenting a similar pattern to that seen with colonic diverticulosis.[22] The haemorrhage results from ulceration at the diverticular neck, where the blood vessels penetrate the bowel wall and are vulnerable due to the lack of muscularis.[23]

Vascular abnormalities

Vascular anomalies account for fewer than 1% of patients presenting with haematemesis and/or melaena,[24] but as they are so difficult to diagnose, they account for a larger percentage of those patients in whom the diagnosis remains obscure. Fortunately lesions such as arteriovenous malformation,

angiodysplasia, phlebectasia and intestinal telangiectasia have become increasingly recognized.[25] The proportion of gastrointestinal vascular anomalies (including angiodysplasia) causing haemorrhage increases with age,[26,27] although such lesions have been encountered in the very young and are reported in association with congenital lesions such as Meckel's diverticulum.[28] Angiodysplasia is predominantly a colonic condition and is almost invariably located in the caecum and ascending colon.[26,29] Telangiectatic lesions in the small bowel are not uncommon causes of iron deficiency anaemia. Although they may be part of hereditary conditions such as the Osler–Weber–Rendu syndrome, they are more commonly found as isolated flat intramucosal telangiectasia or as true haemangiomas (Figure 54.5). Haemangiomas may be diffuse and occupy the whole thickness of the bowel wall, or cavernous and simple with the potential to become polypoid. Phlebectasiae are small bluish submucosal lesions caused by anomalies of the mesenteric veins. Angiomatosis is a diffuse vascular abnormality and can lead to massive haemorrhage.[30]

Diagnosis is always made easier in conditions such as the Osler–Weber–Rendu syndrome and the blue rubber naevus syndrome, in which there are cutaneous as well as visceral

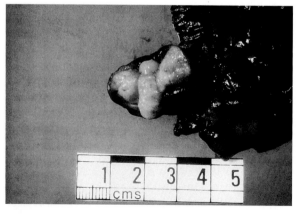

Figure 54.3
Ectopic gastric and pancreatic mucosa in a Meckel's diverticulum.

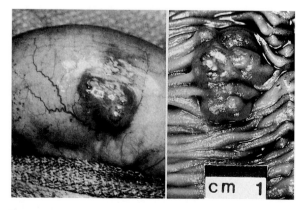

Figure 54.5
A benign haemangioma of the small bowel demonstrating the serosal aspect (left) and the mucosal aspect (right). (By kind permission of *World J Surgery*.)

vascular malformations. In hereditary haemorrhagic telangiectasia, multiple dilatations of capillaries and vessels are seen on the skin, buccal mucosa and gastrointestinal tract. Gastrointestinal bleeding occurs in 20% of cases,[31] and by its very nature is usually treated conservatively.

Vasculitis can lead to chronic gastrointestinal haemorrhage. Although such cases are uncommon, evidence should be sought for systemic disease such as systemic lupus erythematosus, rheumatoid arthritis, polyarteritis nodosa, Ehlers–Danlos syndrome, dermatomyositis, Henoch–Schönlein purpura and amyloidosis.

Any patient who has undergone previous aortic surgery and presents with obscure gastrointestinal haemorrhage should be assumed to have an aortoenteric fistula until proved otherwise (see also Chapter 49). This fistula tends to develop in about 1–2% of prosthetic graft reconstructions,[32] but can also occur after endarterectomy.[33] The diagnosis is primarily a clinical one[34] but other causes of haemorrhage, such as peptic ulceration, often coexist with vascular disease and should be sought.[35] However, even if other bleeding sources are found, it is essential to exclude an aortoenteric fistula as it carries a mortality of up to 45% in some series.[36]

Tumours

Any tumour of the small bowel may be responsible for some degree of gastrointestinal haemorrhage. Such lesions include carcinoid tumours (Chapter 59), adenocarcinoma, leiomyosarcoma, lymphoma (Chapter 50) and benign tumours (Chapter 58). Tumours rarely account for more than 2–3% of cases of gastrointestinal bleeding. When bleeding does occur, the tumour is usually an adenocarcinoma.[37,38] Carcinoid and lymphoma are almost as common in the small bowel as adenocarcinoma,[39] but these tumours are more likely to perforate or obstruct than to cause haemorrhage. Leiomyomas may also present with recurrent haemorrhage,[40] whereas any benign lesion or polyp can initiate an intussusception. If the intussusception becomes chronic or recurrent without causing overt obstruction, it may result in enteric ulceration and occult bleeding.

Occult bleeding can also result from other polypoid conditions such as the Peutz–Jeghers syndrome (Figure 54.6), where the classical melanin pigmentation of the oral mucocutaneous junction provides a valuable clue to the underlying diagnosis. However, there are two potential clinical pitfalls: Peutz–Jeghers polyps have been described without the pigmentation,[41] and gastrointestinal adenocarcinoma can be associated with the syndrome in about 2–3% of cases.[42] Other polyposis conditions, such as familial polyposis, Gardner's syndrome, juvenile polyps and benign lymphoid polyps, may also present with some degree of gastrointestinal haemorrhage.

Miscellaneous causes of haemorrhage

Patients with clotting disorders, such as thrombocytopenic purpura, thrombocythaemia, Von Willebrand's disease, haemophilia or poorly controlled anticoagulation, may also present with acute gastrointestinal bleeding. It must be stressed

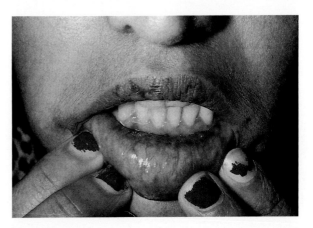

Figure 54.6

The mucocutaneous junction of a patient with Peutz–Jeghers syndrome.

that up to 25% of these patients have a coexisting organic lesion of the gastrointestinal tract,[43] and occasionally such a lesion is found within the small bowel. The presence of a clearly defined bleeding diathesis does not therefore exclude an organic lesion within the gut, indeed there is a definite clinical association between Von Willebrand's disease and an increased incidence of angiodysplasia.

Other disorders, such as endometriosis, postirradiation ileitis (Chapter 52) or uraemia, may present as uncommon causes of small bowel bleeding. Certain conditions may masquerade as small bowel bleeding in those patients in whom no gastroduodenal or colonic cause is found. These include cases of haemobilia, such as a ruptured hepatic artery aneurysm,[44] or occult bleeding from pseudoaneurysm formation in cases of chronic pancreatitis.[45]

Finally there are cases in which patients suffer from iron deficiency anaemia with positive occult bloods for which no cause can be identified. The author has encountered two such cases in a series of 53 cases of recurrent obscure gastrointestinal haemorrhage.[46] A similar picture has been described in marathon runners who may develop iron deficiency anaemia with occult gastrointestinal blood loss; no precise mechanism for this phenomenon has yet been delineated.[47]

Diagnosis

History

An accurate and detailed history is essential in all cases of small bowel haemorrhage. All too often valuable clues to the underlying pathology may be missed by failure to recognize the importance of symptomatic minutiae; thus attention to detail is vital. Even if an accurate history alone does not provide a definitive diagnosis in the majority of cases, it will often indicate which investigations are likely to be most productive.

The age of the patient is important: certain conditions, such as Meckel's diverticulum,[15] are more likely to present in children or young adults, while vascular anomalies are more common in the elderly.[26] In neonates, certain congenital abnormalities, such as intestinal atresia, ectopic gastric mucosa and intestinal reduplications, may be associated with haemorrhage and ulceration.

Any abdominal discomfort should be recorded, and its site and nature ascertained. Central abdominal colicky pain may indicate an element of obstruction caused by some form of small bowel stricture, such as a tumour, Crohn's disease or intussusception. Severe postcibal pain and weight loss may indicate mesenteric ischaemia in a patient with severe cardiac or peripheral vascular disease; mesenteric atheroma can result in ischaemic small bowel ulceration.[2] Rarely a cyclical pattern of colicky pain and positive faecal occult blood may indicate a diagnosis of small bowel endometriosis.

Accompanying symptoms such as nausea, vomiting, altered bowel habit and weight loss may provide further clues to the level and nature of the lesion.

Great attention should be paid to the *pattern of bleeding*. Three broad clinical groups have been defined in this connection:[46] (1) those patients in whom bleeding is occult throughout their clinical presentation, simply presenting with iron deficiency anaemia and positive faecal occult blood; (2) those in whom the bleeding is initially occult and then subsequently and intermittently overt; and (3) those in whom the bleeding is overt and often sudden and dramatic from the outset. As the pattern of bleeding will often reflect the nature of the underlying pathology, it tends to indicate the sequence of investigations, and in this context it is the most important part of the history.

An accurate past medical history should be taken. Any evidence of past systemic or gastrointestinal disease should be sought because ulceration of the small bowel occurs in such a wide spectrum of clinical conditions (Table 54.1). A history of travel abroad should be ascertained because in certain parts of the world parasitic infestation is a common cause of chronic gastrointestinal blood loss; stool samples should be examined for ova and cysts. A history of foreign body ingestion or trauma should also be excluded.

Attention should be focused on any history of recent medication. Drugs such as enteric-coated potassium,[9] corticosteroids, non-steroidal anti-inflammatory agents and immunosuppresive regimens have been associated with small bowel ulceration.[11] Anticoagulant therapy or bleeding diatheses may aggravate any potential bleeding lesion, and a history of alcohol abuse should be sought, since this may have led to cirrhosis, portal hypertension or chronic pancreatitis. Chronic pancreatitis has occasionally been associated with recurrent obscure gastrointestinal haemorrhage that results from pseudoaneurysm formation.[45] The aneurysm can leak into the pancreatic duct or directly into the gut.

Any past abdominal operations may be relevant. Suture-line haemorrhage should be rare as long as careful attention is given to surgical technique, but regrettably it still occurs from time to time. Operations remote in time may also be of importance, particularly in the case of aortic reconstruction. *Secondary aortoenteric fistulas* have become more common with the great increase in vascular surgery over the last two decades. This condition presents the characteristic clinical picture of secondary haemorrhage. The bleeding is initially occult,

eventually becomes overt and usually ends up as massive rapid haemorrhage than can be fatal. The initial sentinel bleeds should be recognized as warning signs, and it is essential that surgical intervention is undertaken before the final massive haemorrhage occurs. In spite of this well-recognized clinical picture, a worrying feature with nearly all published series of aortoenteric fistulas is the delay in diagnosis, which varies from 24 hours to 3 months.[34] It is to be hoped that a greater awareness of this condition amongst non-surgical clinicians will decrease this delay in diagnosis.

Examination

Examination of the patient may reveal clinical evidence of anaemia, telangiectasia, stigmata of portal hypertension, pigmentation of Peutz–Jeghers syndrome, scars of previous surgery and abdominal tenderness or masses. It will also demonstrate any clinical evidence of acute blood loss. Rectal examination may confirm the presence of melaena, and sigmoidoscopy and proctoscopy may exclude any lower rectal lesion. It must be pointed out that although melaena usually indicates upper gastrointestinal haemorrhage, red rectal bleeding may also originate high in the small bowel if the rate of bleeding is rapid enough, although in this case the indices of acute blood loss, such as tachycardia and hypotension, should be obvious.

Investigations

In patients with an established diagnosis of iron deficiency anaemia, one of the first priorities is to confirm that this is indeed due to gastrointestinal haemorrhage. Faecal occult blood testing was initially designed to screen for colonic cancer,[48] but it is also applicable to bleeding from small bowel lesions. It has been calculated that in normal controls blood loss into the bowel is 0.5 ± 0.4 ml ($\pm$ SD) per day or 2 mg haemoglobin/g stool (equivalent to 2 ml/day for a stool weight of 150 g).[49] Early tests for faecal occult blood developed a poor reputation because of the high frequency of false-positive reactions.[50,51] A modification of these tests using Haemoccult, which is less sensitive than the standard guaiac test, produces positive results with an excess of 10 mg haemoglobin/g stool.[50] However, this threshold tends to lead to an increase in false-negative results,[52] which can be as high as 30% even in known cases of overt colorectal cancer.[49,53] To overcome the false-negative rate, some workers have recommended a rehydration technique,[49] but this is not officially advised as it increases the false-positive rate to an unacceptable level. Nevertheless, rehydration reduces the false-negative level from 30 to 9%. Other workers suggest that extending the 3-day sample to 6 days reduces the false-positive level to 10%.[53] In spite of these adjustments, Haemoccult still has its limitations; immunofluorescent techniques have been devised to overcome them.[52] These techniques employ fluorescein-labelled rabbit antihuman haemoglobin serum, and this undoubtedly increases the specificity of the test. Its advantage includes the absence of cross-reaction with animal haemoglobin, minimal observer error and, in particular, the ability to adjust the sensitivity.

Once it has been confirmed that a patient is suffering from gastrointestinal haemorrhage, the rest of the investigation should be specifically planned to localize the source of bleeding. Standard investigations should be utilized to exclude upper and lower gastrointestinal bleeding; undoubtedly oesophagogastroduodenoscopy and total colonoscopy are the investigations of choice in this respect. Once a source of bleeding has been confidently excluded from the upper gastrointestinal tract and colon, attention is turned to the small bowel. The following investigations are particularly described with reference to their sensitivity and their reliability in demonstrating small bowel sources of haemorrhage. The reader should consult Chapter 45 for further detail of the various radiological techniques.

Barium studies Barium contrast studies have long been the mainstay of imaging of the small intestine.[54] Radiologists have traditionally relied on the follow-through technique, but this has now been found to be inadequate in many patients, especially for delineating cases of small bowel ulceration.[5,55] It has been suggested that it is only the infrequency of small bowel lesions that has disguised the inadequacies of the barium follow-through for so long.[56] Barium enemas are also inadequate for examination of the terminal ileum because reflux through the ileocaecal valve only occurs in about 25% of patients.[57]

Enteroclysis, or small bowel enema, is now the technique of choice for radiological examination of the small bowel and has significantly improved the diagnostic yield of small bowel abnormalities.[58] It involves the passage of a 12 Fr tube to the duodenojejunal flexure,[59] and infusion of barium at pressure until all segments of the small bowel are moderately distended. Intermittent compression fluororadiography is undertaken, looking at each segment of jejunum and ileum in turn. The diagnostic rate can be further improved by the simultaneous infusion of methylcellulose, water or air down the tube. It can be a time-consuming investigation and may be uncomfortable for the patient,[60] but those workers involved in performing a considerable number of small bowel enemas stress that it is easy to perform, safe and quick.[59]

Enteroclysis has yielded over 90% positive diagnosis in certain series[60] and is frequently successful in situations in which a follow-through study has failed to reveal any pathological features.[59] A barium follow-through should now be reserved for patients in whom duodenal intubation cannot be achieved.

A small bowel enema may be instrumental in identifying such lesions as small bowel tumours, ulcers, strictures (Figure 54.7) or jejunal diverticula, but it is unreliable for demonstrating vascular anomalies or Meckel's diverticulum. It is therefore an investigation worth considering if the patient presents with any symptoms suggestive of an obstructive element, such as central abdominal colicky pain. However, it is important to avoid barium studies if angiography or computed tomography (CT) is being considered, as residual barium within the intestine obscures angiographic detail and produces distortion on scanning; barium may remain in the bowel for several days.

Angiography In many centres angiography is rapidly becoming the most effective investigation for identifying the source of

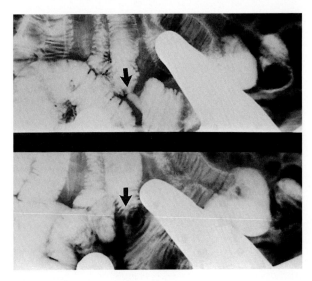

Figure 54.7
Distal small bowel stricture demonstrated by enteroclysis (arrowed).

small bowel haemorrhage or obscure haemorrhage from an unknown site.[26] All patients presenting for angiography should have had both upper and lower gastrointestinal endoscopy to exclude common recognizable bleeding sources. The role of angiography depends on the nature of the bleeding. In acute blood loss angiography seeks to demonstrate the actual site of bleeding by the confirmation of intraluminal extravasation of contrast medium, while in chronic haemorrhage abnormal vascular patterns are sought that may represent tumours or vascular anomalies.

Acute haemorrhage Small bowel haemorrhage may account for up to 30% of patients presenting with acute rectal bleeding with a negative nasogastric aspirate.[61] Unfortunately all too often the bleeding has stopped by the time the patient undergoes angiography, but if bleeding is active at the time of the investigation it can be shown to originate from arteriovenous malformations, diverticula, ulcers, tumours, Meckel's diverticulum and surgical suture lines. Intraluminal extravasation may be seen in the superior mesenteric artery series (Figure 54.8), and very occasionally extravasated contrast can be seen pooling in the adjacent diverticulum that led to the haemorrhage.

It is important to attempt to localize whereabout in the small bowel the haemorrhage originates. With care and patience, a side-winder catheter can often be manipulated into most of the jejunal arteries and the inferior pancreaticoduodenal arcade. Such selective catheterization is not only helpful in localizing a lesion but it also increases the success rate for demonstrating intraluminal extravasation.

For an aortic injection, a lesion needs to be bleeding at a rate of 5–6 ml/min to be identified,[62] but for selective visceral catheterization the rate required falls to 0.5–2 ml/min.[63] This technique is frequently limited by the intermittent nature of the bleeding. In cases of massive haemorrhage the success rate is high, but the pick-up rate falls off as the bleeding rate diminishes or the actual haemorrhage becomes intermittent. In one

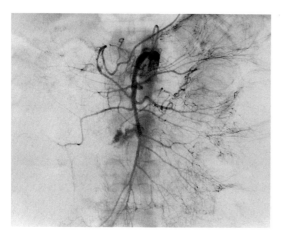

Figure 54.8
Intraluminal extravasation demonstrated by selective visceral angiography. (By kind permission of Professor A. P. Hemingway.)

recent series only 7% of patients had evidence of active haemorrhage during angiography.[26]

In certain cases of active bleeding, angiographic techniques may be of therapeutic value in helping to stop the haemorrhage. In the past, local infusion of vasopressin directly into the feeding artery often resulted in the cessation of bleeding. However, the use of vasopressin has diminished due to doubts as to its efficacy and because of its systemic vasoconstrictor effects. Newer agents, such as the long-acting synthetic analogues of somatostatin (octreotide, lanreotide) act more specifically on the smooth muscle of splanchnic vessels to reduce flow. Furthermore, in carefully selected cases, embolization can be of value. Such embolization is not recommended in the large bowel where the collateral supply is poor, but in the small bowel adequate collaterals usually prevent infarction. In a review of all reported cases up to 1984,[64] four of 18 patients embolized developed some degree of ischaemic damage, but in spite of this many authorities still recommend embolization over vasopressin infusion.[65] Embolization is also of particular value in dealing with certain cases of haemobilia or sources of haemorrhage arising from the coeliac or hepatic artery, as intrahepatic or pancreatic bleeding can present a daunting surgical prospect. Other indications for embolization include cases of small bowel pathology in which vasopressin is known to be ineffective, such as tumours, abscesses and trauma.[66]

Chronic haemorrhage When there is no active bleeding at the time of angiography, attempts are made to identify a tumour blush (Figure 54.9) or a vascular malformation (Figure 54.10). In these cases it is recommended that the inferior mesenteric artery is catheterized first to allow good views of the sigmoid colon and rectum before the urinary bladder becomes filled with contrast, thus obscuring the view of this area. This step is followed by selective catheterization of the superior mesenteric artery and the coeliac axis. Some vascular anomalies, namely venous abnormalities (phlebectasia), may not be picked up by this technique and sometimes are only diagnosed by intraoperative enteroscopy.

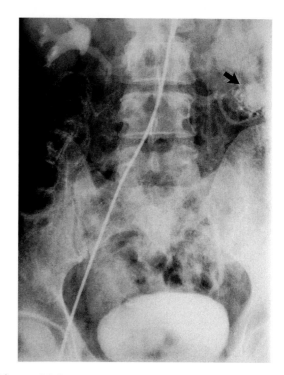

Figure 54.9
Small bowel tumour blush demonstrated by angiography (arrowed).

Even when a lesion has been identified by angiography, it may still prove difficult to identify at laparotomy. In some cases, therefore, it may be worthwhile leaving a selective angiography catheter in situ and transferring the patient to the

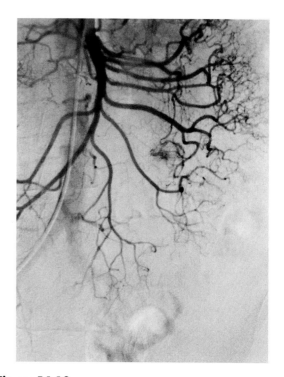

Figure 54.10
Intestinal vascular malformation. (By kind permission of Professor A. P. Hemingway.)

operating theatre immediately. This manoeuvre allows on-table angiography with marker clips or the injection of a dye such as methylene blue, which may facilitate the identification of the lesion.

Radionuclide scanning Radionuclide scanning techniques have recently gained in popularity, since they appear to have no morbidity and are becoming increasingly reliable in demonstrating sources of recurrent gastrointestinal bleeding (see also Chapter 44). Such techniques may be used for measurement of gastrointestinal blood loss, localization of the source of bleeding or looking for specific lesions such as Meckel's diverticulum.

Measurement of gastrointestinal blood loss Autologous red blood cells may be labelled with about 1 MBq of ^{51}Cr and reinjected intravenously. Stool samples are then collected for several days. A blood sample is taken 10 minutes after injection and then again at the end of the investigation. As the half-life of ^{51}Cr is 28 days, the blood loss over a period of 5 days can be calculated by comparing the radioactivity of the stool samples with those of the two blood samples. A normal individual may lose up to 3 ml of blood per day into the bowel, but the figure is usually much less.

Localization of blood loss The localization of bleeding is of far greater clinical value than the mere knowledge of the rate of blood loss. Localization depends on the patient actively bleeding at the time of investigation, as any radioactivity present in the circulation at the time of haemorrhage will appear in the lumen of the bowel. Therefore any colloid suitable for reticuloendothelial scintigraphy would be effective. The technique has changed little since first described by Alavi et al. in 1977.[67] The principle of the colloid test is that labelled colloidal particles of ^{99m}Tc-sulphur colloid are actively cleared by the reticuloendothelial system within 10–15 min. Thus any blush of radioactivity in the mid- or lower abdomen outside the liver, spleen or bone marrow would represent a site of haemorrhage. The lesion-to-background ratio at the bleeding site will depend on the rate of haemorrhage. It has been estimated that bleeding rates below 1 ml/min can be regularly detected,[68] and rates as low as 0.1 ml/min have sometimes been reported.[69]

The circulating level of radioactivity may be prolonged by labelling autologous red blood cells either in vivo or in vitro. Once securely bound to red cells the radioactive label is retained within the blood compartment for several hours. This method can allow extended studies for up to 24 hours, and any accumulation of blood within the bowel lumen will eventually produce an area of abnormal activity against the background of the normal abdominal blood pool. The technique of in vivo labelling is simple, and the patient requires no special preparation.[70] A reducing agent such as stannous chloride is injected intravenously, followed by 400–600 MBq of sodium pertechnetate. In the presence of stannous chloride the pertechnetate is bound within the red cells, but such binding takes a few minutes and some of the free pertechnetate will be excreted by the kidneys and some taken up in gastric mucosa. Other labelling techniques have been used, involving ^{51}Cr as sodium chromate, ^{99m}Tc-methylene disphosphonate or [111]In.

Once labelled, the patient lies under a gamma camera with a large field of view and images are recorded over the next hour. If necessary, further images can be obtained up to 24 hours.

Using such extended methods, some workers claim up to 100% success rates for identifying bleeding sites,[71] as compared with 65% with conventional angiography. This superior success rate with labelled red cells over both colloid scanning and angiography is due to its ability to demonstrate intermittent bleeding.[72] It is also more sensitive than angiography in detecting venous bleeding, but the precision of siting this source of haemorrhage is diminished. Nevertheless it can direct the angiographer or surgeon to the area under suspicion.

Meckel's diverticulum Meckel's diverticulum is an important cause of small bowel bleeding, both acute[15] and chronic,[16] and yet it is rarely demonstrated on barium studies (see also Chapter 57). The incidence in the general population, based on autopsy studies, is up to 2%, but only a minority of cases are symptomatic. However, in children and adolescents Meckel's diverticulum is an important source of intestinal haemorrhage, and in this age range scintigraphic detection plays a useful role. Scintigraphic studies have the advantage of not depending upon active bleeding but upon the trapping of ^{99m}Tc-pertechnetate by ectopic gastric (oxyntic) mucosa found in a Meckel's diverticulum. It is the acid produced from such mucosa that causes ulceration of the adjacent small intestinal mucosa, thereby resulting in small bowel haemorrhage.

The patient should be starved for 12 hours to reduce gastric acid secretion, and then 100–200 MBq of sodium pertechnetate is injected intravenously. Gamma-camera images are recorded sequentially for up to 1 hour. Activity is usually visible in the stomach within 2 minutes. Within 15–30 minutes activity is seen in the small bowel, and this may be enough to obscure a Meckel's diverticulum. However, if a diverticulum is present it is usually represented by an area of activity which is located below and to the right of the midline and appears within 5 minutes (Figure 54.11). The rate of development of activity can be compared with that of the parietal

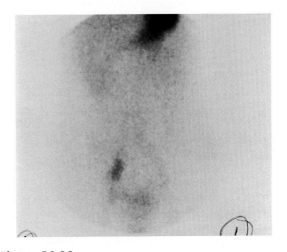

Figure 54.11

A positive technetium scan consistent with a Meckel's diverticulum. (By kind permission of *Current Practice in Surgery*.)

cell population of the stomach (Figure 54.12), as ectopic gastric mucosa has a similar rate of uptake to that of normal stomach. This comparison will help to distinguish a diverticulum from other areas of activity, such as the renal areas, ureters and bladder. False-positive results include other sites of ectopic gastric mucosa or uptake in lesions other than a Meckel's diverticulum, such as reduplication, intussusception and infarction. Further false-positive results are seen occasionally representing the ureter or the uterus during certain phases of the cycle in young women. Other false positives remain unexplained (Figure 54.13).

Pertechnetate imaging of a Meckel's diverticulum gives a reported sensitivity of 75%,[73] but the ease of visualization may be further improved by the simultaneous administration of a number of other agents.[74] Pertechnetate is not only extracted by the gastric mucosa but also secreted into the lumen of the stomach. Transmission of such radioactivity along the bowel lumen is likely to cause confusing results. Some workers have advocated the use of pentagastrin to increase the uptake of pertechnetate, but this also accelerates gastric emptying and thus exacerbates the problem of on excessive amount of activity in the bowel. As glucagon reduces gastric motility, these workers have given the two agents together[75] and found the accuracy of the technique to be improved. H_2-receptor blocking agents reduce acid secretion and intraluminal release of pertechnetate without impairing its uptake, and so have become the agents of choice.[76]

Using such techniques, the accuracy of Meckel's diverticulum imaging in children was said to be about 90% in one report.[77] This figure is open to debate, as the series contained several children in whom the absence of a Meckel's diverticulum was not surgically confirmed. In spite of this, the investigation is a valuable diagnostic tool as it is non-invasive, cheap, simple to perform and administers a much smaller radiation dose than enteroclysis or angiography.

Radionuclide scanning therefore can play a useful role in these patients with melaena or dark red stools in whom the source of bleeding has not been identified endoscopically.

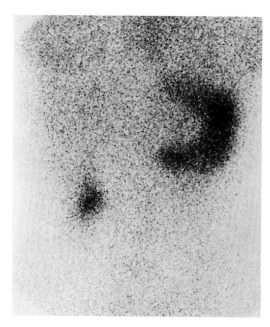

Figure 54.13
A false-positive Meckel's scan. Laparotomy was negative.

Negative scintigraphy may indicate that the patient has temporarily stopped bleeding, but positive scintigraphy can provide a quick, inexpensive and non-invasive localization of the bleeding source. Such techniques are of particular value in younger patients, in whom a Meckel's diverticulum is suspected. The major limiting feature in most cases is the need for an active on-call service to be available out-of-hours, as in some instances these patients need to be investigated urgently.

Endoscopic techniques The value of endoscopy in investigating gastrointestinal blood loss is well established. Indeed oesophagogastroduodenoscopy will demonstrate the cause of bleeding in the vast majority of cases of upper gastrointestinal haemorrhage, whereas colonoscopy will exclude or confirm a bleeding source in the large bowel. Endoscopy of the small bowel is fraught wih problems, however. The jejunum and ileum are relatively inaccessible to standard endoscopic techniques, yet they can harbour bleeding ulcerated lesions representing a wide variety of clinical conditions, many of which cannot be identified by any of the imaging techniques already described. In ideal circumstances the gastroscope may be advanced into the proximal jejunum and the colonoscope passed into the distal 50 cm of the terminal ileum,[78] but this still leaves most of the small bowel unexamined.

Three types of instrument have now been designed to traverse the whole length of the small bowel, with the aim of examining the lumen during withdrawal:[78,79]

- The 'push-type' endoscope is simply an extremely long end-viewing duodenoscope that is advanced as far as possible, but even under ideal circumstances this only allows visualization of the proximal 90 cm of jejunum.

- The 'rope-way' endoscope depends on a previously passed transintestinal string which is retrieved per anum, and this pulls the endoscope through the intestine. However, this

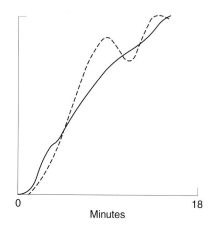

Figure 54.12
Rate of pertechnetate uptake (corrected curves) in Meckel's diverticulum (----) compared with gastric parietal cell (—). (By kind permission of *Current Practice in Surgery*.)

technique can only be performed under general anaesthesia as it is most uncomfortable for the patient and there is a danger of damaging the bowel by a 'cheese-wire' mechanism.

- The 'sonde-type' endoscope works on the same principle as the Miller–Abbott or Cantor tube. The patient swallows the endoscope and once it reaches the distal duodenum a distal balloon cuff is inflated. The endoscope is then allowed to migrate distally through the small bowel; unfortunately this technique not only takes time but is sometimes unsuccessful.

All three methods are unreliable, time-consuming and not routinely available.

Intraoperative endoscopy is now growing in its applications and practice,[80,81] and it is proving particularly useful in identifying vascular anomalies within the small bowel. It provides the advantage of detecting occult lesions not apparent on gross examination or palpation of the bowel. It can confirm that any clinically apparent lesion is actually the source of bleeding. When multiple lesions are present, it will identify which lesion or lesions are the source of haemorrhage, thus indicating the extent of enteric resection required. The results of intraoperative enteroscopy can be most rewarding, but only if certain practical considerations are observed.

Adequate bowel preparation is essential. If there is any question as to the adequacy of bowel clearance, the author has found total gut irrigation to be of great value. In the unexpected or emergency situation, in which intraoperative enteroscopy is required without adequate prior bowel preparation, then it is possible to carry out total gut irrigation intraoperatively, but this manoeuvre is not recommended unless absolutely necessary as it can leave the bowel very moist and it also takes time. The patient is then operated on in the lithotomy position, and a thorough laparotomy is performed.

Once it has been deemed necessary to proceed to enteroscopy, a colonoscope is introduced via the mouth and the operating surgeon helps the endoscopist to pass the instrument to its full length, feeding the small bowel over it in a concertina manner. The furthest limitation should be marked with a stay stitch, and the lumen of the bowel is examined during withdrawal of the instrument. The endoscope can then be introduced into the remainder of the bowel by means of an enterotomy, but this technique is messy, and the author finds it preferable to introduce it via the anus and pass it up the remainder of the small bowel. Some workers prefer to introduce the endoscope initially through the anus as there is more room to work at that end of the table, but this technique requires another clean colonoscope to be introduced via the mouth if the distal examination is unproductive or inadequate.

During examination it is advisable to turn off the main lights in the theatre. This step is advantageous to the endoscopist, but it also allows the operating surgeon to get a good view of the transilluminated bowel wall, which is particularly useful for identifying small vascular anomalies.[46] As soon as any lesion is identified, a marking suture is inserted from the serosal aspect.

If the patient has had preoperative angiography in which a lesion has been identified, it is possible to leave in situ a superselective arterial catheter for intraoperative injection of methylene blue. This technique often facilitates the localization of a lesion endoscopically, while occasionally it may even obviate the need for endoscopy. It is of particular value when intraoperative enteroscopy is impossible due to marked adhesions, strictures, extraluminal tumour deposits or other pathology that may limit the passage of the scope without being the actual source of bleeding.

Intraoperative enteroscopy is thus a valuable addition to the diagnostic modalities available to the gastrointestinal surgeon and endoscopist faced with obscure bleeding in the small bowel. It requires patience and care. It is important that both endoscopist and operating surgeon are aware of the pitfalls and problems. When introducing the endoscope via the mouth, care must be taken not to allow a large loop to form along the greater curvature, as this can enlarge very quickly without either operator being aware of it. This problem can lead to gastric damage or even bleeding due to tearing of the short gastric vessels. Great care must be taken in passing the scope through the small bowel, otherwise small artefactual ulcers or breaches of the mucosa may occur. Finally, it is important to decompress the bowel on withdrawal of the endoscope or it will prove difficult to close the abdomen.

Miscellaneous diagnostic techniques Other forms of imaging have a limited role in investigation of small bowel haemorrhage. The application of ultrasonography is growing rapidly, but at present it remains unreliable when examining the bowel owing to luminal gas. CT may help pick up lesions within the liver or pancreas, and its main role is in excluding extraenteric causes of bleeding.

Staining techniques have been employed in the past.[82] The staining test involves the passage of a weighted string by mouth and screening the patient until the weight reaches the distal small bowel. An intravenous injection of fluoroscein is then administered, the string is retrieved and the level of fluoroscein staining is identified. The distance from the mouth will give a very approximate level of any bleeding lesion. The sensitivity and specificity of angiography and the availability of interoperator endoscopy have tended to render such staining techniques obsolete.

Intraoperative staining with methylene blue has already been mentioned, and it is used to help identify the segment of bowel in which the abnormality lies. Other workers have used indigo–carmine solution injected into the relevant small bowel artery for such segmental staining.[83] The success of this technique depends on superselective catheterization preoperatively, but it may give valuable information and allow easy recognition and resection of the affected segment.

Treatment

It has been estimated that 80% of episodes of severe bleeding from the bowel will stop spontaneously.[84] However, this figure can lull the clinician into a false sense of security. It should be remembered that in every situation adequate blood replacement is essential to maintain a good circulating blood volume and urine output.

In cases of rapid and massive haemorrhage, resuscitation and investigations should proceed simultaneously. Investigations should never take priority over resuscitation, yet all too often patients have to be rescued from exsanguination as various forms of imaging are being attempted. In such cases of massive haemorrhage, which are fortunately uncommon, a wide-bore cannula should be inserted intravenously; it is also advisable to have a central venous line for the monitoring of central venous pressure. Adequate transfusion and resuscitation should be undertaken before a patient is allowed to be taken down to the radiology department.

In cases of slow or occult haemorrhage, any iron deficiency anaemia should be corrected before operation. The treatment required will then depend on the underlying cause of the haemorrhage. When the bleeding results from any systemic disease, bleeding disorder or drug-induced lesion, appropriate steps should be taken specifically to treat that disease or correct the haemorrhagic tendency.

When a vascular anomaly, tumour, stricture, ulcer or Meckel's diverticulum has been identified preoperatively, the management of the patient is usually straightforward. Surgical excision of the lesion is generally curative, unless the lesion recurs or, in the case of a tumour, has disseminated.

In patients with bleeding from a Meckel's diverticulum, resection of the diverticulum should include its neck and the feeding artery. It is most inadvisable to treat a Meckel's diverticulum like the appendix and to invert the stump. In most cases the base of the diverticulum is too wide, and even if it is narrow, much of the ulceration occurs in the neighbouring small bowel mucosa due to peptic ulceration. Furthermore, at the site at which a Meckel's diverticulum occurs any inverted base can so easily form the basis for an intussusception.[85] Therefore formal diverticulectomy is necessary, taking care to ligate and divide the diverticular artery coming from the ileal mesentery.

In the case of multiple lesions, such as jejunal diverticula, when all the lesions cannot be excised, it is essential to ensure that the lesion responsible for the haemorrhage is included in the excised segment. Intraoperative enteroscopy is particularly helpful in this situation.

In cases of aortoenteric fistula, simple disconnection of the fistula is inadequate. Three main treatment options are available[34] (Figure 54.14). The fistula can be repaired by closing the defect in the duodenum and simple repair of the vascular defect, but this must be accompanied by interposition of the omentum. This technique will not be applicable in most cases.

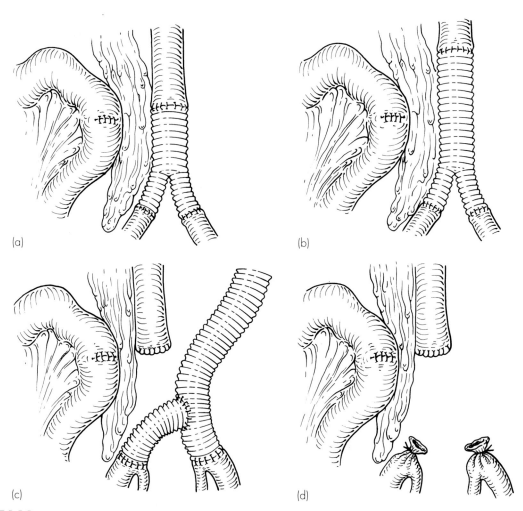

(a)

(b)

(c)

(d)

Figure 54.14
Operative procedures for the treatment of aortoenteric fistulas.

Excision of any previous graft is usually required, either with more proximal grafting or an extra-anatomic reconstruction such as an aortobifemoral graft. If the graft is grossly infected then the latter treatment option is recommended. Simply to excise the old graft and to leave alone with no vascular reconstruction is rarely appropriate.

In those patients in whom laparotomy should be avoided if possible, or in those cases of rapid exsanguinating bleeding identified at angiography, superselective intra-arterial vasopressin infusion or embolization[63,64] should be considered. The choice of embolic material is usually determined by both clinical and technical considerations. Sterile absorbable gelatin sponge (Gelfoam) has been commonly employed,[86] whereas in cases of life-threatening haemorrhage isobutyl-2-cyanoacrylate has been utilized. In the light of recent health scares, human dura mater (Lyodura) has fallen from favour.

The major therapeutic challenge is in those cases where no preoperative diagnosis has been achieved, or when laparotomy reveals no obvious bleeding pathology. A thorough laparotomy examination by an experienced surgeon is required, not only to examine the serosal surface of the small bowel but also to feel the texture of the bowel. This examination may reveal small luminal polyps or thickened ulcerated areas. Kocherization of the duodenum and mobilization of the duodenojejunal flexure is required to exclude a diverticulum or small luminal tumour. When such manoeuvres prove unproductive, one should proceed to intraoperative enteroscopy, which requires both an experienced surgeon and endoscopist.

If technical considerations preclude this course of action and the patient is bleeding at the time of operation, then intraoperative angiography may be considered. This is not an easy option, however, unless there is already an angiographic catheter in situ and the patient is undergoing operation on a suitable table. Therefore unless the surgeon has predicted the need for angiography and taken the appropriate steps, such a course of action is rarely feasible or productive.

Certain lesions that are multiple, such as telangiectasia, and are also within endoscopic range may be amenable to endoscopic treatment using laser or heater probes. This technique is more applicable to lesions within the stomach and duodenum rather than within the small bowel. However, any suitable lesion found by intraoperative enteroscopy may also be dealt with along these lines.

Finally, in certain cases the surgeon may be faced with the situation in which no apparent cause for bleeding can be found in spite of careful pre- and intraoperative investigations. The management of such cases remains controversial. If the patient is suffering from rapid bleeding at the time of operation, this will usually mean that there was no time for preoperative angiography, as such an investigation should have demonstrated a rapidly bleeding lesion. In these cases, clamping the bowel into segments using soft non-crushing clamps will usually identify the guilty segment. Some workers have utilized temporary enterotomies or even temporary stomas. Others have advocated a 'blind' right hemicolectomy because an undetected bleeding lesion, such as a bleeding diverticulum

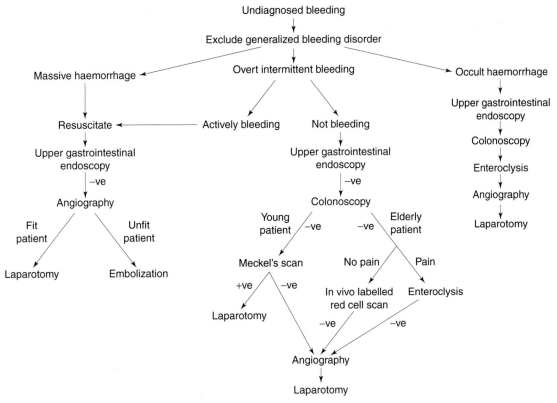

Figure 54.15

Suggested course of action for investigating obscure gastrointestinal haemorrhage.

or angiodysplasia, may lurk in the caecum. These practices are unsatisfactory, and it is to be hoped that with improved angiography and intraoperative enteroscopy the need for such surgical options will become increasingly rare.

In cases in which the bleeding is occult and slow and no demonstrable cause is found, it may be adequate simply to treat the patient with iron. In two cases in the author's series, no cause has been found for occult bleeding, and at a follow-up of 4–8 years both patients remain in apparent good health.[46]

Conclusion

It can be seen that small bowel haemorrhage can occur from a wide variety of pathological conditions and present in a wide variety of clinical manifestations. It is therefore helpful to have a plan of action that is dependent upon the pattern of bleeding and the clinical picture. Figure 54.15 presents a suggested course of action based on the author's experience of over 80 cases of obscure gastrointestinal bleeding. It is not intended to be followed slavishly but more to act as a guideline for investigation. Once a laparotomy has been decided upon, if the diagnosis remains elusive intraoperative enteroscopy should be performed.

Regrettably, even after such extensive and meticulous investigations about 5% of cases remain undiagnosed. Once a diagnosis has been achieved, however, local resection is usually curative, unless a generalized disorder underlies the clinical presentation, in which case the prognosis will depend on the nature of this disorder.

SMALL BOWEL PERFORATION

Causes

Many of the causes of small bowel perforation (Table 54.2) are also causes of small bowel ulceration or haemorrhage (see Table 54.1). The final presenting feature is usually that of peritonitis, but this may be superimposed on other clinical features that offer clues to the underlying pathology. The cause may be obvious in cases of trauma, such as stabbing or shotgun injuries, or only become apparent at the time of laparotomy, for example perforation of a jejunal diverticulum. However, in some cases no underlying or precipitating cause can be found, and such cases are labelled as idiopathic small bowel perforations.[87] In certain cases contributing factors may be present, such as those cases of spontaneous focal perforations in children of exceptionally low birth weight.[88] Otherwise, spontaneous perforation is both rare and of diverse causation.

Congenital abnormalities

Congenital abnormalities of the small bowel causing perforation usually present in the neonatal period or in childhood. Duplications, abnormalities of rotation or meconium ileus can occasionally lead to ulceration and perforation, but the most common cause of perforation is due to ecotopic gastric mucosa such as in a Meckel's diverticulum (see also Chapter 57).[15] The incidence of diverticulitis in a Meckel's diverticulum is much

Table 54.2   Causes of small bowel perforation

Congenital
Meconium peritonitis
Reduplication
Ectopic gastric mucosa
Meckel's diverticulum

Acquired
Infective
Typhoid
Tuberculosis
Amoebiasis
Ascaris
Cytomegalovirus

Traumatic
Blunt
Penetrating
Luminal
    Exogenous – foreign body
    Endogenous – gallstone ileus

Vascular
Mesenteric infarction

Inflammatory
Crohn's disease
Jejunal diverticulitis
Neonatal necrotizing enterocolitis

Hormonal
Zollinger–Ellison syndrome

Neoplastic
Lymphoma
Adenocarcinoma
Secondary tumour (ovary, melanoma, lung, breast)

Metabolic
Amyloid

Mechanical
Obstruction
Stangulated hernia (external, internal)
Bands and adhesions
Intussusception

Iatrogenic
Operative injury
Anastomotic dehiscence
Endoscopic injury
Radiation enteritis
'Cheese-wire' injury from abdominal closure sutures

Drug – induced
Chemotherapy
Steroids
Non-steroidal anti-inflammatory drugs
Slow release potassium

Idiopathic (spontaneous)

lower than acute inflammation of the appendix, as the diverticulum tends to have a wider mouth and it contains little lymphoid tissue.[89] However, when diverticulitis does occur it can be complicated by perforation (Figure 54.16), fistulation to adjacent intestine or acute peridiverticulitis. Perforation may also be precipitated by enteroliths, foreign bodies[90] or simple

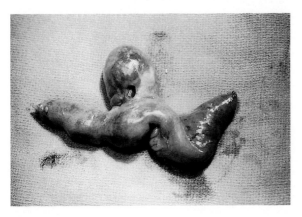

Figure 54.16
A perforated Meckel's diverticulum. (By kind permission of *World J Surgery*.)

peptic ulceration of the adjacent ileal mucosa owing to acid secreted from the ectopic gastric mucosa. Slow-release potassium has also been implicated in perforation of a Meckel's diverticulum.[91]

Small bowel ulceration

Any type of small bowel ulceration has the potential to perforate, although fortunately this is an uncommon complication. Idiopathic ulcers usually present with obstruction or occult haemorrhage, but earlier reports described a high incidence of perforation.[12,13]

Peptic ulceration For the purposes of this discussion, classical duodenal ulceration is excluded. However, peptic ulceration can occur distal to the duodenojejunal flexure, either in relation to ectopic gastric mucosa, as in a Meckel's diverticulum (Chapter 57), or secondary to excessive gastric acid production, as in the Zollinger–Ellison syndrome (Chapter 36).[92] In this syndrome patients may suffer from diarrhoea and weight loss, with a known history of peptic ulceration or bleeding, and then present with sudden peritonitis.

In gastrinoma patients with peritonitis laparotomy may reveal multiple perforations.[93] In such cases it is essential to look for hypergastrinaemia and any other factors, such as hypercalcaemia, that may suggest that the patient is suffering from multiple endocrine neoplasia (MEN type I). Often the fulminating form of the Zollinger–Ellison syndrome does not develop until after gastric surgery or some physiological event such as childbirth. In these cases perforation usually occurs in a recurrent ulcer, often in the early postoperative period. This syndrome should be considered in any patient presenting with jejunal ulceration in whom there is no other obvious cause.[94]

Inflammatory ulceration Perforation can occur in neonates with necrotizing enterocolitis[95] and may present with multiple perforations in a segment of necrotic bowel (Chapter 62). The basic aetiology of the patchy necrosis of both large and small intestine remains unknown, but it is associated with low birth weight, prematurity and neonatal shock. The mortality and morbidity rates are reduced by early diagnosis, and perforation is an absolute indication for operation.

In adults, inflammatory perforation is an established complication of jejunoileal diverticula (Chapter 57). Perforation and diverticulitis account for up to 50% of the complications arising in jejunal diverticula.[20,96] Perforation itself is usually easy to recognize as a clinical diagnosis,[97,98] but some patients present with suppurative peritonitis with an acutely inflamed diverticulum and a local abscess but no overt diverticular perforation.[22] Conversely, some patients with perforation of a diverticulum present only with a localized abscess,[99] although most perforations result in generalized peritonitis[100] and are misdiagnosed as acute appendicitis, acute colonic diverticulitis or a perforated peptic ulcer. Therefore it is essential to examine the small bowel when laparotomy (usually via a gridiron incision) has been performed for supposed appendicitis and the appendix is found to be normal. Occasionally perforation of a diverticulum is precipitated by foreign bodies, parasites, enteroliths or even food particles, such as a rolled-up tomato skin.[101] The overall mortality rate of perforation of a jejunal diverticula can be as high as 30%,[102] so early diagnosis and operative treatment is essential.

Perforation of a segment of small bowel Crohn's disease is uncommon[103] and only occurs in 1–2% of patients with this disease.[104,105] It usually occurs at a site of chronic but active disease, often associated with a distal stenosis. In some cases of perforation histological examination of the specimen does not reveal any granulomas, but their absence should not detract from the diagnosis in patients with known Crohn's disease.[93,106] Perforation is seldom a complication of acute ileitis.

Infective ulceration Worldwide, the most common cause of small bowel perforation is typhoid fever,[107,108] but fortunately the disease is very uncommon in Western society. Likewise, perforation of tuberculous enteritis is rare in the West, but it continues to be associated with a high morbidity rate and a mortality rate of up to 45%.[109] Other forms of infective ulceration and perforation are rare (see also Chapter 52), but cases have been reported associated with *Ascaris lumbricoides* infestation[110] although this is debated,[111] and cytomegalovirus infection in patients with the acquired immunodeficiency syndrome (HIV).[112]

Strangulation

Most enteric perforations in Western countries occur in association with intestinal obstruction, strangulation or trauma.[103] Strangulation is usually secondary to either an internal or external hernia or bands and adhesions (see Chapter 53), but it can also occur with intussusception (see Chapter 62). Strangulation is notoriously difficult to detect clinically in the early stages and can never be completely excluded without laparotomy. All too often patients with a strangulating obstruction are neglected, with dire consequences from perforation of the gangrenous bowel. This is particularly true for rather obese patients with a femoral hernia, in whom the hernia is overlooked because of inadequate examination of the groins.

A high suspicion of strangulation should always be entertained in patients with intestinal obstruction who complain of constant pain with tenderness and guarding. The suspicion should be increased in patients who are more ill than might be anticipated and show pallor, toxicity and signs of early shock. The examining clinician should always be aware of the diagnostic pitfall of a Richter's hernia, in which only a portion of the circumference of the intestine is strangulated.[113] This condition can lead to gangrene of the bowel wall without signs of intestinal obstruction. It usually occurs in association with a femoral hernia or rarely an obturator hernia.

Vascular insufficiency

In the past, the classical case of acute mesenteric ischaemia was due to an embolus arising as a complication of rheumatic heart disease. This is now an extremely rare condition; most patients with acute intestinal ischaemia do not have emboli, although this phenomenon can still occur in patients who have had a recent myocardial infarct. Most patients with intestinal ischaemia have atheromatous plaques at the origin of the superior mesenteric artery, but in up to one-third of fatal cases no vascular occlusion is found (see also Chapter 55).[114] In many cases acute occlusion of the superior mesenteric artery will result in intense small bowel spasm,[115] causing severe pain, and this is followed by the bowel becoming immobile and the abdomen distended. Necrosis supervenes, proceeding from the mucosa outwards to the serosa. The patient becomes extremely ill, restless, cyanosed and shocked. Often, if the ischaemia is widespread, the patient will die from renal failure, dehydration, acidosis and coma. However, if the ischaemic segment is limited, then perforation may occur. It is in this limited group of patients that an accurate diagnosis is required to allow surgical intervention before such a perforation occurs.

Perforation of the small bowel can also occur from vasculitis, which may be secondary to systemic disease (Table 54.3). Evidence of the underlying disease should be apparent in these patients.

Table 54.3 Systemic diseases causing small bowel perforation

Vasculitis
  Polyarteritis
  Systemic lupus erythematosus
  Rheumatoid disease
  Polymyositis
  Takayasu's disease
  Fabry's disease
Ehlers–Danlos syndrome
Behçet's syndrome
Leukaemia
Neurofibromatosis

Trauma

A history of trauma always provides a strong diagnostic clue in any case of small bowel perforation. Blunt trauma typically causes perforation of the jejunum just distal to the fixed point of the duodenojejunal flexure, and this area requires careful inspection (Chapter 47). Occasionally such perforation may

become sealed off, only to present at a later date as high small bowel obstruction due to a local abscess at that site or a foreign body granulomatous reaction resulting in a local stricture. All penetrating wounds must be treated with great caution, and care should be taken to look for multiple entry and exit holes. Penetrating wounds may initially present with minimal physical signs, especially if the patient is obese,[93] so laparotomy is recommended for all penetrating wounds.

Foreign bodies are commonly ingested but rarely cause small bowel perforation. The vast majority (over 90%) pass per rectum without any obvious complication developing.[116,117] However, certain objects such as nails[118] can lead to perforation, so patients with sharp ingested objects should be admitted for observation and serial radiography. Occasionally unexpected objects, such as rolled-up tomato skins,[119] can lead to perforation, although this event usually occurs when the object lodges in a blind pouch, such as Meckel's diverticulum or jejunal diverticula (Chapter 57).[101] Endogenous luminal objects can also lead to perforation, for example in gallstone ileus. This complication of a condition which is itself fairly uncommon is fortunately rare, but it can occur if the ileus is neglected and the stone ulcerates through the bowel wall. Perforated gallstone obturation carries a high morbidity and mortality rate, since it tends to occur in elderly female patients who often have associated cardiorespiratory disease.

Neoplasia

Any tumour of the small bowel has the potential to perforate, but this is exceedingly uncommon in the case of benign tumours such as leiomyomas.[120] Lymphomas appear to be more likely to perforate than carcinomas (Figure 54.17), with a perforation rate of 27% in one series of lymphomas.[39] Malignant sarcomas of the small bowel may also present with perforation (Figure 54.18), as can metastatic deposits from malignant melanoma[121] and carcinoma of the ovary, breast and lung.[122] In many cases the perforation is either a terminal or a very late complication of disseminated disease, but in some primary tumours perforation may be the first indication of any intra-abdominal pathology (see also Chapter 60).

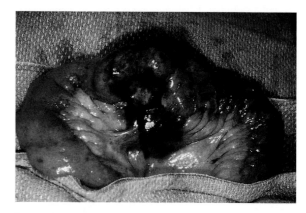

Figure 54.17
A perforated small bowel lymphoma.

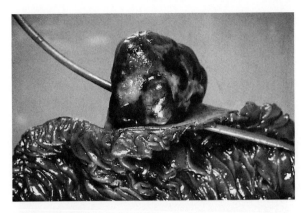

Figure 54.18
A perforated ileal leiomyosarcoma.

Iatrogenic perforations

Operation Operative injury or perforation of the small bowel should be apparent at the time of laparotomy, but occasionally in operations for severe adhesions small serosal tears can occur, that may become full-thickness without the surgeon realising it. In recent years the advent of minimal access surgery has brought with it a spate of iatrogenic perforations associated with the injudicious use of the Verres needle and trocars. Anastomotic dehiscence should be a rare event in the small intestine, but it may occur in patients who are markedly catabolic and hypoproteinaemic. One preventable cause of operative perforation is that caused by 'cheese-wiring' of abdominal sutures through the small bowel. This problem occurs if a lax loop of suture inadvertently catches a loop of small bowel and is then pulled taut. There is a particular risk when deep tension sutures are used.

Endoscopy Upper gastrointestinal endoscopy can occasionally be associated with iatrogenic perforation of the proximal gastrointestinal tract, especially the oesophagus. Only rarely will the standard endoscope be passed far enough into the jejunum to produce a small bowel perforation. However, this risk is much increased if some of the newer and more experimental small-bowel endoscopes are used.[78,79] In certain cases endoscopy can lead to spontaneous pneumoperitoneum without peritonitis or a 'clinical' perforation.[123] This event is usually associated with the transmural passage of air through the semipermeable membrane of thin-walled duodenal or small bowel diverticula.[124,125] It can result in a rather alarming radiological picture following a straightforward endoscopic procedure, but it should be treated conservatively as long as the patient exhibits no signs of a perforation or peritonitis.

Drugs Many and various medications have been implicated in perforations of the small bowel (see Chapter 52). Often the perforation appears to be directly related to such agents as steroids[126] and non-steroidal anti-inflammatory drugs.[127] In other reports the administered drug may act in a secondary capacity, potentiating any tendency of a pre-existing lesion to perforate: for example, perforations occurring in Crohn's disease after slow release potassium administration[128] or gastrointestinal neoplasms perforating during aggressive chemotherapy.[129]

Radiation Radiation for abdominal or pelvic malignancy can damage the small bowel and lead to radiation enteritis (see Chapter 52). The risk of developing complications depends on the radiation dosage, and the small bowel is more sensitive than the rest of the gastrointestinal tract. A dose of 4000 rad (40 Gy) to the small bowel may be associated with a risk of radiation enteritis of 5% within 5 years.[130] The usual presentation is with pain, nausea, vomiting and abdominal distension; barium studies may demonstrate generalized narrowing of the small bowel lumen, irregularity and mucosal swelling. When the damage is severe, necrosis of the gut can occur with free perforation into the peritoneal cavity, but more commonly there is fistulation to other adjacent organs, such as other loops of bowel, bladder or vagina.

Other causes of perforation

There are a number of conditions in which intestinal perforation rarely develops, for example amyloid disease or Degos' disease, in which perforations may be multiple.[131] In Degos' disease vasculitic skin lesions are associated with multiple infarcts of the gastrointestinal tract; it is often called the 'fatal cutaneointestinal syndrome'.

Clinical features

Small bowel perforation presents a totally different diagnostic problem to that of small bowel haemorrhage. In most cases perforation causes diffuse peritonitis, and any diagnostic failure lies in not being able to identify or recognize the precise underlying cause of the perforation until it is revealed at the time of operation.

The speed of development of signs of peritonitis will depend on the nature of the contents of the perforated segment of intestine. The physical signs of peritonitis will be slower to develop if the intestine is empty, as is usually the case with the jejunum (Latin *jejunum*, empty).[93] In most cases, perforation will present with sudden onset of abdominal pain and will usually progress to diffuse peritonitis. This presentation may be superimposed on the clinical picture of an underlying systemic disease, a past history of radiation, trauma or operation, diffuse vascular insufficiency or drug ingestion. The variability of the clinical picture emphasizes the importance of an accurate history and examination.

Occasionally perforation may be occult and present late as an intra-abdominal or interloop abscess.[118] This event may result from the actual perforation being sealed by the greater omentum, which causes symptoms and signs similar to those of an appendix mass.

Sometimes the inflammatory phlegmon may settle slowly, but this will usually lead to an interloop abscess. In these patients, both diagnosis and treatment are delayed, with the potential for more serious complications such as septicaemia, portal pyaemia and hepatic abscess formation.[132]

Investigation

In many situations, no specific investigation is required. Most patients will present with overt clinical peritonitis requiring urgent laparotomy, and the only preoperative investigations required will be those necessary for the purpose of administration of a general anaesthetic, such as investigations related to fluid balance and the cardiorespiratory system.

Occasionally there will be preoperative diagnostic uncertainty in differentiating a small bowel perforation from acute pancreatitis. Serum amylase may be raised in small bowel perforation and thus not be of particular value. Plain erect abdominal and chest radiographs may reveal a pneumoperitoneum,[133] but the amount of air is likely to be slight and the signs minimal (Figure 54.19). It must be stressed that in many cases the films will be normal, as pneumoperitoneum is only seen in 25–40% of cases of small bowel perforation.[103,109] The absence of intraperitoneal air must not therefore be construed as excluding intestinal perforation.

Barium studies are not recommended for confirming small bowel perforation because they can lead to barium peritonitis,[134] which can be extremely difficult to clear at laparotomy. Barium peritonitis causes a granulomatous peritoneal reaction with microabscesses, which may be persisting foci of sepsis. Even with assiduous peritoneal lavage, it is virtually impossible to remove all the barium crystals from the peritoneal cavity. Furthermore, in certain cases barium studies may turn an incipient small bowel perforation or a localized walled-off perforation into overt diffuse peritonitis.

After ingestion of a foreign body, if there is no evidence clinically or radiologically of perforation or obstruction, patients who have swallowed sharp objects such as nails should be admitted for observation. Serial plain abdominal radiography is undertaken to follow progress and exclude an occult perforation.

Intra-abdominal abscesses may show as a mottled soft tissue swelling on a plain abdominal film; occasionally a fluid level may be seen. Other features include a small sympathetic pleural effusion or displacement of normal soft tissue structure or planes, such as the psoas muscle outline. Abdominal ultrasonography has an accuracy of localization of 60–90%, while CT has a published accuracy of up to 97%[135] (Figure 54.20). Radionuclide scanning may also be used to demonstrate occult intra-abdominal abscesses, using either ^{67}Ga or ^{111}In to label leucocytes. The value of this technique is limited because, unlike ultrasonography and CT, it does not allow route planning and

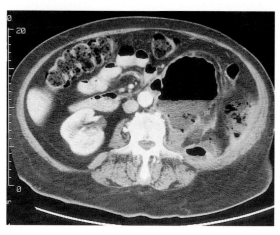

Figure 54.20
An intra-abdominal abscess demonstrated by CT.

isolation for percutaneous drainage. The role of nuclear magnetic resonance in the imaging of ultraabdominal abscesses requires further investigation.

Treatment

Laparotomy is recommended for all cases of small bowel perforation that present with clinical peritonitis. An accurate preoperative diagnosis will not be available in many situations. The differential diagnosis will include such conditions as a perforated gastric or duodenal ulcer, perforated appendicitis, perforated caecal carcinoma, perforated colonic diverticulitis and perforated pyosalpinx.

The diagnosis at laparotomy usually causes little problem. The site of perforation is obvious in most cases, but care must be taken to examine the entire bowel, as perforations can be multiple.[93] Surgical resection is curative in all but a few cases, and in these the outcome depends on the underlying pathology. Perforated malignant tumours or widespread ischaemic necrosis carry an extremely poor prognosis. Other conditions may prove troublesome if the precipitating cause or underlying pathology, such as irradiation damage, infections or inflammatory conditions, systemic disease or an undiagnosed gastrinoma, is not eradicated.

In cases of penetrating trauma, such as stab or gunshot wounds, great care should be taken to look for multiple entry and exit holes in several loops of small bowel. In blunt trauma special attention must be paid to the fixed points of the bowel, especially just distal to the duodenojejunal flexure. Any tear in the mesentery must be viewed with suspicion in case it could lead to vascular insufficiency of a small segment of bowel and a delayed perforation.

In the vast majority of cases, surgical excision of any perforated lesion and end-to-end anastomosis is adequate treatment.

Intra-abdominal abscesses

In cases in which the underlying pathology or the perforation does not require immediate resection, an intra-abdominal or intrahepatic abscess may be drained percutaneously under ultrasonographic or CT guidance. This step may allow formal

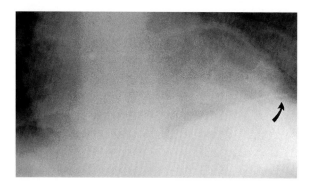

Figure 54.19
Pneumoperitoneum from small bowel perforation: bilateral thin slithers of air (arrowed).

surgical exploration to be delayed or even occasionally avoided in very ill patients. Straight line percutaneous drainage is preferred, avoiding vital organs, and an extraperitoneal route is recommended.[135]

A 'pigtail' catheter may be left in situ to allow continuous drainage. It also provides access for irrigation, antibiotic instillation and sinograms if indicated. Subsequent laparotomy is necessary if resolution does not occur after percutaneous drainage or if the primary pathology requires resection.

Complications

Acute

The morbidity rate following small bowel perforation depends on the nature of the underlying lesion and the delay in diagnosis. The mortality rate of generalized peritonitis has been reported as being of the order of 15%.[136] Although this figure is significantly less than for generalized faecal peritonitis from perforated colonic diseases (which causes a mortality rate of up to 70%), it rises at the extremes of age and with intercurrent disease.

Any delay in surgical exploration for generalized peritonitis may result in an increased incidence of pulmonary, renal or hepatic complications in the early postoperative period, as well as an increase in the incidence of wound infections (>40%) and subsequent intra-abdominal abscesses (30%).[136] The risks of septicaemia and shock are also increased by delay in treatment, and appropriate resuscitation and antibiotic therapy are essential.

Chronic

The widespread fibrinous exudate caused by generalized peritonitis from a small bowel perforation often results in the formation of dense fibrous intraperitoneal adhesions. Over subsequent years these adhesions may be responsible for causing multiple episodes of small bowel obstruction, possibly requiring further surgical intervention.

Good surgical techniques should not ordinarily allow the development of an anastomotic stricture unless the underlying pathology, such as Crohn's disease or malignancy, recurs. Occasionally foreign body granulomas present at a later date, having arisen in response to material extruded through the initial perforation. These lesions can also present as intestinal obstruction.

Perforated malignancies, particularly adenocarcinoma, may result in disseminated peritoneal tumour deposits (carcinomatosis peritonei), while serosal implantations of mucigenic cells may result in pseudomyxoma peritonei. This is a rare condition in which vast quantities of mucinous gelatinous material is found in the peritoneal cavity. It usually follows perforation of a mucocele of the appendix, but it has been reported after perforation of mucinous adenocarcinomas of the small bowel or the vitellointestinal duct.[137]

Resection of short segments of small bowel are usually accompanied by no chronic sequelae with regard to malabsorption unless the ileum, which is the site of active absorption of bile salts and vitamin B_{12}, is removed. However, if more than 50% of the small intestine is resected, the resulting nutritional deficiencies can lead to a severe malabsorption syndrome. This state of affairs is unlikely to result from resection for perforation, unless a long segment is excised because of multiple perforations or widespread ischaemia.

Conclusion

Perforation of the small bowel results from a diversity of pathological conditions and presents in a similarly diverse manner. The presentation may be either sudden and dramatic or slow and insidious. In the very early stages, if the bowel is empty, symptoms and signs may be minimal and accurate assessment can be hindered especially by obesity.[93] An increased awareness of small bowel disease will lead to earlier diagnosis and surgical correction, which in turn will result in a decrease in the morbidity and the excessive mortality rates noted in some series.[103]

REFERENCES

1. Boydstun JS, Gaffey TA & Bartholomew LG. Clinicopathologic study of non-specific ulcers of the small intestine. *Dig Dis Sci* 1981; **26**: 911.
2. Glynn MJ, Pendower J, Shousha S & Parkins RA. Recurrent bleeding from idiopathic ulceration of the small bowel. *BMJ* 1984; **288**: 975.
3. Baer AM, Bayless TM & Yardley JH. Intestinal ulceration and malabsorption syndromes. *Gastroenterology* 1980; **79**: 754.
4. Robertson DAF, Dixon MF, Scott BB, Simpson FG & Losowsky MS. Small intestinal ulceration: diagnostic difficulties in relation to coeliac disease. *Gut* 1983; **24**: 565.
5. Thomas WEG & Williamson RCN. Non-specific small bowel ulceration. *Postgrad Med J* 1985; **61**: 587.
6. Guest JL Jr. Non-specific ulceration of the intestine. *Int Abst Surg* 1963; **117**: 409.
7. Baillie M. *The Morbid Anatomy of Some of the Most Important Parts of the Human Body*, 1st American edn. Albany: Barber & Southwick, 1795. Cited by Guest[6].
8. Morgenstern L, Freilich M & Parish JF. The circumferential small-bowel ulcer: clinical aspects in 17 patients. *JAMA* 1965; **191**: 637.
9. Campbell JR & Knapp RW. Small bowel ulceration associated with thiazide and potassium therapy: review of 13 cases. *Ann Surg* 1966; **163**: 291.
10. Boley SJ, Schultz L, Krieger H, Schwartz S, Elguezabal A & Allen AC. Experimental evaluation of thiazides and potassium as a cause of small bowel ulcer. *JAMA* 1965; **192**: 763.
11. Lang J, Bjarnason I, Levi AJ & Price AB. Pathology of iatrogenic ileal strictures caused by non-steroidal anti-inflammatory drugs. *Gut* 1985; **26**: A542.
12. Watson MR. Primary non-specific ulceration of the small intestine. *Arch Surg* 1963; **87**: 600.
13. Evert JA, Black BM & Dockerty MB. Primary non-specific ulcers of the small intestine. *Surgery* 1948; **23**: 185.
14. Grosfield JL, Schiller M, Weinberger M & Clatworthy HW. Primary non-specific ileal ulcers in children. *Am J Dis Child* 1970; **120**: 447.
15. Mackey WC & Dineen P. A fifty year experience with Meckel's diverticulum. *Surg Gynecol Obstet* 1983; **156**: 56.
16. Williamson RCN, Cooper MJ & Thomas WEG. Intussusception of invaginated Meckel's diverticulum. *J R Soc Med* 1984; **77**: 652.
17. Neuss MN, Garbutt JT, Leight GS et al. Intraluminal thrombus and bowel obstruction in acute leukaemia due to bleeding Meckel's diverticulum. *Am J Med* 1986; **80**: 1194.
18. Long BW. Early diagnosis and management of bleeding Meckel's diverticulum. *J Miss State Med Assoc* 1986; **27**: 149.
19. Thomas CS, Tinsley EA & Brockman SK. Jejunal diverticula as a source of massive upper gastrointestinal bleeding. *Arch Surg* 1967; **95**: 89.
20. Geroulakis G. Surgical problems of jejunal diverticulosis. *Ann R Coll Surg Engl* 1987; **69**: 266.
21. Taylor MT. Massive hemorrhage from jejunal diverticulosis. *Am J Surg* 1969; **118**: 117.
22. Jones P.F. Jejunal and ileal diverticula. In *Emergency Abdominal Surgery*. Oxford: Blackwell, 1974: 550.

23. Shackelford RT & Marcus WY. Jejunal diverticula – a cause of gastrointestinal haemorrhage. A report of three cases and review of the literature. *Ann Surg* 1960; **151**: 930.

24. Forrest JAH. Gastrointestinal bleeding. In Shearman DJC & Finlayson NDC (eds) *Diseases of the Gastrointestinal Tract and Liver.* Edinburgh: Churchill Livingstone, 1982: 204.

25. Beaton HL. Small intestinal bleeding. *N Y State J Med* 1982; **82**: 171.

26. Thompson JN, Salem RR, Hemingway AP et al. Specialist investigations of obscure gastrointestinal bleeding. *Gut* 1987; **28**: 47.

27. Boley SJ, Sammartano R, Adams A et al. On the nature and aetiology of vascular ectasias of the colon (degenerative lesions of ageing). *Gastroenterology* 1977; **72**: 650.

28. Hemingway AP & Allison DJ. Angiodysplasia and Meckel's diverticulum: a congenital association? *Br J Surg* 1982; **69**: 600.

29. Baum S, Athanasoulis CA, Waltman AC et al. Angiodysplasia of the right colon: a cause of gastrointestinal bleeding. *AJR* 1977; **129**: 789.

30. Pierce WS & Davis AV. Massive bleeding from a diffuse vascular malformation of the small intestine. *Arch Surg* 1969; **98**: 336.

31. Driscoll JE & Rabe MA. Haemorrhagic telangiectasis of the gastrointestinal tract; an obscure source of gastrointestinal bleeding. *Am Surg* 1954; **20**: 1281.

32. Sheil AGR, Reeve TS, Little JM et al. Aorto-intestinal fistulas following operations on the abdominal aorta and iliac artery. *Br J Surg* 1969; **56**: 840.

33. Lamerton AJ. Iliaco-appendiceal fistula complicating endarterectomy alone. *Br J Surg* 1984; **71**: 501.

34. Thomas WEG & Baird RN. Secondary aorto-enteric fistulae: towards a more conservative approach. *Br J Surg* 1986; **73**: 875.

35. Crowson M, Fielding JWL, Black J et al. Acute gastrointestinal complications of infrarenal aortic aneurysm repair. *Br J Surg* 1984; **71**: 825.

36. Reilly LM, Altman H, Lusby RJ et al. Late results following surgical management of vascular graft infection. *J Vasc Surg* 1984; **1**: 36.

37. Schiller KFR, Truelove SC & Williams DG. Haematemesis and melaena with special reference to factors influencing the outcome. *BMJ* 1970; **2**: 7.

38. Forrest JAH & Finlayson NDC. The investigation of acute upper gastrointestinal haemorrhage. *Br J Hosp Med* 1974; **12**: 160.

39. Williamson RCN, Welch CE & Malt RA. Adenocarcinoma and lymphoma of the small intestine. *Ann Surg* 1983; **197**: 172.

40. Huntley BF, Laurain AR & Stephenson WH. Haemorrhage from leiomyomas of the gastrointestinal tract. *Arch Intern Med* 1960; **106**: 245.

41. Bartholomew LG, Dahlin DC & Waugh JM. Intestinal polyposis associated with muco-cutaneous melanin pigmentation (Peutz–Jeghers syndrome). Review of literature and report of 54 cases with special reference to pathologic findings. *Gastroenterology* 1957; **32**: 434.

42. Bussey HJR. Gastrointestinal polyposis. *Gut* 1970; **11**: 970.

43. Forbes CD, Barr RD, Prentice CRM & Douglas A. Gastrointestinal bleeding in haemophilia. *Q J Med* 1973; **42**: 503.

44. Thomas WEG & May RE. Hepatic artery aneurysm following cholecystectomy. *Postgrad Med J* 1981; **57**: 393.

45. Hall RI, Lavelle MI & Venables CW. Chronic pancreatitis as a cause of gastrointestinal bleeding. *Gut* 1982; **23**: 250.

46. Thomas WEG. Recurrent obscure gastrointestinal haemorrhage. *Curr Pract Surg* 1989; **1**: 17.

47. Stewart JG, Ahlquist DA, McGill DB et al. Gastrointestinal blood loss and anemia in runners. *Ann Intern Med* 1984; **100**: 843.

48. Gnauck R. Occult blood tests. *Lancet* 1980; **i**: 822.

49. Macrae FA & St John DJB. Relationship between patterns of bleeding and hemocult sensitivity in patients with colorectal cancer or adenoma. *Gastroenterology* 1982; **82**: 891.

50. Ostrow JD, Mulvaney CA, Hansell UR & Rhodes RS. Sensitivity and reproducibility of chemical tests for fecal occult blood with an emphasis on false positive reactions. *Am J Dig Dis* 1973; **18**: 930.

51. Irons GV & Kirsner JB. Routine chemical tests of the stool for occult blood: an evaluation. *Am J Med Sci* 1965; **249**: 247.

52. Vellacott KD, Baldwin RW & Hardcastle JD. An immunofluorescent test for faecal occult blood. *Lancet* 1981; **i**: 18.

53. Doran J & Hardcastle JD. Bleeding pattern in colorectal cancer: the effect of aspirin and the implications for faecal occult blood testing. *Br J Surg* 1982; **69**: 711.

54. Nolan DJ. Barium examination of the small intestine. *Gut* 1981; **22**: 682.

55. Reid J, Gilmour HM & Holt S. Primary non-specific ulcer of the small intestine. *J R Coll Surg Edinb* 1982; **27**: 228.

56. Maglinte DD & Antley RM. Radiology of the small bowel: enteroclysis and the conventional follow-through. *Gastroenterology* 1984; **86**: 383.

57. Gurian L, Jendrzejewski J, Katon R, Bilbao M, Cope R & Melnyk C. Small bowel enema. An underutilised method of small bowel examination. *Dig Dis Sci* 1982; **27**: 1101.

58. Sellink JL. Radiologic examination of the small intestine by duodenal intubation. *Acta Radiol (Diagn)* 1974; **15**: 318.

59. Maglinte DDT, Hall R, Miller RE et al. Detection of surgical lesions of the small bowel by enteroclysis. *Am J Surg* 1984; **147**: 225.

60. Keddie N, Watson-Baker R & Saran M. The value of the small bowel enema to the general surgeon. *Br J Surg* 1982; **69**: 611.

61. Briley CA, Jackson DC, Johnsrude IS & Mills SR. Acute gastrointestinal haemorrhage of small bowel origin. *Radiology* 1980; **136**: 317.

62. Jaffe BF, Youker JE & Margoulis AR. Aortographic localisation of controlled gastrointestinal haemorrhage in dogs. *Surgery* 1965; **58**: 984.

63. Balint JA & Sarfeh IJ. *Gastrointestinal Bleeding. Diagnosis and Management.* New York: Wiley, 1977: 31–41.

64. Palmaz JC, Walter JF & Cho KJ. Therapeutic embolisation of the small bowel arteries. *Radiology* 1984; **152**: 377.

65. Chalmers AG, Robinson PJ & Chapman AH. Embolisation in small bowel haemorrhage. *Clin Radiol* 1986; **37**: 379.

66. Athanasoulis CA. Therapeutic applications of angiography. *N Engl J Med* 1980; **302**: 1117.

67. Alavi A, Dann RW, Baum S & Biery DN. Scintigraphic detection of acute gastrointestinal bleeding. *Radiology* 1977; **124**: 753.

68. Alavi A. Detection of gastrointestinal bleeding with Tc99m sulphur colloid. *Semin Nucl Med* 1982; **12**: 126.

69. Merrick MV. The small intestine. In Rhys Davies E & Thomas WEG (eds) *Nuclear Medicine: Applications to Surgery.* Tunbridge Wells: Castle House, 1988, 69.

70. Pavel DG, Zimmer AM & Patterson VN In vivo labelling of red blood cells with Tc99m: a new approach to blood pool visualisation. *J Nucl Med* 1977; **18**: 305.

71. Winzelberg GG, McKusick KA, Froelich JW et al. Detection of gastrointestinal bleeding with Tc99m-labelled red blood cells. *Semin Nucl Med* 1982; **12**: 139.

72. Bunker SR, Lull RJ, Tanasescu DE et al. Scintigraphy of gastrointestinal haemorrhage; superiority of ^{99m}Tc red blood cells over ^{99m}Tc sulphur colloid. *AJR* 1984; **143**: 543.

73. Berquist TH, Nolan NG, Stephens DH et al. Specificity of ^{99m}Tc-pertechnitate in scintigraphy diagnosis of Meckel's diverticulum. Review of 100 cases. *J Nucl Med* 1976; **17**: 465.

74. Anderson GF, Sfakianakis G, King DR et al. Hormonal enhancement of technetium-99m pertechnitate uptake in experimental Meckel's diverticulum. *J Pediatr Surg* 1980; **15**: 900.

75. Yeker D & Buyukunal C. Radionuclide imaging of Meckel's diverticulum: cimetidine versus pentagastrin plus glucagen. *Eur J Nucl Med* 1984; **9**: 316.

76. Baum S. Pertechnitate imaging following cimetidine administration in Meckel's diverticulum of the ileum. *Am J Gastroenterol* 1981; **76**: 464.

77. Sfakianakis GN, Anderson GF & King DR. The effect of intestinal hormones on the Tc99m pentechnitate imaging of ectopic gastric mucosa in experimental Meckel's diverticulum. *J Nucl Med* 1981; **22**: 678.

78. Shinya H & McSherry C. Endoscopy of the small bowel. *Surg Clin North Am* 1982; **62**: 821.

79. Tada M & Kawai K. Small bowel endoscopy. *Scand J Gastroenterol* 1984; **19**: (Suppl.102): 39.

80. Lau WY, Fan ST, Chu KW et al. Intra-operative fibre optic enteroscopy for bleeding lesions in the small intestine. *Br J Surg* 1986; **73**: 217.

81. Apelgren KM, Vargish T & Al-Kawas F. Principles for use of intra-operative enteroscopy for haemorrhage from the small bowel. *Am Surg* 1988; **54**: 85.

82. Haynes WF, Pittmann FE & Christakis G. Localisation of site of upper gastrointestinal tract haemorrhage by the fluorescein string test. *Surgery* 1960; **48**: 421.

83. Crawford ES, Roehm JOF & McGavran MH. Jejuno-ileal arteriovenous malformation. Localisation for resection by segmental bowel staining techniques. *Ann Surg* 1980; **191**: 404.

84. Hardcastle JD. Bleeding from the small or large intestine. In Misiewicz JJ, Pounder RE & Venables CW (eds) *Diseases of the Gut and Pancreas.* Oxford: Blackwell, 1987: 456.

85. Dowse JLA. Meckel's diverticulum. *Br J Surg* 1961; **48**: 392.

86. Allison DJ, Hemingway AP & Cunningham DA. Angiography in gastrointestinal bleeding. *Lancet* 1982; **ii**: 30.

87. Scharf GM, Van Rensburg PJ & Mieny CJ. Idiopathic small bowel perforations. *S Afr J Surg* 1987; **25**: 53.

88. Aschner JL, Deluga KS, Metlay LA et al. Spontaneous focal gastrointestinal perforations in very low birth weight infants. *J Pediatr* 1988; **113**: 364.

89. Rutherford RB & Akers DR. Meckel's diverticulum – a review of 148 pediatric patients with special reference to the pattern of bleeding and to mesodiverticula bands. *Surgery* 1966; **59**: 618.

90. Rosswick RP. Perforation of Meckel's diverticulum by foreign body. *Postgrad Med J* 1965; **41**: 105.

91. Layer GT, Scott-Jupp RH, Maitra TK et al. Slow release potassium and perforation of Meckel's diverticulum. *Postgrad Med J* 1987; **63**: 211.

92. Ellison EH & Wilson SD. The Zollinger–Ellison syndrome: re-appraisal and evaluation of 260 registered cases. *Ann Surg* 1964; **160**: 512.

93. Thomas WEG & Williamson RCN. Enteric ulceration and its complications. *World J Surg* 1985; **9**: 876.

94. Watson CG, Moseley RV & Wheeler HB Perforated jejunal ulcer and the Zollinger–Ellison syndrome. *Arch Surg* 1986; **96**: 274.

95. Frey EE, Smith W, Franken EA et al. Analysis of bowel perforation in necrotizing enterocolitis. *Pediatr Radiol* 1987; **17**: 380.

96. Nobles ER. Jejunal diverticula. *Arch Surg* 1971; **102**: 172.

97. Herrington JL. Perforation of acquired diverticula of jejunum and ileum. *Surgery* 1962; **51**: 426.

98. Smith JS. Jejunal diverticula – subtle cause of acute abdomen. *Pa Med* 1976; **79**: 60.

99. Brown RJ & Thompson RL. Perforated jejunal diverticulum presenting with a psoas abscess. *Ulster Med J* 1985; **54**: 78.

100. Pyper PC & Hood JM. Perforation of jejunal diverticula. *JR Coll Surg Edinb* 1987; **32**: 248.

101. Phillips JHC. Jejunal diverticulitis. Some clinical aspects. *Br J Surg* 1953; **40**: 350.

102. Babcock T, Hutton J & Salander J. Perforated jejunal diverticulitis. *Am Surg* 1976; **42**: 568.

103. Rajagopalan AE & Pickleman J. Free perforation of the small intestine. *Ann Surg* 1982; **196**: 576.

104. Steinberg DM, Cooke WT & Alexander-Williams J. Free perforation in Crohn's disease. *Gut* 1973; **14**: 187.

105. Greenstein AJ, Mann D, Sachar DB et al. Free perforation in Crohn's disease: survey of 99 cases. *Am J Gastroenterol* 1985; **80**: 682.

106. Kyle J, Cardis T, Duncan T et al. Free perforation in regional enteritis. *Am J Dig Dis* 1968; **13**: 275.

107. Archampong EQ. Operative treatment of typhoid perforation of the bowel. *BMJ* 1969; **3**: 273.

108. Eggleston FC, Santoshi B & Singh CM. Typhoid perforation of the bowel. *Ann Surg* 1979; **190**: 31.

109. Kakar A, Aranya RC & Nair SK. Acute perforation of small intestine due to tuberculosis. *Aust N Z J Surg* 1983; **53**: 381.

110. Ihekwaba FN. *Ascaris lumbricoides* and perforation of the ileum; a critical review. *Br J Surg* 1979; **66**: 132.

111. Efem SEE. *Ascaris lumbricoides* and intestinal perforation. *Br J Surg* 1987; **74**: 643.

112. Houin HP, Gruenberg JC, Fisher EJ et al. Multiple small bowel perforations secondary to cytomegalovirus in a patient with acquired immunodeficiency syndrome. *Henry Ford Hosp Med J* 1987; **35**: 17.

113. Efem EE. Strangulated Richter's hernia presenting as Fournier's gangrene. *Postgrad Doct Afr* 1985; **7**: 181.

114. Marston A. Ischaemia of the gut. In Misiewicz JJ, Pounder RE & Venables CW (eds) *Diseases of the Gut and Pancreas*. Oxford: Blackwell, 1987: 1029.

115. Marston A. Causes of death in mesenteric arterial occlusion. *Ann Surg* 1963; **158**: 952.

116. Gross RE. Foreign bodies in the alimentary tract. In *The Surgery of Infancy and Childhood*. Philadelphia: WB Saunders, 1953; 246.

117. Ashby BS & Hunter-Craig ID. Foreign body perforation of the gut. *Br J Surg* 1967; **54**: 382.

118. Ani AN & Itayeni SO. Intestinal perforation in an adult. *JR Coll Surg Edinb* 1982; **27**: 186.

119. Lumsden AB & Dixon JM. Tomato skins penetrating the small bowel. *Br J Surg* 1984; **71**: 648.

120. Laursen E. Leiomyomas of the small intestine: a rare cause of abdominal emergency. *Acta Chir Scand* 1987; **153**: 391.

121. Klausner JM, Skornick Y, Lelcuk S et al. Acute complications of metastatic melanoma to the gastrointestinal tract. *Br J Surg* 1982; **69**: 195.

122. Pang JA & King WK. Bowel haemorrhage and perforation from metastatic lung cancer. Report of 3 cases and a review of the literature. *Aust N Z J Surg* 1987; **57**: 779.

123. Brown MW, Brown RC & Orr G. Pneumoperitoneum complicating endoscopy in a patient with duodenal and jejunal diverticula. *Gastrointest Endosc* 1986; **32**: 120.

124. Dunn Y & Nelson JA. Jejunal diverticula and chronic pneumoperitoneum. *Gastrointest Radiol* 1979; **4**: 165.

125. Madura MJ & Craig RM. Duodenal and jejunal diverticula causing a pneumoperitoneum. *J Clin Gastroenterol* 1981; **3**: 61.

126. Fadul CE, Lemann W, Thaler HT et al. Perforation of the gastrointestinal tract in patients receiving steroids for neurologic disease. *Neurology* 1988; **38**: 348.

127. Day TK Intestinal perforation associated with osmotic slow release indomethacin capsules. *BMJ* 1983; **287**: 1671.

128. Brower RA. Jejunal perforations possibly induced by slow release potassium in a patient with Crohn's disease. *Dig Dis Sci* 1986; **31**: 1387.

129. Randall J, Obeid ML & Blackledge GR. Haemorrhage and perforation of gastrointestinal neoplasms during chemotherapy. *Ann R Coll Surg Engl* 1986; **68**: 286.

130. Rowsit B, Malsky SJ & Reid CB. Severe radiation injuries of the stomach, small intestine, colon and rectum. *AJR* 1972; **114**: 460.

131. Evans GH & Ribeiro BF. Dego's disease. A rare cause of multiple intestinal perforations. *J R Coll Surg Edinb* 1987; **32**: 371.

132. Pedersen VM, Geerdsen JP, Bartholdy J et al. Foreign body perforation of the gastrointestinal tract with formation of liver abscess. *Ann Chir Gynaecol* 1986; **75**: 245.

133. Winek TG, Mosely HS, Grout G et al. Pneumoperitoneum and its association with ruptured abdominal viscus. *Arch Surg* 1988; **123**: 709.

134. Kapote S, Nazareth HM & Bapat RD. Barium peritonitis. *J Postgrad Med* 1988; **34**: 103.

135. Thomas WEG, Virjee J & Leaper DJ. Intra-abdominal abscesses. *Surgery* 1986; **34**: 803.

136. Hutchinson GH. Diseases of the peritoneum. In Misiewicz JJ, Pounder RE & Venables CW (eds) *Diseases of the Gut and Pancreas*. Oxford: Blackwell, 1987: 1056.

137. Long RT, Spratt JS & Dowling E. Pseudomyxoma peritonei. *Am J Surg* 1969; **117**: 162.

55

MESENTERIC VASCULAR DISEASES

RN Kaleya
SJ Boley

Mesenteric vascular diseases (MVDs) result from inadequate blood flow to all or part of the small intestine and right half of the colon. Irrespective of the cause of the ischaemic insult, the end-results are similar: a spectrum of bowel injury ranging from completely reversible alterations of bowel function to transmural haemorrhagic necrosis of the intestinal wall. Depending on the degree of ischaemia and the length of bowel involved, a wide variety of clinical presentations is observed. With the heightened awareness of these clinical syndromes, a greater understanding of the pathophysiological basis of mesenteric ischaemia and improvements in medical technology, a cogent and effective approach to the diagnosis and treatment of MVDs has been formulated over the past 30 years.

CLASSIFICATION

Mesenteric vascular disease can be broadly classified into acute and chronic forms and into conditions of venous or arterial origin (Figure 55.1). In the chronic forms of mesenteric ischaemia, the viability of the bowel is not compromised, but the blood flow is inadequate to support the functional demands of the intestine, while with the acute forms of mesenteric ischaemia,

intestinal viability is threatened. Atherosclerotic narrowing or occlusion of the mesenteric arteries, producing intestinal angina, and gradually evolving mesenteric venous thrombosis (MVT) are the common forms of chronic ischaemia. Acute mesenteric ischaemia (AMI) is much more common than chronic, and ischaemia of arterial origin is much more frequent than venous disease. The arterial forms of AMI include superior mesenteric arterial embolus (SMAE), non-occlusive mesenteric ischaemia (NOMI), superior mesenteric artery thrombosis (SMAT) and those cases of focal segmental ischaemia resulting from local atherosclerotic emboli or vasculitides. Acute MVT and focal segmental ischaemia caused by strangulation obstruction of the small intestine or by localized venous thrombosis comprise the venous forms of AMI.

DEMOGRAPHICS AND INCIDENCE

Due, in part, to an absolute rise in the incidence of this family of diseases, but also to a familiarity with the syndromes produced by vascular insufficiency of the intestines, MVDs have been increasingly diagnosed in the past 30 years. The higher incidence has been attributed to the ageing of the population as MVD occurs predominantly, but not exclusively, in geriatric patients, especially those with serious cardiovascular and systemic disorders. Similarly, the widespread use of coronary and surgical intensive care units and other extraordinary means of cardiopulmonary support has salvaged patients, who would previously have died rapidly of cardiovascular conditions, only to have them go on to develop AMI as a later consequence of their primary disease.

The exact incidence of MVD is difficult to determine but as the number of elderly individuals in the population grows, disorders affecting the mesenteric circulation will continue to increase. In our large metropolitan medical centre, MVD is responsible for approximately 0.1% of all admissions.

Acute mesenteric ischaemia

There has been a changing distribution of causes of AMI over the past 50 years (Figure 55.2). Acute MVT was believed to

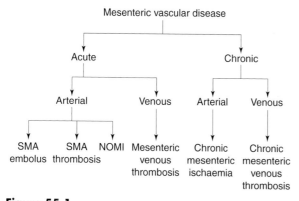

Figure 55.1

Classification of mesenteric vascular diseases. SMA, superior mesenteric artery; NOMI, non-occlusive mesenteric ischaemia.

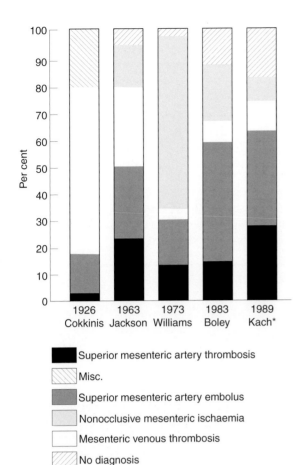

Figure 55.2

Changing patterns of mesenteric vascular disease. SMAT, superior mesenteric artery thrombosis; SMAE, superior mesenteric artery embolus; MVT, mesenteric venous thrombosis; Misc, miscellaneous; NOMI, non-occlusive mesenteric ischaemia; No Dx, no diagnosis.

Legend:
- ■ Superior mesenteric artery thrombosis
- ▨ Misc.
- ▥ Superior mesenteric artery embolus
- ▨ Nonocclusive mesenteric ischaemia
- □ Mesenteric venous thrombosis
- ▨ No diagnosis

be the major cause of AMI in the early studies, e.g. in 1926 Cokkinis[1] reported that 60% of his patients presenting with AMI had MVT. However, after Ende[2] described the non-occlusive form of AMI in 1958, it was recognized that many patients considered to have MVT before Ende's report were, in actuality, suffering from NOMI. This observation was reflected in Jackson's[3] report in 1963, in which MVT accounted for only 25% of the cases of AMI. As the diagnosis of NOMI by angiography became standard, the incidence of MVT fell to under 10% by 1973[4] and to under 5% at our institution by 1983.

In most recent series, SMAE and NOMI were responsible for 70–80% of cases of AMI. More recently, we have noted a decline in the incidence of non-occlusive ischaemia, possibly owing to the increasing use of systemic vasodilators, such as the calcium channel blocking agents and nitrates, in coronary intensive care units. In addition, the more common use of left ventricular assist devices in the treatment of cardiogenic shock has decreased the period of profound hypotension associated with left ventricular failure and, presumably, has attenuated its affect on the mesenteric circulation.

Arterial forms

Emboli to the superior mesenteric artery (SMA) are responsible for 40–50% of episodes of AMI. The emboli usually originate from a left atrial or ventricular mural thrombus. The thrombus embolizes after being dislodged or fragmented during a period of an arrhythmia. Many patients with SMAE have a history of previous peripheral artery embolism, and approximately 20% have synchronous emboli in other arteries. Emboli to the SMA tend to lodge at points of normal anatomical narrowings, usually immediately distal to the origin of a major branch (Figure 55.3). In 10–15% of patients the emboli lodge peripherally in branches of the SMA or in the SMA itself, distal to the origin of the ileocolic artery. The embolus may completely occlude the arterial lumen, but more commonly it only partially occludes the vessel. After a period of partial occlusion and diminution of blood flow distal to the embolus, vasoconstriction develops in arteries both proximal and distal to the embolus (Figure 55.4); this vasoconstriction can impair collateral blood flow to the SMA and its branches distal to the embolus, exacerbating the ischaemic insult.

NOMI causes 20–30% of episodes of AMI and is thought to result from splanchnic vasoconstriction initiated by a period of decreased cardiac output associated with hypotension caused by arrhythmias, cardiogenic shock, hypovolaemic shock or vasoactive medications. The vasoconstriction may persist even

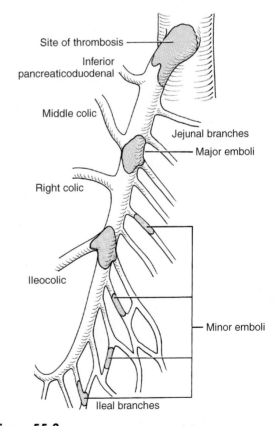

Figure 55.3

Common sites of superior mesenteric artery (SMA) emboli. Emboli distal to the ileocolic branch or in segmental arteries are considered minor emboli. Thrombosis usually occurs near the origin of the SMA.

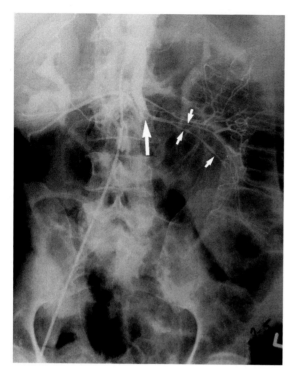

Figure 55.4
Arteriogram showing embolus completely occluding the superior mesenteric artery (Large arrow) with associated vasoconstriction in the arterial bed distal to the embolus (small arrows). (Reproduced with permission from Brandt LJ & Boley SJ. In McLean LD (ed.) *Advances in Surgery*. Chicago: Year Book, 1981.

after the precipitating cause has been eliminated or corrected. Predisposing factors for NOMI include acute myocardial infarction, congestive heart failure, aortic insufficiency, hepatic diseases, renal diseases, especially in patients requiring haemodialysis, and major cardiac or intra-abdominal operations. In addition, a more immediate precipitating cause such as acute pulmonary oedema, cardiac arrhythmia or shock is usually present, although the consequent intestinal ischaemia may not become manifest until hours or days later.

SMAT occurs at areas of severe atherosclerotic narrowing, most often at the origin of the SMA (see Figure 55.3). The acute ischaemic episode is commonly superimposed on chronic mesenteric ischaemia, hence approximately 20–50% of these patients have a history of abdominal pain with or without evidence of malabsorption and weight loss during the weeks to months preceding the acute episode. Additionally, most patients with SMAT have severe and diffuse atherosclerosis with a prior history of coronary, cerebrovascular or peripheral arterial insufficiency.

Venous forms

Approximately two patients per 100 000 admissions to our institution have had operative or pathological confirmation of MVT. This represents less than 5% of all cases of AMI. While reviews of the literature report a male predilection of up to 1.5 : 1,[5,6] our series showed no such preference. In our review

of the literature the mean age was 48 years, whereas it was 60 years in our series. We have attributed these differences to the higher proportion of geriatric patients seen at our medical centre as compared with most other institutions.

Many conditions have been associated with MVT (Table 55.1). Although all of the causes listed have been implicated in patients with MVT, in 20–35% of patients no contributing or associated factors can be identified. However, many of the cases cited in retrospective reviews were reported before haematological diseases such as antithrombin III, protein C and protein S deficiencies were described. It is expected that the number of cases of MVT in which no cause can be found will decrease as we uncover newer aetiologies and test for those that have already been identified.

Table 55.1 Conditions associated with mesenteric venous thrombosis

Primary
Portal hypertension
  Cirrhosis
  Congestive splenomegaly
  Following sclerotherapy for oesophageal varices
Inflammation
  Peritonitis (e.g. perforated viscus, appendicitis)
  Inflammatory bowel disease
  Pelvic or intra-abdominal abscess
  Diverticular disease
Traumatic injury
  Blunt abdominal trauma
  Operative trauma (especially splenectomy)
'Hypercoagulable states'
  Neoplasms (e.g. pancreatic or colonic)
  Antithrombin III deficiency
  Protein C deficiency
  Protein S deficiency
  Dysfibrinogenaemia
  Plasminogen activator deficiency
  Myeloproliferative syndromes
  Sickle cell disease
  Pregnancy
  Oral contraceptive use
  Deep venous thrombosis
Other
  Volvulus
  Decompression sickness

Oral contraceptive-related MVT accounts for about 9% of females in our series and approximately 4% of our total study population. This finding was corroborated by Abdu et al.[6] who also reported a 5% incidence in their total study population. There was, however, an 18% incidence in the female population they reviewed. The differences in these two series possibly reflects the older population seen at our institution. In addition, there has been a spate of isolated case reports relating oral contraceptives to MVT, and these may skew the composition of cases reported in the literature reviews.

Chronic mesenteric ischaemia

The exact incidence of the chronic forms of MVDs is unknown, largely because there are no specific tests for these diseases.

Chronic mesenteric ischaemia usually presents in the sixth or seventh decade in patients with signs of advanced atherosclerotic vascular disease. There is a 3:1 female predominance.

Although the majority of patients with MVT present acutely, up to one-third will present with symptoms of more than 1 month's duration.[7] The therapy remains the same as for the acute presentation, although the diagnosis is more obscure.

MESENTERIC CIRCULATION AND PATHOPHYSIOLOGY OF MESENTERIC VASOCONSTRICTION

The intestines are protected from ischaemia by their abundant collateral circulation. Communications between the coeliac, superior mesenteric and inferior mesenteric vascular beds are numerous, and it has become axiomatic over the years that at least two of these vessels must become compromised to produce symptomatic chronic intestinal ischaemia.

Collateral flow around occlusions of smaller arterial branches in the mesentery of the small intestine and right colon is made possible by the branching primary, secondary and tertiary arcades. Within the bowel wall there is a network of communicating submucosal vessels that can maintain the viability of short segments of intestine where the extramural arterial supply has been compromised.

Collateral pathways open immediately upon occlusion of a major vessel in response to arterial hypotension distal to the obstruction. Increased blood flow through the collateral pathways continues as long as the pressure in the vascular bed distal to the obstruction remains below systemic pressure. If, however, vasoconstriction develops in the distal arterial bed, the arterial pressure rises due to increased resistance, which ultimately impairs collateral flow to the dependent segment.

Despite adequate collateral vasculature in most cases, acute interruption or diminution of blood flow in the mesenteric circulation caused by emboli or hypotension results in intestinal ischaemia secondary to persistent vasospasm. A decrease in SMA flow initially produces local mesenteric vascular responses that tend to maintain intestinal blood flow, but if the diminished flow is prolonged, active vasoconstriction develops and may persist even after the primary cause of decreased flow is corrected. We[8] have shown that following an acute 50% reduction in SMA blood flow in anaesthetized dogs, the mesenteric arterial pressure (MesAP) in the peripheral mesenteric arteries falls to 49% of mean control values. When the SMA flow is maintained at 50% of normal, the MesAP returns to control values in 1–6 hours, while the coeliac flow, which had initially increased, falls to control levels. The increased vascular resistance caused by vasoconstriction ultimately results in decreased collateral perfusion from the coeliac and inferior mesenteric systems. If the flow restrictor is removed from the SMA as soon as the MesAP rises to control values, the flow through the SMA also returns to normal. However, if the SMA occlusion is maintained for 30–240 minutes after the MesAP has returned to control levels, the flow in the SMA never returns to normal. It remains at 30–50% of control because of persistent arterial vasoconstriction despite the removal of the

SMA flow restrictor. This decreased flow continues for up to 5 hours of observation but can be corrected by direct infusion of papaverine into the SMA. In this manner, mesenteric vasoconstriction plays a significant role in the development of ischaemia both in the acute occlusive and non-occlusive arterial forms of mesenteric ischaemia.

When papaverine is infused during the 50% flow restriction, the MesAP remains low throughout 4 hours of observation and the SMA flow returns to normal upon release of the obstruction. Based on these observations, the use of intra-arterial papaverine infusions is recommended in the management of both the occlusive and non-occlusive forms of AMI. Intra-arterial papaverine is also recommended for some patients with the venous forms of MVDs, because venous thrombosis has been shown, experimentally, to cause arterial spasm.[9]

In NOMI it had been presumed that the bowel injury occurs during the period of diminished cardiac output or hypotension, and that with correction of these cardiovascular problems the mesenteric blood flow returns to normal. This simplistic concept is contradicted by operative findings of persistent bowel ischaemia when no arterial or venous obstruction is found and cardiac function has been optimized. It is known that in patients with NOMI the onset of abdominal signs and symptoms caused by intestinal ischaemia may actually begin after the correction of the primary systemic problem. This paradox can be explained by the experimental observations that an episode of low mesenteric flow, as short as 2 hours in duration, can produce mesenteric ischaemia as a result of vasoconstriction, and that the vasoconstriction and ischaemia may continue after correction of the initiating problem.

The end-result of an ischaemic episode depends on many factors. Thus the extent of intestinal injury is a function of the:

1. State of the systemic circulation;
2. Degree of functional or anatomical compromise;
3. Number and calibre of vessels affected;
4. Response of the vascular bed to diminished perfusion;
5. Nature and capacity of the collateral circulation to supply the needs of the dependent segment of bowel;
6. Duration of the insult;
7. Metabolic needs of the dependent segment as dictated by its function and bacterial population.

TREATMENT OF SPECIFIC MESENTERIC VASCULAR DISEASES

Arterial forms of acute mesenteric ischaemia

Clinical aspects

Early identification of AMI requires a high index of suspicion by the clinician in those patients who have significant risk factors associated with this disease. AMI occurs most frequently in patients over 50 years of age who have chronic heart disease and long-standing congestive heart failure, especially those poorly controlled with diuretics or digitalis. Cardiac arrhythmias, commonly atrial fibrillation, recent myocardial infarction or hypotension due to burns, pancreatitis or haemorrhage all predispose the patient to AMI. Previous or synchronous arterial emboli increase the likelihood of an acute SMAE. The development of sudden abdominal pain in a patient with any or all of these risk factors should suggest the diagnosis of AMI.

A history of abdominal pain, often after meals, for weeks to months before the onset of an acute episode has been considered a frequent finding in patients with AMI. This misconception was based on reports by Dunphy[10] in 1936 and again by Mavor et al.[11] in 1962, who found that 50% of patients with AMI had antecedent abdominal symptoms. The prodromal abdominal pain occurred, however, only in patients with acute SMAT superimposed on chronic mesenteric ischaemia – the cause of AMI in less than 25% of patients. Thus a history of postprandial abdominal pain in the weeks to months preceding the acute onset of severe abdominal pain occurs in only a small fraction of patients with AMI.

Acute abdominal pain varying in severity, nature and location occurs in 75–98% of patients with intestinal ischaemia. Characteristically, in early AMI the pain experienced by the patient is markedly out of proportion to the physical findings. Therefore, sudden severe abdominal pain accompanied by rapid and often forceful bowel evacuation, especially with minimal or no abdominal signs, strongly suggests an acute arterial occlusion in the mesenteric circulation.

Unexplained abdominal distension or gastrointestinal bleeding may be the only indications of acute intestinal ischaemia, especially in non-occlusive disease, since pain is absent in up to 25% of these patients. Patients surviving cardiopulmonary resuscitation who develop culture-proven bacteraemia and diarrhoea without abdominal pain should be suspected of having NOMI.[12] Distension, while absent early in the course of mesenteric ischaemia, is often the first sign of impending intestinal infarction. The stool contains occult blood in 75% of patients, and this bleeding may precede any other symptom of ischaemia. Right-sided abdominal pain associated with the passage of maroon or bright-red blood in the stool, though characteristic of colonic ischaemia, also suggests the diagnosis of AMI.

Although there are no abdominal findings early in the course of intestinal ischaemia, as infarction develops, increasing tenderness, rebound tenderness and muscle guarding reflect the progressive loss of intestinal viability and the presence of transmural gangrene. Marked abdominal findings strongly indicate the presence of infarcted bowel. Nausea, vomiting, haematochezia, haematemesis, massive abdominal distension, back pain and shock are other late signs.

Diagnosis

Leucocytosis exceeding 15 000 cells/mm^3 occurs in approximately 75% of patients with AMI, whereas about 50% will present with a metabolic acidaemia. Elevations of serum amylase and phosphate as well as peritoneal fluid intestinal alkaline phosphatase and inorganic phosphate have been described, but the sensitivity and specificity of these markers of intestinal ischaemia have not been established. Leucocytosis out of proportion to the clinical findings, an elevated haemoglobin and haematocrit and blood-tinged peritoneal fluid, often with an elevated amylase content are not specific for AMI but suggest advanced intestinal necrosis and sepsis.

Plain abdominal radiographs are usually normal in early mesenteric ischaemia, before infarction occurs. Late in the course of the disease, formless loops of small intestine or small intestinal 'thumbprinting' can suggest the diagnosis of AMI. Less commonly, isolated 'thumbprinting' of the right colon may be the only indication of AMI. Even if colonoscopy reveals the haemorrhagic bullae characteristic of colonic ischaemia, the finding of colonic ischaemia confined to the right colon may be the result of disease in the main SMA rather than simply interference of colonic blood flow.

Several interesting techniques utilizing radioisotopic scintigraphy[13,14] have been developed in animal models to detect intestinal ischaemia, but have yet to prove reliable in clinical practice. ^{99m}Tc-pyrophosphate or diphosphate and ^{99m}Tc-sulphur colloid labelled leucocytes are the most promising techniques. These and other materials are undergoing clinical trials.

Another experimental modality for the detection of mesenteric ischaemia is ^{31}P magnetic resonance spectroscopy using surface coils.[15,16] In rodent systems, occlusion of either the superior mesenteric artery or vein resulted in pathologically confirmed transmural bowel ischaemia which was detected non-invasively with magnetic resonance spectroscopy. This method has not been sufficiently refined to detect early ischaemia that remains confined to the muscosa.

Laparoscopy[17] may be useful in patients whose clinical status precludes angiography. SMA blood flow decreases profoundly, however, with intraperitoneal pressures exceeding 20 mmHg, making laparoscopy potentially dangerous in the setting of suspected AMI.[18] Lower intraperitoneal pressures for brief periods produce only minimal alterations in mesenteric perfusion. Laparoscopic examination of the bowel is limited to the serosal surface, making it unreliable for diagnosing early mucosal necrosis at a time when the serosa still appears relatively normal.

Duplex scanning has been of some value in identifying portal and superior mesenteric venous thrombosis, and, in a few patients, SMA occlusion. The flow in the SMA can be reproducibly determined by this method, but the wide range of normal SMA blood flow from 300 to 600 ml/min[19] limits the value of this test in diagnosing ischaemia. As the capabilities of this modality improve and clinical trials determine its sensitivity and specificity, it may become a reliable screening method for the detection of the occlusive forms of AMI. Computerized tomography (CT) has also been used to identify arterial and venous thromboses as well as ischaemic bowel, but only in the late stages of the disease.

Historically, angiography was limited to identifying arterial occlusions by embolus or thrombosis. Currently, selective angiography is the mainstay of both the diagnosis and initial treatment of AMI[20] (see also Chapter 45). Based on experimental and retrospective studies of patients undergoing abdominal angiography, Siegelman et al.[21] identified four reliable angiographic criteria for the diagnosis of mesenteric vasoconstriction (Figure 55.5):

1. Narrowing of the origins of multiple branches of the SMA.
2. Irregularities in the intestinal branches.
3. Spasm of the arcades.
4. Impaired filling of intramural vessels.

While mesenteric vasoconstriction occurs in hypotensive patients and in those with pancreatitis, its presence in patients with suspected intestinal ischaemia who are not in shock, do not have pancreatitis and are not receiving vasopressors is diagnostic of NOMI. Therefore, if angiography is performed sufficiently early in the disease, patients with occlusive and non-occlusive AMI can be identified before bowel infarction develops, and before clinical and radiological signs of infarction make the diagnosis of intestinal ischaemia evident.

General principles of management

Patients over 50 years of age with any of the previously enumerated risk factors for AMI, who develop the sudden onset of abdominal pain severe enough to call it to the attention of a physician and which lasts for more than 2 hours, should be suspected of having AMI. These patients should be managed according to an aggressive radiological and surgical algorithm (Figures 52.6 and 52.7). Less absolute indications for inclusion into this protocol include unexplained abdominal distension, colonoscopic evidence of isolated right-sided colonic ischaemia or acidosis without an identifiable cause. Because the presence of diagnostic clinical or radiological signs usually indicates irreversible intestinal injury, broad selection criteria are essential if early diagnosis and successful treatment are to be achieved. Some negative studies must be accepted in order to identify and salvage patients who do have AMI.

Preoperative management Initial treatment is directed towards both resuscitation and correction of the predisposing or precipitating causes of the ischaemia. Relief of acute congestive heart failure and correction of hypotension, hypovolaemia and cardiac arrhythmias must precede any diagnostic evaluation. Efforts to improve mesenteric blood flow will be futile if low cardiac output, hypovolaemia or hypotension persist. Frequently, these patients are septic with low systemic vascular resistence and sequestration of fluid into the 'third space'. Optimal cardiac performance can best be achieved under these circumstances with the aid of a Swan–Ganz

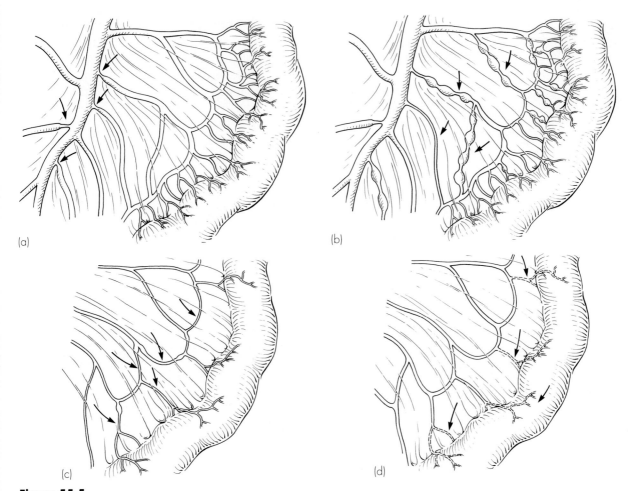

Figure 55.5
Angiographic criteria of acute mesenteric ischaemia: (a) narrowing of multiple branches; (b) alternate spasm and dilatation of intestinal branches (string of sausages sign); (c) spasm of arcade; (d) impaired filling of intramural vessels.

catheter, using serial cardiac profiles to insure maximal systemic perfusion. After resuscitation is accomplished, plain radiographs of the abdomen are obtained. These are taken not to establish the diagnosis of AMI but rather to exclude other identifiable causes of abdominal pain, e.g. a perforated viscus with free intraperitoneal air. A normal plain radiograph does not exclude AMI; indeed, ideally patients will be stud-

ied before radiological signs are present, as such findings indicate the presence of infarcted bowel. If no alternative diagnosis is made on the basis of the plain abdominal radiographs, selective SMA angiography is performed immediately. Based on the angiographic findings and the presence or absence of peritoneal signs, the patient is treated according to the algorithm in Figure 55.6.

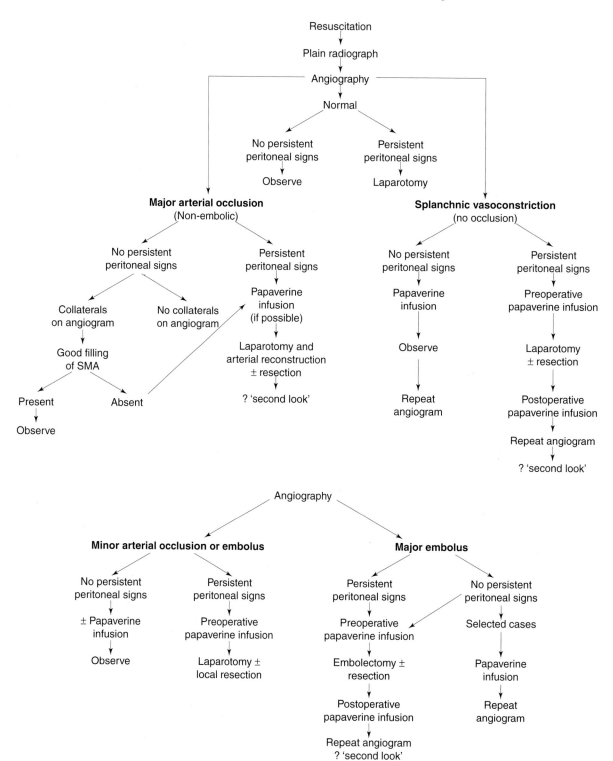

Figure 55.6
Diagnosis and treatment of acute mesenteric ischaemia. SMA, superior mesenteric artery.

Even when the decision to operate has been made based on clinical grounds, a preoperative angiogram should be obtained to manage the patient properly at laparotomy. Moreover, relief of mesenteric vasoconstriction is essential for proper treatment of emboli and thromboses as well as the non-occlusive 'low-flow' states. Intra-arterial infusion of papaverine through an angiography catheter placed percutaneously in the origin of the SMA is the best method of relieving mesenteric vasoconstriction pre- and post-operatively. It is infused at a constant rate of 30–60 mg/h using an infusion pump. Although almost all of the papaverine infused into the mesenteric circulation is cleared during one passage through the liver, in some cases this dose may have systemic effects; therefore, the systemic arterial pressure and cardiac rate and rhythm must be monitored constantly during the papaverine infusion. The clinical and angiographic responses of the patient to the vasodilator therapy determines the duration of the papaverine infusion.

Management at laparotomy Laparotomy is indicated in AMI to restore intestinal arterial flow after an embolus or thrombosis and/or to resect irreparably damaged bowel. Revascularization should precede evaluation of intestinal viability because bowel that initially appears infarcted may show surprising recovery after restoration of adequate blood flow.

After revascularization, intestinal viability can be assessed by several methods. Traditionally, the bowel is placed in warm, saline-soaked laparotomy pads and observed over a period of 10–20 minutes for return of normal colour, peristalsis and the presence or absence of pulsations in the intestinal arteries. This clinical assessment is of limited accuracy, however, and a more sensitive and specific evaluation depends on technological aids. Techniques that have been proposed include surface fluorescence,[22] perfusion fluorimetry,[23] Doppler measurements of arterial flow,[24] electromyography,[25] surface temperature, serosal pH, surface oxygen consumption and radioisotope uptake determinations. Only Doppler pulse determinations, fluorescence using an ultraviolet light after an intravenous injection of fluorescein and perfusion fluorimetry have gained wide clinical acceptance. Surface fluorescence increases the accuracy of differentiating viable from non-viable bowel, the equipment is inexpensive and the dye is safe, but the technique remains subjective. Perfusion fluorimetry is more objective, allows repeated estimations and is more accurate, in general, than surface fluorescence; However, the equipment is expensive and only small areas of the bowel can be evaluated at one time. Although Doppler probes are available in most operating rooms, this modality is again limited to examining small areas of the intestine. A practical solution is the initial use of surface fluorescence, with either perfusion fluorimetry or Doppler examination reserved for evaluation of the equivocal areas when diffuse patchy involvement is seen, or at the margins of unresected bowel.

Short segments of bowel that are non-viable or questionably viable after revascularization are resected and a primary anastomosis is performed. If extensive portions of the bowel are involved, only the clearly necrotic bowel is resected, and a planned re-exploration (second look) is performed within 12–24 hours. The ends of the questionable bowel can simply be closed or a double ostomy performed. The decision to perform a second-look operation is made during the initial laparotomy if major portions or multiple segments of intestine are of questionable viability, and the second-look laparotomy must be carried out irrespective of the patient's subsequent clinical course. The purpose of the second-look laparotomy, as proposed by Shaw,[26] is 'not just to allow a clear definition between dead and live bowel to take place, but also to allow time for the institution of supportive measures which may render more of the bowel viable'. Such measures may include, among others, optimizing cardiac output, SMA infusion of papaverine, antibiotic therapy and anticoagulant therapy.

If, at laparotomy, there is obvious infarction of all or most of the small bowel, with or without a portion of the right colon, then the surgeon is faced with a philosophical decision about whether to do anything at all. Resection of all of the involved bowel will inevitably produce a patient with short bowel syndrome with its attendant problems (Chapter 46) and, almost certainly in these older patients, a commitment to life-long parenteral nutrition. A preoperative discussion with the patient and the patient's family concerning this problem is warranted, so that an acceptable decision can be reached if this situation is encountered at operation.

Postoperative management The use of anticoagulants in the management of AMI remains controversial. Heparin anticoagulation may cause intestinal, submucosal or intraperitoneal haemorrhage and, except in the case of MVT, we have not used it in the immediate postoperative period. Late thrombosis following embolectomy of arterial reconstruction, however, occurs frequently enough that anticoagulation 48 hours postoperatively seems advisable. Some authors have advocated immediate anticoagulation in all patients, or especially when a second look is required.

Both systemic and locally administered antibiotics have been shown to improve the survival of ischaemic bowel.[27] For this reason, and because of the high incidence of positive blood cultures in patients with AMI, broad-spectrum systemic antibiotics are begun as soon as the diagnosis is entertained and are continued throughout the postoperative period as dictated by the findings at laparotomy.

Management of specific types

Superior mesenteric artery embolus Upon identification of an SMAE at angiography, a papaverine infusion is begun through the catheter placed selectively in the origin of the SMA, proximal to the occlusion. The patient is then managed according to the algorithm in Figure 55.6, based on the site of the embolus, the presence or absence of peritoneal signs, the extent of the collateral blood flow and the degree of vasospasm in the vascular beds both proximal and distal to the embolus, as determined by an angiogram repeated following a selective intra-arterial bolus injection of 25 mg tolazoline.

Minor emboli are those limited to the branches of the SMA or to the SMA distal to the origin of the ileocolic artery (see Figure 55.3). Patients with minor emboli whose pain is relieved by the vasodilator therapy can be managed expectantly. However, patients with major emboli selected for non-operative therapy must fulfil certain criteria. They must have: (1) a major contraindication to operation; (2) no peritoneal signs; and (3) adequate perfusion of the vascular beds distal to the embolus following the introduction of a bolus of a vasodilator into the SMA. Direct infusion of thrombolytic agents through selectively placed catheters has been employed successfully by others in a few patients, but this approach must still be considered experimental.

Embolectomy is always performed before assessing intestinal viability. The embolus is approached directly or, less optimally, through a proximal arteriotomy (Figure 55.7). The proximal SMA is exposed by drawing the transverse colon cephalad and anteriorly, as the small intestine is retracted inferiorly. The inferior leaf of the transverse mesocolon is incised and the proximal SMA is dissected free between the pancreas and the fourth portion of the duodenum. The SMA is exposed for 2–3 cm proximal and distal to the origin of the middle colic artery. The SMA is palpated gently to determine the most distal extent of arterial pulsation, or the artery may be examined directly with a Doppler probe to identify the site of the embolus. Once the site of the embolus is found, the SMA and its branches are controlled proximally and distally with vessel loops or gentle vascular clamps. A longitudinal arteriotomy is made over the embolus or just proximal to it, and the embolus is removed and residual clots are flushed out of the artery by briefly releasing the vessel loops. A Fogarty balloon catheter is then passed proximally and distally to remove all remaining

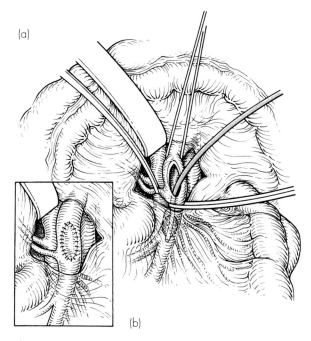

(a)

(b)

Figure 55.7

Technique of superior mesenteric artery (SMA) embolectomy: (a) The artery at the site of the embolus is identified at the base of the transverse mesocolon; a longitudinal arteriotomy is made and the vessel is cleared of debris; (b) The arteriotomy is closed primarily or with a vein patch (shown).

clots. The arteriotomy is closed with or without a vein patch.

After embolectomy, bowel viability is determined. If no second look is planned, the papaverine infusion is continued for an additional 12–24 hours. An arteriogram is then obtained to exclude persistent vasospasm before the arterial catheter is removed (Figure 55.9). If a second look is performed, the infusion is continued through the second procedure and until no vasoconstriction is present on a follow-up angiogram.

Non-occlusive mesenteric ischaemia NOMI is diagnosed when the angiographic signs of mesenteric vasoconstriction are seen in a patient who has the clinical picture of mesenteric ischaemia and is neither in shock nor receiving vasopressors. The angiographic findings may vary from the previously described local signs to a pruned appearance of the entire mesenteric vasculature (Figure 55.8). A selective SMA infusion of papaverine is begun in all patients with NOMI as soon as the diagnosis is made. In patients with persistent peritoneal signs the infusion is continued during and after exploration. At operation, manipulation of the SMA is minimized. Overtly necrotic bowel is resected, and a primary anastomosis is performed only if no second look is planned. We believe it is better to leave bowel of questionable viability than to perform a massive enterectomy, because frequently the bowel will improve with supportive measures or demarcate more clearly by the time of the second look.

When a papaverine infusion is used as the primary treatment for NOMI it is continued for approximately 24 hours, after which the infusion is changed to normal saline for 30 minutes prior to a repeat angiogram. Based on the clinical course of the patient and the presence or absence of vasoconstriction on the repeat angiogram, the infusion is either discontinued or maintained for an additional 24 hours. Angiography is repeated daily until there is no radiographic evidence of vasoconstriction (Figure 55.8) and the patient's clinical symptoms and signs are gone. Infusions have usually been discontinued after 24 hours, but have been maintained for as long as 5 days.

When papaverine is used in conjunction with surgery for non-occlusive disease, a second-look operation is frequently necessary. In such cases, the infusion is continued as previously described for second-look operations following embolectomy. The arterial catheter is removed when no angiographic signs of vasoconstriction are seen 30 minutes after cessation of vasodilator therapy.

Acute superior mesenteric artery thrombosis SMAT is most often identified on a flush aortogram showing complete occlusion of the SMA within 1–2 cm of its origin. Some filling of the SMA distal to the obstruction via collateral pathways is almost always present. Branches both proximal and distal to the obstruction may show local spasm or diffuse vasoconstriction. Differentiation between thrombosis and an embolus can be difficult, and in such cases the patients are treated initially for SMAE. A more difficult problem arises in patients with abdominal pain without abdominal signs and complete occlusion of the SMA on aortogram. In these cases it is important to differentiate between an acute and a long-standing occlusion, as the

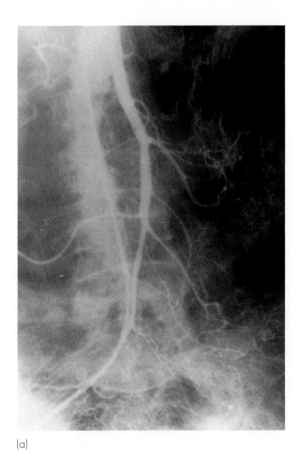

(a)

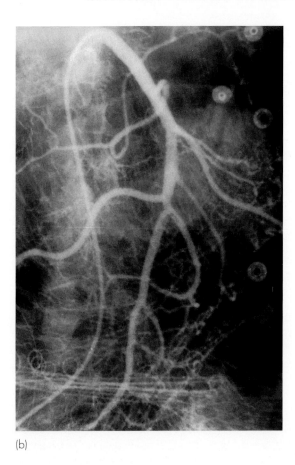

(b)

Figure 55.8

Patient with non-occlusive mesenteric ischaemia managed with papaverine for 3 days. (a) Initial angiogram showing spasm of the main superior mesenteric artery, origins of the branches and the intestinal arcades. (b) Angiogram after 36 hours of papaverine infusion. The study was obtained 30 minutes after papaverine was replaced with saline. At this time the patient's abdominal symptoms had resolved. (Reproduced with permission from Boley SJ, Brandt LJ & Veith FJ. *Curr Probl Surg* 1978).

latter may be coincidental to an unrelated presenting illness. Prominent collateral vessels between the superior mesenteric and the coeliac and/or inferior mesenteric circulations are characteristic of chronic SMA occlusion. If large collaterals are present and there is good filling of the SMA on the late films during the angiogram, the occlusion can be considered to be chronic and the abdominal pain is probably unrelated to MVD. In the absence of peritoneal signs, such patients are treated expectantly. The absence of collateral vessels or the presence of collaterals with inadequate filling of the SMA indicates an acute occlusion. In the latter instance the middle colic artery is probably occluded, interrupting the collateral circulation to an already marginal system. Prompt intervention is indicated irrespective of the abdominal findings in these cases.

An angiographic catheter is placed in the proximal SMA and a papaverine infusion is begun. If the origin of the SMA cannot be identified or cannulated at angiography, a small Silastic catheter should be advanced proximally into the SMA through a jejunal artery at the time of operative revascularization to treat the associated vasospasm. This catheter is brought out through a separate incision in the abdominal wall and is used for postoperative papaverine infusion.

Revascularization procedures for SMAT are similar to those used for chronic mesenteric ischaemia, in which thrombectomy

and endarterectomy or some form of bypass graft to the SMA distal to the obstruction are employed. Although a short graft from the aorta to the SMA is the simplest procedure, extensive aortic atherosclerotic disease often precludes this option. The internal or external iliac artery may be the best source of inflow in these cases. Although autologous reversed saphenous vein is the preferred conduit, polytetrafluoroethylene (PTFE) has been used successfully, even in the presence of peritoneal contamination. Percutaneous balloon and laser angioplasty of the SMA also have been reported.[28] Because there is presently no good method to monitor end-organ injury and because of the danger of rethrombosis with irreparable bowel loss (as was the case with one of our patients), we do not recommend these techniques for acute SMA occlusions.

Results of therapy

Traditional methods of managing AMI,[29,30] have resulted in mortality rates between 70 and 90%. Using the aggressive approach outlined above, this catastrophic mortality has been substantially reduced. Overall, 50% or more of the patients presenting with AMI and treated according to the present algorithm survive, and approximately 70–90% lose less than a metre of intestine.[31,32]

Venous forms of acute mesenteric ischemia

Clinical aspects

MVT has long been known as the 'great imitator' of other abdominal disorders. These varied presentations contribute to the infrequency of a correct preoperative diagnosis. As can be seen in Table 55.2, the symptoms reported in patients with MVT are non-specific. Except for abdominal pain, which is present in more than 90% of patients, no clinical symptom would clearly point to the diagnosis of MVT. Moreover, even the nature, severity and location of the pain can vary widely. In our series, the two patients without abdominal pain developed MVT in the postoperative period.

Table 55.2 Symptoms associated with mesenteric venous thrombosis

SYMPTOM	%
Abdominal pain	91
Vomiting	71
Nausea	66
Diarrhoea	35
Constipation	28
Haematochezia	14
Haematemesis	8

The mean duration of pain before admission is more than 5 days. Survivors in our series tend to have a longer interval before admission than do those patients with a fatal outcome (6 versus 4.4 days). This unexpected finding can be explained by the possibility that patients with a more indolent course have less extensive bowel infarction and, hence, a better prognosis.

Other prominent symptoms include nausea and vomiting, which occur in more than half of the patients. Bloody diarrhoea in up to 15% of patients and haematemesis in 13% are indications of bowel infarction and are non-specific for MVT. The presence of haematemesis, however, should alert the physician to the possibility of a mesenteric ischaemic catastrophe. Half the patients have occult blood in their stool.

Although almost all patients present with abdominal tenderness (Table 55.3), the remainder of the physical examination varies greatly. Most have decreased bowel sounds and abdominal distension, but only two-thirds manifest clear signs of peri-

Table 55.3 Physical findings in mesenteric venous thrombosis

FINDING	%
Abdominal tenderness	97
Abdominal distension	80
Decreased bowel sounds	77
Guarding/rebound	53
Stool positive for blood	54
Temperature >38°C	47
Blood pressure <90 mmHg systolic	23

tonitis. The majority have temperatures greater than 38°C, but only one-quarter of patients present with clinical signs of septic shock.

Laboratory studies for the diagnosis of all forms of intestinal ischaemia have proved to have a low sensitivity and low specificity. Numerous serum markers have been described, but none has been shown to be of great clinical value. In our series of 22 patients with MVT, only an elevated white blood count of 12 000 or more and an increased proportion of polymorphonuclear cells were present in the majority of patients. At present, laboratory studies can support – but not confirm or exclude – the diagnosis of intestinal ischaemia.

Diagnosis

The absence of any reliable specific symptoms, signs or laboratory studies in patients with MVT makes the diagnosis very difficult. Moreover, the variability in the course of the disease further obscures the diagnosis: some patients have an indolent course of days to weeks and others have a relatively acute onset and progressive course. In the past, radiographic studies were the only helpful preoperative tests. However, plain radiographs of the abdomen, when abnormal, always reflect the presence of infarcted bowel. In our series fewer than 25% of plain radiographic studies suggested the presence of some form of AMI, 25% were normal and 50% showed a non-specific ileus pattern. Barium enemas are usually of little value because the colon is rarely involved. An upper gastrointestinal tract contrast study can demonstrate some 'thumbprinting' of the proximal bowel, supporting the diagnosis of acute intestinal ischaemia.

More recently, special radiological studies such as selective mesenteric angiography and CT,[31,33] have established the diagnosis of MVT preoperatively (see also Chapter 45). In our experience, selective mesenteric angiography, when performed preoperatively established the diagnosis in most cases, and in the remainder the diagnosis of some form of mesenteric ischaemia was made. Angiography may reveal a thrombus within the vein, with partial or complete occlusion of the superior mesenteric vein and reconstitution of the portal system closer to the liver. Another angiographic finding suggesting MVT is the failure of the arterial arcades supplying a portion of the bowel to empty even during the venous phase of the study. CT may show a thrombus in the superior mesenteric vein (Figure 55.9) itself or a thickening of the wall of the small bowel, with perhaps the presence of ascites, suggesting a diagnosis of intestinal ischaemia.

Other diagnostic modalities that have been used in a small number of patients include echography, duplex scanning and magnetic resonance imaging. Ultrasonography (Figure 55.10), magnetic resonance imaging and CT can demonstrate thrombus within the superior mesenteric vein. Doppler ultrasonography can demonstrate the length of the superior mesenteric vein that is occluded as well as show reconstitution of the portal flow above the thrombus. Perhaps the most important contribution of these newer and non-invasive diagnostic studies is the ability to recognize patients with MVT who have chronic

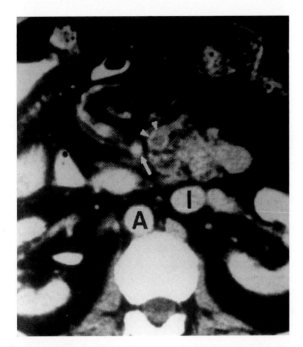

Figure 55.9
Thrombosis of superior messenteric vein (arrowheads) as seen on CT. Arrow, superior mesenteric artery; A, aorta; I, inferior vena cava. (Reproduced with permission from Rosen A, Korobkin M, Silverman PM et al. *AJR* 1984; **143**: 83.)

symptomatology. As these diagnostic modalities become more refined, the diagnosis of MVT may increase substantially. Gastroscopy and colonoscopy are of little value in MVT. Laparoscopy has been successful in a small number of patients.[17] Evaluation of the proximal jejunum with a long endoscope has established the diagnosis in a few cases.[32]

The correct diagnosis of MVT is usually made at laparotomy. The diagnosis has been made preoperatively in only 5–10% of reported patients. However, 30–40% of patients had the diagnosis of some form of AMI before operation.

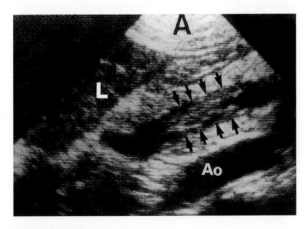

Figure 55.10
Longitudinal ultrasonographic section obtained on admission shows thrombus (arrows) in the distended superior mesenteric vein. A, abdominal wall; Ao, aorta; L, liver. (Reproduced with permission from Kidambi H, Herbert R & Kidami AV. *JCU* 1986; **14**: 199

Increasing the ability to diagnose MVT earlier requires a high index of suspicion and a rapid and aggressive work-up of the patient. In all patients suspected of having MVT, the same protocol used for all other forms of acute mesenteric ischaemia is initiated. This protocol calls first for prompt resuscitation. A plain X-ray of the abdomen is then performed to exclude other causes of abdominal pain. If no other cause is found, selective SMA angiography is performed. Depending upon the angiographic findings and the presence or absence of peritoneal signs the patients is treated according to the algorithm for MVT (Figure 5.11).

Management

When MVT is suspected or diagnosed on angiography, CT, ultrasonography or magnetic resonance imaging, prompt laparotomy is indicated. In the past, therapy was limited to resection of infarcted bowel and possibly the immediate institution of anticoagulant therapy with intravenous heparin. In several studies, including our own, a clear benefit of the immediate use of heparin was demonstrated. Anticoagulated patients had recurrence or progression of the disease in only 13% and a similar mortality rate of 13%, as compared with a 20–25% recurrence rate and a 50% mortality rate in those who did not receive postoperative heparin.

Other therapeutic options are mesenteric venous thrombectomy, which has been used successfully in a few reported cases. Intra-arterial papaverine infused through the catheter placed angiographically into the SMA has also been successful. The limited experience with these latter two modalities makes it impossible to recommend their use wide use in the treatment of MVT.

A logical application of the information available would suggest the following approach. If at operation a short segment of ischaemic bowel is found, then local resection followed by prompt heparinization should be performed (Figure 55.11). At the opposite end of the spectrum, if at operation there is obvious infarction of all or most of the small bowel with or

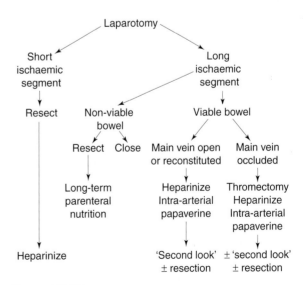

Figure 55.11
Treatment of mesenteric venous thrombosis.

without a portion of the right colon, then one is faced with a philosophical dilemma of whether to do anything at all. Resection of all the involved bowel will produce a short bowel syndrome and a requirement for life-long parenteral nutrition. In such a situation it would appear that the possibility should be discussed with the patient before operation, or with the family when the abdomen is opened, and an acceptable decision may then be reached.

The more difficult problem comes when one finds extensively involved bowel which is of questionable viability. In such situations the angiographic findings may be essential to make a reasonable decision as to how to proceed. If the angiogram demonstrates that the major vein is open or reconstituted, indicating that blood is flowing through the vein or around the obstruction, then a second-look operation should be performed 12–18 hours later, utilizing the intervening time to improve circulation with papaverine infused into the SMA. In one instance where this situation was noted upon opening the abdomen, the surgeon found almost all of the small bowel to be blue, but at a second look 18 hours later, after infusing papaverine and starting heparin therapy, the entire small bowel was pink and viable. The basis for this vasodilator therapy is that MVT has been shown experimentally to be associated with arterial spasm, which contributes to the ischaemia. Relief of the arterial vasoconstriction may improve the blood supply sufficiently to preserve viability.

If at laparotomy a long segment of questionable bowel is found and the angiogram or operative findings indicate complete thrombosis of the superior mesenteric vein at its junction with the portal vein, with or without extension into the portal vein, then venous thrombectomy is indicated. A second-look operation should be performed 18–24 hours after thrombectomy if the bowel is not clearly viable. Again, heparin therapy is promptly instituted. Intra-arterial papaverine may be beneficial if there appears to be arterial vasoconstriction after thrombectomy.

This approach to the management of the various surgical findings that one might encounter is aimed at salvaging the maximum length of bowel. Thrombectomy is not indicated when short segments of bowel are involved, nor is there any evidence that it is advantageous when venous flow is reconstituted around a thrombus.

Results of therapy and prognosis

The mortality rate of MVT is lower than that encountered in the other forms of AMI, varying from 32% in our series to approximately 50% in the literature. Our lower mortality rate may be a reflection of our aggressive approach to AMI. The overall recurrence rate has been about 20–25% but, as mentioned previously, after heparin therapy this falls to approximately 13%.

Almost all patients diagnosed with MVT have had some infarcted bowel. This was true in all patients in our own series. However, the amount of bowel resected was significantly less than in patients with arterial forms of AMI. The mean length of bowel resected in our series was 151 cm (range 43–450 cm).

There was no correlation between the length of involved bowel and the risk of death. Ninety-five per cent of our patients had segmental involvement of the jejunum and/or ileum, and 5% had involvement of the terminal ileum and right colon.

When compared with other forms of AMI, MVT occurs in younger patients, typically has a more indolent and non-specific course, involves shorter segments of bowel and has a lower mortality rate. In contradistinction to our recommended therapy in other forms of AMI, immediate anticoagulation is indicated for mesenteric venous thrombosis. Second-look operations are used, as in other forms of AMI, whenever portions of bowel of questionable viability are not resected at the primary operation.

The continuing difficulty in diagnosing MVT was graphically described by Anane-Sehaf and Blair[34] in the statement: 'Perhaps the best overall finding was an uneasy feeling on the part of the examining physician that his patient looks sick but that he could not say why or from what.'

Chronic mesenteric ischaemia

Clinical aspects

Chronic mesenteric ischaemia results from inadequate perfusion of the midgut during periods of increased oxygen demand. The oxygen requirements of the bowel increase significantly in the postprandial period owing to rises in motility, secretion and absorption, which are all energy-dependent functions of the bowel. Although experimental studies have shown increases in mesenteric blood flow after meals, vascular resistance also increases during peristalsis, impairing intramural perfusion. In the normal individual these changes in blood flow are well tolerated and lead to no untoward effects. However, in patients with impairment of mesenteric circulation resulting from atherosclerotic disease of the vessels feeding the intestines, the oxygen requirements often exceed the ability to meet these demands, and feeding causes cellular hypoxia. This hypoxic injury is manifested either by ischaemic visceral pain and/or abnormalities in gastrointestinal absorption or motility. The pain is similar to that arising in the myocardium with angina pectoris or in the calf with intermittent claudication.

Atherosclerotic involvement of the mesenteric vessels is almost always the cause of this form of intestinal ischaemia, but the various small vessel diseases, such as thromboangiitis obliterans (Buerger's disease) or polyarteritis nodosa, may also produce chronic intestinal ischaemia. Although partial or complete occlusion of the coeliac artery, the SMA or the inferior mesenteric artery is fairly common, relatively few patients have documented chronic intestinal ischaemia. Moreover, there are many patients with occlusion of two or even all three of these vessels who remain asymptomatic.

The one consistent feature of chronic mesenteric ischaemia is abdominal discomfort or pain. Most commonly this occurs 10–15 minutes after meals, gradually increasing in severity, finally reaching a plateau and then slowly dissipating over the course of 1–3 hours. The pain pattern is so intimately associated with eating that the patients reduce their food intake and have massive weight loss. Bloating, flatulence and derangements in motility with constipation or diarrhoea also occur.

The physical findings are rarely helpful, although the presence of an abdominal bruit has been reported in up to 75% of the patients. Occasionally the patient will have occult blood in the stool. Weight loss in the setting of occult faecal blood often leads to an evaluation for gastrointestinal malignancy.

Diagnosis

The failure to demonstrate a cause for postprandial abdominal pain associated with weight loss should strongly suggest chronic intestinal ischaemia. Up to now there has been no specific reliable diagnostic test for abdominal angina. Absorption studies have not been dependable, nor has indirect measurement of blood flow. However, we have employed an objective provocative test[33] for intestinal angina that might accurately identify patients requiring revascularization. The test is based upon experimental studies demonstrating that, in the presence of limited splanchnic arterial inflow, the intramural pH of the small intestine determined indirectly by a tonometer positioned in the jejunum, falls when a test meal is placed into the stomach. In our initial clinical trial the tonometer was introduced endoscopically, and a prompt fall in intramural pH accompanied by pain occurred with the test meal. After operative revascularization there was no change in intramural pH and no pain

when the test meal was given. If further trials demonstrate similar results, this test may enable us both to prove the presence of chronic mesenteric ischaemia and to evaluate the success of therapy. In the absence of an objective test the diagnosis has been based on the clinical symptoms, the arteriographic demonstration of occlusion of at least two of the splanchnic arteries and to a great degree on the exclusion of other gastrointestinal diseases.

Angiographic evaluation includes flush aortography in the frontal and lateral views and selective injections of the superior mesenteric, coeliac and inferior mesenteric arteries. The degree of occlusion of the three major arteries can best be assessed on the lateral projections, while the collateral circulation and patterns of flow are best evaluated on the frontal views (Figure 55.12). The presence of prominent collateral vessels not only indicates a significant stenosis of a major vessel but connotes a chronic process. Stenosis or occlusion of one or more of the major visceral vessels demonstrated on an angiogram does not by itself establish the diagnosis of arterial insufficiency.

In the absence of symptoms, occlusion even of all three major splanchnic arteries is not necessarily an indication for revascularization. There is one special case in which reconstruction or bypass of obstructed visceral arteries is recommended in the absence of abdominal pain. This occurs in patients who are undergoing aortic reconstructions for peripheral vascular disease, in whom aortography demonstrates

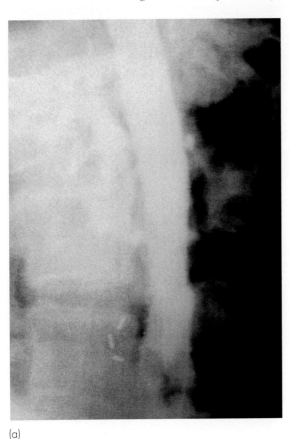

(a)

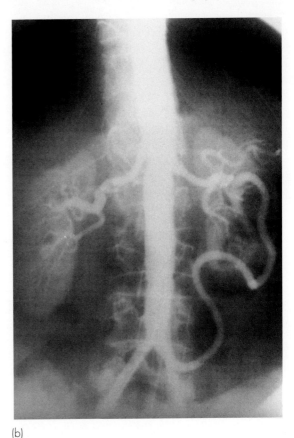

(b)

Figure 55.12
Chronic versus acute superior mesenteric artery occlusion: (a) lateral projection showing occlusion of major vessels;
(b) Chronic occlusion with large meandering vessel.

occlusive disease of the SMA or coeliac artery and the presence of a large 'meandering artery'.

In patients with intestinal angina, there is a real risk of acute occlusion of either a stenotic main artery or of the entrance of a major collateral inflow source into the mesenteric bed, e.g., acute thrombosis of the origin of the middle colic artery which provided collateral circulation to the SMA distribution from the inferior mesenteric artery via the 'meandering artery'. Hence, there is an urgency in identifying and treating patients suspected of having chronic mesenteric ischaemia.

Management

The previous difficulty in establishing an unequivocal diagnosis of chronic mesenteric ischaemia, the fragility of these elderly patients and the risks of a major operation for revascularization of the gut has made the selection of patients for operation a difficult matter. More recently, limited success with balloon angioplasty,[31] which can be performed with much less morbidity, has made it less critical to establish a definitive diagnosis before undertaking treatment.

With no available method for measuring intestinal blood flow accurately, precise criteria to define the need for operative arterial reconstruction are lacking. There is agreement that a patient with the typical pain of abdominal angina and unexplained weight loss, whose diagnostic evaluation has excluded other gastrointestinal diseases and whose angiogram shows occlusive involvement of at least two of the three major mesenteric arteries, should benefit from revascularization. The issue is less clear if only one major vessel is involved or if the clinical presentation is atypical. Until a quantitative test, such as we have described, is proved to be reliable, the patient with atypical symptoms should be observed. Revascularization is indicated in those patients whose pain and weight loss does not respond to other treatment and in whom balloon angioplasty is unsuccessful, even if only one vessel is occluded.

The patients suffering from chronic intestinal ischaemia are often severely malnourished and generally require a period of parenteral alimentation before revascularization. Serum albumin and prothrombin time should also be corrected. In addition, vitamin deficiencies may be apparent, and supplementation with parenteral folate, vitamin C, vitamin K, thiamine and B_{12} should be considered if they have lost more than 10% of their lean body weight.

Several procedures[32,35] have been advocated for restoring normal flows and pressures distal to an occlusion of the SMA or coeliac artery, including reimplantation, endarterectomy and bypass. Presently, the most commonly performed procedure is bypass to the SMA distal to the occlusion, although several surgeons believe that both the SMA and coeliac artery must be revascularized if they are both occluded.

Reimplantation Reimplantation is performed by transecting the artery distal to the occlusion and creating an anastomosis directly to the aorta. This procedure is technically difficult owing to the short length of available vessel and the presence of severe aortic atherosclerotic disease in the region of the origins of the coeliac and SMA trunks. It should be reserved for those situations in which the aorta is being replaced and the revascularization is undertaken prophylactically.

Endarterectomy (Figure 55.13) Endarterectomy has been attempted both through the diseased vessel and through the aorta itself. Both are technically difficult and can result in embolization of atheromatous fragments into the distal visceral and systemic circulation. The transarterial approach is usually unsuccessful because the most proximal extent of the occlusion is difficult to remove safely. The transaortic 'trapdoor'[36] endarterectomy requires cross-clamping the aorta in the supracoeliac position, which increases the possibility of ischaemic injury to the kidneys and distal circulation. Although this approach offers the theoretical advantage of clearing both the visceral and renal vessels and is completely autogenous, it is a much more major operation than a bypass operation.

Bypass (Figure 55.14) Mesenteric bypass from the aorta or the iliac artery to the side of the SMA distal to the occlusion is the procedure of choice. Reversed autologous saphenous vein is the preferred graft material if, after gentle distension, the vein is at least 5 mm in its smallest diameter. PTFE or knitted Dacron are suitable substitutes if the saphenous vein is unavailable or inadequate.

The optimal site of origin of the graft has been disputed. Because of the mobility of the SMA, grafts originating from the infrarenal aorta may be occluded with the movement of the mesentery of the small intestine. In addition, late failure due to progressive atherosclerotic disease of the infrarenal aorta has led some surgeons to use the supracoeliac aorta as the inflow for the graft. Occasionally the common, external or internal iliac arteries are the only non-calcified vessels, and we have successfully used these as the source of inflow.

Results

Patency rates with such bypass grafts to the SMA and coeliac artery have been generally good, and symptomatic relief in

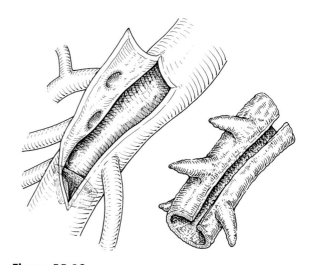

Figure 55.13

Combined visceral and renal endarterectomy with sleeve aortic endarterectomy.

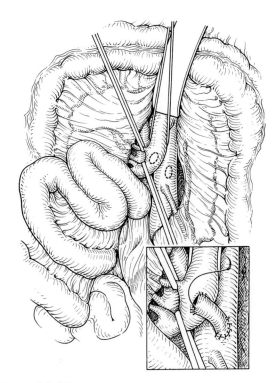

Figure 55.14
Technique of aorta-to-superior mesenteric artery (SMA) bypass. An incision in the retroperitoneum has been made over the aorta and carried superiorly to divide the ligament of Treitz. This provides exposure of the aorta and the SMA in the region of the middle colic artery. Sites of anastomoses are shown. Insert left shows the fine suture technique of anastomosis. Inset right shows completed bypass.

properly selected patients has been excellent. Stoney and associates[35] have recently reported poor results with retrograde bypasses. They attribute this finding to an unusual and rapidly progressive form of atherosclerosis that involves the subdiaphragmatic aorta and that occurs more commonly in females and in relatively young subjects. On the basis of their extensive experience, they advocate either an antegrade prosthetic bypass from the supracoeliac aorta via transabdominal approach or a thoracoabdominal retroperitoneal 'trapdoor' endarterectomy.

The future of this type of surgery will almost certainly be influenced by the application of tonometry balloon and possibly laser angioplasty as well as the newer thrombolytic agents.

Focal intestinal ischaemia

Ischaemic insults localized to short segments of the small intestine produce a broad spectrum of clinical features without the life-threatening systemic consequences associated with more extensive portions of the gut. The most frequent causes are atheromatous emboli, strangulated hernias, blunt abdominal trauma and segmental venous thrombosis. During the late 1960s enteric-coated thiazide – potassium chloride preparations were the most common cause (see also Chapter 52). Lesions associated with systemic diseases may occur late in the course

of the illness or may be the heralding event of the generalized disorder.

Pathophysiology

Focal intestinal ischeamia usually occurs in the presence of adequate collateral circulation to prevent transmural haemorrhagic infarction. Lesions are commonly infected infarcts resulting from partial necrosis of the bowel wall and secondary invasion by the intestinal bacterial flora. Limited tissue necrosis may result in complete healing, a chronic enteritis simulating Crohn's disease, or a stricture with partial or complete intestinal obstruction. Transmural necrosis with perforation or localized peritonitis may follow a severe local insult.

Clinical aspects

Patients with short segment ischaemic bowel injury present differently, depending on the severity of the infarct. In the acute presentation, seen with transmural necrosis, there is a sudden onset of abdominal pain that often simulates an acute appendicitis. These patients manifest clinical signs of peritonitis and sepsis. Another common presentation is that of chronic enteritis with crampy abdominal pain, diarrhoea, occasional fever and weight loss. This clinical picture may be indistinguishable from Crohn's disease of the small intestine (Chapter 50).

The most common presentation, however, is that of chronic small bowel obstruction, with or without a history of some antecedent episode of trauma, pain or hernia incarceration. Intermittent abdominal pain, distension and vomiting are the direct results of the obstruction, and bacterial overgrowth in the dilated loop proximal to the obstruction may lead to the metabolic and clinical derangements usually associated with the blind-loop syndrome, i.e. anaemia, diarrhoea and steatorrhoea. A preoperative diagnosis of focal ischaemia is difficult to make. A previous episode of transient pain, trauma, incarcerated hernia or a known systemic illness can suggest the correct diagnosis.

Diagnosis and management

The treatment of acute focal intestinal ischaemia is usually surgical, but some patients without signs of peritonitis can be managed expectantly. In those instances the diagnosis is based on the radiological findings of 'thumbprints' indicative of acute ischaemia. Serial studies should reveal a changing pattern. Both clinical and radiological findings must resolve or the nonoperative approach is abandoned.

Patients who present with chronic enteritis or obstruction should undergo exploration immediately upon diagnosis and after proper preparation. Awareness of these lesions of segmental ischaemia is essential because a limited resection is the procedure of choice for both focal enteritis and obstructing lesions.

REFERENCES

1. Cokkinis AJ. *Mesenteric Venous Occlusion*. London: Baillière Tindall, 1926.
2. Ende N. Infarction of the bowel in cardiac failure. *N Engl J Med* 1958; **258**: 879.

3. Jackson BB. Occlusion of the superior mesenteric artery. Monograph in *American Lectures in Surgery*. Springfield, IL: C C Thomas, 1963.

4. Wittenberg J, Athanasoulis CA, Shapiro JH & Williams LF. A radiological approach to the patient with acute extensive bowel ischemia. *Radiology* 1973; **106**: 13.

5. White R & Boley SJ. Mesenteric venous thrombosis (MVT): an unusual cause of acute mesenteric ischemia. Read before the *50th Annual Scientific Meeting of the American College of Gastroenterology*, 9–11 October 1985, Philadelphia.

6. Abdu RA, Zakhour BJ & Dalis DJ. Mesenteric venous thrombosis, 1911–1984. *Surgery* **101**: 383, 1987.

7. Font VE, Hermann RE & Longworth DL. Chronic mesenteric venous thrombosis: difficult diagnosis and therapy. *Cleve Clin J Med* 1989; **56**: 823.

8. Boley SJ, Regan JA, Tunick PA, Everhard ME, Winslow PR & Veith FJ. Persistent vasoconstriction – a major factor in nonocclusive mesenteric ischemia. *Curr Top Surg Res* **3**: 1971; 425.

9. Laufman H. *Significance of vasospasm in vascular occlusion.* Thesis, Northwestern University Medical School, Chicago, 1948.

10. Dunphy JE. Abdominal pain of vascular origin. *Am J Med Sci* 1936; **192**: 109.

11. Mavor GE, Lyall AD & Chrystal KMR & Tsapogasi M. Mesenteric infarction as a vascular emergency: the clinical problems. *Br J Surg* 1962; **50**: 219.

12. Gaussorgues P, Guerugniand PY, Vedrinne JM, Salord F, Mercatello A & Robert D. Bacteremia following cardiac arrest and cardiopulmonary resuscitation. *Intensive Care Med* 1988; **14**: 575.

13. Bardfeld PA, Boley SJ, Sammartano RJ & Bontemps R. Scientigraphic diagnosis of intestinal ischemia with technetium 99m sulfur colloid labelled leukocytes. *Radiology* 1977; **124**: 439.

14. Ortiz VN, Sfanianakis G, Haase GM & Boles ET. The value of radionuclide scanning in early diagnosis of intestinal infarction. *J Pediatr Surg* 1978; **13**: 616.

15. Blum H, Chance B & Buzby GP. In vivo noninvasive observation of acute mesenteric ischemia in rats. *Surg Gynecol Obstet* 1987; **164**: 409.

16. Kass DA, Banville DL, Gooding CA & James TL. ^{31}P magnetic resonance spectroscopy of mesenteric ischemia. *Magn Reson Med* 1987; **4**: 83.

17. Serreyn RF, Schoofs PR, Baetens PR & Vandekerckhove D. Laparoscopic diagnosis of mesenteric venous thrombosis. *Endoscopy* 1986; **18**: 249.

18. Kleinhaus S, Sammartano RJ & Boley SJ. Variations in blood flow during laparoscopy. *Physiologist* 1976; **19**: 255.

19. Qamar MI, Read AE, Skidmore R, Evans JM & Wells PNT. Transcutaneous Doppler ultrasound measurements of superior mesenteric artery blood flow in man. *Gut* 1986; **27**: 100.

20. Boley SJ, Sprayregen S, Siegelman SS & Veith FJ. Initial results from an aggressive roentgenological and surgical approach to acute mesenteric ischemia. *Surgery* 1977; **82**: 898.

21. Segelman SS, Sprayregen S & Boley SJ. Angiographic diagnosis of mesenteric arterial vasoconstriction. *Radiology* 1974; **122**: 533.

22. Stolar CJ & Randolph JG. Evaluation of ischemic bowel viability with a fluorescent technique. *J Pediatr Surg* 1978; **13**: 221.

23. Carter M, Fantini G, Sammartano RJ, Mitsudo SM, Silverman D & Boley SJ. Qualitative and quantitative fluorescein fluorescence for determining intestinal viability. *Am J Surg* 1984; **147**: 117.

24. Shah S & Andersen C. Prediction of small bowel viability using Doppler ultrasound. *Ann Surg* 1981; **194**: 97.

25. Brolin RE, Semmelow JL & Koch RA. Myoelectric assessment of bowel viability. *Surgery* 1987; **102**: 32–38.

26. Shaw RS. The 'second look' after superior mesenteric arterial embolectomy or reconstruction for mesenteric infarction. In Ellison EH, Fieser SR & Mulholland JH (eds) *Current Surgical Management*. Philadelphia: WB Saunders, 1965: 509.

27. Cohn I, Floyd CE, Dresden CF & Bornside GH. Strangulation obstruction in germ-free animals. *Ann Surg* 1962; **156**: 692.

28. Becker GJ, Katzen BT & Dake MD. Noncoronary angioplasty. *Radiology* 1989; **170**: 921.

29. Hibbard JS, Swenson JC & Levin AG. Roentgenology of mesenteric vascular occlusion. *Arch Surg* 1933; **26**: 20.

30. Koveker G, Reichow W & Becker HD. Ergebnisse der Therapie des akuten Mesenterialgefassverschlusses. *Langenbecks Arch Chir* 1985; **366**: 536.

31. Odurny A, Sniderman KW & Colapinto RF. Intestinal angina: percutaneous transluminal angioplasty of the celiac and superior mesenteric arteries. *Radiology* 1988; **167**: 59.

32. Stoney RJ, Ehrenfeld WKL & Wylie EJ. Revascularization methods in chronic mesenteric visceral ischemia caused by atherosclerosis. *Ann Surg* 1977; **186**: 468.

33. Brandt LJ & Boley SJ. A new provocative test for intestinal angina. Presented at the *Annual Meeting of the American College of Gastroenterology*, 27 October 1990, San Francisco.

34. Anane-Sehaf JC & Blair E. *Surg Gynecol Obstet* 1975; **741**: 740–741.

35. Stoney RJ, Reilly IM & Ehrenfeld WR. Chronic mesenteric ischemia and surgery for chronic visceral ischemia. In Wilson SE, Veith FJ, Hobson RW & Williams RA (eds) *Vascular Surgery*. New York: McGraw-Hill, 1986: 672.

36. Wylie EJ, Stoney RJ & Ehrenfeld WK. *Manual of Vascular Surgery*, vol. I. New York: Springer, 1980: 210.

56

SMALL BOWEL STOMAS AND CONDUITS

RJC Steele
HB Devlin

The small bowel is a versatile organ. If handled properly, it can compensate for loss of the entire stomach, colorectum and bladder. After total gastrectomy, a patient can survive quite comfortably with a direct anastomosis between the oesophagus and the jejunum, which can be fashioned into a simple loop, a Roux loop or even a pouch on a vascular pedicle to allow oesophagoduodenal continuity and provide a food reservoir. Following colectomy good results can be obtained with ileorectal anastomosis, and after panproctocolectomy the patient with an ileostomy or pelvic pouch with ileoanal anastomosis can expect a good quality and quantity of life. A loop ileostomy is a useful means of defunctioning the colon or a portion of the small bowel, and after total cystectomy the ureters can be implanted into an isolated small bowel conduit.

In this chapter we shall deal with those small bowel conduits that are of importance to the surgical gastroenterologist and are not covered elsewhere in the book. These conduits include the end ileostomy, the diverting (loop) ileostomy, the Kock continent ileostomy and the ileal pelvic pouch. Each section consists of a discussion of the indications for the procedure, the technical aspects of the operation involved, and the short-term and long-term complications. To finish, there is a brief section on the role of the stoma clinic and the stoma nurse.

END (BROOKE) ILEOSTOMY

Indications

By far the most common indication for a permanent end ileostomy is a panproctocolectomy for inflammatory bowel disease. Since the introduction of restorative proctocolectomy with ileal reservoir, surgery for ulcerative colitis is no longer an absolute indication for a permanent ileostomy. However, after a full discussion some patients will still opt for an ileostomy, and those with poor anal sphincter function are better served by this simpler option. When panproctocolectomy is required for Crohn's disease, permanent ileostomy is considered mandatory in view of the risk of developing disease in a pelvic pouch. An end ileostomy may also be used as a temporary measure in the patient undergoing emergency operation for severe ulcerative colitis, especially when high-dose steroids are being used. Primary construction of a pelvic ileal reservoir is hazardous under these circumstances, and it is usual to preserve the rectum and bring out an end ileostomy with the intention of performing proctectomy and pouch construction at a later stage.

Other occasional indications for an end ileostomy are multiple malignant tumours of the colon (when the rectum has to be removed) and familial adenomatous polyposis. It should be stressed, however, that polyposis is more often treated by colectomy and ileorectal anastomosis or restorative proctocolectomy. A temporary end ileostomy may also be required after breakdown of an ileocolonic anastomosis, as attempts at repair are likely to be fruitless in the presence of sepsis.

Technique

Technique can be divided into siting, formation of the trephine, construction of the spout, dealing with the lateral space and postoperative management. Each will be covered in turn.

Siting

Correct siting is critical to the patient's future well-being, and every effort should be made to identify the ideal position for the ileostomy before operation. Even before this stage, however, detailed and sensitive counselling is necessary, and patients often feel that they have been given inadequate information regarding the effect that a stoma will have on their lives.[1,2] Ideally, all patients having an ileostomy should be seen by a stomatherapist or appropriately trained nurse before operation, and, if possible, they should speak to an ileostomy patient. This requirement can be difficult in the emergency situation, however; as around 30% of ileostomies are performed as urgent procedures, the tasks of explaining and siting may sometimes fall to the surgeon.

It is important to realize that the ideal position for an ileostomy will vary greatly from one patient to another. The skin around the stoma should be flat, to allow easy placement of appliances, and should be easily accessible to the patient. The ideal site is therefore the summit of the infraumbilical mound, well away from scars, skin creases, the umbilicus and the iliac crest (Figure 56.1). It should also be positioned so that the ileum will cross the rectus muscle, to minimize the risk of prolapse or hernia.

Once a reasonable site has been identified, the patient should wear an appliance at that site and test it both empty and full of water while fully clothed, standing and sitting.[3] When the site has been optimized it should be marked, usually on the skin with indelible ink. It has been suggested that injection of methylene blue deep into the abdominal wall is helpful to ensure that a straight course is achieved during construction of the trephine.[4]

Formation of the trephine

This is commonly done towards the end of the operation, but we have recommended construction of the trephine before the abdomen has been opened to ensure a straight course through the abdominal wall.[5] The first step is to lift up the skin at the centre of the siting mark with a pair of tissue forceps, and to cut out a disc of skin and cylinder of subcutaneous tissue down to the anterior rectus sheath. The sheath is then opened with a cruciate incision, and the underlying rectus muscle fibres one split longitudinally, carefully avoiding damage to the inferior epigastric vessels. The posterior rectus sheath is opened, also with a cruciate incision, and stretched with two fingers to allow the ileum to pass through easily but snugly.

Construction of the spout

The terminal small bowel mesentery is prepared so that an adequate arcade is preserved to ensure good perfusion right to

the cut end of the ileum. The ileum is divided as close to the caecum as possible, traditionally between De Martel's or Zachary Cope's clamps. An alternative technique is to divide the bowel with a linear cutting and stapling (GIA-type) device. Not only does this manoeuvre obviate the risk of contamination from slippage of the clamp, but it is also very useful for delivering the ileum through an obese abdominal wall.

When the ileum has been brought through the trephine and the abdomen and skin have been closed, the clamp is taken off or the staple line excised. Four 3/0 Vicryl sutures are then placed from the skin edge through the seromuscular surface of the ileum as it emerges from the anterior rectus sheath, taking great care not to penetrate the mucosa for fear of skin-level fistulas, and then to the cut edge of the ileum (Figure 56.2). When these sutures are tied, the ileum automatically everts to form a spout, which should be 2–3 cm long (Figure 56.3). Further sutures are then placed between the skin and the ileum to secure the mucocutaneous junction. This eversion technique was first described by Brooke in 1952;[6] it largely overcame the problems of skin excoriation and ileostomy stenosis seen with a flush stoma.

Dealing with the lateral space

The space between the terminal ileal mesentery and the lateral abdominal wall can be closed by means of a purse-string suture inserted into the lateral parietal peritoneum and the cut edge of the terminal ileal mesentery, but this procedure can be technically difficult and may not achieve a secure closure. It is better to suspend the terminal small bowel from a ventral

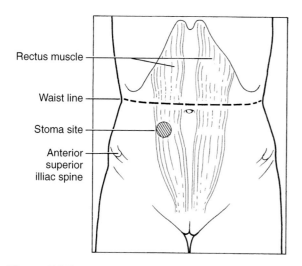

Figure 56.1
The ideal site for an ileostomy.

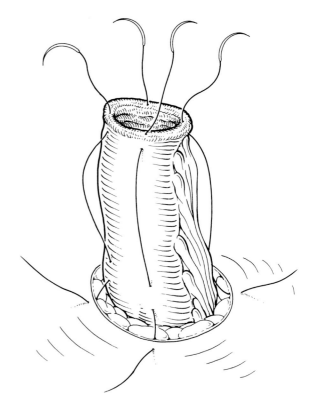

Figure 56.2
Construction of the Brooke end ileostomy.

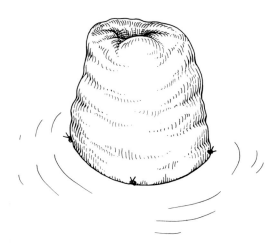

Figure 56.3
Completed Brooke end ileostomy.

mesentery fashioned by suturing this cut edge to the anterior abdominal wall. Alternatively, the peritoneum can be left intact during formation of the trephine, and the ileum can be delivered to the trephine through an extraperitoneal tunnel.[7] It has to be said, however, that there is little evidence to support obliteration of the lateral space conclusively, and many surgeons deliberately leave the space open.

Postoperative management

When the stoma has been fashioned, the surgeon fits a drainable bag appliance, which is usually a one-piece system at first. It is very important to use a transparent bag in the first instance so that the ileostomy can be inspected easily in the immediate postoperative period. Preferably, the appliance should be left undisturbed except for emptying for the first week, as changing it at this stage will be very uncomfortable for the patient. Usually the ileostomy will start to function on the second or third postoperative day, and as soon as this occurs a rapid increase of oral intake to full fluids and light diet can be achieved. It is very important to measure the ileostomy output and to replace this volume with intravenous normal saline (plus potassium 40 mmol/l) in addition to normal fluid requirements. When the patient is on full oral intake, fluid balance regulation is not normally a problem, but occasionally excessive ileostomy loss will require prolonged intravenous supplementation.

As soon as possible after operation the patient must become accustomed to the stoma and learn how to drain the appliance. A stoma therapist or experienced nurse is invaluable in this respect, and a decision as to the long-term appliance to be used must be made fairly quickly. To protect the skin from the digestive action of ileostomy effluent and to minimize the risk of leakage, an effective sealant is necessary which will adhere firmly to skin without causing damage or allergic reactions. The two most widely available sealants are karaya gum and Stomahesive.

Karaya gum is a naturally occurring polysaccharide collected from the *Sterculia urens* tree in India.[8] At concentrations of 20–50% in water it has strong adhesive properties, and as it

avidly absorbs water it retains its strength in a damp environment. It is normally used blended with a mild alkali to improve its adhesive properties, and by combining it with gelatine it can be moulded into solid flat rings which can be attached to the base of an appliance. In addition, karaya gum powder can be applied directly to protect excoriated skin around a stoma.

Stomahesive is a gelatin-based synthetic product which is adherent and resistant to moisture, heat and ileostomy effluent;[9] it can remain on the skin around the stoma for up to 15 days.[10] Stomahesive is less irritant to skin than karaya[11] and needs replacing less frequently.[12] Another substance similar to Stomahesive is a synthetic cellulose derivative called Comfeel. This is very elastic and can be helpful in physically active patients.

The actual appliance consists of a base of adherent sealant with an aperture for the stoma leading to a pouch, which must have a capacity of around 500 ml. For the ileostomy patient, the pouch must be drainable for convenient emptying, and such pouches are usually sealed by clips or seal strips. The appliance can be constructed either in one piece or it may consist of a base and a detachable pouch. The two-piece system has the advantage that the base can usually be left on the skin for about a week,[13] but the locking device used to achieve a tight seal between the base and the bag can be difficult to use and is painful in the early postoperative period.

The final choice of appliance has to be the patient's personal preference, guided by the stoma therapist; before the patient leaves hospital he or she must be adept at using the device.

The Ileostomy Association provides help and support for many patients, and information regarding its activities should be provided. The patient must know about the local stoma clinic or equivalent, and common complications that might arise should be explained. Finally, it is important to keep the patient's general practitioner informed, and arrangements with the district nurse to visit the patient at home must be made before discharge.

Complications

Short-term complications

Complications of ileostomy seen in the immediate postoperative period include bleeding, oedema, necrosis, retraction and obstruction.

Bleeding It is common to have a small amount of oozing of blood at the mucocutaneous junction, but this nearly always stops spontaneously. Occasionally a brisk bleed from a small vessel in the subcutaneous tissue or the mesentery of the terminal ileum will necessitate local reoperation.

Oedema Swelling of the ileostomy is almost inevitable. As long as it is not associated with ileostomy obstruction or necrosis, it can be safely disregarded as it will always settle.

Necrosis True necrosis of the stoma is very rare, but not infrequently it may appear very dark blue or even black in the immediate postoperative period. In this situation it is best to adopt an expectant policy with careful, regular inspection; a normal colour will usually be seen within 3–4 days. If the ischaemia is severe, stenosis of the stoma may develop at a later stage, but early reoperation for gangrene of the ileum is hardly ever necessary.

Retraction Retraction in the early postoperative period can be a problem as it causes severe skin excoriation, which can be difficult to manage with standard skin protection techniques. It is therefore advisable to refashion the stoma at an early stage, and this can usually be done quite simply. The stoma can be re-everted by grasping the ileum about 2 cm below the skin surface with tissue forceps, and it is held in place with absorbable sutures passed through both the emergent and reflected layers of the stoma. Alternatively, a linear stapler without a blade may be used to keep the two walls together.[14]

Ileostomy obstruction If the ileostomy does not function in the first few days and the patient develops distension and vomiting, there may be either obstruction to the ileostomy as it crosses the abdominal wall, adhesions or volvulus around the stoma. Other possibilities include ileus due to intrabdominal sepsis, retroperitoneal haematoma or small bowel ischaemia. Initial management should include nasogastric aspiration and careful assessment of fluid and electrolyte balance together with appropriate intravenous replacement. A soft catheter should be placed into the stoma as this will overcome any local stomal occlusion. If resolution has not occurred within about a week, then total parenteral nutrition should be instituted and plans made for laparotomy.

Long-term complications The long-term complications of ileostomy are legion. They can be subdivided into local stomal complications, systemic complications and social complications (Table 56.1). Each of these will be taken in turn.

Skin problems Excoriation of the skin around the ileostomy site is the most common complication,[2] and this can be divided into effluent dermatitis, which is due to the digestive action of ileostomy effluent, and contact dermatitis, which is due to sensitivity to the appliance. Effluent dermatitis can be quickly distinguished by its irregular outline from contact dermatitis which exhibits a regular pattern conforming to the shape of the appliance (Figure 56.4).

Effluent dermatitis is commonly due to poor construction or poor siting of the stoma. When severe, it may necessitate reconstruction or resiting, but in many instances conservative management will be successful. Firstly, the skin must be swabbed to look for secondary bacterial or fungal infection. The affected area is then cleaned with soap and water and carefully dried. Creases around the stoma predispose to contamination, and these can be filled with karaya paste to protect the skin from leaking effluent. If the skin is flat, then sheets of Stomahesive or Comfeel can be used.

In severe cases, when the skin becomes soggy and hyperaemic, it may be necessary to use short courses of local corticosteroid preparations; these can be combined with antibiotics or antifungal agents as appropriate. Corticosteroids are also useful to alleviate the itching produced by contact dermatitis, but the root of this problem is hypersensitivity to the adhesive sealant being used, and an alternative has to be found.

Leakage Leakage is essentially due to an ill-fitting appliance, and, as such, the problem and its solutions are closely tied up with effluent dermatitis. The most likely underlying causes are poor siting or poor stoma construction, hence resiting is frequently required for severe leakage.

Retraction Retraction of an ileostomy will cause leakage and consequent excoriation of the skin,[15] and revision is usually necessary. If the retraction occurs early, then local re-eversion and fixation is often successful (see above), but in later cases this procedure is usually not possible. The options are then to mobilize the stoma fully and refashion it at the same site or to perform a laparotomy and completely resite the stoma. Many authorities favour the latter approach of resiting, largely because after mobilization the trephine is much wider than the ileum, making recurrent retraction likely. Todd,[16] however, favours careful fixation of the stoma to the rectus sheath followed by excision and suturing of three wedges of skin, in the so-called 'Mercedes' manoeuvre, in order to produce a snug skin closure at the mucocutaneous junction (Figure 56.5).

Prolapse Prolapse of an ileostomy is less common than with a colostomy, but it can present troublesome problems when it does occur. It is usefully classified into fixed and sliding varieties,[15] according to whether or not the degree of prolapse varies intermittently. The fixed prolapse is basically an error of construction where the spout has been made too long. This type can be treated relatively easily by dividing the junction between the mucosa and skin without disturbing the emerging ileum, straightening out the everted stoma, excising an appropriate length of ileum and refashioning the everted spout.

Table 56.1 Long-term complications of end ileostomy

LOCAL	SYSTEMIC	SOCIAL
1. Skin problems	9. Fluid and electrolyte disorders	13. Odour and flatus
2. Leakage	10. Haematological sequelae	14. Sexual problems
3. Retraction	11. Urolithiasis	15. Psychological problems and social activity
4. Prolapse	12. Cholelithiasis	
5. Stenosis		
6. Parastomal herniation		
7. Fistula		
8. Bleeding		

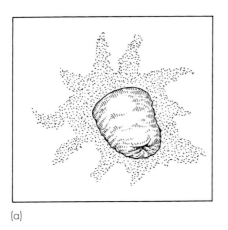

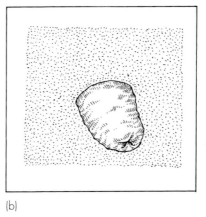

(a)　　　　　　　　　　　　　　(b)

Figure 56.4
Ileostomy dermatitis. (a) Pattern seen with effluent dermatitis. (b) Pattern seen with contact dermatitis.

The sliding prolapse is a more challenging problem. Here the ileum is not attached to the deep layers of the abdominal wall so that the spout can vary in length enormously. Essentially the same approach can be used as for fixed prolapse, but the ileum should be anchored carefully to the rectus sheath and the two walls of the spout should be sutured or stapled together. It has been suggested that, before this is done, the ileum should be pulled as taut as possible and the redundant bowel excised,[16] but this can result in loss of a substantial segment of the terminal ileum, with possible metabolic sequelae.

Stenosis Prior to the development of the eversion ileostomy by Brooke, stenosis at the mucocutaneous junction was common, owing to inflammation and subsequent fibrosis of the surrounding skin, and this will still occur with the retracted stoma which goes uncorrected. Stenosis at the level of the abdominal wall may occur due to too tight an opening, and stenosis of the spout itself may follow severe ischaemia or may indicate recurrent Crohn's disease.

In general, stenosis will require full mobilization of the ileostomy, with or without laparotomy, resection of the spout and full reconstruction. Treatment of stenosis at the level of the abdominal wall by subcutaneous fasciotomy has been described,[17] but this approach has not been widely adopted.

Parastomal herniation Parastomal herniation usually occurs when the ileostomy has been brought out through the abdominal wall outside the rectus muscle, and is particularly likely if a stoma has been constructed through the main abdominal incision.[18,19] Such hernias can be troublesome as they can interfere with secure placement of an appliance, and small bowel obstruction with or without strangulation can supervene.

Owing to perceived difficulties with local repair, many parastomal hernias are left undisturbed unless the patient becomes severely symptomatic. As the cause of the problem is usually poor siting, repair is best effected by taking the stoma down via a laparotomy and constructing a new stoma on the other side of the abdomen through healthy rectus muscle. Local repair can be achieved successfully if the original position is reasonable,[20] but this is a rare situation.

Fistula Paraileostomy fistula can result from recurrent Crohn's disease or from chronic sepsis related to a suture on the anterior or posterior rectus sheath which has discharged into the ileum and to the skin surface (Figure 56.6). This latter complication is why absorbable sutures should always be used for constructing the ileostomy in the first instance.

The Crohn's fistulas are inevitably associated with active disease with sepsis and abscess cavities; as a result the tracks are

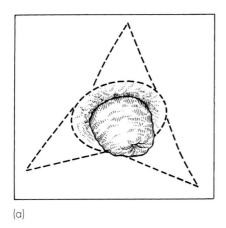

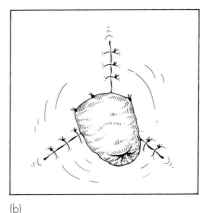

(a)　　　　　　　　　　　　　　(b)

Figure 56.5
The 'Mercedes' manoeuvre for refashioning a retracted ileostomy.

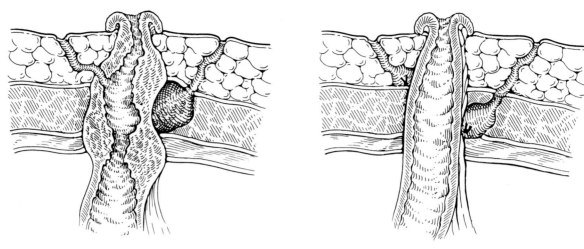

Figure 56.6
Paraileostomy fistulas: (a) Due to Crohn's disease; (b) Due to stitch abscesses.

often complex and multiple. Fistulas occurring from discharge of stitch abscesses, on the other hand, are usually straight and associated with an otherwise healthy stoma. Whatever the cause, paraileostomy fistulas cause difficulties with stoma management because the discharge will seep under the base of the appliance and tend to lift it off the skin. In addition, as the discharge consists of ileostomy effluent, severe skin excoriation will ensue.

The most effective means of dealing with fistulas is to take down the ileostomy completely, resect the affected segment and refashion the spout. This procedure should be done via a laparotomy, especially when Crohn's disease is suspected, because a fairly extensive resection may be required and abscess cavities will have to be drained. If there is appreciable sepsis, the original trephine site will be unsuitable, and the stoma will need to be resited, preferably on the other side of the abdomen. Occasionally, a simple fistula track will respond to a conservative approach of cleaning and phenolization.[21]

Bleeding Late-onset bleeding can be due to traumatic ulceration, polyps, recurrent Crohn's disease or peristomal varices associated with portal hypertension (see also Chapter 54). Ulceration is usually associated with prolapse or a long stoma that rubs against the appliance; if severe, it necessitates stoma revision. Polyps may occur in patients with familial adenomatous polyposis, and, if isolated, may be locally excised. Polypoid granulation tissue can also occur at the mucocutaneous junction in any patient, and this condition may respond to diathermy or silver nitrate.

Peristomal varices in the patient with hepatic cirrhosis or other cause of portal hypertension is the most dangerous cause of bleeding. A caput medusae forms from the shunting of blood from the ileal veins to the abdominal wall veins. Although this shunt may protect against the development of oesophageal varices,[22] bleeding from the peristomal varices themselves can be profuse and life threatening. Immediate control can be achieved by local pressure, and the immediate risk of continued bleeding can be removed by discon-

necting the stoma at the mucocutaneous junction to interrupt the portasystemic communication, oversewing both divided edges and resuturing the ileostomy.[23] Unfortunately, recurrent bleeding is common,[24] and if this is troublesome portasystemic shunting may be advisable.[25]

Fluid and electrolyte disorders (Table 56.2) The normal subject loses only about 150 ml water and 5 mmol sodium in the faeces each day, whereas the accepted daily losses for an ileostomy patient are in the region of 600 ml water and 80 mmol sodium. Thus, owing to the absence of the absorptive capacity of the colon, even the healthy ileostomy patient is in a chronic water and sodium depletion state.[26] This state is made possible by renal homeostasis mediated by the renin–angiotensin mechanism; it has been shown that basal levels of both renin and aldosterone are elevated in the presence of an ileostomy.[27] Potassium loss is a particular potential problem as the kidney conserves sodium at the expense of potassium, and the urinary sodium : potassium ratio is low in ileostomy

Table 56.2 Typical daily urine and faecal losses in normal individuals and healthy ileostomy patients

	AVERAGE LOSSES/DAY	
	NORMAL INDIVIDUAL	ILEOSTOMATE
Urine		
Volume (ml)	1500	800–1000
Sodium (mmol)	110–240	93
Potassium (mmol)	35–90	114
Faeces		
Sodium (mmol)	10	38–40
Potassium (mmol)	12	3–6
Magnesium (mmol)	3–3.5	3.5–4.5
Calcium (mmol)	5.5	7.5–20
Nitrogen (mmol)	107	43–171
Fat (mmol)	11–18	5–13
Bilirubin (μmol)	—	118–166
Stercobilinogen (μmol)	35–420	5–52
Volume (ml)	100–150	350–700

patients.[27] In addition, there is loss of potassium in the ileostomy effluent, again in exchange for sodium.[28]

Remarkably few patients have clinical fluid and electrolyte problems, but when profuse ileostomy diarrhoea does occur it poses serious problems. Ileostomy 'flux', as it is sometimes known, may be precipitated by gastroenteritis, bacterial overgrowth, recurrent Crohn's disease and systemic sepsis,[29] but in many cases it remains idiopathic. Patients who develop this complication become rapidly depleted of water, sodium and potassium, and they may even slip into an addisonian crisis if they have recently been on steroid therapy.

The patient feels weak and thirsty, will have noticed a marked increase in the volume of the ileostomy effluent and runs the risk of developing a cardiac arrhythmia. An intravenous infusion of saline with added potassium (40 mmol/l) must be started without delay, and the patient is catheterized to monitor urine output. Daily estimations of plasma urea and electrolyte levels are necessary, and a sample of the effluent should be sent for microbiological examination. It is also better to monitor the urine concentrations of sodium and potassium during the acute phase. If the patient has been on steroids in the recent past, intravenous hydrocortisone should be administered at 100 mg g.d.s.

In a severe attack the patient may lose 3–4 litres a day, but the volumes usually start to tail off after 2–3 days. Nevertheless, until fairly normal volumes are observed, it is best to avoid oral fluids as these will tend to exacerbate the ileal losses.[30] Steroids may help to reduce water and sodium losses by a mineralocorticoid effect.[31] Oral intake should start with a glucose–electrolyte solution, and drugs such as codeine, Lomotil (co-phenotrope) and loperamide may contribute by reducing the ileostomy output.[32,33] It should be noted that bulking agents such as Fybogel (ispaghula) are not indicated, as these can make the situation worse.

In patients with persistent idiopathic ileostomy diarrhoea, operation has been recommended by some groups. The most common operation has been reversal of a 12 cm segment of terminal ileum some 30 cm proximal to the ileostomy,[34,35] but there is a fine line between producing inadequate reduction in small bowel transit time and precipitating intestinal obstruction. Because of this fact and because of the risk of producing or exacerbating a short bowel syndrome, such operations are not widely popular.

Haematological sequelae Although major haematological abnormalities do not occur, when corrected for dehydration low haemoglobin levels are found in ileostomy patients.[36] Low mean corpuscular volume and mean corpuscular haemoglobin values are also found, suggesting mild iron deficiency anaemia. No evidence of vitamin B_{12} or folate deficiency has been demonstrated, although ileostomy patients with Crohn's disease may have reduced absorption of vitamin B_{12}.[36]

Urolithiasis There is some debate as to whether or not ileostomy subjects are at particular risk of developing urinary stones. The prevalence of calcified urinary stones in the UK population at large is believed to be in the region of 4%,[37] whereas the reported incidence of urolithiasis in ileostomy

patients varies between 1.3%[38] and 10.3%;[1] an even higher incidence has been reported from the USA.[39] It is possible that the length of small bowel resected is of some importance, with an increased incidence in those who have lost a marked amount,[40] and it is likely that length of follow-up is crucial.

Ileostomy patients have a high incidence of uric acid stones,[41] and this is presumably related to their high uric acid levels.[42] Another important factor is the low urine volume produced by these patients and their persistently acid urine, which favours the precipitation of uric acid.[39]

Cholelithiasis Again, there is controversy over the increased incidence of gallstones in ileostomy patients, and it is thought that this is only the case where more that 10 cm of terminal ileum has been resected.[43] This outcome might be expected, as loss of the terminal ileum is known to compromise reabsorption of bile salts, and by reducing the bile acid pool this decreases the solubility of cholesterol in bile.[44,45] It is not surprising, therefore, that many patients with an ileostomy do have gallstones,[46,47] particularly those who have had their operation for Crohn's disease (see Chapter 50).[48]

Odour and flatus Odour and flatus cause less of a problem with an ileostomy than they do with a colostomy. They do occur, however, and can be both embarrassing and troublesome; excessive flatus can distend and even dislodge the bag from the appliance. Activated charcoal filters are available which can be fitted to stoma bags and may reduce smell, but diet is really the key to minimizing this problem. It is also important to warn patients that flatus and bag 'blow off' can be a problem when flying in pressurized aircraft.

Flatus is largely caused by carbohydrates which are not digested and absorbed, but fermented by gut bacteria. Thus it is less of a problem when the colon is missing, but some bacteria do colonize the terminal ileum in ileostomy patients. Common foods that tend to produce gas and smell include beans, eggs, onions, cabbage and other bulky green vegetables such as broccoli or sprouts. Patients should be given appropriate advice on diet, but it usually comes down to trial and error for individual subjects.

Sexual problems Sexual problems can be divided into physical disability caused by the rectal dissection that has often accompanied the formation of the ileostomy and problems of a psychological and emotional nature. Damage to the autonomic nervous supply to the bladder, seminal vesicles, prostate or penis can result in impotence or retrograde ejaculation,[49,50] but recent studies of rectal excision for inflammatory bowel disease have found a low incidence of such problems.[1,51] Physical sexual problems in women are less easy to define, but both dyspareunia and decreased libido have been reported.[49,50] Chronic perineal discomfort is a common problem after rectal excision,[52] and there may be vaginal stenosis or a vaginoperineal fistula.

Quite apart from such physical problems, however, patients with an ileostomy may develop understandable sexual inhibitions. Many male patients who have not become impotent have difficulties with sexual intercourse,[1] and as such difficulties are not seen after colectomy with ileorectal anastomosis,[53] it may be assumed that the ileostomy itself is at least partially responsible. In general, women appear to be more affected than men, as fewer women than men marry after proctocolectomy and ileostomy.[54]

Women with ileostomies need special advice regarding contraception. Oral contraceptives may be inadequately absorbed, especially if there has been extensive loss of small bowel, and the margin of safety from pregnancy is much less with an ileostomy than in the normal subject.[55] Tubal ligation in the postproctectomy patient is fraught with hazards, and insertion of an intrauterine device may be difficult if the uterus has become retroverted as a result of pelvic surgery. All in all, therefore, it is better for the male partner to take responsibility for contraception in a stable relationship where the woman has an ileostomy. Pregnancy does not usually pose particular problems for the ileostomy patient,[50,56] but displacement of the ileostomy site by the enlarging abdomen may make management difficult, and there is a tendency towards an increased incidence of intestinal obstruction. Furthermore, the anaemia of pregnancy can be exacerbated by the presence of a stoma, as iron supplements may cause stoma dysfunction and there may be difficulties in absorbing vitamin B_{12}, especially in patients with Crohn's disease.

Psychological problems and social activity In general, although the complications of ileostomy cause psychological and social problems, most ileostomy patients report an improvement in well-being and life-style limitations after being relieved of the symptoms of their original disease.[57,58] Although over 50% of patients have minor complications such as skin irritation, flatus and odour, less than 10% develop disabling complications.[57] Whates and Irving[59] carried out a survey through the Ileostomy Association and found that most patients returned to work after ileostomy, despite the fact that about one-third had to give up work through ill health before operation. Not all studies have been so encouraging, however, and some have found a high incidence of unemployment and a sense of adverse discrimination.[58]

LOOP ILEOSTOMY

Indications

The loop ileostomy is now used mostly as a defunctioning stoma, but it was originally designed as a method of constructing an end ileostomy where technical difficulties were encountered with the formation of a conventional Brooke spout.[60] In this operation the end of the ileum was closed off (see section on Technique), but it soon followed that a loop ileostomy could be done without dividing the bowel and thereby act to defunction the distal ileum and colon.[61] The loop ileostomy is now widely used to protect ileorectal anastomoses and ileoanal pouches,[18,62,63] and it has been proposed as definitive treatment for megacolon.[64]

If the colon has been prepared, loop ileostomy is also an effective method of defunctioning the large bowel to protect a low colorectal anastomosis,[65,66] and there is some evidence to suggest that it may be preferable to transverse colostomy for

this purpose. There may be a lower incidence of sepsis and herniation,[67] but the main argument for its use is the lower incidence of complications following closure.[66] It is important to stress, however, that a loop ileostomy should not be used as a means of decompressing a large bowel obstruction, as this will be ineffective – especially when the ileocaecal valve is competent.

Technique

Formation of the loop ileostomy

A trephine is made in the anterior abdominal wall through the rectus muscle, as for an end ileostomy with the exception that the opening has to be slightly bigger to admit the two limbs of the ileal loop. Before delivering the loop through the bowel wall, it is best to mark the distal limb with a suture so that no mistake is made in making the spout. A Jaques catheter or similar smooth catheter is then introduced between the mesentery and the bowel wall at the proposed apex of the loop: a tape may be used, but this is more difficult to remove as it tends to drag on the tissues. Artery forceps are then introduced through the trephine, and the two ends of the catheter or tape are grasped (Figure 56.7) so that the apex of the bowel loop can be gently coaxed to lie on the anterior abdominal wall (Figure 56.8).

Using a diathermy blade, an enterotomy encompassing

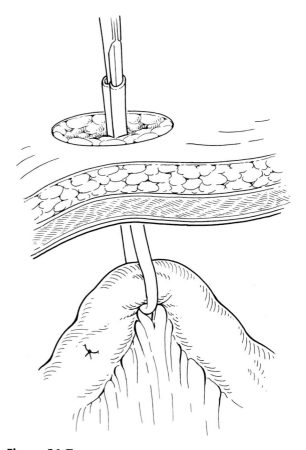

Figure 56.7

Catheter around apex of proposed loop ileostomy ready to bring through abdominal wall trephine.

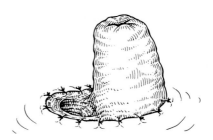

Figure 56.10
Completed loop ileostomy.

chromic catgut mucocutaneous sutures (Figure 56.10). As long as the enterotomy is not too large, the proximal limb spout will remain everted without extra sutures between the skin and the serosal aspect of the bowel.

The temporary use of a rod to prevent retraction of the loop has been advocated,[60] but this is usually unnecessary.[68] If support is felt to be necessary, it is possible to leave a short segment of the rubber catheter used to pull the loop through the trephine sutured to the skin (Figure 56.11).

It has been suggested that orientation of the loop is important, and that the proximal limb should be dependent to prevent overspill into the distal loop.[69] This matter is probably unimportant, however; the ileostomy effluent is only likely to enter the bowel distal to the loop if there has been marked retraction.[70]

Closure of the loop ileostomy

As the loop ileostomy is normally a temporary measure, the technical aspects of its closure are important. As a rule, the ileostomy should be left for at least 6 weeks so that all the local swelling has resolved, and any subclinical distal leaks have had time to heal. A longer period should elapse if there has been clinical evidence of intra-abdominal or pelvic sepsis.

Before closure, it is important to assess the anastomosis that the loop ileostomy has been constructed to protect. Often this assessment will be possible by means of a sigmoidoscope, but, if not, a contrast enema must be performed either per anum or via the distal limb of the ileostomy.

Although the operation is often straightforward, closure of a loop ileostomy should always be regarded as a major procedure and should be performed by an experienced surgeon. Single-dose intravenous antibiotic prophylaxis should be used, as for any gastrointestinal operation in which there is a risk of endogenous infection from opened bowel, and provision

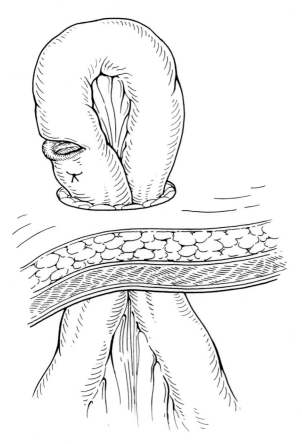

Figure 56.8
Ileal loop brought through anterior abdominal wall and enterotomy made in distal limb of ileal loop.

somewhat less than half of the circumference of the bowel wall is made on the antimesenteric aspect of the distal limb, about 1 cm away from the skin (Figure 56.8). An Allis forceps is then inserted into the enterotomy, and the full thickness of the wall of the ileum near the top of the proximal loop is grasped (Figure 56.9). The proximal limb is then everted by pulling the wall grasped by the Allis forceps through the enterotomy, and the stoma is completed by the insertion of 2/0

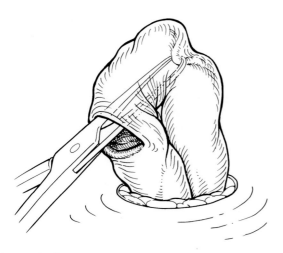

Figure 56.9
Allis forceps used to form proximal spout of loop ileostomy.

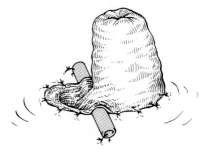

Figure 56.11
Loop ileostomy supported by short segment of catheter.

should be made for a formal laparotomy as this is occasionally necessary.

A useful first step is to place several sutures around the ileostomy, passing through the mucocutaneous junction, and to hold them at one point with artery forceps. This manoeuvre allows even traction of the skin around the ileostomy in any direction and facilitates dissection of the bowel loop from the skin and subcutaneous tissues (Figure 56.12). The skin is then incised very close to the mucocutaneous junction, and the serosa of the bowel is separated from the investing fibrous tissue. Further dissection with fine scissors frees the bowel from the rectus sheath and then the peritoneum, so that the ileum can be returned into the peritoneal cavity after closure.

To close the ileostomy it is sometimes possible to turn back the everted spout by scissor dissection and to excise the attached skin. The enterotomy is then closed with interrupted serosubmucosal 3/0 braided nylon (Figure 56.13), the rectus sheath is closed with interrupted 1 polydioxanone, and the skin is closed with interrupted sutures or staples. Quite often there is so much fibrosis around the bowel wall that a neat, safe closure is not possible, and under these circumstances it is preferable to carry out a formal limited ileal resection. An end-to-end small bowel anastomosis is then carried out using a single layer of interrupted serosubmucosal 3/0 braided nylon (Figure 56.14). A stapled closure can be used, but there is no evidence to suggest that this is any safer or easier.

When closure of a loop ileostomy is particularly difficult, it is sometimes necessary to perform a laparotomy in order to dissect out the loop from inside. Thus the patient should always be warned of the possibility of a laparotomy. It is usually feasible to overcome most difficulties by extending the trephine rather than making a separate incision.

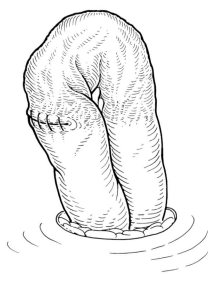

Figure 56.13
Closure of loop ileostomy by reinversion and closure of the enterotomy.

Complications

With the provision that the loop ileostomy is usually a temporary measure, the complications are essentially the same as those seen with the end ileostomy. There are certain specific complications resulting from closure that are worth considering (Table 56.3).

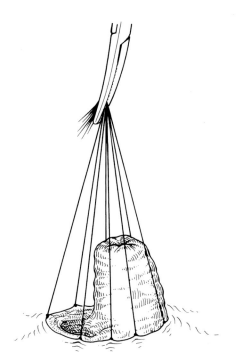

Figure 56.12
Sutures used to retract loop ileostomy during mobilization.

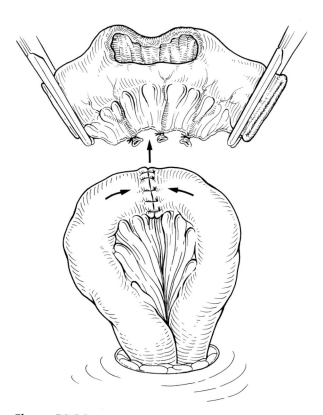

Figure 56.14
Closure of loop ileostomy by resection.

Table 56.3   Specific complications of closure of loop ileostomy

1. Wound infection
2. Suture line dehiscence
3. Intestinal obstruction
4. Hernia

Wound infection This can be minimized by perioperative antibiotics and careful, atraumatic surgery. Some authorities suggest leaving the wound open in all cases, but although this will certainly make infection less likely, it condemns many patients to an unnecessarily long period with an open wound. If infection does occur, the skin sutures or staples can be removed and the wound opened to allow adequate drainage.

Suture line dehiscence If the suture line or anastomosis breaks down, the patient may develop generalized peritonitis and require an urgent laparotomy and refashioning of the ileostomy. This serious complication is unusual as the closed loop is often surrounded by adhesions, and a dehiscence will more commonly present as an abscess and/or a fistula. The patient will usually develop a fever, fairly sudden abdominal pain localized to the area of the previous ileostomy, and may also have the symptoms and signs of intestinal obstruction. If this combination of symptoms suggests a dehiscence, a conservative regimen of intravenous fluids and intravenous antibiotics is commenced. If an abscess develops, it should be drained. A fistula then often results and the patient should be kept nil by mouth and supported by total parenteral nutrition.

Provided that all sepsis is drained and there is no distal intestinal obstruction, the fistula will close spontaneously. If there is a large cavity associated with the fistula, it will be necessary to perform a laparotomy, fully mobilize the affected segment of bowel, excise it and carry out a formal small bowel anastomosis. Alternatively, if there is severe sepsis, a loop ileostomy may have to be brought out at a different site. Likewise, intestinal obstruction that does not resolve will necessitate a laparotomy.

Intestinal obstruction Quite apart from anastomotic problems, intestinal obstruction is fairly common after loop ileostomy closure, and this is particularly true in association with a pelvic pouch. If it occurs, it should be treated conservatively in the first instance. However, if nasogastric suction and intravenous fluids have not brought about resolution within 48 hours, then laparotomy should be considered.

Hernia Herniation at the site of trephine closure can occur, especially if there has been a wound infection. The hernia should be repaired at the first available opportunity owing to the risk of bowel entrapment.

CONTINENT ILEOSTOMY

Indications

Clearly the conventional Brooke ileostomy is incontinent and, although modern appliances are reasonably satisfactory, the unpredictability of ileostomy action can be inconvenient. When the continent or reservoir ileostomy was introduced by Kock in 1969,[71] it was the only alternative to the conventional ileostomy that offered any hope of continence. However, since the development of the ileal pelvic pouch with ileoanal anastomosis, the indications for a continent ileostomy are rather different and probably more infrequent than before.

Patients who have already had a panproctocolectomy and ileostomy, and who are highly motivated towards having a continent stoma that does not require an appliance, may benefit from this procedure. In addition, it may be appropriate for those who have had a pelvic pouch that has not functioned properly. Another group who might benefit are those who have severe acquired or congenital anorectal anomalies requiring a stoma. The continent colostomy has not been particularly successful, and a total colectomy with the formation of a continent ileostomy may prove a satisfactory alternative.

It must be stressed that the formation of a continent reservoir ileostomy is a highly specialized operation and should only be undertaken by surgeons with a special interest, who have been fully trained in the procedure and who are prepared to dedicate considerable time and effort to their patients' postoperative care. There are also several patient-related contraindications to the operation, among which psychological instability, low intelligence and obesity are important.[72–74] Multiple previous operations, particularly if there has been loss of small bowel, should also weigh against performing this procedure, but perhaps the most crucial contraindication is Crohn's disease.

Most experience of the continent ileostomy in patients with Crohn's disease has resulted from the procedure being carried out in the mistaken belief that the underlying disease was ulcerative colitis (see also Chapter 51). In such cases, the complications of Crohn's pouchitis, chronic sepsis and fistula formation have led most authorities to advise strongly against constructing a pouch if Crohn's disease is suspected.[71,74,75] Furthermore, if an appreciable proportion of the small bowel has been taken up by the pouch, subsequent resections for recurrent disease will compromise the patient even more than if a conventional ileostomy had been performed.

Technique

The concept of the continent reservoir ileostomy was introduced in 1969 by Kock.[71] Initial attempts were not particularly successful, but after several modifications it was recognized that internal intussusception of a segment of ileum was the key to obtaining continence.[76] In this section a modern technique of construction will be described, and this will be followed by an account of postoperative management and long-term management.

Construction

The trephine, as for conventional ileostomy, is placed through rectus muscle but is situated just suprapubically. Sixty centimeters of terminal ileum are required for construction of the whole continent ileostomy (Figure 56.15), the proximal 30 cm

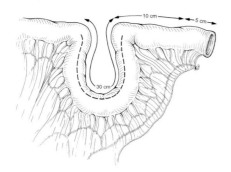

Figure 56.15
Extent of terminal ileum required for continent ileostomy.

for the reservoir and the distal 30 cm for the nipple valve and the exit conduit. The first step is to open the antimesenteric aspect of the proximal loop and to suture the posterior wall of the pouch with a continuous serosubmucosal suture of 3/0 polydioxanone or other similar long-lasting but absorbable material (Figure 56.16). The proximal 10 cm of the distal loop, which is to be used for the nipple valve, is then scarified over its serosal surface with diathermy in an attempt to make the valve more stable.[77,78] The bulk of the mesentery at the level of the nipple valve is then reduced by skeletonization of the mesenteric vessels, as this has been shown to reduce the incidence of desusception.[79,80]

Formation of the nipple valve is created by introducing two Allis forceps into the distal limb through the pouch and grasping the full thickness of the wall at a distance of 5 cm from the pouch. The ileum is then intussuscepted into the pouch (Figure 56.17) and stabilized by means of four rows of staples inserted by a linear stapler without the blade (Figure 56.18). Care must be taken to avoid damage to the intussuscepted mesenteric vessels. This manoeuvre has been instrumental in reducing valve slippage problems to an acceptable level,[76,80,81] and the incidence of this complication can be as low as 3%.[82]

The serosal aspect of the nipple valve is then sutured circumferentially to the exit conduit. In a further attempt to maintain stability, a collar of Marlex mesh can also be introduced

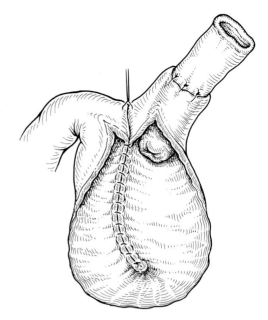

Figure 56.17
Intussusception of the nipple valve into the pouch of the continent ileostomy.

through an ileal window around the ileum at the base of the nipple valve. However, this modification is associated with a high incidence of fistulation,[82] and a strip of anterior rectus sheath may be better.[74]

Once the nipple valve has been constructed, the anterior wall of the reservoir is closed transversely, again using a single layer of continuous serosubmucosal sutures (Figure 56.19). The lateral aspect of the base of the nipple valve is then sutured to the lateral aspect of the trephine, the exit conduit is brought through the trephine, and the medial aspect of the nipple valve is also sutured to the trephine. To finish, the exit conduit is cut flush with the skin and sutured in place with interrupted mucocutaneous sutures (Figure 56.20).

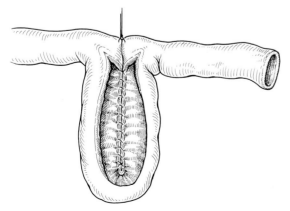

Figure 56.16
Construction of the posterior wall of the continent ileostomy pouch.

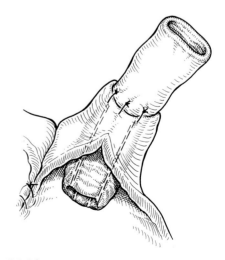

Figure 56.18
Stabilization of the nipple valve by the placement of four staple lines.

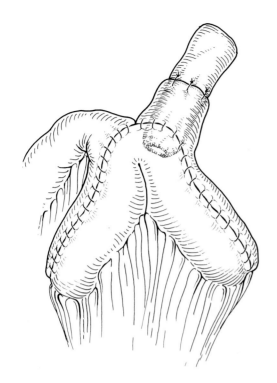

Figure 56.19
Pouch of the continent ileostomy completed.

Postoperative care

As soon as the pouch has been constructed and sutured into place, a Medina catheter is inserted into the pouch and saline is introduced. The catheter is then withdrawn to test the continence of the nipple valve. If this is satisfactory, the catheter is reinserted and the fluid drained, and the catheter is sutured to the abdominal wall so that it is retained at the optimum position within the pouch. A catheter bag is then attached to the catheter.

In the postoperative period the catheter is irrigated with 50 ml saline every 6 hours to prevent occlusion, and on about the third day faeculent material will be seen in the effluent. Oral fluids are then commenced, followed by light diet. Throughout the first week the catheter is kept on free drainage, and the irrigations are continued. The catheter can then be occluded for 3-hour periods, and if the patient can tolerate this, the catheter can be withdrawn and 3-hourly catheterizations started. The patient must then develop a catheterization pattern with increasing periods between catheterizations until a comfortable and convenient routine is established.

Long-term management

The aim of the continent reservoir ileostomy is to provide a stoma that is completely continent of gas and ileostomy effluent and that requires no more than a simple dressing, so that it is invisible beneath all but the most flimsy clothing. Obviously the pouch has to be emptied by catheterization, but this should not be necessary at night and should only be required 3–4 times during the day.

Emptying of the pouch is effected by inserting a lubricated Medina catheter to a depth that will have been worked out in the postoperative period, based on the operative findings. The patient stands in front of a basin or other receptacle, and if the catheter becomes blocked by food particles it can either be irrigated while in situ or removed and washed. the whole process should take no longer than 15 minutes, and it can be assisted by gentle movement of the catheter and suprapubic pressure.

Complications

Complications of the continent ileostomy that are seen in the immediate postoperative period are related to ischaemia and leakage, whereas the longer-term complications tend to be related to the function of the pouch (Table 56.4).

Table 56.4 Complications of the Kock continent ileostomy

SHORT TERM	LONG TERM
1. Ischaemia of the exit conduit	1. Nipple valve dysfunction
2. Ischaemia of the nipple valve	2. Late fistulation
3. Leakage from the pouch	3. Late stricture
	4. Intubation injury
	5. Pouch volvulus
	6. Leakage
	7. Pouchitis

Short-term complications

Ischaemia of the exit conduit Ischaemia of the exit conduit can be due to constriction of the mesenteric vessels as they pass through the trephine or damage to the vessels during the skeletonization procedure. Ischaemia may result in frank gangrene of the efferent limb, requiring complete revision and perhaps sacrifice of the pouch. If the bowel recovers, late stenosis may be a problem.

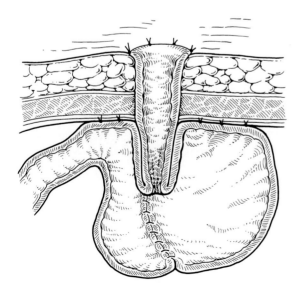

Figure 56.20
Cross-section of the completed Kock continent ileostomy in place.

Ischaemia of the nipple valve This is again due to problems with occlusion of the mesenteric blood supply. It may be caused by injudicious placement of a staple line too close to the intussuscepted mesentery. Complete necrosis will result in leakage with faecal peritonitis, requiring emergency laparotomy and loss of the pouch. If the intussuscepted portion alone sloughs, intestinal continuity will be preserved, but long-term function will of course be compromised.

Leakage from the pouch Catheter damage, suture line dehiscence or development of ischaemic patches may lead to the development of a faecal peritonitis or a faecal fistula. Peritonitis will require laparotomy; if the leakage is minor, local repair with proximal diversion by means of a loop ileostomy may salvage the pouch. A fistula will usually be associated with abscess formation, and although this is best treated by drainage and proximal diversion,[83] sump drainage alone may be effective.[84]

Long-term complications

Nipple valve dysfunction Dysfunction of the nipple valve results from complete desusception of the valve resulting in elongation and possible kinking of the efferent limb (Figure 56.21) or from slippage of the valve on its mesenteric aspect (Figure 56.22).[75] These structural problems lead to varying degrees of incontinence, difficulty in intubation and difficulty in emptying the pouch. Although less common since the introduction of the stapled valve, they can still defeat the object of the procedure.

When nipple dysfunction is suspected, the abnormality should be defined; this is best done by a double-contrast barium pouchogram.[85] It may also be possible to use a flexible sigmoidoscope to obtain a retroflex view of the valve. It may then

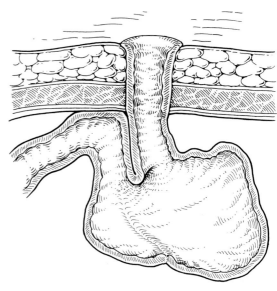

Figure 56.22
Slippage of the nipple valve on its mesenteric aspect.

be feasible to reconstruct the valve; the use of staples is invaluable in this context if they have not been used before.

Late fistulation Fistulation can occur directly from the pouch to the skin and present as peristomal discharge. Alternatively it may occur at the base of the nipple valve (Figure 56.23) and present as sudden incontinence in a patient who has had a previously satisfactory result.[86] Late fistulation can result from erosion of a foreign body, but must raise the suspicion of unrecognized Crohn's disease.

Late stricture Stenosis at the mucocutaneous junction can occur as a result of early ischaemia, or it may be the result of an exit conduit which is too short, especially in an obese patient. Dilatation may be effective but revisional surgery will be required for a long stricture.

Intubation injury Careless intubation may cause perforation of the pouch, with consequent faecal peritonitis. If laparotomy is carried out soon enough, it may be possible to repair the defect and raise a proximal loop ileostomy. In advanced cases, however, pouch sacrifice may be necessary.

Pouch volvulus Volvulus is a rare complication which can result in intermittent obstructive symptoms or ischaemic necrosis of the whole pouch.[87] It is probably due to inadequate fixation of the pouch to the anterior abdominal wall.

Leakage Frank incontinence is usually due to nipple valve dysfunction (see above), but excessive discharge of mucus is sometimes seen. This problem can be extremely troublesome as there is no spout, and it may require formal stoma care to protect the skin. Large amounts of mucus should alert one to the possibility of pouchitis or unrecognized Crohn's disease.

Pouchitis As in pelvic ileal pouches, pouchitis can be a major problem. In the patient with a continent ileostomy, it presents as an influenza-like illness associated with abdominal pain and high volumes of watery effluent on catheterization. It is

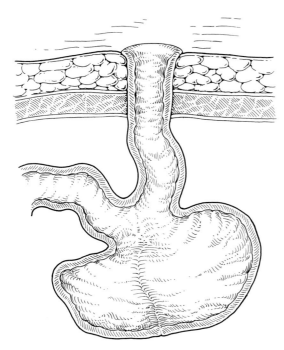

Figure 56.21
Complete desusception of the nipple valve in a continent ileostomy.

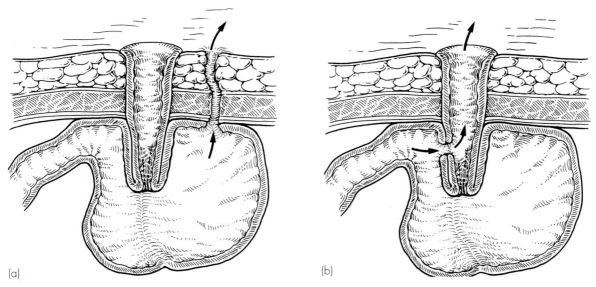

(a)   (b)

Figure 56.23

Fistulation in association with a Kock's continent ileostomy: (a) from pouch to skin; (b) through base of nipple valve.

thought to be due to an overgrowth of anaerobic bacteria within the pouch,[8] specifically *Bacteroides fragilis*. This concept is supported by the rapid resolution of pouchitis seen with metronidazole therapy,[88,89] and by the finding that patients with asymptomatic pouchitis develop vitamin B_{12} deficiency similar to that seen in the blind-loop syndrome.[90,91]

Pouch endoscopy should be performed on any patient suspected of having pouchitis, and this will show an inflamed mucosa which is often haemorrhagic. Histology is non-specific, but villous atrophy is often seen.[88] Treatment consists of continuous pouch drainage to relieve stasis plus metronidazole therapy.

ILEAL PELVIC POUCH

Indications

Ileoanal anastomosis after proctocolectomy ('restorative' proctocolectomy) has been an important surgical goal for many years. It was first seriously attempted by Ravitch,[92] but owing to the high incidence of incontinence, disabling frequency and septic complications, progress in this field was slow until it was realized that some form of reservoir was necessary to achieve acceptable results. Sir Alan Parks was the first to develop this concept; using a triplicate or S ileal pouch, he produced the first series of ileoanal anastomoses with pelvic ileal reservoir.[63,93] The main long-term problem was inability to evacuate the pouch without catheterization, but it was later found that this was related to the length of the efferent spout.[94]

There have been major advances since these early days, and most interested centres now regard restorative proctocolectomy as the surgical treatment of choice for a substantial proportion of patients with ulcerative colitis.[95] It has also been used in megacolon, intractable chronic idiopathic constipation and familial adenomatous polyposis, although many would regard colectomy and ileorectal anastomosis as preferable in

the latter two situations. As in the case of the Kock continent ileostomy, known Crohn's disease represents an absolute contraindication to restorative proctocolectomy because of an unacceptable complication rate, particularly fistulation (see also Chapter 51).[96,97]

Given that ulcerative colitis is the primary indication for restorative proctocolectomy, it is important to compare it with the two other surgical options, namely panproctocolectomy with end ileostomy and colectomy with ileorectal anastomosis. The most obvious advantage of a pelvic pouch over an ileostomy is the avoidance of a stoma. There is good evidence that most patients who have experienced an ileostomy before the formation of a pouch prefer the latter for psychological, social and practical reasons.[98,99] The restorative procedure also avoids a perineal wound; as primary healing of such a wound is by no means the rule,[100] this is an important consideration. Panproctocolectomy, even with intersphincteric rectal excision, is also associated with an appreciable incidence of sexual dysfunction,[101] whereas, in men at least, this is very rare after restorative proctocolectomy,[102,103] Related to this problem is the high incidence of persistent difficulties with micturition after conventional proctocolectomy, which is not seen with pouch formation.[104] These findings are probably due to a lesser degree of nerve and pelvic floor damage when the anal canal is left intact during the course of the operation.

Ileorectal anastomosis after colectomy for ulcerative colitis has been fairly widely used, but this is associated with a continuing risk of developing cancer in the rectal stump[105] – a problem that is all but eliminated with a pouch.[106] There is no evidence that bowel frequency after ileorectal anastomosis is any less than with a pouch, and, indeed, the reverse may be true.[107] Continuing or recurrent proctitis may also be troublesome,[53] and patients with a retained rectum require medication more frequently than pouch patients for this reason.[107] There is good reason, therefore, to prefer a pelvic pouch to an ileorectal anastomosis, and most authorities now take this view.

Technique

The techniques used to perform restorative proctocolectomy are varied, and for the purposes of this chapter we shall deal with them under several headings. Firstly, it is important to consider patient selection and counselling, as without these even the best technician will fail to obtain uniformly good results. We shall then cover the timing of the operation in relation to severity of disease, methods of excising the rectum, the rationale of mucosectomy and the different types of reservoir that are currently constructed. Finally, a reasonably detailed account of the formation of a J pouch and the pouch–anal anastomosis will be provided.

Patient selection and counselling

The main contraindication to restorative proctocolectomy, as discussed above, is any clinical, radiological or histological evidence of Crohn's disease. In addition, a previous small bowel resection will lead to intractable diarrhoea, and a patient with weak anal sphincters will find control very difficult. Age itself is not a contraindication,[108] but assessment of anal function by manometry and electromyography should be carried out in the elderly before reaching a decision. Colonic cancer complicating ulcerative colitis will deter many surgeons, but there is now good evidence that even rectal carcinomas can be treated in this way providing the tumour is mobile and above the sphincters.[109,110]

Before a patient makes a decision regarding a restorative proctocolectomy it is absolutely vital that the alternatives are discussed and the risks of the operation are fully explained. Only if the patient is still determined to go ahead after a full and frank discussion of this nature should the next steps be taken. A stomatherapist should see the patient, both for counselling and to mark a stoma site in case a loop ileostomy or even a permanent ileostomy is required. All patients should have the opportunity to meet a subject who has a functioning pouch, and it is ideal if they can also meet someone who has had a poor result.

Timing of the operation

There is some debate as to whether or not a restorative proctocolectomy should be performed at the same time as the initial colectomy. One of the arguments for not doing so is the possibility of missing Crohn's disease that is only discovered when the resected specimen is subjected to histological examination. Certainly, preoperative biopsy is not foolproof,[111] but even after careful examination of the resected specimen Crohn's disease may declare itself only in the patient's subsequent clinical course.[112]

Clearly, the sick patient who is undergoing an emergency colectomy for severe disease should have an end ileostomy and preservation of the rectum so that a pouch can be constructed at a later stage when the patient is fully recovered. It is also recommended that the patient should have been off steroid therapy for at least 3 months before pouch construction, and if there has been weight loss, this should be normalized. Thus, in many patients there will be a clear indication to carry out a simple colectomy, keeping the pouch in reserve for a later day.

Excision of the rectum

Excision of the rectum, whether it is done at the time of initial colectomy or not, is an important aspect of the whole operation of restorative proctocolectomy and deserves separate consideration. It is now recognized that the entire rectum can be removed to the level of the anorectal ring with preservation of continence and sensation,[113,114] and that preservation of a long tube of rectal muscle confers no benefit.[115] It is therefore likely that the necessary sensation is mediated by stretch proprioceptors in puborectalis or within the wall of the pouch itself.

For benign disease, excision of the mesorectum is not necessary for therapeutic reasons and, to avoid damage to the pelvic nerves and consequent sexual or bladder dysfunction, many surgeons employ a close rectal dissection, preserving the main rectal branch of the inferior mesenteric artery. This is a tedious and potentially bloody operation, however, and it is perfectly feasible to preserve the pelvic nerves by taking the rectum and mesorectum together and keeping to the avascular plane just outside the mesorectum. Those who advocate this approach report a very low incidence of impotence among their male patients.[116]

Mucosectomy

To obtain complete eradication of disease in ulcerative colitis it is necessary to remove the small amount of mucosa that is left above the dentate line after total rectal excision. It has to be said, however, that severe colitis rarely affects the mucosa that makes up the anal transitional zone 2–3 cm above the dentate line,[111] and excision of this zone may adversely affect anal sensation.[117] It may make sense, therefore, to try to preserve this short segment of mucosa, but it is technically easier with a hand sewn pouch–anal anastomosis to put the sutures into the dentate line, so that a total mucosectomy is necessary.[107]

With the advent of the stapled anastomosis, this argument has gone full circle yet again. Many surgeons now cross-staple the upper anal canal so that the transitional zone is preserved, and anal sensation is preserved.[118] From a functional point of view this approach seems to be better than an endoanal anastomosis constructed at the dentate line,[119] but whether this benefit is due to preservation of the transitional zone or related to the relatively prolonged period of anal dilatation required by the sewn anastomosis is open to debate.

Obviously, the main argument in favour of mucosectomy is reduction of cancer risk.[120] However, although the residual mucosa can undergo dysplastic change,[121] development of invasive cancer at this site has not been a clinical problem.

Types of reservoir

An ileal reservoir is basically constructed by plicating the terminal ileum into a multiple loop configuration, opening the anterior aspect of the plicated bowel, suturing (or stapling) the adjacent cut edges together to form the posterior wall of the pouch, and then suturing the free edges to complete the

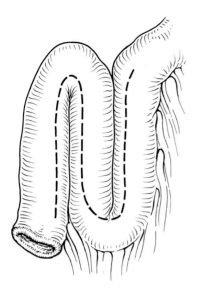

Figure 56.24
Configuration of ileum required for an S pouch. The dotted line shows the position of the enterotomy.

pouch. The first pouch to be used was the three limb or S pouch (Figure 56.24). Early experience with this construction indicated that a long efferent limb resulted in the need for intubation for evacuation in a substantial proportion of patients.[93,122] If an S pouch is to be used, therefore, there should be almost no efferent limb if good functional results are to be obtained.[112]

The two-limb J pouch[123] (Figure 56.25) has become by far the most popular, not least because it can be very simply and quickly constructed using a linear anastomosing stapler.[124] Good results have been generally reported with this pouch,[115,125] but there has been concern that the relatively small capacity makes frequency of defecation less satisfactory than with the S pouch.[122,126] Pouch volume does increase with time, however,[127]

and a progressive improvement of function of the J pouch is observed over 2 years.[128]

The quadruple W pouch (Figure 56.26) was designed to increase the volume of the reservoir without having an efferent limb,[129] and it has been suggested that frequency of defecation, night evacuation and the incidence of pouchitis are less than with other pouches.[130] In a randomized trial comparing W with J pouches, however, no differences in the functional results were seen,[131] even after long-term follow-up.[116]

Other forms of pouch have been used for ileoanal anastomosis, notably the lateral isoperistaltic H pouch[132] and a modification of the Kock pouch.[133] The reported results have been good, but neither of these procedures has gained wide acceptance.

Formation of a J pouch

For restorative proctocolectomy, the patient is positioned in the Lloyd-Davies position to allow good access to the anus. It is usual to make a long midline incision, although some surgeons prefer a transverse incision in the lower abdomen. If a colectomy has not been performed already, this should be done with particular attention to ligation of the blood supply, preserving the entire length of the ileocolic artery, and performing a peripheral ligation of the sigmoid vessels to avoid any damage to the sympathetic supply to the pelvis.

If a previous colectomy has been performed, the first step is to take down all the adhesions and fully mobilize the small bowel by division of the peritoneum over the lateral aspects of the duodenum and the duodenojejunal flexure. If this is not done, an adequate length of small bowel mesentery may not be achieved. The ileostomy must be carefully dissected from the abdominal wall, the spout turned back and the open end of the ileum closed by means of a clamp or staples.

The rectum is then excised as described above, mobilizing

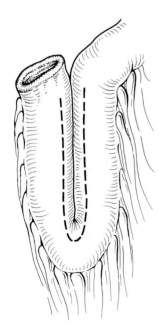

Figure 56.25
Configuration of ileum required for a J pouch.

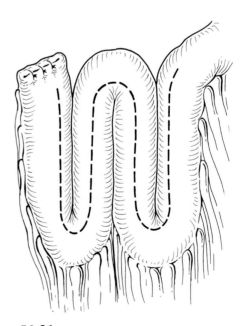

Figure 56.26
Configuration of ileum required for a W pouch.

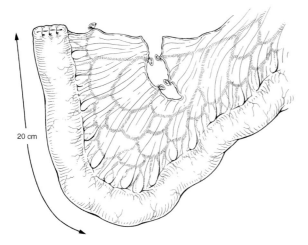

Figure 56.27

Extent of ileum required for J pouch, with typical vascular divisions.

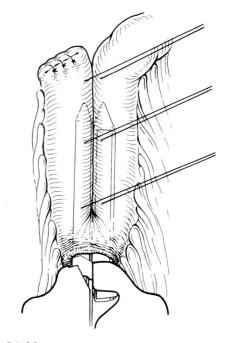

Figure 56.28

Stay suture holding the J loop in place with stapler inserted into J pouch.

the rectum and upper half of the anal canal after dividing Waldeyer's fascia. Before transecting the anal canal it is wise to place a clamp across the proposed site of anastomosis and to carry out a digital examination to check that it is at the correct level (2 cm above the dentate line). If a stapled anastomosis is to be carried out, the anal canal is transected by firing a linear stapler across the anal canal and cutting across just above it. Otherwise, the bowel is transected with scissors. It is also possible to carry out a complete mucosectomy at this stage by just cutting through the muscle of the rectum and excising the anal mucosa down to the dentate line in continuity with the rectum.

The apex of the J pouch should be 20 cm proximal to the closed end of the ileum (Figure 56.27). To obtain adequate length it may be necessary to divide some of the arterial supply, making sure that a good blood supply to the terminal ileum is preserved by the peripheral arcades. Once the appropriate length has been achieved, the J loop is formed, and a decision has to be made regarding a stapled or sewn anastomosis. This is largely down to personal preference, but stapling is certainly quicker.

If the pouch is to be stapled, three stay sutures are placed on the antimesenteric aspect of the bowel (Figure 56.28). A small enterotomy is then made at the apex of the pouch, and a long (75 or 90 mm) linear anastomosing stapler is inserted so that the two limbs of the stapler enter the adjacent bowel loops (Figure 56.28). The stapler is then fired after the bowel has been advanced as far as possible, but this will only complete a portion of the pouch. It is then necessary to reload the stapler, concertina the ileum over the stapler and fire it again. This manoeuvre is usually repeated twice with a 90 mm stapler and three times with a 75 mm device. A purse-string suture of 0 polypropylene is then inserted around the enterotomy, the proximal ileum is occluded with a soft bowel clamp and the pouch is filled with saline by means of a Foley catheter to check for leaks.

If a sewn pouch is preferred, the end of the ileum is oversewn with continuous 3/0 polydioxanone. The two limbs of

the pouch are then approximated with stay sutures, and a long enterotomy is made along the anterior aspect of the loop. Using a single layer of continuous serosubmucosal 3/0 polydioxanone, the posterior wall of the pouch is formed by suturing the adjacent ileal walls together (Figure 56.29). The anterior wall of the pouch is constructed by suturing together the remaining cut edges of ileum in the same way (Figure 56.30). An enterotomy is then made at the apex of the pouch, and leak testing is carried out as above.

When a stapled anastomosis is to be performed, a 28 or 29 mm anvil from a circular stapler is detached from the main instrument and inserted into the enterotomy of the pouch, and

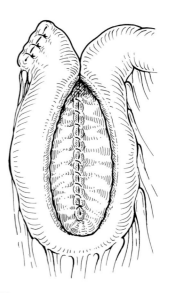

Figure 56.29

Posterior wall of J pouch completed by suturing.

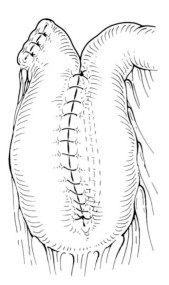

Figure 56.30
Completed sutured **J** pouch.

the purse-string suture is tightened (Figure 56.31). The head of the stapling device is then inserted into the cross-stapled anal stump so that the head impinges on the staple line. With the abdominal operator ensuring correct alignment of the head, the central pin is advanced so that it penetrates the centre of the staple line (Figure 56.32). When the central pin has been advanced to its full extent, the anvil shaft, which is now emerging from the apex of the pouch, is attached. The circular stapling device is then closed to the correct position (as shown on the thickness gauge) and fired. This manoeuvre applies two

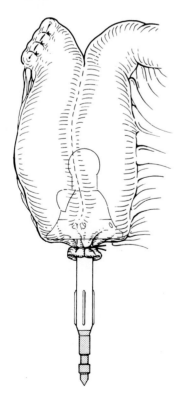

Figure 56.31
Detached stapler anvil in apex of **J** pouch.

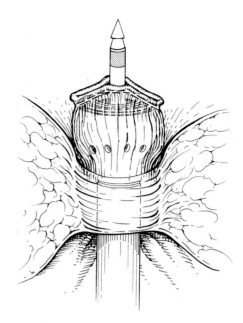

Figure 56.32
Head of stapling device in anal stump with central pin penetrating the staple line.

concentric staple rings and cuts a hole through the anal stump and the apex of the pouch within the inner ring. The stapling device is then opened, rotated gently to ensure that the blade has divided the bowel all the way round, and removed. The completeness of the resected bowel rings or 'doughnuts' is checked, and the anastomosis is palpated through the anus. To check finally for leaks, the pelvis can then be filled with saline and the pouch insufflated with air through the anus, with occlusion of the proximal ileum.

If a hand-sewn anastomosis is preferred, this must be done from within the anal canal (which of course will not have been stapled). An anal retractor is placed into the anal canal, and two stay sutures are placed on either side of the enterotomy at the apex of the pouch. If an abdominal mucosectomy has not been performed, this is now done by infiltrating 1 in 100 000 adrenaline solution in the submucosal plane and excising the mucosa above the dentate line with scissor dissection. The stay sutures are then passed through the anal canal, and the apex of the pouch is gently brought down to the dentate line (Figure 56.33). The edge of the enterotomy is then sutured to the dentate line with 10–12 interrupted sutures.

When the pouch anal anastomosis is complete, it is usual to place two suction drains in the pelvis to prevent the formation of a haematoma. Many surgeons will then routinely perform a defunctioning loop ileostomy, but if everything appears to be satisfactory after careful checking at the end of the procedure, some feel that this is unnecessary.[116] If a loop ileostomy is to be performed, the segment chosen must not place any tension on the pouch.

Complications

The short-term complications of a pelvic ileal reservoir are largely related to sepsis secondary to local problems with

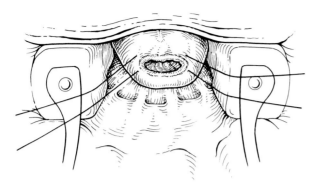

Figure 56.33

J pouch brought down into anal canal by stay sutures, ready for anastomosis.

healing and to intestinal obstruction. The longer-term complications are due to functional disorders of the pouch and the sequelae of the whole operation (Table 56.5).

Table 57.5 Complications of the pelvic ileal reservoir

SHORT TERM	LONG TERM
1. Bleeding	1. Incontinence
2. Pelvic sepsis	2. Sexual dysfunction
3. Fistula	3. Pouchitis
4. Stenosis	
5. Intestinal obstruction	

Short-term complications

Bleeding When bleeding from the pouch occurs soon after operation it is usually due to a vessel that has not been caught in the suture or staple line. It may also be due to suture line dehiscence and accompanying sepsis. If bleeding is encountered, a wide-bore Foley catheter should be placed into the pouch and left to drain, with regular irrigation to prevent blockage. If the bleeding does not settle, an examination under anaesthetic should be carried out, and any accessible bleeding point is sutured. As this is usually impossible, a balloon inflated within the pouch can control the situation. Occasionally, the pouch has to be taken down.

Pelvic sepsis Pelvic sepsis may be due to an infected haematoma or, more frequently, leakage from a pouch suture line or the ileoanal anastomosis. The patient will feel unwell, have a low-grade fever and may exhibit anal or vaginal purulent discharge. Under these circumstances an examination under anaesthetic should be carried out. If there is disruption of the ileoanal anastomosis it may be possible to drain the abscess by placing a catheter through the defect into the collection. If the collection is large, it is better to carry out a laparotomy, take down the pouch and drain the pelvis from above. Unless the pouch is badly damaged it is not necessary to sacrifice it, and it can be brought out as a mucous fistula for later reanastomosis.

Fistula Fistulas can occur between the pouch and the vagina, anal canal or skin. Although the fistula is often related to

anastomotic problems, it may take many months to declare itself, especially if a defunctioning ileostomy has been performed.[134] Fistulas between the pouch and the vulva usually result from the ileoanal anastomosis, whereas high pouch–vaginal fistulas may be secondary to pelvic sepsis, ischaemia, catching the vagina in the staple gun or unrecognized Crohn's disease. Low fistulas may be treated by fistulotomy if the sphincter mechanism is not compromised, but pouch advancement may be more satisfactory.[135]

Anal fistulas from the ileoanal anastomosis to the perineum can occur, and these can be managed by a fistulotomy or, if the external sphincters are involved, by a seton. Pouch–cutaneous fistula can often be managed by diverting the ileal content by a loop ileostomy and excising the fistula. If Crohn's disease is present, however, the pouch has to be removed and the patient given a permanent ileostomy.

Stenosis Stenosis at the pouch–anal junction is quite common, particularly if a loop ileostomy is used. It can be readily diagnosed by digital examination and treated by dilatation with a series of Hegar's dilators. Persistent stricture may be treated by pouch advancement,[135] but if this is not feasible the patient might require to intubate the pouch or even revert to ileostomy.

Intestinal obstruction Unfortunately, owing to the extensive nature of the operation, intestinal obstruction after restorative proctocolectomy is common. It is usually due to adhesions, but volvulus at the loop ileostomy site may be responsible.[136] Reoperation is avoided if possible, treating the patient with nasogastric suction and intravenous fluids or even total parenteral nutrition. If resolution does not occur within a week, however, or if the abdomen becomes tender, a laparotomy becomes necessary for fear of intestinal ischaemia.

Long-term complications

Incontinence and frequency Complete incontinence (where the patient cannot control the pouch effluent) is unusual, occurring in only about 3% of patients.[98] However, up to 34% of patients may be incontinent of flatus,[137] and soiling is very common, necessitating the use of a pad in around 50% of subjects.[98] Soiling is often associated with dermatological problems, and the patients may have excoriation and pruritus ani.[138]

Frequency of defecation is very variable and improves with time. On average, the patient can expect to have eight stools per day in the first month, six at 6 months and five by 9 months.[102] Although it is difficult to predict, frequency is inversely related to mouth-to-pouch transit times,[139] and the volume of the pouch is an important determinant.[128] Excessive stool frequency can be alleviated by constipating agents such as loperamide, diphenoxylate and ispaghula.

Sexual dysfunction Presumably owing to the avoidance of pelvic floor damage and the careful rectal dissection that accompanies pouch construction, sexual dysfunction in men is very rare.[98,107,115] Women, however, are more prone to sexual problems, mainly dyspareunia and leakage during intercourse.[128] Pregnancy is certainly not contraindicated with a pouch, but pregnant women often have increased frequency of defecation.

There has been some debate as to whether or not caesarean section is advisable to protect pouch function, but in fact vaginal delivery can be achieved in most patients without compromising continence.[140]

Pouchitis Pouchitis is inflammation of the ileal reservoir, and it affects about 35% of patients within 5 years of operation.[141] The aetiology is unknown, but it is thought that bacterial overgrowth in the pouch may be responsible. There is no definite evidence that the bacterial flora in pouchitis differs from that in the normal pouch,[142,143] but anaerobe counts correlate with the degree of inflammatory change in the pouch.[139] In addition, pouchitis exhibits a rapid clinical response to metronidazole, and such treatment is associated with a fall in the numbers of *Bacteroides* spp.[144,145]

It is also possible that ischaemia plays a part in the aetiology of pouchitis. There is evidence that mucosal blood flow is reduced in pouchitis,[146] and the subsequent development of the condition may be associated with low blood flow rates in the ileum at the time of operation.[116] Another theory is that pouchitis is, in fact, a form of the original disease process that caused the colitis. Colonic metaplasia is thought to occur in the pouch epithelium, and this allows the colitis to reassert itself.[147] Against this idea is the fact that pouchitis can affect patients who have had the operation for familial adenomatous polyposis,[148,149] and the risk of pouchitis is unrelated to the presence of backwash ileitis.[150]

The patient who develops pouchitis becomes pyrexial, feels generally unwell and has diarrhoea, often with blood. Not infrequently the patient will also suffer from some of the extraintestinal manifestations of colitis, such as arthritis, eye complications and skin problems.[141,151] A flexible sigmoidoscopy after an enema should be carried out, and biopsies taken. The appearances are of an oedematous and often haemorrhagic mucosa, and the biopsies show an acute inflammatory infiltrate, as opposed to the mild chronic inflammatory infiltrate which is normal in the healthy pouch.[152] It is also important for the pathologist to look for signs of Crohn's disease, and stool culture must be performed to exclude pathogens such as *Clostridium difficile* or *Campylobacter* spp.

Once the diagnosis has been made, the first-line therapy is metronidazole 200 mg three times daily; this treatment is effective in around 90% of patients. If it fails, then topical application of steroids may be helpful.[153] Systemic steroids may be required if the patient becomes unwell with extraintestinal manifestations.

THE STOMATHERAPIST AND THE STOMA CLINIC

Any surgeon whose practice involves stomas or pelvic ileal reservoirs should work closely with a qualified stomatherapist. A stomatherapist is a nurse who has been on an appropriate training course and who has a wide knowledge and experience of stoma care and the problems encountered by stoma and pouch patients. He or she must be skilled in communication with patients, relatives and medical and nursing colleagues, and must be prepared to give help and advice at all times.

The stomatherapist should interview the patient and relatives well before the operation, if possible, and find out about the severity of the illness and the social background. The stomatherapist will then provide a detailed explanation of the operation and its consequences, and arrange for the patient to meet someone who has had the procedure done already. The patient must then be introduced to the appliances and their function, and the stomatherapist will help the patient to find the ideal site for a stoma.

It is also important for the stomatherapist to see the patient immediately preoperatively so that the stoma site can be marked. This marking is very useful for the surgeon because it is impossible to estimate the ideal site in an anaesthetized patient who has not had preoperative counselling and marking. If at all possible, the surgeon should arrange for the stomatherapist to visit any emergency patient who is likely to require a stoma – a point that is often forgotten, to the detriment of the patient.

Although a proportion of the work is in the community, for the stomatherapist to operate efficiently it is best to have a formal stoma clinic in the hospital that generates the most work. Ideally, there should be secretarial support for answering the telephone, keeping records and making sure that communication with patients, relatives, general practitioners, district nurses and surgeons is adequate. The clinic may be run from the usual clinic rooms in the hospital, but this is not ideal because the nature of a stoma service is such that patients need to be seen at short notice at any time. It is therefore better to have a dedicated clinic area, and it may be best to have this situated close to the surgical gastroenterology wards so that the stomatherapist can be available for both ward-based and clinic-based problems without too much inconvenience.

The clinic itself should have at least one area with facilities for examination, washing and waste disposal. The area should be large enough for the patient to practice stoma care procedures, and it should have adequate ventilation to dispel odours. Nearby there should be a consultation area, which should be comfortable and have a relaxed atmosphere suitable for prolonged counselling sessions with patients and their relatives. A selection of the various appliances should be kept in this area for illustrative purposes, and it is very useful to have a blackboard and explanatory charts or diagrams.

Record-keeping can be a problem in a stoma clinic. If the main hospital records are used, these may not be available when needed, especially if the patients are offered open access to the clinic. It is therefore probably better for the clinic to keep its own records, which will be sufficient for continuing stoma care. Reordering stoma appliances can also be a problem for the patient, and the stoma clinic should carry a wide variety of appliances for emergencies, in addition to being able to issue prescriptions as appropriate. It should also be remembered that the cheapest appliances may not turn out to be economical if they do not suit the patient; it is therefore a false economy to stock a limited range.

Although a single stomatherapist can often manage the bulk of the work created by a stoma service and clinic, it has to be remembered that the commitment is continuous and help must be available 24 hours a day, 7 days a week. For this reason it is important for the stomatherapist to carry a pager or mobile telephone, and to arrange adequate cover by properly trained nurses. Although medical staff play a subsidiary role in the provision of a stoma service, it is crucial for the success of such an enterprise for an interested and experienced surgeon or group of surgeons to be involved and available to give surgical advice and help where necessary. However, when a stoma service covers a number of hospitals and the activity of a number of surgeons it is very important that the original operating surgeon is contacted whenever there are problems.

All patients should be put in contact with the voluntary associations that deal with stoma problems. While they do not suit everyone, these associations offer support to many thousands of stoma patients, offering counselling, advice on a wide variety of problems and a chance to meet other people with stomas. They also provide a home visiting service, and the stoma association visitor can play a crucial role in an individual's rehabilitation.

Addresses that are useful in this context are given below:

- The Ileostomy Association of Great Britain and Ireland
  Amblehurst House
  Black Scotch Lane
  Mansfield
  Nottinghamshire NG18 4PF

- The British Colostomy Association
  38/39 Eccleston Square
  London SW1V 1PB

- The United Ostomy Association
  1111 Wilshire Boulevard
  Los Angeles
  California 90017

- The International Ostomy Association,
  10 Carteret Street
  Queen Ann's Gate
  London SW1H 9DR

Although we have mentioned some specific products for stoma care, there are many other excellent products that we have not had space to detail. A comprehensive list is available in the *British National Formulary*, Appendix 8.

REFERENCES

1. Kennedy HJ, Lee EGS, Claridge G & Truelove SC. The health of subjects living with permanent ileostomy. *Q J Med* 1982; **203**: 341–357.
2. Phillips R, Pringle W, Evans C & Keighley MRB. Analysis of a hospital-based stomatherapy service. *Ann R Coll Surg Engl* 1985; **67**: 37–40.
3. Devlin HB. Stomas and stoma care. In Bouchier IA, Allan RN, Hodgson H & Keighley MRB (eds) *Textbook of Gastroenterology*. London: Baillière Tindall, 1981: 1009–1021.
4. Turnbull RB & Weekley FL. *An Atlas of Intestinal Stomas*. St Louis: CV Mosby, 1967: 97.
5. Devlin HB. Stoma therapy review (part II). *Coloproctology* 1982; **4**: 250–259.
6. Brooke BN. The management of an ileostomy including its complications. *Lancet* 1952; **ii**: 532–536.
7. Goligher JC. Extraperitoneal colostomy or ileostomy. *Br J Surg* 1958; **46**: 97–103.
8. Whistler RL. Exudate gums. In Whistler RL & Bemiller JN (eds) *Industrial Gums, Polysaccharides and Their Derivatives*, 3rd edn. New York: Academic Press, 1973: 318–326.
9. Evans G, Wood RAB & Hughes LE. Comparative trial of two enterostomy sealants. *BMJ* 1976; **1**: 1510–1511.
10. Beernaerts J, Bouffioux C, Chantrie M et al. The management of abdominal wall stomata skin, particularly peritoneal wound healing and support for the collecting bag. *Acta Chir Belg* 1977; **76**: 533–537.
11. Marks R, Evans E & Clarke TK. The effects on normal skin of adhesives from stoma appliances. *Curr Med Res Opin* 1978; **5**: 720–725.
12. Devlin HB & Plant HA. Disposal of disposable colostomy appliances. *BMJ* 1975; **4**: 705.
13. Hell LG & Pickford IR. A new appliance for collecting ileostomy and jejunostomy fluid in the postoperative period. *Br J Surg* 1979; **66**: 203–206.
14. Winslet MC, Alexander-Williams J & Keighley MRB. Ileostomy revision with a GIA stapler under intravenous sedation. *Br J Surg* 1990; **77**: 647.
15. Goldblatt MC, Corman ML, Haggitt RC, Coller JA & Veidenheimer MC. Ileostomy complications regarding revision: Lahey Clinic experience 1964–1973. *Dis Colon Rectum* 1977; **20**: 209–214.
16. Todd IP. The resolution of stoma problems. In Allan RN, Keighley MRB, Alexander-Williams J & Hawkins C (eds) *Inflammatory Bowel Disease*. London: Churchill Livingstone, 1983: 256–261.
17. Malt RA, Bartlett MK & Wheelock FC. Subcutaneous fasciotomy for relief of stricture of the ileostomy. *Surg Gynecol Obstet* 1984; **159**: 175–176.
18. Hulten L, Fasth S. Loop ileostomy for protection of the newly constructed ileostomy reservoir. *Br J Surg* 1981; **68**: 11–13.
19. Leslie D. The parastomal hernia. *Surg Clin North Am* 1984; **64**: 407–415.
20. Weaver RM, Alexander-Williams J & Keighley MRB. Indications and outcome of reoperations for ileostomy complications in inflammatory bowel disease. *Int J Colorectal Dis* 1988; **3**: 38–42.
21. Greatorex RA. Simple method of closing a paraileostomy fistula. *Br J Surg* 1988; **75**: 543.
22. Hamlyn AN, Lanzer MR, Morris JS et al. Portal hypertension with varices in unusual sites. *Lancet* 1974; **ii**: 1531–1534.
23. Beck DE, Fazio VW & Grundfest-Broniatowski S. Surgical management of bleeding stomal varices. *Dis Colon Rectum* 1988; **31**: 343–346.
24. Askerman NB, Graeber GM & Fey J. Enterstomal varices secondary to portal hypertension. *Arch Surg* 1980; **115**: 1154–1155.
25. Ricci RL, Lee KR & Greenberger NJ. Chronic gastrointestinal bleeding from ileal varices after total proctocolectomy for ulcerative colitis: correction of mesocaval shunt. *Gastroenterology* 1980; **78**: 1053–1069.
26. Clarke AM, Chirnside A, Hill GL & Pope G. Chronic dehydration and sodium depletion with established ileostomies. *Lancet* 1967; **ii**: 740–743.
27. Kennedy HJ, Al-Dujaili EAS, Edwards CRW & Truelove SC. Water and electrolyte balance in subjects with a permanent ileostomy. *Gut* 1983; **24**: 702–705.
28. Ladas SD, Isaacs PET, Murphy GM & Sladen GE. Fasting and postprandial ileal function in adapted ileostomates and normal subjects. *Gut* 1986; **27**: 906–912.
29. Hill GL, Mair WS & Goligher JC. Cause and management of high volume output salt-depleting ileostomy. *Br J Surg* 1975; **62**: 720–726.
30. Lennard-Jones JE. Effects of different drinks on fluid and electrolyte losses from a jejunostomy. *J R Soc Med* 1985; **78**: 27–34.
31. Feretis CB, Vyssoulis GP, Pararas BM et al. The influence of corticosteroids on ileostomy discharge of patients operated for ulcerative colitis. *Am Surg* 1984; **50**: 433–436.
32. Newton CR. Effect of codeine phosphate, Lomotil and Isogel on ileostomy function. *Gut* 1978; **19**: 377–383.
33. Tytgat GN & Huibregtse K. Loperamide and ileostomy output: placebo controlled double-blind crossover study. *BMJ* 1975; **2**: 667.
34. Cohen SE, Matolo NM, Michas CA & Wolfman EF Jr. Anti-peristaltic ileal segment in the prevention of ileostomy diarrhoea. *Arch Surg* 1975; **110**: 829–832.
35. Matolo NM & Wolfman EF Jr. Reversed ileal segment for treatment of ileostomy dysfunction. *Arch Surg* 1976; **11**: 891–892.
36. Kennedy HJ, Callender ST, Truelove SC & Warner GT. Haematological aspects of life with an ileostomy. *Br J Haematol* 1982; **52**: 445–454.
37. Scott R, Freeland R, Mowat W et al. The prevalence of calcified urinary tract stone disease in a random population: Cumbernauld Health Survey. *Br J Urol* 1977; **49**: 589–595.
38. Goligher JC. *Surgery of the Anus, Rectum and Colon*, 5th edn. London: Baillière Tindall, 1984: 912.

39. Gelzayd EA, Brener RI & Kirsner JB. Nephrolithiasis in IBD. *Am J Dig Dis* 1968; **13**: 1027–1034.
40. Bambach CP, Robertson WG, Peacock M & Hill GL. Effect of intestinal surgery on the risk of urinary stone formation. *Gut* 1981; **22**: 257–263.
41. Bennett RC & Hughes ESR. Urinary calculi and ulcerative colitis. *BMJ* 1972; **2**: 494–496.
42. Clarke AM & McKenzie RG. Ileostomy and the risk of urinary acid stones. *Lancet* 1969; **ii**: 395–397.
43. Hill GL, Mair WSJ & Goligher JC. Gallstones after ileostomy and ileal resection. *Gut* 1975; **16**: 932–936.
44. Cohen S, Kaplan M, Gottlieb C & Patterson J. Liver disease and gall stones in regional enteritis. *Gastroenterology* 1971; **60**: 237–245.
45. Dowling RH, Bell GD & White J. Lithogenic bile in patients with ileal dysfunction. *Gut* 1972; **13**: 415–420.
46. Jones MR, Evans GKT & Rhodes J. The prevalence of gallbladder disease in patients with ileostomy. *Clin Radiol* 1976; **27**: 561–562.
47. Kurchin A, Ray JE, Bluth EI et al. Cholelithiasis in ileostomy patients. *Dis Colon Rectum* 1984; **27**: 585–588.
48. Baker A, Kaplan MM, Norton A & Paterson J. Gallstone in inflammatory bowel disease. *Dig Dis Sci* 1974; **19**: 109–112.
49. Watts J McK, De Dombal FT & Goligher JC. Long term complications and prognosis following major surgery for ulcerative colitis. *Br J Surg* 1966; **53**: 1014–1023.
50. Burnham WR, Lennard-Jones JE & Brooke BN. Sexual problems among married ileostomists. Survey conducted by the Ileostomy Association of Great Britain and Ireland. *Gut* 1977; **18**: 673–677.
51. Leicester RJ, Ritchie JK, Wadsworth J, Thomson JPS & Hawley PR. Sexual function after intersphincteric excision of the rectum for inflammatory bowel disease. *Dis Colon Rectum* 1984; **27**: 244–248.
52. Devlin HB & Plant JA. Sexual function in aspects of stoma care. *Br J Sex Med* 1979; **6**: 33–37.
53. Jones PF, Munro A & Ewan SWB. Colectomy and ileorectal anastomosis for colitis: report on a personal series, with critical review. *Br J Surg* 1977; **64**: 615–623.
54. Gruner OPN, Nass R, Fretheim B & Gjone E. Marital status and sexual adjustment after colectomy. Results in 178 patients operated on for ulcerative colitis. *Scand J Gastroenterol* 1977; **12**: 193–197.
55. Hudson CN & Lennard-Jones JE. Sexual relationships and childbirth. In Todd IP (ed.) *Intestinal Stomas*. London: Heinemann, 1978: 200–220.
56. Bone J & Sorensen FH. Life with a conventional ileostomy. *Dis Colon Rectum* 1974; **17**: 194–199.
57. McLeod RS, Lavery IC, Leatherman JR et al. Patient evaluation. *Dis Colon Rectum* 1985; **28**: 152–154.
58. McLeod RS, Lavery IC, Leatherman JR et al. Factors affecting quality of life with a conventional ileostomy. *World J Surg* 1986; **10**: 474–480.
59. Whates PD & Irving M. Return to work following ileostomy. *Br J Surg* 1984; **71**: 619–622.
60. Turnbull RB & Weekley FL. Ileostomy techniques and indications for surgery. *Rev Surg Year Book* 1966; 310–314.
61. Alexander-Williams J. Loop ileostomy and colostomy for faecal diversion. *Ann R Coll Surg Engl* 1974; **54**: 141–148.
62. Avlett SO. 300 cases of diffuse ulcerative colitis treated by total colectomy and ileorectal anastomosis. *BMJ* 1966; **1**: 1001–1005.
63. Parks AG & Nicholls J. Proctocolectomy without ileostomy for ulcerative colitis. *BMJ* 1978; **1**: 85–88.
64. Raimes SA, Mathew VV & Devlin HB. Temporary loop ileostomy. *J R Soc Med* 1984; **77**: 738–741.
65. Fasth S, Hulten L & Palselius I. Loop ileostomy: an attractive alternative to a temporary transverse colostomy. *Acta Chir Scand* 1980; **146**: 203–207.
66. Williams NS, Masmyth DG, Jones D & Smith AH. Defunctioning stomas: a prospective controlled trial comparing loop ileostomy with loop transverse colostomy. *Br J Surg* 1986; **73**: 566–570.
67. Fazio VW. Invited commentary: loop ileostomy. *World J Surg* 1984; **8**: 405–407.
68. Shirley F, Kodner IJ & Fry RD. Loop ileostomy technique and indications. *Dis Colon Rectum* 1984; **27**: 382–386.
69. Utley RJ & Macbeth WAAG. The split ileostomy. *J R Coll Surg Edinb* 1984; **29**: 93–95.
70. Winslet MC, Droll Z, Allan A & Keighley MFB. Assessment of the defunctioning efficiency of the loop ileostomy. *Dis Colon Rectum* 1991; **34**: 699–703.
71. Kock NG, Intra-abdominal 'reservoir' in patients with permanent ileostomy. *Arch Surg* 1969; **99**: 223–231.
72. Golden HK. Psychiatric casualties following revision to the 'continent' Kock ileostomy. *Am J Dig Dis* 1976; **21**: 969–972.
73. Gelernt IM, Bauer JJ & Kreel I. The reservoir ileostomy: early experience with 54 patients. *Ann Surg* 1977; **185**: 179–184.
74. Falles DG. The continent ileostomy – an 11 year experience. *Aust N Z J Surg* 1984; **54**: 345–352.
75. Goldman SL & Rombeau JL. The continent ileostomy: a collective review. *Dis Colon Rectum* 1978; **21**: 594–599.
76. Kock NG, Myrvold HE, Nilsson LO et al. Construction of a stable valve for the continent ileostomy. *Ann Chir Gynaecol* 1980; **69**: 132–143.
77. Barker WF. A modification in the technique of making the Kock ileostomy pouch. *Surg Gynecol Obstet* 1978; **147**: 761–764.
78. Cranley B & McKelvey STD. The Kock ileostomy reservoir: an experimental study of methods of improving valve stability and competence. *Br J Surg* 1981; **68**: 545–550.
79. Kock NG, Myrvold HE, Nilsson LO & Philipson BM. Continent ileostomy. An account of 314 patients. *Acta Chir Scand* 1981; **147**: 67–72.
80. Cohen Z. Evolution of the Kock continent reservoir ileostomy. *Can J Surg* 1982; **25**: 509–514.
81. Steichen FM. The creation of autologous substitute organs with stapling instruments. *Am J Surg* 1977; **134**: 659–673.
82. Hulten L & Svaninger G. Facts about the Kock continent ileostomy. *Dis Colon Rectum* 1984; **27**: 553–557.
83. Halvorsen JF, Heimann P, Hoel R & Nygaard K. The continent reservoir ileostomy; review of a collective series of 36 patients from 3 surgical departments. *Surgery* 1978; **83**: 252–258.
84. Palmu A & Sivula A. Kock's continent ileostomy: results of 51 operations and experiences with correction of nipple valve insufficiency. *Br J Surg* 1978; **65**: 646–648.
85. Standertskjold-Nordenstam C-G, Palmu A & Sivula A. Radiological assessment of nipple valve insufficiency in Kock's continent reservoir ileostomy. *Br J Surg* 1979; **66**: 269–272.
86. Thompson JS & Williams SM. Fistula following continent ileostomy. *Dis Colon Rectum* 1984; **27**: 193–195.
87. Cranley B. The Kock reservoir ileostomy: a review of its development, problems and role in modern surgical practice. *Br J Surg* 1983; **70**: 94–99.
88. Kelly DG, Phillips SF, Kelly KA, Weinstein WM & Gilchrist MJR. Dysfunction of the continent ileostomy: clinical features and bacteriology. *Gut* 1983; **24**: 193–201.
89. Schjonsby H, Halvorsen JF, Hofstad T & Hovdenak N. Stagnant loop syndrome in patients with continent ileostomy (intra-abdominal ileal reservoir). *Gut* 1977; **18**: 795–799.
90. Varel VH & Bryant MP. Nutritional features of *Bacteroides fragilis* subsp. *fragilis*. *Appl Microbiol* 1974; **28**: 251–257.
91. Loeschke K, Balkert T, Kiefhaber P et al. Bacterial overgrowth in ileal reservoirs (Kock pouch): extended functional studies. *Hepatogastroenterology* 1980; **27**: 310–316.
92. Ravitch MM & Sabiston DC. Anal ileostomy with preservation of the sphincter. *Surg Gynecol Obstet* 1947; **84**: 1095–1109.
93. Parks AG, Nicholls RJ & Belliveau P. Proctocolectomy with ileal reservoir and anal anastomosis. *Br J Surg* 1980; **67**: 533–538.
94. Nicholls RJ. Restorative proctocolectomy with ileal reservoir. *Ann R Coll Surg Engl* 1983; **66**: 42–45.
95. Williams NS. Restorative proctocolectomy is the first choice elective surgical treatment for ulcerative colitis. *Br J Surg* 1989; **76**: 1109–1110.
96. Koltun WA, Schoetz DJ Jr, Roberts PL, Murray JJ, Coller JA & Veidenheimer MC. Indeterminate colitis predisposes to perineal complications after ileal pouch-anal anastomosis. *Dis Colon Rectum* 1991; **34**: 857–860.
97. Deutsch AA, McLeod RS, Cullen J & Cohen Z. Results of the pelvic-pouch procedure in patients with Crohn's disease. *Dis Colon Rectum* 1991; **34**: 475–477.
98. Wexner SD, Jensen L, Rothenberger DA, Wong WD & Goldberg SM. Long term functional analysis of the ileoanal reservoir. *Dis Colon Rectum* 1989; **32**: 275–281.
99. Skarsgard ED, Atkinson KG, Bell GA, Pezim ME, Seal AM & Sharp FR. Function and quality of life results after ileal pouch surgery for chronic ulcerative colitis and familial polyposis. *Am J Surg* 1989; **157**: 467–471.
100. Irvin TT & Goligher JC. A controlled clinical trial of three different methods of perineal wound management following excision of the rectum. *Br J Surg* 1975; **62**: 287–291.
101. Keighley MRB, Winslet MC, Pringle W & Allan RN. The pouch as an alternative to permanent ileostomy. *Br J Hosp Med* 1987; **35**: 286–294.

102. Cohen Z, McLeod RS, Stern H et al. The pelvic pouch and ileoanal anastomosis procedure: surgical technique and initial results. *Am J Surg* 1985; **150**: 601–607.

103. Dozois RR. Ileal **J** pouch–anal anastomosis. *Br J Surg* 1985; **72** (Suppl.): S80–S82.

104. Neal DE, Parker AJ, Williams NS & Johnston D. The long term effect of proctocolectomy on bladder function in patients with inflammatory bowel disease. *Br J Surg* 1982; **69**: 349–352.

105. Madden MV, Neale KF, Nicholls RJ et al. Comparison of morbidity and function after colectomy with ileorectal anastomosis or restorative proctocolectomy for familial adenomatous polyposis. *Br J Surg* 1991; **78**: 789–792.

106. Wiltz O, Hashmi HF, Schoetz DR Jr et al. Carcinoma and the ileal pouch–anal anastomosis. *Dis Colon Rectum* 1991; **34**: 805–809.

107. Nicholls RJ, Pescatori M, Motson RW & Pezim ME. Restorative proctocolectomy with a three loop ileal reservoir for ulcerative colitis and familial adenomatous polyposis. *Ann Surg* 1984; **199**: 383–388.

108. Perry TG, Strong SA, Fazio VW et al. Ileal pouch–anal anastomosis: is it ever too late? *Dis Colon Rectum* 1992; **35**: 14.

109. Strong SA, Oakley JR, Fazio VW, Lavery IC, Church JM & Milson JW. Ileal pouch–anal anastomosis: a safe option in advanced colon carcinoma. *Dis Colon Rectum* 1992; **35**: 22.

110. Fozard JBJ, Nelson H, Pemberton JH & Dozois RR. Primary ileal pouch–anal anastomosis and colorectal cancer – results and contraindications. *Dis Colon Rectum* 1992; **35**: 22.

111. Dixon JB & Riddell RH. Histopathology of ulcerative colitis. In Allan RN, Keighley MRB, Alexander-Williams J & Hawkins C (eds) *Inflammatory Bowel Disease*, 2nd edn. Edinburgh: Churchill Livingstone, 1990: 287–300.

112. Poppen B, Svenberg T, Bark T et al. Colectomy–proctomucosectomy with **S**-pouch: operative procedures, complications, and functional outcome in 69 consecutive patients. *Dis Colon Rectum* 1992; **35**: 40–47.

113. O'Connell PR, Pemberton JH & Kelly KA. Motor function of the ileal **J** pouch and its relation to clinical outcome after ileal pouch anal anastomosis. *World J Surg* 1987; **11**: 735–741.

114. Keighley MRB, Yoshioka K, Kmiot W & Heyen F. Physiological parameters influencing function in restorative proctocolectomy and ileo pouch anal anastomosis. *Br J Surg* 1988; **75**: 997–1002.

115. McHugh SM, Diamant NE, McLeod R & Cohen Z. **S** pouches vs **J** pouches. A comparison of functional outcomes. *Dis Colon Rectum* 1987; **30**: 671–677.

116. Keighley MRB. Restorative proctocolectomy and ileal pouch anal anastomosis. In Keighley MRB & Williams NS (eds) *Surgery of the Anus, Rectum and Colon*. London: WB Saunders, 1993: 1488–1591.

117. Miller R, Lewis GT, Bartolo DCC, Cervero F & Mortensen NJMcC. Sensory discrimination and dynamic activity in the anorectum: evidence using a new ambulatory technique. *Br J Surg* 1988; **75**: 1003–1007.

118. Lavery IC, Tuckson WB & Easley KA. Internal anal sphincter function after total abdominal colectomy and stapled ileal pouch anal anastomosis without mucosal proctectomy. *Dis Colon Rectum* 1989; **32**: 950–953.

119. Holdsworth PJ & Johnston D. Anal sensation after restorative proctocolectomy for ulcerative colitis. *Br J Surg* 1988; **75**: 993–996.

120. Ambroze WL, Pemberton JH, Dozois RR & Carpenter HA. Does retaining the anal transition zone (ATZ) fail to extirpate chronic ulcerative colitis (CUC) after ileal pouch–anal anastomosis (IPAA)? *Dis Colon Rectum* 1991; **34**: 20 (abstract).

121. Schmitt SL, Wexner SD, James K, Lucas F, Nogueras JJ & Jagelman DG. The fate of retained mucosa after non-mucosectomy ileoanal reservoir. *Dis Colon Rectum* 1992; **35**: 13.

122. Nicholls RJ & Pezim ME. Restorative proctocolectomy with ileal reservoir for ulcerative colitis and familial adenomatous polyposis: a comparison of 3 reservoir designs. *Br J Surg* 1985; **72**: 470–474.

123. Utsunomiya J, Iwama T, Imajo M et al. Total colectomy, mucosal proctectomy and ileoanal anastomosis. *Dis Colon Rectum* 1980; **23**: 459–466.

124. Taylor BA & Dozois RR. The **J** ileal pouch anal anastomosis. *World J Surg* 1987; **11**: 727–734.

125. Taylor BM, Beart RW, Dozois RR, Kelly KA, Wolff BG & Ilstrup DM. The endorectal ileal pouch–anal anastomosis: current clinical results. *Dis Colon Rectum* 1984; **27**: 347–350.

126. Williams NS & Johnston D. The current status of mucosal proctectomy and ileo-anal anastomosis in the surgical treatment of ulcerative colitis and adenomatous polyposis. *Br J Surg* 1985; **72**: 159–168.

127. Chaussade S, Michopoulos S, Hautefeuille M et al. Clinical and physiological study of anal sphincter and ileal pouch before preileostomy closure and 6 and 12 months after closure of loop ileostomy. *Dig Dis Sci* 1991; **36**: 161–167.

128. Oresland T, Fasth S, Norkgren S & Hulten L. The clinical and functional outcome after restorative proctocolectomy. A prospective study in 100 patients. *Int J Colorectal Dis* 1989; **4**: 50–56.

129. Nicholls RJ, Moskowitz RL & Shepherd NA. Restorative proctocolectomy with ileal reservoir. *Br J Surg* 1985; **72**: S76–S79.

130. Nicholls RJ & Lubowski DZ. Restorative proctocolectomy: the four loop **W** reservoir. *Br J Surg* 1987; **74**: 564–566.

131. Keighley MRB, Yoshioka K & Kmiot W. Prospective randomised trial to compare the stapled double lumen pouch and the sutured quadruple pouch for restorative proctocolectomy. *Br J Surg* 1988; **75**: 1008–1011.

132. Fonkalsrud EW. Update on clinical experience with different surgical techniques of the endorectal pull-through operation for colitis and polyposis. *Surg Gynecol Obstet* 1987; **165**: 309–316.

133. Kock NG, Hulten L & Myrvold HE. Ileoanal anastomosis with interposition of the ileal 'Kock pouch'. Preliminary results. *Dis Colon Rectum* 1989; **32**: 1050–1054.

134. Keighley MRB, Grobler S & Bain I. An audit of restorative proctocolectomy. *Gut* 1993; **34**: 680–684.

135. Fazio VW & Tjandra JJ. Pouch advancement and neoileoanal anastomosis for anastomotic stricture and anovaginal fistula complicating restorative proctocolectomy. *Br J Surg* 1992; **79**: 694–696.

136. Marcello PW, Roberts PL, Schoetz DJ Jr, Murray JJ, Coller JA & Veidenheimer MC. Obstruction after ileal pouch–anal anastomosis (IPAA) – a preventable complication? *Dis Colon Rectum* 1992; **35**: 12.

137. Pescatori M, Mattana C & Castagneso M. Clinical and functional results after restorative proctocolectomy. *Br J Surg* 1988; **75**: 321–324.

138. Moller P, Lohmann M & Brynitz S. Cholestyramine ointment in the treatment of perianal skin irritation following ileoanal anastomosis. *Dis Colon Rectum* 1987; **30**: 106–107.

139. Santavirta J. Lactulose hydrogen and [¹⁴C]xylose breath tests in patients with ileoanal anastomosis. *Int J Colorectal Dis* 1991; **6**: 208–211.

140. Nelson H, Dozois RR, Kelly KA, Malkasian GD, Wolff BG & Ilstrup DM. The effect of pregnancy and delivery on the ileal pouch–anal anastomosis functions. *Dis Colon Rectum* 1989; **32**: 384–388.

141. Lohmuller JL, Pemberton JH, Dozois RR, Ilstrup D & Van Heerden J. Pouchitis and extraintestinal manifestations of inflammatory bowel disease after ileal pouch–anal anastomosis. *Ann Surg* 1990; **211**: 622–629.

142. O'Connell PR, Rankin DR, Weiland LH & Kelly KA. Enteric bacteriology, absorption, morphology and emptying after ileal pouch–anal anastomosis. *Br J Surg* 1986; **73**: 909–914.

143. Nasmyth DG, Godwin DGR, Dixon MF et al. Ileal ecology after pouch–anal anastomosis or ileostomy: a study of mucosal morphology, fecal bacteriology, fecal volatile bile acids and their interrelationship. *Gastroenterology* 1989; **96**: 817–824.

144. Luukkonen P, Valtonen V, Sivonen A, Sipponen P & Jarvinen H. Faecal bacteriology and reservoir ileitis in patients operated on for ulcerative colitis. *Dis Colon Rectum* 1988; **31**: 864–867.

145. Tytgat GNJ & Van Deventer SJH. Pouchitis. *Int J Colorectal Dis* 1988; **3**: 226–228.

146. Perbeck L, Lindquist K & Liljeqvist L. The mucosal blood flow in pelvic pouches in man. A methodological study of fluorescein flowmetry. *Dis Colon Rectum* 1985; **28**: 931–936.

147. Lerch MM, Braun J, Harder M et al. Postoperative adaptation of the small intestine after total colectomy and pouch–anal anastomosis. *Dis Colon Rectum* 1989; **32**: 600–608.

148. Kmiot WA, Williams MR & Keighley MRB. Pouchitis following colectomy and ileal reservoir construction for familial adenomatous polyposis. *Br J Surg* 1990; **77**: 1283.

149. Madden MV, Farthing MJG & Nicholls RJ. Inflammation in ileal reservoirs: 'pouchitis'. *Gut* 1990; **31**: 247–249.

150. Gustavsson S, Weiland LH & Kelly KA. Relationship of backwash ileitis to ileal pouchitis after ileal pouch–anal anastomosis. *Dis Colon Rectum* 1987; **30**: 25–28.

151. Nicholls RJ, Belliveau P, Neill M, Wilks M & Tabaqchali S. Restorative proctocolectomy with ileal reservoir: a pathophysiological assessment. *Gut* 1981; **22**: 462–468.

152. Moskowitz RL, Shepherd NA & Nicholls RJ. An assessment of inflammation in the reservoir after restorative proctocolectomy with ileoanal ileal reservoir. *Int J Colorectal Dis* 1986; **1**: 167–174.

153. Rauh SM, Schoetz DJ Jr, Roberts PL, Murray JJ, Coller JA & Veidenheimer MC. Pouchitis – is it a wastebasket diagnosis? *Dis Colon Rectum* 1991; **34**: 170–187.

57

SMALL BOWEL DIVERTICULA

MG Wyatt
MJ Cooper

A small bowel diverticulum is an abnormal outpouching from the bowel wall and can be either congenital or acquired.

Congenital diverticula contain all three layers of the bowel wall and are considered to be 'true diverticula', developing from an embryonic structure. The most common example of this condition is a Meckel's diverticulum, which develops from the vitellointestinal or omphalomesenteric duct. More rarely, duplication of the gut can form a true diverticulum, the most common site being in the ileum.

Acquired or 'false' diverticula consist of mucosal and submucosal pouches only, and their walls contain no muscle. Although the definitive mechanism of formation is not known, most are considered to be pulsion diverticula due to some form of deranged intestinal motility. They tend to develop at sites of weakness in the muscle wall, where blood vessels (vasa brevia) pierce the muscularis. Traction diverticula are rare outside the oesophagus.

Acquired diverticula can also develop secondary to long-standing ulceration and fibrosis, i.e. in the duodenal cap of patients with chronic peptic ulceration. Patients with Crohn's disease can also develop these lesions in the distal small bowel. Secondary diverticula consist of all three layers of the bowel wall and are simply the result of adjacent cicatrization.

MECKEL'S DIVERTICULUM

Incidence and position

Meckel's diverticulum is a true diverticulum of the midgut and was first described by Johann Friedrich Meckel[1] in 1809. It arises from embryonic failure of regression of the omphalomesenteric (vitellointestinal) duct. This duct connects the primitive intestinal loop of the midgut with the exterior and usually becomes completely involuted by the end of the fifth week of gestation. When the duct persists in its entirety, an omphalomesenteric fistula is formed which opens externally at the umbilicus. Obliteration at the midgut end results in the formation of an umbilical sinus, and if both ends are obliterated an umbilical cyst or intra-abdominal enterocystoma develops. By far the most common remnant of the omphalomesenteric

duct is the Meckel's diverticulum, a partial persistence of the proximal duct at the central portion of the embryonic midgut loop (Figure 57.1, see colour plate also).

About 90% of Meckel's diverticula are situated within the terminal 100 cm of ileum, but they have also been found more proximally in the small bowel up to a distance of 180 cm from the ileocaecal valve (see also Chapter 42).[2,3] In 10% of cases a fibrous band connects the apex of the diverticulum to the undersurface of the umbilicus (mesodiverticular band), or to the ileal mesentery.[3,4]

Meckel's diverticulum is the most frequent anomaly of the gastrointestinal tract. It is found in between 0.3 and 4% of autopsy series, although an average incidence of 2% is quoted in most texts.[5-10] It is more common in those possessing other congenital malformations, particularly oesophageal atresia, anorectal atresia or exomphalos (see also Chapter 62). The sex incidence is the same in most autopsy series, although there does appear to be a male preponderance to the development of complications.

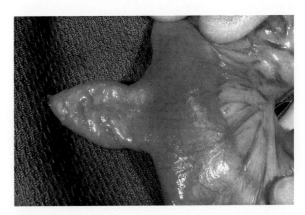

Figure 57.1
Meckel's diverticulum found incidentally at laparotomy in a child of 10 years. The diverticulum was resected uneventfully, although a wide-mouthed diverticulum such as this is unlikely to cause symptoms during life (photograph supplied by Professor RCN Williamson).

Pathology

Histologically this true diverticulum of the ileum is composed of all three layers of the gastrointestinal tract. In addition, in 30–50% of Meckel's diverticula the mucosa contains heterotopic tissue; in symptomatic cases this incidence may rise to 72%.[11,12] This heterotopic tissue takes the form of gastric, duodenal, jejunal or colonic epithelium, or occasionally pancreatic tissue (Figure 57.2) Gastric tissue is the most common variety (52%). The presence of aberrant gastric glands capable of producing both acid and pepsin under the same control mechanisms as for the stomach can be responsible for peptic ulceration within or adjacent to the diverticulum. Pancreatic tissue (5%) and a combination of the two (8%) are found less frequently, and in 35% ileal mucosa alone is present.[13] When present, heterotopic tissue usually lines the greater part of the diverticulum, often involving the neck of the pouch and frequently extending into the nearby ileum. The presence of ectopic mucosa is often the main risk factor in the development of the complications associated with Meckel's diverticula.[12]

Presentation

Most Meckel's diverticula remain asymptomatic and are incidental findings at autopsy (45%), at laparotomy (35%) or on barium studies of the small intestine (2%).[14] Only 4% ever become symptomatic and this figure diminishes with age.[15] The presenting features of the complications of Meckel's diverticulum are related to obstruction, inflammation, herniation, fistula formation, haemorrhage, neoplasia or malabsorption. Less frequently Meckel's diverticulum can present as intermittent or partial band obstruction or chronic peptic ulceration (dyspepsia Meckelii), resulting in a confusing clinical picture.[3]

Intestinal obstruction

The most common presenting feature of Meckel's diverticulum is intestinal obstruction, which occurs in approximately a third of symptomatic cases.[3,14,15] It may occur as a result of volvulus of the bowel, when the apex of the diverticulum is attached

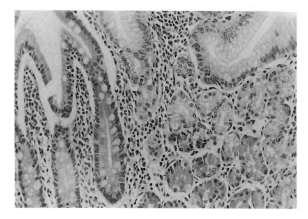

Figure 57.2

Photomicrograph of the wall of a Meckel's diverticulum showing ectopic gastric mucosa as well as normal ileal mucosa.

directly or via a fibrous omphalodiverticular band to the undersurface of the umbilicus. It can also occur due to entrapment of a bowel loop under a mesodiverticular band, inflammatory adhesions, intussusception or entrapment in a Littre's hernia.[6,9,11,14,16,17] On rare occasions calculi or faecoliths can form within the Meckel's diverticulum and, if dislodged, these can produce bolus obstruction (see also Chapter 53).[18,19]

The presentation is usually that of classical small bowel obstruction with abdominal pain, distension and vomiting and can be confirmed on plain radiological examination. Typically there is no obvious underlying cause for the obstruction. However, when intussusception occurs, overt small bowel obstruction is often absent and the diagnosis is not immediately apparent.[20,21]

Involvement of a Meckel's diverticulum in an external hernia is not uncommon.[14,22] It was first described by Littre in 1742 and has been described in all age groups. It has a male predominance, is especially common on the right and is found in approximately 1 in 200 groin hernias.[23] The majority (50%) are found within inguinal hernias, with femoral and umbilical hernias accounting equally for 40% of cases. Although small bowel obstruction can be the presenting feature, intestinal obstruction is fairly uncommon in association with a Littre's hernia, unless the hernia strangulates or the ileum becomes wrapped around the hernial neck.[24]

Haemorrhage

A 'peptic ulcer' of the ileum or diverticulum close to a patch of ectopic gastric mucosa may bleed. This can result in severe haemorrhage, especially if a remnant of the vitellointestinal artery (which crosses the base of the diverticulum) becomes eroded. Approximately 25% of patients with symptomatic Meckel's diverticula will have lower gastrointestinal haemorrhage. It is the most common cause of severe intestinal bleeding in childhood, half of these patients being under 2 years of age.[14] The usual presentation is with episodes of painless rectal bleeding with characteristically dark-red blood.[17] A previous history of gastrointestinal bleeding can be elicited in 40% of patients, but in some the initial bleed is so brisk as to be life threatening and rapid diagnosis is essential (see also Chapter 54).[25]

Inflammation

Meckel's diverticula can become inflamed and give rise to symptoms not dissimilar to those of acute appendicitis. However, the percentage of acute inflammation in a Meckel's diverticulum is considerably lower than in the appendix, due to both the wide-mouthed neck of the Meckel's diverticulum and the relative lack of lymphoid tissue, resulting in more efficient self-emptying.[16]

When acute inflammation does occur in a Meckel's diverticulum it is usually secondary to neck obstruction due to oedema, enteroliths, tumours, foreign bodies or ectopic mucosa.[26] The signs and symptoms are often difficult to distinguish from acute appendicitis, although characteristically the tenderness is more central and there may occasionally be cellulitis of the umbilicus.[3]

Perforation is a common complication of diverticulitis, but it may also be precipitated by enteroliths, foreign bodies (e.g. fish bones) or peptic ulceration with respect to ectopic gastric mucosa (see also Chapter 54).[27]

Tumours

Tumours related to Meckel's diverticulum are uncommon and occur in only 2% of cases.[3] Pathologically they can be either small bowel in type or can arise in ectopic mucosal elements within the diverticulum. Malignant tumours are three times more common than benign lesions (see also Chapters 58 and 60). They may present with intussusception or volvulus,[28-30] but by far the majority are incidental findings at post mortem or laparotomy.[31]

Carcinoids can also develop within a Meckel's diverticulum but are usually small (<1 cm),[31-33] occurring at a mean age of 55 years. They are four times as common in men and rarely metastasize or produce the carcinoid syndrome (see also Chapter 59).

Other rare tumours include malignant melanoma, neurovascular hamartoma, leiomyoma and leiomyosarcoma.[29,34-38]

Fistula

Complications related to the omphalomesenteric duct may also occur. Usually this problem will present as a fistula in a newborn child with a mucoid, purulent or faecal discharge and excoriation around the umbilicus (see also Chapter 62).[14] Occasionally fistulas can appear in adult life, when they usually develop from an area of recurrent periumbilical cellulitis or a deep-seated abdominal wall abscess representing an infected enterocystoma.

Miscellaneous

Other rare presentations of Meckel's diverticulum include malabsorption and exomphalos.[39]

Diagnosis

The diagnosis of a Meckel's diverticulum is often difficult and is usually made at laparotomy or autopsy. Plain abdominal radiographs are unhelpful, unless they confirm the presence of intestinal obstruction.[23] Barium studies are usually unhelpful, with only about 1–2% of diverticula diagnosed incidentally on follow-through examinations. This low figure is usually due to inadequate visualization of the suspect area because of overlying barium-filled loops.[40] However, in cases of intussusception, the diagnosis is readily made if a filling defect can be observed.[17] If a Meckel's diverticulum is complicated by haemorrhage, superior mesenteric artery angiography can be of use (see also Chapter 45).[40,41] Usually extravasation of contrast or a slight blush can be demonstrated, although the latter can be misinterpreted as a leiomyoma[17] (Figure 57.3; Figure 57.4, see colour plate also).

Perhaps the most accurate way of diagnosing a Meckel's diverticulum is to use scintigraphic methods.[42] The technique requires the use of ^{99m}Te-pertechnetate and is able to demonstrate the ectopic gastric mucosa within these diverticula. The pertechnate anion is selectively taken up and excreted into the

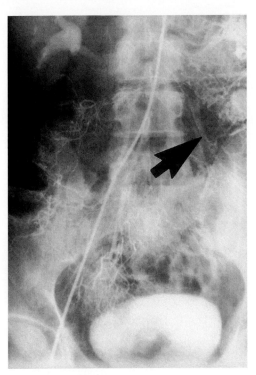
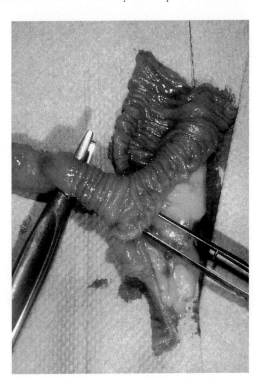

Figure 57.3 and Figure 57.4

A 55-year-old man had recurrent episodes of colicky abdominal pain. He showed evidence of iron-deficiency anaemia with stools that were persistently positive for occult blood. Visceral angiography (Figure 57.3) shows a blush in the mid small bowel that was interpreted as a leiomyoma. At operation the bleeding lesion proved to be an invaginated Meckel's diverticulum (Figure 57.4), which had led to ulceration of the mucosa and intussusception into the ileum.

lumen of the diverticulum by the mucoid cells that line the surface of the ectopic gastric mucosa (Figure 57.5).

A technetium or Meckel's scan will show up a Meckel's diverticulum containing ectopic gastric mucosa as a 'hot' spot in the lower abdomen, often on the right of the midline. Although false-negative and false-positive results do occur, primarily due to renal tract obstruction, angiomas or leiomyomas, the sensitivity of a Meckel's scan in the detection of ectopic gastric mucosa in a bleeding Meckel's diverticulum is 85%, with a specificity of 95% and on accuracy of 90%. This test is now the method of choice for the diagnosis of a Meckel's diverticulum.[43]

Meckelian diverticulectomy

The role of meckelian diverticulectomy in the treatment of an asymptomatic Meckel's diverticulum found incidentally at laparotomy is controversial. Although many surgeons have advocated routine excision, there is as yet no consensus view among British surgeons. As over 75% of Meckel's diverticula are found incidentally at laparotomy, there is a great need for accurate surgical guidelines.[44]

It has been calculated that to prevent one death it would be necessary to remove 800 uncomplicated Meckel's diverticula. Attempts have thus been made to define which diverticula are most at risk of developing complications. Such risk factors include bands, ectopic tissue, enteroliths and narrow necks. The age of the patient is also of use, and a suggested working policy is that diverticulectomy should only be considered for a diverticulum with the above risk factors found incidentally in a young child.[23] However, when a wide-mouthed diverticulum with no band or palpable ectopic tissue is found in an adult, it should be left alone.

For a complicated Meckel's diverticulum, resection is always required. Occasionally an acute bleed may be controlled with H₂-receptor antagonists, but this is uncommon and emergency operation is usually indicated.

The technique of diverticulectomy usually involves simple excision and closure in layers in either the transverse or oblique axis of the ileal lumen.[23] Care is taken to identify, ligate and divide the diverticular artery which arises from the ileal mesentery. Occasionally ileal resection is required, usually when the base of the diverticulum is wide but also in cases of diverticulitis with adjacent ileal inflammation or for malignancy. Ligation–excision and invagination of the stump as for appendicectomy is not recommended as the neck is usually too wide and can initiate intussusception.

DUODENAL DIVERTICULUM

Diverticula of the duodenum are of two types, intraluminal and extraluminal.

Intraluminal diverticula

These were first described by Boyd[45] in 1845 and are extremely rare. The sac is congenital and lined with duodenal mucosa. It lies entirely within the lumen, often adjacent to the ampulla of Vater. Its embryonic development is not yet established, and it is regarded by some as a variety of duodenal diaphragm rather than a diverticulum in its own right. On barium examination, it appears as a pear-shaped, intraluminal, barium-filled abnormality; it has been likened to a 'wind sock or the thumb of a glove'.[46]

Extraluminal diverticula

This type of duodenal diverticulum is relatively common and usually acquired. It may be primary or secondary in nature.

Primary extraluminal duodenal diverticula are generally found in the elderly, and most are located on the inner or medial wall of the second part of the duodenum. They usually arise at sites of weakness in the duodenal wall, presumably at the site of entry of blood vessels or around the common bile duct as it runs within the duodenal wall. Endoscopic retrograde cholangiopancreatography (ERCP) can be difficult in the presence of these lesions, as the ampulla of Vater often lies on the edge of the diverticulum or buried in its depths (Figure 57.6, see colour plate also). Although usually solitary, they can be multiple or multilocular and are a coincidental finding in 2–5% of barium meals.[47,48] At autopsy this incidence can reach 22%.[49]

Secondary extraluminal duodenal diverticula are almost always the result of long-standing peptic ulceration with its associated chronic scarring and fibrous deformity. They are usually found in the duodenal cap and present with the complications of peptic ulceration. An unusual case in which the

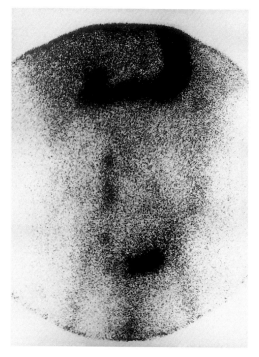

Figure 57.5
Technetium scan showing a pool of isotope in the lower midline region of the abdomen, consistent with a Meckel's diverticulum. The isotope is taken up by the ectopic gastric mucosa in the diverticulum but also by the orthotopic gastric mucosa in the stomach, which explains the black shadow in the upper abdomen.

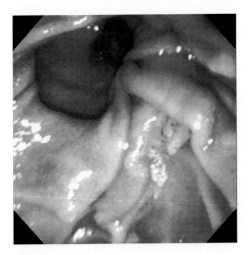

Figure 57.6
Endoscopic photograph showing a large duodenal diverticulum that arises in the typical position in the medial wall just above the papilla.

diverticulum arose on the lateral wall of descending duodenum at the site of a previous incision is shown in Figure 57.7 (see colour plate also).

Presentation

Although most duodenal diverticula are asymptomatic, some may present with vague symptoms of weight loss, nausea, vomiting and abdominal pain or discomfort. Major complications are rare, but when they occur the mortality rate is high (33%).[50] This high figure is probably because the patients are old, but it may also reflect delayed diagnosis due to failure to recognize the importance of this condition.

Perforation

Perforation is one of the most common complications of duodenal diverticula and tends to occur retroperitoneally,

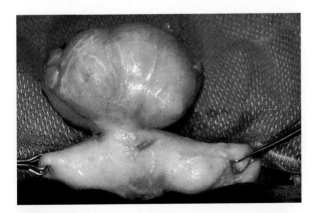

Figure 57.7
A large diverticulum on the antimesenteric border of the descending duodenum was found at laparotomy in a 68-year-old woman with chronic epigastric pain after meals. There was a healed incision in the bowel at this site following an obscure operation forty years earlier (photograph supplied by Professor RCN Williamson).

producing an oedematous bile-stained phlegmon (with oedema and emphysema) lateral to the duodenum.[51] The condition can develop into an abscess and can be identified on an abdominal radiograph by a small fluid level in the vicinity of the duodenum. Intraperitoneal perforation either produces biliary peritonitis or fistulation into an adjacent structure such as the small bowel, colon or gall bladder.

The mechanism of perforation is usually stasis. It results from erosion of an enterolith through the thin mucosal and submucosal wall of the diverticulum. Peptic ulceration and acute diverticulitis are less frequently implicated. Although duodenal diverticulitis is uncommon, when it does occur it presents with epigastric symptoms of inflammation which are easily mistaken for peptic ulceration, cholecystitis or pancreatitis. Although in most cases there are no pathognomonic signs of duodenal diverticulitis, subsequent perforation can present with erythema of the flanks;[52] this is readily mistaken for the discoloration found in acute pancreatitis (Grey Turner's sign). Failure to recognize such a perforation is the main cause of death from duodenal diverticula.[47]

Perforation can occur as a complication of endoscopic sphincterotomy. If the ampulla lies adjacent to or within a diverticulum, the muscle wall of the duodenum may be deficient, and if sphincterotomy is attempted the risk of perforation is high.

Haemorrhage

Haemorrhage from a duodenal diverticulum is usually severe and life-threatening.[53] The common cause is bleeding from an area of ulceration and erosion into an adjacent artery, such as the gastroduodenal. Although repeated small bleeds can occur, they are usually not recognized as originating from such lesions, but may be the cause of chronic gastrointestinal blood loss resulting in an iron deficiency anaemia of unknown aetiology.

Obstruction

Duodenal diverticula can be associated with obstruction to the duodenum and small intestine, or to the pancreatic or common bile ducts. Intraluminal duodenal diverticula can fill with food debris and directly occlude the lumen of the duodenum. Although extraluminal diverticula rarely obstruct locally, large enteroliths can occasionally be extruded into the bowel lumen and cause downstream bolus obstruction, usually in the mid-ileum.

When a diverticulum lies in the vicinity of the ampulla of Vater, both bile and pancreatic duct obstruction can occur due directly to kinking, or blockage by food debris or enteroliths. Obstruction results in either obstructive jaundice or acute pancreatitis, and these complications can even occur in association with an intraluminal diverticulum.[54] Chronic pancreatitis has also been recorded in association with an intraluminal diverticulum and an annular pancreas.[55] In addition, patients with diverticula in the second part of the duodenum have a higher incidence of gallstones when compared with the general population. The explanation for this fact is uncertain,[56] but it may relate to dysmotility of the adjacent bile duct.

Metabolic disturbances

Rarely duodenal diverticula can become extensively colonized by bacteria, with resultant metabolic abnormalities.[57,58]

Diagnosis

Duodenal diverticula are usually diagnosed by barium studies or at endoscopy. A barium meal will clearly delineate both intraluminal and extraluminal diverticula, and side-viewing scopes are excellent for examining the interior of these diverticula in the search for bleeding points or enteroliths.

The diagnosis of perforation of a diverticulum is usually made at operation unless the presence of such diverticula is already known. The diagnosis is often confused with that of a perforated duodenal ulcer or acute pancreatitis. A plain abdominal radiograph may be helpful if it shows free gas or a localized collection of retroperitoneal air relating to the upper pole of the right kidney or the duodenum.[59] A retroperitoneal phlegmon can often be shown on ultrasonography, but it is usually impossible to exclude the diagnosis of acute pancreatitis as an elevated serum amylase can occur in either condition.

Treatment

By far the majority of duodenal diverticula are asymptomatic, and treatment should be conservative. Only a minority will ever require surgical intervention. Intraluminal diverticula may cause duodenal obstruction and should be treated either surgically or endoscopically.[60] Surgical treatment usually involves subtotal resection of the diverticulum via a duodenotomy with preservation of the ampulla.[61] Alternatively endoscopic resection can be attempted using a diathermy snare to evert and resect the apex of the diverticulum.[62]

Extraluminal diverticula should only be treated if complications ensue. Perforation usually requires resection, but when this is not possible a tube duodenostomy can be performed.[63] If difficulty is encountered in closing the perforation without narrowing the lumen, a Roux-en-Y loop of jejunum may be constructed over the defect.

In patients with obstruction of the common bile duct a choledochoduodenostomy or choledochojejunostomy should be performed. If the patient has gallstones, cholecystectomy and exploration of the common bile duct is inadequate[64,65] because in 85% of patients the disease will recur if the diverticulum is left in situ.[66] In these patients, if excision is impractical, a duodenojejunostomy can be performed.[67] The procedure involves dividing the duodenum just distal to the pylorus, closing the distal end and anastomosing the proximal end to a Roux loop of jejunum. In this way, the diverticulum is removed from the food stream, thus reducing the risk of recurrent cholangitis and pancreatitis caused by food debris.

In all cases of surgical treatment of duodenal diverticula, exposure can be greatly improved by initial kocherization of the duodenum. Often these lesions, which are situated on the medial wall of the duodenum, are difficult to visualize unless distended with air, fluid or food debris. If surgical excision is indicated, great care must be taken in identifying and preserving both the common bile duct and the ampulla before excision. Both the pancreatic and bile ducts should be cannulated before closure to ensure that they are not compromised. A two-layer closure of the duodenal wall is usual, and this may be reinforced by an omental patch.

JEJUNOILEAL DIVERTICULA

Jejunoileal diverticula have historically been regarded as rare and curious anomalies of little clinical significance.[68] Their first description is credited to Summerling in 1794,[69] and Osler[70] reported the initial series of patients in 1881. The first operation on a patient with jejunoileal diverticula was reported in 1906; this involved the resection of a section of jejunal diverticulosis for the treatment of intestinal obstruction.[71]

Incidence and distribution

Jejunoileal diverticula are acquired thin-walled sacs consisting of mucosa and submucosa. They are found on the mesenteric border of the small bowel. The diverticula are often associated with abnormal intestinal motility,[72] and the muscle of the adjacent jejunal wall can be hypertrophied.[73] They are usually multiple and are found in greatest number in the proximal jejunum. They tend to occur at the point in the jejunal wall where the vasa recta or vasa brevia pierce the muscle (Figure 57.8, see colour plate also). Often they can extend into the mesentery and may not be seen unless the jejunum is deliberately distended with air.[74] Only rarely is the ileum involved.[75] Jejunoileal diverticulosis is more common in men than in women (M : F = 2 : 1).[76,77] It is a disease of the elderly, showing an increasing incidence with age, and is rarely diagnosed before the age of 40 years.[76,78-81] The true incidence is difficult to ascertain. At autopsy an overall figure of 0.7% is quoted,[82] whereas the frequency of radiological detection ranges from 0.07 to 2.3%.[83-86]

Aetiology

Various theories have been proposed concerning the aetiology of these lesions. Baskin and Mayo[78] suggested that some could be congenital, and specifically that solitary diverticula in

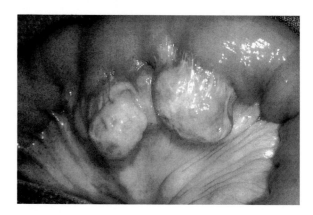

Figure 57.8
Multiple jejunal diverticula found incidentally at laparotomy in an elderly woman. The diverticula arose in the typical site on the antimesenteric border of the bowel.

younger patients may represent partial reduplication of the small bowel. The majority are acquired, especially when multiple and identified in patients over 40. It has been suggested that most diverticula begin as a pair of small pouches on either side of the mesentery where the vessels pierce the muscular and serosal coats. These pouches then enlarge and coalesce to form a single thin-walled diverticulum (Figure 57.9, see colour plate also). This outpouching may result from raised intraluminal pressure and deranged intestinal motility,[72] due possibly to visceral myopathy caused by abnormal small bowel function and structure.[87] In addition, some are secondary to small bowel pathology such as Crohn's disease, scleroderma and non-specific ulceration,[88] whereas some follow operative intervention.[86]

Presentation

Most patients with jejunal diverticula have no symptoms and no treatment is required. In about 40% of cases, patients present with chronic non-specific symptoms including abdominal discomfort, flatulence, borborygmi and pseudo-obstruction.[81] About 10% of patients experience complications requiring surgical intervention.[78] These complications include diverticulitis, perforation and peritonitis, intestinal obstruction, haemorrhage, stasis or 'blind-loop' syndrome, and in rare cases neoplastic transformation: fibroma, carcinoma and sarcoma.[86]

Diverticulitis and perforation

Approximately half of all the complications related to jejunal diverticulosis involve diverticulitis or perforation (see Chapter 54).[82,89] It is often difficult to separate these two conditions. Although perforation in the absence of inflammation is well recognized,[90,91] perforation in the presence of diverticulitis may be complicated by sequelae of the diverticulitis process itself, such as localized peritonitis and abscess formation[92,93] (Figure 57.10, see colour plate also).

In the absence of acute diverticulitis, jejunal diverticula perforation can be caused by enteroliths, parasitic overgrowth of foreign bodies.[73] The mortality of acute perforation can be 30%, making both early diagnosis and operative treatment vital if results are to be improved.

Occasionally spontaneous pneumothorax can be found

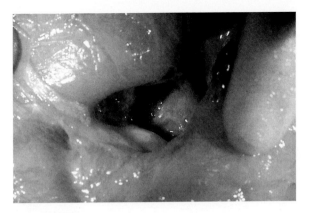

Figure 57.10
Operative findings in a patient with perforated jejunal diverticulitis (photograph supplied by Professor RCN Williamson).

without peritonitis.[94,95] This complication is thought to be due to the transmural passage of air through the semipermeable membrane of a thin-walled diverticulum, and it can complicate an otherwise uneventful gastrointestinal endoscopy.[96]

Intestinal obstruction

There are several mechanisms for the development of intestinal obstruction in the presence of jejunal diverticulosis (see also Chapter 53). The diverticulum may initiate an intussusception[97] or act as a pivot for a volvulus, especially if previous attacks of diverticulitis have produced an adhesion band.[23] Jejunal diverticulitis can also result in the formation of an extrajejunal peridiverticular adhesion, which may produce obstruction directly by kinking the involved segment of bowel, or indirectly by allowing a separate piece of bowel to become trapped and obstructed beneath the adhesion.[64,98]

Enteroliths may also be the cause of small bowel obstruction.[99] They are usually composed of choleic acid and cause obstruction either at the site of the diverticulum, or by migrating into the lumen and impacting distally to produce a bolus obstruction.[82,100–103]

Patients with jejunoileal diverticulosis can also present with chronic intestinal pseudo-obstruction[73] due to abnormal intestinal motility and an instrinsic muscular abnormality, rather than a mechanical blockage.[87] However, both the clinical and radiological picture make it difficult to identify these patients as they may present with abdominal pain and vomiting, have visible peristalsis on examination and show small bowel fluid levels and distension on abdominal radiographs.

Haemorrhage

Gastrointestinal haemorrhage from a jejunal diverticulum is rare and difficult to diagnose. Bleeding may be acute and severe[104] or chronic, presenting with vague symptoms of abdominal pain or an iron deficiency anaemia in the presence of normal endoscopy and barium studies of the large bowel.[23] Most patients present with melaena stool or an acute massive rectal bleed,[98,105,106] but haematemesis may also occur on occasions.[81,107] The pattern of bleeding is similar to that found in

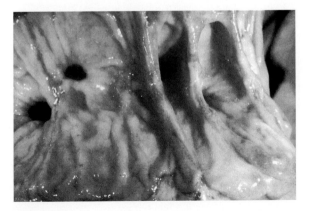

Figure 57.9
Mucosal aspect of a resected segment of jejunum showing multiple jejunal diverticula.

association with acute colonic diverticulitis,[92] and in a quarter of acute bleeds a history of chronicity before the major haemorrhage can be elicited (see also Chapter 54).[106]

Malabsorption

Patients with jejunal diverticula may present with symptoms attributable to malabsorption due to a 'blind-loop' or 'stagnant-loop' syndrome. The reasons why only some patients with jejunal diverticula develop this complication are unclear, but achlorhydria may permit jejunal colonization.[108]

In the normal jejunum the bacterial count is low (10^1–10^4 organisms/ml), whereas in the 'blind-loop' syndrome counts of up to 10^{12} organisms/ml have been reported.[109] Multiple organisms of varied type are found but the bacterial population resembles that of the colon, prompting Gracey[110] to refer to this condition as 'contaminated small bowel syndrome'.

As in other forms of blind-loop syndrome the metabolic products of bacterial overgrowth in the diverticula are thought to be toxic to the small bowel, thereby leading to malabsorption. Patients with this condition can have either steatorrhoea or anaemia, which is either macrocytic or microcytic, since malabsorption of both vitamin B_{12} and iron can occur. The steatorrhoea is caused by retention of intestinal contents in the diverticula, as well as 'functional stagnation' related to altered jejunal motility.[68] Other absorptive problems result in mineral deficiencies and oedema due to hypoproteinaemia.[111]

Diagnosis of 'blind-loop' syndrome depends on the finding of steatorrhoea (faecal fat elevated) and a low vitamin B_{12} level (see also Chapter 44). A lactulose hydrogen breath test can confirm bacterial overgrowth,[112] but it may give false-positive and false-negative results.[23] If the diagnosis is suspected, attempts should be made to demonstrate the jejunal diverticula. A trial of broad-spectrum antibiotics is indicated as this can relieve the chronic gastrointestinal symptoms, such as steatorrhoea, bloating and anaemia, that are associated with jejunal diverticulosis.[113,114]

Diagnosis

The diagnosis of jejunal diverticulosis is usually made by upper gastrointestinal barium studies as these lesions are inaccessible to standard endoscopes. Occasionally a plain abdominal radiograph may show multiple fluid levels in the jejunal diverticula (Figure 57.11), pneumoperitoneum in the case of perforation or a fluid level in an abscess. However, these appearances are not specific for jejunal diverticulosis, and laparotomy is often required to confirm the diagnosis.

The first antemortem demonstration of jejunal diverticula using barium follow-through examination was by Case[83] in 1920, and to the present day this has remained the first-line investigation. However, although most cases of jejunal diverticulosis are picked up by barium follow-through examination, many are missed.[86] Barium may not enter some small diverticula with narrow necks, and in others the diverticulum may be so large that the barium is not retained and the diverticulum rapidly empties. A refinement of the technique is enteroclysis, in which the lumen of the jejunum is distended, thus allowing

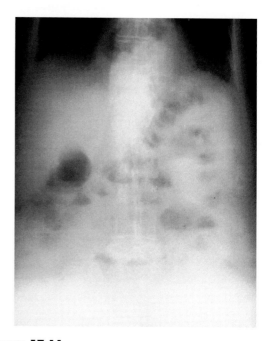

Figure 57.11
Erect abdominal x-ray showing multiple fluid levels in a patient with jejunal diverticulosis. The patient showed no clinical features of intestinal obstruction.

distension of even the smallest diverticulum. The technique of enteroclysis involves intubation of the duodenojejunal junction followed by instillation of barium and methylcellulose under pressure. Single-and double-contrast views of the bowel are obtained by continued insufflation of the bowel, usually with associated external pressure.[115] The use of this technique has resulted in a fourfold increase in the detection of jejunal diverticula, indicating that the prevalence of acquired jejunal diverticula is greater than previously reported.[86,116] Disadvantages of enteroclysis include both the need to intubate the small bowel and the inability to combine this method with upper gastrointestinal examination, as can be done with the standard small bowel follow-through study.

Other diagnostic techniques include selective mesenteric angiography and ^{99m}Tc–sulphur colloid scanning (see also Chapters 45 and 54). These are of use in cases of undiagnosed gastrointestinal blood loss, where gastroscopy and barium enema examination have been negative. For patients who are actively bleeding, selective mesenteric artery catheterization can detect a bleeding source providing that the rate of blood loss exceeds 0.5 ml/min.[117] For those with a blood loss of 0.1–0.5 ml/min, a ^{99m}Tc-labelled red cell scan detects bleeding with a high degree of accuracy.[118]

Treatment

For most asymptomatic jejunoileal diverticula found by chance at laparotomy, no treatment is required. For blind-loop syndrome, operation is only required if the condition is complicated by intestinal obstruction, perforation, diverticulitis haemorrhage or malignancy. In all other instances, the treatment of choice is broad-spectrum antibiotic therapy.

For complicated jejunal diverticulosis, simple excision with end-to-end anastomosis is the surgical treatment of choice.[64,119] When the diverticulosis is extensive and resection is not feasible, resection of individual diverticula is reasonable, particularly if bleeding or perforated areas can be identified. Unfortunately the involved diverticulum is not always easy to find and on some occasions a blind resection may be necessary.[120] In patients in whom blind resection is not possible (extensive disease), on-table endoscopy of the small bowel via a transverse enterotomy may be of benefit. Occasionally a peroral endoscope can be milked to the ileocaecal valve at laparotomy.

When jejunal diverticulitis is associated with intestinal obstruction, resection is usually indicated. Exceptions are band obstructions, which can usually be divided, and localized volvulus, which can be untwisted. Enteroliths should be removed locally,[103] and if pseudo-obstruction is suspected metoclopramide may be of use.[121]

REFERENCES

1. Meckel JF. Uber das Divertikel am Darmkanal. *Arch Physiol* 1809; **9**: 421–453.
2. Dowse JL. Meckel's diverticulum. *Br J Surg* 1961; **48**: 392–399.
3. Williams RS. Management of Meckel's diverticulum. *Br J Surg* 1981; **68**: 477–480.
4. Johns TN, Wheeler JR & Johns FS. Meckel's diverticulum and Meckel's diverticular disease. *Ann Surg* 1959; **150**: 241–256.
5. Christie A. Meckel's diverticulum: a pathological study of 63 cases. *Am J Dis Child* 1931; **42**: 544–557.
6. Harkins HH. Intussusception due to invaginated Meckel's diverticulum: report of two cases with a study of 160 cases collected from the literature. *Ann Surg* 1933; **98**: 1070–1095.
7. Kittle CF, Jenkins HP & Dragstedt LR. Patent omphalomesenteric duct and its relationship to the diverticulum of Meckel. *Arch Surg* 1947; **54**: 10–31.
8. Jay GD, Margulis RR, McGraw AR et al. Meckel's diverticulum: a survey of 109 cases. *Arch Surg* 1950; **61**: 158–169.
9. Seagram CG, Louch RE, Stephens A et al. Meckel's diverticulum; a 10 year review of 218 cases. *Can J Surg* 1968; **2**: 369–373.
10. Michas CA, Cohen SE & Wolfman EF. Meckel's diverticulum. *Am J Surg* 1975; **129**: 682–685.
11. Soderlund S. Meckel's diverticulum: a clinical and histological study. *Acta Chir Scand* 1959; **248**: 1–233.
12. Artigas V, Calabuig R, Badia F et al. Meckel's diverticulum: value of ectopic tissue. *Am J Surg* 1986; **151**: 631–634.
13. Gross RE. *The Surgery of Infancy and Childhood*. Philadelphia: WB Saunders, 1953.
14. Mackey WC & Dineen P. A fifty year experience with Meckel's diverticulum. *Surg Gynecol Obstet* 1983; **156**: 56–64.
15. Soltero MJ & Bill AH. The natural history of Meckel's diverticulum and the relation to incidental removal. *Am J Surg* 1976; **132**: 168–171.
16. Rutherford RB & Akers DR. Meckel's diverticulum: a review of 148 paediatric patients with special reference to the pattern of bleeding and to mesodiverticular bands. *Surgery* 1966; **59**: 618–626.
17. Williamson RC, Cooper MJ & Thomas WE. Intussusception of invaginated Meckel's diverticulum. *J R Soc Med* 1984; **77**: 652–655.
18. Moran KT, Flynn JR & McCormack M. Unusual presentation of a stone in a Meckel's diverticulum in association with acute appendicitis. *Irish Med J* 1985; **78**: 320–321.
19. Barr H. Meckel's diverticulum. *Br J Surg* 1986; **40**: 301–302.
20. Moore T & Johnston AO. Complications of Meckel's diverticulum. *Br J Surg* 1976; **63**: 453–454.
21. Yamagüchi M, Takeuchi S & Awazu S. Meckel's diverticulum. Investigation of 600 patients in Japanese literature. *Am J Surg* 1978; **136**: 247–249.
22. Weinstein EC, Cain JC & Remine WM. Meckel's diverticulum. *JAMA* 1962; **182**: 251–253.
23. Thomas WEG. Complications of small bowel diverticula. In Williamson RC & Cooper MJ (eds) *Emergency Abdominal Surgery*. Edinburgh: Churchill Livingstone, 1990; **13**: 191–208.
24. Payson BA, Schneider KM & Victor MB. Strangulation of a Meckel's diverticulum in a femoral hernia (Littre's). *Ann Surg* 1956; **144**: 277–281.
25. Long BW. Early diagnosis and management of bleeding Meckel's diverticulum. *J Miss State Med Assoc* 1986; **27**: 149–154.
26. Boothroyd IS. The odd Meckel's diverticulum. *Can Med Assoc J* 1967; **96**: 45–49.
27. Rosswick RP. Perforation of Meckel's diverticulum by foreign body. *Postgrad Med J* 1965; **41**: 105–107.
28. Lie JT. Leiomyosarcoma of Meckel's diverticulum. *Br J Surg* 1966; **53**: 336–339.
29. Niv Y, Abu-Avid S, Kopelman C et al. Torsion of leiomyosarcoma of Meckel's diverticulum. *Am J Gastroenterol* 1986; **81**: 288–291.
30. Sayfan J, Borowsky A, Halevy A et al. Volvulus due to a tumour of Meckel's diverticulum. *J Clin Gastroenterol* 1985; **7**: 314–317.
31. Jones EL, Thompson H & Alexander Williams J. Argentaffin tumour of Meckel's diverticulum. a report of 2 cases and review of the literature. *Br J Surg* 1972; **59**: 213–219.
32. Weitzner S. Carcinoid of Meckel's diverticulum. Report of a case and review of the literature. *Cancer* 1969; **23**: 1436–1440.
33. Payne-James JJ, Law NW & Watkins RM. Carcinoid tumour arising in Meckel's diverticulum. *Postgrad Med J* 1985; **61**: 1009–1011.
34. Hertzog MS, Chacko AK & Pitts CM. Leiomyoma of terminal ileum producing false positive Meckel's scan. *J Nucl Med* 1985; **26**: 1278–1282.
35. Blamey SL & Woods SD. Leiomyoma of Meckel's diverticulum. *Med J Aust* 1986; **45**: 232–234.
36. Saadia R & Decker GA. Leiomyosarcoma of Meckel's diverticulum: a case report and review of literature. *J Surg Oncol* 1986; **32**: 86–88.
37. Bloch T, Tejada E & Brodhecker C. Malignant melanoma in Meckel's diverticulum. *Am J Clin Pathol* 1986; **86**: 231–234.
38. Stewart IC. Neurovascular hamartoma in a Meckel's diverticulum. *Br J Clin Pract* 1985; **39**: 411–412.
39. Simms MH & Corkery JJ. Meckel's diverticulum: its association with congenital malformation and the significance of atypical morphology. *Br J Surg* 1980; **67**: 216–219.
40. Hall TJ. Meckel's bleeding diverticulum diagnosed by mesenteric arteriography. *Br J Surg* 1975; **62**: 882–884.
41. Faris JG & Whitley JC. Angiographic demonstration of Meckel's diverticulum: case report and review of literature. *Radiology* 1973; **108**: 285–286.
42. Jewett TC, Duszynski DO & Allen JE. The visualisation of Meckel's diverticulum with ^{99m}Tc pertechnetate. *Surgery* 1970; **68**: 467–470.
43. Petrokubi RJ, Baum S & Rohrer GU. Cimetidine administration resulting in improved pertechnetate imaging of Meckel's diverticulum. *Clin Nucl Med* 1978; **3**: 385–388.
44. Editorial. Meckel's diverticulum. Surgical guidelines at last? *Lancet* 1983; **ii**: 1438–1439.
45. Boyd R. Description of malformation of the duodenum. *Lancet* 1845; **i**: 648.
46. Silcock AQ. Epithelioma of ascending colon, entero-colitis, and congenital duodenal septum with internal diverticulum. *Trans Pathol Soc Lond* 1885; **36**: 207.
47. Neill SA & Thompson NW. The complications of duodenal diverticula and their management. *Surg Gynecol Obstet* 1965; **120**: 1251–1258.
48. Wilk PJ, Mollura J & Danese CA. Jaundice and pancreatitis caused by duodenal diverticulum. *Am J Gastroenteral* 1973; **60**: 273–279.
49. Ackerman W. Diverticula and variations of the duodenum. *Ann Surg* 1943; **117**: 403–413.
50. Munnell ER & Preston WJ. Complications of duodenal diverticula. *Arch Surg* 1966; **92**: 152–156.
51. Juler GL, List JW, Stemmer EA et al. Perforated duodenal diverticulitis. *Arch Surg* 1969; **99**: 572–578.
52. Stebbings WS & Thompson JP. Perforated duodenal diverticulum. A report of two cases. *Postgrad Med J* 1985; **61**: 839–840.
53. Sonnenfeld T, Alveryd A & Nyberg B. Jejunal diverticula causing massive haemorrhage. *Acta Chir Scand* 1986; **530**: 101–102.
54. Fleming CR, Newcomer AD, Stephens DH et al. Intraluminal duodenal diverticulum. Report of two cases and review of the literature. *Mayo Clin Proc* 1975; **50**: 244–248.
55. Hirsch F, Halet W & Piront A. Diverticule interne du duodenum: forme de duplication. *Arch Mal Appar Dig* 1964; **53**: 839–844.
56. Leinkram C, Roberts-Thompsons IC & Kune GA. Juxta papillary duodenal diverticula: association with gallstones and pancreatitis. *Med J Aust* 1980; **1**: 209–210.

57. Goldstein F, Cozzolino HJ & Wirts CW. Diarrhoea and steatorrhoea due to a large solitary duodenal ulcer. Report of a case. *Am J Dig Dis* 1963; **8**: 937–943.

58. Gorbach SL & Levitan R. Intestinal flora in health and in gastrointestinal disease. In Glass GBJ (ed.) *Progress in Gastroenterology*, vol. II. New York: Grune & Stratton, 1970; 252–270.

59. Wolfe RD & Pearl MJ. Acute perforation of duodenal diverticulum with roentgenographic demonstration of localised retroperitoneal emphysema. *Radiology* 1972; **104**: 301–302.

60. Adams DB. Management of the intraluminal duodenal diverticulum: endoscopy or duodenotomy. *Am J Surg* 1986; **151**: 524–526.

61. Howard JW, Wynn OB, Lenhart FM et al. Intraluminal duodenal diverticulum: an unusual cause of acute pancreatitis. *Am J Surg* 1986; **151**: 505–508.

62. Hajiro K, Yamamoto H, Matsui H et al. Endoscopic diagnosis and excision of intraluminal duodenal diverticulum. *Gastrointest Endosc* 1979; **25**: 151–154.

63. Beech RR, Friesen DL & Shield CF. Perforated duodenal diverticulum: treatment by tube duodenostomy. *Curr Surg* 1985; **42**: 462–465.

64. Donald JW. Major complications of small bowel diverticula. *Ann Surg* 1979; **190**: 183–188.

65. Manny J, Muga M & Eyal Z. The continuing clinical enigma of duodenal diverticula. *Am J Surg* 1981; **142**: 596–600.

66. Lotveit T, Osnes M & Larsen S. Recurrent biliary calculi – duodenal diverticulum as a predisposing factor. *Ann Surg* 1982; **196**: 30–32.

67. Critchlow JF, Shapiro ME & Silen W. Duodenojejunostomy for the pancreaticobiliary complications of duodenal diverticula. *Ann Surg* 1985; **202**: 56–58.

68. Wilcox RD & Shatney CH. Surgical implications of jejunal diverticula. *South Med J* 1988; **11**: 1386–1391.

69. Localio SA & Stahl WM. Diverticular disease of the alimentary tract. part II. *Curr Probl Surg* 1968; **5**: 1–47.

70. Osler W. Notes on intestinal diverticula. *Ann Surg* 1881; **4**: 202–207.

71. Gordinier HC & Samson JA. Diverticulitis (not Meckel's) causing intestinal obstruction. Multiple mesenteric (acquired) diverticula of the small intestine. *JAMA* 1906; **46**: 1463–1470.

72. Edwards HC. Intestinal diverticulosis and diverticulitis. *Ann R Coll Surg Engl* 1954; **14**: 371–388.

73. Phillips JH. Jejunal diverticulitis. Some clinical aspects. *Br J Surg* 1953; **40**: 350–354.

74. Welsh JD, Rohrer GV & Porter MG. The Baker–Hughes gastrointestinal biopsy tube. *Am J Dig Dis* 1966; **11**: 559–563.

75. Cocks JR & Zinco FJ. Acute diverticulitis of the terminal ileum. *Br J Surg* 1968; **55**: 45–49.

76. Rankin FW & Martin WJ. Diverticula of the small bowel. *Ann Surg* 1934; **100**: 1123–1135.

77. Benson RE, Dixon CF & Waugh JW. Nonmeckelian diverticula of the jejunum and ileum. *Ann Surg* 1943; **118**: 377–393.

78. Baskin RH & Mayo CW. Jejunal diverticulosis. A clinical study of 87 cases. *Surg Clin North Am* 1952; **32**: 1185–1196.

79. Williams RA, Davidson DD, Serota AI et al. Surgical problems of diverticula of the small intestine. *Surg Gynecol Obstet* 1981; **152**: 621–626.

80. Shackelford RT & Marcus WY. Jejunal diverticula – a cause of gastrointestinal haemorrhage. A report of three cases and review of the literature. *Ann Surg* 1960; **151**: 930–938.

81. Altemeier WA, Bryant LR & Wulsin JH. The surgical significance of jejunal diverticulosis. *Arch Surg* 1963; **86**: 732–744.

82. Geroulakis G. Surgical problems of jejunal diverticulosis. *Ann R Coll Surg Engl* 1987; **69**: 266–268.

83. Case JT. Diverticula of the small intestine other than Meckel's diverticulum. *JAMA* 1920; **75**: 1463–1470.

84. Caplan HH & Jacobson HG. Small intestine diverticulosis. *AJR* 1964; **92**: 1048–1060.

85. Parulekar SG. Diverticulum of terminal ileum and its complications. *Radiology* 1972; **103**: 283–287.

86. Maglinte DDT, Chernish SM, Deweese R et al. Acquired jejuno-ileal diverticular disease; subject review. *Radiology* 1986; **158**: 577–580.

87. Krishnamurthy S, Kelly MM, Rohrman CA et al. Jejunal diverticulosis. *Gastroenterology* 1983; **85**: 538–547.

88. Thomas WEG & Williamson RCN. Non-specific small bowel ulceration. *Postgrad Med J* 1985; **61**: 587–591.

89. Nobles ER. Jejunal diverticula. *Arch Surg* 1971; **102**: 172–174.

90. Herrington JL. Perforation of acquired diverticula of jejunum and ileum. *Surgery* 1962; **51**: 426–433.

91. Smith JS. Jejunal diverticula – subtle cause of acute abdomen. *Pa Med* 1976; **79**: 60–63.

92. Jones PF. Jejunal and ileal diverticula. In *Emergency Abdominal Surgery*. Oxford: Blackwell, 1974: 550–552.

93. Brown RJ & Thompson RL. Perforated jejunal diverticulum presenting with a psoas abscess. *Ulster Med J* 1985; **54**: 78–79.

94. Dunn Y & Nelson JA. Jejunal diverticula and chronic pneumoperitoneum. *Gastrointest Radiol* 1979; **4**: 165–168.

95. Madura MJ & Craig RM. Duodenal and jejunal diverticula causing a pneumo-peritoneum. *J Clin Gastroenterol* 1981; **3**: 61–63.

96. Brown MW, Brown RC & Orr G. Pneumoperitoneum complicating endoscopy in a patient with duodenal and jejunal diverticula. *Gastrointest Endosc* 1986; **32**: 120–121.

97. Soofi R & Abouchedid C. Intussusception of small bowel secondary to jejunal diverticulosis. *N Engl J Med* 1986; **83**: 309–312.

98. Eckhauser FE, Zelenok GB & Freider DT. Acute complications of jejuno-ileal pseudo-diverticulitis: surgical implications and management. *Am J Surg* 1979; **138**: 320–323.

99. King PM, Bird DR & Eremin O. Enterolith obstruction of the small bowel. *J R Coll Surg Edinb* 1985; **30**: 269–270.

100. Bewes PC. Surgical complications of jejunal diverticulosis. *Proc R Soc Med* 1967; **60**: 225–226.

101. Ottinger LW & Carter EL. Obstruction of the ileum by a jejunal diverticular enterolith. *Gastroenterology* 1975; **68**: 1596–1597.

102. Svanes K & Halvorsen JF. Enterolith obstruction of the ileum as a complication of jejunal diverticulosis. *Acta Chir Scand* 1975; **141**: 816–819.

103. Clarke PJ & Kettlewell MGW. Small bowel obstruction due to an enterolith originating in a jejunal diverticulum. *Postgrad J Med* 1985; **61**: 1019–1020.

104. Thomas CS, Tinsley E & Brockman SK. Jejunal diverticula as a source of massive upper gastrointestinal bleeding. *Arch Surg* 1967; **95**: 89–92.

105. Civetta JM & Daggett WM. Gastrointestinal bleeding from jejunal diverticula. *Ann Surg* 1967; **166**: 976–979.

106. Taylor MT. Massive haemorrhage from jejunal diverticulosis. *Am J Surg* 1969; **118**: 117–129.

107. Miller RE, McCabe RE, Salomon PF et al. Surgical complications of small bowel diverticula exclusive of Meckel's. *Ann Surg* 1970; **171**: 202–210.

108. Murray-Lyon IM, Finlayson NDC & Shearman DJC. Studies on two patients with concomitant intrinsic factor secretory defect and jejunal diverticulosis. *Scand J Haematol* 1968; **5**: 383–389.

109. Draser BS & Hill MJ. *Human Intestinal Flora*. London: Academic Press, 1974.

110. Gracey M. Intestinal absorption in the 'contaminated small bowel syndrome'. *Gut* 1971; **12**: 403–410.

111. Tabaqchali S & Booth CC. Bacteria and the small intestine. In Card WI & Creane B (eds) *Modern Trends in Gastroenterology*, vol. 4. London: Butterworth, 1970: 143.

112. Rhodes IM, Middleton P & Jewell DP. The lactulose hydrogen breath test as a diagnostic test for small bowel bacterial overgrowth. *Scand J Gastroenterol* 1979; **14**: 333–336.

113. Knaver M & Svoboda A. Malabsorption and jejunal diverticulosis. *Am J Med* 1968; **44**: 606–610.

114. Christiansen M. Jejunal diverticulosis. *Am J Surg* 1969; **118**: 612–618.

115. Maglinte DDT, Hall R, Miller RE et al. Detection of surgical lesions of the small bowel by enteroclysis. *Am J Surg* 1984; **147**: 225–229.

116. Salomonowitz E, Wittich G, Hajek P et al. Detection of intestinal diverticula by double contrast small bowel enema: differentiation from other intestinal diverticula. *Gastrointest Radiol* 1983; **8**: 271–278.

117. Balint JA, Sarfeh IJ & Fried MB. In *Gastrointestinal Bleeding: Diagnosis and Management*. New York: Wiley, 1977: 33–41.

118. Winzelberg GG, McKusick KA, Froelich JW et al. Detection of gastrointestinal bleeding with 99Tc labelled red blood cells. *Semin Nucl Med* 1982; **12**: 139–146.

119. McGrew V, Patel J & Miller P. Jejunal diverticulosis: medical and surgical management. *S Afr Med J* 1985; **78**: 533–535.

120. Thomas WEG & Williamson RCN. Enteric ulceration and its complications. *World J Surg* 1985; **9**: 876–886.

121. Albibi R & McCallum RW. Metoclopramide: pharmacology and clinical applications. *Ann Intern Med* 1983; **98**: 86–95.

58

BENIGN TUMOURS OF THE SMALL BOWEL

JGN Studley
RCN Williamson

The small bowel, comprising duodenum, jejunum and ileum, provides 75% of the length of the gastrointestinal tract and 80–90% of its absorptive surface.[1] The duodenum is approximately 25 cm in length and the jejunoileum 500 cm, of which 40% represents the jejunum and 60% the ileum, although the transformation between them is indistinct. The length of small bowel is extremely variable, however, from as little as 300 cm up to 850 cm (see also Chapter 42).[2]

Accepting these facts, one might predict that the majority of gastrointestinal neoplasms would arise from the small intestine. In reality the converse is true: tumours are rare in the small bowel but common in the oesophagus, stomach and colorectum, although the discrepancy is more pronounced for malignant lesions than it is for benign tumours.

Overall only 1.5–6.0% of all intestinal tumours arise in the small bowel.[3] Benign small bowel tumours are reported in 0.1–0.8% of post-mortem and surgical studies.[4] Within the small intestine there is a concentration of both benign and malignant tumours in the duodenum, which harbours approximately 20–25% of the total number.[3,5,6]

PRESENTATION

Small bowel tumours present predominantly in the sixth and seventh decades of life.[7] Mean time to diagnosis varies from 6 to 8 months.[7] Several reasons account for the delay in diagnosis: (1) difficulty in interpreting vague gastrointestinal symptoms; (2) the fact that small intestinal lesions are rare and may therefore be considered late; (3) the investigations that are available, with special reference to the jejunum and ileum, are not as definitive as those available for in the rest of the gastrointestinal tract (which is much more accessible to endoscopy).

In contrast to malignant lesions, which almost all become symptomatic with time, over 50% of benign lesions are asymptomatic and are found incidentally during radiological investigations or at laparotomy or post-mortem.[7] Some tumours present with features of obstruction or haemorrhage.[6] The remainder fall into the elusive group of those with vague gastrointestinal symptoms.[6]

Among symptomatic patients, *obstruction* is reported in 40–70% of cases.[8,9] Recurrent episodes may occur, and the obstruction can be either partial or complete.[6] The mechanism leading to obstruction is usually a local mass effect, but sometimes the tumour predisposes to the development of an intussusception.[8] In 80% of adults with intussusception a clear-cut causative lesion will be found,[10] which is a much greater proportion than in children (see Chapter 62).

Haemorrhage occurs in 20–50% of symptomatic patients (see also Chapter 54).[8,9,11,12] Occult bleeding is much more common than major haemorrhage.[6] It is important to keep this presentation in perspective as over 90% of cases of gastrointestinal haemorrhage will originate from the oesophagus, stomach, duodenum or large bowel, and these sources of bleeding must be considered initially.[13]

A variety of *vague symptoms* has been reported: loss of energy, loss of weight, nausea, a feeling of fullness, dyspepsia and upper abdominal discomfort.[8] It is these non-specific symptoms that are often associated with a delay in diagnosis.

Tumours in the periampullary region may present with *obstructive jaundice* or *acute pancreatitis*.[14] Other unusual presentations include a palpable abdominal mass[6] and tumours that perforate, form fistulas or cause intraperitoneal haemorrhage.[9]

Skin changes are sometimes associated with small intestinal abnormalities: café au lait spots with neurofibromatosis, telangiectasia in Osler–Weber–Rendu syndrome and mucocutaneous pigmentation in Peutz–Jegher's syndrome.

INVESTIGATION

The diagnosis of small bowel lesions has been described fully in Chapters 44 and 45. In brief, lesions in the first and second part of the duodenum can be identified by upper gastrointestinal endoscopy; this method has the advantage of permitting biopsy and subsequent histological diagnosis. The whole duodenum may be examined by contrast studies, hypotonic duodenography being preferable to barium meal.

The jejunum and ileum are the most difficult areas of the small intestine to evaluate. Contrast studies are the established techniques. Intubated small bowel meals are generally favoured over barium meal and follow-through studies. The terminal ileum may be demonstrated on barium enema radiographs and also in 20–30% of colonoscopic examinations.[9] A new technique that is currently being developed is small bowel enteroscopy[15,16] (see Chapter 54).

Identification of bleeding points in the bowel may necessitate isotope scanning or angiography, since many of these lesions lie within the wall of the small bowel precluding identification by intraluminal contrast studies. Advantages of angiography over isotope scanning include precise identification of the area of blood loss. In addition, the intra-arterial catheter can be advanced into the vascular tree and left in situ to allow identification of abnormal areas at laparotomy by the injection of dye. If all else fails, either laparoscopy or formal laparotomy may be necessary to diagnose a small bowel tumour. Most lesions will be self-evident, but others require enteroscopy by introducing a colonoscope into the small bowel lumen via the mouth or through the bowel wall itself. Lesions may be identified by the endoscopist or within the wall by means of transillumination.[17,18]

Among the other modalities in common use, computed tomography (CT) scan is of most value. The main indications for CT scan are the evaluation of duodenal lesions and the differentiation of lipomas from other tumours.[3,19–21] The role of ultrasound scan is limited by bowel gas, and the efficacy of magnetic resonance imaging is reduced by movement of the abdominal contents and peristalsis.

CLASSIFICATION

For the purpose of this chapter benign small bowel tumours are classified as epithelial or non-epithelial neoplasms, hamartomas, heterotopic tissues and duplications (Table 58.1). Differences of opinion arise in two areas of this classification. The first is the categorization of some lesions as benign

tumours as opposed to hamartomas. A hamartoma may be defined as 'an excessive focal overgrowth of mature normal cells and tissues in an organ, composed of identical cellular elements'.[22] Some authorities consider Brunner's gland adenomas, certain neurogenic tumours, haemangiomas and lymphangiomas to be hamartomas, whereas others classify these as benign tumours. In this chapter these lesions are considered to be benign tumours.

The second area of contention lies in the categorization of neoplasms as benign or malignant, because the nature of some lesions is unclear. Previously, we have described these lesions as 'intermediate tumours.[7,13,23] Endocrine tumours are considered by some to be benign neoplasms with a potential to become malignant,[13] whereas others classify them all as malignant.[9] Endocrine tumours are discussed fully in Chapter 59 and are therefore not considered further here. Villous adenomas have a strong malignant potential and can therefore be regarded as intermediate tumours. The behaviour of leiomyomas (stromal tumours) is also unclear, as the nature of the lesion is difficult for the histopathologist to classify as clearly benign or malignant. Both these tumours are considered as benign for the purpose of this chapter.

BENIGN NEOPLASMS

Adenomas represent 10–30% of benign small bowel tumours. Within this group the majority are tubular; villous adenomas and Brunner's gland adenomas occur less frequently. Of the non-epithelial tumours, the commonest types are leiomyomas (15–45%) and lipomas (15–25%). In most series vascular, neurogenic and lymphatic tumours, as well as fibromas, each represent less than 10% of the total.[6,8,9,24]

Adenoma

Two main types of adenoma are described: tubular and villous (papillary). Tubular adenoma usually presents as a polypoid lesion, whereas villous adenoma has a sessile appearance. Some adenomas have features of both types and can be termed tubulovillous lesions, a situation akin to that in the large bowel.[24,25]

Tubular adenomas are relatively common benign tumours, which are usually found in the duodenum as opposed to the more distal small bowel.[24,26] Single lesions are more frequent than multiple tumours and commonly measure 1–3 cm in size.[4,27] By contrast, villous adenomas are relatively uncommon,[6,9,24] although they have been reported more frequently in recent years.[25] The second part of the duodenum is the main site of occurrence for villous adenoma, the mean size of the tumour at presentation being approximately 4 cm in diameter[25,28–30] (Figure 58.1, see colour plate also).

Symptoms of both types of adenoma depend not only on the size of the lesion, but also on its position. Abdominal pain, obstruction and occult (or overt) haemorrhage are reported.[24] Obstructive jaundice may occur with tumours near the ampulla,[24] but it is sometimes minimal or absent (Figure 58.2, see colour plate also).

Malignant change has been reported in each type of adenoma with increasing frequency. This situation is comparable

Table 58.1 Classification of benign tumours

Benign neoplasms	Epithelial	– Adenoma
		Tubular
		Villous
		– Polyposis syndromes (adenoma)
		– Brunner's gland adenoma
	Non-epithelial	– Leiomyoma
		– Lipoma
		– Vascular tumours
		– Neurogenic tumours
		– Lymphatic tumours
		– Fibroma
Hamartomas:	Peutz–Jegher's syndrome	
	Other hamartomatous conditions	
Heterotopic tissue	Ectopic pancreas etc.	
Duplications		

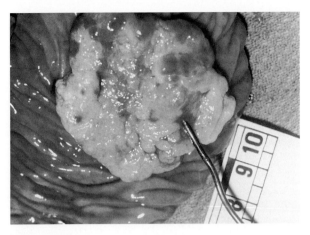

Figure 58.1
Tubulovillous adenoma (5 cm diameter) arising in the second part of the duodenum and surrounding the orifice of the major papilla, which is marked by a probe. There was no evidence of invasive carcinoma. The patient was a woman of 66 years who had presented with acute cholangitis and Gram-negative septicaemia, and the lesion was observed at ERCP. The lesion was excised by means of pylorus-preserving proximal pancreatoduodenectomy.

to the adenoma–carcinoma sequence in the colon. Risk factors in both the small and large bowel include the histological type, size, number and site of the lesion. Villous tumours have a greater tendency to become malignant, carcinoma occurring in 35–63% of cases.[29,31] Size is an important predictor in tubular adenomas, but not so much in villous lesions.[27,28] In one study, the average diameters were as follows: benign polyps 2.65 cm, polyps containing both adenoma and carcinoma 3.7 cm, jejunal carcinomas 4.3 cm and ileal carcinomas 4.7 cm.[24] Adenomas in the periampullary region have a particular predisposition to malignant transformation, and so do multicentric adenomas.[24]

Management is governed by the propensity to malignant

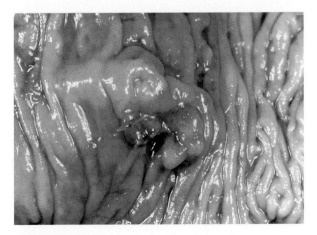

Figure 58.2
Sessile villous adenoma showing histological evidence of moderate-to-severe epithelial dysplasia. The patient was a man of 65 years who had presented with non-specific abdominal pain and heartburn. The lesion was observed during upper gastrointestinal endoscopy and was excised by means of pylorus-preserving proximal pancreatoduodenectomy.

change. In most instances the diagnosis is made by endoscopy as the lesions are most commonly situated in the duodenum. To obtain an accurate histological diagnosis and remove the risk of malignant change, polyps must be excised in their entirety. Tubular adenomas in the duodenum that are less than 2 cm in diameter can be snared and removed endoscopically.[32] Larger tumours will require open operation, duodenotomy and local excision. Jejunal and ileal polyps may be removed by formal resection of the segment (with end-to-end anastomosis) or local enterotomy with excision of the polyp alone.[8,24]

Villous adenomas in the duodenum represent more of a challenge and are fortunately rare. Excision of the whole lesion is mandatory in order to obtain a histological diagnosis. Endoscopic biopsy has a false negative rate of 25–56% presumably owing to the sampling error implicit in detecting a small area of carcinomatous change in these sizeable lesions.[25,31] At one end of the spectrum, small lesions may be excised by endoscopic snare removal, but this approach is exceptional as most are over 4 cm in diameter. At the other extreme, malignant disease may be indicated by the presence of secondaries in the liver or a CT scan indicating infiltration of surrounding tissues.

Most villous adenomas of the duodenum require laparotomy. If no obvious metastatic spread is present, the tumour should be palpated and any infiltrating, hard or indurated areas are biopsied. If malignant change is present, radical resection should be carried out by means of pancreatoduodenectomy, nowadays with preservation of the pylorus and duodenal cap. If the lesion feels soft, duodenotomy is performed to expose the tumour which may then be excised by submucous resection; unfortunately a local recurrence rate of 46% is reported following this procedure.[25] Consequently radical resection may be advocated for almost all villous tumours[28] (Figures 58.1 and 58.2, see colour plates also). A complicating factor in some cases is the proximity of the ampulla to the tumour. Options include local excision of the ampulla with reimplantation of the ducts, sphincteroplasty or radical resection.[33] In unfit subjects alternative procedures to be considered include endoscopic removal[32,34] or laser ablation.[35] If the ampulla is compromised, a stent may be inserted.[25] Villous adenomas distal to the ampulla in the duodenum or jejunoileum should be removed by segmental resection.[30]

Continued surveillance of these patients is determined by the final histology and the procedure undertaken. Clearly, locally excised lesions must be followed by regular upper gastrointestinal endoscopy. Tumours that have undergone malignant transformation are considered further in Chapter 60.[59]

Polyposis syndromes

Familial adenomatous polyposis (FAP, polyposis coli) is an autosomal dominant condition manifested by multiple adenomatous polyps in the colon and rectum. It has recently become clear that polyps can occur throughout the gastrointestinal tract, hence the use of the term familial adenomatous polyposis to describe the condition.[36] One variant of the disease is Gardner's syndrome in which additional (extraintestinal) manifestations are apparent, including desmoid tumours within the abdominal cavity, soft tissue tumours of the skin and osteomas in the skull and mandible. Another rare variant is Turcot's syndrome, in which brain tumours occur as well as polyposis.[37]

Adenomatous polyps occur within the small intestine in 24–93% of these patients, especially in the duodenum.[38,39] They are usually multiple and have an affinity for the periampullary region.[36,39,40] There is now considerable evidence that these polyps can become malignant.[36,41,42] Periampullary carcinoma occurs in 2–12% of FAP patients,[39,42–44] and in those who have had a colectomy this tumour may occur more frequently than a carcinoma in the remaining rectum.[36]

Adenomas also develop, albeit rarely, in the jejunum and ileum. The natural history is unclear,[40,45–47] but the relative risk of malignancy seems low.[45] Polyps are also reported to occur in the stomach, but most are hyperplastic in nature (fundal gland polyps).[38,40,43] Carcinoma of the stomach is unusual in this condition, but we have treated one patient with metachronous gastric and duodenal cancers.[48]

It is important that patients with this inherited condition should undergo investigation for upper gastrointestinal polyps. Endoscopy usually suffices, but contrast studies are indicated in some patients.[36,38]

The optimum management of these polyps is uncertain as the natural history is not clearcut.[49] Microscopic adenomas may be present in the 'normal' duodenum, and biopsies should be taken from the periampullary region.[39,40,50] It would seem prudent to remove polyps greater than 0.5 cm in diameter, but smaller ones may be kept under review[38] or destroyed by endoscopic ablation.[36] Patients with FAP should have regular follow-up endoscopy.[36,38]

The approach to jejunal and ileal polyps is also unclear. However, it would seem reasonable to excise those with an increased risk of malignant change as suggested by the size or histological type.[47]

Brunner's gland adenoma

These glands are located in the submucosa of the proximal duodenum. Some consider the lesions to be hamartomas. Tumours arising from Brunner's glands take one of three forms: polypoid, isolated nodular hyperplasia and diffuse nodular hyperplasia.[51]

Polypoid lesions are usually single and less than 1 cm in diameter, although sizes up to 12 cm in diameter can occur.[52,53] Tumours may be found incidentally during routine investigations or manifest themselves with bleeding or vague upper gastrointestinal symptoms or (sometimes) obstruction.[5,54] Only one report has suggested malignancy developing in Brunner's glands.[55] Small lesions can be removed endoscopically, but large tumours may require operation.[56]

Nodular hyperplasia occurs in two forms, both having sessile projections on the surface. The isolated variety appears in the first part of the duodenum, whereas the diffuse form can involve the whole duodenum.[5] The condition has been observed in patients with chronic renal failure, although the reason is obscure.[57] These lesions are usually asymptomatic. If endoscopy and biopsy can confirm the diagnosis, no treatment is required in asymptomatic patients.[23]

Leiomyoma

Leiomyomas, also called stromal tumours, are one of the commonest benign small bowel neoplasms representing 15–45% of the total. There may be a slight male predisposition, and typically they present in the fifth and sixth decades.[4,8,58,59] These tumours are usually single. They can develop in any part of the small intestine but may be a little more frequent in the jejunum and ileum.[4,60] Within the duodenum they occur predominantly in the second part.[5] The macroscopic appearances are varied. Extraluminal lesions are the commonest, but intramural, dumbbell and intraluminal forms also occur.[61]

The commonest presenting symptom is bleeding from mucosal ulceration, which may be manifest as anaemia or frank haemorrhage (Figure 58.3, see colour plate also). Extraluminal tumours can present as large masses and be palpable through the abdominal wall. Necrosis within these tumours leads to haemorrhage, perforation or abscess formation. Intraluminal tumours can precipitate intussusception and obstruction. Rarely volvulus or fistula formation can develop.[6,8,9] Leiomyomas can be difficult to classify as benign or malignant by the histopathologist.[58] The mitotic index is usually indicative, but not invariably pathognomonic.[62]

The diagnosis can be suggested by various investigations. As most tumours are extraluminal, CT scanning is helpful.[8] Intraluminal lesions typically have a central crater which can be demonstrated by contrast studies.[9] These tumours are often very vascular and can be depicted by selective mesenteric angiography.[63] Treatment is by excision. The malignant potential of these tumours should be kept in mind, and reasonable clearance is desirable. Satisfactory clearance can be achieved fairly easily in the jejunum and ileum by segmental resection. In the duodenum clearance may be limited. If malignant change has occurred more radical surgery should be entertained, as discussed in Chapter 59.

Lipoma

This tumour is relatively common in the small bowel, representing 15–25% of benign lesions. As with leiomyomas, there may be a slight male preponderance.[5] Age of presentation is mainly in the sixth and seventh decade.[6,8,9] Lipomas can develop in any part of the small bowel, but they favour the ileum.[6,60] Usually arising in the submucosa, they can grow into a pedunculated intraluminal lesion of 0.5–8.0 cm in diameter.[6,9,58]

Small tumours are usually discovered incidentally,[3] but as size increases they are more likely to become symptomatic. Obstruction can arise from intussusception or obturation.[3,8,58,64] Haemorrhage from ulceration can occur even in tumours less than 1 cm in size.[65] Duodenal lesions may also cause epigastric pain.[20] Malignant change is considered a rare event, though one case of an ileal liposarcoma has been reported.[66]

Most tumours turn up incidentally during radiological investigation, at operation or at autopsy. CT helps to differentiate lipomas from other tumours.[21] Symptomatic tumours should be

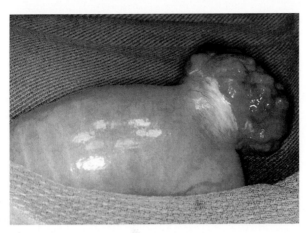

(a)

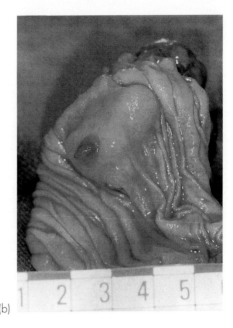

(b)

Figure 58.3

Leiomyoma (stromal tumour) of the jejunum. This lesion was found and resected at emergency laparotomy in a 55-year-old man who presented with shock and the passage of red blood per rectum. (a) Serosal aspect of the bowel with an exophytic tumour; (b) blood clot in a small ulcer on the mucosal surface.

excised. Proximal duodenal lesions may be removed endoscopically, whereas more distal tumours require operation. Removal of all duodenal lipomas has been advocated to prevent the possibility of obstruction, haemorrhage or jaundice.[20]

Vascular tumours

These tumours represent less than 10% of benign small bowel neoplasms. It is contentious whether they are neoplastic or hamartomatous. Three types of vascular tumour are described: capillary haemangioma, cavernous haemangioma and multiple phlebectasia.[9] They all arise in the submucosa.

Capillary haemangiomas tend to occur in the young. Single and multiple forms exist, and large lesions cause intraluminal swellings.[58] Cavernous haemangiomas are reported from the second decade onwards. They may be solitary, but can also present as large and diffusely infiltrating tumours.[4,9,58,60] Multiple telangiectasia presents between the fourth and seventh decades.[58] The condition, which may be either sporadic or hereditary (Osler–Weber–Rendu disease), is characterized by numerous haemangiomas, 1–5 mm in diameter, which can affect the whole bowel but occur predominantly in the jejunum.[4] The gastrointestinal lesions may also occur as part of a generalized haemangiomatosis.[58]

The dominant presenting feature of capillary and cavernous haemangiomas is haemorrhage (Figure 58.4, see colour plate also), but large tumours can cause obstruction.[59,60] Telangiectasia is usually symptomless.[58] Malignant change is rare.[67] Multiple lesions can lead to an erroneous diagnosis of a malignant vascular lesion with metastases. The diagnosis of vascular lesions has already been discussed. Intraluminal contrast studies can identify large lesions, but selective mesenteric angiography is indicated for small, intramural abnormalities. Laparotomy with intraoperative endoscopy should not be delayed in patients who are bleeding (see

Chapter 54). From a clinical point of view these tumours usually present in a similar manner to vascular malformations.

Solitary vascular tumours should be excised. If there are multiple lesions involving large amounts of bowel, only symptomatic abnormalities should be resected so as to prevent or reduce the risk of malabsorption.

Neurogenic tumours

These lesions develop from the nerve sheath, paraganglia or ganglia. Certain forms of neurogenic tumour may be hamartomas. All varieties make up less than 10% of all benign small bowel tumours. Neurofibromas are the commonest form. Gangliocytic paragangliomas, paragangliomas (Figure 58.5, see colour plate also, and Figure 58.6) and ganglioneuromas are other rarer variants.[58,68–70]

Neurofibromas are typically solitary lesions that particularly affect the ileum rather than the rest of the small bowel.[4] However, 11–25% of patients with Von Recklinghausen's disease have multiple gastrointestinal lesions.[71,72] In this condition

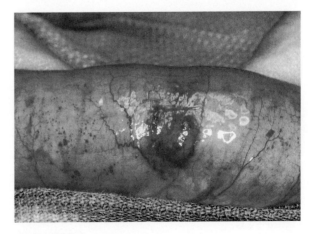

Figure 58.4

Capillary haemangioma of the upper ileum in a 64-year-old woman who presented with persistent iron-deficiency anaemia.

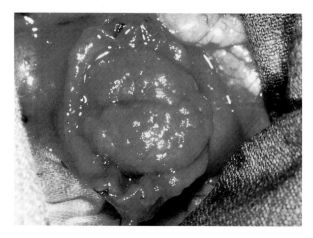

Figure 58.5
Duodenal paraganglioma. The pedunculated lesion which arose in the third part of the duodenum was excised via a duodenotomy.

the jejunum and stomach are primarily involved as opposed to the ileum and duodenum.[71] The tumours are often subserosal, but intramural and intraluminal forms can also occur.[4,6,73] Bleeding is the commonest presenting feature and follows mucosal ulceration.[6] More rarely, obstruction occurs.[4] The diagnosis may be suspected in Von Recklinghausen's disease by café au lait spots or cutaneous neurofibromas. An important feature of these tumours is their malignant predisposition, which is reported in 15–20% of cases. Thus segmental excision is indicated.

Gangliocytic paragangliomas preferentially arise in the second part of the duodenum, although they can also develop in the distal duodenum and jejunum. They form a polypoid mass.[68] Presentation is usually in the sixth decade, with haemorrhage and sometimes abdominal pain.[68] Treatment is by simple excision.

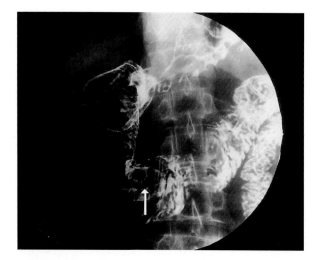

Figure 58.6
Duodenal paraganglioma. The lesion arose in the third part of the duodenum and was demonstrated on a barium meal examination carried out for indigestion.

Lymphatic tumours

Three lesions can develop from small bowel lymphatics: lymphatic cysts, lymphangiomas and lymphangiectasia. All are rare.

Lymphatic cysts are often multiple. They originate in the submucosa and appear as fluid-filled swellings up to 1 cm in diameter projecting into the bowel lumen.[58] Lymphangiomas (Figure 58.7, see colour plate also) consist of multiple lymphatic channels, which lead to luminal swellings.[74] Both lesions are usually asymptomatic and considered benign. Treatment, if necessary, is by simple excision.

Lymphangiectasia is more serious. In this abnormality the lymphatics of the small bowel become abnormally dilated.[58] Affected bowel may have a brown discoloration.[58] The disease is characterized by protein loss.[58,74] Lymphangiectasia is thought to arise from a congenital defect of the lymphatic vessels.[58] A secondary form may result from acquired lymphatic obstruction, associated with diseases such as lymphoma, carcinoma and sarcoidosis.[58,74]

Fibroma

This rare tumour arises in the wall of the small intestine.[6] It is possible that many are fibroid polyps. In the past some may have been misdiagnosed as smooth muscle or neurogenic tumours.[57,58] Fibromas are almost all asymptomatic, but large lesions may precipitate intussusception and obstruction.[4,6] Treatment is by local excision or segmental resection.

HAMARTOMAS

Peutz–Jegher's syndrome

This syndrome is an autosomal dominant disease manifested by gastrointestinal polyps and mucocutaneous pigmentation. The polyps appear throughout the small bowel but preferentially in the jejunum as opposed to the ileum or duodenum.[27] Colonic and gastric polyps are also well recognized. The lesions are multiple and may or may not be pedunculated.[27] Although size is variable, most are 0.5–1.0 cm in diameter.[60] Polyps may grow sequentially in different anatomical sites.[27,60]

Age of presentation is usually the first three decades of life. The diagnosis should always be considered in children with small bowel polyps. The two main features are recurrent colic due to intussusception (Figure 58.8, see colour plate also) and occult bleeding leading to anaemia.[60] Peutz–Jegher's syndrome should be suspected by the pigmentation that occurs on the lips, buccal mucosa, palms, soles and web spaces. The buccal changes remain throughout life, but the others may fade at puberty.[4,60]

In contrast to familial adenomatous polyposis, malignant change is thought to be rare in hamartomatous polyps,[75] but a recent study has indicated cancer developing in up to 6% of small bowel lesions.[76] Carcinoma is more frequent in the duodenum than in the jejunum and ileum. Cancer also develops in the large bowel in Peutz–Jegher's syndrome and may be due to malignant change in a coexisting adenomatous polyp; this sequence is not proven for the small bowel.[75] Interestingly, patients with this disease are at increased risk of dying of

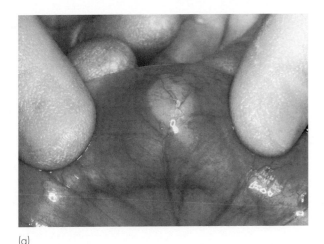
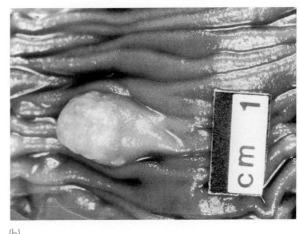

(a)   (b)

Figure 58.7
Lymphangioma of the upper ileum. The lesion was found incidentally at laparotomy. The serosal (a) and mucosal (b) aspects are shown.

carcinoma at a young age, not only from gastrointestinal malignancies, but also from apparently unrelated tumours.[76]

Treatment should be aimed at preserving small bowel as problems may occur throughout life requiring multiple operations.[8] Duodenal lesions causing symptoms should be removed endoscopically if possible, but more distal hamartomas require operative excision. One study reported 54 laparotomies in 23 patients over a 44-year period.[77] To reduce early reoperation, peroperative endoscopy and removal of polyps has been recommended.[77]

Other hamartomatous conditions

Juvenile polyposis can affect the whole gastrointestinal tract. Presentation is in childhood in the form of gastrointestinal haemorrhage, obstruction or intussusception. Malignant change is not reported in the small bowel.[27] Another rare familial hamartomatous disease is Cowden's syndrome; hamartomas occur in the gastrointestinal tract and are associated with

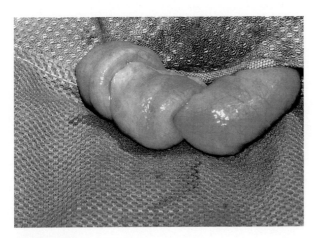

Figure 58.8
Intussusception of the jejunum in a young man with Peutz–Jeghers syndrome who had presented with intermittent attacks of subacute intestinal obstruction.

orocutaneous hamartomas, thyroid and breast disease. Gastrointestinal symptoms are unusual.[78]

Hamartomatous polyps also occur in the gastrointestinal tract in the Cronkhite–Canada syndrome, which is an acquired non-familial condition. Clinical manifestations are diarrhoea and steatorrhoea leading to weight loss and malnutrition. The diagnosis may be suggested by the associated features of alopecia, nail dystrophy and skin hyperpigmentation.[27]

HETEROTOPIC TISSUE

Heterotopic tissue refers to a cluster of specialised cell types being located in unusual sites. In the gastrointestinal tract, the commonest tissues involved are gastric mucosa and exocrine pancreas.

Heterotopic *gastric* mucosa has been identified in the duodenum, Meckel's diverticulum and small bowel duplications.[79] The lesions are usually unremarkable in appearance, though duodenal lesions can take the unusual form of a polyp or prominent fold and ulceration can develop in a Meckel's diverticulum.[60,80–83] Symptoms occasionally rise from a duodenal polyp in the duodenum,[60,80] and peptic ulceration in a Meckel's diverticulum leads to bleeding and perforation (see also Chapter 57).[60] Symptomatic lesions are managed by endoscopic removal (duodenal polyp) or operative excision (Meckel's diverticulum).

Heterotopic *pancreatic* tissue occurs not only in the duodenum and Meckel's diverticulum, but also in the proximal jejunum.[79,84] The macroscopic appearance is of a submucosal nodule or less often a polyp.[5,85] Most of these lesions are asymptomatic, but ampullary lesions can cause jaundice, and both small bowel obstruction and haemorrhage have been described. Only symptomatic lesions require removal.

Rarely pancreatic and gastric tissue exist concurrently in the duodenum or in a Meckel's diverticulum.[79,86]

Endometriosis may also be considered a heterotopic condition. The gastrointestinal tract is involved in 12% of patients, especially the sigmoid colon and rectum. The small bowel (particularly the ileum) is involved in only 7%.[87,88] Endometriosis usually occurs on the serosal surface of the bowel. At the end of the endometrial cycle engorgement and sloughing leads to haemorrhage. The subsequent inflammatory response causes dense adhesions. The peak incidence is between the ages of 30 and 40 years. Small bowel involvement is usually asymptomatic, but it may be indicated by features suggesting impending obstruction. The symptoms tend to be cyclical in nature.[88] The main problem is not so much the endometriotic plaques but obstruction that results from the adhesions. The condition should be considered in patients with known endometriosis. It is diagnosed, either incidentally or in symptomatic patients, by laparoscopy or laparotomy. Treatment of asymptomatic patients is debatable, and expert gynaecological advice should be sought.[88] Symptomatic lesions require resection.[89]

DUPLICATIONS

These interesting developmental abnormalities are rare. Approximately half of them involve the jejunum or ileum.[90,91] The appearances are of a swelling in the small bowel mesentery, which may be cystic (containing mucosal secretions) or tubular, communicating proximally or distally with the lumen of the bowel.[92] The abnormal segment is lined with intestinal epithelium,[79,92,93] gastric heterotopia is recognized in 15–36% of cases.[90,93]

Presentation occurs in most instances in infancy (see Chapter 62), although the abnormality can also be diagnosed in later years.[90,92,93] The condition is manifest by an abdominal mass or obstruction; bleeding and perforation are rare.[94–97] The diagnosis may be suspected by abdominal radiographs and contrast studies.[91] Ultrasound scan may demonstrate the cystic variety.[91]

Treatment of small lesions is by resection of the duplication together with the associated bowel. Longer lesions are not so easily dealt with, as they have a common blood supply with the normal bowel and extensive resection may lead to long-term problems.[90,91] Options include removal or destruction of the mucosa, with or without partial resection of the abnormality, or anastomosis of both ends of the duplication into the normal bowel lumen.[90,98,99]

REFERENCES

1. Zollinger RM Jr, Sternfeld WC & Schreiber H. Primary neoplasms of the small intestine. *Am J Surg* 1986; **151**: 654.
2. Adkins RB Jr & Daview J. Cross and microscopic anatomy of the stomach and small intestine. In Scott HWJ, Sawyers JL (eds) *Surgery of the Stomach, Duodenum and Small Intestine*. Boston: Blackwell Scientific Publications, 1987: 45.
3. Jennings BS & Doerr RJ. Duodenal lipoma causing intussusception. *Surgery* 1989; **105**: 560.
4. Dial P & Cohn I Jr. Tumors of the jejunum and ileum. In Scott HW Jr, Sawyers JL (eds) *Surgery of the Stomach, Duodenum and Small Intestine*. Boston: Blackwell Scientific Publications, 1987: 937.
5. Perey BJ. Neoplasms of the duodenum. In Scott HW Jr, Sawyers JL (eds). *Surgery of the Stomach, Duodenum and Small Intestine*. Boston: Blackwell Scientific Publications, 1987: 571.
6. Wilson JM, Melvin DB, Gray G & Thorbjarnarson B. Benign small bowel tumor. *Am Surg* 1975; **181**: 247.
7. Studley JGN & Williamson RCN. Small bowel tumours. *Surgery* (Oxford) 1991; **95**: 2263.
8. Ashley SW & Wells SA Jr. Tumors of the small intestine. *Semin Oncol* 1988; **15**: 116.
9. Herbsman H, Wetstein L, Rosen Y et al. Tumors of the small intestine. *Curr Probl Surg* 1980; **17**: 127.
10. Ketonen P, Virkkula L, Ketonen L & Mattila S. Recurrent small bowel obstruction caused by a benign tumour. *Acta Chir Scand* 1978; **144**: 261.
11. Lowenfels AB. Why are small bowel tumours so rare? *Lancet* 1973; **i**: 24.
12. Ebert PA & Zuidema GD. Primary tumours of the small intestine. *Arch Surg* 1965; **91**: 452.
13. Williamson RCN. Small bowel tumours. *Surgery* (Oxford) 1984; **1**: 340.
14. Burt RW, Rikkers LF, Gardner EJ, Lee RG & Tolman KG. Villous adenoma of the duodenal papilla presenting as necrotizing pancreatitis in a patient with Gardner's syndrome. *Gastroenterology* 1987; **92**: 532.
15. Lewis BS & Waye JD. Chronic gastrointestinal bleeding of obscure origin: role of small bowel enteroscopy. *Gastroenterology* 1988; **94**: 1117.
16. Frimberger E, Hagenmuller F & Classen M. Endostomy: a new approach to small-bowel endoscopy. *Endoscopy* 1989; **21**: 86.
17. Lau WY, Wong SY, Yuen WK & Wong KK. Intraoperative enteroscopy for bleeding angiodysplasias of small intestine. *Surg Gynecol Obstet* 1989; **168**: 341.
18. Flickinger EG, Stanforth AC, Sinar DR, MacDonald KG, Lannin DR & Gibson JH. Intraoperative video panendoscopy for diagnosing sites of chronic intestinal bleeding. *Am J Surg* 1989; **157**: 137.
19. Farah MC, Jafri SZH, Schwab RE et al. Duodenal neoplasms: role of CT. *Radiology* 1987; **162**: 839.
20. Michel LA, Ballet T, Collard JM, Bradpiece HA & Haot J. Severe bleeding from submucosal lipoma of the duodenum. *J Clin Gastroenterol* 1988; **10**: 541.
21. Kang JY, Chan-Wilde C, Wee A, Chew R & Ti TK. Role of computed tomography and endoscopy in the management of alimentary tract lipomas. *Gut* 1990; **31**: 550.
22. Cotran RS, Kumar V & Robbins SL. Diseases of infancy and childhood. In Robbins SL (ed) *Pathologic Basis of Disease*, 4th edn. Philadelphia: WB Saunders, 1989: 515.
23. Studley JGN & Williamson RCN. Hamartomas and benign neoplasms of the small bowel. In Morris PJ, Malt RA (eds), *Oxford Textbook of Surgery*. Oxford: Oxford University Press, 1994: 999.
24. Perzin KH & Bridge MF. Adenomas of the small intestine: a clinicopathologic review of 51 cases and a study of their relationship to carcinoma. *Cancer* 1981; **48**: 799.
25. Galandiuk S, Hermann RE, Jagelman DG, Fazio VW & Sivak MV. Villous tumors of the duodenum. *Ann Surg* 1988; **207**: 234.
26. Hancock RJ. An 11-year review of primary tumours of the small bowel including the duodenum. *Can Med Assoc J* 1970; **103**: 1177.
27. Morson BC, Dawson IMP, Day DW, Jass JR, Price AB & Williams GT. Benign epithelial tumours and polyps. In: Morson BC & Dawson IMP (eds) *Morson & Dawson's Gastrointestinal Pathology*, 3rd edn. Oxford: Blackwell Scientific Publications, 1990: 351–359.
28. Chappuis CW. Divincenti FC & Cohn I Jr. Villous tumors of the duodenum. *Ann Surg* 1989; **209**: 593.
29. Schulten MF Jr, Oyasu R & Beal JM. Villous adenoma of the duodenum. A case report and review of the literature. *Am J Surg* 1976; **132**: 90.
30. Braga M, Stella M, Zerbi A, Staudacher C, Sironi M & Di Carlo V. Giant villous adenoma of the duodenum. *Br J Surg* 1986; **73**: 924.
31. Ryan DP, Shapiro RH & Warshaw AL. Villous tumours of the duodenum. *Ann Surg* 1986; **203**: 301.
32. Ghazi A, Ferstenberg H & Shinya H. Endoscopic gastroduodenal polypectomy. *Ann Surg* 1984; **200**: 175.
33. Krukowski ZH, Ewen SWB, Davidson AI & Matheson NA. Operative management of tubulovillous neoplasms of the duodenum and ampulla. *Br J Surg* 1988; **75**: 150.
34. Haubrich WS, Johnson RB & Foroozan P. Endoscopic removal of a duodenal adenoma. *Gastrointest Endosc* 1973; **19**: 201.
35. Paraf F, Naveau S, Zourabichvili O, Poynard T & Chaput JC. Endoscopic laser therapy for duodenal villous adenoma. *Dig Dis Sci* 1989; **34**: 1466.
36. Sarre RG, Frost AG, Jagelman DG, Petras RE, Sivak MV & McGannon E. Gastric and duodenal polyps in familial adenomatous polyposis: a prospective study of the nature and prevalence of upper gastrointestinal polyps. *Gut* 1987; **28**: 306.
37. Clark ML, Price AB & Williams CB. Tumours of the gastrointestinal tract. In: Weatherall DJ, Ledingham JGG & Warrell DA (eds) *Oxford Textbook of Medicine*, 2nd edn. Oxford: Oxford University Press. 1987; **12**: 146.
38. Kurtz RC, Sternberg SS, Miller HH & Decosse JJ. Upper gastrointestinal neoplasia in familial polyposis. *Dig Dis Sci* 1987; **32**: 459.

39. Yao T, Iida M, Ohsato K, Watanabe H & Omae T. Duodenal lesions in familial polyposis of the colon. *Gastroenterology* 1977; **73**: 1086.

40. Ranzi T, Castagnone D, Velio P, Bianchi P & Polli EE. Gastric and duodenal polyps in familial polyposis coli. *Gut* 1981; **22**: 363.

41. Sugihara K, Muto T, Kamiya J, Konishi F, Sawada T & Morioka Y. Gardner's syndrome associated with periampullary carcinoma, duodenal and gastric adenomatosis. *Dis Colon Rectum* 1982; **25**: 766.

42. Jones TR & Nance FC. Periampullary malignancy in Gardner's syndrome. *Ann Surg* 1977; **185**: 565.

43. Burt RW, Berenson MM, Lee RGD, Tolman KG, Freston JW & Gardner EJ. Upper gastrointestinal polyps in Gardner's syndrome. *Gastroenterology* 1984; **86**: 295.

44. Bussey HJR. Extracolonic lesions associated with polyposis coli. *Proc R Soc Med* 1972; **65**: 294.

45. Hamilton SR, Bussey HJR, Mendelsohn G et al. Ileal adenomas after colectomy in nine patients with adenomatous polyposis coli/Gardner's syndrome. *Gastroenterology* 1979; **77**: 1252.

46. Ojerskog B, Myrvold HE, Nilsson LO, Philipson BM & Ahren C. Gastroduodenal and ileal polyps in patients treated surgically for familial polyposis coli with proctocolectomy and continent ileostomy. *Acta Chir Scand* 1987; **153**: 681.

47. Beart RW Jr, Fleming CR & Banks PM. Tubulovillous adenomas in a continent ileostomy after proctocolectomy for familial polyposis. *Dig Dis Sci* 1982; **27**: 553.

48. Desa LA, Williamson RCN, Grace PA & Denham P. Metachronous gastric and duodenal carcinoma in Gardner's syndrome. *Coloproctology* 1990; **12**: 190.

49. Iida M, Yao T, Itoh H et al. Natural history of duodenal lesions in Japanese patients with familial adenomatosis coli (Gardner's syndrome). *Gastroenterology* 1989; **96**: 1301.

50. Bulow S, Lauritsen KB, Johansen A, Svendsen LB & Sondergaard JO. Gastroduodenal polyps in familial polyposis coli. *Dis Colon Rectum* 1985; **28**: 90.

51. Feyrter F. Überwucherungen der Brunnerschen Drüsen. *Virchows Arch* 1934; **293**: 509.

52. De Silva S & Chandrasoma P. Giant duodenal hamartoma consisting mainly of Brunner's glands. *Am J Surg* 1977; **133**: 240.

53. Maglinte DDT, Mayes SL, Ng AC & Pickett RD. Brunner's gland adenoma: diagnostic considerations. *J Clin Gastroenterol* 1982; **4**: 127.

54. Hedges AR. Hamartoma of Brunner's gland causing pyloric obstruction and a biliary fistula. *Acta Chir Scand* 1988; **154**: 475.

55. Christie AC. Duodenal carcinoma with neoplastic transformation of the underlying Brunner's glands. *Br J Cancer* 1953; **7**: 65.

56. Khawaja HT, Deakin M & Colin-Jones DG. Endoscopic removal of a large ulcerated Brunner's gland adenoma. *Endoscopy* 1986; **18**: 199.

57. Paimela H, Tallgren LG, Stenman S, Numers H & Scheinin TM. Multiple duodenal polyps in uraemia: a little known clinical entity. *Gut* 1984; **25**: 259.

58. Morson BC, Dawson IMP Day DW, Jass JR, Price AB & Williams GT. Non-epithelial tumours. In: Morson BC & Dawson IMP (eds.) *Morson & Dawson's Gastrointestinal Pathology*, 3rd edn. Oxford: Blackwell Scientific Publications, 1990; 372.

59. Riggle KP & Boeckman CR. Duodenal leiomyoma: a case report of hematemesis in a teenager. *J Paediatr Surg* 1988; **23**: 850.

60. Slavin G. Tumours and tumour-like conditions. In: Booth CC & Neale G (eds) *Disorders of the Small Intestine*, Oxford: Blackwell Scientific Publications, 1985; 363.

61. Starr GF & Dockerty MB. Leiomyomas and leiomyosarcomas of the small intestine. *Cancer* 1955; **8**: 101.

62. Akwari OE, Dozois RR, Weiland LH & Beahrs OH. Leiomyosarcoma of the small and large bowel. *Cancer* 1978; **42**: 1375.

63. Cho KJ & Reuter SR. Angiography of duodenal leiomyomas and leiomysarcomas. *AJR* 1980; **135**: 31.

64. Weiss A, Mollura JL, Profy A & Cohen R. Two cases of complicated intestinal lipoma. *Am J Gastroenterol* 1979; **72**: 83.

65. Sarma DP, Weilbaecher TG, Basavaraj A & Reina RR. Symptomatic lipoma of the duodenum. *J Surg Oncol* 1984; **25**: 133.

66. Mohandas D, Chandra RS, Srinivasan V & Bhaskar AG. Liposarcoma of the ileum with secondaries in the liver. *Am J Gastroenterol* 1972; **58**: 172.

67. Murray–Lyon IM, Doyle D, Philpott RM & Porter NH. Haemangiomatosis of the small and large bowel with histological malignant change. *J Pathol* 1971; **105**: 295.

68. Damron TA, Rahman D & Cashman MD. Gangliocytic paraganglioma in association with a duodenal diverticulum. *Am J Gastroenterol* 1989; **84**: 1109.

69. Gemer M & Feuchtwanger MM. Ganglioneuroma of the duodenum. *Gastroenterology* 1966; **51**: 689.

70. Goldman RL. Ganglioneuroma of the duodenum. Relationship to non-chromaffin paraganglioma of the duodenum. *Am J Surg* 1968; **115**: 716.

71. Wander JV & Das Gupta TK. Neurofibromatosis. *Curr Probl Surg* 1977; **14** (2): 1.

72. Davis GB & Berk RN. Intestinal neurofibromas in Von Recklinhausen's disease. *Am J Gastroenterol* 1973; **60**: 410.

73. Sivak MV, Sullivan BH & Farmer RG. Neurogenic tumours of the small intestine. *Gastroenterology* 1975; **68**: 374.

74. Davis M, Fenoglio–Preiser C & Haque AK. Cavernous lymphangioma of the duodenum: case report and review of the literature. *Gastrointest Radiol* 1987; **12**: 10.

75. Reid JD. Intestinal carcinoma in the Peutz–Jeghers syndrome. *JAMA* 1974; **229**: 833.

76. Spigelman AD, Murday V & Phillips RKS. Cancer and the Peutz–Jeghers syndrome. *Gut* 1989; **30**: 1588.

77. Spigelman AD, Thomson JPS & Phillips RKS. Towards decreasing the relaparotomy rate in the Peutz–Jegher syndrome: the role of peroperative small bowel endoscopy. *Br J Surg* 1990; **77**: 301.

78. Weinstock JV & Kawanishi H. Gastrointestina polyposis with orocutaneous harmatomas (Cowden's disease). *Gastroenterology* 1978; **74**: 890.

79. Morson BC, Dawson IMP, Day DW, Jass JR, Price AB & Williams GT. Normal embryology and fetal development; developmental abnormalities. In Morson BC, Dawson IMP (eds) *Morson & Dawson's Gastrointestinal Pathology*, 3rd edn. Oxford: Blackwell Scientific Publications, 1990; 216.

80. Bayerdortfer E, Voeth C & Ottenjann R. Antral mucosa heterotopy in the duodenal bulb. *Hepatogastroenterology* 1986; **33**: 278.

81. Rosch W & Hoer PW. Hyperplasiogenic polyp in the duodenum. *Endoscopy* 1983; **15**: 117.

82. Tsadilas T. Duodenal polyp composed of ectopic gastric mucosa. *Dig Dis Sci* 1984; **29**: 475.

83. Remele W, Hartmann W, Von der Laden U et al. Three other types of duodenal polyps: mucosal cysts, focal foveolar hyperplasia and hyperplastic polyp originating from islands of gastric mucosa. *Dig Dis Sci* 1989; **34**: 1468.

84. Coupland RM, Aukland P, Harrison DA. Heterotopic pancreas: a rare cause of obstructive jaundice. *J R Coll Surg Edinb* 1987; **32**: 168.

85. Barbosa JJ, Dockerty MB & Waugh IM. Pancreatic heterotopia. *Surg Gynecol Obstet* 1946; **82**: 527.

86. Tanemura H, Uno S, Suzuki M et al. Heterotopic gastric mucosa accompanied by aberrant pancreas in the duodenum. *Am J Gastroenterol* 1987; **82**: 685.

87. MacAfee CHG & Greer HL. Intestinal endometriosis. *J Obstet Gynaecol Br Emp* 1960; **67**: 539.

88. Stahl C & Grimes EM. Endometriosis of the small bowel. Case reports and review of the literature. *Obstet Gynecol Surv* 1987; **42**: 131.

89. Perry EP & Peel ALG. The treatment of obstructing intestinal endometriosis. *J R Soc Med* 1988; **81**: 172.

90. Bower RJ, Siber WK & Kiesewetter WB. Alimentary tract duplications in children. *Ann Surg* 1978; **188**: 669.

91. Harmel RP Jr & Clatworthy HW Jr. Intestinal obstruction in infants and children. In Scott HW Jr, Sawyers JL (eds) *Surgery of the Stomach, Duodenum, and small Intestine*. Boston: Blackwell Scientific Publications, 1987: 859.

92. Walker Smith J & Wright V. Congenital anatomical abnormalities. In Booth CC, Neale G (eds) *Disorders of the Small Intestine*. Oxford: Blackwell Scientific Publications, 1985 : 43.

93. Gross RE, Holcomb GW Jr & Farber S. Duplications of the alimentary tract. *Pediatrics* 1952; **9**: 449.

94. Royle SG & Doig CM. Perforation of the jejunum secondary to a duplication cyst lined with ectopic gastric mucosa. *J Paediatr Surg* 1988; **23**: 1025.

95. Newmark H, Ching G, Halls J & Levy IJ. Bleeding peptic ulcer caused by ectopic gastric mucosa in a duplicated segment of jejunum. *Am J Gastroenterol* 1981; **75**: 158.

96. Scully RE, Galdabini JJ & McNeely BU. Case records of the Massachusetts General Hospital. *N Engl J Med* 1980; **302**: 958.

97. Collins CD. Perforation of a peptic ulcer in duplicated ileum. *Br J Surg* 1972; **59**: 159.

98. Schwartz DC, Becker JM, Schneider KM & So HB. Tubular duplication with autonomous blood supply: resection with preservation of adjacent bowel. *J Paediatr Surg* 1980; **15**: 341.

99. Wrenn EL Jr. Tubular duplication of the small intestine. *Surgery* 1962; **52**: 49.

59

CARCINOID AND OTHER APUDOMAS OF THE SMALL INTESTINE

MC Aldridge

Carcinoids are solid tumours arising from enterochromaffin cells. These cells are one component of a diffuse neuroendocrine system of cells scattered throughout the body, with similarities in ultrastructure, function and histochemical characteristics. The cells of the neuroendocrine system synthesize and release a variety of active substances, mainly polypeptides, which mediate many physiological actions such as gut motility, vascular tone and gastric secretion (see Chapter 43). They are very similar to certain elements of the nervous system such as the postganglionic fibres of the sympathetic system. The differences between the various neuroendocrine cells reflect the differences and the enormous variety of active constituents that they produce. Nearly 40 polypeptides have now been identified, but gut hormone-producing tumours remain rare with an overall incidence of approximately 1 per 200 000 population in the UK.

One of the biochemical pathways of neuroendocrine cells – amine precursor uptake and decarboxylation – has led to their designation as the APUD system of cells. All tumours from these different cell types are descriptively lumped together as APUDomas. It was once believed that these cell types had a common embryonic origin in the neural crest, but this is now disputed.[1]

The main neuroendocrine tumours found in the small intestine are carcinoids, gastrinomas (which usually occur in the pancreas but may also arise within the duodenum and lead to enteric effects) and somatostatinomas. The clinical problems associated with carcinoid tumours occur mainly as a result of hepatic metastases, whereas the primary tumour often causes little in the way of symptoms. This pattern is in contrast with most other neuroendocrine tumours, which cause symptoms in the absence of metastases.

CARCINOID TUMOURS

Incidence and distribution

Primary gastrointestinal carcinoid tumours are not rare. They are probably the most common tumour of the small intestine, representing a quarter of all small bowel neoplasms[2] and between 17 and 46% of all malignant tumours of the small bowel.[3] The annual age-adjusted incidence of carcinoids (all sites) per 100 000 of the white population in the USA has been reported as 1.31 in men and 1.63 in women.[4] The incidence of small bowel carcinoids in the same groups was 0.48 and 0.28 per 100 000, respectively.

The overall incidence of carcinoid tumours in the UK is unknown.[5] In the Trent Region abdominal carcinoids have an incidence of 0.7 per 100 000 of the population with the small bowel being the most common site and accounting for 36% of the tumours.[6] In Northern Ireland there is an annual incidence of gastrointestinal carcinoids of 1.3 per 100 000.[7]

Carcinoid tumours may occur in the foregut (including bronchus, stomach, first part of duodenum and pancreas), midgut (second, third and fourth parts of duodenum, jejunum, ileum and right colon) or hindgut (transverse colon, left colon and rectum). They may also occur in rarer sites such as the thymus, ovary, testis, parotid, breast, kidney or bladder. Midgut carcinoids account for 75% of all gastrointestinal carcinoid tumours (those in the appendix and ileum alone account for 70%) with only 10% occurring in the foregut and 15% in the hindgut (rectum).[8] The incidence of hepatic metastases varies with the location of the primary tumour but is highest for small bowel carcinoids. In a study of nearly 4000 patients with carcinoid tumours, Maton and Hodgson[8] reported hepatic metastases in 35% of ileal and jejunal carcinoids but in only 2% of carcinoids of the appendix.

Not all patients with hepatic metastases develop symptoms of the carcinoid syndrome, and for those with metastasizing carcinoids of the ileum it is only a quarter. Overall, the carcinoid syndrome occurs in less than 10% of patients with carcinoid tumours and is most common in small bowel carcinoids.[9]

Pathological aspects

Carcinoid tumours originate in the enterochromaffin cell. These cells are situated in the lamina propria of the gut near the base of crypts, where they are called Kulchitsky cells. They are termed 'enterochromaffin' cells because their contained secretory product (5-hydroxytryptamine or serotonin) causes them to stain with potassium chromate. They are also termed 'argentaffin' cells as they take up silver salts, this being the classical staining reaction of neuroendocrine cells. Foregut carcinoids are argentaffin negative and have a low content of serotonin (5-hydroxytryptamine; 5-HT) whereas midgut carcinoids are argentaffin positive and have a high serotonin content.

Serotonin is not the only secretory product of midgut carcinoids. Histamine, substance P, prostaglandins and neuropeptide K can also be produced and may be implicated in the clinical manifestations of the carcinoid syndrome.

Although carcinoids are classically tumours of enterochromaffin and argentaffin cells of the gastrointestinal tract, the term **carcinoid tumour** is expanded by some pathologists to cover gut tumours of paracrine and endocrine-like cells of unknown function. These tumours are of neuroendocrine origin, derive from a primitive stem cell and then may differentiate into one of a variety of endocrine-secreting cells such as α cells (glucagonoma), β cells (insulinoma), δ cells (somatostatinoma), the pancreatic polypeptide cells (PPoma) or cells capable of secreting adrenocorticotrophin growth hormone-releasing factor, vasoactive intestinal polypeptide, (VIP), substance P, gastrin releasing factor, calcitonin and the enterochromaffin cell which is able to secrete serotonin and motilin.

Macroscopic features

Most small bowel carcinoids (at least 80%) are found within 60 cm of the ileocaecal valve and a third of patients have multiple tumours. The primary tumour is usually submucosal and has a yellow colour as a result of its high lipid content (Figure 59.1, see colour plate also). The tumour tends to spread outwards and only rarely ulcerates.

All carcinoid tumours have malignant potential but the risk of developing metastases to regional lymph nodes, liver and bone varies with the site and the size of the primary tumour. Liver metastases occur in 35% of small bowel carcinoids but in only 2% of carcinoids of the appendix.[8] When the primary tumour is less than 1 cm in size, the incidence of metastases is under 2%; this figure rises to 100% in those tumours greater than 2 cm. It follows, therefore, that all primary tumours greater than 2 cm should be considered as malignant. In the case of midgut carcinoids, however, evidence from Sweden[10] would suggest that all primary tumours arising in this site should be considered malignant irrespective of size. In a study of 51 midgut carcinoids treated surgically, primary tumours less than 0.5 cm in diameter were associated with regional lymph node metastases in 69% and liver metastases in 46% whereas for tumours between 0.5 and 1 cm the figures were 94 and 50%, respectively.[10] These authors also reported the incidence of multiple midgut carcinoids as 39%. Such additional tumours may be due to luminal implantation and lymphatic spread within the bowel wall.[11,12]

Spread of the tumour through the wall of the bowel evokes

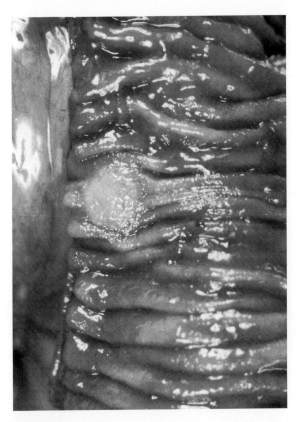

Figure 59.1
A small carcinoid tumour in the ileum. This benign tumour was an unexpected finding in the ileal wall at laparotomy and was treated by local resection.

an intense desmoplastic or fibroplastic reaction, at first around the tumour itself and then spreading into the mesentery (Figure 59.2a, see colour plate also). There may be contraction and adherence of adjacent small bowel loops and it is this which causes partial or complete obstruction of the bowel rather than the primary tumour itself. Ischaemic enteritis and small bowel gangrene (Figure 59.2b, see colour plate also) may occur as a result of compromise of the intestinal blood supply secondary to either mesenteric fibroplasia or periadventitial hyperelastosis and occlusive changes in small to moderate-sized mesenteric arteries.[13] Transmural spread of the tumour and invasion of lymphatics results in metastasis to regional lymph nodes which precedes spread to the liver.

Microscopic features

Carcinoid tumours are not encapsulated. The constituent cells are uniform and often polygonal in shape with a central nucleus containing speckled chromatin and basal granules. Three patterns of cells have been decribed:[14] alveolar clusters, ribbons and cell columns. A fourth scirrhous pattern is only rarely seen.

Natural history and clinical features

Small bowel carcinoids are slow-growing tumours[15] and may be present for years without giving rise to symptoms. In the early stages, vague abdominal pain may be ascribed to irritable

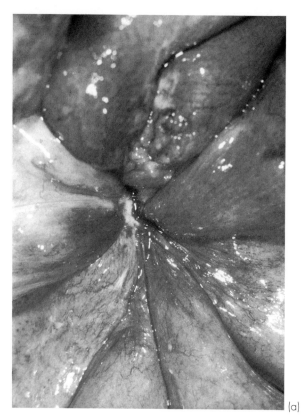

(a)

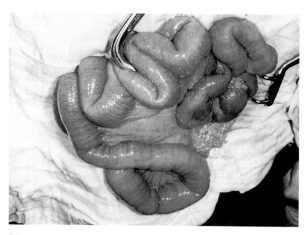

(b)

Figure 59.2
Multiple carcinoid tumours of the ileum with local lymph node metastases in 69-year-old man who presented with symptoms of small bowel colic and underwent elective laparotomy.
(a) Desmoplastic reaction involving the ileal mesentery. (b) Purplish discoloration of the tumour-bearing segment of bowel following simple handling at laparotomy, presumably due to the local release of vasoactive substances.

bowel syndrome and it is well recognized that at least a third of patients with small bowel carcinoids present with years of intermittent non-specific abdominal pain,[16] diarrhoea and weight loss. Carcinoid may present because of symptoms attributable to the primary tumour or because of the effects of liver metastases (see Carcinoid Syndrome below). A primary small bowel carcinoid may present as a mass lesion causing either partial or complete intestinal obstruction, gastrointestinal haemorrhage or more rarely small bowel ischaemia (see above). These tumours may also present more insidiously with a malabsorption syndrome, which is thought to occur secondary to impaired intestinal venous drainage.[17] Partial obstruction of the small bowel secondary to mesenteric lymph node metastases and the intense fibrous reaction around them, together with oedema and compromise of the venous or arterial circulation appears to be the most frequent cause of disturbed intestinal function in these patients and probably contributes to the severe diarrhoea that may be a presenting feature.

Liver metastases may be found incidentally on routine investigation of patients presenting with primary small bowel carcinoids, or may cause symptoms in their own right. Local symptoms of hepatic metastases are uncommon except when they bleed or undergo spontaneous necrosis.

Diagnosis

The diagnosis of small bowel carcinoid tumours depends on a strong clinical suspicion in patients with a long history of intermittent abdominal pain, diarrhoea, malabsorption, flushing, wheezing and symptoms of right heart disease. In such patients, further investigation should be by biochemical laboratory investigations and localization studies.

Laboratory investigations

There is no tumour marker universally present in the serum in carcinoid tumours, but various polypeptides may occasionally be detected: neurotensin is elevated in 43% of cases, substance P in 32%, motilin in 14% and somatostatin in 5%. The best screening test for the diagnosis of midgut carcinoid tumours is the measurement of the urinary metabolite 5-hydroxyindoleacetic acid (5-HIAA) in a 24 hour urine specimen. 5-HIAA is the breakdown product of serotinin (5-HT) following action by the enzyme monoamine oxidase and by aldehyde dehydrogenase. The normal range for 5-HIAA excretion is 2–8 mg per 24 hours. Levels of greater than 30 mg (90 mmol) per 24 hours are usually considered as diagnostic. Mild elevations, however, may also be seen in other conditions such as the blind loop syndrome, Whipple's disease and coeliac disease. False-positive results can also occur if the patient has eaten large amounts of serotonin-enriched foods (such as bananas, pineapples, kiwi fruits, walnuts, pecans or avocados) or is taking reserpine, acetanilide, methysergide or cough medicines containing glyceryl guaiacolate (guaiphenesin). False negatives can also occur in patients taking salicylates or L-dopa.

Liver function tests such as alkaline phosphatase may be abnormal in the presence of hepatic metastases.

Localization studies

Small bowel carcinoids are probably the most difficult of all primary carcinoids to localize. They are generally small tumours which are not readily identified on either a small bowel meal or barium enema. The tumour size is also often below the resolution capacity of both computed tomography

(CT) and ultrasonography. Refinements in contrast radiography, such as the small bowel enema with additional fluoroscopy and compression[18] may increase the detection rate of small bowel carcinoids (Figure 59.3). Similarly, improvements in ultrasonographic technique and resolution may make the diagnosis of larger carcinoid tumours a possibility (see also Chapter 45).[19]

Several types of radiological investigation have been used in the diagnosis of carcinoid tumours, including barium examination, CT, [131I]metaiodobenzylguanidine (MIBG) scanning, 111In-labelled diethylenetriamine penta-acetate-D-Phe-octreotide scintigraphy, angiography and venous sampling. Barium examinations are little used these days but they may demonstrate fixation, separation, thickening and angulation of bowel loops (Figure 59.3). CT is particularly useful for tumour staging;[20] it allows assessment of the extent of tumour spread in the bowel wall and into the mesentery as well as identifying lymph node and liver metastases. The typical CT appearance of mesenteric invasion by carcinoid tumour is of a mesenteric mass with radiating linear densities representing thickened neurovascular bundles. The combination of CT and MIBG scanning has been advocated as the most useful screening test for the diagnosis of carcinoid tumours[21] but this may soon be superseded by octreotide scintigraphy.

The use of angiography to localize carcinoid tumours has to some extent been superseded by the newer imaging methods. Diagnostic angiography is usually employed when other imaging studies are equivocal and operation is planned. The arteriographic appearances of malignant carcinoid tumours with mesenteric involvement are retraction, tortuosity and occlusion of the mesenteric arteries. Percutaneous transhepatic portal and systemic venous sampling is a useful technique for the localization of carcinoid tumours when other imaging modalities have failed. Venous samples are obtained from the portal, hepatic, jugular, subclavian and gonadal veins for hormone assay.

The use of [131I]MIBG for the localization of carcinoid tumours has been available for more than 10 years.[22] It is routinely used in the diagnosis of phaeochromocytoma, but it is also concentrated in many other neuroendocrine tumours of the APUD type (including carcinoid tumours) and in platelets by the same mechanism as serotonin uptake.[23] The overall sensitivity for this investigation has been calculated at 55%.[24] MIBG scintigraphy may be particularly useful in patients who have had previous surgery and in whom there is either distorted anatomy or the presence of metallic clips which interfere with CT.

Carcinoid tumours have a high expression of somatostatin receptors and this fact has been exploited in the development of somatostatin receptor scintigraphy. The long-acting somatostatin analogue, octreotide, is a well-established treatment modality and when radiolabelled can localize carcinoid tumours that express somatostatin receptors.[25,26] Recent experience from Sweden, has shown that scintigraphy using 111In-labelled diethylenetriamine penta-acetate-D-Phe-octreotide in 19 patients with disseminated midgut carcinoids detected tumours in 27 locations previously unrecognized by other forms of imaging.[27] Octreotide scintigraphy was also shown to have a diagnostic sensitivity superior to that of CT and ultrasonography. This technique can certainly detect primary midgut carcinoids and also hepatic and lymph node metastases. In the future, it may find a place in the detection of recurrent disease in patients considered to be in remission and also in the targeting of tumours likely to respond to treatment with octreotide.

Localization of hepatic carcinoid metastases

The techniques for imaging hepatic carcinoid tumours have been reviewed by Adam.[28]

Ultrasonography Metastases of 1 cm or greater may be detected on liver ultrasonography. They are more often hyperechoic but may occasionally be hypoechoic; sometimes both appearances occur in the same patient.

Computed tomography CT can detect liver metastases of 0.5 cm or greater, especially if intravenous contrast-enhancement is employed. The lesions are usually of low attenuation (Figure 59.4).

Angiography Angiography is the most sensitive of the imaging modalities in the detection of carcinoid liver metastases. Four patterns may be seen, which correspond to the nature of the deposits;[29] diffuse fine nodular, diffuse coarse nodular, single masses or a combination. Carcinoid hepatic metastases are highly vascular lesions and show up as a blush on the angiogram. Angiography is an essential investigation in the assessment of respectability of metastases and is used in combination with CT and ultrasonography in this regard. Rarely, the selective superior mesenteric angiogram may also show up a primary carcinoid tumour of the small bowel.

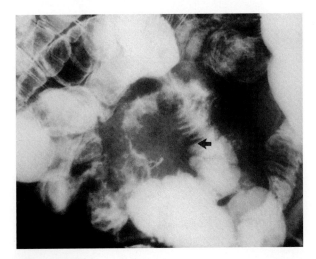

Figure 59.3
Small bowel enema examination in a patient with malignant carcinoid syndrome arising from multiple primary tumours of the distal ileum. There is a soft tissue mass (arrowed), with stretching and ulceration of the mucosa and fixity of the surrounding loops of bowel. (Reproduced from Williamson *Surgery* 1985; **15**: 340–342, by kind permission of The Medicine Group (UK) Ltd.)

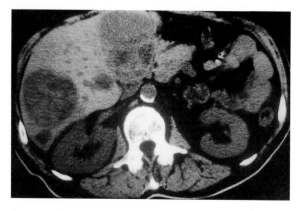

Figure 59.4
Carcinoid hepatic metastases in a patient with severe, intractable symptoms of the carcinoid syndrome. CT scan showing replacement of the majority of the right liver by multiple metastases of various sizes. (Reproduced by kind permission of Professor IS Benjamin.)

Magnetic resonance imaging (MRI) MRI is a very sensitive technique for the detection of liver metastases but is probably less sensitive than CT in the detection of extrahepatic disease. MRI needs further evaluation before it is used as a screening modality for the diagnosis and extent of carcinoid tumours.[30]

Carcinoid syndrome

Carcinoid syndrome occurs in less than 10% of patients with carcinoid tumours but is most common in small bowel carcinoids.[9] The syndrome occurs when the tumour produces active substances that reach the systemic circulation, resulting in the characteristic symptoms of flushing, diarrhoea, sweating, wheezing, abdominal pain and heart disease. In the case of gut carcinoids, 95% of patients with the carcinoid syndrome have liver metastases[9] (Figure 59.5). Occasionally, primary midgut carcinoids with extensive nodal involvement resulting in direct access to

the systemic venous circulation will produce the syndrome in the absence of hepatic metastases.[31]

Not all carcinods metastatic to the liver will produce the carcinoids syndrome. Although approximately a third of patients with small bowel carcinoids will develop liver metastases, only a quarter of such patients will go on to develop the carcinoid syndrome.[32]

Carcinoid syndrome may occur in patients of either sex and at any age, although the sixth decade is the most common time of presentation. The syndrome may be the first presentation of the tumour, the primary itself having remained asymptomatic. At least 50% of patients, however, have the symptoms and signs of advanced metastatic disease at the time of their first presentation.

Not all patients present all of the symptoms of the carcinoid syndrome. Diarrhoea is found in 83% of cases, flushing in 49%, dyspnoea in 20% and bronchospasm in 6%.[33] The relationship between diarrhoea and flushing is variable – one can occur without the other and there may be no temporal relationship between the two. The substances responsible for the many components of the carcinoid syndrome are unknown, but serotonin, prostaglandins, 5-hydroxytryptophan, substance P, kallikrein, histamine, dopamine and neuropeptide K have all been implicated at one time or another.

Components of the carcinoid syndrome

Flushing Over 90% of patients with the carcinoid syndrome will experience flushing attacks. These are of two types. (1) The flush that occurs with midgut carcinoids is usually a faint pink or red colour and involves the face and upper trunk as far as the nipples. It may be provoked by alcohol, or tyramine-containing foods such as blue cheese, chocolate and red wine. The flush only lasts a few minutes and may occur many times over the course of the day. (2) The flush that occurs with foregut tumours is more intense and may last several hours.

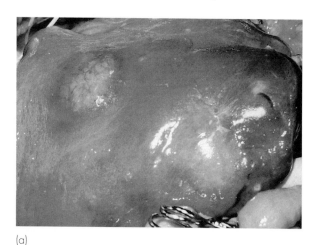
(a)

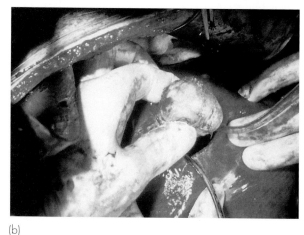
(b)

Figure 59.5
Carcinoid hepatic metastases in a patient with severe, intractable symptoms of the carcinoid syndrome. A debulking procedure was performed by both enucleation and subsegmental resection of the metastases and led to marked clinical improvement. (Figures reproduced by kind permission of Professor IS Benjamin) (a) The appearance of the liver at surgery prior to resection of the metastases. (b) Enucleation of a metastasis.

There may be a purplish discoloration of the skin, and the limbs are involved as well as the upper trunk.

The pentagastrin provocation test has been advocated in the diagnosis of flushing due to the carcinoid syndrome in patients with midgut carcinoids and hepatic metastases.[34]

Diarrhoea Diarrhoea occurs in approximately 75% of patients with the carcinoid syndrome.[35] Most frequently attributed to circulating peptides and a secretory state in the small bowel,[36] it may also occur as a result of a primary tumour causing subacute small bowel obstruction, bacterial overgrowth or lymphatic obstruction.

Secretory diarrhoea tends to persist despite fasting. The differential diagnosis includes the following: Verner–Morrison syndrome (watery diarrhoea, hypokalaemia, hypochlorhydria and acidosis (WDHHA) secondary to a tumour secreting VIP, Zollinger–Ellison syndrome, medullary cell carcinoma of the thyroid, villous adenoma of the rectum and laxative abuse. A history of improvement in the diarrhoea with the administration of H_2 receptor antagonists or omeprazole is strongly suggestive of the Zollinger–Ellison syndrome. Hypocalcaemia is frequent with VIPomas, and steatorrhoea in general only occurs with the Zollinger–Ellison syndrome. Marked metabolic acidosis is usually only a feature of VIPomas. Large villous adenomas of the rectum result in the production of profuse mucous discharge with watery diarrhoea and hypokalaemia.

Cardiac manifestations Fewer than 50% of patients with the carcinoid syndrome develop heart disease. It results from fibrosis of the endocardium of the right side of the heart and leads to progressive right heart failure[37] with associated tricuspid valve disease.

Treatment of carcinoid

Prognosis

Prognosis appears to be determined largely by the extent of tumour involvement and in particular the presence or absence of nodal and/or hepatic metastases at the time of diagnosis. In a study of 188 patients with gastrointestinal carcinoid tumours, McDermott and colleagues[38] found that 5-year survival was 43% for those with lymph node metastases and 94% in those who were node-free. The presence of liver metastases had a similar effect: 5-year survival was 88% in those with metastases at diagnosis but only 25% in patients with liver involvement. These workers also found that prognosis varied with tumour site: 5-year survival was 60% in patients with small bowel carcinoids and 100% for carcinoids of the appendix. Patients with colorectal carcinoid tumours fared worse with only 44% surviving 5 years. In view of the indolent behaviour of these tumours, surgical palliation is warranted in patients with symptomatic bowel obstruction or ischaemia, even in the presence of liver metastases.[39] In patients with hepatic metastases, an aggressive approach to tumour reduction by a combination of surgery and hepatic arterial embolization has recently been shown to result in a 5-year survival of almost 60%.[40]

The treatment of carcinoid tumours of the small bowel can be considered under two main headings: the treatment of the primary tumour and the treatment of hepatic metastases in patients with or without carcinoid syndrome.

Treatment of the primary tumour

Surgical resection of the primary tumour should be the aim in all small bowel carcinoids, even in the presence of diffuse hepatic metastases.[41] This is usually possible when the tumour is small and well localized but may be impossible when there is extensive mesenteric fibroplasia and nodal involvement. In the latter situation, a debulking procedure may be all that can be done and this may be combined with either an ileoileo or ileocolic bypass. In a series of 51 patients with midgut carcinoids, Makridis and colleagues[10] reported that local radical removal of the primary tumour was only possible in 20 patients (39%) and in the remaining 61%, extensive fibrosis and advanced tumour growth into the mesentery, often to the origin of the mesenteric vessels, precluded radical resection of the primary tumour.

Treatment of hepatic metastases and the carcinoid syndrome

Treatment of the carcinoid syndrome may be either by a direct attack on the liver metastases themselves (surgically or radiologically) or by indirect (medical) means aimed at the inhibition of the peripheral actions of 5-HT, the release of kallikrein or the generation of other vasoactive substances.[42]

Hepatic resection Resection of carcinoid liver metastases serves a useful purpose by reducing tumour mass (and hence alleviating local symptoms if they are present) and also by reducing the release of 5-HT and other vasoactive substances. Workers from the Mayo Clinic have stated that 'there seems little doubt that resection may have long-term benefits for patients with localized carcinoid hepatic metastases.[43] In a review (1984–1992) of their patients,[44] 74 underwent hepatic resection with a 4-year survival of 73%. However, almost two thirds of the operations were palliative but symptomatic response to hepatic resection was seen in 90% with a mean duration of response of 19.3 months. The normal 'rules' for the resection of liver metastases can be relaxed to a certain degree in the case of carcinoid because, even if a 'curative' resection cannot be achieved, debulking has definite therapeutic advantages. Enucleation of metastases (Figure 59.5b), segmental and subsegmental resections may be combined with contralateral hepatectomy in this regard.

Operations in patients with the carcinoid syndrome are potentially hazardous since handling of lesions may lead to the sudden release of 5-HT into the circulation and this in turn may cause rapid alteration in blood pressure, bronchial constriction, hyperpnoea and hyperglycemia. Agents that precipitate flushing should be avoided by the anaesthetist, and nerve blockers, acetylcholine and morphine should all be used with caution. An intravenous infusion of somatostatin should be commenced before operation and continued into the early postoperative period. Other pharmacological agents such as chlorophenylalanine, cyproheptadine and nicotinamide may be used to block the actions of released 5-HT. Hypotensive episodes should be treated with angiotensin and blood transfusion (not catecholamines), and hydralazine should be used for hypertension.

Hepatic dearterialization Liver tumours (both primary and secondary) derive their blood supply primarily from the hepatic artery, whereas normal liver tissue is supplied by the portal vein.[45-52] Dearterialization aims to interrupt arterial inflow to the liver while maintaining portal venous flow, thus depriving the metastases of their blood supply. Carcinoid hepatic metastases are highly vascular lesions and are particularly sensitive to this form of treatment. Dearterialization may be either permanent (hepatic artery ligation) or temporary, when an occluding device placed around the hepatic artery is used to provide intermittent arterial occlusion. The early results of hepatic artery ligation were disappointing,[53,54] possibly as a result of the early formation of collaterals.[55] In an effort to delay collateral formation, Bengmark and coworkers[56] developed the technique of total hepatic dearterialization, the aim of which was to completely mobilize the liver by dividing all its attachments with the exception of the hepatic artery, hepatic veins, portal vein and bile duct. When combined with intermittent occlusion of the hepatic artery by slings (temporary hepatic dearterialization) and regional chemotherapy, this procedure results in useful palliation with a low operative mortality rate.[57] The results have been particularly impressive in the case of carcinoid hepatic metastases, possibly because of the highly vascular nature of these lesions.[58]

The technique of hepatic dearterialization was first described in detail by Bengmark and his associates[56] who have since published a number of modifications including the introduction of the concept of temporary dearterialization.[57-60] Briefly, the liver is fully mobilized by disconnection of all ligamentous attachments and dissection of all structures within the hepatoduodenal ligament. The hepatic artery is surrounded by either silastic occluding slings (which are brought out through the abdominal wall) or an inflatable arterial occluder. These devices allow temporary occlusion of the hepatic artery to be performed on a regular basis once the patient has recovered from the operation. The first such treatment is usually commenced 4 weeks after operation. Hepatic ischaemia is induced by either traction on the silastic slings or inflation of the arterial occluder for a period of 16 hours. Colour flow Doppler ultrasonography can be used to ensure that all arterial inflow to the liver has ceased on clamping. Two hours after release of the arterial clamp, systemic chemotherapy may be administered in the form of streptozotocin (500 mg/m²) and 5-fluorouracil (400 mg/m²) which are continued daily for 5 days. The cycle of hepatic ischaemia followed by chemotherapy is repeated every 4 weeks.

Interruption of the arterial blood supply to the liver and its metastases has evolved as a form of therapy over the last 30 years.[61] Hepatic artery ligation (permanent dearterialization) has been shown to give symptomatic relief in about 50% of patients with the carcinoid syndrome but the procedure has been beset with a high operative mortality rate[62] and the early re-establishment of collaterals.[55] Temporary hepatic dearterialization was aimed at achieving the same symptomatic results but with a lower operative mortality rate. When used for colorectal liver metastases, temporary hepatic dearterialization is no better than single agent intra-arterial chemotherapy,[63] and it is only in the case of carcinoid hepatic metastases that it has a beneficial effect.[64] Bengmark and his associates[59] have reported no operative deaths and a 6% 60-day mortality rate in their first 16 patients to undergo this procedure. All but one of the 16 patients had relief of their symptoms of the carcinoid syndrome but they only remained asymptomatic for a mean of 3 months. Four patients, however, were symptom-free for between 24 and 62 months. The same group have reported their experience in a total of 19 patients with the carcinoid syndrome and found that after 6 months of treatment by temporary dearterialization, 79% of patients had either stability or regression of hepatic metastases (assessed angiographically); at 1 year the figure was 58%.[64]

The future of hepatic dearterialization for the treatment of carcinoid hepatic metastases depends on further investigation of its mechanism of action and on the accurate timing of chemotherapy. The main effect of vascular occlusion and tissue ischaemia occurs after release of the circulation rather than during the ischaemic period itself, and therefore rapid restoration of the circulation may be important in the success of this technique. Temporary dearterialization may thus be expected to produce superior results to those obtained by hepatic artery embolization (see below) because, in the former technique, rapid restoration of the circulation is possible, whereas embolization leads to irreversible arterial occlusion. The death of tumour cells following vascular occlusion probably acts as a stimulus for the surviving cells to divide and grow, with the peak of mitosis occurring between 24 and 48 hours after the release of the circulation.[59] This would seem the most logical time to administer chemotherapy to obtain maximum efficacy.

The length of time of hepatic arterial occlusion for optimal results remains unknown. It is possible that the 16 hour occlusion recommended by Dahl and colleagues[68] is too long. The interval between treatments has also been reached quite arbitrarily, and a time interval of 1 month may be excessive. Occlusion for 1 hour was advocated by El Domeiri and Mojab[65] in an early study, and it has since been shown that there is no induction of arterial collaterals following such a short period of vascular occlusion.[66] Bengmark's group[67] have suggested ultra short-term vascular occlusion (45–60 minutes) repeated twice daily for as long as the patient survives.

Hepatic artery embolization This is an alternative form of permanent dearterialization which is performed without the need for an open operation. The method has been described in detail by workers from the Hammersmith Hospital.[68] Briefly, selective arteriography of both the coeliac axis and the hepatic artery is performed. The arterial phase shows the distribution of metastases and the venous phase the degree of patency of the portal vein. If the portal vein is patent, embolization of one or more branches of the hepatic artery is performed using a variety of material, such as pieces of gelatin sponge (Gelfoam; 1–3 mm) or steel coils. Necrosis of tumour deposits may lead to the release of large amounts of vasoactive substances and therefore blocking agents are administered both before and after the procedure (as for operation: see above). Antibiotics are given at the time of the procedure and for up to 10 days afterwards (or as long as the fever lasts) to prevent superinfection of necrotic tumour deposits.

The results of this procedure are variable and patient selection is important. Embolization has a beneficial effect in controlling the symptoms of the carcinoid syndrome and also in reducing local symptoms from the tumour. In the early series reported from the Hammersmith,[68] 12 patients with the carcinoid syndrome underwent embolization and nine had a dramatic improvement in their symptoms with abolition of flushing, abdominal pain and wheezing and reduction in diarrhoea. Relief of symptoms lasted for between 1 and 24 months, but only four of the nine patients were still asymptomatic 6 months after embolization. There was a 30-day mortality rate of 17% in this series. Carrasco and colleagues[69] have reported 23 patients with the carcinoid syndrome, 20 of whom responded to embolization by a symptomatic improvement, the response lasting a median of 11 months. In these patients the symptomatic response correlated with a reduction in the extent of liver involvement and a decrease in urinary 5-HIAA levels. Again, two patients (9%) died from complications attributable to the embolization. Bengmark and his colleagues[60] in Lund have reported the most recent series of ten patients with carcinoid syndrome treated by hepatic artery embolization. Tumour regression occurred in 70% at 6 months and in 40% at 1 year, but relief of the symptoms of carcinoid syndrome was less impressive. All ten patients initially had relief of symptoms, but these returned in seven patients (within 6 months in five) and four were still symptomatic at the time of death.

Liver transplantation Liver transplantation may provide long-term symptomatic relief and sometimes cure, in patients with disabling symptoms of the carcinoid syndrome whose disease is confined to the liver and in whom current therapy such as temporary dearterialization, hepatic artery embolization, chemotherapy, somatostatin and other pharmacological blocking agents has failed. The reported worldwide experience of liver transplantation for carcinoid hepatic metastases is very limited.[70–74] The Cambridge group led by Calne has described two patients, one who had relief of symptoms and remained well 20 months after transplantation and one who also had relief of carcinoid symptoms but died (asymptomatic) from chronic graft failure at 8 months after transplantation.[70] The most recent series has been reported from France[75] and describes transplantation in nine patients with liver metastases from a variety of neuroendocrine tumours (four carcinoids). There were three early deaths; one from primary non-function of the graft and two as a result of portal vein thrombosis. A fourth patient died at day 7 from fulminant septicaemia. There were two late deaths at 8 and 17 months; the first shortly after re-transplantation for chronic rejection and the second from metastatic disease. Three patients transplanted for carcinoid hepatic metastases were currently alive at 15, 24 and 62 months, although the latter patient had recently been diagnosed as having bone and liver metastases. After a critical review of their indications for transplantation, the authors concluded that only three of the nine patients should have undergone liver transplantation as many had extrahepatic spread of their tumour. At this early stage in the world experience, it is still unclear as to what part liver transplantation should play in the management of patients with the carcinoid syndrome.

Chemotherapy A number of chemotherapeutic agents have been used in the treatment of carcinoid tumours both singly, and in combination, but there is little evidence of benefit in terms of symptomatic relief or increased survival, and toxicity is also a problem.[76] Streptozotocin and 5-fluorouracil are the agents most commonly used; adriamycin, cyclophosphamide and doxorubicin have also been used. The combination of streptozotocin and 5-fluorouracil is the most frequently used but shows a response rate of only about 30%.[77] In a review of the place of chemotherapy in patients with metastatic carcinoid, Bukowski and colleagues[78] evaluated 56 patients treated with a combination of 5-fluorouracil, adriamycin, cyclophosphamide and streptozotocin (FAC-S). In those with small bowel carcinoids, a complete response occurred in only 5% with 27% having a partial response. In the future, chemotherapy may find a place when used in combination with ischaemic therapy, either temporary hepatic dearterialization or hepatic artery embolization (see above). It would seem that chemotherapy alone is ineffective.

Somatostatin and somatostatin analogue (SMS 201-995/octreotide) Somatostatin is a peptide synthesized in a variety of tissues which can inhibit the secretion of hormones or other cell products. It probably exerts its beneficial effect in the carcinoid syndrome as a 5-HT antagonist. Over the last ten years, a long-acting analogue of somatostatin (octreotide, SMS 201–995; Sandostatin) with similar biological effects as the naturally occurring hormone has been introduced into clinical practice. Octreotide can be self-administered over prolonged periods of time with minimal adverse side-effects.

Kvols and colleagues[76,79] evaluated the effects of octreotide in 25 patients with the carcinoid syndrome treated by thrice daily subcutaneous injections, each of 150 µg. Flushing and diarrhoea were rapidly relieved in 22 patients (88%), and 5-HIAA levels decreased by over 50% in 18 (72%). The median duration of response was over 12 months. Up until November 1987, 80 patients with the carcinoid syndrome treated by octreotide had been reported in the world literature.[80] Symptoms (flushing, diarrhoea or both) improved in 54 of 59 patients (92%) for whom data were available. Urinary 5-HIAA decreased in 66% but in no patient did it fall to within the normal range. Several subsequent large series have confirmed these good results[80–86] and octreotide is now considered to be one of the most effective drugs available in the control of the symptoms of carcinoid syndrome. The effect on tumour size is less clear; current data suggest that only a small proportion of patients respond by reduction in tumour size.[80]

A second somatostatin analogue, RC-160, has also been evaluated in patients with the carcinoid syndrome. Mathé and colleagues[87] showed that administration of RC-160 in doses of 100–400 µg three times daily to 21 patients caused a complete relief of flushing, diarrhoea and abdominal pain and reduced levels of urinary 5-HIAA, but it had no effect on tumour size.

At the present time, it is considered that the main clinical use of somatostatin analogues is in the control of the symptoms of the carcinoid syndrome, particularly in the acute situation of the 'carcinoid crisis' and in 'covering' patients undergoing resection, temporary hepatic dearterialization or hepatic artery embolization.

Human leucocyte interferon Interferon (IFN) is a naturally occurring protein produced by leucocytes in response to viral infections. Administration of large doses of IFN has been shown to inhibit the growth of a variety of cancers including carcinoid.[88] The exact mechanism of action of IFN on carcinoid tumour growth is unknown, but it is most likely to act as a direct inhibitor of cell proliferation and hormone synthesis.[89–91] Early clinical results suggested that IFN could reduce levels of hormones and other tumour-associated peptides as well as control symptoms in patients with midgut carcinoid tumours and the carcinoid syndrome.[92] These same workers subsequently reported their experience in 36 patients and also provided detailed long-term results.[93] Twenty nine patients had midgut carcinoids. Objective tumour responses (>50% reduction in tumour markers and/or tumour size on CT) were seen in 17 of 36 patients (47%) treated with IFN. Patients with midgut carcinoids had a response rate of 48%. Stable disease (a reduction of tumour markers and/or tumour size by <50% and no appearance of new metastases) was recorded in 14 of the 36 patients (39%), all of whom had midgut carcinoids. Two patients had a complete remission. The median duration of objective response was 34 months, and the median duration of stable disease was 25 months. Of the 14 patients with midgut carcinoids who showed an objective response 13 had a >50% reduction in urinary 5-HIAA levels, and two patients showed a significant reduction in tumour size on CT. Subjective responses were recorded in 21 of 29 patients (72%) with midgut carcinoids. All these patients showed less frequent flushing episodes, which were of shorter duration and less intensity, whereas 14 had fewer episodes of diarrhoea.

In a controlled study, Oberg and colleagues[94] compared treatment with human leucocyte IFN with that by combination chemotherapy (streptozotocin plus 5-fluorouracil) in 20 patients with malignant midgut carcinoids. Ten patients received IFN and ten chemotherapy. After 6 months of treatment, an objective response was recorded in five patients (50%) treated with IFN and in none treated with chemotherapy. Stable disease was recorded in 50% of the patients on IFN and 40% of those on chemotherapy. Progressive disease was not seen in any of the patients on IFN whereas six of the patients (60%) on chemotherapy progressed. Three of eight patients who had initially been treated with chemotherapy and were later treated with IFN also showed an objective response. The objective responses were mainly in the form of a reduction in tumour markers, but two patients did show a significant reduction in tumour size on CT. Subjective responses were recorded in 72% of patients treated with IFN but in only 9% of those treated with chemotherapy. The results of this small study suggest that IFN is associated with a higher response rate than the combination of streptozotocin and 5-fluorouracil. No survival data are available.

Treatment with IFN is not without its side-effects. In order of frequency these include 'flu-like' symptoms with fever, malaise and fatigue; anaemia; leucopenia; increases in transaminase and alkaline phosphatase; increase in serum triglycerides and fatty change in the liver. All of these effects are dose dependent and reversible. More serious side-effects are the autoimmune phenomena seen in a minority of patients: autoimmune thyroiditis, pernicious anemia and systemic lupus erythematosus.

At the present time neither optimal doses nor dose intervals of IFN have been worked out. Regional intra-arterial infusion may be more effective than subcutaneous injections and there may be some advantage in combining IFN treatment with chemotherapy. IFN is probably the treatment of choice for malignant carcinoid tumours, having a better response rate than chemotherapy or somatostatin analogues.

Additional medical therapy A number of other drugs are in use for the control of symptoms of the carcinoid syndrome.

- *Ketanserin.* This is a 5-HT antagonist which is effective in reducing both diarrhoea and flushing. It is given in a dose of 20 mg four times daily.
- *Cyproheptadine.* This drug acts by blocking the effect of 5-HT on smooth muscle. Its main use is in the treatment of diarrhoea and it is one of the principal drugs in the medical treatment of the carcinoid syndrome. It is given in a dose of 4 mg four times daily.

OTHER NEUROENDOCRINE TUMOURS OF THE MIDGUT

Carcinoid tumours are by far the most common primary APUDomas or neuroendocrine tumours of the midgut. Other primary neuroendocrine tumours are much more commonly found within the pancreas but may rarely be found within the midgut or may cause enteric effects as a result of the actions of their secretory peptides. Gastrinomas can occur in the duodenum (or more rarely the jejunum); somatostatinomas may occur in the duodenum, at the ampulla of Vater or within the small bowel. Secretory diarrhoea and other enteric effects may be associated with the Zollinger–Ellison syndrome (gastrinoma), the Verner–Morrison syndrome (VIPoma) and medullary cell carcinoma of the thyroid.

Gastrinoma and the Zollinger–Ellison syndrome

Pathology

Gastrinomas are usually small tumours, less than 2 cm in diameter. Until recently, it was considered that 80–90% of gastrinomas arose within the pancreas but a detailed study of failed operations for the Zollinger–Ellison syndrome (ZES) has highlighted the fact that small gastrinomas may occur in the duodenum[95] (Figure 59.6, see colour plate also). The incidence of duodenal gastrinomas has been reported as 38%.[96] Even more

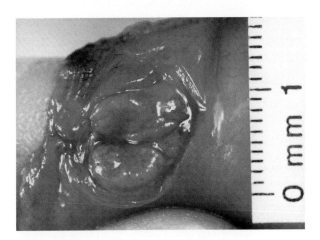

Figure 59.6
Duodenal gastrinoma. This lesion is seen incorporated in the total gastrectomy specimen from a patient who presented with duodenal and oesophageal ulceration and stenosis.

rarely, gastrinomas may be found in the stomach, periduodenal lymph nodes and jejunum. Nearly 90% of gastrinomas can be found within the boundaries of the so-called 'gastrinoma triangle' formed by the junction of the cystic and common bile duct superiorly, the junction of the second and third parts of the duodenum inferiorly, and the junction of the neck and body of the pancreas medially (see also Chapter 36).[97]

Macroscopically, gastrinomas are oval or round lesions with a smooth tan appearance. They are solid tumours with a thin fibrous capsule surrounding a reddish-brown core of tumour and may look strikingly similar to carcinoids. Almost all gastrinoma cells give a positive reaction to Grimelius silver stain but immunocytochemistry is the only reliable technique for diagnosis. Approximately 50% of gastrinomas contain cells producing additional peptides to gastrin.

Although it is generally considered that 60% of gastrinomas are malignant,[98,99] there is confusion over how malignancy should be defined. Histological appearances are of little help and the presence of either lymph node or liver metastases should be the sole criterion. There is increasing evidence that the biological behaviour of extrapancreatic malignant gastrinomas may be more favourable than that of tumours arising within the pancreas. Kaplan and colleagues[96] found that malignancy was present in only four of 11 patients (36%) with duodenal gastrinomas but in five of seven (71%) of those with sporadic pancreatic gastrinomas. In addition, none of the malignant duodenal gastrinomas had liver or other distant metastases (all four had nodal metastases only), whereas liver metastases were present in four of the seven pancreatic gastrinomas.

Clinical features

Peptic ulcer symptoms are present in almost all patients with the Zollinger–Ellison syndrome and may be long-standing (see also Chapter 36). Severe abdominal pain is the most common specific symptom, occurring in 70–80% of patients overall and complicated by gastrointestinal haemorrhage in 30–40%.[96]

It is now recognized that diarrhoea may be the presenting symptom in approximately a third of patients with gastrinoma.[96] The diarrhoea, which may be very profuse, results from severe acid jejunitis secondary to the upper small bowel being exposed to a persistently low pH which inactivates pancreatic lipase and deconjugates bile salts. Control of acid secretion, whether by omeprazole or total gastrectomy, will abolish the diarrhoea, and this helps differentiate this form of secretory diarrhoea from that due to other APUDomas such as carcinoid syndrome, the Verner–Morrison syndrome, or medullary cell carcinoma of the thyroid.

Diagnosis

The diagnosis of gastrinoma is made by demonstrating *gastric acid hypersecretion* and a *raised serum gastrin level*. Basal acid output is normally less than 5 mmol/h; for the diagnosis of gastrinoma it should be greater than 15 mmol/h (or greater than 5 mmol/h if the patient has had previous gastric surgery). Fasting serum gastrin should be less than 50 pmol/l. Values between 50 and 100 pmol/l are abnormal and values greater than 100 pmol/l in association with gastric hypersecretion are strongly suggestive of gastrinoma.

Imaging and localization

Once the diagnosis of Zollinger–Ellison syndrome is established, the gastrinoma should be localized if possible before operating to remove it.

Preoperative imaging The main imaging modalities used in the preoperative localization of gastrinomas are ultrasonography, CT, selective arteriography, portal venous sampling and MRI. *Ultrasonography* has a low sensitivity for localizing primary gastrinomas.[100] The recent introduction of *endoscopic ultrasonography* has increased the usefulness of ultrasonography as it can provide high-resolution images of the pancreatic parenchyma and duodenum.[101] *Computed tomography* has a poor record in the detection of gastrinomas. In a collective review,[102] CT only detected 35–59% of primary gastrinomas. *Selective arteriography* has a higher sensitivity than CT in the detection of both primary and secondary gastrinomas[103] and is the investigation of choice.

Peroperative imaging Localizing investigations comprise intraoperative ultrasonography and intraoperative endoscopy. *Intraoperative ultrasonography* with a 7 MHz transducer is an extremely useful adjunct to palpation during laparotomy for gastrinoma. Although in experienced hands most pancreatic and duodenal gastrinomas should be palpable, intraoperative ultrasonography has been shown in several prospective studies to change operative strategy in as many as 10% of patients, either by detecting non-palpable tumours or by detecting nodal or liver metastases.[104,105] *Intraoperative endoscopy* with transillumination of the duodenal wall has been advocated in the detection of duodenal gastrinomas. Frucht and colleagues[106] were able to detect six out of seven duodenal gastrinomas using this technique among patients in whom CT and arteriography had only detected two tumours and palpation and intraoperative ultrasonography only one.

Treatment of the Zollinger–Ellison syndrome

The optimal treatment for the Zollinger–Ellison syndrome is surgical excision of the gastrinoma for cure. Surgical cure can be defined as resection of all gastrinoma tumour such that the patient is rendered eugastrinaemic, requires no antiulcer medication and has no evidence of recurrent disease on long-term follow-up.

Once the diagnosis is made, the first objective is to render the patient 'safe' for operation by effective medical treatment with omeprazole. During this period, preoperative localizing investigations are performed to show the site of primary disease and the presence or absence of liver metastases. The presence of liver metastases should not deter the surgeon, as a debulking procedure may still be worthwhile in the control of the Zollinger–Ellison syndrome.

The abdomen is opened and a full and detailed laparotomy is carried out. If hepatic metastases are found and confirmed on biopsy, a decision must be taken as to whether to perform total gastrectomy or to close the abdomen and treat the patient with omeprazole. This decision will depend on the ease with which preoperative symptoms were controlled on medical treatment and the patient's compliance plus the extent of carcinomatosis and thus the expectation of survival. An aggressive surgical approach to metastatic gastrinoma has been proposed with limited success[107] (see below).

If there are no hepatic metastases, a detailed search is undertaken for both primary gastrinoma and regional nodal metastases. The search is concentrated within the 'gastrinoma triangle' (see above), but the stomach, small bowel, retroperitoneum and ovary must also be examined. The pancreas is fully mobilized to allow full palpation and the use of intraoperative ultrasonography. The duodenum is fully Kocherized to allow examination of the head of pancreas and exposure of the posterior surface of the duodenum, a frequent site for nodal metastases. Any enlarged nodes are excised and sent for frozen section. The duodenum is carefully palpated between finger and thumb to identify small microadenomas which can often be felt as small 'millet seeds' in the duodenal wall. If at this point no tumour has been found, a longitudinal duodenotomy should be performed in the second part of the duodenum to allow careful evaluation of the mucosa by direct inspection and then with the index finger inside the lumen and the thumb outside. Eversion of the mucosa is crucial for the identification of microadenomas which may be as small as 2 mm.[95] Small gastrinomas discovered in this way may simply be enucleated from the mucosa.

Despite all attempts before and during the operation, no tumour will be found in some patients (perhaps up to a third). Intraoperative ultrasonography and routine exploration of the duodenum for microgastrinomas are likely to reduce the percentage of negative laparotomies, but the situation will still arise in which no tumour is found. Classically there are then two options: either to close the abdomen and treat the patient with antisecretory medication, such as omeprazole, or to perform a total gastrectomy, thus removing the target organ (see Chapter 36). The availability of omeprazole certainly reduces the need for total gastrectomy, although the long-term effects of this drug are not yet known. A possible alternative is to perform a lesser gastric resection (i.e. subtotal) with vagotomy, thereby reducing the amount of medical treatment required.

Treatment of metastatic gastrinoma

Between 25 and 40% of patients with the Zollinger–Ellison syndrome have metastatic disease.[108] The most recent figures suggest an actuarial 5-year survival rate of around 20% in this group.[107]

If gastric acid hypersecretion is adequately controlled (either surgically or medically or both), patients with metastatic gastrinoma may remain asymptomatic until late in the course of the disease. Thus, patients with metastases may only require treatment if the lesions are painful or enlarging. Options include chemotherapy, hepatic artery embolization, aggressive surgical resection of all gross disease, hormonal therapy with octreotide and treatment with IFN; the best form of treatment remains unclear.

Chemotherapy This can involve streptozotocin with or without 5-fluorouracil, or 5-fluorouracil plus doxorubicin: response rates of 20–60% have been reported.[102] The value of chemotherapy is uncertain. In one study of ten patients, streptozotocin and 5-fluorouracil with or without doxorubicin resulted in a 40% response rate,[109] but in another study of 22 patients receiving the same therapy the response rate was only 5%.[110]

Hepatic artery embolization and temporary hepatic dearterialization Both of these techniques have been used with some success in the treatment of carcinoid hepatic metastases (see above), but experience with metastatic gastrinoma is limited.[68,111,112] In the most recent of these studies, hepatic artery embolization combined with chemotherapy resulted in an excellent symptomatic response in 50% of patients, a good response in 30% and no response in 20%.[112]

Aggressive surgical resection of metastatic gastrinoma This has been shown by Zollinger and colleagues[113] to prolong average survival from 3 years to 9 years. Norton and colleagues[107] reported their results of complete surgical resection plus chemotherapy (streptozotocin, doxorubicin and 5-fluorouracil) in five patients with extensive metastatic gastrinoma confined to the abdomen. Complete resection was possible in four of the five, and all four showed improvement, with a reduction in their requirements for antiacid therapy and a return to a normal working life. Three of the four patients had no detectable tumour on follow-up and two were eugastrinaemic at 14 and 32 months. This aggressive approach may lead to a survival benefit in a small selected number of patients with resectable disease but requires further evaluation before it can be uniformly recommended.

Somatostatin and octreotide Somatostatin and its long-acting analogue, octreotide, are potent inhibitors of hormone secretion from both normal and tumour tissue and have been shown to be effective in relieving symptoms from a variety of islet cell tumours including gastrinomas.[114] The original suggestion that hepatic metastases from gastrinoma can sometimes regress during treatment with octreotide[115,116] has not been confirmed by other workers.[117,118] There is a need to further evaluate somatostatin analogues, including the more potent RC-160 (see above) in the treatment of metastatic gastrinoma.

Human leucocyte interferon IFN has been shown to produce an objective response in patients with metastatic islet cell tumours including gastrinoma.[119,120] In a study from Sweden,[119] 12 patients with malignant endocrine pancreatic tumours refractory to chemotherapy were treated with IFN. Ten of the 12 patients showed an objective response as defined by a reduction in tumour markers and a greater than 50% reduction in tumour mass on CT or ultrasonography. One of three patients with gastrinoma responded. These early results suggested that IFN was as effective as chemotherapy but had fewer side-effects.

Somatostatinoma

Somatostatin was originally isolated from the hypothalamus and later from other parts of the central nervous system. It is also to be found in the δ-cells of the pancreas and in the upper gastrointestinal tract. Somatostatin inhibits the secretion of many hormones, including growth hormone, thyrotropin, insulin, glucagon, gastrin and renin. It also inhibits exocrine pancreatic and gastric secretion.

Pathology

Although most somatostatinomas occur within the pancreatic head, they may also be found in the small bowel,[121] duodenum and the ampulla of Vater.[122] They arise from δ-cells and are usually solitary tumours. About 50% of somatostatinomas are malignant, and most of these have hepatic metastases at the time of diagnosis.

Clinical features

The clinical presentation is characterized by dyspepsia, mild diarrhoea (usually steatorrhoea), wasting, fatigue, anaemia, diabetes and gallstones.[123] Some of these symptoms may be explained by the inhibitory action of somatostatin on gastrin, secretion, insulin and cholecystokinin.

Investigation

Plasma concentrations of somatostatin are markedly raised. As the clinical presentation is so vague, it is unlikely that less advanced disease will be detected unless all diabetics are screened by somatostatin assay.

Treatment

Surgical removal of the tumour has relieved symptoms in a few patients. Streptozotocin may be used in patients with metastatic disease.

VIPoma and the WDHA (Verner–Morrison) syndrome

Primary VIPomas are usually found within the pancreas, but their clinical presentation is with profuse watery diarrhoea due to the enteric effects of their peptide product. The terms Verner–Morrison syndrome,[124] WDHA-syndrome[125] (watery diarrhoea, hypokalaemia, achlorhydria), and pancreatic cholera[126] are all used synonymously. The syndrome consists of diarrhoea with motions of a very fluid consistency, free of blood and mucus and with a volume of over 20 ml/kg per day; diarrhoea precipitates hypokalaemia, and there is either hypochlorhydria or complete achlorhydria. Some two thirds of patients complain of abdominal pain and there is often marked loss of weight. One third of patients have hypoglycaemia and/or flushing attacks.[127]

Between 10 and 20% of VIPomas are extrapancreatic, occurring in the retroperitoneal sympathetic chain and the adrenal medulla[128] and 50–75% of all VIPomas are malignant.

The diagnosis of a VIPoma requires the demonstration of an elevated fasting concentration of plasma VIP in a patient with the typical clinical picture. All patients with circulating VIP exceeding 60 pmol/1 have been found to have VIPomas.[127]

Treatment

All patients with the VIPomas syndrome should undergo operation, and the tumour should be resected if at all possible. In the case of a malignant VIPoma with hepatic metastases, debulking is indicated to decrease VIPoma symptoms and allow more effective medical treatment.[129] Treatment with octreotide may provide relief of intractable diarrhoea in patients with metastatic VIPoma.[130]

Postoperatively, serial determination of plasma VIP levels will help detect recurrent disease. Patients with benign VIPomas can be cured by operation. The average survival time for those with malignant VIPoma syndrome is approximately 12 months.[131]

Medullary cell carcinoma of the thyroid

Medullary cell carcinoma of the thyroid is a rare tumour accounting for less than 7% of all thyroid malignancies. It arises from parafollicular C cells which are part of the APUD system.

Medullary cell carcinoma may present with diarrhoea, and indeed almost a third of patients with this tumour have diarrhoea at some stage during their illness.[132] Most pass less than five loose stools per day but occasionally stool frequency may be twice this figure. Other features of the syndrome relate mainly to local invasion and the effects of the endocrine secretion. Hypocalcaemia as a result of calcitonin hypersecretion is very rare.

The diagnosis of this tumour is based on the detection of high levels of calcitonin. Most patients have fasting calcitonin levels above 0.38 ng/ml. In all patients the calcitonin level rises over 1 ng/ml in response to a calcium infusion. The pentagastrin provocation test can also be used when peak calcitonin levels are reached within 5 minutes of the intravenous pentagastrin injection (0.5 μg/kg).

Treatment

Total thyroidectomy with lymph node clearance of the central cervical and upper mediastinal nodes is the treatment of choice. Mediastinal clearance is probably not justified if CT shows hepatic metastases, although solitary metastases may be amenable to local removal.

REFERENCES

1. Stevens DR & Moore GE. Inadequacy of APUD concept in explaining production of peptide hormones by tumours. *Lancet* 1983; **i**: 118.
2. O'Rourke MGE, Lancashire RP & Vattoune JR. Carcinoid of the small intestine. *Aust NZ J Surg* 1986; **56**: 405.
3. Buchanan KD, Johnston CF, O'Hare MMT et al. Neuroendocrine tumours. A European view. *Am J Med* 1986; **81**: (Suppl. 6b): 14.
4. Godwin JD. Carcinoid tumours. An analysis of 2837 cases. *Cancer* 1975; **36**: 560–569.
5. Payne-James JJ, de Gara CJ, Lovell D, Silk DBA & Misiewicz JJ. Gastrointestinal carcinoid tumours in a district general hospital. *J R Coll Surg Edinb* 1989; **34**: 94.
6. Woods HF, Bax ND & Ainsworth I. Abdominal carcinoid tumours in Sheffield. *Digestion* 1990; **45** (Suppl. 1): 17.
7. Watson RG, Johnston CF, O'Hare MMT et al. The frequency of gastrointestinal endocrine tumours in a well-defined population – Northern Ireland 1970–1985. *Q J Med* 1989; **72**: 647–657.
8. Maton PN & Hodgson HJF. Carcinoid tumours and the carcinoid syndrome. In Bouchier IAD, Allan RN, Hodgson HJF & Keighley MRB (eds) *Textbook of Gastroenterology*. London: Baillière Tindall, 1984.
9. Davis Z, Moertel CG & McLirath DC. The malignant carcinoid syndrome. *Surg Gynecol Obstet* 1973; **137**: 637.
10. Makridis C, Oberg K, Juhlin C et al. Surgical treatment of mid-gut carcinoid tumours. *World J Surg* 1990; **14**: 377.
11. Warner TF, O'Reilly G & Power G. Carcinoid diathesis of the ileum. *Cancer* 1979; **43**: 1900.
12. Strodel WE, Talpos G, Eckhauser F & Thompson N. Surgical therapy for small bowel carcinoid tumors. *Arch Surg* 1983; **118**: 391.
13. Eckhauser FE, Argenta LC, Strodel WE et al. Mesenteric angiopathy, intestinal gangrene and midgut carcinoids. *Surgery* 1981; **90**: 720.
14. Soga J & Tazawa K. Pathologic analysis of carcinoids. *Cancer* 1971: **28**: 990.
15. Moertel CG, Sauer WG, Dockerty MB & Baggenstoss AH. Life history of the carcinoid tumour of the small intestine. *Cancer* 1961; **14**: 901.
16. Vinik AI & Moattari AR. The use of somatostatin analogue in the management of the carcinoid syndrome. *Am J Dig Dis* 1989; **34**: 14s.
17. Knowlessar OD, Law DH & Sleisinger MH. Malabsorption syndrome associated with metastatic carcinoid tumor. *Am J Med* 1959; **27**: 673.
18. Jeffree MA & Nolan DJ. Multiple ileal carcinoid tumours. *Br J Radiol* 1987; **60**: 402.
19. Skaane P. The ultrasonic demonstration of carcinoid tumor of the ileocecal valve. *Am J Gastroenterol* 1987; **82**: 168.
20. Gould M & Johnson RJ. Computed tomography of abdominal carcinoid tumour. *Br J Radiol* 1986; **59**: 881.
21. Adolph JMG, Kimming BN, Georgi P et al. Carcinoid tumours: CT and I-131 Meta-iodobenzylguanidine scintigraphy. *Radiology* 1987; **164**: 199.
22. Fischer M, Kamanabroo D, Sonderkamp H et al. Scintigraphic imaging of carcinoid tumours with I-131-metaiodobenzylguanidine. *Lancet* 1984; **ii**: 165.
23. Feldman JM, Frankel N & Coleman RE. Platelet uptake of the phaeochromocytoma-scanning agent I-131-meta-iodobenzylguanidine. *Metabolism* 1984; **33**: 397.
24. Vinik AI, McLeod MK, Fig LM, Shapiro B, Lloyd RV & Cho K. Clinical features, diagnosis and localization of carcinoid tumours and their management. *Gastroenterol Clin North Am* 1989; **18**: 865.
25. Kenning EP, Bakker WH, Brennan WAP et al. Localization of endocrine related tumours with radioiodinated analogue of somatostatin. *Lancet* 1990; **i**: 242–244.
26. Lamberts SWJ, Bakker WH, Reubi JC & Kenning EP. Somatostatin-receptor imaging in the localization of endocrine tumours. *N Eng J Med* 1990; **323**: 1246–1249.
27. Ahlman H, Wangberg B, Tidell LE et al. Clinical efficacy of octreotide scintigraphy in patients with midgut carcinoid tumours and evaluation of intraoperative scintillation detection. *Br J Surg* 1994; **81**: 1144–1149.
28. Adam A. Carcinoid syndrome – radiology. *Br J Hosp Med* 1986; **35**: 154.
29. Sato T, Sakai Y, Sonoyama A et al. Radiological spectrum of rectal carcinoid tumors. *Gastrointest Radiol* 1984; **9**: 23.
30. Kressel HY. Strategies for magnetic resonance imaging of focal liver disease. *Radiol Clin North Am* 1988; **26**: 607.
31. Feldman JM & Jones RS. Carcinoid syndrome from gastrointestinal carcinoid without liver metastasis. *Ann Surg* 1982; **196**: 33–37.
32. Hodgson HJ & Maton PN. Carcinoid and neuroendocrine tumours of the liver. *Baillière's Clin Gastroenterol* 1987; **1**: 35.
33. Strodel W, Vinik AI, Thompson NW et al. Carcinoid tumours of the small intestine. In Thompson NW & Vinik AI (eds) *Endocrine Surgery Update*. New York: Grune & Stratton, 1983: 293–320.
34. Ahlman H, Dahlstrom A, Gronstad K et al. The pentagastrin test in the diagnosis of the carcinoid syndrome. *Ann Surg* 1985; **201**: 81.
35. Thorson A. Studies on carcinoid disease. *Acta Med Scand* 1958; **334** (Suppl.) 7.
36. Donowitz M & Binder HJ. Jejunal fluid and electrolyte secretion in carcinoid syndrome. *Am J Dig Dis* 1975; **20**: 1115.
37. Roberts WC & Sjoerdsma A. The cardiac disease associated with the carcinoid syndrome (carcinoid heart disease). *Am J Med* 1964; **36**: 5.
38. McDermott EWM, Guduric B & Brennan MF. Prognostic variables in patients with gastrointestinal carcinoid tumours. *Br J Surg* 1994; **81**: 1007–1009.
39. Makridis C, Rastad J, Oberg K & Akerstrom G. Progression of metastases and symptom improvement from laparotomy in midgut carcinoid tumours. *World J Surg* 1996; **20**: 900–907.
40. Wangberg B, Westberg G, Tylen U et al. Survival of patients with disseminated midgut carcinoid tumours after agressive tumour reduction. *World J Surg* 1996; **20**: 892–899.
41. Partensky C, Landraud R, Velecela E & Souquet JC. Resection of carcinoid tumours of the small intestine is still indicated in the presence of disseminated hepatic metastases. *Ann Chir* 1990; **44**: 34.
42. Coupe M, Levi S, Ellis M et al. Therapy for symptoms in the carcinoid syndrome. *Q J Med* 1989; **73**: 1021.
43. Martin JK, Moertel CG, Adson MA & Schutt AJ. Surgical treatment of functioning metastatic carcinoid tumors. *Arch Surg* 1983; **118**: 537.
44. Que FG, Nagorney DM, Batts KP, Linz LJ & Kvols LK. Hepatic resection for metastatic neuroendocrine carcinomas. *Am J Surg* 1995; **169**: 36.
45. Segall HN. An experimental anatomical investigation of the blood and bile channels of the liver. *Surg Gynecol Obstet* 1923; **37**: 152.
46. Breedis C & Young G. The blood supply of neoplasms in the liver. *Am J Pathol* 1954; **30**: 969.
47. Ackerman NB. The blood supply of experimental liver metastases. IV. Changes in vascularity with increasing tumour growth. *Surgery* 1974; **75**: 589.
48. Conway JG, Popp JA, Sungchul J & Thurman RG. Effect of size on portal circulation of hepatic nodules from carcinogen-treated rats. *Cancer Res* 1983; **43**: 3374.
49. Lin G, Lunderquist A, Hagerstrand I & Boijsen E. Postmortem examination of the blood supply and vascular pattern of small liver metastases in man. *Surgery* 1984; **96**: 517.
50. Ackerman NB. Experimental studies on the role of the portal circulation in hepatic tumour vascularity. *Cancer* 1986; **58**: 1653.
51. Ridge JA, Bading JR, Gelbard AS, Benua RS & Daly JM. Perfusion of colorectal hepatic metastases, relative distribution of flow from the hepatic artery and portal vein. *Cancer* 1987; **59**: 1547.
52. Archer SG & Gray BN. Vascularisation of small liver metastases. *Br J Surg* 1989; **76**: 545.
53. Nilsson LAV. Therapeutic hepatic artery ligation in patients with secondary liver tumours. *Rev Surg* 1966; **23**: 374.
54. Koudahl G & Funding J. Hepatic artery ligation in primary and secondary hepatic cancer. *Acta Chir Scand* 1972; **138**: 289.
55. Bengmark S & Rosengren K. Angiographic study of the collateral circulation to the liver after ligation of the hepatic artery in man. *Am J Surg* 1970; **119**: 620.
56. Bengmark S, Fredlund P, Hafstrom L & Vang J. Present experiences with hepatic dearterialisation in liver neoplasm. *Prog Surg* 1974; **13**: 141.
57. Bengmark S & Fredlund PE. Palliative treatment of primary and secondary malignant liver neoplasms. In Calne RY (ed.) *Liver Surgery*. Padua: Piccin, 1982: 157–185.
58. Dahl EP, Fredlund PE, Tylen U & Bengmark S. Transient hepatic dearterialization followed by regional intra-arterial 5-fluorouracil infusion as treatment for liver tumours. *Ann Surg* 1981; **193**: 82.
59. Bengmark S, Ericsson M, Lunderquist A, Martensson H, Nobin A & Sako M. Temporary liver dearterialisation in patients with metastatic carcinoid disease. *World J Surg* 1982; **6**: 46.
60. Bengmark S, Jeppsson B & Nobin A. Arterial ligation and temporary dearterialization. In Blumgart LH (ed.) *Surgery of the Liver and Biliary Tract*. Edinburgh: Churchill Livingstone, 1988: 1219–1235.

61. Almersjo O, Bengmark S, Engevik L et al. Hepatic artery ligation as pre-treatment for liver resection of metastatic cancer. *Rev Surg* 1966; **23**: 377.

62. Farndon JR. The carcinoid syndrome: methods of treatment and recent experience with hepatic artery ligation and infusion. *Clin Oncol* 1977; **3**: 365.

63. Ekberg H, Tranberg K-G, Lundstedt C et al. Determinants of survival after intraarterial infusion of 5-fluorouracil for liver metastases from colorectal cancer: a multivariate analysis. *J Surg Oncol* 1986; **31**: 246.

64. Bengmark S & Jeppsson B. Status of ischaemic therapy for hepatic tumours. *Surg Clin North Am* 1989; **69**: 411.

65. El-Domeiri AA & Mojab K. Intermittent occlusion of the hepatic artery and infusion chemotherapy for carcinoma of the liver. *Am J Surg* 1978; **135**: 771.

66. Persson B, Andersson L, Jeppsson B, Ekelund L, Strand SE & Bengmark S. The prevention of arterial collaterals after repeated temporary blockade of the hepatic artery in pigs. *World J Surg* 1987; **11**: 672.

67. Bengmark S, Jeppsson B, Lunderquist A, Tranberg K-G & Persson B. Tumour calcification following repeated hepatic de-arterialization in patients: a preliminary communication. *Br J Surg* 1988; **75**: 525.

68. Maton PN, Camilleri M, Griffin G, Allison DJ, Hodgson HJF & Chadwick VS. Role of hepatic arterial embolisation in the carcinoid syndrome. *BMJ* 1983; **287**: 932.

69. Carrasco CH, Charnsangavej, Ajani J, Samaan NA, Richi W & Wallace S. The carcinoid syndrome: palliation by hepatic artery embolization. *Am J Radiol* 1986; **147**: 149.

70. Arnold JC, O'Grady JGO, Bird GL, Calne RY & Williams R. Liver transplantation for primary and secondary hepatic apudomas. *Br J Surg* 1989; **76**: 248.

71. Makowka L, Tzakis AG, Mazzaferro V et al. Transplanation of the liver for metastatic endocrine tumors of the intestine and pancreas. *Surg Gynecol Obstet* 1989; **168**: 107.

72. Bizouarn P, Villalon L, Campion JP, Saint-Marc C & Launois B. Liver transplantation in metastases of carcinoid tumour. *Ann Fr Anesth Reanim* 1990; **9**: 180.

73. Lehello C, Auvray S, Letellier P & Segol P. Transplantation orthotopique hepatique pour metastases d'une tumeur carcinoide bronchique. *Gastroenterol Clin Biol* 1992; **16**: 281.

74. LeTreut YP, Delpero JR, Houssin D et al. Que peut-on penser de la transplantation hepatique pour metastases des tumeurs neuroendocrines? Resultats d'une serie multicentrique de 28 cas. *Gastroenterol Clin Biol* 1992; **19**: A4.

75. Dousset B, Saint-Marc O, Pitre J, Soubrane O, Houssin D & Chapuis Y. Metastatic endocrine tumours: medical treatment, surgical resection or liver transplantation. *World J Surg* 1996; **20**: 908–915.

76. Kvols LK. Metastatic carcinoid tumors and the carcinoid syndrome. *Am J Med* 1986; **81** (Suppl. 6B): 49.

77. Moertel CG & Hanley JA. Combination chemotherapy trials in metastatic carcinoid tumors and the malignant carcinoid syndrome. *Cancer Clin Trials* 1979; **2**: 327.

78. Bukowski RM, Johnson KG, Peterson RF et al. A phase II trial of combination chemotherapy in patients with metastatic carcinoid tumours: a Southwest Oncology Group study. *Cancer* 1987; **60**: 2891.

79. Kvols LK, Moertel CG, O'Connell J, Schutt AJ, Rubin J & Hahn RG. Treatment of the malignant carcinoid syndrome. *N Engl J Med* 1986; **315**: 663.

80. Maton PN. Use in patients with gut neuroendocrine tumors, pp 41–44. In Gorden P (moderator). Somatostatin and somatostatin analogue (SMS 201–995) in treatment of hormone-secreting tumors of the pituitary and gastrointestinal tract and non-neoplastic diseases of the gut. *Ann Intern Med* 1989; **110**: 35.

81. Maton PN. The use of the long-acting somatostatin analogue, octreotide acetate, in patients with islet tumors. *Gastroenterol Clin North Am* 1989; **18**: 897.

82. Souquet JC, Sassolas G, Forichon J, Champetier P, Partensky C & Chayvialle JA. Clinical and hormonal effects of a long-acting somatostatin analogue in pancreatic endocrine tumors and in carcinoid syndrome. *Cancer* 1987; **59**: 1654.

83. Lamberts SWJ, Koper JW & Reubi JC. Potential role of somatostatin analogues in the treatment of cancer (editorial). *Eur J Clin Invest* 1987; **17**: 281.

84. Schally A. Oncological applications of somatostatin analogues. *Cancer Res* 1988; **48**: 6977.

85. Chayvialle JA. Sandostatin and carcinoid tumours in France: experience in the Lyon area. *Digestion* 1990; **45** (Suppl 1): 23.

86. Grosman I & Simon D. Potential gastrointestinal uses of somatostatin and its synthetic analogue octreotide. *Am J Gastroenterol* 1990; **85**: 1061.

87. Mathé G, Gastiaburu J, Comaru-Schally AM et al. Octastatine, an agonist of somatostatin. In *Second International Conference of the Metastasis Research Society*, September, 1988, Heidleberg.

88. Evers BM, Hurlbut SC, Tyring SK, Townsend CM, Uchida T & Thompson JC. Novel therapy for the treatment of human carcinoid. *Ann Surg* 1991; **213**: 411.

89. Quesada JR & Gutterman JU. Interferons and cell growth regulation. *Eur J Cancer Clin Oncol* 1981; **24**: 1213.

90. Inglot A. The hormonal concept of interferon. *Arch Virol* 1983; **76**: 1.

91. Wilander E, Bengtsson A, Norheim I et al. Interferon induced nuclear DNA alterations in malignant carcinoid tumors in vivo. *J Natl Cancer Inst* 1986; **76**: 429.

92. Oberg K, Funa K & Alm G. Effects of leucocyte interferon on clinical symptoms and hormone levels in patients with mid-gut carcinoid tumors and the carcinoid syndrome. *N Engl J Med* 1983; **309**: 129.

93. Oberg K, Norheim I, Lind E et al. Treatment of malignant carcinoid tumors with human leukocyte interferon: long-term results. *Cancer Treat Rep* 1986; **70**: 1297.

94. Oberg K, Norheim I & Alm A. Treatment of malignant carcinoid tumors: a randomized controlled study of streptozotocin plus 5-FU and human leukocyte interferon. *Eur J Cancer Clin Oncol* 1989; **25**: 1475.

95. Thompson, NW, Vinik AI & Eckhauser E. Microgastrinomas of the duodenum. A cause of failed operations for the Zollinger–Ellison syndrome. *Ann Surg* 1989; **209**: 396.

96. Kaplan EL, Horvath K, Udekwu A et al. Gastrinomas: a 42-year experience. *World J Surg* 1990; **14**: 365.

97. Stabile BE, Morrow DJ & Passaro E Jr. The gastrinoma triangle: operative implications. *Am J Surg* 1984; **147**: 25.

98. Zollinger RM, Martin EW, Carey LC et al. Observations on the postoperative tumor growth of certain islet tumors. *Ann Surg* 1976; **184**: 525.

99. Wolfe MM, Alexander RV & McGuigan JE. Extrapancreatic extraintestinal gastrinoma effective treatment by surgery. *N Engl J Med* 1982; **306**: 1533.

100. Norton JA, Doppman JL, Collen MJ et al. Prospective study of gastrinoma localisation and resection in patients with Zollinger–Ellison syndrome. *Ann Surg* 1986; **204**: 468.

101. Boyce GA & Sivak MV. Endoscopic ultrasonography in the diagnosis of pancreatic tumours. *Gastrointest Endosc* 1990; **36**: 528.

102. Vinayek R, Frucht H, Chiang H-C V, Maton PN, Gardner JD & Jensen RT. Zollinger–Ellison syndrome. Recent advances in the management of gastrinoma. *Gastroenterol Clin North Am* 1990; **19**: 197.

103. Maton PN, Miller DL, Doppman JL et al. Role of selective angiography in the management of Zollinger–Ellison syndrome. *Gastroenterology* 1987; **92**: 913.

104. Norton JA, Cromack DT, Shawker TH et al. Intraoperative ultrasonographic localisation of islet cell tumours. *Ann Surg* 1988; **207**: 160.

105. Cromack DT, Norton JA, Sigel B et al. The use of high-resolution intraoperative ultrasound to localise gastrinomas: An initial report of a prospective study. *World J Surg* 1987; **11**: 648.

106. Frucht H, Norton JA, Maton PN et al. Intraoperative endoscopy (IOE) detects a high frequency of duodenal gastrinomas in patients with Zollinger–Ellison syndrome (abstract). *Gastroenterology* 1988; **94**: 137.

107. Norton JA, Doppman JL, Gardner JD et al. Aggressive resection of metastatic disease in selected patients with malignant gastrinoma. *Ann Surg* 1986; **203**: 352.

108. Fox PS, Hofmann JW, Wilson SD & DeCossee JJ. Surgical management of the Zollinger–Ellison syndrome. *Surg Clin North Am* 1974; **54**: 395.

109. von Schrenck T, Howard JM, Doppman JL et al. Prospective study of chemotherapy in patients with metastatic gastrinoma. *Gastroenterology* 1988; **96**: 431.

110. Ruszniewski P, Rowgier P, Andre-David F et al. Prospective multicentric study of chemotherapy with streptozotocin (STZ) and 5-fluorouracil (5FU) for liver metastases (LM) in Zollinger–Ellison syndrome (ZES) (abstract). *Gastroenterology* 1989; **96**: 431.

111. Carrasco CH, Chuang VP, Wallace S et al. Apudoma metastatic to the liver: treatment by hepatic artery embolization. *Radiology* 1983; **149**: 79.

112. Moertel CG, May GR, Martin JK et al. Sequential hepatic artery occlusion (HAO) and chemotherapy for metastatic carcinoid tumor and islet cell tumor (ICC). *Proc Am Soc Clin Oncol* 1985; **4**: 80 (abstract).

113. Zollinger RM, Ellison EC, Fabri PJ et al. Primary peptic ulcerations of the jejunum associated with islet cell tumors. *Ann Surg* 1980; **192**: 422.

114. Ellison EC, Woltering EA, O'Dorisio TM et al. Efficacy of long-acting analogue (SMS 201-995) in the ulcerogenic syndrome. *Gastroenterology* 1985; **88**: 1873.

115. Shepherd JJ & Senator GB. Regression of liver metastases in patients with gastrin secreting tumours treated with SMS 201–995. *Lancet* 1986; **ii**: 574.

116. Maton PN, Gardner JD & Jensen RT. The use of the long-acting analogue SMS 201–995 in patients with pancreatic islet cell tumors. *Dig Dis Sci* 1989; **34** (Suppl.): 285.

117. Williams G, Anderson JV & Bloom SR. Treatment of gut-associated neuroendocrine tumours with the long-acting somatostatin analogue SMS 201–995. In Reichlin S (ed.) *Somatostatins: Basic and Clinical Status.* New York: Plenum Press, 1984: 343–356.

118. Kvols LK, Buck M, Moertel CG et al. Treatment of metastatic islet cell carcinoma with somatostatin analogue (SMS 201–995). *Ann Intern Med* 1987; **107**: 162.

119. Eriksson B, Oberg K, Alm G et al. Treatment of malignant endocrine pancreatic tumours with human leukocyte interferon. *Cancer Treat Rep* 1987; **71**: 31.

120. Oberg K, Eriksson B & Norheim I. Interferon treatment of neuroendocrine tumors of pancreas and gut. In: Revel M (ed.) *Clinical Aspects of Interferons.* Boston; Kluwer, 1988: 195–211.

121. Wood SM, Polak JM & Bloom SR. Gastrointestinal endocrine tumours. In Hodgson HJF & Bloom SR (eds) *Gastrointestinal and Hepatobiliary Cancer.* London: Chapman & Hall, 1983: 207–227.

122. Marcial MA, Pinkus GS, Skarin A, Hinrichs HR & Warhol MJ. Ampullary somatostatinoma – an immunohistochemical and ultrastructural study. *Am J Clin Pathol* 1983; **80**: 755.

123. Krejs GJ, Orci L & Conlon M. Somatostatinoma syndrome. Biochemical, morphological and clinical features. *N Engl J Med* 1979; **301**: 285.

124. Verner JV & Morrison AB. Non-B islet tumours and the syndrome of refractory watery diarrhoea and hypokalaemia. *Am J Med* 1958; **25**: 374.

125. Marks IN, Bank S & Louw JH. Islet cell tumour of the pancreas with reversible watery diarrhoea and achlorhydria. *Gastroenterology* 1967; **52**: 695.

126. Matsumoto KK, Peter JB, Schultze RG, Hakim AA & Franck PT. Watery diarrhoea and hypokalaemia associated with pancreatic islet cell adenoma. *Gastroenterology* 1966; **50**: 231.

127. Bloom SR & Polak JM. Glucagonomas, VIPomas and somatostatinomas. *Clin Endocrinol* 1980; **9**: 285.

128. Long RG, Bryant MG, Mitchell SJ, Adrian TE, Polak JM & Bloom SR. Clinicopathologic study of pancreatic and ganglioneuroblastoma tumours secreting vasoactive intestinal polypeptide (VIPomas). *BMJ* 1981; **282**: 1767.

129. Nagorney DM, Bloom SR, Black JM & Blumgart LH. Resolution of recurrent Verner-Morrison syndrome by resection of metastatic VIPoma. *Surgery* 1983; **93**: 348.

130. Maton PN, O'Dorisio TM, Howe BA et al. Effect of a long-acting somatostatin analogue (SMS 201–995) in a patient with pancreatic cholera. *N Engl J Med* 1985; **312**: 17.

131. Smale BF & Reber HA. Vasoactive intestinal polypeptide (VIP) producing tumors. In Howard JM, Jordan GL & Reber HA (eds) *Surgical Diseases of the Pancreas.* Philadelphia: Lea & Febiger, 1987: 860–864.

132. Steinfeld CM, Moertel CG & Woolner LB. Diarrhoea and medullary cell carcinoma of the thyroid. *Cancer* 1973; **31**: 1237.

60

MALIGNANT TUMOURS OF THE SMALL BOWEL

JGN Studley
RCN Williamson

The small intestine varies in length between 300 and 850 cm in normal adults and its villous pattern further increases the mucosal surface available for malignant change,[1,2] yet cancer of the duodenum, jejunum and ileum are decidedly uncommon. To appreciate the perspective, large bowel tumours are 40–60 times more frequent than small bowel tumours.[3,4]

Between 1 and 2% of gastrointestinal malignancies occur in the small bowel.[1,5] The duodenum, which is approximately 5% of the length of the small bowel, harbours 20–25% of malignant lesions, indicating a predisposition for this segment.[6,7] It is difficult to be certain of the relative numbers of benign and malignant lesions: at least 50% of benign lesions are asymptomatic and are detected incidentally during investigation, laparotomy or autopsy,[6] whereas virtually all malignant lesions will eventually become symptomatic.

It is interesting to consider the reasons for the rarity of small bowel neoplasia. Several hypotheses are well recognized: exposure to carcinogens may be reduced by rapid transit, formation of carcinogens may be limited by low bacterial counts and an alkaline pH, detoxification of harmful substances may result from enzyme secretions (including benzopyrene hydroxylase) and finally the secretion of immune factors by the small bowel may be relevant.[8–10]

Malignant disease of the small bowel may be classified into the following groups:

1. *Primary malignancy*: adenocarcinoma, neuroendocrine tumours, lymphoma, sarcoma;

2. *Secondary malignancy*: carcinoma, melanoma, lymphoma, leukaemia, sarcoma;

3. *Malignancy associated with immune deficiency syndrome (AIDS)*: Kaposi's sarcoma, lymphoma.

The relative frequency of each primary malignancy is shown in Table 60.1.[5,9,11–16] Each group will now be considered with the

exception of neuroendocrine tumours, which have been discussed fully in Chapter 59.

Table 60.1 Relative frequency of primary malignant tumours of the small bowel

Adenocarcinoma	32–54%
Neuroendocrine tumours	16–39%
Lymphoma	7–24%
Sarcoma	7–22%

PRIMARY MALIGNANCY
Adenocarcinoma

Incidence

This is the commonest small bowel malignancy representing between one third and one half of the total. Peak incidence is in the seventh decade,[17,18] and the disease is slightly more common in males.[17,19]

Pathology

There is a markedly uneven distribution of adenocarcinoma in the small bowel, with a concentration proximally and frequency decreasing towards the terminal ileum (Table 60.2).[5,11,13,14,17–21]

Between 80 and 90% of cancers in the duodenum are adenocarcinomas, indicating a clear preponderance of this

Table 60.2 Relative frequency of adenocarcinomas within the small intestine

Duodenum	40–50%
Jejunum	35–40%
Ileum	20–25%

histological type at this site.[20] Duodenal carcinomas may be further classified according to their position in relation to the papilla, though this varies between reports. Up to half (42–56%) lie distal to the papilla, 32–48% are in the peri-ampullary region and 7–10% arise proximal to the papilla.[22,23] Supra-ampullary lesions are usually in the upper part of the descending duodenum, with lesions in the first part of the duodenum being extremely rare.[17] In our own series, however, the greatest proportion of duodenal carcinomas lay in the periampullary segment (82%) with the potential to obstruct the bile duct; none were present in the first part, with the remainder spread equally between the third and fourth parts.[24] In the polyposis syndromes (Gardner's syndrome) there is a similar concentration of lesions around the ampulla.[25]

Macroscopic appearances are varied: most tumours are annular and constricting, but polypoid and fungating lesions can occur.[9,14,17] Multiple lesions are present in 15–25% of cases.[5,13] Histological features demonstrate a preponderance of moderately differentiated lesions with mucin secretion.[3,5,9,17,19,26,27]

Malignant spread is common at presentation, over 50% of carcinomas having metastasized.[5,11,13,17] Lymph nodes are generally involved, but transperitoneal spread and hepatic metastases can also occur.[3,17,26]

In the duodenum, as in the large intestine, *adenomas* have a particular predisposition to malignant change.[11,18,28,29] Thus the adenoma–carcinoma sequence probably occurs throughout the gastrointestinal tract. The risk of malignancy depends on the histological type of adenoma as well as the size, site and number of lesions.

Aetiology (Table 60.3)

Both tubular and villous adenomas are recognized; differentiation between these types can be difficult, as some have both tubular and villous elements (tubulovillous adenoma). Villous adenomas have a much greater propensity to malignant change than the tubular variety. These lesions develop mainly in the second part of the duodenum (Figure 60.1, see colour plate also). The mean age at presentation of benign villous adenoma is 60 years, with no sex preponderance.[31] Between 35 and 63% of tumours are reported to contain carcinomatous foci.[32,33] Thus approximately half of duodenal villous adenomas have already undergone malignant change by the time of presentation. In our series dysplasia was evident in the adjacent mucosa in 60% of patients, supporting a true duo-

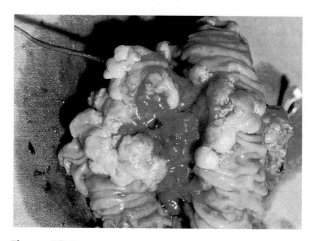

Figure 60.1

Carcinoma of the duodenum in a 71-year-old man treated by pylorus-preserving proximal pancreatoduodenectomy (PPPP). As is frequently the case with primary duodenal cancer, the carcinoma had arisen in an underlying villous adenoma.

denal origin of the tumours (as opposed to an origin from biliary epithelium at the papilla).[24]

For tubular adenomas the risk of malignant change increases with the size of the tumour. In one series purely benign polyps measured 2.7 cm in diameter, whereas those with coincident malignant change measured 3.7 cm. The mean size of carcinomas in the jejunum was 4.3 cm and in the ileum 4.7 cm.[29] Periampullary adenomas have a greater propensity to malignant change than those elsewhere in the small bowel.[18,29]

Familial adenomatosis polyposis is an autosomal dominant disease characterized by multiple adenomatous polyps in the colon and rectum. The disease is also known as familial polyposis coli; Gardner's syndrome is a variant, said to be due to variable penetration of abnormal genes, which includes additional extracolonic manifestations including various mesodermal tumours (sebaceous cysts, osteomas of the skull and mandible and desmoid tumours of the abdomen). In this condition, adenomatous polyps have been reported in the duodenum in 24–93% of patients,[34,35] the wide discrepancy probably reflecting the diligence with which upper gastrointestinal endoscopy is carried out in those without symptoms. Adenomas are usually multiple and occur in the second part of the duodenum, predominantly surrounding the papilla.[35–38] Periampullary carcinoma is reported to occur in 2–12% of these patients.[35,39–41] Indeed, follow-up of patients who have received abdominal colectomy for familial adenomatous polyposis has revealed that carcinoma of the duodenum is commoner than carcinoma of the rectum. Jejunoileal polyps have also been reported in this condition.[42] The natural history of lesions at this site is unclear, but the risk of carcinoma appears to be very low.[42–45]

Brunner's gland adenomas are benign lesions found within the duodenum (see Chapter 58). Malignant change is rare but has been reported.[46]

Peutz–Jegher's syndrome is an autosomal dominant inherited disease in which hamartomatous polyps occur throughout the intestinal tract but especially in the jejunum (see Chapter

---

Table 60.3 Conditions predisposing to adenocarcinoma of the small bowel

Adenomas
  Tubular
  Villous (Tubulovillous)
Familial adenomatous polyposis
Peutz–Jeghers syndrome
Crohn's disease
Coeliac disease
Rare associations (see text)

58). Malignant change has been reported in up to 6% of cases; it affects the small bowel, predominantly the duodenum.[47] Thus the preferential site for carcinoma may not be the site of maximum involvement by the hamartomas.

Crohn's disease of the small intestine is associated with malignant change in approximately 0.3–0.6% of cases.[18,20,48,49] The mean age of presentation of Crohn's carcinoma is within the fifth decade.[20,48–50] The main site of occurrence is the ileum, reflecting the dominant location of enteric Crohn's disease (Chapter 51). Approximately 70% of Crohn's cancers affect the ileum and 30% the jejunum; the duodenum is rarely involved.[48,50–54] In 30–40% of cases the disease develops in defunctioned loops of bowel,[48,50,55,56] possibly reflecting the influence of stagnant bowel contents and bacterial contamination. Tumours can also develop in association with fistulas and their tracts.[56] Dysplasia has been reported in surrounding tissues, which presumably accounts for the occasional occurrence of multifocal tumours.[49,53] Carcinoma may arise in parts of the bowel separate from overt inflammatory disease.[55] In most patients there has been a 15–30-year history of Crohn's disease before the development of malignant change,[5,28,48–51,56] although cancer can be present with short histories or even with undiagnosed Crohn's disease.[21,48]

Coeliac disease is also associated with malignant change in the small intestine, but here lymphoma is the commonest tumour (see below). Adenocarcinoma may also occur, the dominant sites being in the pharynx, oesophagus, stomach, rectum and (within the small intestine) the duodenum and jejunum.[5,57,58] The disease has often been present for 10–30 years before malignancy occurs.[5,57]

Other rare associations include neurofibromatosis (Von Recklinghausen's disease),[59,60] Torre's syndrome, a variant of familial adenomatous polyposis in which multiple sebaceous adenomas co-exist with primary malignant tumours of the viscera[61,62] and radiation enteritis[63] (Chapter 52). An association between Lynch syndrome II and adenocarcinoma of the small bowel has also been reported.[64] This condition is one of the variants of hereditary non-polyposis colorectal cancer, in which multiple carcinomas develop.[65] Carcinoma can also arise sporadically in ileum used to create a urinary conduit or reconstruction of the bladder.[66]

Clinical features

Unlike benign tumours of the small bowel, all malignant lesions will eventually become symptomatic. However, an important feature of these neoplasms is the delay in diagnosis, which is a major factor in their poor outcome. The mean time from onset of symptoms to diagnosis is 6–9 months.[9,21,27,67] The duodenum is more accessible to investigation, so the diagnosis of duodenal tumours tends to be earlier than it is for more distal lesions.[19] The diagnostic delay may be due to several factors: vague symptoms, absence of clinical signs, the difficulty in investigating the distal small bowel and the rarity of these tumours.

Carcinomas of the duodenum and jejunoileum present with different features. In the duodenum, there may be vague

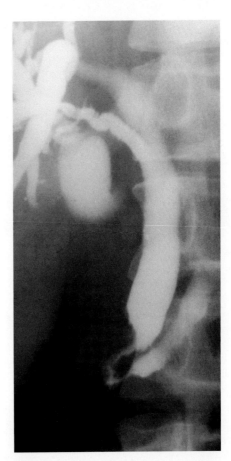

Figure 60.2
Percutaneous transhepatic cholangiography in a 34-year-old man with primary duodenal cancer causing obstructive jaundice. There is dilatation of the comon bile duct and the main pancreatic duct with strictures in the terminal segment of each duct.

symptoms of nausea, intermittent vomiting, epigastric discomfort, which may be associated with meals and suggest peptic ulcer disease, and weight loss.[28,68,69] Eventually obstruction will supervene if no diagnosis is made.[17,25] Occult bleeding and its manifestations occur in 25–50% of patients; overt haemorrhage is unusual.[17,24,25] One third of patients have weight loss, and in one quarter a mass is evident.[17,25] Jaundice is the presenting feature in 20–55% of cases[5,17,21,24,28] (Figure 60.2). The frequency of presenting features in a personal series is shown in Table 60.4. In the jejunoileum, symptoms leading up to obstruction are the commonest feature (Figure 60.3, see colour plate also). Initial complaints may include nausea, vomiting and discomfort related to meals, which is associated with weight loss.[11,15,17,19] Obstruction may eventually result either from a stenosing lesion or sec-

Table 60.4 Symptoms of duodenal carcinoma

Jaundice	55%
Epigastric pain	32%
Anaemia	27%
Vomiting	27%

Data from Scott-Coombes and Williamson.[24]

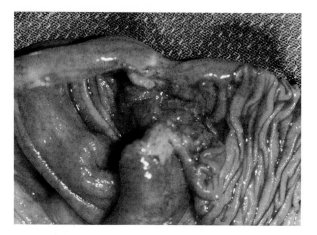

Figure 60.3
Annular carcinoma of the jejunum treated by local excision. The patient had presented with chronic small bowel obstruction, and there is an obvious disparity in size between the obstructed proximal bowel (left) and the collapsed distal bowel (right).

ondary to intussusception of a polypoid tumour.[11,15,17,28] Alternatively, anaemia may result from occult bleeding;[5,15,17,28] overt bleeding is uncommon (Figure 60.4, see colour plate also). A mass may be palpable in up to one third of patients.[15,17] Fistula formation and perforation are both rare presentations.[3,11,14,15,28]

Diagnosis

Particular features are summarized below. Investigation of the small bowel is fully discussed in Chapters 44 and 45.

Detection of duodenal lesions is more straightforward than for those in the jejunum and ileum. Upper gastrointestinal endoscopy can readily detect tumours in the first and second parts of the duodenum, and it allows biopsy of tissue. Radiographic contrast studies are complementary. A barium meal examination may demonstrate abnormalities, but the false negative rates can be as high as 40%.[5] Hypotonic duodenography allows more thorough visualization (Figure 60.5).

The jejunoileum may be investigated by barium meal and follow-through or by an intubated small bowel meal, which

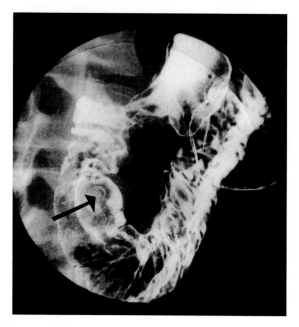

Figure 60.5
Hypotonic duodenogram showing a periampullary carcinoma on the medial wall of the descending duodenum (arrow).

will detect 80–90% of lesions.[5,11] The intubated meal is preferable as better imaging is achieved with the introduction of contrast directly into the jejunum through a transduodenal tube (Figure 60.6). The terminal ileum may be visualized in 20–30% of barium enemas or colonoscopies. Tumours that are bleeding can be demonstrated by isotope scan; either ^{99m}technetium-labelled red cells or ^{99m}technetium-labelled sulphur colloid may be used. Rates of haemorrhage as low as 0.1 ml/min may be detected using this technique. An alternative approach is selective mesenteric angiography, although bleeding rates of 0.5–1.0 ml/min are necessary to facilitate detection.[19] However, angiography will sometimes demonstrate the vascular blush of a tumour that is not bleeding at the time.

Small bowel enteroscopy is a new approach to the diagnosis of small bowel tumours. In this technique a 5 mm diameter endoscope is introduced into the bowel transnasally. Using this technique in 60 patients, visualization of the distal ileum and colon was achieved in over 50% of cases.[70] Another technique currently being evaluated is percutaneous endoscopy. Access to the bowel is achieved through the stomach or caecum using the technique described for the insertion of a percutaneous feeding gastrostomy.[71] These latter techniques remain experimental at the present time.

CT scanning and, to a lesser extent, ultrasound scanning may be helpful in defining the size, extent and spread of malignant lesions.[72-74] MRI scanning is not at present an established technique for investigating small bowel tumours; resolution is poor and motion artefacts limit its efficacy. Advances in technology may resolve these problem.[73,74]

Finally laparotomy may be necessary to diagnose and treat lesions that cause symptoms attributable to the small bowel, but have not been defined by other investigative methods. A high index of suspicion is necessary and operation should not

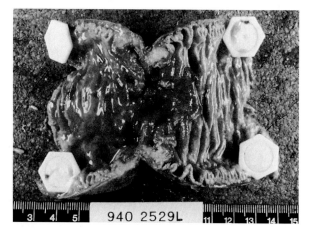

Figure 60.4
Resected carcinoma of the jejunum in an elderly man who had presented with melaena.

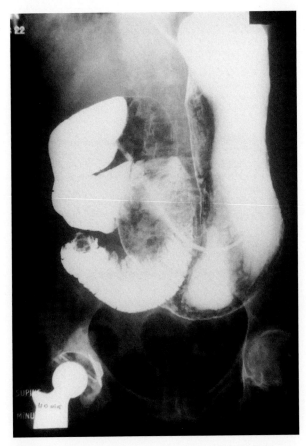

Figure 60.6
Intubated small bowel meal showing complete obstruction above a high jejunal carcinoma. The patient was a woman of 80 years with previous total hip replacement who presented with vomiting and a succussion splash.

be delayed.[75] Laparoscopy is a new modality that permits thorough inspection of the entire mesenteric small bowel.

Treatment

A cure can only be achieved by surgical excision. Mucin-producing adenocarcinomas are relatively radioresistant, and radiotherapy has no defined role at present.[1,6,8,21,35] Similarly chemotherapy has also proved very disappointing, although minimal response has been reported.[23,76,77]

Both palliative and curative operations must be considered. Unfortunately early lesions confined to the mucosa and submucosa are rare,[3] and laparotomy generally shows that the tumour has extended through the bowel wall; overall, 50% of patients will have metastases.[3,5,11,13]

In the duodenum potential curative operations are possible in 50–80% of cases.[22,28,68,69,78] In our own series 77% of duodenal carcinomas were resected.[24] Appropriate procedures are pancreatoduodenectomy for periampullary lesions and segmental duodenal resection for more distal tumours. Sparing of the duodenal cap means that a pylorus-preserving approach can be considered for pancreatoduodenectomy. Alternative approaches are local excision of a small ampullary tumour and local excision of polyps provided the tumour is confined and

does not invade the stalk. Frozen-section analysis is necessary to confirm complete removal.

The surgical approach to an ampullary lesion must be carefully considered. Determination of its exact tissue of origin may be difficult. The resection rate for carcinoma of the pancreas varies between 15 and 30%,[78,79] but for carcinoma of the ampulla, bile duct or duodenum the rates are higher, ranging from 50 to 90%.[68,69,78,79] These facts should be taken in context with the results of resection for these different carcinomas: in carcinoma of the head of the pancreas the overall 5 year survival is less than 10%, whereas other tumours in this region offer a better outlook with rates of 15–45%.[69,79–81] If distant metastases are present the results of major resection are poor, so palliative bypass is generally indicated unless haemorrhage has been a problem.[18] Involved local lymph nodes may be resected en bloc.[68–82]

Palliative surgical procedures generally involve both biliary and duodenal bypass. An alternative approach for lesions causing obstructive jaundice is stenting of the tumour, which can be achieved endoscopically or percutaneously.[83] However, the endoscopic route may be technically impossible with a florid tumour obscuring the ampulla. The disadvantages of stenting are subsequent dislodgement of the stent or the possibility of blockage and cholangitis.[82]

An irresectable advanced tumour of the duodenum may be defunctioned by an antrectomy and gastroenterostomy. This approach has the advantage of total diversion of both acid and gastric contents from the ulcerated duodenum. Haemorrhage from such tumours may be reduced by ligation of the gastroduodenal artery.[24] Median survival following palliative operation is 6–7 months.[24,69]

In the jejunum and ileum curative resection should be aimed at wide local excision to include the regional lymph nodes. The mesenteric dissection may be limited by the proximity of the superior mesenteric artery. Distal ileal lesions may require right hemicolectomy for adequate excision.[17,19] Potentially curative operations may be performed in approximately 80% of jejunal tumours and 70% of ileal tumours.[18] For lesions that are clearly not curable by resection, local excision is preferable to bypass. Tumours left in situ may bleed, perforate or erode into other structures.[11]

Prognosis

Survival rates for small bowel carcinoma are disappointing. This fact reflects the biological behaviour of the tumours, and the delay that so often occurs in diagnosis explains the widespread disease found at operation.

In the duodenum overall 5-year survival rates usually vary from 15 to 30%.[18,26,28] For patients having potentially curative pancreatoduodenectomy, most reports indicate that 5-year survival lies between 15 and 45%.[15,25,69] The operative mortality rate of pancreatoduodenal resection must be remembered when considering resection for patients with a poor prognosis. Although hospital death has been recorded in up to 24% of these operations,[17,81,84] this risk is greatly reduced (to 5% or below) in centres with experience in the technique.[79,81,84]

The results of segmental duodenal resection vary widely, with 5-year survival rates raging between 20 and 70%.[22,85] The results appear to be superior for distal tumours, compared with those at or above the papilla (5-year survival rate 87% versus 20%).[85] Local resection of the ampulla is associated with survival up to 80% at 2 years[86] and 40% at 5 years.[80] Morbidity and mortality rates are probably lower for the lesser procedures compared to pancreatoduodenectomy.[22,78,87] Simple polypectomy for suitable lesions appears to have good results, with up to 87% 5-year survival.[88] A poor prognosis of duodenal carcinoma is indicated by extensive local disease, distal nodal involvement and poor differentiation of the lesion.[18,68,79,85,89] The overall 5-year survival rate for jejunoileal carcinomas is 20–30%,[11,15,26,28] jejunal carcinomas have a slightly better prognosis than ileal carcinomas (44–62% versus 20–36%.[5,15,18] If there is no nodal involvement at operation, survival is increased up to 50–70%.[15,18,28] Ileal carcinoma secondary to Crohn's disease has a particularly poor prognosis, with a mean survival of only 6–11 months.[28,48–51,56]

Lymphoma

The gastrointestinal tract is the commonest site of primary extranodal lymphoma, which comprises 5–10% of all lymphomas.[17,90] Secondary involvement of the small bowel is approximately ten times more common than the primary disease.[11] Primary intestinal lymphoma represents 7–24% of small bowel malignant tumours (Table 60.1). Within the gastrointestinal tract 40–55% of tumours occur in the stomach, 30–33% in the small bowel and 8–18% in the large intestine.[91–93] Features defining primary lymphoma of the gut are shown in Table 60.5.[94,95]

Table 60.5 Features defining primary lymphoma of bowel

1. No palpable lymphadenopathy
2. Normal white cell count and marrow
3. Normal chest radiograph and CT scan excluding mediastinal lymphadenopathy
4. Tumour mass confined mainly to bowel, as defined by imaging or laparotomy
5. No lymphadenopathy apart from local and retroperitoneal nodes
6. No hepatic or splenic enlargement

Classification

This complicated subject has undergone many reviews in recent years with increasing knowledge of the subject. Isaacson et al.[96] defined one approach which covers the broad categories (Table 60.6).

The main groups of lymphoma to be considered are.[97]

1. 'Western' lymphoma
   (a) Europe and North America
   (b) Lesions develop in previously small bowel
   (c) B cell tumours
2. Lymphoma associated with coeliac disease or lymphoid nodular hyperplasia

Table 60.6 Lymphomas of the small bowel

B cell	Low grade (mucosa associated lymphoid tissue)
	High grade (mucosa associated lymphoid tissue)
	(± evidence of low grade component)
	Mediterranean (immunoproliferative small intestinal disease)
	(low, mixed or high grade)
	Lymphomatous polyposis
	Burkitt
	Others
T cell	Various grades

   (a) Developing in abnormal bowel
   (b) T cell tumour
3. 'Mediterranean' lymphoma
   (a) North Africa and Middle East
   (b) Associated with immunoproliferative small intestinal disease
   (c) B cell tumours
4. Lymphomatosis polyposis
   (a) Rare
   (b) B cell tumours

Western lymphoma

The disease may present either in childhood or in adults within the fifth or sixth decades.[76,90] There is a slight male preponderance.[76,90,93] In children the tumours are predominantly in the ileocaecal region, whereas in adults they are distributed throughout the small bowel.[97,98] The caecum may be involved with ileal disease.[99,100]

Macroscopic appearances are varied. Lesions are generally localized and annular, but there may be nodular, polypoid, ulcerative, aneurysmal or strictured areas; a more diffuse infiltrative form is also recognized. Multiple lesions occur in approximately 8–20% of cases.[11,17,76,91,97,98,101,102] Ulceration can lead to haemorrhage, and lesions may fistulate, perforate or obstruct.[11,91,98] Tumours usually spread early to regional nodes. Eventually the disease disseminates to involve the liver spleen and lungs.[98]

Clinical features Presentation is variable and includes symptoms suggestive of impending obstruction in 60–70% of patients: anorexia, nausea and vomiting, abdominal pain, weight loss and diarrhoea.[17,90,91,98,99,101] Bleeding occurs in approximately 50% of cases, leading to anaemia.[17,91,97] An abdominal mass may be present in 30–40% of cases[5,91] (Figure 60.7, see colour plate also). Presentation may occur in 30% with perforation, haemorrhage or obstruction due to intussusception or stenosis Table 60.7.[98,99] Protein-losing enteropathy can also be in evidence.[91]

Diagnosis The mainstays for elucidating the nature of a small bowel tumour are endoscopy and biopsy for proximal lesions and contrast studies for more distal lesions. Occasionally terminal ileal tumours can be biopsied via the colonoscope. Ultrasonography and computed tomography (CT) scanning can define the extent of the lesion. Operation may often be required to make a definitive diagnosis, as well as to determine the extent and therefore stage of the tumour.

Table 60.7 Presenting symptoms of carcinoma and lymphoma of small bowel

	CARCINOMA OF DUODENUM	CARCINOMA OF JEJUNUM	CARCINOMA OF ILEUM	LYMPHOMA (ALL SITES)
Number	17	10	3	8
Cramps and vomiting	10	5	1	7
Bleeding				
Overt	3	2	0	7
Occult	7	5	0	1
Jaundice	6	0	0	1
Weight loss > 5 kg	10	9	3	5

Data from Williamson et al.[5]

Investigation of an intestinal lymphoma includes routine haematological and biochemical tests. Chest radiographs may show evidence of hilar lymphadenopathy, but a CT scan is the definitive investigation to rule out mediastinal lymphadenopathy. CT scan of the abdomen is invaluable for determining intra-abdominal involvement. The role of magnetic resonance imaging (MRI) is being assessed.[91]

Possible underlying conditions such as coeliac and Crohn's disease should be considered. Immunological defects, whether drug-induced, congenital or acquired, also require thorough investigation.[98]

Treatment Management of this disease is determined by the stage.[91,98] Localized small bowel lymphomas should be excised together with their contiguous lymph nodes plus a margin of normal tissue. Even with disseminated disease the primary lesion should be removed, since both radiotherapy and chemotherapy may be indicated and these can lead to perforation or haemorrhage of the tumour.[91] If resection is not possible bypass should be undertaken to prevent obstruction.

Adjuvant therapy includes radiotherapy and chemotherapy,[91,98] although the optimal treatment is not yet known. Radiotherapy is tending to be replaced by combination chemotherapy, including vincristine, cyclophosphamide and doxorubicin[97] (Figure 60.8, see colour plate also).

Prognosis The overall 5-year survival rate is 10–40%,[28,90,98] although children often do worse.[90] The prognosis depends on the stage of the disease[98] and the histological type of tumour may also affect the outcome.[90,102–105] Advanced tumours and those that perforate (and thus disseminate) do badly.[105,106] Curative resection has been reported to result in a 48% 5-year survival.[107]

Lymphoma associated with coeliac disease

Enteropathy-associated T cell lymphoma accounts for approximately one-third of tumours in this group.[108] Presentation is usually between the sixth and seventh decade, although the disease can occur in children.[109] Tumours may be single or multiple.[98] They affect the jejunum more frequently than the ileum,[101] thus reflecting the pattern of the underlying coeliac disease. Macroscopic appearances are often of a diffusely infiltrative tumour with ulceration and stricture formation.[101] Ulcerative jejunitis may be in evidence before the development of lymphoma.[97]

The tumour may present in several ways. In patients with long-standing coeliac disease, malignancy may be suggested by the recurrence of symptoms such as abdominal pain, weight loss and diarrhoea[57,101] despite the patient adhering to a gluten-free diet. The time factor is usually 5–10 years after the first diagnosis of coeliac disease.[57,98] Alternatively, in patients who have recently diagnosed disease, lymphoma may be suspected if the condition does not respond to treatment.[57,98,101] Acute presentations include perforation, obstruction or gastrointestinal bleeding.[57,101] The diagnosis may be difficult in patients with non-specific symptoms, and laparotomy may be required.[97] At operation widespread dissemination is

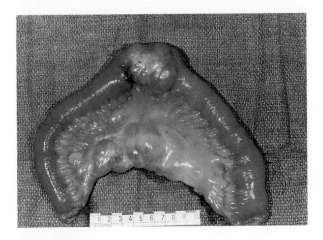

Figure 60.7
Non-Hodgkin's lymphoma involving the ileum in a 37-year-old man who presented with an enormous lower abdominal mass which disappeared after a course of combination chemotherapy. His residual obstructive symptoms were cured by small bowel resection, but he died of cerebral metastases one year later.

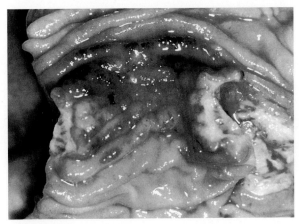

Figure 60.8
Healed stricture resulting from a lymphoma that had been successfully treated with radical chemotherapy four years earlier. There was no evidence of residual tumour in the resection specimen.

common with involvement of mesenteric nodes, the liver, spleen and bone marrow.[110,111] Treatment has been discussed in the previous section. Prognosis is poor, with few patients surviving a year.[57]

Mediterranean lymphoma

Small bowel lymphoma is the commonest gastrointestinal malignancy in many middle eastern countries.[101] This so-called Mediterranean lymphoma is a disease that occurs mainly in young adults, often males, in their third and fourth decades.[10,112–114] It was first described along the Mediterranean littoral and occurs in low socioeconomic groups.[101,114]

The underlying abnormality appears to be a diffuse infiltration of the small bowel mucosa and mesenteric nodes with plasma cells. Over a period of years the abnormality progresses to malignancy.[11] The abnormal cells lead to a defective IgA in which alpha light chains are not produced, leaving the alpha heavy chain alone, which can be detected in the serum.[11,115] The term immunoproliferative small intestinal disease (IPSID) is often applied to these lesions.

The whole of the small bowel may be affected, although the duodenum and jejunum are most commonly involved.[17,91] Macroscopic appearances are of multiple lesions forming thickened areas in the bowel with subsequent stenosis and obstruction.[101] Malignant spread is primarily to the lymph nodes which are usually involved.[113] Histological examination shows abnormal villous patterns,[113] as well as infiltrates of plasma cells around which multifocal malignancy develops.[116] The cellular infiltrate deforms the crypts and villi.[101]

Clinical features Mediterranean lymphoma typically presents with a history of abdominal pain, diarrhoea and steatorrhoea, weight loss and anaemia.[91,101,113,114] An abdominal mass may also be palpable.[109] Acute presentations can also occur with obstruction and intussusception, bleeding or perforation.[98,101] Finger clubbing may be evident.[97]

Diagnosis Investigations will reveal malabsorption which, in turn, leads to megaloblastic anaemia due to vitamin B_{12} and folate deficiency.[117] Electrophoresis may demonstrate an abnormal protein.[109] Enteric parasitic infections can be shown in 50% of patients.[118] Endoscopy and biopsy may lead to diagnosis, especially if the disease occurs predominantly in the small bowel. In other cases contrast studies may be suggestive of the diagnosis by demonstrating abnormalities including mucosal thickening.[119]

Treatment and prognosis Three grades of disease have been described:[116]

1. Early disease – infiltration with plasma cells

2. Intermediate disease

3. Malignant disease

Early disease may be treated with the appropriate therapy for parasites if present. Otherwise tetracycline or metronidazole with ampicillin may be helpful, leading to a 40% cure.[109] In those unresponsive to antibiotics and patients with grade B

and C disease, chemotherapy and possibly radiotherapy is indicated. Unfortunately the prognosis in these groups is poor, the majority of patients dying within two years.[114,120]

Lymphomatous polyposis

This rare form of lymphoma is a B cell tumour. It particularly affects the elderly. Multiple tumour nodules develop in the bowel between the pylorus and rectum. Prognosis is poor.[101]

Sarcoma

Leiomyosarcomas are the commonest type of connective tissue malignancy in the small bowel, representing over 95% of tumours in this group.[9,121] Neurofibrosarcoma is probably the most frequent member of the other occasional variants.[25,122,123] Rare tumours reported include neurogenic sarcomas, i.e. malignant schwannoma and ganglioneuroma,[19,124,125] angiosarcoma and haemangiosarcomas,[19,121,126–128] liposarcoma[19,129] and rhabdomyosarcoma.[130]

Leiomyosarcoma

Incidence This lesion makes up 7–22% of small bowel malignancies.[9,11–14] Evidence suggests a slight male preponderance.[10,11] Presentation is usually between the fifth and eighth decades.[11,17,19,25,76,101,131]

Pathology There are no known aetiological factors.[101] These lesions can be found throughout the small bowel. The jejunoileum harbours 80–90% of leiomyosarcomas and the duodenum 10–25%.[9,25,76] Duodenal lesions most commonly arise from the second part, with a few arising in the third part.[25] The tumour has also been reported as an occasional finding in jejunal diverticula or Meckel's diverticulum.[76,101] A rare association is the development of the tumour in the leiomyomas that occasionally complicate Von Recklinghausen's disease.[132]

Macroscopic appearances vary considerably: extraluminal, intramural, intraluminal and 'dumbbell' lesions can all exist.[133] Most lesions are extraluminal appearing as firm white or grey tumours[19] that grow by expansion and can develop into a substantial mass (Figure 60.9, see colour plate also). About 10% of tumours are intraluminal.[25] Leiomyosarcomas tend to be slow-growing. As they enlarge, they may outgrow the blood supply and develop central necrosis with haemorrhage or cystic degeneration.[17,19,25] Infection can supervene and lead to abscess formation.[25] Perforation of extraluminal lesions will cause peritonitis[25] and tumours can ulcerate into adjacent viscera to produce a fistula.[17]

The histological characteristics are of spindle-shaped cells interspersed with connective tissue.[17] The lesions usually arise from the circular or longitudinal muscle coats of the bowel as opposed to the muscularis mucosa. Development from vascular smooth muscle has also been reported.[17,19,76] Leiomyomas and leiomyosarcomas are sometimes termed benign and malignant stromal tumours.

An important feature of this tumour is the difficulty in defining benign or malignant characteristics.[101] Some lesions are clearly malignant as shown by local invasion or distant meta-

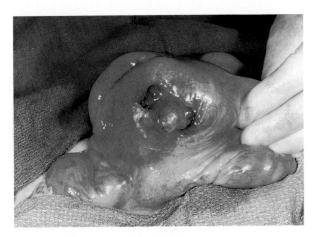

Figure 60.9
Leiomyosarcoma of the jejunum. The patient, a 64-year-old woman, had presented with high small bowel obstruction. Lymph node metastases were present at operation, and she died of disseminated disease two years later.

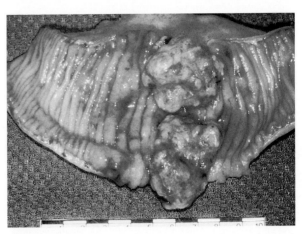

Figure 60.10
Epithelial leiomyosarcoma of the ileum in a 53-year-old man who had symptoms of intermittent small bowel obstruction.

stasis. However, the distinction on a histological basis is not clear cut: the frequency of mitoses is an important indicator, but is not always pathognomonic.[134] High-grade and low-grade tumours can be distinguished by mitotic activity, high-grade lesions having more than 10 mitoses per 10 high power fields; low grade tumours have a better prognosis (see below). Other factors suggesting malignancy include a size of over 5 cm and areas of haemorrhage or necrosis.[3]

Malignant spread into surrounding tissues is a common feature of this disease. Lymph node secondaries are unusual. Liver, lung and bone may be involved by haematogenous spread, though secondaries outside the abdomen are rare.[28,101]

Clinical features Leiomyosarcomas quite often present with bleeding from ulceration of a lesion.[17,76,131] The bleeding is often occult in nature leading to anaemia, but major haemorrhage can also occur. Haematemesis results from duodenal tumours and melaena from those sited in the jejunum or ileum.[11,76] Abdominal discomfort may be associated with nausea and vomiting. Obstruction is another potential presentation and results either from a large tumour or one that is intraluminal in site and causes intussusception[17,25,76] (Figure 60.10, see colour plate also). These tumours can be big enough to be palpable as an abdominal mass.[11,17,25,101,135]

Unusual manifestations include perforation,[25] fistula formation[17] or more rarely pyrexia (associated with tumour necrosis and infection) or retroperitoneal haemorrhage.[76]

Diagnosis Extramural lesions may be detected by CT scanning.[19,135] Intraluminal lesions may be evident on small bowel contrast studies, which typically demonstrate a tumour with a central crater. Another useful approach is angiography as these tumours tend to be extremely vascular.[135,136]

Treatment Unfortunately 25–35% of patients have metastases at operation.[11] In these instances, primary resection of the lesion is preferable to bypass (if feasible) so as to prevent the complications of local disease. In potentially curative cases, wide local 'en-bloc' resection is indicated to include all tissue involved. If this clearance is not achieved, local recurrence will occur.[101] Resection of local lymph nodes is not usually necessary as spread tends to be via the bloodstream.[17,19]

Most duodenal lesions arise in the second part and therefore require pancreatoduodenal resection to obtain adequate clearance. Localized tumours in the third part may be excised adequately by segmental resection. In the jejunoileum a limiting factor in achieving wide clearance may be the superior mesenteric artery. In distal ileal lesions right hemicolectomy may be required.

Adjunctive therapeutic options include radiotherapy and chemotherapy. Many reports indicate that these lesions are radioresistant,[17,19,28] but irradiation can be effective therapy for sarcomas in extra-abdominal sites.[137] The place of chemotherapy is also uncertain. It may be of value in palliation, although results are not overly encouraging.[138,139] Rational treatment protocols are hampered by the rarity of the disease.

Prognosis These lesions tend to be slow-growing, and their prognosis is better than for other small bowel malignancies.[19] Overall 5-year survival rate varies from 20 to 50%[28,76,121] rising to 35–50%, in lesions that appear to have been completely excised.[11]

Factors consistent with a good prognosis include a long history (of more than one year, indicating that the tumour is slow-growing), the absence of metastases at operation and a tumour diameter of less than 9 cm,[140] or less than 5 cm in another series.[11] Poor prognosis is indicated by extraintestinal invasion or presentation with intra-abdominal perforation.[11] High-grade tumours have a poorer prognosis: median survival in patients with low-grade lesions is 98 months whereas those with high-grade tumours only survive approximately 25 months.[141]

SECONDARY MALIGNANCY

Metastatic tumours may involve the small intestine by direct spread from local structures or by lymphatic, bloodstream or transcoelomic spread from further afield. Malignancies may be considered in the following groups: carcinoma, melanoma, lymphoma, leukaemia and sarcoma.

Carcinoma

Intra-abdominal malignancies that commonly give rise to secondaries involving the small bowel include carcinoma of the stomach, pancreas, colon, kidney, adrenal, cervix, uterus and ovary.[11,17,19,25,26,28] Spread from these structures may occur either directly, through involved nodes or by migration of cells across the peritoneal cavity. Common extra-abdominal primaries include the breast, lung (Figure 60.11, see colour plate also) and testis plus malignant melanoma.[11,25,142] These lesions metastasize to the abdominal cavity by lymphatic or haematogenous routes.

Metastases may declare their presence in several ways. Direct invasion into surrounding structures is common. Thus the second and third part of the duodenum may be invaded by carcinoma of the head of the pancreas, hepatic flexure, biliary tract or right kidney. The first part of the duodenum may be invaded by cancers of the stomach or pancreatic head, and the fourth part (or the duodenojejunal flexure) by cancer of the pancreatic body.[17,28] The jejunoileum may be invaded by organs in close proximity such as the colon, uterus and ovaries. Either solitary (or a few) isolated deposits may occur, or the bowel may adhere to malignant lymph nodes. Carcinomatosis peritonei heralds generalized intra-abdominal disease. In this condition, multiple discrete localized secondaries are found on the serosa of the small bowel and throughout the peritoneal cavity.[26,28]

A rare condition referred to as Linitis plastica has also been described. The tumour is present in the submucosa and muscular coats of the small intestine, often in continuity with the stomach. The bowel appears diffusely thickened and rigid: single or multiple strictures may be produced suggesting Crohn's disease.

Clinical features

Localized lesions are usually manifest by intestinal obstruction.[28] Intussusception is very unusual, though it has been reported with an intraluminal polypoid secondary from the kidney.[143] Lesions do not usually penetrate the whole of the bowel wall, but if they do, then bleeding, perforation, and abscess or fistula

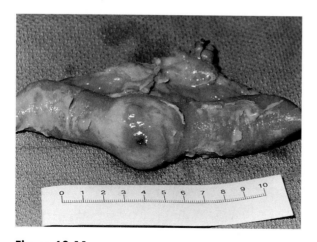

Figure 60.11
Jejunal metastasis from a primary carcinoma of the bronchus. The patient presented with perforation and peritonitis.

formation can result.[26,28] Carcinomatosis peritonei is associated with profuse ascites, which is often bloodstained.

In patients who are known to have a primary tumour, new symptoms may suggest the possibility of secondary spread. Isolated secondaries causing specific symptoms and signs may be confused with primary small bowel lesions. Laparotomy is often indicated for obstruction, and the diagnosis will then be made. In patients with malignant ascites, paracentesis and examination of the fluid will confirm the diagnosis and indicate the possible site of the primary tumour. Laparoscopy may assist in making a diagnosis.

Treatment

Management of a locally invasive carcinoma depends on which organ is involved. If resection of the tumour mass is possible, e.g. carcinoma of the colon infiltrating a loop of small bowel or duodenum, this should be performed.[17,28,144,145] Carcinoma of the pancreas infiltrating the duodenum can provide greater difficulty. Resection may be undertaken if cure is thought possible, but palliative bypass will often be the only option.[28]

Solitary metastases do occasionally present, usually secondary to carcinoma of the kidney or melanoma.[19] If possible these should be excised with a margin of normal tissue. In most cases multiple lesions are present.[11] These may be discovered at laparotomy for the primary condition, the secondaries themselves being asymptomatic. The primary tumour may be treated to relieve symptoms, but palliative surgery is usually all that can be offered.[11,17] In the case of obstruction local excision is indicated, but if not resectable, bypass should be undertaken. Bleeding lesions should be excised if possible, as should tumours that have perforated or caused fistulas.

Prognosis

Survival is related to the nature of the primary lesion and the extent of dissemination.[11] Locally invasive lesions that are removed en bloc can have a reasonable outcome. This fact is demonstrated by reports of long-term survivors following resection of colonic tumours invading the duodenum.[144]

Malignant melanoma

This condition is noteworthy because of its uncharacteristic behaviour. Over half of patients with terminal metastatic melanoma have secondaries involving the small bowel, and a quarter may have tumours in the stomach or colon. By contrast reports of small bowel melanoma presenting during life are rare[146,147] (Figure 60.12, see colour plate also). Two main forms are reported; the multiple polypoid form is common whereas the solitary infiltrating form is rare.[146,148] Complications seldom arise, but obstruction can result from stenosis or intussusception of polypoid lesions, and these tumours can bleed or perforate.[146-148]

Operative treatment is indicated for solitary lesions or those causing complications. Mean survival after operation for complications is 9 months.[147] The prognosis of multiple metastases is poor, most patients failing to survive beyond 3 months.[146] Solitary lesions are more favourable, with isolated reports of patients being alive for up to 5 years after resection.[146-148]

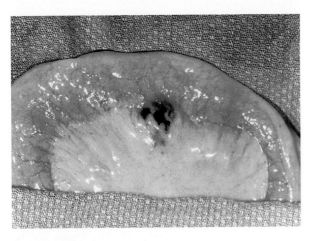

Figure 60.12
Malignant melanoma of the mid small bowel. The patient had iron-deficiency anaemia and stools that were persistently positive for occult blood.

Lymphoma

Metastatic involvement of the gastrointestinal tract is approximately 10 times commoner than primary lymphoma.[91,101] The bowel is involved in approximately 50% of terminal disseminated non-Hodgkins lymphoma[90,91,149,150] and 20% of Hodgkin's lymphoma.[12] The commonest site of involvement is the stomach.[90]

Macroscopic appearances are usually of multiple infiltrative nodules.[101] Symptoms develop only in the minority; pain, bleeding and obstruction are the commonest features.[90,101,149] Treatment is along conventional lines with radiotherapy and chemotherapy. Palliative surgery is indicated for complications. Prognosis is poor due to disseminated disease, and average survival is only nine months.[90]

Leukaemia

Approximately 15% of patients dying of leukaemia demonstrate infiltration of the gastrointestinal tract at autopsy.[101,151] In the small bowel, lesions are most commonly found in the ileum. Other common sites are the stomach and colon.[101]

Macroscopic appearances are of polyploid or thickened areas in the mucosa or submucosa, but diffuse infiltrative forms can also occur. Histologically, there is diffuse infiltration of the submucosa and lamina propria. Necrosis may lead to infection.[101]

Other asymptomatic small bowel lesions may present with haemorrhage, perforation or obstruction, often due to intussusception.[101] Treatment may be considered in the form of chemotherapy, but there is a risk of enterocolitis and intestinal perforation.[101,152] Palliative surgery should be considered for complications.

Sarcoma

Metastatic sarcoma involving the small bowel is almost invariable due to spread from contiguous structures. This aspect has been discussed in the section on primary sarcoma.

MALIGNANCY ASSOCIATED WITH AIDS

Malignant disease has been reported in approximately 40% of patients with AIDS.[153] Kaposi's sarcoma and B-cell lymphomas make up 95% of these cancers,[154] and each type of tumour can affect the small bowel. Carcinoma of the small bowel has not been described, although carcinoma has been reported in the stomach and colon.[155]

Kaposi's sarcoma

This disease is present in up to one third of patients dying of AIDS.[11,153,156] The skin is predominantly affected, but 45–50% of patients have part of the gastrointestinal tract involved.[11,157] The disease is found in the oesophagus, stomach, duodenum and colon.[158] Macroscopic appearances are of small telangiectatic lesions or nodular or polypoid masses.[159–161]

Most lesions are asymptomatic, but bleeding and obstruction can occur.[11,153,158] The diagnosis may not emerge until the bowel is investigated, often for diarrhoea. If lesions are asymptomatic, no treatment is indicated.[153] Complications such as haemorrhage or obstruction necessitate local resection.[11] Radiotherapy and chemotherapy may be considered but with care in view of their appreciable morbidity.[153]

The prognosis is poor due to the fact that the patient has defective immune status. Involvement of the viscera is a bad prognostic sign and indicates advanced immune deficiency. Death in this disease is usually due to opportunistic infection.[153]

Lymphoma

Non-Hodgkin's lymphoma and rarely Hodgkin's lymphoma can develop in patients with AIDS.[153] In non-Hodgkin's disease, 90% of tumours are extranodal in site.[162] The commonest organ is the central nervous system, but bone marrow, liver, spleen, lungs and skin can also be affected.[153]

Approximately 20% of patients with AIDS with lymphoma have gastrointestinal disease.[11,162] Within the bowel, lymphoma is commoner in the mouth and rectum, but the small intestine can also be affected.[153]

The clinical features of small bowel disease are of abdominal pain and diarrhoea. Perforation can occur.[11,153,156] In contrast to Kaposi's sarcoma, lymphoma is often the terminal disease in these patients. Treatment options include radiotherapy or chemotherapy; operation is reserved for complications.

Overall, the prognosis in patients with AIDS who have developed lymphoma is extremely poor. Over half the tumours are high-grade and lead to an early demise.[162] Mean survival in aggressive tumours is approximately 3 months.[153]

REFERENCES

1. Zollinger RM Jr, Sternfeld WC & Schreiber H. Primary neoplasms of the small intestine. *Am J Surg* 1986; **151**: 654–658.
2. Adkins RB Jr & Davies J. Gross and microscopic anatomy of the stomach and small intestine. In Scott HW Jr & Sawyers JL (eds) *Surgery of the Stomach, Duodenum and Small Intestine.* Boston: Blackwell Scientific Publications, 1987; 45–60.
3. Slavin G. Tumours and tumour-like conditions. In Booth CC & Neale G (eds). *Disorders of the Small Intestine.* Oxford: Blackwell Scientific Publications, 1985; 363–375.

4. Darling RC & Welch CE. Tumours of the small intestine. *N Engl J Med* 1959; **260**: 397–408.

5. Williamson RCN, Welch CE & Malt RA. Adenocarcinoma and lymphoma of the small intestine. *Ann Surg* 1983; **197**: 172–178.

6. Studley JGN & Williamson RCN. Hamartomas and benign neoplasms of the small bowel. In Morris PJ & Malt RA (eds) *Oxford Textbook of Surgery*. Oxford: Oxford Medical Publications, 1994; 999–1007.

7. Wilson JM, Melvin DB, Gray G & Thorbjarnarson B. Benign small bowel tumor. *Ann Surg* 1975; **181**: 247–250.

8. Wattenburg LW. Studies of polycyclic hydrocarbon hydroxylases of the intestine possibly related to cancer. *Cancer* 1971; **28**: 99–106.

9. Wilson JM, Melvin DB, Gray GF & Thorbjarnarson B. Primary malignancies of the small bowel: a report of 96 cases and review of the literature. *Ann Surg* 1974; **180**: 175–179.

10. Lowenfels AB. Why are small bowel tumours so rare? *Lancet* 1973; **i**: 24–26.

11. Dial P & Cohn I Jr. tumors of the jejunum and ileum. In Scott HW Jr & Sawyers JL (eds) *Surgery of the Stomach, Duodenum and Small Intestine*. Boston: Blackwell Scientific Publications, 1987; 937–951.

12. Mittal VK & Bodzin JH. Primary malignant tumors of the small bowel. *Am J Surg* 1980; **140**: 396–399.

13. Lanzafame RJ, Long JE & Hinshaw JR. Primary cancer of the small bowel. *NY State J Med* 1982; **82**: 1325–1329.

14. Awrich AE, Irish CE, Vetto RM & Fletcher WS. A twenty-five year experience with primary malignant tumors of the small intestine. *Surg Gynecol Obstet* 1980; **151**: 9–14.

15. Bridge MF & Perzin KH. Primary adenocarcinoma of the jejunum and ileum: a clinicopathologic study. *Cancer* 1975; **36**: 1876–1887.

16. Ciccarelli O, Welch JP & Kent GG. Primary malignant tumors of the small bowel. The Hartford Hospital experience, 1969–1983. *Am J Surg* 1987; **153**: 350–354.

17. Herbsman H, Wetstein L, Rosen Y et al. Tumors of the small intestine. *Curr Probl Surg* 1980; **17**: 127–182.

18. Ouriel K & Adams JT. Adenocarcinoma of the small intestine. *Am J Surg* 1984; **147**: 66–71.

19. Ashley SW & Wells SA Jr. Tumors of the small intestine. *Semin Oncol* 1988; **15**: 116–128.

20. Reiner MA. Primary malignant neoplasms of the small bowel. *Mt Sinai J Med* 1976; **43**: 274–280.

21. Cooper MJ & Williamson RCN. Enteric adenoma and adenocarcinoma. *World J Surg* 1985; **9**: 914–920.

22. Spira IA, Ghazi A & Wolff WI. Primary adenocarcinoma of the duodenum. *Cancer* 1977; **39**: 1721–1726.

23. Sakker S & Ware CC. Carcinoma of the duodenum: comparison of surgery, radiotherapy, and chemotherapy. *Br J Surg* 1973; **60**: 867–872.

24. Scott-Coombes DM & Williamson RCN. Surgical treatment of primary duodenal carcinoma – a personal series. *Br J Surg* 1984; **81**: 1472–1474.

25. Perey BJ. Neoplasms of the duodenum. In Scott HW Jr & Sawyers JL (eds) *Surgery of the Stomach, Duodenum and Small Intestine*. Boston: Blackwell Scientific Publications, 1987; 571–584.

26. Morson BC, Dawson IMP, Day DW, Jass JR, Price AB & Williams GT. Malignant epithelial tumours. In Morson BC & Dawson IMP (eds) *Morson and Dawson's Gastrointestinal Pathology*, 3rd edn. Oxford: Blackwell Scientific Publications, 1990; 360–371.

27. Morgan DF & Busuttil RW. Primary adenocarcinoma of the small intestine. *Am J Surg* 1977; **134**: 331–333.

28. Williamson RCN. Cancer of the small intestine. In Misiewicz JJ, Pounder RE & Venables CW (eds) *Diseases of the Gut and Pancreas*. Oxford: Blackwell Scientific Publications, 1994; 713–722.

29. Perzin KH & Bridge MF. Adenomas of the small intestine: a clinicopathologic review of 51 cases and a study of their relationship to carcinoma. *Cancer* 1981; **48**: 799–819.

30. Galandiuk S, Hermann RE, Jagelman DG, Fazio VW & Sivak MV. Villous tumors of the duodenum. *Ann Surg* 1988; **207**: 234–239.

31. Chappuis CW, Divincenti FC & Cohn I Jr. Villous tumors of the duodenum. *Ann Surg* 1989; **209**: 593–599.

32. Schulten MF Jr, Oyasu R & Beal JM. Villous adenoma of the duodenum. A case report and review of the literature. *Am J Surg* 1976; **132**: 90–96.

33. Ryan DP, Shapiro RH & Warshaw AL. Villous tumours of the duodenum. *Ann Surg* 1986; **203**: 301–306.

34. Kurtz RC, Sternberg SS, Miller HH & Decosse JJ. Upper gastrointestinal neoplasia in familial polyposis. *Dig Dis Sci* 1987; **32**: 459–465.

35. Yao T, Iida M, Ohsato K, Watanabe H & Omae T. Duodenal lesions in familial polyposis of the colon. *Gastroenterology* 1977; **73**: 1086–1092.

36. Sarre RG, Frost AG, Jagelman DG, Petras RE, Sivak MV & McGannon E. Gastric and duodenal polyps in familial adenomatous polyposis: a prospective study of the nature and prevalence of upper gastrointestinal polyps. *Gut* 1987; **28**: 306–314.

37. Ranzi T, Castagnone D, Velio P, Bianchi P & Polli EE. Gastric and duodenal polyps in familial polyposis coli. *Gut* 1981; **22**: 363–367.

38. Gerritsen RTh, Spoelstra P & Breeuwsma NG. Carcinoma of the papilla of Vater in a brother and sister with familial adenomatous polyposis. *Neth J Med* 1993; **43**: 22–25.

39. Burt RW, Berenson MM, Lee RGD, Tolman KG, Freston JW & Gardner EJ. Upper gastrointestinal polyps in Gardner's syndrome. *Gastroenterology* 1984; **86**: 295–301.

40. Jones TR & Nance FC. Periampullary malignancy in Gardner's syndrome. *Ann Surg* 1977; **185**: 565–573.

41. Bussey HJR. Extracolonic lesions associated with polyposis coli. *Proc R Soc Med* 1972; **65**: 294.

42. Iida M, Itoh H, Matsui T, Mibu R, Iwashita A & Fujishima M. Ileal adenomas in postcolectomy patients with familial adenomatosis coli/Gardner's syndrome. Incidence and endoscopic appearance. *Dis Colon Rectum* 1989; **32**: 1034–1038.

43. Hamilton SR, Bussey HJR, Mendelsohn G et al. Ileal adenomas after colectomy in nine patients with adenomatous polyposis coli/Gardner's syndrome. *Gastroenterology* 1979; **77**: 1252–1257.

44. Ross JE & Mara JE. Smallbowel polyps and carcinoma in multiple intestinal polyposis. *Arch Surg* 1974; **108**: 736–738.

45. Roth JA & Logio T. Carcinoma arising in an ileostomy stoma, an unusual complication of adenomatous polyposis coli. *Cancer* 1982; **49**: 2180–2184.

46. Christie AC. Duodenal carcinoma with neoplastic transformation of the underlying Brunner's glands. *Br J Cancer* 1953; **7**: 65–67.

47. Reid JD. Intestinal carcinoma in the Peutz–Jeghers syndrome. *JAMA* 1974; **229**: 833–834.

48. Fresko D, Lazarus SS, Dotan J & Reingold M. Early presentation of carcinoma of the small bowel in Crohn's disease. *Gastroenterology* 1982; **82**: 783–789.

49. Michelassi F, Testa G, Pomidor WJ, Lashner BA & Block GE. Adenocarcinoma complicating Crohn's disease. *Drs Colon Rectum* 1993; **36**: 654–661.

50. Hawker PC, Gyde SN, Thompson H & Allen RN. Adenocarcinoma of the small intestine complicating Crohn's disease. *Gut* 1982; **23**: 188–193.

51. Hoffman JP, Taft DA, Wheelis RF et al. Adenocarcinoma in regional enteritis of the small intestine. *Ann Surg* 1977; **112**: 606–611.

52. Savoca PE, Ballantyne GH & Cahow CE. Gastrointestinal malignancies in Crohn's disease. A 20-year experience. *Dis Colon Rectum* 1990; **33**: 7–11.

53. Rubio CA, Befritz R, Poppen B, Svenberg T & Slezak P. Crohn's disease and adenocarcinoma of the intestinal tract. Report of four cases. *Dis Colon Rectum* 1991; **34**: 174–180.

54. Slezak P, Rubio C, Blomqvist L, Nakano H & Befrits R. Duodenal adenocarcinoma in Crohn's disease of the small bowel: a case report. *Gastrointest Radiol* 1991; **16**: 15–17.

55. Greenstein AJ, Sachar DB, Smith H, Janowitz HD & Aufses AH. Patterns of neoplasia in Crohn's disease and ulcerative colitis. *Cancer* 1980; **46**: 403–407.

56. Ribeiro MB, Greenstein AJ, Heimann TM, Yamazaki Y & Aufses AH. Adenocarcinoma of the small intestine in Crohn's disease. *Surg Gynecol Obstet* 1991; **173**: 343–349.

57. Cooper BT, Holmes GKT, Ferguson R & Cooke WT. Celiac disease and malignancy. *Medicine (Baltimore)* 1980; **59**: 249–261.

58. O'Brien CJ, Saverymuttu S, Hodgson HJF & Evans DJ. Coeliac disease, adenocarcinoma of the jejunum and *in situ* squamous carcinoma of the oesophagus. *J Clin Pathol* 1983; **36**: 62–68.

59. Jones TJ & Marshall TL. Neurofibromatosis and small bowel adenocarcinoma: an unrecognised association. *Gut* 1987; **28**: 1173–1176.

60. McGlinchey JJ, Santer GJ & Haqqani MT. Primary adenocarcinoma of the duodenum associated with cutaneous neurofibromatosis (von Recklinghausen's disease). *Postgrad Med J* 1982; **58**: 115–116.

61. Ryan TJ. Diseases of the skin. In Weatherall DJ, Ledingham JGG & Warrell DA (eds) *Oxford Textbook of Medicine*, 2nd edn, Oxford: Oxford Medical Publications, 1988: 20–79.

62. Panday SCN, Go IH, Mravunac M & de Koning RW. Obstructive jejunal adenocarcinoma in the Muir-Torre syndrome. *Neth J Med* 1993; **43**: 116–120.

63. Gajraj H, Davies DR & Jackson BT. Synchronous small and large bowel cancer developing after pelvic irradiation?. *Gut* 1988; **29**: 126–128.

64. Lynch HT, Smyrk TC, Lynch PM et al. Adenocarcinoma of the small bowel in lynch syndrome II. *Cancer* 1989; **64**: 2178–2183.

65. Lynch HT, Kimberling W, Albano WA et al. Hereditary nonpolyposis colorectal cancer (Lynch syndromes I and II). *Cancer* 1985; **56**: 934–938.

66. Shousa S, Scott J & Polak J. Ileal loop carcinoma after cystectomy for bladder extrophy. *BMJ* 1978; **2**: 397–398.

67. Adler SN, Lyon DT & Sullivan PD. Adenocarcinoma of the small bowel. Clinical features, similarity to regional enteritis and analysis of 338 documented cases. *Am J Gastroenterol* 1982; **77**: 326–330.

68. Lai ECS, Doty JE, Irving C & Tompkins RK. Primary adenocarcinoma of the duodenum: analysis of survival. *World J Surg* 1988; **12**: 695–699.

69. Rotman N, Pezet D, Fagniez P-L et al. Adenocarcinoma of the duodenum: factors influencing survival. *Br J Surg* 1994; **81**: 83–85.

70. Lewis BS & Waye JD. Chronic gastrointestinal bleeding of obscure origin: role of small bowel enteroscopy. *Gastroenterology* 1988; **94**: 117–120.

71. Frimberger E, Hagenmuller F & Classen M. Endostomy: a new approach to small-bowel endoscopy. *Endoscopy* 1989; **21**: 86–88.

72. Farah MC, Jafri SZH, Schwab RE et al. Duodenal neoplasms: role of CT. *Radiology* 1987; **162**: 839–843.

73. Moss AA & Margulis AR. Stomach and duodenum: overview. In Margulis AR & Burhenne HJ (eds) *Alimentary Tract Radiology*, 4th edn, St Louis: CV Mosby, 1994: 691–708.

74. Goldberg HI, Jeffrey RB. Small Bowel: overview. In Margulis AR & Burhenne HJ (eds) *Alimentary Tract Radiology*, 4th edn, St Louis: CV Mosby, 1994: 857–868.

75. Desa LAJ, Bridger J, Grace PA, Krauz T & Spencer J. Primary jejunoileal tumors: a review of 45 cases. *World J Surg* 1991; **15**: 81–87.

76. Bouchier IAD, Allan RN, Hodgson HJF & Keighley MRB (eds) *Textbook of Gastroenterology* London: Ballière Tindall; 1984;

77. Jigyasu D, Bedikian AY & Shroehlein JR. Chemotherapy for primary adenocarcinoma of the small bowel. *Cancer* 1984; **53**: 23–25.

78. Lillemoe K & Imbembo AL. Malignant neoplasms of the duodenum. *Surg Gynecol Obstet* 1980; **150**: 822–826.

79. Michelassi F, Erroi F, Dawson PJ et al. Experience with 647 consecutive tumors of the duodenum, ampulla, head of the pancreas, and distal common bile duct. *Ann Surg* 1989; **210**: 544–554.

80. Tarazi RY, Hermann RE, Vogt DP et al. Results of surgical treatment of periampullary tumors: a thirty-five year experience. *Surgery* 1986; **100**: 716–723.

81. Moossa AR & Lavelle-Jones M. Whipple for pancreatoduodenectomy. In Blumgart LH (ed) *Surgery of the Liver and Biliary Tract.* London: Churchill Livingstone, 1988: 869–879.

82. Blumgart LH. Cancer and the bile ducts. In: Blumgart LH (ed) *Surgery of the Liver and Biliary Tract.* London: Churchill Livingstone, 1988: 829–853.

83. Cotton PB. Nonsurgical palliation of jaundice in pancreatic cancer. *Surg Clin North Am* 1989; **69**: 613–627.

84. Braasch JW. Periampullary and pancreatic cancer. In: Blumgart LH (ed) *Surgery of the Liver and Biliary Tract.* London: Churchill Livingstone, 1988: 855–868.

85. Joesting DR, Beart RW, van Heerden JA & Weiland LH. Improving survival in adenocarcinoma of the duodenum. *Am J Surg* 1981; **141**: 228–231.

86. Goldberg M, Zamir O, Hadary A & Nissan S. Wide local excision as an alternative treatment for periampullary carcinoma. *J Gastroenterol* 1987; **82**: 1169–1171.

87. van Ooijen B & Kalsbeek HL. Carcinoma of the duodenum. *Surg Gynecol Obstet* 1988; **166**: 343–347.

88. Alwmark A, Andersson A & Lasson A. Primary carcinoma of the duodenum. *Ann Surg* 1980; **191**: 13–18.

89. Cohen JR, Juchta N, Geller N, Shines GT & Dineen P. Pancreatoduodenectomy. A 40 year experience. *Ann Surg* 1982; **195**: 608–617.

90. Herrmann R, Panahon AM, Barcos MP, Walsh D & Stutzman L. Gastrointestinal involvement in non-Hodgkin's lymphoma. *Cancer* 1980; **46**: 215–222.

91. Timothy A, Sloane J & Selby P. Lymphomas. In: Sikora K & Halnan KE (eds) *Treatment of Cancer*, 2nd edn. London: Chapman and Hall Medical, 1990: 695–736.

92. Lewin KJ, Ranchod M & Dorfman RF. Lymphomas of the gastrointestinal tract. *Cancer* 1978; **42**: 693–707.

93. Green JA, Dawson AA, Jones PF & Brunt PW. The presentation of gastrointestinal lymphoma. *Br J Surg* 1979; **66**: 798–801.

94. Dawson MP, Coones S & Morson BC. Primary malignant lymphoid tumours of the intestinal tract. *Br J Surg* 1961; **49**: 80–89.

95. Thomas CR & Share R. Gastrointestinal lymphoma. *Med Pediatr Oncol* 1991; **19**: 48–60.

96. Isaacson PG, Spencer J & Wright DH. Classifying primary gut lymphomas. *Lancet* 1988; **ii**: 1148–1149.

97. Calam J & Williamson RCN. Neoplastic and miscellaneous disease of the small intestine. In Misiewicz JJ, Pounder RE & Venables CW (eds). *Diseases of the Gut and Pancreas*, 2nd edn. Oxford: Blackwell Scientific Publications, 1994: 649–673.

98. Cooper BT & Read AE. Small intestinal lymphoma. *World J Surg* 1985; **9**: 930–937.

99. Auger MJ & Allan NC. Primary ileocecal lymphoma. A study of 22 patients. *Cancer* 1990; **65**: 358–361.

100. Sweetenham JW, Mead GM, Wright DH et al. Involvement of the ileocaecal region by non-Hodgkin's lymphoma in adults: clinical features and results of treatment. *Br J Cancer* 1989; **60**: 366–369.

101. Morson BC, Dawson IMP, Day DW, Jass JR, Price AB & Williams GT. Non-epithelial tumours. In Morson BC & Dawson IMP, (eds) *Morson & Dawson's Gastrointestinal Pathology*, 3rd edn. Oxford: Blackwell Scientific Publications, 1990: 372–387.

102. Contreary K, Nance FC & Becker WF. Primary lymphoma of the gastrointestinal tract. *Ann Surg* 1980; **191**: 593–598.

103. Filippa DA, Lieberman PH, Weingrad AN, Decosse JJ & Bretsky SS. Primary lymphomas of the gastrointestinal tract. Analysis of prognostic factors with emphasis on histologic type. *Am J Surg Pathol* 1983; **7**: 363–372.

104. Domizio P, Owen RA, Shepherd NA, Talbot IC & Norton A. Primary lymphoma of the small intestine. A clinicopathological study of 119 cases. *Am J Surg Pathol* 1993; **17**: 429–442.

105. Blackledge G, Bush H, Dodge OG & Crowther D. A study of gastrointestinal lymphoma. *Clin Oncol* 1979; **5**: 209–219.

106. Fu YS & Perzin KH. Lymphosarcoma of the small intestine. *Cancer* 1972; **29**: 645–659.

107. Taggart DP, McLatchie GR & Imrie CW. Survival of surgical patients with carcinoma, lymphoma and carcinoid tumours of the small bowel. *Br J Surg* 1986; **73**: 826–828.

108. Editorial. Primary gut lymphomas. *Lancet* 1991; **337**: 1384–1385.

109. Smith MSH. Gastrointestinal lymphoma. In Misiewicz JJ, Pounder RE & Venables CW (eds) *Diseases of the Gut and Pancreas*, 2nd edn. Oxford: Blackwell Scientific Publications, 1994: 979–987.

110. Isaacson P & Wright DH. Intestinal lymphoma associated with malabsorption. *Lancet* 1978; **i**: 67–70.

111. Isaacson P & Wright DH. Malignant histiocytosis of the intestine. Its relationship to malabsorption and ulcerative jejunitis. *Hum Pathol* 1978; **9**: 661–677.

112. Nasr K, Haghighi P, Bakhshandeh K, Abadi P & Lahimgarzadeh A. Primary upper small intestinal lymphoma. *Am J Dig Dis* 1976; **21**: 313–323.

113. Al-Bahrani Z, Al-Saleem T, Al-Monhiry M et al. Alpha heavy chain disease. *Gut* 1978; **19**: 627–631.

114. Salem PA, Nassar VH, Shahid MJ et al. Mediterranean abdominal lymphoma or immunoproliferative small intestinal disease. Part I: Clinical aspects. *Cancer* 1977; **40**: 2941–2947.

115. Rambaud J-C, Modigliani R, Nguyen Phuoc BK & Lejeune R. Non-secretory alpha-chain disease in intestinal lymphoma. *N Engl J Med* 1980; **303**: 53.

116. Galian A, Lecestre MJ, Scotto J, Bognel C, Matuchansky C & Rambaud J. Pathological study of α chain disease with special emphasis on evolution. *Cancer* 1977; **39**: 2081–2101.

117. Khojasteh A, Haghshenass M & Haghighi P. Current concepts – immunoproliferative small intestinal disease. A third world lesion. *N Engl J Med* 1983; **308**: 1401–1405.

118. Jacobs P. The malignant lymphomas in Africa. *Haemat Oncol Clin NA* 1991; **5**: 953–982.

119. Vessal K, Dutz W, Kohout E et al. Immunoproliferative small intestinal disease with duodenojejunal lymphoma: radiologic changes. *Am J Roent* 1980; **135**: 491–497.

120. Rambaud JC. Small intestinal lymphomas and a chain disease. *Clin Gastroenterol* 1983; **12**: 743–766.

121. Pagtalunan RJG, Mayo CW & Dockerty MB. Primary malignant tumors of the small intestine. *Am J Surg* 1964; **108**: 13–18.

122. Wander JV & Das Gupta TK. Neurofibromatosis. *Curr Probl Surg* 1977; **14**(2): 1–81.

123. Sivak MV, Sullivan BH & Farmer RG. Neurogenic tumours of the small intestine. *Gastroenterology* 1975; **68**: 374–380.

124. *Arch Pathol* 1972; **93**: 549–551.

125. Ostermiller W, Joergenson EJ & Weibel L. A clinical review of tumours of the small bowel. *Am J Surg* 1966; **111**: 403–409.

126. Murray-Lyon IM, Doyle D, Philpott RM & Porter NH. Haemangiomatosis of the small and large bowel with histological malignant change. *J Pathol* 1971; **105**: 295–297.

127. Chen KTK, Hoffman KD & Hendricks EJ. Angiosarcoma following therapeutic irradiation. *Cancer* 1979; **44**: 2044–2048.

128. Hwang T-L, Sun C-F & Chen MF. Angiosarcoma of the small intestine after radiation therapy: Report of a case. *J Formosan Med Assoc* 1993; **92**: 658–661.

129. Mohandas D, Chandra RS, Srinivasan V & Bhaskar AG. Liposarcoma of the ileum with secondaries in the liver. *Am J Gastroenterol* 1972; **58**: 172–176.

130. Moses I & Coodley EL. Rhabdomyosarcoma of duodenum. *Am J Gastroenterol* 1969; **51**: 48–54.

131. Hansen CP, Colstrup H & Mogensen AM. Recurrent gastrointestinal bleeding due to leiomyosarcoma of the small intestine. *Eur J Surg* 1991; **157**: 227–229.

132. Ishizaki Y, Tada Y, Ishida T et al. Leiomyosarcoma of the small intestine associated with von Recklinghausen's disease: report of a case. *Surgery* 1992; **111**: 706–710.

133. Starr GF & Dockerty MB. Leiomyomas and leiomyosarcomas of the small intestine. *Cancer* 1955; **8**: 101–111.

134. Akwari OE, Dozois RR, Weiland LH & Beahrs OH. Leiomyosarcoma of the small and large bowel. *Cancer* 1978; **42**: 1375–1384.

135. Tarraza HM, Smith WG, Granai CO, DeCain M & Jones MA. Leiomyosarcoma of the small intestine presenting as a pelvic mass: four cases. *Gynecol Oncol* 1991; **41**: 167–171.

136. Cho KJ & Reuter SR. Angiography of duodenal leiomyomas and leiomyosarcomas. *AJR* 1980; **135**: 31–35.

137. Suit HD, Russell WO & Martin RG. Management of patients with sarcoma of soft tissue in an extremity. *Cancer* 1973; **3**: 1247–1255.

138. Gottlieb JA, Baker LH, O'Bryan RM et al. Adriamycin (NSC-123127) used alone and in combination for soft tissue and bony sarcomas. *Cancer Chemother Rep* part 3 1975; **6**: 271–278.

139. Gottlieb JA. Combination chemotherapy for metastatic sarcoma. *Cancer Chemother Rep* 1974; **58**: 265–270.

140. Chiotasso PJP & Fazio VW. Prognostic factors of 28 leiomyomas of the small intestine. *Surg Gynecol Obstet* 1982; **155**: 197–202.

141. Evans HL. Smooth muscle tumours of the gastrointestinal tract: A study of 56 cases followed for a minimum of 10 years. *Cancer* 1985; **56**: 2242–2250.

142. McNeill PM, Wagman LD & Neifeld JP. Small bowel metastases from primary carcinoma of the lung. *Cancer* 1987; **59**: 1486–1489.

143. Haynes IG, Wolverson RL & O'Brien JM. Small bowel intussusception due to metastatic renal carcinoma. *Br J Urol* 1986; **58**: 460.

144. Ellis H, Morgan MN & Wastell C. Curative surgery in carcinoma of the colon involving duodenum. *Br J Surg* 1972; **59**: 932–935.

145. Das Gupta TK & Brasfield RD. Metastatic melanoma of the Gastrointestinal tract. *Arch Surg* 1964; **88**: 969–973.

146. Willbanks OL & Fogelman MJ. Gastrointestinal melanosarcoma. *Am J Surg* 1970; **120**: 602–606.

147. Jorge E, Harvey HA, Simmonds MA, Lipton A & Joehl RJ. Symptomatic malignant melanoma of the gastrointestinal tract. *Ann Surg* 1984; **199**: 328–331.

148. Klausner JM, Skornick Y, Lulcuk S, Baratz M & Merhave A. Acute complication of metastatic melanoma to the gastrointestinal tract. *Br J Surg* 1982; **69**: 195–196.

149. Rosenberg SA, Diamond HD, Jaslowitz B & Carven LF. Lymphosarcoma: a review of 1269 cases. *Medicine (Baltimore)* 1961; **40**: 31–34.

150. Cornes JS. Hodgkin's disease of the gastrointestinal tract. *Proc R Soc Med* 1967; **60**: 732–733.

151. Prolla JC & Kirschner JB. The gastrointestinal lesions and complications of the leukaemias. *Ann Intern Med* 1964; **61**: 1084–1103.

152. King A, Rampling A, Wight DGD & Warren RF. Neutropenic enterocolitis due to *Clostridium septicum* infection. *J Clin Pathol* 1984; **37**: 335–343.

153. Stewart JS & Munro AJ. Aids and cancer. In: Sikora K, Halnan KE (eds) *Treatment of Cancer* 2nd edn. London: Chapman and Hall Medical, 1990: 777–790.

154. Levine AM. Non-Hodgkin's lymphomas and other malignancies in the acquired immune deficiency syndrome. *Semin Oncol* 1987; **14** (Suppl 3): 34–39.

155. Ravalli S, Chabon AB & Koan AA. Gastrointestinal neoplasia in young HIV antibody positive patients. *Am J Clin Pathol* 1989; **9**: 458–461.

156. Potter DA, Danforth DN Jr, Macher AM, Longo DL, Stewart L & Masur H. Evaluation of abdominal pain in the AIDS patient. *Ann Surg* 1984; **199**: 332–339.

157. Krigel RL & Fredman-Klein AE. Kaposi's sarcoma in AIDS. In DeVita VT, Hellman S & Rosenberg SA (eds) *AIDS: Aetiology, Diagnosis, Treatment and Prevention*. Philadelphia; JB Lippincott, 1985; 1214–1282.

158. Weller IVD. Aids and the gut. *Scand J Gastroenterol* 1985; **20** (Suppl 114): 77–82.

159. Safia B. Clinical manifestation of Kaposi's sarcoma. In: Ma P, Armstrong D (eds) *Aids and Infections of Homosexual Men* 2nd edn. New York: Butterworth, 1989: 251–264.

160. Bayley AC. Aggressive Kaposi's sarcoma in Zambia. *Lancet* 1983; **i**: 1318–1320.

161. Friedman-Kien A, Laubenstein LJ, Rubinstein P et al. Disseminated Kaposi's sarcoma in homosexual men. *Ann Intern Med* 1982; **96**: 693–700.

162. Ziegler JL, Beckstead JA, Volberding PA et al. Non-Hodgkin's lymphoma in 90 homosexual men. *N Engl J Med* 1984; **311**: 565–570.

61

MISCELLANEOUS CONDITIONS OF THE SMALL INTESTINE

DM Scott-Coombes

WILKIE SYNDROME (SUPERIOR MESENTERIC ARTERY SYNDROME)

Definition

At the level of the first lumbar vertebra, the root of the superior mesenteric artery arises from the aorta at an angle of 38–41.25°.[1] Immediately inferior to the origin of the superior mesenteric artery, the third part of the duodenum traverses the abdominal aorta; therefore any disorder that may bring about a narrowing of the angle subtended between the superior mesenteric artery and the aorta could theoretically result in duodenal compression. In 1842 Rokitansky[2] became the first clinician to describe such an organic vascular duodenal compression in a patient whose symptoms were relieved in the knee–chest or recumbent position lying on the left side. This condition has latterly become eponymously referred to as Wilkie syndrome in recognition of Wilkie's studies on duodenal ileus.[3] Although this condition tends to be overdiagnosed,[1] its incidence has been estimated to be 0.2% of the population from a series of 6000 patients who underwent barium meal examination. Several small series have been reported in the literature, but some clinicians still deny its existence.[1,4,5]

Any condition that results in a more acute angle (6–16°) between the aorta and superior mesenteric artery predisposes to Wilkie syndrome (Table 61.1), whether a primary anatomical anomaly or disorders that secondarily narrow the vascular

Table 61.1 Risk factors for superior mesenteric artery compression of the duodenum

Congential acute angle
Short ligament of Treitz
Loss of the fat pad (emaciation)
Low origin of the superior mesenteric artery
Lumbar lordosis
Positional – prolonged period in a supine state
         – body cast

angle, particularly illnesses necessitating a long hospitalization. Recumbency not only confines the patient to a supine position for prolonged periods of time but often results in loss of the fat pad, which is believed to keep the angle open. Defects in the myenteric plexus and duodenal smooth muscle may result in a 'megaduodenum', which can mimic Wilkie syndrome.[4]

Clinical aspects

Patients with chronic disease, typically women in the second and third decades of life, are at greatest risk of developing Wilkie syndrome. Symptoms are often intermittent in nature and range from postprandial or positional discomfort to high intestinal obstruction with bile-stained vomiting and weight loss. This condition is diagnosed by barium meal examination, but owing to its intermittent nature the diagnosis may be missed if the patient is asymptomatic at the time of the investigation. Typical radiological features include to-and-fro peristalsis in the second and third parts of the duodenum with an abrupt, but incomplete hold-up in the third part combined with proximal duodenal dilatation.[1,4] The differential diagnosis of Wilkie syndrome (Figure 61.1) includes scleroderma, malignant involvement of local lymph nodes and primary retroperitoneal tumours. In a series of 12 patients with a radiological diagnosis of Wilkie syndrome, one-quarter were ultimately found to have an underlying malignancy.[4]

Management

A conservative approach to this condition includes nutritional support and attention to the position of the patient, making attempts to prevent the patient lying supine for long periods of time. Between 55 and 100% of patients come to operation. Division of the ligament of Treitz after mobilization of the right colon (Strong's procedure) effectively relieves duodenal obstruction. Where intra-abdominal adhesions predominate, the simplest procedure would be to bypass the obstruction via a duodenojejunostomy. For those patients in whom gastric dilatation is prominent, and when other procedures are

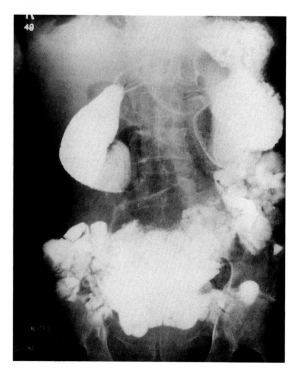

Figure 61.1

Barium meal examination in a cachectic man of 67 years who was thought to have Wilkie syndrome of duodenal compression by the superior mesenteric artery. The radiograph shows gross dilatation of the second and proximal third parts of the duodenum. Laparotomy revealed that the obstruction was caused by an adherence of the third part of the duodenum to an aortic Dacron graft that had been used to replace an aortic aneurysm 3 years earlier. (Professor Williamson's case.)

technically difficult, a gastrojejunostomy would be the operation of choice. This may be combined with a vagotomy in the presence of associated peptic ulceration. The preferred operation is Strong's procedure because it obviates the need to breach the bowel. A recent modification to this technique, which is effectively a derotational procedure, involves delivering the duodenojejunal segment behind the superior mesenteric vessels.[6]

ANNULAR PANCREAS

Pathogenesis

Two theories have been proposed for the development of this anatomical anomaly. Tieken[7] described two elements to the ventral moiety of the pancreas and suggested that as the right element rotated in a clockwise rotation around the duodenal axis, so the left element became extruded around the duodenum separately, forming a circumduodenal rim of pancreatic tissue. Should the tip of the ventral moiety remain attached to the ventral duodenum, as proposed by Lecco,[8] pancreatic tissue will remain attached to the right side of the duodenum following rotation. There is a bimodal distribution to this condition, which either presents in the neonatal period or during the fourth and fifth decades of life. Over a 20-year period the Mayo Clinic reported equal numbers of patients presenting in

both the infantile and adult stages.[9] Approximately 1 in 20 000 adults are affected.[10] Infantile annular pancreas is discussed in Chapter 62.

Clinical aspects

The principal presenting symptom is pain, which may arise from either peptic ulceration or chronic pancreatitis (Figure 61.2, see colour plate also). Peptic ulceration occurs in 29–48% of affected patients.[10] The aetiology is uncertain, but is thought to be related to antral distension and consequent hypergastrinaemia.[11] Chronic pancreatitis is reported to affect between 14 and 50% of patients and is usually confined to the annular moiety of the pancreas.[12,13] Again the aetiology is obscure; favoured theories include poor ductal drainage of the annular pancreas and local pancreatic trauma secondary to its close proximity to the duodenum.[12] Vomiting is usually bile stained because the biliary opening is proximal to the duodenal constriction. Jaundice is rarely observed, but the common bile duct may become narrowed secondary to pancreatitic oedema.[10]

Annular pancreas may be easily overlooked at laparotomy. Although the double-bubble sign on a plain abdominal radiograph is usually diagnostic in the neonate, contrast studies are required in adults. The classical changes observed on hypotonic duodenography include the presence of a smooth annular defect in the descending duodenum and evidence of duodenal obstruction, e.g. symmetrical proximal luminal dilatation and reverse peristalsis. Computerized tomography (CT) has also proven useful as long as careful attention is given to oral contrast delivery and patient positioning.[10] Nevertheless, both these modes of imaging may fail to establish the diagnosis, which is often confused in the presence of peptic ulceration.[13] Alternatively, endoscopic retrograde pancreatocholangiography should diagnose adult annular pancreas. Exceptions include the presence of severe duodenal obstruction (hindering passage of the endoscope), obstruction of the annular pancreatic duct, and cases in which this duct does not drain into the main pancreatic duct.[13]

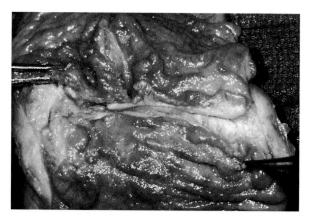

Figure 61.2

Chronic pancreatitis in a 43-year-old man with annular pancreas. The circumferential duct has been opened in the pancreatoduodenectomy specimen. (Professor Williamson's case.)

Treatment

Surgery is the only therapeutic approach, and the choice is between division and bypass. Previous published experience dictates that the annulus should be left untouched, although safe division of the pancreatic ring has been reported when the ring was not closely adherent to the duodenum.[14] Many surgical bypass techniques have been advocated. As with infants, duodenoduodenostomy remains the most attractive option, offering low morbidity and mortality rates while preserving normal intestinal continuity.[15]

NODULAR LYMPHOID HYPERPLASIA

Definition

Nodular lymphoid hyperplasia is a reaction by intestinal lymphatic tissue to specific inflammatory stimuli, characterized by the presence of hyperplastic nodules of lymphoid cells within the lamina propria and submucosa of the gastrointestinal tract. In the small intestine these nodules are 1–3 mm in diameter and are similar to the germinal centres of lymph nodes. Normal villi are stretched over these nodules.

Clinical aspects

In children, nodular lymphoid hyperplasia occurs as a transient phenomenon affecting the terminal ileum, which spontaneously regresses at adolescence.[16] In adults, it is commonly associated with immunodeficiency.[17] Most patients (up to 60%) have common variable hypogammaglobulinaemia, an acquired immunoglobulin deficiency that results in impairment (to differing degrees) of immunoglobulin synthesis affecting serum IgG and IgA levels.[18] This reduction in immunoglobulin levels is thought to be a consequence of a defect in the maturation of B cells, possibly due to suppression by T-suppressor cells, the activity of which is frequently raised in this condition. Although cell-mediated immune function is preserved, affected patients usually suffer with recurrent intestinal infections resulting in diarrhoea, weight loss and failure to thrive. Histological examination reveals villous stunting, which in extreme cases can resemble coeliac disease and be associated with malabsorption. The most common infectious agent is the protozoon *Giardia lamblia*, which itself can predispose to steatorrhoea and should be considered in the absence of histological evidence of villous atrophy.[19] Other recognized pathogens include salmonella, mycobacterial species and *Campylobacter jejuni*.

An association between nodular lymphoid hyperplasia and small bowel lymphoma has been reported in immunocompetent patients, suggesting a susceptibility to malignant transformation, although nodular lymphoid hyperplasia is rarely seen in the absence of immunodeficiency.[16] Histological examination has detected nodular lymphoid hyperplasia close to intestinal lymphomas, with a gradual transition between the hyperplastic and neoplastic areas. Furthermore, Matuchansky et al.[17] have provided very suggestive evidence for a cytogenic relationship between lymphoma and nodular lymphoid hyperplasia on the basis of similar patterns of monoclonality in the two areas.

There are, however, increasing reports of small intestinal lymphoma arising in immunocompromised patients with nodular lymphoid hyperplasia, providing further evidence that it may be a premalignant entity.[20] Nodular lymphoid hyperplasia has also been reported in human immunodeficiency virus infection.[21]

Diagnosis

This condition is usually diagnosed either by jejunal biopsy or radiologically. Intestinal biopsies may reveal giardia trophozoites in addition to the hyperplastic lymphoid nodules. Barium contrast studies reveal multiple nodular filling defects between 2 and 4 mm in diameter with a segmental, focal or diffuse distribution (Figure 61.3).

Treatment

Treatment in nodular lymphoid hyperplasia is only indicated when patients are symptomatic; these are usually patients with associated common variable hypogammaglobulinaemia. Gluten-mediated enteropathy should first be excluded from the diagnosis. Diarrhoea is typically associated with giardiasis and responds to appropriate antimicrobial therapy, usually metronidazole. For those patients who suffer recurrent and or debilitating infections, intravenous immunoglobulin replacement is indicated.

COELIAC DISEASE

Pathology

Coeliac disease is defined as an abnormal jejunal mucosa which improves morphologically on a gluten-free diet and then deteriorates following reintroduction of gluten. It is otherwise termed gluten-sensitive enteropathy. The disease may become manifest at any stage of life, but it is most commonly diagnosed around the fourth decade. Approximately 1 in 2000 individuals in the UK are affected, and it is the most common cause of malabsorption in the Western world. Its peak prevalence (1/300) occurs in Galway, Ireland. Boys and girls are

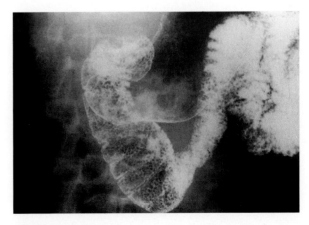

Figure 61.3

Hypotonic duodenogram showing nodular lymphoid hyperplasia of diffuse type. (Courtesy of Dr J Virjee, Bristol Royal Infirmary.)

equally affected, but a preponderance of females is reported among adults.[22]

Genetics

The exact mode of inheritance of coeliac disease is unknown, but it is probably polygenic. Siblings and offspring of sufferers have a 2–5% risk of developing the disease, whereas 10% of asymptomatic first-degree relatives have subtotal villous atrophy. There is strong association between coeliac disease and the HLA class II D region marker HLA-DR3, and an even closer association has been shown with DQw2.[23] These genes code for cell surface molecules critical to the immune response (see below). Although 90% of coeliac patients possess the HLA DR3, DQw2 haplotype, 25–30% of normal individuals within the same population have the same haplotype and do not have coeliac disease. Furthermore, less than 0.1% of individuals with the serological markers HLA-DR3 and DQw2 develop coeliac disease. Using restriction fragment length polymorphism analysis of these HLA class II antigens, it has been possible to distinguish between normal individuals and those individuals with coeliac disease, all of whom possess DR3/DQw2. It has emerged that susceptibility genes for coeliac disease are encoded in the HLA-DP subregion.[24]

Pathophysiology

Gluten is a protein constituent of wheat flour found in wheat, rye, barley and oats. The substance toxic to the intestinal mucosa of coeliac patients has been identified as gliadin, the alcohol-soluble portion of gluten. Gliadin exists in four subfractions (α, β, γ, ω), and there is continuing debate as to the relative toxicity of these individual subfractions. It is generally agreed, however, that α-gliadin is the most active. The exact mechanism by which gliadin leads to the manifestations of coeliac disease remains obscure. The two favoured mechanisms are (1) an enzyme deficiency, and (2) a primary local immunological reaction.[22] It has been postulated that gluten is enzymatically digested to a non-toxic product, and therefore a mucosal enzyme deficiency could lead to accumulation of toxic material. However, no consistent deficiency has yet been identified, and this problem is compounded as many enzyme deficiencies may be secondary phenomena consequent upon mucosal damage. The favoured mechanism involves an aberrant immunological response.[22] Circumstantial evidence for this hypothesis includes the frequent detection of serum antigliadin antibodies, the association with other autoimmune diseases, reduced serum concentration of IgM in 75% of sufferers and hyposplenism (splenic atrophy) in 30–50% of patients. One theory incriminates the production of a gluten antibody with antigen–antibody complexes activating a cytotoxic immune response, but an antigluten antibody has yet to be identified. Alternatively, a cross-reaction between gliadin and class II major histocompatability antigens may occur, leading to an autoimmune-directed mucosal cell injury. It has been suggested that the particular haplotype associated with coeliac disease allows gliadin peptide to be presented in such a way that T-helper cells in the small intestinal mucosa are specifically stimulated to produce an immunological reaction, leading to the typical pathological changes of coeliac disease.

Histopathology

The universal pathological feature of coeliac disease is loss of normal villous architecture with consequent flattening of the mucosal surface.[25] Microscopic examination reveals loss of villi, elongated crypts and a chronic inflammatory infiltrate within the lamina propria. Intraepithelial lymphocytes account for the greater proportion of the cell population owing to a 3–5-fold increase within the hyperplastic crypts. There may be squamous or cuboidal epithelial metaplasia and loss of the microvillous brush border.

Clinical aspects

The presenting symptoms of coeliac disease are typically nonspecific. Children usually present within the first 3 years of life with loss of appetite, abdominal distension, pale bulky stools and irritability. With progression of the disease, wasting and poor growth become apparent. Adults may have watery diarrhoea, often intermittent, associated with a combination of steatorrhoea, weight loss, lassitude and generalized abdominal pains. However, some patients may have no gastrointestinal symptoms and indeed may even be asymptomatic. Anaemia may present, with angular stomatitis and mouth ulcers. Hypogonadism affects between 5 and 10% of male patients. At all ages there may be other associated autoimmune diseases.

Clinical examination is often unrewarding, but may reveal the signs of malnutrition and folate deficiency anaemia. In severe cases, ascites and dependent oedema will be associated with hypoalbuminaemia. Serum tests may reveal macrocytosis from folate deficiency, but this can be masked by a coexistent iron deficiency. A blood film examination may reveal Howell–Jolly bodies secondary to hyposplenism. The definitive test is a jejunal biopsy obtained using a Crosby capsule sited just distal to the duodenojejunal flexure, although the diagnosis can often be clinched from a duodenal biopsy. Barium meal and follow-through studies usefully define the anatomy of the small intestine and exclude the presence of other pathologies, in particular Crohn's disease.

Treatment

In severe cases, patients require resuscitation from their malnourished state. In all patients a gluten-free diet must be taken indefinitely. The exclusion of wheat, barley rye and oats imposes a severe restriction on the patient, and the support of a dietician is essential; patients may require supplementation with vitamins and iron. In children, a subsequent biopsy should be taken to demonstrate recovery of the villous architecture and thus exclude the differential diagnosis of milk intolerance. For adults, a repeat biopsy in the responders is not obligatory. Patients who do not respond to a gluten-free diet do not, by definition, have coeliac disease. For this minority (about 15% of new patients with a flat biopsy), steroids or azathioprine chemotherapy or zinc supplements may be tried.

In non-responders and those who relapse, consideration should be given to the development of lymphoma.

Malignancy

There is an 8% incidence of malignancy among coeliac disease sufferers.[22] There is an increased incidence of carcinoma of the mouth, pharynx and oesophagus, but the most common malignancy is small bowel lymphoma. Lymphoma typically occurs in patients over 50 years of age, who present with vague abdominal pains, fever, or failure to respond to a gluten exclusion diet. The diagnosis is often made at laparotomy when the tumour is irresectable, and patients generally respond poorly to adjuvant oncotherapy. A gluten-free diet is believed to protect against the development of lymphoma, but this benefit may be reserved for those diagnosed in infancy.

Dermatitis herpetiformis

This subepidermal blistering disease of the skin is a chronic and persistent disorder which may occur at any age, but onset is rare in children and the elderly.[26] The rash is due to gluten, and about 80% of patients have small intestinal enteropathy akin to coeliac disease. However, the mucosal abnormality is usually less pronounced than in coeliac disease and takes the form of a partial villous atrophy. There are few clinical manifestations associated with this mucosal abnormality: occasionally a mild degree of malabsorption and associated iron and folate deficiencies. There is a high incidence of associated autoimmune diseases. Dermatitis herpetiformis is strongly associated with the HLA-DR3 histocompatability antigen, and some authorities have postulated that this condition and coeliac disease are two separate entities that are genetically linked. The diagnosis is established by a skin biopsy, which shows (using immunofluorescence staining techniques) IgA deposits in the dermal papillae of uninvolved skin. Patients respond to a gluten-free diet. Although response can take up to 6 months, this treatment not only clears the rash but improves the enteropathy and reduces the risk of lymphoma (about half of that for coeliac disease).

AMYLOIDOSIS

Pathology

Amyloid is a proteinaceous substance deposited between cells in various tissues and organs of the body in a wide variety of clinical settings. Amyloidosis is a group of diseases sharing in common the deposition of similar appearing proteins. Macroscopically amyloid has an amorphous appearance, which under the light microscope classically stains pink/red with a Congo red stain and exhibits apple-green birefringence under polarizing light (Figure 61.4, see colour plate also). Electron microscopy has revealed that amyloid is composed of two subunits: strands of fibrils 7.5–10 nm in diameter (90%) and pentagonal doughnut-shaped units (P component, 10%) bound together in a β-pleated sheet. Progressive extracellular accumulation of amyloid encroaches on adjacent cells, with resultant pressure atrophy; however, an inflammatory reaction is not observed.

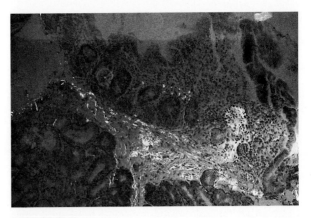

Figure 61.4
A 50-year-old female with chronic intra-abdominal sepsis developed protein-losing enteropathy. A biopsy of the duodenum stained with Congo red revealed amyloid deposits within the duodenal submucosa. Under polarized light these deposits demonstrate apple-green birefringence (250 ×). (Courtesy of Dr EM Thompson, Hammersmith Hospital.)

Classification

Historically amyloidosis was classified as follows: primary disease, when no underlying cause could be identified, which affects the heart, gastrointestinal tract, skin, nerves and tongue; and secondary disease, which classically complicates chronic inflammatory disease states and involve the liver, spleen, kidneys and adrenals. Amyloidosis has been reclassified following the discovery of two antigenically distinct classes of fibrils.[27] Amyloid light chain (AL) fibrils are derived from immunoglobulin light chains, mainly κ, but occasionally λ. Amyloid-associated (AA) fibrils constitute a unique non-immunoglobulin protein. Its precursor, serum amyloid associated protein (SAA), is synthesized by the liver during inflammation. Five subtypes of amyloidosis are now recognized:[28]

1. Immunocyte-derived (AL) amyloidosis complicates any immunocyte dyscrasia, of which multiple myeloma is the archetypal disease as the AL fibrils have been shown to be derived from the circulating light chains (Bence Jones proteins).

2. Reactive systemic (AA) amyloidosis is the sequel to chronic inflammatory or infectious disease states, including rheumatoid arthritis, scleroderma and inflammatory bowel disease.

3. Heredofamilial amyloidosis is very rare, confined to certain geographical areas and includes familial Mediterranean fever.

4. Senile amyloidosis, in which the fibrils are derived from serum prealbumin.

5. Amyloid deposition is now a recognized complication of long-term haemodialysis. In these patients the fibril is derived from β_2-microglobulin from the light chain of the HLA class I antigen.

The historic primary and secondary amyloidoses seem to conform with the modern immunocyte-derived and reactive systemic subtypes respectively. The pathophysiology of amyloidosis remains unresolved, but it is thought to be secondary either to overproduction of precursor proteins, such as λ light chains and SAA, or to defective degradation of these proteins.

Amyloidosis of the small intestine

The gastrointestinal tract is commonly affected in patients with amyloid (70–100%), although clinical manifestations are infrequently seen.[29,30] Amyloid may be found anywhere from mouth to anus, but the small bowel is the most commonly affected site.[29,31] From its perivascular origin, amyloid extends to the submucosa and permeates through to involve the muscularis propria and subserosa. Ultimately these lesions coalesce to form plaques. Disturbances of digestion, malabsorption and diarrhoea are the main clinical manifestations of small bowel involvement. Motility disturbances, including pseudo-obstruction, are reported in about 7% of patients with amyloidosis and are thought to be due either to involvement of the autonomic nerves and ganglia or secondary to a myopathy.[32,33] Malabsorption is seen in 5% of patients and is believed to be secondary to a bacterial overgrowth, possibly as a result of intestinal dysmotility.[27] The perivascular infiltration can occasionally result in intestinal ischaemia, with consequent perforation or mucosal ulceration. Other rare complications include gastrointestinal haemorrhage secondary to multiple mucosal nodules and intestinal obstruction secondary to large submucosal amyloid 'pseudotumours'.[27,30]

Diagnosis

A rectal biopsy is positive in 80% of all cases of amyloidosis, and a radioisotope scan of labelled P component may prove even more useful.[34] Small intestine barium studies characteristically show fine granular mucosal elevations, thickening of intestinal folds, delay in the passage of barium and dilatation of small bowel loops. Thickening of the folds of intestine is thought to be secondary to the bowel wall oedema that follows prolonged intestinal ischaemia from the perivascular deposits. Some radiologists can recognize the different chemical subtypes of amyloid according to the barium findings;[31] AA amyloid classically produces the granular mucosal appearance, whereas AL amyloid is typically associated with polypoid protrusions measuring 4–15 mm in diameter.

Treatment

There is no effective treatment for amyloid except for resection of tumour masses and the treatment of end-stage renal failure.[28] Attention has therefore been directed to treatment of the underlying disease and nutrient replacement in the malnourished. Alkylating agents have been tested with little effect, although colchicine has been found to effectively suppress the abdominal pain associated with familial Mediterranean fever.

INTESTINAL LYMPHANGIECTASIA

This pathological condition is characterized by the presence of distended and leaky mucosal lymphatics in the intestine, believed to be caused by lymphatic obstruction. It produces not only a protein-losing enteropathy but a concomitant lymphocyte loss, which results in an immunodeficient state. This disease has been subclassified into a primary congenital form and an acquired secondary phenomenon. Primary intestinal lymphangiectasia is very rare and may be associated with a variety of congenital conditions including Milroy's disease, and Noonan's and Turner's syndromes. Even though primary intestinal lymphangiectasia is associated with abnormal limb lymphatic drainage, no identifiable structural lymphatic abnormality has yet been identified.[35] The causes of secondary intestinal lymphangiectasia are legion (Table 61.2). They are secondary *either* to direct blockage of the lymphatics from (1) disorders that raise central venous pressure and thus impair thoracic duct drainage into the subclavian vein and (2) obstruction of the intraperitoneal lymphatics (Figure 61.5, see colour plate also), *or* to indirect lymphatic obstruction resulting from overwhelming lymph drainage, e.g. in systemic lupus erythematosus when interstitial venulitis increases vascular permeability.[36]

Pathology

Macroscopically the surface of the intestine possesses thickened villi coated in a white chylous substance. The microscopic hallmark is the presence of dilated intestinal lymphatics, most pronounced at the tip of the villi, leading to their distortion (Figure 61.6). Lipid droplets accumulate both in the intercellular spaces and within the enterocytes.

Table 61.2 Causes of secondary intestinal lymphangiectasia

Direct lymphatic obstruction

Impaired drainage of thoracic duct	– constrictive pericarditis	
	– atrial septal defect	
	– tricuspid valve regurgitation	
	– major vein thrombosis	
Intraperitoneal lymphatic obstruction	– inflammatory cell infiltration of lymphatics	– infective: bacteria, parasites, fungi
		– Whipple's disease
		– Crohn's disease
	– malignant disease	
	– postradiation	
	– inflammatory processes impinging upon lymphatics	– mediastinitis, sclerosing mesenteritis, retroperitonitis

Indirect lymphatic obstruction

Overload of the lymphatic system	– systemic lupus erythematosus

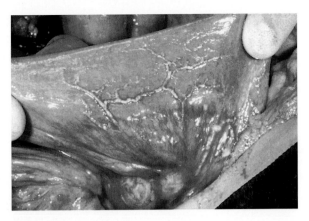

Figure 61.5
Intestinal lymphangiectasia secondary to malignant mesenteric nodes in a young woman with carcinomatosis. Dilated lymphatics are seen on the serosal aspect of the bowel. (Professor Williamson's case.)

Clinical aspects

Intestinal lymphangiectasia may present at one of three stages.[36] The primary disease typically presents before the age of 30 years, with an equal sex distribution. Affected neonates and infants younger than 3 months develop massive oedema together with malabsorption and usually succumb to overwhelming sepsis. Older children suffer growth retardation, and sexual and mental development is usually impaired. Most commonly, however, the disease manifests itself in adolescence or early adulthood with a mixture of impaired lymphatic drainage and immunodeficiency. The most common symptoms stem from oedema, which may be present in the limbs – indicating a primary abnormality of lymphatic drainage – or present as a generalized oedema secondary to the hypoalbuminaemic state, with ascites and pleural effusions. Patients therefore complain of fatigue, abdominal swelling or dyspnoea (50% of patients). Gastrointestinal symptoms are common but mild and include abdominal pain (15%), which may either be secondary to oedema or possibly to intestinal dysmotility. Diarrhoea and steatorrhoea are uncommon. The coexistent lymphopenia results in a mild impairment of humoral immunity; for example, patients are exposed to chronic viral infections such as persistent warts. In addition to signs of ascites, pleural effusions and viral warts, clinical examination may reveal asymmetric limb oedema and characteristics of an underlying genetic disorder, or perhaps evidence of a secondary predisposing disease, e.g. a rash in systemic lupus erythematosus or a raised jugular venous pressure in restrictive pericarditis.

Diagnosis

The definitive diagnosis can only be made from a jejunal biopsy, but the distribution of the disease is patchy and some biopsy samples may be normal. Barium contrast studies demonstrate small bowel dilatation with thickened bowel walls secondary to oedema[37]. Protein loss can be assessed from the serum albumin and IgG concentrations or more accurately by recording $^{51}CrCl_3$-labelled protein 5-day stool collections. The lymphopenia predominantly affects long-lived cells circulating in the vascular and lymphatic circulations.[38] Most of these lymphocytes are T cells, and consequently there is a reduction in T-cell count, particularly CD4 cells.

Treatment

The management of primary intestinal lymphangiectasia is supportive and consists of diuretics and a low-fat diet. Restriction of dietary fat intake reduces lymph flow, but the diet may be supplemented with medium chain triglycerides which are preferentially absorbed by the venous system rather than the lymphatics.[36] Surgical excision of affected segments is rarely advantageous and can lead to complications.[39] Where an underlying disorder leads to secondary lymphangiectasia, it is frequently possible to remedy the lymphatic obstruction, e.g. pericardiectomy in patients with constrictive pericarditis. The supportive nature of the management of primary intestinal lymphangiectasia necessitates an exhaustive search for a secondary cause for this disease. Intestinal lymphangiectasia is also associated with an increased incidence of malignancy, particularly lymphoma, probably as a consequence of either defective immunosurveillance or defective T-cell regulation of B-cell proliferation.[36]

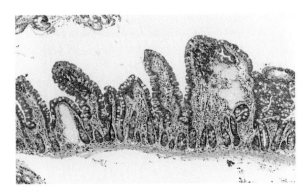

Figure 61.6
Intestinal lymphangiectasia. Biopsy of small intestine from a 57-year-old man with diarrhoea. Dilated lymphatics are observed in the lamina propria with associated mild villous atrophy (72.5 x.) (Courtesy of Dr EM Thompson, Hammersmith Hospital.)

ENDOMETRIOSIS

Aetiology

Endometriosis is defined as the presence of endometrial tissue outside the myometrium. Several theories have been advanced to explain the pathogenesis of endometriosis, but Sampson's[40] proposed mechanism of retrograde menstruation and subsequent implantation remains the most keenly supported.[41] Other aetiological theories include peritoneal metaplasia, possibly secondary to chronic irritation by menstrual blood, and direct implantation from other sites of endometriosis.

Incidence

The overall incidence of endometriosis is thought to be rising, but this may be explained in part by the increased use of diagnostic laparoscopy. Nevertheless, incidences reported in the literature range from 10 to 50% of women.[41,42] The intestine constitutes only 12% of all cases, and the small intestine is involved in only 1–7% of all intestinal endometriosis.[43–45] As with pelvic endometriosis, women most commonly present in the third decade of life.

Clinical aspects

The symptoms of small intestinal endometriosis are as vague as they are wide ranging and commonly include nausea, vomiting, abdominal pain and bloating. The diagnosis may therefore be confused with irritable bowel syndrome, regional enteritis and acute appendicitis. However, symptoms tend to be clustered around menstruation, and infertility may be an associated complaint. Furthermore, these patients usually experience symptoms of pelvic endometriosis. Rarely, small intestine endometriosis may be complicated by obstruction or perforation. Intestinal obstruction can develop from adhesions or a stricture arising from a desmoplastic response to endometriotic tissue, or from intussusception of a lesion. Perforation may be precipitated by the presence of an intraluminal foreign body proximal to a stenosis.

Diagnosis

In the presence of pelvic endometriosis, rectovaginal examination will disclose tender nodules behind the uterine cervix, enlarged and possibly fixed ovaries and a bulky uterus. Abdominal examination, however, is likely to be unrewarding in the absence of intestinal obstruction. Barium meal and follow-through is the mainstay of preoperative diagnosis, and the classical features are those of a long constant filling defect with an intact mucosa and fixation of the intestine.[46] These features are highlighted at the time of menstruation. A barium enema should also be performed to exclude the coexistence of colonic endometriosis.

The diagnosis is usually apparent at laparotomy, particularly in the presence of pelvic involvement. Endometrial deposits are usually less than 5 cm in diameter and are sited in the submucosa and muscularis propria. Tiny haemorrhagic areas are characteristic. In other circumstances, small intestinal endometriosis may mimic carcinoma. The distinguishing features of endometriosis are an absence of enlarged nodes; if a stricture is found, it is usually non-circumferential and the lesion is not usually tethered to its mesentery. Other differential diagnoses include regional ileitis and carcinoid tumours.

Treatment

An awareness of this diagnosis should allow some patients initially to be managed medically, without recourse to operation. For those women who proceed to laparotomy, resection is indicated either in the presence of the complications of obstruction or perforation, or when there is doubt over the possibility of malignancy. Ideally, frozen section should be available to the surgeon. Extensive involvement of the ileum necessitates either excision of the lesion or resection of a segment of intestine with end-to-end anastomosis. For women over 35 years who have finished their family, consideration

should also be given towards a total hysterectomy and bilateral salpingo-oophorectomy. Removal of the ovaries should stimulate regression of small lesions in the bowel. For the remainder, hormonal therapy directed at ovarian suppression is employed. Treatment regimens include either pseudo-pregnancy with continuous high doses of progestagens or oral contraceptives, or the use of danazol, a modified androgen.

PNEUMATOSIS INTESTINALIS

Definition

Pneumatosis intestinalis is a condition involving submucosal or subserosal gas-containing cysts of the wall of the gastrointestinal tract, most commonly the small intestine. It is a rare entity which generally occurs between the third and fifth decades of life without a clear sex predominance. Cysts may be primary (idiopathic) or secondary to another disease. Necrotizing enterocolitis is classified as a secondary pneumatosis intestinalis and is covered in Chapter 62.

Aetiology

A number of potential pathophysiological mechanisms for the development of this condition have been proposed. There remain, however, patients presenting with this condition who do not have any obvious underlying cause. The two favoured mechanisms are:[47]

- *Bacterial.* Infection may arise either by penetration of the mucosa or serosa by micro-organisms which then form cysts secondary to fermentation, or by permeation of the gas through the intestinal wall from remote sites, for example along the muscular planes from limbs infected with gas-forming organisms, typically clostridial species. This possibility is supported by the experimental production of pneumatosis by contamination of rats with *Clostridium perfringens.*[48]

- *Mechanical.* Gas either gains entry from the lumen of the bowel or from without the intestine. A combination of mucosal injury and raised intraluminal pressure must exist to enable pneumatosis intestinalis to occur. The common predisposing causes for this combination are listed in Table 61.3. Inspired air has been proposed as the extraintestinal gas that gains entry into the intestinal wall from the lungs via dissection along the retroperitoneal and perivascular

Table 61.3 Mechanical predisposing factors for pneumatosis cystoides intestinalis

Mucosal injury
Ulcer (benign/malignant)
Radiation
Ischaemia
Inflammation (inflammatory bowel disease, connective tissue disorders)

Raised intraluminal pressure
Bowel obstruction
Gastrointestinal endoscopy
Paralytic ileus

planes. Patients at risk from this route are those receiving mechanical lung ventilation and those with chronic obstructive airways disease who leak secondary to alveolar rupture.

Clinical aspects

There are no pathognomonic symptoms; the condition is typically diagnosed as an incidental radiological finding on a plain abdominal radiograph (Figure 61.7). Where there is an associated disease, its symptoms usually overshadow the pneumatosis; in the absence of any associated disease, patients are typically asymptomatic. Symptoms usually arise only as a result of complications. Bowel obstruction can arise from extrinsic compression of the cyst upon the bowel lumen, and severe gastrointestinal haemorrhage has been reported.[47] In addition to a plain abdominal film, the diagnosis can be confirmed using CT, which is more sensitive in demonstrating both the pneumatosis and its complications. However, no radiological characteristics are regarded as pathognomonic for the underlying cause of the pneumatosis.[49]

Treatment

If a primary cause of pneumatosis intestinalis has been diagnosed, then appropriate therapy should be directed towards that pathology. The need for therapeutic intervention of pneumatosis intestinalis *per se* is dictated by the presence of symptoms. Therefore, in patients in whom the cause is believed to

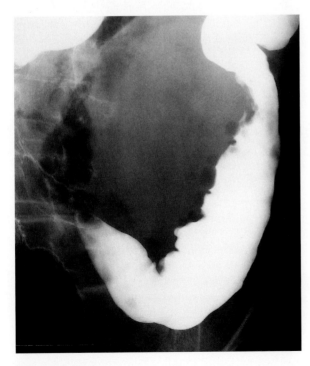

Figure 61.7
Pneumatosis intestinalis in a 52-year-old male who presented with lower gastrointestinal haemorrhage. Single contrast barium enema. A localized view of the distal descending colon demonstrating multiple gas-filled 'cysts' in the wall of the large bowel. (Courtesy of Dr M Roddie, Kingston Hospital NHS Trust.)

be mechanical with no symptoms, it is reasonable to observe the patient. Methods of treatment in symptomatic cases include hyperbaric oxygen, antibiotics and (in severe cases) resection of the diseased part of the intestine. Hyperbaric oxygen may theoretically encourage gas resorption from the cysts secondary to an increased gas pressure gradient from cyst to tissues.[47] Furthermore, oxygen may assist in the elimination of anaerobic gas-forming bacteria. For the same reason antibiotics may be used, but they must include an antianaerobic spectrum of activity.

Operative treatment is reserved for serious complications including haemorrhage, obstruction and infarction. Haemorrhage should be investigated as for any gastrointestinal bleed, including upper and lower endoscopy and possibly visceral angiography or red cell radionucleotide scanning. The affected area demonstrated to be bleeding should be resected. Failure to respond to conservative treatment, together with abdominal pain and tenderness, metabolic acidosis and hyperamylasaemia all conspire towards surgical intervention.[50]

ENTEROLITHS

Formation

Enteroliths, endogenous intestinal concretions, are rare in humans. They can either be true or false, the latter being more common. True enteroliths are derived from precipitation of substances normally found in solution within the gastrointestinal tract; they are composed of either bile salts or mineral salts. The more commonly encountered bile salt enterolith tends to form in proximal small bowel, where a change to a more acid pH promotes the transformation of soluble bile salts to the insoluble choleic acid. The alkaline distal small bowel prevents this bile salt reaction and favours precipitation of calcium phosphate and carbonate mineral salts.[51] False enteroliths arise out of a combination of nidus crystallization and subsequent inspissation of intestinal contents (enteroliths and meconium) around the nidus. A nidus may be derived in a variety of ways, including the presence of indigestible material (e.g. bezoars, fruit skins), dehydration of suspensions of insoluble salts (e.g. aluminium or magnesium salts in antacids) or by precipitation of substances secondary to absorption of their solvents (e.g. varnish stones in varnish drinkers).[52] The main aetiological factor common to all varieties of enterolith is intestinal stasis, and the major predisposing anatomical pathologies are diverticula (including Meckel's), blind loops and strictures secondary to Crohn's disease, tuberculosis or previous trauma.[53]

Enterolith ileus

The main complication arising from enterolith formation is the development of small bowel obstruction, first described by Phillips in 1921.[54] Obstruction occurs either as a result of expulsion of an enterolith from its diverticulum or by local encroachment within the diverticulum, or when an intraluminal enterolith (proximal to a stricture) grows to a diameter equal to that of the intestine. Many enteroliths form without ever being expelled from their diverticula,[52] and enterolith intestinal obstruction remains a rare phenomenon.[51–53] The mechanism of enterolith obstruction remains an enigma because, although these diverticula are relatively wide-mouthed, their walls lack a muscular coat.

The clinical presentation of enterolith ileus is similar to that of gallstone ileus, and the diagnosis should be suspected in the presence of known small bowel diverticula in combination with a normal ultrasonographic scan of the gall bladder. However, fewer than one-third of enteroliths are radiopaque[53] and the diagnosis is usually made at laparotomy. The optimal way to manage this condition is to crush the enterolith externally without performing an enterotomy and then milk the fragments into the proximal colon. A thorough search of the small intestine should now be made for the presence of further enteroliths. If attempts to crush the enterolith fail, it should be milked in a retrograde direction away from the oedematous mucosa and then extracted via a small enterotomy. The diverticulum should be left untouched as recurrence of this condition is unknown, the diverticulum itself has been asymptomatic and resection can be hazardous in patients who are often elderly. In the rare instance in which intestinal obstruction arises from local encroachment of the diverticulum, resection is unavoidable.

MESENTERIC LYMPHADENITIS

This is an inflammatory condition of childhood resulting in enlargement of the mesenteric nodes. The aetiology remains unknown and has been blamed on unspecified viruses. Certainly it is often associated with upper respiratory tract infections, commonly tonsillitis. Children typically present with symptoms of non-specific abdominal colic, generalized malaise and associated vomiting.[55] The pain is usually referred to the umbilicus with pain-free intervals. Often there is an associated upper airways infection, and enquiry will reveal similarly affected children in the family or at school. On examination the child is listless and anorexic and is usually pyrexial (often above 38°C). The fauces may be enlarged and reddened, and there is tender cervical lymphadenopathy particularly in the jugulodigastric nodes. Abdominal tenderness is variable and can be shifted by laying the patient on the left side for a few minutes (Klein's sign). However, tenderness is typically sited at McBurney's point and may mimic acute appendicitis, from which the illness may be indistinguishable.

Diagnosis

Mesenteric adenitis has gained important prominence as its overlapping clinical presentation with acute appendicitis accounts for the high negative appendicectomy rate observed in children (15–30%).[56,57] For this reason a variety of diagnostic modalities have been studied in an attempt to distinguish between these two pathologies more accurately.[57] Laparoscopy can accurately differentiate between the many causes of right iliac fossa pain;[58] but it is invasive and requires a general anaesthetic. On the other hand an inflamed appendix can be successfully removed during this examination.[59] Enlarged mesenteric nodes can be identified using ultrasonography, but

a careful search must be made by the radiologist to exclude other pathology, especially an inflamed appendix.[56] A preliminary study has shown elevated levels of serum interferon-α in children with right iliac fossa pain, including mesenteric adenitis,[60] underlying the viral aetiology of the disease. Further studies are awaited on the role of cytokine assay as a diagnostic tool in this group of patients. In problematic cases, white cell scanning has also been advocated.[61]

MESENTERIC PANNICULITIS

Mesenteric panniculitis is an uncommon non-specific inflammatory process involving the adipose tissue of the mesentery which may present an alarming clinical picture. In a collected review of 68 cases there is a slight male predominance and the peak age of presentation is between the sixth and seventh decades.[62]

Pathology

In the early stages of the disease there is an acute/subacute inflammatory process. Ultimately fibrosis becomes an irreversible and predominant component, and the disease becomes referred as retractile mesenteritis. It differs from retroperitoneal fibrosis in that obstruction of retroperitoneal organs is seldom seen. Macroscopically the mesentery may possess single, multiple or even diffuse mass-like fatty lesions. The histological criteria for a diagnosis of mesenteric panniculitis include: (1) degeneration of adipose cells and fat necrosis; (2) the presence of lipid-laden macrophages; (3) a chronic lymphocytic infiltration; (4) occasional foreign body granulomas; and (5) varying degrees of fibrosis.[62,63] The aetiology of this condition remains obscure. No pathogen has been identified, and it is widely believed that either previous intraperitoneal pathology or laparotomy indirectly stimulates a non-specific inflammatory process. Other theories implicated in its aetiology include prior abdominal trauma, ulcerative disease, retained suture material and resolving appendicitis.[63,64]

Clinical aspects

In their review of the literature, Durst et al.[62] reported the main presenting symptoms to be pain (67%), vomiting (32%) and the presence of a mass or swelling (16%). Rarely patients may develop an acute abdomen. On examination a mass can be palpated in half of all patients and tenderness elicited in one-third. The diagnosis rests on identifying histologically confirmed lesions within the mesenteric adipose tissue, in the absence of inflammatory bowel disease, extra-abdominal fat necrosis (Weber–Christian disease) and especially pancreatitis.[64,65] Barium meal series demonstrate partial obstruction and displacement of bowel loops by an extrinsic mass in 30% of cases.[62] CT can usually identify a mesenteric mass with a well-defined fibrous wall and a calcified (fat necrosis) cystic core.[64,65] After long-standing fibrosis, this core may adopt a soft tissue density. Angiography reveals either a hyper- or hypovascular mass, according to the stage of the disease progression. Recently, magnetic resonance scanning has been able to distinguish lesions from the surrounding mesenteric fat and is likely to become the preferred investigation.[66] At laparotomy the surgeon may encounter a spectrum of diseases ranging from a solitary mass in the root of the mesentery, to the presence of several masses, through to a diffusely thickened and contracted, rubbery mesentery. The clinical, radiological and surgical differential diagnoses include lymphoma, mesenteric metastases, liposarcoma and teratoma.

Diagnostic uncertainty may therefore lead to laparotomy. Surgical measures should be confined to biopsy alone, except in the rare instances when bypass is indicated for either bowel obstruction (which has failed to respond to conservative treatment) or involvement of retroperitoneal structures (intestine, ureter, great vessels).[62,63] Resection of the 'tumour' does not appear to be justified.

Outcome

There are some reports of clinical remission following the administration of steroids, but this benefit has probably been confined to cases before fibrosis has become established.[67] Other non-surgical treatments, including antibiotics, radiotherapy and azathioprine, have been tried with little benefit. However, the overall prognosis is good. In some cases spontaneous resolution with near complete recovery occurs, but recurrence of nodules has been reported and follow-up is recommended. In other cases the disease progresses towards a fibrotic process, but most patients endure an indolent course; obstruction of lymphatics and mesenteric veins, which can bring about a fatal outcome, is rare.[62,63,65]

MESENTERIC VARICES

Pathology

In the presence of portal hypertension collaterals develop between the portal and systemic circulations, predisposing to the development of varices. Although the vast majority of patients typically develop varices in the region of the gastro-oesophageal junction, other anatomical sites can be involved in association or in isolation. These sites include rectal, paravertebral, periureteric, abdominal wall, falciform ligament and retroperitoneal veins, and, in patients who have undergone prior laparotomy, intra-abdominal adhesions and stoma sites (see Chapter 56). The mechanism for the development of varices remains unknown, but it is postulated that either embryological channels are opened up, or in the case of adhesions and stomas, new portasystemic collaterals are created at operation.[68]

Clinical aspects

Mesenteric varices may either be an incidental finding at laparotomy or present as a gastrointestinal haemorrhage following erosion of a submucosal varix. In the presence of portal hypertension, such bleeding is usually secondary to gastro-oesophageal varices; there are very few cases in the literature reporting mesenteric variceal haemorrhage. However, mesenteric varices should be considered in the differential diagnosis of gastrointestinal haemorrhage in patients with portal hypertension, particularly in the *absence* of gastro-oesophageal

varices. Mesenteric varices may also develop in the presence of chronic mesenteric venous thrombosis without involvement of the splenic or portal veins.[69] Although mesenteric vein thrombosis is usually an acute event which precedes bowel infarction, some cases have been reported of a chronic superior mesenteric vein thrombosis in association with mesenteric varices.

Diagnosis

Identification of varices

Mesenteric varices have traditionally been diagnosed in the venous phase of visceral angiography (Figure 61.8). Three criteria establish the diagnosis[70]:

1. Visualization of the varices.
2. Retrograde (hepatofugal) flow in the superior and inferior mesenteric veins, whose diameter is typically greater than that of the main portal vein.
3. Visualization of systemic veins following mesenteric catheterization in the absence of gastro-oesophageal varices.

Direct cannulation of the portal vein employing percutaneous transhepatic portography delineates the entire portal venous system better than arterial portography and allows access for intervention (see below).[68] More recently, mesenteric varices have been successfully identified by colour Doppler and magnetic resonance angiography.[71]

Localization of the source of bleeding

In a patient with mesenteric varices, identifying the source of bleeding radiographically is very difficult. In addition to the above modalities, selective scintigraphic angiography has successfully localized mesenteric variceal haemorrhage,[72] but as the source of the bleeding is venous and often intermittent, nuclear medicine scans and angiography often fail. In these circumstances, the source of bleeding may only become apparent at the time of laparotomy using peroperative enteroscopy.

Management of mesenteric variceal haemorrhage

The rarity of this condition has prohibited accurate assessment of pharmacological measures to reduce the portal hypertension. Until recently, the only option was surgical, and there is no clear benefit between portasystemic shunting or small bowel resection.[70] Shunt formation is favoured in the presence of widespread varices in order to preserve the small intestine. If mesenteric thrombosis is present, there must be a sufficient length of superior mesenteric vein proximal to the occlusion to allow the creation of a shunt. Variceal embolization has been successfully carried out using the transhepatic approach,[73] with the advantage of avoiding operation in these technically challenging patients.

MESENTERIC CYSTS AND TUMOURS

Mesenteric cysts are seen in approximately 1 in every 100 000 admissions. Over two-thirds are observed in adults, the peak

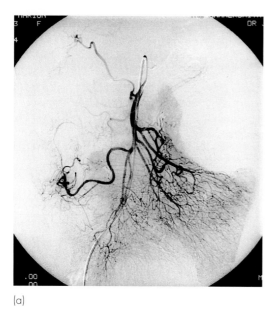

(a)

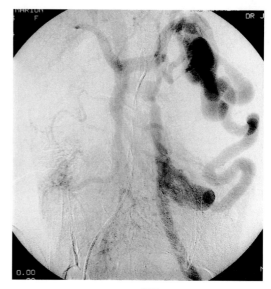

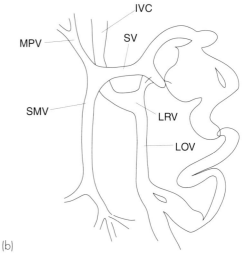

(b)

Figure 61.8

Mesenteric varices in a 71-year-old female who had portal hypertension. (a) Arterial phase from selective superior mesenteric arteriogram. An accessory right hepatic artery is present. The proximal jejunal vessels are displaced inferomedially by an enlarged spleen. (b) The late venous phase of the same study demonstrates antegrade filling of the superior mesenteric vein (SMV) and the main portal vein (MPV). Note that the MPV is of smaller calibre than the SMV. There is retrograde filling of the splenic vein (SV) and thence of massive varices which finally drain via the left ovarian vein (LOV) into the left renal vein (LRV) and inferior vena cava (IVC). (Courtesy of Dr J Jackson, Hammersmith Hospital.)

incidence occurring in the fourth decade. They are found anywhere between the descending duodenum and the rectosigmoid junction, but one half are located in the mesentery of the ileum.[74]

Classification

The classification of these cysts is summarized in Table 61.4.[75] Congenital cysts share their histological features with those of the underlying tissue from which they are derived. The most common congenital cyst is derived from ectopic lymphatic tissue that lacks an efferent communication with the rest of the lymphatic system. These chylolymphatic cysts are therefore lined by simple epithelium and filled with clear lymph. They are usually solitary, commonly arising from the ileal mesentery. By contrast, enterogenous cysts possess a mucous membrane lining and a mucinous fluid content. It is believed that they arise from either duplication of the intestine or sequestration of a diverticulum from the mesenteric border of the intestine. Elements of the mesonephros are to be found in urogenital cysts.

Traumatic cysts arise from a forceful injury to the peritoneal cavity causing either haemorrhage or rupture of a lacteal and

resulting in extravasation of blood or chyle into the surrounding tissues. These cysts are not true cysts as they lack an epithelial lining, and the wall of these pseudocysts comprises

Table 61.4 Classification of mesenteric cysts

Congenital	
Enterogenous	
Chylolymphatic	
Urogenital	
Dermoid	
Acquired	
Traumatic	– serous
	– serosanguinous
	– chylous
Infective/degenerative	– fungal
	– parasitic
	– tuberculous
	– tissue degeneration: lymph nodes, pancreas
Neoplastic	
Benign	– lymphangioma
Malignant	– lymphangioendothelioma
	– adenocarcinoma

mainly fibrous tissue. Such cysts are usually unilocular and can become calcified. Infective and degenerative cysts are also pseudocysts which arise out of walled-off infections or degeneration of tissues, e.g. lymph nodes and pancreas.

Neoplastic mesenteric cysts are extremely rare. The benign lymphangioma is the product of hyperplasia of lymph vessels. Sarcomas of the mesodermal elements of the mesentery are the more common type of malignancy, giving rise to a (usually) low-grade lymphangioendothelioma. Adenocarcinomas are exceptionally rare[76].

Diagnosis

Owing to the rarity of these cysts, their diagnosis is seldom made before laparotomy. Affected patients may be asymptomatic, but they often present with symptoms of an intra-abdominal mass: pain, fullness after a meal, nausea and vomiting. Compression of neighbouring structures may lead to leg oedema or hydronephrosis. Severe pain usually heralds a catastrophic event such as infection, rupture, torsion or haemorrhage into the cyst. Abdominal palpation may reveal a mass which has lateral mobility (perpendicular to the line of the mesentery).[77]

A plain abdominal radiograph will usually reveal no more than a diffuse haziness suggestive of ascites. Barium contrast studies demonstrate displacement of the intestine around the cyst, with possible attenuation and narrowing of the lumen. Ultrasonography will determine the cystic nature of the mass, but CT (Figure 61.9) provides the most accurate information regarding the shape and anatomical relationship to adjacent structures. The differential diagnosis includes metastatic carcinoma, which can present as a solitary cyst.

Treatment

Operation remains the mainstay of managing these cysts as aspiration is associated with both a high recurrence rate and a mortality rate.[74] The exact surgical approach is determined by the size and location of the cyst and its relationship to non-resectable structures. In benign cases resection of the entire cyst without the need for bowel resection is usually attempted,

except for enterogenous cysts when a common blood supply is shared with intestine, necessitating a limited bowel resection. Whenever possible, malignant cysts should be excised with a wide margin in an attempt to achieve nodal clearance. For those cysts that cannot be resected, internal drainage is performed usually via a Roux-en-Y loop.

REFERENCES

1. Hines JR, Gore RM & Ballantyne GH. Superior mesenteric artery syndrome. Diagnostic criteria and therapeutic approaches. *Am J Surg* 1984; **148**: 630–632.
2. Rokitansky C. *Handbuch der pathologischen Anatomie*, vol. 3. Vienna: Braumüller & Seidl, 1842: 187.
3. Wilkie DPD. Chronic duodenal ileus. *Br J Surg* 1921; **9**: 204–214.
4. Anderson JR, Earnshaw PM & Fraser GM. Extrinsic compression of the third part of the duodenum. *Clin Radiol* 1982; **33**: 75–81.
5. Lundell L & Thulin A. Wilkie's syndrome – a rarity? *Br J Surg* 1980; **67**: 604–606.
6. Tocchi A, Basso L, Costa G et al. Derotation of the mid gut for the treatment of chronic duodenal ileus. *Eur J Surg* 1992; **158**: 431–433.
7. Tieken T. Annular pancreas. *Am J Med* 1901; **2**: 826.
8. Lecco TM. Zur Morphologie des Pankreas annulare. *Sher Akad Wiss Wein* 1917; **119**: 391.
9. Kiernan PD, ReMine SG, Kiernan PC & ReMine WH. Annular pancreas. Mayo experience from 1957 to 1976 with review of the literature. *Arch Surg* 1980; **115**: 46–50.
10. Dowsett JF, Rode J & Russell RCG. Annular pancreas: a clinical, endoscopic, and immunohistochemical study. *Gut* 1989; **30**: 130–135.
11. Johnston DWB. Annular pancreas: a new classification and clinical observations. *Can J Surg* 1978; **21**: 241–244.
12. Gilinsky NH, Lewis JW, Flueck JA & Fried AM. Annular pancreas associated with diffuse pancreatitis. *Am J Gastroenterol* 1987; **82**: 681–684.
13. Dharmsathaphorn K, Burrell M & Dobbins J. Diagnosis of annular pancreas with endoscopic retrograde cholangiopancreatography. *Gastroenterology* 1979; **77**: 1109–1114.
14. McGuinness CL, Choy A, Gajraj H & Chilvers AH. Stapling technique for annular pancreas. *Br J Surg* 1993; **80**: 758.
15. Kimura K, Tsugawa C, Ogawa K, Matsumoto Y, Yamamoto T & Asada S. Diamond-shaped anastomosis for congenital duodenal obstruction. *Arch Surg* 1977; **112**: 1262–1263.
16. Fieber SS & Schaefer HJ. Lymphoid hyperplasia of the terminal ileum: a clinical entity? *Gastroenterology* 1980; **78**: 1587–1592.
17. Matuchansky C, Morichau-Beauchant M, Touchard G et al. Nodular lymphoid hyperplasia of the small bowel associated with primary jejunal malignant lymphoma. *Gastroenterology* 1980; **78**: 1587–1592.
18. Castellano G, Moreno D, Galvao O et al. Malignant lymphoma of jejunum with common variable hypogammaglobulinaemia and diffuse nodular hyperplasia of the small intestine. *J Clin Gastroenterol* 1992; **15**: 128–135.
19. Ward H, Jalan KN, Maitra TK, Agarwal SK & Mahalanabis D. Small intestinal nodular lymphoid hyperplasia in patients with giardiasis and normal serum immunoglobulins. *Gut* 1983; **24**: 120–126.
20. Perez Aguilar FP, Alfonso V, Rivas S, Lopez Aldeguer J, Portilla J & Berenguer J. Jejunal malignant lymphoma in a patient with adult-onset hypo-gammaglobulinaemia and nodular lymphoid hyperplasia of the small bowel. *Am J Gastroenterol* 1987; **5**: 472–475.
21. Levendoglu H & Rosen Y. Nodular lymphoid hyperplasia of gut in HIV infection. *Am J Gastroenterol* 1992; **9**: 1200–1202.
22. Ciclitira PJ. Coeliac disease and related disorders. In Bouchier IAD, Allan RN, Hodgson HJF & Keighley MRB (eds) *Gastroenterology, Clinical Science and Practice*. London: WB Saunders, 1993: 537–562.
23. Howdle PD & Blair GE. Molecular biology and coeliac disease. *Gut* 1992; **33**: 573–575.
24. Kagnoff MF. Understanding the molecular basis of coeliac disease. *Gut* 1990; **31**: 497–499.
25. Robbins SL, Cotran RS & Kumar V. The small intestine. In Robbins SL, Cotran RS & Kumar V (eds) *Pathologic Basis of Disease*. London: WB Saunders, 1984: 847–848.
26. Fry L. Bullous disorders. In *Dermatology: An illustrated Guide*, 3rd edn. London: Butterworth, 1984: 91–92.
27. Kyle RA. Amyloidosis. *Clin Haematol* 1982; **11**: 151–180.
28. Pepys MB. Amyloidosis. In Weatherall DJ, Ledingham JGG & Warrell DA

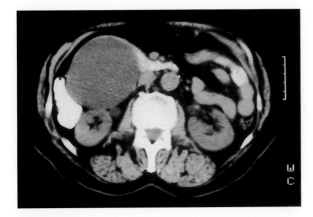

Figure 61.9
Large congenital mesenteric cyst shown on CT scan. (Courtesy of Mr J Spencer, Hammersmith Hospital.)

(eds) *Oxford Textbook of Medicine.* Oxford: Oxford University Press, 1987: 145–157.

29. Gilat T, Revach M & Sohar E. Deposition of amyloid in the gastrointestinal tract. *Gut* 1969; **10**: 98–104.

30. O'Doherty DP, Neoptolemos JP, Bouch DC & Wood KE. Surgical complications of amyloid disease. *Postgrad Med J* 1987; **63**: 281–286.

31. Tada S, Lida M, Yao T et al. Gastrointestinal amyloidosis: radiologic features by chemical types. *Radiology* 1994; **190**: 37–42.

32. Wald A, Kichler J & Mendelow H. Amyloidosis and chronic intestinal pseudo-obstruction. *Dig Dis Sci* 1981; **26**: 462–465.

33. Tada S, Yao T, Kitamoto T & Fujishima M. Intestinal pseudo-obstruction in patients with amyloidosis: clinicopathologic differences between chemical types of amyloid protein. *Gut* 1993; **34**: 1412–1417.

34. Hawkins PN, Myers MJ, Lavender JP & Pepys MB. Diagnostic radionucleotide imaging of amyloid: biological targeting by circulating human serum amyloid P component. *Lancet* 1988; **i**: 1413–1418.

35. Bujanovir Y, Liebman WM & Goodman JR. Primary intestinal lymphangiectasia: case report with radiological and ultrastructural study. *Digestion* 1981; **21**: 101–114.

36. Strober W. Protein losing enteropathy. In Bouchier IAD, Allan RN, Hodgson HJF & Keighley MRB (eds) *Gastroenterology Clinical Science and Practice.* London: WB Saunders, 1993: 618–629.

37. Shimkin PM, Waldmann TA & Krugman RL. Intestinal lymphangiectasia. *Am J Roentgenol Radium Ther Nucl Med* 1970; **110**: 827–841.

38. Weiden PL, Blaese RM, Strober W & Waldmann TA. Impaired lymphocyte transformation in intestinal lymphangiectasia. Evidence for at least two functionally distinct lymphocyte populations in man. *J Clin Invest* 1972; **51**: 1319–1325.

39. Kinmouth JB & Cox SJ. Protein losing enteropathy in primary lymphoedema: mesenteric lymphography and gut resection. *Br J Surg* 1974; **61**: 589–593.

40. Sampson JA. Peritoneal endometriosis due to the menstrual dissemination of endometrial tissue into the peritoneal cavity. *Am J Obstet Gynecol* 1927; **14**: 422–469.

41. Haney AF. Etiology and histogenesis of endometriosis. *Progr Clin Res* 1990; **323**: 1–14.

42. Boles RS & Hodes PJ. Endometriosis of the small and large intestine. *Gastroenterology* 1958; **34**: 367–380.

43. Clark CE. Small intestinal obstruction due to endometriosis. *Am Surg* 1951; **17**: 1145–1154.

44. Martimbeau PW, Pratt JH & Gaffey TA. Small bowel obstruction secondary to endometriosis. *May Clin Proc* 1975; **50**: 239–243.

45. Macafee CHG & Greer HLH. Intestinal endometriosis. *J Obstet Gynaecol Br Commonw* 1960; **67**: 539–555.

46. Townell NH, Vanderwalt JD & Jagger GM. Intestinal endometriosis: diagnosis and management. *Br J Surg* 1984; **71**: 629–630.

47. Eastwood M & Gillon J. Pneumatosis cystoides intestinalis. In Misiewicz JJ, Pounder RE & Venables CW (eds) *Diseases of the Gut and Pancreas.* London: Blackwell, 1994: 1061–1064.

48. Yale CE & Balish E. Pneumatosis cystoides intestinalis. *Dis Colon Rectum* 1976; **19**: 107–111.

49. Feczko PJ, Mezwa DG, Farah MC & White BD. Clinical significance of pneumatosis of the bowel wall. *Radiographics* 1992; **12**: 1069–1078.

50. Knechtle SJ, Davidoff AM & Rice RP. Pneumatosis intestinalis; surgical management and outcome. *Ann Surg* 1990; **212**: 160–165.

51. Yang HK & Fondacaro PF. Enterolith ileus: a rare complication of duodenal diverticula. *Am J Gastroenterol* 1992; **87**: 1846–1848.

52. Crane PW, Crocker PR, Levison DA & Gilmore OJA. Enterolith ileus. *J R Soc Med* 1988; **81**: 292–294.

53. Lopez PV & Welch JP. Enterolith intestinal obstruction owing to acquired and congenital diverticulosis. *Dis Colon Rectum* 1991; **34**: 941–944.

54. Phillips J. Two cases of intestinal obstruction due to an enterolith, with reports of the chemical analysis. *Br J Surg* 1921; **8**: 378–379.

55. Meadows N. Disorders of the gastrointestinal system. In Levene MI (ed.) *Jolly's Diseases of Children.* London: Blackwell, 1991: 206.

56. Ooms HWA, Koumans RKJ, Ho Kang You PJ & Puylaert JBCM. Ultrasonography in the diagnosis of acute appendicitis. *Br J Surg* 1991; **78**: 315–318.

57. Hoffman J & Rasmussen O. Aids in the diagnosis of acute appendicitis. *Br J Surg* 1989; **76**: 774–779.

58. Leape LL & Ramenofsky ML. Laparoscopy in infants and children. *J Pediatr Surg* 1977; **12**: 928–938.

59. Cox MR, McCall JL, Wilson TG, Padbury RTA, Jeans PL & Toolui J. Laparoscopic appendicectomy: a prospective analysis. *Aust N Z J Surg* 1993; **63**: 840–847.

60. Chia YW, Carachi R, Armstrong AA, McGarry GW & Carrington D. Serum alpha interferon in children with right iliac fossa pain. *J Soc Med* 1993; **86**: 259–260.

61. Achong DM, Oates E & Harris B. Mesenteric lymphadenitis depicted by indium 111-labeled white blood cell imaging. *J Pediatr Surg* 1993; **28**: 1550–1552.

62. Durst AL, Freund H, Rosenmann E & Birnbaum D. Mesenteric panniculitis: review of the literature and presentation of cases. *Surgery* 1977; **81**: 203–211.

63. Gudinchet F & Schnyder P. Mesenteric panniculitis. *Acta Radiol* 1987; **28**: 727–729.

64. Katz ME, Heiken JP, Glazer HS & Lee JKT. Intraabdominal panniculitis: clinical, radiographic, and CT features. *AJR* 1985; **145**: 293–296.

65. Cooper CJ, Silverman PM, Forer L & Stull MA. Case 3: Mesenteric panniculitis. *AJR* 1990; **154**: 1328–1329.

66. Kobayashi S, Takeda K, Tanaka N, Hirano T, Nakagawa T & Matsumoto K. Mesenteric panniculitis: MR findings. *J Comput Assist Tomogr* 1993; **17**: 500–502.

67. Kikiros CS & Edis AJ. Mesenteric panniculitis resulting in bowel obstruction: response to steroids. *Aust N Z J Surg* 1989; **59**: 287–290.

68. Matsunaga N, Hayashi K, Amamoto Y, Itoh S, Furuwaka M & Maeda S. Mesenteric varices demonstrated by transhepatic portography. *Gastrointest Radiol* 1986; **11**: 280–282.

69. Soper NJ, Rikkers LF & Miller FJ. Gastrointestinal haemorrhage associated with chronic mesenteric venous occlusion. *Gastroenterology* 1985; **88**: 1964–1967.

70. Ostrow B & Blanchard RJW. Bleeding small bowel varices. *Can J Surg* 1984; **27**: 88–89.

71. Zimmer W & Yucel EK. Mesenteric varices: evalution with color flow doppler and magnetic resonance angiography. *Magn Reson Imaging* 1993; **11**: 1063–1066.

72. George JKSt & Pollak JS. Acute gastrointestinal hemorrhage detected by selective scintigraphic angiography. *J Nucl Med* 1991; **32**: 1601–1604.

73. Ozaki CK, Hansen M & Kadir S. Transhepatic embolization of superior mesenteric varices in portal hypertension. *Surgery* 1989; **105**: 446–448.

74. Vanek VW & Phillips AK. Retroperitoneal, mesenteric, and omental cysts. *Arch Surg* 1984; **119**: 838–842.

75. Bearhs OH, Judd ES & Docherty MD. Chylous cysts of the abdomen. *Surg Clin North Am* 1951; **30**: 1081–1096.

76. Walker AR & Putnam TC. Omental, mesenteric and retroperitoneal cysts: a clinical study of 33 new cases. *Ann Surg* 1973; **178**: 13–19.

77. Warfield JO. A study of mesenteric cysts with a report of two cases. *Ann Surg* 1932; **96**: 329.

PART

FOUR

Paediatric

edited by A Watson, TV Taylor and RCN Williamson

62

PAEDIATRIC ASPECTS OF UPPER DIGESTIVE SURGERY

CM Doig

INTRODUCTION

Although many of the conditions described elsewhere in this volume occur in children and have similar aetiology and treatment, the physiology of children, in particular neonates, is very different. Important points in the care of these children must be mentioned before discussion of individual conditions.

Many of the more common conditions can be operated upon in a district general hospital by a surgeon who has had some training in paediatric surgery. In fact, 75% of surgery in children in the UK is carried out in such hospitals. Teamwork with a trained paediatric anaesthetist and suitably trained nurses is essential. All general surgeons must be aware of the conditions in which it is advisable to transfer the child to the care of a specialist paediatric surgeon in a specialist unit, or paediatric hospital. Such specialist care is necessary for neonates, infants and older children with uncommon conditions.

Paediatric surgery is not so much system orientated as bounded by age limits. Concentration of surgical neonates under specialist paediatric surgical care has helped improve long-term outlook, especially in the premature baby[1] (Table 62.1). Since transportation of neonates is now possible over many miles with experienced call-out teams of paediatricians and anaesthetists with up-to-date incubators, with the baby arriving in excellent condition, there should be no argument for neonatal conditions being in a specialized unit. There is perhaps more controversy when we discuss the older child. The Confidential Enquiry of Peri-operative Deaths (CEPOD) has shown that if good results are to be achieved, surgeons should not operate on conditions that they see and treat rarely. This is especially true in children.

Neonatal surgery

Despite the advances in antenatal diagnoses, more than two-thirds of babies with congenital abnormalities will be born outwith a regional obstetric unit with an associated neonatal surgical unit. Satisfactory transfer of these often premature babies becomes a major factor in long-term prognosis. In the North-West Regional Paediatric Surgical Unit at St Mary's hospital in Manchester, which serves a population of 4.5 million, over 200 neonates per annum are admitted to the surgical unit; of these, over half have upper gastrointestinal problems (Table 62.2).

Transfer

The maintenance of temperature is important, whether during transfer in an incubator, on the unit, or, more importantly, in the neonatal theatre. Heat loss is proportional to surface area, which is large in relation to the baby's weight, as compared to heat production, which is proportional to body weight. Since heat dissipates by evaporation and as the neonate does not have the ability to maintain or increase body temperature by shivering, the environmental temperature must be kept high at 28–30°C. A warm environmental temperature is maintained with the use of a water blanket, warm sterile wet swabs, warm sterile Gamgee to wrap the areas not in use, exposing only the areas necessary for surgery, as well as a water bath for blood before transfusion. A temperature probe, preferably in the child's oesophagus or anus, monitors the temperature. With the increased risk of aspiration, the gastrointestinal tract must be kept deflated by a nasogastric tube left on free drainage. Of

Table 62.1 Mortality figures from the Neonatal Surgical Unit at St Mary's Hospital, Manchester

YEAR	NO. OF PATIENTS	MORTALITY
1978	106	13 (12.3)
1983	146	20 (13.7)
1986	158	10 (6.3)
1990	180	20 (11.1)
1994	254	10 (4)

Values in parentheses are percentages.
Reproduced with permission of Churchill Livingstone, Edinburgh.

Table 62.2 Admissions to the Neonatal Surgical Unit, St Mary's Hospital, Manchester for gastrointestinal conditions: 1979–1994

CONDITION	1980	1982	1984	1986	1988	1990	1994
Tracheo-oesophageal fistula	11	9	17	16	12	16	14
Diaphragmatic hernia	8	16	17	19	10	17	12
Pyloric stenosis	3	3	1	2	2	1	8
Duodenal atresia	5	10	4	9	7	3	6
Malrotation and volvulus	2	5	4	14	5	7	3
Ileal and jejunal atresia	3	8	6	6	14	1	2
Necrotizing enterocolitis	12	18	17	5	15	5	6
Functional obstruction	3	9	13	8	4	7	24
Meconium ileus	9	1	1	2	8	8	5
Exomphalos	8	3	11	5	13	3	19
Gastroschisis	6	3	5	6	9	11	17
Hirschsprung's disease	5	6	8	5	11	18	14
High rectal atresia/ imperforate anus	17	13	11	23	12	22	21
Cleft lip/palate				11	10	4	5
Miscellaneous	27	23	24	31	30	37	98
TOTAL	119	130	144	167	178	180	254

Reproduced with permission of Churchill Livingstone, Edinburgh.

much less importance is fluid balance as a normal newborn has little intake in the first 24 hours, and unless there is a great loss of fluid from the gastrointestinal tract in relation to blood volume, intravenous fluid is not necessary.

It may be necessary to ventilate the baby during transfer, especially if the baby is pre-term with respiratory problems associated with idiopathic respiratory distress syndrome. It should be remembered that these children are sometimes being transported long distances, and as much information as possible should be sent with them, as well as a consent form for surgery.

Physiology

In the transition from fetus to child, various physiological changes occur. Most of the organ systems, even in a full-term baby, are immature. One already mentioned is thermal imbalance. Others include respiration, circulation and energy metabolism. Gas exchange no longer happens at the placenta and fluid has to be removed from the immature lungs. By 36 weeks gestation, surfactant production reduces surface tension to help gas exchange and prevent atelectasis. Persistence of the ductus arteriosus means that shunting can occur, leading to heart failure. The kidneys are immature and so there is a real risk of overloading these babies with intravenous fluids given injudiciously. A low urine output does not necessarily mean dehydration. The kidneys can cope with a certain amount of milk orally, but not the same amount of fluid intravenously. When renal failure in the newborn occurs, treatment by peritoneal dialysis is possible.[2]

The body water has a different distribution from that in an adult, comprising 80% of the total weight, with 45% in the extracellular and 35% in the intracellular compartment, compared with adult values of 60% of body weight, with 20% extracellular and 40% intracellular. A rough calculation for the

blood volume of a neonate is weight (kg) × 80 ml, e.g. in a 3 kg baby the blood volume would be approximately 240 ml. The daily water turnover for a child may be twice that of an adult and varies from none in the newborn, due to large reserves, to 100 ml/kg per 24 hours at 1 year of age, to 50 ml/kg per 24 hours at 12 years. Calculations for fluid replacement in a surgical neonate are not the same as for a baby with dehydration due to gastroenteritis. Weight gain postoperatively consists of increases in both fat tissue and body water.[3]

In summary, it is better to have a dry baby, but if fluids are required they must be calculated to meet losses as well as for maintenance.

Calories are often more important than fluid because these babies are growing rapidly with a high energy metabolism. Because of these requirements, parenteral feeding of additional protein, carbohydrate and fat may be necessary if there is delay in oral feeding. However, such intravenous fat infusions run the risk of fat deposits in brain and liver, especially if a bolus is given at once.[4] Parenteral feeding also has complications of overloading with fluid and of sepsis.

An increased amount of protein is required (110–65 kcal/kg per day), and increased requirements for glucose and calcium, especially in the very pre-term baby, if not met, lead to hypoglycaemia and hypocalcaemia. More sodium is lost, so more is required, as well as adequate amounts of potassium, magnesium, zinc, copper, phosphates[5] and vitamins, especially those associated with blood clotting factors, so vitamin K must be given before surgery.[6] These requirements are despite the losses which may be incurred as a result of surgery. The hormonal and metabolic response to surgery in a neonate is proportional to the surgical stress, which can be measured.[7] The sucking–swallowing reflex is not established until 34–36 weeks gestation, so problems can arise in the very small pre-term infant who cannot swallow and requires tube feeding.

Irrespective of the surgical condition which exists, the baby (premature or small-for-dates) will have problems associated with these conditions, e.g. idiopathic respiratory distress syndrome requiring ventilation, jaundice requiring phototherapy or even exchange transfusions, renal failure requiring peritoneal dialysis,[8] sepsis because of the low IgM and IgA factors (although IgG is high),[9] and even septicaemia leading to disseminated intravascular coagulation syndrome, intraventricular haemorrhage, with sometimes a doubtful outcome, and necrotizing enterocolitis, whether surgery has been performed or not. Wound infections are common, especially in neonates.[10,11] Postoperative mortality depends on how many other stresses are present.[12]

It is common for more than one abnormality to occur, sometimes constituting a specific syndrome. Geneticists should be involved to help determine prognosis. One gastrointestinal abnormality may be associated with another, or with renal, cardiac or skeletal problems. Screening for other abnormalities should only be done when there is a reasonable chance of occurrence.[13] It may be necessary to make a decision not to operate on a neonate on occasion.[14] Unfortunately, intellectual development may be reduced, especially in children who have had major neonatal surgery and have a continuing need for surgery.[15,16]

Antenatal diagnosis

The development of antenatal diagnosis has meant a possible change in prognosis and a need to determine when and where a particular baby with a known abnormality should be born. Although accuracy is not complete, the different methods used – ultrasonography, amniocentesis, and occasionally molecular genetic and biochemical techniques[17] – means that abnormalities can be diagnosed earlier. This does not necessarily mean that abortion is then offered. Most babies can go to term and may be delivered normally. However, in many cases the delivery should be close to the neonatal surgical unit. Transport in utero leads to better prognosis than transport after birth. Some gastrointestinal abnormalities can be diagnosed before the child is born but, at present, less than half of the abnormalities seen on antenatal ultrasonography are gastrointestinal. If an abnormality is detected early, there is need for support and discussion with the prospective parents and for up-to-date information as to what the diagnosis means, what the treatment involves and what the likely outcome is.[18] Such advice can be provided by a fetal abnormality team consisting of a paediatric surgeon, a neonatologist, an obstetrician, a geneticist and a radiologist with special expertise in ultrasonography, as is provided at St Mary's Hospital, Manchester.

Fetal surgery

Fetal surgery has been performed both experimentally in animals and in humans, but at present results are poor. Only correction of diaphragmatic herniation has been attempted.[19] Recent work demonstrates that fetal wounds heal quicker and without scar formation.[20] The future lies in further experimental work[21] to prevent as well as treat major congenital abnormalities before birth.

Infants and children

Any surgeon associated with the care of children must remember that they are dealing with more than one person; it is important that the parents as well as the patient are fully involved. If the child is old enough he or she must be involved in any discussion as to the diagnosis and treatment. A brief anatomy lesson will often help the parents understand not only what is wrong, but also how it is treated and why complications may arise. Although 70% of paediatric surgery is of an emergency nature, preparation of the child for admission as well as for surgery will help reduce the psychological trauma which haunts some children. If they wish, parents should be allowed into the anaesthetic room; 80% of elective surgery can be performed on a day-case basis if there is careful choice of patient, and district liaison nurses are used for follow-up at home. A suitably relaxed environment, both in the ward and the anaesthetic room, is important.

In an older child, dehydration of 10% requires urgent replacement (a lethargic child has lost more than 5% of blood volume, and by the time there is poor capillary return more than 10% has been lost). The correct type of intravenous fluids is important: normal saline is too hypertonic and gives too many sodium ions, and 0.5% dextrose does not give adequate carbohydrate. The usual intravenous replacement fluid is 0.18% sodium chloride with 4% dextrose.

Paediatric anaesthesia has progressed to the extent that very few babies or children are too ill or too small for the ministrations of a skilled paediatric anaesthetist, who will also provide anaesthesia for radiology, endoscopy and day-case surgery as well as the more major work. Analgesia should not be forgotten in children. Just because the baby cannot speak does not mean he or she is not in pain. Relief can be by local infiltration, regional block on by intravenous or oral route.[22] It must be both adequate and appropriate.[23]

Laparoscopic surgery in children[24] is not commonplace. Short length of hospital stay and small incisions are not obvious benefits as they are normal in paediatric surgery.

THE OESOPHAGUS

OESOPHAGEAL ATRESIA

Embryology

The trachea develops at 4–6 weeks as an offshoot of the foregut in close relationship to the oesophagus. Abnormalities are thought to occur because of faulty development of the tracheo-oesophageal septum; however, such a septum has never been demonstrated. It is likely that the usual form of tracheo-oesophageal atresia with fistula is a primary foregut abnormality and that the rarer and more unusual types are of secondary origin.[1] Apart from atresia, associated abnormalities of the trachea and respiratory tract are not uncommon: laryngeal clefts with incomplete separation of the trachea and pharynx; fistulas into the upper or lower oesophageal pouches (very common); and tracheomalacia (also very common), which can give problems postoperatively. Associated pulmonary abnormalities, such as sequestration or agenesis, also occur.

Physiology

Although much of the physiology of the oesophagus has already been discussed (see pages 5–11, in the premature infant especially, due to immaturity of the system, the oesophagus does not behave as in the adult. The fetus starts mouthing at 18 weeks and swallows less than 10 ml of amniotic fluid; which increases to 20 ml/day by 20 weeks.[2] This helps to regulate the production of amniotic fluid. Superficial glands appear in the oesophagus at 20 weeks, followed by squamous cells at 28 weeks. The sucking–swallowing reflex does not occur until 33–36 weeks. At the same time the development of oesophageal motility occurs, starting with poor tertiary biphasic contractions and progressing to organized peristaltic waves initiated by swallowing. This change is probably due to the maturation of nerve fibres. These immature tertiary contractions can be seen later in children with reflux oesophagitis.[3] Sucking appears to be a conditioned reflex and can improve distal motility and so weight gain, even if the sucking is not nutritive. Thus, in a pre-term baby, irrespective of the presence of an abnormality of the oesophagus, feeding cannot proceed normally, necessitating tube feeding.

Disorders of motility can occur after surgery for oesophageal atresia; whether this is due to delay in swallowing or an inherent motility disorder is uncertain. The lower oesophageal sphincter in the infant has a low pressure which increases with age, so that reflux is common in the young and especially in the premature infant. The actual clinical significance of this reflux is uncertain.[4]

Types of atresia

The most common variety of oesophageal atresia is that found in association with a lower pouch fistula from the trachea, occurring in approximately 80% of cases (Figure 62.1). A further 10% will have an atretic oesophagus with no fistulous connection[5] and the remaining 10% will have fistulas from the upper pouch, with or without lower pouch fistulas. When an H-type fistula occurs, there is an intact normal oesophagus with a fistulous connection between this and the trachea.[6] Webs or overlapping pouches are less common.[7] The inci-

dence of such anomalies is about 1 in 4500 births. Other abnormalities, often multiple, may be associated, occurring in over 50% of children. The grouping of abnormalities into syndromes, e.g. the VATER syndrome, helps determine the prognosis,[8] there being an increased mortality rate with the presence of more than one abnormality.[9] The association with duodenal atresia and rectal atresia is especially lethal.[10] Many atretic babies also have problems because of being small for dates, due perhaps to the lack of swallowing in utero.[11]

Presentation and diagnosis

When a mother has had hydramnios and/or the baby at birth is 'mucusy', the diagnosis of oesophageal atresia should be considered. The baby cannot swallow amniotic fluid, hence the hydramnios, and after birth the baby is unable to swallow saliva. In those with a fistula into the trachea, air passes into the stomach with each breath so that the abdomen is distended, unlike those with only an atresia or upper pouch fistula in whom the abdomen is scaphoid, due to the lack of swallowed air. In an ideal world every newborn baby should have a nasogastric tube passed to exclude atresia, and the fluid aspirated should be tested by means of litmus paper to ensure

(a)

(b)

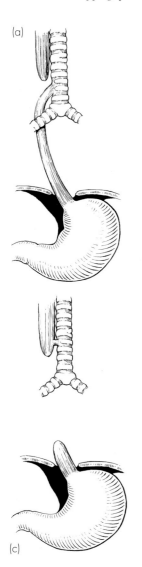
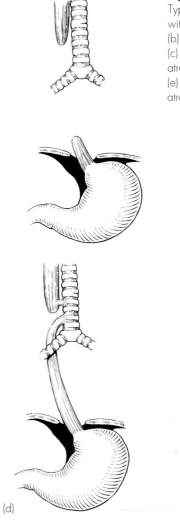
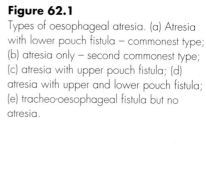
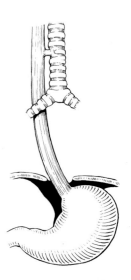

Figure 62.1

Types of oesophageal atresia. (a) Atresia with lower pouch fistula – commonest type; (b) atresia only – second commonest type; (c) atresia with upper pouch fistula; (d) atresia with upper and lower pouch fistula; (e) tracheo-oesophageal fistula but no atresia.

(c)

(d)

(e)

that the tube is in the stomach. Babies should ideally not be fed until oesophageal atresia has been excluded by these means. Radiopaque fluid must not be used to delineate the oesophagus because it spills over into the lungs and produces infection. If necessary, a chest radiograph will show the extent of the upper pouch with the radiopaque tube in situ; the stomach, with or without air, can also be visualized. The diagnosis is more difficult in those with a fistula only. In these babies, specialist contrast radiology with an anaesthetist present may be necessary to delineate the connection.[12] However, in such children, and in all children with any form of oesophageal atresia, we prefer to perform tracheoscopy before proceeding to definitive surgery. The fistula can be visualized, and even catheterized with a ureteric catheter to help delineate it at surgery[13] (Figure 62.2, see colour plate also). If there is more than one fistula, i.e. from upper and lower pouches, these are seen, and involvement of a main bronchus can be observed. Unfortunately, the child with only a fistula and an intact oesophagus is often diagnosed late and may have developed an upper lobe pneumonia, and cyanotic attacks, associated with feeding.

Treatment

Transport of such babies can be difficult due to the risk of inhalation of saliva, and with a large lower pouch fistula acid may also regurgitate from the stomach into the lungs. A Replogle double-lumen tube (or sump catheter)[14] sited in the upper pouch will aspirate saliva and prevent overspill. Positioning the child in the jack-knife position will keep stomach contents out of the bronchi. Should the child have problems with aspiration of saliva or if, unfortunately, the baby has been fed because of delay in diagnosis, physiotherapy and antibiotics will be necessary before surgery can be contemplated.

Operative details: Primary anastomosis

As long as there is no associated rectal agenesis causing a distal obstruction, operative treatment is not urgent. Problems may occur if the fistula is large. A skilled paediatric anaesthetist is essential in such cases as co-operation between the surgeon

and anaesthetist will almost inevitably be necessary. Because of the fistulous connection between trachea and oesophagus, anaesthesia is difficult. Once the baby is anaesthetized, tracheoscopy is performed to determine the presence, number and position of fistulas.[15]

The child is positioned on the left side with a roll under the thorax to assist exposure. The right arm is brought up over the head to give clear access to the axilla. Should a right-sided aorta be present, it may be advantageous to make the approach through the left side.[16] Although a routine thoracotomy incision extending posteriorly can be used, this gives an unsightly scar. The author's practice is to make a vertical axillary incision behind the anterior fold of the axilla. This leaves a much more acceptable scar. Access is good and there is no risk of damage to nerves. The chest is opened through the fourth, or occasionally the third, intercostal space, depending on the position of the pouches as gauged from the chest radiograph. Keeping as far as possible in the extrapleural plane, the pleura is cleared by means of small wet pledglets so that the posterior mediastinum can be visualized. A Denis Browne retractor can be used so that the rakes will retract the ribs. A special adjustable screw retractor will slowly separate them so that an excellent view can be achieved. The lung is retracted using a wet swab under a malleable retractor. Once the posterior mediastinum is cleared of pleura, the azygos vein is visualized and dissected using a Waterston devulsor. Ligation and division of this vein opens up the mediastinum and allows the lower pouch to be dissected free. The fistula must be cleared to the trachea and then transfixed before division (Figure 62.3a–f). A useful check is to clamp the fistula temporarily before ligation and ask the anaesthetist to inflate the lungs. This will prevent inadvertent ligation of a main bronchus should the fistula arise abnormally. A tube passed down into the distal portion of the lower oesophagus will allow deflation of the stomach. Proof of this is achieved by leaving the end of the tube under water. Transfixation of the fistula must be close to the trachea to prevent subsequent tracheal problems. The efficacy of the tracheal suture is checked by filling the thorax with water before forceful ventilation by the anaesthetist to disrupt the suture. The upper pouch can now be dissected clear to match the dissection of the lower pouch. Again, the anaesthetist aids the procedure by displaying the upper pouch with a tube already in situ. It is probably easier to have a red rubber tube split down the side with a smaller transanastomotic tube inside it, so that the latter can be grasped and brought into position through the anastomosis without further intubation of the pouch. Care must be taken whilst dissecting the upper pouch due to its close proximity to the trachea, as tracheal damage can easily result. Stay sutures in the two pouches can be approximated to determine whether a primary anastomosis will be possible. If that is the case, the upper pouch is opened, care being taken to open both muscle and mucosa. The sutures are passed between the two pouches so that knots will end up on the outside[17] of the oesophagus, and are held before tying. Vicryl or PDS sutures (4/0 or 6/0) may be used, only one layer of interrupted sutures being necessary. Once the posterior row is completed and it is confirmed that the anastomosis is possible with little tension,

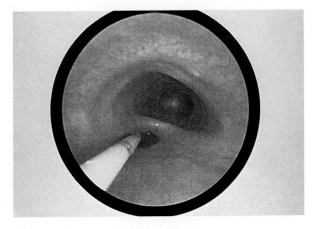

Figure 62.2
Tracheoscopy showing fistula into oesophagus.

(a)

(b)

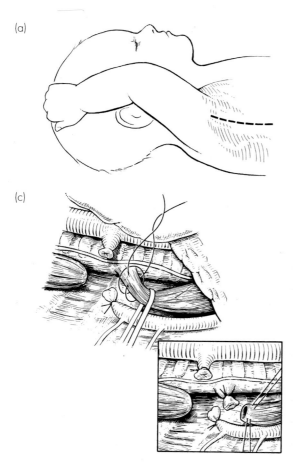

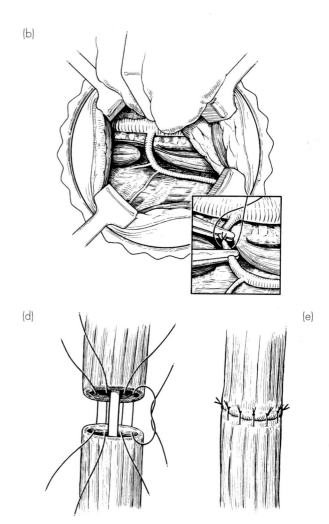

(c)

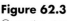

(d)

(e)

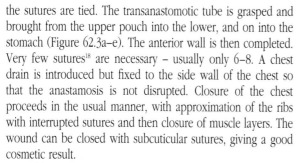

Figure 62.3
Operative stages in repair of oesophageal atresia. (a) Incision
and position. (b) Ligation of azygos vein. (c) Transfix ligation of
fistula. (d) Partial completion of anastomosis. (e) Completed
anastomosis.

the sutures are tied. The transanastomotic tube is grasped and
brought from the upper pouch into the lower, and on into the
stomach (Figure 62.3a–e). The anterior wall is then completed.
Very few sutures[18] are necessary – usually only 6–8. A chest
drain is introduced but fixed to the side wall of the chest so
that the anastamosis is not disrupted. Closure of the chest
proceeds in the usual manner, with approximation of the ribs
with interrupted sutures and then closure of muscle layers. The
wound can be closed with subcuticular sutures, giving a good
cosmetic result.

Problems can occur when the pleura is inadvertently
opened. A transpleural approach means that if there is leakage
it is less likely to resolve. Since the blood supply to the lower
pouch may run with the fistula,[19] ligation and division of the
fistula may devascularize the anastomotic site on the lower
pouch, leading to breakdown of the anastomosis.

Postoperatively, if there is doubt about anastomosis elective
ventilation may be continued for 3–7 days to prevent tension
on the anastomosis.[20] However, if the anastomosis appears
satisfactory, the child should be allowed to breathe spontaneously, with only the addition of postoperative physiotherapy.
Pharyngeal suction in the proximal pharynx must be carried
out carefully so that the anastomosis is not disrupted. Feeding

may commence 24–48 hours postoperatively through the
transanastomotic tube. If the anastomosis is intact, feeding by
mouth starts at 5–7 days. Some workers advocate prior confirmation of anastomotic integrity by contrast barium swallow.
The chest drain is removed once it has been established that
there is no leak, i.e. between the third and fifth days. Most of
these anastomoses result in some stricturing in the early weeks;
it is advisable, to perform a barium meal before discharge from
hospital. These anastomotic strictures usually resolve
spontaneously, but some may require dilatation. The above
description is the routine procedure for children with
oesophageal atresia and lower pouch fistula.

Complications

The main complications of surgery are anastomotic leakage and
stricture, occurring in 75% of children, although many have no
permanent problems.[21] If leakage of saliva is small and there is a
chest drain in situ, conservative management is possible, especially if the approach has been extrapleural. A stricture may
develop at the site of leakage. Intravenous feeding may be
necessary until healing occurs. If there is almost total disruption, a further thoracotomy and conversion to oesophagostomy

and gastrostomy is necessary. Some surgeons perform gastrostomy as a routine to allow feeding early and prevent tension on the anastomosis, but this is probably only necessary if there is serious doubt about the anastomosis.

Although most anastomoses do need at least one dilatation, a few need a series of dilatations before an adequate lumen is achieved and normal feeding is possible. It is only rarely necessary to resect a stricture after a primary anastomosis. If there is difficulty in approximating the two ends, the lower pouch may be pulled up, so producing a reflux, or even a hiatus hernia.[22] This may require surgical correction of the reflux. Since a portion of the oesophagus is missing in atresia, incoordination of the oesophagus with associated motility problems can occur.[23] Most of these improve with time as the child grows.

Another major problem which may improve with time is tracheomalacia. Because of the close development of the oesophagus and trachea, the trachea is frequently abnormal, having either very soft or even no cartilaginous rings. The result of this is that during inspiration, instead of the normal D-shaped trachea, the trachea collapses and the walls are opposed.[24] Approximation of the walls of the trachea during respiration means that there is, at the very least, stridor, and often the risk of respiratory arrest. This worrying phenomenon improves as the child gets older, but the risk of death in one of these apnoeic attacks in high. Prolonged hospitalization may be necessary. Alternatively, some form of aortopexy[25] to relieve tracheal compression has been performed but with mixed success. The insertion of new cartilage rings formed from the costal cartilages into the trachea would seem more logical.[26]

A more worrying and sometimes late complication is that of recurrent fistula,[27] which should always be borne in mind when a child who has had previous oesophageal atresia repair develops recurrent chest infections. The diagnosis is made, as in primary fistulas, by endoscopic catheterization.[28] Closure is not easy and interposition of other tissue, such as pericardium,[29] between the oesophagus and the trachea can help reduce the risk of further recurrence. Endoscopic diathermy has been suggested as a means of obliterating the fistula,[30] but this has yet to be tested extensively.

After thoracotomy in children, chest deformities[31] and scoliosis can occur, even without associated vertebral anomalies.

Other surgical procedures

In circumstances where it is not possible to approximate the two ends of the oesophagus without tension there is a risk of anastomotic dehiscence; various procedures have been devised to overcome this problem.

Cervical myotomy

One or a series of myotomies[32,33] may be made in the upper pouch to provide additional length (Figure 62.4). These may be performed in the neck or the thorax. The underlying mucosa is left intact, and up to 4 cm may be gained. Few problems[34] have been encountered but subsequent diverticula[35] have been observed.

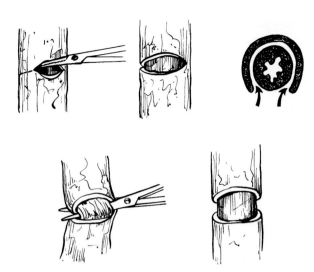

Figure 62.4
Lividatis cervical myotomy.

Delayed primary anastomosis

If the two ends will not approximate, the fistula is ligated and divided and the chest closed with a view to performing a delayed primary anastomosis. Especially in a very premature child[36] or one with other abnormalities, waiting until the baby has gained weight may allow growth of the two ends towards each other. A delayed primary anastomosis[37,38] may then be feasible. A Replogle double-lumen tube is left in the upper pouch to suck it clear of saliva and prevent spillage into the lungs. Although dilatation and stretching of the pouch can be performed daily,[39] the presence of the tube itself may stretch the pouch. If the fistula into the lower pouch is large, it may be difficult to ventilate such a child. In very premature babies, surgery to close the fistula is not always possible initially. In such circumstances a water-seal gastrostomy[30] may be used to allow gastric decompression, or a transgastric balloon may be applied in an attempt to block the air leak temporarily.[41] Anastomosis is then performed at about 3 weeks, when the child has grown and the two ends are closer together. During that time the child can be fed through the gastrostomy tube if the lower pouch has been oversewn at thoracotomy. Cervical myotomy may be added to aid construction of the anastomosis.[42] This delayed method can also be used when there is atresia without fistula, in which case thoracotomy will not have been performed.

Irrespective of whether primary or delayed anastomoses are performed, premature infants with long defects tend to have more problems with respiration and swallowing.[43] With improvement in paediatric intensive care, however, there is less place for such delayed surgery[44] and results are improving, even in very premature babies.[45]

Flap of upper pouch

Since the upper pouch is often very large, it is possible to raise a posteriorly-hinged flap on the base of the pouch, which can then be tubulated, which both narrows and elongates the pouch. This extra portion of upper pouch can then allow a satisfactory anastomosis without tension.[46,47]

End-to-side anastomosis

By anastomosing the end of the upper pouch to the side of the lower oesophagus, and only ligating the fistula, leaving it in continuity with the trachea, it was hoped that the consequent reduction in tension would improve results. However, although some authors have reported good results, there is a suggestion of an increased risk of recurrent fistula.[48]

Oesophagostomy and gastrostomy

If primary anastomosis is thought to be unlikely, e.g. when there is only atresia, some other means of achieving continuity will have to be considered at a later stage. In the meantime, aspiration of saliva must be prevented by oesophagostomy, and feeding established by gastrostomy. A left oesophagostomy can be performed so that the oesophagus is brought out behind the major vessels and the carotid sheath. Care is taken not to damage the thoracic duct, and the opened oesophagus is sutured to the skin. Unfortunately, this often becomes infected with *Pseudomonas* species owing to the continuous discharge of saliva.

Gastrostomy is performed through a separate incision in the epigastrium. The siting of the gastrostomy is important as the greater curvature of the stomach may be used later to make a new oesophagus (see below). A midline vertical incision is made in the epigastrium and the greater curvature of the stomach brought out. A position near the antrum, but not occluding the pylorus, is chosen and a purse-string suture placed. The stomach is opened, care being taken to open all layers as it is easy to miss the mucosa. A Malecot catheter of suitable size, usually 10–12 Fr, is placed into the stomach and the suture tied and left attached with its needle. A further purse-string suture is placed so as to 'ink-well' the first one in the manner of a Stamm gastrostomy. An incision is made in the left side of the upper abdomen and the gastrostomy tube brought out. The remaining portions of the two purse-string sutures are used to fix the stomach to the parietal peritoneum near the gastrostomy opening. Closure of the abdominal incision is then completed. The tube must be anchored on the outside, by means of sticky foam on to the tube itself close to the abdomen, or some other means of stabilization used. This is to ensure that the tube remains vertical at all times, keeping the lumen circular and not elliptical. No sutures are necessary to fix it to skin, but the position is of utmost importance if subsequent problems with leakage of gastric contents and difficulty in spontaneous closure are to be avoided. Apart from these problems, the greatest danger is separation of the stomach from the peritoneum, allowing milk to enter the peritoneal cavity – a lethal situation. If incorrectly anchored, it is possible for the tube to dislodge and migrate into the pylorus, resulting in obstruction. Percutaneous gastrostomy[49] can be performed with the aid of an endoscope, reducing the need for laparotomy.

While waiting for the child to grow, feeding is via the gastrostomy. The establishment of sham feeding by mouth and out via the oesophagostomy is important to establish normal feeding reflexes when oesophageal continuity is re-established.

Less common varieties of oesophageal atresia

Atresia with proximal fistula

Although a proximal fistula can occur in association with a lower fistula, it may also occur in isolation. In both types the diagnosis is easily made at tracheoscopy so that at surgery special care is taken in dissecting the upper pouch. If not previously diagnosed, tracheal damage may result during this dissection, with an air leak being the first indication of the presence of a fistula. If two fistulas are present, the oesophageal ends are frequently held far apart, necessitating a later reconstruction,[50] even three have been found.[51]

Fistula alone

Presentation is usually at an older age and should be suspected when the child has a history of cyanotic attacks when being fed or of recurrent upper lobe pneumonia.[52] As it is a rare occurrence there is often delay in making the diagnosis.[53] Once demonstrated on endoscopy or by specialized radiology the fistula is approached either through the neck or thorax, depending on its position. Ligation and division should be all that is necessary[54] but interposition of other tissue can prevent recurrence. Attempts to use diathermy on the fistula through the endoscope have met with variable results.[30] Even after apparently successful treatment for oesophageal atresia with fistula, a recurrent fistula may occur many years later, giving rise to repeated chest infections. A recurrent fistula should be remembered in the differential diagnosis of recurrent chest infections.

Atresia alone

The diagnosis is made on clinical grounds because of the scaphoid abdomen, while the radiograph shows a gasless abdomen. In such cases, the two ends of oesophagus may be so far apart that thoracotomy need not be carried out and gastrostomy and oesophagostomy are performed as a primary procedure, followed by a later reconstruction. However, after gastrostomy has been performed,[55] anastomosis should be attempted if possible, with preoperative and perioperative delineation of upper and lower pouches by radiology. Metal bougies inserted into the upper pouch and via the gastrostomy into the lower pouch can also be used to estimate the gap.

Results

In the long term, 90% of all children with oesophageal atresia, with or without a fistula, are able to undergo primary anastomosis with very few problems,[56] even in the small preterm babies with other anomalies.[57] The deaths (about 30%) still occur mostly in this latter group (Waterston group C[58]).

It has been shown that children with oesophageal atresia grow up to adulthood with minimal problems,[59] the majority exhibiting catch-up growth.[60] Only a few have respiratory infections on a recurrent basis,[61,62] preventing normal growth. These tend to be due to oesophageal reflux or strictures.[63] The other 10% have major problems necessitating dismantling of the anastomosis and replacement with a neo-oesophagus.

Reconstruction of the oesophagus

Although most paediatric surgeons would allow the children who survive with gastrostomies and oesophagostomies to grow until they weigh about 10 kg before undertaking major reconstructive surgery, the operation can be performed earlier with success if the social circumstances so dictate.[64] These children do well at home once the mother has been shown how to cope with the stomas and perform sham feeding.

Colon transplant

Waterston designed the colon transplant in the early 1950s for strictures associated with caustic swallowing, but realized that the technique could be used to replace an absent oesophagus. A portion of the transverse colon is used to replace the oesophagus,[65] the blood supply being on the middle or left colic artery pedicle. The portion of colon used must be long enough to lie comfortably in the chest and yet not be so long as to cause kinking. The colon left behind is reanastomosed, care being taken not to occlude the blood supply when closing the mesentery. This tenuous blood supply and colon is then brought up behind the stomach and in front of the pancreas. At this point, there are variations in the technique. Classically, Waterston[66] brought the colon into the chest through a separate incision in the diaphragm to allow the conduit to lie behind the root of the lung (Figure 62.5). However, by bringing the colon up in the anterior mediastinum, dissection and anastomosis are not performed in the thorax, the lower anastomosis being made to the anterior wall of the stomach in the abdomen. Freeman has suggested a more anatomical position for the colon, i.e. lying in the posterior mediastinum in the bed of the original oesophagus.[67]

The lower anastomosis of the colon, either to stomach or the lower pouch of the oesophagus, is performed first, with the colon lying in either an isoperistaltic or retroperistaltic manner. Since the colon acts only as a conduit, the direction of peristalsis is unimportant, the direction being dictated by the blood supply. If the oesophageal stump is not used, oesophagitis can subsequently develop within it.[68] Creating the passage for the conduit from the thorax can be hazardous because it is made in an area of major vessels and much of the dissection is blind. The oesophagostomy is taken down and the upper pouch dissected free. The route through the dome of the pleura is dilated so that the colon is not compressed and the distal colon and oesophagus are anastomosed in the neck in a single layer. A tube is left in the neo-oesophagus to keep it deflated, as acute dilatation can impair the viability of the colon.

The major problem with a colon transplant is that the blood supply is very tenuous and the anastomosed end in the neck may stricture because of ischaemia. More seriously, the whole colon may become necrotic, necessitating urgent thoracotomy to remove the gangrenous bowel. If the bowel is lying anteriorly, it is exceedingly difficult to anastomose to the posteriorly lying oesophagus, and dilatation of a stricture is almost impossible, even with flexible endoscopes. In view of the disparity in diameter between the colon and oesophagus, the upper anastomosis often leaks. There are fewer problems with the lower anastomosis but, as the child grows, overgrowth of the colon may produce redundancy and kinking may cause an obstruction to the passage of food into the stomach. Although only a conduit,[69] if the child has been properly trained with sham feeding, normal feeding can commence soon and the child will grow and develop normally. Although in the past this was a staged procedure, it is now possible to complete the procedure as a single stage. The long-term results are reasonably good, with satisfactory normal feeding in most children,[70,71] although redundancy of the colon may lead to stagnation and poor growth.[72]

Colon interposition may be used also for replacing the strictured oesophagus after caustic ingestion, oesophagitis or carcinoma of the oesophagus, but a possible late complication of such an interposition may be carcinoma.[73] More recently an approach through the right chest has been attempted, with the anastomosis of the ends within the mediastinum, giving apparently good results with few complications.[74]

Gastric sleeve

In an attempt to overcome the problems of blood supply of colonic conduits, the greater curvature of the stomach has been used to make a sleeve,[75] initially to replace the oesophagus after removal for carcinoma. In the Heimlich operation,[76] the gastric sleeve so formed is swung up on the fundus of the stomach and into the chest through a separate incision in the diaphragm. Two rows of staples with a dividing knife can be used to make the sleeve starting near the antrum; the proximal anastomosis is, as before, in the neck. Although long, this conduit and its anastomosis rarely give rise to problems, and with preservation of the gastroepiploic vessels ischaemia should not arise. Kinking at the pivotal point of sleeve and remaining stomach can, however, necessitate further surgery. As in the colon, this neo-oesophagus acts as a conduit only.

Some surgeons prefer to bring the whole stomach into the thorax, which gives reasonable results,[77] although the long-term results of this technique are still in doubt.

Other methods

Free grafts of jejunum and ileum to replace the oesophagus, both with and without microvascular techniques,[78] have been used. Experimental work has been performed using Silastic, pericardium and various meshes to replace the missing oesophagus. A more unusual suggestion from the USA has been the use of a high-power magnet in conjunction with metal bougies to stretch and approximate the two pouches.[79] Approximation of the two ends by suture material to allow fistulization to occur has been successful in selected cases[80,81] and is more commonly in use in Europe.

The complexity of these various operations emphasizes the desirability of using the child's own oesophagus wherever possible. It has been shown that the child's own oesophagus functions better than interposition of another portion of the gastrointestinal tract, hence the use of myotomies and flaps. It

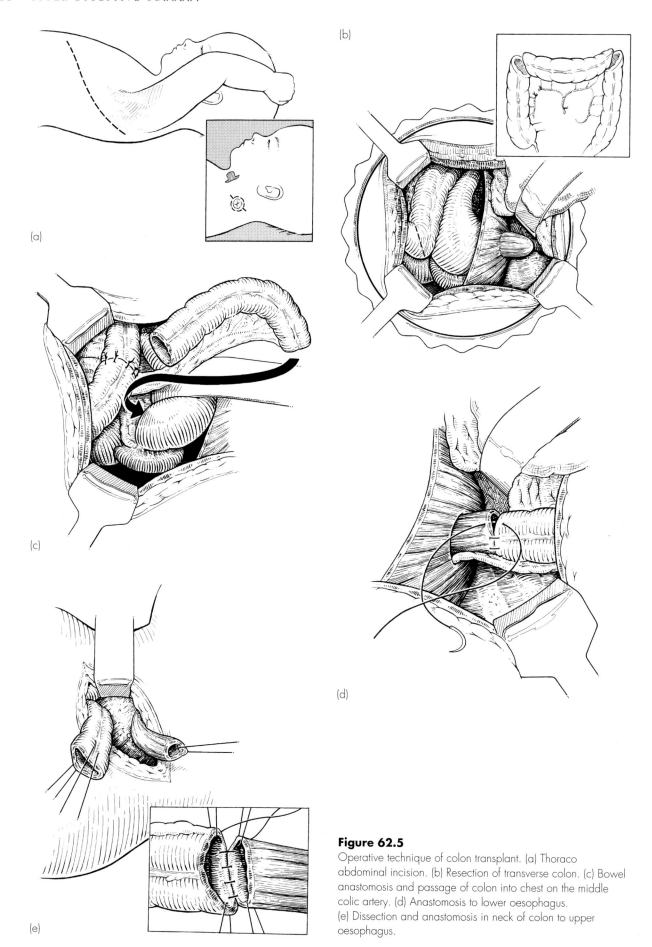

(a)

(b)

(c)

(d)

(e)

Figure 62.5

Operative technique of colon transplant. (a) Thoraco abdominal incision. (b) Resection of transverse colon. (c) Bowel anastomosis and passage of colon into chest on the middle colic artery. (d) Anastomosis to lower oesophagus. (e) Dissection and anastomosis in neck of colon to upper oesophagus.

is certainly worth persevering with a rather doubtful anastomosis in the hope that it will at least eventually make a normal oesophagus.

GASTRO-OESOPHAGEAL REFLUX

Most newborn babies have a lax oesophagogastric junction and reflux is common.[1] However, this tendency diminishes with age so that by a few months old reflux is minimal. For such infants who may vomit after feeds and fail to thrive, conservative treatment by thickening feeds, antacids and advice about positioning the child after feeds is all that is necessary. No investigations need be performed. However, a small percentage (sometimes premature infants)[2] will continue to vomit and will not thrive. In these circumstances, further investigation is necessary. The presence of a hiatus hernia does not necessarily imply the presence of gastro-oesophageal reflux. The presence of reflux is more important than an anatomical hiatus hernia in determining whether surgical treatment is necessary.[3] Reflux does not necessarily give problems.[4]

Presentation

Troublesome reflux should be considered when vomiting after food, sometimes undigested, leads to loss of weight and failure to thrive. Occasionally, haematemesis or anaemia will be the first indication of problems. If undiagnosed, stricture formation may result in dysphagia with further loss of weight. Some children present with respiratory problems of pneumonia, asthma or even apnoeic attacks due to aspiration. A complication of repair of oesophageal atresia[8] and diaphragmatic hernia[9] may be the production of reflux which requires aggressive treatment. Reflux can also complicate congenital pyloric stenosis and malrotation.[10]

Investigation

Barium swallow may not necessarily demonstrate mild reflux but it will show gross reflux and any associated anatomical anomalies, such as hiatus hernia or stricture. Similarly, endoscopy may not necessarily be helpful[11] unless there is either macroscopic or histological evidence of oesophagitis. Endoscopy may be performed with the child anaesthetized; biopsy should always be taken even if the mucosa looks normal.[12] Rarely, inflammatory polyps are seen. Scintigraphy using a radioisotope can be a useful investigation, especially when respiratory problems predominate;[13] pH monitoring over a 24-hour period[14] or less[15] is possible with portable equipment, even in a very small baby,[16] and is more useful than manometry, which has only a limited use in the few children with incoordination problems.[17] A decision on treatment can be made based on severity of acid exposure in the oesophagus, length of time the acid remains and the frequency and severity of reflux episodes.[18] Different patterns of reflux are seen in children, not all of whom necessarily require treatment.

Medical treatment

In mild cases, advice about thickening feeds with Carobel may be all that is necessary, improvement usually following the introduction of weaning diet. The addition of Gaviscon or an antacid may also help. H_2-receptor antagonists and cisapride[19] (a prokinetic agent) have proved useful adjuncts. Monitoring progress by oesophagoscopy, pH studies and the percentile weight chart will allow a decision to be made as to the necessity for and timing of surgery, or whether to continue with intensive medical therapy. Only 10% of children with reflux require an antireflux operation,[20] although some may require admission for agressive medical therapy. Part of the evaluation should include gastric emptying studies, especially in mentally retarded children.[21] Delay in proceeding to surgery may lead to stunted growth,[22] but an operation should not be the first treatment in children with reflux.

Haematemesis due to marked oesophagitis caused by reflux necessitates surgery, as does stricture formation. The presence of a hiatus hernia is not necessarily an absolute indication for operative treatment; other criteria for surgery must also be met. Many of the 10% of children who only have reflux necessitating antireflux surgery have cerebral palsy and other neurological abnormalities.[23] A reduced lower oesophageal sphincter pressure in these children increases the likelihood and severity of reflux. Gastrostomy was often performed in the past to help with feeding of such children, but actually makes reflux worse.[24] The effects of successful antireflux surgery include the abolition of acid reflux and vomiting and resumption of the ability to thrive. There is less chance of stricture formation but, more importantly, the nursing problem for the mother in caring for such a child is eased.[25] Children with respiratory problems require operative management.

Surgical treatment

Preoperative measures include assessment of the respiratory state and occasionally aggressive treatment, and rarely parenteral nutrition, if the nutritional state is particularly compromised. Although antireflux surgery can be performed by a thoracic or abdominal approach, the latter is preferable due to the possible complication of respiratory problems. As in adults (see Chapter 10), a variety of antireflux procedures has been used in infants and children.

Nissen fundoplication

This procedure can be performed satisfactorily in children.[26,27] It is necessary to achieve adequate length of oesophagus in the abdomen, which can prove difficult in the presence of a stricture. A complete wrap is favoured, although some prefer a partial wrap to avoid problems of 'gas bloat'.[28] It has been shown that an adequately sized bougie will prevent too tight a repair.[29] Intraoperative manometry[30] has no place in repair in children. Pyloroplasty may also be added if there is thought to be outlet obstruction.[31] Despite the associated problems, some surgeons will also add a gastrostomy.[32] The operation may be performed laparoscopically.[33]

As in adults, problems of too tight a wrap lead to 'gas bloat' and an inability of the child to belch or vomit.[34] This can sometimes be treated by dilatation. To avoid this problem, incomplete wraps have been suggested but this may lead to problems with recurrent reflux. A few children will have recurrent problems due to disruption of the repair and so require further surgery. Other problems with a Nissen fundoplication can be hyperglycaemia caused by the dumping syndrome,[35] obstruction[36] and ischaemia of the stomach.[37] Paraoesophageal herniation is a particularly dangerous complication.[38]

Boerema gastropexy

Simple fixation of stomach to the abdominal wall, although having the appeal in children of being a relatively minor procedure, is not widely favoured[39] and has a poor long-term prognosis.

Thal fundoplication

Because of problems arising from the Nissen fundoplication, other antireflux operations have found favour with paediatric surgeons.[40] In the Thal operation, the fundus is wrapped anteriorly; it is especially useful in children in whom a stricture has been divided, as the wrap then covers this area.

Boix–Ochoa repair

In children the problem is one of a displaced, incompetent but otherwise healthy lower oesophageal sphincter, as opposed to the adult situation where the sphincter function may be intrinsically damaged. This operation[41] restores anatomical relationships and physiological action to allow restoration of function, unlike the Nissen fundoplication where a new valve is created. The main steps include: restoration of intra-abdominal oesophageal length; tightening the hiatus and fixing the oesophagus to it; restoring the angle of His; and, finally, opening up the fundus by suspending it from the diaphragm (Figure 62.6). This is similar to the procedure described by Watson two years earlier.[42]

Reflux strictures

In most children, reflux-induced oesophageal strictures can be dilated using bougies or Eder-Puestow metal olives. This will restore the oesophagus to a reasonable calibre before surgical correction of the reflux.[43]

The possibility of a reflux-induced stricture should not be forgotten in a child with long-standing swallowing problems or recalcitrant asthma. A paediatrician wondered why a slightly mentally-handicapped boy of 12 who had had asthma for many years failed to grow, hence the investigation. The stricture, although long and tight, was treated successfully by dilatation, followed by repair of his long-standing reflux.

Results

Most children benefit from the surgery, with few operative deaths and remarkably little postoperative morbidity.[44] Reflux occurring after oesophageal atresia repair[45] is more difficult to correct and the Nissen operation only gives good short-term results.[46,47] All have problems of recurrent reflux, but whether

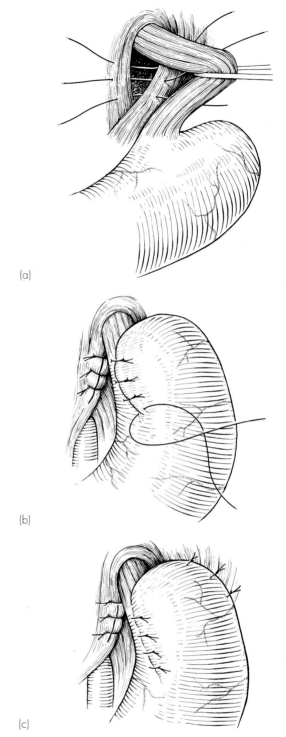

(a)

(b)

(c)

Figure 62.6
Operative details of Boix–Ochoa fundoplasty.

that necessarily requires operative treatment must be determined in individual circumstances. Postoperative investigations are imperative to allow evaluation of the different operations and to determine whether further surgery is needed. Such investigations include pH monitoring and manometry.[48] As yet, the significance of incoordinate peristalsis in infants with continuing problems is unclear.[49]

OTHER OESOPHAGEAL PROBLEMS

Although many conditions occur in both adult and paediatric populations, particular problems either in investigation or treatment of children necessitates some mention of them here. Some conditions are peculiar to childhood.

The investigation of children should be carried out as non-invasively as possible so that the child is not unduly upset. Endoscopy should be performed on a day-case basis, but under general anaesthesia, by an endoscopist accustomed to children and their diseases.[1,2] Paediatric radiology departments are accustomed to dealing with frightened, small children in a happy relaxed atmosphere.

Stricture

Other causes of stricture in children, apart from reflux oesophagitis, need to be assessed by means of radiology but, more importantly, by endoscopy.

Unfortunately, children swallow a variety of corrosive substances which cause oesophagitis and stricture (Figure 62.7), and the possible risk of late malignant change.[3] We offer a service of urgent endoscopy (within 48 hours) to all children with a suspicion of ingestion of a potentially dangerous substance so that an assessment can be made of the extent of any damage to the pharynx, oesophagus or stomach. Immediate medical treatment with steroids and H_2-receptor antagonists may prevent stricture formation and thus the need for dilatations. Once stricture formation is established, treatment is difficult as the tissue is hard and fibrous, increasing the risk of perforation during dilatation. Conservative management of such a perforation is possible in children, with drainage to the area and intravenous alimentation for 2–3 weeks. The residual stricture may require further dilatation or surgery.

Although there is evidence[4] that steroids have little place in preventing strictures, most paediatricians will use them, together with antibiotics.[5] If severe oesophagitis is present,[6] stenting may prevent later stricture formation without the need for steroids. Dilatation can be performed using either tapered plastic bougies, Eder-Puestow metal olives or, more recently developed, balloon dilators.[7] In paediatric practice the use of balloon dilators (Figure 62.8) has replaced the more traditional bougienage because of a reduced incidence of perforation with the former.

Although in most cases it is possible to dilate the stricture,[8] occasionally this is not possible, in which case resection of the stricture should be performed, followed by colon transplant to replace the missing oesophagus. Cervical myotomy may allow the resection and anastomosis of a short stricture.[9]

Surgery of this magnitude leads to a less than satisfactory outcome in many cases: prevention of such strictures is of paramount importance. Education of parents about the importance of labelling bottles of such chemicals and keeping them out of reach of children is very important.

Congenital strictures do occur but are rare and their treatment is the same as for other strictures. Pharyngeal pouches are also rare in children. Disorders of oesophageal motility (without previous surgery, e.g. oesophageal atresia) may necessitate manometry[10] to determine the true nature, and

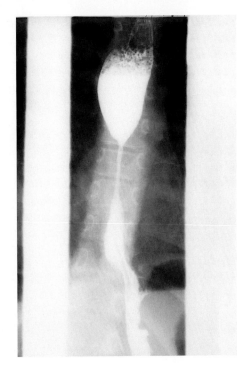

Figure 62.7
Barium study showing long corrosive stricture.

therefore treatment, for the dysphagia. Early dilatations may help with symptomatic relief.[11]

Foreign bodies

As with caustic substances, children swallow a variety of objects, most of which will pass through the intestinal tract without hold-up. However, in babies, an open swallowed safety pin must be closed and removed under anaesthesia, hopefully by means of forceps and manipulation via an endoscope, although open surgery may be necessary. If there has been no previous oesophageal disease or surgery, most objects (usually coins) will pass into the stomach and beyond. The majority should have moved by 24 hours and it is therefore

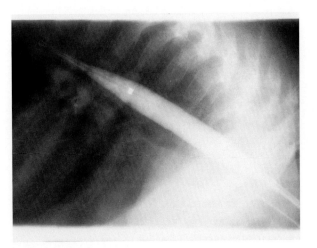

Figure 62.8
Barium study showing stricture dilatation using balloon dilator.

sufficient to keep the child under observation.[12] Problems with an impacted swallowed object may require endoscopy and bougienage[13] or the use of a Foley catheter[14] to help with removal of a difficult object.

The only indication for removal of swallowed foreign bodies is in the case of disc batteries because of the potential for erosion[15] and perforation if they remain static.[16]

Although most foreign bodies, whether in the oesophagus or elsewhere in the gastrointestinal tract, will cause few problems if left in situ, they may lead to occult perforation.[17] Even more difficult is the radiopaque object, especially when there is no clear history of ingestion.[18] Endotracheal tubes carelessly inserted in the newborn may damage the oesophagus extensively.[19] Even if the oesophagus is not perforated, the dislodged tube left in the oesophagus causes problems.[20] Tomography as well as conventional radiology may be necessary to diagnose the trauma[21] and allow conservative treatment, with the addition of a covering gastrostomy.[22]

Achalasia

Achalasia, although less common than in the adult population, does occur in children.[23] The author has treated eight children between 6 and 13 years of age. The classical presentation is with dysphagia and vomiting; but respiratory problems, e.g. late presentation asthma or bronchiectasis, are not uncommon. Some children have been diagnosed as having psychiatric problems, e.g. anorexia nervosa. No child should be so diagnosed without having had radiological studies first. Interestingly, achalasia can occur in families.[24]

An abnormal chest radiograph showing a large dilated oesophagus may suggest achalasia, which can be confirmed by barium meal (Figure 62.9). Endoscopy reveals a large flaccid oesophagus full of recognizable food and debris. It is not surprising that overspill into the lungs occurs, leading to bronchiectasis. Manometry may be useful in the child with a less classical picture, in which the characteristic manometric features (see Chapter 4) enable the diagnosis to be made.[25]

Treatment by forcible pneumatic dilatation, although attractive in children because of being relatively non-invasive, is less likely to offer permanent relief because of their good regenerative powers.[26] For long-term relief of symptoms operative treatment is necessary.[27] A modified Hellér's myotomy, either through the chest[28] or transabdominally,[29] is the preferred treatment. Because of the risk of reflux following myotomy, a loosely wrapped total, or a partial fundoplication procedure may be added.[30] It may take some time (2–3 years) for these often very intense children to improve, despite obvious radiological and manometric improvement. The problem may be more difficult in those children where there is a familial cause and an association with genetic disease, e.g. dysautonomia or glucocorticoid insufficiency.[31] Other operations have been tried,[32] and some surgeons have even resorted to oesophagectomy.[33]

Haematemesis

The main causes of haematemesis in children are nosebleeds and gastro-oesophageal reflux. Mallory–Weiss tears caused by vomit-

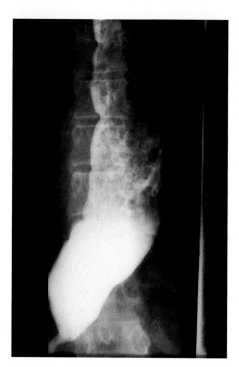

Figure 62.9
Barium study showing achalasia of cardia.

ing are rare in children, as is peptic ulceration with erosion into major vessels. Oesophageal varices, however, do occur in childhood and cause haematemesis, the portal hypertension being caused by portal vein thrombosis, either from umbilical sepsis, congenital portal vein anomalies or cirrhosis due to metabolic causes, such as cystic fibrosis or biliary atresia.[34] The preferred means of treatment of oesophageal varices in children is by endoscopic sclerotherapy[35] with ethanolamine oleate (see Chapter 17). Frequent injection may be necessary to achieve thrombosis of the varices. Endoscopic ligation of varices has been attempted to overcome the problems of ulceration and stenosis which can follow repeated sclerotherapy.[36] Oesophageal transection may need to be performed if such treatment does not prevent massive bleeding. Shunt procedures are rarely performed in the very young as they are associated with a poor prognosis.

Cysts

Mediastinal masses may arise from the bronchi[37] or from the foregut as duplication cysts.[38] Radiological investigation includes a chest radiograph, barium swallow and isotope scanning to determine if there is any connection with the gut. Even extralobular sequestrations of the lung may connect with the upper gastrointestinal tract. Surgery is necessary to prevent respiratory distress.

DIAPHRAGMATIC HERNIA

Congenital diaphragmatic hernia

Embryology

The diaphragm is formed during the eighth week of fetal life from three main areas: (1) the intercostal muscles, (2) the pericardium, giving rise to the central tendon, and (3) the pleuroperitoneal membrane. As a result of either failure of development or failure of fusion of the various parts during the ensuing formation of the diaphragm, a hole allows communication between the abdominal cavity and the thorax (Figure 62.10).[1] These factors account for the different times and different types of presentation. Herniation occurs through the dome of the diaphragm or, more rarely, anteriorly behind the xiphisternum through the foramen of Morgagni. Left-sided herniation is more common, although it can occur on the right side, especially in the older child. Agenesis of the hemidiaphragm can occur,[2] but the prognosis does not differ from that of other types. Pulmonary hypoplasia results, perhaps as result of failure of a feedback mechanism from the kidneys.[3] Bilateral hernias can occur; although they are usually fatal, occasional survivors have been reported.[4] It has been suggested that these defects occur early on in the embryo and not in the fetus.[5]

Pathophysiology

As a result of the presence of a communication between the thorax and the abdomen, the gastrointestinal tract and the cardiovascular and respiratory systems are all affected. If the herniation is a result of failure of fusion, the hole may be only a potential space. As a result there may be no effect for some time, until the child is older[6] when, for example, the overarm movement in swimming opens up the space and allows entry of the bowel into the chest. In most children there is a definite space and the bowel enters the chest some time before birth. To allow this to happen, the bowel must be malfixed and malrotated. Only if the hole in the diaphragm is small is there a risk of a blind loop leading to possible necrosis of the bowel. Such strangulation is more common in the older child who presents late, and may lead to a fatal outcome.[7] The whole of the small bowel, most of the colon, and the stomach and spleen may be in the left thorax (Figure 62.11). Occasionally, mobile kidneys, testes, ovaries and the liver may also be in the chest.

If the thorax is filled with bowel at an early stage of development, the ipsilateral lung cannot develop and remains small

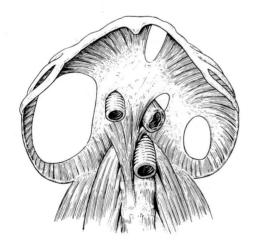

Figure 62.10
Position of defects in diaphragm.

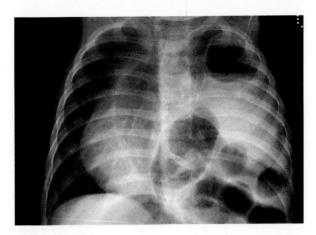

Figure 62.11
Chest radiograph showing late-presenting diaphragmatic hernia with bowel in the chest.

and underweight. Even when the bowel is returned to the peritoneal cavity, the underdeveloped lung does not expand to fill the space. If the hernia develops later, the lung has had time to develop and so will reinflate and behave normally. In the hypoplastic lung, the perfusion : ventilation ratio is abnormal, allowing shunting of blood from right to left via a patent ductus.[8] It is these problems with shunting and ventilation, rather than compression of the lung by herniated bowel, which account for the high morbidity and mortality in babies with diaphragmatic hernia.[9]

If the left side of the chest is filled with bowel, the mediastinum will be shifted to the right, thus reducing the capacity for the right lung, which will also be smaller than normal. Normal lung weights in neonates are about 80 g in total, but in the child with diaphragmatic hernia the ipsilateral lung weighs around 6 g and the contralateral one about 12 g. The total lung weight is therefore abysmally low, at less than 20 g. The venous return of blood to the heart will be compromised due to the mediastinal shift, thus increasing the problems with perfusion.

When the herniation is on the right side (in 35% of these children), usually only the liver enters the chest and there may be delay in the diagnosis.[10]

Experimental work in fetal lambs[11,12] has helped elucidate the pathophysiology and has pointed the way to possible treatment in utero, e.g. by plugging the upper airway to allow fetal lung growth.[13] This is still at the experimental stage, although interuterine repairs have been carried out with varying success.[14-16]

Incidence and presentation

Diaphragmatic hernia occurs in 1 in 4000 livebirths[17] but probably accounts for a further number of stillbirths. Some occur in family groups and in these the chance of a hernia in siblings is 25%.[18] Improvements in obstetric practice have led to an apparent deterioration in survival of these babies because those who previously would have died now survive to be transported earlier.[19] Late presentations occur, most commonly at a few months of age, although some occur years later.[20]

The most common presentation is a cyanosed baby who is difficult to resuscitate at or soon after birth. Such early respiratory problems suggest a poor prognosis. A less common presentation is a chance finding of bowel loops on plain radiography. Intestinal problems with obstruction, necrosis of the bowel[21] and massive gastric enlargement[22,23] are rare, occurring in the older child or adult.[24] Some children (40%) will have associated anomalies, e.g. hypoplastic heart,[25] which will have an impact on the final outcome.

Diagnosis

The diagnosis is easily made by chest radiography as the bowel loops are seen to traverse the area of the diaphragm. Physical examination is rarely helpful because breath sounds can be transmitted easily in the young; the empty scaphoid abdomen may suggest the condition. In the older child, bowel sounds in the chest are obviously diagnostic. A chest radiograph taken very early in the neonatal period may only show a white-out as sufficient air may not have been swallowed to outline the bowel. A lateral view is helpful in differentiation from lung cysts, in that the gas shadows do not enter the abdomen. In the more unusual types of herniation, for example through the foramen of Morgagni, in which obstructed bowel is common, a barium study will be helpful.[26] Antenatal ultrasonography may help decide the type and location of delivery. Hydramnios is frequently present but such early diagnosis does not necessarily result in reduced mortality.[27]

Treatment

The initial treatment depends on whether presentation is early or late. Children or adults presenting late require urgent surgery through an abdominal incision to return the bowel to the abdominal cavity before it becomes ischaemic.[28] The associated malrotation also requires correction (see below). Unless the vascularity of the bowel is already in jeopardy, little in the way of resuscitation is usually required as the lungs are normal. Once the chest is empty the lungs can reinflate. Few postoperative problems are encountered.

In the neonate, however, as already explained, the problem is different and resuscitation is more important than the actual operation. In the past, emergency surgery on these babies did not improve outcome, and even with expert anaesthetic support[29] more than 50% died[30] despite such surgery. The risk to bowel viability is minimal, and a nasogastric tube will help keep it deflated. The main problems are the shunting, poor perfusion and ventilation. Time spent in improving the ventilation[31] by various means[32] to enable correction of hypoxia and acidosis can make all the difference to survival. However, over-enthusiastic ventilation may result in a pneumothorax[33] or interstitial emphysema.[34] It is probable that over-rapid inflation of the hypoplastic lungs contributes to maintenance of the fetal circulation.[35] Some babies initially improve (termed the 'honeymoon period') but later become impossible to ventilate despite various manoeuvres.[36] However, that is not a reason to operate. Vasodilators, e.g. tolazoline, are used to try to reverse the shunting by lowering pulmonary resistance.[37] However,

problems with renal failure can occur and mortality is not necessarily reduced. Recently, inhaled nitric oxide (a selective pulmonary vasodilator) has been used but it is uncertain how long any benefits last.[38]

There is now no place for urgent surgery in the repair of neonatal diaphragmatic hernia.[39] Time spent in resuscitating the baby with positive pressure ventilation and pharmacological support will lead to better prognosis.[40] Pulmonary function tests performed both before and after operation may help predict those children likely to recover.[41]

The period of resuscitation, even up to 72 hours or more, will tide the baby over the 'honeymoon period' and will obviate a false sense of security produced by apparent improvement. In Manchester, delaying surgery has not resulted in death in babies who would otherwise have survived and, in fact, there has been a fall in mortality (Table 62.3).

Table 62.3 Results of treatment of neonatal diaphragmatic hernia in the Neonatal Surgical Unit, St Mary's Hospital

YEAR	NO. OF PATIENTS	MORTALITY
1978	7	3(43)
1982	16	8(50)
1986	19	4(21)
1989	7	1(14.3)
1990	17	6(35)

Values in parentheses are percentages.
Reproduced with permission of Churchill Livingstone, Edinburgh.

A further development has been the use of extracorporeal membrane oxygenation to aid babies with respiratory failure[42,43] during this period of changing ventilation and perfusion.[44,45] Reasonable results can be achieved.[46] In selected cases of severe respiratory failure[47,48] this may be a useful method of maintaining ventilation and circulation until the child's own systems start to work.[49,50] However, its use is exceptional,[51] with only a modest improvement in survival.[52] High-frequency ventilation also has been used to stabilize the patient.[53]

Operative technique

Once the child is stable, surgery can be performed as a second stage in management. As already stated, surgery should be through the abdomen using an upper transverse incision (Figure 62.12). On opening the peritoneum, the abdominal contents should be returned gently from the chest to the abdomen, care being taken not to damage the viscera (Figure 62.12a–c). The liver is often deformed if partially in the chest and may present problems. In the infrequent event of a sac being present, this can be grasped and opened. Usually there is no sac, and the nubbin of hypoplastic lung can be seen in the distant apex of the thorax. The edges of the defect must be delineated (Figure 62.12b) and often the posterior lip is fused with the colon or costal margins. In most circumstances both anterior and posterior lips of the muscle defect can be enlarged to allow

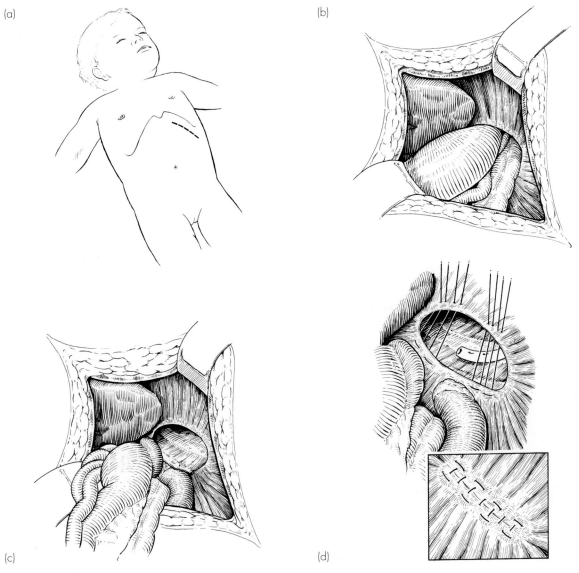

Figure 62.12
Operative details of repair of diaphragmatic hernia. (a) Site of incision; (b) hole in diaphragm with small and large bowel and stomach in chest; (c) contents returned to abdominal cavity and hole in diaphragm visible; (d) closure of hole in diaphragm.

closure of the defect with fairly strong non-adsorbable interrupted sutures (Figure 62.12c), a chest drain normally being left in situ to help allow expansion of the ipsilateral lung.

Sometimes, however, the lips are not well developed or only one can be dissected out. In these cases the anterior abdominal wall musculature or the costal margin can be dissected free to allow closure of a small defect, but this will lead to some chest wall deformity, even pectus excavatum in later life. An artificial patch, such as Gore-tex or Silastic mesh[2,54] has been used but, as with foreign materials used in other circumstances, they may be rejected or become infected. For larger defects, the use of a latissimus dorsi flap works well.[55] Since the muscle has a double blood supply, it can be swung on the lower pedicle into the thorax through an intercostal space and provide adequate cover of the defect.

Very rarely problems may arise on returning the gut to the peritoneum because of insufficient space. In these infants the peritoneal cavity may be enlarged, using a Silastic patch[56] or dura[57] to close the abdominal wall. A right-sided herniation is the only case in which it might be permissible to operate via the thorax to replace the liver. The resulting deformity of the liver can make this manoeuvre very difficult, whether approached from the chest or transabdominally.

Postoperatively, it may take some time to wean the child off the ventilator because of lung dysplasia. Another rare problem is the collection of secretions within the empty left thoracic cavity – sometimes lymph, owing to damage to the thoracic duct.[58] Drainage of the thorax, sometimes for a long period, is all that is necessary for resolution.

Results

If lung function is adequate, results are excellent, with very few sequelae, although some patients may have reduced respiratory capacity due to a persistence of neonatal differences in development.[59] However, despite a successful operation some children will die usually within a few days of surgery, because they have inadequate lung capacity.[60] Postoperative chest radiographs may indicate hypoplasia of the lungs.[61] Improvement in mortality will not come from early diagnosis,[62] although perinatal diagnosis may in time lead to antenatal intervention. However, if diagnosed antenatally the baby can be born at the treatment centre so that transportation problems are avoided. Other major congenital abnormalities account for late deaths.[63] These include major heart conditions, e.g. left ventricular hypoplasia,[64] and other lethal congenital anomalies,[65] making improvement in mortality difficult. Mortality is currently around 35–40%. Recurrence of congenital diaphragmatic hernias can occur as a result of tension on and breakdown of the repair,[66] but there is less chance of bowel problems. Results in the late presenters are good as there is no problem with respiratory function or ventilation difficulty in weaning postoperatively.[67] Even in delayed surgery, there is no change to the neurodevelopment of these children,[68] but there may be problems with hearing, growth and nutrition.[69]

Further improvement in the treatment of congenital diaphragmatic herniation depends on the improvement and further development of fetal surgery. Pulmonary lobar transplantation has been suggested but is not a viable proposition at present.[70]

Traumatic rupture of the diaphragm giving a herniation is rare, despite the fact that 10% of blunt injuries in children involve the chest.[71]

Other variants of diaphragmatic hernia

Another type of herniation is that through the anterior foramen at the ziphisternum – foramen of Morgani. There is a high risk of bowel strangulation because the hole is small and the bowel malfixed so that a blind loop occurs easily.[28] Although barium studies are used to make the diagnosis, the possibility may be raised by the appearance of a bowel shadow overlying the heart. As long as the bowel is not compromised, these children do well.[72]

Eventration of the diaphragm also presents later and is due to a laxity in the muscle so that the diaphragm rises up to allow the bowel still contained within the abdominal cavity to lie in the thorax. Surgery merely consists of plicating the muscle, as for phrenic nerve palsy,[73] with excellent long-term results.[74]

REFERENCES

Introduction

1. Donovan EF. Peri-operative care of the surgical neonate. *Surg Clin North Am* 1985; **65**: 1060.
2. Matthews DE, West KW, Rescorla FJ et al. Peritoneal dialysis in the first 60 days of life. *J Pediatr Surg* 1990; **25**: 110.
3. Winthrop AL, Jones PJH, Schoeller DA et al. Changes in the body composition of the surgical infant in the early postoperative period. *J Pediatr Surg* 1987; **22**: 546.
4. Pierro A, Carnielli V, Filler RM & Heim T. Metabolism of intravenous fat emulsion in the surgical neonate. *J Pediatr Surg* 1989; **24**: 95.
5. Wilkinson AW. Pre- and post-operative treatment. *Recent Advances in Paediatric Surgery*. London: Churchill, 1969; **2**: 40.
6. Najmaldin A, Francis J, Postle A et al. Vitamin K coagulation status in surgical newborns and the risk of bleeding. *J Pediatr Surg* 1993; **28**: 138.
7. Anand KJS & Aynsley-Green A. Measuring the severity of surgical stress in newborn infants. *J Pediatr Surg* 1988; **23**: 297.
8. Huber R, Fuchshuber A & Huber P. Acute peritoneal dialysis in preterm newborns and small infants: surgical management. *J Pediatr Surg* 1994; **29**: 400.
9. Madden NP, Levinsky RJ, Bayston R et al. Surgery, sepsis and non-specific immune function in neonates. *J Pediatr Surg* 1989; **24**: 562.
10. Davenport M & Doig CM. Wound infection in paediatric surgery: a study in 1094 neonates. *J Pediatr Surg* 1993; **28**: 26.
11. Bhattacharyya N, Kosloske AM & Macarthur C. Nosocomial infections in pediatric surgical patients: a study of 608 infants and children. *J Pediatr Surg* 1993; **28**: 338.
12. Chwals WJ, Fernandez ME, Jamie AC & Charles BJ. Relationship of metabolic indexes to postoperative mortality in surgical infants. *J Pediatr Surg* 1993; **28**: 819.
13. Knight PJ & Clatworthy HW. Screening for latent malformations: cost effectiveness in neonates with correctable anomalies. *J Pediatr Surg* 1982; **17**: 123.
14. Hazelbroek FWJ, Tibboel D, Mourik M et al. Withholding and withdrawal of life support from surgical neonates with life-threatening congenital anomalies. *J Pediatr Surg* 1993; **28**: 1093.
15. Kato T, Kanto K, Yoshino H et al. Mental and intellectual development of neonatal surgical children in a long-term follow-up. *J Pediatr Surg* 1993; **28**: 123.
16. Ludman L, Spitz L & Landsdown R. Intellectual development at 3 years of age of children who underwent major neonatal surgery. *J Pediatr Surg* 1993; **28**: 130.
17. Clayton-Smith J, Farndon PA, KcKeown CM & Donnai D. Examination of fetuses after induced abortion for fetal abnormality. *BMJ* 1990; **300**: 295.
18. Joint Study Group on Fetal Abnormalities. Recognition and management of fetal abnormalities. *Arch Dis Child* 1989; **64**: 971.
19. Harrison MR, Langer JC, Adzick NS et al. Correction of congenital diaphragmatic hernia in utero, V. Initial clinical experience. *J Pediatr Surg* 1990; **25**: 47.
20. Longaker MT, Whitby DJ, Adzick NS et al. Studies in fetal wound healing: VI. Second and early third trimester fetal wounds demonstrate rapid collagen deposition without scar formation. *J Pediatr Surg* 1990; **25**: 63.
21. Jennings RW, Adzick NS, Longaker MT et al. New techniques in fetal surgery. *J Pediatr Surg* 1992; **27**: 1329.
22. Hendrickson M, Myre L, Johnson DG et al. Post-operative analgesia in children; a prospective study of intermittent intramuscular injection versus continuous intravenous infusion of morphine. *J Pediatr Surg* 1990; **25**: 185.
23. Dilworth NM & MacKellar A. Pain relief for the pediatric surgical patient. *J Pediatr Surg* 1987; **22**: 264.
24. Rogers DA, Lobe TE & Schropp KT. Evolving uses of laparoscopy in children. *Pediatr Surg* 1992; **72**: 1299.

Oesophageal atresia

1. Kluth D & Habenicht R. The embryology of usual and unusual types of esophageal atresia. *J Pediatr Surg* 1987; **2**: 223.
2. Pritchard JA. Fetal swallowing and amniotic fluid volume. *Obstet Gynecol* 1966; **28**: 606.
3. Bissett WM. Intestinal motor activity in the pre-term infant. In *Disorders of Gastrointestinal Motility in Childhood*. Chichester: Wiley, 1988; 29.
4. Newell SJ. Development of the lower oesophageal sphincter in the pre-term infant. *Disorders of Gastrointestinal Motility in Childhood*. Chichester: Wiley, 1988; 39.
5. Ein SH, Shandling B & Heiss K. Pure esophageal atresia: outlook in the 1990s. *J Pediatr Surg* 1993; **28**: 1147.
6. Pai GK, Pai PK, Kini AU & Rao J. Membranous type of esophageal atresia at the cardiac end of the esophagus: a case report. *J Pediatr Surg* 1987; **22**: 986.
7. Myers NA. Unusual varieties of oesophageal atresia. *Pediatr Surg* 1987; **2**: 195.
8. Touloukian RJ & Keller MS. High proximal pouch esophageal atresia with vertebral rib and sternal anomalies; an additional component of the VATER association. *J Pediatr Surg* 1988; **23**: 76.
9. Ein SH, Shandling B, Wesson D & Filler RM. Esophageal atresia with distal tracheo-esophageal fistula; associated anomalies and prognosis in the 1980s. *J Pediatr Surg* 1989; **24**: 1055.

10. Spitz L, Ali M & Brereton RJ. Combined esophageal and duodenal atresia: experience of 18 patients. *J Pediatr Surg* 1981; **16**: 4.

11. Jolleys A. An examination of the birth weights of babies with some abnormalities of the alimentary tract. *J Pediatr Surg* 1981; **16**: 160.

12. Beasley SW & Myers NA. The diagnosis of congenital tracheo-esophageal fistula. *J Pediatr Surg* 1988; **23**: 415.

13. Spitz L, Kiely E & Brereton RJ. Esophageal atresia; five year experience with 148 cases. *J Pediatr Surg* 1987; **22**: 103.

14. Ohkawa H, Ochi G, Yamazaki S & Sawaguchi S. Clinical experience with a sucking sump catheter in the treatment of esophageal atresia. *J Pediatr Surg* 1989; **24**: 333.

15. Holzki J. Bronchoscopic findings and treatment in congenital tracheo-oesophageal fistula. *Paediatr Anaesth* 1992; **2**: 297.

16. Harrison MR, Weitzman JJ & de Lormier AA. Localization of the aortic arch prior to repair of esophageal atresia. *J Pediatr Surg* 1980; **15**: 312.

17. Carachi R, Stokes KB, Brown TCK & Kent M. Esophageal anastomosis – an experimental model to study the anastomotic lumen and the influence of a transanastomatic tube. *J Pediatr Surg* 1984; **19**: 90.

18. Kullendorff CM, Okmian L & Jonsson N. Technical consideration of experimental esophageal anastomosis. *J Pediatr Surg* 1981; **16**: 979.

19. Lister J. The blood supply of the oesophagus in relation to oesophageal atresia. *Arch Dis Child* 1964; **39**: 131.

20. Louhimo I, Sulamaa M & Suutarinen T. Postoperative intensive care of esophageal atresia patients. *J Pediatr Surg* 1970; **5**: 633.

21. Sillen U, Hagberg S, Rubenson A & Werkmaster K. Management of esophageal atresia; review of 16 years' experience. *J Pediatr Surg* 1988; **23**: 805.

22. Jolley SG, Johnson DG, Roberts CC et al. Patterns of gastro-esophageal reflux in children following repair of esophageal atresia and distal tracheo-esophageal fistula. *J Pediatr Surg* 1980; **15**: 857.

23. Romeo G, Zuccarello B, Proietto F & Romeo O. Disorders of the esophageal motor activity in the esophagus. *J Pediatr Surg* 1987; **2**: 120.

24. Kosloske AM, Jewell PF & Cartwright KC. Crucial bronchoscopic findings in esophageal atresia and tracheo-esophageal fistula. *J Pediatr Surg* 1988; **23**: 466.

25. Applebaum H & Woolley M. Pericardial flap aortopexy for tracheomalacia. *J Pediatr Surg* 1990; **25**: 30.

26. Bianchi A & Greenhaugh S. Repair of long segment tracheomalacia with free autologous cartilage ring grafts. *Pediatr Surg Int* 1992; **7**: 236.

27. Ein SH, Stringer DA, Stephens GA et al. Recurrent tracheo-esophageal fistulas: 17 year review. *J Pediatr Surg* 1983; **18**: 436.

28. Filston HC, Rankin JS & Kirks DR. The diagnosis of primary and recurrent tracheo-esophageal fistulas: value of selective catheterization. *J Pediatr Surg* 1982; **17**: 144.

29. Botham MJ & Coran AG. The use of pericardium for the management of recurrent tracheo-esophageal fistula. *J Pediatr Surg* 1986; **21**: 164.

30. Rangecroft L, Bush GH, Lister J & Irving IM. Endoscopic diathermy obliteration of recurrent tracheo-esophageal fistulae. *J Pediatr Surg* 1984; **19**: 41.

31. Chetcuti P, Myers NA, Phelan PD et al. Chest wall deformity in patients with repair esophageal atresia. *J Pediatr Surg* 1989; **24**: 244.

32. Lividatis A. Cervical circular myotomy in esophageal atresia. *Kinderchirurgie* 1976; **19**: 409.

33. Lindahl H & Louhimo L. Lividatis myotomy in long gap esophageal atresia. *J Pediatr Surg* 1987; **22**: 109.

34. Schneeberger AL, Scott RB, Rubin SZ & Machida H. Esophageal function following Lividitis repair of long gap esophageal atresia. *J Pediatr Surg* 1987; **22**: 779.

35. Otte JB, Gianello P, Wese FX et al. Diverticulum formation after circular myotomy for esophageal atresia. *J Pediatr Surg* 1984; **19**: 68.

36. Schaarschmidt K, Willital GH, Jorch G & Kerreman SJ. Delayed primary reconstruction of an esophageal atresia with distal esophagotracheal fistula in an infant weighing less than 500 g. *J Pediatr Surg* 1992; **27**: 1529.

37. Ito T, Sugito T & Nagaya M. Delayed primary anastomosis in poor risk patients with esophageal atresia associated with tracheo-esophageal fistula. *J Pediatr Surg* **19**: 243.

38. Hight DW, McGowan G, Smith J et al. Atresia of the esophagus. New trends in the management of high risk neonates. *Arch Surg* 1987; **122**: 421.

39. Thomasson BH. Congenital esophageal atresia; mercury bag stretching of the upper pouch in a patient without tracheo-esophageal fistula. *Surgery* 1972; **71**: 661.

40. Fann JI, Hartman GE & Shochat J. 'Waterseal' gastrostomy in the management of premature infants with tracheo-esophageal fistula and pulmonary insufficiency. *J Pediatr Surg* 1988; **23**: 29.

41. Kanowaki H, Nakahira M, Umeda K et al. A method of delayed esophageal anastomosis for high risk congenital atresia with additional intra-abdominal anomalies; transgastric balloon 'Fistulectomy'. *J Pediatr Surg* 1982; **17**: 230.

42. Kimura K, Nishijima E, Tsugawa C & Matsumoto Y. A new approach for the salvage of unsuccessful esophageal atresia repair: a spiral myotomy and delayed definitive surgery. *J Pediatr Surg* 1987; **22**: 981.

43. Hands J & Dudley NE. Comparision between gap-length and Waterson classification as guides to mortality and morbidity after surgery for esophageal atresia. *J Pediatr Surg* 1986; **21**: 404.

44. Pohlson EC, Schaller RT & Tapper D. Improved survival with primary anastomosis in the low birth weight neonate with esophageal atresia and tracheo-esophageal fistula. *J Pediatr Surg* 1988; **23**: 418.

45. Alexander F, Johanningman J & Martin LW. Staged repair improves outcome of high-risk premature infants with esophageal atresia and tracheoesophageal fistula. *J Pediatr Surg* 1993; **28**: 151.

46. Bar-Maor JA, Shoshany D & Sweed Y. Wide gap esophageal atresia; a new method to elongate the upper pouch. *J Pediatr Surg* 1989; **24**: 882.

47. Davenport M & Bianchi A. Early experience with oesophageal flap oesophagoplasty for repair of oesophageal atresia. *Pediatr Surg Int* 1990; **5**: 332.

48. Louhimo I & Lindahl H. Esophageal atresia. Primary results of 500 consecutively treated patients. *J Pediatr Surg* 1983; **18**: 217.

49. Gauderer MWL & Izant RJ. Gastrostomy without laparotomy: a percutaneous endoscopic technique. *J Pediatr Surg* 1980; **15**: 872.

50. Cass D & Auldist A. Oesophageal atresia with proximal tracheo-oesophageal fistula. *J Pediatr Surg* 1987; **2**: 212.

51. Yun KL, Hartman GE & Shochat SJ. Esophageal atresia with triple congenital tracheoesophageal fistulae. *J Pediatr Surg* 1992; **27**: 1527.

52. Myers NA & Egami K. Congenital tracheo-oesophageal fistula. *Pediatr Surg* 1987; **2**: 198.

53. Eckstein HB, Aberdeen E, Chrispin A et al. Tracheo-oesophageal fistula without oesophageal atresia. *Kinderchirurgie* 1979; **9**: 43.

54. Grochowski J, Bilski J, Krysta M & Kobylarz K. H-type tracheoesophageal fistula: diagnosis and treatment. *Surg Child Int* 1993; **1**: 24.

55. Myers NA, Beasley SW, Auldist AW et al. Oesophageal atresia without fistula-anastomosis or replacement? *Pediatr Surg* 1987; **2**: 216.

56. Depaepe A, Dolk H, Lechat MF & EUROCAT Working Group. The epidemiology of tracheo-oesophageal fistula and oesophageal atresia in Europe. *Arch Dis Child* 1993; **68**: 743.

57. Wise WE, Caniano DA & Harmel DP. Tracheo-esophageal anomalies in Waterston C neonates: a 30 year perspective. *J Pediatr Surg* 1987; **22**: 526.

58. Waterston DJ, Bonham Carter RE & Aberdeen E. Congenital tracheo-oesophageal fistula in association with oesophageal fistula. *Lancet* 1963; **ii**: 55.

59. Chetcuti P, Myers NA, Phelan PD & Beasley SW. Adults who survived repair of congenital oesophageal atresia and tracheo-oesophageal fistula. *BMJ* 1988; **297**: 344.

60. Andrassy RJ, Patterson RS & Mahour GH. Long-term nutritional assessment of patients with esophageal atresia and/or tracheo-esophageal fistula. *J Pediatr Surg* 1983; **18**: 431.

61. LeSouef PN, Myers NA & Landau LI. Etiological factors in long-term respiratory function abnormalities following esophageal atresia repair. *J Pediatr Surg* 1987; **22**: 918.

62. Chetcuti P & Phelan PD. Respiratory morbidity after repair of oesophageal atresia and tracheo-oesophageal fistula. *Arch Dis Child* 1993; **68**: 167.

63. Chetcuti P & Phelan PD. Gastrointestinal morbidity and growth after repair of oesophageal atresia and tracheo-oesophageal fistula. *Arch Dis Child* 1993; **68**: 163.

64. Gomez MV. Esophageal replacement in patients under 3 months of age. *J Pediatr Surg* 1994; **29**: 487.

65. Sherman CD & Waterston DJ. Oesophageal reconstruction in children using intrathoracic colon. *Arch Dis Child* 1956; **32**: 11.

66. Waterston DJ. Colonic replacement of esophagus (intra-thoracic). *Surg Clin North Am* 1964; **44**: 1441.

67. Freeman NV & Cass DT. Colon interposition. A modification of the Waterson technique using normal oesophageal route. *J Pediatr Surg* 1982; **17**: 12.

68. Shamberger RC, Eraklis AJ, Kozakewich PW & Hendren WH. Fate of the distal esophageal remnant following esophageal replacement. *J Pediatr Surg* 1988; **23**: 1210.

69. Sieber AM & Sieber WK. Colon transplants as esophageal replacements: cine radiographic and manometric evaluation in children. *Ann Surg* 1968; **168**: 116.

70. Mitchell IM, Goh DW, Roberts KD & Abrams LD. Colon interposition in children. *Br J Surg* 1989; **76**: 681.

71. Carneiro PMR & Doig CMD. Colon interposition for wide gap oesophageal atresia. *East Afr Med J* 1993; **70**: 682.

72. Sutton RK, Sutton H, Ackery DM & Freeman NV. Functional assessment of colonic interposition with ^{99m}Tc-labelled milk. *J Pediatr Surg* 1989; **24**: 874.

73. Adzick NS, Fisher JH, Winter HS et al. Esophageal adenocarcinoma 20 years after esophageal atresia repair. *J Pediatr Surg* 1989; **24**: 741.

74. Martinez-Frontanilla LA, Janik JS & Meagher DP. Colon esophagoplasty in the orthoptic position. *J Pediatr Surg* 1988; **23**: 1215.

75. Heimlich HJ. Esophageal replacement with a reversed gastric tube. *Dis Chest* 1959; **36**: 478.

76. Lindahl H, Louhimo I & Virkola K. Colon interposition or gastric tube? Follow-up study of colon–esophagus and gastric tube–oesophagus patients. *J Pediatr Surg* 1983; **18**: 1858.

77. Atwell JD & Harrison GSM. Observations on the role of esophago-gastrostomy in infancy and childhood with particular reference to the long-term results and operative mortality. *J Pediatr Surg* 1980; **15**: 303.

78. Oesch I & Bettex M. Small bowel esophagoplasty without vascular microanastomosis: a preliminary report. *J Pediatr Surg* 1987; **22**: 877.

79. Hendren WH & Hale RJ. Esophageal atresia treated by electromagnetic bougienage and subsequent repair. *J Pediatr Surg* 1976; **11**: 713.

80. Booss D, Hollwarth M & Sauer H. Endoscopic esophageal anastomosis. *J Pediatr Surg* 1982; **17**: 138.

81. Marshal DG. An alternative to an interposition procedure in esophageal atresia. *J Pediatr Surg* 1987; **22**: 775.

Oesophageal reflux

1. Carre IJ. Clinical significance of gastro-oesophageal reflux. *Arch Dis Child* 1984; **59**: 911.

2. Hrabovsky ER & Mullet MD. Gastro-esophageal reflux and the premature infant. *J Pediatr Surg* 1986; **21**: 583.

3. Jewett TC & Siegel M. Hiatal hernia and gastro-oesophageal reflux. *J Pediatr Gastroenterol Nutr* 1984; **3**: 340.

4. Booth IW. Silent gastro-oesophageal reflux: how much do we miss? *Arch Dis Child* 1992; **67**: 1325.

5. Foglia RP, Fonkalsrud EW, Ament ME et al. Gastro-esophageal fundoplication for the management of chronic pulmonary disease in children. *Am J Surg* 1980; **140**: 72.

6. Ramenofsky ML & Leape LL. Continuous upper esophageal pH monitoring in infants and children with gastroesophageal reflux, pneumonia and apneic spells. *J Pediatr Surg* 1981; **16**: 374.

7. MacFayden UM, Hendry GMA & Simpson H. Gastro-oesophageal reflux in near miss sudden infant death syndrome or suspected recurrent aspiration. *Arch Dis Child* 1983; **58**: 87.

8. Fonkalsrud EW. Gastroesophageal fundoplication for reflux following repair of esophageal atresia. *Arch Surg* 1979; **114**: 48.

9. Koot VCM, Bergmeijer JH, Bos AP & Molenar JC. Incidence and management of gastroesophageal reflux after repair of congenital diaphragmatic hernia. *J Pediatr Surg* 1993; **28**: 48.

10. Kumar D, Brereton RJ, Spitz L & Hall CM. Gastroesophageal reflux and intestinal malrotation in children. *Br J Surg* 1988; **75**: 533.

11. Meyers WF, Roberts CC, Johnson DG & Herbst JJ. Value of tests for evaluation of gastroesophageal reflux in children. *J Pediatr Surg* 1985; **20**: 515.

12. Leape LL, Bhjan I & Ramenofsky ML. Esophageal biopsy in the diagnosis of reflux esophagitis. *J Pediatr Surg* 1981; **16**: 379.

13. Zona JZ, Sty JR & Glicklich M. Simplified radio-isotope technique for assessing gastroesophageal reflux in children. *J Pediatr Surg* 1981; **16**: 114.

14. Varty K, Evans D & Kapila L. Paediatric gastro-oesophageal reflux: prognostic indicators from pH monitoring. *Gut* 1993; **34**: 1478.

15. Jolley SG, Tunnell WP, Carson JA et al. The accuracy of abbreviated esophageal monitoring in children. *J Pediatr Surg* 1984; **19**: 848.

16. Evans DF, Haynes J, Jones JA et al. Ambulatory esophageal pH monitoring in children as indicator for surgery. *J Pediatr Surg* 1986; **21**: 221.

17. Arana J & Tovar JA. Motor efficiency of the refluxing esophagus in basal conditions and after acid challenge. *J Pediatr Surg* 1989; **24**: 1049.

18. Haase G, Ross MN, Gance-Cleveland B & Kolack KE. Extended four-channel esophageal pH monitoring: the importance of acid reflux patterns at the middle and proximal levels. *J Pediatr Surg* 1988; **23**: 32.

19. Rode H, Stunden RJ, Millar AJW & Cwyes S. Esophageal pH assessment of gastroesophageal reflux in 18 patients and the effect of two prokinetic agents: cisapride and metoclopromide. *J Pediatr Surg* 1987; **22**: 931.

20. Jewett TC & Waterson DJ. Surgical management of hiatal hernia in children. *J Pediatr Surg* 1975; **10**: 757.

21. Fonkalsrud EW, Foglia RP, Ament ME et al. Operative treatment for the gastroesophageal reflux in children. *J Pediatr Surg* 1989; **24**: 525.

22. Johnson DG, Jolley SG, Herbst JJ & Cordell LJ. Surgical selection of infants with gastroesophageal reflux. *J Pediatr Surg* 1981; **16**: 587.

23. Spitz L, Roth K, Kiely EM et al. Operation for gastro-oesophageal reflux associated with severe mental retardation. *Arch Dis Child* 1993; **68**: 347.

24. Grunow JE, Al-Hafidh A-S & Tunnell WP. Gastroesophageal reflux following percutaneous endoscopic gastrostomy in children. *J Pediatr Surg* 1989; **24**: 42.

25. Spitz L. Surgical treatment of gastroesophageal reflux in severely mentally retarded children. *J R Soc Med* 1982; **75**: 525.

26. Druker DEM, Michna BA, Krummel TM et al. Transthoracic Nissen fundoplication for gastroesophageal reflux in patients with severe kypho-rota-scoliosis. *J Pediatr Surg* 1989; **24**: 46.

27. Fonkalsrud EW, Ament ME, Byrne WJ & Rachlefsky GS. Gastroesophageal fundoplication for the management of reflux in infants and children. *J Thorac Cardiovasc Surg* 1978; **76**: 655.

28. Kim SH, Hendren WH & Donahoe PK. Gastroesophageal reflux and hiatus hernia in children: experience with 70 cases. *J Pediatr Surg* 1980; **15**: 443.

29. Opie JC, Chaye H & Fraser GC. Fundoplication and pediatric esophageal manometry: actuarial analysis over 7 years. *J Pediatr Surg* 1987; **22**: 935.

30. Noble HGS, Christie DL & Cahill JL. Follow-up on patients undergoing Nissen fundoplication utilizing intra-operative manometry. *J Pediatr Surg* 1982; **17**: 490.

31. Campbell JR, Gilchrist BF & Harrison MW. Pyloroplasty in association with Nissen fundoplication in children with neurological disorders. *J Pediatr Surg* 1989; **24**: 375.

32. Stringle G, Delgado M, Guertin L et al. Gastrostomy and Nissen fundoplication in neurologically impaired children. *J Pediatr Surg* 1989; **24**: 1044.

33. Lobe T, Schropp KP & Lunsford K. Laparoscopic Nissen fundoplication in childhood. *J Pediatr Surg* 1993; **28**: 358.

34. Jolley SG, Tunell WP, Leonard JC & Smith EI. Gastric emptying in children with gastroesophageal reflux. II. The relationship to retching symptoms following anti reflux. *J Pediatr Surg* 1987; **22**: 927.

35. Hirsig J, Baals H, Tuchschmid P et al. Dumping syndrome following Nissen's fundoplication: a cause for refusal to feed. *J Pediatr Surg* 1984; **19**: 155.

36. Wilkins BM & Spitz L. Adhesion obstruction following Nissen fundoplication in children. *Br J Surg* 1987; **74**: 777.

37. Glick PL, Harrison MR, Adzick NS et al. Gastric infarction secondary to small bowel obstruction: a preventable complication after Nissen fundoplication. *J Pediatr Surg* 1987; **22**: 941.

38. Alrabeeah A, Giacomantonio M & Gillis DA. Paraesophageal hernia after Nissen fundoplication: a real complication in pediatric patients. *J Pediatr Surg* 1988; **23**: 766.

39. De Laet M & Spitz L. A comparison of Nissen fundoplication and Boerema gastropexy in the surgical treatment of gastroesophageal reflux in children. *J Pediatr Surg* 1983; **70**: 125.

40. Ashcraft KW, Holder TM, Amoury RA et al. The Thal fundoplication for gastroesophageal reflux. *J Pediatr Surg* 1984; **19**: 480.

41. Boix-Ochoa J. Address of honoured guest: the physiological approach to the management of gastroesophageal reflux. *J Pediatr Surg* 1986; **21**: 1032.

42. Watson A. A clinical and pathophysiological study of a simple and effective operation for the correction of gastrooesophageal reflux. *Br J Surg* 1984; **71**: 991.

43. Bremner CG. Current management of benign oesophageal strictures. *J R Coll Surg Edinb* 1989; **34**: 297.

44. Bettex M & Oesch I. The hiatus hernia saga. Ups and downs in gastroesophageal reflux: past, present and future prospects. *J Pediatr Surg* 1983; **18**: 670.

45. Kazerooni NL, VanCamp J, Hirschl RB et al. Fundoplication in 160 children under 2 years of age. *J Pediatr Surg* 1994; **29**: 677.

46. Lindahl H, Rintala R & Louhimo I. Failure of the Nissen fundoplication to control gastroesophageal reflux in esophageal atresia patients. *J Pediatr Surg* 1989; **24**: 985.

47. Wheatley MJ, Coran AG & Wesley JR. Efficacy of the Nissen fundoplication in the management of gastroesophageal reflux following esophageal atresia repair. *J Pediatr Surg* 1993; **28**: 53.

48. Jolley SG, Tunnell WP, Hoelzer DJ & Smith EI. Intra-operative esophageal manometry and early post-operative esophageal pH monitoring in children. *J Pediatr Surg* 1989; **24**: 336.

49. Arana J, Tovar JA & Garay J. Abnormal pre-operative and post-operative esophageal peristalsis in gastroesophageal reflux. *J Pediatr Surg* 1986; **21**: 711.

Other oesophageal problems

1. Doig CM & Miller V. Upper gastrointestinal endoscopy. *Kinderchirurgie* 1985; Congress vol. 61.

2. Caulfield M, Wyllie R, Sivak MV et al. Upper gastrointestinal tract endoscopy in the pediatric patient. *J Pediatr* 1989; **115**: 339.

3. Benirschk K. Time bomb of Lye. *Am J Dis Child* 1981; **135**: 17.

4. Hawkins DB, Demeter MJ & Barnett TE. Caustic ingestion: controversies in management. Review of 214 cases. *Laryngoscope* 1980; **90**: 98.

5. Adam JS & Birck HG. Pediatric caustic ingestion. *Ann Otol Rhinol Laryngol* 1982; **91**: 656.

6. Wijburg FA, Heymans HSA & Urbanus NAM. Caustic esophageal lesions in childhood: prevention of stricture formation. *J Pediatr Surg* 1989; **24**: 171.

7. Sato Y, Frey YY, Smith WL et al. Balloon dilatation of oesophageal stenosis in children. *AJR* 1988; **150**: 639.

8. Gandhi RP, Cooper A & Barlow BAS. Successful management of oesophageal strictures without resection or replacement. *J Pediatr Surg* 1988; **23**: 371.

9. Al-Samaarai AYI. Circular myotomy for esophageal stricture. *J Pediatr Surg* 1988; **23**: 371.

10. Greenholz SK, Hall RJ, Sondheimer JM et al. Manometric and pH consequence of esophageal endosclerosis in children. *J Pediatr Surg* 1988; **23**: 38.

11. Dinari G, Danziger Y, Mimouni M et al. Cricopharyngeal dysfunction in childhood: treatment by dilatations. *J Pediatr Gastroenterol Nutr* 1987; **6**: 212.

12. O'Neill JA, Holcomb GW & Neblett WW. Management of tracheobronchial and esophageal foreign bodies in childhood. *J Pediatr Surg* 1983; **18**: 475.

13. Bonadio WA, Jonza JZ, Glicklich M & Cohen R. Esophageal bougienage technique for coin ingestion in children. *J Pediatr Surg* 1988; **23**: 917.

14. Kelley JE, Leech MH & Carr MG. A safe and cost-effective protocol for the management of esophageal coins in children. *J Pediatr Surg* 1993; **28**: 898.

15. Sigalet D & Lees G. Tracheoesophageal injury secondary to disc battery ingestion. *J Pediatr Surg* 1988; **23**: 996.

16. Gordon AC & Gough MH. Oesophageal perforation after button battery ingestion. *Ann R Coll Surg Engl* 1993; **75**: 362.

17. Janik JS, Bailey WC & Burrington JD. Occult coin perforation of the esophagus. *J Pediatr Surg* 1986; **21**: 794.

18. Fernandes ET, Hollabaugh RS & Boulden T. Mediastinal mass and radiolucent esophageal foreign body. *J Pediatr Surg* 1989; **24**: 1135.

19. Krasna IH, Rosenfeld D, Benjamin BG et al. Esophageal perforation in the neonate: an emerging problem in the newborn nursery. *J Pediatr Surg* 1987; **22**: 784.

20. Dickson JAS & Fraser GC. 'Swallowed' endotracheal tube: a new neonatal emergency. *BMJ* 1967; **2**: 811.

21. Ben-Ami T, Rozenson J, Yahav J et al. Computed tomography in children with esophageal and airway trauma. *J Pediatr Surg* 1988; **23**: 919.

22. Molitt DL, Schullinger JN & Santulli TV. Selective management of iatrogenic esophageal perforation in the newborn. *J Pediatr Surg* 1981; **16**: 989.

23. Mayberry JF & Mayell M. Epidemiological study of achalasia in children. *Gut* 1988; **29**: 90.

24. Freiling T, Berges W, Borchard F et al. Family occurrence of achalasia and diffuse spasm of the oesophagus. *Gut* 1988; **29**: 1595.

25. Berquist WE, Byrne WJ, Ament ME et al. Achalasia: diagnosis, management and clinical course in 16 children. *Pediatrics* 1983; **71**: 798.

26. Nakayama DK, Shorter NA, Boyle T et al. Pneumatic dilatation and operative treatment of achalasia in children. *J Pediatr Surg* 1987; **22**: 619.

27. Vane DW, Crosby K, West K & Grosfled JL. Late results following esophagomyotomy in children with achalasia. *J Pediatr Surg* 1988; **23**: 515.

28. Lemmer JH, Coran AG, Wesley JR et al. Achalasia in children: treatment by anterior esophageal myotomy (modified Heller operation). *J Pediatr Surg* 1985; **20**: 333.

29. Ballantine TVN, Fitzgerald JF & Grosfeld JL. Transabdominal esophagomyotomy for achalasia in children. *J Pediatr Surg* 1980; **15**: 457.

30. Emblem R, Stringer MD, Hall CM & Spitz L. Current results of surgery for achalasia of the cardia. *Arch Dis Child* 1993; **68**: 749.

31. Nihoul-Fekete C, Bawab S, Lortar-Jacob S et al. Achalasia of the esophagus in childhood: surgical treatment in 35 cases with special reference to familial cases and glucocorticoid deficiency association. *J Pediatr Surg* 1989; **24**: 1060.

32. Allen KB & Ricketts RR. Surgery for achalasia of the cardia in children: the Dor–Gavriliu procedure. *J Pediatr Surg* 1992; **27**: 1418.

33. Gerard UU, Beale PG & Davies MRQ. Oesophagectomy for achalasia in a child. *Pediatr Surg Int* 1993; **8**: 335.

34. Stringer MD, Howard ER & Mowat AP. Endoscopic sclerotherapy in the management of esophageal varices in 61 children with biliary atresia. *J Pediatr Surg* 1989; **24**: 438.

35. Howard ER, Stringer MD & Mowat AP. Assessment of injection sclerotherapy in the management of 152 children with oesophageal varices. *Br J Surg* 1988; **75**: 404.

36. Hall RJ, Lilly JR & Steigmann GV. Endoscopic esophageal varix ligation: technique and preliminary results in children. *J Pediatr Surg* 1988; **23**: 1222.

37. Bagwell CE & Schiffman RJ. Subcutaneous bronchogenic cysts. *J Pediatr Surg* 1988; **23**: 993.

38. Fowler CL, Pokorny WJ, Wagner ML & Kessler MS. Review of bronchopulmonary foregut malformations. *J Pediatr Surg* 1988; **23**: 793.

Diaphragmatic hernia

1. Cullen ML, Klein MD & Philippart AI. Congenital diaphragmatic hernia. *Surg Clin North Am* 1985; **65**: 1115.

2. Valente A & Brereton RJ. Unilateral agenesis of the diaphragm. *J Pediatr Surg* 1987; **22**: 848.

3. Hosoda Y, Rossman JE & Glick PL. Pathophysiology of congenital diaphragmatic hernia. IV. Renal hyperplasia is associated with pulmonary hypoplasia. *J Pediatr Surg* 1993; **28**: 464.

4. Bruce J & Doig CM. Survival in bilateral congenital diaphragmatic hernias. *J R Coll Surg Edin* 1990; **35**: 389.

5. Kluth D, Tenbrink R, von Ekesparre M et al. The natural history of congenital diaphragmatic hernia and pulmonary hypoplasia in the embryo. *J Pediatr Surg* 1993; **28**: 356.

6. Wiseman NE & MacPherson RI. 'Acquired' congenital diaphragmatic hernia. *J Pediatr Surg* 1977; **12**: 657.

7. Berman L, Stringer D, Ein SH & Shandling B. The late presenting pediatric Bochdalek hernia: a 20 year review. *J Pediatr Surg* 1988; **12**: 735.

8. Harrison MR & de Lorimer AA. Congenital diaphragmatic hernia. *Surg Clin North Am* 1981; **61**: 1023.

9. Collins DL, Pomerance JJ, Travis KW et al. A new approach to congenital postero-lateral diaphragmatic hernia. *J Pediatr Surg* 1977; **12**: 149.

10. Khwaja MS, Al-Arfaj AL & Dawoodu AH. Congenital right-sided diaphragmatic hernia: a heterogeneous lesion. *J R Coll Surg Edinb* 1988; **34**: 219.

11. Pringle KC, Turner JW, Schofield JC & Soper RT. Creation and repair of diaphragmatic hernia in the fetal lamb: lung development and morphology. *J Pediatr Surg* 1984; **19**: 131.

12. Soper RT, Pringle KC & Scofield JC. Creation and repair of diaphragmatic hernia in the fetal lamb: techniques and survival. *J Pediatr Surg* 1984; **19**: 33.

13. Hedrick MH, Estes JM, Sullivan KM et al. Plug the lung until it grows (PLUG): a new method to treat congenital diaphragmatic hernia in utero. *J Pediatr Surg* 1994; **29**: 612.

14. Harrison MR, Langer JC, Adzick NS et al. Correction of congenital diaphragmatic hernia in utero. Initial clinical experience. *J Pediatr Surg* 1990; **25**: 47.

15. Harrison MR, Adzick NS, Flake AW et al. Correction of congenital diaphragmatic hernia in utero. VI. Hard-earned lessons. *J Pediatr Surg* 1993; **28**: 1411.

16. Harrison MR, Adzick NS, Flake AW & Jennings RW. The CDH two-step: a dance of necessity. *J Pediatr Surg* 1993; **28**: 813.

17. Butler N & Claireaux AE. Congenital diaphragmatic hernia. *Lancet* 1962; **i**: 659.

18. Hitch DC, Carson JA, Smith EI et al. Familial congenital diaphragmatic hernia is an autosomal recessive variant. *J Pediatr Surg* 1989; **24**: 860.

19. Simson JNL & Eckstein HB. Congenital diaphragmatic hernia: a 20 year experience. *Br J Surg* 1985; **72**: 733.

20. Reed MWR, de Silva PHPD, Mostafa SM & Collins FJ. Diaphragmatic hernia in pregnancy. *Br J Surg* 1987; **74**: 435.

21. Woolley MM. Delayed appearance of a left posterolateral diaphragmatic hernia resulting in significant small bowel necrosis. *J Pediatr Surg* 1977; **12**: 673.

22. Brill PW, Gershwind ME & Kransa IH. Massive gastric enlargement with delayed presentation of congenital diaphragmatic hernia: report of three cases and review of the literature. *J Pediatr Surg* 1977; **12**: 667.

23. Grant H, Rode H & Cywes S. Potential danger of 'trial of life' approach to congenital diaphragmatic hernia. *J. Pediatr Surg* 1994; **29**: 399.

24. Sutton PP & Longrigg N. Strangulated Bochdalek hernia in an adult. *J R Coll Surg Edinb* 1982; **27**: 58.

25. Fauza DO & Wilson JM. Congenital diaphragmatic hernia and associated anomalies: their incidence, identification, and impact on prognosis. *J Pediatr Surg* 1994; **29**: 1113.

26. Pokorny WJ, McGill CW & Harberg FJ. Morgagni hernias during infancy: presentation and associated anomalies. *J Pediatr Surg* 1984; **19**: 394.

27. Adzick NS, Harrison MR, Glick PL et al. Diaphragmatic hernia in the fetus: pre-natal diagnosis and outcome in 94 cases. *J Pediatr Surg* 1985; **20**: 357.

28. Manning PB, Murphy JP, Raynor SC & Ashcraft KW. Congenital diaphragmatic hernia presenting due to gastrointestinal complications. *J Pediatr Surg* 1992; **27**: 1225.

29. Marshall A & Sumner E. Improved prognosis in congenital diaphragmatic hernia: experience of 62 cases over 2 year period. *J R Soc Med* 1982; **75**: 607.

30. Johnson DG, Deaner RM & Koop CE. Diaphragmatic hernia in infancy: factors affecting the mortality rate. *Surgery* 1967; **62**: 1082.

31. Reynolds M, Luck SR & Lappen R. The 'critical' neonate with diaphragmatic hernia: a 21 year perspective. *J Pediatr Surg* 1984; **19**: 364.

32. Vacanti JP, Crone RK, Murphy JD et al. The pulmonary hemodynamic response to peri-operative anaesthesia in the treatment of high risk infants with congenital diaphragmatic hernia. *J Pediatr Surg* 1984; **19**: 672.

33. Gibson C & Fonklasrud EW. Iatrogenic pneumothorax and mortality in congenital diaphragmatic hernia. *J Pediatr Surg* 1983; **18**: 555.

34. Srouji MN, Buck B & Downes JJ. Congenital diaphragmatic hernia: deleterious effects of pulmonary interstitial emphysema and tension extra-pulmonary air. *J Pediatr Surg* 1981; **16**: 45.

35. Cloutier R, Fournier L & Levasseur L. Reversion to fetal circulation in congenital diaphragmatic hernia: a preventable post-operative complication. *J Pediatr Surg* 1983; **18**: 551.

36. Bohn DJ, James I, Filler RM et al. The relationship between $Paco_2$ and ventilation parameters in predicting survival in congenital diaphragmatic hernia. *J Pediatr Surg* 1984; **19**: 666.

37. Sumner E & Frank JD. Tolazoline in the treatment of congenital diaphragmatic hernias. *Arch Dis Child* 1981; **56**: 350.

38. Shah N, Jacob T, Exler R et al. Inhaled nitric oxide in congenital diaphragmatic hernia. *J Pediatr Surg* 1994; **29**: 1010.

39. Langer JC, Filler RM, Bohn DJ et al. Timing of surgery for congenital diaphragmatic hernia: is emergency operation necessary? *J Pediatr Surg* 1988; **23**: 731.

40. Ein SH, Barker G, Olley P et al. The pharmacological treatment of newborn diaphragmatic hernia – a 2 year evaluation. *J Pediatr Surg* 1980; **15**: 384.

41. Tracy TF, Bailey PV, Sadiq F et al. Predictive capabilities of preoperative and postoperative pulmonary function tests in delayed repair of congenital diaphragmatic hernia. *J Pediatr Surg* 1994; **29**: 265.

42. O'Rourke PP, Stolar CJH, Zwischenberger JB et al. Extracorporeal membrane oxygenation: support for overwhelming pulmonary failure in the pediatric population. Collective experience from the extracorporeal life support organization. *J Pediatr Surg* 1993; **28**: 523.

43. Hirschl RB, Schumacher RE, Snedecor SN et al. The efficacy of extracorporeal life support in premature and low birth weight newborns. *J Pediatr Surg* 1993; **28**: 1336.

44. Stolar C, Dillon P & Reyes C. Selective use of extra-corporeal membrane oxygenation in the management of congenital diaphragmatic hernia. *J Pediatr Surg* 1988; **23**: 207.

45. Johnston PW, Bashner B, Liberman R et al. Clinical use of extra-corporeal membrane oxygenation in the treatment of persistent pulmonary hypertension following surgical repair of congenital diaphragmatic hernia. *J Pediatr Surg* 1988; **23**: 908.

46. Adolph V, Ekelund C, Smith C et al. Developmental outcome of neonates treated with extra-corporeal membrane oxygenation. *J Pediatr Surg* 1990; **24**: 43.

47. Breaux CW, Rouse TM, Cain WS & Georgeson KE. Congenital diaphragmatic hernia in an era of delayed repair after medical and/or extracorporeal membrane oxygenation stabilization; a prognostic and management classification. *J Pediatr Surg* 1992; **27**: 1192.

48. vd Staak FHJ, Thiesbrummel A, de Haan AFJ et al. Do we use the right entry criteria for extracorporeal membrane oxygenation in congenital diaphragmatic hernia? *J Pediatr Surg* 1993; **28**: 1003.

49. Minifee PK, Daeschner CW, Griffin MP et al. Decreasing blood donor exposure in neonates on extra-corporeal membrane oxygenation. *J Pediatr Surg* 1990; **25**: 38.

50. Stolar CJH & Dillon PW. Modification of cardiopulmonary hemodynamics and vasoactive mediators by extracorporeal membrane oxygenation in newborn lambs. *J Pediatr Surg* 1990; **25**: 33.

51. Cloutier R. Congenital diaphragmatic hernia and extra-corporeal membrane oxygenation. *Int J Pediatr Surg Sci* 1992; **6**: 51.

52. Steimle CN, Meric F, Hirschl RB et al. Effect of extra-corporeal life support on survival when applied to all patients with congenital diaphragmatic hernia. *J Pediatr Surg* 1994; **29**: 997.

53. Tamura M, Tsuchida Y, Kawano T et al. Piston pump type high frequency oscillatory ventilation for neonates with congenital diaphragmatic hernia: a new protocol. *J Pediatr Surg* 1988; **23**: 478.

54. Geisler F, Gotlieb A & Fried D. Agenesis of the right diaphragm repaired with Marlex. *J Pediatr Surg* 1977; **12**: 587.

55. Bianchi A, Doig CM & Cohen SJ. The reverse lattisimus dorsi flap for congenital diaphragmatic hernia repair. *J Pediatr Surg* 1983; **18**: 560.

56. Michalevicz D & Chaimoff C. Use of a silastic sheet for widening the abdominal cavity in the surgical treatment of diaphragmatic hernia. *J Pediatr Surg* 1989; **24**: 265.

57. Hutson JM & Azmy AF. Preserved dura and pericardium for closure of large abdominal wall and diaphragmatic hernia defects in children. *Ann R Coll Surg Engl* 1985; **67**: 107.

58. Mercer S. Factor involved in chylothorax following repair of congenital postero-lateral diaphragmatic hernia. *J Pediatr Surg* 1986; **21**: 809.

59. Nielsen OH & Henriksen O. Regional lung function after repair of congenital diaphragmatic hernia. *Kinderchirurgie* 1980; **29**: 9.

60. Nielsen OH & Jorgensen AF. Congenital postero-lateral diaphragmatic hernia factors affecting survival. *Kinderchirurgie* 1978; **24**: 201.

61. Cloutier R, Allard V, Fournier L et al. Estimation of lungs' hypoplasia on postoperative chest X-rays in congenital diaphragmatic hernia. *J Pediatr Surg* 1993; **28**: 1086.

62. Adzick NS, Vacanti JP, Lillehei CW et al. Fetal diaphragmatic hernia: ultrasound diagnosis and clinical outcome in 38 cases. *J Pediatr Surg* 1989; **24**: 654.

63. Benjamin DR, Juul S & Siebert JR. Congenital posterolateral diaphragmatic hernia: associated malformations. *J Pediatr Surg* 1988; **23**: 899.

64. Siebert JR, Haas JE & Beckwith JB. Left ventricular hypoplasia in congenital diaphragmatic hernia. *J Pediatr Surg* 1984; **19**: 567.

65. Puri P & Gorman F. Lethal non-pulmonary anomalies associated with congenital diaphragmatic hernia: implications for early intra-uterine surgery. *J Pediatr Surg* 1984; **19**: 29.

66. Cohen D & Reid IS. Recurrent diaphragmatic hernia. *J Pediatr Surg* 1981; **16**: 42.

67. McCue J, Ball A, Brereton RJ et al. Congenital diaphragmatic hernia in older children. *J R Coll Surg Edinb* 1985; **30**: 305.

68. Davenport M, Rivlin E, D'Souza SW & Bianchi A. Delayed surgery for congenital diaphragmatic hernia: neuro-development outcome in later childhood. *Arch Dis Child* 1992; **67**: 1353.

69. Lund DP, Mitchell J, Kharasch V et al. Congenital diaphragmatic hernia: the hidden morbidity. *J Pediatr Surg* 1994; **29**: 258.

70. Crombleholme TM, Adzick NS, Hardy K et al. Pulmonary lobar transplantation in neonatal swine: a model for treatment of congenital diaphragmatic hernia. *J Pediatr Surg* 1990; **25**: 11.

71. West K, Weber TR & Grosfeld JL. Traumatic diaphragmatic hernia in childhood. *J Pediatr Surg* 1981; **16**: 392.

72. Berman L, Stringer D, Ein SH & Shandling B. The late presenting pediatric Morgagni hernia: a benign condition. *J Pediatr Surg* 1989; **24**: 970.

73. Langer JC, Filler RM, Coles J & Edmonds JF. Plication of the diaphragm for infants and young children with phrenic nerve palsy. *J Pediatr Surg* 1988; **23**: 749.

74. Kizilcan F, Tanyel FC, Hicsonmez A & Buyukpamukcu N. The long-term results of diaphragmatic plication. *J Pediatr Surg* 1993; **28**: 42.

STOMACH AND DUODENUM

STOMACH

Physiology

Little is known about the acid state of the neonatal or premature stomach. Basal acid output is low at birth and thought to be even lower in the preterm infant[1-3] but increases to adult level at one month.[4] Perhaps enteral feeding stimulates the maintenance of gastric secretions and motility.[5,6] In association with other host defence mechanisms this acid acts as a barrier in the stomach to the entry of unwanted substances and helps digestion. There is doubt as to normal levels of gastrin in newborn infants[7,8] and the very sick preterm infant[9] although levels in the older child[10] are known. In the very preterm baby delay in gastric emptying can lead to abdominal distension and difficulty in feeding, especially if there is a high calorific load.[11] Such intolerance decreases with increasing gestational age but if there is morbidity in the neonate this tolerance reduces. Also, with increasing gestational age there is an increase in gastric antral pressure which affects the power of antral activity and degree of motor coordination.[12]

CONGENITAL ABNORMALITIES

Pyloric atresia

This is an exceedingly uncommon congenital abnormality, presenting in the newborn period with gross distension of the stomach and complete absence of distal gas.[1,2] It is often associated with other abnormalities, especially of the dermis.[3-7] Treatment involves anastomosis between bowel, duodenum and stomach in a partial gastrectomy type operation. Another rarity is a double pylorus.[8,9] Antral webs also occur, presenting sometimes in the older child and mimicking pyloric stenosis.[10,11] Treatment is by pyloroplasty and gastrostomy. If only partial there may be delay in the diagnosis, even into adult life.[12]

Microgastria

Impairment of normal development of the foregut can lead very rarely to microgastria, often associated with other defects like malrotation, asplenia and pulmonary abnormalities. It must not be mistaken for a small stomach due to a hiatus hernia with most of the stomach in the chest. Death due to malnutrition has been the outcome but recently a few patients have survived by means of a double lumen Roux-en-Y loop creating an artificial food reservoir (Hunt–Lawrence pouch).[13]

Other congenital abnormalities

A gastric duplication may cause obstruction,[14] similar to the signs found in an acute abdomen.[15] A parasitic twin,[16] an extremely rare occurrence, or even the liver[17] can also obstruct the gastric outlet.

Congenital hypertrophic pyloric stenosis

The thickened circular pyloric muscle obstructs the outlet of the stomach, causing projectile vomiting and failure to thrive. The exact aetiology is unknown. Suggestions of a neuropathy[18-20]

have yet to be proved. Gastrin has also been implicated[21,22] but gastrin levels and responses are normal[23,24] although indirect effects may still be possible.[25] Differing results have been obtained by workers seeking to elucidate the cause by investigating prostaglandins,[26] basal acid secretion[27] and immunochemistry.[28] Pyloric stenosis, not of the congenital type, has occurred after transpyloric tube feeding.[29]

The incidence is generally reported as 5 per 1000 live births with an increased incidence in siblings of up to 12 times. this strong hereditary influence suggests an environmental or genetic cause.[30] Thus it may occur especially in the first male child of parents who have had the problem in infancy, especially if the mother had the same diagnosis. It is less common in small for dates babies.[31] Hypertrophic pyloric stenosis is very rare in Chinese, Indians and Africans.

Associated abnormalities of the genitourinary tract occur in 20% of such children[32] although these do not necessarily require treatment. There appears to be an increased incidence in children who have survived oesophageal atresia surgery[33,34] as well as an association with other gastrointestinal abnormalities.[35,36]

Presentation and diagnosis

The usual presentation is with forceful projectile vomiting, the vomitus often landing some feet away from the mother and child. Vomitus may be blood stained due to gastritis,[37] but does not contain bile. It may, however, be yellowish in colour due to the digestive process in the stomach. Although vomiting after feeds the baby will be keen to feed. Left undiagnosed the child may become marasmic developing metabolic alkalosis and hypochloraemia.[38]

A clinical diagnosis can be made by observing peristaltic waves crossing the upper abdomen with a test feed to confirm the pyloric 'tumour' by palpation. However, if this is small and under the liver it may not be possible to palpate. Ultrasonography[39,40] and a barium meal can aid the diagnosis. Such investigations should be performed in all vomiting children if and when a clear diagnosis cannot be made;[41] it will delineate pyloric stenosis but will also show oesophageal reflux, duodenal stenosis and malrotation – other major surgical causes of vomiting in infancy.

It has been suggested that prenatal gastric dilatation seen on ultrasonography may indicate later development of pyloric stenosis.[42]

Treatment

Medical treatment alone is rarely successful. Preoperative treatment necessitates rehydration and correction of the electrolyte imbalance by treating the alkalosis. Replacement of sodium and chloride allows excretion of bicarbonate. Potassium must also be added to the intravenous fluid.[43] The gastritis should be treated by washing out the stomach until it is clear of food debris. Oral feeds are stopped. Once the blood chemistry has improved, surgery should be performed.

Operative treatment

With modern paediatric anaesthesia there is no place for local anaesthesia when operating on a baby with pyloric stenosis.[44]

Although most infants can satisfactorily be treated in a district general hospital,[45] with the very small preterm patient or one with respiratory problems, referral to a paediatric surgeon will result in a better prognosis.[46]

A right upper transverse incision in the pyloric plane[47] will lead to the recti muscles, the fibres of which are separated. Once the peritoneum is opened the liver can be reflected upwards and the stomach grasped. If difficulty is encountered, by pulling on the omentum and transverse colon, the stomach will become visible. The pylorus must be delivered into the wound. Since the pylorus bulges into the duodenum, if the former is grasped between the thumb and index finger of the left hand, the muscle can be divided transversely in the avascular area with a knife without damaging the duodenum. Separation of the fibres by Spencer Wells forceps allows bulging of mucosa. Care should be taken to separate all fibres and also to divide the tumour completely. The extent of the muscle hypertrophy has no correlation with the duration or severity of symptoms.[48,49] However, there is still a danger of opening the duodenum but as long as this is recognized a suture can close the perforation, although feeding will be delayed. Perforation can be checked by insufflating the stomach with air (by the anaesthetist) so that if perforation has occurred, air will bubble through the blood present at the site. To ensure an adequate myotomy, some surgeons formally open the duodenum and then close it. The wound is then closed in layers with subcutaneous wound closure. Another approach through the umbilical region[50] gives a good cosmetic scar but a potential risk of infection. Within 6 hours (if the duodenum is not perforated) the baby can be fed with increasing amounts and sent home within 2–3 days.[51]

Results

Recurrent vomiting rarely indicates incomplete myotomy but more commonly a residual gastritis which will be cleared with further stomach washouts. In some infants the vomiting is due to reflux oesophagitis[52] so that sitting the babies at an angle of 60° may help.[53] Because of prolonged preoperative dehydration and malnutrition, some babies develop wound infection[54] and dehiscence can be a problem. In view of this the baby should be kept for 3–5 days in hospital so that if the wound does break down it can be repaired. Although the results of this operation are generally satisfactory with normal feeding, there is a 20% risk of complications overall,[55] with an increased risk of duodenal reflux later.[56] Whether this leads to dyspepsia in adult life is uncertain. The use of endoscopic balloons to treat adult pyloric stenosis[57,58] may suggest a future development for the treatment of congenital hypertrophic pyloric stenosis.

PEPTIC ULCERATION

Peptic ulceration does occur in children, but usually there is a strong family history[1] or other associated problems, e.g. hypergastrinaemia.[2]

Although the presentation is of abdominal pain, the pain is not always of the typical dyspeptic type and 'tummy-ache' is a common problem in children. In the very young, acute stress ulcers occur, often perforating.[3,4] The stress may be as a result of a serious illness, after a severe burn (Cushing ulcer) or as a result of treatment, e.g. steroids.

Haematemisis may be the first indication of ulceration, especially in the young[5,6] although perforation is uncommon. The importance of chronic peptic ulceration in children is to exclude it as a cause of abdominal pain. Many children may appear to have dyspeptic symptoms and a barium meal may be highly suggestive of duodenal ulcer. However, the duodenum in a child is very irritable so that such a radiograph is not diagnostic. The only way to diagnose peptic ulcer disease in children is to visualize the area endoscopically.[7–9] Since endoscopy has been used routinely there appears to have been a threefold increase in the incidence of ulceration:[10] whether this is a true increase remains to be seen. The finding of *Helicobacter pylori* in children[11,12] with gastritis indicates that this is likely to be the causal agent in their peptic ulceration.[13–15] It may prove difficult to eradicate this organism.[16]

Treatment with antacids may improve the symptoms initially but in many[17] these return. The treatment of choice in those where the pyloris is present is to attempt to eradicate the organism. Triple therapy with a colloidal bismuth preparation, tetracycline and metronidazole is the first line treatment; omeprazole and amoxycillin or clarithromycin are alternative agents.[3,18]

Furthermore, medical therapy with, for example anticholinergic or H_2-histamine receptor antagonist drugs,[19] like cimetidine, will improve their symptoms[20] and further endoscopy is normal. Should complications of ulceration develop some children will require surgery[21] – highly selective vagotomy being the least destructive which gives reasonable results.[22] It is still uncertain whether childhood peptic ulceration leads on to adult disease[23,24] but there is a percentage of children who continue to have recurrent problems,[25] which in all probability relates to persistent *Helicobacter pylori* infection.

OTHER STOMACH PROBLEMS
Perforation of stomach

Apparently spontaneous perforation of the stomach occurs in newborn babies.[1] This is sometimes caused by a large gastric tube being passed carelessly, leading to perforation of the oesophagus or stomach. Overvigorous hand ventilation has also been implicated. Many of these children are premature. The child presents collapsed and shocked with a grossly distended tympanitic abdomen[2] The stomach usually perforates along the greater curvature and the serosa, retracts rather like the peel on an orange leaving a very large defect. Surgery involves closing the defect after resuscitation of the baby. Drainage by means of a gastrostomy tube may be effected through the perforation. This particular problem has the highest mortality rate for neonatal perforations at 60%.[3]

In the older child, pathological air swallowing can occur[4] leading to massive dilation of the stomach and rarely perforation. Treatment is difficult, involving counselling and gastric decompression. Most children grow out of the problem.

Foreign bodies

Mention has already been made of the problems that follow ingestion of corrosive substances in the oesophagus. Although the oesophagus is the area mostly involved in ingestion damage, it may be spared and the stomach is involved when acid is ingested. This leads to massive fibrosis or necrosis of the stomach, in turn leading to complete obstruction due to pooling of the acid as a result of pylorospasm.[5,6] If not too severe, resting the gut by giving parenteral feeding and histamine blockers may allow resolution.[7] If necessary, surgery involves a partial gastrectomy.

The infant and older child may, however, swallow a variety of different foreign objects. As most foreign objects pass on down the gastrointestinal tract,[8] an expectant policy should be employed with check x-ray examination performed at 2–3 weeks. Only if there is no movement out of the stomach should an attempt be made to remove the object endoscopically with grasping forceps. A magnet may be necessary to remove a small object, for example, a battery. Open removal is rarely necessary. Occasionally a hair grip or similar object may stick in the first part of the duodenum. Once beyond that point it is very unusual for the object not to pass out through the gut normally. Rubber teats, especially if they are made in two parts, may block the small intestine causing a 'wind sock' and require surgery. Pieces of glass will pass through, rarely causing damage, and if the child is asymptomatic a conservative approach is advisable.

The only exception to such conservative treatment are small mercury button batteries of the type used in hearing aids etc. Since the gastric contents may erode such an object so releasing the chemicals,[9] it is reasonable to remove the battery by means of endoscopy within 12–24 hours if they have not progressed.[10]

Aspiration of foreign bodies also occurs and should be remembered if there is no evidence of the object within the gastrointestinal tract. Although respiratory problems arise these may be late.[11]

Of more serious importance are bezoars. Disturbed children with pica may swallow anything from wool or hair to wallpaper. The child becomes anorexic with weight loss and a mass palpable in the epigastrium.[12] Differential diagnosis includes malignancy. As well as forming in the stomach bezoars can also occur further down the gastrointestinal tract.[13,14] Abdominal radiography, barium meal and ultrasonography are diagnostic.[15] Treatment involves removal usually by open gastrostomy of utmost importance is the psychiatric follow-up so that a recurrence does not occur.

Tumours

Tumours of the stomach are a rare occurrence in children; they comprise benign teratoma, especially in the newborn,[16,17] and malignant lymphomas. Unusual tumours are found: like rhabdomyosarcoma and leiomyosarcoma.[18] Diagnosis is made on a space occupying lesion in the stomach on barium studies. Treatment depends on the histological diagnosis but involves resection and reconstruction with or without chemotherapy. Prognosis is poor in the malignant type.

Gastric volvulus

Gastric volvulus, with a distended stomach as predisposing cause, leads to collapse. The inability to pass a gastric tube should lead to the suspicion of the diagnosis.[19] Barium studies confirm the diagnosis and at laparotomy fixation of the stomach should prevent further problems. This should not be misdiagnosed as the more common acute dilatation of the stomach occurring after trauma.

DUODENUM

Embryology

The duodenum develops from terminal foregut and proximal midgut to form a loop which moves to the right and dorsally with gastric growth. The mesentery fuses with the dorsal peritoneum and so the duodenum lies in the retroperitoneum. In the meantime the midgut increases in length at variance with the fore and hind gut and their anterior and posterior mesenteries. It forms another loop with the vitellointestinal duct at the apex. This increase necessitates the bowel herniating out through the umbilicus at 5–10 weeks, returning at 12 weeks having rotated in an anticlockwise fashion through 270°. Fixation occurs so that the dorsal mesentery becomes the mesentery of the small bowel. The mesenteries of the ascending and descending colon also fuse with the posterior peritoneum, whereas that of the transverse bowel fuses with the greater omentum.

Abnormalities occur because of failure of the endoderm of the yolk sac and the notocord to separate at 3 weeks – leading to: reduplications of the gut; continuing presence of the vitellointestinal duct or part of it beyond 5 weeks, e.g. Meckel's diverticulum; or failure of reduction of the herniation giving an exomphalos, or failure of fixation between 5 and 12 weeks leading to malrotation.[1] Other problems arise from incomplete canalization[2] especially in the duodenum and damage to the blood supply during its return to the abdomen causing atresia in the small bowel.[3]

Histological development starts with a single layer of cells changing at about 8–10 weeks to a columnar pattern with villi in a craniocaudal direction. By 12 weeks the cells resemble mature enterocytes.[4] The nerve supply also proceeds in a craniocaudal fashion so that neuroblasts have reached the midgut by 8 weeks and innervation should be complete by 12 weeks. Arrest of this mechanism leads to Hirschsprung's disease.

Physiology

The small bowel is involved in the absorption of nutrients from the gut. To this end various enzymes[5] are secreted into the lumen to aid active transport of fat, carbohydrates and protein into the body's systems.[6,7] The small bowel also has an important immunological function. Little is known about neonatal gastrointestinal motility; it is assumed that it is similar to that of the adult which has been well researched. However, we have no clear understanding of when activity starts and why problems arise.[8] The baby piglet has proved to be a useful model[9] so that further research should be possible.

A child that loses more than 75% of the small bowel will not survive without artificial feeding. Adaptation occurs in time even if there is only a small amount of small bowel left.

Presentation and diagnosis

Most small bowel problems relate to malabsorption or obstruction (complete or incomplete), therefore, failure to grow, vomiting and constipation are usual presentations. Depending on the anatomical level of the obstruction, the vomiting may or may not be bile stained, there may be abdominal distension and the patient may have colicky abdominal pain.

Diagnosis is made by examination to determine the state of the bowel: tenderness suggests that the bowel is becoming ischaemic, whereas tinkling bowel sounds indicate total obstruction.

Radiographs of the abdomen, both erect and supine, help define the degree and site of obstruction and will also show the presence of free gas indicating perforation. If there is no evidence of perforation, barium studies (a meal and follow through, small bowel enema or colonic enema) may make the diagnosis clear. A gastrografin enema[10] may be therapeutic as well as diagnostic in some newborns. In children with bleeding, double-contrast studies and endoscopy are helpful. Rarely in the newborn are blood estimations useful in making a diagnosis, but they help in determining the degree of dehydration.

The surgery involved usually consists of resection with anastomosis – using a single layer extramucosal suture[11] – or the formation of stomas. Bypass of the area rarely works in children and in fact leads to more problems.

DUODENAL ATRESIA AND STENOSIS

If the duodenum fails to recanalize completely, duodenal atresia results with a diaphragm either at, above or below the ampulla of Vater.[1] A similar diaphragm can occur at the third part of the duodenum which will be discussed with high jejunal atresias (p. 1012). Sometimes a 'wind-sock' develops[2] so that the stretched diaphragm becomes floppy and appears to obstruct more distally, leading to incorrect surgery being performed. An incomplete diaphragm gives a stenosis (Figure 62.13). In the atretic duodenum the pancreas frequently develops abnormally so that of the two portions, instead of rotating to lie posteriorly on the left of the duodenum, the uncinate lobe crosses anteriorly to envelop the duodenum, giving an appearance of an annular pancreas. However, it is not the pancreas that obstructs the bowel – it merely indicates the pathology within the duodenum. The diagnosis of duodenal obstruction (?duodenal atresia) can be made antenatally.[3,4] Maternal hydramnios should alert one to the possible diagnosis. The incidence varies from 1 : 10 000 to 1 : 40 000 livebirths.[5]

The baby presents with vomiting, and, depending on the site of obstruction, this may or may not be bile stained. Little abdominal distension will occur because the blockage is high, although a fullness in the epigastrium, i.e. the grossly distended stomach may be noted. Plain abdominal radiography will show a large stomach and the erect film is classically that of a 'double bubble' appearance of the fluid levels in distended

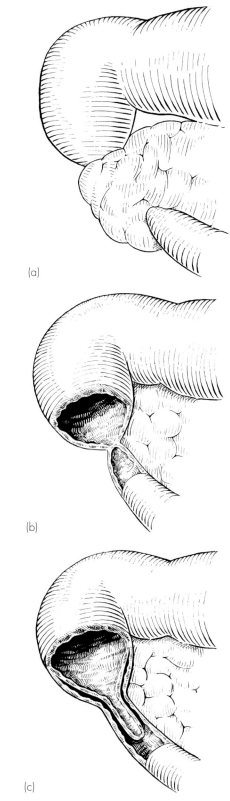

(a)

(b)

(c)

Figure 62.13

a–c Types of duodenal atresia/stenosis. (a) Annular pancreas with complete atresia of duodenum; (b) internal diaphragm; (c) wind-sock type of diaphragm. Types (b) and (c) may have a small hole in the diaphragm leading to stenosis.

stomach and duodenum (Figure 62.14). These only indicate an obstruction at the second part of the duodenum and may also be present in malrotation with volvulus. No gas is seen distally. If a nasogastric tube has been passed, it may be necessary to instil air into the stomach to confirm the diagnosis.

In infants with stenosis the diagnosis may be delayed and a misdiagnosis of pyloric stenosis may be made. Radiological appearances are similar to the atretic case but now there is distal gas. A barium study will show the site and type of the diaphragm.

Associated abnormalities

These are common[6] especially chromosomal abnormalities. Trisomy 21 (Down syndrome) occurs in 40–50% of duodenal obstructions whether complete or not.[7] Cardiac abnormalities may be associated with this chromosomal abnormality. Since there is much musculoskeletal development at the time when such abnormalities occur, it is not surprising that such abnormalities are equally common – in 37%.[8] The triad of oesophageal atresia, cardiac anomalies and duodenal atresia is usually fatal.[9]

Treatment

Resuscitation is necessary before surgery in view of the gross disturbance in electrolytes following excessive vomiting or

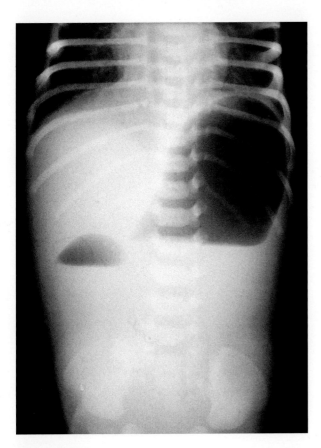

Figure 62.14
Plain erect abdominal radiography showing 'double bubble' of dilated stomach and duodenum.

fluid lying in the stomach and duodenum. The treatment is the same whether dealing with a complete atresia or a stenosis: to bypass the obstruction as close as possible so that a blind loop is not left.

At laparotomy via a transverse upper abdominal incision, the large stomach is visible with collapsed distal bowel. The duodenum is kocherized to allow mobilization. The upper jejunum and third part of the duodenum are freed and brought through the transverse mesocolon to lie close to the proximal duodenum. No effort should be made to dissect the annular pancreas if present. The posterior layer of the two portions of duodenum are stitched together. The proximal bowel is opened and confirmation of the site and type of obstruction made by means of a probe. When the distal bowel is opened, further confirmation is necessary to check on the position of the obstruction. If such care is not taken it is possible to anastomose the bowel above the diaphragm, especially when a 'wind-sock' is present.[10] The entire posterior wall and part of the anterior wall is closed in a single layer before a transanastomotic tube (tat) is passed, either via the nose or by a gastrostomy in the stomach to lie through the anastomosis into the upper jejunum. It should be remembered that such a tube slips back into the upper bowel so that a long enough portion should be threaded into the distal bowel. The anastomosis is completed and, if the gastric distension is gross, a gastrostomy tube may be placed in preference to a nasogastric tube. Both the gastrostomy and transanastomotic tube can be brought out through a separate incision, care being taken to fix the gastrostomy tube before closure of the abdomen.

Due to the gross gastric and duodenal distension it may take some time, up to 3 weeks, for the bowel to start normal peristalsis and return to a more normal configuration. Oral feeding has to be delayed because of large gastric aspirates leading to dehydration. To avoid metabolic disturbances[11] and to allow normal growth, milk feeding via the transanastomotic tube can commence within 24–48 hours of surgery.[12] However, it is wise to check the position of the end of the tube by instillation of a small amount of contrast before starting feeding. Once the stomach has been deflated by the gastrostomy tube left on low reflux, oral feeding may be introduced between 10 and 21 days.

Such a duodenoduodenostomy[13] (Figure 62.15) has been shown to give better results than a duodenojejunostomy.[14] It is important that the duodenoduodenostomy is as short as possible because a large amount of redundant bowel will not deflate and in time will lead to blind-loop problems – as seen in a 13-year-old who had had a posterior gastroenterostomy performed as a neonate. Undoing this and reconstruction of a duodenoduodenostomy was necessary to correct the problem and to allow the child to grow.

In an attempt to obviate such surgery, both open and closed methods of disrupting the diaphragm have been attempted with varying success. Although endoscopic disruption has been attempted,[15] it has not been evaluated. Open duodenoplasty to remove the diaphragm[16] would appear to allow earlier feeding. Late obstruction of the duodenoduodenostomy suggests that plication of the proximally dilated

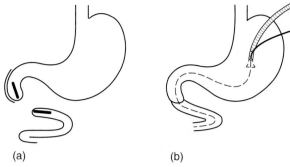

Figure 62.15

(a) Showing incisions in duodenum above and below the obstruction. (b) Anastomosis with TAT tube in situ and gastrostomy.

first part of the duodenum should be included in the initial operation.[17]

Postoperatively, further loss of fluids may lead to electrolyte imbalance, requiring large amounts of intravenous fluids for correction. Although those diagnosed antenatally had earlier surgery and therefore less fluid disturbance, there is little difference in the long-term results.[18]

Results

The association with Down syndrome may affect short-term results[19] but long-term results in any risk groups are excellent.[20] If a baby with this syndrome is vomiting, active measures should be taken early to exclude the diagnosis and treat. These babies are also more likely to require re-exploration because of late complications. There may be repercussions later because of bile reflux so that even in the asymptomatic, gastrointestinal disturbances may eventually cause problems.

Survival is likely in over 70% with death due to other congenital abnormalities[21] and low birth weight.[22] More than a third will have prolonged jaundice.[23]

An annular pancreas is an incidental finding[13] associated with embryological development. As with prepyloric portal veins,[24,25] this does not of itself obstruct. Malrotation may be associated with an intrinsic duodenal obstruction which should be checked.

Other causes of duodenal obstruction

Rarer causes of obstruction of the duodenum in the older child are duplication cysts;[26] tumours[27] – usually malignant – requiring a Whipple procedure; or intramural haematomas[28] caused by trauma[29,30] or a bleeding abnormality associated with Henoch–Schonlein purpura.

Duplication cysts are described later in relation to the small bowel (p. 1023). Duodenal haematomas only require surgery if there is a tender enlarging mass or signs of peritonitis.[31] Ultrasonography helps with observation during conservative management with nasogastric suction and if necessary parenteral nutrition. Coagulation studies as well as serum amylase must be kept under review. Non-accidental injury[32] must not be forgotten as a cause of this problem.

MALROTATION

Another form of duodenal obstruction presenting at any age is malrotation of the bowel,[1] which may lead to volvulus of the small bowel.

Embryology

Malrotation means incomplete or abnormal rotation of the intestine around the superior mesenteric artery and abnormal fixation of this bowel. Antenatally, the bowel develops and rotates in an anticlockwise direction outwith the peritoneal cavity. It returns to the abdominal cavity in the first 3 months of fetal development, the duodenum and proximal jejunum first, to lie in the anatomically normal position with the duodenojejunal flexure on the left side of the abdomen at the level of the lesser curvature of the stomach; the base of the mesentery lies from the left upper quadrant to the right lower quadrant so that the caecum lies in the right iliac fossa. The transverse colon lies anteriorly across the upper abdomen behind the abdominal wall; on the left of the abdomen lies the descending colon (Figure 62.16). Should the bowel fail to rotate or only partially rotate the bowel is malfixed and so malrotated or unrotated. The dorsal mesentery cannot easily fuse with the posterior peritoneum in the right paracolic gutter and so forms a band to reach the right fossa crossing and obstructing the duodenum (Ladd's bands).

Various forms of malrotation (Figure 62.17) occur;[2] the most common are:

(a) non-rotation of all the intestine;

(b) non-rotation of the right colon with normal rotation of the duodenum.

(c) both of these predispose easily to volvulus of the small bowel. Other types are as follows:

(d) occasionally, although the colon rotates normally the duodenum does not, leading to malfixation of the duodenojejunal junction with kinking and obstruction;

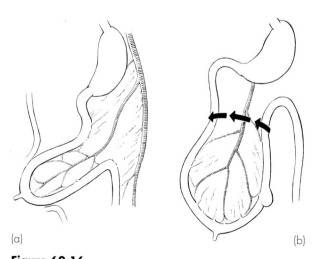

(a)   (b)

Figure 62.16

Embryology and rotation of small bowel.

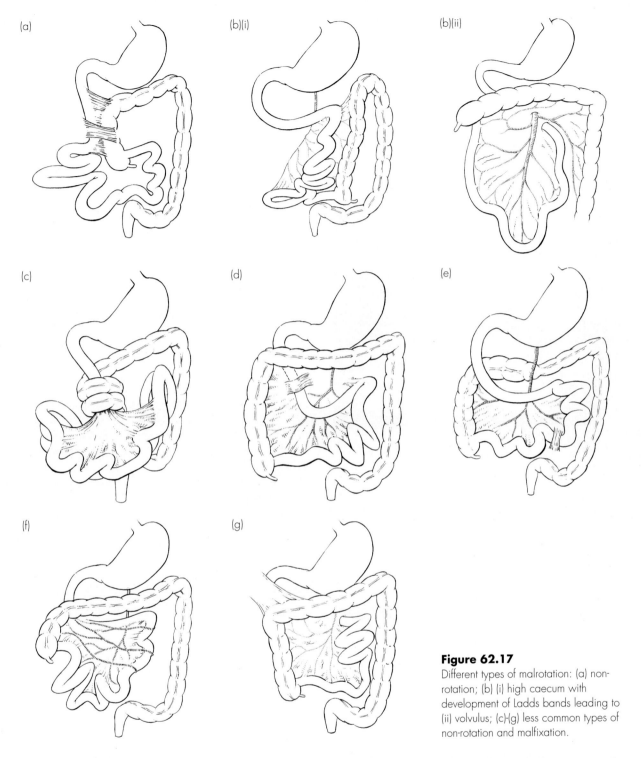

Figure 62.17
Different types of malrotation: (a) non-rotation; (b) (i) high caecum with development of Ladds bands leading to (ii) volvulus; (c)-(g) less common types of non-rotation and malfixation.

(e) rarely a reversed position occurs with the colon lying behind the duodenum but the caecum in the right iliac fossa; here the obstruction in the transverse colon is caused by the superior mesenteric vessels;

(f) a reversed rotation of the duodenum is associated with normal fixation of the colon, a right mesenteric pouch develops allowing for a paraduodenal hernia;[3]

(g) an incomplete fixation of the hepatic flexure causes problems by Ladd's bands obstructing the duodenum to give bile stained vomiting;

(h) a loose or incomplete attachment of the caecum allows for it to be mobile so that the appendix can vary in site.

Presentation

In view of the abnormal development, most children with malrotation will present early in the newborn period. Classically the main problem is bile-stained vomiting due to the obstructed second part of the duodenum with bands. Colicky abdominal pain may suggest intermittent twisting of the bowel. Infants with failure to thrive should be investigated for

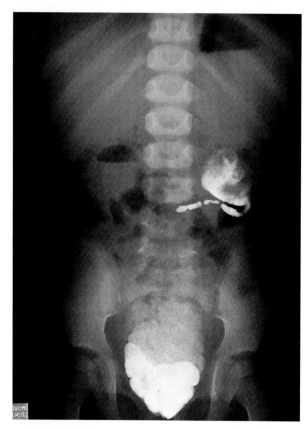

Figure 62.17(h)
Plain x-ray after normal barium enema showing appendix moved to left side.

malrotation as many such children have an associated protein malnutrition.[4]

However, a potential for serious problems exists because in the usual form, the duodenojejunal flexure now lies on the right as does the base of the mesentery. This narrow base allows for midgut volvulus around the blood supply, i.e. the superior mesenteric vessels. Such a volvulus leads to ischaemia and eventual infarction of the whole of the small bowel. If ischaemia occurs, the passage of blood per rectum is associated with shock, collapse and circulatory failure. This will happen regardless of age at presentation.[5]

It is to be hoped that the diagnosis is considered before such a catastrophe. Bile-stained vomiting is an indication of a surgical problem until proved otherwise and demands urgent investigation. Malrotation with or without volvulus can occur in the older child and may be missed.[6] Occasionally the history of intermittent colicky pain in the past leads one to the diagnosis. Often there is little to find on examination unless the bowel has become infarcted.

Diagnosis

If volvulus has occurred, plain abdominal radiographs will show a duodenal obstruction with little or no gas in the distal small bowel – similar to the double bubble described in duodenal atresia. In the malrotated bowel the radiograph may be singularly unimpressive although sometimes the gas shadows will look abnormal. Further elucidation with barium studies should not be delayed if the possibility of malrotation is seriously considered as volvulus can occur at any time.[5] A barium meal and follow through will delineate the position of the duodenojejunal flexure which should be at the level of the lesser curvature of the stomach on the left side of the vertebral column (Figure 62.18). The position of the small bowel can be demonstrated.[7] Minor degrees of malrotation can be more difficult to demonstrate by radiological means. Barium enema will show the position of the caecum and if on the left side indicates malrotation (Figure 62.19). Sometimes a mobile caecum may only show up on a delayed film. Ultrasound examination may show reverse position of superior mesenteric artery and vein.

Associated abnormalities, especially diaphragmatic hernia and defects of the abdominal wall are particularly common in the newborn.[8] However, it is also commonly found with upper gastrointestinal atresia and stenosis as well as Hirschsprung's disease and intussusception.[9]

Surgery

If malrotation alone is present, laparotomy is performed to open up the base of the mesentery to prevent volvulus. Such surgery also helps to fix the bowel so that it is rarely necessary to suture the bowel in each iliac fossa.[10,11] No attempt should be made to return the bowel to the anatomically correct position as the bowel has not developed in this manner and will become ischaemic if this is done. This leaves the caecum and the appendix on the left side. Some surgeons perform appendicectomy to prevent later problems.

If the bowel is twisted around the base of the mesentery it is imperative that it is untwisted – this is usually in a clockwise direction. If volvulus has occurred or there have been recurrent problems over many years, it may be very difficult to undo the loops of bowel, but, if it is not done, the child will be prone to further problems and may lose some bowel. If the bowel is already ischaemic it may or may not recover on undoing the twist. If it remains ischaemic, resection of bowel will be necessary. However, if the entire small bowel is ischaemic – which is likely in view of the blood supply – it may be wiser to undo the volvulus and return the infarcted bowel to the abdominal cavity. If the child survives a second look laparotomy will reveal rather less necrotic bowel to be resected. Even so, the short inadequate length of bowel will cause problems with growth and development.

Results

Results from surgery for malrotation alone are excellent as long as no volvulus had occurred. The chance of recurrent problems is low despite the bowel being in an abnormal position.

Unfortunately over 70% of malrotations presenting in the neonatal period are associated with volvulus and in these, the results are poor.[12] Older children may die because the diagnosis has not been considered. If the entire bowel is necrotic most will die. Even those who survive have a stormy course and may require parenteral nutrition for life.

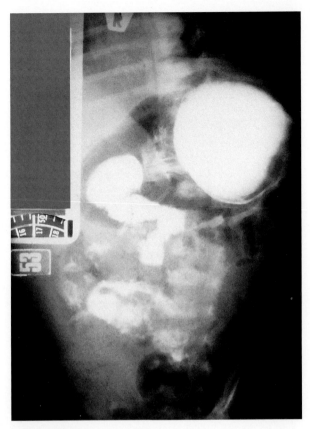

Figure 62.18
Barium meal and follow through indicating duodeno jejunal flexure low on right side of vertebral column.

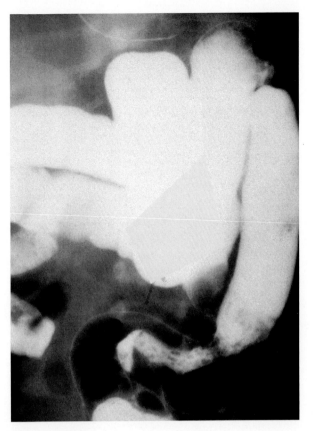

Figure 62.19
Barium enema showing caecum on the left side of the abdomen.

After treatment these children may still vomit because of the continuation of gastro-oesophageal reflux, caused initially by the delay in gastric emptying.[13]

Volvulus can occur without malrotation and may complicate intestinal atresia, meconium ileus or duplication cysts by the excess size allowing the twist to occur. A similar situation occurs in midgut volvulus associated with dilatation of the ileum or in children with intestinal ascariasis.[14]

Situs inversus does not of itself require treatment but it is more likely to cause neonatal obstruction and is usually associated with major abnormalities – biliary atresia, annular pancreas and preduodenal portal vein[15,16] which in itself may cause obstruction.

REFERENCES

Stomach

1. Euler AR, Byrne WJ, Cousins LM, Ament ME, Leake RD & Walsh JH. Increased serum gastrin concentrations and gastric acid hyposecretion in the immediate newborn period. *Gastroenterology* 1977; **72**: 1271.
2. Euler AR, Byrne WJ, Meis PJ et al. Basal and pentagastrin-stimulated acid secretion in newborn human infants. *Pediatr Res* 1979; **13**: 36.
3. Hyman PE, Clarke DD, Everett SL et al. Gastric acid secretory function in preterm infants. *J Pediatr* 1985; **106**: 467.
4. Kopel FB & Barbero GJ. Gastric acid secretion in infancy and childhood. *Gastroenterology* 1967; **52**: 1101.
5. Widstrom AM, Winberg J, Werner S, Svensson K, Posloncec B & Ulnas-Moberg K. Breast feeding induced effects on plasma gastrin and somatostatin levels and their correlation with milk yield in lactating females. *Early Hum Dev* 1988; **16**: 293.
6. Marchini G, Winberg J & Uvnas-Moberg K. Plasma concentrations of gastrin and somatostatin after breast feeding in 4 day old infants. *Arch Dis Child* 1988; **63**: 1218.
7. Salmenpera L, Perheentupa J, Siimes MA, Adrian TE, Bloom SR & Aynsley-Green A. Effects of feeding regimen on blood glucose levels and plasma concentrations of pancreatic hormones and gut regulatory peptides at 9 months of age: comparison between infants fed with milk formula and infants exclusively breast fed from birth. *J Ped Gastroenterol Nutr* 1988; **7**: 651.
8. Widstrom AM, Christensson K, Ransjo Arvidson AB, Matthiesen AS, Winberg J & Uvnas Moberg K. Gastric aspirates of newborn infants: pH volume and levels of gastrin – and somatostatin like immunoreactivity. *Acta Paediatr Scand* 1988; **77**: 502.
9. Marchini G, Lagercrantz H, Milerad J, Winberg J & Uvnas Moberg K. Plasma levels of somatostatin and gastrin in sick infants and small for gestational age infants. *J Pediatr Gastroenterol Nutr* 1988; **7**: 641.
10. Euler AR, Byrne WJ & Campbell MF. Basal and pentagastrin – stimulated gastric acid secretory rates in normal children and in those with peptic ulcer disease. *J Paediatr* 1983; **103**: 766.
11. Siegal M. Gastric emptying time in premature and compromised infants. *J Pediatr Gastroenterol Nutr* 1983; **2**: (suppl 1) S136.
12. Bissett WM, Watt JB, Rivers RPA & Milla PJ. The ontogeny of small intestinal manor motor activity. *Pediatr Res* 1986; **20**: 692.

Congenital abnormalities

1. Bar-Maor JA, Nissan S & Nevo S. Pyloric atresia. A hereditary congenital anomaly with autosomal recessive transmission. *J Med Genet* 1972; **9**: 70.
2. Moore CCM. Congenital gastric outlet obstruction. *J Pediatr Surg* 1989; **24**: 1241.
3. Korber JS & Glasson MJ. Familial pyloric atresia associated with EB. *J Pediatr* 1977; **90**: 600.
4. Pederson PV. Pyloric atresia and epidermolysis bullosa. *J Pediatr* 1977; **91**: 852.

5. DeGroot WG, Postuma R & Hunter AGW. Familial pyloric atresia associated with epidermolysisbullosa. *J Pediatr* 1978; **82**: 429.
6. Swinburne L & Kohler HG. Familial pyloric atresia associated with EB. *J Pediatr* 1979; **94**: 162.
7. Carmi R, Sofer S, Karplus M et al. Aplasia cutis congenita in two sibs discordant for pyloric atresia. *Am J Med Genet* 1982; **11**: 319.
8. Kelly ME, Mohtashemi H, Patel S et al. Report of a case of double pylorus. *Dig Dis Sci* 1979; **24**: 807.
9. Williams RS, Gilmore IT & Johnson AG. Congenital double pylorus: a case report. *Br J Surg* 1981; **68**: 65.
10. Tunnell WP & Smith EI. Antral web in infancy. *J Pediatr Surg* 1980; **15**: 152.
11. Blazek FD & Boeckman CR. Prepyloric antral diaphragm: delays in treatment. *J Pediatr Surg* 1987; **22**: 948.
12. Mitchell KG, McGowan A, Smith DC & Gillespie G. Pyloric diaphragm, antral web, congenital antral membrane – a surgical rarity? *Br J Surg* 1979; **66**: 572.
13. Velasco AKL, Holcomb GW, Templeton JM & Ziegler MM. Management of congenital microgastria. *J Pediatr Surg* 1990; **25**: 192.
14. Gonzales OR, Hardin WD, Issacs H, Lally KP & Brennan LP. Duplication of the hepatopancreatic bud presenting as pyloric stenosis. *J Pediatr Surg* 1988; **23**: 1053.
15. Sieunarine K & Manmohansingh E. Gastric dyuplicationcyst presenting as an acute abdomen in a child. *J Pediatr Surg* 1989; **24**: 1152.
16. Blumberg NA. Abdominal parasitic twin: an unusual case of duodenal obstruction. *Br J Surg* 1980; **67**: 675.
17. Bruce J, Afshand E, Karp MP & Jewett TC. Omphalocele with pyloroduodenal obstruction by extrinsic hepatic compression; a case report. *J Pediatr Surg* 1988; **23**: 1081.
18. Freisen SR, Boley JO & Miller DR. The myenteric plexus of the pylorus: its early development and its changes in hypertrophic pyloris stenosis. *Surgery* 1956; **39**: 21.
19. Friesen SR & Pearse ASE. Pathogenesis of congenital pyloric stenosis: histochemical analysis of pyloric ganglion cells. *Surgery* 1963; **53**: 604.
20. Belding H & Keruohan JW. A morphological study of the mysenteric plexus and musculature of the pylorus. *Surg Gynecol Obstet* 1953; **97**: 322.
21. Rogers JM, Macgillan & Drainer IK. Congenital hypertrophic pyloric stenosis: a gastrin hypothesis pursued. *J Pediatr Surg* 1976; **11**: 173.
22. Docege JA. Production of duodenal ulcers and hypertrophic pyloric stenosis by the administration of pentagastin to pregnant and newborn dogs. *Nature* 1970; **225**: 284.
23. Werlin SL, Grand RJ & Drug DE. Congenital hypertrophic pyloric stenosis – the role of gastin re-evaluated. *Paediatrics* 1978; **61**: 883.
24. Hamburg MA, Miguon M, Ricoor C, Accary J & Pellerin D. Serum gastrin levels in hypertrophic pyloric stenosis of infancy. Response to a gastrin secretion test. *Arch Dis Child* 1979; **54**: 208.
25. Moazam F, Rodgers BM, Talbert JL & Mc Guigan JE. Fasting and post prandial serum gastrin levels in infants with hypertrophic pyloric stenosis. *Ann Surg* 1978; **188**: 623.
26. La Ferla G, Watson J, Fyfe AH & Drainer IK. The role of prostoglandins E_2 and F_2 Alpha in infantile hypertrophic pyloric stenosis. *J Pediatr Surg* 1986; **21**: 410.
27. Rodgers IM, Drainer IK, Dougal AJ, Black J & Logan R. Serum cholecystokin in basal acid secretion and infantile pyloric stenosis. *Arch Dis Child* 1979; **54**: 773.
28. Tam PK. Observations and perspectives of the pathology and possible aetiology of infantile hypertrophic pyloric stenosis. A histological, biochemical, histochemical and immunocytochemical study. *Ann Acad Med* Singapore 1985; **14**: 523.
29. Latchaw LA, Jacir NN & Harris BH. The development of pyloric stenosis during transpyloric feedings. *J Pediatr Surg* 1989; **24**: 823.
30. Czeizel A. Birth weight distribution in congenital pyloric stenosis. *Arch Dis Child* 1972; **47**: 978.
31. Carter CO & Evans KA. Inheritance of congenital pyloric stenosis. *J Med Genet* 1969; **6**: 233.
32. Atwell JD & Levick P. Congenital hypertrophic pyloric stenosis and associated anomolies in the genito-urinary tract. *J Pediatr Surg* 1981; **16**: 1029.
33. Franklin EA & Salchiw RN. Hypertrophic pyloric stenosis complicating oesophageal atresia with tracheo branchial fistula. *Am J Surg* 1969; **117**: 647.
34. Glasson MJ, Bandrevics V & Cohen DH. Hypertrophic pyloric stenosis complicating esophageal atresia. *Surgery* 1973; **74**: 530.
35. Polloch WF, Norris WJ & Gordon HE. The management of HPS and the Los Angeles Children's Hospital: a review of 1422 cases. *Am J Surg* 1949; 335.
36. Ahmed S. Infantile pyloric stenosis associated with major anomalies of the alimentary tract. *J Pediatr Surg* 1970; **5**: 660.
37. Spitz L & Batcup G. Haematemesis in infantile hypertrophic pyloric stenosis: the source of the bleeding. *Br J Surg* 1979; **66**: 827.
38. Breaux CW, Hood JS & Georgeson KE. The significance of alkalosis and hypochloremia in hypertrophic pyloric stenosis. *J Pediatr Surg* 1989; **12**: 1250.
39. Tunell WP & Wilson DA. Pyloric stenosis: diagnosis by real time sonography, the pyloric muscle length method. *J Pediatr Surg* 1984; **19**: 795.
40. Keller E, Waldmann D & Greiner P. Comparison of preoperative sonography with intraoperative findings in congenital hypertrophic pyloric stenosis. *J Pediatr Surg* 1987; **22**: 950.
41. Forman HP, Leonidas JC & Kronfeld GD. A rational approach to the diagnosis of hypertrophic pyloric stenosis: do the results match the claims? *J Pediatr Surg* 1990; **25**: 262.
42. Katz S, Basel D and Branski. Prenatal gastric dilatation and infantile hypertrophic stenosis. *J Pediatr Surg* 1988; **23**: 1021.
43. Spicer RD. Infantile hypertrophic pyloric stenosis: a review. *Br J Surg* 1982; **69**: 128.
44. Rasmussen L, Hansen LP & Pedersen SA. Infantile hypertrophic pyloric stenosis: the changing trend in treatment in a Danish County. *J Pediatr Surg* 1987; **22**: 953.
45. Saunders MP & Williams CR. Infantile hypertrophic pyloric stenosis: experience in a district general hospital. *J R Coll Surg Edinb* 1990; **35**: 36.
46. McDonald PJ. Ramstedt's operation in district hospitals – is it safe? *J R Soc Med* 1986; **79**: 17.
47. Beynon J, Brown R, James C & Fernando R. Pyloromyotomy: can the morbidity be improved? *J R Coll Surg Edinb* 1987; **32**: 291.
48. Dodge JA. Infantile hypertrophic pyloric stenosis in Belfast. *Arch Dis Child* 1975; **50**: 171.
49. Ukabiala O & Lister J. The extent of muscle hypertrophy in infantile hypertrophic pyloric stenosis does not depend on age and duration of symptoms. *J Pediatr Surg* 1987; **22**: 200.
50. Tan KC & Bianchi A. Circmumbilical incision for pyloromyotomy. *Br J Surg* 1986; **73**: 399.
51. Foster ME & Lewis WG. Early postoperative feeding – a continuing controversy in pyloric stenosis. *J R Soc Med* 1989; **82**: 532.
52. Spitz L. Vomiting after pyloromyotomy for infantile hypertrophic pyloric stenosis. *Arch Dis Child* 1979; **54**: 886.
53. Spitz L & MacKinnon AE. Posture in the postoperative management of infantile pyloric stenosis. *Br J Surg* 1984; **71**: 643.
54. Gray DW, Gear MW & Stevens DW. The results of Ramstedt's operation: room for complacency? *Ann R Coll Surg Engl* 1984; **66**: 280.
55. Bristol JB & Bolton RA. The results of Ramstedt's operation in a district general hospital. *Br J Surg* 1981; **68**: 590.
56. Tam PKH, Saing H, Koo J, Wong J & Ong GB. Pyloric function five to eleven years after Ramstedt's pyloromyotomy. *J Pediatr Surg* 1985; **20**: 236.
57. Griffin SM, Chung SCS, Leung JWC & Li AKC. Pepticpyloric stenosis treated by endoscopic balloon dilatation. *Br J Surg* 1989; **76**: 1147.
58. Heymans HSA, Bartelsman WFM & Herweijer TJ. Endoscopic balloon dilatation as treatment of gastric outlet obstruction in infancy and childhood. *J Pediatr Surg* 1988; **23**: 139.

Peptic ulceration

1. Habbick BF, Melrose AG & Grant JC. Duodenal ulcer in childhood. A study of predisposing factors. *Arch Dis Child* 1968; **43**: 23.
2. Tam PKH. Hypergastrinemia in children with duodenal ulcer. *J Pediatr Surg* 1988; **23**: 331.
3. Seagram CGF, Stephens CA & Cumming WA. Peptic ulceration at the Hospital for Sick Children Toronto, during the 20 year period 1949–1969. *J Pediatr Surg* 1973; **8**: 407.
4. Bell MJ, Keating JP, Ternberg JL & Bower RJ. Perforated stress ulcers in infants. *J Pediatr Surg* 1981; **16**: 998.
5. Tam PKH, Saing H & Lau JTC. Diagnosis of peptic ulcer in children: the past and present. *J Pediatr Surg* 1986; **21**: 15.
6. Rosenlund ML & Koop CE. Diagnosis and treatment. Duodenal ulcer in childhood. *Pediatrie* 1970; **45**: 283.
7. Miller V & Doig CM. Personal practice. Upper gastrointestinal tract endoscopy. *Arch Dis Child* 1984; **59**: 1100.
8. Tam PKH & Saing H. Pediatric upper gastrointestinal endoscopy: a 13 year experience. *J Pediatr Surg* 1989; **24**: 443.
9. Sobala GM, Rathbone BJ, Wyatt JI, Dixon MF, Heatley RV & Axon ATR. Investigating young patients with dyspepsia. *Lancet* 1989; **i**: 50.

10. Murphy MS, Eastham EJ, Jimenez M, Nelson R & Jackson RH. Duodenal ulceration reveiw of 110 cases. *Arch Dis Child* 1987; **62**: 554.
11. Drumm B, Sherman P, Cutz E & Kamali M. Association of *Campylobacter pylori* on the gastric mucosa with antral gastritis in children. *N Engl J Med* 1987; **316**: 1557.
12. Thomas J, Eastham EJ, Elliott TSJ, Dobson CM & Jones DM. *Campylobacter pylori* gastritis in children – a common cause of symptoms? *Gut* 1988; **29**: A707.
13. Persic VN & Sarjanovic L. *Campylobacter pylori*, resistant duodenal ulcers, and antibiotic treatment. *J Pediatr Gastroenterol Nutr* 1988; **7**: 934.
14. Oberda G, Ansaldi N, Boero M, Ponzetto A & Bellis D. *Campylobacter pylori* in families of children with relapsing gastroduodenal disease due to *C. pylori* infection. *Am J Gastroenterol* 1988; **83**: 1437.
15. Tolia V, Thirumoorthi MC, Fleming SI, Chang CH & Newell D. Role of *Campylobacter pylori* (CP) in children with relapsing abdominal pain (RAP). *Gastroenterology* 1988; **94**: A463.
16. Oberda G, Vaira D, Holton J, Ainley C, Altare F & Ansaldi N. Amoxycillin plus tinidazole for *Campylobacter pylori* gastritis in children: assessment by serum IgG antibody, pepsinogen I and gastrin levels. *Lancet* 1989; **i**: 690.
17. Puri P, Boyd E, Blake N & Guiney EJ. Duodenal ulcer in childhood: a continuing disease in adult life. *J Pediatr Surg* 1978; **13**: 525.
18. Mohammed R & Mackay C. Peptic ulceration in adolescence. *Br J Surg* 1982; **69**: 525.
19. Hyman PE & Hassall E. Marked basal gastric acid hyper-secretion and peptic ulcer disease: medical management with a combination H2-histamine receptor antagonist and anticholinergics *J Pediatr Gastroenterol Nutr* 1988; **7**: 57.
20. Curci MR, Little K. Sieber WK & Kieswetter WB. Peptic ulcer disease in childhood reexamined. *J Pediatr Surg* 1976; **11**: 329.
21. Irving AD & Lyall ME. Surgical management of bleeding duodenal ulcer in children. *J R Coll Surg Edinb* 1981; **26**: 360.
22. Mulvihill SJ & Fonklasrud EW. Pyloroplasty in infancy and childhood. *J Pediatr Surg* 1983; **18**: 930.
23. Michener WM, Kennedy RLJ & Du Shane JW. Duodenal ulcer in childhood. Ninety-two cases with follow-up. *Am J Dis Child* 1960; **100**: 36.
24. Baida M, McIntyre A & Deitel M. Peptic ulcer in children and adolescents. A review of 28 cases. *Arch Surg* 1969; **99**: 15.
25. Drumm B, Rhoads J, Stringer DA, Sherman PM, Ellis LE & Durie PR. Peptic ulcer disease in children – etiology, clinical findings and clinical course. *Pediatrie* 1988; **82**: 410.

Other stomach problems

1. Rosser SB, Clark CE & Elechi EN. Spontaneous neonatal gastric perforation. *J Pediatr Surg* 1982; **17**: 390.
2. Robarts FH. Neonatal perforation of the stomach. *Kinderchir* 1968; **S5**: 62.
3. Tan CEL, Kiely EM, Agrawal M, Brereton RJ & Spitz L. Neonatal gastrointestinal perforation. *J Pediatr Surg* 1989; **24**: 888.
4. Gauderer MWL, Halpin TC & Izant RJ. Pathologic childhood aerophagia: a recognizable clinical entity. *J Pediatr Surg* 1981; **16**: 301.
5. Gandhi RK & Robarts FE. Hour-glass stricture of the stomach and pyloric stenosis due to ferrous sulphate poisoning. *Br J Surg* 1962; **218**: 613.
6. Gillis DA, Higgins G & Kennedy R. Gastric damage from ingested acid in children. *J Pediatr Surg* 1985; **20**: 494.
7. Cullen ML & Klein MD. Spontaneous resolution of acid gastric injury. *J Pediatr Surg* 1987; **22**: 550.
8. Webb WA. Management of foreign bodies of the upper gastrointestinal tract. *Gastroenterology* 1988; **94**: 204.
9. Katz L & Cooper MT. Danger of small children swallowing hearing aid batteries. *J Otolaryngology* 1978; **7**: 467.
10. Votteler TP, Nash JC & Rudledge JC. The hazard of ingested alkaline disk batteries in children. *JAMA* 1983; **249**: 2504.
11. Wiseman NE. The diagnosis of foreign body aspiration in childhood. *J Pediatr Surg* 1984; **19**: 531.
12. Shawis RN & Doig CM. Gastric trichobezoar associated with transient pancreatitis. *Arch Dis Child* 1984; **59**: 994.
13. Choi S-O & Kang J-S. Gastrointestinal phytobezoars in childhood. *J Pediatr Surg* 1988; **23**: 338.
14. Swift RI, Wood CB & Hershman MJ. Small bowel obstruction due to phytobezoars in the intact gastrointestinal tract. *J R Coll Surg Edinb* 1989; **34**: 267.
15. Ratcliffe JF. The ultrasonographic appearance of a trichobezoar. *Br J Radiol* 1981; **55**: 166.
16. Atwell JD, CLaireaux AE and Nixon HH. Teratoma of the stomach in the newborn. *J Pediatr Surg* 1967; **2**: 197.
17. Earnshaw JJ. Gastric teratoma in infancy. *J R Coll Surg Edinb* 1985; **30**: 199.
18. Mahour GH, Isaacs H & Chang L. Primary malignant tumors of the stomach in children. *J Pediatr Surg* 1980; **15**: 603.
19. Cameron AEP & Howard ER. Gastric volvulus in childhood. *J Pediatr Surg* 1987; **22**: 944.

Duodenum

1. McCollum JPK & Milla PJ. Prenatal development of structure and function. In Harries JT (ed.) *Essentials of Paediatric Gastroenterology*. Edinburgh: Churchill Livingstone, 1977; 1.
2. Puri P & Fujimoto T. New observations on the pathogenesis of multiple atresias. *J Pediatr Surg* 1988; **23**: 221.
3. Kaga Y, Hayashida Y, Ikeda K, Inokuthi K & Hashimoto N. Intestinal atresia in fetal dogs produced by localized ligation of mesenteric vessels. *J Pediatr Surg* 1975; **10**: 949.
4. Varkonyi T, Gergely G & Varro V. The ultrastructure of the small intestinal mucosa in the developing human fetus. *Scand J Gastroenterol* 1974; **9**: 495.
5. Grand RJ, Watkins JB & Torti FM. Development of the human gastrointestinal tract: a review. *Gastroenterology* 1976; **70**: 790.
6. Koldovsky O, Heringova A, Jirsova V, Jirasek JE & Uher J. Transport of glucose against a concentration gradient in everted sacs of jejunum and ileum of human fetuses. *Gastroenterology* 1965; **48**: 185.
7. Levin RJ, Koldovsky O, Hoskova J, Jirsova V & Uher J. Electrical activity across human foetal small intestine associated with absorption processes. *Gut* 1968; **9**: 206.
8. Milla PJ. Gastrointestinal motility disorders in children. *Pediatr Clin North Am* 1988; **35**: 311.
9. Groner JI, Altschuler SM & Ziegler MM. The newborn piglet: a model of gastrointestinal motility. *J Pediatr Surg* 1990; **25**: 315.
10. Noblett HR. The treatment of uncomplicated meconium ileus by gastrograffin enema. A preliminary report. *J Pediatr Surg* 1962; **4**: 190.
11. Brain AJL & Kiely EM. Use of a single layer extramucosal suture for intestinal anastomosis in children. *Br J Surg* 1985; **72**: 483.

Duodenal atresia and stenosis

1. Boyden EA, Cope JC & Bill AG. Anatomy and embryology of congenital intrinsic obstruction of the duodenum. *Am J Surg* 1967; **114**: 190.
2. Rowe MB, Bichler D & Clatworthy HW. Windsock of the duodenum. *Ann Surg* 1968; **116**: 444.
3. Gee H & Abdulla U. Antenatal diagnosis of fetal duodenal atresia by ultrasound scan. *BMJ* 1978; **2**: 1265.
4. Hancock BJ & Wiseman NE. Congenital duodenal obstruction: the impact of an antenatal diagnosis. *J Pediatr Surg* 1989; **24**: 1027.
5. Lynn HB. Duodenal obstruction: atresia, stenosis and annular pancreas. In Ravitch MM, Welch KJ, Benson CD, Aberdeen E & Randolph JG (eds) *Pediatric Surgery*. Chicago: Chicago Year Book. 1979; 902.
6. Young DG & Wilkinson AWW. Abnormalities associated with neonatal duodenal atresia. *Surgery* 1968; **6**: 832.
7. Bodian M, White IIR, Carter Co & Louw JH. Congenital duodenal obstruction and mongolism. *BMJ* 1952; **1**: 77.
8. Atwell JD & Klidjan AM. Vertebral anomalies and duodenal atresia. *J Pediatr Surg* 1982; **17**: 237.
9. Kawana T, Ikeda K, Nakagawara A, Kajiwara M, Fukazawa M & Hara K. A case of VACTEL syndrome with antenatally diagnosed duodenal atresia. *J Pediatr Surg* 1989; **24**: 1158.
10. Richardson WR & Martin IW. Pitfalls in the surgical management of the incomplete duodenal diaphragm. *J Pediatr Surg* 1969; **4**: 303.
11. Wilkinson AWW, Hughes EA & Stevens LH. Neonatal duodenal obstruction: the influence of treatment on the metabolic effects of operation. *Br J Surg* 1965; **52**: 410.
12. Curet-Scott MJ, Meller JL & Shermeta DW. Transduodenal feedings: a superior route of enteral nutrition. *J Pediatr Surg* 1987; **22**: 516.
13. Girvan DP & Stephens CA. Congenital duodenal obstruction: a twenty-year review of its surgical management and consequences. *J Pediatr Surg* 1974; **9**: 833.
14. Young DG & Wilkinson AWW. Mortality in neonatal duodenal obstruction. *Lancet*. 1966; **ii**: 18.
15. Okamatsu T, Arai K, Yatsuzuka M et al. Endoscopic membranectomy for congenital duodenal stenosis in an infant. *J Pediatr Surg* 1989; **24**: 367.

16. Weber TR, Lewis JE, Mooney D & Connors R. Duodenal atresia: a comparison of techniques of repair. *J Pediatr Surg* 1986; **21**: 1133.
17. Ein SH & Shandling B. The late nonfunctioning duodenal atresia repair. *J Pediatr Surg* 1986; **21**: 798.
18. Kokkonen M-L, Kalima T, Jaaskelainen J & Louhimo I. Duodenal atresia: late follow-up. *J Pediatr Surg* 1988; **23**: 216.
19. Al-Salem AH, Khwaja S, Grant C & Dawodu A. Congenital intrinsic duodenal obstruction: problems in the diagnosis and management. *J Pediatr Surg* 1989; **24**: 1247.
20. Stauffer UG & Irving I. Duodenal atresia and stenosis – long term results. *Prog Pediatr Surg* 1977; **10**: 49.
21. Perrelli L & Wilkinson AWW. Mortality in neonatal duodenal obstruction; a reveiw of 76 cases compared with a previous reveiw of 142 cases. *J R Coll Surg Edinb* 1975; **20**: 365.
22. Baardson A & Knutrud O. Mortality in neonatal duodenal obstruction. *Z Klin Chir* 1971; **9**: 325.
23. Fonkalsrud EW, deLorimer AA & Hayes DM. Congenital atresia and stenosis of the duodenum: a reveiw compiled from the membership of the surgical section of the American Academy of Pediatrics. *Pediatrie* 1969; **43**: 79.
24. Bower RJ & Ternberg JL. Preduodenal portal vein. *J Pediatr Surg* 1972; **7**: 579.
25. Esscher T. Preduodenal portal vein – a cause of intestinal obstruction. *J Pediatr Surg* 1980; **15**: 609.
26. Wold M, Callery M & White JJ. Ectopic gastric-like duplication of the pancreas. *J Pediatr Surg* 1988; **23**: 1051.
27. Marshall DG & Kim F. Leiomyosarcoma of the duodenum. *J Pediatr Surg* 187; **22**: 1007.
28. Vellacott KD. Intramural haematoma of the duodenum. *Br J Surg* 1980; **67**: 36.
29. Chittmittrapap S, Chandrakamol B & Chomdej S. Intramural haematoma of the alimentary tract in children. *Br J Surg* 1988; **75**: 757.
30. Robarts FH. Traumatic intramural haematoma of the proximal jejunal loop. *Arch Dis Child* 1957; **32**: 484.
31. Stevenson RJ. Non-neonatal intestinal obstruction in children. *Surg Clin North Am* 1985; **65**: 1217.
32. Touloukian RJ. Protocol for nonoperative treatment of obstructing intramural duodenal hematoma during childhood. *Am J Surg* 1983; **145**: 330.

Malrotation

1. Gohl ML and DeMeester WR. Midgut nonrotation in adults: an aggressive approach. *Am J Surg* 1975; **129**: 319.
2. Bill AH. Malrotation of the intestine. In Ravitch MM, Welch KJ, Benson CD, Aberdeen E and Randolph JG (eds) *Pediatric Surgery*. Chicago: Chicago Year Book Medical. 1979; 912.
3. Synder WH & Chaffin L. Embryology and pathology of the intestinal tract: Presentation of 40 cases of malrotation. *Ann Surg* 1954; **140**: 368.
4. Dengler WC & Reddy PP. Right paraduodenal hernia in childhood: a case report. *J Pediatr Surg* 1989; **24**: 1153.
5. Filstron HC & Kirks DR. Malrotation – the ubiquitous anomaly. *J Pediatr Surg* 1981; **16**: 614.
6. Howell CG, Vozza F, Shaw S et al. Malrotation, malnutrition and ischemic bowel disease. *J Pediatr Surg* 1982; **17**: 469.
7. Powell DM, Biemann HO & Smith CD. Malrotation of the intestines in children: the effect of age on presentation and therapy. *J Pediatr Surg* 1989; **24**: 777.
8. Wang CA & Welch CE. Anomalies of intestinal rotation in adolescents and adults. *Surgery* 1963; **54**: 839.
9. Kullendorf CM, Mikaelsson C & Ivancev K. Malrotation in children with symptoms of gastrointestinal allergy and psychosomatic abdominal pain. *Acta Paediatr Scand* 1985; **74**: 296.
10. Stewart DR, Colodny AL & Daggett WC. Malrotation of the bowel in infants and children: a 15 year old review. *Surgery* 1976; **79**: 716.
11. Firor HV & Harris VJ. Rotational anomalies of the gut: recognition of a neglected facet – isolated incomplete rotation of the duodenum. *AJR* 1974; **120**: 315.
12. Stauffer UG and Herrmann P. Comparison of late results in patients with corrected intestinal malrotation with and without fixation of the mesentery. *J Pediatr Surg* 1980; **15**: 9.
13. Jolley SG, Tunnell WP, Thomas S, Young J & Smith EI. The significance of gastric emptying in children with intestinal malrotation. *J Pediatr Surg* 1985; **20**: 627.
14. Wiersma R & Hadley GP. Small bowel volvulus complicating intestinal ascariasis in children. *Br J Surg* 1988; **75**: 86.
15. Ruben GD, Templeton JM & Ziegler MM. Situs inversus: the complex inducing neonatal intestinal obstruction. *J Pediatr Surg* 1983; **18**: 751.
16. Adeyemi SD. Combination of annular pancrease and partial situs inversus: a multiple organ malrotation syndrome associated with duodenal obstruction. *J Pediatr Surg* 1988; **23**: 188.

SMALL BOWEL

SMALL BOWEL ATRESIA

Embryology

Although the cause for duodenal atresia has not been fully elucidated, it is accepted that most small bowel atresias are due to some form of vascular catastrophe. The atresia may be: (1) a complete or incomplete diaphragm within the lumen of the gut; (2) a fibrous band in place of bowel; (3) an area of gut missing; or (4) a gap in both bowel and mesentery[1,2] (Figure 62.20). All are caused by varying degrees of vascular damage, from occlusion of a small end artery to infarction of mesentery and associated bowel. In utero the bowel may intussuscept[3] or the blood supply may be obstructed during the return to the abdominal cavity[4]. There appears to be an association with umbilical cord ulceration.[5] These anomalies occur in 1:6000 live births. Fetal accidents, however, cannot account for all atresias; thus hereditary[6] and intrauterine inflammation have been implicated in multiple atresias.[7]

Amniocentesis has also been implicated.[8] Although jejunal and ileal atresias are usually discussed together, it may be that they are not of similar aetiology[9] for example jejunal atresias are commoner in twins[10] due perhaps to a circulatory imbalance between the twins. There is an equal distribution of atresias between jejunum and ileum.[11]

The proximal bowel becomes grossly dilated whereas the distal bowel remains small, especially if the damage occurs early. If the lesion occurs later in development the distal bowel may contain meconium and be nearer normal size. Multiple atresias can be found in about 20% of such children;[12] the more distal ones may be difficult to diagnose if they are of the diaphragm type as there will be no disparity in size. These multiple atresias are usually jejunoileal,[13,14] but associations with duodenal atresias[15] and other gut atresias[16,17] have been reported. If the blood supply to the small bowel is damaged at source, the supply is taken over by the distal vessels, i.e. coming in a retrograde manner from the ileocolic artery. This supply is insufficient, so that the more proximal bowel becomes atretic and avascular. Such an atresia is called 'apple peel'[18,19] because of the appearance of the bowel hanging on the distal blood supply; other names are 'Christmas tree',[20] 'fir tree' or 'barber pole'. The gut is frequently short in length, and the proximal portion often has a very tenuous blood supply making anastomoses doubtful. Small bowel stenosis is found in only 5% of cases.

Presentation

The newborn presents with bile-stained vomiting and usually with failure to pass meconium, although in the late type, the infant may pass some meconium from the distal gut. Distension depends on the site of obstruction. The mother may

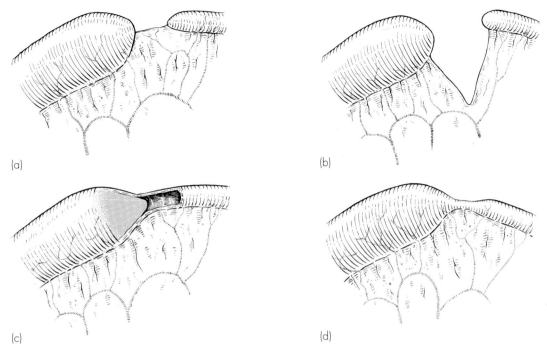

(a)

(b)

(c)

(d)

Figure 62.20
(a–d) Different types of small bowel atresi. (Reproduced with permission of W.B. Saunders.)

have had polyhydramnios. Small bowel atresias, especially of the apple peel or multiple type, can occur in families.[21,22]

Diagnosis

Diagnosis is made by means of erect (or lateral decubitus) and supine abdominal radiographs. A small bowel obstruction will be seen with no colonic gas. The number of fluid levels helps to indicate the level of the atresia. Sometimes the grossly dilated distal portion of the bowel above the obstruction can be seen. Care should be taken to differentiate this problem from that of meconium ileus which also gives a small bowel obstruction. The use of gastrografin[23] will not always help elucidate the problem and urgent laparotomy may be necessary to make the diagnosis.

Operation

At laparotomy the site of the first atresia is obvious. Resection of the proximal portion of the distal collapsed bowel allows for passage of a catheter, so that fluid may be passed distally to delineate the gut and pick up any further atretic areas. It should be possible to watch for the distension also occurring in the colon, as occasionally colonic atresias can occur in conjunction with small bowel atresias.[16,17]

In ileal atresias, it is relatively easy to resect back the proximal dilated bowel until more normal peristaltic bowel is reached without compromising the length of bowel retained. If this procedure is not carried out, the dilated bowel acts like a sump and causes an obstruction.[15] Fish-tailing of the distal bowel is usually necessary on the antimesenteric edge to allow for end-to-end anastomosis. End-to-side anastomosis should not be performed, as this leads later to enlargement of the end of bowel and problems with overgrowth of organisms in the

blind loop. With the more proximal atresias such resection is more difficult especially in high jejunal cases as this would involve the duodenum. Since the ischaemic damage is limited,[24] tailoring of the proximal bowel[25] may allow for an easier and better anastomosis and is preferable to infolding (plication)[26] of the proximal bowel to equate the size of lumen. In any case such high atresias should not be treated with stomas since these would be of the high output type. Lower down the bowel it may be better to form stomas side by side to allow the distillation of the output from the proximal stoma to be instilled via a catheter into the distal stoma, thereby preventing fluid and electrolyte loss and promoting an increase in size.

Results

In the ileal atresias, the results are excellent, as the atresia usually occurs late and primary anastomosis is possible. Jejunal atresias occur in babies with low gestational age and birth weight,[9] thus giving a higher mortality rate. Often the postoperative course is prolonged and complicated. In the high atresias of the 'apple peel' type, the bowel is often already short, so that after operation there may be insufficient length for development. Problems of short gut, either iatrogenic or congenital, will be discussed later. With the apple peel type, stricture at the anastomotic site or breakdown of the anastomosis due to further ischaemia are not uncommon. Another reason for anastomosis failure is distal Hirschsprung's disease.[27]

Overall 85% survival rate can be expected. Apart from an association with meconium ileus in children, with cystic fibrosis other congenital abnormalities are rare.[28] Urgent surgery before perforation has occurred, should ensure reasonable results[29] even in the premature baby. If insufficient of the dilated gut has been resected, further surgery may be necessary.

MECONIUM ILEUS

Cause

Children with cystic fibrosis lack pancreatic enzymes and so have viscid secretions which lead to chronic infection of the lungs and pulmonary damage. In the bowel the meconium is also viscid and blocks the lumen of the bowel, leading to meconium ileus which occurs in 10–15% of these children. The 1:2000 incidence becomes one in four in affected families.[1] Inherited as an autosomal recessive trait, the gene has now been identified.[2]

In the newborn child the viscid meconium causes a small bowel obstruction. The distal bowel remains as a microcolon and the inspissated meconium forms hard pellets which increase the obstruction. Proximal to the terminal ileum the gut is dilated with sticky meconium and may even twist on its mesentery and perforate if the obstruction is not relieved. Not all children with cystic fibrosis suffer from meconium ileus. Indeed a mild form may present only with a meconium plug, removal of which relieves the obstruction.[3] Since older children may present with rectal prolapse, cystic fibrosis should be excluded in all children with rectal prolapse. These gastrointestinal problems are related to exocrine pancreatic function.[4] Symptoms suggestive of motility disorders may present later, for example oesophageal reflux and distal intestinal obstruction syndrome (DIOS).[5]

Children presenting with meconium ileus tend to be less severely affected by lung disease but this is not invariably the case.[6]

Respiratory problems may occur later. Most children (70%) with cystic fibrosis now survive into adult life.

Presentation and diagnosis

As with the small bowel atresia cases, affected children present with abdominal distension and failure to pass meconium. In mild cases occasionally a meconium plug is passed, which relieves the obstruction. Estimation of the proteolytic activity of the meconium and the presence or absence of trypsin is not always accurate. The protein content of the meconium[7] is very high but only in those with pancreatic insufficiency at birth. A family history is not always available.

Plain abdominal radiograph shows uniformly distended bowel but sometimes little gas despite the gross distension. If there is no suggestion of perforation, a gastrografin enema[8,9] will delineate the microcolon and show the meconium pellets. Gastrografin consists of a 76% aqueous solution of sodium methyl glucamine diatrizoate plus a wetting agent. Its high osmolality (1900 mosmol/l as opposed to that of plasma of 300 mosmol/l) gives it its hygroscopic properties, so that it may also loosen the viscid meconium and relieve the obstruction. This therapeutic as well as diagnostic use means that, in the absence of complications, the problem can be treated without operation, allowing medical treatment of the cystic fibrosis to start early.

Sometimes it may take more than one gastrografin enema to relieve the obstruction. Care must be taken to perform this investigation with an intravenous drip in situ, since it is easy for such small babies to become dehydrated[10] as the fluid is drawn into the lumen of the bowel. There is also a danger of perforation of the bowel.[11] If the plain radiograph of the abdomen suggests perforation, then such an enema should not be performed. As the perforation occurs antenatally there is no free gas, rather an increase in extraluminal contents of the abdomen giving an appearance of very little gas within the bowel; the meconium gives a mottled appearance with calcification if the perforation is long standing. Meconium peritonitis is a sterile chemical reaction following intrauterine perforation, causing a dense reaction with calcification and even a meconium pseudocyst.[12] Such calcification does not always mean that the diagnosis[13] is meconium ileus. The perforation is a result of the heavy meconium filling the dilated small bowel which twists and gives rise to ischaemia.

If the child has not been fed, it is possible to test the first passed meconium for trypsin activity. However, this test is rarely possible. Apart from histological examination the diagnosis has to await the result of a sweat test.[14] The child must be old enough and large enough to produce sufficient sweat to allow estimation of the sodium content. High sodium levels above 70 meq/l are abnormal but the test may need to be repeated if doubtful. In the past mothers would comment on the fact that their children tasted salty when kissed! Gene identification can now be undertaken of the child and parents[15].

Not all children with the signs suggestive of meconium ileus have cystic fibrosis[16] and so the sweat test is important for long-term prognosis.[17] A microcolon on contrast studies is not always pathognomonic.[18]

Meconium plug syndrome

The passage of a meconium plug may relieve the obstruction so that the infant continues to pass meconium satisfactorily. Dislodgement of the plug may have been achieved by saline washouts or a gastrografin enema. In all such cases even if they appear well, Hirschsprung's disease and cystic fibrosis must be excluded before discharge, although some may have no abnormal findings.[19]

Operation

Surgical treatment is necessary in one-half to two-thirds of cases. If perforation has occurred or gastrografin enema has been unsuccessful, a laparotomy will reveal the obstruction. When perforation has occurred, the meconium pseudocyst will make dissection difficult. It is necessary to resect the most dilated and necrotic area. Both proximal and distal bowel can be washed out, preferably with gastrografin, to clear the meconium. Alternatively some of the sticky meconium may be milked distally through the microcolon to pass per rectum. Some surgeons advocate reanastomosis[20] after this manoeuvre or only perform enterotomies[21,22] to irrigate the bowel, but there is a high risk of further problems. Most surgeons advocate either doubled-barrelled ileostomy or a Bishop–Koop anastomosis.[23]

Bishop–Koop anastomosis

This operation avoids excessive handling of what may be friable bowel of doubtful viability. In this operation, after resection, the dilated proximal bowel is anastomosed to the side of the narrow terminal ileum, care being taken not to twist the mesentery (Figure 62.21). Contents may pass through the anastomosis into the colon, but if there is still distal obstruction the contents will pass out through the ileostomy which is made from the proximal end of the distal bowel. Gastrografin can be instilled through this stoma to relieve the obstruction.[24] When the bowel is working normally, closure is performed relatively easily, as the continuity of the bowel does not need to be interrupted. The use of the appendix as a stoma has been suggested.[25]

Meconium ileus equivalent (DIOS)[26]

In the older child or adult, a similar problem can obstruct the lumen of the gut with sticky meconium.[27] It sometimes arises when the pancreatic enzyme given to help digestion of food is administered incorrectly or in the wrong dosage.[28] Again gastrografin enema may obviate the need to operate.[29] DIOS is an indication of pancreatic insufficiency.

Postoperative management

Life-long treatment with pancreatic enzymes must be started as soon as feeding is commenced although the risk of breakdown of any anastomosis must be kept in mind. Pancreatic enzymes, such as Pancreax or Creon, are given to aid digestion. Prophylactic antibiotics and daily physiotherapy are needed to control respiratory infection.

Results

It appears that children with cystic fibrosis who present with meconium ileus tend to do rather better than those presenting later with respiratory problems. However, those who have already perforated by the time of diagnosis, do badly and may not survive.[24]

Prolonged jaundice[30] in infancy may complicate recovery. About 5% of patients develop multilobular cirrhosis of the liver,[31] and some go on to portal hypertension. Young adolescents may have obstruction of the biliary tree with stones or sludge.[32] Problems with short bowel and malabsorption may lead to failure to thrive. As well as oesophageal reflux,[33] gastric emptying may be delayed and small bowel transit time prolonged.[34] Infertility is likely in both males[35] and females.[36]

It is best for the child to come under the care of a paediatrician with an interest in the disease so that up-to date treatment and proper surveillance is given. A problem can arise with the late diagnosis of appendicitis[37] in association with their other problems. Genetic counselling must also be given. Although moderate, the long-term prognosis for these children has certainly improved over recent years so that survival into their thirties is possible.

Milk plug syndrome

Inspissated milk curds can block the terminal ileum[38] presenting at about one week of life. The aetiology is unclear, since a variety of different milks including dried powdered milk[39] have been implicated. It does not occur in babies fed on breast milk possibly because 92% of breast milk fat is absorbed in contrast to only 65% of other types, e.g. formula (Ostermilk).[40]

Milk plug syndrome can even mimic necrotizing enterocolitis[41] in that abdominal distension may be associated with blood per rectum. Radiological appearances show an intramural mass with a halo of air.[42] A gastrografin enema will sometimes relieve the obstruction,[43] but it will show a normal-sized colon and not a microcolon as in meconium ileus. If unsuccessful, operation is performed to remove the 'soap' by enterostomy.

NECROTIZING ENTEROCOLITIS (NEC)

Incidence

The main reason for gastrointestinal perforation in the neonate involving the large or small bowel is necrotizing enterocolitis.[1] About 10–20% of admissions to a neonatal surgical unit will be because of necrotizing enterocolitis or its complications. The incidence has increased to 24 per 1000 births[2] as a result of improved neonatal care, especially of the very small premature infant.[3] Although 75% of cases occur in these small and very premature babies, weighing less than 2000 g with an Apgar score of less than 6,[4] necrotizing enterocolitis can occur in full-term or older children[5,6] and sometimes postoperatively.[7,8] It can even occur in adults.[9] Although common in multiple births, not all babies of each pregnancy are necessarily involved.[10] A form of ulcerating enterocolitis can occur in infants.[11]

Pathogenesis

The precise aetiology has still not been fully worked out.[12] Probably the cause is multifactorial in the susceptible infant. Experimental work on pigs[13] and rats[14] has tried to produce an experimental model to study the pathogenesis and also a

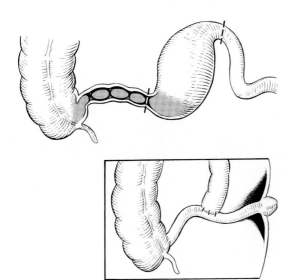

Figure 62.21
Diagrammatic illustration of Bishop Koop anastomosis.

means of modifing or preventing the disease. There is often an anoxic episode either at or after birth leading to a reduction in the microcirculation with ischaemia and cell damage.[15] Haemodynamic changes as seen in exchange transfusions[16] or with a patent ductus arteriosus[17] lead to ischaemic bowel. Whether ischaemia results from anoxia or from direct damage to the vessels[18] (even if temporary[19]), the bowel has no defence to infection which probably stems from its own lumen.

In a full blown case, a mucosal ulcer allows gas from the lumen to enter the wall of the bowel giving the classical appearance of pneumocystis intestinalis.[20] Less severe cases may only exhibit a picture of functional obstruction. As well as prematurity, the stress of a traumatic birth (e.g. the cord round the neck) or respiratory problems are frequently found to precede necrotizing enterocolitis.[21] In the past, the use of umbilical vessel catheters that were incorrectly positioned led to ischaemic gut and so to necrotizing enterocolitis.[22]

At operation the bowel is paper-thin with necrotic patches, inflammatory exudate or areas of perforation. The lumen is filled with haemorrhagic debris, and the mucosa may slough.[23] Considering the complex intestinal flora pattern, it is not surprising that numerous organisms are grown, e.g. anaerobes, especially *Clostridium* sp.[24] or *Escherichia coli*[25] and coagulase negative staphylococci.[26] Quantitative changes have been found in the bacterial flora of the intestine preceding an episode.[27] No one organism can be implicated, but those children in whom clostridia are grown seem to have a more fulminating disease.[28] Although it has been suggested that delaying feeding reduces the chance of necrotizing enterocolitis,[29] the disease may be evident within days of birth before feeding has started.[30] Different feeding regimes may also have a bearing on the aetiology, since they allow for different colonization of the bowel. It has been suggested that breast milk helps reduce the incidence by an immunological mechanism.[31] Although the defence mechanism is poor in such children and the immunological action of immunoglobulins IgM and IgG promote further cell damage,[21,32] necrotizing enterocolitis is not a result of an immature immune mechanism.[33] Other factors may be increased intraluminal pressure and decreased pH.[34] The occurrence of many cases in a unit might suggest an epidemiological cause,[35] but it could also be a reflection on the excellent postnatal care of these infants, since it is not uncommon now for babies of 26 weeks to survive (less than 1 kg in weight). Prevention may depend on modification of the bowel flora.[36] One of the risk factors appears to be gestational age so that there is usually a predisposing factor[37] when the disease occurs in the full-term baby.

Presentation and diagnosis

The full blown picture may not occur in all children. A baby may only have a functional obstruction with vomiting and abdominal distension, sometimes associated with delay in the passage of meconium. Most babies will have abdominal distension with the passage of blood per rectum. If septicaemia occurs, disseminated intravascular coagulation can lead to bleeding problems and eventual death. The area and extent of

bowel involved can vary, but the terminal ileum is frequently affected.

The diagnosis of a mild case is by an abdominal radiograph, which shows only gaseous distension with separation of loops of bowel by intraperitoneal fluid. In the established case the radiograph shows intramural gas, giving an appearance of a target (Figure 62.22). A poor prognostic sign, seen either on abdominal radiograph or ultrasonography, is gas in the portal venous system[38,39] although this is not invariably the case[40] and the gas may last only 24 hours. If perforation has occurred, free gas is seen. Even on the supine radiograph a haziness over the liver or an odd-shaped gas shadow suggests gas outside the bowel. Perforations may be difficult to diagnose on plain radiograph. The use of Omnipaque, which does not irritate when extravasated, may allow early diagnosis.[41] Volvulus which can give a similar picture, and bilious vomiting should alert one to the possibility of this diagnosis.[42] The diagnosis of necrotizing enterocolitis is often made on suspicion alone, and therefore treatment is started empirically.

Treatment

Medical treatment

In the absence of complications, it is better to treat the baby conservatively without operation by resting the bowel and treating the infection. Intravenous feeding is given for 2 to 3 weeks with appropriate antibiotics to treat the Gram-negative

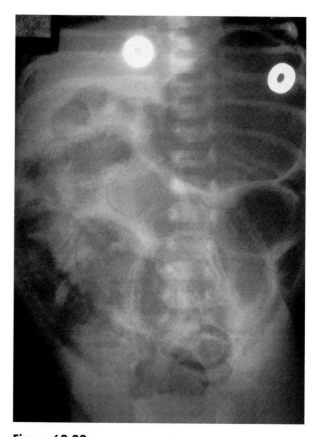

Figure 62.22
Plain abdominal radiograph indicating intramural gas in a neonate with NEC.

infection, especially the anaerobic bacteria. Gentamycin and metronidazole are a suitable combination. In the very ill child, fresh frozen plasma or steroids may be indicated to treat the septicaemia and shock. Experimentally dopamine and other adrenergic amines do not help; in fact they aggravate the intestinal ischaemia.[43] Many very small babies with enterocolitis die with or without operation.[44] Frequent radiographs,[45] even 6 hourly, will help to determine when perforation occurs. It can be surprisingly difficult otherwise to know when perforation has occurred, and the diagnosis may even be missed on radiograph. Perforation of the intestine occurs in about half the cases of necrotizing enterocolitis.[46] Otherwise the disease process may resolve or lead on to late stricture formation.

Surgical treatment

Results with or without early operation[47] show that even if laparotomy is undertaken, when there is no perforation, the results are poor because it can be difficult to know which part of the bowel to remove and how much. Despite aggressive medical treatment, operation may still be necessary especially for the complications. Serial platelet counts and abdominal radiographs help in the decision to operate.[48] Complications in the acute phase are abscess formation or perforation with peritonitis and septicaemia.[49] If these occur, operation is the only hope of saving the child, yet the baby may be too ill to undergo laparotomy. In such infants, a drain inserted into the abdomen may improve the child's condition.[50,51] In the past, most of these babies died before definitive surgery could be carried out, since the septicaemia did not resolve. However, more recent results suggest that this is an effective means of temporizing.[52] In a few cases, there can be complete resolution of the disease,[53] especially in the very small birthweight infant.[54]

At operation it may be necessary to resect large areas of bowel, either colon or small bowel, leaving the child with an insufficient length of intestine. The decision is whether to bring out stomas,[55] which may be high in the small bowel or perform a primary anastomosis.[56,57] By anastomosing the bowel, problems with fluid losses and malabsorption can be avoided but problems with ischaemic anastomoses and breakdown can occur. If stomas are performed – and this is generally preferred[58,59] – these can be closed early[60,61] without problems rather than wait some months until the child has gained weight. Although some surgeons maintain that they can always anastomose the bowel at the initial operation, it is probably better to decide on the correct treatment in individual cases depending on the condition of the child and the extent and state of the diseased bowel.[62] In the very ill baby with numerous areas of diseased bowel, ligation of segments followed by a second look and later resection has been suggested.[63]

Late complications

In a child who has been treated for enterocolitis problems can arise later with the introduction of feeding, bleeding[64] or recurrent abdominal distension. A delayed barium study (either barium meal, follow-through or enema) may then delineate strictures in the large or small bowel.[65] Such strictures occur in a quarter of survivors of medical treatment[66] and especially affect the colon.[67,68] Routine barium studies should therefore be performed in all such children.[69,70] Treatment is by resection and primary anastomosis, although balloon dilatation has been attempted.[71] A further problem can be a fatal fungal infection, especially after an operation and parenteral nutrition and intensive care.[72]

Results

Since not all newborns with necrotizing enterocolitis will be sent to specialized medical or surgical units, it is difficult to gauge the true incidence of the disease or the number of those requiring surgical intervention. Not all babies have the full-blown picture, and milder cases may not be included in any statistics. Other problems of prematurity, such as respiratory disease and intracranial haemorrhage have a bearing on the eventual prognosis, as do other congenital defects or a low platelet count and blood pH.[73] Although survival rates have improved[74] and mortality rates are less than 40%,[75] long-term sequelae are not uncommon, probably reflecting more the prematurity than the poor condition of the child.[76] Although there may be some late gastrointestinal problems, the long-term results in children who survive necrotizing enterocolitis are encouraging.[77] Although total involvement of the intestine is almost uniformly fatal, almost 60% of premature children survive.[78] Postoperative enterocolitis complicating other neonatal surgical conditions should be treated in the same manner. Again the pathogenesis is not clear.

Not all perforations in the newborn period are due to this condition.[79] Localized single perforations may be the cause if there is no evidence of other disease.[80] Maternal obstetric problems are common in such cases.[81] Simple excision of the perforation site and closure is all that is necessary. There is an 80% survival with few sequelae.

Functional obstruction

Mention has already been made of a possible lesser degree of necrotizing enterocolitis presenting as a functional obstruction. Failure to pass meconium associated with abdominal distension and vomiting are common presentations to a neonatal surgical unit.[82]

Some infants will proceed to a full-blown necrotizing enterocolitis especially if there are associated factors of prematurity and respiratory distress. Others will settle after a few days of intravenous fluids and nasogastric suction. In all infants, Hirschsprung's disease, meconium ileus and sepsis should be excluded by suction biopsy, sweat test and an infection screen, respectively. Other causes include hypothyroidism and hypoglycaemia associated with a diabetic mother. In such a child, barium enema appearances can mimic Hirschsprung's disease giving a 'hypoplastic left colon'.[83] Functional obstruction can also complicate malrotation and children with short gut for whatever reason.[84]

COMPLICATIONS OF SMALL BOWEL OPERATION

It has already been mentioned that operations on the small bowel in neonates or the underlying abnormality itself frequently give rise to complications.

Stomas

Stomas can lead to massive fluid and electrolyte loss, especially those created high in the jejunum. Losses can be partially counteracted by instilling the secretions from the proximal stoma into the distal stoma to allow absorption. However in the more distal stomas, electrolyte loss, especially chloride and sodium, can still occur, so that many babies with stomas will require salt supplements. Early closure of stomas will reduce these problems.

If correctly fashioned and brought out separate to the wound, the actual stomas in the small bowel should give few problems. Unlike colostomies in children, they rarely prolapse, and if the bowel is viable they should not retract. Most babies accept a stoma and will even play with it. The problem of acceptance is with the parents, especially in certain ethnic groups.

Disaccharide intolerance[1]

Even when resection has not been carried out, anastomoses without resection have been shown to affect growth and maturation[2] of the gut so that, in duodenal atresia for example, disaccharide intolerance may occur. Profuse diarrhoea produces loss of weight and dehydration. In such children the stools should be immediately checked for acid by using a litmus paper. If positive, a stool specimen can be sent for estimation of the amount and types of sugars present. Changing the child to an appropriate sugar-free feed[3] will lead to thickening of the stool, an increase in weight and a general improvement. As various sugars can be malabsorbed, including lactose, fructose and maltose, it is important to use the correct feed. Since this is an acquired intolerance, in time, the bowel will adapt and the child can be weaned back onto normal feeds some months later. Care must be taken during this process so that a recurrence of the diarrhoea does not occur.

Parenteral nutrition

Even if the neonate has an adequate length of bowel, failure to feed within 2 to 3 days, for whatever reason, necessitates parenteral feeding to allow for normal growth.[4] If the neonate or infant is left with a short length of bowel, malabsorption and malnutrition[5] will occur necessitating parenteral feeding for some time.

Intravenous feeding is by means of a central catheter[6,7] easily inserted either under local anaesthetic in the neonatal unit or under general anaesthetic in theatre.[8] If the catheter is left in situ for any length of time, there is a high complication rate.[9] Sepsis[10,11] may be local at the site of insertion or general, i.e. septicaemia. Even fragments of the line can be left behind requiring surgery for removal.[12] Jaundice, due to cholestasis,[13–15]

Venous thrombosis[16] even of superior vena cava[17] and misplacement of the catheter[18] can also occur. Such problems are minimized by the use of special teams.[19] Metronidazole has helped reduce liver dysfunction by decreasing intestinal anaerobic flora[20] in these children. The actual cause of liver damage is unknown, but it may partly be due to deficiencies in the solutions administered.[21,22] During such treatment, deficiencies of amino acids,[23] vitamins and trace elements[24,25] will develop without the necessary supplements, and careful monitoring is required if the parenteral feeding is prolonged. Hyperlipidaemia[26] can occur, and lipid may be deposited in the brain and liver[27] if it is not given in regulated doses.[28]

In the past this necessitated long-term hospitalization, but with home parenteral nutrition programmes[29,30] it is possible to send these children home. Home parentral nutrition puts a great strain on both the family and the unit supervising the care. It is possible for children to grow and develop normally on such a regime,[31,32] despite the fact that gastrointestinal growth and development is delayed[33] on total parenteral nutrition. Eventually oral feeding can be slowly reintroduced, and the child can be weaned off the parenteral feeding.

Although some intestinal fistulas require long-term parenteral nutrition to heal, the use of long-acting somatostatin can be beneficial in infants and reduce the duration of parenteral feeding.[34]

Short bowel syndrome

Normal intestinal length in premature infants more than doubles[35] during the later weeks of gestation, the average length being 250 cm at birth. Although the actual length of bowel is important and should be measured at operation, the normal process of lengthening should be remembered when dealing with preterm babies. Under 75 cm of small bowel remaining suggests that the child will have problems associated with short gut. Until recently, 20–25 cm of bowel, including an intact ileocaecal valve, was thought to be the minimum length for survival,[36] indicating that the type of bowel preserved and the maintenance of the ileocaecal valve are important for maximum absorption.[37,38] As well as malabsorption of proteins, carbohydrates and fat, trace elements such as zinc, magnesium,[39] cobalt, copper and selenium are low. As these trace elements are important for healing of tissues, breakdown of wounds and anastomoses may occur. Some children also have transient hypothyroidism[40] requiring hormonal treatment. Given time (often months) adaptation[41] occur (see Chapter 46). Although some enteral feeding may then be possible,[42] to allow growth, the child still requires intravenous supplementation with all its attendant problems. With adaptation, physiological and microscopic morphology alter[43] so that by one year the child no longer has diarrhoea and will absorb water-soluble vitamins and electrolytes.[44] The bowel will also have increased in length.[45] The loss of the ileocaecal valve and the terminal ileum will only require vitamin B12 supplements after 2 years, since liver stores of this vitamin are substantial.[46] A variety of factors[47,48] including the H$_2$ receptor antagonist, cimetidine[49] accelerate bowel adaptation.

Even if total parenteral nutriton has not been necessary, children with short bowel require long hospitalization with manipulation of their diet to give an isotonic or hypotonic feed. Comminuted chicken plus some medium chain triglyceride (MCT) are easily absorbed, but each child needs individual dietary attention for up to two years. The outlook is promising and most children eventually grow normally.

Bowel lengthening

To try to reduce the time spent in hospital and the complications associated with such parenteral feeding, various methods[50] have been tried to delay transit or lengthen the bowel. Surgical procedures include reversed intestinal segments and colonic interposition, either isoperistaltic[51] or antiperistaltic,[52] but these attempts have met with little success. The formation of a valve by means of intussuscepting bowel[53] has been suggested, but this may be impractical in children with already insufficient bowel.

Bianchi[54] has developed a means of lengthening the bowel, which is particularly easy in the dilated bowel of an atresia. The blood supply in the mesentery can be separated to supply each half of the bowel which can then be divided into two by means of a stapler; thus each half has its own blood supply (Figure 62.23a–d). The two portions of bowel can then be anastomosed in continuity in a peristaltic fashion, thereby doubling the length of remaining bowel and converting a child with a critically short gut into one who requires little or no parenteral nutrition.[55]

Experimental work to grow small bowel mucosa[56,57] or to transplant the small bowel[58–62] has led to liver and small bowel transplants with improvements in the survival rate in these children.[63–67] Liver failure following long-term parenteral nutrition may respond to isolated liver transplant[68] or even tandem transplantation of liver and bowel.[69]

INTUSSUSCEPTION

Pathogenesis

Intussusception is the commonest cause of bowel obstruction in infancy;[1] if not diagnosed it may lead to long-term problems or even death. When proximal bowel infolds into distal bowel, peristalsis enables it to progress onwards, dragging the mesentery into the intussucepiens. This occurs either with thickening of the bowel due to an increase of lymphatic tissue (Peyer's patches)[2] itself the result of recent infection or because a lesion such as a polyp, tumour or Meckel's diverticulum acts as a target leading on to a secondary intussusception (especially in the older child).[3] In either case, the mesentery becomes oedematous, and venous congestion develops with subsequent

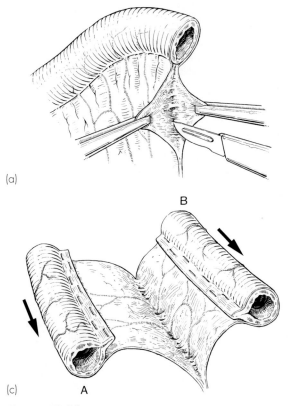

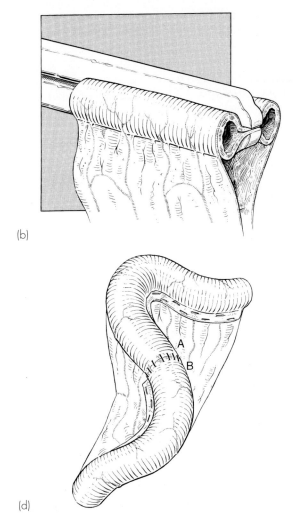

Figure 62.23
Stages of Bianchi bowel lengthening. (a) Splitting of mesentery with vessels either side; (b) stapler used to form two new loops of bowel; (c) completion of separation, with division and stapling of bowel; (d) joining in continuity the two loops of bowel to double the length of bowel available. (Reproduced by permission of W.B. Saunders.)

arterial compression. These changes lead on to ischaemia and infarction of the bowel with resultant perforation and peritonitis. Such events occur over a period of time and, until ischaemia occurs, are reversible. However, the actual progression of the intussusception occurs rapidly.[4] The intussusception may be ileoileal, ileocolic or colocolic or combinations of these as one intussusception may lead to another.

Presentation

Classically occurring in the healthy infant from 4 to 10 months, the intussusception presents with colic, the baby drawing up his legs in distress. There may have been a preceding viral infection.[5] The mass of the intussusceptum may be difficult to feel, especially in an unhappy, irritable child. The sausage-shaped mass may lie below the liver. The association of vomiting and diarrhoea[6,7] which occurred in 11% of our series, suggests the misleading diagnosis of gastroenteritis. Passage of blood per rectum, the typical 'red currant jelly' stools, is pathognomonic but indicates that the intussusceptum is already congested and probably ischaemic. The diagnosis should have been made before the triad of colic, a mass and blood per rectum, are present, since this occurs at a late stage. If intussusception is diagnosed before this stage, it may be possible for it to reduce spontaneously or with assistance. Dehydration and shock occur rapidly to produce a quiet, unresponsive infant. However, the presentation is rarely classical.[8]

In the older child or adult,[9] polyps or tumour may lead to a recurrent, chronic intussusception. They may also be difficult to diagnose.[10] Meckel's diverticulum can also lead to an intussusception but it can also produce bleeding from ulceration of ectopic gastric mucosa. The most likely tumour in a child is lymphosarcoma,[11] and this can also present with bleeding in the absence of intussusception.

Diagnosis

As already stated the triad of pain, mass and bleeding is important but occurs late in the natural history of intussusception and in only 50% of cases.[12] Colic is a common problem in the young so the diagnosis must be kept in mind. The child may be lethargic and disinclined to feed, and may even be shocked.

With a high index of suspicion, a plain radiograph of the abdomen can show an emptiness in the right iliac fossa. This 'signe de Dance' is not a good physical sign but it is helpful on radiographs. If the history is short and the child in reasonable condition, a barium enema performed early will help to confirm the diagnosis and may even, by using increased hydrostatic pressure,[13] reduce the intussusception. This manoeuvre is successful in over three quarters of children if performed early enough.[14,15] Thus the investigation is both diagnostic, visualizing the cup-shaped indentation or corkscrew appearance, and also therapeutic. The risk in performing this manoeuvre is that of perforation of the bowel,[16] which is more likely to occur if the bowel is ischaemic, i.e. if there is blood per rectum, or the infant is shocked with signs of peritonitis. These are the only absolute contraindications. The presence on the radiograph of

fluid levels does not itself preclude a barium study,[17,18] but it diminishes the chances of success in reducing the intussusception.[19] During attempts to reduce the intussusception, barium must flow freely up the ileum to confirm complete reduction. Thereafter the child requires observation for 24 hours in case of a recurrence.[20]

A contrast or air enema should be performed on suspicion as occasionally a long-standing intussusception will be painless.[21] It is also possible, especially in the older child, to misdiagnose appendicitis as a successfully reduced intussusception[22] so that a laparotomy should be performed if doubt exists. A long-standing intussusception[23,24] of over 48 hours with bleeding per rectum and fluid levels on the radiograph is unlikely to reduce.[25] In such cases there is a contraindication to hydrostatic reduction[26,27] since the manoeuvre is unlikely to be successful. More recently air enemas[28] have been used with success especially when used in association with ultrasonography.[29] Saline enemas[30] also have been used. However, if the reduction is to be attempted by a radiologist who infrequently deals with children, barium is the best medium.[31]

Operation

Even if the appearance on barium study suggests reduction, if there is no resultant free flow up the small bowel laparotomy should be performed. This should also be the case in those children in whom a target lesion is suspected, since recurrence of the problem is inevitable.

Preoperative rehydration is mandatory as well as preoperative antibiotics. While the contrast enema is being performed, the surgical team should be ready to operate immediately in case of perforation.

At operation (Figure 62.24) through a small transverse incision, it may be possible by gentle manipulation to milk the bowel and reduce the intussusception, care must be taken not to tear the serosa. It is unwise to attempt this reduction if the bowel is thought to be necrotic. In these cases, resection of the segment is performed, almost always including the ileocaecal valve, followed by primary anastomosis.[32-34] Complications may result when the anastomosis is carried out in the presence of obstruction. Late problems can also arise from the loss of the ileocaecal valve, especially in the very young infant.

Recurrence

If a successful radiological reduction is achieved, recurrence of the intussusception suggests the presence of an underlying polyp or diverticulum and indicates that operation should be undertaken on this second occasion. This is especially true in children over the age of 2 years. If recurrence occurs early, it is more likely to be due to incomplete initial reduction than actual recurrence. Otherwise, recurrence is unusual with an incidence of 5–10%.[35] Recurrence is especially unlikely after operative reduction because adhesions reduce the mobility of the bowel. A rare occurrence is chronic intussusception,[36] which lasts for days and is associated with weight loss as well as an abdominal mass. This condition necessitates laparotomy as there is almost always a precipitating cause.

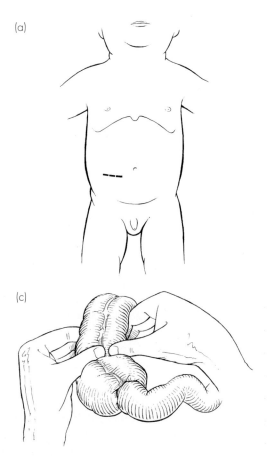

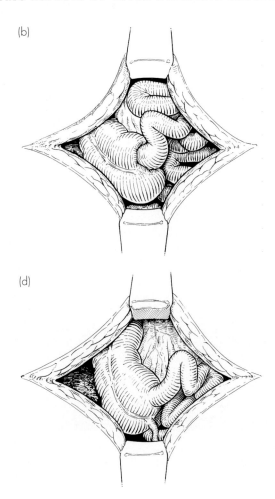

Figure 62.24
(a–d) Operative technique for reducing an intussusception.

Intrauterine intussusceptions may lead to atresia and even ascites.[37] Another type of intussusception is that of a gastrostomy tube pushing gastroduodenal mucosa forwards to block the gastric outlet.[38] It is important to remember this possibility in all babies with gastrostomy tubes.

OTHER SMALL BOWEL CONDITIONS

Recurrent abdominal pain

In the infant and older child abdominal pain or 'little belly achers'[1] is a common problem. It has been said that two out of 500 children under the age of 12 will have abdominal pain serious enough to warrant admission to hospital.[2] The causes are numerous[3] and the pain may be acute or recurrent. Apart from those mentioned later, other common diagnoses[4] to be considered are appendicitis,[5,6] constipation,[7,8] urinary tract infection and mesenteric adenitis as well as rare causes like segmental infarction of the greater omentum[9,10] and primary peritonitis. Medical conditions should not be forgotten, e.g. pneumonia,[11] gastroenteritis, infective hepatitis and sickle cell crisis.[12] Diagnostic investigations[13] include full blood count, erythrocyte sedimentation rate, urinalysis, abdominal radiographs, intravenous urography, gastrointestinal contrast studies, ultrasonography,[14] other types of scans and endoscopy. Exploratory laparotomies[15,16] must not be performed in children to exclude organic disease. If necessary, laparoscopy[17,18] may be used in a difficult case. As a therapeutic measure,

laparoscopic appendicectomy in children is becoming more common.[19,20]

Other small bowel problems present with either a mass, intestinal obstruction or gastrointestinal bleeding. Rare causes of obstruction (Figure 62.25) are congenital bands,[21] fibromatosis,[22] trichobezoar[23] or, in the older girl, a membrane (an abdominal cocoon[24,25] possibly of an infective nature.

Although a high percentage of children with recurrent abdominal pain will have behavioural and psychological problems, care must be taken to make sure that organic disease is not present before the child is so labelled.

Inguinal hernia

The commonest cause of obstruction is an incarcerated inguinal hernia. The anatomy of the groin in young children, especially those under the age of one year, means that an indirect hernia is almost direct.[25] Therefore, it is relatively easy for bowel to become incarcerated in the hernia and cause an obstruction. If the bowel is only partially involved (Richter's hernia)[27] the hernia may not be seen on inspection and is only diagnosed on palpation.

At operation, not only is the gut necrotic but the testis may also be dead.[28] To prevent this complication, infant hernias must be operated on[29] as an emergency as soon as the diagnosis is made, even in the very premature baby.[30] With modern anaesthesia and paediatric trained surgeons results can be excellent.[31,32]

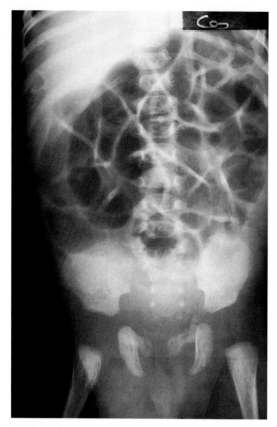

Figure 62.25
Plain abdominal x-ray showing abdominal distension with air in the right scrotum indicating an obstructed hernia.

Once the bowel has become incarcerated, if it is not reduced immediately, the surgeon is faced with a series of difficult decisions often in a very small baby: (1) to deal with infarcted gut by resection followed either by a doubtful anastomosis in obstructed bowel or by a stoma requiring later reanastomosis; (2) an ischaemic testis which should either be removed or left in the hope that it might improve; (3) a very fine and oedematous hernial sac which is likely to tear so increasing the chance of a recurrent hernia.[33] All these problems stand in contrast to simple day-case surgery for herniotomy in an elective case.[34] It is not justified to explore the contralateral side if there is no evidence of a hernia, as damage to the testes is possible.[35]

Direct inguinal hernias with weakness of the fascia are rare.[36] Femoral hernias are also uncommon[37] and often misdiagnosed as inguinal hernias[38] but they rarely strangulate.[39]

Crohn's disease

Inflammatory bowel disease in children is not uncommon, occurring in 3 per 100 000 population in one survey which probably underestimated the problem.[1] Nor is it only a problem of the adolescent as 50% of cases begin before 12 years of age. As in adult series, there appears to be an increase in Crohn's disease.[2,3] In about a quarter of children there is a family history of inflammatory bowel disease, either Crohn's disease or ulcerative colitis, suggesting an environmental or genetic influence.[4]

Presentation

Approximately 50% of children with Crohn's disease have both large and small bowel involvement, 10% have only colonic disease, 20% have diffuse small bowel disease and in a further 10% the disease is confined to the terminal ileum.[5]

Although the presentation is often similar to that in adults with weight loss, anaemia and vague abdominal pain,[6] extra-intestinal manifestations[7] may occur some years before the abdominal signs and symptoms leading to misdiagnosis or a delay of several years, in making the diagnosis.[8] Thus growth retardation, odd rashes and aphthous ulcers,[9] arthritis[10] and conjunctivitis[11] should be treated with suspicion; it is rare for a mass or obstruction to be the initial problem.

Complications of the disease are uncommon, the main problem being stricture formation[12] and obstruction in about a quarter of cases. Spontaneous fistulas are rare. Although fistulas can occur postoperatively,[13] the incidence is less so if the operation has been planned.[6] Toxic megacolon, which is commoner in ulcerative colitis, is associated with abscess formation and potential perforation, thus indicating the need for emergency surgery. The risk of developing cancer in the long term should not be forgotten, although the number of cases is small.[14]

Diagnosis

Diagnosis is mostly by small bowel enema[15], which will show the irregular mucosa and sometimes a stricture ('string sign'). Blood tests[16] are less helpful although evidence of anaemia, raised erythrocyte sedimentation rate and high orosomucoid agglutination tests may indicate active disease. A non-invasive means of indicating active disease is a sucralfate scan,[17] which will indicate ulceration in the bowel, but does not differentiate between ulcerative colitis and Crohn's disease.[18]

Treatment

Medical therapy includes various drugs:[19] antibiotics such as sulphasalazine[20,21] and metronidazole[22] especially for anal disease, and immunosuppressents such as azathioprine[23] and systemic corticosteroids. Most children require treatment with steroids plus dietary manipulation, either an elemental diet[24,25] or even parenteral nutrition.[26] The main problem for children suffering from Crohn's disease is failure to grow[27] and develop, either physically or sexually, rather than obstruction[28] or fistula formation. Whether this failure to grow is a result of the disease causing malabsorption[29] and reduced calorie intake[30] or whether it complicates the actual treatment with steroids is difficult to decide. To estimate such growth retardation and lack of sexual development, these parameters must be carefully recorded. Unfortunately these records are not always kept even in clinics with an interest in inflammatory bowel diseases.[31]

Surgical treatment

Failure to grow means that operation[32] may have to be contemplated earlier in a child than in the adult patient with Crohn's disease.[5] Before operation it is necessary to improve the nutritional state[33] and many trace elements and vitamins will have been depleted.[34] Resection with anastomosis can usually be performed; a right modified hemicolectomy being the commonest operation.[35] A stoma may be necessary in colonic disease especially in the emergency presentation, but it may only be needed for a short time. Children cope with stomas remarkably well.[36] The site of the disease has an influence on the final outcome. The prognosis is better in terminal ileal disease after resection rather than after ileostomy leaving residual disease in situ.[37] Anal disease is difficult to treat but rarely requires operation, either for the local condition or for the proximal bowel.[38] Possibly because operations are seldom performed in the presence of obstructed bowel, few postoperative problems[5] are encountered. The immediate results are gratifying in that a child operated on before puberty will start to grow.[39,40] Even if recurrence occurs,[41] as it does in nearly half these cases the child will have developed normally[42,43] if the operation has been performed early enough.[44] Earlier operative treatment may mean a lower steroid requirement and consequently less stunting of growth. Aggressive surgical treatment for moderate disease (not just severe disease) has lowered the mortality rate and improved the prognosis,[45,46] and reoperation may not be needed at an early stage.[35] Patients who develop Crohn's disease in childhood tend to have a poorer prognosis and quality of life than those with late-onset disease but operation will improve initial well-being, provide symptomatic relief and promote growth, even if further treatment is necessary at a later stage.[37]

Hirschsprung's disease and variants

Cause

Ganglion cells grow into the bowel from the cephalic to caudal end of the gut. In Hirschsprung's disease this ingrowth does not occur. The lack of these cells in the mucosal and submucosal plexuses prevents the normal reflex of propulsive peristalsis, in turn causing either obstruction or constipation. The actual cause of the abnormal nerve fibres is still unclear.[1-3] Normally the area of bowel involved extends proximally from the anus but involves only the large bowel. In less than 10% of children, however, not only the large bowel is involved but also varying lengths of small bowel.[4] Subtotal disease (Jirasek–Zuelzer–Wilson syndrome) is rare, occurring in less than 5% of cases[5,6] and tending to affect families[7,8] as an autosomal recessive gene[9,10] and may be associated with other congenital conditions or various syndromes.[11,12] The risk of the disease in siblings of those with long segment disease is 1 in 10. If most of the small bowel is involved there is little hope of long-term survival.[13-15] If the area involved is only colon and a small area of ileum, survival and eventual well-being is possible.

Presentation and diagnosis

The child will present early with small bowel obstruction but not necessarily in the newborn period, although there will be a history of problems with constipation or intermittent obstruction since birth. The presentation may even be with duodenal obstruction.[16]

Radiology is not always helpful showing only a small bowel obstruction. Faeces may be present in the diseased bowel.

Barium enema may not show the classical cone at the transitional zone since this may lie at the ileocaecal junction, and the colon will be of normal calibre. Immunohistochemistry can help in the diagnosis of Hirschsprung's disease.[17,18]

Operation

At emergency laparotomy the diagnosis may still not be clear,[19] and numerous frozen sections are necessary to make the diagnosis and allow correct positioning of the stoma. It is likely that the stoma will have to be sited high up the bowel, giving major problems with fluid and electrolyte balance.[20]

The definitive operation usually involves side-to-side anastomosis, with the Lester Martin modification[21,22] of the Duhamel pull-through,[23] so that there is a partially aganglionic reservoir for the small bowel contents. However, this modification can cause problems with malabsorption,[24] fluid loss[25] and inadequate emptying.[26] Other procedures involving endorectal techniques have been suggested, with a patch graft of colon sutured onto the bowel that is to be brought down.[37] In subtotal disease, an attempt to produce more normal bowel by means of a Bianchi lengthening has been attempted before the pull-through operation.

Pseudo-obstruction

In some children and adults, there is impaired peristalsis of the gut so that intestinal contents are not advanced by propulsive movements.[1] Symptoms of obstruction recur without any actual mechanical obstruction being present. The term 'pseudo-obstruction' probably covers a mixture of diseases[2] and they can mimic Hirschsprung's disease.[3,4] It may be possible to divide it into myopathic,[5] neuropathic[6] and hormonal groups.

At least some patients appear to have an autsomal recessive trait.[7] Often occurring in families,[8] the first problems can be encountered in the first month of life, although some may develop in late teens.[9] Pseudo-obstruction can affect both small and large bowel, as well as the stomach to cause delayed gastric emptying.[10] Gross abdominal distension, vomiting and constipation are associated with failure to thrive. Diagnosis is often by exclusion, of Hirschsprung's disease for example. Manometry and motility studies[11] may help. Intestinal biopsies may show abnormal plexuses[12] and either degeneration or hypertrophy of muscles.[13] Immunohistological investigations show an abnormal distribution of gut peptides.[14] Disorders of electrical activity also have been reported.[15] In adynamic bowel syndrome[16] no acetylcholinesterase nerve cells have been found.[17] This hypoperistaltic syndrome can be associated with urological problems,[18] notably dilated upper tracts with incomplete emptying of the bladder, indicating a visceral myopathy.[19]

Treatment is difficult. Operation does not lead to cure but may be necessary for biopsies and for decompression.[20,21] Dietary management may involve parenteral nutrition as well as various drugs to stimulate intestinal motility.

Neuronal intestinal dysplasia

Other children presenting with a Hirschsprung-like illness are said to have neuronal intestinal dysplasia. It is possible that some cases of pseudo-obstruction should more correctly be included in this group.

Ganglion cells are seen on biopsy but abnormalities may be found in the smooth muscle (as seen on electron microscopy) and/or in the neurones themselves (by using monoclonal antibodies).[1,2] The characteristics are: (1) hyperplasia of the submucous and myenteric plexuses giving giant ganglia; (2) sometimes isolated ganglion cells in the lamina propria and between muscle layers of the muscularis mucosae (where they should not be present); (3) elevation of acetylcholinesterase activity in the parasympathetic fibres[3] in the lamina propria and circular muscles; and (4) hypoplastic or aplastic sympathetic innervation of the myenteric plexus.[4] Occasionally hyperplasia of the myenteric plexus is associated with von Recklinghausen's disease appearing as nodules in the bowel, which are rarely plexiform,[5] and presenting with constipation.

Although von Recklinghausen's disease affects the sympathetic system, neuronal dysplasia is clearly a disease of the parasympathetic system. Varying degrees are found, some in association with actual Hirschsprung's disease,[6] others localized presenting like Hirschsprung's disease, and others as a more disseminated form.[7] Most present with a functional bowel obstruction soon after birth, and in the disseminated form gross abdominal distension may necessitate operation for possible obstruction. Those cases associated with Hirschsprung's disease make the diagnosis and treatment of that disease difficult, as the gut fails to work after what appeared to be a satisfactory pull-through procedure. The diagnosis requires specialized enzyme, histochemical and immunocytochemical studies and biopsies must include the submucosa.[8] Even so it may prove difficult to decide the amount and portion of bowel to be resected. Treatment of the localized type is similar to that for Hirschsprung's disease although some patients can be managed with dilatations and irrigations. Although morphology does not seem to improve on subsequent rectal biopsy, there is a functional improvement suggesting that maturation of the myenteric ganglion cells may occur.[9] The disseminated type of neuronal dysplasia is more difficult to treat. Ileostomy with or without colectomy does not necessarily improve matters. For some patients there is no cure at present.

Dilatations and duplications

Segmental intestinal dilatation

Segmental dilatations of the intestine, although uncommon, can occur throughout the gut: in the colon,[1,2] duodenum,[3] jejunum[4] but especially in the ileum.[5,6] The cause of this obstruction is unknown but it is possible that it is a form fruste of an atresia; local deficiency of circular muscle with associated proximal dilatation has been described.[7] In the ileum the dysgenesis appears to be an intrinsic abnormality associated with the junction with the yolk sac. Although the bowel is patent the infant presents with obstruction and radiography shows a dilated terminal ileum. Resection of the dilated portion with anastomosis gives excellent results. However long-term evaluation of vitamin B_{12} and folic acid absorption will be necessary. Rarely, diverticulum of the small bowel can produce obstruction.[8]

Duplication cyst

It can be difficult to distinguish duplications of the gut from mesenteric cysts and they may co-exist. During development any area of the bowel[9] from the oesophagus to the rectum can be duplicated by groups of cells separating off. One theory[10] suggests that adhesions between the notochord and the endoderm allows splitting off of some endoderm cells, so leading to a duplication and also accounting for the vertebral anomalies found in some of these patients. The duplications have a complete muscular wall lying along the mesenteric border of the gut and they share the same blood supply as the adjacent bowel. In the foregut above the diaphragm the lining mucosa may be either respiratory or alimentary. Lower down, if the lining of the cyst is that of intestinal type (or is ectopic gastric mucosa) it can ulcerate, leading to bleeding per rectum or even perforation.[11] Although presentation of this congenital anomaly usually occurs in the first year of life, problems may not arise until adult life.[12,13] The usual type is cystic, but tubular duplications[14] of long areas of bowel (e.g. 60–90 cm) may give special problems. The duodenum[15] can be involved, but the mesenteric small bowel is the most frequent site.[16,17]

Abdominal duplications present with a mass or with bleeding.[18] Ultrasound scan or plain radiographs will show displacement and flattening out of the bowel, sometimes causing obstruction. The same appearance may be visualized on barium studies, either small bowel or large bowel enema. An association with vertebral anomalies may also suggest the diagnosis.[9]

Treatment of a small or moderate-sized duplication is by resection and anastomosis. If a large part of the bowel is involved this procedure may not be possible. Mucosal stripping[19,20] of the extra lumen to give a double-barrelled appearance may be the best that can be achieved, but there remains a risk of malignant change later.[21] Rarely is it possible to enucleate the cyst,[22] as the remaining bowel wall and blood supply are closely involved.[23]

Thoracic duplications[24,25] whether bronchogenic or enteric, cause different problems. They are difficult to differentiate from hamartomatous malformations of the lung. An association with oesophageal atresia[26] should be remembered.

Omental cysts

Other cysts are omental, mesenteric or retroperitoneal.[27,28] They are not necessarily congenital[29] but may be traumatic, neoplastic or infective in origin[30–32] and can occur anywhere along the bowel. They are not associated with any particular anatomical structure. Although rare, they may present in adult life but more commonly as an acute abdomen in a child.[33,34] An exact preoperative diagnosis is unusual since there are no distinctive features[35] but ultrasonography[36] can give useful information.

Large cysts can cause volvulus and obstruction. The results of resection are excellent. Aspiration and marsupialization are contraindicated.

Polyps and tumours

Adenomas and hamartomas

Benign polyps occur in the small bowel, usually as part of a syndrome and sometimes in association with polyps elsewhere in the gastrointestinal tract. Peutz–Jaghers syndrome is a familial condition in which the polyps are hamartomatous on histological examination. Thought not to be premalignant,[1] the condition appears to carry an increased risk of neoplastic degeneration in some children and families.[2] Easily recognizable because of the pigmentation in the buccal mucosa these children present with anaemia or abdominal pain due to intussusception. Small bowel enema may delineate the polyps before resection. Endoscopy can be useful in obscure gastrointestinal bleeding.[3] Care must be taken to preserve as much bowel as possible as further surgery is likely during the patients' lifetime. Occasionally if the small bowel lesions are associated with similar polyps in the large bowel, the child will have life-threatening bloody diarrhoea and protein-losing enteropathy.[4]

Less commonly premalignant small bowel polyps may be found in association with large bowel polyps, e.g. in polyposis coli, when they are located especially in the stomach or duodenum.[5,6] In Gardner's syndrome when familial adenomatous polyposis is accompanied by ectodermal lesions (sebaceous cysts, osteomas), duodenal and gastric polyps[7] are particularly common. The duodenal polyps are adenomatous, so regular endoscopy and biopsy of duodenal (and gastric) lesions must be undertaken.[8] There is evidence of a definite malignant risk in such juvenile polyps.[9] Recent genetic advances have helped to pin-point those requiring regular follow-up.[10-12]

The outlook for children with widespread polyps from mouth to anus (Cronkhite–Canada syndrome) is dismal since it is associated with protein-losing enteropathy, hypotonia, finger clubbing, macrocephaly and hepatosplenomegaly.[13]

Sometimes hamartomatous (juvenile-type) polyps coexist with adenomatous polyps.[14] Inflammatory pseudotumours (myofibroblastic tumours) can occur in children.[15] Although not initially malignant, mesenteric fibromatosis[16] can infiltrate and obstruct the gut. An association with polyposis may be present.

Lymphoid hyperplasia

Lymphoid polyps are rare in children[17] but nodular lymphoid hyperplasia occurs as part of the spectrum of lymphoid hyperplasia of the intestinal tract. A diffuse form can also present with malabsorption. Such children present with abdominal pain, obstruction, recurrent intussusceptions[18] or rectal prolapse.[19] Diagnosis is made on histological material. Staining for IgA and IgG shows numerous plasma cells in the lamina propria, and secretory IgA can be found on the luminal surface of the mucosa.[20] There appears to be an association with viral illness and the surgical manifestations as complications.[21]

Another type of lymphoid hyperplasia presents in a less acute fashion with chronic anaemia, moderate abdominal pain and weight loss.[22] As in the acute form, the terminal ileum or appendix is the usual site of involvement, and resection of the area may result in amelioration of symptoms.

Haemangiomas

Other pseudopolyps throughout the intestine may turn out on histological examination to be cavernous haemangiomas. These infiltrate the bowel wall with their vessels. Haemangiomas of the gut are associated with cutaneous haemangiomas in 50% of children.

They present with intestinal bleeding, either as frank blood per rectum or as anaemia and melaena. Although in time (like capillary naevi elsewhere) they will thrombose, fibrose and disappear, they can cause torrential bleeding, enough to warrant transfusion and even operation. The problem then is to determine which is the source of bleeding. Technetium scans may help in pin-pointing the bleeding.[23] There is a limit to the number of enterotomies that can be undertaken to deal with what is in essence a self-limiting condition. However, local excision is the best treatment as recurrence is common after sclerotherapy.[24]

Malignant tumours

Although adenocarcinomas of the colon occur in children, albeit rarely, enteric malignancies tend to arise from the reticular system. Only pre-existing adenoma would lead one to expect adenocarcinoma in the small bowel.[25]

Lymphosarcoma of the bowel presents either with anaemia or acutely as an obstruction or intussusception. Occasionally infiltration of the mesentery leads to ureteric obstruction so that the presentation is that of a hydronephrotic kidney rather than an intestinal problem. The results of surgery and chemotherapy depend on the staging of the malignancy.

Less common still are leiomyosarcomas occurring in the stomach, duodenum[26] or jejunoileum. Besides obstruction, such tumours can lead to perforation. Resection is the only hope of recovery since adjuvant chemotherapy has little to offer.[27] Perforations also occur in association with leukaemic infiltration of the gut in acute lymphoblastic leukaemia.[28]

Infections

Both bacterial and protozoal infections can present as acute abdominal problems. Acute ileitis, caused by *Yersinia, Campylobacter* or *Escherichia coli*[29] can be mistaken for Crohn's disease. Roundworm (*Ascaris lumbricoides*) infestations may lead to obstruction[30] or peritonitis.[31] In the tropics typhoid infection may lead to perforation and peritonitis.[32]

Primary peritonitis in girls requires to be differentiated from other causes, e.g. appendicitis. A focus for the infection is rarely found and the organisms implicated may be *E. coli*, streptococci, meningococci or pneumococci.[33]

Ascites caused by chylous effusion[34] can occur as a result of surgery, e.g. diaphragmatic hernia repair or oesophageal atresia repair, or as a result of obstruction in the mesentery. Mesenteric obstruction may be inflammatory in nature or be due to carcinomatous infiltration. Most cases can be managed conservatively with a low-fat, high-protein diet with or without paracentesis. In a few, peritoneal-venous shunts may be necessary to drain the chyle but these do not always give a cure.

UMBILICAL PROBLEMS

Embryology

During normal development the abdominal contents pass out through the umbilicus, to return later after elongation and rotation. Should the bowel remain outside the abdominal cavity within the umbilical cord varying degrees of exomphalos occur from herniation into the cord to a major exomphalos containing liver as well as large and small intestine. Hence exomphalos is part of normal development. During the period of development of the gut, tethering via the vitello-intestinal duct maintains a connection between mother and child. This duct should atrophy and disappear by the seventh week, but in some infants either all or part of this structure remains and gives rise to a Meckel's diverticulum.

When the gut lies outside the abdominal cavity free in the amniotic fluid, this is not part of normal development. For some reason the mesodermal plates have failed to fuse so that a defect to the side of the umbilicus occurs.

Persistence of the urachus may be due to bladder outlet obstruction.

Vitello-intestinal remnants

The actual vitello-intestinal duct may remain patent so that there is an opening at the umbilicus which may discharge gas and/or faeces[1,2] and even roundworms.[3] This opening may look like an actual stoma but more commonly it presents as a discharging umbilicus that is slow to heal or a polyp.[4]

Although this is a rare anomaly (1 in 15 000 births),[5] an unusual umbilicus should be examined with such an abnormality in mind. A rare occurrence is a fistula from the appendix to the umbilicus.[6] The diagnosis is made by instilling radio-opaque dye into the umbilicus. If operation is not undertaken urgently[7] there is a risk of intussusception of the entire small bowel out through the umbilicus which can prove fatal. Resection and primary anastomoses is curative.[8,9]

Other problems arise if the duct only partially disappears. If a band exists, it may cause an internal hernia. Such bands may also be found in association with Meckel's diverticulum. An enclosed cyst, either at the umbilicus or along the connecting band, may become infected and give rise to an abscess.[10]

Meckel's diverticulum

The commonest abnormality of the vitello-intestinal duct is partial absorption, which leaves a diverticulum (Meckel's diverticulum) about 60 cm proximal to the ileocaecal valve.[11] The diverticulum is of varying length and may or may not have a wide neck. Meckel's diverticulum may be found in association with other congenital abnormalities[12] or even angiodysplasia.[13] The diverticulum can become infected and present like acute appendicitis, especially in adults.[14] Obstruction may result[15] with or without a band which can cause an internal herniation. The commonest presentation, however, is with gastrointestinal bleeding, usually severe enough to lower the child's haemoglobin. The bleeding is characteristically bright red or maroon-coloured rather than a true melaena, but it may be occult.[16]

Bleeding is the result of acid produced in the ectopic gastric mucosa, which ulcerates the adjacent small bowel, which is unprotected by mucus. Pain is not necessarily a feature. *Campylobacter pylori* may be present if gastric mucosa is found.[17] but probably this is not associated with the perforation.[18] Perforation is dangerous and is usually associated with foreign bodies impacted in the diverticulum. Most of these complications occur in infants, under the age of one year.[19] Rarely the diverticulum may be involved in a groin hernia (Littre's hernia).[20]

The diagnosis may be difficult to make and may only be resolved at laparotomy. Barium studies tend to be unhelpful, since the neck of the diverticulum has to be wide for it to fill with contrast. The ectopic gastric mucosa may fill up the lumen so that even lateral projections of the follow-through examination do not show a diverticulum. Occasionally such a view will show tethering when a band is attached to the umbilicus. Nevertheless, barium studies should be part of the work-up of these children.[21] Pertechnetate scans will pinpoint the area if bleeding persists or ulceration has occurred[22] in nearly 90% of cases.[23] The addition of pentagastrin and glucagon enhances the uptake and increases the sensitivity of the scan.[24]

If the diverticulum is the source of bleeding or is inflamed, resection is necessary. It should be carried out by means of a V-shaped incision to resect not only the diverticulum but also the area of adjacent small bowel,[25] since this is the area that ulcerates. If the actual diverticulum invaginates, it may also bleed as part of an intussusception. The diverticulum can be removed laparoscopically.[26]

It is more difficult to know whether or not to resect a Meckel's diverticulum found by chance at laparotomy. The risk of complications in such diverticula is more than 25%.[27] If there is peritonitis (of other causation) and the diverticulum looks unlikely to give problems (i.e. it is wide necked), it should be left in situ.[28] However, even in the presence of pus, if the diverticulum seems likely to give trouble in the future, it should be removed.[29,30] The outcome is excellent.[31]

Other umbilical problems

Umbilical hernias in infants rarely cause obstruction, so that any pain or vomiting is an indication of other pathology. Differentiation must be made in the newborn between umbilical hernia and herniation into the cord, in essence a very minor exomphalos.

Umbilical hernias do not need operation until around three years of age as most close spontaneously, although this is less likely to happen in negro children.[32] Repair consists of a subumbilical incision with suturing of the peritoneum. The muscle defect should be closed with a Mayo type repair followed by subcuticular skin closure. On no account should the umbilicus be removed.

If the umbilical stump fails to heal an umbilical polyp (see above) may require cauterization. Tumours are rare, although haemangiomas can occur and require excision. It is now rare in Western countries for infection of the umbilicus to progress to gangrene[33] and thrombosis of the umbilical vein, leading eventually to portal hypertension.

It is important to excise the umbilical vessels and urachal remnant in cases of periumbilical necrotizing fasciitis.[34]

CONGENITAL DEFECTS OF THE ANTERIOR ABDOMINAL WALL

Pathogenesis

Mention has already been made of the difference between exomphalos and gastroschisis. The defect in the anterior abdominal wall in exomphalos consists of absence of abdominal muscles, fascia and skin at the junction of the umbilical cord with the abdomen.[1] The sac, which varies from a small herniation into the cord to a giant exomphalos, is covered with a membrane of amnion and parietal peritoneum. Exomphalos appears to be persistence of the body stalk with bowel remaining outside the abdominal cavity.[2] In some cases the entire anterior abdominal wall is involved. Here, not only are all the abdominal viscera included, but the heart associated with a diaphragmatic defect is lying free under the skin (ectopia cordis). Other major congenital abnormalities are common such as congenital heart disease, myelomeningocele and abdominal anomalies. Exomphalos may be part of various syndromes, being found in trisomy 13 (Patau's syndrome), trisomy 18 (Edward's syndrome) and trisomy 21 (Down syndrome).[3] The association with macroglossia and gigantism termed Beckwith–Wiedemann syndrome (BWS or EMG), is important as hypoglycaemia may occur.[4] Such an association occurs in 12% of children with exomphalos.

Although it has been suggested that gastroschisis is evidence of an in utero rupture of exomphalos,[5] this has not been completely resolved and it may be an entirely different abnormality. Gastroschisis consists of gut, often short in length, lying free in the amniotic fluid[6] so that it is possible for the amniotic fluid[7] or rather the fetal urine[8] in the amniotic fluid, to cause a fibrinous exudate which covers the bowel, making it rigid and prevents its motility.[9] This fibrinous 'peel' dissolves in time[10] so that at a second laparotomy it has disappeared, probably associated with an improvement in bowel function. A defect in the mesenchyme to the right (very occasionally to the left) of the umbilical cord leads to failure of skin formation at the site of the defect.[7] Associated gastrointestinal abnormalities in 12% of cases[11] include atresias[12] and malrotation and volvulus[13] and can lead to even more problems with short gut. Very occasionally a child is born with hardly any gut at all as the intestine outside the abdomen has twisted and atrophied.[14] As well as bowel and liver, gonads may be found outside the peritoneal cavity.[15] The associated atresia may be due to the compression of bowel loops.[16,17] The baby is often small for dates or premature. Although the combined incidence of these defects is about 1 in 5000 births,[18] the incidence of exomphalos is around 1 in 6000 live births[19] and that of gastroschisis about 1 in 10 000.

There appears to be a recent increase in the incidence of gastroschisis,[20] but this may reflect better obstetric care and survival of children with gross defects. These malformations are rarely familial except when associated with syndromes.[21,22]

Transportation

Antenatal ultrasonographic investigations[23] now mean that the diagnosis is often made before delivery, so that a choice can be made regarding the method and site of delivery. Some indication of intestinal viability can also be gained. If the exomphalos is large, vaginal delivery is contraindicated because of the danger of rupture. Rupture converts a relatively safe covered situation (in exomphalos) into one similar to gastroschisis. However, Caesarean section performed electively does not improve the prognosis in gastroschisis.[24–26] The transport of a newborn with exomphalos is no different from that of any other child apart from care being taken not to damage the membrane and cause rupture. In both anomalies, a nasogastric tube should be passed before transfer to deflate the bowel. Problems can arise during transfer of a neonate with gastroschisis so that delivery is best close to the neonatal surgical unit, i.e. transferring the child in utero.[27] As long as no other major defect is diagnosed, the child may be delivered near term.[28] In the neonate with gastroschisis hypothermia is a problem. The method of transfer appears to influence both this and the final outcome.[29,30] The practice of wrapping the bowel in saline packs only helps to reduce the temperature of the baby as the fluid evaporates. Using a plastic bag strapped to the anterior abdominal wall to contain the bowel will maintain body temperature.

Preoperative management

Time should be taken to exclude major congenital anomalies such as congenital heart disease before operation. With an intact membrane there is no immediate need to operate. Because of exposure of the bowel in a newborn with gastroschisis and the antenatal peritonitis, these babies lose fluid rapidly. Fluid loss requires replacement with colloid in large amounts irrespective of the gestational age or birth weight.[31] This problem with fluid is exacerbated postoperatively with sequestration of fluid in the static bowel and peritoneum, giving an appreciable fall in extracellular fluid volume and a decrease in total body water.[32] Replacement of this fluid is essential.

Exomphalos

Depending on the size of the defect and exomphalos, various treatments have been tried.

Herniation into the cord

If the knuckle of bowel is not fixed in the sac, it is possible to twist the cord and return the loop of bowel to the abdominal cavity. Ligation of the sac and umbilical cord completes the operation, which can be performed on the neonatal unit. Care must be taken to ensure that no bowel is trapped. It is possible for a Meckel's diverticulum to be present and fixed, which makes it impossible to perform this manoeuvre. In such cases a mini-laparotomy is carried out and the umbilicus is remodelled.

Exomphalos

In most children it is possible to open up the defect and return the contents to the abdominal cavity. This manoeuvre is assisted by vigorous stretching of the abdominal cavity and manual emptying of the gastrointestinal tract.[33] There is no need to perform an enterotomy to achieve it.[34] Closure of the wound in layers means that it may be possible to make a new umbilicus. If the defect is large and contains not only bowel but liver[35] it may not be possible to return the contents to the abdominal cavity without prejudicing both respiration and gut viability.[36] Occasionally if the membrane is intact, the conservative measure of painting the membrane with 2% aqueous mercurochrome[37,38] may allow for epithelialization in time. Unfortunately this technique precludes a check for other gastrointestinal abnormalities.[39] There is also a risk of mercury poisoning[40] so that 70% alcohol or 1% aqueous gentian violet have been used.[41]

Closing only the skin over the defect[42] leaves a very large ventral hernia which is difficult to close. The closure is usually left until the child is older with a larger abdominal cavity but the bowel and liver will by then be adherent to the edge of the defect or may even cause obstructive symptoms.[43] In an attempt to prevent this sequel, a polyamide mesh[44] has been used. Various methods have been employed to increase the abdominal cavity of these children, depending on the individual baby.[45] These include making an artifical pneumoperitoneum,[46] using external compression,[47] or making new muscle flaps.[48] Rather than leave the child with a large defect, the use of a silastic silo or pouch has been advocated, as used in the repair of gastroschisis (see later). Although most surgeons remove the amniotic membrane, closure can be performed with it in place[49] and fascial, silo[50,51] or polymer membrane[52] can be placed over the amniotic fluid.

If the membrane has ruptured during or immediately after delivery, the problem is one of transporting the baby with free bowel. Unlike the newborn with gastroschisis the bowel is of adequate length. Unless it is damaged during transit, it will undergo normal peristalsis. Closure is then as described above and the results are satisfactory.[53]

Gastroschisis

Surgical treatment is urgent because of the loss of fluid, the development of hypothermia and the risk of bowel damage. The choice lies between primary closure and the use of a silastic covering. A nasogastric tube or gastrostomy is necessary for deflation until the gut starts to work.

To decide whether primary closure will lead to respiratory and circulatory problems, measurement of intragastric pressure may give some indication if the pressure is above 20 cm water.[54] Respiratory compliance and haemodynamic parameters measured intraoperatively give information on which to base the decision as to the means of closure.[55] Apart from the respiratory embarrassment with diaphragmatic splinting, the inferior vena cava may be compressed giving problems with cardiac output. If the closure is too tight the bowel itself may become ischaemic.[56] This problem can also occur in a staged procedure.[57] Renal impairment may also result.

These problems are avoided by giving the bowel more time to return to the abdominal cavity.[58] The use of a silo (Figure 62.26) to cover the bowel[59,60] as soon as the child is resuscitated allows time and prevents major sepsis. Before attaching the silo or silastic patch to the muscle layer, the actual abdominal defect must be enlarged. By making a silo rather than a patch, gravity can be used to return the bowel to the abdominal cavity. Over the next 10–12 days the silo can be slowly reduced, thereby squeezing the bowel back into the abdominal cavity without prejudicing respiratory function. Reduction in size of the silo can be carried out by means of an umbilical clamp or by suturing the silo, care being taken not to damage the bowel inside.

Such a staged reduction[61] can be carried out on the neonatal unit with only the final closure performed in theatre. Antibiotic powder must be used around the suture line of skin/muscle and silastic sheeting. The treatment of associated atresias is along standard lines (see above).[62] Problems can occur with postoperative malrotation leading to obstruction.[63]

Local infection is common and leads to silo separation, requiring resuturing, or generalized septicaemia.[33,64] Thus primary repair is preferable, since it is attended by less infection.[65–67] It is also more difficult to make a neo-umbilicus when a silo is used.[68] The best treatment must be determined for each individual child, the disproportion between herniated viscera and abdominal cavity being the major deciding factor.[69]

Postoperative management

Ventilation for 24–48 h[70] has helped improve the condition of these patients. The use of parenteral nutrition[71] by means of a central catheter has improved the prognosis of this anomaly since it may take up to three weeks for the gut to resume peristalsis.[72] In the meantime, the infant on parenteral nutrition can grow and develop normally.[73] The resumption of peristalsis appears to be quicker in those undergoing primary repair.[74]

Results

The improvement in the prognosis for this defect is a result of better transport and improved neonatal care.[75] Unfortunately many children have major intestinal defects such as atresia[76] associated with short gut, so this may affect the long-term outlook (although the bowel is probably capable of returning to normal length).[77,78]

Complications of parenteral nutrition (see above) will also affect the mortality rate, the main problems being septicaemia and superior vena cava thrombosis. Although almost 20% of infants may develop necrotizing enterocolitis[79] after closure, the long-term prognosis for survivors is excellent.[56]

In summary, no fetus should undergo termination of pregnancy for either of these abnormalities. The prognosis for gastroschisis is so much improved[80] so that it is now superior to that for exomphalos.[81,82] Further experimental work is necessary to elucidate the cause of these defects, especially gastroschisis.[83]

Recent attempts to close the defect in the special care unit show that anaesthesia involves using the umbilical stump and can give good results (A. Bianci, pers. comm.).

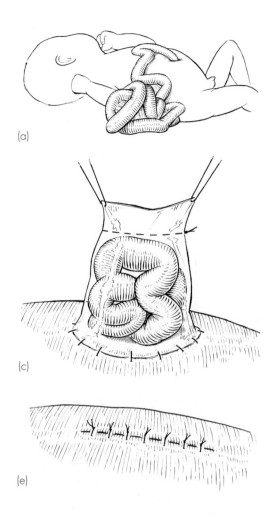

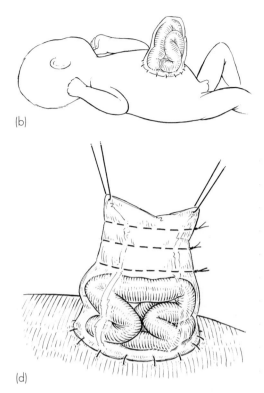

Figure 62.26
(a & b) Formation of silo in theatre for gastroschisis.
(c & d) Completed silo hitched up to incubator to allow gravity to help return the bowel to the peritoneal cavity. (e) End result. (Reproduced by permission of the University of Manchester Department of Medical Illustration.)

Ectopia cordis

This rare pentad anomaly is associated with giant exomphalos, diaphragmatic herniation and congenital heart defects.[84,85] Although closure must be in stages,[86] the results are abysmal due to the life-threatening intracardiac defects.

Vitello-intestinal fissure[87] or cloacal extrophy

The rare anomaly of vitello-intestinal fissure consists of exomphalos, ectopic bladder, anorectal anomalies and occasionally a myelomeningocoele, as a result of a split notochord. These abnormalites all require treatment but at different times: urgent closure of the exomphalos, emergency treatment of the bowel obstruction and later closure of the bladder extrophy. Most eventually require stomas both for the bowel and urinary systems. The most difficult decision is to decide the sexual rearing of the child. In the male infant, since the penis is bifid and underdeveloped, reassignment to the female gender is thought to be best. The long-term outlook by improved aggressive treatment has meant that the quality of life is now better[88] for these children.

Postoperative management

The actual closure can be monitored by the anaesthetist to prevent respiratory embarrassment. Postoperative ventilation for 24–48 h may improve the results. This measure together with parenteral nutrition has improved survival rates to more than 90% if no other abnormality exists.[89]

Results

The prognosis of children with exomphalos depends on whether they have an associated major defect.[90] Low birthweight also affects the outcome.[91] Neither the size of the defect[92] nor the means of repair affect the outcome, although complications are more likely with silo repair, which should therefore be reserved for those in whom a primary repair is not possible.

REFERENCES

Small bowel atresias

1. Martin LW & Zerella JT. Jejunoileal atresia: a proposed classification. *J Pediatr Surg* 1976; **11**: 399.
2. Grosfeld JL. Jejunoileal atresia and stenosis. In Ravitch MM, Welch KJ, Benson CD, Aberdeen E & Randolph JG (eds) *Pediatric Surgery,* Chicago: Chigago Year Book, 1986; 933.
3. Adejuyigbe O & Odesanmi WO. Intrauterine intussusception causing intestinal atresia. *J Pediatr Surg* 1990; **25**: 562.
4. Louw JH. Congenital intestinal atresia and stenosis in the newborn: observations on its pathogenesis and treatment. *Ann Roy Coll Surg Engl* 1959; **25**: 209.
5. Khong TY, Ford WDA & Haan EA. Umbilical cord ulceration in association with intestinal atresia in a child with deletion 13q and Hirschsprung's disease. *Arch Dis Child* 1994; **71**: f21.

6. Rickham PP & Karplus M. Familial and hereditary intestinal atresia. *Helv Paediatr Acta* 1971; **26**: 561.

7. Puri P & Fujimoto T. New observations on the pathogenesis of multiple atresias. *J Pediatr Surg* 1988; **23**: 221.

8. Swift PGF, Driscoll IB & Vowles KDJ. Neonatal small-bowel obstruction associated with amniocentesis. *BMJ* 1979; **1**: 720.

9. Heij HA, Moorman-Voestermans CGM & Vos A. Atresia of jejunum and ileum: is it the same disease? *J Pediatr Surg* 1990; **25**: 635.

10. Moorman-Voestermans CGM, Heij HA & Vos A. Jejunal atresia in twins. *J Pediatr Surg* 1990; **25**: 638.

11. Grosfeld JL, Ballantine TVN & Shoemaker R. Operative management of intestinal atresia and stenosis based on pathologic findings. *J Pediatr Surg* 1979; **14**: 368.

12. DeLorimier AA, Fonkalsrud EW & Hays DM. Congenital atresia and stenosis of the jejunum and ileum. *Surgery* 1969; **65**: 819.

13. El Shafie M & Rickham PP. Multiple intestinal atresia. *J Pediatr Surg* 1970; **5**: 655.

14. Louw JH. Jejunoileal atresia and stenosis. *J Pediatr Surg* 1966; **1**: 8.

15. Nixon HH & Tawes R. Etiology and treatment of small intestinal atresia: analysis of a series of 127 jejunoileal atresias and comparison with 62 duodenal atresias. *Surgery* 1971; **69**: 41.

16. Jackman S & Brereton RJ. A lesson in intestinal atresias. *J Pediatr Surg* 1988; **23**: 852.

17. Weiss RRG, Ryan DP, Iilstad ST, Noseworthy J & Martin LW. A complex case of jejunoileocolic atresias. *J Pediatr Surg* 1990; **25**: 560.

18. Dickson JAS. Apple peel small bowel: an uncommon variant of duodenal and jejunal atresia. *J Pediatr Surg* 1970; **5**: 595.

19. Zivkoric SM & Milonsevic VR. Duodenal and jejunal atresia with agenesis of the dorsal mesentry: 'apple-peel' small bowel. *Am J Surg* 1979; **137**: 767.

20. Weitzman JJ & Vanderhoof RS. Jejunal atresia with agenesis of the dorsal mesentry with 'Christmas tree' deformity of the small intestine. *Am J Surg* 1966; **111**: 443.

21. Al-Awadi SA, Farag TI, Naguib K, Cuschieri A & Issa M. Familial jejunal atresia with 'apple-peel'. *J R Soc Med* 1981; **74**: 499.

22. Gibson MF. Familial multiple jejunal atresia with malrotation. *J Pediatr Surg* 1987; **22**: 1013.

23. Ein SH, Venugopal S & Mancer K. Ileocaecal atresia. *J Pediatr Surg* 1985; **20**: 525.

24. Hamdy MH, Man DWK, Bain D & Kirkland IS. Histochemical changes in intestinal atresia and its implications on surgical management: a preliminary report. *J Pediatr Surg* 1986; **21**: 17.

25. Howard ER & Othersen HB. Proximal jejunoplasty in the treatment of jejunal atresia. *J Pediatr Surg* 1973; **8**: 685.

26. de Lorimier AA & Harrison MR. Intestinal plication in the treatment of atresia. *J Pediatr Surg* 1983; **18**: 734.

27. Lally KP, Chwals WJ, Weitzman JJ, Black T & Singh S. Hirschsprung's disease. *J Pediatr Surg* 1992; **27**: 469.

28. Moore TC & Stokes GE. Congenital stenosis and atresia of the small intestines. *Surg Gynecol Obstet* 1953; **97**: 719.

29. Adeyemi SD. Prognostic factors in neonatal intestinal obstruction: a prospective study of Nigerian newborns with bowel obstruction. *J Pediatr Surg* 1988; **23**: 135.

Meconium ileus

1. Dickson JAS & Mearns MB. Meconium ileus. In Wilkinson AWW (ed.) *Recent Advances Paediatric Surgery*. Edinburgh: Churchill Livingstone, 1975; **3**: 143.

2. Kerem B-S, Rommens JM, Buchanan JA et al. Identification of the cystic fibrosis gene: genetic analysis. *Science* 1989; **245**: 1073.

3. Olsen MM, Luck SR, Lloyd-Still J & Raffensperger JG. The spectrum of meconium disease in infancy. *J Pediatr Surg* 1982; **17**: 479.

4. Gaskin KJ, Gurwitz D, Durie PR, Corey ML & Forstner GG. Improved respiratory prognosis in patients with cystic fibrosis with normal fat absorption. *J Pediatr* 1982; **100**: 857.

5. Durie PR. Gastrointestinal disorders in cystic fibrosis. In Milla PJ (ed.) *Disorders of Gastrointestinal Motility in Childhood*. Chichester: Wiley, 1988; 91.

6. Shwachman H. Meconium ileus: ten patients over 28 years of age. *J Pediatr Surg* 1983; **18**: 570.

7. Schutt WH & Isles TE. Protein in meconium from meconium ileus. *Arch Dis Child* 1968; **43**: 178.

8. Noblett HR. Treatment of uncomplicated meconium ileus by gastrografin enema. *J Pediatr Surg* 1969; **4**: 190.

9. Lille JG & Chrispin AR. Investigation and management of neonatal obstruction by gastrografin enema. *Ann Radiol* 1971; **15**: 237–241.

10. Wagget J, Bishop HC & Koop CE. Experience with gastrografin enema in the treatment of meconium ileus. *J Pediatr Surg* 1970; **5**: 649.

11. Ein SH, Shandling B, Reilly BJ & Stephens CA. Bowel perforation with nonoperative treatment of meconium ileus. *J Pediatr Surg* 1987; **22**: 146.

12. Forouhar F. Meconium peritonitis. *Am J Clin Pathol* 1982; **78**: 208.

13. Miller JP, Smith SD, Newman B & Sukarochana K. Neonatal abdominal calcification: is it always meconium peritonitis? *J Pediatr Surg* 1988; **23**: 555.

14. di Sant'Agnese PA, Darling RC, Perera GA & Shea E. Abnormal electrolyte composition of sweat in cystic fibrosis of the pancreas. *Pediatre* 1953; **12**: 549.

15. Kererm B, Rommens JM, Buchanan JA et al. Identification of cystic fibrosis gene: genetic analysis. *Science* 1989; **245**: 1073.

16. Rickham PP & Boeckmann CR. Neonatal meconium obstruction in the absence of mucoviscidosis. *Am J Surg* 1965; **106**: 173.

17. Shigemoto H, Endo S, Isomoto T, Sano K & Taguchi K. Neonatal meconium obstruction in the ileum without mucoviscidosis. *J Pediatr Surg* 1978; **13**: 475.

18. Leonidas JC. Microcolon in the absence of small bowel obstruction in the newmorn. *J Pediatr Surg* 1989; **24**: 180.

19. Ellis DG & Clatworthy HW. The meconium plug syndrome revisited. *J Pediatr Surg* 1966; **1**: 54.

20. Harberg FJ, Senekijan EK & Pokorny WJ. Treatment of uncomplicated meconium ileus via T-Tube ileostomy. *J Pediatr Surg* 1981; **16**: 61.

21. Nguyen LT, Youssef S, Guttman FM, Laberge J-M, Albert D & Doody D. Meconium ileus: is a stoma necessary? *J Pediatr Surg* 1986; **21**: 766.

22. Docherty JG, Zaki A, Coutts JAP, Evans TJ & Carachi R. Meconium ileus: a review 1972–1990. *Br J Surg* 1992; **79**: 571.

23. Bishop HC & Koop CE. Management of meconium ileus: resection, Roux-en-Y anastomosis and ileostomy irrigation with pancreatic enzymes. *Ann Surg* 1957; **145**: 410.

24. McPartlin JF, Dickson JAS & Swain VAJ. Meconium ileus: immediate and long-term survival. *Arch Dis Child* 1972; **47**: 207.

25. Fitzgerald R & Conlon K. Use of the appendix stump in the treatment of meconium ileus. *J Pediatr Surg* 1989; **24**: 899.

26. Park RW & Grand RJ. Gastrointestinal manifestations of cystic fibrosis. *Gastroenterology* 1981; **81**: 1143.

27. Rosenstein BJ & Langbaum TS. The incidence of distal intestinal obstruction syndrome in cystic fibrosis. *J Pediatr Gastroenter Nutr* 1983; **2**: 299.

28. Copeland G, Waldron R & Wilson WA. Meconium ileus equivalent. *J R Coll Surg Edinb* 1984; **29**: 325.

29. Cordonnier JK & Izant RJ. Meconium ileus equivalent. *J Pediatr Surg* 1963; **54**: 667.

30. Valman HB, France NE & Wallis PG. Prolonged neonatal jaundice in cystic fibrosis. *Arch Dis Child* 1971; **46**: 805.

31. Roy CC Weber AM, Morin CI et al. Hepatobiliary disease in cystic fibrosis: a survey of current issues and concepts. *J Pediatr Gastroenterol Nutr* 1982; **1**: 469.

32. Bass J, Connon JJ & Ho CS. Biliary tree in cystic fibrosis. *Gastroenterology* 1983; **84**: 1592.

33. Bendig DW, Seilheimer DK, Wagner ML, Ferry GD & Harrison GM. Complications of gastroesophageal reflux in cystic fibrosis. *J Pediatr* 1982; **100**: 536.

34. Bali A, Stableforth DE & Asquith P. Prolonged small-intestinal transit time in cystic fibrosis. *BMJ* 1983; **287**: 1011.

35. Valman HB & France NE. The vas deferens in cystic fibrosis. *Lancet* 1969; **ii**: 566.

36. Cohen LF, Di Sant'Agnese PA & Friedlander J. Cystic fibrosis and pregnancy. *Lancet* 1980; **ii**: 842.

37. Coughlin JP, Gauderer MWL, Stern RC, Doershuk CF, Izant RJ & Zollinger RM. The spectrum of appendiceal disease in cystic fibrosis. *J Pediatr Surg* 1990; **25**: 835.

38. Lewis CT, Dickson JAS & Swain VAJ. Milk bolus obstruction in the neonate. *Arch Dis Child* 1977; **52**: 68.

39. Cremin BJ, Smythe PM & Cywes S. The radiological appearance of inspissated milk syndrome. *Br J Radiol* 1970; **43**: 856.

40. Southgate DA, Widdowson EM, Smits BJ, Cooke WT, Walker CHM & Mathers NP. Absorption and excretion of calcium and fat by young infants. *Lancet* 1969; **i**: 487.

41. Berkowitz GP. Milk curd obstruction mimicking necrotizing enterocolitis. *Am J Dis Child* 1980; **134**: 989.

42. Konvolinka CW & Frederick J. Milk curd syndrome in neonates. *J Pediatr Surg* 1989; **24**: 497.
43. Steiner GM. Abnormal meconium and 'Milk inspissation'. *Proc R Soc Med* 1972; **65**: 733.

Necrotizing enterocolitis

1. Tan CEL, Keily EM, Agrawal M, Brereton RJ & Spitz L. Neonatal gastrointestinal perforations. *J Pediatr Surg* 1989; **24**: 88.
2. Ryder RW, Shelton JD & Guinan ME. Necrotizing enterocolitis. A prospective multicenter investigation. *Am J Epidemiol* 1980; **12**: 113.
3. Pokorny WJ, Garcia-Prats JA & Barry YN. Necrotizing enterocolitis: incidence, operative care and outcome. *J Pediatr Surg* 1986; **21**: 1149.
4. O'Neill JA. Neonatal necrotizing enterocolitis. *Surg Clin North Am* 1981; **61**: 1013.
5. Takayanagi K & Kapila L. Necrotizing enterocolitis in older infants. *Arch Dis Child* 1981; **56**: 468.
6. West KW, Rescorla FJ, Grosfeld JL & Vane DW. Pneumotosis intestinalis in children beyond the neonatal period. *J Pediatr Surg* 1989; **24**: 819.
7. Shanbhogue LKR, Tam PKH & Llyod DA. Necrotizing enterocolitis following operation in the neonatal period. *Br J Surg* 1991; **78**: 1045.
8. Stringer MD, Brereton RJ & Wright VM. Necrotizing enterocolitis in infants with esophageal atresia awaiting delayed primary repair. *Pediatr Surg Int* 1992; **7**: 353.
9. Pujari BD & Deodare SG. Necrotising enteritis. *Br J Surg* 1980; **67**: 254.
10. Powell RW, Dyess DL, Luterman A, Simon NP & Ramenofsky ML. Necrotizing enterocolitis in multiple-birth infants. *J Pediatr Surg* 1990; **25**: 319.
11. Sanderson IR, Risdon RA & Walker-Smith JA. Intractable ulcerating enterocolitis of infancy. *Arch Dis Child* 1990; **65**: 295.
12. Touloukian RJ. Neonatal necrotizing enterocolitis: an update on etiology, diagnosis and treatment. *Surg Clin North Am* 1976; **56**: 281.
13. Cohen IT, Nelson SD, Moxley RA, Hirsh MP, Counihan TC & Martin RF. Necrotizing enterocolitis in a neonatal piglet model. *J Pediatr Surg* 1001; **26**: 598.
14. Musemeche C, Caplan M, Hsueh W, Sun X & Kelly A. Experimental necrotizing enterocolitis: the role of polymorphonuclear neutrophils. *J Pediatr Surg* 1991; **26**: 1047.
15. Harrison MW, Connell RS, Campbell JR & Webb MC. Microcirculatory changes in the gastrointestinal tract of the hypoxic puppy: an electron microscope study. *J Pediatr Surg* 1975; **10**: 599.
16. Orme RL & Eades SM. Perforation of the bowel in the newborn as a complication of exchange transfusion. *BMJ* 1968; **4**: 349.
17. Palder SB, Schwartz MZ, Tyson KRT & Marr CC. Association of closure of patent ductus arteriosus and development of necrotizing enterocolitis. *J Pediatr Surg* 1988; **23**: 422.
18. Krasna IH, Howell C, Vega A, Zeigler M & Koop CE. A mouse model for the study of necrotizing enterocolitis. *J Pediatr Surg* 1986; **21**: 26.
19. Tibboel D, van Nie CJ & Molenaar JC. The effects of temporary general hypoxia and local ischaemia on the development of the intestines: an experimental study. *J Pediatr Surg* 1980; **15**: 57.
20. Stone HH, Webb HW & Kovalchik Mt. Pneumatosis intestinalis of infancy. *Surgery* 1971; **130**: 806.
21. Wijesinha SS. Neonatal necrotizing enterocolitis : new thoughts for the 'eighties. *Ann R Coll Surg Eng* 1982; **64**: 406.
22. Alloway AJ & Young DG. Umbilical vessel catheters. *J R Coll Surg Edinb* 1982; **27**: 174.
23. Santulli TV, Schullinger JN, Heird WD et al. Acute enterocolitis in infancy: a review of 64 cases. *Pediatre* 1975; **55**: 376.
24. Thomas DFM. Pathogenesis of neonatal necrotizing enterocolitis. *J R Soc Med* 1982; **75**: 838.
25. Bell MJ, Sheckelford P, Feigin RD, Sternberg JL & Brotherton T. Epidemiologic and bacteriologic evaluation of neonatal necrotizing enterocolitis. *J Pediatr Surg* 1979; **14**: 1.
26. Mollitt DL, Tapas JJ & Talbert JL. The role of coagulase-negative staphylococcus in neonatal necrotizing enterocolitis. *J Pediatr Surg* 1988; **23**: 60.
27. Hoy C, Millar MR, MacKay P, Godwin PGR, Langdale V & Levene MI. Quantitative changes in faecal microflora preceding necrotising enterocolitis in premature neonates. *Arch Dis Child* 1990; **65**: 1057.
28. Kosloske AM & Ulrich JA. A bacteriologic basis for the clinical presentations of necrotizing enterocolitis. *J Pediatr Surg* 1980; **15**: 558.
29. McCormack CJ, Emmens RW & Putman TC. Evaluation of factors in high risk neonatal necrotizing enterocolitis. *J Pediatr Surg* 1987; **22**: 488.
30. Marchidon MB, Buck BE & Abdenour G. Necrotizing enterocolitis in the unfed infant. *J Pediatr Surg* 1982; **17**: 620.

31. Barlow B, Santulli TV, Heird WC, Pitt J, Blanc WA & Schullinger JN. An experimental study of acute neonatal enterocolitis: the importance of breast milk. *J Pediatr Surg* 1974; **9**: 587.
32. Wijesinha SS, Steer HW, Dudley NE & Gough MH. Neonatal necrotising enterocolitis: the role of the intestinal immune system. *Ceylon Med J* 1982; **27**: 25.
33. Dykes EH, Liddell RHA, Galloway E & Azmy AF. Immune competence in necrotizing enterocolitis. *J Pediatr Surg* 1986; **21**: 211.
34. Garstin WIH, Kenny BD, McAneaney DS, Patterson CC & Boston VE. The role of intraluminal tension and pH in the development of necrotizing enterocolitis: an animal model. *J Pediatr Surg* 1987; **22**: 205.
35. Stein H, Beck J, Solomon A & Schmaman A. gastroenteritis with necrotizing enterocolitis in premature babies. *BMJ* 1972; **2**: 616.
36. Musemeche CA, Kosloske AM, Bartow SA & Umland ET. Comparative effects of ischaemia, bacteria and substrate on the pathogenesis of intestinal necrosis. *J Pediatr Surg* 1986; **21**: 536.
37. Beeby PJ & Jeffery H. Risk factors for necrotising enterocolitis: the influence of gestational age. *Arch Dis Child* 1992; **67**: 432.
38. Lindley S, Mollitt D, Seibert JJ & Golladay ES. Portal vein ultrasonography in the early diagnosis of necrotizing enterocolitis. *J Pediatr Surg* 1986; **21**: 530.
39. Griffiths DM & Gough MH. Gas in the hepatic portal veins. *Br J Surg* 1986; **73**: 172.
40. Donoghue V & Kelman CG. Transient portal venous gas in necrotizing enterocolitis. *Br J Radiol* 1982; **55**: 681.
41. Clarke EA and Dutton NE. Use of Iohexol in the early determination of gastrointestinal perforation. *J Pediatr Surg* 1988; **23**: 1027.
42. Boulton JE, Ein SH, Reilly BJ, Smith BT & Pape KE. Necrotizing enterocolitis and volvulus in the premature neonate. *J Pediatr Surg* 1989; **24**: 901.
43. Lobe TE, Dobkin ED, Gore D, Bhatia J Linares HA & Traber DL. Comparative effects of dopamine, naloxone and prostacylin in the resuscitation of fecal – *Escherichia coli* peritonitis – induced septic shock in neonatal swine. *J Pediatr Surg* 1986; **21**: 539.
44. Lister J, Asopa H, Cardenas F & Gill B. Neonatal necrotising enterocolitis. *Prog Pediatr Surg* 1978; **10**: 75.
45. Beasley SW, Auldist AW, Ramanujan TM & Campnell NT. The surgical management of neonatal necrotizing enterocolitis, 1975–1984. *Pediatr Surg* 1986; **1**: 210.
46. Mazzoni G, Doig CM, Bianchi A & Gough DCS. Neonatal necrotising enterocolitis: the surgical complications. *It J Pediatr Surg* 1987; **1**: 13.
47. Martin LW & Neblett WW. Early operation with intestinal diversion for necrotizing enterocolitis. *J Pediatr Surg* 1981; **16**: 252.
48. O'Neill JA, Stahlman MT & Meng HC. Necrotizing enterocolitis in the newborn: operative indications. *Ann Surg* 1975; **182**: 274.
49. Hofmann S, Baumann H, Emmrich P & Schreiber E. Surgical problems in necrotizing enterocolitis in childhood. *Prog Pediatr Surg* 1978; **11**: 87.
50. Janik JS & Ein SH. Peritoneal drainage under local anaesthesia for necrotizing enterocolitis (NEC) perforation: a second look. *J Pediatr Surg* 1980; **15**: 565.
51. Cheu HW, Sukarochana K & Llyod DA. Peritoneal drainage for necrotizing enterocolitis. *J Pediatr Surg* 1988; **23**: 557.
52. Ein SH, Shandling B, Wesson D & Filler RM. A 13 year experience with peritoneal drainage under local anesthesia for necrotizing enterocolitis perforation. *J Pediatr Surg* 1990; **25**: 1034.
53. Takamatsu H, Akiyama H, Ibara S, Seki S, Kuraya K & Ikenoue T. Treatment for necrotizing enterocolitis perforation in the extremely premature infant (weighing <1000g). *J Pediatr Surg* 1992; **27**: 741.
54. Morgan LJ, Shochat SJ & Hartman GE. Peritoneal drainage as primary management of perforated NEC in the very low birth weight infant. *J Pediatr Surg* 1994; **29**: 310.
55. O'Neill JA & Holcmb GW. Surgical experience with neonatal necrotizing enterocolitis. *Ann Surg* 1979; **189**: 612.
56. Harberg FJ, McGill CW, Saleem MM, Halbert R & Anastassiou P. Resection with primary anastomosis for necrotizing enterocolitis. *J Pediatr Surg* 1983; **18**: 743.
57. Griffiths DM Forbes DA, Pemberton PJ & Penn IA. Primary anastomosis for necrotizing enterocolitis: a 12-year experience. *J Pediatr Surg* 1989; **24**: 515.
58. Musemche CA, Kosloske AM & Ricketts RR. Enterostomy in necrotizing enterocolitis: an analysis of techniques and timing of closure. *J Pediatr Surg* 1987; **22**: 479.
59. Festen C, Severijnen RSVM & Staak FHJvd. Early closure of enterostomy after exteriorization of small intestine for abdominal catastrophies. *J Pediatr Surg* 1987; **22**: 144.

60. Ross MN, Wayne ER, Janik JS, Hanson JB, Burrington JD & Chang JHT. A standard of comparison for acute surgical necrotizing enterocolitis *J Pediatr Surg* 1989; **24**: 999.

61. Gertler JP, Seashore JH & Touloukian RJ. Early ileostomy closure in necrotizing enterocolitis. *J Pediatr Surg* 1987; **22**: 140.

62. Cooper A, Ross AJ, O'Neill JA & Schnaufer L. Resection with primary anastomosis for necrotizing enterocolitis: a contrasting veiw. *J Pediatr Surg* 1988; **23**: 64.

63. Schneider PA & Harrison MR. Sausage resection of ischaemic intestine. *J Pediatr Surg* 1987; **22**: 1011.

64. Nanjundiah P, Lifschitz CH, Gopalakrishna GS, Cochran WJ & Klish WJ. Intestinal strictures presenting with gastrointestinal blood loss. *J Pediatr Surg* 1989; **24**: 174.

65. Born M, Holgersen LO, Shahrivar F, Stanley-Brown E & Hilfer C. Routine contrast enemas for diagnosing and managing strictures following nonoperative treatment of necrotizing enterocolitis. *J Pediatr Surg* 1985; **20**: 461.

66. Schwartz MZ, Hayden CK, Richardson CJ, Tyson KRT & Lobe TE. A prospective evaluation of intestinal stenosis following necrotizing enterocolitis. *J Pediatr Surg* 1982; **17**: 764.

67. Stein H, Kavin I & Faerber EN. Coloni strictures following nonoperative management of necrotizing enterocolitis. *J Pediatr Surg* 1975; **10**: 943.

68. Keily E & Eckstein HB. Colonic stricture and enterocolic fistulae following necrotizing eneterocolitis. *Br J Surg* 1984; **71**: 613.

69. Hartman GE, Drugas GT & Shochat SJ. Post-necrotizing enterocolitis strictures presenting with sepsis or perforation: risk of clinical observation. *J Pediatr Surg* 1988; **23**: 562.

70. Radhakrishnan J, Blechman G, Shrader C, Patel MK & Mangurten HH. Colonic strictures following successful medical management of necrotizing enterocolitis: a prospective study evaluating early gastrointestinal contrast studies. *J Pediatr Surg* 1991; **26**: 1043.

71. Ball WS, Kosloske AM, Jewell PF, Seigel RS & Bartow SA. Balloon catheter dilatation of focal intestinal strictures following necrotizing enterocolitis. *J Pediatr Surg* 1985; **20**: 637.

72. Smith SD, Tagge EP, Miller J, Cheu H, Sukarochana K & Rowe MI. The hidden mortality in surgically treated necrotizing enterocolitis: fungal sepsis. *J Pediatr Surg* 1990; **25**: 1030.

73. Dykes EH, Gilmour WH & Azmy AF. Prediction of outcome following necrotizing enterocolitis in a neonatal surgical unit. *J Pediatr Surg* 1985; **20**: 3.

74. Freeman RB, Lloyd DJ, Miller SS & Duffy P. Surgical treatment of necrotizing enterocolitis: a population-based study in the Grampian region, Scotland. *J Pediatr Surg* 1988; **23**: 942.

75. Jackman S, Brerton RJ & Wright VM. Results of surgical treatment of neonatal necrotizing enterocolitis. *Br J Surg* 1990; **77**: 146.

76. Cirkit D, West KW, Schreiner R & Grosfeld JL. Long-term follow-up after surgical management of necrotizing enterocolitis: sixty-three cases. *J Pediatr Surg* 1986; **21**: 533.

77. Stevenson DK, Kernr JA, Malechowski N & Sunshine P. Late morbidity among survivors of necrotizing enterocolitis. *Pediatre* 1980; **66**: 925.

78. Rowe MI, Reblock KK, Kurchubasche AG & Healy PJ. Necrotizing enterocolitis in the extremely low birth weight infant. *J Pediatr Surg* 1994; **29**: 987.

79. Meyer CL, Payne NR & Roback SA. Spontaneous, isolated intestinal perforations in neonates with birth weight < 1000g not associated with necrotizing enterocolitis. *J Pediatr Surg* 1991; **26**: 714.

80. Weinberg G, Kleinhaus S & Boley SJ. Idiopathic intestinal perforations in the newborn: an increasingly common entity. *J Pediatr Surg* 1989; **24**: 1007.

81. Zamir O, Goldberg M, Udassin R, Peleg O, Nissan S & Eyal F. Idiopathic gastrointestinal perforation in the neonate. *J Pediatr Surg* 1988; **23**: 335.

82. Howat JM & Wilkinson AWW. Functional intestinal obstruction in the neonate. *Arch Dis Child* 1970; **45**: 800.

83. Lassmann G, Kees A, Korner K & Wurnig P. Transient functional obstruction of the colon in neonates: an investigation by rectal manometry and biopsy. *J Pediatr Surg* 1986; **21**: 244.

84. Shawis RN, Rangecroft I, Cook RCM & Gough DCS. Functional obstruction associated with malrotation and short small-bowel. *J Pediatr Surg* 1984; **19**: 172.

Complications of small bowel operation

1. Howat JM & Aaronson I. Sugar intolerance in neonatal surgery. *J Pediatr Surg* 1971; **6**: 719.

2. Stringel G, Uauy R & Guertin L. The effect of intestinal anastomosis on gut growth and maturation. *J Pediatr Surg* 1989; **24**: 1086.

3. Clayton BE, Arthur AB & Francis DEM. Early dietary management of sugar intolerance in infancy. *BMJ* 1966; **2**: 679.

4. Hughes EA, Stevens LH & Wilkinson AWW. Some aspects of starvation in the newborn baby. *Arch Dis Child* 1964; **39**: 598.

5. McCance RA & Wilkinson AWW. Experimental resection of intestine in newborn pigs. *Br J Nutr* 1967; **21**: 731.

6. Newman BM, Jewett TC, Karp MP & Cooney DR. Percutaneous central venous catheterisation in children: first line choice for venous access. *J Pediatr Surg* 1986; **21**: 685.

7. Warner BW, Gorgone P, Schilling S, Farrell M & Ghory MJ. Multiple purpose central venous access in infants less than 1000 grams. *J Pediatr Surg* 1987; **22**: 820.

8. Lally KP, Hardin WD, Boettcher M, Shah SI & Mahour GH. Broviac catheter insertion: operating room or neonatal intensive care unit. *J Pediatr Surg* 1987; **22**: 823.

9. Roberts JP & Gollow IJ. Central venous catheters in surgical neonates. *J Pediatr Surg* 1990; **25**: 632.

10. King DR, Komer M, Hoffman J et al. Broviac catheter sepsis: the natural history of an iatrogenic infection. *J Pediatr Surg* 1985; **20**: 728.

11. Nahata MC, King DR, Powell DA, Marx SM & Ginn-Pease ME. Management of catheter-related infections in pediatric patients. *J Parenter Nutr* 1988; **12**: 58.

12. Gamba PG, Zanon GF, Fabris S, Midrio P, Orzali A & Guglielmi M. Fragments of central venous line in the heart of neonates and pediatric patients. *Ital J Pediatr Surg* 1993; **7**: 21.

13. Manginello FP & Javitt NB. Parental nutrition and neonatal cholestasis. *J Pediatr* 1979; **94**: 296.

14. Hodes JF, Grosfeld JL, Weber TR, Schreiner RL, Fitzgerald JF & Mirkin LD. Hepatic failure in infants on total parenteral nutrition (TPN): clinical and histopathologic observations. *J Pediatr Surg* 1982; **17**: 463.

15. Hughes CA, Talbot IC, Ducker DA & Harran MJ. Total parenteral nutrition in infancy: effect on the liver and suggested pathogenesis. *Gut* 1983; **24**: 241.

16. Grisoni ER, Mehta SK & Connors AF. Thrombosis and infection complicating central venous catheterization in neonates. *J Pediatr Surg* 1986; **21**: 772.

17. Mollitt DL & Golladay ES. Complications of TPN catheter-induced vena caval thrombosis in children less than one year of age. *J Pediatr Surg* 1983; **18**: 462.

18. Groff DB. Complications of intravenous hyperalimentation in newborns and infants. *J Pediatr Surg* 1969; **4**: 460.

19. Mughal MM. Complications of intravenous feeding catheters. *Br J Surg* 1989; **76**: 15.

20. Kubota A, Okado A, Imura K et al. The effect of Metronidazole on TPN-associated liver dysfunction in neonates. *J Pediatr Surg* 1990; **26**: 618.

21. Tibboel D, Delemarre FMC, Przyrembel H, Bos AP, Affourtit MJ & Molenaar JC. Carnitine deficiency in surgical neonates receiving total parenteral nutrition. *J Pediatr Surg* 1990; **25**: 418.

22. Whalen GF, Shamberger RC, Perez-Atayde A & Folkman J. A proposed cause for the hepatic dysfunction associated with parentral nutrition. *J Pediatr Surg* 1990; **25**: 622.

23. Pierro A, Carnielli V, Filler RM, Smith J & Heim T. Characteristics of protein sparing effect of total parenteral nutrition in the surgical infant. *J Pediatr Surg* 1988; **23**: 538.

24. Weber TR, Sears N, Davies B & Grosfeld JL. Clinical spectrum of zinc deficiency in pediatric patients receiving total parenteral nutrition (TPN). *J Pediatr Surg* 1981; **16**: 236.

25. Suita S, Ikeda K, Hayashida Y, Naito K, Handa N & Doki T. Zinc and copper requirements during parenteral nutrition in the newborn. *J Pediatr Surg* 1984; **19**: 126.

26. Filler RM, Takada Y, Carreras T & Heim T. Serum lipids in neonates during parenteral nutrition: the relation to gestational age. *J Pediatr Surg* 1980; **15**: 405.

27. Barson AJ, Chiswick ML & Doig CM. Fat embolism in infancy after intravenous fat infusions. *Arch Dis Child* 1978; **53**: 218.

28. Bedrick AD. Metabolic tolerance of parenteral lipid in neonates. *Am J Dis Child* 1988; **142**: 135.

29. Liston L. Paediatric HTPN: a father's view. *Intens Ther Clin Monitor* 1987; **8**: 186.

30. Lin CH, Rossi TM, Heitlinger LA, Lerner A, Riddlesberger MM & Lebenthal E. Nutritional assessment of children with short-bowel syndrome receiving home parenteral nutrition. *Am J Dis Child* 1987; **141**: 1093.

31. Suita S, Ikeda K, Nagasaki A et al. Follow-up studies of children treated with a long-term intravenous nutrition (IVN) during the neonatal period. *J Pediatr Surg* 1982; **17**: 37.

32. Cooper A, Floyd TF, Ross AJ, Bishop HC, Templeton JM & Ziegler MM. Morbidity and mortality of short bowel syndrome acquired in infancy: an update. *J Pediatr Surg* 1984; **19**: 711.

33. Morgan W, Yardley J, Luk G, Niemiec P & Dudgeon D. Total parenteral nutrition and intestinal development: a neonatal model. *J Pediatr Surg* 1987; **22**: 541.

34. Wallace AM & Newman K. Successful closure of intestinal fistulae in an infant using the somatostatin analogue SMS 201–995. *J Pediatr Surg* 1991; **26**: 1097.

35. Touloukian RJ & Smith GJW. Normal intestinal length in preterm infants. *J Pediatr Surg* 1983; **18**: 720.

36. Wilmore DW. Factors correlating with a successful outcome following extensive resection in newborn infants. *J Pediatr* 1972; **80**: 88.

37. Kurz R & Sauer H. Treatment and metabolic findings in extreme short-bowel syndrome with 11cm jejunal remnant. *J Pediatr Surg* 1983; **18**: 257.

38. Postuma R, Moroz S & Friesen F. Extreme short bowel syndrome in an infant. *J Pediatr Surg* 1983; **18**: 264.

39. Wilkinson AWW. Magnesium in paediatric surgery. *Acta Paediatr Biol* 1973; **27**: 133.

40. Puri P & Guiney EJ. Transient hypothyroidism associated with short gut syndrome. *J Pediatr Surg* 1982; **17**: 22.

41. Rickham PP, Irving I & Shmerling DH. Long term results following extensive small intestinal resection in the neonatal period. *Prog Pediatr Surg* 1977; **10**: 65.

42. Levy E, Frileux P, Sandrucci S et al. Continous enteral feeding during the adaptive stage of the short bowel syndrome. *Br J Surg* 1988; **75**: 549.

43. Sigalet DL, Lees GM, Aherne F et al. The physiology of adaption to small bowel resection in the pig: an integrated study of morphological and functional changes. *J Pediatr Surg* 1990; **25**: 650.

44. Valman HB. Diet and growth after resection of ileum in childhood. *J Pediatr* 1976; **88**: 41.

45. Reiquam CW, Allen RP & Akers DR. Normal and abnormal small bowel lengths: an analysis of 389 autopsy cases in infants and children. *Am J Dis Child* 1965; **109**: 447.

46. Valman HB & Roberts PD. Vitamin B_{12} absorption after resection of the ileum in childhood. *Arch Dis Child* 1974; **49**: 932.

47. Weaver LT, Austin S & Cole TJ. Small intestinal length: a factor essential for gut adaption. *Gut* 1991; **32**: 1321.

48. Chaet MS, Arya G, Ziegler MM & Warner BW. Epidermal growth factor enhances intestinal adaption after massive small bowel resection. *J Pediatr Surg* 1994; **29**: 1035.

49. Goldman CD, Rudloff MA & Ternberg JL. Cemetidine and neonatal small bowel adaption: an experimental study. *J Pediatr Surg* 1987; **22**: 484.

50. Mitchell A, Watkins RM & Collin J. Surgical treatment of the short bowel syndrome. *Br J Surg* 1984; **71**: 329.

51. Garcia VF, Templeton JM, Eichelberger MR, Everett CE & Vinograd I. Colon interposition for the short bowel syndrome. *J Pediatr Surg* 1981; **16**: 994.

52. Lloyd DA. Antiperistaltic colonic interposition following massive small bowel resection in rats. *J Pediatr Surg* 1981; **16**: 64.

53. Grieco GA, Reyes HM & Ostrovsky E. The role of a modified intussusception jejunocolic valve in short-bowel syndrome. *J Pediatr Surg* 1983; **18**: 354.

54. Bianchi A. Intestinal loop lengthening – a technique for increasing small intestinal length. *J Pediatr Surg* 1980; **15**: 145.

55. Boeckman CR & Taylor R. Bowel lengthening for short gut syndrome. *J Pediatr Surg* 1981; **16**: 996.

56. Lillimoe KD, Berry WR, Harmon JW, Tai YH, Weichbrod RH & Cogen MA. Use of vascularised abdominal wall pedicle flaps to grow small bowel neomucosa. *Surgery* 1982; **91**: 293.

57. Kimura K & Soper RT. Isolated bowel segment (model 1): creation by myoenteropexy. *J Pediatr Surg* 1990; **25**: 512.

58. Shimazu R, Raju S, Fujwara H & Grogan JB. Experimental small-bowel transplantation: alternative strategies for graft prolongation. *J Pediatr Surg* 1989; **24**: 1253.

59. Taguchi T, Zorychta E, Sonnino RE & Guttman FM. Small intestinal transplantation in the rat: effect on physiological properties of smooth muscle and nerves. *J Pediatr Surg* 1989; **24**: 1258.

60. Kelnar S, Herkomer C, Bae S & Schumacher U. Allogenic transplantation of fetal rat intestine: anastomosis to the normal bowel of the host. *J Pediatr Surg* 1990; **25**: 415.

61. Hale DA, Waldorf KA, Kleinschmidt J, Pearl RH & Seyfer AE. Small intestinal transplantation in nonhuman primates. *J Pediatr Surg* 1991; **26**: 914.

62. Revillon Y, Jan D, Sarnacki S, Goulet O. Brousse N & Ricour C. Intestinal transplantation in the child: experimental and clinical studies. *J Pediatr Surg* 1993; **28**: 292.

63. Maeda K, Oki K, Nakumura K & Schwartz MZ. Small intestinal transplantation: a logical solution for short bowel syndrome? *J Pediatr Surg* 1988; **23**: 10.

64. Wood RFM. Small bowel transplantation. *Br J Surg* 1992; **79**: 193.

65. Kellnar S, Schreiber C, Rattanasouwan T & Trammer A. Fetal intestinal transplantation: a new therapeutic approach in short-bowel syndrome. *J Pediatr Surg* 1992; **27**: 799.

66. Clark CI. Recent progress in intestinal transplantation. *Arch Dis Child* 1992; **67**: 976.

67. Meijssen MAC & Heineman E. Functional aspects of small bowel transplantation: past, present, and future. *Gut* 1994; **35**: 1338.

68. Lawrence JP, Dunn SP, Billmire DF, Falkenstein K, Vinocur CD & Weintraub WH. Isolated liver transplantation for liver failure in patients with short bowel syndrome. *J Pediatr Surg* 1994; **29**: 751.

69. Williams JW, Sankary HN & Foster PF. Technique for splanchnic transplantation. *J Pediatr Surg* 1991; **26**: 79.

Intussusception

1. Dennison WM & Shaker M. Intussusception in infancy and childhood. *Br J Surg* 1970; **57**: 679.

2. Perrin WS & Lindsay EC. Intussusception: monograph based on 400 cases. *Br J Surg* 1921; **9**: 46.

3. Ong NT & Beasley SW. The leadpoint in intussusception. *J Pediatr Surg* 1990; **25**: 640.

4. Ong NT & Beasley SW. Progression of intussusception. *J Pediatr Surg* 1990; **25**: 644.

5. Nicolas JC, Ingrand D, Fortier B & Bricout F. A one-year virological survey of acute intussusception in childhood. *J Med Viral* 1982; **9**: 267.

6. Winstanley JHR, Doig CM & Brydon H. Intussusception: the case for barium reduction. *J R Coll Surg Edinb* 1987; **32**: 285.

7. Wilson-Storey D, MacKinlay GA, Prescott S & Hendry GMA. Intussusception: a surgical condition. *J R Coll Surg Edinb* 1988; **33**: 270.

8. Bruce J, Huh YS, Cooney DR, Karp MP, Allen JE & Jewett TC. Intussusception: evolution of current management. *J Pediatr Gastroenterol* 1987; **6**: 663.

9. Carter CR & Morton AL. Adult intussusception in Glasgow, UK. *Br J Surg* 1989; **76**: 727.

10. Turner D, Rickwood AMK & Brereton RJ. Intussusception in older children. *Arch Dis Child* 1980; **55**: 544.

11. Ein SN, Stephens CA, Shandling B & Filler RM. Intussusception due to lymphoma. *J Pediatr Surg* 1986; **21**: 786.

12. Butchinson IR, Olayiwola B & Young DG. Intussusception in infancy and childhood. *Br J Surg* 1980; **67**: 209.

13. Ravitch MM & McCune RM. Intussusception in infants and children: Analysis of 152 cases with a discussion of reduction by barium enema. *J Pediatr* 1950; **37**: 153.

14. Minami A & Kiyosho F. Intussusception in children. *Am J Dis Child* 1975; **129**: 346.

15. Eklof OA, Johanson L & Lohr G. Childhood intussusception: hydrostatic reducibility and incidence of leading points in different age groups. *Pediatr Radiol* 1980; **10**: 83.

16. Humphry A, Ein SH & Mok PM. Perforation of the intussuscepted colon. *Am J Radiol* 1981; **137**: 1135.

17. Ein SH, Mercer S, Humphrey A & MacDonald P. Colonic perforation during attempted barium enema reduction of intussusception. *J Pediatr Surg* 1981; **16**: 313.

18. Liu KW, MacCarthy J, Guiney EJ & Fitzgerald RG. Intussusception – current trends in management. *Arch Dis Child* 1986; **61**: 75.

19. Potts SR & Murphy N. The obstructed intussusception in childhood. *Ulster Med J* 1984; **53**: 140.

20. Daneman A & Reilly BJ. Intussusception. *Am J Rediol* 1982; **139**: 299.

21. Ein SH, Stephens CA & Minor A. The painless intussusception. *J Pediatr Surg* 1976; **11**: 563.

22. Goh DW & Chapman S. False positives diagnosis of intussusception in the older child by contrast enema. *J Roy Coll Edinb* 1990; **35**: 188.

23. Rosenkrantz JG, Cox JA, Silverman FN & Martin LW. Intussusception in the 1970's: indications for operation. *J Pediatr Surg* 1977; **12**: 367.

24. Sparnon AL, Little KET & Morris LL. Intussusception in childhood: a review of 139 cases. *Aust N Z J Surg* 1984; **54**: 353.

25. Ein SH & Stephens CA. Intussusception: 354 cases in 10 years. *J Pediatr Surg* 1971; **6**: 16.

26. Auldist AW. Intussusception in a children's hospital: a review of 203 cases in seven years. *Aust N Z J Surg* 1970; **40**: 136.

27. Reijnen JAM, Festen C & van Roosmalen RP. Intussusception: factors related to treatment. *Arch Dis Child* 1990; **65**: 871.

28. Tamanaha K, Wimbish K, Talwalkar YB & Ashimini K. Air reduction of intussusception in infants and children. *J Pediatr* 1987; **111**: 733.

29. Bowerman RA, Silver TM & Jaffe MH. Real time ultrasound diagnosis of intussusception in children. *Radiology* 1982; **143**: 527.

30. Wang GD & Liu SJ. Enema reduction of intussusception by hydrostatic pressure under ultrasound guidance: a report of 377 cases. *J Pediatr Surg* 1988; **23**: 814.

31. Franken EA. Nonsurgical treatment of intussusception. *Am J Radiol* 1988; **150**: 1353.

32. Ching E, Ching LT, Lynn HB & O'connell EJ. Intussusception in children *Mayo Clin Proc* 1970; **45**: 742.

33. Newman J & Schuh S. Intussusception in babies under 4 months of age. *Can Med Assoc J* 1987; **136**: 266.

34. Schuh S & Wesson DE. Intussusception in children 2 years of age or older. *Can Med Assoc J* 1987; **136**: 269.

35. Ein SC. Recurrent intussusception in children. *J Pediatr Surg* 1975; **10**: 751.

36. Reijnen JAM, Festen C & Joosten HJM. Chronic intussusception in children. *Br J Surg* 1989; **76**: 815.

37. Woodall DL, Birken GA, Williamson K & Lobe TE. Isolated fetal-neonatal abdominal ascites: a sign of intrauterine intussusception. *J Pediatr Surg* 1987; **22**: 506.

38. Galea MH & Mayell MJ. Gastroduodenal mucosal intussusception causing gastric outlet obstruction: a complication of gastrostomy tubes. *J Pediatr Surg* 1988; **23**: 980.

Other small bowel problems

1. Apley J. *The Child with Abdominal Pain*, 2nd edn. Oxford: Blackwell Oxford, 1975.

2. Winsey HS & Jones PF. Acute abdominal pain: analysis of a year's admissions. *BMJ* 1967; **1**: 653.

3. Bain HW. Chronic vague abdominal pain in children. *Pediatr Clin North Amer* 1974; **21**: 991.

4. Drake DP. Acute abdominal pain in children. *J R Soc Med* 1980; **73**: 641.

5. Puri P & O'Donnell B. Appendicitis in infancy. *J Pediatr Surg* 1978; **13**: 173.

6. Lund DP & Murphy EU. Management of perforated appendicitis in children: a decade of aggressive treatnent. *J Pediatr Surg* 1994; **29**: 1130.

7. Dimson SB. Transit time related to clinical findings in children with recurrent abdominal pain. *Pediatr* 1971; **47**: 666.

8. Doig CM. Constipation in childhood. *Update* 1988; **36**: 2366.

9. Soussi MM & Mufarrij AA. Primary segmental infarction of the greater omentum in children. *Pediatr Surg Int* 1988; **3**: 437.

10. Shanbogue LKR & Doig CM. Primary segmental infarction of the greater omentum in children. *Pediatr Surg Int* 1990; **5**: 224.

11. Jona JZ & Belin RP. Basilar pneumonia simulating acute appendicitis in children. *Arch Surg* 1976; **111**: 552.

12. Bonadio WA. Clinical features of abdominal painful crisis in sickle cell anemia. *J Pediatr Surg* 1990; **25**: 301.

13. Lebenthal E. Recurrent abdominal pain in childhood. *Am Dis Child* 1980; **134**: 347.

14. Meiser G & Meissner K. Intermittent incomplete intestinal obstruction: a frequently mistaken entity: ultrasonographic diagnosis and management. *Surg Endosc* 1989; **3**: 46.

15. Stickler G & Maryly DB. Recurrent abdominal pain. *Am Dis Child* 1979; **133**: 486.

16. Johnson LF, Vanderhoof JA & Black S. The role of exploratory laparotomy for chronic abdominal pain in children. *Nebr Med J* 1974; **59**: 430.

17. Gans SL, Johnson DG & Berci G. Laparoscopy in infants and children. In Berci G (ed.) *Endoscopy*. New York: Appleton–Century–Crofts, 1976; 411.

18. Leape LL & Ramenofsky ML. Laparoscopy for questionable appendicitis: can it reduce the negative appendectomy rate? *Ann Surg* 1980; **191**: 410.

19. Sackier JM. Laparoscopy in pediatric surgery. *J Pediatr Surg* 1991; **26**: 1145.

20. El Ghoneimi A, Valla JS, Limonne LV et al. Laparoscopic appendicectomy in children: report of 1379 cases. *J Pediatr Surg* 1994; **29**: 786.

21. Akgur FM, Tanyel FC, Buyukpamukcu N & Hicsonmez A. Anomalous congenital bands causing intestinal obstruction in children. *J Pediatr Surg* 1992; **27**: 471.

22. Chang WWL & Griffith KM. Solitary intestinal fibromatosis: a rare cause of intestinal obstruction in neonate and infant. *J Pediatr Surg* 1991; **26**: 1406.

23. Sharma V & Sharm ID. Intestinal trichobezoar with perforation in a child. *J Pediatr Surg* 1992; **27**: 518.

24. Foo KT, Ng KC, Rauff A, Foong WC & Sinniah R. Unusual small bowel obstruction in adolescent girls: the abdominal cocoon. *Br J Surg* 1978; **65**: 427.

25. Macklin J, Hall C & Feldman MA. Unusual cause of small bowel obstruction in adolescent girls: the abdominal cocoon. *J R Coll Surg Edin* 1991; **36**: 50.

26. Viidik T & Marshall DG. Direct inguinal hernias in infancy and early childhood. *J Pediatr Surg* 1980; **15**: 645.

27. Shanbogue LKR & Miller SS. Richter's hernia in the neonate. *J Pediatr Surg* 1986; **21**: 881.

28. Puri P, Guiney EJ & O'Donnell B. Inguinal hernia in infants: the fate of the testis following incarceration. *J Pediatr Surg* 1984; **19**: 44.

29. Doig CM. In Walker WF (ed.) *Inguinal Hernias and Hydroceles in Infants and Children*. Netherlands: Wolfe Medical Publ 1983.

30. Krieger NR, Shochat SJ, McGowan V & Hartman GE. Early hernia repair in the premature infant: long-term follow-up. *J Pediatr Surg* 1994; **29**: 978.

31. Harvey MH, Johnstone MJS & Fossard DP. Inguinal herniotomy in children: a five year survey. *Br J Surg* 1985; **72**: 485.

32. Morecroft JA, Stringer MD, Higgins M, Holmes SJK & Capps SNJ. Follow-up after inguinal herniotomy or surgery for hydrocele in boys. *Br J Surg* 1993; **80**: 1613.

33. Grosfeld JL, Minnick K, Shedd F, West KW, Rescorla FJ & Vane DW. Inguinal hernia in children: factors affecting recurrence in 62 cases. *J Pediatr Surg* 1991; **26**: 283.

34. Mejdahl S, Gyrtrup HJ & Kvist E. Out-patient operation of inguinal hernia in children. *Br J Surg* 1989; **76**: 406.

35. Surana R & Puri P. Is contralateral exploration necessary in infants with unilateral inguinal hernia? *J Pediatr Surg* 1993; **28**: 1026.

36. Abela M & Sanges G. Direct inguinal hernia in childhood. Case report and literature review. *Ital J Ped Surg* 1993; **7**: 19.

37. Zaman K, Taylor JD & Fossard DP. Femoral herniae in children. *J R Coll Surg Engl* 1985; **67**: 249.

38. Marshall DG. Femoral hernias in children. *J Pediatr Surg* 1983; **18**: 160.

39. Bourke JB. Strangulated femoral hernia in a female child of three years and nine months. *Br J Surg* 1968; **53**: 880.

Crohn's disease

1. Ferguson A, Rifkind EA & Doig CM. Prevalence of chronic inflammatory bowel disease in British children. *Front Gastrointest Res* 1986; **11**: 68.

2. Postuma R & Moroz SP. Pediatric Crohn's disease. *J Pediatr Surg* 1985; **20**: 478.

3. Barton JR, Gillon S & Ferguson A. Incidence of inflammatory bowel disease in Scottish children between 1968 and 1983: marginal fall in ulcerative colitis, three-fold rise in Crohn's disease. *Gut* 1989; **30**: 618.

4. Gelfand MD & Krone CL. Inflammatory bowel disease in family: observations related to pathogenesis. *Ann Intern Med* 1970; **73**: 903.

5. Doig CM. Surgery of inflammatory bowel disease in children, with reference to Crohn's disease. *J R Coll Surg Edinb* 1989; **34**: 189.

6. O'Donoghue DP & Dawson AM. Crohn's disease in childhood. *Arch Dis Child* 1977; **52**: 627.

7. Pettei MJ & Davidson M. Extra-gastrointestinal manifestations of inflammatory bowel disease. *J Pediatr Gastroenterol Nutr* 1985; **4**: 689.

8. Burgibe EJ, Huang SH & Bayless TM. Clinical manifestations of Crohn's disease in children and adolescents. *Pediatre* 1975; **55**: 866.

9. Greenstein AJ, Janowitz HD & Sachar DB. The extra-intestinal complications of Crohn's disease and ulcerative colitis: a study of 700 patients. *Medicine* 1976; **55**: 401.

10. Passo MH, Fitzgerald JF & Brandt KD. Arthritis associated with inflammatory disease in children: relationship of joint disease to activity and severity of bowel lesion. *Dis Dig Sci* 1986; **31**: 492.

11. Farmer RG & Michener WN. Prognosis of Crohn's disease with onset in adolescence. *Dig Dis Sci* 1979; **24**: 752.

12. Gryboski JD & Spiro HM. Prognosis in children with Crohn's disease. *Gastroenterology* 1978; **74**: 807.

13. Poley JR. Chronic inflammatory bowel disease in children and adolescents. *South Med J* 1978; **71**: 935.

14. Gillen CD, Walmsley RS, Prior P, Andrews HA & Allan RN. Ulcerative colitis and Crohn's disease: a comparision of the colorectal cancer risk in extensive colitis. *Gut* 1994; **35**: 1590.

15. Macfarlane PI, Miller V & Ratcliffe JF. Clinical and radiological diagnosis of Crohn's disease in children. *J Pediatr Gastroenterol Nutr* 1986; **5**: 87.

16. Macfarlane PI, Miller V, Wells F & Richards B. Laboratory assessment of disease activity in childhood Crohn's disease and ulcerative colitis. *J Pediatr Gastroenterol Nutr* 1986; **5**: 93.

17. Dawson DJ, Khan AN, Miller V, Ratcliffe RF & Shreeve DR. Detection of inflammatory bowel disease in adults and children revaluation of a new isotope technique. *BMJ* 1985; **291**: 1227.

18. George A, Merrick MV, Palmer KR & Millar AM. ⁹⁹ᵐTc-sucralfate scintigraphy and colonic disease. *BMJ* 1987; **295**: 578.

19. Sanderson IR & Walker-Smith JA. Crohn's disease in childhood. *Br J Surg* 1985; **72**: s87.

20. Singleton JW, Summers RW, Kern F et al. Trial of sulphasalazine as adjunctive therapy in Crohn's disease. *Gastroenterology* 1979; **77**: 887.

21. Kirschner BS. Inflammatory bowel disease in children. *Pediatr Clin North Am* 1988; **35**: 189.

22. Ursing B & Kamme C. Metronidazole for Crohn's disease. *Lancet* 1975; **i**: 775.

23. Lennard-Jones JE. Azathioprine and 6-mercaptopurine have a role in the treatment of Crohn's disease. *Dig Dis Sci* 1981; **26**: 364.

24. Sanderson IR, Udeen S, Davies PSW, Savage MO & Walker-Smith JA. Remission induced by an elemental diet in small bowel Crohn's disease. *Arch Dis Child* 1987; **61**: 123.

25. Belli DC, Seidmen E, Bouthillier L et al. Chronic intermittent elemental diet improves growth failure in children with Crohn's disease. *Gastroenterology* 1988; **94**: 603.

26. Strobel CT, Byrne WJ & Ament ME. Home parentral nutrition in children with Crohn's disease: an effective management alternative. *Gastroenterology* 1979; **76**: 272.

27. Kirshner BS, Voinchet O & Rosenberg IH. Growth retardation in inflammatory bowel disease. *Gastroenterology* 1978; **75**: 504.

28. Raine PAM. BAPS collective review: Chronic inflammatory bowel disease. *J Pediatr Surg* 1984; **19**: 18.

29. Beeken WL. Absorptive defects in young people with regional enteritis. *Pediatre* 1973; **52**: 69.

30. Kirschner BS, Klich JR, Kalman SS, de Favaro MV & Rosenberg IH. Reversal of growth retardation in Crohn's disease with therapy emphasizing oral nutritional restitution. *Gastroenterology* 1981; **80**: 10.

31. Lennard-Jones JE. Nutrition in Crohn's disease. *Ann R Coll Surg Engl* 1990; **72**: 152.

32. Barton JR and Ferguson A. Failure to record variables of growth and development in children with inflammatory bowel disease. *BMJ* 1989; **298**: 865.

33. Blair GK, Yaman M & Wesson DE. Preoperative home elemental enteral nutrition in complicated Crohn's disease. *J Pediatr Surg* 1986; **21**: 769.

34. Miller V & Thomas AG. Disease activity, growth and nutrition – paediatric aspects. In Allan RN & Hodgson HJF (eds) *Inflammatory Bowel Disease: Frontiers in Aetiology*. Smith Kline & French, 1987; 46.

35. Fonkalsrud EW, Ament ME, Fleisher D & Byrne W. Surgical management of Crohn's disease in children. *Am J Surg* 1979; **13**: 15.

36. Lask B, Jenkins J, Nabarro L & Booth I. Psychosocial sequelae of stoma surgery for inflammatory bowel disease in childhood. *Gut* 1987; **28**: 1257.

37. Davies G, Evans CM, Shand WS & Walker-Smith JA. Surgery for Crohn's disease in childhood: influence of site of disease and operative procedure on outcome. *Br J Surg* 1990; **77**: 891.

38. Orkin BA & Telander RL. The effect of intra-abdominal resection or fecal diversion on perianal disease in pediatric Crohn's disease. *J Pediatr Surg* 1985; **20**: 343.

39. Hyams JS, Grand RJ, Colodny AH, Schuster SR & Eraklis A. Course and prognosis after colectomy and ileostomy for inflammatory disease in childhood and adolescence. *J Pediatr Surg* 1982; **17**: 400.

40. Doig CM. Crohn's disease. In: O'Neill JA, Rowe MI, Glosfeld JL, Fonkalsreid EW, Coran AG (eds). *Pediatric Surgery*. Chapter 88. St Louis: Mosby, 1998.

41. Castile RG, Telander RL, Cooney DR et al. Crohn's disease in children: assessment of the progression of disease, growth, and prognosis. *J Pediatr Surg* 1980; **15**: 462.

42. Coran AG, Klein MD & Sarahan TM. The surgical management of terminal ileal and right colon Crohn's disease in children. *J Pediatr Surg* 1983; **18**: 592.

43. Puntis J, McNeish AS & Allan RN. Long term prognosis of Crohn's disease with onset in childhood and adolescence. *Gut* 1984; **25**: 329.

44. Alperstein G, Daum F, Fisher SE et al. Linear growth following surgery in children and adolescents with Crohn's disease: relationship to pubertal status. *J Pediatr Surg* 1985; **20**: 129.

45. Homer DR, Grant RJ & Colodny AH. Growth, course and prognosis after surgery for Crohn's disease. *Pediatrie* 1977; **59**: 717.

46. Inflammatory bowel disease. In: Atwell J. (ed) *Paediatric Surgery*. Chapter 40. London: Arnold 1998.

Hirschsprung's disease and variants

1. Ram PKH & Boyd GP. Origin, course, and endings of abnormal enteric nerve fibres in Hirschsprung's disease defined by whole-mount immunohistochemistry. *J Pediatr Surg* 1990; **25**: 457.

2. Hardy SP, Smith PM, Bayston R & Spitz L. Electrogenic colonic ion transport in Hirschsprung's disease: reduced secretion to the neural secretagogues acetylcholine and iloprost. *Gut* 1993; **34**: 1405.

3. Kobayashi H, Hirakawa H, O'Briain DS & Puri P. Nerve growth factor receptor staining of suction biopsies in the diagnosis of Hirschsprung's disease. *J Pediatr Surg* 1994; **29**: 1224.

4. Ikeda K & Goto S. Total colonic aganglionosis with or without small bowel involvement: an analysis of 137 patients. *J Pediatr Surg* 1986; **21**: 319.

5. Kleinhaus S, Boley SJ, Sheran M & Sieber WK. Hirschsprung's disease: a survey of members of the Surgical Section of the American Academy of Pediatrics. *J Pediatr Surg* 1979; **14**: 588.

6. Ikeda K & Goto S. Diagnosis and treatment of Hirschsprung's disease in Japan. *Ann Surg* 1984; **19**: 400.

7. Schiller M, Levy P, Shawa RA, Abu-d-Dalu K Gorenstein A & Katz S. Familial Hirschsprung's disease – a report of 22 siblings in four families. *J Pediatr Surg* 1990; **25**: 322.

8. Engum SA, Petrits M, Rescorla FJ, Grosfeld JL, Morrison AM & Engels D. Familial Hirschsprung's disease: 20 cases in 12 kindreds. *J Pediatr Surg* 1993; **28**: 1286.

9. MacKinnon AE & Cohen SJ. Total intestinal aganglionosis, an autosomal recessive condition. *Arch Dis Child* 1977; **52**: 898.

10. Cohen IT & Gadd MA. Hirschsprung's disease in a kindred: a possible clue to the genetics of the disease. *J Pediatr Surg* 1982; **17**: 632.

11. Shah KN, Dalal SJ, Desai MP, Sheth PN, Joshi NC & Ambani LM. White forelock, pigmentary disorder of irides, and long segment Hirschsprung's disease: possible variant of Waardenburg syndrome. *J Pediatr* 1981; **99**: 432.

12. Caniano DA, Teitelbaum DH & Qualman SJ. Management of Hirschsprung's disease in children with Trisomy 21. *Am J Surg* 1990; **159**: 402.

13. Coran AG, Bjordal R, Eek S & Knutrud O. The surgical management of total colonic and partial small intestinal ganglionosis. *J Pediatr Surg* 1969; **4**: 531.

14. Saperstein L, Pollack J & Beck AR. Total intestinal aganglionosis. *Mt Sinai J Med* 1980; **47**: 72.

15. Ziegler MM, Ross AJ & Bishop HC. Total aganglionosis: a new technique for prolonged survival. *J Pediatr Surg* 1987; **22**: 82.

16. Ahmed S, Chen SJ & Jacobs SI. Total intestinal aganglionosis presenting as duodenal obstruction. *Arch Dis Child* 1971; **46**: 868.

17. Kato H, Yamamoto T, Yamamoto H, Ohi R, So N & Iwasaki Y. Immunocytochemical characterization of supporting cells in the enteric nervous system in Hirschsprung's disease. *J Pediatr Surg* 1990; **25**: 514.

18. Yamataka A, Miyano T, Urao M & Nishiye H. Hirschsprung's disease: diagnosis using monoclonal antibody 171B5. *J Pediatr Surg* 1992; **27**: 820.

19. Caniano DA, Ormsbee HS, Polito W, Sun C-C, Barone FC & Hill JL. Total intestinal aganglionosis. *J Pediatr Surg* 1985; **20**: 456.

20. Senyuz OF, Buyukunal C, Danismend N, Erdogan E, Ozbay G & Soylet Y. Extensive intestinal aganglionosis. *J Pediatr Surg* 1989; **24**: 453.

21. Prevot J, Joly A & Babut JM. The treatment of total aganglionosis of the colon according to Lester Martin. *Ann Chir Int* 1976; **17**: 103.

22. Ein SH, Shandling B & So H. A new look at an old operation for aganglionosis. *J Pediatr Surg* 1994; **29**: 1228.

23. N-Fekete C, Ricour C, Martelli H, Jacob SL & Pellerin D. Total colonic aganglionosis (with or without ileal involvement): a review of 27 cases. *J Pediatr Surg* 1986; **21**: 251.

24. Heath AL, Spitz L & Milla PJ. The absorptive function of colonic aganglionic intestine: are the Duhamel and Martin procedures rational? *J Pediatr Surg* 1985; **20**: 34.

25. Ross MN, Chang JHT, Burrington JD, Janik JS, Wayne ER & Clevenger P. Complications of the Martin procedure for total colonic aganglionosis. *J Pediatr Surg* 1988; **23**: 725.

26. Davies MRQ & Cywes S. Inadequate pouch emptying following Martin's pull-through procedure for intestinal aganglionosis. *J Pediatr Surg* 1983; **18**: 14.

27. Jordan FT, Coran AG & Wesley JR. Modified endorectal procedure for management of long segment aganglionosis. *Ann Surg* 1981; **94**: 70.

28. Stringel G. Extensive intestinal aganglionosis including the ileum: a new surgical technique. *J Pediatr Surg* 1986; **21**: 667.
29. Boley SJ. A new operative approach to total aganglionosis of the colon. *Surg Gynecol Obstet* 1984; **159**: 481.
30. Shandling B. Total colon aganglionosis – a new operation. *J Pediatr Surg* 1984; **19**: 503.
31. Kimura K, Nishijami E, Muraji T, Tsugawa C & Matsumoto Y. A new surgical approach to extensive aganglionosis. *J Pediatr Surg* 1981; **16**: 840.

Pseudo-obstruction

1. Hyman PE, Tomomasa T & Mc Diarmid SV. Intestinal pseudo-obstruction in childhood. In Milla PJ (ed.) *Disorders of Gastrointestinal Motility in Childhood*. Chichester: Wiley, 1988; 73.
2. Christensen J. The syndromes of pseudo-obstruction. *J Pediatr Gastroenterol Nutr* 1988; **7**: 319.
3. Doig CM. Hirschsprung's disease – a review. *Int J Colorect Dis* 1991; **6**: 52.
4. Doig CM. Hirschsprung's disease and mimicking conditions. *Dig Dis* 1994; **12**: 106.
5. Milla PJ, Lake BD, Spitz L, Nixon HH, Harris JT & Fenton TR. Chronic idiopathic intestinal pseudo-obstruction in infancy: a smooth muscle disease. In Labo G & Bortolitti M (eds) *Gastrointestinal Motility*. Verona: Cortina Int. 1983; 125.
6. Schuffler HO, Bird TD, Sumi SM & Cook A. A familial neuronal disease presenting as intestinal pseudo-obstruction. *Gastroenter* 1978; **75**: 889.
7. Tanner MS, Smith B & Lloyd JK. Functional intestine obstruction due to deficiency of argyophil neurones in the myenteric plexus. *Arch Dis Child* 1978; **51**: 837.
8. Vargas JH, Sachs P & Ament ME. Chronic intestinal pseudo-obstruction syndrome in pediatrics: results of a national survey by members of the North American Society of Pediatric Gastroenterology and Nutrition. *J Pediatr Gastroenterol Nutr* 1988; **7**: 323.
9. Shaw A, Shaffer H, Teja K, Kelly T, Grogan E & Bruni C. A perspective for pediatric surgeons: chronic idiopathic pseudo-obstruction. *J Pediatr Surg* 1979; **14**: 719.
10. Mayer EA, Elashoff J, Hawkins R, Berquist W & Taylor IL. Gastric emptying of mixed solid-liquid meal in patients with intestinal pseudo-obstruction. *Dig Dis Sci* 1988; **33**: 10.
11. Wozniak ER, Fenton TR & Milla PJ. The development of fasting small intestinal motility in the human neonate. In Roman C. (ed.) *Gastrointestinal Motility*. Lancaster: MTP Press, 1984: 1.
12. Smith B. Changes in the myenteric plexus in pseudo-obstruction. *Gut* 1968; **9**: 726.
13. Yamagiwa I, Ohta M, Obata K & Washio M. Intestinal pseudo-obstruction in a neonate caused by idiopathic muscular hypertrophy of the entire small intestine. *J Pediatr Surg* 1988; **23**: 866.
14. Taguchi T, Ikeda K, Shono T et al. Autonomic innervation of the intestine from a baby with megacystitis microcolon intestinal hypoperistalsis syndrome; I. immunohistochemical study. *J Pediatr Surg* 1989; **24**: 1264.
15. Waterfall WE, Cameron GS, Sarna SK, Lewis TD & Daniel DEE. Disorganised electrical activity in a child with pseudo-obstruction. *Gut* 1981; **22**: 77.
16. Kapila L, Haberkorn S & Nixon HH. Chronic adynamic bowel simulating Hirschsprung's disease. *J Pediatr Surg* 1975; **10**: 885.
17. Puri P, Lake BD & Nixon HH. Adynamic bowel syndrome: a report with disturbance of the cholinergic innervation. *Gut* 1977; **18**: 754.
18. Rodriques CA, Shepherd NA, Lennard-Jones JE, Hawley PR & Thompson HH. Familial visceral myopathy: a family with at least six involved members. *Gut* 1989; **30**: 1285.
19. Puri P, Lake BD, Gorman F, O'Donnell B & Nixon HH Megacystis-microcolon-intestinal hypoperistalsis syndrome: a visceral myopathy. *J Pediatr Surg* 1983; **18**: 64.
20. Pitt HA, Mann LL, Berquist WE, Ament ME, Fonkalsrud EW & Denbesten L. Chronic intestinal pseudo-obstruction: management with total parental nutrition and a venting enterostomy. *Arch Surg* 1985; **120**: 614.
21. Shaw A, Shuffler HA & Anuras S. Familial visceral myopathy: the role of surgery. *Am J Surg* 1985; **150**: 102.

Neuronal intestinal dysplasia

1. Kluck P, Tibboel D, Leendertse-Verloop K, van der Kamp AWM, ten Kate FJW & Molenaar JC. Diagnosis of congenital neurogenic abnormalities of the bowel with monoclonal anti-filament antibodies. *J Pediatr Surg* 1986; **21**: 132.
2. Puri P & Fujimoto T. Diagnosis of allied functional bowel disorders using monoclonal antibodies and electronmicroscopy. *J Pediatr Surg* 1988; **23**: 546.
3. Meier-Ruge W, Lutterbeck PM, Herzog B, Moerger R, Moser R & Scharli A. Acetylcholinesterase activity in suction biopsies of the rectum in the diagnosis of Hirschsprung's disease. *J Pediatr Surg* 1972; **7**: 11.
4. Scharli AF. Neuronal intestinal dysplasia. *Pediatr Surg Int* 1992; **7**: 2.
5. Ternberg JL & Winters K. Plexiform neurofibromatosis of the colon as a cause of congenital megacolon. *Am J Surg* 1965; **109**: 663.
6. Puri P, Lake BD, Nixon HH, Mishalany H & Claireaux AE. Neuronal colonic dysplasia: an unusual association of Hirschsprung's disease. *J Pediatr Surg* 1977; **12**: 681.
7. Scharli A and Meier-Ruge W. Localised and disseminated forms of neuronal intestinal dysplasia mimicking Hirschsprung's disease. *J Pediatr Surg* 1981; **16**: 164.
8. MacMahon RA, Moore CCM & Cussen LJ. Hirschsprung-like syndromes in patients with normal ganglion cells on suction biopsies. *J Pediatr Surg* 1981; **16**: 835.
9. Munakata K, Morita K, Okabe I & Sueoka H. Clinical and histologic studies of neuronal intestinal dysplasia. *J Pediatr Surg* 1985; **20**: 231.

Dilatations and duplications

1. De Lorimer AA, Benzian RR & Gooding CA. Segmental dilatation of the colon. *AJR* 1971; **112**: 100.
2. Brawner J & Shafer AD. Segmental dilatation of the colon. *J Pediatr Surg* 1973; **8**: 957.
3. Rovira J, Morales L, Parri FJ, Julia V & Claret I. Segmental dilatation of the duodenum. *J Pediatr Surg* 1989; **24**: 1155.
4. Rossi R & Giocomino MA. Segmental dilatation of the jejunum. *J Pediatr Surg* 1973; **8**: 335.
5. Irving IM & Lister J. Segmental dilatation of the ileum. *J Pediatr Surg* 1977; **12**: 103.
6. Bell MJ, Ternberg JL & Bower RJ. Ileal dysgenesis in infants and children. *J Pediatr Surg* 1982; **17**: 395.
7. Humphrey A, Mancer K & Stephens CA. Obstructive circular-muscle defect in the small bowel in a one-year-old child. *J Pediatr Surg* 1980; **15**: 197.
8. Kuzaat M, Carneiro PMR & Spitz L. Jejunal diverticulum in a child presenting with small bowel obstruction. *J R Coll Surg Edinb* 1992; **37**: 195.
9. Howat JM & Grant JC. Non-vitelline accessory enteric formations. *Br J Surg* 1970; **57**: 205.
10. Fallon M, Gordon ARG & Lendrum AC. Mediastinal cysts of the foregut origin associated with vertebral anomalies. *Br J Surg* 1954; **41**: 520.
11. Royle SG & Doig CM. Perforation of the jejunum secondary to a duplication cyst lined with ectopic gastric mucosa. *J Pediatr Surg* 1988; **23**: 1025.
12. Mair WSJ & Abbott CR. Perforation of ileal duplication in old age. *BMJ* 1976; **2**: 621.
13. Wig JD, Chowdhary A, Suri S & Joshi K. Left duplication in an adult. *Br J Surg* 1984; **71**: 20.
14. Schwartz DL, Becker JM, Schneider KM & So HB. Tubular duplication with autonomous blood supply: resection with preservation of adjacent bowel. *J Pediatr Surg* 1980; **15**: 341.
15. Ross ERS, Larkworthy W & Hutter FHD. A cyst of the second part of the duodenum. *J R Coll Surg Edinb* 1987; **32**: 170.
16. Beach PD, Brascho J, Hein WR, Nichol WW & Geppert LJ. Duplication of the primitive hindgut of the human being. *Surgery* 1961; **49**: 477.
17. Hocking M & Young DG. Duplications of the alimentary tract. *Br J Surg* 1981; **68**: 92.
18. Murty TVM, Bhargava RK & Rakas FS. Gastroduodenal duplication. *J Pediatr Surg* 1992; **27**: 515.
19. Bishop HC & Koop CE. Surgical management of duplications of the alimentary tract. *Am J Surg* 1964; **107**: 434.
20. Nixon HH. Congenital abnormalities of the gut. *Br J Hosp Med* 1977; **19**: 202.
21. Orr MM & Edwards AJ. Neoplastic change in duplications of the alimentary tract. *Br J Surg* 1975; **62**: 269.
22. Norris RW, Brereton RJ, Wright VM & Cudmore RE. A new approach to duplications of the intestine. *J Pediatr Surg* 1986; **21**: 167.
23. Basu R, Forshall I & Rickham PP. Duplications of the alimentary tract. *Br J Surg* 1960; **47**: 477.
24. Ramenofsky ML, Leape LL & McCauley RGK. Bronchogenic cyst. *J Pediatr Surg* 1979; **14**: 219.

25. Superina RA, Ein SH & Humphreys RP. Cystic duplications of the esophagus and neurenteric cysts. *J Pediatr Surg* 1984; **19**: 527.

26. Hemalatha V, Batcup G, Brereton RJ & Spitz L. Intrathoracic foregut cyst (foregut duplication) associated with esophageal atresia. *J Pediatr Surg* 1980; **15**: 178.

27. Adejuyigbe O, Lawal OO, Akinola DO & Nwosu SO. Omental and mesenteric cysts in Nigerian children. *J R Coll Surg Edinb* 1990; **35**: 181.

28. Chung MA, Brandt ML, St-Vil D & Yazbeck S. Mesenteric cysts in children. *J Pediatr Surg* 1991; **26**: 1306.

29. Bearhs OM, Judd ES & Dockerty MB. Chylous cysts of the abdomen *Surg Clin North Am* 1950; **30**: 1081.

30. Hardin WJ & Hardy JD. Mesenteric cysts. *Am J Surg* 1970; **119**: 640.

31. Walker AR & Putman TC. Omental, mesenteric and retroperitoneal cysts. *Ann Surg* 1973; **178**: 13.

32. Vanek VW & Phillips AK. Retroperitoneal, mesenteric and omental cysts. *Arch Surg* 1984; **119**: 838.

33. Christensen JA, Fuller JW, Hallock JA & Sherman RT. Mesenteric cysts: a cause of small bowel obstruction in children. *Am J Surg* 1975; **41**: 352.

34. Mollitt DL, Ballantine TVN & Grosfeld JL. Mesenteric cysts in infancy and childhood. *Surg Gynecol Obstet* 1978; **147**: 182.

35. Molander ML, Mortensson W & Uden R. Omental and mesenteric cysts in children. *Acta Paediatr Scand* 1982; **71**: 227.

36. Geer LL, Mittelstaedt CA, Staab EV & Gaisie G. Mesenteric cyst: sonographic appearance with CT correlation. *Pediatr Radiol* 1984; **14**: 102.

Polyps, tumours and infections

1. Anderson CM & Burke V. *Paediatric Gastroenterology*. Oxford: Blackwell Scientific, 1975; 482.

2. Tovar JA, Eizaquirre I, Albert A & Jimenez J. Peutz – Jeghers syndrome in children: report of two cases and a review of the literature. *J Pediatr Surg* 1983; **18**: 1.

3. Lewis BS, Kornbluth A & Waye JD. Small bowel tumours: yield of enteroscopy. *Gut* 1991; **32**: 763.

4. Soper RT & Kent TH. Fatal juvenile polyposis in infancy. *Surgery* 1971; **64**: 692.

5. Jarvinen H, Nyberg M & Peltokallio P. Upper gastro-intestinal tract polyps in familial adenomatosis coli. *Gut* 1983; **24**: 333.

6. Spigelman AD, Crofton-Sleigh C, Venitt S & Phillips RKS. Mutagenicity of bile and duodenal adenomas in familial adenomatuos polyposis. *Br J Surg* 1990; **77**: 878.

7. Steger AC, Galland RB, Burdett-Smith P & Spencer J. Gardner's syndrome: a spectrum of clinical presentations. *J R Coll Surg Edinb* 1986; **31**: 289.

8. Sarre RG, Frost AG, Jagelman DG, Petras RE, Sivak MV & McGannon E. Gastric and duodenal polyps in familial adenomatous polyposis: a prospective study of the nature and prevalence of upper gastrointestinal polyps. *Gut* 1987; **28**: 314.

9. Heiss KF, Schaffner D, Ricketts RR & Winn K. Malignant risk in juvenile polyposis coli: increasing documentation in the pediatric age group. *J Pediatr Surg* 1993; **28**: 1188.

10. Spigelman AD. Familial adenomatous polyposis: recent genetic advances. *Br J Surg* 1994; **81**: 321.

11. Burn J, Chapman PD & Eastham EJ. Familial adenomatous polyposis. *Arch Dis Child* 1994; **71**: 103.

12. Campbell WJ, Spence RAJ & Parks TG. Familial adenomatous polyposis. *Br J Surg* 1994; **81**: 1722.

13. Scharf GM, Becker JHR & Laage NJ. Juvenile gastrointestinal polyposis or the infantile Cronkhite–Canada syndrome. *J Pediatr Surg* 1986; **21**: 953.

14. Velcek FT, Coopersmith IS, Chen AK, Kasser EG, Klotz DH & Kottmeier PK. Familial juvenile adenomatous polyposis. *J Pediatr Surg* 1976; **11**: 781.

15. Stringer MD, Ramani P, Yeung CK, Capps SNJ, Keily EM & Spitz L. Abdominal inflammatory myofibroblastic tumours in children. *Br J Surg* 1992; **79**: 1357.

16. Suarez V & Hall C. Mesenteric fibromatosis. *Br J Surg* 1985; **72**: 976.

17. Louw JH. Polypoid lesions of the large bowel in children with particular reference to benign lymphoid polyposis. *J Pediatr Surg* 1968; **3**: 195.

18. Fieber SS & Schaefer HJ. Lymphoid hyperplasia of the terminal ileum. *Gastroenterology* 1966; **50**: 83.

19. Atwell JD, Burge D & Wright D. Nodular lymphoid hyperplasia of the intestinal tract in infancy and childhood. *J Pediatr Surg* 1985; **20**: 25.

20. Johnson BL, Goldberg LS, Pops MA & Weiner M. Clinical and immunological studies in a case of nodular lymphoid hyperplasia of the small intestine. *Gastroenterology* 1971; **61**: 369.

21. Swartley RN & Stayman JW. Lymphoid hyperplasia of the intestinal tract requiring surgical intervention. *Ann Surg* 1962; **155**: 238.

22. Jona JZ, Belin RP & Burke JA. Lymphoid hyperplasia of the bowel and its surgical significance in children. *J Pediatr Surg* 1976; **11**: 997.

23. Wesselhoeft CW, DeLuca FG & Luke M. Positive ^{99m}Tc-pertechnetate scan in a child with intestinal arteriovenous malformation. *J Pediatr Surg* 1986; **21**: 71.

24. Stevenson RJ. Gastrointestinal bleeding. *Surg Clin North Am* 1985; **65**: 1475.

25. Tankel JW & Galasko CSB. Adenocarcinoma of the small bowel in a 12 year old girl. *J R Soc Med* 1984; **77**: 693.

26. Riggle KP & Boeckman CR. Duodenal leiomyoma: a case report of hematemesis in a teenager. *J Pediatr Surg* 1988; **23**: 850.

27. McGrath PC, Neifeld JP, Kay S & Salzberg AM. Principles in the management of pediatric intestinal leiomyosarcomas. *J Pediatr Surg* 1988; **23**: 939.

28. Moore TC, Finklestein JZ, Lachman R & Hirose F. Spontaneous perforation and closure of the small intestine in association with childhood leukemia. *J Pediatr Surg* 1975; **10**: 955.

29. Sonnino RE, Laberge J-M, Mucklow MG & Moir CR. Pathogenic *Escherichia coli*: a new etiology for acute ileitis in children. *J Pediatr Surg* 1989; **24**: 812.

30. Surendran N & Paulose MO. Intestinal complications of round worms in children. *J Pediatr Surg* 1988; **23**: 931.

31. Rao PLN, Satyanarayana G & Venkatesh A. Intraperitoneal ascariasis. *J Pediatr Surg* 1988; **23**: 936.

32. Efem SEE, Asindi AA & Aja A. Recent advances in the management of typhoid enteric perforation in children. *J R Coll Surg Edinb* 1986; **31**: 214.

33. Ein SH, Stringel G & Bannaatyne RM. Primary peritonitis in infants and children. *Pediatr Surg Int* 1987; **2**: 235.

34. Man DWK & Spitz L. The management of chylous ascites in children. *J Pediatr Surg* 1985; **20**: 72.

Umbilical problems

1. Kittle CF, Jenkins HP & Dragstedt LR. Patent omphalo mesenteric duct and its relation to diverticulum of Meckel. *Arch Surg* 1947; **54**: 10.

2. Scalettar HE, Mazarsky MM & Rascoff H. Congenital entero-umbilical fistula due to patent vitelline duct. *J Pediatr Surg* 1952; **40**: 310.

3. Surendran N, Kumar R & Nassir A. Unusual presentation of patent vitello-intestinal duct with round worms emerging from the umbilicus. *J Pediatr Surg* 1988; **23**: 1061.

4. Kutin ND, Allen JE & Jewett TC. The umbilical polyp. *J Pediatr Surg* 1979; **14**: 741.

5. Brown KL & Glover DM. Persistent omphalomesenteric duct anomalies. *Am J Surg* 1952; **83**: 680.

6. Kadzombe E & Currie ABM. Neonatal fistula from the appendix to the umbilicus. *J Pediatr Surg* 1988; **23**: 1059.

7. Kling S. Patent omphalomesenteric duct – a surgical emergency. *Arch Surg* 1968; **96**: 545.

8. Mustafa R. Double intussusception of the small bowel through a patent vitello-intestinal duct. *Br J Surg* 1976; **63**: 4525.

9. Pinter A, Schubert W, Pilaszanovich I & Szemledy F. Patent vitelline duct: a survey of 38 patients. *Z Kinderchir* 1978; **23**: 386.

10. Grosfeld JL & Franken EA. Intestinal obstruction in the neonate due to vitelline duct cysts. *Surg Gynecol Obstet* 1974; **138**: 527.

11. Pinter A, Szemledy F & Pilaszanovich I. Remnants of vitelline duct: analysis of 66 cases. *Acta Paediatr Acad Sci Hung* 1977; **19**: 113.

12. Simms MH & Corkery JJ. Meckel's diverticulum: its association with congenital malformation and the significance of atypical morphology. *Br J Surg* 1980; **67**: 216.

13. Hemingway AP & Allison DJ. Angiodysplasia and Meckel's diverticulum: a congenital association? *Br J Surg* 1982; **69**: 493.

14. Diamond T & Russell CFJ. Meckel's diverticulum in the adult. *Br J Surg* 1985; **72**: 480.

15. Koudelka J, Kralova M & Preis J. Giant Meckel's diverticulum. *J Pediatr Surg* 1982; **27**: 1589.

16. Farthing MG, Griffiths NJ, Thomas JM & Todd IP. Occult bleeding from Meckel's diverticulum. *Br J Surg* 1981; **68**: 176.

17. Morris A, Nicholson G, Zwi J & Vanderwee M. *Campylobacter pylori* infection in Meckel's diverticula containing gastric mucosa. *Gut* 1989; **30**: 1233.

18. Kumar S, Small P, Nawroz I & Mohammed R. *Helicobacter pylori* and Meckel's diverticulum. *J R Coll Surg Edinb* 1991; **36**: 225.

19. Meguid M, Canty T & Eraklis AJ. Complications of Meckel's diverticulum. *Surg Gynecol Obstet* 1974; **139**: 541.

20. Perlman JA, Hoover HC & Safer PK. Femoral hernia with strangulated Meckel's diverticulum (Littre's hernia): case report and review of the literature. *Am J Surg* 1980; **139**: 286.

21. Craig O & Murfitt J. Radiological demonstration of Meckel's diverticulum. *Br J Surg* 1980; **67**: 881.

22. Dawson DJ, Khan An, Nutall P & Shreeve DR. Technetium 99m-labelled-sucralphate isotope scanning in the detection of peptic ulceration. *Nucl Med Commun* 1985; **6**: 319.

23. Cooney DR, Duszynski DO, Camboa E, Karp MP & Jewett TC. The abdominal technetium scan (a decade of experience). *J Pediatr Surg* 1982; **17**: 611.

24. Anderson GF, Stakianakis G, King DR & Boles ET. Hormonal enhancement of technetium-99m pertechnetate uptake in experimental Meckel's diverticulum. *J Pediatr Surg* 1980; **15**: 900.

25. Williams RS. Management of Meckel's diverticulum. *Br J Surg* 1981; **68**: 477.

26. Attwood SEA, McGrath J, Hill ADK & Stephens RB. Laparoscopic approach to Meckel's diverticulectomy. *Br J Surg* 1992; **79**: 211.

27. Hutchison GH & Randall PE. Meckel's diverticulum: a study in the north Manchester area. *J R Coll Surg Edinb* 1981; **26**: 86.

28. Leijonmarck C-E, Bonman-Sandelin K, Frisell J & Raf L. Meckel's diverticulum in the adult. *Br J Surg* 1986; **73**: 146.

29. Lang-Stevenson A. Meckel's diverticulum: to look or not to look: to resect or not to resect. *Ann R Coll Surg Engl* 1983; **65**: 218.

30. St-Vil D, Brandt ML, Panic S, Bensoussan AL & Blanchard H. Meckel's diverticulum in children: a 20-year review. *J Pediatr Surg* 1991; **26**: 1289.

31. Mackey WC & Dineen P. A fifty year experience with Meckel's diverticulum. *Surg Gynecol Obstet* 1983; **156**: 56.

32. James T. Umbilical hernia in Xhosa infants and children. *J R Soc Med* 1982; **75**: 537.

33. Stunden RJ, Brown RA, Rode H, Millar AJW & Cywes S. Umbilical gangrene in the newborn. *J Pediatr Surg* 1988; **23**: 130.

34. Kosloske AM & Bartow SA. Debridement of periumbilical necrotizing fasciitis: importance of excision of the umbilical vessels and urachal remnant. *J Pediatr Surg* 1991; **26**: 808.

Anterior abdominal wall defects

1. Duhamel B. Embryology of exomphalos and allied malformations. *Arch Dis Child* 1963; **38**: 142.

2. deVries PA. The pathogenesis of gastroschisis and omphalocele. *J Pediatr Surg* 1980; **15**: 245.

3. Warkany J, Passarge E & Smith LB. Congenital malformations in autosomal trisomy syndromes. *Am J Dis Child* 1966; **112**: 502.

4. Sommer A, Cutler EA, Cohen BL, Harper D & Backes C. Familial occurrence of the Wiedemann-Beckwith syndrome and persistent fontanel. *Am J Med Genet* 1977; **1**: 59.

5. Glick PL, Harrison MR, Adzick NS, Filly RA, deLorimer AA & Callen PW. The missing link in the pathogenesis of gastroschisis. *J Pediatr Surg* 1985; **20**: 406.

6. Moore TC & Stokes GE. Gastroschisis. *Surgery* 1953; **33**: 112.

7. Langer JC, Longaker MT, Crombleholme TM et al. Etiology of intestinal damage in gastroschisis. I: Effects of amniotic fluid exposure and bowel constriction in a fetal lamb model. *J Pediatr Surg* 1989; **24**: 992.

8. Kluck P, Tibboel D, van der Kamp AWM & Molenaar JC. The effect of fetal urine on the development of the bowel in gastroschisis. *J Pediatr Surg* 1983; **18**: 47.

9. O'Neil JA & Grosfeld JL. Intestinal malfunction after antenatal exposure of viscera. *Am J Surg* 1974; **127**: 129.

10. Amoury RA, Beatty EC, Wood WG et al. Histology of the intestine in human gastroschisis-relationship to intestinal malfunction: dissolution of the 'peel' and its ultrastructural characteristics. *J Pediatr Surg* 1988; **23**: 950.

11. Caniano DA, Brokaw B & Ginn-Pease ME. An individualized approach to the management of gastroschisis. *J Pediatr Surg* 1990; **25**: 297.

12. Mud HJ, Bax NMA & Molenaar JC. Gastroschisis: factors affecting prognosis. *Z Kinderchir* 1981; **32**: 214.

13. Martin LW & Torres AM. Omphalocele and gastroschisis. *Surg Clin North Am* 1985; **65**: 1235.

14. Grosfeld JL & Clatworthy HW. Intrauterine midgut strangulation in a gastroschisis defect. *Surgery* 1970; **67**: 519.

15. Gauderer MWL. Gastroscisis and extraabdominal ectopic testis: simultaneous repair. *J Pediatr Surg* 1987; **22**: 657.

16. Tibbeol D, Raine P, McNee M et al. Developmental aspects of gastroschisis. *J Pediatr Surg* 1986; **21**: 865.

17. Shah R & Woolley MM. Gastroschisis and intestinal atresia. *J Pediatr Surg* 1991; **26**: 788.

18. Leader. Congenital defects of the anterior abdominl wall. *BMJ* 1975; **1**: 701.

19. Rickham PP. Rupture of exomphalos and gastroschisis. *Arch Dis Child* 1963; **38**: 138.

20. Torfs C, Curry C & Roeper P. Gastroschisis. *J Pediatr* 1990; **116**: 1.

21. Osuna A & Lindham S. Four cases of omphalocele in two generations of the same family. *Clin Genet* 1976; **9**: 354.

22. Grosfeld JL & Weber TR. Congenital abdominal wall defects: gastroschisis and omphalocele. *Curr Prob Surg* 1982; **19**: 159.

23. Bond SJ, Harrison MR, Filly RA, Callen PW, Anderson RA & Golbus MS. Severity of intestinal damage in gastroschisis: correlation with prenatal sonographic findings. *J Pediatr Surg* 1988; **23**: 520.

24. Kirk EP & Wah RM. Obstetric management of the fetus with omphalocele or gastroschisis: a review and report of one hundred twelve cases. *Am J Obstet Gynecol* 1983; **146**: 512.

25. Bethel CAI, Seashore JH & Touloukian RJ. Cesarean section does not improve outcome in gastroschisis. *J Pediatr Surg* 1989; **24**: 1.

26. Lafferty PM, Emmerson AJ, Fleming PJ, Frank JD & Noblett HR. Anterior abdominal wall defects. *Arch Dis Child* 1989; **64**: 1029.

27. Carpenter MW, Curci MR, Dibbins AW & Haddow JE. Perinatal management of ventral wall defects. *Obstet Gynecol* 1984; **64**: 646.

28. Nakayama DK, Harrison MR, Gross BH et al. Management of the fetus with an abdominal wall defect. *J Pediatr Surg* 1984; **19**: 408.

29. Stringer MD, Brereton RJ & Wright VM. Controversies in the management of gastroschisis: a study of 40 patients. *Arch Dis Child* 1991; **66**: 34.

30. Swift RI, Singh MP, Ziderman DA, Silverman M, Elder MA & Elder MG. A new regime in the management of gastroschisis. *J Pediatr Surg* 192; **27**: 61.

31. Mollitt DL, Ballantine TVN & Grosfeld JL. A critical assessment of fluid requirements in gastroschisis. *J Pediatr Surg* 1978; **13**: 217.

32. Coran AG & Drongowski RA. Body fluid compartment changes following neonatal surgery. *J Pediatr Surg* 1989; **24**: 829.

33. Canty TG & Collins DL. Primary fascial closure in infants with gastroschisis and omphalocele: a superior approach. *J Pediatr Surg* 1983; **18**: 707.

34. Denes J, Leb J & Lukacs FU. Gastroschisis. *Surgery* 1968; **63**: 701.

35. Towne BH, Peters G & Chang JHT. The problem of 'giant' omphalocele. *J Pediatr Surg* 1980; **15**: 543.

36. Campbell TJ, Campbell JR & Harrison MW. Selective management of omphalocele. *Am J Surg* 1982; **143**: 572.

37. Soave F. Conservative treatment of giant exomphalos *Arch Dis Child* 1963; **38**: 130.

38. Gough DCS & Auldist AW. Giant exomphalos – conservative treatment or operative treatment? *Arch Dis Child* 1979; **54**: 441.

39. Mahour GH. Intact omphalocele: perennial dilemma of operative or 'conservative' management *Am J Surg* 1974; **128**: 419.

40. Fagan DG, Pritcard JS, Clarkson TW & Greenwood MR. Organ mercury levels in infants with omphaloceles treated with organic mercurial antiseptic. *Arch Dis Child* 1977; **52**: 902.

41. Chan MC. Giant exomphalos – conservative or operative treatment? *Arch Dis Child* 1980; **55**: 167.

42. Gross RE. New method for surgical treatment of large omphaloceles. *Surgery* 1948; **24**: 277.

43. Bruce J, Afshani E, Karp MP & Jewett TC. Omphalocele with pyloroduodenal obstruction by extrinsic hepatic compression: a case report. *J Pediatr Surg* 1988; **23**: 1020.

44. Yazbeck S. The giant omphalocele: a new approach for a rapid and complete closure. *J Pediatr Surg* 1986; **21**: 715.

45. Wesselhoeft CW & Randolph JR. Treatment of omphalocele based on individual characteristics of the defect. *Pediatrie* 1969; **44**: 101.

46. Ravitch MM. Second stage repair with the aid of pneumoperitoneum. *JAMA* 1963; **185**: 42.

47. Otherston HB & Hargest TS. A pneumatic reduction device for gastroschisis and omphalocele. *Surg Gynecol Obstet* 1977; **144**: 243.

48. Knope S, Srinivasa SK, Anath PK, Venkateswara RC & Rao PLNG. Omphalocele: secondary repair of ventral hernia – a new operative technique. *J Pediatr Surg* 1989; **24**: 1142.

49. Stringel G & Blocker SH. Omphalocele closure: surgical technique with preservation of the amniotic sac. *J Pediatr Surg* 1986; **21**: 1081.

50. Barlow B, Cooper A, Gandhi R & Niemirska M. External silo reduction of the unruptured giant omphalocele. *J Pediatr Surg* 1987; **22**: 75.

51. de Lorimier AA, Adzick NS & Harrison MR. Amnion inversion in the treatment of giant omphalocele. *J Pediatr Surg* 1991; **26**: 804.

52. Ein SH & Shandling B. A new nonoperative treatment of large omphaloceles with polymer membrane. *J Pediatr Surg* 1978; **13**: 255.

53. Knutrud O, Bjordal RI, Ro J & Bo G. Gastroschisis and omphalocele. *Prog Pediatr Surg* 1979; **13**: 51.
54. Wesley JR, Drongowski R & Coran AG. Intragastric pressure measurement: a guide for reduction and closure of the silastic chimney in omphalocele and gastroschisis. *J Pediatr Surg* 1981; **16**: 264.
55. Yaster M, Scherer TLR, Stone MM et al. Prediction of successful primary closure of congenital abdominal wall defects using intraoperative measurements. *J Pediatr Surg* 1989; **24**: 1217.
56. Ein SH, Superina R, Bagwell C & Wiseman N. Ischemic bowel after primary closure for gastroschisis. *J Pediatr Surg* 1988; **23**: 728.
57. King DR, Savrin R & Boles ET. Gastroschisis update. *J Pediatr Surg* 1980; **15**: 553.
58. Stone HH. Immediate permanent fascial prosthesis for gastroschisis and massive omphalocele. *Surg Gynecol Obstet* 1981; **1153**: 221.
59. Thomas DFM & Atwell JD. The embryology and surgical management of gastroschisis. *Br J Surg* 1976; **63**: 893.
60. Aaronson JA & Eckstein HB. The role of the silastic prosthesis in the management of gastroschisis. *Arch Surg* 1977; **112**: 297.
61. Schwartz MZ, Tyson KRT, Milliorn K & Lobe TE. Staged reduction using a silastic sac is the treatment of choice for large congenital abdominal defects. *J Pediatr Surg* 1983; **18**: 713.
62. Gornall P. Management of intestinal atresia complicating gastroschisis. *J Pediatr Surg* 1989; **24**: 522.
63. Lloyd DA. Gastroschisis, malrotation, and chylous ascites. *J Pediatr Surg* 1991; **26**: 106.
64. Filston MC. Gastroschisis – primary fascial closure: the goal for optimal management. *Ann Surg* 1983; **197**: 260.
65. Ein SH & Rubin SZ. Gastroschisis: primary closure or silon pouch. *J Pediatr Surg* 1980; **15**: 549.
66. Gierup J Olsen L & Lundkuist K. Aspects on the treatment of omphalocele and gastroschisis: twenty year's experience. *Z Kinderchir* 1982; **35**: 3.
67. Di Lorenzo M, Yazbeck S & Ducharme J-C. Gastroschisis: a 15-year experience. *J Pediatr Surg* 1987; **22**: 710.
68. Wesson DE & Baesi TJ. Repair of gastroschisis with preservation of the umbilicus. *J Pediatr Surg* 1986; **21**: 764.
69. Fonkalsrud EW. Selective repair of neonatal gastroschisis based on degree of visceroabdominal disproportion. *Ann Surg* 1980; **191**: 139.
70. Bower RJ, Bell MJ, Ternberg JL & Cobb ML. Ventilation support and primary closure of gastroschisis. *Surgery* 1982; **91**: 52.
71. Filler RM, Eraklis AJ, Das JB & Schuster SR. Total intravenous nutrition: an adjunct to the management of infants with a ruptured omphalocele. *Am J Surg* 1971; **121**: 454.
72. Binnington HB, Keating JP & Ternberg JL. Gastroschisis. *Arch Surg* 1974; **108**: 455.
73. Wilmore DW & Dudrick SJ. Growth and development of an infant receiving all nutrients exclusively by vein. *JAMA* 1968; **203**: 140.
74. Luck SR, Sherman JO, Raffensperger JG & Goldstein IR. Gastroschisis in 106 cosecutive newborn infants. *Surgery* 1985; **98**: 677.
75. Hrabovsky EE, Boyd JB, Savrin RA & Boles ET. Advances in the management of gastroschisis. *Ann Surg* 1980; **192**: 244.
76. Pokorny WJ, Harberg FJ & McGill CW. Gastroschisis complicated by intestinal atresia. *J Pediatr Surg* 1981; **16**: 261.
77. Toulouian RJ & Spackman TJ. Gastrointestinal function and radiographic appearance following gastroschisis repair. *J Pediatr Surg* 1971; **6**: 427.
78. Aoki Y, Ohshio T & Komi N. An experimental study on gastroschisis using fetal surgery. *J Pediatr Surg* 1980; **15**: 252.
79. Oldham KT, Coran AG, Drongowski RA, Baker PJ, Wesley JR & Polley TZ. The development of necrotizing enterocolitis following repair of gastroschisis: a surprisingly high incidence. *J Pediatr Surg* 1989; **23**: 945.
80. Muraji T, Tsugawa C, Nishijima E, Tanano H, Matsumoto Y & Kimura K. A 17-year experience. *J Pediatr Surg* 1989; **24**: 343.
81. Mayer T, Black R, Matlak ME & Johnson DG. Gastroschisis and omphalocele: an eight year review. *Ann Surg* 1980; **192**: 783.
82. Mann L, Ferguson-Smith MA, Desai M, Gibson AAM & Raine PAM. Prenatal assessment of anterior abdominal wall defects and their prognosis. *Prenat Diagn* 1984; **4**: 427.
83. Phillips JD, Kelly RE, Fonkalsruf EW, Mirzayan A & Kim CS. An improved model of experimental gastroschisis in fetal rabbits. *J Pediatr Surg* 1991; **26**: 784.
84. Cantrell JR, Haller JA & Ravitch MM. A syndrome of congenital defects involving the abdominal wall, sternum, diaphragm, pericardium and heart. *Surg Gynecol Obstet* 1958; **107**: 602.
85. Toyama WM. Combined congenital defects of the anterior abdominal wall, sternum, diaphragm, pericardium and heart. *Pediatrie* 1972; **50**: 778.
86. Dobell ARC, Williams HB & Long RW. Staged repair of ectopia cordis. *J Pediatr Surg* 1982; **17**: 363.
87. Rickham PP. Vesico-intestinal fissure. *Arch Dis Child* 1960; **35**: 97.
88. Sukarochana K & Sieber WK. Vesicointestinal fissure revisited. *J Pediatr Surg* 1978; **13**: 713.
89. Yazbeck S, Ndoye M & Khan AH. Omphalocele: a 25-year experience. *J Pediatr Surg* 1986; **21**: 761.
90. Hadziselimovic F, Duckett JW, Snyder HM, Schnaufer L & Huff D. Omphalocele, cryptorchidism, and brain malformations. *J Pediatr Surg* 1987; **22**: 854.
91. Stringel G & Filler RM. Prognostic factors in omphalocele and gastroschisis. *J Pediatr Surg* 1979; **14**: 515.
92. Knight PJ, Sommer A & Clatworthy HW. Omphalocele: a prognostic classification. *J Pediatr Surg* 1981; **16**: 599.

INDEX

Note: To find a particular condition, the reader is advised to look up the type of condition and not the portion of the GI tract in which it is found (e.g. 'oesophageal web' is found under 'Web' and not 'Oesophagus' or 'Oesophageal web'). The reader will find only conditions covered by at least whole chapters listed as subentries under the part of the GI tract in which they are found, and these will, in the main, be cross-referenced out to a main entry for the specific condition (e.g Oesophagus, varices, see Varices, oesophageal). Abbreviations used: GOR(D), gastro-oesophageal reflux (disease).